Older Americans
Information Resource

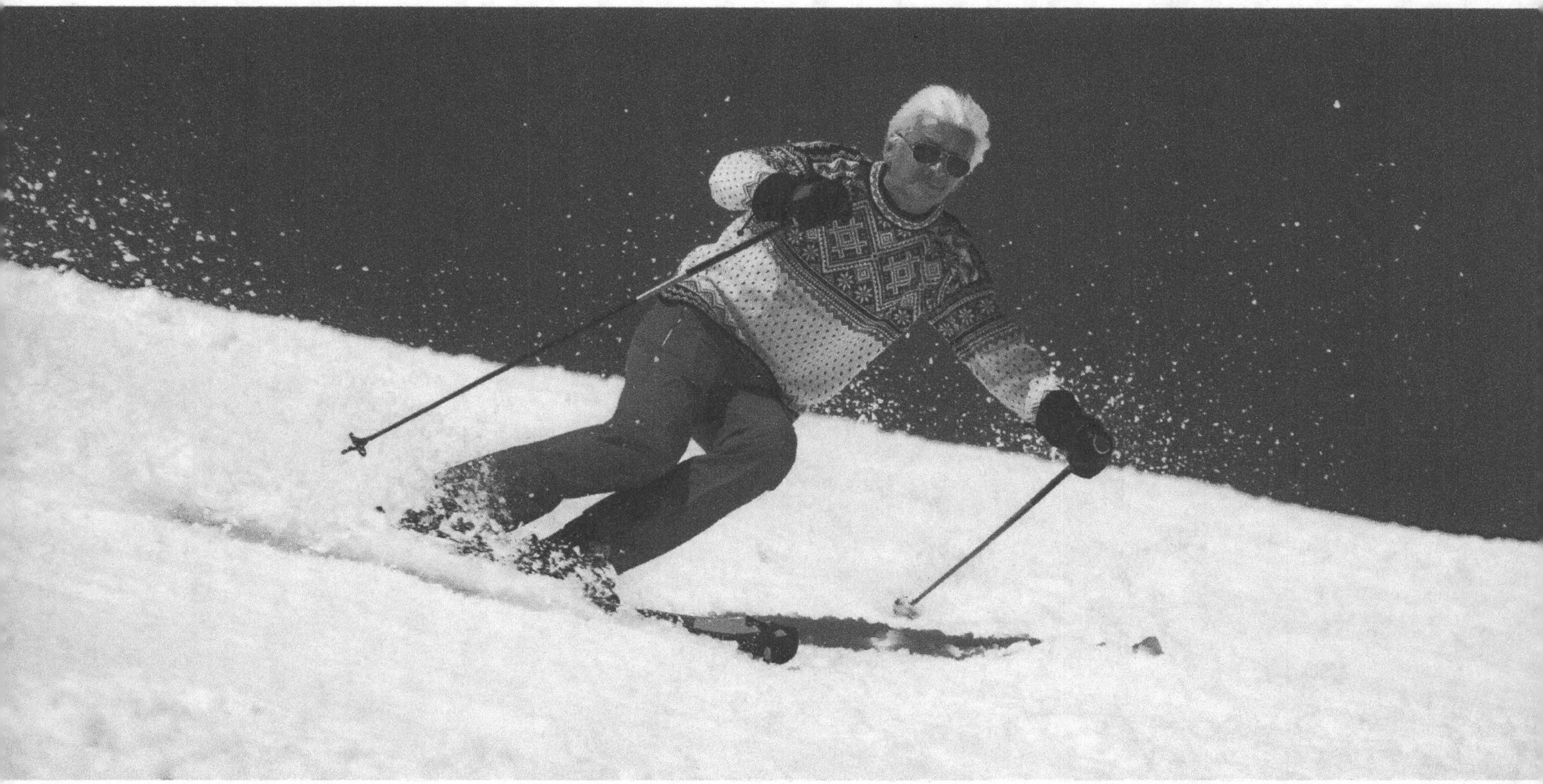

2018/2019
TWELFTH EDITION

Older Americans
Information Resource

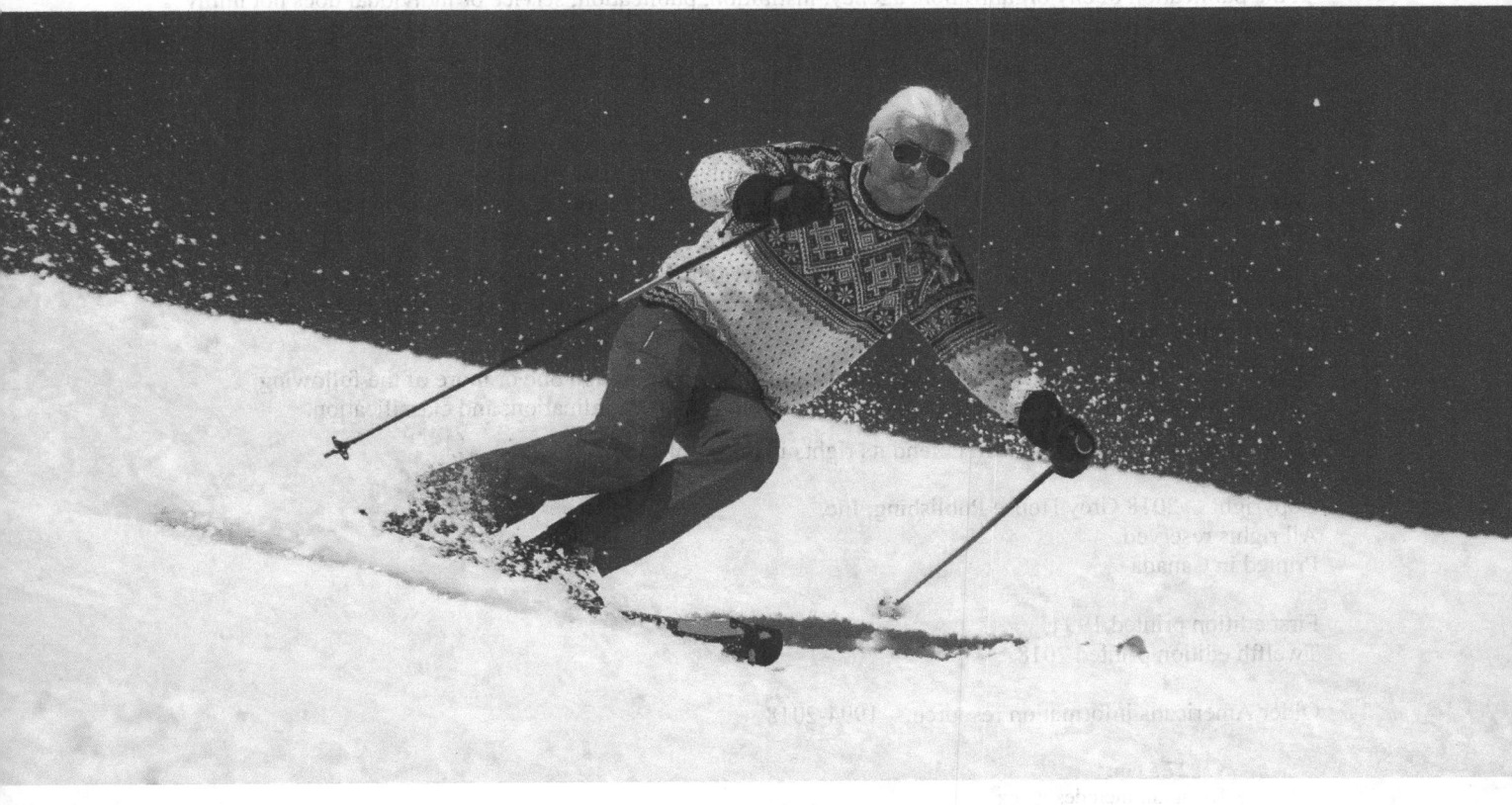

GREY HOUSE PUBLISHING

PUBLISHER:	Leslie Mackenzie
EDITOR:	Richard Gottlieb
EDITORIAL DIRECTOR:	Laura Mars
PRODUCTION MANAGER, COMPOSITION:	Kristen Hayes
PRODUCTION ASSISTANT:	Geoff Graves
MARKETING DIRECTOR:	Jessica Moody

Grey House Publishing, Inc.
4919 Route 22
Amenia, NY 12501
518.789.8700
Fax 518.789.0545
www.greyhouse.com
E-mail: books@greyhouse.com

First edition printed 1994
Twelfth edition printed 2018

Older Americans information resource. – 1994-2018

      v. ; 27.5 cm.
      Biennial, includes index
      ISSN: 1072-477X

1.   Aged-Services for—United States—Directories. 2. Aged—United States—Information services—Directories
I. Gale Research Inc. II. Grey House Publishing, Inc,
Information Services—United States—Directories. 6. Rehabilitation—United States—Directories. I. Title:
DCI

HV1457.O42
362.6/025/73   94660686
ISBN: 978-1-68217-734-1

Table of Contents

Introduction

This twelfth edition of *Older Americans Information Resource* is designed for one of America's largest growing populations, with resources to help aging Americans lead happy and productive lives. It includes 10,000 listings, two glossaries, and three indexes, and is a repeat winner of the **National Mature Media Award**, recognized as "the best in advertising, marketing and educational materials for older adults."

Praise for previous editions:

" . . . *an excellent resource and is of use to seniors looking for continuing education courses, travel opportunities, and ways to improve their quality of life. It also should be of great value to children caring for elderly parents. This resource brings together in one volume a wealth of information to assist elderly Americans. Highly recommended . . .*"

American Reference Book Annual

"*Current, comprehensive, and accessible. . . . a solid directory . . .*"

Library Journal

Following this Introduction, a detailed **Profile of Older Americans: 2016** from the Administration on Aging defines America's seniors by 14 categories, including future growth, income, employment and care giving. This 16-page report is enhanced by tables, charts, and maps. Highlights of the report include:

- Over the past 10 years, the population 65 and over increased from 36.6 million to 47.8 million in 2015, and is projected to more than double to 98 million in 2060;
- The 85+ population is expected to triple from 6.3 million in 2015 to 14.6 million in 2040;
- About one in seven is an older American;
- Persons reaching age 65 have a life expectancy of an additional 19.4 years;
- Older women outnumber older men by 5.6 million;
- California, Florida, and Texas have the highest number of Americans 65 and over.

Detailed Listings

Listings in *Older Americans Information Resource* include name, address, phone, fax, web sites, key personnel, and brief descriptions. Thoughtfully organized into 12 major chapters, content includes *Organizations, Awards, Continuing Education, Disability Aids, Health Conditions, Living Facilities, Legal Resources, Libraries* and *Print Resources*.

The chapter on *Health Conditions* includes 18 specific conditions including *AIDS, Depression, Hypertension, Stroke* and *Visual Impairment*. The listings under each condition include associations, publications, research centers, web sites and more.

Valuable Glossaries

Older Americans Information Resource includes two helpful glossaries. The first is a *Glossary of Health & Medical Terms,* with 65 terms that define language found throughout this and other publications, as well as terms used by professionals in the field. The second is a *Glossary of Legal Terms,* that includes 22 in-depth definitions designed to demystify terms used by lawyers and others regarding legal situations in which older Americans may find themselves.

Helpful Indexes
Three indexes offer additional ways to access this resource's content. The *Entry Index* is an alphabetical list of all entries herein. The *Geographic Index* lists all Agencies, Associations, Facilities, and Organizations by state. The *Subject Index* organizes appropriate listings by more than 100 categories, from Elder Abuse to Wills.

For even easier access to data, *Older Americans Information Resource* is available on our online database platform, http://gold.greyhouse.com. Finding resources for older Americans has never been faster or easier. With our keyword search and quick search, users can pinpoint just the right resource in just a few clicks of the mouse. Plus, users can print out organization listings, save lists of resources, or download data onto their own computer for easy reference.

A Profile
of
Older Americans: 2016

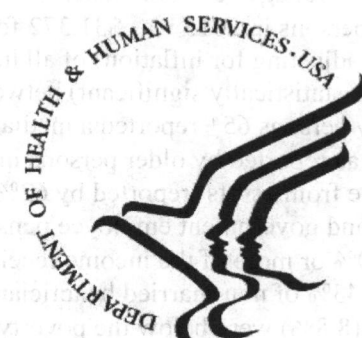

Administration on Aging

Administration for Community Living

U.S. Department of Health and Human Services

Highlights*

- Over the past 10 years, the population 65 and over increased from 36.6 million in 2005 to 47.8 million in 2015 (a 30% increase) and is projected to more than double to 98 million in 2060.
- Between 2005 and 2015 the population age 60 and over increased 34% from 49.8 million to 66.8 million.
- The 85+ population is projected to triple from 6.3 million in 2015 to 14.6 million in 2040.
- Racial and ethnic minority populations have increased from 6.7 million in 2005 (18% of the older adult population) to 10.6 million in 2015 (22% of older adults) and are projected to increase to 21.1 million in 2030 (28% of older adults).
- The number of Americans aged 45-64 – who will reach 65 over the next two decades – increased by 14.9% between 2005 and 2015.
- About one in every seven, or 14.9%, of the population is an older American.
- Persons reaching age 65 have an average life expectancy of an additional 19.4 years (20.6 years for females and 18 years for males).
- There were 76,974 persons aged 100 or more in 2015 (0.2% of the total 65+ population).
- Older women outnumber older men at 26.7 million older women to 21.1 million older men.
- In 2015, 22% of persons 65+ were members of racial or ethnic minority populations--9% were African-Americans (not Hispanic), 4% were Asian or Pacific Islander (not Hispanic), 0.5% were Native American (not Hispanic), 0.1% were Native Hawaiian/Pacific Islander, (not Hispanic), and 0.7% of persons 65+ identified themselves as being of two or more races. Persons of Hispanic origin (who may be of any race) represented 8% of the older population.
- Older men were much more likely to be married than older women---70% of men, 45% of women. In 2016, 34% older women were widows.
- About 29% (13.6 million) of noninstitutionalized older persons live alone (9.3 million women, 4.3 million men).
- Almost half of older women (46%) age 75+ live alone.
- The median income of older persons in 2015 was $31,372 for males and $18,250 for females. Median money income (after adjusting for inflation) of all households headed by older people increased by 4.3% (which was statistically significant) between 2014 and 2015. Households containing families headed by persons 65+ reported a median income in 2015 of $57,360.
- The major sources of income as reported by older persons in 2014 were Social Security (reported by 84% of older persons), income from assets (reported by 62%), earnings (reported by 29%), private pensions (reported by 37%), and government employee pensions (reported by 16%).
- Social Security constituted 90% or more of the income received by 33% of beneficiaries in 2014 (21% of married couples and 43% of non-married beneficiaries).
- Over 4.2 million older adults (8.8%) were below the poverty level in 2015. This poverty rate is statistically different from the poverty rate in 2014 (10.0%). In 2011, the U.S. Census Bureau also released a new Supplemental Poverty Measure (SPM) which takes into account regional variations in living costs, non-cash benefits received, and non-discretionary expenditures but does not replace the official poverty measure. In 2015, the SPM shows a poverty level for older persons of 13.7% (almost 5 percentage points higher than the official rate of 8.8%). This increase is mainly due to including medical out-of-pocket expenses in the poverty calculations.

*Principal sources of data for the Profile are the U.S. Census Bureau, the National Center for Health Statistics, and the Bureau of Labor Statistics. The Profile incorporates the latest data available but not all items are updated on an annual basis.

The Older Population

The population age 65 years or older numbered 47.8 million in 2015 (the most recent year for which data are available). They represented 14.9% of the U.S. population, about one in every seven Americans. The number of older Americans increased by 11.1 million or 30% since 2005, compared to an increase of 5.7% for the under-65 population.

Between 2005 and 2015, the number of Americans aged 45-64 (who will reach age 65 over the next two decades) increased by 14.9% and the number of Americans age 60 and over increased by 34.2% from 49.8 million to 66.8 million.

In 2015, there were 26.7 million older women and 21.1 million older men, or a sex ratio of 126.5 women for every 100 men. At age 85 and over, this ratio increases to 189.2 women for every 100 men.

Since 1900, the percentage of Americans 65+ has more than tripled (from 4.1% in 1900 to 14.9% in 2015), and the number has increased over fifteen times (from 3.1 million to 47.8 million). The older population itself is increasingly older. In 2015, the 65-74 age group (27.6 million) was more than 12 times larger than in 1900 (2,186,767); the 75-84 group (13.9 million) was more than 17 times larger (771,369), and the 85+ group (6.3 million) was 51 times larger (122,362).

In 2015, persons reaching age 65 had an average life expectancy of an additional 19.4 years (20.6 years for females and 18 years for males). A child born in 2015 could expect to live 78.8 years, more than 30 years longer than a child born in 1900 (47.3 years). Much of this increase occurred because of reduced death rates for children and young adults. However, the period of 1990-2007 also has seen reduced death rates for the population aged 65-84, especially for men – by 41.6% for men aged 65-74 and by 29.5% for men aged 75-84. Life expectancy at age 65 increased by only 2.5 years between 1900 and 1960, but has increased by 4.2 years from 1960 to 2007. Nonetheless, some research has raised concerns about future increases in life expectancy in the US compared to other high-income countries, primarily due to past smoking and current obesity levels, especially for women age 50 and over (National Research Council, 2011).

In 2015, 3.5 million persons celebrated their 65th birthday. Census estimates showed an annual net increase between 2014 and 2015 of 1.6 million in the number of persons age 65 and over.

Between 1980 and 2015, the centenarian population experienced a larger percentage increase than did the total population. There were 76,974 persons aged 100 or more in 2015 (0.2% of the total 65+ population). This is more than double the 1980 figure of 32,194.

Sources: U.S. Census Bureau, Population Division, Annual Estimates of the Resident Population for Selected Age Groups by Sex for the United States, States, Counties, and Puerto Rico Commonwealth and Municipios: April 1, 2010 to July 1, 2015. Release Date: June 2016; Table 1. Intercensal Estimates of the Resident Population by Sex and Age for the United States: April 1, 2000 to July 1, 2010. Release Date: September 2011; Annual Estimates of the Resident Population by Single Year of Age and Sex for the United States, States, Counties, and Puerto Rico Commonwealth and Municipios: April 1, 2010 to July 1, 2015. Release Date: July 1, 2016; 2010 Census Special Reports, Centenarians: 2010, C2010SR-03, 2012; Hobbs, Frank and Nicole Stoops, Census 2000 Special Reports, Series CENSR-4, Demographic Trends in the 20th Century, Table 5. Population by Age and Sex for the United States: 1900 to 2000, Part A; National Center for Health Statistics, Xu JQ, Murphy SL, Kochanek KD, Arias E. Mortality in the United States, 2015. NCHS data brief, no 267. Hyattsville, MD: 2016; and National Research Council, Crimmins EM, Preston SH, Cohen B, editors. Explaining Divergent Levels of Longevity in High-Income Countries. Panel on Understanding Divergent Trends in Longevity in High-Income Countries, 2011.

Future Growth

The older population will continue to grow significantly in the future (Figure 1). This growth slowed somewhat during the 1990's because of the relatively small number of babies born during the Great Depression of the 1930's. But the older population is beginning to burgeon as the first wave of the "baby boom" generation is reaching age 65.

The population age 65 and over has increased from 36.6 million in 2005 to 47.8 million in 2015 (a 30% increase) and is projected to more than double to 98 million in 2060. By 2040, there will be about 82.3 million older persons, over twice their number in 2000. People 65+ represented 14.9% of the population in the year 2015 but are expected to grow to be 21.7% of the population by 2040. The 85+ population is projected to more than double from 6.3 million in 2015 to 14.6 million in 2040.

Racial and ethnic minority populations have increased from 6.7 million in 2005 (18% of the older adult population) to 10.6 million in 2015 (22% of older adults) and are projected to increase to 21.1 million in 2030 (28% of older adults). Between 2015 and 2030, the white (not Hispanic) population 65+ is projected to increase by 43% compared with 99% for older racial and ethnic minority populations, including Hispanics (123%), African-Americans (not Hispanic) (81%), American Indian and Native Alaskans (not Hispanic) (82%), and Asians (not Hispanic) (90%).

Figure 1: Number of Persons 65+: 1900-2060 (numbers in millions)

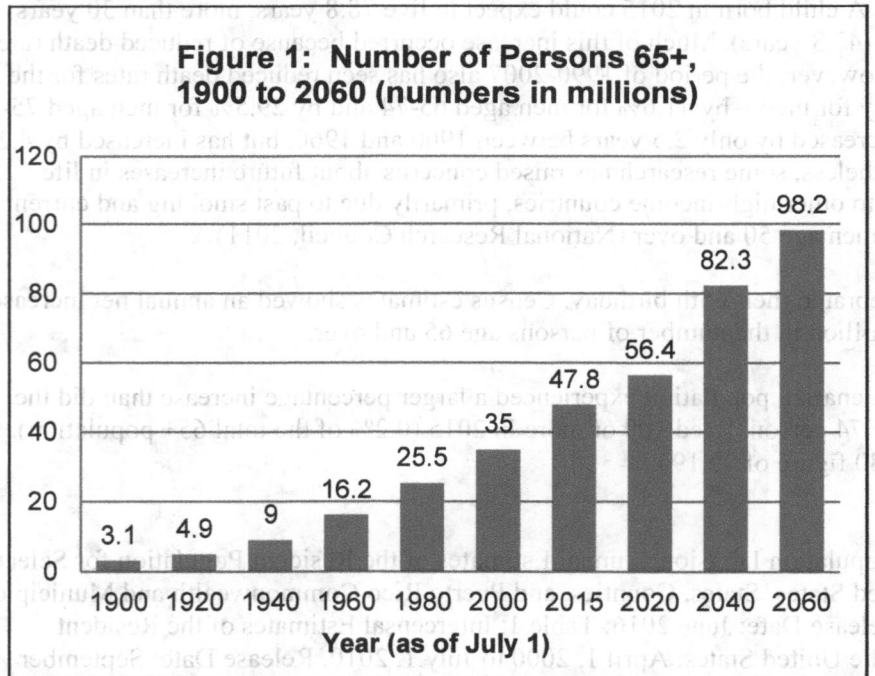

Figure 1: Number of Persons 65+, 1900 to 2060 (numbers in millions)

Note: Increments in years are uneven.
Source: U.S. Census Bureau, Population Estimates and Projections.

Sources: U.S. Census Bureau, Population Division, Annual Estimates of the Resident Population for Selected Age Groups by Sex for the United States, States, Counties, and Puerto Rico Commonwealth and Municipios: April 1, 2010 to July 1, 2015, Release Date: June 2016; Intercensal Estimates of the Resident Population by Sex and Age for the United States: April 1, 2000 to July 1, 2010. Release Date: September 2011; Intercensal Estimates of the White Alone Resident Population by Sex and Age for the United States: April 1, 2000 to July 1, 2010; 2014 National Population Projections: Summary Tables, Table 3. Projections of the Population by Sex and Selected Age Groups for the United States: 2015 to 2060, released December 10, 2014; and NP2014_D1: Projected Population by Single Year of Age, Sex, Race, and Hispanic Origin for the United States: 2014 to 2060.

Marital Status

In 2016, older men were much more likely to be married than older women--70% of men, 45% of women (Figure 2). Widows accounted for 34% of all older women in 2016. There were more than three times as many widows (8.8 million) as widowers (2.6 million).

Divorced and separated (including married/spouse absent) older persons represented only 14% of all older persons in 2016. However, this percentage has increased since 1980, when approximately 5.3% of the older population were divorced or separated/spouse absent.

Figure 2: Marital Status of Persons 65+, 2016

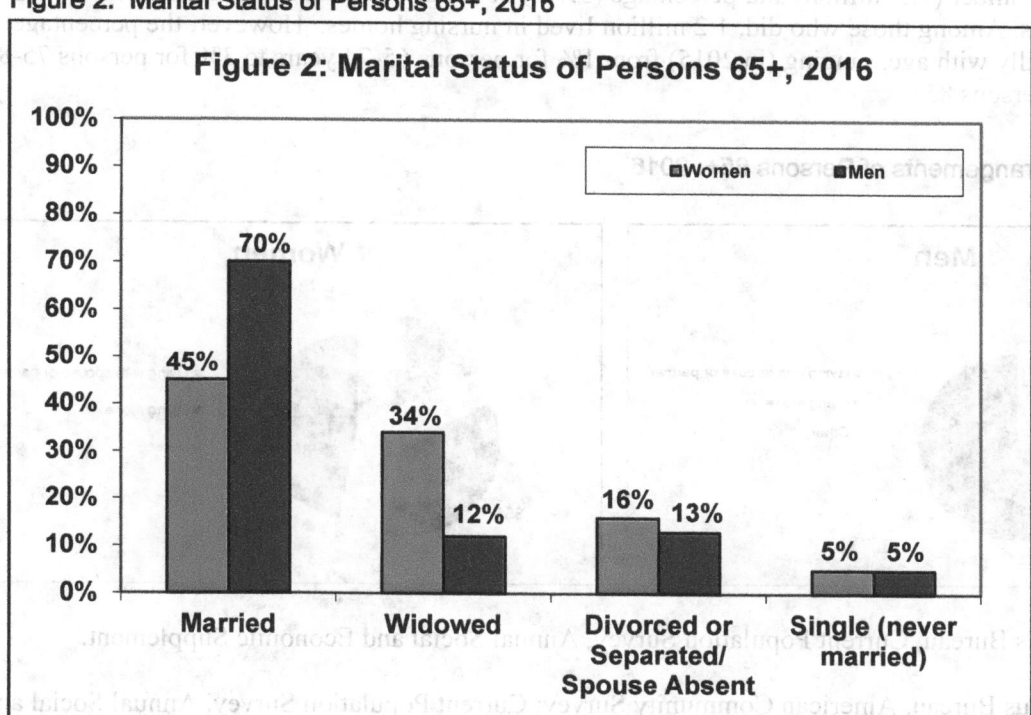

Source: U.S. Census Bureau, Current Population Survey, Annual Social and Economic Supplement.

Source: U.S. Census Bureau, Current Population Survey, Annual Social and Economic Supplement, Table A1. Marital Status of People 15 Years and Over, by Age, Sex, and Personal Earnings: 2016.

Living Arrangements

Over half (59%) of older noninstitutionalized persons age 65+ lived with their spouse (including partner) in 2016. Approximately 15.5 million or 73% of older men, and 12 million or 47% of older women, lived with their spouse (Figure 3). The proportion living with their spouse decreased with age, especially for women. Only 34% of women 75+ years old lived with a spouse.

About 29% (13.6 million) of all noninstitutionalized older persons in 2016 lived alone (9.3 million women, 4.3 million men). They represented 35% of older women and 20% of older men. The proportion living alone increases with advanced age. Among women aged 75 and over, for example, almost half (46%) lived alone.

A relatively small number (1.5 million) and percentage (3.1%) of the 65+ population in 2015 lived in institutional settings. Among those who did, 1.2 million lived in nursing homes. However, the percentage increases dramatically with age, ranging (in 2015) from 1% for persons 65-74 years to 3% for persons 75-84 years and 9% for persons 85+.

Figure 3: Living Arrangements of Persons 65+: 2016

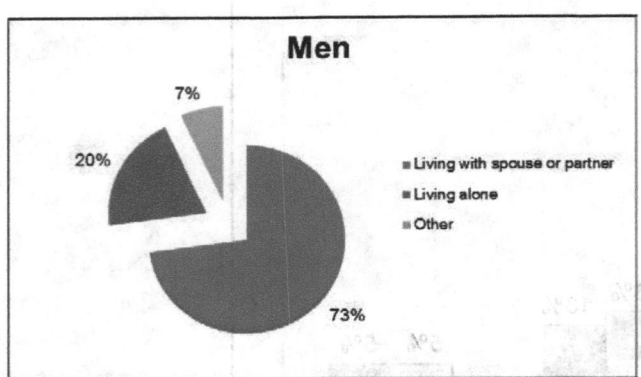 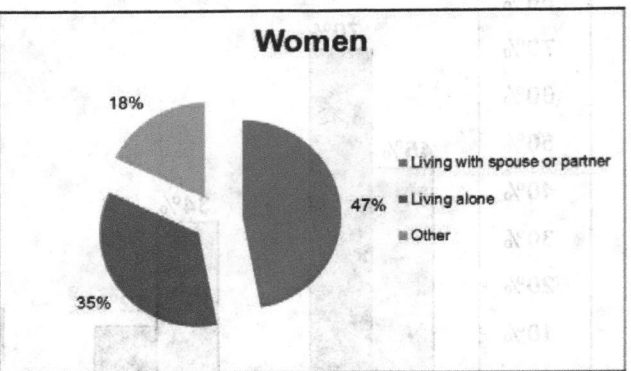

Source: U.S. Census Bureau, Current Population Survey, Annual Social and Economic Supplement.

Sources: U.S. Census Bureau, American Community Survey; Current Population Survey, Annual Social and Economic Supplement 1967 to present; Table AD3. Living arrangements of adults 65 to 74 years old, 1967 to present; Table AD3. Living arrangements of adults 75 and over, 1967 to present.

Racial and Ethnic Composition

In 2015, 22% of persons age 65+ were members of racial or ethnic minority populations—9% were African-Americans (not Hispanic), 4% were Asian or Pacific Islander (not Hispanic), 0.5% were Native American (not Hispanic), 0.1% were Native Hawaiian/Pacific Islander, (not Hispanic), and 0.7% of persons age 65+ identified themselves as being of two or more races. Persons of Hispanic origin (who may be of any race) represented 8% of the older population.

Only 9% of all the people who were members of racial and ethnic minority populations were 65+ in 2015 compared with 19% of non-Hispanic whites. The percentage of people age 65 and over within each racial and ethnic minority group are as follows: 11% of African-Americans (not Hispanic), 12% of Asians (not Hispanic), 8% of Native Hawaiian and Other Pacific Islanders (not Hispanic), 10% of American Indian and Native Alaskans (not Hispanic) and 7% of Hispanics.

Source: U.S. Census Bureau, Population Division, Annual Estimates of the Resident Population by Sex, Age, Race, and Hispanic Origin for the United States and States: April 1, 2010 to July 1, 2015. Release Date: June 2016.

Geographic Distribution

The proportion of older persons in the population varies considerably by state with some states experiencing much greater growth in their older populations (Figures 4 and 5). In 2015, more than half (54%) of persons 65+ lived in 10 states: California (5.2 million); Florida (3.9 million); Texas (3.2 million); New York (3.0 million); Pennsylvania (2.2 million); Ohio (1.8 million); Illinois (1.8 million); Michigan (1.6 million); North Carolina (1.5 million); New Jersey (1.3 million); and Georgia, Virginia, Arizona, Massachusetts, Washington and Tennessee each had well over 1 million (Figure 6).

Persons 65+ constituted approximately 18% or more of the total population in three states in 2015: Florida (19.4%); Maine (18.8%); and West Virginia (18.2%).

In 5 states, the 65+ population increased by 50% or more between 2005 and 2015: Alaska (63%); Nevada (55%); Colorado (54%); Georgia (50%); and South Carolina (50%).

The 10 jurisdictions with poverty rates over 10% for older adults during 2015 were: District of Columbia (15.2%); Louisiana (12.8%); Mississippi (12.5%); Kentucky (11.2%); New York (11.2%); New Mexico (11.1%); Arkansas (10.3%); Florida (10.3%); Rhode Island (10.3%); and Texas (10.3%).

Older adults are less likely to change residence than other age groups. From 2015 to 2016, only 3% of older persons moved as opposed to 13% of the under 65 population. Most older movers (62%) stayed in the same county and 22% remained in the same state (different county). Only 16% moved out-of-state or abroad.

Sources: Administration for Community Living agid.acl.gov. Data Source: Population Estimates 2005, accessed December 12, 2016. U.S. Census Bureau, American Community Survey; Current Population Survey, Annual Social and Economic Supplement; Table 1. General Mobility, by Race and Hispanic Origin, Region, Sex, Age, Relationship to Householder, Educational Attainment, Marital Status, Nativity, Tenure, and Poverty Status: 2015 to 2016; Annual Estimates of the Resident Population for Selected Age Groups by Sex for the United States, States, Counties, and Puerto Rico Commonwealth and Municipios: April 1, 2010 to July 1, 2015. Release date June 2016.

Figure 4: Persons 65+ as a Percentage of Total Population, 2015

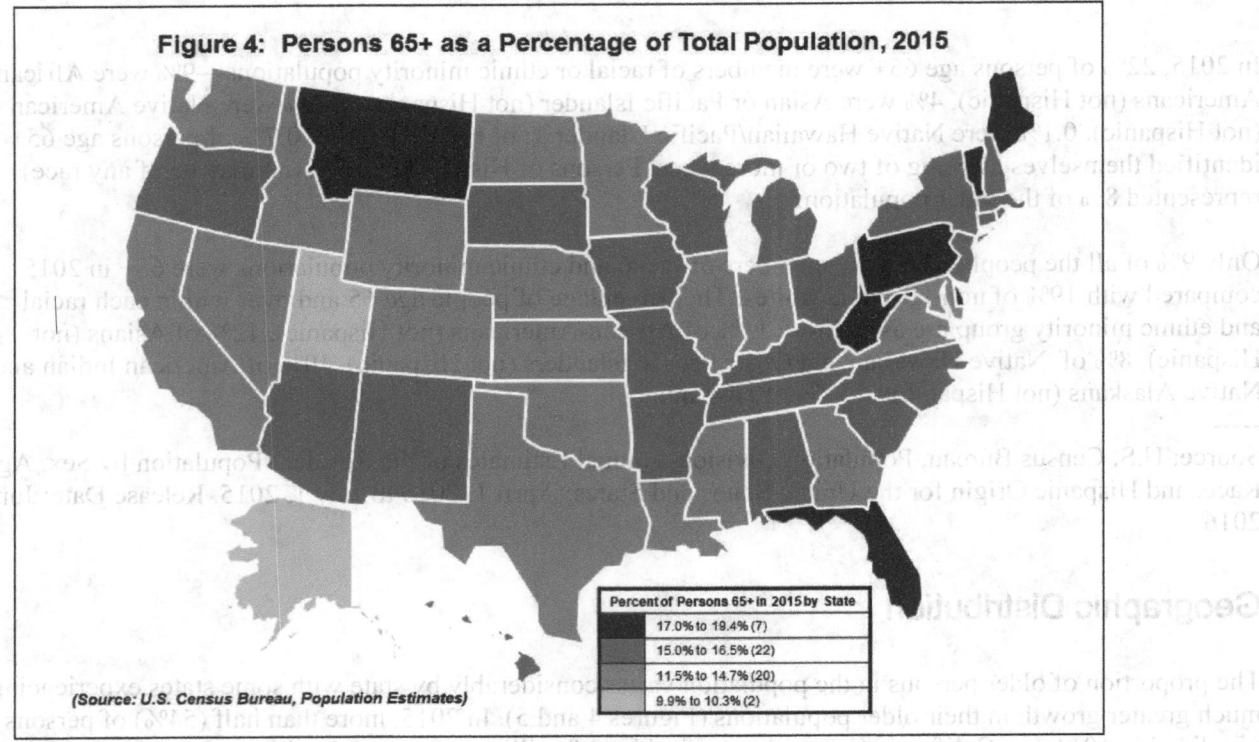

Figure 4: Persons 65+ as a Percentage of Total Population, 2015

Percent of Persons 65+ in 2015 by State
- 17.0% to 19.4% (7)
- 15.0% to 16.5% (22)
- 11.5% to 14.7% (20)
- 9.9% to 10.3% (2)

(Source: U.S. Census Bureau, Population Estimates)

Figure 5: Percent Increase in Population 65+, 2005 to 2015

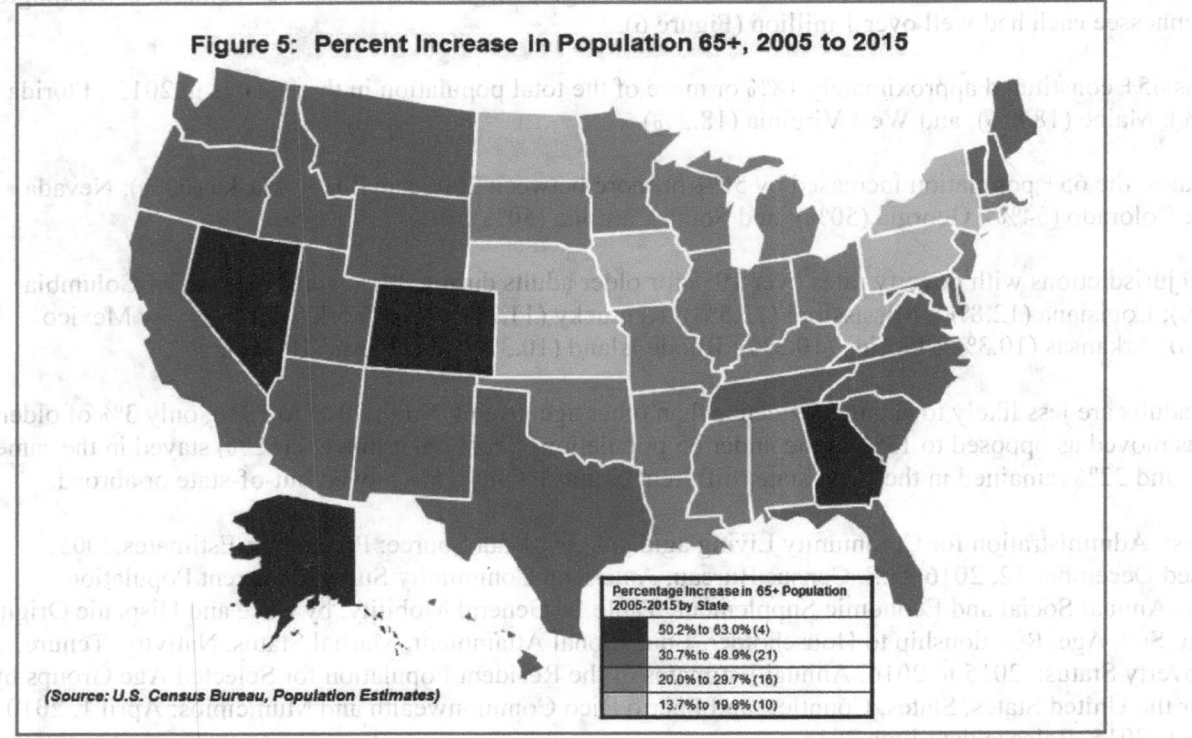

Figure 5: Percent Increase in Population 65+, 2005 to 2015

Percentage Increase in 65+ Population 2005-2015 by State
- 50.2% to 63.0% (4)
- 30.7% to 48.9% (21)
- 20.0% to 29.7% (16)
- 13.7% to 19.8% (10)

(Source: U.S. Census Bureau, Population Estimates)

Figure 6: The 65+ Population by State, 2015

State	Number of Persons 65 and Older (1)	Percent of All Ages	Percent Increase from 2005 to 2015	Percent Below Poverty 2015 (2)
US Total (50 States + DC)	47,760,852	14.9%	30.3%	8.8%
Alabama	764,162	15.7%	27.1%	9.9%
Alaska	72,837	9.9%	63.0%	4.5%
Arizona	1,120,054	16.4%	48.0%	9.0%
Arkansas	477,149	16.0%	24.2%	10.3%
California	5,188,754	13.3%	35.2%	9.9%
Colorado	711,625	13.0%	53.8%	7.0%
Connecticut	566,806	15.8%	19.3%	7.2%
Delaware	160,515	17.0%	43.2%	6.2%
District of Columbia	77,004	11.5%	15.8%	15.2%
Florida	3,942,468	19.4%	32.3%	10.3%
Georgia	1,304,924	12.8%	50.2%	9.7%
Hawaii	236,914	16.5%	35.4%	7.8%
Idaho	243,494	14.7%	47.8%	8.7%
Illinois	1,830,277	14.2%	20.6%	8.5%
Indiana	966,127	14.6%	24.4%	7.2%
Iowa	502,877	16.1%	15.1%	7.0%
Kansas	426,410	14.6%	19.6%	7.3%
Kentucky	672,765	15.2%	27.5%	11.2%
Louisiana	653,094	14.0%	22.7%	12.8%
Maine	250,536	18.8%	30.7%	8.8%
Maryland	849,571	14.1%	33.1%	7.3%
Massachusetts	1,045,222	15.4%	23.1%	9.2%
Michigan	1,570,671	15.8%	25.1%	7.8%
Minnesota	805,643	14.7%	29.7%	6.9%
Mississippi	439,701	14.7%	23.5%	12.5%
Missouri	954,922	15.7%	23.5%	8.5%
Montana	178,011	17.2%	37.3%	7.6%
Nebraska	278,711	14.7%	18.9%	7.4%
Nevada	422,118	14.6%	55.3%	8.4%
New Hampshire	218,942	16.5%	38.6%	6.1%
New Jersey	1,343,626	15.0%	20.0%	7.9%
New Mexico	330,405	15.8%	39.7%	11.1%
New York	2,964,315	15.0%	19.0%	11.2%
North Carolina	1,516,824	15.1%	43.2%	9.2%
North Dakota	107,281	14.2%	13.7%	8.9%
Ohio	1,842,952	15.9%	20.7%	7.6%
Oklahoma	576,250	14.7%	23.4%	8.4%
Oregon	660,876	16.4%	40.4%	7.3%
Pennsylvania	2,179,788	17.0%	15.5%	7.8%
Rhode Island	169,976	16.1%	14.5%	10.3%
South Carolina	794,795	16.2%	48.9%	9.3%
South Dakota	134,420	15.7%	22.6%	8.3%
Tennessee	1,016,552	15.4%	35.3%	9.8%
Texas	3,225,168	11.7%	42.9%	10.3%
Utah	307,867	10.3%	44.0%	6.8%
Vermont	109,893	17.6%	34.4%	6.6%
Virginia	1,188,393	14.2%	38.0%	7.3%
Washington	1,036,046	14.4%	45.0%	7.4%
West Virginia	336,288	18.2%	19.8%	8.5%
Wisconsin	902,134	15.6%	24.3%	7.1%
Wyoming	84,699	14.5%	36.1%	8.0%
Puerto Rico	626,962	18.0%	27.4%	41.0%

Notes: (1) Population Estimates (2) Poverty data for US are from the Current Population Survey, Poverty data for States and Puerto Rico are from the American Community Survey.

Data Sources: U.S. Census Bureau, Current Population Survey, Annual Social and Economic Supplement; Population Estimates; and American Community Survey.

Income

The median income of older persons in 2015 was $31,372 for males and $18,250 for females. From 2014 to 2015, median money income (after adjusting for inflation) of all households headed by older people increased by 4.3% which was statistically significant. Households containing families headed by persons 65+ reported a median income in 2015 of $57,360 ($60,266 for non-Hispanic Whites, $42,334 for Hispanics, $43,855 for African-Americans, and $64,688 for Asians). About 5% of family households with an older adult householder had incomes less than $15,000 and 72% had incomes of $35,000 or more (Figure 7).

Figure 7: Percent Distribution by Income: 2015

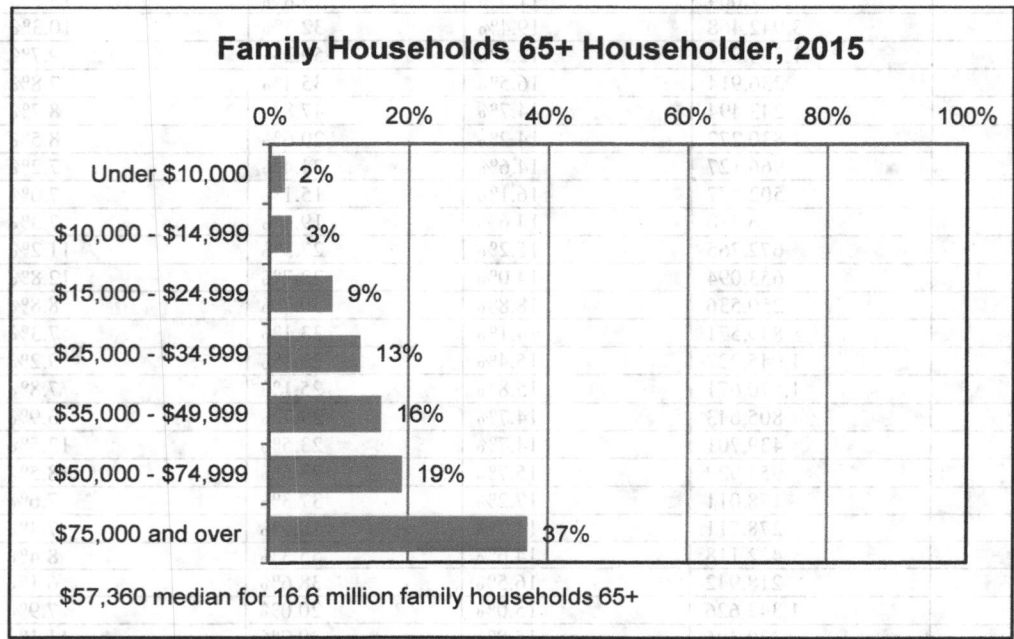

Family Households 65+ Householder, 2015

Income	Percent
Under $10,000	2%
$10,000 - $14,999	3%
$15,000 - $24,999	9%
$25,000 - $34,999	13%
$35,000 - $49,999	16%
$50,000 - $74,999	19%
$75,000 and over	37%

$57,360 median for 16.6 million family households 65+

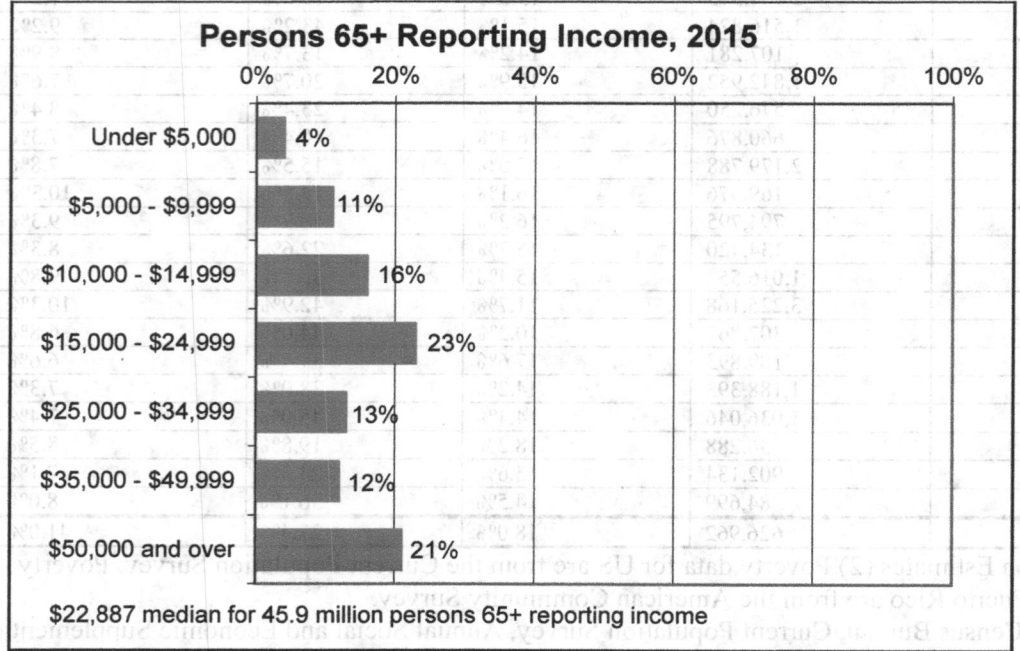

Persons 65+ Reporting Income, 2015

Income	Percent
Under $5,000	4%
$5,000 - $9,999	11%
$10,000 - $14,999	16%
$15,000 - $24,999	23%
$25,000 - $34,999	13%
$35,000 - $49,999	12%
$50,000 and over	21%

$22,887 median for 45.9 million persons 65+ reporting income

Note: Percentages may not add to 100 due to rounding.
Source: U.S. Census Bureau, Current Population Survey, Annual Social and Economic Supplement.

For all older persons reporting income in 2015 (45.9 million), 15% reported less than $10,000 and 46% reported $25,000 or more. The median income reported was $22,887.

The major sources of income as reported by older persons in 2014 were Social Security (reported by 84% of older persons), income from assets (reported by 62%), earnings (reported by 29%), private pensions (reported by 37%), and government employee pensions (reported by 16%). In 2014, Social Security benefits accounted for 33% of the aggregate income[1] of the older population. The bulk of the remainder consisted of earnings (32%), asset income (10%), pensions (21%) and other (4%). Social Security constituted 90% or more of the income received by 33% of beneficiaries (21% of married couples and 43% of non-married beneficiaries).

Sources: U.S. Census Bureau, Current Population Survey, Annual Social and Economic Supplement, FINC-01. Selected Characteristics of Families by Total Money Income in 2015; PINC-01. Selected Characteristics of People 15 Years Old and Over by Total Money Income in 2015, Work Experience in 2015, Race, Hispanic Origin, and Sex; and U.S. Census Bureau, Income and Poverty in the United States: 2015, Current Population Reports, P60-256(RV), issued September 2016. Social Security Administration, "Fast Facts and Figures About Social Security, 2016."

Poverty

Over 4.2 million people age 65 and over (8.8%) were below the poverty level in 2015.[2] This poverty rate is statistically different from the poverty rate in 2014 (10.0%). Another 2.4 million or 5% of older adults were classified as "near-poor" (income between the poverty level and 125% of this level).

Just over 2.4 million older Whites (alone, not Hispanic) (6.6%) were poor in 2015, compared to 18.4% of older African-Americans (alone), 11.8% of older Asians (alone), and 17.5% of older Hispanics (any race).

Older women had a higher poverty rate (10.3%) than older men (7%) in 2015. Older persons living alone were much more likely to be poor (15.4%) than were older persons living with families (5.7%). The highest poverty rates were experienced among older Hispanic women who lived alone (40.7%).

In 2011, the U.S. Census Bureau released a new Supplemental Poverty Measure (SPM). The SPM methodology shows a significantly higher number of older persons below poverty than is shown by the official poverty measure. For persons 65 and older this poverty measure shows a poverty level of 13.7% in 2015 (almost 5 percentage points higher than the official rate of 8.8%). Unlike the official poverty rate, the SPM takes into account regional variations in the cost of housing etc. and, even more significantly, the impact of both non-cash benefits received (e.g., SNAP/food stamps, low income tax credits, and WIC) and non-discretionary expenditures including medical out-of-pocket (MOOP) expenses. For persons 65 and over, MOOP was the major source of the significant differences between these measures. The SPM does not replace the official poverty measure.

Sources: U.S. Census Bureau, Current Population Survey, Annual Social and Economic Supplement; POV01: Age and Sex of All People, Family Members and Unrelated Individuals Iterated by Income-to-Poverty Ratio and Race: 2015; "Income and Poverty in the United States: 2014," P60-256, issued September, 2016; Poverty Thresholds for 2015 by Size of Family and Number of Related Children Under 18 Years; and "The Supplemental Poverty Measure: 2015," P60-258(RV), revised September 2016.

---

[1] Aggregate income refers to the total income of couples and nonmarried persons aged 65 or older.
[2] The poverty threshold in 2015 was $11,367 for householders age 65 and over living alone.

Housing

Of the 11.9 million households headed by persons age 75 and over in 2015, 76% were owners and 24% were renters. The median family income of older homeowners was $31,000. The median family income of older renters was $17,400. In 2015, almost 44% of older householders spent more than one-third of their income on housing costs - 36% for owners and 78% for renters.

For older homeowners age 75 and over in 2015, the median construction year was 1969 compared with 1978 for all homeowners. Among the homes owned by people age 75 and older, 3.5% had moderate to severe problems with plumbing, heating, electric, wiring, and/or upkeep. In 2015, the median value of homes owned by older persons was $150,000 (with a median purchase price of $53,000). In comparison, the median home value all homeowners was $180,000 (with a median purchase price of $127,000). About 78% of older homeowners in 2015 owned their homes free and clear.

Source: Department of Housing and Urban Development, American Housing Survey, National Tables: 2015.

Employment

In 2015, 8.8 million (18.9 %) Americans age 65 and over were in the labor force (working or actively seeking work), including 4.8 million men (23.4%) and 4 million women (15.3%). They constituted 5.6% of the U.S. labor force. About 3.8% were unemployed. Labor force participation of men 65+ decreased steadily from 63.1% in 1900 to 15.8% in 1985; then stayed at 16%-18% until 2002; and has been increasing since then to over 20%. The participation rate for women 65+ rose slightly from 8.3% in 1900 to 10.9% in 1956, fell to 7.3% in 1985, and then stayed at 8%-9% during the 1990s. Beginning in 2000, labor force participation of older women started to gradually rise from 9.7% to the 2015 level. This increase is especially noticeable among the population aged 65-69.

Source: Bureau of Labor Statistics, Current Population Survey, Labor Force Statistics,

Education

The educational level of the older population is increasing. Between 1970 and 2016, the percentage of older persons who had completed high school rose from 28% to 85%. About 28% in 2016 had a bachelor's degree or higher. The percentage who had completed high school varied considerably by race and ethnic origin in 2016: 90% of Whites (not Hispanic), 80% of Asians (not Hispanic), 77% of African-Americans (not Hispanic), 71% of American Indian/Alaska Natives (not Hispanic), and 54% of Hispanics. The increase in educational levels is also evident within these groups. In 1970, only 30% of older Whites and 9% of older African-Americans were high school graduates.

Source: U.S. Census Bureau, Current Population Survey, Annual Social and Economic Supplement.

Health and Health Care

In 2015, 39% of noninstitutionalized people age 75 and over assessed their health as excellent or very good (compared to 54% for persons aged 45-64 years). Most older persons have at least one chronic condition and many have multiple conditions. In 2015, the most frequently occurring conditions among older persons age 75 and over were: diagnosed arthritis (53%), all types of heart disease (35%), any cancer (32%), diagnosed diabetes (22% in 2011-2014), and hypertension (high blood pressure or taking antihypertensive medication) (72% among men age 75 and over and 80% among women age 75 and over in 2011-2014).

In January-June 2016, 70% of people age 65 and over reported that they received an influenza vaccination during the past 12 months and 68% reported that they had ever received a pneumococcal vaccination. About 30% (of persons 60+) reported height/weight combinations that placed them among the obese. Slightly under half (45%) of persons aged 65-74 and 29% of persons 75+ reported that they engaged in regular leisure-time physical activity. Only 9% reported that they are current smokers and 8% reported excessive alcohol consumption. Less than 3% reported that they had experienced serious psychological distress during the past 30 days.

In 2015, 7.1 million people age 65 and over stayed in a hospital overnight at least one night during the year. Among this group of older adults, 10% stayed overnight 1 time, 3% stayed overnight 2 times, and 2% stayed overnight 3 or more times. This is approximately double the number of overnight hospital stays for the population age 45 to 64; 6% had stayed overnight 1 time, 1% stayed overnight 2 times, and 1% stayed overnight 3 or more times. Older persons averaged more office visits with doctors than younger persons in 2015. Among people age 75 and over, 23% had 10 or more visits to a doctor or other health care professional in the past 12 months compared to 15% among people age 45 to 64.

In January-June 2016, 97% of older persons reported that they did have a usual place to go for medical care and only 2% said that they failed to obtain needed medical care during the previous 12 months due to financial barriers.

In 2015 older consumers averaged out-of-pocket health care expenditures of $5,756, an increase of 37% since 2005 ($4,193). In contrast, the total population spent considerably less, averaging $4,342 in out-of-pocket costs. Older Americans spent 12.9% of their total expenditures on health, as compared with 7.8% among all consumers. Health costs incurred on average by older consumers in 2015 consisted of $3,893 (68%) for insurance, $967 (17%) for medical services, $672 (12%) for drugs, and $224 (4%) for medical supplies.

Sources: National Center for Health Statistics, National Health Interview Survey, Early Release of Selected Estimates Based on Data from the January-June 2016; Tables of Summary Health Statistics for U.S. Adults: 2015. Bureau of Labor Statistics, Consumer Expenditure Survey, Table 1300. Age of Reference Person: Annual Expenditures Means, Shares, Standard Errors, and Coefficient of Variation, 2015.

Health Insurance Coverage

In 2015, almost all (93%) non-institutionalized persons age 65+ were covered by Medicare. Medicare covers mostly acute care services and requires beneficiaries to pay part of the cost, leaving about half of health spending to be covered by other sources. About half of older adults (52%) had some type of private health insurance, 7% had military-based health insurance, 7% were covered by Medicaid, and 1% had no coverage (Figure 8).

Figure 8: Percentage of Persons 65+ by type of Health Insurance Coverage, 2015

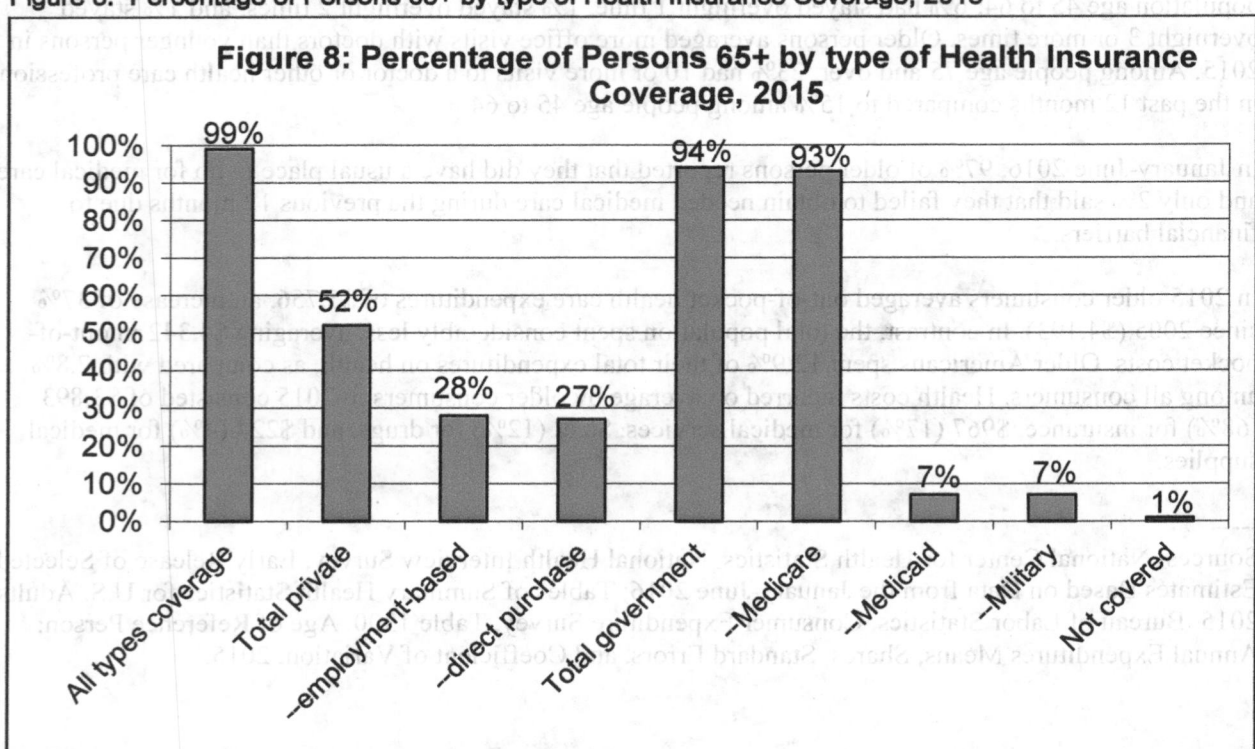

Figure 8: Percentage of Persons 65+ by type of Health Insurance Coverage, 2015

Note: A person can be represented in more than one category.
Source: U.S. Census Bureau, Current Population Survey, Annual Social and Economic Supplement.

Sources: U.S. Census Bureau, Current Population Survey, Annual Social and Economic Supplement; and Health Insurance in the United States: 2015," P60-257, issued September, 2016.

Disability and Activity Limitations

According to the U.S. Census Bureau's American Community Survey, some type of disability (i.e., difficulty in hearing, vision, cognition, ambulation, self-care, or independent living) was reported by 35% of people age 65 and over in 2015. The percentages for individual disabilities ranged from almost one quarter (23%) having an ambulatory disability to 7% having a vision difficulty (Figure 9).

Figure 9: Percentage of persons 65+ with a disability, 2015

Figure 9: Percentage of Persons 65+ with a disability, 2015

Category	Percentage
Independent living difficulty	15%
Self-care difficulty	8%
Ambulatory difficulty	23%
Cognitive difficulty	9%
Vision difficulty	7%
Hearing difficulty	15%
Any disability	35%

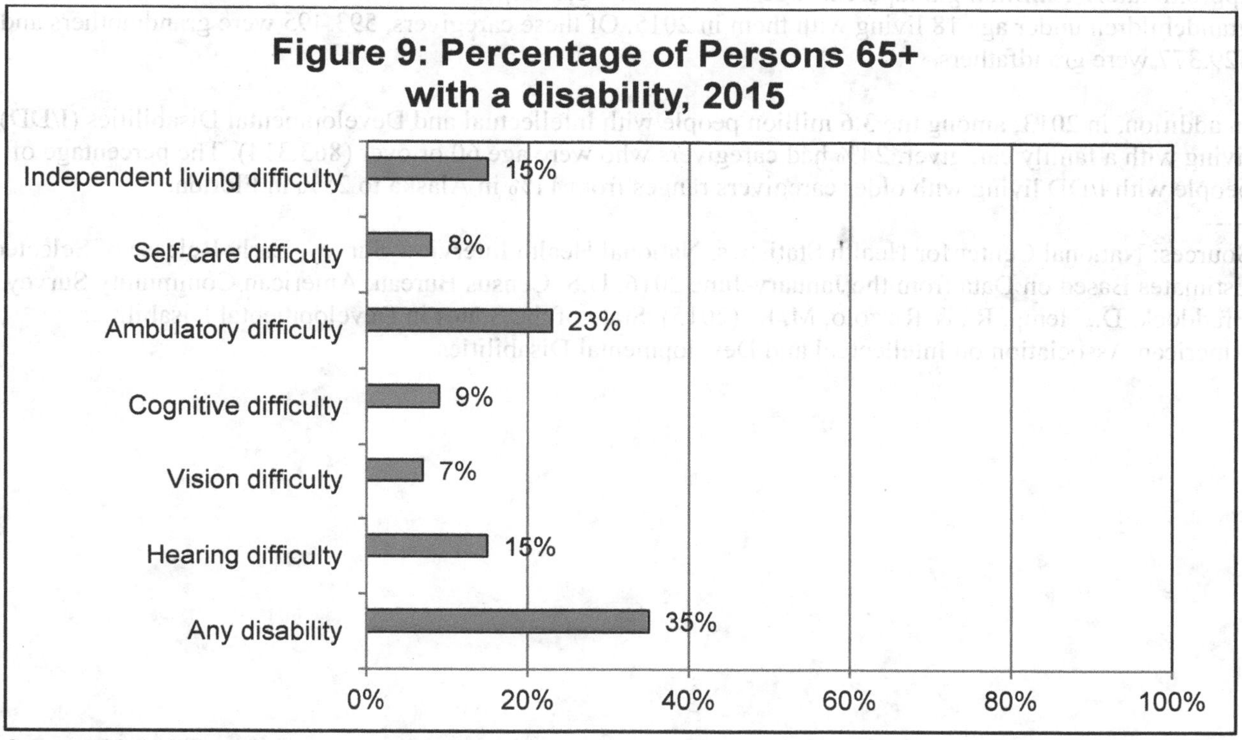

Source: U.S. Census Bureau, American Community Survey.

Using limitations in activities of daily living (ADLs) and instrumental activities of daily living (IADLs) to measure disability, in 2013, 30% of community-resident Medicare beneficiaries age 65+ reported difficulty in performing one or more ADLs and an additional 12% reported difficulty with one or more IADLs. By contrast, 95% of institutionalized Medicare beneficiaries age 65 and over had difficulties with one or more ADLs and 81% of them had difficulty with three or more ADLs. [ADLs include bathing, dressing, eating, and getting around the house. IADLs include preparing meals, shopping, managing money, using the telephone, doing housework, and taking medication.] Limitations in activities because of chronic conditions increase with age.

Sources: U.S. Census Bureau, American Community Survey. Centers for Medicare and Medicaid Services, Medicare Current Beneficiary Survey.

Caregiving

The need for caregiving increases with age. In January-June 2016, older adults aged 85 and over were more than twice as likely (20%) as adults age 75–84 (7%) to need help with personal care from other persons, and adults age 85 and over were more than six times as likely as adults age 65–74 (3%) to need help with personal care from other persons. Among older adults age 85 and over, women were more likely (23%) than men (14%) to need help with personal care from other persons.

Older adults not only need care, but often also provide care to younger family members. For example, approximately 1 million grandparents age 60 and over were responsible for the basic needs of one or more grandchildren under age 18 living with them in 2015. Of these caregivers, 593,495 were grandmothers and 429,377 were grandfathers.

In addition, in 2013, among the 3.6 million people with Intellectual and Developmental Disabilities (I/DD)[3] living with a family caregiver, 24% had caregivers who were age 60 or over (863,314). The percentage of people with I/DD living with older caregivers ranges from 11% in Alaska to 25% in Florida.

Sources: National Center for Health Statistics, National Health Interview Survey, Early Release of Selected Estimates Based on Data from the January-June 2016. U.S. Census Bureau, American Community Survey. Braddock, D., Hemp, R., & Rizzolo, M. K. (2015). State of the States in Developmental Disabilities. American Association on Intellectual and Developmental Disabilities.

---

[3] The total number of people with Intellectual and Developmental Disabilities (I/DD) is estimated to be 5 million.

Notes

Principal sources of data for the Profile are the U.S. Census Bureau, the National Center for Health Statistics, and the Bureau of Labor Statistics. The Profile incorporates the latest data available but not all items are updated on an annual basis.

Age-adjusted estimates are used when available.

The data presented in this report refer to the noninstitutionalized population except where noted.

A Profile of Older Americans: 2016 was developed by the Administration on Aging (AoA), Administration for Community Living, U.S. Department of Health and Human Services.

AoA serves as an advocate for older adults within the federal government and is working to encourage and coordinate a responsive system of family and community based services throughout the nation. AoA helps states develop comprehensive service systems which are administered by 56 State Units on Aging, 629 Area Agencies on Aging, 244 Tribal organizations, and 2 Native Hawaiian organizations.

National Organizations & Federal Agencies

General

1 50Plus.org

www.50plus.org

Fifty Plus is a nonprofit organization whose mission is to promote an active lifestyle for older people. The organization started at Stanford University as an outgrowth of some medical research on the value of exercise for older persons. Fifty Plus sponsors fitness activities such as walks, runs and hikes for seniors. It organized runs, walks and get-togethers in various regions.

Year Founded: 1979; Number of Members: 2,000

2 Administration for Community Living (ACL)

330 C Street SW
Washington, DC 20201
202-401-4634
www.acl.gov

Lance Robertson, Administrator
Mary Lazare, Principal Deputy Administrator
Edwin Walker, Deputy Assistant Secretary

The ACL is part of the U.S. Department of Health and Human Services. It is committed to designing and implementing policies and programs that ensure older Americans and persons with disabilities are able to fully participate in their communities. The organization includes the Administration on Aging (AoA) and the Administration on Disabilities (AoD).

Year Founded: 2012

3 Air Force Aid Society

241 18th Street S
Suite 202
Arlington, VA 22202
703-972-2650
Fax: 703-972-2646; *Toll Free:* 800-769-8951
afas@afas-hq.org
www.afas.org

Lt Gen John D. Hopper Jr, CEO
Col Linda Egentowich, COO
Col Sidney Heetland, CFO

The Air Force Aid Society is the official charity of the United States Air Force, providing world wide emergency assistance, sponsoring education assistance programs and offering an array of base community enhancement programs that improve quality of life for Airmen and their families.

Year Founded: 1942

4 Alzheimer's Disease Demonstration GrantProgram
Administration on Aging

330 C Street SW
Washington, DC 20201
202-401-4634
www.aoa.acl.gov

Fosters the development of innovative models of care for persons with Alzheimer's disease and their caregivers..

Year Founded: 1992

5 America's Health Insurance Plans

601 Pennsylvania Avenue NW
South Building, Suite 500
Washington, DC 20004
202-778-3200
Fax: 202-331-7487
ahip@ahip.org
www.ahip.org

Trade association representing America's health insurance industry.

Number of Members: 1,300

6 American Academy of Ambulatory Care Nursing

East Holly Avenue Box 56
Pitman, NJ 08071-0056
Fax: 856-589-7463; *Toll Free:* 800-262-6877
aaacn@aaacn.org
www.aaacn.org

Cynthia Hnatiuk, CEO
Tom Greene, Marketing Director
Pat Reichart, Director of Association Services

Membership includes nurses in direct practice, education, and research roles as well as those in management and administration. AAACN is the only specialty nursing association that focuses on excellence in ambulatory care, providing a forum for nursing organizations to dialogue, collaborate, and facilitate policy formulation on professional practice and national health.

7 American Academy of Nursing

1000 Vermont Avenue NW
Suite 910
Washington, DC 20005-4903
202-777-1170
Fax: 202-777-0107
info@aannet.org
www.aannet.org

Cheryl G. Sullivan, CEO
Jocelyn Cunic, COO

The Academy serves the public and the nursing profession by advancing health policy and practice through the generation, synthesis, and dissemination of nursing knowledge. Members are nursing's most accomplished leaders in education, management, practice and research.

Year Founded: 1973

8 American Academy of Oral & Maxillofacial Radiology

3086 Stevenson Drive
Suite 200
Springfield, IL 62703
303-724-7117
Fax: 303-724-7109
ed@aaomr.org
www.aaomr.org

Dr. Jie Yang, President
Dr. Robert Cederberg, Executive Director

The AAOMR aims to promote and advance the art and science of radiology in dentistry, and to provide a forum for communication among its members, to the healthcare community and to the public. The AAOMR conducts continuing education programs, including the annual scientific session, sponsors a scientific journal publications, has a newsletter, issues guidelines, and pursues additional activities consistent with the purpose of the Academy.

Year Founded: 1945

9   American Academy of Otolaryngology - Head and Neck Surgery

1650 Diagonal Road
Alexandria, VA 22314-2857
703-836-4444
Fax: 703-683-5100
info@entnet.org
www.entnet.org

Sujana S. Chandrasekhar, President
Scott P. Stringer, Secretary/Treasurer

Representing specialists who treat the ear, nose, throat and related structures of the head and neck. The AAO-HNS Foundation works to advance the art, science, and ethical practice of otolaryngology-head and neck surgery through education, research, and lifelong learning.

10   American Assembly for Men in Nursing

PO Box 7867
Philadelphia, PA 19101-7867
215-243-5813
Fax: 215-387-7497
aamn@aamn.org
www.aamn.org

Karen Mota, Account Executive

The nation's oldest and largest multipurpose state professional association for registered nurses. Works with members to meet their needs through representation in the workplace, advocacy in the halls of government, and provision of quality continuing education and practice standards.

Year Founded: 1901

11   American Association for Adult and Continuing Education

1827 Powers Ferry Road
Building 14, Suite 100
Atlanta, GA 30339
678-271-4319
Fax: 678-229-2777
aaace10@aol.com
www.aaace.org

Margaret Eggleston, President
Jill Zarestky, Secretary
Chad Hoggan, Treasurer

To honor the learner who serves as an exemplar for adult education students throughout the nation. See Continuing Education chapter for specific opportunities by state.

12   American Association for Respiratory Care

9425 North MacArthur Boulevard
Suite 100
Irving, TX 75063-4706
972-243-2272
Fax: 972-484-2720
info@aarc.org
www.aarc.org

Allied health society of respiratory care technicians and therapists employed by hospitals, skilled nursing facilities, home care companies, group practices, educational institutions, and municipal organizations. To encourage, develop, and provide educational programs for persons interested in the profession of respiratory care; and to advance the science of respiratory care.

Year Founded: 1947; Number of Members: 37,000

13   American Association of Colleges of Nursing

One Dupont Circle NW
Suite 530
Washington, DC 20036
202-463-6930
Fax: 202-785-8320
info@aacn.nche.edu
www.aacn.nche.edu

Deborah Trautman, President & CEO
Jennifer Ahearn, COO

Institutions offering baccalaureate and/or graduate degrees in nursing. Seeks to advance the practice of professional nursing by improving the quality of baccalaureate and graduate programs, promoting research, and developing academic leaders. Works with other professional nursing organizations and organizations in other health professions to evaluate and improve health care. Conducts educational programs on masters and doctoral nursing education and faculty practice; sponsors executive development series for new and aspiring deans of nursing.

14   American Association of Colleges of Osteopathic Medicine

5550 Friendship Boulevard
Suite 310
Chevy Chase, MD 20815
301-968-4100
Fax: 301-968-4101
www.aacom.org

Stephen C. Shannon, President & CEO
John R. Roane, COO

Supporting and assisting the nation's osteopathic medical schools, and serving as a unifying voice for osteopathic medical education. The association is actively involved in all areas of osteopathic medical education, developing national initiatives to promote and raise awareness of osteopathic medicine.

15   American Association of Critical-Care Nurses

101 Columbia
Aliso Viejo, CA 92656-4109
949-362-2000
Fax: 949-362-2020; *Toll Free:* 800-809-2273
info@aacn.org
www.aacn.org

AACN is the largest specialty nursing organization in the world, representing the interests of nurses who are charged with the responsibility of caring for acutely and critically ill patients. The association is dedicated to providing members with the knowledge and resources necessary to provide optimal care to critically ill patients.

Number of Members: 100,000

16   American Association of Managed Care Nurses

4435 Waterfront Drive
Suite 101
Glen Allen, VA 23060
804-747-9698
Fax: 804-747-5316
sreed@aamcn.org
www.aamcn.org

Jacquelyn Smith, President

Non-profit organization representing Registered Nurses, Nurse Practitioners, Licensed Practical/Vocational Nurses and Social Workers. AAMCN seeks to offer those nurses the opportunity to become more successful, both in their workplace and their community, through interactive membership services, quality educational resources and unparalleled networking with other managed care nurses throughout the industry.

Year Founded: 1994

17   American Association of Nurse Anesthetists
222 South Prospect Avenue
Park Ridge, IL 60068-4001
847-692-7050
Fax: 847-692-6968; Toll Free: 855-526-2262
info@aana.com
www.aana.com

Wanda Wilson, Executive Director & CEO
Margaret S. Jung, COO

AANA advances patient safety, practice excellence, and its members' profession.

Year Founded: 1931

18   American Association of Nurse Practitioners
PO Box 12846
Austin, TX 78711
512-442-4262
Fax: 512-442-6469
admin@aanp.org
www.aanp.org

Cindy Cooke, President
Joyce M. Knestrick, Treasurer

National membership organization for NPs of all specialties.

Year Founded: 2013; Number of Members: 205,000

19   American Association of Occupational Health Nurses
7794 Grow Drive
Pensacola, FL 32514
850-474-6963
Fax: 850-484-8762; Toll Free: 800-241-8014
aaohn@internationalamc.com
www.aaohn.org

Jeannie Tomlinson, President
Ronda Weiss, Secretary

Registered professional nurses employed by business and industrial firms; nurse educators, nurse editors, nurse writers, and others interested in occupational health nursing. Promotes and sets standards for the profession. Provides and approves continuing education; maintains governmental affairs program; offers placement service.

20   American Association of Retirement Communities
PO Box 10981
Southport, NC 28461
Toll Free: 866-531-5567
info@the-aarc.org
the-aarc.org

Andre Nabors, Chairperson
Rachel Baker, Vice-Chairperson
Kristy Peters, Secretary

Works to promote the economic enhancement of communities through the promotion of retiree attraction as an economic development strategy. The AARC communicates the benefits of attracting migrating retirees to communities and assists those interested in marketing to this ever increasing portion of the American population.

Year Founded: 1994

21   American Baptist Homes and Caring Ministries
PO Box 239
Southworth, WA 98386
www.abhcm.org

Rev. Bill Painter, Board President

Retirement facilities (80), nursing homes and hospitals (31), and children's homes and special services (23). Provides special programs and educational events for member institutions. Offers consulting network program for member facilities. Compiles statistics.

Year Founded: 1930

22   American Bar Association
321 N Clark Street
Chicago, IL 60654
312-988-5000; *Toll Free: 800-285-2221*
www.americanbar.org

Paulette Brown, President
Mary T. Torres, Secretary
G. Nicholas Casey Jr., Treasurer

National representative of the legal profession.

Year Founded: 1878

23   American Benefits Council
1501 M Street NW
Suite 600
Washington, DC 20005
202-289-6700
Fax: 202-289-4582
info@abcstaff.org
www.americanbenefitscouncil.org

James A. Klein, President
Lynn D. Dudley, SVP, Retirement & Comp Policy
Katy Spangler, SVP, Health Policy

Represents Fortune 500 companies on federal employee benefits policy issues. Serving as a technical resource on benefits issues for lawmakers, the media and other industry trade association. Also leading other public policy organizations in developing and communicating a collective business community position and forge alliances on benefits issues.

Year Founded: 1967

24   American Board of Internal Medicine
510 Walnut Street
Suite 1700
Philadelphia, PA 19106-3699
Fax: 215-446-3590; Toll Free: 800-441-2246
www.abim.org

Richard J. Baron, President & CEO
Richard G. Battaglia, Chief Medical Officer
Suzanne Biemiller, Chief of Staff

Certification board established to determine the qualifications of, administer examinations to, and certify as specialists in internal medicine those doctors meeting its standards of clinical competence. Board members are elected from certified leaders in internal medicine. The board has certified approximately 121,000 internists and 54,000 subspecialist diplomates and issued 10,000 recertification certificates.

Year Founded: 1936

25 American Board of Perianesthesia Nursing Certification
475 Riverside Drive
6th Floor
New York, NY 10115-0089
Fax: 212-367-4256; *Toll Free:* 800-622-7262
abpanc@proexam.org
cpancapa.org

Linda Lakdawala, President

ABPANC is responsible for developing, sponsoring and managing the CPAN and CAPA nursing certification programs. These national professional certification programs are designed for registered nurses caring for patients who have experienced sedation, analgesia and anesthesia in a hospital or ambulatory care facility.

Year Founded: 1985

26 American College Health Association
1362 Mellon Road
Suite 180
Hanover, MD 21076
410-859-1500
Fax: 410-859-1510
contact@acha.org
www.acha.org

Matt J. Granato, Executive Director

Institutions (930) and individuals (2500). Provides an organization in which institutions of higher education and interested individuals may work together to promote health in its broadest aspects for students and all other members of the college community. Offers continuing education programs for health professionals. Maintains placement listings for physicians and other personnel seeking positions in college health. Compiles statistics. Conducts seminars and training programs. See Continuing Education chapter for specific educational opportunities.

Year Founded: 1920

27 American College of Clinical Pharmacology
PO Box 1758
Ashburn, VA 20146
571-291-3493
Fax: 571-918-4167
www.accp1.org

Krista L. Levy, Executive Director

Seeks to address the educational needs of its diverse membership and all healthcare professionals, covering a range of topics that span the entire area of the interaction between drugs and humans. Working to advance the science of clinical pharmacology in all its phases and to engage in appropriate educational efforts in the public interest, improve health by optimizing therapeutics, and provide innovative leadership and interdisciplinary education that will enable the generation, integration and translation of scientific knowledge to optimize research, development and utilization of medication for the benefit of all.

Year Founded: 1969

28 American College of Legal Medicine
9700 W Bryn Mawr Avenue
Suite 210
Rosemont, IL 60018
847-447-1713
Fax: 847-447-1150
info@aclm.org
www.aclm.org

Thomas R. McLean, President
Laurie Krueger, Executive Director

For persons interested in degrees in medicine, dentistry, and law. Promotes and advances the field of legal medicine or medical jurisprudence; arranges for meetings with medical, legal, and professional groups and legislative, judicial, and enforcement bodies interested in any province where law and medicine are contiguous; fosters and encourages centers for study and research in the field of legal medicine and publishes materials pertaining to legal medicine.

Year Founded: 1960

29 American College of Physicians
190 North Independence Mall West
Philadelphia, PA 19106-1572
215-351-2400; *Toll Free:* 800-523-1546
www.acponline.org

Steven E. Weinberger, Executive Vice President & CEO
Wayne H. Bylsma, COO
Ralph L. Hibbs Jr., CFO

National organization of internists - physicians who specialize in the prevenion, detection and treatment of illnesses in adults. ACP is the largest medical-specialty organization and second-largest physician group in the United States. Working to enhance the quality and effectiveness of health care by fostering excellence and professionalism in the practice of medicine.

Year Founded: 1915

30 American College of Trust and Estate Counsel
901 15th Street NW
Suite 525
Washington, DC 20005
202-684-8460
Fax: 202-684-8459
www.actec.org

Bruce Stone, President
Cynda C. Ottaway, President-Elect
Susan T. House, Vice-President

Attorneys specializing in probate law. Sends delegates to American Bar Association's Real Property, Probate, and Trust Law Section; maintains liaison with other organizations involved in probate law. See Legal Resources chapter for specific legal resources by state.

31 American Correctional Health Services Association
250 Gatsby Place
Alpharetta, GA 30022
Fax: 770-650-5789; *Toll Free:* 877-918-1842
admin@achsa.org
www.achsa.org

Members share the unique vocation of providing medical, mental health and dental health care for incarcerated individuals in our nation's jails, detention facilities, and prisons and within our communities. Includes the administrators, nurses, physicians, psychiatrists, nurse practitioners and physician assistants, mental health professionals, medical assistants, administrative personnel and ancillary personnel who work in a correctional setting, as well as those individuals and companies that support the associations' efforts.

Year Founded: 1976

32 American Council of Life Insurers
101 Constitution Avenue NW
Suite 700
Washington, DC 20001-2133
202-624-2000; *Toll Free: 877-674-4659*
contact@acli.com
www.acli.com

Dirk Kempthorne, President & CEO
Larry Burton, COO
Brian Waidmann, Chief of Staff

National trade association that represents the interests of legal reserve life insurance companies in legislative, regulatory and judicial matters at the federal, state and municipal levels of government and at the NAIC. Its member companies hold more than 90 percent of the life insurance force in the United States.

Number of Members: 300+

33 American Council on Education
One Dupont Circle NW
Washington, DC 20036
202-939-9300
comments@acenet.edu
www.acenet.edu

Renu Khator, Chair
John J. DeGioia, Vice Chair/Chair-elect

Professional educators providing support and guidance in the development of policies, procedures and evaluation for post secondary educational institutions. See Coninuing Education chapter for specific opportunities by state.

Year Founded: 1918

34 American Counseling Association
6101 Stevenson Avenue
Alexandria, VA 22304
703-823-9800
Fax: 703-823-0252; Toll Free: 800-347-6647
membership@counseling.org
www.counseling.org

Thelma Duffey, President

Counseling professionals in elementary and secondary schools, higher education, community agencies and organizations, rehabilitation programs, government, industry, business, private practice, career counseling, and mental health counseling. Conducts professional development institutes and provides liability insurance.

Year Founded: 1952; Number of Members: 50000

35 American Dental Society of Anesthesiology
211 E Chicago Avenue
Suite 780
Chicago, IL 60611
312-664-8270
Fax: 312-224-8624; Toll Free: 877-255-3742
adsahome@icloud.com
www.adsahome.org

Kenneth L. Reed, President
Daniel S. Sarasin, Vice President
Michael Rollert, President Elect

Members are dentists and physicians interested in the study and advancement of dental anesthesiology.

Year Founded: 1953; Number of Members: 5000

36 American Federation of School Administrators
1101 17th Street NW
Suite 408
Washington, DC 20036
202-986-4209
Fax: 202-986-4211
afsa@afsaadmin.org
afsaadmin.org

Diann Woodard, President
Ernest A. Logan, Executive Vice President
Leonard Pugliese, Secretary-Treasurer

Provides labor relations and professional and occupational services to public school principals, vice principals, administrators and supervisors in diverse school districts across the US, Puerto Rico and the US Virgin Islands.

Year Founded: 1976; Number of Members: 20000

37 American Health Care Association
1201 L Street NW
Washington, DC 20005
202-842-4444
Fax: 202-842-3860
www.ahcancal.org

Mark Parkinson, President & CEO

Federation of state associations of long-term health care facilities. Promotes standards for professionals in long-term health care delivery and quality care for patients and residents in a safe environment. Focuses on issues of availability, quality, affordability, and fair payment. Operates as liaison with governmental agencies, Congress, and professional associations. Compiles statistics.

Number of Members: 12,000

38 American Holistic Nurses Association
100 SE 9th Street
Suite 3A
Topeka, KS 66612-1213
785-234-1712
Fax: 785-234-1713; Toll Free: 800-278-2462
info@ahna.org
www.ahna.org

Terri Roberts, Executive Director
Nicole Malcom, Director of Operations

Members of the AHNA embrace holistic nursing as a lifestyle and as a profession. Realizing that true healing comes from within, holistic nurses must first heal themselves before they can facilitate the healing of others. Members work in all arenas of nursing to facilitate the integration of holistic nursing principles into nursing education, clinical practice and nursing research.

Year Founded: 1981

39 American Kinesiotherapy Association
118 College Drive
Suite 5142
Hattiesburg, MS 39406
Fax: 216-615-3355; Toll Free: 800-296-2582
info@akta.org
akta.org

Cynthia Howell, President

The AKTA is working to promote Kinesiotherapy and improve recognition of the profession through the pursuit of legislaion and public relations. The AKTA will serve the interests of its members and will work to enhance the standard of care provided by Kinesiotherapists through educational opportunities.

Year Founded: 1946

40   American Medical Association Alliance
550 M Ritchie Highway
Suite 271
Severna Park, MD 21146
312-464-4470
Fax: 312-464-5020; *Toll Free:* 800-549-4619
admin@amaalliance.org
www.amaalliance.org

Julie Newman, President

Representing the family of medicine in the United States. The Alliance network of physicians and physicians' spouses represents all stages of the medical lifestyle, from the training years to retirement.

Year Founded: 1922

41   American Medical Informatics Association
4720 Montgomery Lane
Suite 500
Bethesda, MD 20814
301-657-1291
Fax: 301-657-1296
mail@amia.org
www.amia.org

Douglas B. Fridsma, President & CEO
Karen Greenwood, Executive Vice President & COO

Medical personnel, physicians, physical scientists, engineers, data processors, researchers, educators, hospital administrators, nurses, medical record administrators, and computer professionals. Objectives are: to apply advanced systems and information technologies to scientific, literary, and educational activities; to promote excellence in health care; to promote patient care, teaching, research, and health administration.

Year Founded: 1990; Number of Members: 5,000

42   American Medical Rehabilitation Providers Association
1710 N Street NW
Washington, DC 20036
202-223-1920
Fax: 202-223-1925; *Toll Free:* 888-346-4624
www.amrpa.org

David Stover, President & CEO

AMRPA has emerged from the traditions of medical rehabilitation and stands poised to renew the power of collective advocacy.

43   American Mental Health Counselors Association
675 N Washington Street
Suite 470
Alexandria, VA 22314
703-548-6002
Fax: 703-548-4775; *Toll Free:* 800-326-2642
www.amhca.org

Joel E. Miller, Executive Director & CEO
James K. Finley, Assoc. Executive Director

A growing community of clinical mental health counselors making a critical impact on the lives of Americans. AMHCA succeeds in giving a voice to the profession nationwide and in helping serve professionals and their colleagues in their individual states.

44   American Nephrology Nurses' Association
East Holly Avenue
PO Box 56
Pitman, NJ 08071
856-256-2320
Fax: 856-589-7463; *Toll Free:* 888-600-2662
anna@annanurse.org
www.annanurse.org

Mike Cunningham, Executive Director

Registered nurses, physicians, dietitians, social workers, and technicians. Promotes continuing education of members at national, regional, and local levels.

Year Founded: 1969; Number of Members: 10,000+

45   American Nurses Association
8515 Georgia Avenue
Suite 400
Silver Spring, MD 20910-3492
301-628-5000
Fax: 301-628-5001; *Toll Free:* 800-274-4262
www.nursingworld.org

Pamela F. Cipriano, President
Ernest J. Grant, Vice President
Patricia Travis, Treasurer

Represents the interests of the nation's 3.1 million registered nurses through its constituent and state nurses associations and its organizational affiliates. The ANA advances the nursing profession by fostering high standards of nursing practice, promoting the rights of nurses in the workplace, projecting a positive and realistic view of nursing, and by lobbying the Congress and regulatory agencies on health care issues affecting nurses and the public.

Year Founded: 1911

46   American Occupational Therapy Association
4720 Montgomery Lane
Suite 200
Bethesda, MD 20814-3449
301-652-6611
Fax: 301-652-7711; *Toll Free:* 800-729-2682
www.aota.org
TDD 800-377-8555

Representing the interests and concerns of occupational therapy practitioners and students of occupational therapy and to improve the quality of occupational therapy services.

Year Founded: 1917; Number of Members: 42,000

47   American Physiological Society
9650 Rockville Pike
Bethesda, MD 20814-3991
301-634-7164
Fax: 301-634-7241
www.the-aps.org

Martin Frank, Executive Director
Scarletta Whitsett, Executive Assistant
Esther Samuel, Administrative Assistant

Devoted to fostering education, scientific research, and dissemination of information in the physiological sciences.

Year Founded: 1887; Number of Members: 10,500

48   American Psychiatric Nurses Association

3141 Fairview Park Drive
Suite 625
Falls Church, VA 22042
571-533-1919
Fax: 855-883-2762; *Toll Free:* 855-863-2762
info@apna.org
www.apna.org

Mary Ann Nihart, President
Joyce Shea, Secretary
Susan Dawson, Treasurer

The largest professional membership organization committed to the specialty practice of psychiatric-mental health (PMH) nursing and wellness promotion, prevention of mental health problems, and the care and treatment of persons with psychiatric disorders.

Year Founded: 1986

49   American Psychoanalytic Association

309 E 49th Street
New York, NY 10017
212-752-0450
Fax: 212-593-0571
info@apsa.org
www.apsa.org

Dean K. Stein, Executive Director

Focusing on education, research and membership development. An affiliate of the American Association for the Advancement of Science.

Year Founded: 1911

50   American Society for Laser Medicine andSurgery

2100 Stewart Avenue
Suite 240
Wausau, WI 54401
715-845-9283
Fax: 715-848-2493; *Toll Free:* 877-258-6028
information@aslms.org
www.aslms.org

Dianne Dalsky, Executive Director

Physicians, physicists, and other scientists; nurses, dentists, podiatrists, veterinarians, and other paramedical personnel; technicians and commercial representatives concerned with the medical applications of lasers. Facilitates exchange of information concerning lasers.

Year Founded: 1979

51   American Society for Parenteral and Enteral Nutrition

8630 Fenton Street
Suite 412
Silver Spring, MD 20910
301-587-6315
Fax: 301-587-2365; *Toll Free:* 800-727-4567
aspen@nutritioncare.org
www.nutritioncare.org

Debra BenAvram, CEO
Lowell Aplebaum, COO

Dedicated to improving patient care by advancing the science and practice of clinical nutrition and metabolism. AS-PEN is an interdisciplinary organization whose members are involved in the provision of clinical nutrition therapies, including parenteral and enteral nutrition. Members are dietitians, nurses, pharmacists, physicians, scientists, students and other health professionals from every facet of nutrition support clinical practice, research and education.

Year Founded: 1975

52   American Society of Colon and Rectal Surgeons

85 West Algonquin Road
Suite 550
Arlington Heights, IL 60005
847-290-9184
Fax: 847-290-9203
ascrs@fascrs.org
www.fascrs.org

Charles E. Littlejohn, President
Tracy L. Hull, Secretary
Neil H. Hyman, Treasurer

The premier society for colon and rectal surgeons and other surgeons dedicated to advancing and promoting the science and practice of the treatment of patients with diseases and disorders affecting the colon, rectum and anus. Assuring high quality patient care and advancing the science through research and education for prevention and management of disorders.

53   American Society of General Surgeons

4582 S Ulster Street
Suite 201
Denver, CO 80237
303-771-5948
Fax: 303-771-2550; *Toll Free:* 800-998-8322
www.theasgs.org

G. Kevin Gillian, President
Kwan Albert, Secretary/Treasurer

The ASGS seeks to serve as a knowledgeable and respected advocate for General Surgeon specialists, and also seeks to enhance General Surgery as a specialty. Dedicated to maintaining the highest standards of practice for the specialty of General Surgery, and the highest quality of care for patients.

54   American Society of Maxillofacial Surgeons

500 Cummings Center
Suite 4550
Beverly, MA 01915
978-927-8330
Fax: 978-524-0498
admin@maxface.org
maxface.org

Arun Gosain, President

Representing maxillofacial surgeons who are devoted to improving and promoting the highest levels of patient care. Maxillofacial and Craniofacial surgeons specialize in bone and soft tissue reconstruction and enhancement of the face. Advancing the science and practice of surgery of the facial region and craniofacial skeleton through excellence in education and research and through advocacy on behalf of patients and practitioners.

55   American Society of Neuroradiology

800 Enterprise Drive
Suite 205
Oak Brook, IL 60523

630-574-0220
Fax: 630-574-0661
www.asnr.org

James B. Gantenberg, Executive Director/CEO

Neuroradiologists who spend at least half of their time practicing neuroradiology. Fosters education, basic science research, and communication in neuroradiology.

Year Founded: 1962

56 American Society of PeriAnesthesia Nurses
90 Frontage Rd
Cherry Hill, NJ 08034
856-616-9600
Fax: 856-616-9601; *Toll Free:* 877-737-9696
aspan@aspan.org
www.aspan.org

Kevin Dill, CEO

Nurses practicing in all phases of ambulatory surgery, preanesthesia and post anesthesia care. Promotes quality and cost effective care for patients, their families, and the community through public and professional education, research and standards of practice. Offers continuing education programs.

Year Founded: 1980; Number of Members: 15,000

57 American Society of Plastic Surgeons
444 E Algonquin Road
Arlington Heights, IL 60005
847-228-9900
Fax: 847-228-7485
www.plasticsurgery.org

Michael D. Costelloe, Executive Vice President

Working to advance quality care to plastic surgery patients by encouraging high standards of training, ethics, physician practice and research in plastic surgery. The Society is a strong advocate for patient safety and requires its members to operate in accredited surgical facilities that have passed rigorous external review of equipment and staffing.

Year Founded: 1931

58 American Society of Tropical Medicine and Hygiene
One Parkview Plaza
Suite 800
Oakbrook Terrace, IL 60181
847-686-2238
Fax: 847-686-2251
info@astmh.org
www.astmh.org

Karen A. Goraleski, Executive Director

Worldwide organization of scientists, clinicians, and program professionals whose mission is to promote global health through the prevention and control of infectious and other diseases that disproportionately afflict the global poor. Research, health care and education are the central activities of ASTMH members, whose work bridges basic laboratory research to international field work and clinics to countrywide programs.

Year Founded: 1903

59 American Thoracic Society
25 Broadway
New York, NY 10004

212-315-8600
Fax: 212-315-6498
atsinfo@thoracic.org
www.thoracic.org

Atul Malhotra, President
Marc Moss, Vice President
Polly Parsons, Secretary-Treasurer

Dedicated to advancing clinical and scientific understanding of pulmonary diseases, critical illnesses and sleep-related breathing disorders.

Year Founded: 1905

60 American Yoga Association
PO Box 19986
Sarasota, FL 34276
941-927-4977
Fax: 941-921-9844
info@americanyogaassociation.org
www.americanyogaassociation.org

Alice Christensen, Founder

Goal is to provide the highest quality yoga instruction and educational resources to anyone interested in yoga.

61 Armed Forces Benefit Association
909 N Washington Street
Alexandria, VA 22314
703-549-4455
Fax: 703-706-5961; *Toll Free:* 800-776-2322
info@afba.com
www.afba.com

Ralph E. Eberhart, President & Chairman

Active and retired military personnel. Informs members of current legislation and benefits for military staff. Sponsors group insurance, discounts on merchandise, and group medical and dental care. Bestows honorary memberships.

Year Founded: 1947

62 Army Distaff Foundation
6200 Oregon Avenue NW
Washington, DC 20015
202-541-0149
Fax: 202-364-2856; *Toll Free:* 800-541-4255
armydistaff.org

MG Stephen Rippe, President & CEO
Barbara D'Agostino, COO
Enrico Santos, CFO

Provides retirement housing and health care services to active and retired military officers, and their relatives. Operates Knollwood, a military retirement community with independent apartment, as well as assisted living and nursing care.

Year Founded: 1959

63 Army Emergency Relief
200 Stovall Street
Room 5S33
Alexandria, VA 22332
703-428-0000
Fax: 703-325-7183; *Toll Free:* 866-878-6378
aer@aerhq.org
www.aerhq.org

Gen Dennis Reimer, President

Nonprofit organization created for the purpose of collecting and holding funds to relieve distress of members of the Army and their dependents.

Year Founded: 1942

64   Asian Americans Advancing Justice
1620 L Street NW
Suite 1050
Washington, DC 20036
202-296-2300
Fax: 202-296-2318
www.advancingjustice-aajc.org

Mee Moua, President & Executive Director

National nonprofit advocating for the civil and human rights of Asian Americans and ensuring their full participation in society.

Year Founded: 1991

65   Assisted Living Federation of America
1650 King Street
Suite 602
Alexandria, VA 22314
703-894-1805
Fax: 703-894-1831
info@alfa.org
www.alfa.org

James Balda, President & CEO
Maribeth Bersani, COO & SVP, Public Policy

ALFA serves as the voice for operators of senior living communities and the seniors and families those communities serve.

Year Founded: 1990

66   Association for Gerontology in Higher Education
1220 L Street NW
Suite 901
Washington, DC 20005
202-289-9806
Fax: 202-289-9824
aghe@aghe.org
www.aghe.org

Donna L. Wagner, President
Christine A. Fruhauf, Treasurer
Lydia Manning, Secretary

Higher education institutions which offer, on a national level, gerontological education and research programs. Promotes and encourages education and training of persons preparing for research or careers in gerontology, and works to increase public awareness of the needs of such training. Provides base for continuing cooperation with public officials, voluntary organizations, national associations, and others interested in aging and education. See Continuing Education chapters for specific state opportunities.

Year Founded: 1974

67   Association for Professionals in Infection Control and Epidemiology
1275 K Street NW
Suite 1000
Washington, DC 20005-4006
202-789-1890
Fax: 202-789-1899; Toll Free: 800-650-9570
www.apic.org

Susan A. Dolan, President
Linda McKinley, Secretary
Marc-Oliver Wright, Treasurer

Physicians, microbiologists, nurses, epidemiologists, medical technicians, sanitarians, and pharmacists. Purpose is to improve patient care by improving the profession of infection control through the development of educational programs and standards. Promotes quality research and standardization of practices and procedures. Develops communications among members, and assesses and influences legislation related to the field. Conducts seminars at local level.

Year Founded: 1972; Number of Members: 14,000

68   Association for Radiologic & Imaging Nursing
2201 Cooperative Way
Suite 600
Herndon, VA 20171
703-884-2229
Fax: 703-884-2229; Toll Free: 866-486-2762
info@arinursing.org
www.arinursing.org

Mary Sousa, President
Kristy L. Reese, Secretary
Christine Keough, Treasurer

A network of dynamic professionals who are committed to the development and growth of nurses who advance the standard of care in the imaging environment.

Year Founded: 1981

69   Association for Spiritual, Ethical and Religious Values in Counseling
www.aservic.org

Elizabeth O'Brien, President
Rick Gressard, Secretary
Amanda Giordano, Treasurer

A division of American Counseling Association. Counselors and other human development professionals who are convinced that religious, spiritual and other human values are essential to the full development of the person and to the discipline of counseling. Strives to understand and find ways to integrate religious, spiritual and other values in counseling and other developmental processes.

Year Founded: 1993

70   Association of Black Nursing Faculty
PO Box 580
Lisle, IL 60532
630-969-0221
Fax: 630-969-3895
abnf.secretary@gmail.com
www.abnf.net

Diana P. Jones, President
Voncella McCleary-Jones, Vice President
Patsy R. Smith, Secretary

Black nursing faculty teaching in nursing programs accredited by the National League for Nursing. Works to promote health-related issues and educational concerns of interest to the black community and ABNF. Serves as a forum for communication and the exchange of information among members; develops strategies for expressing concerns to other individuals, institutions, and communities. Assists members in professional development; develops and sponsors continuing education activities; fosters networking and guidance in employment and recruitment activities. Promotes health-related issues of legislation, government programs, and community activities. Supports black consumer advocacy issues. Encourages research. Maintains speakers' bureau and hall of fame. Offers charitable program and placement services. Compiles statistics, offers a computer-assisted job bank and research group information.

Year Founded: 1987

71 Association of Former Intelligence Officers

7700 Leesburg Pike
Suite 324
Falls Church, VA 22043
703-790-0320
Fax: 703-991-1278; *Toll Free:* 800-234-6717
afio@afio.com
www.afio.com

M.E. Spike Bowman, Chairman
Elizabeth Bancroft, Executive Director

US citizens who have served in any agency or department involved in US intelligence; individuals of good character who support the position that the US needs an adequate intelligence capability. Promotes public understanding and support of a strong and responsible national intelligence establishment. Believes reliable intelligence is essential to the cause of peace and national security. Provides research assistance to writers and scholars in the field; provides speakers for schools and professional and civic groups. Encourages the teaching of intelligence at high schools, universities, and colleges. Offers interviews on intelligence and intelligence-related issues. Maintains placement service and speakers' bureau.

Year Founded: 1975

72 Association of Personal Historians

3208 E 25th Street
Minneapolis, MN 55406
www.personalhistorians.org

Bill Horne, President
Solomon Kahn, Treasurer
Deborah Wilbrink, Secretary

The Association of Personal Historians is an organization whose members are dedicated to helping others preserve their personal histories and life stories. The purpose of the Association is to advance the profession of assisting individuals, organizations and communities to preserve their histories, life stories and memories.

Year Founded: 1995

73 Association of Retired Americans

6505 E 82nd Street
Suite 130
Indianapolis, IN 46250
317-915-2500
Fax: 317-915-2510; *Toll Free:* 800-806-6160
ara@ara-usa.org
www.ara-usa.org

John K. Smith, President & CEO
Terri Geralds, Secretary
Gary Watson, Treasurer

Senior Americans, age 45 or more interested in enhancing their lives through group benefits. Purpose is to offer a program of high quality, low-cost benefits and services to members. Services available through ARA are: discounts on prescriptions, eyeglasses, and hearing aids; low interest credit cards; discounts on lodging, car rental, tours, cruises, and airfare; insurance benefits.

Year Founded: 1972

74 Association of the United States Army

2425 Wilson Boulevard
Arlington, VA 22201
703-841-4300
Fax: 703-525-9039; *Toll Free:* 800-336-4570
membersupport@ausa.org
www.ausa.org

Gordon Sullivan, President
Swan Guy, VP, Education
Sinn Jerry, VP, Finance & Administration

Professional society of: active, retired, and reserve military personnel; West Point and Army ROTC cadets; civilians interested in national defense. Seeks to advance the security of the United States and consolidate the efforts of all who support the United States Army as an indispensable instrument of national security. Conducts industrial symposia for manufacturers of Army weapons and equipment, and those in the Department of the Army who plan, develop, test, and use weapons and equipment. Symposia subjects have included guided missiles, army aviation, electronics and communication, telemedicine, vehicles, and armor. Sponsors monthly PBS TV series America's Army.

Year Founded: 1950

75 B'nai B'rith International

1120 20th Street NW
Suite 300 N
Washington, DC 20036
202-857-6600
Fax: 202-857-1099; *Toll Free:* 888-388-4224
info@bnaibrith.org
www.bnaibrith.org

Gary P. Saltzman, President
Peter Perlman, Chairman of the Executive
A. Michael Gellman, Treasurer

This national center for Housing and Services sponsors housing and travel for senior citizens.

Year Founded: 1843

76 CARF International

6951 E Southpoint Road
Tucson, AZ 85756-9407
Fax: 520-318-1129; *Toll Free:* 888-281-6531
www.carf.org

Herb Zaretsky, Board Chair

Nonprofit accreditor of health and human services facilities.

Year Founded: 1966

77 Caregiver Action Network

1130 Connecticut Avenue NW
Suite 300
Washington, DC 20036
202-454-3970
info@caregiveraction.org; www.caregiveraction.org

John Schall, Chief Executive Officer
Lisa Winstel, Chief Operating Officer

Practical help, support and information for more than 90 million family caregivers.

Year Founded: 1993

78 Catholic Charities USA
2050 Ballenger Avenue
Suite 400
Alexandria, VA 22314
703-549-1390
Fax: 703-549-1656; *Toll Free:* 800-919-9338
info@catholiccharitiesusa.org
www.catholiccharitiesusa.org

Sister Donna Markham, President & CEO
Keith Styles, COO & General Counsel

CCUSA is a network of organizations offering nationwide services to older people, including counseling, homemaker and caregiver services, emergency assistance, group homes, and institutional care.

Year Founded: 1910

79 Catholic Golden Age
PO Box 249
Olyphant, PA 18447
Toll Free: 855-586-1091
www.catholicgoldenage.org

CGA sponsors charitable work and helps older people meet their social, physical, economic, intellectual and spiritual needs.

Year Founded: 1975

80 Centers for Medicare and Medicaid Services
7500 Security Boulevard
Baltimore, MD 21244
410-786-3000; *Toll Free:* 877-267-2323
www.cms.gov
TTY: 866-226-1819

Andy Slavitt, Acting Administrator
Dr. Mandy Cohen, COO & Chief of Staff

CMS, part of the Federal Government, administers health insurance through Medicare and Medicaid. CMS regulates hospitals, nursing homes, and home health agencies.

Year Founded: 1965

81 Christian Association of Primetimers
PO Box 282
Iola, WI 54945
Fax: 630-443-0087; *Toll Free:* 800-443-0227
customerservice@capmemberbenefits.org
capmemberbenefits.org

The purpose of this ministry is to provide money-saving values for its members while promoting traditional values in our society, including superior products and services. It encourages prime-timers (seniors) to use their talents and acquired wisdom for the benefit of their community. The Christian Association of PrimeTimers has been referred to as the Christian alternative to the American Association of Retired Persons.

Year Founded: 1994

82 Church of the Brethren
1451 Dundee Avenue
Elgin, IL 60120
847-742-5100
Fax: 847-742-6103; *Toll Free:* 800-323-8039
cobweb@brethren.org
www.brethren.org

Stanley J. Noffsinger, General Secretary

The Association of Brethren Caregivers fosters the ministry of giving and receiving care through the development of resources, programs, events and leadership that connect persons and communities in their lifelong journeys toward wholeness.

Year Founded: 1708

83 City of Hope
1500 East Duarte Road
Duarte, CA 91010
626-256-4673
Fax: 626-301-8115; *Toll Free:* 800-826-4673
www.cityofhope.org

Supports the National Pilot Medical Center and the Beckman Research Institute, which are engaged in treatment, research, and medical education in catastrophic diseases including cancer; leukemia; blood, heart and lung diseases; certain hereditary maladies; and metabolic disorders, such as diabetes. Patient care is available on a national and nonsectarian basis. Provides physician referrals. Offers free consulting service to doctors and hospitals. Seeks to influence medicine and science through 80 pilot research programs. From its staff and 200 laboratories, during the past decade over 3000 original findings have emerged in diseases treated as well as studies in diabetes, Alzheimer's disease, AIDS, Huntington's disease, genetics, and brain and nerve function. Receives nationwide support from nearly 500 chartered auxiliaries in over 230 cities, 32 states and Washington, DC, and from management, labor, fraternal and benevolent organizations, individuals, and special campaigns.

Year Founded: 1913

84 Clearinghouse on Abuse and Neglect of the Elderly
Center for Drug and Health Studies
257 E Main Street, Suite 110
Newark, DE 19716
302-831-3525
Fax: 302-831-6081; *Toll Free:* 800-677-1116
cane-ud@udel.edu
www.cane.udel.edu

CANE, funded by the Administration on Aging, is a database of elder abuse materials and resources operated by the University of Delaware's National Center on Elder Abuse.

85 Coalition for Economic Survival
514 Shatto Place
Suite 270
Los Angeles, CA 90020
213-252-4411
Fax: 213-252-4422
contactces@earthlink.net
www.cesinaction.org

Larry Gross, Executive Director
Carlos Aguilar, Director of Organizing
Lourdes Soto, REAP Tenant Outreach Coordinator

Supports senior citizens in economic concerns such as affordable housing, rent control, repairs and tenants rights.

Year Founded: 1973

86 Commission on Disability Rights
American Bar Association
1050 Connecticut Avenue NW
Suite 400
Washington, DC 20036

202-662-1570
Fax: 202-442-3439
cdr@americanbar.org

Amy L. Allbright, Director

87 Commission on Law and Aging
American Bar Association
1050 Connecticut Avenue NW
Suite 400
Washington, DC 20036
202-662-8690
Fax: 202-662-8698
aging@americanbar.org
www.americanbar.org/aging

Charles P. Sabatino, Director

The Commission examines and responds to law-related needs of older people. It makes referrals and maintains a listing of legal aid offices where older people can get free or low-cost legal assistance. See Legal Resources chapter for specific state resources.

88 Compassion & Choices
PO Box 101810
Denver, CO 80250
Fax: 866-312-2690; *Toll Free:* 800-247-7421
www.compassionandchoices.org

Barbara Coombs Lee, President
Marcia Campbell, CFO
Trish Bernstein, COO

Working to expand choice at the end of life.

Number of Members: 400,000

89 Corporation for National & Community Service
250 E Street SW
Washington, DC 20525
e-mail: info@cns.gov
www.nationalservice.gov
TTY: 800-833-3722

Wendy Spencer, CEO

Empowering Americans to address the nation's challenges through service.

Year Founded: 1993

90 Council for Health & Human Services Ministries
700 Prospect Avenue
Cleveland, OH 44115
216-736-2260
Fax: 216-736-2251; *Toll Free:* 866-822-8224
www.chhsm.org

Michael Readinger, President & CEO

Health and human service institutions related to the United Church of Christ. Seeks to study, plan, and implement a program in health and human services; assist members in developing and providing quality services and in financing institutional and noninstitutional health and human service ministries; stimulate awareness of and support for these programs; inform the UCC of policies that affect the needs, problems, and conditions of patients; cooperate with inter-denominational agencies and others in the field. Maintains placement service and hall of fame. Compiles statistics; provides specialized education programs.

Year Founded: 1982

91 Council of Better Business Bureaus
3033 Wilson Boulevard
Suite 600
Arlington, VA 22201
703-276-0100
Fax: 703-525-8277
www.bbb.org/council

Mary E. Power, President & CEO
Beverly Baskin, SVP, BBB Services
Genie Barton, VP & Director

BBBOnLine's mission is to promote trust and confidence on the Internet through the BBBOnLine Reliability and Privacy Seal Programs. BBBOnLine's web site seal programs allows companies with web sites to display the seals once they have been evaluated and confirmed to meet the program requirements.

92 Dermatology Nurses' Association
435 N Bennett Street
Southern Pines, NC 28387
Fax: 910-246-2361; *Toll Free:* 800-454-4362
dna@dnanurse.org
www.dnanurse.org

Linda Markham, Executive Director
Dorothy Caputo, Director of Education

Established to develop and foster the highest standards of dermatologic nursing care, enhance professional growth through education and research, facilitate communication among members, and promote interdisciplinary collaboration.

Year Founded: 1981; Number of Members: 3,000

93 Devonshire Acres Nursing and Rehabilitation Center
Chancellor Health Care
1330 North Sidney Avenue
Sterling, CO 80751
970-522-4888
Fax: 970-522-4892
www.chancellorhealthcare.com

Management of long-term care facilities for the elderly.

Year Founded: 1992

94 Diplomatic and Consular Officers, Retired
DACOR Bacon House
1801 F Street NW
Washington, DC 20006
202-682-0500
Fax: 202-842-3295
dacor@dacorbacon.org
www.dacorbacon.org

Susan Cimburek, Executive Director
Meg Beitz, Director of Operations

Active and retired Foreign Service members who have served in officer positions.

Year Founded: 1950

95 Eldercare Initiative in Consumer Law
National Consumer Law Center
7 Winthrop Square
Boston, MA 02110-1245
617-542-8010
Fax: 617-542-8028
consumerlaw@nclc.org
www.nclc.org

Richard Dubois, Executive Director

The Initiative provides assistance on legal issues of older people. See Legal Resources for specific resources by state.

Year Founded: 1992

96   **Eldercare Locator**
U.S. Department of Health and Human Services
Toll Free: 800-677-1116
www.eldercare.gov

Eldercare Locator links those who need assistance with state and local area agencies on aging and community-based organizations that serve older adults and their caregivers.

97   **Emergency Nurses Association**
915 Lee Street
Des Plaines, IL 60016-6569
Toll Free: 800-900-9659
enainfo@ena.org
www.ena.org

Registered nurses, licensed practical nurses, and licensed vocational nurses; emergency medical technicians or nurses and members of allied health fields engaged or interested in emergency patient care. Objectives are: to promote emergency nursing and to establish standards in the field; to work with other health-related organizations toward the improvement of emergency care; to serve as a resource for emergency nursing education and research. Seeks to identify and address emergency nursing issues. Disseminates educational and research information in the field. Sponsors: Emergency Nursing Core Curriculum; Standards of Emergency Nursing Practice; Emergency Nursing Pediatric Course; Trauma Nursing Core Course.

Year Founded: 1970

98   **Employee Benefits Security Administration**
U.S. Department of Labor
Frances Perkins Building
200 Constitution Avenue NW
Washington, DC 20210
202-254-7013; *Toll Free: 866-444-3272*
www.dol.gov/ebsa
TTY: 877-889-5627

Thomas E. Perez, Secretary of Labor
Christopher Lu, Deputy Secretary of Labor

EBSA protects the integrity of pensions, health plans, and other employee benefits for more than 150 million people.

Year Founded: 2004

99   **Employment Discrimination: Age**
U.S. Equal Employment Opportunity Commission
131 M Street NE
Washington, DC 20507
Toll Free: 800-669-4000
info@eoc.gov
www.eeoc.gov/laws/types/age.cfm
TTY: 800-669-6820

Jenny R. Yang, Chair
David Lopez, General Counsel

To prohibit arbitrary age discrimination of people over the age of 40, in hiring and other employment practices, promote the employment of older workers based on ability rather than age, and help employers and employees find ways to meet problems arising from the impact of age on employment.

100   **Employment Discrimination: Disabled**
U.S. Equal Employment Opportunity Commission
131 M Street NE
Washington, DC 20507
Toll Free: 800-669-4000
info@eeoc.gov
www.eeoc.gov/laws/types/disability.cfm
TTY: 800-669-6820

Jenny R. Yang, Chair
David Lopez, General Counsel

To provide for enforcement of the Federal prohibition against employment discrimination by private employers and state and local governments against qualified individuals with disabilities.

101   **Equal Employment Opportunity Commission**
131 M Street NE
Washington, DC 20507
Toll Free: 800-669-4000
info@eeoc.gov
www.eeoc.gov
TTY: 800-669-6820

Jenny R. Yang, Chair
David Lopez, General Counsel

Provides information on and accepts and investigates charges of discrimination based on age, sex, race, color, etc. Spanish-speaking operator available.

102   **Experience Works**
4401 Wilson Boulevard
Suite 1100
Arlington, VA 22203
703-522-7272
Fax: 703-522-0141; Toll Free: 866-397-9757
www.experienceworks.org

Roger Noonan, Chairman
Sally A. Boofer, President & CEO
Richard Schorr, CFO

Experience Works helps low-income seniors, with multiple barriers to employment, get the training they need to find good jobs in their local communities.

Year Founded: 1965

103   **Families USA**
1201 New York Avenue NW
Suite 1100
Washington, DC 20005
202-628-3030
Fax: 202-347-2417
info@familiesusa.org
familiesusa.org

Ron Pollack, Executive Director

Works with those involved in health care and long-term care reform through reports and other materials.

104   **Family Caregiver Alliance**
785 Market Street
Suite 750
San Francisco, CA 94103
415-434-3388
Fax: 414-434-3508; Toll Free: 800-445-8106
info@caregiver.org
www.caregiver.org

Kathleen Kelly, Executive Director

Good information with resources and hotline numbers. Family Caregiver Alliance supports and assists caregivers of brain-impaired adults through education services, research and advocacy.

Year Founded: 1977

105 Federal Trade Commission
600 Pennsylvania Avenue NW
Washington, DC 20580
202-326-2222; *Toll Free: 877-382-4387*
www.ftc.gov
Edith Ramirez, Chairwoman
David B. Robbins, Executive Director

The FTC site includes news and alerts, consumer protection and anti-trust information, including how these issues apply to older Americans.

Year Founded: 1938

106 Federal-Postal Coalition
National Active & Retired Federal Employees Assoc.
606 N Washington Street
Alexandria, VA 22314
703-838-7760
Fax: 703-838-7785
www.narfe.org
Richard G. Thissen, President
Jon Dowie, Secretary/Treasurer

Founded as the Fund for Assuring an Independent Retirement (FAIR), the coalition now includes 30 national organizations, such as the National Association of Letter Carriers.

Year Founded: 1921

107 Food Distribution Programs
USDA Food and Nutrition Service
3101 Park Center Drive
Alexandria, VA 22302
703-305-2062
Fax: 703-305-2908
www.fns.usda.gov
Audrey Rowe, Administrator

To improve the diets of school and preschool children, the elderly, needy persons in charitable institutions, and other individuals in need of food assistance, and to increase the market for domestically produced foods acquired under surplus removal or price support operations.

108 Foster Grandparents Program
Corporation for National and Community Service
250 E Street NW
Washington, DC 20525
202-606-5000
Fax: 202-606-3472; Toll Free: 800-942-2677
info@cns.gov
www.nationalservice.gov
TTY: 800-833-3722
Wendy Spencer, CEO
Kim Mansaray, Chief of Program Operations

The Foster Grandparents Program connects volunteers age 60 and over with children and young people with exceptional needs. Volunteers mentor, support and help some of the most vulnerable children in the United States.

109 Foundation Aiding the Elderly
PO Box 254849
Sacramento, CA 95865-4849
916-481-8558
Fax: 916-481-2239; Toll Free: 877-481-8558
caroleh@4fate.org
www.4fate.org
Carole Herman, President
Harris Herman, Secretary/Treasurer

Assists the public with relatives and friends in long-term care nursing homes. Provides awareness of the existence of, and potential for abuse, neglect, and lack of dignity of the elderly in nursing homes. Initiates action to make improvements. Raises funds for the grassroots efforts to end nursing home abuse.

Year Founded: 1980

110 Genesis Institute
1220 N Howard Street
Spokane, WA 99201
509-467-7913
Fax: 509-467-0344
genesisinstitute.org
Dave Hutchins, Executive Director
Linda Depew, Development Director

Exists to care for human souls, guided by the fixed point of biblical revelation. All Genesis training ministries seek to enable and encourage the Christian Community to this end. Offers a variety of courses designed for Christian leaders and layworkers, including the elderly population.

111 Grandparents Rights Organization
1760 S Telegraph Road
Suite 300
Bloomfield Hills, MI 48302
248-646-7177
rvictor@hertzschram.com
www.grandparentsrights.org
Richard S Victor, Founder/Executive Director

Conducts educational and advocacy activities aimed at preserving and fostering the child-grandparent relationship in cases where grandparents have been denied the right to visit their grandchildren. Conducts research programs; compiles statistics.

Year Founded: 1984

112 Gray Panthers NYC
244 Madison Avenue
Suite 396
New York, NY 10016
917-535-0457
jkupferman@aol.com
graypanthersnyc.org
Jack Kupferman, President

Consciousness-raising activist group of older adults and young people. Aims to combat ageism - the discrimination against persons on the basis of chronological age. Believes that both the old and the young have much to contribute to make our society more just and humane. Advises, acts as catalyst for, and organizes local groups of young, middle-aged, and older persons to work on issues of their choosing.: national health care, affordable housing, environmental preservation, peace, ending discrimination, education, economic and tax justice and social justice.

Year Founded: 1970

113 Greater Washington Urban League
2901 14th Street NW
Washington, DC 20009
202-265-8200
Fax: 202-265-6122
www.gwul.org

George H. Lambert Jr., President & CEO

Offers companionship and volunteer opportunities for those 60 years of age or older. Provides services to low-income elderly through mental healthcare of the terminally ill and acute care.

Year Founded: 1938

114 HEATH Resource Center at the National Youth Transitions Center
The George Washington University
2134 G Street NW
Suite 308
Washington, DC 20052-0001
202-994-1000
askheath@gwu.edu
www.heath.gwu.edu

Sponsored by the President's Committee on Employment of People with Disabilities. Provides information on education and accommodations for the disabled in work settings. Also offers referral to local sources. Newsletter and resource papers available.

Year Founded: 2000

115 Healing Arts Initiative
33-02 Skillman Avenue
1st Floor
Long Island City, NY 11101
212-575-7676
Fax: 212-575-7669
outreach@hainyc.org
hainyc.org

D. Alexandra Dyer, Executive Director

Service recipients include people with mental and physical disabilities, the frail elderly, youth at risk of HIV and violence or in detention, mentally retarded/developmentally disabled persons, homeless single adults and families, and persons with HIV/AIDS. Promotes the cultural enrichment of these individuals by arranging access to cultural experiences, and by presenting music, dance, and theater events for people from health/human service facilities. Develops daily living skills through hands-on participation in the arts. Provides prevention education/skill building to persons at high risk regarding critical public health issues, such as HIV/AIDS and youth violence.

Year Founded: 1969

116 HealthyWomen
PO Box 430
Red Bank, NJ 07701
732-530-3425
Fax: 732-865-7225; Toll Free: 877-986-9472
info@healthywomen.org
www.healthywomen.org

Beth Battaglino, Co-Founder
Marcia Mangum Cronin, Senior Managing Editor

Award-winning website educating and empowering women to make smart health choices.

117 Home Healthcare Nurses Association
228 7th Street SE
Washington, DC 20003
202-547-7424
Fax: 202-547-3540
www.hhna.org

Elaine D. Stephens, Chair

Works to develop and promote the specialty of home healthcare nursing. Provides a forum for members to exchange information; influences public policy affecting the practice; fosters excellence in practice.

Year Founded: 1993

118 Hospice Association of America
228 Seventh Street SE
Washington, DC 20003
202-546-4759
Fax: 202-547-9559
www.nahc.org/haa

Val J. Halamandaris, President

Hospices, home health agencies, community cancer centers, and interested health care professionals. Promotes concept of hospice, a philosophy of health care which is expressed through the provision of a variety of medical and nonmedical services to terminally ill patients and their families. Technical assistance, educational programs, publications, and representation of industry issues to state and federal governments. Maintains speakers' bureau. Compiles statistics.

119 Hospice Foundation of America
1710 Rhode Island Avenue NW
Suite 400
Washington, DC 20036
202-457-5811; *Toll Free: 800-854-3402*
hospicefoundation.org

Amy Tucci, President & CEO

Works to promote the philosophy and application of hospice care for terminally ill people and improve the American health system. Advocates the hospice concept of care; offers professional development and educational programs; sponsors research on ethical issues; participates in public policy initiatives; provides technical assistance to hospices.

Year Founded: 1982

120 International Association for the Study of Pain
1510 H Street NW
Suite 600
Washington, DC 20005-1020
202-524-5300
Fax: 202-524-5301
iaspdesk@iasp-pain.org
iasp-pain.org

Matthew D'Uva, Executive Director

Scientists, physicians, and other health professionals interested in pain research and therapy. Encourages research on pain mechanisms and syndromes; seeks to improve management of patients with acute and chronic pain. Promotes education and training in the field of pain; informs the public of results of current research. Fosters development of an international data bank, adoption of a uniform classification and definition regarding pain and pain syndromes, and creation of a uniform records system on information relating to pain mechanisms, syndromes, and management. Promotes the formation of national associations for the study and treatment of pain.

Year Founded: 1974; Number of Members: 6,500

121 International Psychogeriatric Association

555 E Wells Street
Suite 1100
Milwaukee, WI 53202
414-918-9889
Fax: 414-276-3349
ipa-info@ipa-online.org
www.ipa-online.org

Health care professionals and scientists with an interest in the behavioral and biological aspects of mental health in the elderly. Works to keep members abreast of developments in research and clinical practice in the field of geriatric mental health. Conducts research programs.

Year Founded: 1982

122 International Society for Quality-of-Life Studies

www.isqols.org

Rhonda Phillips, President
Jill Johnson, Executive Director

Seeks to stimulate research in quality of life studies. Conductional resarch and educational programs.

123 International Society for Traumatic Stress Studies

One Parkview Plaza
Suite 800
Oakbrook Terrace, IL 60181
847-686-2234
Fax: 847-686-2251
info@istss.org
www.istss.org

Rick Koepke, Executive Director

Professionals who treat individuals suffering from traumatic stress. (Traumatic stress is a medical term applied to persons who experience severe mental or emotional reactions to extraordinary stressful situations such as war, crime, natural disasters, and high-stress occupations.) Conducts research in the treatment of these cases; disseminates information. Holds seminars. Bestows awards.

Year Founded: 1985

124 International Society of Psychiatric-Mental Health Nurses

2424 American Lane
Madison, WI 53704-3102
608-443-2463
Fax: 608-443-2474
info@ispn-psych.org; www.ispn-psych.org

Elizabeth Bonham, President
Margaret Plunkett, Treasurer

Nurses engaged in the practice of, or with an interest in, psychiatric consultation liaison nursing. Promotes development of psychiatric consultation nursing as a subspecialty of psychiatric and mental health nursing. Seeks to advance understanding of mind-body interaction in healing and wellness. Facilitates communication among members and serves as a clearinghouse on psychiatric consultation liaison nursing. Makes available networking opportunities and professional conference discounts to members.

Year Founded: 1999

125 Judge Advocates Association

c/o The Army Navy Club
901 17th Street
Washington, DC 20006
e-mail: jaa@jaa.org
jaa.org

MG Daniel Wright (Ret.), President

Active, reserve, retired and former Judge Advocates of the Army, Navy, Air Force, Marine Corps, and Coast Guard. Assists in developing of military law and an efficient military legal and judicial system.

Year Founded: 1943

126 Latino Center of Aging

576 Fifth Avenue
Suite 903
New York, NY 10036
212-330-8120
info@gerolatino.org
www.gerolatino.org

Mario E Tapia, President and CEO

The LCA was established to improve the lives of Latino seniors through advocacy and education. The LCA Media Initiative is an ongoing project that achieves the organization's goal through electronic and print media.

Year Founded: 1991

127 Meals on Wheels America

1550 Crystal Drive
Suite 1004
Arlington, VA 22202
Fax: 703-548-5274; Toll Free: 888-998-6325
www.mealsonwheelsamerica.org

Ellie Hollander, President & CEO
Don Miller, Chief Financial & Admin. Officer

Provides home delivery of meals, improving the quality of life for low-income, elderly, homebound and disabled.

Year Founded: 1973

128 MedicAlert Foundation

2323 Colorado Avenue
Turlock, CA 95382
Toll Free: 800-432-5378
www.medicalert.org

David Leslie, President & CEO

Provides information on registering with MedicAlert (personal medical emergency services) and ordering alert emblem (bracelet). Free registration form and catalog are available.

Year Founded: 1956

129 Medical Library Association

65 East Wacker Place
Suite 1900
Chicago, IL 60601-7246
312-419-9094
Fax: 312-419-8950
websupport@mail.mlahq.org
www.mlanet.org

Kevin Baliozian, Executive Director

A nonprofit, educational organization of more than 1,100 institutions and 3,600 individual members in the health sciences information field, committed to educating health information professionals, supporting health information research, promoting access to the world's health sciences information, and working to ensure that the best health information is available to all. See Libraries chapter for state listings.

Year Founded: 1898

130   Men's Health Network
PO Box 75972
Washington, DC 20013
202-543-6461
www.menshealthnetwork.org

Mike Leventhal, Executive Director

Health awareness and disease prevention messages and tools for men and boys.

131   Mental Health America
2000 N Beauregard Street
6th Floor
Alexandria, VA 22311
703-684-7722
Fax: 703-684-5968; Toll Free: 800-969-6642
www.mentalhealthamerica.net

Paul Gionfriddo, President & CEO

Promoting mental health as part of overall wellness.

Year Founded: 1909

132   Military Benefit Association
14605 Avion Parkway
PO Box 221110
Chantilly, VA 20153-1110
703-968-6200
Fax: 703-968-6423; Toll Free: 800-336-0100
www.militarybenefit.org

Michael Reyna, President
Glenda Lee, Vice President
G. Thomas Collins Jr., Secretary & Treasurer

The objects and purposes of this Association shall be the promotion of the welfare of its members; the advancement and safeguarding of their economic interets; and generally to encourage and promote better financial conditions for its members through cooperative enterprises.

Year Founded: 1956

133   Military Officers Association of America
703-549-2311; *Toll Free: 800-234-6622*
msc@moaa.org
www.moaa.org

LG Dana Atkins (Ret.), President & CEO

Men and women who are or have been commissioned or warrant officers in any component of the Army, Navy, Air Force, Marine Corps, Coast Guard, National Oceanic and Atmospheric Administration, and Public Health Service. Supports strong national defense and represents and assists members and their dependents and survivors with retirement issues and benefits. Sponsors educational assistance program, survivor assistance, travel, and insurance.

Year Founded: 1929; Number of Members: 370,000+

134   Military Order of the World Wars
435 N Lee Street
Alexandria, VA 22314-2301
703-683-4911
Fax: 703-683-4501
www.moww.org

BG A.B. Morrill III (Ret.), Chief of Staff

Commissioned officers and warrant officers who served in the active or reserve components of any of the uniformed services. Promotes patriotic education in schools. Supports Junior and Senior ROTC programs and Boy Scouts and Girl Scouts of America.

Year Founded: 1919

135   Mobility International USA
132 E Broadway
Suite 343
Eugene, OR 97401
541-343-1284
Fax: 541-343-6812
www.miusa.org

Susan Sygall, CEO & Co-founder
Cindy Lewis, Director of Programs

Project of U.S. Department of State Bureau of Educational and Cultural Affairs to increase participation of people with disabilities in international "travel with a purpose" - study, volunteer and more.

136   NIH Osteoporosis & Related Bone DiseasesNational Resource Center
National Institutes of Health
2 AMS Circle
Bethesda, MD 20892-3676
202-223-0344
Fax: 202-293-2356; Toll Free: 800-624-2663
nihboneinfo@mail.nih.gov
www.bones.nih.gov
TTY: 202-466-4315

The NIH/Osteoporosis and Related Bone Diseases National Resource Center provides patients, health professionals, and the public with an important link to resources and information on metabolic bone diseases such as osteoporosis. Paget's disease of bone, osteogenesis imperfecta, and primary hyperarathyroidism. Specific populations include the elderly, men, women, adolescents, and minorities. The Resource Center offers materials in English, Spanish, Chinese, Korean, Lao, Cambodian and Vietnamese. The center offers links to selected resources, information packet publications, electronic newsletters and support groups.

137   National Academy of Elder Law Attorneys
1577 Spring Hill Road
Suite 310
Vienna, VA 22182
703-942-5711
Fax: 703-563-9504
naela@naela.com
www.naela.org

Shirley Berger Whitenack, President

Practicing attorneys, law professors, and others interested in the provision of legal services to the elderly. Promotes technical expertise and education for legal services addressing the needs of the elderly and their families.

Year Founded: 1987; Number of Members: 4,200+

138   National Active and Retired Federal Employees Association
606 N Washington Street
Alexandria, VA 22314

703-838-7760
Fax: 703-838-7785
www.narfe.org
Richard G. Thissen, President
Jon Dowie, Secretary/Treasurer

Retired US Government civilian and District of Columbia employees, their spouses, persons drawing annuities as survivors of retired US government employees, present employees eligible for optional retirement, and federal employees. Seeks to: serve annuitants and potential annuitants and their survivors under the retirement laws; sponsor and support beneficial legislation; promote the general welfare of civil service annuitants and their families. Association is also interested in preretirement programs, especially in federal and district government agencies, and in broad field of problems of the aged and aging.

Year Founded: 1921

139 National Adult Day Services Association
1421 E Broad Street
Suite 425
Fuquay Varina, NC 27526
Fax: 919-825-3945; *Toll Free:* 877-745-1440
info@nadsa.org
www.nadsa.org

Lisa Peters-Beumer, Chair
Corinne Jan, Treasurer
Keith Anderson, Secretary

Adult daycare practitioners; health and social service planners; individuals involved in planning and providing services for older persons. Promotes and enhances adult daycare programs; provides services and activities for disabled older persons on a long-term basis; provides training and technical assistance and consultation services for daycare personnel; organizes funding; develops statndards and guidelines for adult daycare programs; encourages adult daycare centers to participate in local area health planning activities to heighten the effectiveness of adult daycare. Plans and conducts training events for annual meeting and related conferences; maintains annotated bibliography; lobbies for approved public policy positions; surveys state adult daycare regulations and legislation.

Year Founded: 1979

140 National Association for Hispanic Elderly
234 E Colorado Boulevard
Suite 300
Pasadena, CA 91101
626-564-1988
Fax: 626-564-2659
www.anppm.org

Carmela G. Lacayo, President & CEO

Established to serve the needs of Hispanic and low income elderly.

Year Founded: 1975

141 National Association for Home Care and Hospice
228 Seventh Street SE
Washington, DC 20003
202-547-7424
Fax: 202-547-3540
www.nahc.org

Val J. Halamandaris, President

Providers of home health care, hospice, and homemaker-home health aide services; interested individuals and organizations. Develops and promotes high standards of patient care in home care services. Seeks to affect legislative and regulatory processes concerning home care services; gathers and disseminates home care industry data; develops public relations strategies; works to increase political visibility of home care services. Interprets home care services to governmental and private sector bodies affecting the delivery and financing of such services. Provides legal and accounting consulting services; conducts market research and compiles statistics. Offers members insurance discounts. Sponsors educational programs for organizations and individuals concerned with home care services.

142 National Association for Practical Nurse Education and Service, Inc. (NAPNES)
2071 N Bechtle Avenue
PMB 307
Springfield, OH 45504-1583
703-933-1003
Fax: 703-940-4089
support@napnes.org
www.napnes.org

Ann Bauer LPN, President
Roy Wilson, LPN, Treasurer
Lola Crum LPN, Vice President

NAPNES is the oldest association that advocates the practice, education and regulation of practical and vocational nurses.

Year Founded: 1941

143 National Association of Activity Professionals
3604 Wildon Street
Eau Claire, WI 54703
913-748-7288
office@naap.info
www.naap.info

Alisa Tagg, President

An organization of individuals who provide activity programming for the residents of long-term care facilitites, retirement living communities, adult day care centers, and other primarily geriatric setting. Members provide individualized therapeutic and restorative activities. NAAP provides excellence in support services to activity professionals through education, advocacy, technical assistance, promotion of standards, fostering of research, and peer and industry relations. NAAP represents the interests of activity directors, assistants, educators, and consultants certified for practice by a variety of certification bodies.

144 National Association of Area Agencies on Aging
1730 Rhode Island Avenue NW
Suite 1200
Washington, DC 20036
202-872-0888
Fax: 202-872-0057
www.n4a.org

Sandy Markwood, CEO

NoA is the umbrella organization for the AoA-funded Area Agencies on Aging. The association administers the AoA sponsored Eldercare Locator. See State chapter for state agencies.

Year Founded: 1973

145 National Association of Directors of Nursing Administration in Long Term Care
513-791-3679; *Toll Free: 800-222-0539*
info@nadona.org
www.nadona.org
Sherrie Dornberger, Executive Director

Directors, assistant directors, and former directors of nursing in long term care. Goals are: to create and establish an acceptable ethical standard for practices in long term care nursing administration; to promote and encourage research in the profession; to develop and provide a consistent program of education and certification for the positions of director, associate director, and assistant director; to promote a positive image of the long term health care industry. Encourages members to share concerns and experiences; sponsors research programs. Advocates legislation pertaining to the practice of professional nursing. Maintains speakers' bureau.

Year Founded: 1986

146 National Association of Nutrition and Aging Services Programs
1612 K Street NW
Suite 400
Washington, DC 20006
202-682-6899
Fax: 202-223-2099
pcarlson@nanasp.org
www.nanasp.org
Robert Blancato, Executive Director

NANASP, a membership organization, supports a broad range of nutrition and related services for community-dwelling older people by training nutrition providers and advocating for older people.

Year Founded: 1977

147 National Association of State Retirement Administrators
449 Lewis Hargett Circle
Suite 290
Lexington, KY 40503-3590
www.nasra.org
Dana K. Bilyeu, Executive Director

Administrators of statewide public employee retirement systems. Encourages nationwide review of pension and retirement programs; sponsors conferences; provides technical and information services.

Year Founded: 1947

148 National Association of State Veterans Homes
www.nasvh.org
William Peterson, President

State supported veterans homes. Seeks to: maintain high standards of domiciliary, nursing home, and hospital care for veterans and eligible family members; provide a clearinghouse for techniques and expertise in veteran care and in the management of these institutions; represent the veterans' needs before Congress and the Veterans Administration. Encourages continued federal financial support for building state facilities and for providing care for veterans currently living in state homes. Works to sustain current veterans' benefits. Assists other states in establishing homes. Compiles statistics.

Year Founded: 1952

149 National Association of States United for Aging and Disabilities
1201 15th Street NW
Suite 350
Washington, DC 20005
202-898-2578
Fax: 202-898-2583
info@nasuad.org
www.nasuad.org
Martha Roherty, Executive Director
Camille Dobson, Deputy Executive Director
Bryan Proctor, COO

Represents the nation's 56 state and territorial agencies on aging and disabilities.

Year Founded: 1964

150 National Association of Veterans' Program Administrators
www.navpa.org
Mark Baker, President

Devoted to promoting professional competency and efficiency through an association of members and others associated with and involved in Veterans Education Assistance Programs. Offers membership to those directly employed in veterans affairs or those genuinely interested in and supportive of the goals of the Association.

Year Founded: 1975

151 National Board for Certified Counselors
3 Terrace Way
Greensboro, NC 27403-3660
336-547-0607
Fax: 336-547-0017
nbcc@nbcc.org
www.nbcc.org
Dr. Thomas Clawson, President & CEO
Sherry Allen, Executive Director

Sets professional counselor credentialing standards.

Year Founded: 1982

152 National Caucus & Center on Black Aging
1220 L Street NW
Suite 800
Washington, DC 20005
202-637-8400
Fax: 202-347-0895
www.ncba-aged.org
Karyne Jones, President & CEO
Elias Hussein, Executive Vice President

Seeks to improve living conditions for low-income elderly Americans, particularly blacks. Advocates changes in federal and state laws in improving the economic, health, and social status of low-income senior citizens. Promotes community awareness of problems and issues effecting low-income aging population. Operates an employment program involving 2000 older persons in 14 states. Sponsors, owns, and manages rental housing for the elderly. Conducts training and intern programs in nursing home administration, long-term care, housing management, and commercial property maintenance.

Year Founded: 1970

153 National Committee for Quality Assurance
1100 13th Street NW
Suite 1000
Washington, DC 20005
202-955-3500
Fax: 202-955-3599
www.ncqa.org

Margaret E. O'Kane, President

Coalition of health care professionals and organizations
principally involved in the health care industry; includes
hospitals, physicians, health maintenance organizations,
nursing homes, manufacturers of health care equipment, investment bankers, architects, contractors, and accountants.
Works to maintain and strengthen quality health care in the
US.

Year Founded: 1990

**154 National Committee for Responsive
Philanthropy**
1331 H Street NW
Suite 200
Washington, DC 20005
202-387-9177
Fax: 202-332-5084
info@ncrp.org
www.ncrp.org

Aaron Dorfman, Executive Director

Organization representing low income, minorities, women,
consumers, environmentalists, older Americans, youth, and
others working for social change and the public interest
who are concerned about the lack of philanthropic giving to
organizations working for social change or progressive issues. Works with leaders in the philanthropic community
and the recipients of philanthropic giving to increase public
accountability by philanthropies. Also works to increase
access to philanthropy's monies for those groups representing critical public needs. Initiates efforts to facilitate access
to charity drives in the workplace. Is concerned with the
giving patterns of private foundations, United Way, and
corporations with philanthropic programs. Conducts research; compiles statistics; publicizes reports; organizes
local alternatives to United Way.

Year Founded: 1976

**155 National Committee for the Prevention of Elder
Abuse**
1730 Rhode Island Avenue NW
Suite 1200
Washington, DC 20036
202-464-9481
Fax: 202-872-0057
info@preventelderabuse.org
www.preventelderabuse.org

Patricia Brownell, President

An association of researchers, educators, and advocates
dedicated to protecting the safety and well-being of older
people and adults with disabilities.

Year Founded: 1988

**156 National Committee to Preserve Social Security
& Medicare**
10 G Street NE
Suite 600
Washington, DC 20002

202-216-0420
Fax: 202-216-0446; Toll Free: 800-998-0180
www.ncpssm.org

Max Richtman, President & CEO

An advocacy and education membership organization,
works to protect and enhance Federal programs vital to seniors' health and economic well-being.

Year Founded: 1982

**157 National Conference on Public Employee
Retirement Systems**
444 N Capitol Street NW
Suite 630
Washington, DC 20001
202-624-1456
Fax: 202-624-1439; Toll Free: 877-202-5706
info@ncpers.org
www.ncpers.org

Hank H. Kim, Executive Director & Counsel

Dedicated to the protection and preservation of retirement
benefits for all public sector employees and retirees.
Founded to protect public employees against an action by
the federal government that would have wiped out public
pension systems, namely, mandatory Social Security coverage of non-covered state and local government employees.

Year Founded: 1941

**158 National Council of Social Security
Management Associations**
Greystone Group LLC
3303 S Wakefield Street
Arlington, DC 22206
202-547-8530
Fax: 202-547-8532
ncssma@ncssma.org
www.ncssma.org

Rick Warsinskey, President

Managers and supervisors of the 1350 Social Security field
offices and teleservice centers in the US and Puerto Rico.
Purposes are to represent the interests of members before
Congress, the media, and agency heads and to improve the
image and professionalism of federal employees. Has conducted research on federal employee pay and retirement
benefits. Maintains speakers' bureau.

Number of Members: 3,200

**159 National Council on Child Abuse & Family
Violence**
1025 Connecticut Avenue NW
Suite 1000
Washington, DC 20036
202-429-6695
Fax: 202-521-3479
info@nccafv.org
www.nccafv.org

Works to prevent elder abuse and all forms of family violence including child abuse and spouse/partner abuse.
NCCAFI provides information through its website and referrals for services upon request.

Year Founded: 1984

160   National Council on Disability
1331 F Street NW
Suite 850
Washington, DC 20004
202-272-2004
Fax: 202-272-2022
ncd@ncd.gov
www.ncd.gov
TTY: 202-272-2074

Rebecca Cokley, Executive Director

Federal agency led by 15 members appointed by the President of the United States and confirmed by the United States Senate. The overall purpose of the National Council is to promote policies, programs, practices and procedures that guarantee equal opportunity for all people with disabilities, regardless of the nature of severity of the disability; and to empower people with disabilities to achieve economic self-sufficiency, independent living and integration into all aspects of society.

Year Founded: 1978

161   National Emergency Medicine Association
PO Box 1039
Edgewood, MD 21040
443-922-7533
Fax: 888-682-7947
info@nemahealth.org
www.nemahealth.org

Thomas Blair, Chair
Patricia Brookhart, Treasurer
Suzanne Levin, Secretary

Nonprofit organization committed to trauma prevention and the delivery of quality medical services at each stage of trauma with an emphasis on first response.

Year Founded: 1982

162   National Endowment for the Arts
400 7th Street SW
Washington, DC 20506-0001
202-682-5400
www.arts.gov
TTY: 202-682-5496

Jane Chu, Chairman

Offer cultural organizations information on how to make programs accessible to older adults and individuals with various disabilities.

Year Founded: 1965

163   National Eye Institute
31 Center Drive
MSC 2510
Bethesda, MD 20892-2510
301-496-5248
Fax: 301-402-1065
2020@nei.nih.gov
nei.nih.gov

As part of the federal government's National Institutes of Health (NIH), the National Eye Institute's mission is to "conduct and support research, training, health information dissemination, and other programs with respect to blinding eye diseases, visual disorders, mechanisms of visual function, preservation of sight, and the special health problems and requirements of the blind."

Year Founded: 1968

164   National Federation of Licensed Practical Nurses
3801 Lake Boone Trail
Suite 190
Raleigh, NC 27607
919-779-0046
Fax: 919-779-5642; *Toll Free:* 800-948-2511
nflpn@caphill.com
www.nflpn.org

Promoting high standards of nursing care and lifelong learning.

Year Founded: 1949

165   National Gerontological Nursing Association
3493 Lansdowne Drive
Suite 2
Lexington, KY 40517
859-977-7453
Fax: 859-271-0607; *Toll Free:* 800-723-0560
info@ngna.org
www.ngna.org

Mary Rita Hurley,RN,MPA, President
Joanne Alderman,MSN,RN,BC, Vice President
Jean M Gaines,RN,PhD, Treasurer

An organization of nurses specializing in care of older adults, informs the public on health issues affecting older people, supports education for nurses and other health care practitioners, and provides a forum to discuss topics such as nutrition in long-term care facilities and elder law for nurses.

Year Founded: 1984

166   National Health Information Center
Office of Disease Prevention and Health Promotion
1101 Wootton Parkway
Suite LL100
Rockville, MD 20852
Fax: 240-453-8282
odphpinfo@hhs.gov
health.gov

Don Wright, Director, ODPHP

Aids consumers and health professionals in locating health information; provides referrals to national organizations. Free literature is available; some publications for sale.

167   National Heart, Lung, & Blood Institute
NHLBI Health Information Center
PO Box 30105
Bethesda, MD 20824-0105
301-592-8573
nhlbiinfo@nhlbi.nih.gov
www.nhlbi.nih.gov

Gary H. Gibbons, Director

The mission is to improve meaning of one American people by supporting and understanding research to prevent, detect, diagnose and treat diseases of heart, lungs, blood vessels, and sleep disorders.

Year Founded: 1887

168   National Hispanic Council on Aging
734 15th Street NW
Suite 1050
Washington, DC 20005

202-347-9733
Fax: 202-347-9735
www.nhcoa.org

Yanira Cruz, President & CEO

Leading national organization working to improve the lives of Hispanic older adults.

Year Founded: 1980

169 National Hospice and Palliative Care Organization

1731 King Street
Alexandria, VA 22314
703-837-1500
Fax: 703-837-1233
www.nhpco.org

J. Donald Schumacher, President & CEO
John Mastrojohn III, EVP & COO

Caring Connections, a program of the National Hospice and Palliative Care Organization (NHPCO), is a national consumer engagement initiative to improve care at the end of life, supported by a grant from The Robert Wood Johnson Foundation. Caring Connections provides free brochures on a wide range of end-of-life topics including advance care planning, caregiving, hospice and palliative care, grief and loss, and pain. State-specific advance directives for all 50 states and the District of Columbia are also available. Consumers can access the free brochures and state-specific advance directives by calling our Helpline or by visiting our website.

Year Founded: 1978

170 National Indian Council on Aging

10501 Montgomery Boulevard NE
Suite 210
Albuquerque, NM 87111
505-292-2001
Fax: 505-292-1922
nicoa.org

Randella Bluehouse, Executive Director

Advocating for American Indian and Alaska Native Elders.

Year Founded: 1976

171 National Indian Council on Aging (NICOA)

8500 Menaul Boulevard NE
Albuquerque, NM 87112
505-292-2001
Fax: 505-292-1922
www.nicoa.org

Randella Bluehouse, Executive Director
James De La Cruz, Sr., Chairman
Eddie Tullis, Vice Chairman

Seeks to bring about improved, comprehensive services to the Indian and Alaska native elderly. Objectives are to act as a focal point for the articulation of the needs of the Indian elderly; to disseminate information on Indian aging programs; to provide technical assistance and training opportunities to tribal organizations in the development of their programs. Conducts research on the needs of Indian elderly.

Year Founded: 1976

172 National Institute of Dental and Craniofacial Research

National Institutes of Health
Bethesda, MD 20892-2190
301-496-4261; *Toll Free: 866-232-4528*
nidcrinfo@mail.nih.gov
www.nidcr.nih.gov

Focuses on the information needs of special care patients — persons with medical or disabling conditions that can affect their oral health. Staff responds to inquiries from patients, health care providers, and the public; produces and distributes professional and patient education materials on special care and oral health; and also provides information on general oral health topics.

Year Founded: 1948

173 National Institute of Environmental Health Sciences

National Institutes of Health
111 T.W. Alexander Drive
Research Triangle Park, NC 27709
919-541-3345
Fax: 301-480-2978
www.niehs.nih.gov

Conducts and supports research on potential environmental contributors to human illnesses and dysfunction, including asthma, alzheimer's, bronchitis, cancer, lead poisoning.

174 National Institutes of Health

9000 Rockville Pike
Bethesda, MD 20892
301-496-4000
nihinfo@od.nih.gov
www.nih.gov
TTY: 301-402-9612

Francis S. Collins, Director

The nation's medical research agency.

Year Founded: 1887

175 National Jewish Health

1400 Jackson Street
Denver, CO 80206
303-388-4461; *Toll Free: 877-225-5654*
www.nationaljewish.org

Michael Salem, President & CEO
Robin Chotin, Secretary
Larry Silverstein, Treasurer

Care for lung, heart and immune diseases.

Year Founded: 1899

176 National Law Housing Project

703 Market Street
Suite 2000
San Francisco, CA 94103
415-546-7000
Fax: 415-546-7007
nhlp@nhlp.org
www.nhlp.org

Stephen Knight, Interim Co-Director
Susan Stern, Interim Co-Director

HUD originally made direct loans and subsequently made capital grants to nonprofit sponsors for the construction or substantial rehabilitation of rental housing for elderly people or persons with disabilities. In 1990, this program was revised into the supportive housing for elderly people and for persons with disabilities programs. Financial assistance is now in the form of a capital advance for 40 years that is non-repayable and interest-free so long as the project is available for low-income elderly persons and rental assistance is provided through a 20-year renewable contract to subsidize shortfalls in project income from dwelling unit rents.

177 National Long-Term Care Ombudsman Resource Center
1001 Connecticut Avenue, NW
Suite 632
Washington, DC 20036
202-332-2275
Fax: 202-332-2949
ombudcenter@theconsumervoice.org
www.ltcombudsman.org

Lori Smetanka, Executive Director
Amity Overall-Laib, Director
Robyn Grant, Director, Public Policy

The Center provides support, technical assistance and training to the 53 State Long-Term Care Ombudsman Programs and their statewide networks of almost 600 regional (local) programs. The Center's objectives are to enhance the skills, knowledge, and management capacity of the State programs to enable them to handle residents' complaints and represent resident interests.

Year Founded: 1972

178 National Organization for Albinism and Hypopigmentation
PO Box 959
East Hampstead, NH 03826-0959
603-887-2310
Fax: 800-648-2310; *Toll Free:* 800-473-2310
info@albinism.org
www.albinism.org

Michael McGowan, Executive Director

NOAH provides information and support regarding albinism and related conditions, promotes public and professional education about these conditions, and encourages research and funding that will lead to improved diagnosis and management of albinism. NOAH provides networking for those with special interests related to albinism, such as minority groups and Hermansky-Pudlak syndrome.

Year Founded: 1982

179 National Organization for Victim Assistance
510 King Street
Suite 424
Alexandria, VA 22314
703-535-6682
Fax: 703-535-5500; *Toll Free:* 800-879-6682
www.trynova.org

CJ Richard Barajas (Ret.), Executive Director

NOVA's mission is to promote rights and services for victims of crime and crisis everywhere.

Year Founded: 1975

180 National Organization on Disability
77 Water Street
Suite 204
New York, NY 10005

646-505-1191
Fax: 646-505-1184
info@nod.org
www.nod.org

Carol Glazer, President

A resource for businesses seeking to access the talent pool of working-age people with disabilities.

Year Founded: 1981

181 National Osteoporosis Foundation
251 18th Street S
Suite 630
Arlington, VA 22202
703-647-3000
Fax: 703-414-3742; *Toll Free:* 800-231-4222
info@nof.org
nof.org

Amy M. Porter, Executive Director

Health organization dedicated to promoting strong bones for life.

Year Founded: 1984

182 National People's Action
810 N Milwaukee
Chicago, IL 60642
312-243-3035
npa-us.org

National direct action organization for economic and racial justice.

Year Founded: 1972

183 National Prison Hospice Association
npha.org

Fleet Maull, President

Promotes hospice care for terminally ill inmates and those facing the prospect of dying in prison. Hospice is a comfort-oriented care that allows seriously ill and dying patients to die with dignity and humanity with as little pain as possible.

Year Founded: 1991

184 National Rehabilitation Information Center
8400 Corporate Drive
Suite 500
Landover, MD 20785
Fax: 301-459-4263; *Toll Free:* 800-346-2742
naricinfo@heitechservices.com
www.naric.com

Mark X Odum, Project Director

Gateway to disability- and rehabilitation-oriented information.

Year Founded: 1995

185 National Resource Center on Native American Aging
501 N Columbia Road MS 9037
Grand Forks, ND 58202-9037
701-777-6780
Fax: 701-777-6779; *Toll Free:* 800-896-7628
info@nrcnaa.org
www.nrcnaa.org

Paula Carter, Director

The Resource Center, funded by the Administration on Aging, provides support, advocacy, and information for older Native Americans, including American Indians, Alaska Natives, and Native Hawaiians.

Year Founded: 1994

186 National Resource Center on Supportive Housing & Home Modification
USC Andrus Gerontology Center
3715 McClintock Avenue
Los Angeles, CA 90089
213-740-1364
Fax: 213-740-7069
gero.usc.edu

Jon Pynoos, Director

Contact the center for information on government-assisted housing, assisted living policies, home modifications for older people, training and education courses, and technical assistance.

187 National Retired Teacher's Association
AARP
601 E Street NW
Washington, DC 20049
202-434-3525; *Toll Free: 888-687-2277*
member@aarp.org
www.aarp.org
TTY: 877-434-7598

Jo Ann Jenkins, CEO

Retired or current teachers who are 50 years of age or older.

Year Founded: 1958

188 National Rural Health Association
4501 College Boulevard
Suite 225
Leawood, KS 66211-1921
816-756-3140
Fax: 816-756-3144
mail@NRHArural.org
www.ruralhealthweb.org

Alan Morgan, CEO
Rob McVay, Director of Operations/CFO
Gabriela Boscan, Director of Program Services

Non-profit, professional organization targeting healthcare problems unique to rural areas and serving as a liaison between rural health care providers and older people.

Year Founded: 1978; Number of Members: 20,000

189 National Senior Corps Association
1316 E McKinney
Denton, TX 76209
940-383-1508
www.nscatogether.org

Gary C. Goosman, President

Volunteers from all different backgrounds of at least 55 years of age, involved in community needs. Local projects are organized and include healthcare, schools, courts and day dare.

Year Founded: 1993

190 National Senior Games Association
PO Box 82059
Baton Rouge, LA 70884

225-706-5101
Fax: 225-766-9115
nsga@nsga.com
www.nsga.com

Marc T. Riker, CEO

Non-profit organization promoting healthy lifestyles for older people through education, fitness, and sports.

Year Founded: 1985

191 National Tax Association
725 15th Street NW
Suite 600
Washington, DC 20005-2109
202-737-3325
Fax: 202-737-7308
natltax@aol.com
www.ntanet.org

Peter Brady, President

Government and corporate tax officials, accountants, consultants, economists, attorneys, teachers, and others interested in the field of taxation. Promotes scientific, nonpolitical study of taxation; encourages better understanding of the common interests of national, state, and local governments in matters of taxation and public finance. Membership benefits: National Tax Journal, Annual Conference on Taxation, Spring Symposium, NTA Forum and Special Conferences and Symposiums.

192 National Urban League
120 Wall Street
New York, NY 10005
212-558-5300
Fax: 212-344-5332
info@nul.org
nul.iamempowered.com

Marc H. Morial, President & CEO

Non-profit, community service organization helping older African Americans through advocacy and service programs which include health awareness, nutrition, housing, and intergenerational activities.

Year Founded: 1910

193 National Women's Health Network
1413 K Street NW
4th Floor
Washington, DC 20005
202-682-2640
Fax: 202-682-2648
nwhn@nwhn.org
www.nwhn.org

Cindy Pearson, Executive Director

An advocacy organization giving women a greater voice in the health care system in the United States. It is the only such membership organization and has a 20-year history of accomplishments on behalf of all women. Its clearinghouse of women's health information helps women make well-informed decisions. Also monitors federal legislation to ensure that women's needs are not overlooked.

Year Founded: 1974

194 Navy Seabee Veterans of America Inc.
555 Fairview Street
Creve Coeur, IL 61610

203-843-5513; *Toll Free: 800-732-2335*
nsvasec@gmail.com
www.nsva.org

Nancy Staples, President
Betty Nelson, Vice President
Linda Schmuck, Treasurer

A national organization comprised of veterans of the Naval Construction Forces and the Civil Engineer Corps of the United States Navy, whose objectives are to preserve and support the National Defense; to promote patriotism; to fosyer and strengthen comradeship; to support fellow veterans, widows, widowers; and to assist in the rehabilitation and welfare of veterans.

Year Founded: 1948

195 OWL: The Voice of Women 40+
1627 Eye Street NW
Suite 600
Washington, DC 20006
202-450-8986
info@owl-national.org
www.owl-national.org

Bobbie Ann Brinegar, Executive Director

Advocating on economic security and quality-of-life issues affecting women over 40.

Year Founded: 1980

196 Old Lesbians Organizing for Change
PO Box 5853
Athens, OH 45701
Toll Free: 888-706-7506
info@oloc.org
www.oloc.org

Alix Dobkin, Co-Director
Sally Tatnall, Co-Director

Lesbians over 60 confronting ageism in our communities.

197 Oley Foundation for Home Parenteral and Enteral Nutrition
43 New Scotland Avenue
MC-28, Albany Medical Center
Albany, NY 12208-3478
518-262-5079
Fax: 518-262-5528
bishopj@amc.edu
www.oley.org

Mary Patnode, President
Joan Bishop, Executive Director
Roslyn Dahl, Communications Director

The Oley Foundation is a national, nonprofit organization that strives to enrich the lives of patients dependent on home intravenous nutrition and tube feeding through education, advocacy, and networking.

Year Founded: 1983

198 Over the Hill Gang International
2121 North Weber Street
Colorado Springs, CO 80907
719-471-0222
Fax: 719-389-0024
www.othgi.com

Physically active seniors enjoying discounts on ski trips and other outdoor activities.

Number of Members: 3,000

199 Pension Research Council
Wharton School, University of Pennsylvania
3620 Locust Walk
3000 Steinberg Hall-Dietrich Hall
Philadelphia, PA 19104-6302
215-898-7620
Fax: 215-573-3418
prc@wharton.upenn.edu
www.pensionresearchcouncil.org

Olivia S. Mitchell, Executive Director

Sponsors nonpartisan, interdisciplinary research on the entire range of private and social retirement security and related benefit plans in the United States and around the world. Affiliated with the Wharton School of the University of Pennsylvania, and is supported by contributions from industry, insurance companies, banks, and pension consultants. Conducts interpretive studies of broad scope.

Year Founded: 1952

200 Pension Rights Center
1350 Connecticut Avenue NW
Suite 206
Washington, DC 20036
202-296-3776
Fax: 202-833-2472; Toll Free: 888-420-6550
www.pensionrights.org

Karen Ferguson, Director

Public interest group whose purpose is to protect and promote the pension rights of workers, retirees, and their families and to develop solutions to the nation's retirement income problems. Represents workers and retirees' interests before government agencies and Congress.

Year Founded: 1976

201 People. Animals. Love.
731 8th Street SE
Suite 202
Washington, DC 20003
202-966-2171
Fax: 202-966-2172
info@peopleanimalslove.org
peopleanimalslove.org

Autumn Young, Executive Director
Lillian Knudsen, Deputy Director

PAL is a nonprofit organization that brings people and animals together, brightening the lives of the lonely, easing the pain of the sick, and enriching the world of at-risk children.

Year Founded: 1982

202 Plan Sponsor Council of America
200 S Wacker Drive
Suite 3100
Chicago, IL 60606
312-419-1863
Fax: 703-516-9308
psca@psca.org
www.psca.org

Jack Towarnicky, Executive Director
Tobi Davis, Director of Operations
Hattie Greenan, Dir., Research/Communications

Sponsors sharing information and working together to preserve a favorable regulatory environment for profit sharing and 401(K) plans. Collects best practices information and shares it with members through faxes, publications, conferences and a technical assistance hotline. Also, supports plan sponsors and participants in Washington through Congressional lobbying.

Year Founded: 1947

203 Points of Light: New York

35 West 35th Street
6th Floor
New York, NY 10001
212-850-4170
www.pointsoflight.org

Tracy Hoover, CEO
Alison Doerfler, Executive Director

Mobilizing people to take action on the causes they care about.

204 Pride Foundation

2014 E Madison Street
Suite 300
Seattle, WA 98122
206-323-3318; *Toll Free: 800-735-7287*
www.pridefoundation.org

Kris Hermanns, Executive Director

Regional nonprofit advancing equality for LGBTQ people in the Northwest.

Year Founded: 1985

205 Pride Foundation: Idaho

PO Box 1827
Boise, ID 83701
208-914-0442
www.pridefoundation.org

Steve Martin, Regional Development Organizer

Regional nonprofit advancing equality for LGBTQ people in the Northwest.

206 Pride Foundation: Montana

PO Box 772
Helena, MT 59624
406-546-7017
www.pridefoundation.org

Kim Leighton, Regional Development Organizer

Regional nonprofit advancing equality for LGBTQ people in the Northwest.

207 Pride Foundation: Oregon

PO Box 12093
Portland, OR 97212
541-603-8626
www.pridefoundation.org

Katie Carter, Regional Development Organizer

Regional nonprofit advancing equality for LGBTQ people in the Northwest.

208 Pride Foundation: Washington

PO Box 30700
Spokane, WA 99223
509-481-0402
www.pridefoundation.org

Farand Gunnels, Regional Development Organizer

Regional nonprofit advancing equality for LGBTQ people in the Northwest.

209 ProLiteracy Worldwide

104 Marcellus Street
Syracuse, NY 13204
315-422-9121
Fax: 315-422-6369; Toll Free: 888-528-2224
info@proliteracy.org
www.proliteracy.org

Kevin Morgan, President & CEO

Supports worldwide adult literacy. Programs include speaking, reading, writing and computational skills. Provides reading materials and resources for those with limited reading abilities.

Year Founded: 2002

210 Railroad Retirement Board

844 N Rush Street
Chicago, IL 60611-1275
312-751-4300; *Toll Free: 877-772-5772*
secure.rrb.gov
TTY: 312-751-4701

Adminisisters comprehensive retirement-survivor and unemployment-sickness benefit programs for the Nation's railroad workers and their families. Participates in the administration of the Social Security Act and the Health Insurance for the Aged Act insofar as they affect railroad retirement beneficiaries. Note: Any local chapter can be reached by calling the 800# above.

Year Founded: 1935

211 Rebuilding Together

1899 L Street NW
Suite 1000
Washington, DC 20036
Toll Free: 800-473-4229
info@rebuildingtogether.org
togetherwetransform.org

Caroline Blakely, President & CEO

Revitalizing communities by helping low-income homeowners improve the safety and health of their homes.

Year Founded: 1988

212 Respiratory Nursing Society

www.respiratorynursingsociety.org

Ashok Patel, President

Association of nurses who care for patients with respiratory problems.

Year Founded: 1990

213 Retired Enlisted Association

1111 S Abilene Court
Aurora, CO 80012
303-752-0660
Fax: 303-752-0835; Toll Free: 800-338-9337
treahq@trea.org
trea.org

Deirdre Parke Holleman, Executive Director

Association works to stop the erosion of earned benefits for service personnel and their families.

Year Founded: 1963

214 Retired Military Police Officers Association

PO Box 25343
Fayetteville, NC 28314-5005

703-508-9552
www.rmpo.org

Retired military police personnel. Works with active duty military police and civilian police during catastrophes. Conducts reunions and special events. Performs volunteer work and charitable services.

215 SPRY Foundation
3916 Rosemary Street
Chevy Chase, MD 20815
301-656-3405
Fax: 301-656-6221
morganr@spry.org
www.spry.org

Richard Browdie, Chair
Russell E. Morgan, President
Sandy Markwood, Vice Chair, Secretary/Treasurer

Non-profit foundation that develops research and education programs to help older adults plan for a healthy and financially secure future.

216 Senior Job Bank
PO Box 508
Marlborough, MA 01752
www.seniorjobbank.org

Gene Burnard, Publisher

Online resource for employers and over-50 job seekers.

Year Founded: 1975

217 Senior Service America
8403 Colesville Road
Suite 1200
Silver Spring, MD 20910
301-578-8900
contact@ssa-i.org
www.seniorserviceamerica.org

Gary A Officer, President/CEO
Donna Satterhwaite, Director, Workforce Development
Lynn Woo, Director, Finance

A nonprofit that provides community service and employment opportunities for adults organization that provides community service and employment opportunities for adults age 55 and over.

Year Founded: 1961

218 Social Security Administration
Office of Public Inquiries
1100 West High Rise, 6401 Security Boulevard
Baltimore, MD 21235
Toll Free: 800-772-1213
www.ssa.gov

Carolyn W. Colvin, Acting Commissioner

The Social Security Administration administers a national program of contributory social insurance whereby employees, employers, and the self-employed pay contributions which are pooled in special trust funds. When earnings stop or are reduced because the worker retires, dies, or becomes disabled, monthly cash benefits are paid to partially replace the earnings the family has lost.

219 Society of Health and Physical Educators (SHAPE America)
1900 Association Drive
Reston, VA 20191-1598

703-476-3400
Fax: 703-476-9527; *Toll Free:* 800-213-7193
evp@aahperd.org
www.aahperd.org

Steve Jefferies, President
E. Paul Roetert, Chief Executive Officer

National organization of health and physical education professionals providing leadership, professional development and advocacy.

Year Founded: 1885

220 Society of Military Widows
www.militarywidows.org

Patricia Walker, President

Formed to serve the interests of women whose husbands died while on active duty, of a service connected illness, during disability, or regular retirement from the armed forces.

Year Founded: 1968

221 Special Care Dentistry Association
2800 W Higgins Road
Suite 440
Hoffman Estates, IL 60169
312-527-6764
Fax: 847-885-8393
scda@scdaonline.org
www.scdaonline.org

Beth Weinstein, Executive Director
Sam Swetchkenbaum, President
David Miller, Vice President

A unique international organization of oral health professionals and other individuals who are dedicated to promoting oral health and well being for people with special needs; including dentists, dental hygienists and assistants, non-dental healthcare providers, health program administrators, residents, students and hospitals.

Year Founded: 1987

222 Supportive Older Women's Network
4100 Main Street
Suite 403
Philadelphia, PA 19127
215-487-3000
Fax: 215-487-3111
info@sown.org
www.sown.org

Merle Drake, Executive Director

Helps women (60+) to cope with aging issues through support groups, leadership training, consultation and newsletters. Telephone support groups for homebound women are also provided.

223 Tax Counseling for the Elderly
Internal Revenue Service
www.irs.gov

IRS program offering free tax help to seniors.

224 Teachers Insurance and Annuity Association of America
PO Box 1259
Charlotte, NC 28201
Fax: - - 0; *Toll Free:* 800-842-2252
www.tiaa.org

Roger Ferguson, President & CEO

TIAA CREP provides a nationwide portable pension system for over 2 million employees of some 8,000 colleges, universities, independent schools, and related nonprofit educational and research institutions.

Year Founded: 1918

225   Therapeutic Touch International Association
Box 310
Delmar, NY 12054
518-325-1185
Fax: 509-693-3537
info@therapeutic-touch.org
therapeutic-touch.org

Sue Conlin, President

Official organization of Therapeutic Touch, sets the standards for the practice and teaching of Therapeutic Touch. An international network of members interested in healing. It facilitates the exchange of research findings, teaching strategies, and new developments in this area. The human being is viewed as a complex, dynamic whole, and healing is seen as the means of restoring the integrity of the mind, body and spirit.

Year Founded: 1979

226   U.S. Commission on Civil Rights
1331 Pennsylvania Avenue NW
Suite 1150
Washington, DC 20425
202-376-7700
www.usccr.gov
TTY: 202-376-8116

Martin R. Castro, Chair

Informing the development of civil rights policy in the United States.

Year Founded: 1957

227   U.S. Department of Education Office of Civil Rights
400 Maryland Avenue SW
Washington, DC 20202
Toll Free: 800-872-5327
www2.ed.gov/ocr

Catherine E. Lhamon, Assistant Secretary

Prohibits discrimination on the basis of disability in programs and activities funded by the Department of Education. Investigates complaints and provides technical assistance to individuals and entities with rights and responsibilities under Section 504.

228   U.S. Department of Health & Human Services
200 Independence Avenue SW
Washington, DC 20201
Toll Free: 877-696-6775
www.hhs.gov

Sylvia Mathews Burwell, Secretary
Mary K. Wakefield, Acting Deputy Secretary

The Secretary advises the President on health, welfare, and income security plans, policies, and programs of the Federal Government. The Secretary directs Department staff in carrying out the approved programs and activities of the Department and promotes general public understanding of the Department's goals, programs, and objectives. The Sec-

retary administers these functions through the Office of the Secretary and the 4 Operating Divisions.

229   U.S. Department of Housing & Urban Development Office of Fair Housing & Equal Opportunity
U.S. Dept. of Housing & Urban Development
451 7th Street SW
Washington, DC 20410
www.hud.gov

Gustavo Velasquez, Assistant Secretary

Working to eliminate housing discrimination by enforcing federal fair housing policies and laws.

Year Founded: 1937

230   U.S. Department of Justice: Civil RightsDivision
950 Pennsylvania Avenue NW
Washington, DC 20530-0001
202-514-4609
www.justice.gov
TTY: 202-514-0716

Vanita Gupta, Deputy Asst. Attorney General

Coordinates the implementation by federal agencies of section 504 of the Rehabilitation Act of 1973, as amended, which prohibits discrimination on the basis of handicap in federally assisted programs and in programs and activities conducted by federal executive agencies.

231   U.S. Department of Veterans Affairs
Toll Free: 800-488-8244
www.va.gov

Robert A. McDonald, Secretary

The US Department of Veterans Affairs provides patient care and federal benefits to veterans and their dependents.

232   U.S. Office of Personnel Management
1900 E Street NW
Washington, DC 20415-1000
202-606-1800
www.opm.gov
TTY: 800-877-8339

Beth F. Cobert, Acting Director

Establishes policies for employment of the handicapped within the federal service. Administers a merit system for federal employment that includes recruiting, examining, training, and promoting people on the basis of knowledge and skills, regardless of sex, race, religion or other factors.

233   U.S. Senate Special Committee on Aging
G31 Dirksen Senate Office Building
Washington, DC 20510-6050
202-224-5364
Fax: 202-224-9926
www.aging.senate.gov

Susan M. Collins, Chairman

The committee has no legislative authority. It studies and debates issues relating to older Americans and makes recommendations to the Senate.

Year Founded: 1961

234   U.S. Small Business Administration
409 3rd Street SW
Washington, DC 20416

Toll Free: 800-827-5722
www.sba.gov

Maria Contreras-Sweet, Administrator

To utilize the management experience of retired and active business executives to counsel and train potential and existing small businesses. The business must be independently owned and operated, not dominant in its field, and conform to SBA size standards.

Year Founded: 1953

235 Vestibular Disorders Association

5018 NE 15th Avenue
Portland, OR 97211
Fax: 503-229-8064; *Toll Free:* 800-837-8428
info@vestibular.org
vestibular.org

Cynthia Ryan, Executive Director

Serving people suffering from disorders of the inner ear.

Year Founded: 1985

236 Visiting Nurse Associations of America

2121 Crystal Drive
Suite 750
Arlington, VA 22202
571-527-1520
Fax: 571-527-1521; *Toll Free:* 888-866-8773
vnaa@vnaa.org
www.vnaa.org

Tracey Moorhead, President & CEO

Voluntary, nonprofit home health care agencies. Develops competitive strength among community-based nonprofit visiting nurse organizations; works to strengthen business resources and economic programs through contracting, marketing, governmental affairs and publications.

Year Founded: 1983

237 WomenHeart: The National Coalition for Women with Heart Disease

1100 17th Street NW
Suite 500
Washington, DC 20036
202-728-7199
Fax: 202-728-7238
mail@womenheart.org
www.womenheart.org

Mary McGowan, CEO

Advocating for women at risk of heart disease.

Year Founded: 1999

238 Workmen's Benefit Fund of the USA

399 Conklin St
Suite 310
Farmingdale, NY 11735-2614
516-938-6060
Fax: 516-706-9020
info@wbfusa.com
www.wbfusa.org

Charles J Borg, National President

The WBF is a fraternal benefit society offering affordable life insurance and competitive annuity products to people of all ages. WBF is committed to helping its membership, their families and local communities in the spirit of fraternalism.

Year Founded: 1884; Number of Members: 8,000

239 World Institute on Disability

3075 Adeline Street
Suite 155
Berkeley, CA 94703
510-225-6400
Fax: 510-225-0477
wid@wid.org
www.wid.org

Anita Shafer Aaron, Executive Director
Sheridan Gates, Treasurer
Eli Gelardin, Secretary

the World Institute on Disability (WID) is a nonprofit that works to fully integrate people with disabilities into the communities around them through employment opportunities, disability benefits, financial planning, and healthcare access.

Year Founded: 1983

240 Aging Life Care Association

3275 W Ina Road
Suite 130
Tucson, AZ 85741-2198
520-881-8008
Fax: 520-325-7925
info@aginglifecare.org
www.aginglifecare.org

Thomas A Kube, CEO
Julie Wagner, Director of Administration
Sarah Garcia, Member Services Assistant

The Aging Life Care Association is a holistic, client-centered approach to caring for older adults or others facing ongoing health challenges. The Association provides families with guidance in areas including health and disability, finances, housing, legal, crisis intervention, and local resources. The Association also helps people who have physical disabilities, developmental disabilities, brain injuries, mental health problems, and chronic illnesses.

Year Founded: 1985; Number of Members: 2,000+

International

241 Advocacy Centre for the Elderly

2 Carlton Street
Suite 701
Toronto, ON M5B 1J3
416-598-2656
Fax: 416-598-7924; *Toll Free:* 855-598-2656
www.advocacycentreelderly.org

Irene Carriere, Chair
Susan Bryson, Vice-Chair
Graham Webb, Executive Director

Provides legal services to low income seniors in the Greater Metropolitan Toronto Area. Also provides public legal education & law reform services provincially.

Year Founded: 1984

242 Age & Opportunity: Support Services

200-280 Smith Street
Winnipeg, MB R3C 1K2
204-956-6440
Fax: 204-946-5667

info@aosupportservices.ca
www.aosupportservices.ca

Vernon De Pape, Chair
Laryssa Sawchuk, 1st Vice Chair
Gabrielle Marrin, Treasurer

A & O: Support Services for Older Adults is a
not-for-profit organization that provides specialized services for older Manitobans across the province. The goal of
these programs is to empower and support older adults in
the community.

Year Founded: 1957

243 **Association of Mature Canadians**
366 Bay Street
7th Floor
Toronto, ON M5H 4B2
416-601-0429
Fax: 416-601-0429; Toll Free: 800-667-0429
service@maturecanadians.ca
www.maturecanadians.ca

Robert Bruce, Executive Director

The Associatio of Mature Canadians is a nonprofit, member controlled organisation dedicated to supporting the
community of mature canadians, through education and
communication, by addressing their changing lifestyle and
healthcare needs in a socially and financially responsible
way.

244 **Canada Association for Retired Persons
(CARP)**
64 Jefferson Avenue
Toronto, ON M6K 1Y4
416-363-2277
Fax: 416-363-8748; Toll Free: 888-363-2279
advocacy@carp.ca
www.carp.ca

Moses Znaimer, President
Wanda Morris, Vice President, Advocacy
Laas Turnbull, Chief Operating Officer

Canada's largest advocacy association for older Canadians,
CARP promotes the rights & quality of life through advocacy, education, information & other services.

Year Founded: 1985; Number of Members: 300,000

245 **Carefirst Seniors & Community Services
Association**
300 Silver Star Boulevard
Scarborough, ON M1V 0G2
416-502-2323
Fax: 416-502-2382
info@carefirstseniors.com
www.carefirstseniors.com

Helen Leung, Executive Director

Carefirst Seniors & Community Services Association is a
non-profit charitable community services agency whose
mission is to ensure that seniors and others in need of services, living in Toronto and surrounding areas, enjoy a high
quality of life in their communities.

Year Founded: 1976; Number of Members: 350

246 **Help the Aged**
1300 Carling Avenue
Ottawa, ON K1Z 7L2

613-232-0727
Fax: 613-232-7625; Toll Free: 800-648-1111
info@helpagecanada.ca
www.helpagecanada.ca

Jacques Bertrand, Executive Director
Rosalie Gelderman, Secretary
Don Hefler, Treasurer

To improve the quality of life of the elderly poor, support
their independence and inclusion, and provide services and
programs to relieve distress, poverty and sickness.

Year Founded: 1975

247 **Institute for Life Course and Aging**
University of Toronto
246 Bloor Street W
Room 238
Toronto, ON M5S 1V4
416-978-0377
aging@utoronto.ca
www.aging.utoronto.ca

Prof Esme Fuller-Thomson, Director
Susan Murphy, Administration
Nina Carlton, Reception

To conduct interdisciplinary research on the biological,
psychological and social dimensions of the life course and
aging; to provide graduate and post-graduate education on
the life course and aging.

Year Founded: 1979

248 **NWT Senior's Society**
102, 4916 46th Street
Yellowknife, NT X1A 1L2
867-920-7444
Fax: 867-920-7601; Toll Free: 800-661-0878
ed@seniorsnwt.ca
www.nwtseniorssociety.ca

Mary Pat Short, President
Barb Hood, Executive Director
Tom Makepeace, Secretary

The Society provides information, acts as a resource and
support for seniors and elders across the NWT. The Society
is the only voluntary agency representing the individual
and collective interests of all seniors and elders in the
NWT.

Year Founded: 1983

249 **National Institute for the Care of the Elderly
(NICE)**
246 Bloor Street W
Room 234
Toronto, ON M5S 1V4
416-978-7037
nicenetadmin@utoronto.ca
www.nicenet.ca

Dr. Barry Goldlist, Chair
Raza M Mirza, Network Manager
Lynn McDonald, Scientific Director

NICE is an international network of researchers, practitioners, students and seniors dedicated to improving the care
of older adults, both in Canada and abroad.

250 National Pensioners & Senior Citizens Federation

2186 Stanfield Road
Mississauga, ON L4Y 1R5
519-350-3221
info@@npfmail.ca
nationalpensionersfederation.ca

Herb John, Past President
Patrick Brady, Secretary
Mary Forbes, Treasurer

The National Pensioners and Senior Citizens Federation is an organization devoted entirely to the welfare and best interests of Canada's elderly.

Year Founded: 1945; Number of Members: 1,000,000

251 Older Women's Network

115 The Esplanade
Toronto, ON M5E 1Y7
416-214-1518
info@olderwomensnetwork.org
olderwomensnetwork.org

Mary Hynes, Chair

OWN is a voice for mid-life and older women in Canada, one that challenges discrimination on the basis of age, gender, religion, or disability. OWN is an educational organization that embraces a feminist perspective in order to empower women to overcome injustices and inequities of gender in the home, the workplace and in society at large.

Year Founded: 1986

State Organizations & Government Agencies

Alabama

252   Alabama Client Assistance Program
400 South Union Street
Suite 465
Montgomery, AL 36104
334-263-2985
Fax: 334-230-9765; *Toll Free:* 800-228-3231
sacap.alabama.gov

Rachel Hughes, Director/Advocate
Kerri Butler, Administrative Support

Mission is to enable Alabama's disabled population to achieve their maximum potential.

253   Alabama Department of Education: Disability Determination Service
50 North Ripley Street
PO Box 302101
Montgomery, AL 36104
334-242-9700
www.alsde.edu

Thomas R Bice, State Superintendent
Warren Craig Pouncy, Chief of Staff
Sherrill Parris, Deputy State Superintendent

Assessment department for learning disabilities.

254   Alabama Department of Public Health
201 Monroe Street
Montgomery, AL 36104
334-206-5300; *Toll Free:* 800-272-1818
www.alabamapublichealth.gov

Donald Williamson, State Health Officer

The purpose of the Alabama Department of Public Health is to provide caring, high quality and professional services for the improvement and protection of the public's health through disease prevention and the assurance of public health services to resident and transient populations of the state regardless of social circumstances or the ability to pay.

255   Alabama Department of Rehabilitation Services
602 S Lawrence Street
Montgomery, AL 36104
334-293-7500
Fax: 334-293-7383; *Toll Free:* 800-441-7607
www.rehab.alabama.gov

Jane E Burdeshaw, Commissioner
Stephen Kayes, District 1, Mobile
Jimmy Vernado, District 2, Montgomery

The Alabama Department of Rehabilitation Services (ADRS) is the state agency that serves people with disabilities from birth to old age through a "continuum of services," including Early Intervention, Children's Rehabilitation, Vocational Rehabilitation, and Independent Living.

Year Founded: 1994

256   Alabama Department of Retirement Systems
201 South Union Street
Montgomery, AL 36104

334-517-7000
Fax: 334-517-7001; *Toll Free:* 877-517-0020
field.services@rsa-al.gov
www.rsa-al.gov

Kay Ivey, Chair
Clinton Carter, State Finance Director
Young Boozer, State Treasurer

It is the mission of the Retirement Systems of Alabama to serve the interests of its members by preserving the excellent benefits and soundness of the Systems at the least expense to the state of Alabama and all Alabama taxpayers.

257   Alabama Department of Revenue
50 N Ripley Street
Montgomery, AL 36104
334-242-1175
revenue.alabama.gov

Vernon Barnett, Commissioner
Michael D Gamble, Deputy Co-Commissioner
Brenda R Coone, Deputy Co-Commissioner

Mission is to efficiently and effectively administer the revenue laws in an equitable, courteous and professional manner to fund the governmental services for the citizens of Alabama.

258   Alabama Department of Senior Services
201 Monroe Street
Suite 350
Montgomery, AL 36104
334-242-5743
Fax: 334-242-5594; *Toll Free:* 877-425-2243
ageline@adss.alabama.gov
alabamaageline.gov

Todd Cotton, Commissioner
Thomas Ray Edwards, Chairman
Horace Patterson, Vice Chairman

A cabinet level state agency that administers programs for senior citizens and people with disabilities. The department was originaly establised by the Alabama Legislature in 1957 as the Alabama Commission on Aging.

259   Alabama Department of Veteran Affairs
334-242-5066; *Toll Free:* 800-273-8255
www.va.state.al.us

W Clyde Marsh, Commissioner
Kay Ivey, Chairwoman
Chad Richmond, Vice-Chairman

Mission is to promote awareness, assist eligible veterans, their families, and survivors to receive from the US Federal and State Governments and and all benefits to which they may be entitled under existing or future laws to be enacted.

260   Alabama Developmental Disability Council
RSA Union Building
100 N Union Street
PO Box 301410
Montgomery, AL 36130-1410
334-242-3976
myra.jones@mh.alabama.gov
www.acdd.org

Elmyra Jones-Banks, Executive Director
Sophia Whitted, Fiscal Manager
Holli C Zukowski, Contracts Manager

Serves Alabama's disabled population and representatives of all service provider agencies that serve people with disabilities. The Council generates a state plan and identifies priority areas for service planning.

Number of Members: 36

261 Alabama Disabilities Advocacy Program
P.O. Box 870395
Tuscaloosa, AL 35487-0395
205-348-4928
Fax: 205-348-3909; Toll Free: 800-826-1675
adap@adap.ua.edu
adap.ua.edu

Barbara Lawrence, Senior Staff Attorney
James Tucker, Director
Nancy Anderson, Associate Director

The Alabama Disabilities Advocacy Program (ADAP) is the federally mandated, statewide, 'Protection, and Advocacy' system serving eligible individuals with disabilities in Alabama. ADAP has four program components: protection and advocacy for persons with developmental disabilities (PADD), protection and advocacy for individuals with mental illness (PAIMT), protection and advocacy of individual rights (PAIR), and protection and advocacy for assistive technology (PAAT).

262 Alabama Radio Reading Service Network
650 11th Street South
Birmingham, AL 35233
205-934-2606
Fax: 205-934-5075; Toll Free: 800-444-9246
info@wbhm.org
www.wbhm.org

Chuck Holmes, General Manager
Michael Krall, Program Director
Darrell McCalla, Chief Operator/Engineer

The objectives and activities of the Service is to bring printed matter to all in the state of Alabama that are physically handicapped or physically impaired.

263 Alabama State Department of Human Resources
50 North Ripley Street
Gordon Persons Bldg, Suite 2104
Montgomery, AL 36130
334-242-1310
Fax: 334-353-1115
barry.spear@dhr.alabama.gov
www.dhr.state.al.us

Barry Spear, Public Information Officer
Nancy T Buckner, Commissioner

The mission of the Alabama Department of Human Resources is to partner with communities to promote family stability and provide for the safety and self sufficency Alabamians.

Year Founded: 1935

264 Alabama Tombigbee Regional Commission
107 Broad Street
Camden, AL 36726-2122
334-682-4234
cynthia.agee@atrc.net
www.atrcregion6.com

Cynthia Agee, Case Manager
Ann Alford, Revolving Loan Fund Manager
Fred Armstead, Rural Transportation Director

the Alabama-Tombigbee Regional Commission promotes area-wide progress through regional planning and development concepts in such areas as local planning, economic and community development and human resources coordination. The Commission was formed by voluntary actions of county and municipal officials and other community leaders from the ten county area in cooperation with various federal and state agencies.

Year Founded: 1969

265 Alabama Workers Compensation Division
Department of Labor
649 Monroe Street
Montgomery, AL 36131
334-353-0430; *Toll Free: 800-528-2546*
mary.jorgensen@labor.alabama.org
labor.alabama.gov

Steve Garrett, Director

This division humanizes the Alabama workplace through its protective effort for employees and employers. It administers the Alabama Workers' Compensation (WC) law providing compensation for job related injuries and occupational diseases. In doing so, safety in the workplace is encouraged and expanded for all workers.

266 East Alabama Commission: Agency on Aging
Quintard Tower, Suite 300
1130 Quintard Avenue
Anniston, AL 36201
256-237-6741
Fax: 256-237-6763; Toll Free: 800-239-6741
www.earpdc.org

Tony Wilkie, Chairman
Paul J Perrett, Vice Chairman
Albertha F Grant, Executive Director

The Area Agency on Aging (AAA) is designated by the State of Alabama to develop and administer an Area Plan providing a comprehensive and coordinated service delivery system for older Alabamians in the 10 county service area.

267 Governor's Committee on Employment of Persons with Disabilities
Division of Rehabilitation Service
602 South Lawerence Street
Montgomery, AL 36104
205-290-4457; *Toll Free: 800-671-6837*
leslie.dawson@rehab.alabama.gov
rehab.alabama.gov

Jane E Burdeshaw, Commissioner
Stephen Kayes, Board Member District 1
Jimmie Varnado, Board Member District 2

The committee's goals are to educate the public about the benefits of hiring people with disabilities and promoting a greater independence for people with disabilities. The committee provides information and resources on workplace accessibility, the Americans with Disabilities Act, rehabilitation services, and coordinating awareness events.

268 Lee Russell Council of Governments: Area Agency on Aging
2207 Gateway Drive
Opelika, AL 36801-6834
334-749-5264
Fax: 334-749-6582; Toll Free: 800-243-5463

sburnette@lrcog.com
www.lrcog.com

Mayor Bill Ham, Jr., Chair
Suzanne G. Burnette, Executive Director
Van Vanoy, Finance Director

Services offered through the Area Agency on Again inclue: Medicaid Waiver Program, home delivered meals, legal assistance, State Health Insurance Program, Senior Medicare Patrol Program, preventive health coordination and assistance, senior workers, SenioRx Prescription Drug Program, Medicare Part D assistance, Alabama Cares Referral and Resource Program, and Alzheimer's Support Group coordination.

269 Montgomery Area Council on Aging

115 E Jefferson Street
Montgomery, AL 36104-3654
334-263-0532
Fax: 334-240-6769
macoa@macoa.org
www.macoa.org

Donna Marietta, Executive Director
Chacolby Burns-Johnson, Director of Development
Jennifer Dvorak, RSVP Director

MACOA promotes independent, dignified, and meaningful living for senior citizens through a variety of programs that offer hope, care, sustenance, and opportunity to more than 2,500 seniors each month. MACOA's activities provide the warmth of family and home along with hope, motivation, enjoyment, and means to live independently.

270 North Central Alabama Regional Council of Governments: Area Agency on Aging

216 Jackson Street SE
Decatur, AL 35601
256-355-4515; *Toll Free:* 800-682-8604
cathleen.mcculloch@adss.alabama.gov
www.narcog.org

Jeffrey A Pruitt, AICP, Executive Director
Cathleen McCulloch, Program Administrative Assistant
Carol Lindsey, Accounting Coordinator

NARCOG is the North-central Regional Council of Governments. NARCOG's Board of Directors consists of representatives from 7 participating member governments.

271 Northwest Alabama Council of Governments: Area Agency on Aging

103 Student Drive
Muscle Shoals, AL 35661
256-389-0500
Fax: 256-389-0599; *Toll Free:* 800-838-5845
kjones@nwscc.edu
www.nacolg.com

Keith Jones, Executive Director
Mayor Mickey Haddock, Chairman
Shelia Bentley, Medicaid Waiver Case Manager

The Northwest Alabama Council of Local Governments is not a municipal government, county government, a part of the federal government or a regulator agency. NACOLG is a regional council of governments established to deal with problems that cross the city lines, country lines or the whole region such as transportation, aging services, community/economic development and planning.

272 RSVP Athens Limestone County

409 West Washington Street
Athens, AL 35611
256-232-7207
Fax: 256-232-8842
bruth@al-rsvp.com
www.al-rsvp.com

Betty Ruth, Executive Director
Marilyn Posey, Transportation Coordinator
Willa Dean Morgan, Secretary and Office Assistant

RSVP offers men and women exciting opportunities for personal development and satisfaction by providing volunteer programs that offer outlets for their energy and creativity while serving in their community.

273 RSVP Baldwin County
Kiwanis Club of Bay Minette

300 N Hoyle Avenue
Bay Minette, AL 36507
251-580-0385
bcvoad@gmail.com

Faye Robinson, Director

8-10 senior volunteers helping with beach clean up yearly at Gulf Shores. This benefits not only the residents but visitors also. Our senior volunteers also plant and maintain gardens and trees, and are involved in recycling, environmental education, local museums, and working with the handicapped.

274 RSVP Etowah County

800 Forrest Avenue
Room 219
Gadsden, AL 35901-3672
256-549-8147
Fax: 256-549-5351; *Toll Free:* 866-314-7660
tpondick@etowahcounty.org
www.etowahcounty.org

Traci Pondick, Director

The Retired and Senior Volunteer Program (RSVP) provides opportunities for people 55 and over to make a difference in their community through volunteer service. RSVP volunteers contribute anywhere from a few to over forty hours a week, serving through schools, day care centers, police departments, hospitals and other nonprofit and public organizations to help meet critical community needs. RSVP offers maximum flexibility and choice to its volunteers. RSVP matches the personal interests and skills of older Americans with opportunities to help solve community problems and offers supplemental insurance while on duty, and on-the-job training from the agency or organization where volunteers are placed.

275 Railroad Retirement Board: Alabama District Office

950 22nd Street N
Suite 426
Birmingham, AL 35203-1134
Fax: 205-731-0026; *Toll Free:* 877-772-5772
www.rrb.gov

Martin J Dickman, Inspector General

The Railroad Board is an independent agency in the executive branch of the Federal Government. The primary function is to administer comprehensive retirement-survivor and unemployment sickness benefit programs for the nation's railroad workers and their families.

276 TARCOG: Area Agency on Aging
5075 Research Drive NW
Huntsville, AL 35805-5912
256-830-0818
tarcog.us

Nancy Robertson, Executive Director
Helen Cartner, President
Mary Caudle, Vice President

TARCOG provides many services to the region's elderly population. The AAA plans and manages a system of in-home and community services to help seniors maintain their independence and dignity, and it administers federal, state, local and private funds to support those services.

Year Founded: 1968

277 Volunteer Center of Morgan County
811 2nd Avenue SE
Suite 1
Decatur, AL 35601
256-355-8628
Fax: 256-355-8726
vcomc@vcomc.org
www.vcomc.org

Connie Larkin, Staff Member
Quay Lively, Staff Member
Priscilla Nunnelee, Staff Member

Recruits, trains, and interviews volunteers and refers them to qualified community agencies requesting such services. Volunteers of all ages, abilities and backgrounds are mobilized to feed the hungry, serve seniors, protect the environment, mentor children and make a difference in our community in many other ways.

Year Founded: 1970

278 Volunteers of America Southeast
1204 Hillcrest Road
Mobile, AL 36609
251-300-3500
Fax: 251-666-2836; *Toll Free:* 800-859-4431
voase.org

Cheryl Williams, Chair
Patsy Dow, Vice Chair
Charles Story, Treasurer

Volunteers of America Southeast makes every effort to create a community of care that enables individuals to live as independently as possible for as long as possible. We provide for individuals who are 62 years of age and older with a low income an opportunity to live in a safe, comfortable, and affordable setting.

Year Founded: 1896

Alaska

279 Alaska Client Assistance Program (CAP)
Disability Law Center of Alaska
3330 Arctic Boulevard
Suite 103
Anchorage, AK 99503
907-565-1002
Fax: 907-565-1000; *Toll Free:* 800-478-1234
akpa@dlcak.org
www.dlcak.org

Tracy Barbee, President
Kim Rion, Vice President
Sarah Randolph-Andrew, Secretary

CAP is Alaska's Client Assist Program. An ombudsman/advocacy service that provides information, help and individualized advocacy.

280 Alaska Commission on Aging
240 Main Street
P.O. Box 110693
Juneau, AK 99811-0693
907-465-3030
Fax: 907-465-1398
hss.acoa@alaska.gov
dhss.alaska.gov/acoa

Lesley Thompson, H&SS Planner

The mission of the Alaska Commission on Aging is to promote the dignity and independence of senior Alaskans, and to assist them in leading useful and meaningful lives.

281 Alaska Department of Military and Veterans Affairs
907-428-6003
Fax: 907-428-6019
dmva.alaska.gov

Laurel Hummel, Commissioner
Robert Doehl, Deputy Comissioner
Verdie Bowen, Director, State Veterans Office

Provides services such as healthcare, employment, and education benefits to veterans.

282 Alaska Department of Revenue
PO Box 110400
Juneau, AK 99811-0400
907-465-2300
Fax: 907-465-2389
www.revenue.state.ak.us

Sheldon Fisher, Commissioner

The mission of the Department of Revenue is to collect and invest funds for public purposes. The mission of the Office of the Commissioner is to provide support and policy direction to the divisions in the department.

283 Alaska Division of Retirement & Benefits
P.O. Box 110203
6th Floor State Office Bldg
Juneau, AK 99811-0203
907-465-4460
Fax: 907-465-3086; *Toll Free:* 800-821-2251
doa.alaska.gov/drb/
TDD 907-465-2805

Ajay Desai, Director
Kathy Lea, Chief Pension Officer
Michele Michaud, Chief Health Officer

Mission is to deliver beneifits to members in accordance with legal requirements.

284 Alaska Division of Vocational Rehabilitation
Department of Labor and Workforce Development
P.O. Box 115516
Juneau, AK 99811-5516
907-465-2814
Fax: 907-465-2856; *Toll Free:* 800-478-2815
dol.dvr.info@alaska.gov
labor.alaska.gov

John Cannon, Director

Mission is to assist individuals with disabilities to obtain and maintain employment.

285 Alaska Statewide Independent Living Council
1057 West Fireweed Lane
Suite 206
Anchorage, AK 99501
907-263-2011
Fax: 907-263-2012; *Toll Free:* 888-392-4560
heidi@alaskasilc.org
www.alaskasilc.org

Michael Christian, Chair
Richard K O'Donnell, Vice Chair
Joan O'Keefe, Treasurer

The Alaska Statewide Independent Living is committed to promoting a philosophy of consumer control, peer support, self help, self determination, equal access, and individual and systems advocacy, in order to maximize leadership, empowerment, independence, productivity, and to support full inclusion and integration of individuals with disabilities into the mainstream of American society.

286 Alaska Workers Compensation Board
Department of Labor
1111 West 8th Street, Room 305
P.O. Box 115512
Juneau, AK 99801
907-465-2790
Fax: 907-465-2797; *Toll Free:* 877-783-4980
workerscomp@alaska.gov
labor.alaska.gov/wc/

Marie Marx, Director

Workers' Compensation is a system which requires an employer to pay an injured employee's work-related medical and disability benefits. Workers' Compensation also requires the payment of benefits to dependents in the case of work-related death.

287 Alaska's Intellectual and Developmental Disabilities Unit
Senior & Disabilities Services
550 W 8th Avenue
Anchorage, AK 99501-3574
907-269-3666
Fax: 907-269-3639; *Toll Free:* 800-478-9996
dhss.alaska.gov

Senior and Disabilities Services promotes health, well being and safety for individuals with disabilities, seniors and vulnerable adults by facilitating access to quality services and supports that foster independence, personal choice and dignity.

288 Alaskans Commission on Aging
240 Main Street
P.O. Box 110693
Juneau, AK 99811-0693
907-465-4793
Fax: 907-465-1398
hss.acoa@alaska.gov
dhss.alaska.gov

Denise Daniello, Executive Director
Lesley Thompson, H&SS Planner

Statewide services for Alaskans aged 60 and older.

289 Assistive Technology of Alaska
3330 Arctic Boulevard
Suite 101
Anchorage, AK 99503
907-563-2599
Fax: 907-563-0699; *Toll Free:* 800-723-2852
atla@atlaak.org
www.atlaak.org
TTY: 907-561-2592

Kathy Privratsky, Executive Director

Statewide program that provides demonstrations, information, and device loans to help Alaskans make informed decisions and select the AT that best meets their needs.

290 Disability Law Center of Alaska
3330 Arctic Boulevard
Suite 103
Anchorage, AK 99503
907-344-1002
Fax: 907-565-1000; *Toll Free:* 800-478-1234
akpa@dlcak.org
www.dlcak.org

Tracy Barbee, President
Kim Rion, Vice President
Sarah Randolph-Andrew, Secretary

An independent non-profit organization that provides legal advocacy services for people with disabilities anywhere in Alaska. DLC is designated under federal law as the Sate of Alaska's Protection and Advocacy (P&A) agency.

291 Fairbanks Senior Center
North Star Council on Aging
1424 Moore Street
Fairbanks, AK 99701
907-452-1735
Fax: 907-451-9974
nscoa.newsletter@alaska.net
fairbanksseniorcenter.org

Pat Ivey, President
Darlene Supplee, Executive Director
Natalie Gaskins, Vice President

Provides community service opportunities for persons age 55 and older. Provide community service opportunities for seniors to work with children one on one.

292 Pride Foundation: Alaska
3201 C
Suite 110
Anchorage, AK 99503
907-249-6628
www.pridefoundation.org

Josh Hemsath, Regional Development Organizer

Regional nonprofit advancing equality for LGBTQ people in the Northwest.

293 Social Security: Disability Determination Services
709 W 9th RM 231
Juneau, AK 99501
907-777-8100; *Toll Free:* 800-577-3334
labor.alaska.gov

Patty Trott, Executive Director

Determination committee for disability and social security benfits in Alaska.

294 State of Alaska, Department of Health & Social Services Division of Senior & Disabilities Services
3601 C Street
Suite 902
Anchorage, AK 99503
907-269-7800
dhss.alaska.gov

Valerie Nurr'araaluk Davidson, Commissioner
Shawnda O'Brien, Assistant Commissioner

The mission of the Division Of Senior and Disabilities Services is to promote independence of Alaska seniors and people with physical and developmental disabilites.

Arizona

295 Arizona Area Agency on Aging: Region One
1366 E Thomas Road
Suite 108
Phoenix, AZ 85014-5739
602-264-4357; *Toll Free: 888-783-7500*
info@aaaphx.org
www.aaaphx.org

Mary Lynn Kasunic, President & CEO
Debby Elliott, VP, Programs & Services
David Diaz, Chief Financial Officer

The Area Agency on Aging serves senior citizens and adults 18 to 59 with disabilities through a variety of home and community based programs including home delivered meals, adult day health care, home care, trasportation and legal assistance.

296 Arizona Center on Aging
1807 E Elm Street
Tucson, AZ 85719
520-626-5800
Fax: 520-626-5801
info@aging.arizona.edu
aging.arizona.edu

Mindy Fain, MD, Co-Director
Janko Nikolich-Zugich, MD, Co-Director
Jane Mohler MSN, FNP, PhD, Associate Director, RD

Long-term care, retirement communities, minority elderly, health and long-term care policy, and aging. Conducts applied research in service delivery system development and provides technical assistance and research dissemination.

297 Arizona Department of Economic Security
1789 W Jefferson Street
Phoenix, AZ 85007
602-542-1290
des.az.gov

Michael Trailor, Director

The Department of Economic Security is a human service agency providing services in six areas: Aging and Community Services, Benefits and Medical Eligibility, Child Support Enforcement, Children and Family Services, Developmental Disabilities and Employment and Rehabilitation Services.

298 Arizona Department of Family Health Services
150 N 18th Avenue
Phoenix, AZ 85007-2670

602-542-1025
Fax: 602-542-0883
www.azdhs.gov

Cara Christ, Director

The Arizona Department of Health Services promotes and protects the health of Arizona's children and adults. Its mission is to set the standard for personal and community health through direct care, science, public policy, and leadership. The department operates programs in behavioral health, disease prevention and control, health promotion, community public health, environmental health, maternal and child health, emergency preparedness and regulation of childcare and assisted living centers, nursing homes, hospitals, and emergency services.

299 Arizona Department of Revenue
P.O. Box 29070
Phoenix, AZ 85038-9070
602-255-3381
Fax: 602-716-7990; Toll Free: 800-352-4090
www.azdor.gov

David Briant, Director

The mission of the Arizona Department of Revenue is to administer tax lawas fairly and efficiently for the people of Arizona. It is their vision that they set standard for tax services

300 Arizona Department of Veterans Services
3839 N 3rd Street
Phoenix, AZ 85012
602-255-3373
www.azdvs.gov

Wanda Wright, Director
John Scott, Interim Deputy Director

Provides direct services to Veterans through the administration of 19 Veterans Benefits Offices throughout the state - helping Veterans connect with their VA benefits, Veterans' Home facilities, providing short and long-term care, and Veterans' Memorial cemeteries.

301 Arizona Division of Againg and Adult Services
1789 W Jefferson Street
Mail Drop 6288
Phoenix, AZ 85007-3202
602-542-4446
Fax: 602-542-6575; Toll Free: 800-432-4040
contactdaas@azdes.gov
www.azdes.gov

Priscilla Kadi, Assistant Director
Frank Migali, Bureau Chief
Cynthia Saverino, Aging/Disability Services Admin.

Arizona's designated State Unit on Aging. The Older Americans Act provides the Division of Aging and Adult Services with its authority. Works to advocate for and on behalf of at-risk and older persons. Also develops and impliments a comprehensive service delivery system that most accurately reflects the needs of their local communities.

302 Arizona Inter Tribal Council
2214 N Central Avenue
Suite 100
Phoenix, AZ 85004
602-258-4822
Fax: 602-258-4825

info@itcaonline.com
www.itcaonline.com

Maria Dadgar, Executive Director
Travis L Lane, Assistant Director
Verna Monenerkit, Office Manager

The pupose of the ITCA is to provide the member tribes with the means for action on matters that affect them collectively and individually, to promote tribal sovereignty and to strengthen tribal governments.

Year Founded: 1952

303 Arizona Public Safety Personnel Retirement System

3010 E Camelback Road
Suite 200
Phoenix, AZ 85016-4416
602-255-5575
Fax: 602-255-5572; Toll Free: 877-925-5575
benefitsgroup@psprs.com
www.psprs.com

Jared A Smout, Administrator
Dave DeJonge, Deputy Administrator
Ryan Parham, Chief Investment Officer

PSPRS provides retirement benefits and programs to nearly 59,000 active members, retired members and surviving beneficiaries, and to more than 250 employers groups (municipalities, agencies and districts) throughout the state.

304 Arizona Retirement System

3300 N Central Avenue
Phoenix, AZ 85012-0250
602-240-2000
www.azasrs.gov

Paul Matson, Director
Anthony Guarino, Deputy Director/COO
Karl Polen, Chief Investment Officer

A leading state benefit plan administrator in the areas of core member service funded status, investment performance, and operational effectiveness.

305 Arizona Workers Compensation Board Industrial Commission

800 W Washington Street
Phoenix, AZ 85007
602-542-4411
Fax: 602-542-7889
kara.dimas@azica.gov
www.azica.gov

James Ashley, Director
Melinda Poppe, Deputy Directory
Kara Dimas, Commission Secretary

The mission statement of the Industrial Commission is to efficiently administer and effectively enforce all applicable laws and regulations not specifically delegated to others, relative to the protection of life, health, safety, and welfare of employees within the State.

306 Northern Arizona Council of Governments Area Agency on Aging

119 E Aspen Avenue
Flagstaff, AZ 86001
928-774-1895
Fax: 928-773-1135
nacog@nacog.org
www.nacog.org

Kenneth Hall, Executive Director

The NACOG Area Agency on Aging, Region III, serves clients in the four Northern Counties of Arizona, excluding the reservations. We are part of a national network of organizations, established under the Older Americans Act of 1965 to respond to the needs of Older Adults. There are more then 650 Area Agencies on Aging throughout the United States.

307 Pima Council on Aging

8467 E Broadway Boulevard
Tucson, AZ 85710
520-790-7262
Fax: 520-790-7577
help@pcoa.org
www.pcoa.org

W Mark Clark, President & CEO
Debra Adams, SVP, Chief Operating Officer
Donna Burrows, VP, Chief Financial Officer

Mission is to promote dignity and respect for aging, and to advocate for independence in the lives of Pima County's older adults and their families, now and for generations to come.

308 Pinal/Gila Council for Senior Citizens

8969 W McCartney Road
Casa Grande, AZ 85194
520-836-2758; *Toll Free: 800-293-9393*
info@pgcsc.org
www.pgcsc.org

Olivia Guerrero, President & CEO

PGCSC responds to community needs through a comprehensive planning process. PGCSC provides services and programs directly or through contracts with local service providers to assist older adults and adults with disabilities to remain in their home for as long as possible.

Year Founded: 1974

309 RSVP East Valley Retired & Senior Volunteer Program
East Valley Adult Resources

45 West University
Mesa, AZ 85201
480-964-9014
info@evadultresources.org
www.evadultresources.org

Deborah B Schaus, Chief Executive Officer
Carol Dopudja, Director, Program Operations
Phil Contino, Finance Director

RSVP links the skills and talents of persons 55 and over with needs in the East Valley communities of Chandler, Gilbert, Guadalupe, Mesa and Tempe. Volunteers serve hospitals, schools, food banks, museums, literacy programs, police and fire departments, libraries, etc. Volunteers who register with RSVP receive supplemental accident/liability insurance while traveling to volunteer assignments and mileage and meal reimbursement.

310 RSVP Tucson

8467 E Broadway Boulevard
Tucson, AZ 85710
480-874-2500
tucson.rsvppublications.com

Scott Rubel, Director

The Retired and Senior Volunteer Program (RSVP) provides opportunities for people 55 and over to make a difference in their community through volunteer service. RSVP volunteers contribute anywhere from a few to over forty hours a week, serving through schools, day care centers, police departments, hospitals and other nonprofit and public organizations to help meet critical community needs. RSVP offers maximum flexibility and choice to its volunteers. RSVP matches the personal interests and skills of older Americans with opportunities to help solve community problems and offers supplemental insurance while on duty, on-the-job training from the agency or organization where volunteers are placed. The following County is served: Pima.

311 SEAGO Area: Agency on Aging
SouthEaster Arizona Governments Organization
1403 W Highway 92
Bisbee, AZ 85603
520-432-5301
info@seago.org
www.seago.org

Tedd Soltis, Chair
Matthew Williams, Vice Chair
Horatio Skeete, Secretary

Operates home and community based services through contract providers. Assist individuals seeking information about services for disabled and elders. Assist with Medicare and other benefit programs.

Year Founded: 1972

312 Senior Citizens of Patagonia
P.O. Box 241
Patagonia, AZ 85624
520-394-7750
www.patagoniaaz.com

The mission of the Senior Citizens of Patagonia is to provide transportation, social, educational and nutritional support for the senior citizens of the Patagonia/Sonoita area.

313 Verde Valley Senior Citizens Association
500 E Cherry Street
P.O. Box 681
Cottonwood, AZ 86326
928-634-5450
info@verdevalleyseniorcenter.org
www.verdevalleyseniorcenter.com

Lara Wilson, Executive Admin. Assistant
Geri Manzella, Volynteer Coordinator

The Verde Valley Senior Center's primary objective is to enrich the lives of senior citizens and Verde Valley communities by providing wholesome meals, safe, convenient transportation and promoting a variety of social and recretional activities for all to enjoy.

314 Western Arizona Council of Governments: Area Agency on Aging
1235 S Redondo Center Drive
Yuma, AZ 85365
928-782-1886
Fax: 928-329-4248
www.wacog.com

Provides referrals for care giver assistance, intake and application guidance for financial or food assistance, transportationa assistance, elder rights assistance and health care assistance.

Arkansas

315 Arkansas Advocates for Nursing Home Residents
32 Lexington Drive
Conway, AR 72034
501-450-9619
marthadeaver@sbcglobal.net
www.aanhr.org

Martha Deaver, President

AANHR is a nonprofit organization dedicated to protecting and improving the quality of care and life for Arkansas residents in long term care facilities.

316 Arkansas Department of Finance and Administration
Little Rock, AR
501-682-2242
Fax: 501-682-1029
rachel.jones@dfa.arkansas.gov
www.dfa.arkansas.gov

Rachel Jones, Director

317 Arkansas Department of Human Services: Division of Aging and Adult Services
PO Box 1437, Slot S-530
Little Rock, AR 72203-1437
501-682-2441; *Toll Free: 866-801-3435*
aging.services@arkansas.gov
www.daas.ar.gov

The mission of the Division Of Aging and Adult Services is to promote the health, safety, and independence of older Arkansans and adults with physical disabilities.

Year Founded: 1985

318 Arkansas Department of Public Employees Retired Systems
124 W Capitol
Suite 400
Little Rock, AR 72201
501-682-7800; *Toll Free: 800-682-7377*
www.apers.org

Gail Stone, Executive Director
Jay Wills, Deputy Director
Jason Willett, Chief Financial Officer

APERS' mission is to provide income to retired members, to survivors and to disabled members of the system.

319 Arkansas Department of Veterans Affairs
501 Woodlane Drive
Suite 230C
Little Rock, AR 72201
501-683-1787
www.veterans.arkansas.gov

Nathaniel Todd, Director

The mission of the Arkansas Department of Veterans Affairs is to provide assistance to veterans and their dependents in acquiring state and federal benefits to which they are entitled to by virtue of ther service to this country. We maintain a claims and appeals section in the VA Regional Office and operate two veterans' homes and one veterans' cemetary. We also provide support and training to the seventy-five (75) county veterans' service officers.

Year Founded: 1925

320 Arkansas Developmental Disability Council
1515 W 7th Street
Suite 320
Little Rock, AR 72201
501-682-2897
ddcstaff@dfa.arkansas.gov
gcdd.ar.gov

Eric Munson, Executive Director
Diana Wilson, Program Manager
Assiah Lewellen, Grants/Outreach Coordinator

The Arkansas Governor's Developmental Disabilities
Council supports people with developmental disabilities in
the achievement of independence, productivity, integration,
and inclusion in the community.

321 Arkansas Disability Determinations for SSA
701 Pulaski Street
Little Rock, AR 72201-3926
501-682-3049
Fax: 501-682-7553
arthur.boutiette@ssa.gov
www.arkansas.gov/ddssa

Arthur Boutiette, Executive Director

The Arkansas Disability Determination for Social Security
Administration has an agreement with the federal Social
Security Administration to determine eligibility for Social
Security disability for individuals in Arkansas.

**322 Arkansas Division of Developmental Disabilities
Services**
Donaghey Plaza
P.O. Box 1437
Little Rock, AR 72203
501-682-1001
humanservices.arkansas.gov
TDD 501-682-8820

Cindy Gillespie, Director
Marci Manley, Deputy Chief of Communication
Keesa Smith, Deputy Director

State agency to assist persons with developmental disabilities and their family in obtaining appropriate assistance and
services.

323 Arkansas Division of Services for the Blind
700 Main Street
Little Rock, AR 72203
501-682-5463
Fax: 501-682-0366
humanservices.arkansas.gov/dsb

Terry Sheeler, Chairman
William Johnson, Vice Chairman
Sandy Edwards, Secretary

Dedicated to the independence of Arkansans who are blind
or visually impaired and is committed to the principal that
these individuals have the right to make informed choices
regarding where they live, where they work, how they participate in the community, and how they interact with
others.

324 Arkansas Rehabilitation Services
525 W Capitol Avenue
Little Rock, AR 72201
501-296-1600
Fax: 501-296-1141
ACECommunications@arkansas.gov

www.arcareereducation.org
TDD 501-296-1669

Alan McClain, Commissioner
Angela Heard, Program Coordinator
Joseph Baxter, DeputyCommissioner

Offers total rehabilitative care making the patient understand the problems to which they will need to adjust, what
abilities they have and what types of assistance or equipment they will need, and what resources in the community
can help with their return to independent living. The staff is
dedicated to providing the kind of specialized treatment
necessary for those constantly changing needs.

Year Founded: 1927

325 Arkansas Teacher Retirement System
1400 W Third Street
Little Rock, AR 72201
501-682-1517
Fax: 501-682-2359; *Toll Free:* 800-666-2877
info@artrs.gov
www.artrs.gov

George Hopkins, Executive Director
Gail Bolden, Deputy Director
Curtis Carter, Chief Fiscal Officer

The Arkansas Teacher Retirement System was established
to provide retirement benefits to the employees of the
state's education community. Operation of the system began as a reserve system, whereby a financial base derived
from employer and employee contributions, and income
from investments, pay future benefits.

Year Founded: 1937

326 Central Arkansas Area: Agency on Aging
P.O. Box 5988
North Little Rock, AR 72119
501-372-5300
info@care-link.org
www.care-link.org
TDD 800-482-6359

John Davis, Chair
Luke Mattingly, President and CEO
Joy Scates, Vice President, Finance

Services include home care, hospice, information and assistance, case management, home-delivered meals, senior
centers, transportation, employment, and adult day care.

327 East Arkansas Area: Agency on Aging
2005 E Highland Drive
Jonesboro, AR 72401
Toll Free: 800-467-3278
referral@eaaaa.org
www.e4aonline.com

The mission of the East Arkansas Area Agency on Aging is
to provide leadership relative to aging issues on behalf of
older persons in East Arkansas, and to carry out a wide
range of functions in planning, coordination, and service
delivery such as that the older persons are assisted in leading independent, meaningful, and dignified lives in their
own homes and communities as long as possible.

328 Northwest Arkansas Area: Agency on Aging
1510 Rock Springs Road
PO Box 1795
Harrison, AR 72602-1795

870-741-1144
Fax: 870-741-6214; *Toll Free:* 800-432-9721
info@aaanwar.org
www.aaanwar.org
TDD 870-741-1346

A private, nonprofit organization dedicated to enhancing the lives of senior citizens and helping them to continue living at home as long as possible. The agency offers a wide array of home and community based services with a mix of federal and state funding, private contributions and private pay.

329 RSVP Greater Texarkana Arkansas
216 Walnut Street
Texarkana, AR 71854
870-779-4952
Fax: 870-774-3170
arkansas.txkusa.org

The Retired and Senior Volunteer Program (RSVP) provides opportunities for people 55 and over to make a difference in their community through volunteer service. RSVP volunteers contribute anywhere from a few to over forty hours a week, serving through schools, day care centers, police departments, hospitals and other nonprofit and public organizations to help meet critical community needs. RSVP offers maximum flexibility and choice to its volunteers. RSVP matches the personal interests and skills of older Americans with opportunities to help solve community problems and offers supplemental insurance while on duty, on-the-job training from the agency or organization where volunteers are placed. The following Counties are served: Hempstead, Howard, Little River, Lafayette, Miller, Nevada, Sevier.

330 RSVP of Central Arkansas
16117 Hwy 365S
Wrightsville, AR 72183
501-897-0793
ddgrace11@live.com; www.rsvpcenark.org

Denise Grace, Project Director
Lisa Strain, Volunteer Coordinator
Ed Merck, Webmaster

The Retired and Senior Volunteer Program (RSVP) provides opportunities for people 55 and over to make a difference in their community through volunteer service. RSVP volunteers contribute anywhere from a few to over forty hours a week, serving thourgh schools, day care centers, police departments, hospitals and other nonprofit and public organizations to help meet critical community needs. RSVP offers maximum flexibility and choice to its volunteers. RSVP matches the personal interests and skills to older Americans with opportunities to help solve community problems and offer supplemental insurance while on duty, on-the-job training from the agency or organization where volunteers are placed.

Year Founded: 1972

331 Railroad Retirement Board: Arkansas District Office
1200 Cherry Brook Drive
Suite 500
Little Rock, AR 72211-4113
Fax: 501-225-6782; *Toll Free:* 877-772-5772
littlerock@rrb.gov
www.rrb.gov

Retirement benefit assistance.

332 Senior Specialists Agency on Aging
905 W Grand Avenue
Hot Springs, AR 71913-3438
501-321-2811; *Toll Free:* 800-467-2170
info@seniorspecialists.org
www.seniorspecialists.org

Barbara Flowers, Executive Director
Missy Masterson, Director, In-Home Services
James White, Director, Finance

Serves seniors in the counties of Clark, Conway, Garland, Hot Spring, Johnson, Montgomery, Perry Pike, and Yell in West Central Arkansas. They provide information and assistance, in-home personal care, hospice care, a Senior Companion Volunteer Program, and are the primary funding source for 15 senior adult centers. Their goal is to assist seniors to lead independent, meaningful and dignified lives.

Year Founded: 1974

333 Southeast Arkansas Area: Agency on Aging
709 East Eighth Avenue
Pine Bluff, AR 71601
870-543-6300
Fax: 870-534-2152; *Toll Free:* 800-264-3260
www.aaasea.org
TTY: 870-543-6339

Tony Barr, EEO Director
James Word, ADA and Section 504 Coordinator

Quality home and community services throughout Southeast Arkansas. Services include skilled and personal home care, transportation, senior center services, home delivered meals, case management and housing.

334 Southwest Arkansas Area: Agency on Aging
600 Columbia 11 E
P.O. Box 1863
Magnolia, AR 71753
870-234-7410
Fax: 870-234-6804; *Toll Free:* 800-272-2127
www.agewithdignity.com

A nonprofit organization serving adults age 60 or older, family caregivers, agencies and organizations working with seniors. It is part of a national netowork of more then 650 area agencies on aging throughout the United States.

335 Western Arkansas Area: Agency on Aging
524 Garrison Avenue
PO Box 1724
Fort Smith, AR 72902-1724
479-783-4500; *Toll Free:* 800-320-6667
www.agingwest.org
TDD 866-235-7995

A non-profit, home-based and dedicated to helping you and your loved one realize a better quality of life through individually tailored care. To assist older individuals in maintaining desired lifestyles through accessible and affordable alternatives.

Year Founded: 1974

336 White River Area: Agency on Aging
3998 Harrison Street
Po Box 2637
Batesville, AR 72503
870-612-3000; *Toll Free:* 800-382-3205
www.wraaa.com

A non-profit organization that provides services to older persons to help them remain independent and in their own homes.

California

337 Alameda County Area: Agency on Aging
Department of Adult and Aging Services
6955 Foothill Boulevard, Suite 100
Oakland, CA 94605
510-383-5300
www.alamedasocialservices.org

Lori Jones, Director

The Alameda County Social Services Department of Adult and Aging Servicese strives to be consumer focused and accessible to the community. The Department offers a coordinated service delivery system that protects, supports, and advocates for an aging population, particularly those with disabilities.

338 All People Community Center
822 East 20th Street
Los Angeles, CA 90011-1104
213-747-6357
Fax: 213-747-0541
allpeoples@allpeoplescc.org
www.allpeoplescc.org

Seth Walworth, Chair
Saundra Bryant, Executive Director
Amanda Trefethen, Vice Chair

To provide social services and programs that empower individuals and promote community respect and self determination for all. The services and activities are designed with the propose of helping children succeed, strenghtening relationships, preventing violence and crime in the community, addressing the root causes of gang involvement, providing job training and creating job opportunities, and helping seniors stay active and engaged.

339 Area 1 Agency on Aging
434 Seventh Street
Eureka, CA 95501
707-442-3763
Fax: 707-442-3714
www.a1aa.org

George Ingraham, Chair
Maggie Rose, Executive Director
Diane Lehman, Secretary

Area 1 Agency on Aging (A1AA) advocates, plans, coordinates, develops, and delivers a range of senior, information, volunteer and caregiver services in Humboldt and Del Norte Counties. Our mission is to provide leadership and guidance in supporting an older person's ability to lead a dignified, safe, healthy and independent life and to provide leadership and resources that support volunteers as they make positive changes in our community.

340 Area 12 Agency on Aging
19074 Standard Road
Sonora, CA 95370
209-532-6272; *Toll Free:* 800-510-2020
info@area12.org
www.area12.org

Kristin Millhoff, Executive Director
Tracey Sawyer, Assistant Director
James Maltese, Fiscal Officer

The responsibility of the area 12 Agency on Aging is to serve all of the five counties 60 plus population, including those with different social and cultural needs; support self-determination and independence among the older population; and provide leadership in the development of a community-based system of care. This mission is accomplished through a network of education, advocacy, problem solving, program planning and funding.

Year Founded: 1987

341 Area 4 Agency on Aging
1401 El Camino Avenue
4th Floor
Sacramento, CA 95825
916-486-1876
Fax: 916-486-9454; *Toll Free:* 800-211-4545
contactus@agencyonaging4.org
agencyonaging4.org

Pam Miller, Executive Director
Will H Tift, Assistant Director

Our mission is to provide leadership on issues which affect the quality of life for older persons and to promote citizenship involvement in planning and delivering programs and services necessary to ensure maximum independence and dignity for older individuals and functionally impaired adults.

342 Arthritis Foundation: Northern California Chapter
90 New Montgomery Street
Suite 710
San Francisco, CA 94105
415-356-1230
Fax: 415-356-1240
www.arthritis.org

Dave Hill, Chair
Laurie Stewart, Vice Chair
Bruce Ashcroft, Secretary

Provides a wide range of services to persons with arthritis and their families. Offers physician referral and assistance in locating medical aids and self-help devices for arthritis. Classes by Arthritis Foundation certified instructors in self-help, exercise and aquatics.

343 California Agency of Health & Welfare: Department of Rehabilitation
1600 Ninth Street
Room 460
Sacramento, CA 95814
916-654-3454
www.chhs.ca.gov

Jim Suennen, Director

The California Department of Rehabilitation works in partnership with consumers and other stakeholders to provide services and advocacy resulting in employment, independent living and equality for individuals with disabilities.

344 California Agency of Health and Welfare: Department of Aging
1300 National Drive
Suite 200
Sacramento, CA 95834-1992

916-419-7500
Fax: 916-928-2267
webmaster@aging.ca.gov
www.aging.ca.gov
TDD 800-735-2929

Lora Connolly, Director

The California Department of Aging (CDA) administers programs that serve older adults, adults with disabilities, family caregivers, and residents in long-term care facilities throughout the state.

345 California Association of Area Agencies on Aging
980 Ninth Street
Sacramento, CA 95814
916-443-2800
Fax: 916-554-0111
aging@c4a.info
www.c4a.info

Derrell Kelch, Executive Director
Diane Kaljian, President
Pam Miller, Vice President

Lead in developing a statewide, comprehensive, and integrated home and community-based service system that supports dignity, diversity, and choice for older persons and persons with disabilities, their caregivers, and families.

346 California Commission on Aging
1300 National Drive
Suite 173
Sacramento, CA 95834
916-419-7591
Fax: 916-419-7596
ccoa@ccoa.ca.gov
www.ccoa.ca.gov

Sandra K Fitzpatrick, Executive Director

Principal Advocacy Organization for California seniors and advisor to the governor, state legislature and state departments on senior issues.

Year Founded: 1973

347 California Department of Aging
1300 National Drive
Suite 200
Sacramento, CA 95834-1992
916-419-7500
Fax: 916-928-2267
webmaster@aging.ca.gov
www.aging.ca.gov
TDD 800-735-2929

Lora Connolly, Director

The California Department of Aging (CDA) administers programs that serve older adults, adults with disabilities, family caregivers, and residents in long-term care facilities throughout the State. The Department administers funds allocated under the federal Older Americans Act, the Older, Californians Act, and throughout the Medi-Cal program.

348 California Department of Aging and Adult Services
385 N Arrowhead Avenue
San Bernardino, CA 92415
909-891-3900; *Toll Free: 888-818-8918*
www.sbcounty.gov

Robert A Lovingood, Chair
Curt Hagman, Vice Chair

The Department of Aging and Adult Services offer a wide variety of programs designed to help the senior, disabled, and at-risk adults in our county.

349 California Department of Rehabilitation
721 Capitol Mall
Sacramento, CA 95814-3510
916-324-1313; *Toll Free: 800-952-5544*
externalaffairs@dor.ca.gov
www.rehab.cahwnet.gov
TDD 844-729-2800

Joe Xavier, Director

Assists people with disabilities, particularly those with severe disabilities, in obtaining and retaining meaningful employment and living independently in their communities. The Department develops, purchases, provides and advocates for programs and services in vocational rehabilitation, habilitation and independent living with a priority on serving persons with all disabilities, especially those with the most severe disabilities.

350 California Department of Veterans Affairs
1227 O Street
Sacramento, CA 95814
Toll Free: 800-952-5626

The mission of the California Department of Veterans Affairs is to promote and administer the benefits, programs, and services provided by the grateful state of California to its deserving veterans, their dependents and survivors.

351 California Developmental Disability Council
1507 21st Street
Suite 210
Sacramento, CA 95811
916-322-8481
Fax: 916-443-4957; *Toll Free: 866-802-0514*
council@scdd.ca.gov
www.scdd.ca.gov
TTY: 916-324-8420

Aaron Carruthers, Executive Director
Cindy Smith, Chief Deputy Director
Vicki Smith, Deputy Director

The State Council on Developmental Disabilities (SCDD) is established by state and federal law as an independent state agency to ensure that people with developmental disabilities and their families receive the services and support they need.

Number of Members: 31

352 California Franchise Tax Board
3321 Power Inn Road
Suite 250
Sacramento, CA 95826-3893
916-845-6500; *Toll Free: 800-383-0505*
www.ftb.ca.gov
TTY: 800-822-6268

Betty T Yee, State Controller And Chair
George Runner, Chairman
Michael Cohen, Director of Finance

The purpose of the Franchise Tax Board is to collect the proper amount of tax revenue, and operate other programs entrusted to us, at the least cost; serve the public by continually improving the quality of our products and services;

and perform in a manner warranting the highest degree of public confidence in our integrity, efficiency and fairness.

353 California Governor's Committee on Employment of People with Disabilities
721 Capitol Mall
Sacramento, CA 95814
916-558-5698; *Toll Free: 855-894-3436*
CCEPD@dor.ca.gov
www.dor.ca.gov/boards-and-comittees

Maria Aliferis-Gjerde, Executive Officer

To consult with and advise the Secretary of the Labor and Workforce Development Agency and the Secretary of the California Health and Human Services Agency on all issues related to full inclusion in the workforce of persons with disabilities.

354 California Latino Council of the Deaf and Hard of Hearing
P.O. Box 65591
Los Angeles, CA 90065
562-634-4112
Fax: 562-630-5391
CLCDHH@aol.com
www.deafvision.net/aztlan/resources
TTY: 562-634-4112

Mark D Apodaca, President

CLCDHH's mission is to promote leadership, advocacy, education, and to address the needs of the Deaf and Hard of Hearing Latino Community.

355 California Public Employees' Retirement System
Lincoln Plaza Complex
400 Q Street
Sacramento, CA 95811
Toll Free: 888-225-7377
www.calpers.ca.gov

Priya Mathur, President
Rob Feckner, Vice President
Marcie Frost, Chief Executive Officer

Provides retirement and health benefits programs and services, and administers other programs dedicated to protecting the financial security of our members.

356 California Seniors Council
234 Santa Cruz Avenue
Aptos, CA 95003
831-688-0400
clayk@seniorscouncil.org
www.seniorscouncil.org

Clay Kempf, Executive Director
Bob Campbell, Program Director
Patty Talbott, Associate Director

It is the mission of the Seniors Council to enable older persons to function with independence and dignity in their homes and in the community to their fullest capacity.

357 California State Board of Equalization
3321 Power Inn Road
Suite 210
Sacramento, CA 95826-3889
916-227-6600
Fax: 916-227-1883
www.boe.ca.gov

Betty T Yee, California State Controller
David J Gau, Executive Director
George Runner, Board Member, 1st District

The mission of the State Board of Equalization is to serve the public through fair, effective, and efficient tax administration.

358 California State Teachers Retirement System
100 Waterfront Place
West Sacramento, CA 95605
916-414-1099
Fax: 916-414-5040; Toll Free: 800-228-5453
www.calstrs.com

Jack Ehnes, Chief Executive Officer
Cassandra Lichnock, Chief Operating Officer
Robin Madsen, Chief Financial Officer

Mission is to seure the financial future and sustain the trust of California's educators.

359 California Workers Compensation Board
455 Golden Gate Avenue, 2nd Floor
San Francisco, CA 94102-7014
415-703-5020; *Toll Free: 800-736-7401*
SFO@dir.ca.gov
www.dir.ca.gov/dwc

Division of Workers' Compensation mission is to minimize the adverse impact of work related injuries on California employees and employers.

360 Central Coast Commission for Senior Citizens
528 S Broadway
Santa Maria, CA 93454-5109
805-925-9554; *Toll Free: 800-510-2020*
www.centralcoastseniors.org

The Central Coast Commission for Senior Citizens-Area Agency on Aging (AAA) is a non-profit organization responsible for allocating federal and state dollars to local agencies to insure their supportive, nutrition and health promotion services to older adults in San Luis Obispo and Santa Barbara Counties are availiable.

Year Founded: 1975

361 Central County United Way
418 E Florida Avenue
Hemet, CA 92543
951-929-9691
Fax: 951-652-0064
donor@ccuw.org
www.ccuw.org

Becky Polk, RSVP Director
Bob Duistermars, President & CEO
Connie Hall, Vice President of Operations

RSVP offers meaningful volunteer opportunities for the active senior 55 and better. There are many volunteer opportunities to serve your interest right in the community in which you live.

362 City of Los Angeles Department of Aging
221 N Figueroa Street
Suite 500
Los Angeles, CA 90012
213-482-7252
Fax: 213-482-7256; Toll Free: 800-510-2020
age.webinfo@lacity.org
www.aging.lacity.org

Laura Trejo, General Manager
James Don, Assistant General Manager
Marco Perez, Deputy Director

Mission is to improve the quality of life, independence, health and dignity of the City's older population by managing community based senior programs that are comprehensive, coordinated and accessible, and to advocacte for the needs of older citizens.

363 Costa Mesa Senior Center

695 West 19th Street
Costa Mesa, CA 92627
714-327-7550
cmseniorcenter@costamesaca.gov
costamesaca.gov

Yvette Aguilar, Sr Recreation Program Admin.
Justin Martin, Dir., Parks & Community Services
Charu Mody, Social Services

The Costa Mesa Senior Center is dedicated to improving the lives of older adults by creating a place that offers opportunity to become more educated about health and wellness, share skills and talents with peers, interact and develop communication with friends, family, and others, and be advocates for older adults.

364 Diablo Valley Foundation for the Aging

140 Gregory Lane
Suite 170
Pleasant Hill, CA 94523
925-945-8040
Fax: 925-945-8025
contactus@dv-fa.org
dv-fa.org

Joe Bettencourt, Chairman
Jeff Patton, Acting Executive Director
Laverne Gordon, Secretary

Our mission is to provide that support as your professional relative, enabling you to live with optimal independence and freedom. Whatever they might be, DVFA has the solutions to keep you or the one you love living in comfort.

Year Founded: 1975

365 Elder Care Alliance

1301 Marina Village Parkway
Suite 210
Alameda, CA 94501
510-769-2700
Fax: 510-769-2735
learnmore@eldercarealliance.org
www.eldercarealliance.org

Celia Zavala, Acting Executive Officer

A nonprofit, faith-centered organization dedicated to providing care services to meet the needs of older adults. We are committed to serving and enriching the physical, emotional, and spiritual well-being of older adults through a network of professional, faith-centered care communities and services.

366 Fresno Madera Area: Agency on Aging

3837 N Clark Street
Fresno, CA 93726
559-600-4405
Fax: 559-243-5651; *Toll Free:* 800-510-2020
www.fmaaa.org

Jean Robinson, Exective Director
Paul Bustamante, Director of Finance
Sandi Martin, Programs/Operations Manager

Provides leadership in addressing issues that relate to older Californians; to develop community based systems of care that provide services which support independence within California's interdependent society, and which protect that quality of life of older persons and persons with functional impairments; and to promote citizen involvement in the planning and delivery of service.

Year Founded: 1980

367 HomeAid Orange County

24 Executive Park
Suite 100
Irvine, CA 92614
949-553-9510
www.homeaidoc.org

Scott Larson, Executive Director
Evan Miles, Project Manager
Julia Ung, Administrative Manager

HomeAid Orange County is a nonprofit organization that builds and renovates shelters for those in Orange County who find themselves homeless due to sudden job loss, catastrophic illness, spousal desertion, and domestoc violence.

368 Imperial County: Area Agency on Aging

778 W Street
El Centro, CA 92243
442-265-7000
www.aaa24.org

Our mission is to provide leadership at the local level in developing systems of home and community based services that maintain 'least restrictive' home like environments. In particular, emphasis shall be placed on coordinating with local systems to enable individuals to live with maximum independence and dignity in their homes and communities through the development of comprehensive and coordinated systems of home and community care.

369 Kern County Aging and Adult Services

5357 Truxtun Avenue
Bakersfield, CA 93309
661-868-1000
Fax: 661-868-1001; *Toll Free:* 800-510-2020
aginginfo@kerncounty.com
www.kerncounty.com/aas

Lito Morillo, Director
Kathy Lemon, Manager

Committed to providing community-based services to ensure seniors and disabled adults remain safely in their homes. We strive to preserve the dignity of older adults and persons with disabilities.

370 Kings Tulare Area: Agency on Aging

Visalia, CA
Toll Free: 800-321-2462
ktaaa@tularehhsa.org
www.ktaaa.org

Craig Pedersen, Chair
Amy Shuklian, Vice Chair

The Area Agency on Aging coordinates senior programs for Kings and Tulare County residents 60 years of age and older.

Year Founded: 1965

371 La Quinta Senior Center
78-495 Calle Tampico
La Quinta, CA 92253
760-777-7000
www.laquintaca.gov

The Wellness Center is a community focal point offering a wide range of services to everyone in the community. The Center offers a variety of classes, seminars, special events and weekly programs for adults 55 years of age or older. Seminars and special events are open to all adults.

372 Los Angeles County: Area Agency on Aging
3175 West 6th Street
Los Angeles, CA 90020
Toll Free: 800-510-2020
wdacs.lacounty.gov

Cynthia D Banks, Director
Otto Solorzano, Deputy Director
Joyce Washington, Administrative Services Branch

The Area Agency on Aging plans, develops and delivers services for seniors (60 years and older) and for adults (18-59 years) with disabilities and long-term care needs.

373 Marin Senior Coordinating Council (Whistlestop)
930 Tamalpais Avenue
San Rafael, CA 94901-3325
415-456-9062
Fax: 415-456-1008
whistlestop.org

Dennis D Ryan, Board President
Joe O'Hehir, Chief Executive Officer
Etta Allen, Board Vice President

Founded as Marin Senior Coordinating Council, Whistlestop promotes the independence, well-being and quality of life for older adults and people living with disabilities in Marin County. Whistlestop's Active Aging Center provides delicious meals, educational classes, multicultural gatherings and helpful information and referral services. Whistlestop also provides special needs transportation services through Marin Access, a partnership of Whistlestop, Marin Transit and Golden Gate Transit.

Year Founded: 1954

374 Merced County: Area Agency for Aging
2222 M Street
Merced, CA 95340
209-385-7434; *Toll Free: 800-510-2020*
www.co.merced.ca.us/aaa

James L Brown, County Executive Officer
James N Fincher, County Counsel

Mission is to work in partnership with the community to provide for the protection, care and support of families and individuals, and to promote personal responsibility and self-sufficiency.

375 Monterey County Department of SocialServices, Aging and Adult Services
1000 S. Main Street
Salinas, CA 93901
831-755-4466
Fax: 831-784-5695; Toll Free: 800-510-2020
mcdss.co.monterey.ca.us

Elliot Robinson, Director
Henry Espinosa, Deputy Director
Diana Jimenez, Deputy Director, Aging/CalWORKS

The Aging and Adult Services branch provides health and social work services to the elderly and people with disabilities; promoting the health and safety of individuals in need of support and assistance due to illness, disability or frailty.

376 North Coast Opportunities: Area Agency on Aging
413 North State Street
Ukiah, CA 95482
707-467-3200; *Toll Free: 800-606-5550*
info@ncoinc.org
www.ncoinc.org

Ross Walker, Chair
John Goldsmith, Vice Chair
Desiree Perez, Treasure/Secretary

North Coast Opportunities (NCO) pledges to be a leader in developing and providing human services that strengthen our community.

377 Orange County Area: Agency on Aging
1300 S Grand Avenue
Building B
Santa Ana, CA 92705-4434
714-567-5021; *Toll Free: 800-510-2020*
areaagencyonaging@occr.ocgov.com
www.officeonaging.ocgov.com

Orange Countie's Office on Aging serves as the lead advocate for 400,000 older adults residing in the county, with a specific focus on low-income ethnic minorities. As an advocate, the Office on Aging is responsible for understanding the needs of Orange County's older adults and utilizing the federal funding and programs availiable to meet those requirements. In addition, the office on Aging is charged with directing or participating in coalitions to drive new ideas, services, and legislation in support of Older Adults.

378 RSVP Oxnard County
350 N C Street
Oxnard, CA 93030
805-385-8019
Fax: 805-385-7494
rsvp@oxnard.org
www.oxnard.org

The City of Oxnard Senior Services sponsors the Oxnard Retired and Senior Volunteer Program (RSVP). Through RSVP, men and women 55 and older are putting their life experience to work for their communities.

379 RSVP Sacramento County
3727 Marconi Avenue
Sacramento, CA 95821
916-875-3631
SVS-RSVP@saccounty.net
www.dhhs.saccounty.net

Volunteer assignments for persons 55 years of age and older with nonprofit and public agencies within the community. Staff assists volunteers in finding an assignment consistent with their interests and skills. RSVP volunteers are covered (during volunteer activities) under a supplemental accident and liability insurance. They may also receive limited mileage reimbursement if needed. Any public agency or private nonprofit organization may request volunteers through RSVP. The following Counties are served: Placer, Sacramento, Yolo.

380 Rancho Bernardo Joslyn Senior Center
18402 W Bernardo Drive
San Diego, CA 92127-3018
858-487-9324
edbrowncenter@gmail.com
www.edbrowncenter.org

Lynn Wolsey, President
Marla Cruz, Vice President
Laura Barish, Treasurer

A member-supported, non-profit organization dedicated to enhancing the well-being and quality of life of men and women 50 years of age and older. It has been serving the RB area for 12 years. The Center offers a wide range of activities and services.

Year Founded: 1989

381 San Francisco Commission on the Aging
P.O. Box 7988
San Francisco, CA 94120-7988
415-355-3555; *Toll Free: 800-510-2020*
DAAS@sfgov.org
www.sfhsa.org
TTY: 415-355-6756

Shireen McSpadden, Executive Director
Jill Nielsen, Deputy Director of Programs

The Department of Aging and Adult Services (DAAS) is the Area Agency on Aging for the City and County of San Francisco. In this capacity, DAAS is specifically charged with planning, coordinating, providing and advocactingfor community-based services for older adults and adults with disabilities.

382 Santa Cruz Volunteer Center
1740 17th Avenue
Santa Cruz, CA 95062
831-427-5070
volunteer@scvolunteercenter.org
scvolunteercenter.org

Karen Delaney, Executive Director
Lois Connell, Associate Director
Jan Brady, Office Manager

The mission is accomplished by operating two types of programs: those designed to recruit and orient volunteers for placement in other nonprofit agencies; and those providing direct services to address specific needs by the Board, using volunteer services.

383 Seacrest Village Retirement Communities
211 Saxony Road
Encinitas, CA 92024
760-632-0081
Fax: 760-942-0894
pferris@seacrestvillage.org
www.seacrestvillage.org

Pam Ferris, President/CEO
Robin Israel, Chief Foundation Officer
Brad Blose, Chief Financial Officer

A nonprofit senior housing and healthcare organization with communities in both Encinitas and Rancho Bernardo, California.

Year Founded: 1944

384 Senior Gleaners
1951 Bell Avenue
Sacramento, CA 95838-3039
916-925-3240
gmcdonald@seniorgleaners.org

Our mission is to alleviate hunger among the poor and elderly and to glean surplus foods, at low or no cost, from every available source, for distribution among the needy members and other charitable organizations in a fair and equitable manner.

Year Founded: 1976

385 Solano Napa: Agency on Aging
400 Contra Costa Street
Vallejo, CA 94590-5721
707-644-6612
Fax: 707-644-7905
www.aaans.org

Carolyn Wrage, Chair
Bruce Wagstaff, Interim Executive Director
Heather Stanton, Treasurer

Our Area Agency on Aging (AAA) serves Napa and Solano counties. It is one of 33 similar programs in California. Our role is to plan, coordinate and advocate for the development of local programs to meet the needs of older persons.

386 Sonoma County Task Force for the Homeless
3315 Airway Drive
Santa Rosa, CA 95403
707-575-4484
sonomacohomeless@gmail.com
www.sonomacountyhomeless.org

The Sonoma County Task Force for the Homeless is a catalyst and leadership resource bringing the community together to: promote affordable housing; prevent homelessness; assist people who are homeless.

387 Sunset Hall
504 N Berendo
Suite 500
Los Angeles, CA 90004
323-660-5277
Fax: 323-660-5207
sunsethall@sunsethall.org
www.sunsethall.org

Wendy Caputo, Executive Director

A non-profit program for free thinking elders who continue to share independence fo spirit and involvement in the world. Our mission is to create a sense of community and a caring supportive environment.

Year Founded: 1923

388 Ventura County Area: Agency on Aging
646 County Square Drive
Suite 100
Ventura, CA 93003
805-477-7300
lois.vcaaa@ventura.org
vcaaa.org

Victoria Jump, Executive Director

The responsibility of the Ventura County Area Agency on Aging is to Ventura County's sixty-plus population including those with different social and cultural needs; to foster and support self-determination and independence among the older population; and to provide leadership in the development of community-based system of care. The mission is accomplished through a network of education, advocacy, problem solving, program planning, and funding.

Year Founded: 1873

389 Volunteer Center Orange County
1901 E 4th Street
Suite 100
Santa Ana, CA 92705-3918
714-953-5757
www.oneoc.org

Peter Duncan, Board Chair
Daniel McQuaid, President/CEO
Tim Strauch, Chief Operating Officer

The Volunteer Centers of California and its network of Volunteer Centers participate in Citizens Corps and Homeland Security in collaboration with emergency first responders and statewide disaster organizations. Volunteer Centers specialize in practicing spontaneous volunteers in recovery and clean-up volunteer positions during a disaster.

Year Founded: 1958

390 Volunteer Center of Kern County
1311 Eye Street
Bakersfield, CA 93301
661-395-9787
Fax: 661-395-9780
www.volunteercenter.info

Barbara Goodlow, President
Debra Banks, Vice President
Brenda Ratliff, Executive Director

To promote volunteerism as a means of fostering increased citizen involvement in the community and enabling public and private nonprofit agencies to enhance or maintain needed human services.

Colorado

391 Agency on Aging: Region 10
300 N Cascade Avenue
Suite 1
Montrose, CO 81401
970-249-2436
Fax: 970-249-2488
admin@region10.net
www.region10.net

Michelle Haynes, Executive Director
Eva Veitch, Dir., Community Living Services
Amy Rowan, Dir., AAA Options Counselor

Region 10 is a six county collective effort to get community and small business resources for Delta, Gunnison, Hinsdale, Montrose, Ouray, and San Miguel county. The nonprofit organization focuses on elderly care, small business development, and providing county news.

392 Alpine: Area Agency on Aging
NW Colorado Council of Governments
249 Warren Avenue
P.O. Box 2308
Silverthorne, CO 80498-2308
970-468-0295
Fax: 970-468-1208
aaa12@nwccog.org
www.nwccog.org

Jon Stavney, Executive Director
Erin Fisher, Director
Nate Walowitz, Broadband Director

NWCCOG's Alpine Area Agency on Aging (AAAA) is the designated regional planning and service agency for services to seniors in Region 12. Federal Older Americans Act funds are used in conjunction with state, county, and local funds to develop and implement a comprehensive and coordinated system of service to the elderly in the region.

393 Boulder County Area Agency on Aging
3482 Broadway Street
Boulder, CO 80304
303-441-3570
bcaaa@bouldercounty.org
www.bouldercountyaging.org

Sherry Leach, Manager

Boulder County Area Agency on Aging (BCAAA) Region 3B, is part of the aging network established by the Older Americans Act to serve as advocates for older persons and to be focal points for accessing services. BCAAA also serves as the State Health Insurance Program (SHIP) for the Region. BCAAA provides leadership in assessing the strengths and needs of older adults; facilitates strategic planning and implementation; funds and provides services tobenefit older adults and their family caregivers, and convenes community conversations. Services include ARCH Aging & Disability Resource Center, Aging Resource Consultation, Long Term Care Ombudsman, Medicare Counseling, LGBT programs including Project Visibility, respite and caregiver services, financial assistance, and evidence-based wellness and nutrition education.

394 Colorado Aging and Adult Services
Colorado Department of Human Services
1575 Sherman Street
8th Floor
Denver, CO 80203-1714
303-866-5700
Fax: 303-866-5563
cdhs_communications@state.co.us
www.colorado.gov

David Ervin, Chair

The Division of Aging and Adult Services (AAS) will efficiently and effectively provide human services in support of independent living, self sufficiency, safety and dignity goals. These goals are on behalf of adults age 18 and over who have disabilities or functional impairments or are otherwise at risk. As a Division, we act upon Colorado Department of Human Service's vision to be the nation's leader in helping individuals, families and communities to be safe and independent.

395 Colorado Association of Homes & Services for the Aging
303 East 17th Avenue
Suite 880
Denver, CO 80203
303-837-8834
Fax: 303-837-8836
info@leadingagecolorado.org
www.leadingagecolorado.org

Laura Landwirth, President & CEO
Sarah McVeigh, Member Development
David Smart, Baord Chair

The Colorado Association of Homes and Services for the Aging (CAHSA) is the state's largest and oldest nonprofit organization representing providers of housing and health-related service options to Colorado's elderly. CAHSA advocates public policy initiatives that support individual rights, quality care, equitable access and reimbursement for seniors. CAHSA is the state affiliate for two national organizations, the Assisted Living Federation of America (ALFA) and the American Association of Homes and Services for the Aging (AAHSA).

Year Founded: 1975; Number of Members: 250

396 Colorado Department of Revenue

1375 Sherman Street
Denver, CO 80261
303-205-8411
www.colorado.gov

Michael Hartman, Executive Director
Heidi Humphreys, Deputy Director

397 Colorado Department of Social Services: Division of Vocational Rehabilitation

1575 Sherman Street
8th Floor
Denver, CO 80203-1714
303-866-5700
Fax: 303-866-5563
cdhs_communications@state.co.us
www.colorado.gov/cdhs

The Colorado DVR is committed in helping employer partners find candidates who are skilled, loyal, and committed to your success. Even after placement, employers and employees get ongoing support from DVR's professional staff, including job training, guidance on ADA regulations, and information on disability and employment guidelines.

398 Colorado Developmental Disability Council

1120 Lincoln Avenue
Suite 706
Denver, CO 80203
720-941-0176
cdhs_cddpc_email@state.co.us
www.coddc.org

Marcia Tewell, Executive Director
Mackenzie Helton, Fiscal Manager
Sue Fager, Planner

The mission of the CDDC is to advocate in collaboration with and on behalf of peple with developmental disabilities for the establishment and implimention of public policy which will further their independence, productivity and integration.

399 Colorado Disability Determination Services

1575 Sherman Street
8th Floor
Denver, CO 80203-1714
303-366-5700
Fax: 303-866-5563
cdhs_communications@state.co.us
www.colorado.gov/cdhs

Disability Determination Services (DSS) is the State Agency that makes the disability decisions for Social Security.

Year Founded: 1954

400 Colorado Public Employees Retirement Association

1301 Pennsylvania Street
Denver, CO 80203
Toll Free: 800-759-7372
www.copera.org

Timothy M O'Brien, Chairman
Marcus Pennell, Vice Chair
Will Bain, Board Member

Mission is to promote long-term financial security for our members while maintaining the stability of the fund.

401 Colorado Workers Compensation Board

633 17th Street
Suite 400
Denver, CO 80202
303-318-8000
Fax: 303-318-8710; *Toll Free:* 888-390-7936
www.colorado.gov

The Colorado Division of Worker's Compensation is the state office responsible for administering and enforcing the worker's compensation law in this state. In doing so, it recognizes the intent of the Colorado General Assembly to ensure the quick and efficient delivery of disability and medical benefits to injured workers, at a resonable cost to employers.

402 Denver Regional Council of Governments: Area Agency on Aging

1290 Broadway
Suite 100
Denver, CO 80203-5606
303-455-1000
Fax: 303-480-6790
drcog@drcog.org
www.drcog.org

Douglas Rex, Executive Director
Steve Erickson, Dir., Communications/Marketing
Roxie Ronsen, Administrative Officer

The Denver Regional Council of Governments (DRCOG) is proud of its focus on quality-of-life issues. These include mobility, service to older adults, environmental concerns, planning for the future, public safety, and the provision of information for sound decision-making.

403 East Central Colorado: Area Agency on Aging

128 Colorado Avenue
P.O. Box 28
Stratton, CO 80836-1152
719-348-5562
Fax: 719-348-5887; *Toll Free:* 800-825-0208
aging@prairiedevelopment.com
ecaaa.tripod.com

Terry Baylie, Dir., Senior & Transit Services
Angela Brinkhoff, Senior Services Data Coordinator
Debby Conrads, Nutrition Program Manager

The East Central Area on Aging, is among 16 designated Area Agencies on Aging within the state of Colorado. Through federal Older Americans Act grant funds, allocated to the Region via the East Central Council of Local Governments (ECCOG) the area agencies utilizes these funds in conjunction with state, county, and local funds to plan for, monitor and fund an array of home and community based services and programs.

404 Eastern Colorado Services for the Disabled
617 South 10th Avenue
Sterling, CO 80751
970-522-7121
Fax: 970-522-1173
rhonda@ecsdd.org
www.ecsdd.org

Rhonda Roth, Executive Director
Traci Schrade, Finance Director
Melissa Dassaro, Case Management Director

Eastern Colorado Services for the Developmentally Disabled Inc. is a community centered board serving developmentally disabled persons in 10 rural counties, covering 17,514 square miles. Programs include infant/toddler services, adult community integrated employment, community participation vocational training, sheltered employment, personal and social skills training, residential services supporting life services, and family resource services.

405 Elderhaus
6813 S College Avenue
Fort Collins, CO 80525
970-221-0406
joanne@elderhaus.org
elderhaus.org

Gordon Thayer, President
Joanne Vande Walle, Executive Director
Reesa Hanck, Assistant Director

Providing quality affordable day programs and services to adults with special needs in a safe, pleasant environment through qualified staff and to provide relief and support to caregivers.

406 High Country RSVP
Colorado Mountain College
1402 Blake Avenue
Glenwood Springs, CO 81601-3934
970-947-8460
Fax: 970-947-8488
gw-rsvp@coloradomtn.edu
www.highcountryrsvp.org

Patty Daniells, Program Director
Elisabeth K Worrell, Volunteer Manager

The Mission of RSVP is to enrich the lives of men and women age 55 and older through meaningful opportunities that use their skills, abilities, and life experiences in service to their communities.

Year Founded: 1978

407 Huerfano Las Animas: Area Agency on Aging
300 S Bonaventure Avenue
Trinidad, CO 81082
719-845-1133; *Fax:* 719-845-1130
www.colorado.gov

Walt Boulden, Executive Director
Kelly M Smith, Finance Director
Dawn Williamson, Administrative Assistant

The purpose of the South Central Council of Governments (SCCOG) is to benefit the citizens of Huerfano and Las Animas Counties by serving as the local government vehicle to identify needs, develop responses, implement solutions, eliminate duplication, and promote the efficient and accountable use of public resources and improve the quality of life.

Year Founded: 1975

408 Longmont Meals on Wheels
910 Longs Peak Avenue
Longmont, CO 80501
303-772-0540
info@lmow.org
www.longmontmeals.org

Jay Fernandez, President
Karla Hale, Executive Director
Michael Laurenz, Kitchen Manager / Chef

Longmont Meals on Wheels' primary focus is to provide hot, nutritious meals and a daily check to older adults and people with disabilities that reside in the communities of Longmont and Niwot.

Year Founded: 1969

409 Lyons Golden Gang
P.O. Box 426
Lyons, CO 80540
303-823-8813
www.lyons-colorado.com

Bronwyn Muldoon, President
Jeralyn Berner, Vice President
Craig Ferguson, Treasurer

Lyons Golden Gang provides nutritious meals to the homes of those who are ill, disabled or elderly on Tuesday through Friday.

410 Pikes Peak Area Council of Government:
Agency on Aging
15 S Seventh Street
Colorado Springs, CO 80905-1501
719-471-7080

The Pikes Peak Area Council of Governments (PPACG) serves as the Area Agency on Aging for El Paso, Park and Teller counties and provides programs and services for older adults and thier caregivers.

Year Founded: 1967

411 RSVP Jefferson County Seniors Resource Center
3227 Chase Street
Denver, CO 80212
303-235-6937
volunteer@srcaging.org
www.srcaging.org

Deborah Brackney, Chair
Monica Roers, President & CEO
Chris Lynn, Vice Chair

The Retired and Senior Volunteer Program (RSVP) helps people age 55 and older put their skills and life experiences to work in their communities. RSVP is a network of non-profit agencies in Jefferson County that helps older adults find opportunities to address community needs through volunteer service.

Year Founded: 1978

412 RSVP Otero Bent-Crowley Counties
13 W 3rd Street, Room 110
P.O. Box 494
La Junta, CO 81050-0494
719-383-3166
Fax: 719-383-4607; *Toll Free:* 800-438-3752
jhinkle@oterogov.org
www.oterogov.com

Jean Hinkle, County Administrator
Tina Mascarenas, Finance Officer

Our senior volunteers plant and maintain vegetable and flower gardens and work with the Forest Service to identify plants along trails and keep the trails clean.

413 RSVP Pueblo

230 N Union Avenue
Pueblo, CO 81003
719-545-8900
nawrocki@srda.org
www.srda.org

Steve Nawrocki, Executive Director
George Chintala, Operations Manager
Evie Densford, Controller

The Retired and Senior Volunteer Program (RSVP) provides opportunities for people 55 and over to make a difference in their community through volunteer service. RSVP volunteers contribute anywhere from a few to over forty hours a week, serving through schools, day care centers, police departments, hospitals and other nonprofit and public organizations to help meet critical community needs. RSVP offers maximum flexibility and choice to its volunteers. RSVP matches the personal interests and skills of older Americans with opportunities to help solve community problems and offers supplemental insurance while on duty, on-the-job training from the agency or organization where volunteers are placed. The following County is served: Pueblo.

414 RSVP VOA Colorado Branch

2660 Larimer Street
Denver, CO 80205
303-297-0408
info@voacolorado.org; www.voacolorado.org

Dianna Kunz, President & CEO
Mary Beth Heller, Executive Vice President
Bradley Gulley, Director of Volunteer Programs

The Retired and Senior Volunteer Program (RSVP) provides opportunities for people 55 and over to make a difference in their community through volunteer service. RSVP volunteers contribute anywhere from a few to over forty hours a week, serving thourgh schools, day care centers, police departments, hospitals and other nonprofit and public organizations to help meet critical community needs. RSVP offers maximum flexibility and choice to its volunteers. RSVP matches the personal interests and skills to older Americans with opportunities to help solve community problems and offer supplemental insurance while on duty, on-the-job training from the agency or organization where volunteers are placed.

415 RSVP Weld County
University of Northern Colorado

501 20th Street
Greeley, CO 80639
970-351-2588; *Fax:* 970-351-2581
RSVP@unco.edu
www.unco.edu/nhs/rsvp

Marcia Shafer, Director

Provides opportunities for persons over 55 to become involved in significant and worthwhile volunteer service to their communities and administers serveral community service programs.

Year Founded: 1973

416 Railroad Retirement Board: Colorado District Office

721 19th Street, Room 177
P.O. Box 8869
Denver, CO 80201
Fax: 303-844-2609; *Toll Free:* 877-772-5772
www.rrb.gov/field-office-locator-denver

Steven J Anthony, Manager

The Railroad Retirement Board (RRB) is an independent agency in the executive branch of the Federal Government. The RRB's primary function is to administer comprehensive retirement-survivor and unemployment-sickness benefit programs for the nation's railroad workers and their families, under the Railroad Retirement and Railroad Unemployment Insurance Acts.

417 San Juan Basin Area: Agency on Aging

954 E 2nd Avenue
Suite 102
Durango, CO 81301
970-264-0501
Fax: 888-290-3566
www.sjbaaa.org

The Area Agency on Aging develops and delivers services for seniors (60 years and older) and for adults (18-59 years) with disabilities and long-term care needs.

418 Teller Senior Coalition

750 E Highway 24
Building 2, Suite 100
Woodland Park, CO 80866
719-687-3330
www.tellerseniorcoalition.org

Kathy Lowry, Office Manager
Leni Stevenson, Case Manager
Kimberly Burleson, Marketing/Program Assistant

The Teller Senior Coalition (TSC) was organized when the Teller County Commissioners decided that senior services be privatized. TSC was organized by interested seniors and community leaders to continue vital programs: daily hot meals, transportation, education, information and handy man services.

Year Founded: 1996

419 The Senior Hub

9025 Grant Street
Suite 150
Thornton, CO 80229
303-426-4408
Fax: 303-426-0014
info@seniorhub.org
www.seniorhub.org

Jennifer Pepper, Executive Director
Calina Bowman, Business Manager
Nancy Kingsbury, Adult Day Services Director

A nonprofit resource center for seniors. Our mission is to advance the quality of life for older adults through advocacy, community partnerships, and a variety of direct services planned to sustain their independence.

Year Founded: 1986

420 Upper Arkansas Area: Agency on Aging

139 E 3rd Street
Salida, CO 81201-2612

719-539-3341; *Toll Free: 877-610-3341*
aaareg13@uaacog.com
www.uaaaa.org

Stephen Holland, Director

The Upper Arkansas Area Agency on Aging will assist seniors (60+) through the region in maintaining health, dignity, independence, and quality of life through education, advocacy, coordination and delivery of services and programs.

Year Founded: 1973

Connecticut

421 Bureau of Rehabilitation Services: Disability Determination Services

55 Farmington Avenue
12th Floor
Hartford, CT 06105
860-424-5055
Fax: 860-424-4850; Toll Free: 800-772-1213
kathleen.sullivan@ct.gov
www.ct.gov/dors
TTY: 800-325-0778

Amy Porter, Commissioner

Provides vocational rehabilitation, independent living and social security disability determination services to persons with disabilities.

Year Founded: 1973

422 Connecticut Board of Education and Services for the Blind

184 Windsor Avenue
Windsor, CT 06095-4536
860-602-4000
Fax: 860-602-4020; Toll Free: 800-842-4510
brian.sigman@ct.gov
www.ct.gov/besb/site

Brian Sigman, Director

Provides quality educational and rehabilitative services to all people who are legally blind or deaf-blind and children that are visually impaired at no cost to the clients or their families.

423 Connecticut Commission On Again

55 Farmington Avenue
12th Floor
Hartford, CT 06105-3730
860-424-5274
Fax: 860-424-5301; Toll Free: 866-218-6631
aging.sda@ct.gov
www.ct.gov/agingservices/cwp

Elizabeth B Ritter, Commissioner

The mission is to advocate on behalf of elderly persons in Connecticut by regularly monitoring their status, assessing the impact of current and proposed initiatives, and conducting activities which promote the interest of these individuals and to report to the Govenor and the Legislature.

424 Connecticut Council On Developmental Disabilities

460 Capitol Avenue
Hartford, CT 06106
860-418-8737
Fax: 860-418-6003; Toll Free: 800-653-1134

walter.glomb@ct.gov
www.ct.gov/ctcdd/cwp
TTY: 860-418-6172

Walter Glomb, Executive Director
Cathleen Adamczyk, Disability Policy Specialist
Donna Devin, Program Assistant

Promotes education for children, meaningful work for adults, community living for all people with disabilities, and self-advocacy by people with disabilities and parents.

Year Founded: 1998

425 Connecticut Department of Revenue

450 Columbus Boulevard
Hartford, CT 06103
860-297-5962; *Toll Free: 800-382-9463*
www.ct.gov/drs
TTY: 860-297-4911

Kevin B Sullivan, Commissioner

The mission of the Connecticut Department of Revenue Services (DRS) is to administer the tax laws of the State of Connecticut and collect the tax revenues in the most cost effective manner.

426 Connecticut Teachers Retirement Board

765 Asylum Avenue
Hartford, CT 06105-2822
860-241-8400; *Toll Free: 800-504-1102*
darlene.perez@ct.gov
www.ct.gov/trb

Clare H Barnett, Chair
Darlene Perez, Administrator
Kathy Demsey, Chief Financial Officer

Mission is to adequate funding to pay all benefits, to effectively administer the Retirement System; to protect and administer the statutory rights and benefits of members of the State Teacher's Retirement System; and to provide pre/post retirement services.

427 Disability Rights Connecticut

846 Wethersfield Avenue
Hartford, CT 06114
860-297-4300; *Toll Free: 800-842-7303*
info@disrightsct.org
www.disrightsct.org

Gretchen Knauff, Executive Director
Nancy Alisberg, Legal Director
Megan Collins, Staff Attorney

Disability Rights Connecticut, Inc. (DRCT) is an advocacy organization that is dedicated to identifying and eliminating the barriers that people with disabilities face in exercising their civil, legal and human rights. As Connecticut's protection and advocacy system (P&A), we work to improve the quality of life for individuals with disabilities, their families and our community as a whole using the activities and programs below.

428 Eastern Connecticut Area: Agency on Aging

19 Ohio Avenue
Suite 2
Norwich, CT 06360-2315
860-887-3561
Fax: 860-886-4736; Toll Free: 800-690-6998
seniorinfo@seniorresourcesec.org
www.seniorresourcesec.org

Joan Wessell, Executive Director
Nancy Lisee, Director of Education & Training
Laura Crews, Director of Benefits Access

Mission is to provide information and services to the aging population, their families and care providers.

Year Founded: 1976

429 LeadingAge Connecticut
110 Barnes Road
Wallingford, CT 06492
203-678-4477
ncarrero@leadingagect.org
www.leadingagect.org

James Rosenman, Chair
Mag Morelli, President
Yurka Carrero, Office Manager

LeadingAge Connecticut promotes and advocates for a vision of the world in which every community offers an integrated and coordinated continuum of high quality, affordable health care, housing and community based services.

Year Founded: 1991

430 North Central Area Agency on Aging
151 New Park Avenue
Box 75
Hartford, CT 06106
860-724-6443; *Toll Free: 800-994-9422*
info@ncaaact.org
www.ncaaact.org

North Central Area Agency on Aging, Inc's. (NCAAA) mission is to provide aging resources to help enhance the quality of life for older adults, individuals with disabilities, and their caregivers in North Central Connecticut by ensuring that they have access to quality and cost-effective services.

431 South Central Connecticut: Agency on Aging
One Long Wharf Drive
Suite 1L
New Haven, CT 06511
203-785-8533
www.aoascc.org

Joanne McGloin, Chair
Robert Haley, Vice Chair
Edward Konowitz, Secretary

Care management, volunteer opportunities, CHOICES, funding, planning and advocacy on behalf of older americans in New Haven-Fairfield County.

432 Volunteer Center of United Way for Capital Area
30 Laurel Street
Hartford, CT 06106-1374
860-493-6800
www.uwcact.org

Raymond P Necci, Chair
Sean Egan, Secretary

Referral service for potential volunteers. Works to train volunteer managers, develop volunteer programs for the corporate community, and broker noncash resources of for-profit organizations to nonprofit agencies.

433 Western Connecticut Area: Agency on Aging
84 Progress Lane
Waterbury, CT 06705-3859
203-757-5449
Fax: 203-757-4081; Toll Free: 800-994-9422
info@wcaaa.org
www.wcaaa.org

Pat Bria, President
Joseph DeMayo, Vice President
Dolores Winans, Secretary

The Western CT Area Agency on Aging develops, manages and provides comprehensive services for seniors, caregivers and individuals with disabilities in order to maintain their independence and quality of life.

Delaware

434 Delaware Assistive Technology Initiative
University of Delaware
461 Wyoming Road
Newark, DE 19716
302-831-0354
Fax: 302-831-4690; Toll Free: 800-870-3284
www.dati.org

Funded by the US Department of Education, National Institute on Disability and Rehabilitation Research as one of the Tech Act projects, the DATI focuses on improving public awareness, public access to information, funding for assistive technology devices and services, training and technical assistance, and coordination of statewide activities. The project has established Assistive Technology Resource Centers in each of Delaware's three countiesand is open to the public.

Year Founded: 1991

435 Delaware Commission of Veterans Affairs
802 Silver Lake Boulevard
Suite 100
Dover, DE 19904
302-739-2792
Fax: 302-739-2794; Toll Free: 800-344-9900
www.veteransaffairs.delaware.gov

Larence Kirby, Executive Director
Sherri Taylor, Senior Accountant
Arlynne Pineda, Administrative Specialist

The Delaware Commission of Veterans Affairs (DCVA) was established in 1987 to provide assistance to Delaware's veterans, their spouses and dependent children.

436 Delaware Community Legal Aid Society, Inc.
100 W 10th Street
Suite 801
Wilmington, DE 19801
302-575-0660
Fax: 302-575-0840; Toll Free: 800-292-7980
www.declasi.org
TTY: 302-575-0696

Paul Lockwood, President
Daniel G Atkins, Executive Director
James Reynolds, Treasurer

A private, nonprofit law firm dedicated to the equal justice for all. We provide civil legal services to assist clients in becoming self sufficient and meeting basic needs with dignity. Our clients include members of our community who have low incomes, who have disabilities, or who are age 60 and over.

Year Founded: 1946

437 Delaware Council for Persons with Disabiities
410 Federal Street
Suite 1
Dover, DE 19901-3640
302-739-3620
john.mcneal@state.de.us
scpd.delaware.gov

John McNeal, Director
Jo Singles, Contact

The mission of the State Counicl for Persons with Disabilities is to unite, in one Council, disability advocates and State agency policy makers to ensure that individuals with disabilities are empowered to become fully integrated within the community.

438 Delaware Department of Education
401 Federal Street
Suite 2
Dover, DE 19901-3639
302-735-4000
dedoe@doe.k12.de.us
www.doe.k12.de.us

Susan Bunting, Secretary
Karen Field Rogers, Deputy Secretary

A publicly funded state agency that gives information about local facilities and administers supplemental funds for visually handicapped students in local schools. It also maintains special teachers of sight conservation and braille programs for both children and adults.

439 Delaware Department of Health and Social Services: Division for the Visually Impaired
1901 N DuPont Highway
Biggs Bldg
New Castle, DE 19720
302-255-9800
Fax: 302-255-4441
www.dhss.delaware.gov/dhss/dvi

The Division for the Visually Impaired is the State's oldest agency dating from 1909. Mission is to improve the quality of life for Delaware's citizens by promoting health and well being, fostering self-sufficiency, and protecting vulnerable populations.

Year Founded: 1909

440 Delaware Developmental Disability Council
410 Federal Street
2nd Floor
Dover, DE 19901
302-739-3333
Fax: 302-739-2015
pat.maichle@state.de.us
ddc.delaware.gov

Patricia L Maichle, Senior Administrator
Kristin Harvey, Social Service Administrator
Stefanie Lancaster, Administrative Officer

The mission of the Delaware Developmental Disabilities Council is to promote and embrace inclusion, equality and empowerment.

441 Delaware Division of Revenue
820 N French Street
Wilmington, DE 19801
302-577-8200
Fax: 302-577-8202; *Toll Free:* 800-292-7826
revenue.delaware.gov

Kathy Revel, Assistant Director

As the primary revenue collector for the State, the mission of the Division of Revenue is to collect 100% of the taxes and other revenues required by law, no more and no less, and to do so in a manner that creates the highest possible level of satisfaction on the part of the public with the competence, courtesy, effectiveness, and efficiency of the Division.

442 Delaware Division of Services for Aging Adults with Physical Disabilities
1901 N Dupont Highway
Main Building
New Castle, DE 19720
Fax: 302-255-4445; *Toll Free:* 800-223-9074
delawareadrc@state.de.us
www.dhss.delaware.gov/dhss/dsaapd

Carries out a broad range of activities on behalf of older persons and adults with physical disabilities in Delaware.

443 Delaware Workers Compensation Board
4425 N Market Street
Wilmington, DE 19802
302-761-8000
www.delawareworks.com

The Office of Worker's Compensation administers and enforces state laws, rules and regulations regarding industrial accidents and illinesses.

444 Modern Maturity Center
1121 Forrest Avenue
Dover, DE 19904
302-734-1200
Fax: 302-674-1265
www.modern-maturity.org

Allan Angel, Chair
Carolyn Fredricks, President/CEO
Cathy Nacrelli, 1st Vice Chair

The mission of the Modern Maturity Center is to provide programs and services that will enhance the quality of life, with dignity and respect, for older adults.

Year Founded: 1972

District of Columbia

445 District of Columbia Departnment on Disability Services
250 E Street SW
Washington, DC 20024
202-730-1700
Fax: 202-730-1843
dds@dc.gov
dds.dc.gov
TTY: 202-730-1516

Andrew Reese, Director
Ann Simmons, Executive Assistant
Annissa Amegbe, Service Coordinator

DDS insures that residents with intellectual disabilities recieve the services and support they need to lead self-determined and valued lives in the community. DDS achieves this through the delivery of outreach and service coordination services; the development and management of a provider network delivering community residential, day, vocational, employment and individual and family support services.

446 District of Columbia Rehabilitation Services
250 E Street SW
Washington, DC 20024
202-730-1700
Fax: 202-730-1843
dds@dc.gov
dds.dc.gov
TTY: 202-730-1516

Andrew Reese, Director

447 District of Columbia Retirement Board
900 7th Street NW
Second Floor
Washington, DC 20001
202-343-3200
Fax: 202-566-5000
dcrb.agencymailbox@dc.gov
www.dcrb.dc.gov

Sheila Morgan-Johnson, Executive Director
Joseph W Clark, Chairman
Anthony Shelborne, Chief Financial Officer

The mission of DCRB is to prudently invest the Funds for the exclusive benefit of Plan members, while providing those Plan members with total retirement services.

Year Founded: 1979; Number of Members: 19,295

448 District of Columbia Worker Compensation Board
4058 Minnesota Avenue, NE
Washington, DC 20019
202-724-7000
Fax: 202-673-6993
does@dc.gov
www.does.dc.gov
TTY: 202-698-4817

Francis Smith, Executive Director

The Compensation Review Board (CRB) in accordance with Administrative Police Issuance, replaces the Office of the Director in providing administrative appellate review and dispostion of workers' and disability compensation claims arising under the DC Workers' Compensation Act.

449 Generations United
25 E Street NW
3rd Floor
Washington, DC 20001
202-289-3979
www.gu.org

Matthew E Melmed, Chair
Lynette Fraga, Executive Director
Amanda Charlsie Cavaleri, Founder & CEO

Generations United (GU) is the national membership organization focused solely on improving the lives of children, youth, and older people through intergenerational strategies, programs, and public policies. Our mission is to improve the lives of children, youth, and older people through

intergenerational collaboration, public polices, and programs for the enduring benefit of all.

450 LeadingAge
2519 Connecticut Avenue NW
Washington, DC 20008-1520
202-783-2242
info@LeadingAge.org
www.leadingage.org

Amma Addo, Executive Administrator
Majd Alwan, Executive Director
Natasha S Bryant, Managing Director

Serve two million people every day through mission-driven, not-for-profit organizations dedicated to provide continuum of aging services: adult day services, home health, community services, senior housing, assisted living residences, continuing care retirement communities, and nursing homes.

Year Founded: 1961

451 Mayor's Committee on Persons with Disabilities
441 4th Street NW
Suite 729N
Washington, DC 20001
202-724-5055
Fax: 202-727-9484
odr@dc.gov
odr.dc.gov
TTY: 202-727-3363

Derek Orr, Director
Jessica Hunt, Special Projects Coordinator
Sheryll Streets, Staff Assistant

The Committee acts in an advisory capacity to the Mayor on programs, services, facilities and activities which impact on citizens with disabilities in the District of Columbia. The Committee concerns itself with advocacy issues related to an inclusive delivery system for services to persons with disabilities.

452 The National Consumer Voice
1001 Conneticut Avenue NW
Suite 425
Washington, DC 20036
202-332-2275
Fax: 866-230-9789
info@theconsumervoice.org
www.theconsumervoice.org

Bill Lamb, President
Afsoon Namini, Vice President
Paul van Westrienen, Treasurer

Provides information on nursing home reform, promotes quality standards, and works to empower residents.

Year Founded: 1975

Florida

453 ARC Gateway
3932 North 10th Avenue
Pensacola, FL 32503-2806
850-434-2638
Fax: 850-438-2180
info@arc-gateway.org
www.arc-gateway.org

Vincent Andry, President
Charles Brewer, Executive Director
Todd Torgersen, Vice President

To increase the opportunities for all persons with, or at risk of, development disabilities, to choose where, how and with whom, they live, learn, work and play.

Year Founded: 1954

454 Alliance for Aging
760 NW 107th Avenue
Suite 214
Miami, FL 33172
305-670-6500
Fax: 305-670-6516; *Toll Free:* 800-963-5337
www.allianceforaging.org

Max B Rothman, President/CEO
Rhina Jaar, Executive Assistant
Islara Souto, Planning Director

The Alliance for Aging is a private not-for-profit, agency part of a nationwide network of more then 650 Area Agencies on Aging. A volunteer Board of Directors governs the Alliance. Operating funds are received through federal, state and local grants, as well as private donations from individuals, corporations and special initiatives.

Year Founded: 1988

455 Brevard County Community Services Council
3600 West King Street
Cocoa, FL 32926-4150
321-639-8770
Fax: 321-636-8446
info@communityservicescouncil.org
www.communityservicescouncil.org

Cindy Flackmeier, President/CEO
Janice Wiese, Program Director
Mickey Belson, Program Director

Community Services Council of Brevard is a private not for profit organization dedicated to helping seniors enjoy happy, healthy, and secure lives. The mission of Community Services Council is to develop solutions to community problems and to promote and maintain independence and maximize the quality of life for the citizens of Brevard County, particularly the elderly and disabled adults.

Year Founded: 1965

456 Broward County Area: Agency on Aging
5300 Hiatus Road
Sunrise, FL 33351
954-745-9779
Fax: 305-497-1586
www.adrcbroward.org/

Edith Lederberg, Director

The Agency on Aging plans, develops, coordinates, and evaluates programs, funds services, for people 60 years of age and older. A one stop source of information regarding services for seniors, persons with severe and persistent mental illness ages 18 and over, their families, and caregivers.

457 Coalition for Independent Living Options
6800 Forest Hill Boulevard
West Palm Beach, FL 33413
561-966-4288
Fax: 561-641-6619; *Toll Free:* 800-683-7337

www.cilo.org
TTY: 561-641-6538

Scott Shoemaker, President
Genevieve Cousminer, Esquire, Executive Director
Sharon D'Eusanio, Vice President

The purpose is to have an advocacy organization for children and adults with disabilities.

458 Department of Health & Rehabilitative Services
4042 Bald Cypress Way
Tallahassee, FL 32399-1701
850-245-4444
Fax: 850-922-6969
www.doh.state.fl.us/environment

Cynthia Bearer, Chairman
Dick Batchelor, Vice Chairman
J Routt Reigart, Founding Chair

Offers counseling and referrals on rehabilitation facilities.

Year Founded: 1996

459 Elder Services of Okaloosa County
207 Hospital Drive NE
Fort Walton Beach, FL 22548-5066
850-833-9165
Fax: 850-833-9174
mail@elder-services.org

Ruth R. Lovejoy, Director

Providing Meals on Wheels and income support services.

Year Founded: 1971

460 Florida Association of Homes for the Aging
1812 Riggins Road
Tallahassee, FL 32308
904-671-3700
Fax: 850-671-3790
info@fahsa.org
www.fahsa.org

Diane Marcello, Chair
Janegale Boyd, RN, President/CEO
Al Pasini, MPA CAE, Chief Operating Officer

The mission of the Florida Association of Homes for the Aging is to represent and promote the common interests of continuing care retirement communities, assisted living facilities, nursing homes, and affordable supportive housing members through advocacy, education, leadership development and shared services to enhance their ability to serve older or disabled adults.

Number of Members: 500

461 Florida Council on Aging
1018 Thomasville Road
Suite 110
Tallahassee, FL 32303-8701
850-222-8877
Fax: 850-222-2575
moreinfo@fcoa.org
www.fcoa.org

LuMarie Polivka-West, President
Dan Brady, Secretary
Barbara Kauffman, Treasurer

The Florida Council on Aging is committed to serving Florida's diverse aging interests through education, information-sharing and advocacy.x

Year Founded: 1955

462   Florida Department of Aging
4040 Esplanade Way
Tallahassee, FL 32399-7000
850-414-2000
Fax: 850-414-2004
information@elderaffairs.org
elderaffairs.state.fl.us/index.ph
TDD 850-414-2001

Larry Polivka, Assistant Secretary
Chris Shoemaker, Executive Director

463   Florida Department of Children, Families and Elderly Services
1317 Winewood Boulevard
Building 1, Room 202
Tallahassee, FL 32399-6570
850-487-1111
Fax: 850-922-2993
www.myflorida.com/cf_web

Esther Jacobo, Interim Secretary
Drew Parker, General Counsel

The Florida Department of Children and Families' mission is to protect vulnerable children and adults, to promote strong, economically self-sufficient families, and to advance personal and family recovery and resiliency from mental illness and substance addiction. Our Adult Services Program provides services for frail, elderly and disabled adults who are at risk or are victims of abuse, neglect, or exploitation and disabled adults who need assistance to remain in their own homes in the community.

464   Florida Department of Elder Affairs Program of Aging and Adult Services
4040 Esplanade Way
Tallahassee, FL 32399-7000
850-414-2000
Fax: 850-414-2004
information@elderaffairs.org
elderaffairs.state.fl.us
TDD 850-414-2001

Carole Green, Manager
Susan Tucker, Deputy Secretary
Joan L Spainhower, Communications Director

An agency designated by Flordia voters to be in charge of issues concerning older Flordians. Its purpose is to serve elders in every aspect possible to help them keep their self-sufficiency and self determination. The Department implements a variety of innovative programs for long term care. Recognizing that the majority of Flordia's elders are active and independent and want to remain that way aslong as possible.

465   Florida Department of Revenue
5050 West Tennessee Street
Tallahassee, FL 32399
850-414-4615; *Toll Free:* 800-622-5437
EMailDOR@dor.state.fl.us
dor.myflorida.com
TTY: 800-955-8771

Marshall Stranburg, Executive Director
Andrea Moreland, Deputy Executive Director
Blanca Bayo, Chief of Staff

Mission of the Florida Department of Revenue is to serve citizens with respect, concern, and professionalism. To make complying with tax and child support laws easy and understandable. To administer the laws fairly and consis-

tently and to provide excellent service efficiently and at the lowest possible cost.

466   Florida Department of Veterans Affairs
11351 Ulmerton Road
Suite 311-K
Tallahassee, FL 33778-1630
727-518-3202
Fax: 850-488-4001
www.floridavets.org

Mike Prendergast, Executive Director
Al Carter, Deputy Executive Director
Bobby Carbonell, Legislative and Cabinet Affairs

Our mission is to help Florida veterans, their families and survivors to improve their health and economic well-being through quality benefits information, advocacy, education and long term health services.

467   Florida Developmental Disabilities Council
124 Marriott Drive
Suite 203
Tallahassee, FL 32301-2981
850-488-4180
Fax: 850-922-6702; *Toll Free:* 800-580-7801
fddc@fddc.org
www.fddc.org
TDD 888-488-8633

Debra Dowds, Executive Director
Vanda Bowman, Staff Assistant
Rose Coster, Communications Coordinator

Promotes innovative programs and practices that prevent disabilities and improve the quality of life for people with disabilities and thier families. Participates in statewide and nationwide advocacy.

Year Founded: 1971

468   Florida Division of Vocational Rehabilitation
2002 Old Saint Augustine Road
Building A
Tallahassee, FL 32399-7016
850-245-3399
Fax: 850-921-7215; *Toll Free:* 800-451-4327
www.rehabworks.org

Marilyn Campbell, Strategic Planning Coordinator

State agency serving individuals with physical or mental disabilities that interfere with them keeping or maintaining employment.

469   Florida Dog Guides F.T.D.
PO Box 20662
Bradenton, FL 34203
941-748-8245
Fax: 941-747-0969; *Toll Free:* 800-520-4589
adogs@floridadogguidesftd.org
www.floridadogguidesftd.org
TDD 941-748-8245

Deaf and hard of hearing individuals interested in working with and providing trained certified hearing dogs for the deaf. Sponsors state-wide dog shows and canine good citizen testing. Provides deaf awareness and advocacy.

470 Florida Protection & Advocacy for Persons with Disabilities
2728 Centerview Drive
Suite 102
Tallahassee, FL 32301-5069
850-488-9071
Fax: 850-488-8640; *Toll Free:* 800-342-0823
www.disabilityrightsflorida.org/

Catherine Piecora, Chair
Maryellen McDonald, Executive Director
Minerva Vazquez, Vice-Chair

The Advocacy Center for Persons with Disabilities is a non-profit organization providing Protection and Advocacy services in the State of Florida.

Year Founded: 1977

471 Gray Panthers of North Dade
861 N Venetian Drive
Miami, FL 33139-1012
305-374-8240
yanow420@aol.com
www.graypanthers.org

Dorothy Fleisher, Director

A national organization of intergenerational activists dedicated to social change.

472 Gray Panthers of South Dade
10725 SW 82nd Avenue
Miami, FL 33156
305-595-0594
Fax: 305-273-9664
normansaxe@aol.com
www.graypanthers.org

Norman Saxe, Convener

A network of independent activisits bound together by our passion for social justice. We are a loosely coordinated set of networks bound only by our passionate comnnitment to speak truth to power.

473 Heart of Florida United Way Volunteer Center
Dr. Nelson Ying Center
1940 Traylor Boulevard
Orlando, FL 32804-4714
407-835-0900
Fax: 407-835-2805
www.hfuw.org

John Moskos, Chairman
E. Ann McGee, Ed.D., Vice Chair
James B Cross, Treasurer

Affects community-wide change by linking leaders of businesses and nonprofit organization together. Programs include Volunteer Management Training, volunteer recruitment, corporate volunteerism, community involvement projects, volunteer recognition, and educational resources.

474 Meals on Wheels
2801 S Financial Court
Sanford, FL 32773-6418
407-333-8877
Fax: 407-829-2468
www.mealsetc.org

Cpt. Kip Beacham, President
Elizabeth Darwick, 1st Vice President
Dr. Marcia Roman, 2ndVice President

The mission of Meals on Wheels is to enhance the quality of life for elder Seminole County residents by providing appetizing, nutritious meals, and support services which permit seniors to maintain independence and dignity.

Year Founded: 1973

475 Meals on Wheels South Florida
451 North State Road 7
Palnatation, FL 33317
954-731-8770
Fax: 954-714-6950
info@mowsoflo.org
www.mowsoflo.org

Mark Adler, Executive Director
Shelly McCarty, Director of Finance
Howard Ward, Chairman

Meals on Wheels South Florida is a private nonprofit organization providing hunger-relief services, delivering nutritious meals, friendly visits and safety checks that enable South Florida seniors to live nourished lives with independence and dignity. Included in their comprehensive list of programs and services are home meal delivery, community-based dining, meals for companion pets, grocery shopping assistance, nutrition education and emergency meals.

Year Founded: 1984

476 Miami Dade County Retired and Senior Volunteer Program
2525 West 62nd Street
4th Floor
Miami, FL 33147
305-514-6000
Fax: 305-375-4501
Bsosa@miamidade.gov
www.miamidade.gov/dhs

Joe A Martinez, Chairman
Alexander Penelas, CEO

Miami Dade County's Department of Human Services (DHS) provides volunteer service opportunities in their home communities. This program is available to people 55 years and older. Participants serve up to forty hours a week in organizations that range from hospitals and youth recreation centers to local police stations and education facilities. Seniors are matched by their personal interests, skills, and lifelong experiences.

477 North Florida: Area Agency on Aging
2414 Mahan Drive
Tallahassee, FL 32308-5302
850-488-0055
Fax: 850-922-2420; *Toll Free:* 866-467-4624
aaanf@aaanf.org
www.aaanf.org

Janet Dorrier, President
Eddie Fields, 1st Vice President
Janice Means, 2nd Vice President

The mission of the Area Agency on Aging for North Florida is to plan, coordinate and advocate for programs and services which promote the independence, dignity, health and well being of seniors and caregivers.

478 Northeast Florida: Area Agency on Aging
Eldersource
4160 Woodcock Drive
Jacksonville, FL 32207

904-777-2106
Fax: 352-388-6400
www.myeldersource.com

Linda Levin, Chief Executive Officer

To empower individuals to age with independence and dignity by providing leadership direction, advocacy, and support for a comprehensive coordinated continuum of care.

479 Osceola County Council on Aging

Barney E. Veak Center
700 Generation Point
Kissimmee, FL 34744-6107
407-846-8532
Fax: 407-846-8550
info@osceolagenerations.org
www.osceolagenerations.org

Jim Swan, President
Beverly Hoagland, Chief Executive Officer
Connie Benca, Chief Financial Officer

The Osceols County Council on Aging is a private, non-profit agency dedicated to providing services and housing to promote the physical, mental and social well-being of seniors, at risk youth, adults with disabilities and their care givers in our community. Our goals are to help frail citizens maintain their independence and dignity in an effort to avoid being institutionalized and to provide active seniors with volunteer, recreational and socialactivities to keep them involved and fulfilled.

480 Pensacola Retired Activities Office
Naval Personnel Command

Naval Air Station
150 Hase Road
Pensacola, FL 32508
850-452-5990
Fax: 850-452-2596
www.cnic.navy.mil/pensacola

Keith Hoskins, Commanding Officer
David Jasso, Executive Officer
Jeffery Grosso, Command Master Chief, NAS Pensac

The RAO serves as a link between local retired military and the active-duty community which provides assistance to retired military. It provides installation commanders with a means of providing more effective services and improving communication for the local retired community. The RAO is staffed and operated by volunteer retired military personnel who assist other retired members, their families and survivors to receive entitled services andbenefits. Through newsletters and seminars and appreciation days, the RAO supports quality of life issues throughout the retirement years to their fellow service members.

Year Founded: 1826

481 Pinellas Opportunity Council (POC)

St Petersburg, FL
727-823-4101
ksisson@poc-inc.org
www.poc-inc.org

Katie Sisson, RSVP Program Director

Mobilize federal, state, local and private resources to develop programs that deliver services to help individuals and families alleviate conditions of poverty, empower people to move towards economic self-sufficiency, provide opportunities for people to reach their full potential, and revitalize communities.

Year Founded: 1964

482 RSVP Big Bend

2518 W Tennessee Street
Tallahassee, FL 32304
850-921-5554
Fax: 850-921-0082
info@ecsbigbend.org
www.ecsbigbend.org

Mark D Baldino, President & CEO
Wil Brooks, Director, Food Services
Michael Henderson, Vice President and Director, Nut

The Retired and Senior Volunteer Program (RSVP) provides opportunities for people 55 and over to make a difference in their community through volunteer service. RSVP volunteers contribute anywhere from a few to over forty hours a week, serving through schools, day care centers, police departments, hospitals and other nonprofit and public organizations to help meet critical community needs. RSVP offers maximum flexibility and choice to its volunteers. RSVP matches the personal interests and skills of older Americans with opportunities to help solve community problems and offers supplemental insurance while on duty, and on-the-job training from the agency or organization where volunteers are placed. The following Counties are served: Franklin, Gadsden, Jefferson, Leon, Liberty, Madison, Suwannee, Taylor, Wakulla.

483 RSVP Broward County

4701 NW 33rd Avenue
Ft Lauderdale, FL 33309-6807
954-484-7117
Fax: 954-484-8292
info@impactbroward.org
www.seniorvolunteerservices.org

Peter E Weitz, Chair
Andy Szkaradek, Vice-Chair
Deborah Lauer, Secretary

The Retired and Senior Volunteer Program (RSVP) provides opportunities for people 55 and over to apply the skills and wisdom you've acquired throughout your life to make a positive difference in the lives of others via opportunities in disaster services, ecnomic opportunity, education, environmental stewardship, healthy futures or vetrans and military families.

Year Founded: 1970

484 RSVP Citrus County

110 N Apopka Avenue
Inverness, FL 34450
352-341-6560
Fax: 352-341-6584
catherine.pearson@bocc.citrus.fl.us
www.citruscountyfl.org

Laurie Diestler, Project Coordinator
Patty Lascuola, Sr Program Assistant
Sue Carcadden, Sr Companion Assistant

The RSVP mission is to provide meaningful volunteer opportunities for people 55 and over who bring vast experience, skills, and interests from diverse economic, educational and social backgrounds to serve on a regular basis at sites throughout Citrus County.

485 RSVP Flagler County

PO Box 353755
Bunnell, FL 32135

386-597-2950
Fax: 386-597-2953
flaglervolunteer@cfl.rr.com
www.flaglervolunteer.org

Suzy Gamblain, Executive Director
Jean MacAllister, Volunteer Coordinator
Barb Witt, Special Events & Fundraisers

486 RSVP Martin County
10 SE Central Parkway
Suite 101
Stuart, FL 34994-3033
772-220-4472
Fax: 772-220-7771
chodnett@martinvolunteers.org
www.martinvolunteers.org/rsvp

Denise Eldredge, President
Jim Dudziak, Vice President
Teri Weiss, Secretary

The Retired and Senior Volunteer Program (RSVP) provides opportunities for people 55 and over to make a difference in their community through volunteer service. RSVP volunteers contribute anywhere from a few to over forty hours a week, serving through schools, day care centers, police departments, hospitals and other nonprofit and public organizations to help meet critical community needs. RSVP offers maximum flexibility and choice to its volunteers. RSVP matches the personal interests and skills of older Americans with opportunities to help solve community problems and offers supplemental insurance while on duty, on-the-job training from the agency or organization where volunteers are placed. The following County is served: Martin.

487 RSVP Seminole County
Toll Free: 866-851-5518

The Retired and Senior Volunteer Program (RSVP) provides opportunities for people 55 and over to make a difference in their community through volunteer service. RSVP volunteers contribute anywhere from a few to over forty hours a week, serving through schools, day care centers, police departments, hospitals and other nonprofit and public organizations to help meet critical community needs. RSVP offers maximum flexibility and choice to its volunteers. RSVP matches the personal interests and skills of older Americans with opportunities to help solve community problems and offers supplemental insurance while on duty, on-the-job training from the agency or organization where volunteers are placed. The following County is served: Volusia.

488 RSVP St Lucie County
4204 Okeechobee Road
Ft Pierce, FL 34947
772-429-5510
Fax: 772-429-5506

Susan Helms-Smith, Director

Provides opportunities for people 55 and over to make a difference in their community through volunteer service. RSVP volunteers contribute anywhere from a few to over forty hours a week, serving through schools, day care centers, police departments, hospitals and other nonprofit and public organizations to help meet critical community needs. RSVP matches the personal interests and skills of older Americans with opportunities to help solve community problems and offers supplemental insurance while on duty,

and on-the-job training from the agency or organization where volunteers placed.

489 RSVP Volunteer Services of United Way Palm Beach County
2600 Quantum Boulevard
Boynton Beach, FL 33426-8627
561-375-6600
Fax: 561-375-6666
vwaypbc@gate.net
www.unitedwaypbc.org

Joseph B Shearouse, Chairman
Kristen Murtaugh, Ph.D, Secretary
Stephen McDermott, Treasurer

Designed to engage persons 55 and older iun volunteer service to meet critical community needs and to provide a high quality experience that will enrich the lives of volunteers. There is no minimum of time required for volunteering.

490 Railroad Retirement Board: Jacksonville District Office
550 Water Street
Suite 220
Jacksonville, FL 32202-4411
904-232-2546
Fax: 904-232-2874; *Toll Free:* 877-772-5772
jacksonville@rrb.gov
www.rrb.gov

Henry G Crowe, Representative

The Railroad Retirement Board is an independent agency in the executive branch of the Federal Government. The RRB's primary function is to administer comprehensive retirement-survivor and unemployment-sickness benefit programs for the nation's railroad workers and their families, under the Railroad Retirement and Railroad Unemployment Insurance Acts.

491 Sanford Senior Center
401 E Seminole Boulevard
Sanford, FL 32771
407-688-5000
Fax: 407-302-1090
kim.eltonhead@sanfordfl.gov
www.sanfordfl.gov/index.aspx?page=274

Kim Eltonhead, Manager

Meeting the needs of senior citizens.

492 Senior Solutions of Southwest Florida
2285 First Street
Fort Myers, FL 33901-2959
239-332-4233
Fax: 239-332-3596
www.seniorsolutions.org

Leigh Wade, Director

493 Seniors First
5395 L B McLeod Road
Orlando, FL 32811-2952
407-292-0177
Fax: 407-292-2773
mainoffice@seniorsfirstinc.org
www.seniorsfirstinc.org/

Robert Higgins, Chairman
Gordon Arkin, 1st Vice Chair
Craig Moore, 2nd Vice Chair

Senior First enhances the quality of life for Orange County senior citizens by maintaining their independence and dignity through nutrition, home improvement, and support services which assist seniors in need.

494 Social Security: Tallahassee Disability Determination
PO Box 5200
Tallahassee, FL 32314
850-942-8978
Fax: 850-942-8980; *Toll Free:* 800-342-1823
www.ssa.gov

Rosie M Steele, District Manager

Administers the Title II and Title XVII disability programs. To be insured for Title II benefits, applicants must have worked in covered employment for at least five of the last ten years prior to becoming disabled. To be eligible for Title XVII disability benefits, applicants must meet an income and resource test. For retirement Title II beneficiaries must be 65 or 62 for early retirement. Title XVI recipients must be 65.

495 US Railroad Retirement Board: Tampa District Office
Timberlake Federal Building
500 E Zack Street Suite 300
Tampa, FL 33602
813-228-2695
Fax: 813-228-2939; *Toll Free:* 877-772-5772
tampa@rrb.gov
www.rrb.gov

Virginia W Earl, District Manager

This office handles general inquiries from beneficiaries receiving Railroad Retirement benefits. The office takes applications from eligible employees, their spouses, their survivers for retirement and survivor benefits.

496 United Way of Central Florida
5605 US Highway 98 S
PO Box 1357
Highland City, FL 33846
863-648-1500
Fax: 863-648-1535
info@uwcf.org
www.uwcf.org

Terry Worthington, President
Sandi Honeycutt, Executive Assistant
Kandy Stanton, Creative Director

United Way of Central Florida is focused on kids, families and wellness. We deal with social issues collectively, leveraging investments to create solutions that bring results for our community.

497 Volunteer Jacksonville
6817-1902 Southpoint Parkway
Jacksonville, FL 32216-6299
904-332-6767
Fax: 904-332-6722
hojteam@volunteerjacksonville.org
www.volunteerjacksonville.org

Dan Macferran, Chair
Dr. Judith A Smith, President & CEO
LeAnn Daddario, Sr. Vice-President

We inspire, connect, engage, and support volunteers who make a difference in our community.

498 West Central Florida: Area Agency on Aging
5905 Breckenridge Parkway
Suite F
Tampa, FL 33610-4239
813-740-3888
Fax: 813-623-1342; *Toll Free:* 800-336-2226
www.agingflorida.com/

Maureen S Kelly, President and CEO
CharlotteK. McHenry, Senior Vice President
Katie Parkinson, Vice President, ADRC and Program

The West Central Florida Area Agency on Aging is a private, non-profit ccorporation which adminsters public funds, private grants and donations for senior services in Hillsborough, Polk, Manatee, Highlands and Hardee Counties.

499 William Beardall Senior Center
800 S Delaney Avenue
Orlando, FL 32801-3897
407-246-4440
Fax: 407-246-4114
www.cityoforlando.net

Lisa Early, Director
John Perrone, Manager

City recreation center for seniors.

Georgia

500 ADA Technical Assistance Program
1419 Mayson Street
Atlanta, GA 30324
404-541-9001
Fax: 404-541-9002; *Toll Free:* 800-949-4232
ADAsoutheast@law.syr.edu
www.adasoutheast.org/

Amy Oliveras, Administrative Assistant
Joseph Addo, Owner

One of ten regional centers funded by NIDRR, to provide information and technical assistance to assist in voluntary compliance with the Americans with Disabilities Act.

501 Atlanta Regional Commission: Aging Services Division
40 Courtland Street, NE
Atlanta, GA 30303-2538
404-463-3100
Fax: 404-364-9380
www.atlantaregional.com/aging

Shelley Caplan, Project Director

Mission is to serve as a focal point for older adults and caregivers in the delivery and coordination of information, resources, and services that support a healthy and enriched quality of life.

502 Central Savannah River Regional: Area Agency on Aging
3023 Riverwatch Parkway
Suite A
Augusta, GA 30907-2016
706-210-2000
Fax: 706-210-2006
www.csrardc.org/csra

Andy Crosson, Executive Director
Mack Shealy, Chief Financial Officer
Katrina Mauney, Administrative Assistant

The CSRA RDC is a public-sector, non-profit planning and development agency that serves a 13 county and 41 city region in the eastern portion of central Georgia.

503 DHS Division of Aging Services
2 Peachtree Street NW
33rd Floor
Atlanta, GA 30303-3142
404-657-5258
Fax: 404-657-5285; *Toll Free:* 866-552-4464
www.aging.dhs.georgia.gov

Dr James Bulot, Director
Jean O'Callaghan, Deputy Director
J Blake Lanier, Chief Financial Officer

Assists older individuals, at-risk adults, persons with disabilities, their families and caregivers to achieve safe, healthy, independent, and self reliant lives.

504 Georgia Advocacy Office
150 E Ponce De Leon Avenue
Suite 430
Decatur, GA 30030
404-885-1234
Fax: 404-378-0031; *Toll Free:* 800-537-2329
info@thegao.org
www.thegao.org
TDD 800-537-2329

Ruby Moore, Executive Director
Olwyn Mayer, Deputy Director
Donovan Hylton, Comptroller

Protection and advocacy services for Georgians with developmental disabilities.

Year Founded: 1977

505 Georgia Client Assistance Program Division of Rehabilitation Services
123 N. McDonough Street
Decatur, GA 30030
404-373-2040
Fax: 404-373-4110; *Toll Free:* 800-822-9727
GaCAPDirector@georgiacap.com
www.georgiacap.com/
TDD 404-373-2040

Charles L Martin, Director
Ashley Carraway, Assistant Director
Jennifer Page, Counselor

Helps eligible persons with complaints, appeals and understanding available benefits under the 1992 Rehabilitation Act Amendments and Title I of the Americans with Disabilities Act. CAP investigates complaints, mediates conflict, represents complainants in appeals, provides legal services if warranted, advocates for due process, identifies and recommends solutions to system problems, & advises

of benefits available under the 1992 Rehab Act Amendments and Americans with Disabilities Act.

506 Georgia Department of Aging
2 Peachtree Street NW
33rd Floor
Atlanta, GA 30309-3142
404-657-5258
Fax: 404-657-5285; *Toll Free:* 866-552-4464
aging.dhs.georgia.gov

James Bulot, Director
Kathryn Fowler, Council on Aging Director
Melanie McNeill, Ombudsman

Assists older individuals, at-risk adults, persons with disabilities, their families and caregivers to achieve safe, healthy, independent, and self reliant lives.

507 Georgia Department of Labor: Disability Adjudication Section
PO Box 57
1551 Juliette Road
Stone Mountain, GA 30086
678-476-7000
Fax: 678-476-7377
www.vocrehabga.org

Bruce Johnston, Manager Professional Relations

Specialized program of Rehabilitation Services, works with the Social Security Administration to make disability determinations for Georgia citizens who apply for entitlement programs administered by the SSA. The programs include Disability insurance for workers who pay FICA taxes and SSI, a disability needs program.

508 Georgia Department of Revenue
1800 Century Blvd NE
Augusta, GA 30345
706-821-2476
Fax: 706-731-7956
www.etax.dor.ga.gov/

Douglas MacGinnitie, Commissioner
Mark Chandler, Deputy Commissioner

Principal tax collecting agency for the state of Georgia

509 Georgia Department of Veterans Service
Floyd Memorial Building
Suite E-970
Atlanta, GA 30334-4800
404-656-2300
Fax: 404-657-9738
gavetsvc@vs.state.ga.us
sdvs.georgia.gov

Pete Wheeler, Commissioner
Dan Holtz, Assistant Commissioner
Mike Roby, Assistant Commissioner

Mission of the Department of Veterans Service is to serve the some 700,000 plus-veterans residing in Georgia, their dependents and survivors in all matters pertaining to veterans benefits.

510 Georgia Division of Aging Services: AreaAgency on Aging
335 West Society Avenue
Albany, GA 31701
229-432-1124
Fax: 229-483-0995

info@sowegacoa.org
www.sowegacoa.org

Lorie Farkas, President
Nancy Lorber, Vice-President

511 Georgia Office of Aging

2 Peachtree Street NW
33rd Floor
Atlanta, GA 30303-3142
404-657-5258
Fax: 404-657-5285; Toll Free: 866-552-4464
www.aging.dhr.georgia.gov

Dr James Bulot, Director
Jean O'Callaghan, Deputy Director
J Blake Lanier, Chief Financial Officer

The Division of Aging Services (DAS) continuously seeks
to improve the effectiveness and efficiency of services. We
fully comply with the requirements of the Older Americans
Act to ensure that services are properly and effectively
adminstered to meet the needs of elderly Georgians.

512 Georgia State Board of Workers' Compansation

270 Peachtree Street NW
Atlanta, GA 30303-1299
404-656-2048
Fax: 404-651-9467; Toll Free: 800-533-0682
sbwc.georgia.gov

Judge Frank McKay, Chairman
Thomas M Risko, Chief Financial Officer
Delece A Brooks, Chief Operating Officer

The State Board of Workers Compensation serves over a
quarter of a million employers in Georgia and over 3,8 million workers. The State Board is funded by assessments
from insurance companies and self-insured employers. An
employee that is injured on the job and is covered by the
law may be eligible for replacement of a portion of lost
wages, medical payments, vocational rehabilitation
services and other benefits.

Year Founded: 1920

513 Georgia Teachers Retirement System

2 Northside 75 NW
Suite 100
Atlanta, GA 30318-7778
404-352-6500
Fax: 404-352-4885; Toll Free: 800-352-0650
www.trsga.com

Dr. L.C. Evans, Chair
Jeffrey L Ezell, Executive Director
Stephen J Boyers, Chief Financial Officer

TRS administers the fund from which teachers in the state's
public schools, many employees of the University System
of Georgia, and certain others designated employees in ed-
ucational-related work environments receive retirement
benefits.

514 Governor's Council on Developmental Disabilities

2 Peachtree Street
Suite 26-246
Atlanta, GA 30303-3181
404-657-2126
Fax: 404-657-2123; Toll Free: 888-275-4233
eejacobson@dhr.state.ga.us

www.gcdd.org
TDD 404-657-2133

Eric Jacobson, Executive Director
Dottie Adams, Individual and Family Support Di
D'Arcy Robb, Public Policy Director

515 Gwinnett Council for Seniors

186 E Pike St
Po Box 933
Lawrenceville, GA 30046
770-822-5147
Fax: 770-979-9370
www.gwinnettcouncilforseniors.org/

Rosalind Bennett, President
Keith Nabb, Incoming President
Ann Evans, Vice President

Seniors dedicated to helping other seniors in ways vital to
seniors' benefit and welfare.

516 Heart of Georgia Altamaha: Area Agency on Aging

331 W Parker Street
Baxley, GA 31513
912-367-3648
Fax: 912-367-3640
baxley@hogarc.org
www.hogarc.org/

Brett Manning, Executive Director
Janice Jones, Finance Director
Katy Morton, Director of Economic & Communica

The basic mission of the RDC is to provide professional
advice and assistance to its member governments in the areas of comprehensive planning, community and economic
development, historic preservation, local government and
administration, and management, aging, and workforce
investment

517 Henry County Council on Aging

140 Henry Parkway
McDonough, GA 30253
770-288-6000
Fax: 770-954-2164
www.co.henry.ga.us
TTY: 770-288-6819

Elizabeth Mathis, Chairman
Warren Holder, District 1 Commissioner
Brian Preston, District 2 Commissioner

Provides services to seniors.

518 Legacy Link

PO Box 2534
508 Oak Street
Gainesville, GA 30503-2534
770-538-2650
Fax: 770-538-2660; Toll Free: 800-845-5465
pvfreeman@legacylink.org
www.legacylink.org

Pat Freeman, Chief Executive Officer
Steven Leibel, Attorney

Wide variety of services for seniors and persons with disabilities in 13-county region. Volunteer opportunities and
employment training services available for 55 years and
older. The information source for seniors, their families and
others who care. Legacy Link is an Area Agency on Aging.

519 Northeast Georgia Area: Agency on Aging
305 Research Drive
Athens, GA 30605-2725
706-583-2546
Fax: 706-369-5792
jdove@negrc.org
www.negrc.org

Jim Dove, Executive Director
Peggy Jenkins, AAA Director
Carol Rayburn-Cofer, WIA Director

The Area Agency on Aging (AAA) contracts with counties, private organizations, senior centers, attorneys at law, and non-profit organizations to provide services to the elderly.

520 RSVP Albany County
335 West Society Avenue
Albany, GA 31701
229-432-1124
Fax: 229-438-0408; *Toll Free:* 800-282-6612
www.sowegacoa.org

Lorie Farkas, President

The Retired and Senior Volunteer Program (RSVP) provides opportunities for people 55 and over to make a difference in their community through volunteer service. RSVP volunteers contribute anywhere from a few to over forty hours a week, serving thourgh schools, day care centers, police departments, hospitals and other nonprofit and public organizations to help meet critical community needs. RSVP offers maximum flexibility and choice to its volunteers. RSVP matches the personal interests and skills to older Americans with opportunities to help solve community problems and offer supplemental insurance while on duty, on-the-job training from the agency or organization where volunteers are placed.

521 RSVP Northeast Georgia
141 Garrison Street
Homer, GA 30547
706-677-1543
Fax: 706-677-1548
ctucker@inincga.com
www.athenscommunitycouncilonaging.org

Mary Ellen Quinn, President
Michele Pearson, Vice-President
Joseph Frierson III, Treasurer

The Retired Senior Volunteer Program (RSVP) is part of Senior Corps, a network of national service programs that provides older Americans the opportunity to apply to their life experience to meeting community needs. RSVP volunteers serve in a diverse range of nonprofit organizations, public agencies, and faith-based groups. Among other activities, they mentor children, volunteer in hospitals, deliver meals to homebound elderly persons, assist atthe State Botanical Gardens, and lend their business skills to community groups that provide critical social services. The following Counties are served: Barrow, Clarke, Elbert, Greene, Jackson, Madison, Morgan, Oconee, Oglethorpe, Walton.

522 RSVP Savannah
618 W Anderson Street
PO Box 1353
Savannah, GA 31415-5420
843-681-5825
Fax: 912-238-2977

rsvpfgp@earthlink.net
www.savannah.rsvppublications.com/Market

Debbie W Walker, Director

The Retired and Senior Volunteer Program (RSVP) helps seniors age 55 years and older put their skills and life experience to work for their communities. RSVP volunteers serve from a few hours to forty hours a week. RSVP volunteers meet critical community needs. The following Counties are served: Bacon, Bryan, Camden, Chatham, Effingham, Glynn, Liberty, Long, McIntosh, Pierce, Wayne.

Year Founded: 1985

523 Railroad Retirement Board: Georgia District Office
Peachtree Summit Building, Room 1702
401 West Peachtree Street
Atlanta, GA 30308-3519
404-331-2841
Fax: 404-331-1629; *Toll Free:* 877-772-5772
atlanta@rrb.gov
www.rrb.gov/field/do_atla.asp

Michael Schwartz, Chairman
Nancy Pittman, Assistant to the Chairman
Stephen Seiple, Counsel to the Chairman

Office handles inquiries concerning employee & spouse retirement annuities, retirement & survivor disability annuities, surviving widow(er) & child annuities, Medicare and tax liability.

524 ResCare Home Care
3020 N Patterson Street
Valdosta, GA 31602-2797
229-244-8854
Fax: 229-244-0979; *Toll Free:* 800-894-3715
www.rescarehomecare.com

Ellen Goldberg, Regional Director

Southern Home Care Services has provided professional nursing, personal care homemaking and respite services in the home, the hospitals, and long term care facilities. We are committed to providing the quality and attention that our clients deserve. Delivering service with compassion and respect is our goal.

525 SOWEGA Council on Aging: Area Agency onAging
225 West Society Avenue
Albany, GA 31701
229-432-1124
Fax: 229-483-0995
info@sowegacoa.org
www.sowegacoa.org

Kay H. Hind, Executive Director
Debbie Blanton, Assistant Executive Director

The SOWEGA Council on Aging (SCOA)/Area Agency on Aging plans, provides, develops and coordinates services for all people 60 years of age and older in a 14-county, 6,000 square mile area of Southwest Georgia. This area includes the following counties: Baker, Calhoun, Colquitt, Decatur, Dougherty, Early, Grady, Lee, Miller, Mitchell, Seminole, Terrell, Thomas and Worth. SCOA offers services and programs that serve many people including: Alzheimer's Caregivers Time Out (ACTO); Community Care Services Program (CCSP); Extra Mile Ramp Crew; Emergency Response System; Family Caregiver Program;ADRC/Gateway (Information & Referral); Georgia Cares; Home-Delivered Meals; Homemaker Services; Long Term Care Ombudsman; Retired Senior Volunteer Program; Senior Centers; Tax Aide Program and Senior Employment Program.

Year Founded: 1966

526 Social Security: Atlanta Disability Determination
PO Box 57
Stone Mountain, GA 30083-0057
678-639-2100
www.ssa.gov/atlanta/southeast

Evan Lucas, Manager

Social Security and Disability benefits

Hawaii

527 Assistive Technology Resource Centers of Hawaii
200 North Vineyard Blvd
Suite 430
Honolulu, HI 96817
808-532-7110
Fax: 808-532-7120; *Toll Free:* 800-645-3007
atrc-info@atrc.org
www.atrc.org

Barbara Fischlowitz-Leong, President, CEO
Jodi Asato, M.Ed, Vice President / Program Manager
Candice Young, Information and Outreach Special

Provides information and referral to anyone interested in assistive technology devices and services. Operates eight equipment loan banks. Provides training to consumer and professional groups including self-advocacy skills for consumers and family members. Works to ensure that schools, vocational rehabilitation agencies and health insurers provide assessments, funding and training in the use of assistive technology devices and services for their clients. Low-interest loan programs available.

528 Bureau of Naval Personnel: Hawaii Retired Activities Office
Fleet and Family Support Center
4825 Bougainville Drive
Honolulu, HI 96818-3174
808-474-1820
Fax: 808-474-1822
HawaiiHousing@Navy.mil
www.greatlifehawaii.com

Assistance is provided to retirees, their survivors and family members in obtaining their rights and benefits. The office also holds an Annual Retired Activities Seminar; and publishes a Retired Activities Biannual Newsletter.

529 County of Kauai, Agency on Elderly Affairs
4444 Rice Street
Suite 330
Lihue, HI 96766-1386
808-241-4470
Fax: 808-241-5113
elderlyaffairs@kauai.gov
www.kauaidrc.org

Kealoha Takahashi, Executive on Aging

Purpose is to plan, support, and advocate for programs to promote the well-being of Kauai's older adults and to address and respond to the priority needs of all seniors.

530 Disabilities & Communications Access Board
919 Ala Moana Boulevard
Room 101
Honolulu, HI 96814-4920
808-586-8121
Fax: 808-586-8129
dcab@doh.hawaii.gov
hawaii.gov/health/dcab

Francine Wai, Executive Director
Banjamin Cayetano, ADA Coordinator
Debbra Jackson, Planner

The Disability and Communication Access Board is comprised of seventeen volunteer members apponted by the Governor. Members include people with disabilities, parents, or guardians of persons with disabilities, public and private providers, of service, and other professionals with knowledge in the areas for which the Board has rulemaking authority.

531 Disability Determination Branch
State of Hawaii Dept of Human Services
PO Box 2458
Honolulu, HI 96804-2458
808-979-7000
Fax: 888-337-3910; *Toll Free:* 800-362-1526
www.ssa.gov

Vikki Nakamura, Branch Administrator
George Yamashiro, Professional Relations Officer

Determines eligibility for Social Security Disability Insurance benefits and Supplemental Security Income payments. DDb adjudicates and processes disability claims of Hawaii residents for SSDI authorized by Title II of the Social Security Act and SSI authorized by Title XVI of the Act.

532 Hawaii County Office of Aging
101 Aupuni Street
Suite 342
Hilo, HI 96720-4262
808-961-8600
Fax: 808-961-8603; *Toll Free:* 808-643-2372
hcoa@hcoahawaii.org
www.hcoahawaii.org/

Alan Parker, Director

Serves to represent the County of Hawaii in the planning, coordination, advocacy, and administration of programs for older persons in the county.

533 Hawaii Department of Defense: Office of Veterans Services
3949 Diamond Head Road
Honolulu, HI 96819
808-672-1201
Fax: 808-733-4238
dod@hawaii.gov
hawaii.gov/dod

Darryl Wong, Adjutant General

Objectives are to assist veterans in obtaining State and federal entitlements, to supply the latest information on veterans' issues and to provide advice and support to veterans making the transition back into civilian life.

534 Hawaii Department of Health: Commission on Persons with Disabilities
919 Ala Moana Boulevard
Suite 101
Honolulu, HI 96814-4920
808-586-4400
Fax: 808-586-8129
hawaii.gov/health

Loretta Fuddy, Executive Director

Public advocate of persons with disabilities by providing advice and recommendation on legislation, rules, policies, procedures, and plans relating to persons with disabilities and their civil rights or service needs.

535 Hawaii Department of Health: Disability and Communication Access Board
919 Ala Moana Boulevard
Room 101
Honolulu, HI 96814-4920
808-586-8121
Fax: 808-586-8129
dcab@doh.hawaii.gov
www.hawaii.gov/health/dcab
TDD 808-586-8130
TTY: 808-586-8121

Francine Wai, Executive Director

Provides information and referral on services for people with disabilities.

536 Hawaii Disability Rights Center
1132 Bishop Street
Suite 2102
Honolulu, HI 96813
808-949-2922
Fax: 808-949-2928; *Toll Free:* 800-882-1057
info@hawaiidisabilityrights.org
www.hawaiidisabilityrights.org

Louis Erteschik, Executive Director
Ann Collins, Operations Director
Mary Baca, Intake Advocate

HDRC is the designated Client Assist Program (CAP) and Protection and Advocacy (P&A) system for Hawaii's estimated 180,000 residents with disabilities. We strive to serve as many individuals with disabilities with as many different legal rights issues as our resources will allow.

537 Hawaii Planning Council on Developmental Disabilities
919 Ala Moana Boulevard
Suite 113
Honolulu, HI 96814-4920
808-586-8121
Fax: 808-586-8129
dcab@doh.hawaii.gov
www.hawaii.gov/health/dcab
TTY: 808-586-8121

Francine Wai, Executive Director
Susan Kawano, Secretary

Consists of 25 Hawaii residents appointed by the Governor. The council addresses the needs of the people with developmental disabilities: specifically, develops a state plan that sets the priorities for persons with developmental disabilities.

538 Hawaii State Council on Developmental Disabilities
919 Ala Moana Boulevard
Suite 113
Honolulu, HI 96814
808-586-8100
Fax: 808-586-7543
council@hiddc.org
www.hiddc.org

Waynette Cabral, Executive Administrator
Debbie Miyasaka-Gushiken, Community/Legislative Liason

The mission of the Council is to support with developmental disabilities to control their own destiny and determine the quality of life they desire.

539 Honolulu County Elderly Affairs Division
Standard Finance Building
715 South King Street
Suite 200
Honolulu, HI 96813-3021
808-768-7705
Fax: 808-527-6895
www.elderlyaffairs.com
TDD 808-527-6300

Wesley Lum, Director
Trina Adaro, Secretary

The Elderly Affairs Division (EAD) is an area agency on aging established by the Older Americans Act 1965. Serving Oahu, its mission is to develop systems of home and community-based services that assist older persons in leading independent, meaningful, and dignified lives.
Year Founded: 1973

540 Kauai County Office of Elderly Affairs
4444 Rice Street
Suite 150
Lihue, HI 96766-1386
808-241-4917
Fax: 808-241-5127
elderlyaffairs@kauai.gov
www.kauai.gov

Eleanor J Lloyd, Director

541 Maui County Office on Aging: Department of Housing and Human Concerns
2200 Main Street
Suite 547
Wailuku, HI 96793-2155
808-270-7775
Fax: 808-270-7870
www.co.maui.hi.us

Danny Mateo, Chairman
Joseph Pontanillo, Vice Chairman
Robert Carroll, Council Member

An Area Agency on Aging under the madates of the Older Americans Act reauthorized in 2000.

542 RSVP Hawaii County
127 Kamana Street
Hilo, HI 96720
808-961-8730
Fax: 808-961-8709
rsvp@co.hawaii.hi.us
www.hawaii-county.com

Edward Yokoyama, Director
Pamela Mizuno, Deputy Director

The Retired and Senior Volunteer Program (RSVP) provides opportunities for people 55 and over to make a difference in their community through volunteer service. RSVP volunteers contribute anywhere from a few to over forty hours a week, serving thourgh schools, day care centers, police departments, hospitals and other nonprofit and public organizations to help meet critical community needs. RSVP offers maximum flexibility and choice to its volunteers. RSVP matches the personal interests and skills to older Americans with opportunities to help solve community problems and offer supplemental insurance while on duty, on-the-job training from the agency or organization where volunteers are placed.

Idaho

543   CSI Office on Aging
College of Southern Idaho
PO Box 1238
315 Falls Avenue
Twin Falls, ID 83303-1238
208-736-2122
Fax: 208-736-2126; *Toll Free:* 800-574-8656
jfields@ooa.csi.edu
officeonaging.csi.edu/

Suzanne McCampbell, Director

Provides a one-stop service facility, to provide information and access to services for older people in the Magic Valley, which will help them to have a quality and independent life, with choice, dignity, and purpose.

544   Caribou County Senior Citizens Center
159 South Main
Soda Springs, ID 83276-1426
208-547-4324
www.co.caribou.id.us

Ronda South, Executive Director

Senior community center with home cooked meals, fresh baked goods, thrift store, and activities

545   Eastern Idaho Special Services: Area Agency on Aging
935 East Lincoln Road
Idaho Falls, ID 83402
208-522-5391
Fax: 208-522-5453; *Toll Free:* 800-632-4813
info@eicap.org
www.eicap.org

Russell Spain, Executive Director
Jay Doman, Finance Director
Melissa Krieger, Human Resources Director

An agency helping to empower all people in all communities to achieve maximum self-sufficiency and independence.

546   Idaho Commission on Aging
341 West Washington
Boise, ID 83702
208-334-3833
Fax: 208-334-3033; *Toll Free:* 800-926-2588
ICOA@aging.idaho.gov
www.idahoaging.com

Sam Hawes, Administrator

The Idaho Commission on Aging (ICOA) is the sole state agency designated under the Older Americans Act to administer programs and services for Idahoans 60 years of age and older.

Year Founded: 1965

547   Idaho Council on Developmental Disabilities
700 West State Street
1st Floor
Boise, ID 83702-5868
208-334-2178
Fax: 208-334-3417; *Toll Free:* 800-544-2433
info@icdd.idaho.gov
icdd.idaho.gov/
TDD 208-334-2179

Christine Pisani, Executive Director
Tracy Warren, Program Specialist/Planner
Toni Belknap-Brinegar, Program Specialist

The Council provides public education and awareness about developmental disabilities, promotes quality in-service supports for people with disabilities and their families; monitors and evaluates policies, plans and services provided by public agencies; encourages citizen participation in policymaking; and promotes innovative programs and projects through grants.

548   Idaho Developmental Disability Council
450 West State Street
9th Floor
Boise, ID 83720
208-334-0618
Fax: 208-334-3417; *Toll Free:* 800-356-9868
www.healthandwelfare.idaho.gov

Richard Armstrong, Director

Mission is to protect and promote the health, welfare and safety of Idahoans.

549   Idaho Division of Veterans Services
320 Collins Road
Boise, ID 83702
208-334-5000
Fax: 208-334-2627
www.veterans.idaho.gov

Dave Brasuell, Division Administrator

Dedicated to serving Idaho's veterans and their families by providing superior advocacy, excellent assistance with benefits and education, high quality long-term care, and respectful interment services in a dignified final resting place.7

550   Idaho Industrial Commission
PO Box 83720
Boise, ID 83720-0041
208-334-6000
Fax: 208-334-2321
www.iic.idaho.gov

Thomas P Baskin, Chairman

Regulates Idsho workers compensation. Offers rehabilitation to workers injured in idaho.

551   Idaho Mental Health Center
1720 Westgate Drive
PO Box 83720
Boise, ID 83704-7164

208-334-0800
Fax: 208-334-0828; Toll Free: 800-356-9868
www.healthandwelfare.idaho.gov

Richard Armstrong, Director
Leslie Clement, Deputy Director
Drew Hall, Deputy Director

The Idaho Department of Health and Welfare's prgrams and services are designed to help people live healthy and be productive, strengthening individuals, families and communities.

552   Idaho State Tax Commission
PO Box 36
Boise, ID 83722
208-334-7660; *Toll Free: 800-972-7660*
valerie.dilley@tax.idaho.gov
tax.idaho.gov

Rich Jackson, Chairman
Tom Katsilometes, Commissioner
David Langhorst, Commissioner

Mission is to provide courteous, quality services and to administer the state's tax laws in a fair, timely, and cost effective manner to benefit Idaho and its citizens.

553   North Idaho College: Area Agency on Aging
2120 Lakewood Drive
Suite B
Coeur d'Alene, ID 83814
208-667-3179
Fax: 208-667-5938; Toll Free: 800-786-5536
infoassist@aaani.org
www.aaani.org

Pearl Bouchard, AAS Director
Bobbie Sailor, Assistant Director

Dedicated to protection, independence and dignity of individuals through advocacy and service.

554   RSVP Lewiston
1424 Main Street
Lewiston, ID 83501-1907
208-746-7787
Fax: 208-743-9573
www.newlifestyles.com/facility

Eva Mathewson, Director
Barbara Bush, Executive Director

Most of our senior volunteers are involved with recycling, including four who haul recycle materials to drop points. We have several who beautify and educate as Master Gardeners and others who work to keep the public flower beds maintained in a small town. We have volunteers involved and educating at local museums, our county extension agency, and working for Habitat for Humanity. The following Counties are served: Clearwater, Idaho, Latah, Lewis, Nez Perce.

555   RSVP Magic Valley
Souther Idaho College/The Corp Nat'l & Comm. Servi
315 Falls Avenue
PO Box 1238
Twin Falls, ID 83303
208-736-2122
Fax: 208-736-2126; Toll Free: 800-574-8656
Info@ooa.csi.edu
officeonaging.csi.edu/rsvp

Suzanne McCampbell, Director
Edith Ward, RSVP West End Coordinator
Kitty K Andrews, RSVP East End Coordinator

The Retired and Senior Volunteer Program (RSVP) invites adults age 55 and over to use their life experience and job-related skills to answer the call of their neighbors in need. Giving anywhere from a few to over forty hours per week, RSVP volunteers help solve serious problems in their communities.

556   Sage Community Resources
Idaho Council of Governments
125 East 50th Street
Garden City, ID 83714
208-322-7033
Fax: 208-322-3569; Toll Free: 800-859-0324
info@idahocog.com
www.idahocog.com/

Gordon Cruickshank, Chair
Kendra Kenyon, President
Judy Peavey-Derr, Vice-Chair

Serves as an umbrella for a variety of agencies that have a regional forces. Currently houses the Area Agency Task Force, Economic Development Region District Region III, and the Idaho Hunger Task Force

Illinois

557   American Association of Retired Persons: Midwest Region Office
300 West Edwards Street
3rd Floor
Springfield, IL 32704
Fax: 217-552-7803; Toll Free: 866-448-3613
aarpil@aarp.org
www.aarp.org
TTY: 916-446-2680

Judy Comstock, Director

A resource for AARP members in the states of Illinois, Indiana, Iowa, Michigan, Minnesota, Nebraska, North Dakota, Ohio, South Dakota, and Wisconsin. Hours 9-5, Monday through Friday.

558   Attorney General's Office: Disability Rights Bureau
100 W Randolph Street
Chicago, IL 60601-3218
312-814-3000
Fax: 312-814-1656; Toll Free: 800-964-3013
www.ag.state.il.us

Lisa Madigan, Attorney General

Information on Illinois' Comprehensive Health Insurance Plan and architectural accessibility. Enforcement of Illinois' access law and standards. Information on initiatives such as: 'Opening the Courthouse Doors to People with Disabilities;' accessing effective communication in a medical setting and addressing the abuse, neglect or financial exploitation of people with disabilities. Other information and referrals.

559   Coles County Council on Aging
11021 East Co. Road
800 N
Charleston, IL 61920

217-639-5150
Fax: 217-639-5199
lifespancenter@colescouncilonaging.org
www.colescouncilonaging.org

Janet Grove, President
Dee Braden, Executive Director
Michael Murray, Vice President

The mission of the Coles County Council on Aging is to enhance quality of life by promoting independence, dignity, self-fulfillment and health for older adults in Coles County through advocacy, education and provision of appropriate community-based services.

560 Coles County Telecare
Coles County Council on Aging
11021 East Co. Road, 800 N
Charleston, IL 61920
217-639-5150
Fax: 217-639-5199
lifespancenter@colescouncilonaging.org
www.colescouncilonaging.org

Janet Grove, President
Dee Braden, Executive Director
Michael Murray, Vice President

Senior infromation and assistance Assist with filling out forms, giving information and reffering to other agencies.

561 Community Health Charities of Illinois
525 West Monroe Street
Suite 900
Chicago, IL 60661
312-382-0198
Fax: 312-382-0197; *Toll Free:* 800-299-6842
info@healthcharities.org
www.healthcharitiesillinois.org

David Selzer, President/CEO
Elizabeth Stremel, Vice President
Matte Dewyer, Director

The mission of Community Health Charities is to provide every employee the opportunity to support medical research, health education and patient services through charitable giving in the workplace. Our goal is to advise employers and individuals the convenience of 'one-stop' health support, but with the ability to direct donations to the specific member health charities that you want to support. Contributions are used for research, patient services, and education.

562 Dial-A-Ride Rural Public Transportation
Coles County Council on Aging
11021 East Co. Rd, 800 N
Charleston, IL 61920
217-639-5169
Fax: 217-639-5199; *Toll Free:* 800-500-5505
lifespancenter@colescouncilonaging.org
www.colescouncilonaging.org

Janet Grove, President
Dee Braden, Executive Director
Michael Murray, Vice President

Provides transportation not only to older adults, but also to persons with disabilities and all age groups of the general public. The program, which currently owns eleven wheelchair accessible buses, offers Coles County residents access to community resources while promoting independence and mobility.

563 East Central Illinois: Area Agency on Aging
1003 Maple Hill Road
Bloomington, IL 61704-9327
309-829-2065
Fax: 309-829-6021; *Toll Free:* 800-888-4456
aginginfo@eciaaa.org
www.eciaaa.org

Michael J O'Donnell, Executive Director
Susan H Redman, Deputy Director

A non-profit organization authorized to plan and administer services to enable older adults to live in their homes with dignity and safety as long as possible with appropriate supportive services, prevent unnecessary institutionalization and uphold their rights.

564 Egyptian: Area Agency on Aging
200 E Plaza Drive
Carterville, IL 62918-1982
618-985-8311
Fax: 618-985-8315; *Toll Free:* 888-895-3306
www.egyptianaaa.org

John M Smith, Executive Director
K Velarde, Fiscal Manager
G Johnston, Program Manager

As Area Agencies in Illiois it is our mission to promote the well-being of senior adults and assisting them in maintaining their independence in the community.

565 Equip for Equality Central/Southern Illinois
300 East Main Street
Suite 18
Carbondale, IL 62901
618-457-7930
Fax: 618-457-7985; *Toll Free:* 800-758-0464
contactus@equipforequality.org
www.equipforequality.org
TTY: 800-610-2779

Duane C Quaini, Chairperson
Zena Naiditch, President and CEO
Jeannine M Coredero, Vice Chairperson

The mission of Equip for Equality is to advance the human and civil rights of children and adults with physical and mental disabilities in Illinois. It is the only statewide, cross-disability, comprehensive advocacy organization providing self-advocacy assistance, legal services, and disability rights education while also engaging in public policy and legislative advocacy and conducting abuse investigations and other oversight activities.

Year Founded: 1985

566 Equip for Equality Northeastern Region
20 North Michigan Avenue
Suite 300
Chicago, IL 60602
312-341-0022
Fax: 312-541-7544; *Toll Free:* 800-537-2632
contactus@equipforequality.org
www.equipforequality.org
TTY: 800-610-2779

Duane C Quaini, Chairperson
Zena Naiditch, President and CEO
Jeannine M Coredero, Vice Chairperson

The mission of Equip for Equality is to advance the human and civil rights of children and adults with physical and mental disabilities in Illinois. It is the only statewide, cross-disability, comprehensive advocacy organization providing self-advocacy assistance, legal services, and disability rights education while also engaging in public policy and legislative advocacy and conducting abuse investigations and other oversight activities.

Year Founded: 1985

567 Equip for Equality Northwestern Region
1515 Fifth Avenue
Suite 420
Moline, IL 61265
309-786-6868
Fax: 309-797-8710; *Toll Free:* 800-758-6869
contactus@equipforequality.org
www.equipforequality.org
TTY: 800-610-2779

Duane C Quaini, Chairperson
Zena Naiditch, President and CEO
Jeannine M Coredero, Vice Chairperson

The mission of Equip for Equality is to advance the human and civil rights of children and adults with physical and mental disabilities in Illinois. It is the only statewide, cross-disability, comprehensive advocacy organization providing self-advocacy assistance, legal services, and disability rights education while also engaging in public policy and legislative advocacy and conducting abuse investigations and other oversight activities.

Year Founded: 1985

568 Family Caregiver Resource Center
Coles County Council on Aging
11021 East Co. Road
800 N
Charleston, IL 61920
217-639-5150
Fax: 217-639-5199
lifespancenter@colescouncilonaging.org
www.colescouncilonaging.org

Janet Grove, President
Dee Braden, Executive Director
Michael Murray, Vice President

Provides information and support to persons caring for individuals over sixty years of age, and grandparents raising grandchildren, through counseling services, support groups, training workshops, literature and other resources.

569 Homemaker Program
Coles County Council on Aging
11021 East Co. Road
800 N
Charleston, IL 61920
217-639-5150
Fax: 217-639-5199
lifespancenter@colescouncilonaging.org
www.colescouncilonaging.org

Janet Grove, President
Dee Braden, Executive Director
Michael Murray, Vice President

Provides a variety of personal assistance services to eligible individuals. These services include housekeeping, errands, respite, laundry, meal preparation, personal care tasks, and home budgeting and money management. Through the provision of these services older adults are enabled to remain in their homes safely, and prevent or postpone unnecessary or premature institutionalization.

570 Illinios Department of Revenue
101 W Jefferson Street
Springfield, IL 62702-5145
217-782-3128
www.revenue.state.il.us

Brian Hamer, Director
Vacant , Assistant Director
Ruby Taylor, EEO Officer

To maximize the collections of revenues for the state of Illinois and effectively regulate the manufacture, distribution and sale of alcoholic beverages; all in a manner that promotes fair and consistent enforcement of state laws.

571 Illinois Assistive Technology Project
1 West Old State Capitol Plaza
Suite 100
Springfield, IL 62701-1224
217-522-7985
Fax: 217-522-8067; *Toll Free:* 800-852-5110
iatp@iltech.org
www.iltech.org
TTY: 217-522-9966

Wilhelmina Gunther, Executive Director
Shelly Lowe, Finance/Personnel Manager
Barbara Howell, Administrative Assistant

Directed by and for people with disabilities and their family members. As a federally mandated program, IATP strives to break down barriers and change policies that make getting and using technology difficult. IATP offers solutions to help people find what is available in products and services that will best meet their needs, where to find it, and how to get it.

572 Illinois Council on Developmental Disability
100 W Randolph Street
Suite 10-600
Chicago, IL 60601
312-814-2080
Fax: 312-814-7441
sromano@mail.state.il.us
www.state.il.us/agency/icdd
TTY: 888-261-2717

Sheila T Romano EdD, Executive Director
Sandy Thurston Ryan, Director Program/Planning

ICDD is responsible for investing in new programs to improve the delivery of services and supports to individuals with developmental disabilities and their families in Illinois. The Council focuses on education, employment, transportation, community living, health care and other areas so that people with developmental disabilities can enjoy their lives to the fullest extent possible. Just as importantly, ICDD works to build the capabilities of individuals, families and communities, enabling each to become more self-sufficient through the Developmental Disabilities Assistance and Bill of Rights Act (DD Act).

573 Illinois Department of Human Services: Office of Rehabilitation Services
100 South Grand Avenue East
Springfield, IL 62762
217-782-2000
Fax: 217-785-5753; *Toll Free:* 800-843-6154
dhs.ors@illinois.gov
www.dhs.state.il.us
TTY: 217-557-2134

Michelle R B Saddler, Secretary

Mission is to assist our customers to achieve maximum self-sufficiency, independence and health through the provision of seamless, integrated services for individuals, families and communities.

574 Illinois Department of Mental Health and Developmental Disabilities
319 East Madison
Suite 4 N
Springfield, IL 62762
217-524-7065
Fax: 217-557-6856; *Toll Free:* 800-843-6154
www.dhs.state.il.us
TTY: 217-557-2134

Kevin Casey, Director

Provides leadership for the effective management of the design and delivery of quality outcome-based, person-centered services and supports for individuals who have developmental disabilitites. These services and supports will be appropriate to their needs, gifts, talents and strengths; accessible; life-spanning; based on informed choice; and monitored to ensure individual progress, quality of life, and safety.

575 Illinois Department of Rehabilitation Services
PO Box 19250
Springfield, IL 62794-9250
217-782-2000
Fax: 217-785-1574; *Toll Free:* 800-843-6154
dhs.org@illinois.gov
www.dhs.state.il.us
TTY: 800-447-6404

Dorothy Homeier, Chief Program Services

The state's lead agency serving individuals with disabilities. DRS works in partnership with people with disabilities and their families to assist them in making informed choices to achieve full community participation through employment, education, and independent living opportunities.

576 Illinois Department of Veterans Affairs
833 South Spring Street
Po Box 19432
Springfield, IL 62794-9432
217-782-6641
Fax: 217-524-0344; *Toll Free:* 800-437-9824
webmail@dva.state.il.us
www.state.il.us/agency/dva

Erica Borggren, Director
Rodrigo Garcia, Assistant Director

Mission is to assist veterans and their dependents and survivors in obtaining the benefits they are entitled to under the laws of the United States, and the State of Illinois, or any other governmental agency

577 Illinois Department on Aging
One Natural Resources Way
Suite 100
Springfield, IL 62702-1271
217-785-3356
Fax: 217-785-4477; *Toll Free:* 800-252-8966
ilsenior@aging.state.il.us
www.state.il.us/aging
TDD 800-252-8966
TTY: 888-206-1327

John K Holton, Director
Mary Killough, Deputy Director
Vacant , Chief of Staff

Serves and advocates for older Illinoisans and their caregivers by administering programs and promoting partnerships that encourage independence, dignity and quality of life.

578 Life Services Network of Illinois: Springfield
2 Lawrence Square
Springfield, IL 62704-2581
217-789-1677
Fax: 217-789-1778
info@lsni.org
www.lsni.org

Kathy Burke, Director of Business Development
Danyale Coleman, Confidence Satisfaction Surveys
Leslie Green, Director Quality, Advocacy & Tec

Life Services Network of Illinois (LSN), a statewide trade association, has represented providers of the complete continuum of services for older adults, including nursing facilities, assisted living, senior housing and home and community based services. Our success as an association is founded in our commitment to helping our members overcome obstacles while identifying future opportunities for their success. This philosophy is what makes LSN and our members unique and successful.

579 Lifescape Community Services
705 Kilburn Avenue
Rockford, IL 61101-6537
518-430-1218
Fax: 815-963-1627; *Toll Free:* 800-779-1189
marketing@lifescapeservices.com
www.lifescapeservices.com

Carol Green, Executive Director

To promote independent living and enhance the quality of life for individuals by providing affordable nutrition and other services, with an emphasis on the aging population.

580 Lincolnland: Area Agency on Aging
3100 Montvale Drive
Springfield, IL 62704
217-787-9234
Fax: 217-787-6290; *Toll Free:* 800-252-2918
info@aginglinc.org
www.aginglinc.org

Julie Hubbard, Executive Director

The Area Agency on Aging for Lincolnland is dedicated to helping older adults maintain dignity, health, and independence. Many services and programs are offered to support older adults and family caregivers in a twelve county area.

581 Little Brothers: Friends of the Elderly
Chicago Chapter
355 North Ashland Avenue
Chicago, IL 60607-1019
312-455-1000
Fax: 312-455-9674
general@littlebrotherschicago.org
www.littlebrothers.org

Nicholas Delgado, Chairman
Robin Tillotson, Vice President
Marilyn Hennessey, Treasurer

Provides companionship and special assistance to low-income individuals over 70 years of age.

Year Founded: 1959

582 Mattoon Area Senior Center: Coles Council on Aging

204 S 21st Street
Mattoon, IL 61938-3869
217-234-3311
Fax: 217-234-3410
lifespancenter@colescouncilonaging.org
www.colescouncilonaging.org

Janet Grove, President
Dee Braden, Executive Director
Michael Murray, Vice President

The senior centers provide area older adults not only a place to meet, share and learn from others, but also opportunities to grow, develop and achieve. The centers also are a source for information. A wide variety of recreational and educational programs are routinely offered at the two senior centers. Both centers also serve as congregate meal sites for EIU's Peace Meal program.

583 Midland: Area Agency on Aging

PO Box 1420
434 S. Poplar St
Centralia, IL 62801-9121
618-532-1853
Fax: 618-532-5259; *Toll Free:* 800-252-8966
www.midlandaaa.org
TTY: 800-252-8966

Tracy Barczewski, Executive Director
Sylvia Mahle, Community Services Coordinator
Elaine Baker, Fiscal Manager

To determine the service needs of senior citizens, develop programs, provide funding to local community agencies, develop other resources to help meet service needs, serve as the local focal point on senior citizen issues int he area, act as advocates on behalf of senior citizens and disseminate information.

584 Northeastern Illinois: Area Agency on Aging

245 West Roosevelt Road
Bldg 6, Suite 41
West Chicago, IL 60185
815-939-0727
Fax: 815-939-0022; *Toll Free:* 800-528-2000
info@ageguide.org
ageguide.org

Lucia West Jones, Executive Director
Dawn Simon, Office Manager
Linda Williamson, Administrative Assistant

A not-for-profit agency that plans and coordinates a comprehensive network of services for persons 60+ in the fastest growing areas in the State.

Year Founded: 1974

585 Northwestern Illinois: Area Agency on Aging

1111 South Aplpine Road
Suite 600
Rockford, IL 61108-1652
815-226-4901
Fax: 815-226-8984; *Toll Free:* 800-542-8402
info@nwilaaa.org
www.nwilaaa.org

Grant Myhammer, Executive Director

Mission is to enable older persons to live with dignity and independence. NIAAA collaborates with agencies, businesses, faith communities, and individuals to improve the quality of life for older persons and their caregivers.

586 RSVP Joliet

203 N Ottawa Street
Joliet, IL 60432-4006
815-723-3405
Fax: 815-723-3452
www.cc-doj.org

Sr Ellen Thomas, Director
Kathy McGowan, Executive Director

Helping people age 55 and older find volunteer opportunities in their home and communities by matching their personal interests and experience with the needs of an organization. The following Counties are served: Cook, Dupage, Ford, Grundy, Kendall, Kankakee, Iroquois, Will.

Year Founded: 1949

587 RSVP Kane McHenry Counties

3519 North Richmond Road
McHenry, IL 60051
815-344-3555
Fax: 815-344-3593
help@seniorservicesassoc.org
seniorservicesassoc.org

Tom Van Cleave, President
Linda Longmeyer, Vice President

RSVP engages people age 55 and older in a diverse range of volunteer activities including food pantries, transporting homebound seniors, and delivering meals.

Year Founded: 1973

588 RSVP Maple Lawn

700 N Main Street
Eureka, IL 61530-1085
309-467-2337
Fax: 309-467-9011
www.maple-lawn.com

Donald Litwiller, Chairman
Dave Neuhausser, Vice Chair
Chuck Staley, Treasurer

The program is relatively new. Currently, our volunteers are working on doing repairs and weatherizing the homes of elderly and disabled people in our community. The following Counties are served: Livingston, Marshall, Woodford.

589 RSVP Peoria/Tazewell Counties

814 N.E. Madison Avenue
Peoria, IL 61603-1038
309-682-8521
Fax: 309-682-8524
rsvp@rsvpvolunteers.org
www.rsvpvolunteers.org

Jan Sweikert, Director

The Retired and Senior Volunteer Program (RSVP) provides opportunities for people 55 and over to make a difference in their community through volunteer service. RSVP volunteers contribute anywhere from a few to over forty hours a week, serving thourgh schools, day care centers, police departments, hospitals and other nonprofit and public organizations to help meet critical community needs.

RSVP offers maximum flexibility and choice to its volunteers. RSVP matches the personal interests and skills to older Americans with opportunities to help solve community problems and offer supplemental insurance while on duty, on-the-job training from the agency or organization where volunteers are placed.

590 RSVP Triton College Volunteer Program
2000 Fifth Avenue
River Grove, IL 60171-1907
708-456-0300
Fax: 708-583-3778
www.triton.edu/rsvp.aspx

Geraldine Lustro, Program Assistant
Minerva McLaren, Volunteer Coordinator
Kay Frey, Director

RSVP (Triton College Volunteer Program) is a unique nationwide volunteer program sponsored locally by Triton College. It offers active adults the opportunity to use their talents and experience in service to the community. Public and nonprofit organizations urgently need people who are willing to share their interests and skills with others. RSVP members are able to serve on a monthly or weekly basis. You may be able to serve in one or more ongoing efforts. The number of hours you serve is flexible (the average is one to four hours a week). These hours make a big difference to those you help.

591 RSVP YWCA Senior Services
2025 M Street, NW
Suite 550
Washington, DC 20036
202-467-0801
Fax: 202-467-0802
info@ywca.org
www.ywca.org

Paula Penebaker, Chair
Azuri Gonzalez, Vice Chair/Secretary
Janet Marcotte, Treasurer

YWCA-RSVP helps individuals age 55 and older put their skills and life experiences to work for their community. RSVP facilitates senior volunteerism through carefully matched placement and follow-up support.

Year Founded: 1866

592 Rachel's Place Adult Day Care
309 West Park
Aurora, IL 60506
630-896-9022; *Toll Free: 888-787-4619*
answers@ourparents.com
www.ourparents.com

Adult day service provides a protective and stimulating environment for older adults who are in need of daytime supervision. The elderly profit from the array of services offered, while their caregivers receive respite from the pressures and demands of caring for an elderly relative or friend. Participants benefit from a structured environment, companionship, nutritious meals and a variety of activities under the supervision of professional staff.

593 Railroad Retirement Board: Chicago District Office
844 N Rush Street
9th Floor
Chicago, IL 60611-2092

312-751-4500
Fax: 312-751-7136
chicago@rrb.gov
www.rrb.gov
TTY: 312-751-4701

Michael Schwartz, Chairman
Nancy Pittman, Chairman Assistant
Stephen Seiple, Chairman Counsel

An independent agency in the executive branch of the Federal Government. The primary function is to administer comprehensive retirement-survivor and unemployment sickness benefit programs for the nation's railroad workers and their families

594 Railroad Retirement Board: Decatur District Office
132 S Water Street
Suite 517
Decatur, IL 62523-1397
Fax: 217-423-7872; *Toll Free: 877-772-5772*
decatur@rrb.gov
www.rrb.gov

Sherry M Strocher, District Manager

An independent agency in the executive branch of the Federal Government. Its primary function is to administer comprehensive retirement-survivor and unemployment sickness benefit programs for the nation's railroad workers and their families.

595 Railroad Retirement Board: Survivor Division Bureau of Survivor Benefits
844 N Rush Street
Chicago, IL 60611-1275
312-787-3923; *Toll Free: 877-772-5772*
www.rrb.gov

Provides assistance to widows of railroad workers.

596 Retired & Senior Volunteer Program of Northern DuPage Counties
2121 S Goebbert
Arlington Hights, IL 60005-1814
847-228-1320
Fax: 847-228-1327
volunteer@volunteerinfo.net
www.handsonsuburbanchicago.org/

Kevin O'Connell, Board President
Chris Smith, Executive Director
Sarah Maple, Program Support Administrator

Help people age 55 and over find volunteer opportunities in their community. We match skills and interests for meaninful assignments.

597 Senior Services of Central Illinois
701 W Mason Street
Springfield, IL 62702-2498
217-528-4035
Fax: 217-528-9322
www.ssoci.org

Karen Schainker, Executive Director
Angela M Oliver, Development Director
Deborah Murphy, Fiscal Manager

Specializes in non-medical services to individuals age 60+ nutrition, transportation, counseling, information, elder abuse/crime support, volunteer opportunities, and programs/activities, which prevent premature institutionalization. The following Counties are served: Logan, Mason, Menard, Sangamon.

598 Services for Adults Staying in Their Homes (SASI)
1123 Emerson Street
Suite 200
Evanston, IL 60201
847-864-7274
Fax: 847-864-7295
info@sasiathome.org
www.sasiathome.org

Jeanie Ramsey, Executive Director
Torry Hickey, Program Manager, Home Care
Jonathan Tague, Program Manager, Sr. Connections

Provides employee caregivers to older adults who, due to aging, illness, or injury need assistance at home. SASI also has volunteers who are friendly visitors to isolated older adults.

Year Founded: 1976

599 Shawnee Development Council
530 West Washington Street
PO Box 298
Karnak, IL 62956-0298
618-634-2201
Fax: 618-634-9551; Toll Free: 800-526-0844
sdcinc@shawneedevelopment.org
www.shawneedevelopment.org

Cheryl Vanderford, Executive Director

Provides a variety of volunteer opportunities for retired persons aged 55 and older to participate more fully in the life of their community through significant volunteer service. The program encourages older adults to remain active by utilizing their skills, experience and talents to the benefit of others.

600 Southeastern Illinois: Area Agency on Aging
516 Market Street
Mount Carmel, IL 52863-1558
612-262-2306
Fax: 618-262-4967; Toll Free: 800-635-8544
www.seiaoa.com

Shana A Holmes, Executive Director
Rita Palmer, Program Manager
Christine Baize, Fiscal Manager

Our mission is to serve and advocate for older Illinoisans and their caregivers by administering programs and promoting partnerships that encourage independence, dignity, and quality of life. Counties served: Crawford, Edwards, Hamilton, Jasper, Lawrence, Richland, Wabash, Wayne, and White.

601 Southwestern Illinois: Area Agency on Aging
2365 Country Road
Belleville, IL 62221-2571
618-222-2561
Fax: 618-222-2567; Toll Free: 800-326-3221
ask@answersonaging.com
www.answersonaging.com
TTY: 800-222-2570

Joy Paeth, Chief Executive Officer
Tara Stancil, Volunteer Coordinator

Our mission is to serve and advocate for older Illinoisans and their caregivers by administering programs and pro-

moting partnerships that encourage independence, dignity, and quality of life. Counties served: Bond, Clinton, Madison, Monroe, Randolph, St. Clair, and Washington.

602 Springfield Social Security DisabilityDetermination
Dpeartment of Human Services
PO Box 19250
Springfield, IL 62794-9250
217-785-0218; Toll Free: 800-225-3607
www.ssa.gov/chicago/dds.htm
TTY: 217-782-5734

Ann P Robert, Deputy Director

The Social Security Disability program provides benefits to persons with severe disabilities whose impairments prevent them form performing gainful work.

603 U.S. Railroad Retirement Board: Joliet District Office
63 W Jefferson Street
Suite 102
Joliet, IL 60432
Fax: 815-740-2139; Toll Free: 877-772-5772
joliet@rrb.gov
www.rrb.gov

Bernadette Roddy, Claims Representative
Sheila Rucker, Claims Representative
Natalie Horvath, Claims Representative

Federal agency administering the RR Retirement Act N,E, ILL suburbs.

604 West Central Illinois: Area Agency on Aging
639 York Street
PO Box 428
Quincy, IL 62306-0428
217-223-5700
Fax: 217-222-1220; Toll Free: 800-252-9027
info@wciagingnetwork.org
www.wciagingnetwork.org

Lynn Niewohner, Director

Our mission is to serve and advocate for older Illinoisans and their caregivers by administering programs and promoting partnerships that encourage independence, dignity, and quality of life.

605 Western Illinois Area: Agency on Aging
729 34th Avenue
Rock Island, IL 61201-5911
309-793-6800
Fax: 309-793-6807; Toll Free: 800-322-1051
www.wiaaa.org/
TDD 309-793-6800

Greta Brooks, Director

Our mission is to server and advocate for older Illinoisans and their caregivers by administering programs and promoting partnerships that encourage independence, dignity, and quality of life.

Year Founded: 1973

Indiana

606 Adams County Council on Aging
313 W Jefferson Street
Decatur, IN 46733-1656

260-724-5300
accoa@onlyinternet.net
www.co.adams.in.us

Sharon Tester, Director

Provides information and referral, transportation assistance, outreach, and advocacy to individuals over 60 years of age.

607 Aging and Community Service of South Central Indiana
1531 13th Street
Suite G900
Columbus, IN 47201-1302
812-372-6918
Fax: 812-372-7846; *Toll Free:* 866-644-6407
Contact@thrive-alliance.org
www.agingandcommunityservices.org

Diane Cantrell, Director

Plan, develop and coordinate a comprehensive system of services for the elderly and disabled persons at risk of institutionalization.

Year Founded: 1981

608 Aging and In-Home Services
2927 Lake Avenue
Fort Wayne, IN 46805-5414
260-745-1200
Fax: 260-422-4916; *Toll Free:* 800-552-3662
info@agingihs.org
www.agingihs.org

Heidi Adair, Chairperson
Keith Huffman, Elder Law Attorney
Sarah Earls, VP, Controller

The mission of Aging and In-Home Services of Northeast Indiana is to promote independence, dignity, and advocacy for all older adults and persons with disabilities. Counties served: Adams, Allen, DeKalb, Huntington, LaGrange, Noble, Steuben, Wells and Whitley.

609 Area 1 Northwest Indiana Community Action Corp.
5240 Fountain Drive
Crown Point, IN 46307
219-794-1829
Fax: 219-931-5501; *Toll Free:* 800-826-7871
director@nwi-ca.com
www.nwi-ca.com
TTY: 888-814-7597

Dr. Karen Evans, Board President
Gary Olund, President/CEO
Jennifer Malone, Chief Operating Officer

Mission is to help people to be independent and advocate for those who can't.

610 Area 10 Agency on Aging
631 West Edgewood Drive
Ellettsville, IN 47429
812-876-1079
Fax: 812-876-9922; *Toll Free:* 800-844-1010
area10@area10agency.org
www.area10agency.org

Kerry Conway, Executive Director
Mary Boutain, Strategic Initiatives Director
Natalie LeBeau, Financial Director

Multi service agency for Older Americans in Monroe and Owen Counties. Information and Assistance, Home and Community Based Services, Caregiver Support, Transportation, plus Health and Nutrition, Fitness and Housing. Respecting the dignity and independence of each individual.

Year Founded: 1981

611 Area 12 Council on Aging: Lifetime Resources
13091 Benedict Drive
Dillsboro, IN 47018
812-432-6200
Fax: 812-432-3822; *Toll Free:* 800-742-5001
www.lifetime-resources.org

Sally Beckley, Director

Programs are designed to meet the growing needs of people in the communities we serve. Senior citizens, individuals with disabilities, caregivers, concerned neighbors, and the community at large will find services, resources or referrals to meet their needs.

Year Founded: 1974

612 Area 13 Agency on Aging: Generations
1019 N 4th Street
Po Box 314
Vincennes, IN 47591-2355
812-888-5880
Fax: 812-888-4568; *Toll Free:* 800-742-9002
generations@vinu.edu
www.generationsnetwork.org

Laura Holscher, Executive Director
Geri Webster, Fiscal Director
Stacey Kahre, Director of Client Services

Provides case management, information, and referrals to various services for persons who are aging or developmentally disabled.

Year Founded: 1975

613 Area 15 Hoosier Uplands Agency on Aging
500 West Main Street
Mitchell, IN 47446-1410
812-849-4457
Fax: 812-849-6785; *Toll Free:* 800-827-2219
area15@hoosieruplands.org
www.hoosieruplands.org

David Miller, CEO
Barbara Tarr, Aging Director

A local non-profit agency based in southern Indiana that serves as an Area Agency on Aging, Community Action Agency, licensed Home Health Care and Hospital Care and Hospice agency, and Community Housing Development Organization.

Year Founded: 1966

614 Area 2 Agency on Aging: Real Services
1151 S Michigan Street
South Bend, IN 46601
574-284-2644
Fax: 574-284-2691; *Toll Free:* 800-552-7928
info@realservices.org
www.realservicesinc.com

Steven Watts, Chairperson
Becky Zaseck, President / CEO
Mary Downes, Treasurer

Provides in-home and community services to the elderly, disabled and low-income.

Year Founded: 1966

615 Area 5 Agency on Aging and Community Services
1801 Smith Street
Logansport, IN 46947-2152
574-722-4451
Fax: 219-722-3447; *Toll Free:* 800-654-9421
areafive@areafive.com
www.areafive.com

Michael Meagher, Executive Director
Ellen Zimmerman, Aging Director

An independent not-for-profit organization, governed by a volunteer board of directors, dedicated to meeting the needs of the elderly, disabled, and disadvantaged members of the communities we serve.

Year Founded: 1974

616 Area 9 Agency on Aging: Home and Community Services Agency
520 S 9th St
Richmond, IN 47374-4227
765-966-1795
Fax: 765-962-1190; *Toll Free:* 800-458-9345
area9@iue.edu
www.iue.edu/area9/

Tony Shepherd, Executive Director
Kathy Bridgford, Director Of Administration
Brian Weaver, ADRC Director

To assist older persons and disabled individuals of all ages in leading independent, meaningful and dignified lives in their own homes and communities for as long as possible.

Year Founded: 1975

617 Central Indiana Council on Aging
4755 Kingsway Drive
Suite 200
Indianapolis, IN 46205-1560
317-254-5465
Fax: 317-254-5494; *Toll Free:* 800-489-9550
contact@cicoa.org
www.cicoa.org

Mary Beth Tuohy, Chair
Orion Bell IV, President/CEO
Laura Boyle, SVP Client Services

Helps build communities that enable older persons and those of any age with a disability to live with the greatest possible independence, dignity and quality of life.

Year Founded: 1974

618 Environmental Alliance for SeniorInvolvement
PO Box 250
Milford, CT 06460
203-779-0024
Fax: 203-779-0025
easi.org

Kent Lizer, President

This program, made possible by the Corporation for National and Community Service, provides funding and support for selected older Americans to serve as technical and administrative consultants to organizations around the United States in establishing self sufficient Senior Environment Corps.

Year Founded: 1991

619 Indiana Aging Division
PO Box 7083
402 West Washington, MS21 Room W-454
Indianapolis, IN 46207-7083
317-233-4454
Fax: 317-233-4693
www.in.gov/fssa

Faith Laird, Director
Susan Waschevski, Deputy Director
Karen Filler, Deputy Director

The Indiana Division of Aging (IDA) provides a broad range of in-home and community based services to older adults and persons of all ages with disabilities. Services provided focus on prevention, early intervention, protection and advocacy. The Division collaborates with communities, local organizations, and other units of government to provide services to individuals and their families.

620 Indiana Association of Area Agencies on Aging Aging and Community Services
1531 13th Street, Suite G900
Columbus, IN 47201-1302
812-372-6918
Fax: 812-372-7846; *Toll Free:* 866-644-6407
Contact@thrive-alliance.org
www.agingandcommunityservices.org

Diane Cantrell, Executive Director

The Indiana Association of Area Agency on Aging (IAAAA) advocates for quality programs and services for older adults and persons with disabilities.

Year Founded: 1981

621 Indiana Department of Aging and Community Services
1531 13th Street
Suite G900
Columbus, IN 47201
812-372-6918
Fax: 812-372-7846; *Toll Free:* 866-644-6407
Contact@thrive-alliance.org
www.agingandcommunitysevices.org

Cathy Boggs, Executive Director

Offers information on state-wide programs for the elderly.

Year Founded: 1981

622 Indiana Department of Health Veteran's Home
2 North Meridian Street
Indianapolis, IN 46204
317-233-1325
Fax: 765-497-8004
www.in.gov/isdh

Jim Huston, Chief of Staff
Joan Duwve, MD, MPH, Chief Medical Officer
Eric Miller, Deputy Chief of Staff

Supports Indiana's economic prosperity and quality of life by promoting, protecting and providing for the health of Hoosiers in their communities.

623 Indiana Department of Revenue
100 N Senate Avenue
Indianapolis, IN 46204-2253
317-233-4018
Fax: 317-233-2329
www.in.gov/dor
TDD 317-232-4952

John Eckart, Commissioner

The Department of Revenue is responsible for providing
service to Indiana citozens regarding state tax matters. Additionally, the Department administers state tax laws, develops regulations and makes decisions about tax policy.

Year Founded: 1947

624 Indiana Department of Veterans Affairs
302 W Washington Street
Room E120
Indianapolis, IN 46204-2761
844-480-0009
Fax: 317-232-7721; *Toll Free:* 800-400-4520
VetEmployment@dva.IN.gov
www.in.gov/dva

Charles T Applegate, Executive Director

Remains focused on aiding and assisting Hoosier veterans
and qualified family members or survivors, who are eligible for benefits or advantages provided by Indiana and the
US government.

625 Indiana Developmental Disability Council
402 West Washington Street
Indianapolis, IN 46204-2801
317-232-7770
Fax: 317-233-3712
gpcpd@gpcpd.org
www.in.gov/gpcpd
TDD 317-232-7771

Suellen Jackson-Boner, Executive Director
Christine Dahlberg, Deputy Director
Jim Geswein, Chief Financial Officer

Promotes public policy which leads to the independence,
productivity, and inclusion of people with disabilities.

626 Indiana Disability Determination Bureau
402 W. Washington
Suite W451
Indianapolis, IN 46207-7083
317-396-2000
Fax: 317-232-1240; *Toll Free:* 800-545-7763
www.in.gov/fssa/ddrs
TDD 800-252-0573

Patricia Carew-Ceesay, Deputy Director

The Division of Disability and Rehabilitative Services
(DDRS) exists to inform, protect and serve individuals with
disabilities and their families in need of human services, resources, or support to attain employment and self-sufficiency or to maintain independence.

**627 Indiana Governor's Planning Council for
People with Disabilities**
402 West Washington Street
Indianapolis, IN 46204
317-232-7770
Fax: 317-233-3712
gpcpd@gpcpd.org
www.in.gov/gpcpd

Suellen Jackson-Boner, Executive Director
Christine Dahlberg, Deputy Director
Jim Geswein, Chief Financial Officer

Mission is to promote public policy which leads to the independence, productivity and inclusion of people with disabilities in all aspects of society.

628 Indiana Protection & Advocacy Services
4701 North Keystone Avenue
Suite 222
Indianapolis, IN 46205
317-722-5555
Fax: 317-722-5564; *Toll Free:* 800-622-4845
dward@ipas.IN.gov
www.in.gov/ipas

Karen Pedevilla, Education & Training Director

To see that the human, legal and civil rights of people with
disabilities are affirmed. Congress established protection
and advocacy (P&A) systems in each state. Indiana Protection & Advocacy Services provides advocacy for Indiana
citizens. IPAS proudly serves people with disabilities, helping them exercise their rights, as well as providing training
and resources to ensure their inclusion in the life of our
communities.

Year Founded: 1977

629 Indiana Public Employee's Retirement Fund
One North Capitol
Suite 001
Indianapolis, IN 46204
317-232-3882; *Toll Free:* 866-591-9441
www.in.gov/inprs

Steve Russo, Executive Director
Steven Barley, Deputy Director
David Cooper, Chief Investment Officer

Advances the achievement of retirement security for current and future retirees and beneficiaries through the delivery of operational and investment excellence, exemplary
customer service and trusted stakeholder communication

630 Life Stream Services
Po Box 308
Yorktown, IN 47396
765-759-1121
Fax: 765-759-0060; *Toll Free:* 800-589-1121
mail@lifestreaminc.org
www.lifestreaminc.org

Leisal Julian, JD, Board Chairman
Kenneth D Adkins, President/CEO
Jenny Hamilton, MBA, Vice President of Home & Communi

Working together to improve and extend the quality of life
for persons at risk of losing their independence. Services
offered include home delivered meals, transportation, care
management, homemaker, home health aide, senior cafes,
information and assistance.

631 RSVP Dearborn County
PO Box 4194
98 East High Street
Lawrenceburg, IN 47025-4194
812-539-4005
Fax: 812-539-2362
info@myrsvp.org
www.myrsvp.org

Mary Lewis, Executive Director

The Retired and Senior Volunteer Program (RSVP) provides opportunities for people 55 and over to make a difference in their community through volunteer service. RSVP volunteers contribute anywhere from a few to over forty hours a week, serving through schools, day care centers, police departments, hospitals and other nonprofit and public organizations to help meet critical community needs. RSVP offers maximum flexibility and choice to its volunteers. RSVP matches the personal interests and skills of older Americans with opportunities to help solve community problems and offers supplemental insurance while on duty, on-the-job training from the agency or organization where volunteers are placed. The following Counties are served: Dearborn, Ohio, Ripley, Switzerland.

632   RSVP Lake County
6919 Indianapolis Blvd
Hammond, IN 46324-2205
219-844-5174
Fax: 219-844-4885
byurko@catholic-charities.org

Betty A Yurko, Contact

Provides opportunities for people 55 and over to make a difference in their community through volunteer service. RSVP volunteers contribute anywhere from a few to over forty hours a week, serving through schools, day care centers, police departments, hospitals and other nonprofit and public organizations to help meet critical community needs. RSVP matches the personal interests and skills of older Americans with opportunities to help solve community problems and offers supplemental insurance while on duty, on-the-job training from the agency or organization where volunteers are placed.

633   RSVP Putnam County
30 No 7th Street, Suite 105
PO Box 1018
Terre Haute, IN 47808
812-232-1264
Fax: 812-232-9634
www.putnamcountyny.com/rsvp/

Monica Van Hook, Director

Enables adults, 55 and older, to contribute meaningful service in a wide variety of community agencies.

634   RSVP St. Joseph County
1817 Miami Street
South Bend, IN 46613
574-234-3111
Fax: 574-289-1034
www.diocesefwsb.org/charity

Stephen Hughes, Director

The Retired and Senior Volunteer Program (RSVP) provides opportunities for people 55 and over to make a difference in their community through volunteer service. RSVP volunteers contribute anywhere from a few to over forty hours a week, serving through schools, day care centers, police departments, hospitals and other nonprofit and public organizations to help meet critical community needs. RSVP offers maximum flexibility and choice to its volunteers. RSVP matches the personal interests and skills of older Americans with opportunities to help solve community problems and offers supplemental insurance while on duty, on-the-job training from the agency or organization where volunteers are placed.

635   Railroad Retirement Board District Office
50 S Meridian Street
Suite 303
Indianapolis, IN 46204-3538
317-226-6111
Fax: 317-226-5374; *Toll Free:* 877-772-5772
www.rrb.gov/field/do_indi.asp

Robert Braitman, Manager

An independent agency in the executive branch of the Federal Government. The primary function is to administer comprehensive retirement-survivor and unemployment-sickness benefit programs for the nation's railroad workers and their families.

636   South Central Indiana Council for Aging and Aged
Po Box 995
33 State Street, Third Floor
New Albany, IN 47151-0995
812-948-8330
Fax: 812- 94- 014; *Toll Free:* 888-948-8330
information@lsr14.org
www.lifespanresources.org
TTY: 812-542-6895

Steve Meyer, President
Lisa Heideman, Vice President
Annette Roberts, Treasurer

Provides assistance with case management, information and referral to various services for persons who are aging or developmentally disabled. Provides assistance with home health care, personal assistance, home-delivered and congregate meals, adult day care, respite care for families, and prescriptions. Counties served: Clark, Floyd, Harrison, Scott.

637   Southwestern Indiana Regional Council on Aging
16 West Virginia Street
Evansville, IN 47710-1742
812-464-7800
Fax: 812-464-7811; *Toll Free:* 800-253-2188
swirca@swirca.org
www.swirca.org

Rhonda Zuber, Chief Executive Officer
Jeff Wolf, Chief Financial Officer
Jerry Scheidler, VP of Operations

Volunteers aged 60 years or older in Evansville, IN. Provides a variety of opportunities for persons 60 years or older to participate more fully in the life of their community through significant volunteer service. Distributes teddy bears to abused, neglected, disabled, and underprivileged children. The following Counties are served: Gibson, Perry, Posey, Vanderburgh and Warrick.

638   West Central Indiana Economic Development District: Area Agency on Aging and Disabled
PO Box 359
1718 Wabash Avenue
Terre Haute, IN 47808
812-238-1561
Fax: 812-238-1564; *Toll Free:* 800-489-1561
www.westcentralin.com

Gloria Wetnight, Assistant Program Director
Patty Cannoy, Outreavh Coordinator

we serve a 6-county area with only one major metro area; five counties are 80% or more rural. We serve the 60+ population and birth to death disabled providing home and community based services.

Iowa

639 Connections Area Agency on Aging
2301 Pierce Street
Sioux City, IA 51104-3850
712-279-6900
Fax: 712-233-3415; *Toll Free:* 800-432-9209
info@connectionsaaa.org
www.connectionsaaa.org

Terry Amburn, Chairperson,Glenwood
John Twombly, Vice Chair,Greenfield
Barbara Morrison, Executive Director of senior ser

Siouxland Aging enables older Iowans to live with maximum possible dignity, well being, and independence.

640 Elderbridge: Area Agency on Aging
22 N Georgia Avenue
Suite 216
Mason City, IA 50401-3435
641-424-0678
Fax: 641-424-2927; *Toll Free:* 800-243-0678
rthompson@elderbridge.org
www.elderbridge.org

Mick Tagesen, Executive Director

Elderbridge is a non-profit organization funded through federal Older Americans Act and State of Iowa General Revenue funds, and contributions.

641 Hawkeye Valley: Area Agency on Aging
2101 Kimball Ave.
Suite 320
Waterloo, IA 50702
319-272-2244
Fax: 319-272-2455; *Toll Free:* 800-779-8707
www.hvaaa.org

Mike Isaacson, Executive Director

Agency provides planning, advocacy, funding for senior programs and services. Funded services include: Meals on Wheels, Senior Dining, Adult Day Care, Case Management and Transportation.

642 Heritage: Area Agency on Aging
6301 Kirkwood Boulevard SW
Cedar Rapids, IA 52404
319-398-5411
Fax: 319-398-5533; *Toll Free:* 800-332-2055
ask@kirkwood.edu
www.kirkwood.edu

Dr Mick Starcevich, President
Jill Gleason, Associate Director
Michele Boughan, Care Connections Director

Agency provides planning, advocacy, funding for senior programs and services in a seven county area. Funded services include: Meals on Wheels, Senior Dining, Adult Day Care, Case Management and Transportation.

643 Iowa Commission of Veterans Affairs
7105 NW 70th Avenue
Camp Dodge Bldg 3465
Johnston, IA 50131-1824

51- 25- 469
Fax: 515-727-3713; *Toll Free:* 800-838-4692
www.iowava.org

Colonel Robe King, Executive Director
Jill Joseph, Outreach Coordinator
Mari Mielke, Secretary

Dedicated to ensuring Iowa veterans and their dependents recieve the full measure of county, state, and federal, benfits to which they are entitled. Commited to helping the newest veterans with successful reintegration into civilian life.

644 Iowa Commission on Persons with Disabilities
321 E. 12th Street
Lucas State Office Building
Des Moines, IA 50319
515-242-5655
Fax: 515-242-6119; *Toll Free:* 888-219-0471
golsen@graceland.edu
www.state.ia.us/dhr
TTY: 888-219-0471

Dr. Jill Olsen, Chair

The Division of Persons with Disabilities exists to promote the employment of Iowans with disabilities and reduce barriers to employment by providing information, referral, assessment and guidance, training, and negotiation services to employers and citizens with disabilities.

645 Iowa Department of Aging
Jesse M Parker Building
510 E 12th Street, Suite 2
Des Moines, IA 50319-9025
515-725-3333
Fax: 515-242-3300; *Toll Free:* 800-532-3213
contactida@iowa.gov
www.aging.iowa.gov

Donna Harvey, Director

The mission of the Iowa Department on Aging is to provide advocay, educational, prevention and health services for older Iowans, their families and caregivers through partnerships with Area Agencies on Aging and other stakeholders. The Iowa Department on Aging is a Cabinet-level State agency whose director is appointed by the Governor and confimed by the Senate. The agency is responsible for the application and receipt of Federal Older Americans Act funds as well as State appropriations. The Department administers over 40 supports and services through a network of 13 Area Agencies on Aging, utilizing more than $32 million federal and state funds which allows nearly 74,000Iowans 60 and older to remain independent and healthy as they age.

646 Iowa Department of Human Rights: Deaf Services Commissions
Department Of Human Rights, 2nd Floor
Lucas State Office Building
Des Moines, IA 50319
515-281-3164
Fax: 515-242-6119; *Toll Free:* 888-221-3724
lynsie.crawford@iowa.gov
www.iowa.gov/dhr/ds

San Wong, Director
Stephanie Lyons, Consultant
Linda Scott, Secretary

Mission is to serve, represent, and provide greater understanding of deaf and hard of hearing individuals at any age across the state.

647 Iowa Department of Revenue & Finance
Hoover Building
1305 E Walnut
Des Moines, IA 50319
515-281-3114
Fax: 800-572-3943; *Toll Free:* 800-367-3388
idr@iowa.gov
www.iowa.gov/tax

Courtney Kay-Decker, Director

Mission is to serve all Iowans and to support government services in Iowa by collecting all taxes required by law, but no more.

648 Iowa Developmental Disability Council
617 E Second Street
Des Moines, IA 50309
515-725-0151
Fax: 515-725-0437; *Toll Free:* 866-432-2846
www.idaction.com

Becky Maddy Harker, Executive Director
Rick Shannon, Public Policy Manager
Fran Morris, Office Manager

The Council identifies, develops and promotes public policy and support practices through capacity building, advocacy, and systems change activities. The purpose is to ensure that people with developmental disabilities and their families are included in planning, decision making, and development of policy related to services and supports that affect their quality of life and full participation in communities of their choice.

649 Iowa Division of Mental Health: Office of Human Services
Hoover
Des Moines, IA 50319
515-281-5874
Fax: 515-281-4597
www.dhs.state.ia.us

Charles Palmer, Director

Helps individuals and families achieve safe, stable, self-sufficient, and healthy lives, therby contributing to the economic growth of the state

650 Iowa Program for Assistive Technology
Center for Disabilities and Development
100 Hawkins Drive
Iowa City, IA 52242-1011
319-356-0550
Fax: 319-384-5139; *Toll Free:* 800-779-2001
IPAT@uiowa.edu
www.iowaat.org
TTY: 877-686-0032

Jane Gay, Director
Gary Johnson, Community Programs Coordinator
Marlene Phipps, Office Clerk

The Iowa Program for Assistive Technology (IPAT) is Iowa's grant project under the Assistive Technology Act (ATA) of 1998. IPAT's goals are to promote and create systems change in the state with regards to assistive technology (AT) and it's use. IPAT works with consumers and family members, service providers, and state and local

agencies/organizations to promote assistive technology through awareness, training, and policy work. IPAT accomplishes this through five specific goal areas: education, employment, health, community living and recreation, telecommunication and information and technology.

Year Founded: 1989

651 Iowa Workers Compensation
1000 E Grand Avenue
Des Moines, IA 50319-0209
515-281-5387
Fax: 515-281-6501; *Toll Free:* 800-562-4692
iwd.dwc@iwd.iowa.gov
www.iowaworkforce.org/wc

Christopher Godfrey, Workers' Comp Comissioner
Janna E Martin, Assistant Commissioner
Sharon K Ortega, Administrative Secretary

Assistance to eligible employees about their benefits front heir employers when they have injuries arising of and in the course of employment

652 Lucas County Health Center
1200 N 7th Street
Chariton, IA 50049-1210
641-774-3000
Fax: 641-774-3233; *Toll Free:* 800-404-3111
www.lchcia.com

Betty Hansen, Chair
Dr. Manganel , President
Natalie McGee, Vice Chair

Lucas County Health Center Volunteer Services plays an important role in the local community. Volunteer Services has four areas of focus: volunteer placement, a personal emergency response program, insurance education, and low-cost food distribution. LCHC Volunteer Services is designed to match volunteers with opportunities for the mutual benefit of all involved.

Year Founded: 1961

653 RSVP Black Hawk & Fayette County
2101 Kimball Avenue
Suite 121
Waterloo, IA 50702-5057
319-272-2250
Fax: 319-272-1958
rsvpwaterloo1@hotmail.com
www.rsvpserves.com

Sheila Bohr, Director

The Retired and Senior Volunteer Program (RSVP) provides opportunities for people 55 and over to make a difference in their community through volunteer service. RSVP volunteers contribute anywhere from a few to over forty hours a week, serving through schools, day care centers, police departments, hospitals and other nonprofit and public organizations to help meet critical community needs. RSVP offers maximum flexibility and choice to its volunteers. RSVP matches the personal interests and skills of older Americans with opportunities to help solve community problems and offers supplemental insurance while on duty, on-the-job training from the agency or organization where volunteers are placed. The following County is served: Black Hawk.

Year Founded: 1972

654 RSVP Dubuque County
350 N Grandview Avenue
Dubuque, IA 52001-6388
563-582-1881
Fax: 563-557-2813; *Toll Free:* 800-424-3258
www.unitypoint.org/dubuque/Default.aspx

David Brandon, President and CEO
Chad Wolbers, Chief Operating Officer
Diana Batchelor, Chief Nursing Officer

RSVP of Dubuque County provides persons age 55 and older opportunities to enhance their lives and their community through volunteer service.

655 RSVP Fort Dodge
819 1st Avenue South
Municipal Building
Fort Dodge, IA 50501-3811
515-573-7144
Fax: 515-573-5751
webmaster@fortdodgeiowa.org
www.fortdodgeiowa.org

Lori Branderhorst, Director, Parks & Recreation
Timothy Carmody, Police Chief, Police Department
David Fierke, City Manager

The Retired and Senior Volunteer Program (RSVP) provides opportunities for people 55 and over to make a difference in their community through volunteer service. RSVP volunteers contribute anywhere from a few to over forty hours a week, serving through schools, day care centers, police departments, hospitals and other nonprofit and public organizations to help meet critical community needs. RSVP offers maximum flexibility and choice to its volunteers. RSVP matches the personal interests and skills to older Americans with opportunities to help solve community problems and offers supplemental insurance while on duty, on-the-job training from the agency or organization where volunteers are placed. The following County is served: Webster.

656 RSVP Henry County
407 South White Street
Mt Pleasant, IA 52641-2262
319-385-6523
Fax: 319-385-6731
carrk@hchc.org
www.healthyhenrycounty.org

Karen Bates Chabal, Rsvp Director
Nancy Hahn, Program Coordinator

The Retired and Senior Volunteer Program (RSVP) provides opportunities for people 55 and over to make a difference in their community through volunteer service. RSVP volunteers contribute anywhere from a few to over forty hours a week, serving through schools, day care centers, police departments, hospitals and other nonprofit and public organizations to help meet critical community needs. RSVP offers maximum flexibility and choice to its volunteers. RSVP matches the personal interests and skills of older Americans with opportunities to help solve community problems and offers supplemental insurance while on duty, on-the-job training from the agency or organization where volunteer is placed. The following County is served: Henry.

Year Founded: 1999

657 RSVP North Central Iowa
500 College Drive
Mason City, IA 50401
641-585-2450
Fax: 641-585-8194; *Toll Free:* 888-GON-IACC
rsvp@niacc.edu
www.niacc.edu

Dr. Steven Schulz, President
Deb Derr, President, Administrative Service
Kathy Grove, Vice President, Administrative

The Retired and Senior Volunteer Program (RSVP) provides opportunities for people 55 and over to make a difference in their community through volunteer service. RSVP volunteers contribute anywhere from a few to over forty hours a week, serving through schools, day care centers, police departments, hospitals and other nonprofit and public organizations to help meet critical community needs. RSVP offers maximum flexibility and choice to its volunteers. RSVP matches the personal interests and skills of older Americans with opportunities to help solve community problems and offers supplemental insurance while on duty, on-the-job training from the agency and organization where volunteers are placed. The following Counties are served: Poweshiek, Tama.

Year Founded: 1918

658 RSVP North Lee County
811 Avenue E
PO Box 386
Fort Madison, IA 52627-0386
319-372-7700
Fax: 319-372-8661
jbergman@fortmadison-ia.com
www.newlifestyles.com

Jean Bergman, Director

The Retired and Senior Volunteer Program (RSVP) provides opportunities for people 55 and over to make a difference in their community through volunteer service. RSVP volunteers contribute anywhere from a few to over forty hours a week, serving through schools, day care centers, police departments, hospitals and other nonprofit and public organizations to help meet critical community needs. RSVP offers maximum flexibility and choice to its volunteers. RSVP matches the personal interests and skills of older Americans with opportunities to help solve community problems and offers supplemental insurance while on duty, on-the-job training from the agency or organization where volunteers are placed.

659 RSVP Northeast Iowa
202 Winnebago Street
Decorah, IA 52101-1812
563-382-3717
Fax: 563-382-4524
rsvp@decorah.lib.ia.us
www2.decorah.lib.ia.us/RSVP/index.htm

Kathy Barloon, Director of the RSVP Program

The Retired and Senior Volunteer Program (RSVP) provides opportunities for people 55 and over to make a difference in their community through volunteer service. RSVP volunteers contribute anywhere from a few to over forty hours a week, serving through schools, day care centers, police departments, hospitals and other nonprofit and public organizations to help meet critical community needs. RSVP offers maximum flexibility and choice to its volunteers. RSVP matches the personal interests and skills of older Americans with opportunities to help solve community problems and offers supplemental insurance while on duty, on-the-job training from the agency or organization where volunteers are placed. The following Counties are served: Allamakee, Bremer, Chickasaw, Clayton, Fayette, Howard, Winneshiek.

660 RSVP Ottumwa
217 East Main Street
PO Box 308
Ottumwa, IA 52501-0308
641-683-1161
Fax: 641-682-3466
www.newlifestyles.com

Patsy Seals, Director

The Retired and Senior Volunteer Program (RSVP) provides opportunities for people 55 and over to make a difference in their community through volunteer service. RSVP volunteers contribute anywhere from a few to over forty hours a week, serving through schools, day care centers, police departments, hospitals and other nonprofit and public organizations to help meet critical community needs. RSVP offers maximum flexibility and choice to its volunteers. RSVP matches the personal interests and skills of older Americans with opportunities to help solve community problems and offers supplemental insurance while on duty, on-the-job training from the agency or organization where volunteers are placed.

661 RSVP United Way of Central Iowa
1111 Ninth Street
Suite 100
Des Moines, IA 50314-2527
515-246-6500
Fax: 515-246-6522
contactus@unitedwaydm.org
www.unitedwaydm.org

Mary Sellers, President
Elisabeth Buck, Chief CommunityImpact Officer
Sarah Roy, Chief Operating Officer

United Way of Central Iowa will be the leader and catalyst for community change in the business of caring.

662 Railroad Retirement Board: Iowa District Office
844 North Rush Street
Chicago, IL 60611-2092
515-284-4344
Fax: 515-284-4616; *Toll Free:* 877-772-5772
desmonies@rrb.gov
www.rrb.gov
TTY: 312-751-4701

Michael S. Schwartz, Chairman of the Board
George V. Govan, Senior Executive Officer,Executi
Ram Murthy, Chief Information Officer

An independent agency in the executive branch of the Federal Government. Primary function is to administer comprehensive retirement-survivor and unemployment-sickness benefit programs for the nations railroad workers and their families.

663 Scenic Valley: Area Agency on Aging
2101 Kimball Ave
Suite 320
Waterloo, IA 50702
319-272-2244
Fax: 563-588-1952; *Toll Free:* 800-779-8707
mail@scenicvalley.org
www.nei3a.org

Linda McDonald, Manager

Provides information and assistance and to arrange services for seniors age 60 and older.

664 Seneca: Area Agency on Aging
117 North Cooper Street
Suite 2
Ottumwa, IA 52501
641-682-2270
Fax: 641-682-2445; *Toll Free:* 800-642-6522
seneca@seneca-aaa.org
www.seneca-aaa.org

Connie Holland, Chief Executive Officer
Christa Merritt, Chief Operating Officer
Jeri Swisher, Human Resources Director

Our mission is to advocate for and provide assistance to older persons in a non-discriminatory manner, working toward fostering and maintaining independence while preserving the dignity of each individual and focusing on their quality of life.

665 Southeast Iowa Area: Agency on Aging
510 East 12th Street
Jessie M. Parker Building ,Suite 2
Des Moines, IA 50319-9025
515-725-3333
Fax: 319-754-7030; *Toll Free:* 800-532-3213
a.agency@mchsi.com
www.iowaaging.gov/southeast-iowa-area-ag

Donna K. Harvey, Director

A planning and funding agency whose purpose is to fund services which enable older persons to remain as independent as possible in the least restrictive environment.

Year Founded: 1973

Kansas

666 Beach Center on Families and Disability
University of Kansas
1200 Sunnyside Avenue
Room 3136
Lawrence, KS 66045
785-864-7600
Fax: 785-864-7605
www.beachcenter.org
TTY: 785-864-3434

Dr. Rud Turnbull, Co-Founder,Co-Director

A federally funded center that conducts research and training in the factors that contribute to the successful functioning of families with members who have disabilities.

Year Founded: 1988

667 Butler County Department on Aging
205 West Central
El Dorado, KS 67042
316-322-4300
Fax: 316-322-4387; *Toll Free:* 800-822-6104
cnoles@bucoks.com
www.bucoks.com

Crytal Noles, Director
Brenda Louthan, Assistant Director/Program Mgr
Kauffman Brandon, Asstistant Co. Administrator/Fin

The Department on Aging serves nearly 10,000 Butler County citizens, age 60 and older. We are committed to helping the frail and elderly who choose to remain at home, by providing a link to in-home services. Our goal is to promote independence, health, self-care, and self-value for the elders who reside in Butler County.

668   Central Plains: Area Agency on Aging
2622 West Central Avenue
Suite 500
Wichita, KS 67203-3725
316-660-7298
Fax: 316-660-1936; *Toll Free:* 800-367-7298
www.cpaaa.org

Ray Vail, Director of Finace and Support S
Monica Cissell, Director of Information and Comm
Annette Graham, Executive Director

Central Plains Area Agency on Aging is one of eleven Area Agencies on Aging (AAA's) in Kansas. Its service area is Harvey, Sedgwick, and Butler Counties and it has the highest number of older people of any AAA in the state; approximately 84,737 people aged 60 and over. Services provided include case management, in-home and community services, information, assistance and volunteer services.

Year Founded: 1973

669   Disability Rights Center of Kansas
635 South West Harrison Street
Suite 100
Topeka, KS 66603-3726
785-273-9661
Fax: 785-273-9414; *Toll Free:* 877-776-1541
drckansas.org
TDD 877-335-3725

Rocky Nichols, Executive Director
Debbie White, Deputy Director,Administration
Lane Williams, Deputy Director, Legal Division

Legal, administrative and other advocacy to protect the rights of persons with disabilities.

670   East Central Kansas: Area Agency on Aging
117 S. Main
Ottawa, KS 66067-2327
785-242-7200
Fax: 785-242-7202; *Toll Free:* 800-633-5621
eckaaa@eckaaa.state.ks.us
www.eckaaa.org

Elizabeth Maxwell, Executive Director
Sherry Hushka, Fiscal Manager
Leslea Rockers, Special Projects &SHICK Coordin

A non-profit corporation which receives funds from the federal, state and local governments, client fees, and private resources. It was founded in 1973 and has a successful history of meeting the needs of the rural elderly. The Area Agency is responsible for providing and coordinating services for persons age sixty and over.

671   Harvey County Department on Aging
800 North Main Street
PO Box 687
Newton, KS 67114-1807

316-284-6880
Fax: 316-284-6882
www.harveycounty.com

Carmen Reimer, Executive Secretary
Linda Kientz, Personnel Director
Rich Hanley, Director

Provides services to Harvey County's seniors aged 60 and older. Commited to helping the frail and elderly who choose to remain at home by providing home and community based services, their goal is to promote level of choice, independence and self-care.

672   KSDS Assistance Dogs
120 West 7th Street
Washington, KS 66968-2222
785-325-2256
Fax: 785-325-2258
ksds@ksds.org
www.ksds.org

A program which trains and placing dogs with individuals with disabilities

673   KSDS, Inc. Assistance Dogs
120 West 7th Street
Washington, KS 66968-2222
785-325-2256
Fax: 785-325-2258
ksds@ksds.org
www.ksds.org

Glenda Keller, Chief Executive Officer
Roger Post, President
Midge Miller, Secretary
Year Founded: 1990

674   Kansas Client Assistance Program
635 South West Harrison Street
Suite 100
Topeka, KS 66603
785-273-9661; *Toll Free:* 877-776-1541
rocky@drckansas.org
www.drckansas.org
TDD 877-335-3725

Rocky Nichols, Executive Director
Debbie White, Deputy Director,Administration
Lane Williams, Deputy Director, Legal Division

CAP assists anyone with a disability that is interested in applying for and receiving services from rehabilitation programs, projects or facilities funded under the Rehabilitation Act.

675   Kansas Commission on Disability Concerns
900 South West Jackson Street
Suite 100
Topeka, KS 66612-1877
785-296-1722
Fax: 785-296-6809; *Toll Free:* 800-295-5232
www.kcdcinfo.com
TDD 800-295-5232
TTY: 711- -

Martha Gabehart, Executive Director
Kerry Bacon, Legislative Liaison

KCDC believes that all people with disabilities are entitled to be equal partners in Kansas society. The purpose is to involve all sentiments of the Kansas Community through legislative advocacy, education and resource networking to ensure full and equal citizenship for all Kansas with disabilities.

676 Kansas Commission on Veterans Affairs

700 South West Jackson
Jayhawk Tower, Suite 1004
Topeka, KS 66603-3743
785-296-3976
Fax: 785-296-1462; Toll Free: 800-273-8255
www.kcva.ks.gov

Michael Neer, Chairman,Overland Park
Jim Buterbaugh, Vice Chairman, Winfield

Provides Kansas veterans, their relatives, and other eligible dependents with information, advice, direction, and assistance through the coordination of programs and services in the fields of education, health, vocational guidance and placement, and economic security.

677 Kansas Council of DevelopmentalDisability

915 South West Harrison
Dock State Office Building Room 141
Topeka, KS 66612-1570
785-296-2608
Fax: 785-296-2861; Toll Free: 877-431-4604
www.kcdd.org

Steve Gieber, Executive Director
Shelly May, Grants Manager
Charline Cobbs, Senior Administrative Assisstant

Mission is to ensure the opportunity to make choices regarding participation in society and quality of life for individuals with developmental disabilities.

678 Kansas Department for Aging andDisability Services

503 South Kansas Avenue
Topeka, KS 66603-9800
785-296-4986
Fax: 785-296-0256; Toll Free: 800-432-3535
wwwmail@kdads.ks.gov
www.kdads.ks.gov/Advocacy_Legislation/Ad

Shawn Sullivan, Secretary

A grassroots initiative that promotes support of issues involving older adults and intergenerational concerns. It is not a lobbying effort, and policy is not created by a board in a top down manner. It has been designed as an educational effort administered by and for older adults. To serve, you must be at least 60 years old at the time of filing as a candidate for election.

Year Founded: 1997

679 Kansas Department for Aging and Disability Services

New England Building
503 South Kansas Avenue
Topeka, KS 66603-3404
785-296-4986
Fax: 785-296-0256; Toll Free: 800-432-3535
wwwmail@kdads.ks.gov
www.kdads.ks.gov
TTY: 785-291-3167

Shawn Sullivan, Secretary

Mission is to foster an environment which; promotes security, dignity, and independence, while providing the right care at the right time in a place called home

680 Kansas Department of Aging andDisability Services

New England Building
503 South Kansas Avenue
Topeka, KS 66603-3403
785-296-4986
Fax: 785-296-0256; Toll Free: 800-432-3535
www.kdads.ks.gov

Shawn Sullivan, Secretary
Gina Meier-Hummel, Commissioner, Community Service
Craig Kaberline, Commissioner of Aging

This is a state agency whose mission is to foster an environment that promotes security, dignity and independence for all Kansans. We envision a community that empowers Kansas' older adults and persons with disabilities to make choices about their lives.

681 Kansas Department of Health andEnvironment

1000 South West Jackson
Suite 330
Topeka, KS 66612-1365
785-296-0127
Fax: 785-291-3419; Toll Free: 800-332-6262
ksresourceguide@kdheks.gov
www.kdheks.gov/health/servguid.html

Sam Brownback, Governor
Robert Moser, MD,Secretary
Gina Meier-Hummel, Protection Services Director

682 Kansas Department of Social and Rehabilitation Services

1000 South West Jackson
Suite 220
Topeka, KS 66612-1274
785-296-1317
Fax: 785-296-2173; Toll Free: 800-332-6262
ksresourceguide@kdheks.gov
www.ksresourceguide.org/srs.htm

Sam Brownback, Governor
Robert Moser, MD,Secretary
Angela De Rocha, Communications Director

Mission is to protect children and promote adult self-sufficiency

683 Kansas Department on Aging

503 South Kansas Avenue
New England Building
Topeka, KS 66603-9800
785-296-4986
Fax: 785-296-0256; Toll Free: 800-432-3535
wwwmail@kdads.ks.gov
www.kdads.ks.gov

C Sullivan, Secretary

Provides information on services available to seniors within Kansas.

684 Kansas Public Employees Retirement System

611 South Kansas Avenue
Suite 100
Topeka, KS 66603-3803
785-296-6166
Fax: 785-296-6638; Toll Free: 888-275-5737
kpers@kpers.org
www.kpers.org

Alan D. Conroy, Executive Director
Laurie McKinnon, Legal Department
Elizabeth Miller, Investment Services

KPERS provides three statewide defined benfit retirement plans for state and local public employees. The system also oversees the State's Deferred Compensation Plan, a voluntary 457(b) savings plan

685 North Central Flint Hills: Area Agency on Aging
401 Houston Street
Manhattan, KS 66502-6135
785-776-9294
Fax: 785-776-9479; *Toll Free:* 800-432-2703
ncfhaaa@ncfhaaa.com
www.ncfhaaa.com

Julie Govert Walter, Executive Director
Ashley Noll, Long Term Care Supervisor
Karen Mayse, Information & Assistance Supervi

A private, non-profit organization that plans, coordinates and sponsors services in 18 counties to enhance the quality and dignity of life for older Kansans and their families. Programs and services are partially funded by the Older Americans Act through the Kansas department on Aging and voluntary participant contributions.

Year Founded: 1975

686 Northeast Kansas: Area Agency on Aging
1803 Oregon
Hiawatha, KS 66434-2222
785-742-7152
Fax: 785-742-7154; *Toll Free:* 800-883-2549
nekaaa@hotmail.com
www.nekaaa.org

Karen Wilson, Executive Director
Julie Welch, Fiscal Manager
Jon Stallbaumer, Case Manager Supervisor

Northeast Kansas Area Agency on Aging is a single point of entry for senior citizens in a 7 county area. Services range from in-home help, insurance counseling, information to educational programs. We serve senior citizens 60 and over. Some in-home services cost a minimal amount while others are no cost.

687 Northwest Kansas: Area Agency on Aging
510 West 29th Street
Suite B - PO Box 610
Hays, KS 67601
785-628-8204
Fax: 785-628-6096; *Toll Free:* 800-432-7422
nwkaaa@nwkaaa.org
www.nwkaaa.com

Jan Williams, Director

Provides needs and services to Senior Adults. Acts as an advocacte for their interests, and to provide a means for Senior Adults to gain and maintain direct input into decision-making processes.

688 RSVP Butler County
205 West Central
El Dorado, KS 67042
316-322-4300
Fax: 316-322-4387; *Toll Free:* 800-822-6104
www.bucoks.com

Crystal Noles, Director
Brenda Louthan, Assistant Director/Program Mgr
Kauffman Brandon, Asstistant Co. Administrator/Fin

The Retired and Senior Volunteer Program (RSVP) provides opportunities for people 55 and over to make a difference in their community through volunteer service. RSVP volunteers contribute anywhere from a few to over forty hours a week, serving thourgh schools, day care centers, police departments, hospitals and other nonprofit and public organizations to help meet critical community needs. RSVP offers maximum flexibility and choice to its volunteers. RSVP matches the personal interests and skills to older Americans with opportunities to help solve community problems and offer supplemental insurance while on duty, on-the-job training from the agency or organization where volunteers are placed.

689 RSVP Harvey County
800 North Main Street
PO Box 687
Newton, KS 67114-1807
316-284-6806
Fax: 316-284-6811
www.harveycounty.com

John Waltner, Harvey County Administrator
Anthony Swartzendruber, Assistant County Administrator
Carmen Reimer, Executive Secretary

The Retired and Senior Volunteer Program (RSVP) provides opportunities for people 55 and over to make a difference in their community through volunteer service. RSVP volunteers contribute anywhere from a few to over forty hours a week, serving through schools, day care centers, police departments, hospitals and other nonprofit and public organizations to help meet critical community needs. RSVP offers maximum flexibility and choice to its volunteers. RSVP matches the personal interests and skills of older Americans with opportunities to help solve community problems and offers supplemental insurance while on duty, on-the-job training from the agency or organization where volunteers are placed.

690 RSVP Johnson County: Coming of Age
5200 Oak Street
3rd Floor
Kansas City, MO 64112
816-444-1121
Fax: 913-341-0275
www.sccentral.org/coming-of-age-rsvp-joh

Pamela Seymour, Executive Director
Cheryl Brown Henderson, Coordinator COA/RSVP Johnson Cou

RSVP of Johnson County partners with approximately 150 agencies across the metro area. Volunteers are giving their time and expertise by delivering meals to homebound individuals, assisting teachers, making quilts for children in hospitals, cashiering at hospital gift shops, tutoring students, and much more. The following Counties are served: Johnson.

691 RSVP Northwest Kansas
Colby Community College
165 Fike Park
PO Box 803
Colby, KS 67701-2447

785-462-6744
Fax: 785-462-6283
www.newlifestyles.com

Laura Withington, Director

The Retired and Senior Volunteer Program (RSVP) provides opportunities for people 55 and over to make a difference in their community through volunteer service. RSVP volunteers contribute anywhere from a few to over forty hours a week, serving through schools, day care centers, police departments, hospitals and other nonprofit and public organizations to help meet critical community needs. RSVP offers maximum flexibility and choice to its volunteers. RSVP matches the personal interests and skills of older Americans with opportunities to help solve community problems and offers supplemental insurance while on duty, on-the-job training from the agency or organization where volunteers are placed. The following Counties are served: Logan, Phillips, Sheridan, Thomas.

692 RSVP Saline CountyThe Volunteer Connection
239 North Santa Fe Avenue
Salina, KS 67401-2317
785-823-3128
Fax: 785-823-3819
www.allforgood.org/organizations/salina/

Nancy Klostermeyer, Director

The Retired and Senior Volunteer Program (RSVP) provides opportunities for people 55 and over to make a difference in their community through volunteer service. RSVP volunteers contribute anywhere from a few to over forty hours a week, serving through schools, day care centers, police departments, hospitals and other nonprofit and public organizations to help meet critical community needs. RSVP offers maximum flexibility and choice to its volunteers. RSVP matches the personal interest and skills of older Americans with opportunities to help solve community problems and offers supplemental insurance while on duty, on-the-job training from the agency or organization where volunteers are placed. The following County is served: Saline.

693 RSVP Southeast Kansas
3740 South Santa Fe
Chanute, KS 66720
620-431-3902
Fax: 620-431-1409
www.newlifestyles.com/facility/facility.

Patty Allen, RSVP Director

Volunteer Program for those 55 years of age or older. Seventy volunteer stations are available where volunteers can serve to make a positive impact in their community.

694 Railroad Retirement Board: Kansas
601 East 12th Street
Room G47
Kansas City, MO 64106-2818
620-287-5973
Fax: 816-426-5334; *Toll Free:* 877-772-5772
wichita@rrb.gov
www.rrb.gov/field/do_kans.asp
TTY: 816-426-5334

Michael S. Schwartz, Chairman of the Board
George V. Govan, Senior Executive Officer,Executi
Ram Murthy, Chief Information Officer

The Railroad Retirement Board (RRB) is an independent agency in the executive branch of the Federal Government.

The RRB's primary function is to administer comprehensive retirement-survivor and unemployment-sickness benefit programs for the nation's railroad workers and their families, under the Railroad Retirement and Railroad Umemployment Insurance Acts. In connection with the retirement program, the RRB has administrative responsibilities under the Social Security Act for certain benefit payments and railroad workers' Medicare coverage.

695 Senior Center of Finney County
907 N Tenth Street
Garden City, KS 67846-5209
620-275-5566
Fax: 620-275-2285
finneycountyrsvp@sbcglobal.net
www.seniorcenterfc.com/RSVP.html

Janice Parks, Chairman
Shari Brandenburg, Vice Chairman
Marty Dinkel, RSVP Director

The Retired and Senior Volunteer Program (RSVP) provides opportunities for people 55 and over to make a difference in their community through volunteer service. RSVP volunteers contribute anywhere from a few to over forty hours a week, serving through schools, day care centers, police departments, hospitals and other nonprofit and public organizations to help meet critical community needs. RSVP offers maximum flexibility and choice to its volunteers. RSVP matches the personal interests and skills of older Americans with opportunities to help solve community problems and offers supplemental insurance while on duty, on-the-job training from the agency or organization where volunteers are placed. The following County served is: Finney.

Year Founded: 1975

696 South Central Kansas: Area Agency on Aging
304 South Summit street
Po Box 1122
Arkansas City, KS 67005-1122
620-442-0268
Fax: 620-442-0296; *Toll Free:* 800-362-0264
www.agingcare.com/local/South-Central-Ka

Betty Londeen, Executive Director

The role of the agency is to plan, coordinate and to adovocate for the development of comprehensive service delivery system to meet the needs of older persons living in Planning and Service area no 10, Chautauqua, Cowley, Elk, Greenwood, Harper, Kingman, McPherson, Reno, Rice and Summer counties.

697 Southeast Kansas: Area Agency on Aging
1 West Ash
Chanute, KS 66720-1010
620-431-2980
Fax: 620-431-2988; *Toll Free:* 800-794-2440
seksaaa@sekaaa.com
www.sekaaa.com

John L. Green, Executive Director

The general purpose of the Southeast Kansas Area Agency on Aging is to assess the needs of persons 60 years of age or older and plan the delivery of priority service programs.

Year Founded: 1973

698 United Way of Wyandotte County
434 Minnesota Avenue
PO Box 171042
Kansas City, KS 66117
913-371-3674
Fax: 913-371-2718
cedwards@unitedway-wyco.org
community.unitedway-wyco.org/comm

Wendell Maddox, President/CEO
Joy Richardson, Senior Director of Resource Deve
Judy Manning, Director, Campaign

The Retired and Senior Volunteer Program (RSVP) provides opportunities for people 55 and over to make a difference in their community through volunteer service. RSVP
volunteers contribute anywhere from a few to over forty
hours a week, serving through schools, day care centers,
police departments, hospitals and other nonprofit and public organizations to help meet critical community needs.
RSVP offers maximum flexibility and choice to its volunteers. RSVP matches the personal interests and skills of
older Americans with opportunities to help solve community problems and offers supplemental insurance while on
duty, on-the-job training from the agency or organization
where volunteers are placed. The following County is
served: Wyandotte.

Year Founded: 1973

Kentucky

699 Audubon Area Community Services, Inc.
1700 West Fifth Street
PO Box 20004
Owensboro, KY 42304-0004
270-686-1600
Fax: 270-686-1614
cferrell@audubon-area.com
www.audubon-area.com

Cindy Ferrell, Director

The Retired and Senior Volunteer Program (RSVP) provides opportunities for people 55 and over to make a difference in their community through volunteer service. RSVP
volunteers contribute anywhere from a few to over forty
hours a week, serving through schools, day care centers,
police departments, hospitals and other nonprofit and public organizations to help meet critical community needs.
RSVP offers maximum flexibility and choice to its volunteers. RSVP matches the personal interests and skills of
older Americans with opportunities to help solve community problems and offers supplemental insurance while on
duty, on-the-job training from the agency or organization
where volunteers are placed. The following Counties are
served: Daviess, Hancock, Henderson, McLean, Ohio,
Union, Webster.

700 Barren River Area Development District
177 Graham Avenue
Bowling Green, KY 42101
270-781-2381
Fax: 270-842-0768; *Toll Free:* 800-598-2381
www.bradd.org

Rodney Kirtley, Executive Director
Jolynn Vincent, Office Manager
Peggy Thompson, Director Human Services

Area Agency on Aging programs

701 Big Sandy Area Development District
110 Resource Court
Prestonsburg, KY 41653
606-886-2374
Fax: 606-886-3382; *Toll Free:* 800-737-2723
sandy.runyon@bigsandy.org
www.bigsandy.org

Sandy Runyon, Executive Director
Kelly Callaham, Martin county Judge-Executive
Wayne T. Rutherford,, Johnson County Judge-Executive

A Æmulti-county organization charged with planning, promoting, and coordinating programs for regional economic
and social development.

**702 Bluegrass Area Agency on Aging
andIndependent Living**
699 Perimeter Drive
Lexington, KY 40517
859-269-8021
Fax: 859-269-7917; *Toll Free:* 866-665-7921
cclark@bgadd.org
www.bgaaail.com

Celeste Collins, Aging Director
Mary Crowley-Schmidt, Assistant Director/Homecare Coor
Jeff Roback, Aging Program/Computer Specialis

As a part of a national network, our role is to develop and
coordinate a comprehensive service delivery system to
meet the needs of seniors in Central Kentucky. Counties
served: Anderson, Bourbon, Boyle, Clark, Estill, Fayette,
Franklin, Garrard, Harrison, Jessamine, Lincoln, Madison,
Mercer, Nicholas, Powell, Scott and Woodford.

703 Buffalo Trace: Area Agency on Aging
201 Government Street
PO Box 460, Suite 300
Maysville, KY 41056
606-564-6894
Fax: 606-564-0955; *Toll Free:* 800-998-4347
www.btadd.com
TDD 800-648-6056

Caroline Ullery, Director of Aging Services
Beth Love, Homecare case Manager
Cathie Drury, Caregiver Support Coordinator

Buffalo Trace Area Development District is a state designated Area Agency on Aging and part of a National Network on Aging under the direction of the US
Administration on Aging and under the supervision of the
Kentucky Office of Aging Services. An Area Agency on
Aging holds the responsibility of implementing the Older
Americans Act of 1965, as amended, and charged with the
responsibility of identifying the needs of the elderly, addressing those needs as well as serving as an advocate on
behalf of all Older Americans at the local level. Counties
served: Bracken, Fleming, Lewis, Mason, and Robertson.

**704 Community Action Council: Lexington Fayette
Jessamine Counties**
710 West High Street
PO Box 11610
Lexington, KY 40508
859-223-4600
Fax: 859-244-2219; *Toll Free:* 800-244-2275
www.commaction.org

Jack E Burch, Executive Director

The Retired and Senior Volunteer Program serves community organizations, historic sites, health care facilities, and more by placing volunteers at locations throughout Fayette and Jessamine counties. The volunteers serve as mentors, tutors and caregivers for at-risk children and youth or fill the needs of nonprofits by providing a helping hand.

Year Founded: 1965

705 Cumberland Valley: Area Agency on Aging

Po Box 1740
London, KY 40743-1740
606-864-7391
Fax: 606-878-7361; *Toll Free:* 800-795-7654
cvadd@cvadd.org
www.cvadd.org
TDD 800-648-6057

Mike Patrick, Executive Director
Leigh Powell, Area Agency on Aging Director
Revonda Evans, Aging Case Manager

Home to most of the states human services and health care programs.

706 Department for Disability Determination Services

PO Box 1000
275 East Main Street, 1E-B
Frankfort, KY 40601
502-564-5497
Fax: 502-564-9523; *Toll Free:* 800-928-8050
www.ssa.gov/disability/professionals

Audrey Tayse-Haynes, Secretary

The Kentucky Disability Determination Services (DDS) is a division of the the Department for Income Support fully funded by the Federal Government, and is responsible for developing medical evidence and making the determination on whether residents of Kentucky are or are not disabled under Social Security disability law.

707 Department for the Blind

275 East Main Street
Mailstp 2E-J
Frankfort, KY 40621
502-564-4754
Fax: 502-564-2951; *Toll Free:* 800-321-6668
blind@ky.gov
www.blind.ky.gov/Pages/default.aspx
TDD 502-564-2929

Gerry Slusher, Chairman
Bess Douthitt, Vice Chair
Paul Wiese, Immediate Past Chair

Our mission is to provide opportunities for employment and independence to individuals with visual disabilities. We offer services to assist their effort to become more independent and productive in the workplace, community, school, and home.

708 Disabled American Veterans

3725 Alexandria Pike
Cold Spring, KY 41076-1799
859-441-7300
Fax: 859-441-1416; *Toll Free:* 877-426-2838
www.dav.org

Wallace Tyson, Chairman
Larry Polzin, Vice-Chairman
Arthur H Wilson, Secretary

An organization of disabled veterans who are focused on building better lives for disabled veterans and their families.

709 FIVCO: Area Agency on Aging

32 Fivco Court
Grayson, KY 41143
606-929-1366
Fax: 606-929-1390
www.fivco.org
TTY: 800-648-6056

Clyde Johns, Chairman
Sherry McDavid, Executive Director
John M Clevenger, 1st Vice chairman

Assist in the areas of plannig, transportation, GIS, and economic development
Year Founded: 1968

710 Gateway Area Development District

110 Lake Park Drive
Morehead, KY 40351
606-780-0090
Fax: 606-780-0111
www.gwadd.org

Gail K Wright, Executive Director
Jason Boggs, Public Administration Specialist
Mark Collier, Director of Housing Program

711 Green River: Area Agency on Aging

300 Gradd Way
Owensboro, KY 42301-0200
270-926-4433
Fax: 270-684-0714
www.gradd.com

Jiten Shah, Executive Director
Keith Harpole, Associate Director
Debra James, Associate Director, Finance

The mission of the Green River Area Development District (GRADD) is to afford local governments and citizens a regional forum to identify issues and opportunities, and to provide leadership in planning and implementing programs to improve the quality of life in our district.

712 Kentucky Cabinet for Education, Arts and The Humanities: Commission for the Deaf and Hearing Impaired

700 Capitol Avenue
Room 209
Frankfort, KY 40601-3858
502-573-2604
Fax: 502-573-3594; *Toll Free:* 800-372-2907
www.kentucky.gov
go.hubbiz.com/State-Of-Kentucky-K

Bobbie Beth Scoggine, Executive Director

713 Kentucky Client Assistance Program

275 East Main Street
2nd Floor, Mail Stop 2EJ
Frankfort, KY 40601
502-564-8035
Fax: 502-564-1566; *Toll Free:* 800-633-6283
kycap.ky.gov

Gerry Gordon-Brown, CAP Director

Provides information, advice and advocacy on benefits available from rehabilitation programs to individuals with disabilities.

714 Kentucky Council on Developmental Disabilities

100 Fair Oaks Lane
4E-F
Frankfort, KY 40601
502-564-7841
Fax: 502-564-9826; Toll Free: 877-367-5332
shelley.runkle@ky.gov
chfs.ky.gov/ccdd/

Pat Seybold, Executive Director
Adam Jones, Program Administrator
Raymond Anderson, Internal Policy Analyst

The Kentucky Council on Developmental Disabilities is to create change through visonary leadership and advocacy so that people have choices and control over their own lives.

715 Kentucky Department of Veterans Affairs

1111B Louisville Road
Frankfort, KY 40601
502-564-9203
Fax: 502-564-9240; Toll Free: 800-572-6245
www.veterans.ky.gov

Kenneth Lucas, Commissioner
Margaret Plattner, Deputy Commissioner
Gilda Hill, Executive Director

Goal is to provide excellence in patient care, veteran's benefits and customer satisfaction. We have reformed our department internally and are striving for high quality, prompt and seamless service to veterans. Our department's employees continue to offer their dedication and commitment to help veterans gtet the service they have earned. Our nations veterans deserve NO less.

Year Founded: 1998

716 Kentucky Department of Workers Claims

657 Chamberlain Avenue
Frankfort, KY 40601-6117
502-564-5550
Fax: 502-564-5732
www.labor.ky.gov/workersclaims

Ingrid Bowling, Director, Division of Claims
Fran Davis, Director, Information Research
Connie Morris, Claims Branch Manager

Worker's compenasation claims office

717 Kentucky Office of Aging Services
Cabinet for Families and Children

275 East Main Street
3E-E
Frankfort, KY 40621
502-564-6930
Fax: 502-564-4595; Toll Free: 800-372-2970
www.chfs.ky.gov
TTY: 888-642-1137

Stacy Woodrums, Director, Operation and support
Tonia Wells, Director, Quality Living
Brian Boisseau, Branch Manager, Aging Program

Home to most of the state's human services and health care programs.

718 Kentucky Protection & Advocacy Division

100 Fair Oaks Lane
Third Floor
Frankfort, KY 40601
502-564-2967
Fax: 502-564-0848; Toll Free: 800-372-2988
www.kypa.net

Marsha Hockensmith, Division Director
Heidi Scissler, Legal Director
Necole Newton, Fiscal Officer

Protecting the rights of persons with disabilities in Kentucky providing information and referral, training, and technical assistance.

719 Kentucky Retirement Systems
Perimeter Park West

1260 Louisville Road
Frankfort, KY 40601-6124
502-696-8800
Fax: 502-696-8822; Toll Free: 800-928-4646
krs.mail@kyret.ky.gov
https://kyret.ky.gov/Pages/default.aspx

William A Thielen, Executive Director
Karen Roggenkamp, Chief Operations Officer
Todd E Coleman, Director, Accounting

Kentucky Retirement Systems is responsible for the investment of funds and administration of benefits for over 267,000 state and local governement employees in the Commonwealth of Kentucky. These employees include state employees, state police officers, city and county employees, as well as nonteaching staff of local school boards and regional universities.

720 Kentucky Revenue Cabinet

501 High Street
Frankfort, KY 40620
502-564-4581
Fax: 502-564-3875
www.revenue.ky.gov
TTY: 502-564-3058

Bonnie Lee, Executive Director

the mission of the Finance Cabinet is to be the best possible steward of the taxpayer's dollar by responsibly investing and distributing the Commonwealth's financial resources, effectively administering the collection of state revenues, efficiently managing and procuring all of the Commonwealth's property and attentively operating the state's consolidated technology platforms.

721 Kentucky River: Area Agency on Aging

917 Perry Park Road
Hazard, KY 41701
606-436-3158
Fax: 606-436-2144
stacie@kradd.org
www.kradd.org/Aging/Aging.htm

Sherry Burchell, Program Coordinator
Stacie Noble, Program Director

Serves Lee, Breathett, Ousley, Wolfe, Leidue, Perry, Knott, Letcher counties elderly populations.

722 Kentucky Teachers Retirement System

479 Versailles Road
Frankfort, KY 40601-3868

502-848-8500
Fax: 502-573-0199; *Toll Free:* 800-618-1687
ktrs.info@ky.gov
www.ktrs.ky.gov

Barbara Sterrett, Chairperson
Robert Conley, Vice Chair
Charles Ludwig, Board Committee

An actuarial reserve, joint contributory system, meaning that contributions of the members and employers and the earnings from KTRS investments are placed in reserve to pay for the system's annuity obligation

723 Kentuckyiana Regional Planning & Development Agency
11520 Commonwealth Drive
Louisville, KY 40299-2340
502-266-6084
Fax: 502-266-5047
kipda.trans@ky.gov
www.kipda.org
TDD 800-648-6056

John Lugan Brent, Chairperson
Jack Couch, Executive Director
Jeff Gahan, Vice Chairperson

KIPDA provides regional planning, review and technical services in the areas of public administration, social services and transportation as well as community ridesharing programs. KIPDA also coordinates services for persons 60 years of age and over. KIPDA is designated by the Kentucky State Clearinghouse as the regional review agency for virtually all applications for federal and/or state funds made by organizations or governments within the state of Kentucky.

724 Lake Cumberland Area Development District: Area Agency on Aging
2384 Lakeway Drive
PO Box 1570
Russell Springs, KY 42642-1570
270-866-4200
Fax: 270-866-2044; *Toll Free:* 800-264-7093
info@cadd.org
lcadd.org/manager

Donna Diaz, Executive Director
Donna Little, Finance Officer
Luanne Adams, Executive Assistant

Helps frail and elderly remain at home provding in home and community based services.

725 Lincoln Trail: Area Agency on Aging
613 College Street Road
PO Box 604
Elizabethtown, KY 42702-0604
270-769-2393
Fax: 270-769-2993; *Toll Free:* 800-247-2510
info@ltadd.org
www.ltadd.org
TDD 800-247-2510

Bobby Claycomb, Chairperson
John G. Mattingly, First Vice-Chairperson
David Pace, Second Vice-Chairperson

Our mission is to build the capacity of its members to help older persons and persons with disabilities live with dignity and choices in their homes and communities for as long as

possible. The following Counties are served: Breckinridge, Grayson, Hardin, Larue, Marion, Nelson, Washington.

Year Founded: 1968

726 Metro United Way
334 East Broadway
PO Box 4488
Louisville, KY 40204-0488
502-583-2821
Fax: 502-583-0330; *Toll Free:* 800-541-6882
info@metrounitedway.org
www.metrounitedway.org
TDD 502-589-4259

Joe Tolan, President/CEO
Maggie Elder, Vice President
Gil Betz, Chief Strategy Officer

Improves lives and our community by engaging people to give, advocate, and volunteer

727 Northern Kentucky: Area Agency on Aging
22 Spiral Drive
Florence, KY 41042-1300
859-283-1885
Fax: 859-283-8178; *Toll Free:* 866-766-2372
info@nkadd.org
www.nkadd.org
TDD 859-282-2707

George Zubaty, Chairman
Harold Shorty Tomlinson, First Vice-Chairperson
Rick Skinner, Secretary/Treasurer

Works as advocates, planners, coordinators and developers to ensure the needed services and monitors to citizens of the community who are 60 years of age and older. The agency also contracts with service prodivers in the area to deliver services to older adults. The agency also accesses the services provided and monitors the providers for compliance to predetermined service levels and goals.

Year Founded: 1971

728 Purchase Area Development District
1002 Medical Drive
PO Box 588
Mayfield, KY 42066
270-247-7171
Fax: 270-251-6110
purchase.add@purchaseadd.org
www.purchaseadd.org

Jennifer Beck Walker, Executive Director
Andy Benette, Associate director,Finance
Deana Burkeen, Administrative assistant

The Purchase Area Development District is a partnership organization that offers support to city and county governments in the 8-county region of Western Kentucky. We provide opportunities for community leaders to gather, share common concerns, and create innovative approaches to local and regional challenges.

729 RSVP Brighton Center
741 Central Avenue
PO Box 325
Newport, KY 41072
859-491-8303
Fax: 859-491-8702
Brighton@BrightonCenter.com
www.brightoncenter.com

Tammy Weidinger, President/CEO
Wonda Winker, Vice President
June Mileer, Chief Financial Officer

To create opportunities for individuals and families to reach self-sufficiency through family support services, education and leadership throughout the communities of Northern Kentucky. We will achieve this mission by creating an environment which rewards excellence and innovation, encourages mutual respect and maximizes resources.

Year Founded: 1966

730 RSVP Central Kentucky
617 north Mulberry Street
Suite 4
Elizabethtown, KY 42701-1940
270-737-066
Fax: 270-234-8764
ckrsvp@windstream.net
www.newlifestyles.com

Judy Cedarholm, Director

The Retired and Senior Volunteer Program (RSVP) provides opportunities for people 55 and over to make a difference in their community through volunteer service. RSVP volunteers contribute anywhere from a few to over forty hours a week, serving through schools, day care centers, police departments, hospitals and other nonprofit and public organizations to help meet critical community needs. RSVP offers maximum flexibility and choice to its volunteers. RSVP matches the personal interests and skills of older Americans with opportunities to help solve community problems and offers supplemental insurance while on duty, on-the-job training from the agency or organization where volunteers are placed. The following Counties are served: Breckinridge, Grayson, Hardin, Larue, Nelson.

731 RSVP Hickman-McCracken Counties
217 1/2 East Clay Street
Clinton, KY 42031
270-653-5853
Fax: 270-443-8609
rsvphickmanco@earthlink.net
www.hickmancounty.ky.gov/departments/RSV

Alma Blair, Volunteer Coordinator

Our mission is to provide an affordable and positive comprehensive system of recreation programs designed to enhance the quality of life for the residents of the City of Paducah as well as surrounding communities. We will strive to organize and implement leisure pursuits that promote the mental, social, and physical well being of all actively or passively participating citizens regardless of socioeconomic background, race, creed or religion.

732 RSVP Louisville Metro Community Action Partnership
1200 South 3rd Street
Louisville, KY 40203-2906
502-574-1157
Fax: 502-637-6814
www.louisvilleky.gov

Theresa Reno-Weber, Director
Daro Mott, Deputy director
Mitchell Burmeister, Organisation Performance Analyst

Provides opportunities for persons 55 and over to have a continuing positive impact on their community through meaningful volunteer projects.

Year Founded: 1964

733 Railroad Retirement Board: Kentucky District Office
629 South Fourth Street
Room 301
Louisville, KY 40202
312-751-4300
Fax: 502-582-5518; *Toll Free:* 877-772-5772
louisville@rrb.gov
www.rrb.gov/field/do_loui.asp
TTY: 312- 75- 470

Michael S. Schwartz, Chairman of the Board
Walter A Barrows, Labor Member
Jerome F Kever, Mnagement Member

An independent agency in the executive branch of the Federal Government. The primary function is to administer comprehensive retirement-survivor and unemployment sickness benefit programs for the nation's railroad workers and their families, under the Railroad Retirement and Railroad Unemployment Insurance Act.

734 Senior Citizens of Whitley County
208 South 2nd Street
Williamsburg, KY 40769-1221
606-549-5600
www.yelp.com/biz/senior-citizens-of-whit

Jackie Hake, Executive Director
Carrie Perry, Nutrition Director
Bernie King, WCT Scheduler

Provides information and referral service, meals, transportation, escorts, and domestic services for people over the age of 60.

735 Senior Services of Northern Kentucky
1032 Madison Avenue
Covington, KY 41011-3172
859-491-0522
Fax: 859-491-4590; *Toll Free:* 800-255-7265
INFO@SENIORSERVICESNKY.ORG
www.seniorservicesnky.org

Ken Rechtin, Executive Director
Tricia Watts, Advancement Director
Charles Brewer, Communications Officer

Senior Services of Northern Kentucky provides a vital role in keeping older adults healthy, by providing healthy nutrition (Meals on Wheels), education programs on health and wellness, transportation for medical appointments and a wide array of social services. By keeping the elderly healthy they can remain a vital part of their community and can continue to live in their own home.

Year Founded: 1962

736 Social Security: Louisville Disability Determination
601 West Broadway
Room 101
Louisville, KY 40202
502-582-6690; *Toll Free:* 800-928-3202
www.disability-benefits-help.org/social-
Determines social security benefits for disabled workers

737 The Mason County Democrats
PO Box 1272
Shelton, WA 98584

360-427-2731
Fax: 606-564-5512
www.masoncountydemocrats.com/component/c

Mike Mosbarger, Chairperson
Adreinne Amar, Vice Chairperson
Linda Amar, secretary

RSVP helps people age 55 and older find volunteer service opportunities in their communities. RSVP particiapants serve from a few to over forty hours a week in organizations that range from hospital and youth centers to local service agencies and education facilties. RSVP involves seniors in service that matches their personal interests and makes use of their skills and lifelong experiences.

Louisiana

738 Beauregard Council on Aging
104 Port Street
PO 534
Deridder, LA 70634
337-463-6578
Fax: 337-463-7431
clgbcoa@aol.com
www.caddocouncilonaging.org/index.php?sr

Connie Granger, Director
Richard Nix, EVP
Gina Paddock, VP Sales

The Beauregard Council on Aging is a multipurpose center whose total program is to provide development and delivery of services for persons sixty years of age and over and/or their spouse. The center also serves as a community resource for information, referral and training in the field of aging. We operate under the Governor's Office of Elderly Affairs. The program is funded by both federal and state funds. The BCOA is a non-discriminating agency that encourages participation of low-income, minority, socially needy, and the handicapped. However, anyone sixty years of age or older is eligible for our services.

739 Bienville: Area Agency on Aging
600 Factory Outlet Drive
Suite 15
Arcadia, LA 71001-3617
318-263-8936
Fax: 318-263-9774
biencoa@bayou.com
www.agingcare.com

Triveria Roberson, Director

Provide support services to persons age 60 and over which help maintain their independence and quality of life in a home environment and to serve as a focal point on issues affecting the health and welfare of the aging population.

740 Bossier Council on Aging
706 Bearkat Drive
PO Box 5606
Bossier City, LA 71111-4566
318-741-8302
Fax: 318-741-7490; *Toll Free:* 800-256-8993
bcoamar@suddenlinkmail.com
bossiercoa.org

Mary Anne Rankin, Executive Director

Support service to persons age 60 and over which help maintain their independence and quality of life in a home

environment and to serve as a focal point on issues affecting the health and welfare of the aging population.
Year Founded: 1975

741 Caddo Council on Aging
1700 Buckner Street
Suite 240
Shreveport, LA 71104
318-676-7900
Fax: 318-676-7911; *Toll Free:* 800-256-3003
ccoa@caddocoa.org
www.caddocouncilonaging.org

Mary Alice Rountree, Executive Director

The Caddo Council on Aging serves as both a unifying force for services to seniors and as a focal point for federal, state, and local agencies, which serve the elderly.

742 Cajun: Area Agency on Aging
110 Toledo Drive
Po Box 60850
Lafayette, LA 70596-0850
337-572-8940
Fax: 337-237-7756; *Toll Free:* 800-738-2256
cajnaaa@bellsouth.net
www.cajunaaa.org/site.php

Shannon Broussard, Director

Cajun Area Agency on Aging Inc., is a non-profit corporation, that exists to identify the needs of persons 60 and older and to coordinate agreements for the delivery of services. The agency administers federal and state dollars through contractual agreements with service providers in an eight parish planning and service area.

743 Calcasieu Council on Aging
3950 Highway 14
Lake Charles, LA 70607
337-474-2585
Fax: 337-474-6563; *Toll Free:* 800-223-5872
www.calcoa.org

Sonya Caraway, Director

It is the sole purpose of the Calcasieu Council of Aging to assist older adults in order to remain independent in their own homes.

744 Caldewell Parish Council on Aging
307 Main Street
PO Box 1498
Columbia, LA 71418-1498
318-649-2584
Fax: 318-649-7600
dottie@caldwellcoa.org
www.caldwellcoa.org

Dottie Etheridge, Executive Director
Monica Pauley, Office Manager

Congregate Meals, Home Delivered Meals, Recreation, Information and Assistance, Homemaker Services, Transportation, Medication Mangement, Nutrition Counseling, Nutrition Education, Legal Assistance are some of the services offered.

Year Founded: 1964

745 Cameron Council on Aging
723 Marshall Street
PO Box 421
Cameron, LA 70631

337-775-5668
Fax: 337-775-7877
www.caddocouncilonaging.org
Dinah N Landry, Director

Cameron Council on Aging program helps older people to remain health, find jobs, discover new ways to continue contributing to society after retirement, and take advantage of government and private benefits programs that can improve the quality of their lives.

746   Capital: Area Agency on Aging
6554 Florida Boulevard, Suite 221
PO Box 66038
Baton Rouge, LA 70896-6038
225-922-2525
Fax: 225-922-2528; *Toll Free:* 800-833-9883
caaa@capitalaaa.org
www.capitalaaa.org

James O. Blouin, President,BOD
Linda Beauvais, Executive Director

Mission of the Capital Area Agency on Aging, is to ensure availiability of interrelated supportive and nutrition services to all persons aged 60 and older.

747   Claiborne Voluntary Council on Aging
608 East 4th Street
PO Box 480
Homer, LA 71040-3530
318-927-6922
Fax: 318-927-1070
josreed@bellsouth.net
www.manta.com

Josephine Miller, Executive Director
Cheryl Zeagler, Director

Services are for persons over 60 years of age.

Year Founded: 1975

748   Disability Determination Services
5905 Florida Boulevard, Room 2110
PO Box 96074
Baton Rouge, LA 70806-4335
225-925-3533
Fax: 225-925-1831; *Toll Free:* 800-256-2288
wwwprd.doa.louisiana.gov/laservic

Lonnie Beverly, Manager

Eligibility determination for disability benefits

749   Disability Determination Services: Shreveport Branch
2920 Knight Street, Suite 232
PO Box 4446
Shreveport, LA 71105
318-869-6400
Fax: 318-869-6406
Robbie.Day@ssa.gov
wwwprd.doa.louisiana.gov/laservic

Eligibility determination for disability benefits

750   East Baton Rouge Council on Aging
5790 Florida Boulevard
Baton Rouge, LA 70806-4244
225-923-8000
Fax: 225-923-8030
louise@ebrcoa.org
www.ebrcoa.org

Johnny G. Anderson, Chairman
Julie Cherry, Secretary
Tasha Clark Amar, Executive Director

Mission is to serve the elderly in East Baton Rouge Parish, to enrich and enhance their quality of life through advocacy efforts, creative planning and coordination and provision of needed services, and to make possible for them to live independent lives as long as possible.

Year Founded: 1973

751   Jefferson Council on Aging
6620 Riverside Drive
Suite 216
Metairie, LA 70003
504-888-5880
Fax: 504-828-1596; *Toll Free:* 800-635-1437
hlangley@bellsouth.net
www.jcoa.net

Ms. Anna Toujas, Vice Chairperson
Albert J. Robichaux, Executive Director,CEO
Ms. Lynne Peterson, Treasurer

Mission is to assist the senior citizens of Jefferson Parish to age with dignity and independence in the place and manner of their choice.

752   Lafourche Council on Aging, Inc.
4876 Highway 1
PO Box 500
Mathews, LA 70375
985-532-0457
Fax: 985-532-0462; *Toll Free:* 888-879-4400
laf.coadirector@mobiletel.com
www.lafourchecoa.org

Hamilton Dantin, Chairman
Gail Tolbert, Vice Chairman
Charlene Rodriguez, Executive Director

Service organization for senior citizens in Lafourche Parish, LA. Conducts charitable activities.

753   Lincoln Council on Aging
15 Bedford Road
Po Box 1058
Lincoln, MA 01773
781-259-8811
Fax: 781-259-7990
mdwright@suddenlinkmail.com
www.lincolntown.org

Mary Day, Treasurer/Collector
Colleen Wilkins, Finance Director/Accountant
Veronica Philips, Assistant Finance Director

Mission is to provide a broad range of programs and services which improve the quality of life for older and at-risk senior citizens and enables them to live independently with dignity in the least restrictive environment.

754   Louisiana Client Assistance Program
8325 Oak Street
New Orleans, LA 70118
504-522-2337
Fax: 504-522-5507; *Toll Free:* 800-960-7705
advocacycenter@advocacyla.org
www.advocacyla.org
TTY: 855-861-3577

Dale Higgins, Board President
Rachael Maddox, Community Living Ombudsman
Nell Hahn, Director of Litigation & Systems

Programs in each state provide information and assistance to individuals seeking or receiving service under the Rehabilitation Act of 1973.

Year Founded: 1978

755 Louisiana Department of Revenue
617 North Third Street
PO Box 201
Baton Rouge, LA 70802
225-922-2300
www.rev.state.la.us

Tim Barfield, Secretary of Revenue
Jarrod Coniglio, Deputy Secretary
Jason DeCuir, Executive Counsel

Mission is to administer applicable laws and collect revenues to fund state services.

756 Louisiana Department of Veterans Affairs
PO Box 94095
Baton Rouge, LA 70804-9095
225-922-0500
Fax: 225-219-5590; *Toll Free:* 877-GEA-XVA
veteran@la.gov.
www.vetaffairs.la.gov

Mr Don A. Beasley, Chairman
Rodney Alexander, Secretary
Thomas Burbank, Undersecretary

Mission is to assist Louisiana veterans and their dependents in receiving all federal and state benefits, and deliver quality services.

757 Louisiana Developmental Disability Council
626 Main Street, Suite A
PO Box 3455
Baton Rouge, LA 70821-3455
225-342-6804
Fax: 225-342-1970; *Toll Free:* 800-450-8108
shawn.fleming@la.gov
www.laddc.org

Paige Freeman, Executive Secretary
Sandee Winchell, Executive Director
Shawn Fleming, Deputy Director

The mission of the Council is to assure that all persons with developmental disabilities receive the best services, the most appropriate assistance, and the opportunities necessary to enable them to achieve their maximum potential through increased self determination, independence, producitivity, integration, and inclusion.

Year Founded: 1970

758 Louisiana Employee's Retirement Department
8401 United Plaza Boulevard, 1st Floor
PO Box 44213
Baton Rouge, LA 70804-4213
225-922-0600
Fax: 225-935-2856; *Toll Free:* 800-256-3000
www.lasersonline.org
TDD 225-922-0612

Robert W. Beale, Chief Investment Officer
Cindy Rougeou, Executive Director
Marie Le Blanc, Deputy Director

A defined benefit plan

759 Louisiana Protection & Advocacy for Persons with Disabilities
8325 Oak Street
Suite 2600
New Orleans, LA 70118
504-522-2337
Fax: 504-522-5507; *Toll Free:* 800-960-7705
advocacycenter@advocacyla.org
www.advocacyla.org
TTY: 855-861-3577

Dale Higgins, President
Paget Bazile, Secretary
James Thompson, Treasurer

A protection and advocacy system that protects the rights of persons with mental or physical disabilities.

Year Founded: 1977

760 Louisiana Teachers Retirement System
8401 United Plaza Boulevard, 3rd Floor
Po Box 94123
Baton Rouge, LA 70809-7017
225-925-6446
Fax: 225-925-3944; *Toll Free:* 1 8-7 2-5 87
web.master@trsl.org
trsl.org
TDD 255-925-3653

Charlene Wilson, Chief Financial Officer
Maureen H. Westgard, Director
Dana Lee Haltom, Executive Assistant

The Teacher's Retirement System of Louisiana (TRSL) is a governmental defined benefit plan as a public trust fund to provide retirement benefits for its members. TRSL is the state's largest public retirement system with 160,000 active and retired members.

761 Madison Council on Aging
PO Box 1229
203 South Elm Street
Tallulah, LA 71284-1229
318-574-3666
Fax: 318-574-4113
mcoa@louisiana-internet.net

Mike Rome, Executive Director

762 Morehouse Council on Aging
200 Elm Street
Bastrop, LA 71221-1471
318-283-0845
Fax: 318-283-0835; *Toll Free:* 800-256-3006
reggiedir@bellsouth.net
www.morehousecoa.org

R D DeFreese, Director
Diane DeFreese, Service Manager,Coordinator
Charler Walker, Fitness Center Manager

Provides an array of service choices to peopl in the community age 60 plus.

763 Natchitoches Parish Council on Aging
1016 Keyser Avenue
Natchitoches, LA 71457-5817
318-357-3250
Fax: 318-357-2424
Natchitoches@LouisianaCouncilsOnAging.com
www.louisianacouncilsonaging.com

Alice Barrios, Director
Betty Newman, Administrative Secretary
Shelby Graham, Nutrition Coordinator

provides services for the elderly

Year Founded: 1969

764 New Orleans Council on Aging

2475 Canal Street, Suite 400
PO Box 19067
New Orleans, LA 70179-0067
504-821-4121
Fax: 504-821-1222
administration@nocoa.org
www.nocoa.org
TDD 504-586-4475

Okeyame M Haley, President
So'Nia L. Gilkey, Vice President
Howard L Rodgers, Executive Director

A private, non-profit corporation that services as the Area
Agency on Aging for Orleans parish. As such it is responsible for seeing that a comprehensive and coordinated assortment of social, recreational, educational, employment and
nutritional services are made availiable for all persons aged
60 and over in the city of New Orleans.

765 North Delta: Area Agency on Aging

1913 Stubbs Avenue
Monroe, LA 71201-3617
318-387-2572
Fax: 318-387-9054
office@northdelta.org
www.northdelta.org

David Creed, Executive Director
Louise Collins-Harris, Chief Operations Officer
Lanell Winston, Area Agency on Aging Director

Through the North Delta Area Agency on Aging, we assist
six parishes within our district in administration of programs to assist Senior Citizens. Whether our Senior Citizens receive services from only one program, or from many
of these programs, their quality of life is enhanced through
the dedicated efforts of the Councils on Aging who actually
render these services.

766 Ouachita Council on Aging

2407 Ferrand Street
Monroe, LA 71201-3248
318-387-0535
Fax: 318-322-0545
aging@centurytel.net
www.ouachitacoa.com
TDD 318-324-0607

Lynda McGehee, Executive Director
Ernest Jackson, Chief custodian
Neil Billups, Assistant Custodian

Responsible for carrying out a wide range of functions relative to advocacy, planning, coordination, inter-agency linkage, information sharing, brokering, monitoring, and
evaluation designed to lead to the development or enhancement of comprehensive and coordinated community based
system to serve all areas in Ouachita Parish.

Year Founded: 1967

767 Plaquemines Council on Aging

8056 Highway 23
Suite 200
Belle Chasse, LA 70037
504-564-0600
Fax: 504-274-2463
plaqcoal@bellsouth.net
plaqueminesparish.com

Billy Nungesser, Parish President
Kathy B. Motes, Executive Assistant
Therese M. Wooton, Scheduling Secretary

Plaquemines Council on Aging was established to provide
a variety of services to persons 60 years of age or older residing in Plaquemines Parish.

768 Protection & Advocacy of Individual Rights
Advocacy Center for the Elderly and Disabled

1010 Common Street
Suite 2600
New Orleans, LA 70112
504-522-2337
Fax: 504-522-7705; Toll Free: 800-960-7705
advocacycenter@advocacyla.org
www.advocacyla.org

Lois Simpson, Executive Director
Elizabeth Smith, Controller

The Advocacy Center believes in the dignity of every life,
and in the freedom of all people to experience the highest
degree of self-determination. Embracing this philosophy,
the Advocacy Center protects and advocates for the human
and legal rights of persons living in Louisiana who are
elderly or disabled.

769 RSVP Calcasieu Parish

1015 Pithon Road, 2nd Floor
PO Box 1583
Lake Charles, LA 70602
337-721-3500
Fax: 337-437-3399
administration@cppj.net
www.cppj.net

Jessica D. Williamson, Executive Secretary
Bryan C Beam, Parish Administrator

The mission of this program is to create and maintain senior citizen volunteer service opportunities within the Parish for active and healthy seniors residing in Parish.

Year Founded: 1840

770 RSVP Jefferson Parish

1221 Elmwood Park Boulevard
Suite 402
Harahan, LA 70123-2337
504-736-6410
Fax: 504-736-6413
www.jeffparish.net

John F. Young, President,Chief Administrative
Timothy Palmatier, Finance Director
Jacques L. Molaison, Deputy Chief Operating Officer

RSVP provides a variety of opportunities for retired individuals and seniors to help their community and benefit
from performing useful services. Volunteers work in hospitals, offices, nursing homes, day care centers, schools.
They also receive limited insurance and expense
reimbursement.

Year Founded: 1825

771 RSVP River Parishes
274 Judge Edward Dufresne Pkwy
Luling, LA 70070-2163
985-783-8907
Fax: 985-785-1950
fcairersvp@stcharlesgov.net
www.stcharlesgov.net

Michelle Higgins, Director,RSVP
Kim Boudreaux, Coordinator,RSVP

The purpose of RSVP is to enable older Americans aged 55 and over to contribute to their communities through volunteer service, to enhance the lives of the volunteers and those whom they serve, and to provide communities valuable services. RSVP utilizes the vast talents of older volunteers willing to share their experiences, abilities, and skills in responding to a wide variety of community needs. The following Counties are served: St. Charles, St. James, St. John the Baptist.

772 RSVP St. Tammany Parish
Volunteers of American GNO - North Shore Office
823 Carroll Street
Suite B
Mandeville, LA 70448
985-674-0488
Fax: 985-674-0336
dwild@voagno.org

Dee Wild, RSVP Director

RSVP offers volunteers 55 and older a variety of volunteer opportunities addressing critical needs here in St. Tammany Parish. We are dedicated to helping seniors remain active and involved by providing a high quality volunteer experience. Volunteer assignments offer variety, flexibility, and the opportunity to make a difference right here in your own community.

773 Railroad Retirement Board: District Office
500 Poydras Street
Suite 1045
New Orleans, LA 70130-3399
504-589-2597
Fax: 504-589-4899
www.rrb.gov

Paul Sosricki, Representative

An independent agency in the executive branch of the Federal Government. The RRB's primary function is to administer comprehensive retirement survivor and unemployment sickness benefit programs for the nation's railroad workers and their families.

774 Red River Council on Aging
PO Box 688
1825 Front Street
Coushatta, LA 71019
318-932-5721
Fax: 318-932-9572
rrcoa@bellsouth.net

Mary Wailes, Executive Director

Collects facts and statistics to make special studies of conditions pertaining to the employment, financial status, recreation, social adjustments, mental and physical health or other conditions affecting the welfare of the aging people in the parish.

775 St Charles Council on Aging
626 Pine Street
Suite A
Hahnville, LA 70057-2358
985-783-6683
Fax: 985-783-1996
info@stcharlescoa.com
www.stcharlesgov.net

Margaret Powe, Executive Director

Serve senior citizens sixty and older in St Charles Parish.

776 St John Area: Agency on Aging
214 Regala Park Road
Reserve, LA 70084
985-652-3660
Fax: 985-651-4933
stjohncoa@bellsouth.net
goea.louisiana.gov

Barbara Gralapp, Executive Director

Designated by the state to develop and administer the area plan for a comprehensive and coordinated system of services for older person in a planning and service area.

777 St John Parish Council on Aging
1801 West Airline Highway
La Place, LA 70068
985-652-9569
Fax: 985-651-4933; *Toll Free:* 866-437-5262
info@stjohnla.us
www.stbparish.com

Nickie Monica, Parish President
Stacey Cador, Director Human Resources

Dedicated to improving the health and independence of older persons and increasing their continuing contributions to communities, society, and future generations.

778 St. Bernard Council on Aging
8201A W Judge Perez Drive
Chalmette, LA 70043-1611
504-278-7335
Fax: 504-278-7452
stbernardcoa@yahoo.com
www.sbcoa.org

Joy Pell, Director
Carol Lejeune, Assistant Director

Dedicated to improving the health and independence of older persons and increasing their continuing contributions to communities, society, and future generations.

779 St. James Parish Department of Human Resources
5800 Highway 44
Convent, LA 70723
225-562-2305
Fax: 504-562-2425
humanresources@stjamesla.com
www.stjamesla.com

Michelle Nailor-Octave, Director Of Human Resources
Bedar Warren, Asst. Director Human Resources
Doris Brignac, Financial Officer

Mission is to provide residents with programs and services to help improve their quality of life leading to self-sufficiency.

780 **St. Tammany Council on Aging**
PO Box 171
623 Plaza Drive
Covington, LA 70434
985-892-0377
Fax: 985-892-2014; *Toll Free:* 800-256-2823
coast@coastseniors.org
coastseniors.org

Mary Toti, Executive Director
Irva Amacker, Administrative Director
Len Beech, Seniior Srvs. Operations Dir

Coasts helps seniors stay healthy with nutrition services; stay active with wellness and recreation activities; stay alive with medical alert program; and stay informed with classes and presentations.

781 **Tensas Council on Aging**
PO Box 726
118 Plank Road
Saint Joseph, LA 71366
318-766-3770
Fax: 318-766-3774
Tensas@LouisianaCouncilsOnAging.com
www.louisianacouncilonaging.com

Clarissa C Newman, Executive Director
Clifford Walker, Transportation Coordinator
Elize Williams, Site Manager

Dedicated to improving the lives and independence of senior citizens

782 **Terrebonne Council on Aging**
995 W Tunnel Boulevard
Houma, LA 70360-5557
985-868-8411
Fax: 985-868-7806
tcoainfo@tcoa-la.org
www.tcoa-la.org

Diana N Edmonson, Executive Director

An aging program that provides information and services on a range of assistance for older adults and those who care for them.

783 **The Rapides Parish Council on Aging, Inc.**
204 Chester Street
Alexandria, LA 71301-6511
318-445-7985
Fax: 318-445-7919
www.rapidescouncilonaging.org

Bettyte DeKeyzer, Executive Director
Rebecca Maricle, Program Manager
Al Armstrong, Chore/Transportation Superviser

The Retired and Senior Volunteer Program (RSVP) provides opportunities for people 55 and over to make a difference in their community through volunteer service. RSVP volunteers contribute anywhere from a few to over forty hours a week, serving through schools, day care centers, police departments, hospitals and other nonprofit and public organizations to help meet critical community needs. RSVP offers maximum flexibility and choice to its volunteers. RSVP matches the personal interests and skills of older Americans with opportunities to help solve community problems and offers supplemental insurance while on duty, on-the-job training from the agency or organization where volunteers are placed. The following County is served: Rapides.

Year Founded: 1967

Maine

784 **Aroostook: Area Agency on Aging**
1 Edgemont Drive
Suite 2
Presque Isle, ME 04769
207-764-3396
Fax: 207-764-6182; *Toll Free:* 800-439-1789
information@aroostookaging.org
www.aroostookaging.org

Stephen Farnham, Executive Director

Mission is to improve the quality of life and well-being of older people in the community.

785 **Central Maine: Area Agency on Aging**
Spectrum Generations
89 State House Station
Augusta, ME 04333-0084
207-287-5795
Fax: 207-622-7857; *Toll Free:* 800-639-1553
www.maine.gov

Muriel Scott, Executive Director

A cebtral resource for elder services.

786 **Disability Determination Services**
11 State House Station
19 Union Street
Augusta, ME 04330
207-624-4168
Fax: 207-287-5096
www.maine.gov/dhhs/ofi/services/dds/offi

Scott Mack, Director

Mission is to provide acuurate, timely, and cost effective decisions for Social Security Disabiliy Claims.

787 **Eastern Maine: Area Agency on Aging**
450 Essex Street
Bangor, ME 04401
207-941-2865
Fax: 207-941-2869; *Toll Free:* 800-432-7812
info@eaaa.org
www.eaaa.org
TTY: 207-992-0150

Noelle Merrill, Executive Director
Carol Higgins-Taylor, Director of Community Education
Deborah Poulton, Deputy Director/Director of Fami

It is the mission of Eastern Area agency on Aging to be the best source of information, options and services for seniors, adults with disabilities and caregivers..

788 **Freeport Elders Association**
49 Park Street
PO Box 176
Freeport, ME 04032-1319
207-865-6462

Patricia Guild, President

Senior citizens information and services.

789 **Maine Assistive Technology Projects**
University of Maine System University College
46 University Drive
Augusta, ME 04330

207-621-3195
Fax: 207-629-5429
iweb@mainecite.org
www.mainecite.org

Kathleen Powers, Program Director
Kathy Adams, Training Coordinator
Darcy York, Administrative Assistant

A statewide program promoting assistive technology devices and services for persons of all ages with all disabilities.

790 Maine Association of Retirees

280 Maine Avenue
Farmingdale, ME 04344
207-582-1960
Fax: 207-582-4764; *Toll Free:* 800-535-6555
mgorten@roadrunner.com
www.maineretirees.org

Barbara J. Van Burge, Interim Executive Director
Joseph Pietroski, Legislative & Financial Program
Amelia Cater, Membership Coordinator & Benefit

Nonprofit organization exists solely to work to protect and/or expand the rights and benefits of Maine's retirees.

791 Maine Bureau of Elder and Adult Services

221 State Street
Augusta, ME 04333
207-287-3707
Fax: 207-287-3005; *Toll Free:* 800-262-2232
www.maine.gov/dhhs/beas
TTY: 800-606-0215

Ricker Hamilton, Director
Romaine Turyn, Policy Director
Elizabeth Gattine, Long Term Care Director

The Office of Elder Services promotes programs and services for older adults, their families and for people with disabilities.

792 Maine Department of Defense, Veterans and Emergency Management

Joint Force Headquarters
Maine National Guard Camp Keyes
Augusta, ME 04333-0033
207-626-4271
Fax: 207-626-4509
www.maine.gov/dvem

Robert P McAleer, Commissioner

The Department of Defense, Veterans and Emergency Management coordinates and administers the discharge of Maine State Government's responsibility relating to military, veterans and civil emergency preparedness through the authorization, planning, provision of resources, administration, operation and audit of activities in these areas.

793 Maine Department of Labor: Bureau of Rehabilitation Services

150 State House Station
45 Commerce Drive
Augusta, ME 04333-0150
207-623-6799
Fax: 207-287-5292; *Toll Free:* 800-698-4440
mdol@maine.gov
www.maine.gov/rehab
TTY: 888-755-0023

Jill C Duson, Executive Director

BRS works to bring about full access to employment, independence and community integration for people with disabilities.

794 Maine Department of Labor: Bureau of Employment Security
Veterans' Employment Service

54 State House Station
Augusta, ME 04333
207-623-7981
Fax: 207-623-7900; *Toll Free:* 888-457-8883
mdol@maine.gov
www.maine.gov/labor/bes

Valerie Landry, Director

Provides veterans and transitioning service members with employment and training opportunities, and protects their employment rights.

795 Maine Developmental Disability Council

225 Western Avenue
Suite 4
Augusta, ME 04330-0139
207-287-4213
Fax: 207-287-8001; *Toll Free:* 800-244-3990
jbell@maineddc.org
www.maineddc.org

Julia Bell, Executive Director
Erin Howes, Office Manager
Rachel Dyer, Policy/Planning Specialist

The Maine Developmental Disabilities Council is a partnership of people with developmental disabilities, family members, and state and local agencies and organizations. We work together to bring about the necessary changes to achieve self-determination and independence for persons with developmental disabilities, and full inclusion in their communities of choice.

796 Maine Revenue Services

24 State House Station
Augusta, ME 04333
207-287-2076
Fax: 207-624-9694
www.state.me.us/revenue

Jerome D Gerard, Executive Director

Mission is to serve the citizens of Maine by administering the tax laws of the State effectively and professionally in order to provide the revenues necessary to support Maine government.

797 Maine Worker's Compensation Board

27 State House Station
Augusta, ME 04333-0027
207-287-3751
Fax: 207-287-7198; *Toll Free:* 888-801-9087
maine.gov/wcb
TTY: 877-832-5525

Paul H Sighinolfi, Executive Director
Lindsay Lizotte, Secretary Specialist

The general mission of the Maine Workers' Compensation Board is to serve the employees and employers of the State fairly and expeditiously by ensuring compliance with the workers' compensation laws, ensuring the prompt delivery of benefits legally due, promoting the prevention of disputes, utilizing dispute resolution to reduce litigation and facilitating labor-management cooperation.

798 RSVP Aroostook
1 Edgemont Drive
Suite 2
Presque Isle, ME 04769-1288
207-764-3396
Fax: 207-764-6182; Toll Free: 800-439-1789
information@aroostookaging.org
www.aroostookaging.org

Eleanor Reese, Director

The mission of the Aroostook Agency on Aging is improving the quality of life and promoting the well-being of older people in our communities.

Year Founded: 1974

799 RSVP Penquis
315 Main Street
Suite 205
Rockland, ME 04841
207-596-0361
Fax: 207-594-2695; Toll Free: 800-585-1605
info@penquis.org
www.penquis.org

Tom Lizotte, Chair
Fred Brown, Vice Chair
Jeffers Ashley, Secretary

To engage folks 55+ to volunteer in their communities. Services include: companion outreach, read to children, transport seniors to medical appointments, mentor prisoners, food pantries, soup kitches, clerical help in clinics, hospitals and more.

Year Founded: 1967

800 RSVP Southern Maine
136 US Route One
Scarborough, ME 04074-9055
207-396-6500
Fax: 207-883-8249; Toll Free: 800-427-7411
info@smaaa.org
www.smaaa.org
TDD 207-883-0532
TTY: 207-883-0532

Larry Gross, Executive Director
David Smith, President
Terry Bagley, Vice President

The Retired and Senior Volunteer Program (RSVP) provides opportunities for people 55 and over to make a difference in their community through volunteer service. RSVP volunteers contribute anywhere from a few to over forty hours a week, serving through schools, day care centers, police departments, hospitals and other nonprofit and public organizations to help meet critical community needs. RSVP offers maximum flexibility and choice to its volunteers. RSVP matches the personal interests and skills of older Americans with opportunities to help solve community problems and offers supplemental insurance while on duty, on-the-job training from the agency or organization where volunteers are placed. The following Counties are served: Cumberland, York.

801 Seniors Plus
8 Falcon Road
PO Box 659
Lewiston, ME 04240
207-795-4010
Fax: 207-795-4009; Toll Free: 800-427-1241
info@seniorsplus.org

www.seniorsplus.org
TTY: 207-795-7232

Michael Burke, Chairperson
Annette Nadeau, Vice Chairperson
Betsy Sawyer-Manter, Executive Director

Seniors Plus believes in maintaining the independence, dignity and quality of life of older adults. Seniors Plus will work consistently to remove barriers and strive to provide services in a reliable and coordinated manner.

Year Founded: 1972

802 Southern Maine: Area Agency on Aging
136 Route US One
Scarborough, ME 04074
207-396-6500
Fax: 207-883-8249; Toll Free: 800-427-7411
info@smaaa.org
www.smaaa.org
TTY: 207-883-0532

Larry Gross, Executive Director
David Smith, President
Terry Bagley, Vice President

Mission of Southern Maine Agency on Aging is to assure that older people living in Southern Maine, especially those who are frail, living alone, or have low incomes, receive the support necessary to maintain their independence in the community.

803 Spectrum Generations
One Weston Court
Suite 109
Augusta, ME 04338
207-622-9212
Fax: 207-622-7857; Toll Free: 800-639-1553
Spectrum@spectrumgenerations.org
www.spectrumgenerations.org
TTY: 800-464-8703

Kristin Overton, Chief Operating Officer
Jerry Corey, Chief Financial Officer
Stephanie Hanner, Community Engagement Officer

Central Maine Area Agency on Aging providing information and assistance, respite care, adult day programs, Meals on Wheels, benefits counseling, home care services, and social activities for seniors.

Year Founded: 1972

804 United Way of Eastern Maine
24 Springer Drive
Suite 201
Bangor, ME 04401-3655
207-941-2800
Fax: 207-941-2805
info@unitedwayem.org
www.unitdwayem.org

Andrew Hamilton, Chair
Lannie Moffatt, Vice Chair
John Kuropchak, President/CEO

Our mission is to improve the lives of people in Eastern Maine by mobilizing the caring power of people and communities. We bring together human, financial and strategic resources to strengthen children and families, support seniors, meet people's basic needs, and promote self-sufficiency for all people.

Maryland

805 Allegany County: Area Agency on Aging
125 Virginia Avenue
Cumberland, MD 21502-2309
301-777-5970
Fax: 301-722-0937
anelson@alleganyhrdc.org
www.alleganyhrdc.org
TDD 800-735-2258

Gil Frankenberry, Chair
Nicholas Hadley, Vice Chair
Courtney A Thomas, Executive Director

Full range of aging services: elder support, medical waivers, senior centers, activities, nutrition, transportation and vulnerable adult programs.

Year Founded: 1966

806 Anne Arundel County Department of Aging and Disabilities
44 Calvert Street
2666 Riva Road
Annapolis, MD 21401-7345
410-222-4464
Fax: 410-222-4360; *Toll Free:* 800-492-2499
info_and_assistance@aacounty.org
www.aacounty.org/aging
TDD 410-222-4355
TTY: 410-222-4355

Virginia A Thomas, CFA, Director
Sandra Berkeley, Director I & A Program

The Department of Aging provides a number of programs for both older persons and persons with disabilities.

807 Anne Arundel County: Area Agency on Aging
2666 Riva Road
Suite 400
Annapolis, MD 21401
410-222-4464
Fax: 410-222-4360; *Toll Free:* 800-492-2499
info_and_assistance@aacounty.org
www.aacounty.org
TDD 410-222-6825

Pamela Jordon, Director

Services for persons 60 and older.

808 Baltimore City Commission on Aging, Retirement Education
100 N. Holiday Street
Baltimore, MD 21202
410-396-3835
Fax: 410-576-9425
Lindsey.Hill@baltimorecity.gov
www.baltimorecity.gov

Neetu Dhawn-Gray, Director
Alexannder M Sanchez, Chief of Staff
Stephanie Rawlings-Blake, Mayor

Mission is to provide information, assistance, education, traing and support3 through a broad range of services and activities that enhance the quality of life for caregivers and their loved ones throughout Baltimore.

809 Baltimore County Department of Aging
400 Washington Avenue
Towson, MD 21204-4299
410-887-2450
Fax: 410-887-2159
www.baltimorecountymd.gov
TDD 410-887-3787

Joanne Williams, Director
Donald Mohler, Chief of Staff
Kevin Kamenetz, Country Executive

Provides a wide arraay of services to older seniors: nationally accredited senior centers, information and assistance, outreach, employment, housing, caregiver support, transportation, nutrition sites, and educational and informational booklets.

810 Bureau of Naval Personnel: Maryland Retired Activities Office
Fleet and Family Support Center
58 Bennion Road
Annapolis, MD 21402-5073
410-293-2641
Fax: 410-293-5380
www.cnic.navy.mil

The RAO serves as a link between local retired military and the active-duty community which provides assistance to retired military. It provides installation commanders with a means of providing more effective services and improving communication for the local retired community. The RAO is staffed and operated by volunteer retired military who assist other retired members, their families and survivors to receive entitled services and benefits. Through newsletters, seminars and appreciation days, the RAO supports quality of life issues throughout the retirement years to their fellow service members.

Year Founded: 1851

811 Carroll County Bureau of Aging
125 Stoner Avenue
Westminster, MD 21157-5451
410-386-3800
Fax: 410-840-0436
ccboa@ccg.carr.org
ccgovernment.carr.org
TDD 410-848-5355

Jolene Sullivan, Director

Mission is to provide the highest quality of services, programs, and assistance to promote choice, dignity and independence for older adults, adults with disabilities, and those who care for them.

812 Cecil County Department of Aging
200 Chesapeake Road
Suite 2550
Elkton, MD 21921-5513
410-996-5295
Fax: 410-620-9483
tmoore@ccgov.org
www.ccgov.org

David Trolio, Director
Mary Kahoe, Sr Information Assistance
Tari Moore, County Executive

Serves Cecil county residents sixty years and older

813 Charles County Department of Community Service Aging Division
200 Baltimore Street
PO Box 2150
La Plata, MD 20646
301-645-0550
Fax: 301-934-0126; *Toll Free:* 800-735-2258
www.charlescounty.org

Dina Barclay, Division Chief
Margaret Cheseldine, Director

Provides a wide range of programs and services to promote independence and improve the quality of life for older persons.

814 Department of Disabilities and Special Needs
217 E Redwood Street
Suite 1300
Baltimore, MD 21202
410-767-3660; *Toll Free:* 800-637-4113
mdod@mdod.state.md.us
www.mdod.maryland.gov
TTY: 410-767-3660

Cathy Raggio, Secretary
George P Failla Jr, Deputy Secretary
John Brennan, Chief of Staff

The mission of the Department of Disabilities is to empower individuals with disabilities to achieve their personal and professional goals in the communities where they live.

815 Frederick County Commission on Aging
12 East Church Street
Frederick, MD 21701-5243
301-600-1100
Fax: 301-600-1849
rcherney@FrederickCountyMD.gov
www.frederickcountymd.gov
TDD 301-694-1672

Blaine Young, President
Paul Smith, Vice President
Joyce Grossnickel, Administrative Officer

Local Area Agency on Aging.

816 Harford County Office on Aging
145 N Hickory Avenue
Bel Air, MD 21014-3239
410-638-3025
Fax: 410-893-2371
hcaging@harfordcountymd.gov
www.harfordcountymd.gov/services/aging

Karen Winkowski, Administrator

Serves seniors age 60 plus, their families and caregivers through a variety of programs, activities, services, and information.

817 Maintaining Active Citizens
909 Progress Circle
Salisbury, MD 21804
410-742-0505
Fax: 410-742-0525
macmail@macinc.org
www.macinc.org

Peggy Bradford, Executive Director
Margaret A Bradford, Executive Director
June F Messinger, Fiscal Director

MAC is dedicated to the principal that older persons are entitled to lives of dignity, security, physical, mental, and social well being.

818 Maryland Association of Area Agencies on Aging
Baltimore City Commission on Aging
169 Conduit Street
Annapolis, MD 21401
410-269-0043
Fax: 410-268-1775
msanderson@baltimorecity.gov
www.mdcounties.org

Michael Sanderson, Executive Director
Thomas G Duncan, President
Isiah Leggette, First Vice President

A nonprofit organization representing 19 Area Agencies and all jurisdictions, serves as a visible and effective advocate for older adults within the substate jurisdictions of Maryland, educating about aging issues in order to obtain an adequate and appropriate system of services in Maryland.

Year Founded: 1951

819 Maryland Client Assistance Program
2301 Argonne Drive
Baltimore, MD 21218-1628
410-554-9442
Fax: 410-554-9442; *Toll Free:* 888-554-0334
cap@dors.state.md.us
www.dors.state.md.us

Tom Laverty, Director

Helps individuals with disabilities understand the rehabilitation process and receives appropriate and quality services from the Division of Rehabilitation Services and other programs and facilities providing services under the Rehabilitation Act of 1973.

820 Maryland Department of Aging
301 West Preston Street
Suite 1007
Baltimore, MD 21201-2374
410-767-1100
Fax: 410-333-7943; *Toll Free:* 800-243-3425
www.mdoa.state.md.us

Gloria Gary Lawlah, Aging Secretary

Provides leadership, advocacy, and access to information and services for Maryland seniors, their families, and caregivers.

Year Founded: 1959

821 Maryland Developmental Disabilities Council
217 E Redwood Street
Suite 1300
Baltimore, MD 21202
410-767-3670
Fax: 410-333-3686; *Toll Free:* 800-305-6441
www.md-council.org

Brian Cox, Executive Director
Catherine Lyle, Deputy Director
Angela Castillo-Epps, Director Comunications/Policy

The Maryland Developmental Disabilities Council is a public policy organization comprised of people with disabilities and family members who are joined by state officials, service providers and other designated partners. The

Council is an independent, self-governing organization that represents the interests of people with developmental disabilities and their families.

822 Maryland Developmental Disability Council

217 E Redwood Street
Suite 1300
Baltimore, MD 21202
410-767-3670
Fax: 410-333-3686; *Toll Free:* 800-305-6441
www.md-council.org

Brian Cox, Executive Director
Catherine Lyle, Deputy Director
Angela Castillo-Epps, Director Comunications/Policy

Year Founded: 1971

823 Maryland Disability Determination Services

2301 Argonne Drive
Baltimore, MD 21218-1628
410-554-9442
Fax: 410-554-9442; *Toll Free:* 888-554-0334
md.dd.timonium.dds@ssa.gov
www.dors.state.md.us

Joe Simonik, Director

The Maryland Disability Determination Services (DDS) claims examiners, staff physicians and psychologists determine the eligibility of Maryland applicants for Social Security Administration's (SSA) two disability programs.

824 Maryland Protection & Advocacy Agency
Maryland Disability Law Center

1500 Union Avenue
Suite 2000
Baltimore, MD 21211
410-727-6352
Fax: 410-727-6389; *Toll Free:* 800-233-7201
johnd@mdlclaw.org
www.mdlcbalto.org
TDD 410-235-5387

Virginia Knowlton, Executive Director
Brian DeWitt, President
Vicki Finkelstein, Vice President

MDLC is the Protection and Advocacy organization for Maryland. MDLC mission is to ensure that people with disabilities are accorded the full rights and entitlements afforded to them by state and federal law.

825 Maryland Veterans Commission
Wineland Building

16 Francis Street
4th Floor
Annapolis, MD 21401
410-260-3838
Fax: 410-216-7928; *Toll Free:* 866-793-1577
mdveteransinfo@maryland.gov
www.mdva.state.md.us

Edward Chow Jr, Secretary Of Veterans Affairs
Dana Hendrickson, Director
Edward Chow, Secretary

Provides information and assistance so that veterans recieve all the benefits they have earned.

826 Maryland Workers Compensation Board

10 East Baltimore Street
Baltimore, MD 21202-1641
410-864-5100
Fax: 410-864-5101; *Toll Free:* 800-492-0479
info@wcc.state.md.us
www.wcc.state.md.us

R Karl Aumann, Chairman
Patricia C Adams, Commissioner
Lauren Godwin, Commissioner

Processes and ajudicates workers compensation claims.

827 Montgomery County Government: Division of Elder Affairs

401 Hungerford Drive
5th Floor
Rockville, MD 20850-2580
240-777-4565
ConsumerProtection@montgomerycountymd.gov
www.montgomerycountymd.gov/ocp/
TTY: 301-251-4850

John J Kenney, Chief Executive Officer
Eric Friedman, Director

Promotes and ensures the health and safety of the residents and to build individual and family strength and self-sufficiency.

828 Office of Retirement and Survivors
US Department of Health & Human Services

Windsor Park Building
6401 Security Boulevard
Baltimore, MD 21235
Fax: 410-597-0237; *Toll Free:* 800-772-1213
bso.support@ssa.gov
www.ssa.gov
TTY: 800-325-0778

Thomas Crawley, Sr Agency Privacy Official
Nancy A Berryhill, Deputy Commissioner

The Office of Retirement and Survivors Insurance determines benefits to those ages 62 and older and to members of families where the primary income person is deceased.

829 Office of Supplemental Security Income: Social Security Administration
US Department of Health and Human Services

PO Box 17769
6401 Security Boulevard
Baltimore, MD 21235-7769
410-965-2736
Fax: 410-597-0237; *Toll Free:* 800-772-1213
bso.support@ssa.gov
www.ssa.gov
TTY: 800-325-0778

Jo Anne B Barnhart, Commissioner
Nancy A Berryhill, Deputy Commissioner

To insure a minimum level of income to persons who have attained age 65 or are blind or disabled, whose income and resources are below specified levels.

830 Queen Anne's County Department of Aging

104 Powell Street
Centreville, MD 21617-1027
410-758-0848
Fax: 410-758-4489
www.agingcare.com

Catherine Willis, Director

Supports older adults so they can maintain the highest possible quality of life with independence and dignity, and to assist seniors and their family members with the many challenges of the aging process.

831 RSVP Hagerstown
140 West Franklin Street
Fourth Floor
Hagerstown, MD 21740
301-790-0275
Fax: 301-739-4957; *Toll Free:* 866-802-1212
www.wccoaging.org

Belinda Cobert, Executive Director

The Retired and Senior Volunteer Program (RSVP) provides opportunities for people 55 and over to make a difference in their community through volunteer service. RSVP volunteers contribute anywhere from a few to over forty hours a week, serving thourgh schools, day care centers, police departments, hospitals and other nonprofit and public organizations to help meet critical community needs. RSVP offers maximum flexibility and choice to its volunteers. RSVP matches the personal interests and skills to older Americans with opportunities to help solve community problems and offer supplemental insurance while on duty, on-the-job training from the agency or organization where volunteers are placed.

Year Founded: 1982

832 RSVP Montgomery County
100 Maryland Avenue
Rockville, MD 20850-4154
240-777-7900
Fax: 240-777-7989
county.council@montgomerycountymd.gov
www.montgomerycountymd.gov
TTY: 240-777-7914

Ike Leggette, County Executive
Craig Rice, President
George Leventhal, Vice President

RSVP is a multi-service nonprofit meeting the critical human needs in the community through volunteerism. RSVP's Volunteer Impact Programs focus on the needs of vulnerable populations including disadvantaged preschool children, at-risk youth, the elderly, those with low literacy skills, the unemployed and struggling nonprofit organizations.

833 RSVP Prince George's County
14741 Governor Oden Bowie Drive
Upper Marlboro
Maryland, MD 20772-3050
301-265-8486
Fax: 301-265-8482
www.princegeorgescountymd.gov

Pamela Sharps, Project Director

RSVP helps people aged 55 years and older put their skills and life experiences to work in their communities volunteering from a few hours up to 20 hours weekly in a variety of volunteer jobs.

834 RSVP St. Mary's County
Office on Aging
41780 Baldridge Street
PO Box 653
Leonardtown, MD 20650-0653
301-475-4200
Fax: 301-475-4660

diane.gleissner@stmarysmd.com
www.co.saint-marys.md.us

Norine Rowe, Director

The Retired and Senior Volunteer Program (RSVP) provides opportunities for people 55 and over to make a difference in their community through volunteer service. RSVP volunteers contribute anywhere from a few to over forty hours a week, serving through schools, day care centers, police departments, hospitals and other nonprofit and public organizations to help meet critical community needs. RSVP offers maximum flexibility and choice to its volunteers. RSVP matches the personal interests and skills of older Americans with opportunities to help solve community problems and offers supplemental insurance while on duty, on-the-job training from the agency or organization where volunteers are placed. The following County is served: Saint Mary's.

835 Railroad Retirement Board: Maryland District Office
844 North Rush Street
Chicago, IL 60611-2092
410-962-2550
Fax: 410-962-9835; *Toll Free:* 877-772-5772
www.rrb.gov
TTY: 312-751-4701

Casey N Gresey, Representative

An independent agency in the executive branch of the federal government. Its primary function is to administer comprehensive retirement-survivor and unemployment-sickness benefit programs for the nation's railroad workers and their families.

Year Founded: 1935

836 Social Security: Baltimore Disability Determination
2301 Argonne Drive
PO Box 6338
Baltimore, MD 21218-1628
410-554-9442
Fax: 410-554-9442; *Toll Free:* 888-554-0334
www.dors.state.md.us/dors

Offers programs and service that help people with disabilities go to work or stay independent in their homes and communities.

837 St. Mary's County Office on Aging
41780 Baldridge Street
PO Box 653
Leonardtown, MD 20650
301-475-4200
Fax: 301-475-4660
diane.gleissner@stmarysmd.com
www.co.saint-marys.md.us

Lori Jennings-Harris, Director
Alice Allen, Sr Center Operations
Debbie Barker, Senior I&A Manager

The St. Mary's County Department of Aging provides a wide variety of programs and services to the county's senior residents. Activities range from social and recreational programs to the direct support of essential services, such as nutrition, health, and in-home services.

838 Washington County Commission on Aging
140 W Franklin St
4th Floor
Hagerstown, MD 21740
301-790-0275
Fax: 301-739-4957; *Toll Free:* 866-802-1212
www.wccoaging.org

Belinda Corbett, Executive Director

The Washington County Commission on Aging Inc. is the designated Area Agency on Aging for the county serving over 30,000 seniors, their caregivers and adults with disabilities. We are a cost-effective and trusted resource whose mission is to promote quality aging by meeting the needs, protecting the rights, and preserving the dignity of our citizens.

Year Founded: 1982

Massachusetts

839 Adams Council on Aging
Adams Community Center
3 Hoosac Street
Adams, MA 01220-2300
413-743-8333
Fax: 413-743-8356
www.town.adams.ms.us

Erica Girgenti, Director
Linda Cernik, Outrech Coordinator

The Adams Council on Aging (CoA) is a town department. It was organized to develop a comprehensive network of in-home and community-based services and supportive programs for people sixty years of age and over in the Town of Adams.

840 Baypath Senior Citizens Services
33 Boston Post Road West
Po Box 2625
Marlborough, MA 01752
508-573-7200
Fax: 508-872-6449; *Toll Free:* 800-287-7284
jcarrigan@baypath.org
www.baypath.org

Jeanne McCann, Director

Framingham, Dover, Hudson, Ashland, Marlborough, Wayland, Sherborn, Northborough, Hopkinton, Southboro, Holliston, Natick, Sudbury, Westborough.

Year Founded: 1977

841 Boston Commission on Affairs of the Elderly
One City Hall Square
Room 271
Boston, MA 02201-2010
617-635-4366
Fax: 617-635-3213
Elderly@cityofboston.gov
www.cityofboston.gov/elderly
TDD 617-635-4599
TTY: 617-635-4599

Emily Shea, Commissioner
Martin J Walsh, Mayor

The mission of the Commission on Affairs of the Elderly is to enhance the quality of life for Boston's senior citizens through planning, coordinating, and monitoring the deliv-

ery of services to the elderly in an efficient and effective manner.

842 Bristol Elder Services
1 Father DeValles Blvd
Unit 8
Fall River, MA 02723
508-675-2101
Fax: 508-679-0320
info@bristolelder.org
www.bristolelder.org
TTY: 508-646-9704

Margaret Pilkington, Ombudsman Program Director
Nancy Viverios, Nutrition Program Assist Dir

A private non-profit corporation, designated as an Aging Services Access Point and an Area Agency on Aging. Bristol serves as the entry point for elder services in Southeastern Massachusetts.

Year Founded: 1973

843 Cape & Islands Senior Corps
68 Route 134
South Dennis, MA 02660-3710
508-394-4630
Fax: 508-394-3712; *Toll Free:* 800-244-4630
info@escci.org
www.escci.org
TTY: 508-394-8691

Susan Schneider, Director

Dedicated to promoting the welfare and enhancing the quality of life of elders, as well as helping them to maintain maximum independence and dignity. Our organization works with the community to identify and respond to the needs, problems, and concerns of elders and their families.

Year Founded: 1972

844 Central Massachusetts Agency on Aging
360 W Boylston Street
West Boylston, MA 01583-2365
508-852-5539
Fax: 508-852-5425; *Toll Free:* 800-244-3032
cmaaging@seniorconnection.org
www.seniorconnection.org

Theresa Eckstrom, Chair
Nicholas Kaltsas, President
James Leary, Vice President

Mission is to enhance the quality of life for area seniors and their charegivers, the Central Massachusetts Agency on Aging will provide leadership, informantion and resources, coordination of services and advocacy.

Year Founded: 1974

845 Chelsea-Revere-Winthrop: Area Agency onAging
Chelsea Home Care Center
100 Everett Avenue, Unit 10
PO Box 6427
Chelsea, MA 02150-0008
617-884-2500
Fax: 617-884-7988; *Toll Free:* 800-922-2275
crw@crwelderservices.org
www.crwelderservices.org

James Cunningham Jr, Director

A private non-profit Home Care Corporation dedicated to serving people age 60 years and over in the communities of Chelsea, Revere, and Winthrop, Massachusetts. Assists elders and persons with disabilities to live in their own homes, and in their own community with dignity, independence, safety and to promote a good quality of life through a wide range of long-term support and service options.

Year Founded: 1972

846 Coastline Elderly Services

1646 Purchase Street
New Bedford, MA 02740-6819
508-999-6400
Fax: 508-993-6510; *Toll Free:* 866-274-1643
www.coastlineelderly.org
TDD 508-993-4265

Rita L'Etoile, President
Paula Shiner, CEO
Justin Lees, Fiscal Director

A non-profit organization that provides a wide variety of services to the elders in the Greater New Bedford area, and their families.

847 Community Action Commission of Cape Cod & Islands

372 North Street
Hyannis, MA 02601-2212
508-771-1727
Fax: 508-775-7488; *Toll Free:* 800-845-1999
www.cacci.cc

David B Willard, Chairman
Paul Niedzwiecki, Vice Chairman
Stefanie S Coxe, Executive Director

Senior citizens in the Cape Cod, MA area. Evaluates the quality of senior citizens' lives and advocates their rights regarding transportation, housing, nutrition, entitlements, and nursing home care. Offers public education programs on human service issues. Works to further favorable legislation at the state level, especially concerning health care issues.

Year Founded: 1965

848 Dalton Council on Aging

Dalton Community Center
462 Main Street
Dalton, MA 01226-1605
413-684-6111
Fax: 413-684-6107
daltonaa@bcn.net
www.dalton-ma.gov

John F Boyle, Chair
Mary R Cherry, Vice Chairman
Kelly Pizzi, Director

Appointed board of 11 citizens responsible for providing information to and referral for Dalton, MA residents 60 years of age and older and their families.

849 Elder Service Plan of the North Shore

37 Friend Street
Lynn, MA 01902
781-715-6608
Fax: 781-715-6699
www.pacenorthshore.org

Carol Suleski, Executive Director

Elder Service Plans are part of PACE (Programs of All-inclusive Care for the Elderly). These plans provide comprehensive medical and social services to frail elders so that they can live in their communities instead of in nursing homes.

Year Founded: 1995

850 Elder Services of Berkshire County

66 Wendell Avenue
Pittsfield, MA 01201-6306
413-499-0524
Fax: 413-442-6443; *Toll Free:* 800-544-5242
esbc@esbci.org
www.esbci.org
TDD 413-499-0524

Nicholas Kirchner, Executive Director
Roger Suters, Community Services Director
Amy Muldowney, Client Services Supervisor

Offers in home and community services to provide Berkshire elders the opportunity to live with dignity, independence and self determination, and to achieve the highest possible quality of life.

Year Founded: 1974

851 Elder Services of Cape Cod and the Islands

68 Route 134
South Dennis, MA 02660-3710
508-394-4630
Fax: 508-394-3712; *Toll Free:* 800-244-4630
info@escci.org
www.escci.org

Paula George, President
Leslie Scheer, Executive Director

A private, not-for-profit community based organization. Dedicated to promoting the welfare and enhancing the quality of life of elders, as well as helping them to maintain maximum independence and dignity.

Year Founded: 1972

852 Franklin County Home Care Corporation

330 Montague City Road
Suite 1
Turners Falls, MA 01376-2529
413-773-5555
Fax: 413-772-1084; *Toll Free:* 800-732-4636
info@fchcc.org
www.fchcc.org
TDD 413-772-6566

Roseann Martoccia, Executive Director
Regina Curtis, Board President

Area Agency on Aging and Aging Services Access Point serving the Franklin County and Worth Quabbin region of Massachesetts.

853 Friends of the Pepperell Seniors

37 Nashua Road
PO Box 1555
Pepperell, MA 01463-3555
978-433-0326
Fax: 978-433-0347
coaboard@town.pepperell.ma.us
www.pepperell-mass.com

Cathy Forest, Chair
Dianne H Kazanjian, Secretary
Sandy Dube, Board Member

To better the lives of the senior citizens of Pepperell by raising funds that sponsor and support activities that contribute to their health and well-being and to essential items for the Pepperell Senior Center through the Pepperell Council on Aging.

854 Greater Lynn Senior Services
8 Silsbee Street
Lynn, MA 01901-1485
781-599-0110
Fax: 781-592-7540; *Toll Free:* 800-594-5164
info@glss.net
www.glss.net
TDD 781-477-9632

Kathleen Vidala, President
John Baker, Vice President
Charles Marcou, Treasurer

A non-profit agency established to serve those 60 and older and the disabled.

855 Greater Springfield Senior Services
66 Industry Avenue
Suit 9
Springfield, MA 01104-3362
413-781-8800
Fax: 413-781-0632; *Toll Free:* 800-649-3641
www.gsssi.org
TDD 413-781-8800

Nancy Morales, President
Peter Schmidt, Vice President
Daniel Keenan, Vice President

Mission is to keep people age 60+ living at home safely and independently by providing assistance and access to a comprehensive range of services.

856 Hearing Rehabilitation Foundation
35 Medford Street
Somerville, MA 02143-4242
617-628-4537
hearf@aol.com
www.hearf.org

Geoff Plant, PhD, President

Non-profit organization to provide and promote speech communication training for children and adults with hearing loss.

857 Highland Valley Elder Services
320 Riverside Drive
Suite B
Florence, MA 01062-2700
413-586-2000
Fax: 413-584-7076; *Toll Free:* 800-322-0551
qll@highlandvalley.org
www.highlandvalley.org

Robert Gallant, Director

Mission of the Higland Valley Elder Services (HVES) is to assist people taking charge of their lives and communities for quality long living.

858 Jewish Community Relations Council of Greater Boston
126 High Street
Boston, MA 02110-2700
617-457-8600
Fax: 617-988-6255

info@jcrcboston.org
www.jcrcboston.org

Bill Gabovitch, Executive Director

Human rights organization working on behalf of Jews and political prisoners in the former Soviet Union. Membership is concentrated in New England and upper New York state area, but group operates on a national level. Primary purpose is to work toward the emigration of Jews from the former USSR, and provide Jews remaining in the former Soviet Union with religious, cultural, moral and financial support.

859 Massachusetts Assistive Technology Partnership
MATP Center
1295 Boylston Street
Suite 310
Boston, MA 02215-3407
617-355-7820
Fax: 617-345-6345; *Toll Free:* 800-848-8867
www.matp.org

Judy Brewer, Project Director

A statewide program promoting assistive technology devices and services for persons with all disabilities.

860 Massachusetts Client Assistance Program
1 Ashburton Place
Room 1305
Boston, MA 02108-1518
617-727-7440
Fax: 671-727-0965; *Toll Free:* 800-322-2020

Barbara E Lybarger Esq., Assistant Director

Primary mission is to ensure the full and equal participation of all people with disabilities in all aspects of life by working to advance legal rights, maximum opportunities, supportive services, accomodations and accessability in a manner that fosters dignity and self determination.

861 Massachusetts Department of Elder Affairs
1 Ashburton Place
Room 517
Boston, MA 02108-1518
617-727-7750
Fax: 617-727-9368; *Toll Free:* 800-243-4636
www.mass.gov

Ann Hartstein, Secretary of Elder Affairs

We promote the independence and well being of elders and people needing medical and social supportive services by providing advocacy, leadership, and management expertise to maintain a continuum of services responsive to the needs of our constituents, their families, and caregivers.

862 Massachusetts Department of Revenue
PO Box 7010
Boston, MA 02204
617-887-6367; *Toll Free:* 800-392-6089
www.mass.gov

Amy Pitter, Commissioner
James Reynolds, Senior Deputy Commissioner
Dennis Buckley, Tax Payer Advocate

The mission of the Massachusetts Department of Revenue is to achieve maximum compliance with the tax, child support and municipal finance laws of the Commonwealth. In meeting its mission, the Department is dedicated to enforcing these laws in a fair, impartial and consistent manner by providing professional and courteous service to all its customers.

863 Massachusetts Developmental Disabilities Council
1150 Hancock Street
Third Floor, Suite 300
Quincy, MA 02169-4340
617-770-7676
Fax: 617-770-1987
www.mass.gov/mddc/index2.html
TTY: 617-770-9499

Daniel Shannon, Executive Director
Julie Fitzpatrick, Chairperson

Group of citizens which analyzes needs of people with severe, lifelong disabilities and works to improve public policy. MDDC produces several publications and has committees and a grants program to study and advocate for changes in the service system.

864 Massachusetts Disability Determination Services
One Ashburton Place
11th Floor
Boston, MA 02108
617-573-1600
Fax: 617-654-7575
www.mass.gov

Barbara M Kinney, Assistant Commissioner

DDS determines the initial and continued eligibility for federal SSI and SSDI public benefits. Provides special outreach efforts are made to homeless shelters and individuals diagnosed with HIV.

865 Massachusetts Executive Office of Health and Human Services
Commission for the Deaf and Hard of Hearing
210 South Street
5th Floor
Boston, MA 02111-2725
617-695-7500
Fax: 617-695-7599; *Toll Free:* 800-882-1155
www.mass.gov

JudyAnn Bigby, MD, Secretary

Mission is to explore innovavtive solutions for accessible communication, identify links to resources and supports, and become better prepared for current and future challenges impacting people who are deaf, hard of hearting and late-deafened

866 Massachusetts Executive Office for Administration and Finance
Teacher's Retirement Board
One Charles Park
2nd Floor
Cambridge, MA 02142-1206
617-679-6877
Fax: 617-679-1661
www.mass.gov/mtrs

Joan Schloss, Executive director

Mission is to ensure that members of the Massachusetts Teachers' Retirement System achieve and maintain a successful and secure retirement through responsible benefits administration, financial integrity, and the provision of outstanding services.

Year Founded: 1914

867 Massachusetts Executive Office of Health and Human Services
Commission for the Blind
48 Boylston Street
Boston, MA 02116-4718
617-727-5550
Fax: 617-727-5960; *Toll Free:* 800-392-6450
www.mass.gov

Janet Labreck, Commissioner

Provides the highest quality rehabilitation and social services leading to independence, and economic self-sufficiency through employment, and full community inclusion for the blind.

868 Massachusetts Protection & Advocacy Organization
Disability Law Center
11 Beacon Street, Suite 925
Boston, MA 02108
617-723-8455
Fax: 617-723-9125; *Toll Free:* 800-872-9992
mail@dlc-ma.org
www.dlc-ma.org
TTY: 800-381-0577

To provide legal advocacy on disability issues that promote the fundamental rights of all people with disabilities to participate fully and equally in the social and economic life of Massachusetts.

869 Massachusetts Social Security Region 1 Administration
10 Causeway Street
1st Floor, Room 148
Boston, MA 02222
Fax: 410-965-6503; *Toll Free:* 800-772-1213
www.ssa.gov/boston
TTY: 800-325-0778

Michael Bertrand, Regional Commissioner

To advance the economic security of the nation's people through compassionate and vigilant leadership in shaping and managing America's Social Security programs.

870 Massachussetts Association for the Blind Community Services
200 Ivy Street
Brookline, MA 02446-3907
617-738-5110
Fax: 617-738-1247; *Toll Free:* 800-682-9200
www.mabcommunity.org

Craig Pfannensteihl, President
Norman Lang, Vice President
David Schechter, Treasurer

MAB Community Services is dedicated to working with individuals with disabilities to eliminate barriers and create opportunities.
Year Founded: 1903

871 Mystic Valley Elder Services
300 Commercial Street
Suite 19
Malden, MA 02148-7312
781-324-7705
Fax: 781-324-1369

info@mves.org
www.mves.org
TTY: 781-321-8880

Carolyn E Lightburn, President
Judy Whatley, Vice President
Gene J Ferullo, Treasurer

Programs for the aging

872 New Bedford Council on Aging
133 William Street
Room 220
New Bedford, MA 02740
508-961-3136
Fax: 508-991-6262
www.newbedford-ma.gov
TDD 508-979-1796

Cynthia Wallquist, Director

Agency serves area senior citizens through health education
and recreation programs. Operates 2 senior centers. Outreach Benefits Counselor does home visits to shut-ins to assist with health benefits.

Year Founded: 1787

873 North Shore Elder Services
152 Sylvan Street
Danvers, MA 01923-3568
978-750-4540
Fax: 978-750-8053
info@nselder.org
www.nselder.org
TDD 758-750-4540
TTY: 978-624-2244

Paul Lanzikos, Executive Director
Joan Shea, Chair
Katheribe Walsh, Vice Chair

The North Shore is a rental retirement community offering
a senior living experience for value-conscious seniors that
is truly outstanding. There is no endowment, no long-term
commitment, no paying for assistance services which may
not be necessary. Assisted living services are available
through Regency At Home Care Services, Ltd. as an
option, if needed.

874 Northfield Senior Center
69 Main Street
Northfield, MA 01360
413-498-2901
Fax: 413-498-5115; Toll Free: 800-795-3272
www.northfield.ma.us
TDD 202-720-6382

Suzanne Sweeney, Aging Director
Tom Hutcheson, Administrator

Individuals in Franklin County, MA serving senior citizens.

**875 Old Colony Planning Council: Area Agency on
Aging**
70 School Street
Brockton, MA 02301-4097
508-583-1833
Fax: 508-559-8768
www.ocpcrpa.org

Charles Kilmer, Assisstant Director
Eric Arbeene, Community Planner
Lee Hartman, President

Responsible for the establishment of a comprehensive, coordinated system of community-based supportive services
and nutrition services for the elders in our region.

876 Operation ABLE of Greater Boston
Portland Street
Boston, MA 02114
617-542-4180
Fax: 617-542-4187; Toll Free: 888-470-2253
ABLE@operationable.net
www.operationable.net

Joan Cirillo, President/CEO
Judith Serode, CFO
Mark Gyurina, Treasurer

Helps job seekers 45 and older get back to work. Through
its coaching and counseling, retraining opportunities, job
Fairs and Showcases for mature Workers, networking and
support groups, implementation of the Department of Labor's Senior Community Service Employment Program for
job sekers 55 and older and advocacy for mature workers
on city, state and national levels, has assisted well over
30,000 mature job seekers find work.

Year Founded: 1982

877 PXE International
4301 Connecticut Avenue NW
Suite 404
Washington, DC 20008-2369
202-362-9599
Fax: 202-966-8553
info@pxe.org
www.pxe.org

Patrick F Terry, Opresident
Lionel G Bercovitch, MD
Joe Mass, Treasurer

Offers vital services to those with pseudoxanthoma
elasticum, a connective tissue disorder causing calcification
of connective tissue in various places throughout the body,
often affecting the membrane behind the eye.

Year Founded: 1995

878 Quincy Retirement Board
1250 Hancock Street
Suite 506-S
Quincy, MA 02169
617-376-1075
Fax: 617-376-1149
info@quincyretirement.com
www.quincyretirement.com

Edward J Masterson, Executive Director
Marguerite Lightbourne, Deputy Director
George McCray, Chairperson

Defined benefit pension system.

879 RSVP Berkshire
16 Bartlett Ave
Pittsfield, MA 01201-6302
413-449-9345
Fax: 413-442-0422

Andrew Perenick, President
Carolyn Valli, Vice President
Tammy Gage, Treasurer

The Retired and Senior Volunteer Program (RSVP) provides opportunities for people 55 and over to make a difference in their community through volunteer service. RSVP

volunteers contribute anywhere from a few to over forty hours a week, serving through schools, day care centers, police departments, hospitals and other nonprofit and public organizations to help meet critical community needs. RSVP offers maximum flexibility and choice to its volunteers. RSVP matches the personal interests and skills of older Americans with opportunities to help solve community problems and offers supplemental insurance while on duty, on-the-job training from the agency or organization where volunteers are placed. The following County is served: Berkshire.

880 RSVP Boston
One City Hall Square
Boston, MA 02201-1020
617-635-4500
Fax: 617-635-3213
kelley.stout@cityofboston.gov
www.cityofboston.gov/elderly

Kelley Stout, Director
Anique Langlois, Administrator

The Retired and Senior Volunteer Program (RSVP) provides opportunities for people 55 and over to make a difference in their community through volunteer service. RSVP volunteers contribute anywhere from a few to over forty hours a week, serving through schools, day care centers, police departments, hospitals and other nonprofit and public organizations to help meet critical community needs. RSVP offers maximum flexibility and choice to its volunteers. RSVP matches the personal interests and skills of older Americans with opportunities to help solve community problems and offers supplemental insurance while on duty, on-the-job training from the agency or organization where volunteers are placed. The following County is served: Suffolk.

881 RSVP Chicopee-Holyoke-Ludlow
152 Center Street
Chicopee, MA 01013-1611
413-612-0219
Fax: 413-612-0221

Lorraine Norton, Director

Our volunteers are people who don't want to sit around being bored and growing old. Our paid staff of three, recruit people fifty-five and over to volunteer their time and share their talents in human service programs within their own communities.

882 RSVP Fall River-Taunton
264 Griffin Street
Fall River, MA 02724-2702
508-679-0041
Fax: 508-324-7503
Bleary@cfcinc.org
www.CFCINC.org

Mark A Sullivan Jr, Executive Director
Frank S Sullivan, Deputy Executive Director
James Dolin, President

The Retired and Senior Volunteer Program (RSVP) provides opportunities for people 55 and over to make a difference in their community through volunteer service. RSVP volunteers contribute anywhere from a few to over forty hours a week, serving through schools, day care centers, police departments, hospitals and other nonprofit and public organizations to help meet critical community needs. RSVP offers maximum flexibility and choice to its volun-

teers. RSVP matches the personal interests and skills of older Americans with opportunities to help solve community problems and offers supplemental insurance while on duty, on-the-job training from the agency or organization where volunteers are placed. The following County is served: Bristol.
Year Founded: 1995

883 RSVP Greater Lawrence-Haverhill
264 Essex Street
Lawrence, MA 01840-1516
978-686-0900
Fax: 978-794-9953
office@merrimackvalleychamber.com
www.merrimackvalleychamber.com

Salvatore Lupoli, Chairman
Richard C Dewhirst, Immediate Past Chairman
Peter j Mathews, Member Services

The Retired and Senior Volunteer Program (RSVP) provides opportunities for people 55 and over to make a difference in their community through volunteer service. RSVP volunteers contribute anywhere from a few to over forty hours a week, serving through schools, day care centers, police departments, hospitals and other nonprofit and public organizations to help meet critical community needs. RSVP offers maximum flexibility and choice to its volunteers. RSVP matches the personal interests and skills of older Americans with opportunities to help solve community problems and offers supplemental insurance while on duty, on-the-job training from the agency or organization where volunteers are placed. The following County is served: Essex.

884 RSVP Mayflower of Plymouth County
385 Court Street #104
Plymouth, MA 02360-7320
508-746-7787
Fax: 508-746-7795; *Toll Free:* 877-746-7787
MayflowerRSVP@verizon.net
www.mayflowerrsvp.org

Joan E Thompson, Director

The Retired and Senior Volunteer Program (RSVP) provides opportunities for people 55 and over to make a difference in their community through volunteer service. RSVP volunteers contribute anywhere from a few to over forty hours a week, serving through schools, day care centers, police departments, hospitals and other nonprofit and public organizations to help meet critical community needs. RSVP offers maximum flexibility and choice to its volunteers. RSVP matches the personal interests and skills of older Americans with opportunites to help solve community problems and offers supplemental insurance while on duty, on-the-job training from the agency or organization where volunteers are placed. The following County is served: Plymouth.

885 RSVP Norfolk County
614 High Street
PO Box 310
Dedham, MA 02027
781-461-6105
Fax: 781-326-6480
info@norfolkcounty.org
www.norfolkcounty.org

Jean F McLeish, Director
Francis W O'Brien, Chairman
Peter H Collins, Commissioner

The Norfolk County Retired and Senior Volunteer Program (RSVP) invites adults age 55 and over to use their life experience and skills to answer the call of their neighbors in need.

886 RSVP Senior Care North Shore
49 Blackburn Center
Gloucester, MA 01930-2259
978-281-1750
Fax: 978-281-1753; *Toll Free:* 866-921-1050
srcare@seniorcareinc.org
www.seniorcareinc.org
TDD 978-282-1836

Scott Trenti, Executive Director
Tom Tanous, President

Our mission is to provide and coordinate services to elders, enabling them to live independently at home and remain part of their community.

Year Founded: 1972

887 RSVP Urban League of Springfield
Urban League of Springfield
756 State Street
Springfield, MA 01109-4112
413-739-7211
Fax: 413-732-9364
info@ulspringfield.org
www.ulspringfield.org

Henry Thomas, President/CEO
Yvette M Frisby, VP of Operations
Andrew Cade, VP of Senior Operations

The Retired and Senior Volunteer Program (RSVP) provides opportunities for people 55 and over to make a difference in their community through volunteer service. RSVP volunteers contribute anywhere from a few to over forty hours a week, serving through schools, day care centers, police departments, hospitals and other nonprofit and public organizations to help meet critical community needs. RSVP offers maximum flexibility and choice to its volunteers. RSVP matches the personal interests and skills of older Americans with opportunities to help solve community problems and offers supplemental insurance while on duty, on-the-job training from the agency or organization where volunteers are placed. The following County is served: Hampden.

888 RSVP Worcester Area
128 Providence Street
Suite 305
Worcester, MA 01604-5431
508-791-7787
Fax: 508-791-7780
info@rsvp-worcester.org
www.rsvp-worcester.org

Barbara Drapos, Program Director

RSVP connects people age 55 and over with opportunities that address compelling community needs.

889 Railroad Retirement Board District Office
844 North Rush Street
Chicago, IL 60611

312-751-4300
Fax: 617-223-8551; *Toll Free:* 877-772-5772
boston@rrb.gov
www.rrb.gov

Raymond P Fecteau, Manager

An independent agency in the executive branch of the Federal Government. The RRB's primary function is to administer comprehensive retirement-survivor and unemployment-sickness benefit programs for the nations railroad workers and their families.

Year Founded: 1874

890 Scituate Council on Aging
Catherine McGowan Senior Center
600 Chief Justice Cushing Highway
Scituate, MA 02066-1309
781-545-8700
Fax: 781-545-8704
www.town.scituate.ma.us/coa

Florence Choate, Director
Nancy Lafauce, Social Services Coordinator
Jennifer Gerbis, Outreach Assistant

Promotes and provides social services and activities for senior citizens in Scituate, MA.

Year Founded: 1961

891 Senior Home Care Services
49 Blackburn Centre
Gloucester, MA 01930
978-281-1750
Fax: 978-281-1753; *Toll Free:* 866-927-1050
srcare@seniorcareinc.org
www.seniorcareinc.org
TDD 978-468-1193
TTY: 978-282-1836

Scott Ytrenti, Executive Director
Tom Tanous, President

SeniorCare offers short and long-term services that make it easier for elders to remain in the comfort of their own homes. Services may include: homemaking, shopping, personal care, meal preparation, laundry, caregiver, respite and personal emergency response systems. We also offer several enhanced programs for frail elders who might otherwise be facing long-term institutional placement.

Year Founded: 1972

892 Shrewsbury Senior Center
98 Maple Avenue
Shrewsbury, MA 01545-5349
508-841-8640
Fax: 508-841-8641
syager@th.ci.shrewsbury.ma.us
www.shrewsbury-ma.gov/councilaging

Sharon M Yager, Director

The Shrewsbury Senior Center is under the auspices of the Shrewsbury Council on Aging (SCOA), a human service department of the town, which serves the needs and issues of Shrewsbury's seniors, age 60 and over, or families with senior issues.

893 Somerville Cambridge Elder Services
61 Medford Street
Somerville, MA 02143-3429
617-628-2601
Fax: 617-628-1085

SCES@eldercare.org
www.eldercare.org
TDD 617-628-1705

John O'Neill, Executive Director
Mary Ann Dalton, Assistant Executive Director
Nancy Willbanks, Chief Financial Officer

Offers resources, information, advice, and services to seniors, caregivers, and disabled people.

Year Founded: 1972

894 South Shore Elder Services
1515 Washington Street
Braintree, MA 02184-5203
781-848-3910
Fax: 781-843-8279
eflynn@sselder.org
www.sselder.org

Ed Mulvey, President
John Molloy, Vice President
Connie Laughlin, Treasurer

South Shore Elder Services Inc. (SSES) recommends and coordinates resources for elders to help them to remain as independent as possible. The private non-profit agency also advocactes for elders and their caregivers, always with the goal of promoting an optimal quality of life.

895 Springwell
307 Waverley Oaks Road
Suite 205
Waltham, MA 02452
617-926-4100
Fax: 617-926-9897
springwell@springwell.com
www.springwell.com
TDD 617-923-1562

Ruth Beckerman-Rodau, Interim CEO/COO
Kara Donellon, Chief Financial Officer
Judy Joffe, Community Planning Director

A private, non-profit agency that has been creating, managing, and coordinating services for seniors, individuals with disabilities and those who provide care for them. The agency is the state designated Aging Services Access Point and Area Agency on Aging for the communities of Watertown, Belmont, Brookline, Needham, Newton, Waltham, Wellesly, and Weston.

896 Urban Medical Group
545 Centre Street
Suite A
Jamaica Plain, MA 02130-2075
617-522-5464
Fax: 617-524-2966
www.urbanmedical.org

S Stephen Rosefeld, Chair
Karen M Quigley, Vice Chair

Our mission is to provide a lifetime of compassionate, continuous, high-quality primary care to adults. We strive to ensure every patient's dignity and independence.

897 Wellfleet Council on Aging
300 Main Street
Wellfleet, MA 02667-8013
508-349-0330
Fax: 508-349-0305
www.wellfleetma.org

Suzanne Grout Thomas, Director
Linda Balch, Outreach
Terri Frazier, Office Manager

Dedicated to improving the health and independence of older persons and increasing their continuing contributions to communities, societies, and future generations.

Year Founded: 1654

898 WestMass Elder Care
4 Valley Mill Road
Holyoke, MA 01040-5887
413-538-9020
Fax: 413-532-8537; *Toll Free:* 800-462-2301
www.wmeldercare.org
TDD 800-875-0287

Priscilla Chalmers, Director

Private non-profit agency, its programs are funded by grants and contracts from the Massachusetts Executive Office of Elder Affairs, and a number of other funding sources, including private donations.

899 Workers Compensation Board Massachusetts
1 Congress Street
Suite 100
Boston, MA 02114
617-727-4900
Fax: 617-727-2799; *Toll Free:* 800-323-3249
info2@massmail.state.ma.us
www.mass.gov

Joanne Goldstein, Secretary

Determines eligiblity for workers compensation in the state of Massachusetts.

900 Yarmouth Council on Aging
1146 Route 28
South Yarmouth, MA 02664-4492
508-398-2231
Fax: 508-398-4810
www.yarmouth.ma.us/council_on_aging.htm

Karen Marciante, Director
Robert Isadore, Chairperson

The Council on Aging is in charge of assessing the needs of the elderly, offering programs to seniors, and servicing the Town's aging population.

Michigan

901 Agency on Aging: Area 1B
29100 Northwestern Highway
Suite 400
Southfield, MI 48034-1046
248-357-2255
Fax: 248-262-9971; *Toll Free:* 800-852-7795
www.aaa1b.org
TTY: 248-263-1455

Amin Irving, Chair
Tom Miree, !st Chairman
Andrew Hetzel, 2nd Chairman

A nonprofit organization serving the needs of older adults, persons with disabilities and family caregivers residing in the counties of Livingston, Macomb, Monroe, Oakland, St Clair, Washtenaw. Committed to helping individuals remain living in their own home or residence of choice by providing access to home care services.

Year Founded: 1974

902 Agency on Aging: Region 4
2900 Lakeview Avenue
Saint Joseph, MI 49085-2436
269-983-0177
Fax: 616-983-5218; *Toll Free:* 800-442-2803
www.areaagencyonaging.org

Barbara A Farris, Chairman
Larry Smith, Vice Chair
Don Radde, Treasurer

The Ageny on Aging enhances the lives of older adults and
adults with disabilities in the communties that they serve.

903 Alpena Regional Medical Center Auxiliary
1501 W Chisholm Street
Alpena, MI 49707-1498
989-356-7000
Fax: 989-356-7305; *Toll Free:* 800-556-8842
info@agh.org
www.alpenaregionalmedicalcenter.org

John McVeety, Administrator
Eric Smith, Chairperson
Karmon Bjella, Secretary

Volunteers in northeastern Michigan who assist local hospital with community health programs. Conducts fundraising
activities.

**904 Alzheimer's Association: South Central
Michigan Region**
310 North Main Street
Suite 100
Chelsea, MI 48118
734-475-7043
Fax: 734-677-3091; *Toll Free:* 800-272-3900
info@alz.org
www.alz.org

Jennifer Howard, Executive Director
Stephen Campbell, Program Coordinator
Lori Ezrow, Events Coordinator

Families and friends of Alzheimer's Disease patients, interested others. Provides advocacy, education, and support
services. Supports research efforts. Offers support group
programs, educational workshops, and video rental. Maintains speakers' bureau and lending library.

Year Founded: 1980

905 Area Agency on Aging of Western Michigan
3215 Eaglecrest Dr NE
Grand Rapids, MI 49503-1378
616-456-5664
Fax: 616-456-5692; *Toll Free:* 888-456-5664
www.aaawm.org

Thomas Czerwinski, Executive Director
Commissioner Don Black, Chairperson
Carole Hennessey, Vice Chair

The Area Agency on Aging of Western Michigan exists to
help older adults and persons with disabilities live in their
community with independence and dignity. he agency
serves nine counties in the West Michigan area including
Allegan, Ionia, Kent, Lake, Mason, Mecosta, Montcalm,
Newaygo, and Osceola.

Year Founded: 1974

906 Bay County Council on Aging
1116 Frankford Avenue
Panama City, FL 32401-1861
850-769-3468
Fax: 850-872-2151
baycouncil@bellsouth.net
www.baycouncilonaging.org

Elizabeth N Coulliette, Executive Director
Karen Coffman, Assistant Director
Regina Seamstress, Community Services

The organization provides services to the elderly of Bay
County enabling senior adults to be healthy, active and independent in the lifestyles they choose. Bay County Council on Aging offers numerous programs which assist older
persons in need.

907 Blueprint for Aging
4925 Packard Road
PO Box 995
Ann Arbor, MI 48108
734-926-4655
Fax: 734-971-2730
jkind@csswashtenaw.org
www.blueprintfroaging.org

Chris White, Chair
Amy Ruddock Bleed, Project Assistant
Sue Monet, Volunteer Soecialist

The Blueprint for Aging is a diverse coalition of community members and representatives from over 40 public and
nonprofit organizations who have actively worked for over
five years to assist Washentaw County in becoming more
responsive to its older residents.

**908 Bureau of Naval Personnel: Michigan Retired
Activities Office**
Marine Reserve Center
1200 Navy Pentagon
Washington, DC 20350-1200
313-824-1650
Fax: 313-824-2770
www.navy.mil

The RAO serves as a link between local retired military
and the active-duty community which provides assistance
to retired military. It provides installation commanders with
a means of providing more effective services and improving communication for the local retired community. The
RAO is staffed and operated by volunteer retired military
who assist other retired members, their families and survivors to receive entitled services and benefits. Through
newsletters and seminars and appreciation days, the RAO
supports quality of life issues throughout the retirement
years to their fellow service members.

909 Charlevoix County Commission on Aging
218 West Garfield Street
Charlevoix, MI 49720
231-237-0130
Fax: 231-237-0105; *Toll Free:* 866-428-5185
www.charlevoixcounty.org

Jack Messer, Executive Director
Margo Johnson, Chairperson
Nancy Tritsch, Vice Chair

Adult day services, activities, music and exercise, BINGO,
games, outings, socialization, healthy snacks, personal
care, nail and hair care, foot care.

910 Chicago Social Security Management Association
418 C St
Washington, DC 20002
202-547-8530
Fax: 202-547-8532
Kenneth.Tash@ssa.gov
www.ncssma.org

Billie Armenta, President
Charlene Morales, Treasurer
Jari Frassenei, Secretary

CSSMA is a professional organization of Chicago Region field management staff dedicated to the enhancement and improvement of the overall operation of the programs administered by SSA and to futhering the best interests and general welfare of all field personnel.

911 Council on Aging: Region 14
1609 Park Avenue
P.O Box 5926
Tranverse City, MI 49696-5946
231-947-8920
Fax: 616-739-4452; Toll Free: 800-442-1713
www.aaanm.org/area-agencies

Pam Curtis, Executive Director

The Area Agency on Aging is the place to turn when you need assistance with the complex issues facing older adults and their caregivers. They connect you to a variety of resources that will help you or those you care for live as independently as possible in a community setting.

912 Detroit: Area Agency on Aging
1333 Brewery Park Boulevard
Detroit, MI 48207
313-446-4444
Fax: 313-446-4445
www.daaa1a.org

Paul Bridgewater, Executive Director

The Area on Aging is the place to turn when you need assistance witht he complex issues facing older adults and their caregivers. They connect you to a variety of resources that will help you or those you care for live as independently as possible in a community setting.

913 Gray Panthers Huron Valley
10 G St
NE Suite 600
Washington, DC 20002
202-737-6637; *Toll Free: 800-280-5362*
www.graypanthers.org

June Rusten, Conveyor
Jan Bendoer, Chairperson
Brooke Hollister, VC

Intergenerational social justice group which invites activists of all ages to work together to challenge descrimination based on race, sex or age; to work for social and economic justice, universal health care and peace.

914 Gray Panthers Metro Detroit
PO Box 37033
Oak Park, MI 48237
248-549-5170
randyblock@yahoo.com
www.graypanthersmetrodetroit.org

Randy Block, Convener
Ethel Schwartz, Co-Director

Intergenerational social justice group which invites activists of all ages to work together to: challenge descrimination based on race, sex or age; to work for social and economic justice, universal health care and peace.

915 Mature Minglers Senior Center
7273 Wing Lake Road
Bloomfield Hills, MI 48301-3772
810-932-6235
Fax: 248-932-6243
www.salespider.com

Christine Tvaroha, Supervisor

Community service organization for seniors in Bloomfield Hills, Bloomfield Township, Orchard Lake, and West Bloomfield, MI.

916 Michigan Association of Area Agencies on Aging
6105 West St Joseph
Suite 204
Lansing, MI 48917
517-886-1029
Fax: 517-886-1305
www.mi-seniors.org

Mary Ablan, Director

Provide supportive services that enable older adults to live with independence and dignity in a setting of their choice.

917 Michigan Association of Homes and Services for the Aging
201 North Washington Square
Suite 920
Lansing, MI 48917-8248
517-323-3687
Fax: 517-323-4569
www.mahsahome.org

David Herbel, President/CEO
Deanna Ludlow Mitchell, Senior Vice President
Sheri Deisler, VP Business Development

We create the future of aging services, advocate for service excellence, deliver member value, promote a continuum of service.

918 Michigan Association of Retired School Personnel
PO Box 23214
3645 East Jolly Road
Lansing, MI 48909-3214
517-337-1757
Fax: 517-337-8560
staff-marsp@marsp.org
www.marsp.org

Les Nixon, President
Robert Wiles, Vice President
Fayda Mills, Secretary

Represents and promotes the interests of retired school personnel.

919 Michigan Bureau of Workers' Disability Compensation
7150 Harris Drive, 1st Floor
PO Box 30016
Lansing, MI 48909

517-322-1296
Fax: 517-322-1808; *Toll Free:* 888-396-5041
wcinfo@michigan.gov
www.michigan.gov/wca rcomp

Kevin Elsenheimer, Dwirector
Jack Nolish, Deputy Director
Ted Day, Division Manager

The Bureau of Workers' Disability Compensation's mission is to administer the Act in order to facilitate timely benefit payments to injured employees at a reasonable cost to employers.

920 Michigan Client Assistance Program
Michigan Protection and Advocacy Service
4095 Legacy Parkway
Suite 500
Lansing, MI 48933-1700
517-487-1755
Fax: 517-487-0827; *Toll Free:* 800-288-5923
molson@mpas.org
www.mpas.org

Michelle Huerta, President
Kate Pew Wolters, 1st Vice President
Thomas Landry, 2nd Vice President

Our goal is to advance the dignity, equality, self-determination, and expressed choices of individuals.

921 Michigan Department of Community Health
HIV/AIDS Prevention & Intervention Section
3423 N Logan Martin Luther King Jr Boulevard
Lansing, MI 48901
517-373-3654
Fax: 517-335-8395
www.michigan.gov/mdch

Olga Dazzo, Director Division HI

Gives general public and high-risk education grants supporting educational materials, programs and a hotline.

922 Michigan Department of Health and Human
Services Aging and Adult Services Agency
333 S Grand Avenue
4th Floor
Lansing, MI 48933
517-373-8230
Fax: 517-241-2345
AASADirector@michigan.gov
www.michigan.gov/aasa

Richard Kline, Senior Deputy Director
Carol Dye, Senior Executive Management Ast.
Scott Wamsley, Deputy Director

AASA's mission is to provide statewide leadership, direction, and resources to support Michigan's aging, adult services, and disability networks, with the aim of helping residents live with dignity and purpose.

Year Founded: 1973; Number of Members: 45

923 Michigan Department of Human Services
235 South Grand Avenue
PO Box 30037
Lansing, MI 48909
517-373-2035
Fax: 517-335-6101
dhsweb@michigan.gov
www.michigan.gov/dhs
TDD 517-373-8071

Maura Corrigan, Director
Duane Berger, Chief Deputy Director
Terrence Beurer, Field Operations Director

The Department of Human Services (DHS) is Michigan's public assistance, child and family welfare agency. DHS directs the operations of public assistance and service programs through a network of 100 county Department of Human Service offices around the state.

924 Michigan Department of Management and
Budget: Bureau of Retirement Systems
George W Romney Building
111 South Capitol Avenue
Lansing, MI 48909-7671
517-373-3654
Fax: 517-322-6988; *Toll Free:* 800-381-5111
dtmb@michigan.gov
www.michigan.gov/dmb

John Nixon, Director
Sharon Ellis, Director of Operations
Nancy Duncan, Chief Deputy Director

Mission is to provide vital administrative and technology services and information to enable Michigan's reinvention by making Michigan one of the most innovative, efficient, and responsive governments in the world.

925 Michigan Department of Military Affairs
Bureau of State Operations and Veterans'
Affairs
3423 N Martin Luther King Blvd.
Lansing, MI 48906
517-335-6523
Fax: 517-241-0674
www.michigan.gov/dmva

Maj General Gregory Vadnais, Director/Adjutant General
Brig General Burton Francisco, Assistant Adjutatnt General
Brig General Robert Johnston, Commander

926 Michigan Department of Treasury
430 W Allegan Street
Lansing, MI 48922
517-373-3200; *Toll Free:* 800-487-7000
treaslndTax@michigan.gov
www.michigan.gov/treasury

Andy Dillon, Treasurer

The Michigan Department of Treasury collects, invests, an disburses all states monies. Administers major tax laws, property tax laws, and safe guards the credit of the state and its local units of government. They invest retirement funds of state employees, public school employees, public school employees, state police and judges.

927 Michigan Developmental Disability Council
Capitol View Building
201 Townsend Street
Lansing, MI 48913
517-373-3740
Fax: 517-334-7353
vanhornr@michigan.gov
www.michigan.gov/mdch
TDD 517-334-7354

Vendella Collins, Executive Director
Mitzi Allen, Executive Secretary
Dee Florence, Advocacy Secretary

Our mission is to support people with developmental disabilities to achieve life dreams.

928 Michigan Rehabilitation Services
201 North Washington Square 4th Floor
Po Box 30010
Lansing, MI 48909-7510
517-887-9370
Fax: 517-373-0565; *Toll Free:* 800-605-6722
mrs-customerassistance@michigan.gov
www.michigan.gov/mdcd

Jaye Porter, Director
Marlene Malloy, Executive Director

A state and federally funded program that helps persons with disabilities prepare for and find a job that matches their interests and abilities. Assistance is also available to workers with disabilities who are having difficulty keeping a job. A person is eligible for MRS services if he or she has a disability, is unemployed and needs vocational rehabilitation services to prepare for and find a job.

929 Michigan Society of Gerontology
PO Box 4055
East Lansing, MI 48826-4055
616-887-2920
Fax: 616-887-8586
www.msginfo.org

Joan Llardo, President
Marguerite Linteau, Vice President
Clare Luz, Treasurer

A voluntary organization made up of Michigan citizens who are concerned with education, research, action and service on behalf of older people in Michigan. MSG provides a multi-disciplinary forum for the exchange of ideas among diverse groups of professionals and students.

930 Michigan Workers Compensation Board
7150 Harris Drive 1st Floor B Wing
Po Box 30016
Lansing, MI 48913-1321
517-322-1296
Fax: 517-322-1808
wcinfo@michigan.gov
www.michigan.gov/wca

Kevin Elsenheimer, Director
Jack Nolish, Deputy Director
Sue Bickel, Administration

Effectively administer the Workers' Disability Compensation Act of Michigan.

931 Northeast Michigan: Agency on Aging
2375 Gordon Road
Alpena, MI 49707-4627
989-356-3474
Fax: 989-354-5909; *Toll Free:* 866-484-7077
contact@nemcsa.org
www.nemcsa.org

Laurie Sauer, Director
John Swise, CEO

932 Northeast Michigan: Region 9 Area Agency on Aging
2375 Gordon Road
Alpena, MI 49707-4627
989-356-3474
Fax: 989-358-6604; *Toll Free:* 866-484-7077

sauer1@nemcsa.org
www.nemcsa.org
Laurie Sauer, Director
John Swise, CEO

Services provided to Alcona, Alpena, Arenac, Cheboygan, Crawford, Iasco, Montmorency, Ogemaw, Oscoda, Otsego, Presque Isle and Roscommon Counties.

Year Founded: 1973

933 RSVP Genesee-Shiawassee Counties
2421 Corunna Road
Room 118
Flint, MI 48503-3358
810-760-1092
Fax: 810-760-5388
rsvpfnt@aol.com
www.aol.com

Karen Reid Zimmermann, Director

The Retired and Senior Volunteer Program (RSVP) provides opportunities for people 55 and over to make a difference in their community through volunteer service. RSVP volunteers contribute anywhere from a few to over forty hours a week, serving through schools, day care centers, police departments, hospitals and other nonprofit and public organizations to help meet critical community needs. RSVP offers maximum flexibility and choice to its volunteers. RSVP matches the personal interests and skills of older Americans with opportunities to help solve community problems and offers supplemental insurance while on duty, on-the-job training from the agency or organization where volunteers are placed. The following Counties are served: Genesee, Shiawassee.

934 RSVP Ingham
333 Dahlia
Lansing, MI 48911-5990
517-887-6116
Fax: 517-887-7313
community@rsvp-lansing.com
www.volunteerlansing.com

Janet Clark, Executive Director
Rita Bigelow, Volunteer Coordinator
Diana Hrit, Director, SCP Program

The Retired and Senior Volunteer Program (RSVP) provides opportunities for people 55 and over to make a difference in their community through volunteer service. RSVP volunteers contribute anywhere from a few to over forty hours a week, serving though schools, day care centers, police departments, hospitals and other nonprofit and public organizations to help meet critical community needs. RSVP offers maximum flexibility and choice to its volunteers. RSVP matches the personal interests and skills to older Americans with opportunities to help solve community problems and offer supplemental insurance while on duty, on-the-job training from the agency or organization where volunteers are placed.

935 RSVP Jackson County
407 S Mechanic Street
Jackson, MI 49201-2331
517-782-4616
Fax: 517-782-2693

Pamela McCrum, Director

The Retired and Senior Volunteer Program (RSVP) provides opportunities for people 55 and over to make a difference in their community through volunteer service. RSVP volunteers contribute anywhere from a few to over forty hours a week, serving through schools, day care centers, police departments, hospitals and other nonprofit and public organizations to help meet critical community needs. RSVP offers maximum flexibility and choice to its volunteers. RSVP matches the personal interests and skills of older Americans with opportunities to help solve community problems and offers supplemental insurance while on duty, on-the-job training from the agency or organization where volunteers are placed. The following County is served: Jackson.

936 RSVP Kent County
820 Monroe Avenue NW
Suite 460
Grand Rapids, MI 49503-4150
646-596-4205
Fax: 616-459-9906
ginniblanchard@sbcglobal.net
www.sbcglobaladvisors.com

Ginni Blanchard, Director
Laura Byrd, Development Coordinator
Julie Lake, Wellness Coordinator

The Retired and Senior Volunteer Program (RSVP) provides opportunities for people 55 and over to make a difference in their community through volunteer service. RSVP volunteers contribute anywhere from a few to over forty hours a week, serving through schools, day care centers, police departments, hospitals and other nonprofit and public organizations to help meet critical community needs. RSVP offers maximum flexibility and choice to its volunteers. RSVP matches the personal interests and skills of older Americans with opportunities to help solve community problems and offers supplemental insurance while on duty, on-the-job training from the agency or organization where volunteers are placed. The following County is served: Kent.

Number of Members: 1,100

937 RSVP Macomb
15945 Canal Road
PO Box 380290
Clinton Township, MI 48038
586-756-1430
Fax: 586-759-8789
rsvpkearney@hotmail.com
www.csmacomb.org

Sue Siemaszko, Director

The Retired and Senior Volunteer Program (RSVP) provides opportunities for people 55 and over to make a difference in their community through volunteer service. RSVP volunteers contribute anywhere from a few to over forty hours a week, serving thourgh schools, day care centers, police departments, hospitals and other nonprofit and public organizations to help meet critical community needs. RSVP offers maximum flexibility and choice to its volunteers. RSVP matches the personal interests and skills to older Americans with opportunities to help solve community problems and offer supplemental insurance while on duty, on-the-job training from the agency or organization where volunteers are placed.

938 RSVP Marquette County
215 West Hematite Drive
Ishpeming, MI 49849

906-485-1742
Fax: 906-226-4188
www.co.marquette.ci.mi

Elyse Bertucci, Director

The Retired and Senior Volunteer Program (RSVP) provides opportunities for people 55 and over to make a difference in their community through volunteer service. RSVP volunteers contribute anywhere from a few to over forty hours a week, serving thourgh schools, day care centers, police departments, hospitals and other nonprofit and public organizations to help meet critical community needs. RSVP offers maximum flexibility and choice to its volunteers. RSVP matches the personal interests and skills of older Americans with opportunities to help solve community problems and offer supplemental insurance while on duty, on-the-job training from the agency or organization where volunteers are placed.

939 RSVP Mecosta/Lake/Osceola
14485 Northland Drive
Big Rapids, MI 49307-2368
231-796-4848
Fax: 231-796-7864
rsvp@tucker-usa.com
www.michigan.gov

Sandra Dalrymple, Director

Provides opportunities for people 55 and over to make a difference in their community through volunteer service. RSVP volunteers contribute anywhere from a few to over forty hours a week, serving through schools, day care centers, police departments, hospitals and other nonprofit and public organizations to help meet critical community needs. RSVP matches the personal interests and skills of older Americans with opportunities to help solve community problems and offers supplemental insurance while on duty, on-the-job training from the agency or organization where volunteers are placed.

940 RSVP Oakland County
18310 W 12 Mile Road
Southfield, MI 48076-2670
248-559-1147
Fax: 248-559-2309
mastenh@cssoc.org
www.cssoc.org

Herschell T Masten, Director

The Retired and Senior Volunteer Program (RSVP) provides opportunities for people 55 and over to make a difference in their community through volunteer service. RSVP volunteers contribute anywhere from a few to over forty hours a week, serving through schools, day care centers, police departments, hospitals and other nonprofit and public organizations to help meet critical community needs. RSVP offers maximum flexibility and choice to its volunteers. RSVP matches the personal interests and skills of older Americans with opportunities to help solve community problems and offers supplemental insurance while on duty, on-the-job training from the agency or organization where volunteers are placed. The following County is served: Oakland.

941 RSVP Wayne County
1600 S Second St
Richmond
Detroit, IN 48202-1424

765-983-7309
Fax: 765-983-7386
www.volunteermatch.org

Uneil Smith, Director

The Retired and Senior Volunteer Program (RSVP) provides opportunities for people 55 and over to make a difference in their community through volunteer service. RSVP volunteers contribute anywhere from a few to over forty hours a week, serving through schools, day care centers, police departments, hospitals and other nonprofit and public organizations to help meet critical community needs. RSVP offers maximum flexibility and choice to its volunteers. RSVP matches the personal interests and skills of older Americans with opportunities to help solve community problems and offers supplemental insurance while on duty, on-the-job training from the agency or organization where volunteers are placed. The following County is served: Wayne.

942 Railroad Retirement Board: Michigan District Office
McNaunara Federal Building
447 West Michigan Avenue Room 1199
Detroit, MI 48226-2596
313-226-6221
Fax: 313-226-4233
www.rrb.gov

Michael A Schwartz, Chairman
Walter Barrows, Labor Member

An independent agency in the executive branch of the Federal Government. The RRB'S primary function is to administer comprehensive retirement-survivor and umemployment-sickness benefit programs for the nation's railroad workers and their families.

943 Region Seven: Area Agency on Aging
1615 South Euclid Avenue
Bay City, MI 48706-3319
989-893-4506
Fax: 989-893-2651; *Toll Free:* 800-858-1637
www.region7aaa.org

Andrew Orvash, Executive Director

To advocate, plan, devlop, and support a comprehensive system of quality care and services designed to achieve the optimum level of health, well-being, and independence of peopl as they age.

944 Region Two: Area Agency on Aging
102 North Main Street
PO Box 189
Brooklyn, MI 49230
517-467-2204
Fax: 517-592-1975; *Toll Free:* 800-335-7881
www.r2aaa.org

Lisa Tinsley, Executive Director

The Region 2 Area Agency on Aging office administers programs that help the elderly maintain their health and independence in their homes and communities. Counties served: Jackson, Hillsdale, Lenawee.

945 Right to Life of Michigan
2340 Porter Street SW
PO Box 901
Grand Rapids, MI 49509-0901

616-532-2300
Fax: 616-532-3461
info@rtl.org
www.rtl.org

Barb Listing, President

Right to Life of Michigan is a nonpartisan, nonsectarian, nonprofit organization of diverse and caring people united to protect the precious gift of human life from fertilization to natural death.

946 Senior Companion Program of Macomb
15945 Canal Road
Clinton Township, MI 48038
586-756-1435
Fax: 586-759-8789
csmseniors@csmacomb.org
www.csmacomb.org

Carmen Strong, Director

Volunteer service opportunities with hourly stipend for income-eligible adults age 60 or older; non-medical support for homebound adults.

947 Senior Services
918 Jasper Street
Kalamazoo, MI 49001
269-382-0515
Fax: 269-382-3189
www.seniorservices1.org

Robert W Littke PhD, President/CEO
Ken Greschak, Director Fund Development
John Grib, Director Clinical Programs

A 501(c)(3) Agency to provide over 21 services assisting the elderly to remain living at home, safely, independently and with dignity.

948 Sheltering Arms Adult Day Services
3300 S. Adams Road
Auburn Hills, MI 48326
248-537-3300
Fax: 586-777-8740; *Toll Free:* 855-882-2736
www.ccsem.org

Jason Shanks, CEO
Herschell Maston, Director of Senior Services

Supervised, daytime care and activities for physically and/or memory-impaired adults; respite, monthly support groups. Personal care, medication reminders, incontinence care, wheelchair accessible transportation, flexible schedule.

949 The Senior Alliance: Area Agency on Aging 1-C
3850 Second Street
Suite 100
Wayne, MI 48184-1755
734-722-2830
Fax: 734-722-2836; *Toll Free:* 800-815-1112
info@tsalink.org
www.thesenioralliance.org

Bob Brown, Executive Director
Frank Vaslo, Chairperson
John Pedit, Vice Chairman

The Senior Agency is the Area Agency on Aging for western and southern Wayne County, Michigan. People can call or email the office to talk to an Information & Assistance Specialist regarding services available to residents in our region.

Year Founded: 1980

950 Tri-County Office on Aging
5303 South Cedar Street
Suite One
Lansing, MI 48911-3800
517-887-1440
Fax: 517-887-8071; *Toll Free:* 800-405-9141
info@tcoa.org
www.tcoa.org

Marion Owen, Executive Director
Dee Lamb, Finance Director

Our mission is to promote and preserve the independence and dignity of the aging population.

951 Valley: Area Agency on Aging
225 E Fifth Street
Suite 200
Flint, MI 48502
810-239-7671
Fax: 313-239-8869; *Toll Free:* 800-978-6275
www.valleyaaa.org
TDD 810-233-4242

Kathryn Boles, Director

Answers, action, and advocacy to enhance the lives of elderly and disabled adults with support for caregivers and families

952 Waterford Senior Center
3621 Pontiac Lake Road
Waterford, MI 48328
248-682-9450
Fax: 248-738-4710
www.waterfordk12.mi.us/seniorcenter

John Silveri, Superintendent
Carl Solden, Supervisor

Multi purpose senior center offering programs and services to those 55 years and older. Goal is to assist them to maintain independence and enhance their quality of life.

Minnesota

953 Aging Service of Minnesota
2550 University Avenue West
Suite 350 South
Saint Paul, MN 55114-1900
651-645-4545
Fax: 651-645-0002; *Toll Free:* 800-462-5368
info@agingservicesmn.org
www.agingservicesmn.org

Gayle M Kvenvold, President/CEO
Lori Meyer, Sr Vice President
Barbara Landeen, Director of Membership

Aging Services of Minnesota is Minnesota's largest association of aging services organizations. Today our membership encompasses over 1,000 member organizations including 700+ provider member sites. Together, we work with over 50,000 caregivers throughout the state and serve more than 100,000 seniors each year in settings across the continuum from their home to congregate housing to assisted living to care centers. Aging Services members are diverse but share a common focus on person-directed living, missions of service to their communities and choice in older adult services. Aging Services is the state affiliate of the American Association of Homes and Services for the

Aging (AAHSA) and the Assisted Living Federation of America (ALFA).
Year Founded: 1967

954 Arrowhead RSVP-AEOA
702 Third Avenue South
Virginia, MN 55792
218-749-7328
Fax: 218-749-2944; *Toll Free:* 800-662-5711
bonnie.ebnet@aeoa.org
www.aeoa.org

Bonnie Ebnet, Program Director
Harlan Tardy, AEOA Executive Director

RSVP is America's largest volunteer network for people 55 and over, helping them to apply their skills and wisdom to make a positive difference in the lives of others.
Year Founded: 1972; Number of Members: 1450

955 Arrowhead: Area Agency on Aging
221 West 1st Street
Duluth, MN 55802-2316
218-722-5545
Fax: 218-529-7592; *Toll Free:* 800-232-0707
csampson@ardc.org
www.arrowheadaging.org

Catherine Sampson, Director
Kara Edwards, Secretary
Michele Flatau, Volunteer Coordinator

AAAA is a catalyst in building communities where seniors live with dignity, mutual respect and shared responsibilities across generations and cultures.

956 Bureau of Naval Personnel: Minnesota Retired Activities Office
Naval Reserve Readiness Command Region Sixteen
715 Apollo Avenue
Minneapolis, MN 55450-2113
612-713-1578
www.navyreserve.navy.mil

Capt Victor Yanega, III, Commanding Officer
CDR David H Ryan, Executive Officer

The RAO serves as a link between local retired military and the active-duty community which provides assistance to retired military. It provides installation commanders with a means of providing more effective services and improving communication for the local retired community. The RAO is staffed and operated by volunteer retired military who assist other retired members, their families and survivors to receive entitled services and benefits. Through newsletters, seminars and appreciation days, the RAO supports quality of life issues throughout the retirement years to their fellow service members.

957 Cass County Council on Aging
303,Minnesota Awe,W
P.O Box 3000
Walker, MN 56484
269-445-8110
Fax: 269-445-5595; *Toll Free:* 800-323-0390
www.co.cass.mn.us

Robert Cochrane, Executive Director
Adrienne Glover, Asst Executive Director
Suzanne Beurmann, Adult Day Services

The Council on Aging provides information and referral services with senior services and agencies. The Council deals with issues of concern with seniors and with senior clubs in the area. The Council coordinates transportation services for those 60 years and over who sign up through the Council office and demonstrate need.

958 Central Minnesota Council on Aging
1301 West Saint Germain Street
Suite 101
St. Cloud, MN 56301
320-253-9349
Fax: 320-253-9576; *Toll Free:* 800-333-2433
lori@cmcoa.org
www.cmcoa.org

Lori Vrolson, Executive Director
Linda Gansen, Financial Manager
Lynn Loew, Integration Developer

The Central Minnesota Council on Aging is a non-profit organization and designated by the Minnesota Board on Aging as the Area Agency on Aging, to serve the counties of Benton, Cass, Chisago, Crow Wing, Isanti, Kanabec, Mille Lacs, Morrison, Pine Sherburne, Stearns, Todd, Wadena, and Wright. The Central Minnesota Council on Aging is committed to maintaining the highest level of independence with older people by developing and coordinating community care, reducing isolation and improving access to services.

959 Communicating for Seniors
112 East Lincoln Avenue
Fergus Falls, MN 56538
218-739-3241
Fax: 218-739-3832; *Toll Free:* 800-432-3276
memberbenefits@cainc.org
www.communicatingforamerica.org

Milt Smedsrud, Chairman/CEO
Wayne Nelson, President

Provides general information on health-related matters for the elderly, particularly in the area of insurance. Offers group Medicare supplement to members. Offers free brochure and other materials for sale. Hours: 8:00 a.m. to 4:30 p.m. Monday-Friday.

960 Department of Employment and Economic Development
1st National Bank Building
332 Minnesota Street
Suite E-200
St. Paul, MN 55101
651-259-7114
Fax: 651-259-4721; *Toll Free:* 800-657-3858
deedcustomerservice@state.mn.us
www.positivelyminnesota.com
TTY: 218-723-4725

Mark Phillips, Commissioner
Paul Moe, Deputy Commissioner
Lynne Batzil, Director

Our mission is to support the economic success of individual's, businesses, and communities by improving opportunities for growth.

961 Disability Determination Services
190 5th Street
Suite 800
Saint Paul, MN 55104
651-296-2574
Fax: 651-297-1650; *Toll Free:* 800-772-1213

www.ssa.gov
TTY: 800-325-0778
Cory Kissell, Public Relations Officer

The Disability Determination Services Office assists the federal Social Security Administration (SSA) in determining if Minnesota applicants meet federal criteria for disability cash benefits under the SSA's Social Security Disability Insurance (SSDI) or Supplemental Security Income (SSI) programs.

962 East Central Regional Development Commission Area on Aging
100 Park Street South
Mora, MN 55051
320-679-4065
Fax: 320-679-4120
ecrdc@ecrdc.org
www.ecrdc.org

Bob Voss, Executive Director
Jordan Zeller, Development Director
Penny Simonsen, Sr Resource Coordinator

Provides leadership and direction through problem solving. They do this by imitating projects and programs that lead to create solutions to regional problems., by providing tecnical assistance and by identifying and developing available sources. Their mission is to provide a leadership role as an advocate to brbring about positive change.

963 Eldercircle
Old Central School
1105 NW 4th Street
Grand Rapids, MN 55744
218-999-9233
Fax: 218-999-7543; *Toll Free:* 800-327-1617
ecircle@eldercircle.org
www.eldercircle.org

Kristi Kane, Executive Director

The Retired and Senior Volunteer Program (RSVP) provides opportunities for people 55 and over to make a difference in their community through volunteer service. RSVP volunteers contribute anywhere from a few to over forty hours a week, serving through schools, day care centers, police departments, hospitals and other nonprofit and public organizations to help meet critical community needs. RSVP offers maximum flexibility and choice to its volunteers. RSVP matches the personal interests and skills of older Americans with opportunities to help solve community problems and offers supplemental insurance while on duty, on-the-job training from the agency or organization where volunteers are placed.

964 Gray Panthers of Twin Cities
3249 Hennepin Avenue S
Suite 220
Minneapolis, MN 55408-3493
612-822-1011
sallybrown46@comcast.net
www.graypantherstwincities.org

Sally Brown, Co-Director
Jane Hanger-Seeley, Co-Director

Our mission is work for social and economic justice and peace for all people.

965 Happy Old Timers Senior Center
405 Sixth Street
Hawley, MN 56549-4601
218-483-4681; *Toll Free: 888-565-3828*
answers@ourparents.com
www.ourparents.com

Laurence Legler, President

Promotes and provides social services for senior citizens in
Hawley, MN.

966 Metropolitan: Area Agency on Aging
2365 N McKnight Road
Suite 3
North St. Paul, MN 55109
651-641-8612
Fax: 651-641-8618
maaa@tcaging.org
www.tcaging.org

Dawn Simonson, Executive Director
Bob Anderson, Associate Director
Terry Nielson, Finance Director

The designated area agency on aging for the 7 county metropolitan area. In partnerships with public and private organizations, MAAA helps elders age successfully. It does this
by building community capacity, advocating for aging issues, maximizing service effectiveness and linking people
with information.

967 Mid-Minnesota: Area Agency on Aging
333 W 6th Street
Suite 2
Willmar, MN 56201
320-235-8504
Fax: 612-235-4329; *Toll Free: 800-450-8608*
mmrdc@mmrdc.org
www.mmrdc.org

Don Winckler, Executive Director
Kate Selseth, Aging Director
Ashley Ronglien, Sr Outreach Specialist

Provides technical assistance to government, businesses,
and local organizations; administer state and federal programs, and coordinate multi-jurisdictional activities to
maintain or enhance the quality of life.

968 Minnesota Board on Aging
540 Cedar Street
Po Box 64976
Saint Paul, MN 55155-3843
651-431-2500
Fax: 651-431-7453; *Toll Free: 800-627-3529*
mba@state.mn.us
www.mnaging.org

Jean Wood, Executive Director

A state unit on aging for the state of Minnesota. Funds 14
area agencies on aging throughout the state that provide
services at the local level. The mission is to keep older people in their homes or places of residence for as long as
possible.

969 Minnesota Council on Disability
121 E 7th Place
Suite 107
Saint Paul, MN 55101
651-296-6785
Fax: 651-296-5935; *Toll Free: 800-945-8913*

council.disability@state.mn.us
www.disability.state.mn.us

Joan Willshire, Executive Director
Linda Gremillion, Operations Manager
Tricia Drury, Events Coordinator

Advocates for policies and programs in the public and
orivate sectors that advance the rights of Minnesotans with
disabilities.

**970 Minnesota Department of Labor & Industry
Workers Compensation Division**
443 Lafayette Road North
Saint Paul, MN 55155-4307
651-284-5005
Fax: 651-284-5720; *Toll Free: 800-342-5354*
dli.workcomp@state.mn.us
www.doli.state.mn.us
TTY: 651-297-4198

Ken Peterson, Commissioner
Kris Elden, Deputy Commissioner
Jessica Looman, Labor Standards Commissioner

To reduce the impact of work related injuries for employees and employers. Advice is given and questions answered
on the toll-free number.

971 Minnesota Department of Revenue
600 North Robert Street
Saint Paul, MN 55101
651-296-3781; *Toll Free: 800-652-9094*
dorweb.comm@state.mn.us
www.taxes.state.mn.us

Manages the state's revenue system. We administer 28 different taxes, collecting over 12 billion annually. This
money funds education, local government aid, property tax
relief, social service programs, highways, and other state
programs and operations.

972 Minnesota Department of Veterans Affairs
20 12th Street W
2nd Floor, Room 206-C
Saint Paul, MN 55155-2006
651-296-2562
Fax: 651-296-3954
www.mdva.state.mn.us
TDD 194- -

Larry Shelito, Commissioner
Reggie Worlds, Deputy Commissioner, Programs
Michael Gallucci, Deputy Commissioner, Health Care

An organiazation that is committed to ensuring that Minnesota's veterans, their dependents and survivors receive their
full measure of benefits and services to which they are
entitled.

**973 Minnesota Governor's Council on
Developmental Disabilities**
370 Centennial Office Building
658 Cedar Street
Saint Paul, MN 55155
651-296-4018
Fax: 651-297-7200; *Toll Free: 877-348-0505*
admin.dd@state.mn.us
mn.gov/mnddc
TTY: 800-627-3529

Colleen Wieck, PhD, Executive Director

The mission of the Minnesota Governor's Council on Developmental Disabilities is to provide information, education, and training to build knowledge, develop skills, and change attitudes that will lead to increased independence, productivity, self determination, integration and inclusion (IPSII) for people with developmental disabilities and their families.

Year Founded: 1971; Number of Members: 25

974   Minnesota Indian: Area Agency on Aging
15542 State Hwy 371 NW
Po Box 217
Cass Lake, MN 56633
218-335-8585
Fax: 218-335-6562; *Toll Free:* 888-231-7886
vbrown@mnchippewatribe.org
www.mnchiooewatribe.org

Vera Brown, Contact

Works with Indian reservations with planning and implementation of nutrition and supportive services for persons 60 years of age and older.

975   Minnesota Mental Health Division
475 Cleveland Avenue North
Suite 222
St. Paul, MN 55104
651-493-6634; *Toll Free:* 800-862-1799
info@mentalhealthmn.org
www.mentalhealthmn.org

Ed Eide, Executive Director
Brett Dumke, Education Coordinator
Nancy Paul, Development Associate

Oversees the provision of services to people with mental illness in the state of Minnesota. Services are provided on the local level through a network of 87 county social service departments.

976   Minnesota Public Employees Retirement Association
60 Empire Drive
Suite 200
Saint Paul, MN 55103
651-296-7460
Fax: 651-297-2547; *Toll Free:* 800-652-9026
mary.most.vanek@mnpera.org
www.mnpera.org

Mary Vanek, Executive Director

Mission is to create opportunities for members to achieve a successful and secure retirement by providing the highest quality benefits and services that members will value and trust.

977   Minnesota State Council on Disability
121 E 7th Place
Suite 107
Saint Paul, MN 55101-2188
651-361-7800
Fax: 651-296-5935; *Toll Free:* 800-945-8913
council.disability@state.mn.us
www.disability.state.mn.us

Joan Willshire, Executive Director
Linda Gremillion, Operations Manager
Tricia Drury, Events Coordinator

An agency that collaborates, advocactes, and provides information to expand opportunities, increase the quality of life and empower all persons with disabilities.

978   Minnesota System of Technology to Achieve Results Program
358 Centennial Office Building
658 Cedar Street
Saint Paul, MN 55155
651-201-2640
Fax: 651-282-6671; *Toll Free:* 888-234-1267
star.program@state.mn.us
www.starprogram.state.mn.us
TDD 651-296-9478

Jennie Delisi, Executive Director
Joan Gillum, Program Staff
Kim Moccia, Program Staff

The STAR Program was established as Minnesota's Tech Act Project to plan and coordinate assistive technology (AT) information and services for the citizens of Minnesota with disabilities. The STAR Program serves as an advocate for federal and state assistive technology policy and legislation, builds assistive technology capacity in state government and helps assure statewide assistive technology services.

979   Minnesota Teachers Retirement Association
60 Empire Drive
Suite 400
Saint Paul, MN 55103
651-296-2409
Fax: 651-297-5999; *Toll Free:* 800-657-3669
info.tra@state.mn.us
www.tra.state.mn.us
TTY: 800-627-3529

Laurie Fiori Hacking, Executive Director
Luther Thompson PhD, JD, Assistant Executive Director
John Wicklund, Assistant Executive Director

The mission of the Teachers Retirement Association is to enhance the quality of life for Minnesota teachers and their beneficiaries and to assist them in planning for an independent and financially secure retirement. To this end we are committed to the improvement of our customer services. Among the services provided to our customers are counseling members on retirement issues, maintianing member data, administering funds, communicating accurate information and delivering benefits.

980   Minnestoa Retirement System
60 Empire Drive
Suite 300
Saint Paul, MN 55103-3000
651-296-2761
Fax: 651-297-5238; *Toll Free:* 800-657-5757
info@msrs.us
www.msrs.state.mn.us

David Bergstrom, Executive Director

Administers to ten different retirement plans which provide retirement, survivor, and disability benefit coverage for Minnesota state employees as well as employees of the Metropolitan Council and many non-faculty employees at the State University of Minnesota.

981   Paynesville Area Senior Center
1105 W Main Street
Paynesville, MN 56362-1000

320-243-4799
Fax: 320-243-5146
pacenter@clearwire.net
www.lgfws.com

Inez Jones, Director

Provides services and recreational activities for seniors.

982 RSVP Aiken-Carlton Counties

1003 Cloquet Avenue
Suite 102
Cloquet, MN 55720-1694
218-879-9238
Fax: 218-879-1196
www.aikencountysc.gov

Jill Hatfield, Director

The Retired and Senior Volunteer Program (RSVP) provides opportunities for people 55 and over to make a difference in their community through volunteer service. RSVP volunteers contribute anywhere from a few to over forty hours a week, serving through schools, day care centers, police departments, hospitals and other nonprofit and public organizations to help meet critical community needs. RSVP offers maximum flexibility and choice to its volunteers. RSVP matches the personal interests and skills of older Americans with opportunities to help solve community problems and offers supplemental insurance while on duty, on-the-job training from the agency or organization where volunteers are placed. The following Counties are served: Aiken, Carlton.

Year Founded: 1971

983 RSVP Arrowhead County

702 Third Avenue South
Virginia, MN 55792-2775
218-749-2912
Fax: 218-749-2944; *Toll Free:* 800-662-5711
bonnie.ebnet@aeoa.org
www.aeoa.org

Steve Raukar, Chairman
Year Founded: 1955

984 RSVP Eldercircle
Old Central School

1105 NW 4th Street
Grand Rapids, MN 55744-2660
218-999-9233
Fax: 218-999-7543; *Toll Free:* 800-327-1617
ecircle@eldercircle.org
www.eldercircle.org

Kristi Kane, Executive Director
Kara Sagedahl, Program Director
Cole Perry, Project Director

985 RSVP Greater Twin Cities

7625 Metro Boulevard
Minneapolis, MN 55439
612-617-7833
Fax: 612-331-6772
www.voamm.org

Jyni Koschak, Director

The Retired and Senior Volunteer Program (RSVP) provides opportunities for people 55 and over to make a difference in their community through volunteer service. RSVP volunteers contribute anywhere from a few to over forty hours a week, serving through schools, day care centers,

police departments, hospitals and other nonprofit and public organizations to help meet critical community needs. RSVP offers maximum flexibility and choice to its volunteers. RSVP matches the personal interests and skills of older Americans with opportunities to help solve community problems and offers supplemental insurance while on duty, on-the-job training from the agency or organization where volunteers are placed.

986 RSVP Mahube Community Council

1125 West River Road
Po Box 747
Detroit Lakes, MN 56501-0747
218-847-1385
Fax: 218-847-1388
dloffice@mahube.org
www.mahube.org

Leah Pigatti, Executive Director

The Retired and Senior Volunteer Program (RSVP) helps individuals 55 and older put their skills and life experiences to work for their communities. The following Counties are served: Becker, Clearwater, Hubbard, Mahnomen.

987 RSVP Red River Valley
University of Minnesota

247 Student Center
Crookston, MN 56716-5001
218-281-8288
Fax: 218-281-8250; *Toll Free:* 800-232-6466
www.cik.umn.edu/people/services/rsvp

Jan Aamoth, Director
Deanna Patenaude, Program Specialist
Elizabeth Tollefson, Executive Director

The Retired and Senior Volunteer Program (RSVP) provides opportunities for people 55 and over to make a difference in their community through volunteer service. RSVP volunteers contribute anywhere from a few to over forty hours a week, serving thourgh schools, day care centers, police departments, hospitals and other nonprofit and public organizations to help meet critical community needs. RSVP offers maximum flexibility and choice to its volunteers. RSVP matches the personal interests and skills to older Americans with opportunities to help solve community problems and offer supplemental insurance while on duty, on-the-job training from the agency or organization where volunteers are placed.

988 RSVP Semcac

PO Box 549
204 South Elm Street
Rushford, MN 55971-9123
507-864-7741
Fax: 507-864-2440
semcac@semcac.org
www.semcac.org

Wayne Stenberg, Executive Director

The Retired and Senior Volunteer Program (RSVP) provides opportunities for people 55 and over to make a difference in their community through volunteer service. RSVP volunteers contribute anywhere from a few to over forty hours a week, serving through schools, day care centers, police departments, hospitals and other nonprofit and public organizations to help meet critical community needs. RSVP offers maximum flexibility and choice to its volunteers. RSVP matches the personal interests and skills of older Americans with opportunities to help solve community problems and offers supplemental insurance while on duty, on-the-job training from the agency or organization where volunteers are placed. The following Counties are served: Dodge, Fillmore, Houston, Mower, Stelle.

989 RSVP Southern Tri-County

Skyline Plaza
1659 West Main Street
Albert Lea, MN 56007-1868
507-377-7433
Fax: 507-377-2879
info@seniorresourcesfc.org
www.seniorresourcesfc.org

Beth Spande, Director

The Retired and Senior Volunteer Program (RSVP) provides opportunities for people 55 and over to make a difference in their community through volunteer service. RSVP volunteers contribute anywhere from a few to over forty hours a week, serving through schools, day care centers, police departments, hospitals and other nonprofit and public organizations to help meet critical community needs. RSVP offers maximum flexibility and choice to its volunteers. RSVP matches the personal interests and skills of older Americans with opportunities to help solve community problems and offers supplemental insurance while on duty, on-the-job training from the agency or organization where volunteers are placed. The following Counties are served: Faribault, Freeborn, Martin.

990 RSVP Todd, Wadena, Otter Tail & Wilkin
Otter Tail-Wadena Community Action Council

109 South Walker Avenue
PO Box L
New York Mills, MN 56567-4104
218-385-2900
Fax: 218-385-4544
www.mncaa.org

Katie Baril, RSVP Director

The Retired and Senior Volunteer Program (RSVP) provides opportunities for people 55 and over to make a difference in their community through volunteer service. RSVP volunteers contribute anywhere from a few to over forty hours a week, serving through schools, day care centers, police departments, hospitals and other nonprofit and public organizations to help meet critical community needs. RSVP offers maximum flexibility and choice to its volunteers. RSVP matches the personal interests and skills of older Americans with opportunities to help solve community problems and offers supplemental insurance while on duty, on-the-job training from the agency or organization where volunteers are placed. The following Counties are served: Otter Tail, Todd, Wadena, Wilkin.

991 RSVP Volunteer Services
Crow Wing Social Services

204 Laurel Street
Suite 11
Brainerd, MN 56401-3545
218-824-1345
Fax: 218-824-1346
RSVP@co.crow-wing.mn.us
www.co.crow-wing.mn.us

Mike Koecheler, Executive Director
Mari Jo Renstrom, Program Assistant

Our mission is connecting those in need with those able to help through volunteer service. Enhance the lives of the

volunteers and those whom they serve. Provide communities with valuable services.

992 Railroad Retirement Board: Duluth Minnesota District Office

515 W 1st Street
Duluth, MN 55802-1399
Fax: 218-720-5315; *Toll Free:* 877-772-5772
duluth@rrb.gov
www.rrb.gov

Dawn Barto, Manager

An independent agency in the executive branch of the Federal Government. The RRB's primary function is to administer comprehensive retirement-survivor and unemployment-sickness benefit programs for the nation's railroad workers and their families.

993 Railroad Retirement Board: St. Paul Minnesota District Office

180 E 5th Street
Suite 195
Saint Paul, MN 55101-1640
877-772-5772
Fax: 651-290-3076
stpaul@rrb.gov
www.rrb.gov

Brian P Running, Representative

994 Ready Ride-West Central Minnesota Communities Action

411 Industrial Park Boulevard
Elbow Lake, MN 56531
218-685-4486
Fax: 218-685-6741; *Toll Free:* 800-492-4805
office@wcmca.org
www.wcmca.org

Heather Molesworth, Dir., Family/Community Services
Missy Becker-Cook, Executive Director

Ready Ride provides a safe, easy, and reliable way for those 65+ residing in Douglas, Grant, Pope, Stevens and Traverse counties get where they need to go. This program helps take the worry out of driving and empowers seniors to remain active and independent. Ready Ride is supported, in part, by a Live Well At Home Grant from the MN Department of Human Services.

995 Region Nine: Area Agency on Aging

410 E Jackson Street Suite 400
Po Box 3367
Mankato, MN 56002-3367
507-387-5643
Fax: 507-387-7105; *Toll Free:* 800-450-5643
lindag@rndc.mankato.mn.us
www.rndc.org

Linda Giersdorf, Director
Reggie Edwards, Executive Director

Provides area-wide advocacy and leadership regarding aging on behalf of older persons. Provides information, assistance and referral on services for older adults and their families. Serves the following counties: Sibley County, Le Sueur County, Waseca County, Faribault County, Martin County, Watonwan County, Brown County, Nicollet County, Blue Earth County.

996 Southeast Minnesota Area: Agency on Aging
421 SW First Avenue
Suite 201
Rochester, MN 55902
507-288-6944
Fax: 507-288-4823; *Toll Free:* 800-333-2433
semaaa@semaaarochestermn.org
www.semaaarochestermn.org
TDD 800-657-3529

Connie Bagley, Director

Rochester, Rice County, Steele County, Freeborn County, Goodhue County, Dodge County, Mower County, Wabasha County, Olmsted County, Fillmore County, Winona County, Houston County. Community based services for the frail senior citizen. Meals on wheels, chore, advocates education, information and assistance, health insurance counseling, transportation.

997 Southeast Regional Service Center for Hearing Impaired People
Olmstead County Human Services Building
2116 Campus Drive SE
Suite 32
Rochester, MN 55904-4713
507-285-7295
Fax: 507-280-5531
www.co.olmsted.mn.us/cs
TTY: 507-285-7172

Jeff Erickson, Executive Officer

Sponsors services to the deaf and hard of hearing. Provides interpreter referral, message relay, vocational rehabilitation, assistance in dealing with agencies, and loans of materials.

998 Southeast Senior Federation
PO Box 376
West Concord, MN 55985
507-527-2799
Fax: 507-527-2799; *Toll Free:* 866-851-7755
www.southeastseniors.org

Helen Aase, President

Strives to find solutions to problems confronting elderly persons.

999 Southwest Minnesota: Area Agency on Aging
421 SW 1st Ave
Suite 201
Rochester, MN 55902
507-288-6944
Fax: 507-288-4823; *Toll Free:* 800-333-2433
semaaa@semaaarochestermn.org
www.semaaarochestermn.org

Robin Weis, Executive Director

Slayton, Lincoln County, Lyon County, Murray County, Redwood County, Pipestone County, Cottonwood County, Jackson County, Nobles County, Rock County. Mission is providing professional expertise and leadership to enhance regional opportunities.

1000 United Way 211
424 W Superior Street
Suite 402
Duluth, MN 55802-1590
218-726-4770
Fax: 218-726-4778; *Toll Free:* 800-543-7709

211@unitedwayduluth.org
www.unitedwayduluth.org

Paula Reed, President
Rebecca Ballou-Buck, Finance Director
Lynette Swanberg, Community Services Director

Our mission is to lead a united effort to strengthen our community by mobilizing resources to improve people's lives.

1001 Upper Minnesota Valley: Area Agency onAging
323 W Schlieman Avenue
Appleton, MN 56208-1229
320-289-1981
Fax: 320-289-1983; *Toll Free:* 800-752-1983
umvrdc@umvrdc.org
www.umvrdc.org

Dawn Hegland, Executive Director
Jacki Anderson, Community Development
Arlene Tilbury, Financial Director

A five county development agency providing services to local units of government. Its membership is comprised of representatives of townships, cities, counties, schoo boards, and public interest groups.

1002 West Central Minnesota: Area Agency on Aging
109 South Minnesota Street
Po Box 726
Warren, MN 56762
218-739-4617
Fax: 218-739-4618; *Toll Free:* 800-333-2433
reg4aaa@prtel.com
www.dancingskyaaa.org

Margaret Babcock, Director
Mark Tysver, Manager

Becker County, Clay County, Douglas County, Grant County, Otter Tail County, Pope County, Stevens County, Traverse County, Wilkin County.

Mississippi

1003 Central Mississippi: Area Agency on Aging
1170 Lakeland Drive
PO Box 4935
Jackson, MS 39216-4701
601-981-1511
Fax: 601-981-1515; *Toll Free:* 800-315-3103
www.mdhs.state.ms.us/aas

Chelsea Crittle, Director

Mission is to protect the rights of older citizens while expanding their opportunities ans access to quality services. Vision for each older citizen to live the best life possible.

1004 East Central Mississippi: Area Agency onAging
PO Box 499
Newton, MS 39345
601-683-2401
Fax: 601-683-7873; *Toll Free:* 800-264-2007
www.mdhs.state.ms.us

Rosie Coleman, Director

Area agency on Aging for Clarke, Lasper, Kemper, Lauderdale, Leake, Neshoba, Newton, Scott, and Smith Counties in East Central Mississippi. Provides a comprehensive system of home- and community-based services and elder rights protection at the local level. Services include, but not limited to, congregate and home delivered meals; transportation; homemaker services; information, referral, and outreach; insurance counseling, ombudsman services (long-term care facilities); legal assistance; case managment; emergency response; and Title V employment (55+). Services and programs are designed to meet the needs of priority target groups, including those persons aged 60+; low income 60+; rural 60+; minority 60+; and low-income minority 60+.

1005 Mississippi Association of Area Agencies on Aging
9299 Highway 49
Gulfport, MS 39503
228-868-2311
www.smpdd.com

Robert Moore, Aging Director
Bobbie Black, Outreach
Lydia Davis, Referral Coordinator

The Area Agency on Aging serves as the public advocate for the development and implementation of comprehensive and coordinated home and community based care systems responsive to the current needs and future growth of the aging population.

1006 Mississippi Client Assistance Program: Easter Seals Society
3226 N State Street
Jackson, MS 39216-4005
601-362-2585
www.msdisabilities.com

Presley Posey, Executive Director
Karen Brown, CAP Director

Easter Seals program.

1007 Mississippi Department of Mental Health
1101 Robert E Lee Building
239 North Lamar Street
Jackson, MS 39201-1328
601-359-1288
Fax: 601-359-6295; *Toll Free:* 877-210-8513
www.dmh.state.ms.us
TDD 601-359-6230

Dr. Jim Herzog, Chair
Sampat Shivangi, M.D, VC
Robert Landrum, Council

Provides services of the highest quality through a statewide service delivery system. As one of the major state agencies in Mississippi, the Department of Mental Health provides a network of services to persons who experience problems with mental illness, alcohol and/or drug abuse/ dependence, or who have mental retardation or developmental disabilities.

1008 Mississippi Department of Rehabilition Services for the Blind
PO Box 1698
1281 Highway 51
Jackson, MS 39296-5314
601-364-2700
Fax: 601-364-2677; *Toll Free:* 800-443-1000
www.mdrs.state.ms.us
TTY: 601-853-5100

H.S. Butch McMillian, Executive Director
Richard Sorey, Director
Sheila Browning, Deputy Director

It is the mission of the Mississippi Department of Rehabilitaion Services (MDRS) to provide appropriate and comprehensive services to Mississippians with disabilities in a timely and effective manner. Programs and services assist individuals with disabilities to gain employment, retain employment and/or to live more independently.

1009 Mississippi Division of Aging and Adult Services
Mississippi Department of Human Services
750 N State Street
Jackson, MS 39202
601-359-4500; *Toll Free:* 800-345-6347
www.mdhs.state.ms.us

Donald Taylor, Executive Director

The mission of the Division of Aging and Adult Services is to protect the right of older citizens while expanding their opportunities and access to quality services. Our vision is for each older citizen to live the best life possible. The Division of Aging and Adult Services plans, coordinates and advocates for, and ensures the provision of services to all older Mississippians.

1010 Mississippi Office of Disability & Determination Services
Mississippi Department of Rehabilitation Services
PO Box 1698
1281 Highway 51
Jackson, MS 39215-1698
601-364-2700
Fax: 601-364-2677; *Toll Free:* 800-443-1000
www.mdrs.state.ms.us
TTY: 601-853-5100

H.S. Butch McMillian, Executive Director
Richard Sorey, Director
Sheila Browning, Deputy Director

The Office of Disability Determination Services (ODDS), funded entirely through the Social Security Administration, establishes eligibility of Mississippians with severe disabilities that apply for Social Security Disability Insurance and/or Supplemental Security Income.

1011 Mississippi Public Employees Retirement Systems
429 Mississippi Street
Jackson, MS 39201-1005
601-359-3589
Fax: 601-359-2285; *Toll Free:* 800-444-7377
www.per.state.ms.us

Pat Robertson, Executive Director
Lorrie Tingle, Chief Investment Officer
Greg Gregory, Deputy Adminstrator

Retirement system for nearly all non-federal public employees in the state.

1012 Mississippi State Tax Commission
1577 Springridge Road
PO Box 1033
Jackson, MS 39215-1033
601-923-7000
Fax: 601-923-7318
www.dor.ms.gov

Keith Hicks, Manager

Provides state income and business tax forms and information.

1013 Mississippi State Veterans Affairs Board
Po Box 5947
3466 Highway 80
Pearl, MS 39288-5947
601-765-0519
Fax: 601-765-5045; *Toll Free:* 877-203-5632
grice@vab.state.ms.us
www.vab.ms.gov

Adrian Grice, Manager

Charged with assisting former and current members of the Armed Forces of the United States and their dependents in securing any benefits or privileges to which they are entitled.

1014 Natchez-Adams Council on Aging
800 Washington Street
Natchez, MS 39120-3566
601-442-5082
Fax: 601-445-6650
www.cityofnatchez.net

Sabrina Bartley, Executive Director
Evelyn Hutchins, Operations Manager
Carla Monroe, Sr Programs Coordinator

Plans and renders services to aging citizens in Natchez and Adams Counties.
Year Founded: 1716

1015 North Central Mississippi: Area Agency oN Aging
PO Box 1488
Batesville, MS 38601-1488
662-561-4100
Fax: 662-627-6753; *Toll Free:* 800-844-2433
www.mdhs.state.ms.us/aas_agcy.htm

Darlena Allen, Director
Arnetta Brown, LSW Case Manager

Our mission is to enhance the quality of life for older adults in the following counties: Attala, Carroll, Grenada, Holmes, Leflore, Montgomery, Yalobusha by ensuring that they have access to quality and cost effective services.

1016 North Delta: Area Agency on Aging
PO Box 1488
Batesville, MS 38601-1488
662-561-4100
Fax: 662-627-6753; *Toll Free:* 800-844-2433
www.mdhs.state.ms.us/aas_agcy.htm

Arnetta Brown, LSW Case Manager
Darlena Allen, Director

1017 Northeast Mississippi: Area Agency on Aging
PO Box 600
619 East Parker Drive
Booneville, MS 38829
662-728-6248
Fax: 662-728-2417; *Toll Free:* 800-745-6961
info@nempdd.com
www.nempdd.com

Sharon Gardner, Executive Director
Sadie Harden, Assistant Director
Rick Hargett, System Administrator

Our mission is to make it easier for older persons to live independently in the comfort of their own surroundings - is not only cost effective, it is the preferred choice for millions of older adults nationwide. Counties served: Alcorn, Benton, Marshall, Prentiss, Tippah, and Tishomingo.

1018 Preserve Sight Mississippi
2501 North West Street
Po Box 4417
Jackson, MS 39296-4417
601-984-3200
Fax: 601-987-3892; *Toll Free:* 866-859-4461
sales@msblind.org
www.msblind.org

Michael Chew, Executive Director
Tracy Kane, Deputy Director
Vanice Barnes, HRM

Mission is to train and provide jobs for individuals who are blind or visually impaired who are willing and able to work so that they can become self supporting members of the community.

1019 RSVP Adams County
800 Washington Street
Natchez, MS 39120-3566
601-442-5082
Fax: 601-445-6650

Sabrina Bartley, Director

The Retired and Senior Volunteer Program (RSVP) provides opportunities for people 55 and over to make a difference in their community through volunteer service. RSVP volunteers contribute anywhere from a few to over forty hours a week, serving through schools, day care centers, police departments, hospitals and other nonprofit and public organizations to help meet critical community needs. RSVP offers maximum flexibility and choice to its volunteers. RSVP matches the personal interests and skills of older Americans with opportunities to help solve community problems and offers supplemental insurance while on duty, on-the-job training from the agency or organization where volunteers are placed. The following Counties are served: Adams, Washington.

1020 RSVP Clarksdale
313 Issaquena Ave.
Clarksdale, MS 38614-4385
662-624-4887
Fax: 662-624-4915
mooregale61@yahoo.com

Gale Moore, Director

We have about 33 senior volunteers who regularly recycle cans & newspapers, and plant and maintain gardens for product and beautification of the local community.

1021 RSVP Hancock County
1928 Depot Way
PO Box 248
Bay St Louis, MS 39520-4326
228-467-9204
Fax: 228-466-0300

Jo Ann Lagasse, Director

Provides opportunities for people 55 and over to make a difference in their community through volunteer service. RSVP volunteers contribute anywhere from a few to over forty hours a week, serving through schools, day care centers, police departments, hospitals and other nonprofit and public organizations to help meet critical community needs. RSVP matches the personal interests and skills of older Americans with opportunities to help solve community problems and offers supplemental insurance while on duty, on-the-job training from the agency or organization where volunteers are placed.

1022 RSVP Harrison County

1801 23rd Ave
Gulfport, MS 39501
228-867-6537
Fax: 228-867-6539
rsvp@co.harrison.ms.us
www.co.harrison.ms.us

Connie Rockaro, VP
Alandra Knight, Secretary
Marlin Landerer, President

The Retired and Senior Volunteer Program (RSVP) provides opportunities for people 55 and over to make a difference in their community through volunteer service. RSVP volunteers contribute anywhere from a few to over forty hours a week, serving through schools, day care centers, police departments, hospitals and other nonprofit and public organizations to help meet critical community needs. RSVP offers maximum flexibility and choice to its volunteers. RSVP matches the personal interests and skills of older Americans with opportunities to help solve community problems and offers supplemental insurance while on duty, on-the-job training from the agency or organization where volunteers are placed. The following County is served: Harrison.

1023 RSVP Lafayette County

107 Courthouse Square
Oxford, MS 38655
662-232-2377
Fax: 662-232-2377
rsvp@dixie-net.com
www.oxfordparkcommission.com/r_s_v_p.htm

Arledia Bennett, Director
Rosemary Austin, Secretary

RSVP helps people ages 55 and older find service opportunities in their home communities. RSVP participants serve from a few to over forty hours a week in private nonprofit organizations. RSVP involves seniors in services that match their personal interests and make use of their skills and lifelong experiences.

1024 RSVP Laurel-Jones County

433 Arco Lane
Laurel, MS 39440
601-425-5100
Fax: 601-425-9830
www.seniorservice.org/laurel_jones_rsvp

Elma Portero, Project Director

RSVP volunteers choose how and where they want to serve. Many continue to do the type of work they have enjoyed earlier in life, while others try something completely different. As a RSVP volunteer, you might mentor at-risk youth, make hospital visits, check blood pressure, clean grounds, or help people recover from natural disasters.

1025 RSVP Lowndes County

161 Maple Street
PO Box 5015
Columbus, MS 39704
662-328-2174
Fax: 662-328-7264
rsvpcms@cableone.net

Rosemarie Hughes, Director

The Retired and Senior Volunteer Program (RSVP) provides opportunities for people 55 and over to make a difference in their community through volunteer service. RSVP volunteers contribute anywhere from a few to over forty hours a week, serving through schools, day care centers, police departments, hospitals and other nonprofit and public organizations to help meet critical community needs. RSVP offers maximum flexibility and choice to its volunteers. RSVP matches the personal interests and skills of older Americans with opportunities to help solve community problems and offers supplemental insurance while on duty, on-the-job training from the agency or organization where volunteers are placed. The following County is served: Lowndes.

1026 RSVP Meridian-Lauderdale Counties

1528 12th Avenue
PO Box 5204
Meridian, MS 39301-4353
601-483-4607
Fax: 601-483-7011
msharpe357@aol.com

Mary L Sharpe, Director

The Retired and Senior Volunteer Program (RSVP) provides opportunities for people 55 and over to make a difference in their community through volunteer service. RSVP volunteers contribute anywhere from a few to over forty hours a week, serving through schools, day care centers, police departments, hospitals and other nonprofit and public organizations to help meet critical community needs. RSVP offers maximum flexibility and choice to its volunteers. RSVP matches the personal interests and skills of older Americans with opportunities to help solve community problems and offers supplemental insurance while on duty, on-the-job training from the agency or organization where volunteers are placed. The following County is served: Lauderdale.

1027 RSVP Simpson County

406 Main Street North
Mendenhall, MS 39114-3358
601-847-4612
Fax: 601-847-0111
shrrsvp@bellsouth.net

Billie J Brown, Director

The Retired and Senior Volunteer Program (RSVP) provides opportunities for people 55 and over to make a difference in their community through volunteer service. RSVP volunteers contribute anywhere from a few to over forty hours a week, serving through schools, day care centers, police departments, hospitals and other nonprofit and public organizations to help meet critical community needs. RSVP offers maximum flexibility and choice to its volunteers. RSVP matches the personal interests and skills of older Americans with opportunities to help solve community problems and offers supplemental insurance while on duty, on-the-job training from the agency or organization where volunteers are placed. The following County is served: Simpson.

Year Founded: 1976

1028 South Delta Planning and Development District
PO Box 1776
124 South Broadway Street
Greenville, MS 38702-1776
662-378-3831
Fax: 662-378-3834
www.southdeltapdd.com

William B Haney, Executive Director

Networks with other agencies in order to offer ways and means through which assistance to older Americans can be obtained.

1029 Southern Mississippi: Area Agency on Aging
9299 Highway 49
Gulfport, MS 39503
228-868-2311
Fax: 228-868-2311; *Toll Free:* 800-444-8014
www.smpdd.com

Leslie Newcomb, Executive Director
Robert Moore, Aging Director
Betsy Holmes, Deputy Director

Serves as a public advocate for the development and implementation of comprehensive and coordinated home and community based care systems responsive to the current needs and future growth of the aging population.

1030 Southwest Mississippi: Area Agency on Aging
9299 Highway 49
Gulfport, MS 39503
228-868-2311
Fax: 228-868-2311; *Toll Free:* 800-444-8014
www.smpdd.com

Leslie Newcomb, Executive Director
Robert Moore, Aging Director
Betsy Holmes, Deputy Director

Serves as the public advocate for the development and implementation of comprehensive and coordinated home and community based care systems responsive to the current needs and future growth of the aging population.

1031 Three Rivers: Area Agency on Aging
75 South Main Street
Pontotoc, MS 38863
662-489-2415
Fax: 662-489-6815; *Toll Free:* 877-489-6911
www.trpdd.com

Vernon R Kelly, Executive Director
Cleveland Joseph, Aging Director
Tracy Matthews, Fiscal Director

Administers Older Americans Act Programs.

Year Founded: 1971

Missouri

1032 Able Commission
1008 Holloway Street
Rolla, MO 65401-2734
573-364-4357
Fax: 573-364-0223
www.ok.gov/able

Lynne Brennan-Howk, Administrator
A. Keith Burt, Director
Jim Hughes, Assistant Executive Director

Activities for citizens over 55 in multi-purpose senior center; arts and crafts; telephone reassurance programs for older and handicapped people living alone.

1033 Columbia Area Senior Center
Senior Services of Boone County
1121 Business Loop 70 East
Columbia, MO 65201
573-874-2050
Fax: 573-875-8864
columbiaseniorcenter@socket.net
www.columbiaseniorcenter.com

John Zaring, President
Velma Vemer, Vice President
John Becker, Treasurer

Activity center for seniors.

Year Founded: 1995

1034 Disability Determination Services
1500 Southridge Drive
Suite B
Jefferson City, MO 65109-5674
573-751-2929
Fax: 573-526-3788
dese.mo.gov
TTY: 573-526-4513

Jeff Ripley, District Manager

Determines medical eligibility for Missourians who have filed for Social Security Administration (SSA).

1035 Disability Determination Services: Cape Girardeau
3014 Blattner Drive
Cape Girardeau, MO 63701
573-290-5710
Fax: 573-290-5709
www.ssa.gov

Brian Deuster, District Manager

1036 Disability Determination Services: Kansas City
2820 SW Fairlawn Rd
Topeka, KS 66612
888-369-4777
Fax: 816-322-1260; *Toll Free:* 800-584-4303
www.dcf.ks.gov
TTY: 785-296-1491

Scott Crane, District Supervisor

1037 Disability Determination Services: Saint Louis
7545 South Lindbergh Boulevard
Suite 220
Saint Louis, MO 63125-4843
314-416-2803
Fax: 314-416-2846; *Toll Free:* 877-878-4644

Kimberly Kaemmerer, District Manager

1038 Disability Determination Services: Springfield
2530-i S Campbell Avenue
Springfield, MO 65807-3598
417-888-4070
Fax: 417-888-4069
dese.mo.gov
TTY: 417-888-4075

Regina Grieshaber, District Manager

1039 Greater St. Louis Association of the Deaf
2190 Creve Coeur Mill Road
Maryland Heights, MO 63043
314-236-9048
Fax: 314-869-6161
www.gslad.org
TDD 314-222-0185
TTY: 314-932-2024

Paul Kiel, President
Bill Blank, Vice President
Beth Williams, Secretary

GSLAD's mission is to provide social, charitable, athletic and educational opportunities for members of GSLAD and friends of the Deaf in the Metropolitan St. Louis area.

1040 Heartland RSVP
PO Box 116
201 N Elson Suite 205
Kirksville, MO 63501
660-665-8314
Fax: 660-665-8315
www.seniorservices.org

Pat Selby, Director

Persons 55 years of age and older. Provides opportunities for volunteer service and community involvement; holds annual volunteer recognition banquet.

1041 Long Term Care Ombudsman Program
State Of Long-Term Care Ombudsman Program
Po Box 570
Jefferson City, MO 65102
573-526-0727
Fax: 573-751-6499; *Toll Free:* 800-309-3282
ltcombudsman@dhss.mo.gov
www.dhss.mo.gov/ombudsman

Carol Scott, State LTC Ombudsman

Mission is to improve the quality of life for residents of long term care facilities through advocacy and education.

1042 Mid-America Regional Council of Aging Services
600 Broadway
Suite 200
Kansas City, MO 64105-1659
816-474-4240
Fax: 816-421-7758
www.marc.org/aging

David Warm, Executive Director
Jacquelyn Moore, Aging Director
Cindy Terryberry, Nutrition Coordinator

advocates for, design, and impliment programs to meet the unique needs of older citizens within ghe 5 counties they serve.

1043 Mid-East: Area Agency on Aging
14535 Manchester Road
Manchester, MO 63011-3960
314-962-7999; *Toll Free: 800-243-6060*
www.mid-eastaaa.org

Mary Schaefer, Executive Director
Lisa Knoll, Case Management Director
Gayle McHenry, President

Assisting adults through the jorney of aging.

Year Founded: 1973

1044 Missouri Assisted Living Association
2407 B Hyde Park Road
Jefferson City, MO 65101
573-635-8750
Fax: 573-634-7344
info@malarcf.org
www.malarcf.org

Kevin Edmonds, President
Drew Stubblefield, Vice President
Kerri Hock, Executive Director

MALA provides comprehensive legislative and regulatory representation before the Missouri Legislature and the state agencies that regulate assisted living.

1045 Missouri Council of the Blind
5453 Chippewa Street
Saint Louis, MO 63109-1635
314-832-7172
Fax: 314-832-7796; *Toll Free:* 800-342-5632
moblind@moblind.org
www.moblind.org

Denny Huff, President
Chris Gray, Executive Director
Virginia Drapkin, Administrative Assistant

Blind and visually impaired individuals united to improve conditions for the blind in the areas of employment, cultural opportunities, companionship, financial assistance, rehabilitation, and housing. Conducts legislative advocacy.

Year Founded: 1957; Number of Members: 700

1046 Missouri Department of Mental Health
1706 E Elm Street
Po Box 687
Jefferson City, MO 65101-4130
573-751-4122
Fax: 573-751-8224; *Toll Free:* 800-364-9687
www.dmh.missouri.gov

Keith Schafer, Director
Jan Heckmeyer, Deputy Director
Brent McGinty, Administration Director

Three principal missions are the prevention of mental disorders, developmental disabilities, substance abuse, and compulsive gambling. The treatment, habilitation, and rehabilitation of Missourians who have those conditions. And the improvement of public understanding and attitudes about mental disorders, developmental disabilities, substance abuse, and compulsive gambling.

1047 Missouri Department of Revenue
Harry S Truman State Office Building
301 West High Street
Jefferson City, MO 65101
573-751-4450
dormail@dor.mo.gov
www.dor.state.mo.us

Alana Barragan-Scott, Director

The Missouri Department of Revenue serves as the central collection agency for all state revenues. The departments primary duties include collecting taxes, titling and registering motor vehicles, and issuing drivers licenses.

1048 Missouri Division on Aging
PO Box 570
912 Wildwood
Jefferson City, MO 65102

573-751-6400
Fax: 573-751-6041
info@health.mo.gov
www.health.mo.gov

Margaret T Donnelly, Director
Gail Vasterling, Deputy Director

Leader in promoting, protecting, and partnering for health.

1049 Missouri Employees Retirement System
907 Wildwood Drive
PO Box 209
Jefferson City, MO 65102
573-632-6100
Fax: 573-634-7934; *Toll Free:* 800-827-1063
mosers@mosers.org
www.mosers.org

Donald Martin, Chairman

Mission is to exceed customer expectations by providing outstanding benefit services through professional plan administration and sound investment practices.

1050 Missouri Planning Council For Developmental Disabilities
1716 Four Seasons Drive
Suite 103
Jefferson City, MO 65101
573-751-8611
Fax: 573-526-2755; *Toll Free:* 800-500-7878
shanks@mpcdd.com
www.mpcdd.com

Susan Pritchard, Green Director

A federally funded, 23 member council, appointed by the Governor.

1051 Missouri Protection & Advocacy Services
925 S Country Club Drive
Jefferson City, MO 65109-4510
573-893-3333
Fax: 573-893-4231; *Toll Free:* 866-777-7199
mopasjc@embargmail.com
www.moadvocacy.org

Larry Opinsky, Chairman
Joe Wrinkle, Vice Chairman
Michele Ohmes, Secretary

Advocacy services for persons with disabilities who meet eligibility criteria for any of five programs: Protection & Advocacy for Individuals with Mental Illness (PAIMI); Protection and Advocacy for individuals with Developmental Disabilities (PADD); Client Assistance Program (CAP) for persons encountering problems with rehab act agencies; Protection and Advocacy for Individual Rights (PAIR); and Protection and Advocacy for Assistive Technologyy (PAAT).

1052 RSVP Heartland
PO Box 116
201 N Elson Suite 205
Kirksville, MO 63501
660-665-8314
Fax: 660-665-8315
info@seniorservices.org
www.seniorservices.org

Pat Selby, Director

1053 RSVP Andrew County
101 South 4th Street
PO Box 7
Savannah, MO 64485
816-324-5634
Fax: 816-324-0186
rsvp@ccp.com
www.andrewcountyrsvp.freeservers.com

Linda Lambright, Director
Sandra Beattie, Contact

Provides opportunities for people 55 and over to make a difference in their community through volunteer service. RSVP volunteers contribute anywhere from a few to over forty hours a week, serving through schools, day care centers, police departments, hospitals and other nonprofit and public organizations to help meet critical community needs. RSVP matches the personal interests and skills of older Americans with opportunities to help solve community problems and offers supplemental insurance while on duty, on-the-job training from the agency or organization where volunteers are placed.

1054 RSVP Boone County
1123 Wilkes Boulevard
Suite 100
Columbia, MO 65201
573-443-1111
Fax: 573-874-1821
www.bcca.missouri.org

Jessica Macy, Executive Director
Angela Huntington, RSVP Project Director
Nicole King, Care Coordinator

The Retired and Senior Volunteer Program (RSVP) provides opportunities for people 55 and over to make a difference in their community through volunteer service. RSVP volunteers contribute anywhere from a few to over forty hours a week, serving thourgh schools, day care centers, police departments, hospitals and other nonprofit and public organizations to help meet critical community needs. RSVP offers maximum flexibility and choice to its volunteers. RSVP matches the personal interests and skills to older Americans with opportunities to help solve community problems and offer supplemental insurance while on duty, on-the-job training from the agency or organization where volunteers are placed.

1055 RSVP Douglass Community Services
711 Grand Avenue
Hannibal, MO 63401-4225
573-221-3892
Fax: 573-221-6944
www.douglassonline.opg

Dave Dexheimer, Executive Director
Stacey Nicholas, RSVP Director

Provides opportunities for people 55 and over to make a difference in their community through volunteer service. RSVP volunteers contribute anywhere from a few to over forty hours a week, serving through schools, day care centers, police departments, hospitals and other nonprofit and public organizations to help meet critical community needs. RSVP matches the personal interests and skills of older Americans with opportunities to help solve community problems and offers supplemental insurance while on duty, on-the-job training from the agency or organization where volunteers are placed.

1056 RSVP Dunklin County

313 West Main Street
Malden, MO 63863-1508
573-276-3716
Fax: 573-276-3716

Jeannie Collins, Director

RSVP volunteers choose how and where they want to
serve. Today more than 450,000 seniors participate in
RSVP, making it one of the largest volunteer efforts in the
nation. RSVP, is a cost effective way to solve critical problems in education, public safety, human needs and the
environment.

1057 RSVP Grundy/Sullivan Counties

2901 Hoover Drive
PO Box 173
Trenton, MO 64683-0173
816-359-3836
Fax: 660-359-3058

Edna Foster, Director

RSVP provides volunteer opportunities for persons 55 and
older. The purpose of RSVP is to enrich the lives of older
adults through significant community service work. RSVP
encourages seniors to bring a lifetime of talent, experiences, skills and hobbies to community projects and organizations needing volunteer talent.

1058 RSVP Harrison-Daviess Counties

1402 West Main
Bethany, MO 64424
660-425-7555
Fax: 660-425-6953
hcrsvp@grm.net

Louise Akins, Director

Volunteers plant and maintain flowers for handicapped and
elderly and at locations in the city of Bethany. They also
work with youth, teaching them about gardening, beautification, and flower arranging.

1059 RSVP Jackson-Platte Counties

1080 Washington
Kansas City, MO 64105-1334
816-559-4668
Fax: 816-842-1007
www.rsvpkcmo.org

Betsy Phillips, Director

The Retired and Senior Volunteer Program (RSVP) provides opportunities for people 55 and over to make a difference in their community through volunteer service. RSVP
volunteers contribute anywhere from a few to over forty
hours a week, serving through schools, day care centers,
police departments, hospitals and other nonprofit and public organizations to help meet critical community needs.
RSVP offers maximum flexibility and choice to its volunteers. RSVP matches the personal interests and skills of
older Americans with opportunities to help solve community problems and offers supplemental insurance while on
duty, on-the-job training from the agency or organization
where volunteers are placed. The following Counties are
served: Clay, Jackson, Platte.

1060 RSVP Jasper County

101 N Rangeline Road
Suite 2
Joplin, MO 64801-4132

417-627-0600
Fax: 417-627-9710

Tina Jones, Director

The Retired and Senior Volunteer Program (RSVP) provides opportunities for people 55 and over to make a difference in their community through volunteer service. RSVP
volunteers contribute anywhere from a few to over forty
hours a week, serving thourgh schools, day care centers,
police departments, hospitals and other nonprofit and public organizations to help meet critical community needs.
RSVP offers maximum flexibility and choice to its volunteers. RSVP matches the personal interests and skills to
older Americans with opportunities to help solve community problems and offer supplemental insurance while on
duty, on-the-job training from the agency or organization
where volunteers are placed.

1061 RSVP Livingston County

408B S Washignton
PO Box 445
Chillicothe, MO 64601
660-646-0010
Fax: 660-707-0708
chillirsvp@sbcglobal.net
www.seniorservice.org

Patty Mefford, Director
Theresa Figg, Administrative Assistant

Provides volunteer opportunities for persons age 55 and
older. Our purpose is to enrich the lives of older adults
through significant community sevice. More than 500 volunteers contribute nearly 100,000 hours of their time to
meet community needs each year. The places they work
and the jobs they do are as varied as the volunteers
themselves.

1062 RSVP Mississippi County

106 South Washington Street
East Prairie, MO 63845-1526
573-649-5243
Fax: 573-649-2024

Brenda Brewer, Director

The Retired and Senior Volunteer Program (RSVP) provides opportunities for people 55 and over to make a difference in their community through volunteer service. RSVP
volunteers contribute anywhere from a few to over forty
hours a week, serving through schools, day care centers,
police departments, hospitals and other nonprofit and public organizations to help meet critical community needs.
RSVP offers maximum flexibility and choice to its volunteers. RSVP matches the personal interests and skills of
older Americans with opportunities to help solve community problems and offers supplemental insurance while on
duty, on-the-job training from the agency or organization
where volunteers are placed. The following County is
served: Mississippi.

1063 RSVP Northwest Missouri/Northeast Kansas

200 Cherokee Street
PO Box 4038
Saint Joseph, MO 64504-0038
816-232-4511
Fax: 816-238-3274
www.inter-serv.org

David Lewis htenberg, President
Ron Barbosa, Vice President
Rick Weiser, Treasurer

Allows persons 55 years of age and over to remain an active important part of their community by placing the individual or group in meaningful volunteer positions through out Buchman, Clinton, Dekalb and Holt counties inMissouri and Doniphan County.

Year Founded: 1909

1064 RSVP Pemiscot County
1105 Carleton Avenue
PO Box 542
Caruthersville, MO 63830
573-333-1380
Fax: 573-333-2382

Shirley Lacey, Contact

Provides opportunities for people 55 and over to make a difference in their community through volunteer service. RSVP volunteers contribute anywhere from a few to over forty hours a week, serving through schools, day care centers, police departments, hospitals and other nonprofit and public organizations to help meet critical community needs. RSVP matches the personal interests and skills of older Americans with opportunities to help solve community problems and offers supplemental insurance while on duty, on-the-job training from the agency or organization where volunteers are placed.

1065 RSVP Pettis-Saline Counties
515 S Kentucky Avenue
Sedalia, MO 65301-4263
660-826-4212
Fax: 660-827-0633

Cheri Heeran, Director
Roxanne Parker, Housing Director
Tonya Fennell, RSVP Director

The Retired and Senior Volunteer Program (RSVP) provides opportunities for people 55 and over to make a difference in their community through volunteer service. RSVP volunteers contribute anywhere from a few to over forty hours a week, serving through schools, day care centers, police departments, hospitals and other nonprofit and public organizations to help meet critical community needs. RSVP offers maximum flexibility and choice to its volunteers. RSVP matches the personal interests and skills of older Americans with opportunities to help solve community problems and offers supplemental insurance while one duty, on-the-job training from the agency or organization where volunteers are placed. The following County is served: Pettis.

1066 RSVP Poplar Bluff-Altrusa Club
101 Oak Street
PO Box 666
Poplar Bluff, MO 63902
573-686-8624
Fax: 573-686-8605

Marty Warner, Director

The Retired and Senior Volunteer Program (RSVP) provides opportunities for people 55 and over to make a difference in their community through volunteer service. RSVP volunteers contribute anywhere from a few to over forty hours a week, serving through schools, day care centers, police departments, hospitals and other nonprofit and public organizations to help meet critical community needs. RSVP offers maximum flexibility and choice to its volunteers. RSVP matches the personal interests and skills of older Americans with opportunities to help solve commu-

nity problems and offers supplemental insurance while on duty, on-the-job training from the agency or organization where volunteers are placed. The following County is served: Butler.

1067 RSVP Quad Lakes
206 S Baird Ave.
Clinton, MO 64735-2418
660-885-6512
Fax: 660-885-6522

Carole Sue Hoefer, Director

The Retired and Senior Volunteer Program (RSVP) provides opportunities for people 55 and over to make a difference in their community through volunteer service. RSVP volunteers contribute anywhere from a few to over forty hours a week, serving through schools, day care centers, police departments, hospitals and other nonprofit and public organizations to help meet critical community needs. RSVP offers maximum flexibility and choice to its volunteers. RSVP matches the personal interests and skills of older Americans with opportunities to help solve community problems and offers supplemental insurance while on duty, on-the-job training from the agency or organization where volunteers are placed.

1068 RSVP Scott-Cape Counties
105 N Main Street
Chaffee, MO 63740-1116
573-887-3664
Fax: 573-887-3664

Tina M McDowell, Director

Recruits volunteer aged 55 or older to help expand services in not-for-profit agencies who are stuggling with today's social issues. This agency connects them with volunteers and resources so that they may work as effectively and efficiently as possible to create positive change for our communities. Volunteers have an opportunity to continue to contribute their talents and skills to benefit other, thus, enhancing the quality of life for all.

1069 RSVP Springfield
627 North Glenstone
PO Box 3947
Springfield, MO 65808-3947
417-862-3595
Fax: 417-862-2129

Sharon Bradford, Director

The Retired and Senior Volunteer Program (RSVP) has a dual purpose of engaging persons 55 and older in volunteer service to meet critical community needs and to provide a high quality experience that will enrich the lives of the volunteer.

1070 RSVP St. Charles-Lincoln-Warren Counties
2724 Droste Road
St Charles, MO 63301-1504
636-724-7787
Fax: 636-925-3810; *Toll Free:* 800-748-7865

Steve Lewis, Contact

Volunteers serve in a diverse range of nonprofit organizations, including schools, hospitals, food parties, homeless and abuse shelters, local governments, libraries, courts, law enforcement agencies, senior centers, pet adoption agencies, thrift stores and much more.

1071 RSVP St. Louis

7601 Watson Road
Saint Louis, MO 63119-5001
314-918-2294
Fax: 314-962-4159
aklostermann@ccstl.org

Amy Klostermann, Director

The Retired and Senior Volunteer Program (RSVP) provides opportunities for people 55 and over to make a difference in their community through volunteer service. RSVP volunteers contribute anywhere from a few to over forty hours a week, serving through schools, day care centers, police departments, hospitals and other nonprofit and public organizations to help meet critical community needs. RSVP offers maximum flexibility and choice to its volunteers. RSVP matches the personal interests and skills of older Americans with opportunities to help solve community problems and offers supplemental insurance while on duty, on-the-job training from the agency or organization where volunteers are placed. The following Counties are served: Saint Louis, Saint Louis City.

1072 Railroad Retirement Board: Kansas City
Missouri District Office

601 E 12th Street
G 47
Kansas City, MO 64106-2808
Fax: 816-426-5334; *Toll Free:* 877-772-5772
kansascity@rrb.gov
www.rrb.gov

Ada M Foster, Network Manager
Michael Petry, Representative

An independent agency in the executive branch of the Federal Government. The primary function is to administer comprehensive retirement-survivor and unemployment-sickness benefit programs for the nation's railroad workers and their families.

1073 Railroad Retirement Board: St. Louis
Robert A Young Federal Building

601 E 12th Street
G 47
Kansas City, MO 64106-2808
Fax: 816-426-5334; *Toll Free:* 877-772-5772
stlouis@rrb.gov
www.rrb.gov

Michael Petry, Representative
Ada M Foster, Network Manager

An independent agency in the executive branch of the Federal Government. The RRB's primary function is to administer comprehensive retirement-survivor and unemployment sickness benefit programs for the nation's railroad workers and their families.

1074 Region Ten: Area Agency on Aging

2701 South Bird Street
Po Box 3990
Joplin, MO 64803-3990
417-627-0600
Fax: 417-627-9710
bevscrogg@hotmail.com
www.thevantagepoint.org

Linda Carlson, Director

Provides a wide variety of services to seniors and their families.

1075 Southwest Missouri Office on Aging

1735 S Fort Avenue
Springfield, MO 65807-1204
417-862-0762
Fax: 417-865-2683; *Toll Free:* 800-497-0822
swmoa@swmoa.com
www.swmoa.com

Dorothy K Knowles, Executive Director
Vera Trogdon, Director of Aging Services
June Huff, Community Services Director

Established to receive and distribute tax deductible donations to help fund programs and services for seniors. In addition to sponsoring fundraising events, the Foundation provides information about opportunities for participating in one-time donations, memorial gifts and trust funds.

1076 St. Louis Society for the Blind and Visually Impaired

8770 Manchester Road
Saint Louis, MO 63144-2724
314-968-9000
Fax: 314-968-9003
www.slsbvi.org

Sheila Sweeney, Chairman
Sabra Engelbrecht, Vice Chairman
Greg Levine, Secretary

Offers rehabilitation services for blind and visually impaired adults in St. Louis area. Contracts with local schools for services to school age students.

1077 St. Louis: Area Agency on Aging

1200 Market Street
Room 4086
Saint Louis, MO 63103-1002
314-622-4800
Fax: 314-552-2307
stlouis.missouri.org/government

Barbara Selders, Director

Provides a comprehensible and coordinated system of community-based services for older adults in the City of St. Louis. The Agency's objectives are to secure and maintain maximum independence and dignity in a home environment and encourage economic, social and personal independence of older persons by providing opportunities for employment, socialization, and volunteer activities in the community.

1078 UMKC Institute for Human Development

Health Sciences Building, 3rd Floor
215 W. Pershing Road
Kansas City, MO 64108
816-235-1770
Fax: 888-503-3107; *Toll Free:* 800-444-0821
calkinsc@umkc.edu
www.ihd.umkc.edu
TTY: 800-452-1185

Carl F Calkins PhD, Director
Vim Horn, Associate Director
Christy Miller, Program Development

A statewide program promoting assistive technology devices and services for persons of all ages with all disabilities.

1079 VantAge Point: Area Agency on Aging-Region Ten
2701 South Bird Street
PO Box 3990
Joplin, MO 64803-3990
417-627-0600
Fax: 417-627-9710
www.thevantagepoint.org

Richard Russell, Executive Director

The VantAge Point is the information and resource center of the Area Agency on Aging, Region Ten. The VantAge Point/Area Agency provides a wide variety of services to seniors and their families.

1080 Workers Compensation Board Missouri
301 West High Street Room 530
Po Box 690
Jefferson City, MO 65101
573-751-4126
insurance.mo.gov

John J Hickey, Director

Reviews determinations by an insurer or advisory organization.

Montana

1081 Action for Eastern Montana
2030 North Merrill Ave.
PO Box 1309
Glendive, MT 59330-1309
406-377-3564
Fax: 406-377-3570; *Toll Free:* 800-227-0703
www.aemt.org

Lori Brengle, Executive Director

Community action agency with a variety of assistance programs to low-income families and individuals; Head Start, family planning, employment training, housing, family counseling, crisis intervention, child care referral and training, domestic abuse services and shelter. We are more directly involved in the production of affordable housing. Counties covered: Carter, Custer, Daniels, Dawson, Fallon, Geld, McCone, Phillips, Powder River, Prairie, Richland, Roosevelt, Rosebud, Sheridan, Treasure, Valley and Wilbaux.

1082 Area 1 Agency on Aging
Po Box 1309
2030 N Merril Ave
Glendive, MT 59330-1309
406-377-3564
Fax: 406-377-3570; *Toll Free:* 800-227-0703
www.aemt.org
TDD 406-365-3367

Lori Brengle, Director

Services are availiable to anyone sixty years of age or older and their spouse regardless of age. Services under the Older Americans Act have no income guidelines, all programs are open to and encourage contributions by the participants.

1083 Area 2 Agency on Aging
1502 4th Street W
Roundup, MT 59072
406-323-1320
Fax: 406-323-3859

areatwo@midrivers.com
www.midrivers.com

Karen Erdie, Director

1084 Area 4 Agency on Aging
2260 Park Towne Cir
PO Box 1717
Sacramento, CA 95825
916-486-1876
Fax: 916-486-9454; *Toll Free:* 800-356-6544
smann@a4aa.com
www.a4aa.com

Charles W Briggs, Director

Serves the following counties: Broadwater, Gallatin, Jefferson, Lewis & Clark, Meagher and Park.

1085 Area 5 Agency on Aging
1801,Smith Street
307
Longansport, IN 46947
574-722-4451
Fax: 406-563-3524; *Toll Free:* 800-654-9421
www.areafive.com

Joe Gilboy, Director

1086 Area 7 Agency on Aging
1718 Wabash Ave
Terre Haute, IN 47807
812-238-1561
Fax: 406-252-4812; *Toll Free:* 800-758-4812
www.westcentralin.com

Darrell La Mere, Director

1087 Area 8 Agency on Aging
501 Bay Drive
Great Falls, MT 59404-3208
406-454-6990
Fax: 406-454-6991
aging@co.cascade.mt.us
www.co.cascade.mt.us

Randy Barrett, Director

Aging Services provides services to Cascade County residents 60 and over, such as transportation, home attendants, Senior Companions, Medicaid waivers, Meals on Wheels, Ombudsman, Retired and Senior Volunteer Program, Foster Grandparent Program, insurance counseling, caregiver support, Reverse Annuities and Senior Centers, improving the quality of life in later years.

1088 Area 9 Agency on Aging
715 W 21st St
Connersville, IN 47331
765-827-1502
Fax: 406-758-5732
www.iue.edu/area9/

Tony Shepherd, Executive Director
Kathy Bridgford, Director of Administration
Brian Weaver, Director

1089 Disability Determination Services
10 West 15th Street
Suite 1600
Helena, MT 59604-4189
406-444-3054
Fax: 800-356-4410; *Toll Free:* 800-545-3054
www.ssa.gov

Michelle Thibodeau, Manager

Deliver Social Security services that meet the changing needs of the public.

1090 Highwood Senior Citizens
1477 Otto Road
Box 70
Highwood, MT 59450-9801
406-733-5141; *Toll Free: 888-619-7742*

Promotes and provides social services for senior citizens in Highwood, MT.

1091 Missoula Aging Services
337 Stephens Avenue
Missoula, MT 59801
406-728-7682
Fax: 406-728-7687
senior@missoulaagingservices.org
www.missoulaagingservices.org

Susan Kohler-Hurd, Director

Promotes the independence, dignity and health of older adults and those that care for them through advocacy, education, services and volunteer opportunities.

1092 Montana Advocacy Program
PO Box 1681
400 North Park 2nd Floor
Helena, MT 59624-1681
406-449-2344
Fax: 406-449-2418; Toll Free: 800-245-4743
www.mtadv.org
TDD 800-245-4743

Bernadette Franks-Ongoy, Executive Director
Kelley Kaufmann, Finance Director
Steve Heaverlo, Programs Director

Protects and advocates the human and legal rights of Montanans with mental and physical disabilities while advancing dignity, equality, and self-determination. Designated federal P&A, with AT, CAP, PADD, PAIMI and PAIR programs. Advocacy and legal services for abuse, neglect, rights violations, access, discrimination in employment, accommodations and housing, and assistance with vocational rehabilitation/visual services.

1093 Montana Department of Administration: Teacher's Retirement System
1500 E 6th Avenue
PO Box 200139
Helena, MT 59620-0139
406-444-3134
Fax: 406-444-2641
lad@mt.gov
www.trs.doa.state.mt.us

David Senn, Director
Tammy Rau, Deputy Director

Mission is to promote long-term financial security for our membership while maintaining the stability of the fund. To earn the respect and trust of our members.

1094 Montana Department of Military Affairs: Division of Veteran's Affairs
1900 Williams Street
Po Box 5715
Helena, MT 59604

406-324-3740
Fax: 406-226-7459
lehall@mt.gov
dma.mt.gov/mvad

Joseph Foster, Division Administrator

Mission is the promotion of the general welfare of Montana veterans and their families.

1095 Montana Department of Public Health & Human Services
111 North Sanders Street (SRS Building)
Room 301
Helena, MT 59620
406-444-3136
Fax: 406-444-5900
www.dphhs.mt.gov

Anna Whiting-Sorrell, Director
Bernie Jacobs, Chief Legal Counsel

Administers a wide spectrum of programs and projects including public assistance, medicaid, foster care and adoption, nursing home licensing, long-term care, agency services, alcohol and drug abuse programs, mental health services, vocational rehabilitation, disability services, child support enforcement activities, and public health functions.

1096 Montana Department of Retirement Administration
125 N Roberts St. Rm 155 Mitchell Bldg.
PO Box 200101
Helena, MT 59620-0101
406-444-2511
Fax: 406-444-6194; Toll Free: 800-444-5428
www.doa.mt.govgovt/

Janet Kelly, Director
Sheryl Olsen, Deputy Director
Gretchen Bingman, Project Director

Mission is to serve and satisfy our customers.

1097 Montana Department of Revenue
Sam W. Mitchell Building
125 N Roberts 3rd Floor
Helena, MT 59604-5805
406-444-6900
Fax: 406-444-3696; Toll Free: 866-859-2254
www.mt.gov/revenue
TDD 406-444-2830

Dan Bucks, Manager

Mission is to excel at public service and effective administration of the tax and liquor laws of Montana.

1098 Montana Department of Social and Rehabilitation Services
PO Box 4210
111 North Last Chance Gulch, Suite 4C
Helena, MT 59604-4210
406-444-2590
Fax: 406-444-3632; Toll Free: 877-296-1197
www.dphhs.mt.gov

Anna Whiting Sorrell, Director

Offers services for the disabled.

1099 Montana Developmental Disability Council
PO Box 526
7 W 6th Ave Suite 2A
Helena, MT 59624
406-443-4332
Fax: 406-443-4192; *Toll Free:* 866-443-4332
deborah@mtcdd.org
www.mtcdd.org

Deborah Swingley, Executive Director
Dee Burrell, Grant/Contract Manager

The goal of the Council is to increase the independence, productivity, inclusion and integration into the community of people with developmental disabilities through systemic change, capacity building and advocacy activities. The Council has attempted to meet this goal through a two-prong advocacy approach, our State Plan and our Grant Program.

1100 Montana Protection & Advocacy Agency
Montana Advocacy Program
400 North Park, 2nd Floor
PO Box 1681
Helena, MT 59624
406-449-2344
Fax: 406-449-2418; *Toll Free:* 800-245-4743
bernie@mtadv.org
www.mtadv.org
TDD 406-449-2344

Bernadette Franks-Ongoy, Executive Director
Chanda Hermanson, Advocacy Specialist
Charlie McCarthy, Advocay Specialist

To protect and advocate for the human, legal, and civil rights of Montanans with disabilities while advancing dignity, equality, and self-determination.

1101 North Central Montana: Area Agency on Aging
602 South Main Street
Conrad, MT 59425-2335
406-278-5662
Fax: 406-278-5262; *Toll Free:* 800-332-2272
www.area2aging.org

Deborah Pate, Director

Aging services.

1102 Northern Rocky Mountain Retiree Association
1637 Red Crow Road
Victor, MT 59875
406-961-3959
www.fsx.org

James H Freeman, President

1103 RSVP Butte School District No 1
111 N Montana Street
Butte, MT 59701-9295
406-533-2508
Fax: 406-533-2520
brennickml@butte.k12.mt.us
www.butte.k12.mt.us

Michele L Brennick, Director

Butte School District #1 RSVP offers opportunities for individuals 55 and better to make their communities safer, healthier, and stronger through service. The variety of opportunities for community service allows individuals to share their experiences, abilities and skills for the betterment of their community and themselves.

1104 RSVP Cascade County
PO Box 2486
1801 Benfis Court
Great Falls, MT 59403
406-454-6994
Fax: 406-454-6991
volunteerpower@yahoo.com
www.ncmrsvp.com

Audrey Finlayson, Director
Russell McKinney, Sr Volunteer Coordinator
Jenny Albert, Volunteer Coordinator

AKA Cascade County Aging Services serves residents of Cascade Coundty in areas such as Information Assistance and Referral, State Health Insurance Program, Senior Companion, Foster Grandparents, Commodity Foods (part of the Retired and Senior Volunteer Program), Meals on Wheels, Reverse Annuity Mortgage, Home Attendant, Respite Care, Ombudsman, Senior Centers, Medicaid Waiver and Transportation.

1105 RSVP Dawson-Wibaux
604 Grant
PO Box 1324
Glendive, MT 59330-2305
406-377-4716
Fax: 406-377-2022
rsvp@midrivers.com
www.joinservice.org

Patricia Atwell, Director

The Retired and Senior Volunteer Program (RSVP) provides opportunities for people 55 and over to make a difference in their community through volunteer service. RSVP volunteers contribute anywhere from a few to over forty hours a week, serving through schools, day care centers, police departments, hospitals and other nonprofit and public organizations to help meet critical community needs. RSVP offers maximum flexibility and choice to its volunteers. RSVP matches the personal interests and skills of older Americans with opportunities to help solve community problems and offers supplemental insurance while on duty, on-the-job training from the agency or organization where volunteers are placed. The following Counties are served: Dawson, Wibaux.

1106 RSVP Fallon County
420 W Montana Avenue
PO Box 1025
Baker, MT 59620
406-778-2358
Fax: 406-444-2701
www.mt.gov/mcsn
TDD 406-444-1421

Patricia Madler, Director

The Retired and Senior Volunteer Program (RSVP) provides opportunities for people 55 and over to make a difference in their community through volunteer service. RSVP volunteers contribute anywhere from a few to over forty hours a week, serving through schools, day care centers, police departments, hospitals and other nonprofit and public organizations to help meet critical community needs. RSVP offers maximum flexibility and choice to its volunteers. RSVP matches the personal interests and skills of older Americans with opportunities to help solve community problems and offers supplemental insurance while on duty, on-the-job training from the agency or organization where volunteers are placed. The following Counties are served: Carter, Fallon.

1107 RSVP Helena
Rocky Mountain Development Council
200 South Cruse Avenue
PO Box 1717
Helena, MT 59624
406-447-1680
Fax: 406-447-1680; Toll Free: 800-356-6544
bthowell@rmdc.net
www.rmdc.net/volunteer.html

Bonnie Howell, Director

The Retired and Senior Volunteer Program provides a variety of volunteer opportunities for people 55 or better so they can remain active and involved in their communities. Volunteers serve from a few hours per week doing such things as clerical work, tutoring, preparing bulk mailings and sewing quilts. Volunteers also assist at schools, libraries, hospitals, nursing homes and other nonprofit agencies where help is needed.

1108 RSVP Hill County
Hill County Area Ten Agency on Aging
2 West Second Street
Havre, MT 59501-3434
406-265-5464
Fax: 406-265-3611
www.hccaa.com

Paul Babb, Chief Executive Officer

The Retired and Senior Volunteer Program (RSVP) provides opportunities for people 55 and over to make a difference in their community through volunteer service. RSVP volunteers contribute anywhere from a few to over forty hours a week, serving through schools, day care centers, police departments, hospitals and other nonprofit and public organizations to help meet critical community needs. RSVP offers maximum flexibility and choice to its volunteers. RSVP matches the personal interests and skills of older Americans with opportunities to help solve community problems and offers supplemental insurance while on duty, on-the-job training from the agency or organization where volunteers are placed.

1109 RSVP Miles City
VA Center Room 225
210 South Winchester Avenue
Miles City, MT 59301
406-234-0505
Fax: 406-234-0554; Toll Free: 800-431-3975
rsvp05@midrivers.com
www.rsvpmilescity.org

Betty Vail, Director

The Retired and Senior Volunteer Program (RSVP) provides opportunities for people 55 and over to make a difference in their community through volunteer service. RSVP volunteers contribute anywhere from a few to over forty hours a week, serving through schools, day care centers, police departments, hospitals and other nonprofit and public organizations to help meet critical community needs. RSVP offers maximum flexibility and choice to its volunteers. RSVP matches the personal interests and skills of older Americans with opportunities to help solve community problems and offers supplemental insurance while on duty, on-the-job training from the agency or organization where volunteers are placed.

1110 RSVP Roosevelt County
400 2nd Avenue South
Wolf Point, MT 59201-1603
406-653-6200
Fax: 406-653-6201
rsvp@rooseveltcounty.org
www.rooseveltcounty.org

Diane Hanson, Director

The Retired and Senior Volunteer Program (RSVP) provides opportunities for people 55 and over to make a difference in their community through volunteer service. RSVP volunteers contribute anywhere from a few to over forty hours a week, serving through schools, day care centers, police departments, hospitals and other nonprofit and public organizations to help meet critical community needs. RSVP offers maximum flexibility and choice to its volunteers. RSVP matches the personal interests and skills of older Americans with opportunities to help solve community problems and offers supplemental insurance while on duty, on-the-job training from the agency or organization where volunteers are placed.

Year Founded: 1907

1111 RSVP South Central Montana
315 1/2 Main Street
Suite 1
Roundup, MT 59072-2737
406-323-4403
Fax: 406-323-4403
rdprsvp@midrivers.com

Shirlee Brillhart, Director

Placing individuals 55 of age and older in meaningful job opportunities in the community to do volunteer work.

1112 RSVP Southwest Montana
807 North Tracy
Bozeman, MT 59715-2813
406-587-5444
Fax: 406-582-8499
kwelker@rsvpmt.org
www.rsvpmt.org

Kelly Welker, Director

The Retired and Senior Volunteer Program (RSVP) provides opportunities for people 55 and over to make a difference in their community through volunteer service. RSVP volunteers contribute anywhere from a few to over forty hours a week, serving through schools, day care centers, police departments, hospitals and other nonprofit and public organizations to help meet critical community needs. RSVP offers maximum flexibility and choice to its volunteers. RSVP matches the personal interests and skills of older Americans with opportunities to help solve community problems and offers supplemental insurance while on duty, on-the-job training from the agency or organization where volunteers are placed. The following Counties are served: Gallatin, Park.

1113 RSVP Yellowstone County
1505 Avenue D
PO Box 208905
Billings, MT 59102-3151
406-259-9666
Fax: 406-259-2849
www.yccoa.org

Diane Boyett, Chairman
Marvin Carter, Vice Chairman
Jayne Crocker, Volunteer Coordinator

The Yellowstone County Retired and Senior Volunteer Program connects adults, 55+, to critical identified community needs. Through volunteering, these seniors enjoy social interaction while continuing to use their wisdom, experience and skills to impact their communities.

1114 Railroad Retirement Board: Montana District Office
Judge Jameson Federal Building
844 North Rush Street
Room 101
Chicago, IL 60611-2092
Fax: 406-247-7379; *Toll Free:* 877-772-5772
billings@rrb.gov
www.rrb.gov/field/do_bill.asp

Executive branch federal agency handling social security type benefits for railroad workers and their families.

Year Founded: 1935

1115 Ravalli County Council on Aging
310 Old Corvallis Road
Hamilton, MT 59840-2853
406-363-5690
Fax: 406-363-0401
ptravitz@ravalliccoa.org
www.ravalliccoa.org

Paul Travitz, Executive Director
Jean Mathis, Sr Resource Assistant
Kathy Sital, Sr Program Manager

Individuals over 60 years of age. Promotes the well-being of senior citizens through nutrition programs, in-home and transportation services, legal advice, and friendship. Provides information and referral services. Offers blood pressure checks and hearing checks.

1116 Workers Compensation Court Montana
1625 11th Avenue
Po Box 537
Helena, MT 59624
406-444-7794
Fax: 406-444-7798
cwilson@mt.gov
wcc.dli.mt.gov

James Jeremiah Shea, Judge
Jeanine Blaner, Settlement Master
Richard Bach, Law Clerk

Provides a fair, efficient. and effective forum for the resolution of disputes arising under the Montana Workers' Compensation Act and Occupational Disese Act.

Nebraska

1117 Aging Office of Western Nebraska
Bluff's Business Center
1517 Broadway
Suite 122
Scottsbluff, NE 69361-3184
308-635-0851
Fax: 308-635-2321; *Toll Free:* 800-682-5140
www.aown.org

Victor Walker, Executive Director

Mission is to provide a comprehensive and coordinated service delivery system to assist elderly citizens remain safe and independent in their own home and community.

1118 Aging Partners
1005 O Street
Lincoln, NE 68508-3628
402-441-7070
Fax: 402-441-7160; *Toll Free:* 800-247-0938
agingpartners@lincoln.ne.gov
www.aging.lincoln.ne.gov

June Pederson, Director

Aging Partners is part of the Administration on Aging's national network started by the Older Americans Act. Aging Partners works to maintain the dignity and welfare of those over age 60 in the following eight counties in Nebraska: Butler, Filmore, Lancaster, Polk, Saline, Saunders, Seward and York.Programs include: Being Well (information and guidance on meals, health and fitness), Planning Ahead (offering expertise in financial and insurance matters), Staying Involved (offering a wide range of volunteer, employment, recreation and entertainment opportunities), Living at Home (providing a wide range of options to help an individual age in their home).Aging Partners also provides information and referrals on a wide variety of aging concerns. They publish 'Living Well', a quarterly magazine that keeps seniors in teh area apprised of relevant issues and events. The agency assists with transportation options and outreach to rural areas.

Year Founded: 1971

1119 Blue Rivers: Area Agency on Aging
1901 Court Street
Beatrice, NE 68310-2922
402-223-1376
Fax: 402-228-3546; *Toll Free:* 888-317-9417
www.braaa.org

Larry Ossowski, Director

Mission is to assist older adults to remain independent in thier homes.

1120 Community Action Partnership of Mid-Nebraska Volunteer Services
16 West 11th Street
PO Box 2288
Kearney, NE 68847
308-865-5675
Fax: 308-865-5681; *Toll Free:* 877-335-6422
mnca@mnca.net
www.mnca.net

Karen K Lueck, Executive Director
Ed Butler, Business Manager
Kris Wright, Chief Fiscal Officer

Consists of: Retired and Senior Volunteer, Senior Companion Volunteer Program and Kearney Area Interfaith Caregivers.

1121 Diability Rights Nebraska
134 S 13th Street
Suite 600
Lincoln, NE 68508-1903
402-474-3183
Fax: 402-474-3274; *Toll Free:* 800-422-6691
www.disabilityrightsnebraska.org
TDD 402-474-3183

Timothy F Shaw, Executive Director
Eric Evans, Chief Operating Officer
Brian Craig, Law Clerk

The designated protection and Advocacy agency for the state of Nebraska for people with mental and physical disabilities. Direct assistance provided if issue is within broad case priorities. Sliding scale fee. Information and referral at no cost.

1122 Disability Determinations
PO Box 82530
Lincoln, NE 68501-2530
402-471-2961
Fax: 402-471-3626; *Toll Free:* 800-331-5616

Douglas Willman, Administrator

Delivers Social Security services that meet the changing needs of the public.

1123 Division of Aging & Disability Services
Nebraska Health & Human Services System
3416 Goni Road
Suite D-132
Carson City, NE 89706
775-687-4210
Fax: 775-687-0574; *Toll Free:* 800-942-7830
adsd@adsd.nv.gov
www.nvaging.net

Jane Gruner, Administrator
Janet Murphy, Deputy Administrator
Michele Ferrall, Deputy Administrator

Our mission is we help people live better lives through effective health and human services.

1124 Eastern Nebraska Office on Aging
4223 Center Street
Omaha, NE 68105
402-444-6536
Fax: 402-444-6504; *Toll Free:* 888-554-2711
www.enoa.org

Mary Ann Borgeson, Chairperson
Ron Nolte, Vice Chair
Bob Missel, Secretary

Our mission is to help older Nebraskans live independently and remain for as long as possible in their own homes.

1125 Midland: Area Agency on Aging
2727 West 2nd Street
Suite 440
Hastings, NE 68901
402-463-4565
Fax: 402-463-1069; *Toll Free:* 800-955-9714
info@midlandareaagencyonaging.org
www.midlandareaagencyonaging.org

Casey Muzic, Executive Director

Mission is to advocate for and provide caring, quality services to older adults and their families that enable independent living with dignity in their home and community. These program operations are designed to be preventative, social, or individual assistance services, delivered in a senior center or an in-home setting.

Year Founded: 1973

1126 Midwest Geriatrics
Florence Home Healthcare Center
7915 North 30th Street
Omaha, NE 68112-2418
402-827-6015
Fax: 402-827-6005
cwyatt@shf.org
www.mgi-seniors.org

Robert Bloechle, President/CEO
Phil Christensen, Assistant VP
Ann Erickson, Administrator

Our mission is to provide vision, strategic planning, leadership, and management services for its affiliates and other organizations to ensure the accomplishment of their respective missions.

1127 Nebraska Assistive Technology Partnership
3901 N 27th Street
Suite 5
Lincoln, NE 68521
402-471-0734
Fax: 402-471-6052; *Toll Free:* 888-806-6287
www.atp.ne.gov

Leslie Novacek, Director
David Altman, Program Coordinator
Jaime Galloway, Program Coordinator

The Assistive Technology Partnership (ATP) is dedicated to helping Nebraskan's with disabilities, their families and professionals obtain assistive technology devices and services.

1128 Nebraska Association Area Agencies on Aging
South Central Nebraska Area Agency on Aging
4623 2nd Avenue
Suite 4
Kearney, NE 68847-8348
308-234-1851
Fax: 308-234-1853; *Toll Free:* 800-658-4320
www.agingkearney.org

Rod Horsley, Director
Donna Mayo, Assistant Director/Fiscal Ofcr.
Susan Hutsell, Nutrition Coordinator

To advocate and provide supportive services and programs to the elderly, which will allow them to live as independently, and in their own homes, as long as possible.

1129 Nebraska Client Assistance Program
301 Centennial Mall South
PO Box 94987
Lincoln, NE 68508-2529
402-471-3656
Fax: 402-471-0017; *Toll Free:* 800-742-7594
victoria.rasmussen@cap.ne.gov
www.cap.state.ne.us

Victoria Rasmussen, Director

Nebraska Client Assistance Program (CAP) is a free service to help you find solutions

1130 Nebraska Commission for the Blind and Visually Impaired
4600 Valley Road
Suite 100
Lincoln, NE 68510-4844
402-471-2891
Fax: 402-471-3009

pearl.vanzandt@nebraska.gov
www.ncbvi.ne.gov

Dr. Pearl Van Zandt, Director

Offers services for the totally blind, legally blind, visually impaired, mentally retarded blind and more with health, counseling, educational, recreational, rehabilitation, computer training and professional training services.

1131 Nebraska Department of Aging
PO Box 95026
301 Centennial Mall South
Lincoln, NE 68509-5044
402-471-3121
Fax: 402-471-4619; *Toll Free:* 800-942-7830
vivianne.chaumont@dhhs.ne.gov
www.dhhs.ne.gov

Vivianne Chaumont, Director
Roxie Anderson, Administrator

Aging services.

1132 Nebraska Department of Revenue
Nebraska State Office Building
301 Centennial Mall S, 2nd Floor
PO Box 94818
Lincoln, NE 68508-2529
402-471-5729
www.revenue.ne.gov

Leonard J. Sloup, Tax Commissioner
Kimberly Conroy, Tax Commissioner
Ruth Sorensen, Tax Administator

Mission is to serve the public by administering the state revenue laws with integrity, efficiency, and consistency.

1133 Nebraska Department of Veterans Affairs
PO Box 95083
301 Centennial Mall South 6th Floor
Lincoln, NE 68509-5083
402-471-2458
Fax: 402-471-2491
www.vets.state.ne.us

Billy C. Smith, Chairman
Karen Solc, Secretary
John McNally, Deputy Director

Mission is to provide assistance to Nebraska veterans and their dependents in acquiring county, state, and federal benefits to which they are entitled by virtue of their service to this country.

1134 Northeast Nebraska: Area Agency on Aging
119 West Norfolk Avenue
PO Box 1447
Norfolk, NE 68701
402-370-3454
Fax: 402-370-3279; *Toll Free:* 800-672-8368
connie.cooper@nebraska.gov
www.nenaaa.com

Joann Forster, Director
Connie Cooper, Executive Director

Mission is to assist older adults to remain independent.

1135 Papillion Senior Citizen Center
1001 Limerick Road
Papillion, NE 68046-3023

402-597-2059
laura@sc.omhcoxmail.com
www.papillion.org

Laura Jean O'Connor, Executive Director

Papillion Senior Center serves healthy portions of food, friendship and fun to people age 60 and older and their guests.

1136 RSVP Adams-Webster Counties
Senior Action, Inc
212 West 3rd Street, Suite C
Hastings, NE 68901-5221
402-463-1454
Fax: 877-721-1840
julie@hastingsrsvp.org
www.papillion.org

Julie Nash, Director
Allen Sjuts, Board Director

The Retired and Senior Volunteer Program (RSVP) provides opportunities for people 55 and over to make a difference in their community through volunteer service. RSVP volunteers contribute anywhere from a few to over forty hours a week, serving through schools, day care centers, police departments, hospitals and other nonprofit and public organizations to help meet critical community needs. RSVP offers maximum flexibility and choice to its volunteers. RSVP matches the personal interests and skills of older Americans with opportunities to help solve community problems and offers supplemental insurance while on duty, on-the-job training from the agency or organization where volunteers are placed.

1137 RSVP Chadron
Northwest Community Action Partnership
270 Pine Street
PO Box 587
Chadron, NE 69337-2296
308-432-4200
Fax: 308-432-5799; *Toll Free:* 800-361-3393
rjohnson@ncap.info
www.ncap.info

Rachel Johnson, Ambassador

The Retired and Senior Volunteer Program (RSVP) provides opportunities for people 55 and over to make a difference in their community through volunteer service. RSVP volunteers contribute anywhere from a few to over forty hours a week, serving through schools, day care centers, police departments, hospitals and other nonprofit and public organizations to help meet critical community needs. RSVP offers maximum flexibility and choice to its volunteers. RSVP matches the personal interests and skills of older Americans with opportunities to help solve community problems and offers supplemental insurance while on duty, on-the-job training from the agency or organization where volunteers are placed.

1138 RSVP Lincoln
Aging Partners
1005 O Street
Lincoln, NE 68508-3628
402-441-7070
Fax: 402-441-7160; *Toll Free:* 800-247-0938
agingpartners@lincoln.ne.gov
loncoln.ne.gov

June Pederson, Director

The Retired and Senior Volunteer Program (RSVP) provides opportunities for people 55 and over to make a difference in their community through volunteer service. RSVP volunteers contribute anywhere from a few to over forty hours a week, serving through schools, day care centers, police departments, hospitals and other nonprofit and public organizations to help meet critical community needs. RSVP offers maximum flexibility and choice to its volunteers. RSVP matches the personal interests and skills of older Americans with opportunities to help solve community problems and offers supplemental insurance while on duty, on-the-job training from the agency or organization where volunteers are placed.

1139 RSVP Ogallala City-Keith Counties
411 E 2nd Street
Ogallala, NE 69153-2631
308-284-6464
Fax: 308-284-6565
ginny.steinke@ogallala-ne.gov
www.ogallala-ne.gov

Ginny Steinke, Program Director
Steve Krajewski, City Manager

The Retired and Senior Volunteer Program (RSVP) provides opportunities for people 55 and over to make a difference in their community through volunteer service. RSVP volunteers contribute anywhere from a few to over forty hours a week, serving thourgh schools, day care centers, police departments, hospitals and other nonprofit and public organizations to help meet critical community needs. RSVP offers maximum flexibility and choice to its volunteers. RSVP matches the personal interests and skills to older Americans with opportunities to help solve community problems and offer supplemental insurance while on duty, on-the-job training from the agency or organization where volunteers are placed.

1140 Railroad Retirement Board: Nebraska District Office
1299 Farnam Street
Suite 200
Omaha, NE 68102-1857
402-221-4641
Fax: 402-346-6077; *Toll Free:* 877-772-5772
www.rrb.gov

L J Zward, Manager

An independent agency in the executive branch of the Federal Government. The RRB's primary function is to administer comprehensive retirement-survivor and unemployment-sickness benefit programs for the nation's railroad workers and their families.

1141 South Central Nebraska: Area Agency on Aging
4623 2nd Ave
Suite 4
Kearney, NE 68847-8348
308-234-1851
Fax: 308-234-1853; *Toll Free:* 800-658-4320
www.agingkearney.org

Rod S Horsley, Executive Director
Donna Mayo, Director of Finance
Susan A Hutsell, Nutrition Coordinator

Advocating and providing supportive services andorgrams to older adults, to allow them to live with independence, in their own homes, for as long as possible.

1142 West Central Nebraska: Area Agency on Aging
115 N Vine Street
North Platte, NE 69101-3902
308-535-8195
Fax: 308-535-8190; *Toll Free:* 800-662-2961
info@wcnaaa.org
www.wcnaaa.org

Linda Foreman, Director

Dedicated to making sure that the good life continues for older Nebraskans.

Nevada

1143 Bureau of Disability Adjudication
Dept of Employment, Training and Rehabilitation
500 East Third Street
Carson City, NV 89713
775-684-3849
Fax: 775-684-3850; *Toll Free:* 800-326-6868
Internethelp@nvdetr.org
www.detr.state.nv.us
TTY: 775-687-5353

Frank Woodbeck, Director
Dennis Perea, Deputy Director
William Anderson, Chief Economist

The Bureau of Disability Adjudication evaluates applications from individuals with permanent disabilities to determine if they are eligible for federal Supplemental Security Income (SSI) or Social Security Disability Insurance (SSDI).

1144 Division for Aging Services
3416 Goni Road
Suite D-132
Carson City, NV 89706-7968
775-687-4210
Fax: 775-687-0574
adsd@adsd.nv.gov
www.nvaging.net

Jane Gruner, Administrator
Janet Murphy, Deputy Administrator
Tina Gerber-Winn, Deputy Administrator

Develop, coordinate and deliver a comprehensive support service in order for seniors to lead independent, meaningful and dignified lives.

1145 Division of Mental Health & Developmental Services
4126 Technology Way
2nd Floor
Carson City, NV 89706
775-684-5943
Fax: 775-684-5966
mhds.nv.gov

Richard Whitley, Administrator
Karen Hayes, Exec. Assistant/Office Manager

One of the largest State human services agencies in Nevada, amploying more then 1,900 in 8 agencies located in Las Vegas, Reno, Carson City and each of the rural counties.

1146 Nevada Department of Human Resources Rehabilitation Division: Bureau of Services to the Blind

505 E King Street
Carson City, NV 89701-4761
775-884-6125
Fax: 775-687-5980

1147 Nevada Department of Taxation

1550 College Parkway
Suite 115
Carson City, NV 89706-7939
775-684-2000
Fax: 775-684-2020
tax.state.nv.us

Shannon Silva, Chairman
Dorothy Fowler, Vice Chairman

Mission is to provide Fair, Efficient, and Effective Administration of Tax Programs for the State of Nevada in accordance with applicable statutes, regulations and policies. Serve the Taxpayers, State and Local Government Entities, and enable and recognize Department employees.

1148 Nevada Developmental Disability Council

3416 Goni Road
Suite D-132
Carson City, NV 89706
775-687-4210
Fax: 775-687-4264
adsd@adsd.nv.gov

Richard Weathermon, Executive Director

Mission is to provide resources at the community level which promote equal opportunity and life choices for people with disabilities through which they may positively contribute to Nevada society.

1149 Nevada Division for Aging Services

3416 Goni Road
Suite D-132
Carson City, NV 89706
775-687-4210
Fax: 775-687-0574
adsd@adsd.nv.gov
www.nvaging.net

Carol Sala, Administrator
Marilyn Wills, Deputy Administrator
Tina Gerber-Winn, Deputy Administrator

Services for seniors: In-Home Care, Homemaker, Group Home Care, Case Manager, Elder Abuse Investigations, Subsidized Taxi Cab Fare, Medicare Counseling, Information and Referral.

1150 Nevada Division of Industrial Relations

1301 North Green Valley Parkway
Suite 200
Henderson, NV 89704
702-486-9000
Fax: 775-687-9172
dirweb.state.nv.us

Don Soderberg, Administrator
Jan Rosenberg, Deputy Administrator

Providing workers compensation information, news, facts, and contact information for employees, employers, insurers, and medical providers. Find rules, statutes, forms and

professional help relating to workplace injuries and disabilities in the state of Nevada.

1151 Nevada Protection & Advocacy Agency
Nevada Disability Advocacy and Law Center

6039 Eldora Avenue
Suite C, Box 3
Las Vegas, NV 89146
702-257-8150
Fax: 702-257-8170; *Toll Free:* 888-349-3843
www.ndalc.org
TDD 702-257-8160

Jack Mayes, Executive Director

The Nevada Disability Advocacy & Law Center (NDALC) is a private, nonprofit organization and serves as Nevada's federally-mandated protection and advocacy system for the human, legal, and service rights of individuals with disabilities.

1152 Nevada Public Employees' Retirement System

693 W Nye Lane
Carson City, NV 89703-1527
775-687-4200
Fax: 775-687-5131; *Toll Free:* 866-473-7768
www.nvpers.org/public

Mark R Vincent, Chairman
Chris Collins, Vice Chairman
Vacant , Investment Officer

Created to provide a reasonable base income to qualified employees who have been employed by a public employer and whose earning capacity has been removed or has been substantially reduced by age or disability.

1153 RSVP NV Rural Counties

2621 Northgate Lane
Suite 6
Carson City, NV 89706
775-687-4680
Fax: 775-687-4494; *Toll Free:* 800-992-0900
branded@rsvp.carson-city.nv.us
www.nevadaruralrsvp.org

Jerry Thurman, President
Margaret Lowther, Vice President
Tannis Causey, Program Director

Serves age 55 and older. Commited to helping the frail and elderly who choose to remain at home by providing home and community based services, their goal is to promote level of choice, independence and self care. No charge for services except for lifeline.

1154 RSVP Washoe County

1664 N Virginia Street
Center for Moleculer Medicine
Suite 150
Reno, NV 89509
775-784-1808
Fax: 775-327-5015
www.unr.edu/sanford/volunteer/rsvp/html

Scott Trevithick, Project Director

The Retired and Senior Volunteer Program (RSVP) of Washoe County is committed to volunteerism. It actively recruits and encourages people 55 years and older to volunteer and places them in local nonprofit or public agencies of their choice.

New Hampshire

1155 Disability Determination Unit
PO Box 452
101 Pleasant Street
Concord, NH 03301-3860
603-271-3494
Fax: 603-271-1953
lori.temple@doe.nh.gov
www.education.nh.gov

Peggy Vieira, Administrator
Linda Ellsworth, Disability Examiner
Lisa Beck, Disability Examiner

Disability Determination Unit (DDU) determines whether or not an applicant is eligible for Medicaid benefits. Persons who are disabled or alleged disabled are eligible for DDU determination.

1156 New England Gerontological Association
1 Cutts Road
Durham, NH 03824-3102
603-772-2244
www.negaonline.org

Eugene T Tillock, EdD, Executive Director

Offers a broad range of service to individuals and providers of aging services in the New England Region.

1157 New Hampshire Bureau of Elderly and Adult Services
DEAS Office Park South
40 Terrill Park Drive
Concord, NH 03301-3852
603-271-9203
Fax: 603-271-4643
www.dhhs.state.nh.us
TDD 800-735-2964

Kathleen Otte, Director

State agency on aging services; limited services to incapacitated adults, age 18 and older.

1158 New Hampshire Client Assistance Program
Governor's Commission on Disability
57 Regional Drive
Concord, NH 03301-8518
603-271-4175; *Toll Free:* 800-852-3405
john.richards@nh.gov
www.nh.gov/disability
TTY: 603-271-2774

Charles J Saia, Executive Director

CAP assists anyone with a disability that is interested in applying for and receiving services from rehabilitation programs, projects or facilities funded under the Rehabilitation Act.

1159 New Hampshire Commission for Human Rights
2 Chenell Drive
Unit 2
Concord, NH 03301-8501
603-271-2767
Fax: 603-271-6399
humanrights@nhsa.state.nh.us
www.nh.gov/hrc

Joni N Esperian, Executive Director
Roxanne Juliano, Assistant Director
Deborah Evans, Administrative Secretary

Offers legal help and information for disabled persons who are discriminated against in the housing industry.

1160 New Hampshire Department of Mental Health
129 Pleasant Street
Concord, NH 03301
603-271-5000
Fax: 603-271-5058; *Toll Free:* 800-852-3345
www.dhhs.state.nh.us

Nicholas A Toumpas, Commissioner

The New Hampshire Department of Health and Human Services (DHHS) is the largest agency in New Hampshire state government, responsible for the health, safety, and well being of the citizens of New Hampshire.

1161 New Hampshire Department of Revenue
109 Pleasant Street
PO Box 457
Concord, NH 03302-0457
603-230-5005
Fax: 603-271-6121; *Toll Free:* 800-735-2964
www.nh.gov/revenue

John T Beardmore, Commissioner
Kathryn E Skouteris, Assistant Commissioner

The mission of the Department of Revenue Administration is to collect the proper amount of taxes due, incurring the least cost to the taxpayers, and in a manner that merits the highest degree of public confidence in our integrity, efficiency and fairness. Further, it must provide prompt and constructive assistance to the municipal units of government in matters of budjet, finance, and the appraisal of real estate.

1162 New Hampshire Developmental Disabilities Council
Walker Building
21 South Fruit Street
Suite 22
Concord, NH 03301-2451
603-271-3236
Fax: 603-271-1156; *Toll Free:* 800-852-3345
www.NHDDC.org

Kristen McGraw, Chairman
Susan Hatfield, Vice Chairman

Purpose is to engage in advocacy, capacity building, and systemic change activities that are consistent with the purpose of the DD act and contribute to a coordinated, consumer and family-centered, consumer and family-directed, comprehensive system of community services, individualized supports and other forms of assistance that enable individuals with developmental disabilities to excercise self-determination.

1163 New Hampshire Division of Developmental Services
NH DHHS Division of Community Based Care Services
105 Pleasant Street
Concord, NH 03301-3857
603-271-5034
Fax: 603-271-5166; *Toll Free:* 800-852-3345
meartas@dhhs.state.nh.us
www.dhhs.state.nh.us
TDD 800-735-2964

Paul Gorman, EdD, Director
Susan Fox, Director

The developmental services system will join with local communities to support individuals of all ages with developmental disabilities or acquired brain disorders and their families to experience as much freedom, choice, control and responsibility over the services and supports they receive as desired.

1164 New Hampshire Governor's Commission on Disability

57 Regional Drive
Concord, NH 03301-8518
603-271-2773
Fax: 603-271-2837; *Toll Free:* 800-852-3405
www.nh.gov/disability

Charles J Saia, Executive Director
Maureen Stimpson, Program Specialist

The Commission's goal is to remove the barriers, architectural or attitudinal, which bar persons with disabilities from participating in the mainstream of society.

1165 New Hampshire Health and Human Services: Elderly and Adult Services

129 Pleasant Street
Concord, NH 03301-6510
603-271-9203
Fax: 603-271-4643; *Toll Free:* 800-351-1888
www.dhhs.state.nh.us/dhhs

Nicholas A Toumpas, Commissioner

The Bureau of Elderly and Adult Services provides a variety of social and long-term supports to adults age 60 and older and to adults between the ages of 18 and 60 who have a chronic illness or disability.

1166 New Hampshire Protection & Advocacy for Persons with Disabilities

18 Low Avenue
Concord, NH 03301-4971
603-228-0432
Fax: 603-225-2077
advocacy@drcnh.org
www.drcnh.org
TDD 800-834-1721

Paul Levy, President
Joanne Malloy, Vice President
Arpiar Saunders, Secretary

The Disability Rights Center is dedicated to eliminating barriers existing in New Hampshire to the full and equal enjoyment of civil and other legal rights by people with disabilities.

1167 New Hampshire Retirement System

54 Regional Drive
Concord, NH 03301-8507
603-410-3500
Fax: 603-410-3501; *Toll Free:* 877-600-0158
info@nhrs.org
www.nhrs.org
TDD 800-735-2964

George Lagos, Executive Director

The New Hampshire Retirement System is a public employee pension plan. It is a defined benefit plan, which offers eligible retirees a secure lifetime pension. This website has general information about NHRS and describes the eli-

gibility requirements for each of the benefits. Publishes a Retirement Connection newsletter.

Number of Members: 51,000

1168 New Hampshire Veterans Council

275 Chestnut Street
Room 517
Manchester, NH 03101-2411
603-624-9230
Fax: 603-624-9236; *Toll Free:* 800-622-9230
www.nh.gov/nhveterans
TDD 800-735-2964

Mary Morin, Director
Christine Christine, Administrative Officer

The mission of the State Veterans Council (SVC) is to assist veterans who are residents of New Hampshire or their dependents in securing all benefits or preferences to which they may be entitled under any state or federal laws or regulations.

1169 Northern New England Association of Homes and Services for the Aging

345 Edward J Roy Drive
Suite 201
Manchester, NH 03104-4149
603-626-3479
Fax: 603-626-3763
www.elderweb.com

The mission of NNEAHSA is to promote the interests of its not-for-profit members in Maine, New Hampshire, and Vermont which provide healthy, affordable and ethical long term care to our older citizens through education, advocacy, representation and collaboration.

1170 RSVP Merrimack County

121 South Fruit Street
Concord, NH 03301-3852
603-224-3452
Fax: 603-224-0157

Nancy Spater, Director

The Retired and Senior Volunteer Program (RSVP) provides opportunities for people 55 and over to make a difference in their community through volunteer service. RSVP volunteers contribute anywhere from a few to over forty hours a week, serving thourgh schools, day care centers, police departments, hospitals and other nonprofit and public organizations to help meet critical community needs. RSVP offers maximum flexibility and choice to its volunteers. RSVP matches the personal interests and skills to older Americans with opportunities to help solve community problems and offer supplemental insurance while on duty, on-the-job training from the agency or organization where volunteers are placed.

1171 RSVP Monadnock

64 Main Street
Suite212
Keene, NH 03431
603-357-6893
Fax: 603-355-3833
www.monadnockvolunteercenter.org

Kathy Baird, Director

The Retired and Senior Volunteer Program (RSVP) provides opportunities for people 55 and over to make a difference in their community through volunteer service. RSVP volunteers contribute anywhere from a few to over forty hours a week, serving thourgh schools, day care centers, police departments, hospitals and other nonprofit and public organizations to help meet critical community needs. RSVP offers maximum flexibility and choice to its volunteers. RSVP matches the personal interests and skills to older Americans with opportunities to help solve community problems and offer supplemental insurance while on duty, on-the-job training from the agency or organization where volunteers are placed.

1172 RSVP Southern New Hampshire
40 Pine Street
Manchester, NH 03103
603-668-8010
Fax: 603-641-6054; *Toll Free:* 800-322-1073
www.snhs.org

Richard Delay, Chairman
Dolores Bellavance, Vice Chairman
Jill Mc Laughlin, Secretary

The Retired and Senior Volunteer Program (RSVP) provides opportunities for people 55 and over to make a difference in their community through volunteer service. RSVP volunteers contribute anywhere from a few to over forty hours a week, serving thourgh schools, day care centers, police departments, hospitals and other nonprofit and public organizations to help meet critical community needs. RSVP offers maximum flexibility and choice to its volunteers. RSVP matches the personal interests and skills to older Americans with opportunities to help solve community problems and offer supplemental insurance while on duty, on-the-job training from the agency or organization where volunteers are placed.

1173 RSVP and the Volunteer Center
10 Campbell Street
PO Box 433
Lebanon, NH 03766
603-448-1825
Fax: 603-448-3906; *Toll Free:* 877-711-7787
www.rsvptoday.org

Teresa M Volta, Director
Doreen Bowlin, Assistant Program Director

RSVP and the Volunteer Center build on the values of the past, to address the needs of the present, and strengthen our communities for the future, through volunteer service. Working with local nonprofits, we recruit, place, and support volunteers of all ages throughout northern Windsor County, VT, and Sullivan/Grafton Counties in NH. Our signature programs include: Good Morning! telephone reassurance, Bone Builders low impact lifting for elders.

1174 Service Corp of Retired Executives
195 Commerce Way
Unit A
Portsmouth, NH 03801-3251
603-352-0320
www.score.org

RL Devoucoux, Chairperson

Retired business professionals. Provides free business counseling.

1175 Atlantic County Division of Intergenerational Services, Office of Aging
Department of Health and Human Services
Shoreview Building, Office 218
101 South Shore Road
Northfield, NJ 08225
888-426-9243
Fax: 609-345-5907
www.aclink.org/intergenerational

Marilu Gagnon, Director

The Division of Intergenerational Services addresses the needs of youth, families, disabled and senior citizens. Trained staff are available to provide such services as information and referral, outreach, case management and juvenile/family crisis intervention to eligible individuals.

1176 Bergen County Division of Senior Services
One Bergen County Plaza
2nd Floor
Hackensack, NJ 07601-7076
201-336-7000
Fax: 201-336-7304
seniors@co.bergen.nj.us
www.co.bergen.nj.us/bcdhs/divisions

William J Boylan, Director
Kath Leen Donavan, Director

The Bergen County Division of Senior Services was established with a mission to serve as an advocate for older adults. It is a planning, coordinating and funding agency for senior programs and services.

1177 Burlington County Office on Aging
Mount Holly
49 Rancocas Road
Mount Holly, NJ 08060
609-265-5000
Fax: 609-265-3725; *Toll Free:* 800-792-8890
bcofficeonaging@co.burlington.nj.us
www.co.burlington.nj.us

Jeanne Borkowski, Director

Provides information, assistance and outreachservices to seniors in a variety of areas, including legal assistance, transportation, Meals on Wheels, home health services, respite care, home security, adult day care, and care management.

1178 Cape May County Department of Aging
4 Moore Road
CMCH, NJ 08210
609-465-1000
Fax: 609-889-0344; *Toll Free:* 877-222-3737
www.co.cape-may.nj.us

Elizabeth Bozzelli, Executive Director
Michael Lafley, Director of Opereation

Mission is to promote the well being of older persons in Cape May County by developing and advocating for services which assist older citizens to maintain their independence and quality of life.

1179 Cumberland County Office on Aging & Disabled

790 E Commerce Street
Room 29
Bridgeton, NJ 08302
856-453-2220
Fax: 856-453-8419; *Toll Free:* 877-222-3737
www.co.cumberland.nj.us

Macleod Carre, Executive Director
Barbara Nedohon, Adminstrative Assistant
Kristopher Matkowsky, Sr Accountant

Serves as a focal point for information, planning, coordination, and advocacy for programs and services for sr citizens ages 60 and up and for the disabled, through the Office of Disabled.

1180 Disability Rights New Jersey

210 South Broad Street
3rd Floor
Trenton, NJ 08608-2404
609-292-9742
Fax: 609-777-0187; *Toll Free:* 800-922-7233
advocate@drnj.org
www.drnj.org
TTY: 609-633-7106

Walter Anthony Woodberry, Chairperson
Kathleen F. Wood, Vice Chairperson
Mitchell P. Friedman, Treasurer

The Client Assistance Program (CAP) assists persons with disabilities who are seeking or receiving services from federally funded rehabilitation programs. CAP provides legal and nonlegal individuals and systems advocacy.

1181 Division of Disability Determination Services

PO Box 110
1john fitch plazza
trenton, NJ 08625
Toll Free: 866-920-6997
lwd.dol.state.nj.us
TTY: 973-648-2983

David Ramsay, Director
Dr. Joseph Aaron MD, Determination Physician
Susan Lamorte, Operations Director

To serve our customers by providing accurate and timely disability decisions through efficient use of public resources in accordance with Social Security Administration Regulations.

1182 Gloucester County Division of Senior Services

2 South Broad Street
Po Box 337
Wood bury, NJ 08096
856-232-4646
Fax: 856-232-6709; *Toll Free:* 877-222-3737
www.co.gloucester.nj.us

Anna Docimo, Executive Director
Robert Damminger, Freeholder Director
Lyman Barnes, Freeholder Liason

The Gloucester County Division of Senior Services is an active participant in the New Jersey EASE program, administering a broad range of home and community based services that focus on the needs of senior citizens throughout the County. The Division of Senior Services provides information and assistance to aid residents of Gloucester County 60 years of age or older and their families. Our mission is to promote accessible and high-quality health and senior services to help all seniors in Gloucester County attain optimal health and independence. We promote, support and protect-well being. We encourage informed choices that enhance quality of life for seniors.

1183 Gray Panthers Age and Youth in Action

43 Village of Stoney Run
Apt G
Maple Shade, NJ 08052
856-727-4671
Fax: 202-737-1160
felix.at.play@gmail.com
www.graypanthers.org

Felix Ullrich, Convenor

National organization of intergenerational activists dedicated to social change. Takes on societal issues such as peace, healthcare, jobs and housing from an intergenerational perspective, and fights to change laws and attitudes toward social justice.

1184 Hudson County Office on Aging

595 County Avenue
Bldg 2
Secaucus, NJ 07094-2605
201-271-4322
Fax: 201-271-4366; *Toll Free:* 877-222-3737
www.hudsoncountynj.org/office-on-aging

Sandra Vasquez, Executive Director
Catherine Macchi, Senior Affairs Coordinator

The office acts as the local conduit for the NJ EASE program and provides a range of services to the Hudson County Senior Community. These services include maintaining a service network capable of meeting the health, economic and social needs of older adults in Hudson County, with a particular emphasis on assisting those who are considered frail economically disadvantaged or vulnerable.

1185 Hunterdon County Division of Senior Services

4 Gauntt Place Building 1
PO Box 2900
Flemington, NJ 08822-2900
908-788-1361
Fax: 908-806-4537; *Toll Free:* 877-222-3737
aging@co.hunterdon.nj.us
www.co.hunterdon.nj.us/aging.htm

Mary Ann Rosenberger, Division Head

This office is the focal point for compiling and distributing information pertinent to the county's elderly population, its needs, and services implemented to meet those needs. The Division of Senior Services administers several programs including the State Health Program (SHIP), Care/Case Management, Mr. Fixit Program, Senior Health Services and Prevention Health Services. The Division contracts for the provision of a multitude of additional serices with qualified provider agencies, and diligently monitors the performance of these service providers to insure quality and ease of access by the seniors for these services.

1186 Leading Age New Jersey

13 Roszel Road
Suite C-200
Princeton, NJ 08540-6211
609-452-1161
Fax: 609-452-2907

mkent@leadingagenj.org
www.leadingagenj.org

Michele M Kent, President/CEO
Amy Greenbaum, Professional Development
Darlene Arden, Bookkeeper

The statewide association of not-for-profit senior care organizations and is dedicated to advancing quality aging services through advocacy, education and fellowship.

1187 Monmouth County Office on Aging
PO Box 1225
one east main street
Freehold, NJ 07728
732-308-3770
Fax: 732-303-7649; Toll Free: 877-222-3737
mcdhs@co.monmouth.nj.us
www.co.monmouth.nj.us

Charles Brown III, Executive Director

Main goal is to ensure that our older citizens receive the services that will help them maintain their dignity, independence and quality of life. The office is responsible for planning and coordinating the delivery of services to county residents 60 years of age and older.

1188 New Jersey Council On Developmental Disabilities
Po Box 700
20 West State Street 7th Floor
Trenton, NJ 08625-0700
609-292-3745
Fax: 609-292-7114; Toll Free: 800-792-8858
njcdd@njcdd.org
www.njcdd.org
TDD 609-777-3238

Alison M. Lozano, Executive Director
Shirla Rufo Simpson, Deputy Director
Kyoko Coco, Support Coordiantor

Purpose is to assure that individuals with developmental disabilities and their families, participate in the design and have access to needed community services, individualized supports, and other forms of assistance that promote self determination, independence, productivity, integration, and inclusion in all facets of life through culturally competent programs.

1189 New Jersey Department of Aging
12b Quakerbridge Plaza
PO Box 715
Mercerville, NJ 08625-0715
609-292-7837
Fax: 609-633-6609; Toll Free: 800-792-9745
www.nj.gov/humanservices/doas/home/index

Lowell Arye, Deputy/Interim Commissioner

Administers programs designed to make it easier for seniors to get the help they need to support their well being and maintain themselves in the community for as long as possible with independence, dignity and choice.

1190 New Jersey Department of Community Affairs: Commission on Recreation for the Handicapped
101 South Broad Street
PO Box 811
Trenton, NJ 08625-0811

609-984-6654
Patricia.Swartz@dca.state.nj.us
www.state.nj.us/dca/divisions/dhcr/rec/
TDD 609-278-0175

Susan Bass Levin, Commissioner

The Commission functions to promote and assist in the development and implementation of recreation and leisure services for individuals with disabilities in the communities of New Jersey.

1191 New Jersey Department of Human Services: Commission for the Blind
153 Halsey Street 6th Floor
PO Box 47017
Newark, NJ 07101-4701
973-648-3333
Fax: 973-648-7874; Toll Free: 877-685-8878
askcbvi@dhs.state.nj.us
www.state.nj.us/humanservices/cbvi

Daniel B. Frye, Executive Director

Provides services in the areas of education, employment, independence, and eye health for person who are blind or visually impaired, their families, and the community. It seeks to provide or ensure access to services that will enable consumers to obtain their fullest measure of self-reliance and quality of life and fully integrated into their community.

1192 New Jersey Department of Human Services: Deaf and Hard of Hearing Division
PO Box 074
222 South Warren Street
Trenton, NJ 08625-0074
609-503-4862
Fax: 609-588-2528; Toll Free: 800-792-8339
www.state.nj.us/humanservices/ddhh
TTY: 609-588-2648

David Alexander, Director

The Division of the Deaf and Hard of Hearing (DDHH) advocates for people in New Jersey who are Deaf or hard of hearing. It assists consumers in numerous ways to gain access to programs, services and information routinely availiable to others.

1193 New Jersey Department of Mental Health
PO Box 700
Trenton, NJ 08625-0212
609-292-3717
Fax: 777-083-; Toll Free: 800-382-6717
dmhas@dhs.state.nj.us
www.state.nj.us/humanservices/dmhs

Lynn A. Kovich, Assistant Commissioner

The Division of Mental Health Services (DMHS) serves adults with serious and persistent mental illness. The mission is the fact that these individuals are entitled to dignified and meaningful lives.

1194 New Jersey Division of Taxation
PO Box 281
50 Barrack Street, 1st Floor
Trenton, NJ 08695
609-292-6400
Fax: 609-826-4500; Toll Free: 800-286-6613
www.state.nj.us/treasury/taxation

Andrew P. Sidamon-Eristoff, Treasurer

1195 New Jersey Protection & Advocacy for Persons with Disabilities
210 South Broad Street
3rd Floor
Trenton, NJ 08608
609-292-9742
Fax: 609-777-0187; *Toll Free:* 800-922-7233
advocate@drnj.org
www.drnj.org
TTY: 609-633-7106

Joseph Young, Executive Director
Ellen Catanese, Administrative Director
Andrea Curran, Sr Staff Advocate

New Jersey Protection and Advocacy Inc (NJP&A) is the consumer-directed, non-profit organization that serves as New Jersey's designated protection and advocacy system for people with disabilities in the state.

1196 Ocean County Office of Senior Service
1027 Hooper Ave 1st Floor Bldg 2
PO Box 2191
Toms River, NJ 08754-2191
732-929-2091
Fax: 732-506-5019; *Toll Free:* 800-668-4899
www.co.ocean.nj.us/SeniorServicesMainPag

D Jane Maloney, Director

Leading the way in advancing the well-being of Ocean Counties older citizens.

1197 Passaic County Office on Aging
930 Riverview Drive
Suite 200
Totowa, NJ 07512
973-569-4060
Fax: 973-256-5191; *Toll Free:* 877-222-3737
www.passaiccountynj.org/

Mary Kuzinski, Executive Director

Hawthorne, Passaic County.

1198 RSVP Atlantic County
One South New York Avenue
Suite 501
Atlantic City, NJ 08401-5417
609-348-2590
Fax: 609-345-4651

Deborah Hite-Mercado, Director

The Retired and Senior Volunteer Program (RSVP) provides opportunities for people 55 and over to make a difference in their community through volunteer service. RSVP volunteers contribute anywhere from a few to over forty hours a week, serving thourgh schools, day care centers, police departments, hospitals and other nonprofit and public organizations to help meet critical community needs. RSVP offers maximum flexibility and choice to its volunteers. RSVP matches the personal interests and skills to older Americans with opportunities to help solve community problems and offer supplemental insurance while on duty, on-the-job training from the agency or organization where volunteers are placed.

1199 RSVP Bergen County
64 Passaic Street
Hackensack, NJ 07601-5612
201-489-9454
Fax: 201-489-1995

info@bergenvolunteers.org
www.bergenvolunteers.org/

Janet Sharma, Executive Director
Amanda Missey, Civic & Community Director
Jane He, Director Of Development

The Retired and Senior Volunteer Program (RSVP) provides opportunities for people 55 and over to make a difference in their community through volunteer service. RSVP volunteers contribute anywhere from a few to over forty hours a week, serving thourgh schools, day care centers, police departments, hospitals and other nonprofit and public organizations to help meet critical community needs. RSVP offers maximum flexibility and choice to its volunteers. RSVP matches the personal interests and skills to older Americans with opportunities to help solve community problems and offer supplemental insurance while on duty, on-the-job training from the agency or organization where volunteers are placed.

1200 RSVP Burlington County
Burlington County College
601 Pemberton Browns Mills Rd.
Pemberton, NJ 08068
609-894-9311
Fax: 609-894-0587
volcenter@hotmail.com
www.volunteercenterburlingtoncounty.org/

Karen Bennett, Director

Private non-profit, volunteer organization that provides and promotes volunteer opportunities, programs and services to meet community needs.

1201 RSVP Camden County
2500 McClellan Avenue
Suite 110
Pennsauken, NJ 08109-4205
856-663-4773
Fax: 856-663-5621
camdenrsvp.org

Treina Fletcher, Program Director
Terryama Davis, Volunteer Coordinator
Chimere Dotson, Chronic Disease Coordinator

The Retired and Senior Volunteer Program (RSVP) provides opportunities for people 55 and over to make a difference in their community through volunteer service. RSVP volunteers contribute anywhere from a few to over forty hours a week, serving thourgh schools, day care centers, police departments, hospitals and other nonprofit and public organizations to help meet critical community needs. RSVP offers maximum flexibility and choice to its volunteers. RSVP matches the personal interests and skills to older Americans with opportunities to help solve community problems and offer supplemental insurance while on duty, on-the-job training from the agency or organization where volunteers are placed.

1202 RSVP Cape May Chapter
William E Sturm Jr. Bldg
4 Moore Road
Admin Building
Cape May Court House, NJ 08210-1654
609-465-1000
Fax: 609-465-6189
www.capemaycountygov.net

Gerald M. Thornton, Director
Leonard C. Desiderio, Vice-Director

The Retired and Senior Volunteer Program (RSVP) provides opportunities for people 55 and over to make a difference in their community through volunteer service. RSVP volunteers contribute anywhere from a few to over forty hours a week, serving thourgh schools, day care centers, police departments, hospitals and other nonprofit and public organizations to help meet critical community needs. RSVP offers maximum flexibility and choice to its volunteers. RSVP matches the personal interests and skills to older Americans with opportunities to help solve community problems and offer supplemental insurance while on duty, on-the-job training from the agency or organization where volunteers are placed.

1203 RSVP Cumberland
800 E. Commerce Street
Room 21
Bridgeton, NJ 08302-2269
856-453-2171
Fax: 856-453-2212
www.co.cumberland.nj.us

Judy A. Truman, Project Director

The Retired and Senior Volunteer Program (RSVP) provides opportunities for people 55 and over to make a difference in their community through volunteer service. RSVP volunteers contribute anywhere from a few to over forty hours a week, serving thourgh schools, day care centers, police departments, hospitals and other nonprofit and public organizations to help meet critical community needs. RSVP offers maximum flexibility and choice to its volunteers. RSVP matches the personal interests and skills to older Americans with opportunities to help solve community problems and offer supplemental insurance while on duty, on-the-job training from the agency or organization where volunteers are placed.

1204 RSVP Mercer County
60 South Main Street
Pennington, NJ 08534
609-883-2880
Fax: 609-737-2000
www.contactofmercer.org

Hugh Adams, Director
Eleanor Letcher, Director of Contact
Susan Soennecken, Director of Reassurance

The Retired and Senior Volunteer Program (RSVP) provides opportunities for people 55 and over to make a difference in their community through volunteer service. RSVP volunteers contribute anywhere from a few to over forty hours a week, serving thourgh schools, day care centers, police departments, hospitals and other nonprofit and public organizations to help meet critical community needs. RSVP offers maximum flexibility and choice to its volunteers. RSVP matches the personal interests and skills to older Americans with opportunities to help solve community problems and offer supplemental insurance while on duty, on-the-job training from the agency or organization where volunteers are placed.

1205 RSVP Skylands
53 Stickle Avenue
Suite 2
Rockaway, NJ 07866
973-784-4900
Fax: 973-784-4904; *Toll Free:* 888-387-9830
rsvp@norwescap.org
www.norwescap.org

Nancy Hess, Program Director

The Retired and Senior Volunteer Program (RSVP) provides opportunities for people 55 and over to make a difference in their community through volunteer service. RSVP volunteers contribute anywhere from a few to over forty hours a week, serving thourgh schools, day care centers, police departments, hospitals and other nonprofit and public organizations to help meet critical community needs. RSVP offers maximum flexibility and choice to its volunteers. RSVP matches the personal interests and skills to older Americans with opportunities to help solve community problems and offer supplemental insurance while on duty, on-the-job training from the agency or organization where volunteers are placed.

1206 RSVP Somerset County
PO Box 3000
20 Grove Street
Somerville, NJ 08876-1262
908-704-6358
Fax: 908-231-1813
publicinfo@co.somerset.nj.us
www.co.somerset.nj.us

Patrica L. Walsh, Director
Peter S. Palmer, Deputy Director

The Retired and Senior Volunteer Program (RSVP) provides opportunities for people 55 and over to make a difference in their community through volunteer service. RSVP volunteers contribute anywhere from a few to over forty hours a week, serving thourgh schools, day care centers, police departments, hospitals and other nonprofit and public organizations to help meet critical community needs. RSVP offers maximum flexibility and choice to its volunteers. RSVP matches the personal interests and skills to older Americans with opportunities to help solve community problems and offer supplemental insurance while on duty, on-the-job training from the agency or organization where volunteers are placed.

1207 RSVP Sussex-Warren
350 Marshall Street
Phillipsburg, NJ 08865-3273
908-454-7000
Fax: 908-859-0729
ouellettec@norwescap.org

Carol R Ouellette, Contact
Laurie Cahill, Manager

The Retired and Senior Volunteer Program (RSVP) provides opportunities for people 55 and over to make a difference in their community through volunteer service. RSVP volunteers contribute anywhere from a few to over forty hours a week, serving thourgh schools, day care centers, police departments, hospitals and other nonprofit and public organizations to help meet critical community needs. RSVP offers maximum flexibility and choice to its volunteers. RSVP matches the personal interests and skills to older Americans with opportunities to help solve community problems and offer supplemental insurance while on duty, on-the-job training from the agency or organization where volunteers are placed.

1208 Railroad Retirement Board: New Jersey District Office
Veteran's Administration Building
20 Washington Place
Room 516
Newark, NJ 07102-3127
877-772-5772
Fax: 973-645-3373
www.rrb.gov/field/do_newa.asp

Merideth L Rogers, Representative

An independent agency in the executive branch of the Federal Government. The RRB's primary function is to administer comprehensive retirement-survivor and unemployment-sickness benefit programs for the nation's railroad workers and their families.

1209 Salem County Office on Aging
98 Market Street
Salem, NJ 08079
856-935-7510
Fax: 856-935-9102; Toll Free: 877-222-3737
County.administrator@salemcountynj.gov
salemcountynj.gov

Julie A. Acton, Director
Dale A. Cross, Deputy Director
Ben H. Laury, Chairman-Public Works

Assists with social security, medicare, medicaid, pharmaceutical assistance to the aged and disabled, adult protective services, home delivered meals, home health aide, legal services, matter of balance, project healthy bones, global options, adult day care, congregate nutrition and JACC.

1210 Senior Citizens Council of Union County
2187 Morris Avenue
Union, NJ 07083-5908
908-964-7555
Fax: 908-964-7607

Richard Stone, Executive Director

Senior citizens. Advocates for seniors. Provides information and referral services. Conducts 6 seminars per year; sponsors trips.

1211 Social Service Association
6 Station Plaza
Ridgewood, NJ 07450-3125
201-444-2980
Fax: 201-444-4987
ssa6@verizon.net
www.ssa6.org

Linda Gilman, Executive Director

Volunteers. Provides case management and financial assistance to help make families and individuals independent.

1212 Somerset County Office on Aging
First Floor
27 Warren Street
Somerville, NJ 08876
908-704-6346
Fax: 908-253-0180; Toll Free: 888-747-1122
officeaging@co.somerset.nj.us
www.co.somerset.nj.us
TDD 908-231-7168

Patrick Scaglione, Director
Mark Caliguire, Deputy Director

Assesses needs of older persons and plans programs and services to meet those needs. Offers information and referral services, outreach, senior centers, home delivered meals, wellness and care, legal counseling, and eldercare services.

1213 State of New Jersey Department of Labor and Workforce Development
New Jersey Department of Labor And Workforce Development
Trenton, NJ 08625
609-292-2323
Fax: 609-633-9271
cmycoff@dol.state.nj.us
www.state.nj.us/labor

Harold J Wirths, Commissioner
Aaron Fitchner, Deputy Commissioner
Frederick Zavaglia, Chief of Staff

Helping New Jersey's skilled and productive workforce gain the right job so that they can help high quality employers compete successfully in the world marketplace.

1214 Sussex County Office on Aging
One Spring Street
Newton, NJ 07860
973-579-0555
Fax: 973-579-0550; Toll Free: 877-222-3737
www.sussex.nj.us

Lorraine Hentz, Division Director

Mission is to enable older individuals and/or their caregivers to choose from a coordinated system of services that allow seniors to live as independently as possible in their homes and in their communities while enjoying a dignified quality of life.

1215 Union County Division on Aging
Union County Administration Building
10 Elizabethtown Plaza
Elizabeth, NJ 07207
908-527-4000
Fax: 908-659-7410; Toll Free: 877-424-1234
www.unioncountynj.org/aging

Frances A. Benson, Director
Bernadette McCarthy, Assistant Director

Plans, implements and coordinates services for residents aged 60 and older.

1216 Volunteer Center of Camden County
Office Of Constituent Services
Courthouse,Suite 306
520 Market Street
Camden, NJ 08102
856-663-9356
Fax: 856-663-4879; Toll Free: 866-266-3362
www.camdencounty.com/community/volunteer

Louis Cappelli, Director
Edward T. McDonnell, Deputy Director

Offers information about a variety of volunteer opportunities in Camden County, including serving meals to the homebound, mentoring a child, gardening, clerical work and more.

1217 Warren County Division of Senior Services
165 County Rte 519 South
Belvidere, NJ 07823

908-475-6591
Fax: 908-475-6588; *Toll Free:* 877-222-3737
SeniorServices@co.warren.nj.us
www.co.warren.nj.us
TDD 908-689-6900

Susan Lennon, Director

New Mexico

1218 City of Albuquerque-Bernalillo County: Department of Senior Affairs
714 7th Street SW
Albuquerque, NM 87102-3814
505-764-6469
Fax: 505-764-6465
seniorinformation@cabq.gov
www.cabq.gov/seniors

Jorja Armijo-Brasher, Director

A wide array of services and opportunities to enhance Bernalillo County seniors' quality of life. Providing services for active, healthy seniors and for frail, homebound elderly, the goal is to provide a continuum of care to keep seniors mentally and physically active and in their homes for as long as safely possible. Depending on the particular program, the minimum age varies from ages 50-60 years. Contributions requested for some services.

1219 Disability Determination Services
PO Box 4588
3301 Juan Tabo
Albuquerque, NM 87196-4588
505-841-5600
Fax: 505-841-5724; *Toll Free:* 800-432-5868
www.dvrgetsjobs.com

Stephen Abbott, Ajudicator
Kim Banales, Ajudicator

Helps people with disabilities achieve a suitable employment outcome.

1220 Eastern New Mexico: Area Agency on Aging
901 W 13th Street
Clovis, NM 88101-5552
505-769-1613
Fax: 505-769-3530

Frank White, Director
Nancy Arias, Executive Director

The Aging and Long Term Services Dpeartment provides a direct voice and access to critical resources for older adults, persons with disabilities and their caregivers.

1221 New Mexico Client Assistance Program
1720 Louisiana Boulevard NE
Suite 204
Albuquerque, NM 87110-8004
505-256-3100
Fax: 505-256-3184; *Toll Free:* 800-432-4682
info@drnm.org
www.drnm.org/
TTY: 800-432-4682

Adam Carrasco, President
Deanna DeVore, Vice-President

Advocates for people who have questions or concerns about the services offered by Division of Vocational Reha-

bilitation, the Commission for the Blind, and Centers for Independent Living.

1222 New Mexico Department of Aging
2550 Cerrillos Road
Santa Fe, NM 87505
505-476-4799
Fax: 505-827-7649; *Toll Free:* 866-451-2901
www.nmaging.state.nm.us

Retta Ward, Secretary

Dedicated to promoting the independence and dignity of elders and individuals living with a disability. Our mission is to achieve the highest quality of life for older persons, people with disaiblities and their families by enhancing autonomy, health, economic well-being, community involvement, and personal responsibility.

1223 New Mexico Department of Taxation and Revenue
1100 South St Francis Dr
PO Box 630
Santa Fe, NM 87504
505-827-0369
Fax: 505-827-0469
www.tax.state.nm.us

Demesia Padilla, Secretary

Mission is to administer and enforce New Mexico's tax and revenue laws, and vehicle and driver licensing code in a manner warranting the highest degree of public confidence.

1224 New Mexico Educational Retirement Board
701 Camino De Los Marquez
PO Box 26129
Santa Fe, NM 87502
505-827-8030
Fax: 505-827-1855; *Toll Free:* 866-691-2345
www.nmerb.org

Jan Goodwin, Executive Director
Rick Scroggins, Deputy Director
Bob Jacksha, Chief Investment Officer

Provides secure retirement benefits for thier active and retired memebers from school districts, higher education and educational agencies.

1225 New Mexico Governor's Committee on Concern of the Handicapped
491 Old Santa Fe Trail
Santa Fe, NM 87501-2753
505-476-0412
Fax: 505-827-6328; *Toll Free:* 877-696-1470
gcd@state.nm.us
gcd.state.nm.us

Susan Gray, Vice Chairman

Mission is to ensure that all people, regardless of disability, can participate fully in mainstream society. We accomplish this mission by addressing barriers- physical, programmatic and attitudnal- that may keep a person with a disability from enjoying what society has to offer.

1226 New Mexico Protection & Advocacy for Persons with Disabilities
1720 Louisiana Boulevard NE
Suite 204
Albuquerque, NM 87110-7022

505-256-3100
Fax: 505-256-3184; Toll Free: 800-432-4682
info@drnm.org
www.drnm.org

Adam Carrasco, President
Deanna DeVore, Vice-President

Mission is to protect, promote, aand expand the legal and civil rights of persons with disabilities.

1227 New Mexico Public Employees Retirement Association
33 Plaza La Prensa
PO Box 2123
Santa Fe, NM 87507
505-476-9300
Fax: 505-476-9401; Toll Free: 800-342-3422
judy.olson@state.nm.us
www.pera.state.nm.us

Patria French, Chairperson
Daniel Mayfield, Vice Chairman
James B. Lewis, Treasurer

The mission of the Board of Public Employees Retirement Association is to preserve, protect, and administer the trust to meet its current and future obligations and provide quality services to Association members.

1228 New Mexico Veterans Service Commission
Bataan Memorial Building
407 Galisteo Street, Room 142
Santa Fe, NM 87504
505-827-6300
Fax: 505-827-6372; Toll Free: 866-433-8387
www.dvs.state.nm.us

Timothy Hale, Cabinet Secretary
Alan Martinez, Deputy Secretary
Michele Tyson-March, Field Operations Director

Mission is to assist veterans, widows and children of veterans in establishing the privileges to which they are entitled.

1229 New Mexico Workers Compensation Board
2410 Centre Avenue SE
PO Box 27198
Albuquerque, NM 87125-7198
505-841-6000
Fax: 505-841-6060; Toll Free: 800-255-7965
www.workerscomp.state.nm.us

Ned S Fuller, Director
Darren Childers, General Counsel

Mission is to assure the quick and efficient delivery of indemnity and medical benefits to injured workers at a reasonable cost to employees.

1230 North Central New Mexico: Area Agency on Aging
3900 Paseo del Sol
PO Box 5115
Santa Fe, NM 87507
505-827-7313
Fax: 877-293-3710; Toll Free: 866-699-4927
www.ncnmedd.com/aaa.htm

Tim Armer, Executive Director
Duncan Sill, Planning Manager
Francesca Marteniz, Office Administrator

Purose is for developing a comprehensive and coordinated system of services to the elderly population of PSA II and PSA IV

1231 Railroad Retirement Board: New Mexico
421 Gold Avenue SW
Suite 304
Albuquerque, NM 87103-0334
505-346-6407
Fax: 505-346-6407; Toll Free: 877-772-5772
albuquerque@rrb.gov
www.rrb.gov/field/do_albu.asp
TTY: 312-751-4701

Barbara E Aylaian, Representative

An independent agency in the executive branch of the Federal Government. The RRB's primary function is to administer comprehensive retirement-survivor and unemployment-sickenss benefit programs for the nation's railroad workers and their families.

New York

1232 Allegany County Office for the Aging
County Office Building,
Belmont, NY 14813-1001
585-268-9222
Fax: 585-268-9657; Toll Free: 866-268-9390
ofa@alleganyco.com
www.alleganyco.com

Curtis W. Crandall, Chairman
Dwight R. Fanton, Vice Chairman
Mitchell M Alger, County Administrator

Provides expert information and assistance to older individuals and their caregivers to maintain dignity, respect, and independence.

1233 Association of Belltel Retirees
PO Box 33
Cold Spring Harbor, NY 11724
631-367-3067; *Toll Free: 800-261-9222*
association@belltelretirees.org
www.belltelretirees.org

CW Jones, Contact

Advocactes for more then 220,000 Bell Atlantic, NYNEX, GTE, MCI and VERIZON retirees unfairly treated by the company they helped build. The Association also represents active employees regarding retiree issues, such as cash balance plan conversions and recently announced termination of manangement pensions and healthcare benefits.

1234 Birchwood Volunteers In Partnership
4800 Bear Road
Liverpool, NY 13088-4604
315-457-9946
Fax: 315-457-8290
www.elderwood.com

Kristen Russell, Administrator

a 160-bed facility with a reputation for excellence in skilled nursing, subacute care and rehabilitation.

1235 Broome County Office for Aging
4th Floor Broome County Office Building
60 Hawley Street
Binghamton, NY 13902-1766

607-778-2411
Fax: 607-778-2316
ofa@co.broome.ny.us
www.gobroomecounty.com

Helps caregivers and older adults to get the services they need whether they are looking for information on healthy living or need care in their homes.

1236 Buffalo Senior Center
671 W Fetterman Street
PO Box 941
Buffalo, NY 82834
307-684-9551
Fax: 307-684-5585
bjwalseth@buffaloseniorcenter.com
www.buffaloseniorcenter.com

A J Mock, Executive Director
Sally Frost, Assistant Director
Janice Spratt, Access Care Coordinator

Community service organization providing congregate and home delivered meals, transportation, social activity coordination, adult day care and home care, nursing, and aging resource center.

1237 Cattaraugus County Department of Aging
1701 Lincoln Avenue
Suite 7610
Olean, NY 14760-1121
716-373-8032
Fax: 585-372-4734; Toll Free: 800-462-2901
www.cattco.org/aging
TTY: 716-373-8032

John Searles, Director
Cherianne Wold, Manager

Provides or assures the provision of needed services to county residents who are age 60 and older.

1238 Cayuga County Office of the Aging
County Office Building Basement
160 Gennessee Street
Auburn, NY 13021-3483
315-253-1226
Fax: 315-253-1151
ccofa@co.cayuga.ny.us
www.co.cayuga.ny.us/aging

Nancy L Siefka, Director
Brenda Wiemann, Aging Services Coordinator
Julie Casier, Nutrition Project Director

To promote maximum well-being, independence and dignity for persons 60 years of age and older, the office for the aging works with all of the service agencies in the community and individual elders to connect the services availiable with those who need them.

1239 Center for the Study of Aging of Albany
106 Madison Avenue
Albany, NY 12208-3695
518-465-6927
Fax: 518-462-1339
harriscom@comcast.net
www.members.aol.com/iapaas

Sara Harris, Executive Director

Participants include behavioral scientists, educators, gerontologists, physicians, and other health professionals. Promotes education, research, and training; provides

leadership in the field of health and fitness for older people. Includes: programs for volunteers and professionals in aging, gerontology, geriatrics, wellness, physical fitness, and mental health; consultant services include adult day care, nutrition, physical and mental fitness,nursing home, housing, and retirement; speakers' bureau. Develops national and international conferences on health, fitness, and prevention. Provides expert assistance in research, institutional and community program development, planning, and organization; offers consultation addressing the development of library resource centers and collections of books on aging. Conducts seminars and offers information and referral services.

1240 Chautauqua County Office for the Aging
Hall R Clothier Building
7 N Erie Street
Mayville, NY 14757-1027
716-753-4471
Fax: 716-753-4477; Toll Free: 716-363-4471
www.co.chautauqua.ny.us/ccofa

Dr. Mary Ann Spanos, Director

Provides services for the aging and disabled.

1241 Chemung County Office for the Aging
Human Resource Center
378 S. Main Street
PO Box 588
Elmira, NY 14902-0588
607-737-5475
Fax: 607-737-5499
ofa@co.chemung.ny.us
www.chemungcounty.com
TTY: 607-737-5347

Robert D. Siglin, Commissioner
Linda Forrest, Deputy Commissioner

1242 Clinton County Office for the Aging
135 Margaret Street
Suite 105
Plattsburgh, NY 12901-2994
518-565-4620
Fax: 518-565-4812
carterc@co.clinton.ny.us
www.clintoncountygov.com

Crystal L Carter, Director

The Clinton County Office for the Aging is the advocacy, planning, and coordinating agency for senior citizens. Its mission is to understand and strive to meet the needs of the elderly through direct services and referrals to the various agencies.

1243 Corporate Volunteers of New York
61 Chambers Street
New York, NY 10007-1208
212-332-4075

Nichola Arnett, President
Tamara Kiesa, Vice President
James Ennis, Treasurer

Corporate volunteers.

1244 Cortland County: Area Agency on Aging
County Office Building
60 Central Avenue
Cortland, NY 13045-2746

607-753-5060
Fax: 607-758-5528
ccaaa@cortland-co.org
www.cortland-co.org

Liz Haskins, Director

Services include: informative assistance, advocacy, legal services, senior centers, meals on wheels, benefits counseling, health insurance assistance, in-home services, volunteer services, home repairs, recreation, energy programs, consumer information.

1245 Disability Determination Services
Room 430 Federal Building
11 A Clinton Avenue
Albany, NY 12260-0165
518-473-9320
Fax: 518-473-9286; *Toll Free:* 800-772-1213
www.ssa.gov
TTY: 800-325-0778

James Caseo, Director

SSA determination of benefits.

1246 Division of Disability Determinations
195 Montague Street
7th Floor
Brooklyn, NY 11201-2701
718-522-8015
Fax: 718-522-8272; *Toll Free:* 800-772-1213
www.ssa.gov
TTY: 800-325-0778

Sandra Wapner, Manager

SSA determination of benefits.

1247 Erie County Department of Senior Services
95 Franklin Street, 16th Floor
Room 1329
Buffalo, NY 14202-3968
716-858-8500
Fax: 716-858-6679
seniorinfo@erie.gov
www.erie.gov/depts/seniorservices
TTY: 800-622-1220

Ellen E Grant, Commissioner
Patricia Watson, Case Mgmt Services Supervisor

Brings together the programs, services and supportive facilities which help the 190,000 elderly maintain independence whenever possible. Coordinates existing community services as well as plans, develops and administers needed programs and promotes new and better services for all persons age sixty and over.

Year Founded: 1971

1248 Essex County Office for the Aging
132 Water Street
PO Box 217
Elizabethtown, NY 12932-0217
518-873-3695
Fax: 518-873-3784; *Toll Free:* 877-464-1637
webmaster@co.essex.ny.us
www.co.essex.ny.us

Patricia Bashaw, Director

The Essex County Office for the Aging develops and carries out a comprehensive and coordinated system of health, education, employment, and social services for the Dis-

trict's elderly population, who are 60 years of age and older.

1249 Franklin County Office for the Aging
125 Catherine Street
355 West Main Street Suite 447
Malone, NY 12953-1826
518-481-1526
Fax: 518-481-1635; *Toll Free:* 800-397-8686
frankofa@co.franklin.ny.us
www.franklincony.org

Susan Scott, Director
Thomas D. Soucia, Public Defender
Lorelie Miller, Conflict Defender

The purpose of the Office on Aging is to provide centralized access to diverse programs and individualized services for older adults and their families so they can preserve their independence and quality of life.

1250 Fulton County Office for the Aging
19 N William Street
Johnstown, NY 12095-2115
518-736-5650
Fax: 518-762-0698
fcofa@co.fulton.ny.us
www.fcofa.org

Andrea Fettinger BA, Director

Programs and services for older adults and their families. Meals, transportation, home care, case management, long-term care, employment, housing, information, and caregivers services.

1251 Gray Panthers of New York
244 Madison Avenue
Suite 396
New York, NY 10016
212-799-7572
Fax: 202-737-1160
judylear@aol.com
www.graypanthersnyc.org

Mary Springer, Co-Convenor
Jack Kupferman, Co-Convenor

Quality of life issues: Universal health care, secure and comfortable housing, employment and educational opportunities for all.

1252 Gray Panthers of Suffolk County
244 Madison Avenue
Suite 396
New York, NY 10016
212-799-7572
Fax: 202-737-1160
judylear@aol.com
www.graypanthers.org

Mary Springer, Co-Convenor
Jack Kupferman, Co-Convenor

Mission is to work for social and economic justice and peace for all people.

1253 Greater Rochester Area Partnership for the Elderly
100 McAuley Drive
Suite 2000
Rochester, NY 14610-1670

585-256-4351
Fax: 585-256-4352
info@grapelder.org
www.grapelder.org

Elllen O'Reilly, President
Kathy Scott, President-Elect
Kathleen Krauss, Executive Director

Professionals and interested persons who aspire to improve the quality of services for older people. Our three main objectives are professional development, networking, public and social policy advocacy.

1254 Greene County Department for the Aging

411 Main Street
Catskill, NY 12414-1237
518-719-3555
Fax: 518-719-3798
aging@discovergreene.com
www.greenegovernment.com

Therese McGee Ward, Executive Director
Connie Bentley, Aging Services Coordinator

Provides a network of over thirty distinct services designed to meet the needs of the more then 9800 older residents of Greene County ages 60 and older.

1255 Herkimer County Office for the Aging

109 Mary Street
Suite 1101
Herkimer, NY 13350-2924
315-867-1121
Fax: 315-867-1448
hcofa@herkimercounty.org
www.herkimercounty.org

Mary Scanlon, Director

The Herkimer County Office for the Aging (OFA) plans, funds, and delivers services to people aged 60 and older in Herkimer County.

1256 Jefferson County Office for Aging

175 Arsenal Street
Watertown, NY 13601-2546
315-785-3191
Fax: 315-785-5095
www.co.jefferson.ny.us

Peter Fazio, Executive Director

Services for the aging and disabled.

1257 Jewish Association for Services for the Aged Manhattan District Service

132 W 31st Street
Floor 15
New York, NY 10001-3406
212-273-5272
Fax: 212-695-4206
help@jasa.org
www.jasa.org

David Warren, President
Aileen Gitelson, Chief Executive Officer

JASA's mission is to sustain and enrich the lives of the aging in New York metropolitan area so that they can remain in the community with dignity and autonomy.

1258 Lighthouse International Ruth M. Shellens Library

111 E 59th Street
New York, NY 10022-1264
212-821-9200
Fax: 212-821-9687; *Toll Free:* 800-829-0500
www.lighthouse.org
TTY: 212-821-9713

Tricia Reyes, Director Of Marketing

Research and education related rehabilitation services, orientation and mobility. Independent living services.

1259 Livingston County Office for Aging

8 Livingston County Campus
Mount Morris, NY 14510-1197
585-243-7520
Fax: 585-243-7516
www.co.livingston.state.ny.us/ofta.htm

Kaaren Smith, Director

Offers programs and services to individuals 60 and over in their county.

1260 Madison County Office for the Aging

138 Dominic Bruno Boulevard
Canastota, NY 13032-3528
315-697-1500
Fax: 315-697-5777; *Toll Free:* 866-220-2009
information@ofamadco.org
www.ofamadco.org

Theresa Davis, Director
Julie Harney, Respite Case Manager
Anna Marie Vaughn, Respite Case Manager

Mission is to advocacte, assist, and provide services that enrich the quality of life and promote the independence and dignity of older-individuals and their families.

1261 Meals on Wheels of Buffalo and Erie County Foundation

100 James E Casey Drive
Buffalo, NY 14206
716-822-2002
Fax: 716-822-0932
www.mowbuffalo.com

Tara Ellis, President
Francine Powers, Operations Director
Lisa Woodring, Foundation Director

Dedicated to ensuring the those we serve enjoy the highest level of independence possible.

1262 Monroe County Office for the Aging and Adult Services

435 East Henrietta Road
Room 3rd Floor, West
Rochester, NY 14620-4603
585-753-6280
Fax: 585-753-6282
ccrossdale@monroecounty.gov
www.monroecounty.gov/aging.index.php

Corinda Crossdale, Director

The goal for the Office of the Aging and Adult Services is to promote a safe and independent lifestyle through timely and responsive systems of protective services, long-term care, quality nutrition and supportive in-home services through a consumer-focused and coordinated service delivery system that protects, supports, and advocates for older residents of Monroe County.

1263 Montgomery County Office for the Aging

135 Guy Park Avenue
Amsterdam, NY 12010-1055
518-843-2300
Fax: 518-843-7478
mcofakdenis@nycap.rr.com
www.mcofa.org

Lee Broyles, Interim Director

Mission is to help older New Yorkers to be as independent as possible through advocacy, development and delivery of cost effective policies, programs and services which support and empower the elderly and their families, in partnership with the network of public and private organizations which serve them.

1264 Nassau County Department of Senior Citizen Affairs

60 Charles Lindbergh Boulevard
Suite 260
Uniondale, NY 11553-3691
516-227-8900
Fax: 516-571-5978
seniors@nassaucountyny.gov
www.nassaucountyny.gov/agencies/seniors

Lisa A Murphy, Commissioner

As the Area Agency on Aging for Nassau County, the Department provides more than 90 programs and services for the County's 257,000 senior citizens and their caregivers. These programs are designed to maintain seniors' safety in their homes and communities for as long as possible.

1265 New York City Department for the Aging

2 Lafayette Street
7th Floor
New York, NY 10007-1307
212-442-1322
Fax: 212-442-1095
www.nyc.gov
TTY: 212-504-4115

Lilliam Barrios-Paoli, Commissioner

Mission is to work for the empowerment, independence, dignity, and quality of life of New York City's diverse older adults and for the support of their families through advocacy, education and the coordination and delivery of services.

1266 New York Commission on Quality of Care and Advocacy for Persons with Disabilities

161 Delaware Avenue
Delmar, NY 12054-1354
518-381-7102
Fax: 518-388-2860; *Toll Free:* 800-624-4143
www.cqcapd.state.ny.us
TDD 855-373-2122
TTY: 855-373-2123

Andrew M. Cuomo,, Governor
Jeff Wise Executive Director

The New York State Commission on Quality of Care for the Mentally Disabled (CQC) and the New York State Office of Advocate for Persons with Disabilities (OAP wD) have been merged to form a new agency, the New York State Commission on Quality of Care and Advocacy for

Persons with Disabilities (CQCAPD). CQCAPD serves people with mental disabilities and their families by providing independent oversight of the quality and cost-effectiveness of services provided by all mental hygiene programs in New York State.

1267 New York Department of Aging

2 Empire State Plaza
Albany, NY 12207-2018
518-447-7177
Fax: 518-447-7188; *Toll Free:* 800-342-9871
nysofa@ofa.state.ny.us
www.aging.ny.gov

Greg Olsen, Acting Director

The mission of the New York State Office for the Aging is to help older New Yorkers to be as independent as possible for as long as possible through advocacy, development and delivery of cost effective policies, programs and services which support and empower the elderly and thier families, in partnership with the network of public and private organizations which serve them.

1268 New York Department of Taxation & Finance

Building 9 Room 449
PO Box 4127
Albany, NY 12227
518-457-3512
Fax: 518-457-2486
www.tax.state.ny.us

Thomas H Mattox, Commissioner

Mission is to collect tax revenue and provide associated services in support of government services in New York State.

1269 New York Developmental Disability Planning Council

99 Washington Avenue
12th Floor, Suite 1230
Albany, NY 12210
518-486-7505
Fax: 518-402-3505; *Toll Free:* 800-395-3372
ddpc.sm.pio@ddpc.ny.gov
ddpc.ny.gov/

Andrew M. Cuomo,, Governor
Sheila M Carey, Executive Director
Rose M. Toscano,, Chairperson

The New York State Developmental Disabilities Planning Council (DDPC), in partnership with individuals with developmental disabilities, their families and communities, provides leadership by promoting policies, plans, and practices that: affirm dignity, value and worth; support full participation in society; uphold equality and self-determination; and promote access to research and information needed for informed-decision-making for all individuals with developmental disabilities and their families.

1270 New York Division of Veterans Affairs

5 Empire State Plaza, 28th Floor
Suite 2836
Albany, NY 12223-1551
518-474-6784
Fax: 518-473-0379; *Toll Free:* 888-838-7697
dvainfo@veterans.ny.gov
www.veterans.state.ny.us

William Kraus, Acting Director
William Brennan, Counsel
Mary Quay, Secretary

Mission is to provide quality service and advocacy for New York State veterans, armed forces members, their dependents and survivors, ensuring they receive benefits granted by law for their service to New York and the nation.

1271 New York State Association of Area Agencies on Aging
272 Broadway
Albany, NY 12204-2737
518-449-7080
Fax: 518-449-7055
office@nysaaaa.org
www.nysaaaa.org

Laura A Cameron, Executive Director
Karen Thornton, Member Services Director

1272 New York State Coalition for the Aging
1450 Western Avenue
Suite 101
Albany, NY 12206
518-765-2790
Fax: 518-463-8656
info@coalitionforaging.org
www.coalitionforaging.org

Ann Marie Cook, President
Peggy Osborne, Vice President
Lynn Robinson, Secretary

Training, technical assistance, advocacy for senior services in NYS.

1273 New York State Commission for the Blind
155 Washington Avenue
2nd Floor
Albany, NY 12210-2329
518-473-1698
Fax: 518-474-5819
www.ocfs.state.ny.us

Luis A Mendez, Chairman

Offers services for the totally blind, legally blind, visually impaired, mentally retarded blind and more with health, counseling, educational, recreational, rehabilitation, computer training and professional training services.

1274 New York State Division of Disability Determinations
One Commerce Plaza
99 Washington Avenue
Albany, NY 12210
716-847-5007; *Toll Free: 800-726-1353*
www.otda.state.ny.us

Elizabeth Berlin, Executive Deputy Commissioner
Kevin Kehmna, Director
Nancy Maney, Finance Director

The New York State Division of Disability Determinations adjudicates the claims of persons filing for disability benefits with the Social Security Administration.

1275 New York State Intergenerational Network Generations Child and Adult Day Care
179 Stenson Street
Rochester, NY 14606

585-247-3490
Fax: 585-429-2100
www.generations-care.com

Vickie Jesse, Staff Member/Educator
Linda Hooker, Staff Member/Educator
Patty Hasselberg, Staff Member/Educator

Day care for both children and older adults.

1276 New York State Office for the Aging: Senior Citizens Helpline
Agency
Building 2
Albany, NY 12223
Fax: 518-474-1398; *Toll Free: 800-342-9871*
www.aging.ny.gov

Jody Signoracci, Constituency Liaison

Provides information on statewide services for the elderly.

1277 New York State Office of Mental Health
44 Holland Avenue
Albany, NY 12229
518-474-2568
Fax: 518-474-2149; *Toll Free: 800-597-8481*
www.omh.state.ny.us/omhweb

Michael Hogan, Commissioner
Kristen Woodlock, Executive Deputy Commissioner
Lloyd Sederer, Medical Director

Promoting the mental health of all New Yorkers with a particular focus on providing hope and recovery for adults with serious mental illness and children with serious emotional disturbances.

1278 New York Teachers Retirement System
10 Corporate Woods Drive
Albany, NY 12211
518-465-4400; *Toll Free: 888-693-8779*
communit@nystrs.org
www.nystrs.org

R Michael Kraus, President
David Keefe, Vice President
Paul Farfaglia, Delegates Trustee Member

Committed to developing innovations tht enable TRS to fulfill our mission of providing the efficient collection of contributions, the prudnt investment of retirement funds, the responsible disbursement of member benefits, and the delivery of exceptional levels of member service.

1279 Niagara County Office for the Aging
Golden Triangle Building
111 Main Street, Suite 101
Lockport, NY 14094-3319
716-438-4020
Fax: 716-439-7661
www.niagracounty.com/aging

Kenneth Genewick, Director

The Niagra County Office for the Aging brings together the programs, services and supportive facilities which help our 44,000 elderly maintain independence whenever possible.

1280 Oneida County Office for the Aging
120 Airline Street
Suite 201
Oriskany, NY 13424
315-798-5456
Fax: 315-798-6444

webmaster@ocgov.net
www.ocgov.net

Michael Romano, Director

The purpose of the Oneida County Office for the Aging and Continuing Xare is to serve as the lead planning, funding and advocacy agency for older adults, disabled, their families and caregivers. The mission is based on the goal of maintaining maximum independence through service provision that is guided by the core values of respect, dignity, compassion, honesty. confidentiality, commitment, & informed professionalism.

1281 Onondaga County Department of Aging and Youth
421 Montgomery Street
13th Floor
Syracuse, NY 13202-2923
315-435-2362
Fax: 315-435-3129
www.ongov.net\ay

Lisa D Alford, Commissioner

The Onondago County Department of Aging and Youth is the designated Area Agency for Aging in Onondago County. The Department provides and supports a comprehensive system of services for children and youth, senior citizens, caregivers and families. Our services help individuals and families remain safe and productive members of their communities. Services include; Information and Assistance, Caregiver Services, Institute for Caregivers, In-Home Services, Community Living Program, Health Insurance Information Counseling and Assistance, HEAP (Home Energy Assistance Program), Neighborhood Advisor Program, Senior Employment Assistance, Senior Meals and Nutrition Services, Health Promotion and Medication Management.

1282 Ontario County Office for the Aging
3010 County Complex Drive
Canandaigua, NY 14424-9502
585-396-4040
Fax: 585-396-7490
onofa@co.ontario.ny.us
www.co.ontario.ny.us/aging

Helen P Sherman, Director

Committed to enriching the lives of residents 60 years of age and older and their caregivers.

1283 Orange County Office for the Aging
18 Seward Avenue
2nd Floor
Middletown, NY 10940
845-615-3700
Fax: 845-346-1191
www.co.orange.ny.us

Ann Marie Maglione, Director

The primary goal of the Office for the Aging is maintaining the dignity, well-being, and independence of senior citizens through the Office's distinctive role as advocate and community partner.

1284 Oswego County Office for the Aging
70 Bunner Street
PO Box 3080
Oswego, NY 13126-3357

315-349-3484
Fax: 315-349-8413
schmidla@oswegocounty.com
www.oswegocounty.com

Laurence Schmidt, Director

Provides a wide variety of services to the senior citizens of Oswego County either directly or through contracts with other agencies. These services include: information, referral, assistance, home delivered meals, congregate meals, transportation, legal assistance, home care assistance and more.

Year Founded: 1977

1285 Otsego County Office for the Aging
The Meadows Complex
140 Co Highway 33 West
Suite 5
Cooperstown, NY 13326-1128
607-547-4232
Fax: 607-547-6492
www.otsegocounty.com

Kathleen Clark, Director

Provides assistance to county residents age 60 and over, Caregivers of those age 60 and over and age 60 and over caregivers of children.

1286 Perinton Retired Men's Club
1350 Turk Hill Road
Fairport, NY 14450-8795
585-223-0770
Fax: 585-223-3629
www.perinton.org

James Smith, Town Supervisor
Jeffrey Myers, Recreation/Parks Commissioner

1287 Prevent Blindness America New York City Division
211 West Wacker Drive
Suite 1700
Chicago, IL 60606
212-980-2020
Fax: 203-598-0584; *Toll Free:* 800-331-2020
info@preventblindnesstristate.org
www.preventblindness.org

Individuals interested in preventing blindness and preserving sight through research and education programs.

1288 Putnam County Office for the Aging
110 Old Route 6
Building One
Carmel, NY 10512-2119
845-808-1700
Fax: 845-808-1942
www.putnamcountyny.com/ofa

Pat Sheehy, Director

Vrious programs offered to th aging in their county.

1289 RSVP Auburn
Memorial City Hall
24 South Street
Auburn, NY 13021
315-255-1733
Fax: 315-252-3669
www.ci.auburn.ny.us

Michael Quill, Mayor

The Retired and Senior Volunteer Program (RSVP) provides opportunities for people 55 and over to make a difference in their community through volunteer service. RSVP volunteers contribute anywhere from a few to over forty hours a week, serving thourgh schools, day care centers, police departments, hospitals and other nonprofit and public organizations to help meet critical community needs. RSVP offers maximum flexibility and choice to its volunteers. RSVP matches the personal interests and skills to older Americans with opportunities to help solve community problems and offer supplemental insurance while on duty, on-the-job training from the agency or organization where volunteers are placed.

1290 RSVP Broome County
230 Main Street
Binghamton, NY 13905-2610
607-231-0726
Fax: 607-797-6188

Tammy Hodges, Director

The Retired and Senior Volunteer Program (RSVP) provides opportunities for people 55 and over to make a difference in their community through volunteer service. RSVP volunteers contribute anywhere from a few to over forty hours a week, serving thourgh schools, day care centers, police departments, hospitals and other nonprofit and public organizations to help meet critical community needs. RSVP offers maximum flexibility and choice to its volunteers. RSVP matches the personal interests and skills to older Americans with opportunities to help solve community problems and offer supplemental insurance while on duty, on-the-job training from the agency or organization where volunteers are placed.

1291 RSVP Cattaraugus County
1201 New York Avenue, NW
Washington, DC 20525
202-606-5000
Fax: 716-372-4734
darodkey@cattco.org
www.seniorcorps.gov
TTY: 800-833-3722

Cynthia Everetts, Director

The Retired and Senior Volunteer Program (RSVP) provides opportunities for people 55 and over to make a difference in their community through volunteer service. RSVP volunteers contribute anywhere from a few to over forty hours a week, serving thourgh schools, day care centers, police departments, hospitals and other nonprofit and public organizations to help meet critical community needs. RSVP offers maximum flexibility and choice to its volunteers. RSVP matches the personal interests and skills to older Americans with opportunities to help solve community problems and offer supplemental insurance while on duty, on-the-job training from the agency or organization where volunteers are placed.

1292 RSVP Chautaqua County
715 Falconer Street
Jamestown, NY 14701-1935
716-665-3038
Fax: 716-665-8073

Debra Basile, Director

The Retired and Senior Volunteer Program (RSVP) provides opportunities for people 55 and over to make a difference in their community through volunteer service. RSVP

volunteers contribute anywhere from a few to over forty hours a week, serving thourgh schools, day care centers, police departments, hospitals and other nonprofit and public organizations to help meet critical community needs. RSVP offers maximum flexibility and choice to its volunteers. RSVP matches the personal interests and skills to older Americans with opportunities to help solve community problems and offer supplemental insurance while on duty, on-the-job training from the agency or organization where volunteers are placed.

1293 RSVP Chemung County
911 Stowell Street
Elmira, NY 14901-2730
607-734-4161
Fax: 607-734-4166

Carol Houssock, Director

The Retired and Senior Volunteer Program (RSVP) provides opportunities for people 55 and over to make a difference in their community through volunteer service. RSVP volunteers contribute anywhere from a few to over forty hours a week, serving thourgh schools, day care centers, police departments, hospitals and other nonprofit and public organizations to help meet critical community needs. RSVP offers maximum flexibility and choice to its volunteers. RSVP matches the personal interests and skills to older Americans with opportunities to help solve community problems and offer supplemental insurance while on duty, on-the-job training from the agency or organization where volunteers are placed.

1294 RSVP Chenago County
44 West Main Street
Norwich, NY 13815
607-336-6414
Fax: 607-336-6415
rsvp@ofcinc.org
www.ofcinc.org

Doreen Bates, Director

the retired and senior volunteer program (rsvp) provides opportunities for peopel 55 and over to make a difference in thier community through volunteers service in non-profit agencies & organizations. RSVP volunteers decide how muh they want to serve. Some volunteer service opportunities are: food pantries and soup kitchens, thrift stores, animal shelter, museums, libraries, nursing homes and hospitals, senior meal delivery, Habitat for Humanity.

1295 RSVP Clinton County
46 Flynn Avenue
Plattsburgh, NY 12901-3742
518-566-0944
Fax: 518-566-0945
www.clintoncountygov.com/ofa

Patricia McCaughin, Director

The Retired and Senior Volunteer Program (RSVP) provides opportunities for people 55 and over to make a difference in their community through volunteer service. RSVP volunteers contribute anywhere from a few to over forty hours a week, serving thourgh schools, day care centers, police departments, hospitals and other nonprofit and public organizations to help meet critical community needs. RSVP offers maximum flexibility and choice to its volunteers. RSVP matches the personal interests and skills to older Americans with opportunities to help solve community problems and offer supplemental insurance while on

duty, on-the-job training from the agency or organization where volunteers are placed.

1296 RSVP Columbia County
721 Columbia Street
Hudson, NY 12534-2509
518-828-0251
Fax: 518-828-4614
mbeigel@columbiaopportunities.org
www.rsvpcolumbiacounty.org

Marcella Beigle, Director

1297 RSVP Cortland
60 Central Avenue
Room B2
Cortland, NY 13045-2795
607-753-5057
Fax: 607-756-3478
rsvp@cortland-co.org
www.cortland.co.org/ofa/rsvp

Cindy Stockholm, Director

The Retired and Senior Volunteer Program (RSVP) provides opportunities for people 55 and over to make a difference in their community through volunteer service. RSVP volunteers contribute anywhere from a few to over forty hours a week, serving though schools, day care centers, police departments, hospitals and other nonprofit and public organizations to help meet critical community needs. RSVP offers maximum flexibility and choice to its volunteers. RSVP matches the personal interests and skills to older Americans with opportunities to help solve community problems and offer supplemental insurance while on duty, on-the-job training from the agency or organization where volunteers are placed.

1298 RSVP Dutchess County
84 Cannon Street
Poughkeepsie, NY 12601-3022
845-485-8170
Fax: 845-473-1674

Barbara Adams, Director

Recruits people 55 years of age and older to do volunteer work for nonprofit agencies.

1299 RSVP Erie County
Rath Building
95 Franklin Street
Buffalo, NY 14202-3925
716-858-7548
Fax: 716-858-7259
patricia.dowling@erie.gov
www.erie.gov/rsvp

Carrie Smith, Director

The Retired and Senior Volunteer Program (RSVP) provides opportunities for people 55 and over to make a difference in their community through volunteer service. RSVP volunteers contribute anywhere from a few to over forty hours a week, serving though schools, day care centers, police departments, hospitals and other nonprofit and public organizations to help meet critical community needs. RSVP offers maximum flexibility and choice to its volunteers. RSVP matches the personal interests and skills to older Americans with opportunities to help solve community problems and offer supplemental insurance while on duty, on-the-job training from the agency or organization where volunteers are placed.

1300 RSVP Essex County
38 Park Place
Suite 3
Port Henry, NY 12974-1344
518-546-3565
Fax: 518-546-3079
rsvp@bluemoo.net
bluemoo.net/~rsvp

Patricia McCaughin, Program Director
Dusti Pratt, Program Assistant
Annabelle Waite, Office Aide

The Retired and Senior Volunteer Program (RSVP) provides opportunities for people 55 and over to make a difference in their community through volunteer service. RSVP volunteers contribute anywhere from a few to over forty hours a week, serving though schools, day care centers, police departments, hospitals and other nonprofit and public organizations to help meet critical community needs. RSVP offers maximum flexibility and choice to its volunteers. RSVP matches the personal interests and skills to older Americans with opportunities to help solve community problems and offer supplemental insurance while on duty, on-the-job training from the agency or organization where volunteers are placed.

1301 RSVP Franklin County
125 Catherine Street
Malone, NY 12953-1817
518-481-1528
Fax: 518-481-1878
afleury@co.franklin.ny.us

Victoria Brown, Director

Provides opportunities for people 55 and over to make a difference in their community through volunteer service. RSVP volunteers contribute anywhere from a few to over forty hours a week, serving through schools, day care centers, police departments, hospitals and other nonprofit and public organizations to help meet critical community needs. RSVP matches the personal interests and skills of older Americans with opportunities to help solve community problems and offers supplemental insurance while on duty, on-the-job training from the agency or organization where the volunteers are placed.

1302 RSVP Genesee County
Two Bank Street
Batavia, NY 14020-2202
585-343-1611
Fax: 585-344-8559

Dorian Ely, Director

The Retired and Senior Volunteer Program (RSVP) provides opportunities for people 55 and over to make a difference in their community through volunteer service. RSVP volunteers contribute anywhere from a few to over forty hours a week, serving though schools, day care centers, police departments, hospitals and other nonprofit and public organizations to help meet critical community needs. RSVP offers maximum flexibility and choice to its volunteers. RSVP matches the personal interests and skills to older Americans with opportunities to help solve community problems and offer supplemental insurance while on duty, on-the-job training from the agency or organization where volunteers are placed.

1303 RSVP Greene County

411 Main Street
Catskill, NY 12414-1237
518-719-3555
Fax: 518-719-3798

Barbara Cornelius-Premo, Director

The Retired and Senior Volunteer Program (RSVP) provides opportunities for people 55 and over to make a difference in their community through volunteer service. RSVP volunteers contribute anywhere from a few to over forty hours a week, serving though schools, day care centers, police departments, hospitals and other nonprofit and public organizations to help meet critical community needs. RSVP offers maximum flexibility and choice to its volunteers. RSVP matches the personal interests and skills to older Americans with opportunities to help solve community problems and offer supplemental insurance while on duty, on-the-job training from the agency or organization where volunteers are placed.

1304 RSVP Herkimer County

61 West Street
Ilion, NY 13357-1723
315-894-9917
Fax: 315-894-6313
herkimercountyrsvp.org/

Lydia Sexton, Director

The Retired and Senior Volunteer Program (RSVP) provides opportunities for people 55 and over to make a difference in their community through volunteer service. RSVP volunteers contribute anywhere from a few to over forty hours a week, serving though schools, day care centers, police departments, hospitals and other nonprofit and public organizations to help meet critical community needs. RSVP offers maximum flexibility and choice to its volunteers. RSVP matches the personal interests and skills to older Americans with opportunities to help solve community problems and offer supplemental insurance while on duty, on-the-job training from the agency or organization where volunteers are placed.

1305 RSVP Monroe County
LIFESPAN of Greater Rochester

1623 W. Sterns Rd.
Temperance, MI 48182
734-850-6040
Fax: 585-244-9114
deb.brescol@bedford.k12.mi.us
www.rsvpmi.org/contact.htm

Mary Beth Gueldner, Director

The Retired and Senior Volunteer Program (RSVP) provides opportunities for people 55 and over to make a difference in their community through volunteer service. RSVP volunteers contribute anywhere from a few to over forty hours a week, serving though schools, day care centers, police departments, hospitals and other nonprofit and public organizations to help meet critical community needs. RSVP offers maximum flexibility and choice to its volunteers. RSVP matches the personal interests and skills to older Americans with opportunities to help solve community problems and offer supplemental insurance while on duty, on-the-job training from the agency or organization where volunteers are placed.

1306 RSVP New York City

105 E 22nd Street
Suite 401
New York, NY 10010-5495
212-674-7787
Fax: 212-598-4782
www.cssny.org/rsvp/opportunities.html

Bobbie Futrell, Director

The Retired and Senior Volunteer Program (RSVP) provides opportunities for people 55 and over to make a difference in their community through volunteer service. RSVP volunteers contribute anywhere from a few to over forty hours a week, serving though schools, day care centers, police departments, hospitals and other nonprofit and public organizations to help meet critical community needs. RSVP offers maximum flexibility and choice to its volunteers. RSVP matches the personal interests and skills to older Americans with opportunities to help solve community problems and offer supplemental insurance while on duty, on-the-job training from the agency or organization where volunteers are placed.

1307 RSVP Niagara County

1302 Main Street
Niagara Falls, NY 14301-1118
716-285-8224
Fax: 716-285-8232
www.hanci.com

Prisiclla Dolling, Director

The Retired and Senior Volunteer Program (RSVP) provides opportunities for people 55 and over to make a difference in their community through volunteer service. RSVP volunteers contribute anywhere from a few to over forty hours a week, serving though schools, day care centers, police departments, hospitals and other nonprofit and public organizations to help meet critical community needs. RSVP offers maximum flexibility and choice to its volunteers. RSVP matches the personal interests and skills to older Americans with opportunities to help solve community problems and offer supplemental insurance while on duty, on-the-job training from the agency or organization where volunteers are placed.

1308 RSVP Oneida County

220 Memorial Parkway
Utica, NY 13501
315-223-3973
Fax: 315-223-3975
www.oneida.countyrsvp.org

Kari Johnson, Director

Provides opportunities for people 55 and over to make a difference in their community through volunteer service. RSVP volunteers contribute anywhere form a few to over forty hours a week, serving through schools, day care centers, police departments, hospitals and other nonprofit and public organizations to help meet critical community needs. RSVP matches the personal interests and skills of older Americans with opportunities to help solve community problems and offers supplemental insurance while on duty, on-the-job training from the agency or organization where volunteers are placed.

1309 RSVP Orange County

40 Matthews Street,
Suite 104
Goshen, NY 10924

845-291-4000
Fax: 845-346-1191
ofa@co.orange.ny.us
www.orangecountygov.com

L Stephen Brescia, Chairman
Malissa Bonacic, Majority Leader
Jeffry D. Berkmen, Minority Leader

The Retired and Senior Volunteer Program (RSVP) provides opportunities for people 55 and over to make a difference in their community through volunteer service. RSVP volunteers contribute anywhere from a few to over forty hours a week, serving thourgh schools, day care centers, police departments, hospitals and other nonprofit and public organizations to help meet critical community needs. RSVP offers maximum flexibility and choice to its volunteers. RSVP matches the personal interests and skills to older Americans with opportunities to help solve community problems and offer supplemental insurance while on duty, on-the-job training from the agency or organization where volunteers are placed.

1310 RSVP Putnam County
110 Old Route 6
Building One
Carmel, NY 10512-2119
845-621-0600
Fax: 845-621-0800

Mary White, Director

The Retired and Senior Volunteer Program (RSVP) provides opportunities for people 55 and over to make a difference in their community through volunteer service. RSVP volunteers contribute anywhere from a few to over forty hours a week, serving thourgh schools, day care centers, police departments, hospitals and other nonprofit and public organizations to help meet critical community needs. RSVP offers maximum flexibility and choice to its volunteers. RSVP matches the personal interests and skills to older Americans with opportunities to help solve community problems and offer supplemental insurance while on duty, on-the-job training from the agency or organization where volunteers are placed.

1311 RSVP Rockland County
185 North Main Street
Spring Valley, NY 10977
845-356-6818
Fax: 845-574-4498
gzabusky@sunyrockland.edu
www.sunyrockland.edu/rsvp

Gerri Zabusky, Director

RSVP of Rockland County's mission is to match senior volunteers' skills with the needs of local nonprofit agencies.

1312 RSVP Schuyler County
323 Owego St
Unit 5
Montour Falls, NY 14865-9602
607-535-8242
Fax: 607-535-6270

Dick Evans, Director

The Retired and Senior Volunteer Program (RSVP) provides opportunities for people 55 and over to make a difference in their community through volunteer service. RSVP volunteers contribute anywhere from a few to over forty hours a week, serving thourgh schools, day care centers,

police departments, hospitals and other nonprofit and public organizations to help meet critical community needs. RSVP offers maximum flexibility and choice to its volunteers. RSVP matches the personal interests and skills to older Americans with opportunities to help solve community problems and offer supplemental insurance while on duty, on-the-job training from the agency or organization where volunteers are placed.

1313 RSVP Suffolk County
1 West Main Street
Smithtown, NY 11787-2629
631-979-9490
Fax: 631-979-9320
director@rsvpsuffolk.org
www.rsvpsuffolk.org

Pegi Orsino, Director
Betty Dsimone, Executive Assistant
Monica Hall, Bookkeeper

The Retired and Senior Volunteer Program (RSVP) provides opportunities for people 55 and over to make a difference in their community through volunteer service. RSVP volunteers contribute anywhere from a few to over forty hours a week, serving thourgh schools, day care centers, police departments, hospitals and other nonprofit and public organizations to help meet critical community needs. RSVP offers maximum flexibility and choice to its volunteers. RSVP matches the personal interests and skills to older Americans with opportunities to help solve community problems and offer supplemental insurance while on duty, on-the-job training from the agency or organization where volunteers are placed.

1314 RSVP Tompkins County
Lifelong
121 W Court Street
Ithaca, NY 14850-4105
607-273-1511
Fax: 607-272-8060
rsvp@tclifelong.org
www.tclifelong.org

Lillian Hartman, Director

Helps connect interested adults age 55 and older without volunteer opportunities in Tompkins County. RSVp offers supplemental auto and liability insurance and optional travel reimbursement for volunteers and hosts annual recognition events.

1315 RSVP Wayne-Seneca-Ontario
159 Montezuma Street
Lyons, NY 14489-1228
315-946-7530
Fax: 315-946-7430
carm.krueger@waynecap.org

Annette Hawver, Director

The Retired and Senior Volunteer Program (RSVP) provides opportunities for people 55 and over to make a difference in their community through volunteer service. RSVP volunteers contribute anywhere from a few to over forty hours a week, serving thourgh schools, day care centers, police departments, hospitals and other nonprofit and public organizations to help meet critical community needs. RSVP offers maximum flexibility and choice to its volunteers. RSVP matches the personal interests and skills to older Americans with opportunities to help solve community problems and offer supplemental insurance while on

duty, on-the-job training from the agency or organization where volunteers are placed.

1316 Railroad Retirement Board-New York City

844 North Rush Street
Chicago, IL 60611
212-264-9820
Fax: 212-264-1687; *Toll Free:* 877-772-5772
newyork@rrb.gov
www.rrb.gov
TTY: 312-751-4701

An independent agency in the executive branch of the Federal Government whos primary function is to administer comprehensive retirement-survivor and unemployment-sickness benefit programs for the nations railroad workers and their families.

1317 Railroad Retirement Board: Albany District Office

O'Brien Federal Building Room 264
11 A Clinton Avenue
PO Box 529
Albany, NY 12207-2399
518-431-4004
Fax: 518-431-4000; *Toll Free:* 877-772-5772
albany@rrb.gov
www.rrb.gov/field/do_alba.asp

Daniel Layton, Representative

An independent agency in the executive branch of the Federal Government, whos primary function is to administer comprehensive retirement-survivor and unemployment-sickness benefit programs for the nations railroad workers and their families.

1318 Railroad Retirement Board: Buffalo New York District Office

186 Exchange Street
Suite 110
Buffalo, NY 14202-2303
716-551-4141
Fax: 716-551-3802; *Toll Free:* 877-772-5772
buffalo@rrb.gov

Philip C Dissek, Representative

An independent agency in the executive branch of the Federal Government whos primary function is to administer comprehensive retirement-supervisor and unemployment-sickness benefit programs for the natio's railroad workers and their families.

1319 Railroad Retirement Board: Syracuse New York District Office

1400 Old Country Road
Suite 204
Westbury, NY 11590-5156
516-334-5940
Fax: 516-334-4763
westbruy@rrb.gov

Marie Baran, Representative

Administering retirement/survivor and unemployment/sickness benefot programs for railroad workers and their families.

1320 Ready Willing & Able

The Doe Fund
232 East 84th Street
New York, NY 10028-2902
212-628-5207
Fax: 212-249-5589
www.doe.org

George McDonald, President/Founder
Harriet Karr-Mcdonald, Executive Vice President
John McDonald, Chief Operating Officer

Mission is to develop and impliment cost-effective, holistic programs that meet the needs of a diverse population working to break the cycles of homelessness, addiction, and criminal recidivism.

1321 Rensselaer County Department for the Aging

Ned Pattison Rensselaer County
1600 7th Avenue
Troy, NY 12180-3410
518-270-2730
Fax: 518-270-2736
www.rensco.com/departments_aging.asp

Paul Tazbir, Director
Joseph Cybulski, Manager

The primary goal of the Department is to provide a network of supportive and preventive services, which enable the County's elderly to maintain themselves productively and independently within the community.

1322 Rockland County Center for the Physically Handicapped

Jawonio Vocational Center
260 S Little Tor Road
New City, NY 10956-1616
845-634-4648
Fax: 845-634-7731
jawonio@jawonio.org
www.jawonio.org
TTY: 845-634-4672

Esther White, Contact
Paul Tendler, Administrator

Mission is to advance the independence, well-being and equality of people with disabilities or special needs.

1323 Rockland County Office for the Aging

Dr Robert Yeager Health Center
Building B
Pomona, NY 10970
845-364-2110
Fax: 845-364-2348
www.rocklandgov.com/departments/aging

June F Molof, Director

Serves the senior population of Rockland County by promoting a comprehensive and coordinated system of needed services in a high quality, ethical, courteous, timely and cost effective manner.

1324 Saratoga County Office for the Aging

152 West High Street
Ballston Spa, NY 12020-1029
518-884-4100
Fax: 518-884-4104
scross@saratogacountyny.gov
www.saratogacountyny.gov

Sandra Cross, Director

Provides information designed for Older New Yorkers and their families and those concerned about providing iopportunities and srevices to enrich the lives of older people and support their independence.

1325 Schenectady County Office for the Aging
107 Nott Terrace
Suite 202
Schenectady, NY 12307
518-382-8481
Fax: 518-382-0194
www.schenectadycounty.com

Laurie Bacheldor, Manager

Mission is to help older New Yorkers to be as independent as possible for as long as possible through advocacy, development, and delivery of person-centered, consumer-oriented, and cost-effective policies.

1326 Schoharie County Office for the Aging
113 Park Place
Suite 3
Schoharie, NY 12157
518-295-2001
Fax: 518-295-2015
www.schohairecounty-ny.us

R Carol Coltrain, Director

The Schoharie County Office for the Aging is committed to meeting the special needs of Schoharie County's senior population and friends who care for them. Schoharie County Office for the Aging offers service directly or through sub contracts, designed to maintain the quality of life to those age 60 and over.

1327 Schuyler County Office for the Aging
323 Owego Street
Unit 7
Montour Falls, NY 14865
607-535-7108
Fax: 607-535-6832
ofa@co.schuyler.ny.us
www.schuylercounty.us/aging.htm

Tammy Waite, Director
Sheila LaFever, Deputy Director

Mission is to assist our senior population in enhancing their lives by promoting financial security, physical and emotional well-being, and self-sufficiency throughout their lives. This is achieved through innovative programs and services, education, advocacy, identifying and addressing needs and community collaboration.

1328 Seneca County Office for the Aging
Seneca County Office Building
One DiPronio Drive
Waterloo, NY 13165-1680
315-539-1765
Fax: 315-539-9479; Toll Free: 800-688-7188
www.co.seneca.ny.us

Angela M Reardon, Director

Provides services both directly and subcontract for Seneca County residents 60 years of age and older.

1329 Senior Action in a Gay Environment
307 7th Avenue
15th Floor
New York, NY 10001-6008

212-741-2247
Fax: 212-366-1947
info@sageusa.org
www.sageusa.org

Michael Adams, Executive Director
Kenneth Cox, Sr Director of Development
Robert Espinoza, Sr Director of Communications

The nation's largest and oldest social service and advocacy organization dedicated to LGBT seniors. SAGE serves New York City's senior LGBT population with social services, recreational programs, and community organizing, and provides advocacy and education about LGBT aging issues nationwide.

1330 St. Lawrence County Office for the Aging
80 State Highway 310
Suite 7
Canton, NY 13617
315-386-4730
Fax: 315-386-8636
nrobert@stlawco.org
www.co.st-lawrence.ny.us

Nancy Robert, Department Head

Provides service and advocacy for county residents 60 years and older.

1331 St. Regis Mohawk Office for the Aging
St Regis Mohawk Indian Reservation
29 Business Park Road
Hogansburg, NY 13655
518-358-2963
Fax: 518-358-3071
www.aging.state.ny.us

Cynthia Tarbell, Director

The leader relative to all aging issues on behalf of all persons on the Saint Regis Mohawk Indian Reservation by helping the community plan for an aging poulation. This is done through advocacy, planning, and the development and of the delivery of enhanced services which support and empower the elderly and their families.

1332 Steuben County Office for the Aging
3 E Pulteney Square
Bath, NY 14810-1636
607-664-2298
Fax: 607-776-7813; Toll Free: 866-221-7324
ofainfo@co.steuben.ny.us
www.steubencounty.org

Michael Keane, Director

Designated by the State of New York to plan and coordinate services to meet the needs of our country's older residents.

1333 Suffolk County Office for the Aging
100 Veterans Memorial Highway
PO Box 6100
Hauppauge, NY 11788-5402
631-853-8200
Fax: 031-853-8225
aging.office@suffolkcountyny.gov
www.co.suffolk.ny.us

Holly Rhodes-Teague, Director
Steve Levy, County Executive

The Suffolk County Office for the Aging is the designated Area Agency. For over 30 years, Suffolk County Office for the Aging has administered federal, state and county programs for persons 60 years of age and older.

1334 Sullivan County Office for the Aging
100 North Street
PO Box 5012
Monticello, NY 12701-5192
845-794-3000
Fax: 845-794-7409
james.lyttle@co.sullivan.ny.us

Deborah Allen, Director

The primary objective of the Office of the Aging is be the lead advocate for the older population of Sullivan County.

1335 Tioga Opportunities Department on Aging
231 Main Street
Owego, NY 13827-1628
607-687-4120
Fax: 607-687-4147
www.tiogaopp.org

Kathleen L Horner, Executive Director

Mission is to advance self-sufficiency, well being, and growth of individuals, families and communities through human services, education, advocacy and resources.

1336 Warren Hamilton Counties Office for the Aging
333 Glen Street
Third Floor Suite 306
Glens Falls, NY 12801-3548
518-761-6347
Fax: 518-745-7643; *Toll Free:* 866-805-3931
www.co.warren.ny.us
TTY: 518-662-1220

Christie Sabo, Director
Christine Little, Service Coordinator
Deborah Coalts, Nutrition Coordinator

The Warren-Hamilton Counties Office for the Aging is a bi-county governmental agency dedicated to maintaining seniors' independence and dignity. The OFA advocates for seniors and their families, providing support services, education and assistance in accessing available services.

1337 Washington County Office for the Aging
Municipal Center Building B
383 Broadway
Fort Edward, NY 12828
518-746-2420
Fax: 518-746-2418; *Toll Free:* 800-848-3303
www.co.washington.ny.us

Claire Murphy, Director

1338 Washington County Office for the Aging/Aging + Disabilities Resource Center
Municipal Center Building B
383 Broadway
Fort Edward, NY 12828
518-746-2420
Fax: 518-746-2418; *Toll Free:* 800-848-3303
www.co.washington.ny.us

Gina Cantanucci-Mitchell, Director

Committed to service, education and advocacy to meet the needs of the Washington County Seniors.

1339 Wayne County Department of Aging & Youth
1519 Nye Road
Suite 300
Lyons, NY 14489-9133
315-946-5624
Fax: 315-946-5649
aging@co.wayne.ny.us
www.co.wayne.ny.us

Martin Williams, Deputy Aging Director
Kathy McGonigal, Deputy Youth Director

The Department of Aging and Youth is committed to serve under 21 and over 60 residents of Wayne County. The department's primary goals are to foster independence, mediate problems, and advocate for services to enhance the quality of life for old and young populations with allocated State, County and Federal Funds in accordance to policies and guidelines.

1340 Wyoming County Office for the Aging
8 Perry Avenue
Warsaw, NY 14569-1329
585-786-8833
Fax: 585-786-8832; *Toll Free:* 800-836-0067
officeaging@wyomingco.net
www.wyomingco.net

Sabrina Pribek, Director
A D Berwanger, Chairman/Board

Serve residents of Wyoming County aged 60 and older by helping the frail and elderly who choose to remain at home by providing home and community based services.

1341 Yates County Office for the Aging
417 Liberty Street
Suite 2122
Penn Yan, NY 14527-1100
315-536-5515
Fax: 315-536-8987
socialservices@yatescounty.org
www.yatescounty.org

Nancy Gates, Commissioner

Services for the aging.

North Carolina

1342 Albemarle Commission
512 South Church Street
PO Box 646
Hertford, NC 27944
252-426-5753
Fax: 252-426-8482
www.albemarlecommission.org

Bert Banks, Executive Director
Ruth Mengel, Office Manager
Stephenie Humphries, Finance Director

Funds aging services in Camden, Chowan, Gates, Byde, Pasquotank, Perquimans and Washington counties.

1343 Camden County Senior Center
117 North Highway 343
PO Box 190
Camden, NC 27921
252-338-1919
Fax: 252-331-5621
msawyer@camdencountync.gov
www.camdencountync.gov

Michaelene P Sawyer, Director/Nutrition Site Manager

Sponsors congregate lunches and home delivered lunches five days a week for seniors 60+. Offers a complete exercise room for 50+ along with other activities such as table games, Senior Games, and crafts classes. Information and referral is available for legal aid services, Medicaid and Medicare along with Medicare PDP and health insurance, tax assistance. Telephone reassurance program for Camden County. Offers day trips to local areas of interest and weekend trips.

1344 Centralina Area: Agency on Aging

525 North Tryon Street
12th Floor
Charlotte, NC 28202
704-372-2416
Fax: 704-347-4710
dgartman@centralina.org
www.centralinaaging.org
TDD 704-372-2416

Dawn Gartman, Aging Specialist

Serves North Carolinians 60+ and older in Anson, Cabarrus, Goston, Irechell, Lincoln, Meddenburg, Rowan, Stanley and Union counties. Our goal is to provide assistance for older adults to stay independent as long as possible and identify needed resources to maintain quality of life.

1345 Disability Determination Services

PO Box 243
Raleigh, NC 27602
919-212-3222
Fax: 800-804-5509; *Toll Free:* 800-443-9360
tracy.gray@ssa.gov
www.dds.its.state.nc.us

Tracy Gray, Dtermination Specialist

Ajudicates the claims of persons filing for disability benefits with the Social Security Administration.

1346 Eastern Carolina Council of Governments

P.O. Box 1717
233 Middle Street, 3rd Floor
New Bern, NC 28563-1717
252-638-3185
Fax: 252-638-3187
eccadmin@eccog.org
www.eccog.org

Shane Turney, President
Jay Bender, 1st Vice President
Bill Taylor, 2nd Vice President

Misssion is to improve the region's quality of life by providing planning, economic development and senior servicesto local governments and area residents by maximizing resources and collarborating regionally.

Year Founded: 1977

1347 Granville County Senior Center

119 Hilltop Village
Oxford, NC 27565
919-693-1930
Fax: 919-693-5358
kathy.may@granvillecounty.org
www.granvillecounty.org

Kathy B May, Director/Senior Services

Mission is to provide a sense of community, overall health and independence for older adults.

1348 High Country: Area Agency on Aging

468 New Market Blvd
PO Box 1820
Boone, NC 28607-1820
828-265-5434
Fax: 828-265-5439
regiondcog@regiond.org
www.regiond.org

Rick Herndon, Executive Director
Anita Davie, Director
Beth Norris, Finance Director

The Area Agency on Aging plans, administers and advocates for the development of a comprehensive service delivery system to meet short and long-term needs of the elderly in this region. The following Counties are served: Alleghany, Ashe, Avery, Mitchell, Watauga, Wilkes, and Yancey.

1349 Isothermal Planning & Development Commission

111 West Court Street
Rutherfordton, NC 28139
828-287-2281
Fax: 828-287-2735
www.regionc.org

Laura Lynch, Area on Aging Director
Lori Simpson, Aging Specialist
David Bess, Rehabilitation Specialist

A regional council for Region C in western North Carolina. IPDC seeks to serve its members, and their citizens, by fostering regional collaboration and by providing professional and technical expertise.

1350 Jackson County Department on Aging

100 County Services Park
PO Box 596
Sylva, NC 28779-5411
828-586-8562
Fax: 828-586-1120
aging@jacksonnc.org
www.aging.jacksonnc.org

Helen Bryson, Director

Provides services and assistance to the elderly.

1351 KerrTar Regional: Area Agency on Aging

1724 Graham Avenue
PO Box 709
Henderson, NC 27536
252-436-2040
Fax: 252-436-2055; *Toll Free:* 866-506-6223
info@kerrtarcog.org
www.kerrtarcog.org

Diane Cox, Executive Director
Jillian Hardin, AAA Director
Gina Parham, Office Manager

Offers a wide range of services to help senior citizens live independently in their homes and communities for as long as possible.

Year Founded: 1971; Number of Members: 40

1352 McDowell Council on Aging

County Administration Building
60 East Court Street
Marion, NC 28752-1162
828-652-4240
www.mcdowellgov.com

David Walker, Chairman
Barry McPeters, Vice Chairman

Promotes understanding of the special needs of older persons. Provides advocacy, information and referral, and other services.

1353 Meals on Wheels of Rowan

1918 West Innes Street
Po Box 1914
Salisbury, NC 28145-1914
704-633-0352
Fax: 704-638-6248
mealsonwheels@velocenet.net
www.mowrowannc.org

Kathy Rummage, Executive Administrator

Volunteers working to serve a hot noonday meal to the homebound and elderly.

1354 Mid-Carolina: Area Agency on Aging
Old Cumberland County Courthouse

130 Gillespie Street, 3rd Floor
PO Box 1510
Fayetteville, NC 28302-1510
910-323-4191
Fax: 252-323-9330; *Toll Free:* 800-662-7030
www.mccog.org

James Caldwell, Executive Director
Tracy Honeycutt Davis, Referral Specialist
Denise Day, Development Director

Provides a wide variety of programs and services to their local governments and citizens. Provides technical assistance services to its member governments including land use planning, zoning administration, subdivision and zoning ordinances, water and sewer studies, annexation reviews, and community development workshops on timely issues.

1355 Mid-East Carolina: Area Agency on Aging

1385 John Small Avenue
PO Box 1787
Washington, NC 27889-1787
252-946-8043
Fax: 252-974-1852
cdavis@mideastcom.org
www.mecaaa.org

Annette Eubanks, Director
Carol Ward, Administrative Assistaant
Beth Harrell, Aging Specialist

Established to advocate for older adults through planning, training, technical assistance, and resource development.

1356 North Carolina Assistive Technology Projects

1110 Navaho Drive
Suite 101
Raleigh, NC 27609-7322
919-850-2787
Fax: 919-850-2792
rhiatt@ncatp.org
www.ncatp.org

Toni Hiatt, Executive Director

A federally funded grant whose mission is to improve and expand access to assistive technology for North Carolinians of all ages and disability types. The project works in the areas of training, education, device try out, technical assistance, peer support and access to information. The project works to change systems which impede access to technology for people with disabilities. The project hosts an annual statewide expo featuring vendor exhibiits and training workshops.

1357 North Carolina Association of Long Term Care Facilities

4010 Barrett Drive
Suite 102
Raleigh, NC 27609-6622
919-787-3560
Fax: 919-783-5415; *Toll Free:* 888-622-5823
www.ncaltcf.com

Lou Wilson, Executive Director

Rest home operators and employees, social workers, and other interested persons. Works to improve the care and service given by homes for the aged and family care homes.

1358 North Carolina Association of Nonprofit Homes for the Aging

100 Carolina Meadows
Chapel Hill, NC 27517
919-571-8333
Fax: 919-571-1297
www.leadingagenc.org

David Piner, President
Pat Sprigg, Chief Executive Officer
Anne Moffat, Executive Director

State association of not-for-profit providers dedicated to providing quality care, housing, health, community and related services to the elderly.

1359 North Carolina Client Assistance Program
Division of Rehabilitation Services

2806 Mail Service Center
805 Ruggles Drive
Raleigh, NC 27699-2806
919-855-3600
Fax: 919-715-2456; *Toll Free:* 800-215-7227
nccap@dhhs.nc.gov
cap.state.nc.us

John Marens, Director
Sharon Wisner, Client Advocate
Diane Rawdanowicz, Client Advocate

The North Carolina Client Assistance Program (CAP) is a federally funded program designed to assist individuals with disabilities in understanding and using rehabilitation services.

1360 North Carolina Council on Developmental Disabilities

3125 Polarwood Court
Suite 200
Raleigh, NC 27607-2969
919-850-2901
Fax: 919-850-2915; *Toll Free:* 800-357-6916
info@nccdd.org
www.nc-ddc.org

Holly Riddle, Executive Director
Joann Toomey, Operations Director
Kelly Bohlander, Program Director

Mission is to ensure that people with developmental disabilities and their families participate in the design of and have access to culturally competent services and supports, as well as other assistance and opportunities, which promote inclusive communities.

1361 North Carolina Department of Administration: Advocacy Council for Persons with Disabilities

2626 Glenwood Avenue
Suite 550
Raleigh, NC 27608
919-856-2195
Fax: 877-235-4210; *Toll Free:* 877-235-4210
info@disabilityrightsnc.org
www.gacpd.com
TTY: 888-268-5535

Allison Bowen, Executive Director

Mission is to protect the legal rights of people with disabilities through individual and systems advocacy.

1362 North Carolina Department of Human Resources: Services for the Blind

2601 Mail Service Center
309 Ashe Avenue
Raleigh, NC 27699-2601
919-733-9822
Fax: 919-733-9769; *Toll Free:* 866-222-1546
www.dhhs.state.nc.us

Eddie Weaver, Executive Director
Mary Flanagan, Assistant Director
Marvin Gilmore, Administrator

Provides efficient services that enhance the quality of life of North Carolina individuals and families so that they have opportunities for healthier and safer lives resulting ultimately in the achievement of economic and personal independence.

1363 North Carolina Department of Revenue

PO Box 25000
501 North Wilmington Street
Raleigh, NC 27640-0640
919-733-3991
Fax: 919-733-5750
www.dor.state.nc.us

David Hoyle, Secretary Of Revenue

To administer the tax laws and collect the taxes due the state in an impartial, uniform, and efficient manner.

1364 North Carolina Department of the State: Treasurer Division of Retirement Systems

325 N Salisbury Street
1st Floor
Raleigh, NC 27603-1388
919-508-5176
Fax: 919-508-5350
nc.retirement@nctreasurer.com
www.nctreasurer.com

Janet Cowell, Treasurer

Serves the people of North Carolina through a variety of functions related to the financial health of the state and its citizenry.

1365 North Carolina Industrial Commission

4340 Mail Service Center
Raleigh, NC 27699-4340
919-807-2500
Fax: 919-715-0282
www.ic.nc.gov

Pamela Young, Chairperson
Bernadine Ballance, Commissioner
Linda Cheatham, Commissioner

Mission is to effectively and fairly administer the Workers' Compensation Act for the state of North Carolina.

1366 North Carolina Retired Government Employees Association

528 Wade Avenue
Po Box 10561
Raleigh, NC 27605
919-834-4622
Fax: 919-834-4622; *Toll Free:* 800-356-1190
info@ncrgea.com
www.ncrgea.com

Ed Regan, Executive Director

Protects the general welfare of its members. Conducts lobbying.

1367 North Carolina Senior Citizens Association

PO Box 34
Fayetteville, NC 28302
910-323-3641
Fax: 910-323-4343; *Toll Free:* 800-323-6525
www.ncseniorcitizens.org

Dennis Streets, Director

Mission is building a better quality of life for the 50+ generation in North Carolina.

1368 North Carolina: Area Agency on Aging

2101 Mail Service Center
Taylor Hall, 693 Palmer Drive
Raleigh, NC 27699-2101
919-733-3983
Fax: 919-733-0443
www.ncdhhs.gov/aging

Dennis Streets, Division Director
Nancy Warren, Adult Services Administrator
Leslee Breen, Senior Center Development

Mission is to promote independence and enhance the dignity of North Carolina's older adults, persons with disabilities, and their families through a community-based system of opportunities, services, benefits, and protections, to ready younger generations to enjoy their later years, and to help society and government plan and prepare for the changing demographics.

1369 Piedmont Triad Regional Council

2216 West Meadowview Drive
Suite 201
Greensboro, NC 27407-3480
336-294-4950
Fax: 336-632-0457
info@ptrc.org
www.ptrc.org

Kimberly Dawkins Berry, Executive Director

Mission is to ensure maximum options and opportunities exist for a quality of life for older adults through advocacy, planning, training, resource development and technical assistance.

1370 Railroad Retirement Board: North Carolina District Office
Quorum Business Park
844 North Rush Street
Chicago, IL 60611
212-264-9820
Fax: 212-264-1687; *Toll Free:* 877-772-5772
www.rrb.gov
TDD 312-751-4701

Shelia P Gary, Representative

An independent agency in the executive branch of the Federal Government. The RRB'S primary function is to administer comprehensive retirement-survivor, and unemployment-sickness benefit programs for the nations railroad workers and thier families.

1371 Retired Military Police Association
PO Box 25343
Fayetteville, NC 28314-5005
910-867-4292

Mack H Mullins, Executive Director

An informal group of retired military officers, warrant officers, and their spouses.

1372 Richmond County Council on the Aging
225 S Lawrence Street
PO Box 340
Rockingham, NC 28379-3633
910-997-4491
jacqueline.braddock@ncmail.net
www.ncdhhs.gov

Jacqueline Adkins, Executive Director

Provides services to county residents aged 60 years and older.

1373 Upper Coastal Plain: Area Agency on Aging
1309 S Wesleyan Boulevard
PO Box 2748
Rocky Mount, NC 27802
252-446-0411
Fax: 252-446-5651
ww.ucpcog.org

Greg T Godard, Executive Director

The AAA serves a five-county region; Edgecombe, Halifax, Nash, Northampton and Wilson Counties. Our agency coordinates services that help serve adults that remain in their homes-if that is their preference.

1374 Volunteer Center of Greater Durham
136 E Chapel Hill Street
PO Box 3374
Durham, NC 27701-3202
919-613-5109
main@thevolunteercenter.org
www.thevolunteercenter.org

Kim Shaw, Executive Director
Rebekah Haithcock, Youth Prgrams Coordinator
Betsy Voorhees, Program Coordinator

A non-profit organization that enriches the Durham community and the lives of its residents, through volunteerism. Our mission is to connect people of all ages with opportunities to serve, to provide community agencies with essen-

tial resources and training, and to coordinate programs that raise awareness of and impact local needs.

1375 Western Piedmont Council of Governments
Area Agency on Aging
736 4th Street SW
Po Box 9026
Hickory, NC 28602-3401
828-322-9191
Fax: 828-322-5991
director@wpcog.org
www.wpcogaaa.org

H Dewitt Blackwell, Executive Director

The Western Piedmont Area Agency on Aging (AAA) is an organization working on behalf of older adults and their families in Alexander, Burke, Caldwell, and Catawba Counties, North Carolina.

North Dakota

1376 North Dakota Aging Services
1237 W Divide Avenue
Suite 6
Bismarck, ND 58501
701-328-4601
Fax: 701-328-8744; *Toll Free:* 800-451-8693
dhsaging@nd.gov
www.nd.gov/dhs/services/adultsaging
TTY: 800-366-6888

Jan Engan, Executive Director

Aging services division of the North Dakota Department of Human Services.

1377 North Dakota Client Assistance Program
Wells Fargo Bank Building
400 East Braodway, Suite 409
Bismarck, ND 58501-1208
701-328-2950
Fax: 701-328-3934; *Toll Free:* 800-472-2670
www.nd.gov/cap
TDD 701-328-8968

David Boeck, Director
Judy DeWitz, Advocate
Vickay Gross, Program Coordinator

Assists clients and client applicants of North Dakota Vocational Rehabilitation services, Tribal Vocational Rehabilitation, or Independent Living Services.

1378 North Dakota Department of Veterans Affairs
4201 38th Street SW
Suite 104
Fargo, ND 58106-9003
701-239-7165
Fax: 701-239-7166; *Toll Free:* 866-634-8387
lwangen@nd.gov
www.nd.gov/veterans

Lonnie Wangen, Commissioner

The mission is to assist all veterans of North Dakota and their dependents in obtaining all beneifts to which they are entitled, both federal and state either by direct contact or through the assistance of the County and Tribal Veterans Service Officers.

1379 North Dakota Protection & Advocacy
Wells Fargo Bank Building
400 E Broadway
Suite 409
Bismarck, ND 58501-4071
701-328-2950
Fax: 701-328-3934; *Toll Free:* 800-472-2670
panda@nd.gov
www.ndpanda.org
TDD 800-366-6888

David Boeck, Executive Director

The Protection and Advocacy Project (P&A) is a state agency whose purpose is to advocate for, and protect the legal rights of, people with disabilities.

1380 North Dakota Public Employees Retirement System
4201 38th Street South
Suite 104
Fargo, ND 58106-9003
701-239-7165
Fax: 701-239-7166; *Toll Free:* 866-634-8387
ndpers-info@nd.gov
www.nd.gov.ndpers

Sparb Collins, Executive Director
Kathy Allen, Benefits Manager
Cindy Aaser, Benefits Specialist

Mission is to design, communicate and efficiently administer a viable benefits program within a framework of prudent risk-taking, applicable state and federal laws, and professional and ethical standards so as to provide an employee benefit package that is among the best availiable from public and private employers in the upper Midwest.

1381 North Dakota State Council on Developmental Disabilities
1237 W Divide Ave, Suite 3
Dept 325
Bismarck, ND 58501
701-328-4847
Fax: 701-328-8969
www.ndcpd.org/scdd/

Cheryl Hess, Executive Director
Mary Simonson, Service Provider

The Council advocates for policy changes that promote choice, independence, productivity, and inclusion for all North Dakotans with developmental disabilities. The Council supports projects and activities that maximize opportunities in these areas for consumers and families.

1382 North Dakota State Tax Department
600 E Boulevard Avenue
PO Box 5621
Bismarck, ND 58506-5021
701-328-2770
Fax: 701-328-3700; *Toll Free:* 877-328-7088
taxinfo@nd.gov
www.ndgov/tax
TDD 800-366-6888

Cory Fong, Tax Commissioner

Mission is to fairly and effectively administer the tax laws of North Dakota.

1383 North Dakota Teachers Retirement Fund
1930 Burnt Boat Drive
1930 Burnt Boat Drive
PO Box 7100
Bismarck, ND 58507-7100
701-328-9885
Fax: 701-328-9897; *Toll Free:* 800-952-2970
www.nd.gov/rio

Steve Chochrane, Executive Director

Mission is to advocate for, develop, and administer a comprehensive retirement program for all trust fund members within the resources availiable.

1384 North Dakota Workforce Safety And Insurance
1600 East Century Avenue
Suite 1
Bismarck, ND 58503-0644
701-328-3800
Fax: 701-328-3820; *Toll Free:* 800-777-5033
ndwsi@nd.gov
www.workforcesafety.com
TDD 701-328-3786

Dr. Luis Vilella, Medical Director

Mission is to serve North Dakota workers and employers by innovatively providing superior workers compensation and safety services.

1385 RSVP Central North Dakota
1223 South 12th Street
Suite 4
Bismarck, ND 58504-6626
701-258-5436
Fax: 701-258-6771
julie.eikamp@ndsu.edu
www.rsvp.ndsu.nodak.edu

Mary Silverson, Project Director

The Retired and Senior Volunteer Program (RSVP) provides opportunities for people 55 and over to make a difference in their community through volunteer service. RSVP volunteers contribute anywhere from a few to over forty hours a week, serving thourgh schools, day care centers, police departments, hospitals and other nonprofit and public organizations to help meet critical community needs. RSVP offers maximum flexibility and choice to its volunteers. RSVP matches the personal interests and skills to older Americans with opportunities to help solve community problems and offer supplemental insurance while on duty, on-the-job training from the agency or organization where volunteers are placed.

1386 RSVP Devils Lake Area
315 4th Avenue NE
Devils Lake, ND 58301-2420
701-662-6767
Fax: 701-662-6779
rsvp@stellarnet.com

Amy Hellman, Project Director

Provides opportunities for people 55 and over to make a difference in their community through volunteer service. RSVP volunteers contribute anywhere from a few to over forty hours a week, serving through schools, day care centers, police departments, hospitals and other nonprofit and public organizations to help meet critical community needs. RSVP matches the personal interests and skills of older Americans with opportunities to help solve community problems and offers supplemental insurance while on duty, on-the-job training from the agency or organization where volunteers are placed.

1387 RSVP North Central North Dakota
Trinity Hospital-St. Josephs
5th Avenue Medical Building
307 5th Ave, Suite 301
Minot, ND 58701
701-852-3799
Fax: 701-852-3799

Miriam Smette, Director

The Retired and Senior Volunteer Program (RSVP) provides opportunities for people 55 and over to make a difference in their community through volunteer service. RSVP volunteers contribute anywhere from a few to over forty hours a week, serving thourgh schools, day care centers, police departments, hospitals and other nonprofit and public organizations to help meet critical community needs. RSVP offers maximum flexibility and choice to its volunteers. RSVP matches the personal interests and skills to older Americans with opportunities to help solve community problems and offer supplemental insurance while on duty, on-the-job training from the agency or organization where volunteers are placed.

1388 Railroad Retirement Board: North Dakota District Office
844 North Rush Street
Chicago, IL 60611
212-264-9820
Fax: 212-264-1687; Toll Free: 877-772-5772
fargo@rrb.gov
www.rrb.gov
TDD 312-751-4701

Debbie M Heibling, Representative

An independent agency in the federal branch of the Federal Government. The RRB's primary function is to administer comprehensive retirement-survivor and unemployment-sickness benefit programs for the nation's railroad workers and their families.

Ohio

1389 Agency on Aging, Public Service Area
40 W Second St
Suite 400
Dayton, OH 45402
937-341-3000
Fax: 937-341-3005; Toll Free: 800-258-7277
AAA@info4seniors.org
www.info4seniors.org

Douglas McGarry, Director

Provides information and services to older persons and their caregivers in a nine county area in West Central Ohio.

Year Founded: 1993

1390 Alzheimer's Association: Greater Cincinnati
225 N. Michigan Ave.
Flr. 17
Chicago, IL 60601-7633
312-335-8700
Fax: 866-699-1246; Toll Free: 800-272-3900
blunkerman@alz.org

www.alz.org/cincinnati
TDD 312-335-5886

Paula Kollstedt, Executive Director
Bob Luckerman, Operations Director
Steve Olding, Communications Director

Mission is to eliminate Alzheimer's disease through the advancement of research; to provide and enhance care and support for all affected; and to reduce the risk of dementia through the promotion of brain health.

1391 Association of Ohio Philanthropic Homes for the Aging
855 S Wall Street
Columbus, OH 43206-1921
614-444-2882
Fax: 614-444-2974
www.aopha.org

John Alfano, President

Not-for-profit providers of senior services including senior housing, both subsidized and market rate, adult day care, home and community-based services, assisted living and skilled nursing.

1392 Buckeye Hills: Area Agency on Aging
PO Box 370
Reno, OH 45773
740-373-6400
Fax: 740-373-1594; Toll Free: 800-331-2644
info@buckeyehills.org
www.areaagency8.org

Misty Casto, Executive Director
Rick Hindman, Assistant Executive Director
Jane Skeen, Home Care Director

1393 Buckeye Hills: Area Agency on Aging 8
PO Box 370
Reno, OH 45773
740-373-6400
Fax: 740-373-1594; Toll Free: 800-331-2644
info@buckeyehills.org
www.areaagency8.org

Misty Casto, Executive Director
Rick Hindman, Assistant Executive Dir, AAA8

Advocates for and educates older adults and their caregivers and promotes home and community-based services.

1394 Bureau of Disability Determination
Ohio Rehabilitation Services Commission
400 East Campus View Drive
Columbus, OH 43235-9001
614-438-1200
Fax: 614-438-1504; Toll Free: 800-282-4536
www.rsc.ohio.gov
TTY: 800-282-4536

Kevin Miller, Director

The Bureau of Disability Determination, in agreement with the Social Security Administration, is responsible for determining medical eligibility for Ohioans, Social Security Disability Insurance (SSDI) and Supplemental Security Income (SSI) claims. Although BDD is part of the Ohio Rehabilitation Services Commission, it's federally regulated and receives 100 percent of its funding from the Social Security Administration.

1395 Canton Negro Oldtimers

1844 Ira Turpin Way NE
Canton, OH 44705-1416
330-580-9098

A community-based, non-profit organization offering a
wide variety of services in the greater Stark County area
and beyond.

1396 Carroll County Council on Aging

60788 Southgate Road
Byesville, OH 43723
740-439-4478
Fax: 740-432-1060; *Toll Free:* 800-945-4250
1119@aaa9.org
www.aaa9.org

Susan Henderson, Director

Multi-purpose senior citizen center. Serving the Carrollton,
Ohio area.

1397 Central Ohio: Area Agency on Aging

174 East Long Street
Columbus, OH 43215-4479
614-645-7250
Fax: 614-645-3884; *Toll Free:* 800-589-7277
coaaa@coaaa.org
www.coaaa.org
TTY: 614-645-6200

Cindy Farson, Director
Phillip Rollins, Associate Director/Fiscal Mgr.

Provides information, resources, and education to the community, as well as provide help at home for seniors to continue dependent living in their own homes.

1398 Cincinnati Area Senior Services

2368 Victory Parkway
Suite 300
Cincinnati, OH 45203-1720
513-721-4330
Fax: 513-721-8304
info@cassdelivers.org
www.cassdelivers.org

Tracey Collins, Executive Director
Connie Baker, Assistant Director
Jo Ann Matiingly Kells, Personnel Director

Cincinnati, Butler County, Hamilton County, Warren
County, Clermont County, Clinton County. Mission is to
promote the independence and preserve the dignity of older
adults.

1399 Columbus Volunteer Corps

City Hall W Broad Street
Room 12190
Columbus, OH 43215
614-645-6404
Fax: 614-645-5940

Pamela Farber, Administrator

Senior volunteers working for the city of Columbus, OH.

1400 Council for Older Adults

800 Cheshire Road
Delaware, OH 43015-9661
740-363-6677
Fax: 740-363-7588; *Toll Free:* 800-994-2255
info@growingolder.org
www.growingolder.org

Robert Horrocks, Executive Director
Donna Meyer, Outreach Coordinator

Plans, coordinates, and funds services and events for seniors in Delaware County, OH. Mission of the Council for
Older Adults is to improve the quality of life of the older
population of Delaware County by being a catalyst to develop, sustain and continually improve a comprehensive,
coordinated community based system of effective services
and opportunities.

1401 Disability Rights Ohio

50 West Broad Street
Suite 1400
Columbus, OH 43215-5923
614-466-7264
Fax: 614-644-1888; *Toll Free:* 800-282-9181
mkirkman@disabilityrightsohio.org
www.disabilityrightsohio.org

Michael Kirkman, Executive Director

A 501(c)(3) not for profit corporation.

1402 District 5: Area Agency on Aging

780 Park Avenue West
Mansfield, OH 44906
419-524-4144
Fax: 419-522-9482; *Toll Free:* 800-860-5799
www.agingnorthcentralohio.org

Judi Sauers, Executive Director

Mansfield, Seneca County, Wyandot County, Marion
County, Huron County, Crawford County, Morrow County,
Ashland County, Richland County, Knox County. Mission
is to provide leadership for a collaborative service and resource network that supports individual choice, independence, and dignity for older and disabled adults.

1403 District 7: Area Agency on Aging

F-32 URG
PO Box 500
Rio Grande, OH 45674-0500
740-245-5979
Fax: 740-245-5979; *Toll Free:* 800-582-7277
info@aaa7.org
www.aaa7.org
TTY: 888-270-1550

Pamela Matura, Director

The Area Agency on Aging District 7 (AAA7) administers
programs for the elderly funded by the state and federal
governments. Our mission is to identify the needs of Southern Ohioans age 60 and over. The following ten counties
are included in our District 7: Adams, Brown, Gallia, Highland, Jackson, Lawrence, Pike, Ross, Scioto, and Vinton.

1404 District 9: Area Agency on Aging

60788 Southgate Road
S.R. 209S
Byesville, OH 43723-9533
740-439-4478
Fax: 740-432-1060; *Toll Free:* 800-932-7277
info@coaaa.org
www.coaaa.org

Shirley Blackledge, Director

Assisting individuals to maintain independence and personal choice by prviding resource options and services.

1405 Highland County Senior Citizens

185 Muntz Street
Hillsboro, OH 45133-1421
937-393-4745
Fax: 937-393-8797; Toll Free: 888-350-6551
highlandseniorcenter@gmail.com
www.highlandco.org/senior

Suzanne Hopkins, Executive Director

A non-profit organization open to anyone 50 years or older, spouses may join regardless of age.

1406 Massillon Senior Citizens' Center Massilon Parks & Recreation

39 Lincoln Way West
Massillon, OH 44647-6581
330-837-2784
Fax: 330-830-2868
njohnson@massillonohio.com
www.massillonohio.com/senior/index.html

Nancy A Johnson, Director

The Massillon Senior Center is a social and recreational facility, operated by the City of Massillon, under the Department of Parks & Recreation, for the us of all Senior Citizens in western Stark County who are 55 years and older. Activites include chorus, autobiographical writing class, exercise class, bowling team, monthly membership meetings, motor coach and van trips, hot lunches, volunteer opportunities of many varieties and fun, games andparties for all occasions and seasons. The mission of the Senior Center is: To provide a pleasant place for social and recreational activities for senior citizens, to encourage their wellness and active participation for as long as they want and to provide them opportunities for community involvement.

Year Founded: 1980

1407 Maximum Independent Living

11607 Euclid Avenue
Cleveland, OH 44106-4348
440-231-7221
Fax: 440-231-8008
info@mahohio.org
www.milohio.org

Stephen Hansler, Executive Director
Beth Glas, Assistant Director
Bradley Jarvis, Housing Compliance

Mission is to develop and/or facilitate options in housing for persons with physical disabilities.

1408 Midway Community and Senior Citizens

37358 State Route 800
Graysville, OH 45734
740-934-2221
Senior services center.

1409 Muskingum County Senior Services

200 Sunrise Center Drive
Zanesville, OH 43701-3148
740-454-9761
Fax: 740-452-0984
www.mccfs.org

Terry Dunn, Executive Director
Debi Smith, Supportive Services Director
Earl Stapleton, Food Services Director

Offers services to the senior citizens of Muskingum County, OH. Seeks to alleviate institutionalization.

1410 Northwestern Ohio Area: Agency on Aging

2155 Arlington Avenue
Toledo, OH 43609-1903
419-382-0624
Fax: 419-382-4560; Toll Free: 800-472-7277
jmoor@areaofficeonaging.com
www.areaofficeonaging.com

Billie Johnson, President/CEO

Provides you and your loved ones with the quality services that allow you to be as independent as possible, empowering you to live your life to the fullest.

1411 Ohio Association of Area Agencies on Aging

88 East Broad Street
Suite 870
Columbus, OH 43215-1066
614-481-3511
Fax: 614-481-3566
oaaaa@ohioaging.org
www.ohioaging.org

Joe Ruby, President
Rick Hindman, Vice President
Duana Patton, Secretary

The Ohio Association of Area Agencies on Aging (OAAAA), a non-profit organization, is a statewide network of agencies that provide services for the elderly, as well as advocate on behalf of older Ohioans. The Association addresses issues which have an impact on the aging network, provides services to members, and serves as a collective voice for Ohio's Area Agencies on Aging.

1412 Ohio Client Assistance Program

50 West Broad Street
Suite 1400
Columbus, OH 43215-3414
614-466-7264
Fax: 614-644-1888; Toll Free: 800-282-9181
www.olrs.ohio.gov/cap-program

Carolyn Knight, Administrator

CAP advocated for people who are applying for or receiving services from the Bureau of Vocational Rehabilitation (BVR) or the Bureau of Services for the Visually Impaired (BSVI) and/or the Independent Living Centers throughout Ohio. CAP also provides informatio on Title 1 of the Americans with Disabilities Act.

1413 Ohio Department of Aging

50 W Broad Street
9th Floor
Columbus, OH 43215-3363
614-466-6191
Fax: 614-466-5741; Toll Free: 800-266-4346
odamail@age.state.oh.us
www.goldenbuckeye.com

Bonnie Kantor-Burman, Director

The department serves and represents about 2 million Ohioans age 60 and older. They advocate for the needs of all older citizens with emphasis on improving the quality of life, helping senior citizens live active, healthy, and independent lives, and promoting positive attitudes toward aging and older people. Committed to helping the frail elderly who choose to remain at home by providing home and community based services, the level of choice, inddependence and self-care.

1414 Ohio Department of Taxation
Estate Tax Division
1880 E Dublin Granville Road
Suite 200
Columbus, OH 43229-3523
614-895-6250
Fax: 614-895-6655
www.state.oh.us/tax

Joseph Testa, Treasurer

Administers Ohio's tax laws as efficiently as possible. Provides state income and business tax forms and information.

1415 Ohio Developmental Disability Council
899 East Broad Street
Suite 203r
Columbus, OH 43215-2914
614-466-5205
Fax: 614-466-0298; *Toll Free:* 800-766-7426
david.zwyer@dmr.state.oh.us
www.ddc.ohio.gov
TDD 614-644-5530

Carolyn Knight, Director
Fatica Ayers, Program
Kay Treanor, Program

The Ohio DD Council is a planning and advocacy agency that strives to improve services for people with developmental disabilities and to include them more fully in their communities. Council uses grants to model changes in services, and pursues changes on the public policy level.

1416 Ohio Disabled American Veterans
35 East Chestnut Street Suite 503
PO Box 15099
Columbus, OH 43215-4131
614-221-3582
Fax: 614-221-4822
commander@ohiodav.org
www.ohiodav.org

Dennis Hanneman, Commander
William Caine, Sr. Vice Commander
Philip Alexader, 1st Jr. Vice Commander

Provides information concerning veterans benefits in the state of Ohio.

1417 Ohio Governor's Council on People with Disabilities
400 E Campus View Boulevard
Columbus, OH 43235-4604
614-438-1391
Fax: 614-438-1274; *Toll Free:* 800-282-4536
www.rsc.ohio.gov
TDD 800-282-4536

Kevin Miller, Executive Director

Advisory body to the governor and the legislature on issues that concern Ohioans with disabilities. State liaison to President's Committee on Employment of People with Disabilities and National Organization on Disability.

1418 Ohio Protection & Advocacy Agency
50 West Broad Street
Suite 1400
Columbus, OH 43215-5923

614-466-7264
Fax: 614-644-1888; *Toll Free:* 800-282-9181
mkirkman@olrs.state.oh.us
www.disabilityrightsohio.org/padd-progra

Michael Kirkman, Executive Director

1419 Ohio Public Employees Retirement System
277 E Town Street
Columbus, OH 43215-4642
614-222-5684
Fax: 614-466-5837; *Toll Free:* 800-222-7377
benefitquestions@opers.org
www.opers.org

Karen Carraher, Executive Director
Blake Sherry, Chief Operating Officer
John Lane, Investment Director

OPERS will achieve its vision by acting in the best interest of its participants, maintaining the financial security of the trust fund, and providing exceptional service to our members, benefit recipients and employers.

1420 Ohio School Employees Retirement System
300 E Broad Street
Suite 100
Columbus, OH 43215-3746
614-222-5853
Fax: 614-222-5808; *Toll Free:* 800-878-5853
www.ohsers.org

Lisa Morris, Executive Director
Helen Nino, Deputy Executive Director

Established in 1937, the School Employees Retirement System of Ohio is the $11.6 billion statewide pension fund providing pension benefits and access to post-retirement health care coverage to Ohio's 186,500 active and retired non-teaching public school employees.

1421 Oregon Senior Citizens' Center
5760 Bayshore Road
Oregon, OH 43618-1014
419-698-7078
www.oregonohio.org/Community/senior-citi

Billie Derivan, Executive Director

Senior citizen services center.

1422 RSVP Akron
415 S Portage Path
Akron, OH 44320-2327
330-762-8645
Fax: 330-762-5571

Inez Alrarez, Director

The Retired and Senior Volunteer Program (RSVP) provides opportunities for people 55 and over to make a difference in their community through volunteer service. RSVP volunteers contribute anywhere from a few to over forty hours a week, serving thourgh schools, day care centers, police departments, hospitals and other nonprofit and public organizations to help meet critical community needs. RSVP offers maximum flexibility and choice to its volunteers. RSVP matches the personal interests and skills to older Americans with opportunities to help solve community problems and offer supplemental insurance while on duty, on-the-job training from the agency or organization where volunteers are placed.

1423 RSVP Athensns

409 W Washington Street
PO Box 852
Athens, OH 35611
256-232-7207
Fax: 256-232-8842
bruth@al-rsvp.com
www.al-rsvp.com/aboutrsvp.html

Alice Curtis, Executive Director

The Retired and Senior Volunteer Program (RSVP) provides opportunities for people 55 and over to make a difference in their community through volunteer service. RSVP volunteers contribute anywhere from a few to over forty hours a week, serving thourgh schools, day care centers, police departments, hospitals and other nonprofit and public organizations to help meet critical community needs. RSVP offers maximum flexibility and choice to its volunteers. RSVP matches the personal interests and skills to older Americans with opportunities to help solve community problems and offer supplemental insurance while on duty, on-the-job training from the agency or organization where volunteers are placed.

1424 RSVP Belmont County

410 Fox Shannon Place
St Clairsville, OH 43950
740-695-0293
Fax: 740-695-9255
jhartman@cacbelmont.org
www.cacbelmont.org

Judith Hartman, RSVP Coordinator

The Retired and Senior Volunteer Program (RSVP) provides opportunities for people 55 and over to make a difference in their community through volunteer service. RSVP volunteers contribute anywhere from a few to over forty hours a week, serving thourgh schools, day care centers, police departments, hospitals and other nonprofit and public organizations to help meet critical community needs. RSVP offers maximum flexibility and choice to its volunteers. RSVP matches the personal interests and skills to older Americans with opportunities to help solve community problems and offer supplemental insurance while on duty, on-the-job training from the agency or organization where volunteers are placed.

1425 RSVP Cincinnati Area

100 East 8th Street,
5th Flr
Cincinnati, OH 45202
513-241-7745
Fax: 513-241-4333
ccswoh.org/index.html

Michael Dutle, RSVP Director

RSVP links the skills and experiences of mature human resources with community service organization needs. We partner with mature individuals and community service organizations whose priorities include making a significant and positive difference in our community. We provide opportunities for high quality experiences that enrich the lives of volunteers.

1426 RSVP Gallia County

235 Broadway Street
Jackson, OH 45640-1701
740-286-4918
gallia.osu.edu/

Susan Rogers, Executive Director

The Retired and Senior Volunteer Program (RSVP) provides opportunities for people 55 and over to make a difference in their community through volunteer service. RSVP volunteers contribute anywhere from a few to over forty hours a week, serving thourgh schools, day care centers, police departments, hospitals and other nonprofit and public organizations to help meet critical community needs. RSVP offers maximum flexibility and choice to its volunteers. RSVP matches the personal interests and skills to older Americans with opportunities to help solve community problems and offer supplemental insurance while on duty, on-the-job training from the agency or organization where volunteers are placed.

1427 RSVP Harcatus

1324 3rd Street NW
New Philadelphia, OH 44663-1306
330-364-9251
Fax: 330-343-6526

Gail Baldwin, Director

The Retired and Senior Volunteer Program (RSVP) provides opportunities for people 55 and over to make a difference in their community through volunteer service. RSVP volunteers contribute anywhere from a few to over forty hours a week, serving thourgh schools, day care centers, police departments, hospitals and other nonprofit and public organizations to help meet critical community needs. RSVP offers maximum flexibility and choice to its volunteers. RSVP matches the personal interests and skills to older Americans with opportunities to help solve community problems and offer supplemental insurance while on duty, on-the-job training from the agency or organization where volunteers are placed.

1428 RSVP Jefferson

226 North Fourth Street
Steubenville, OH 43952-4416
740-282-1661
Fax: 740-282-1526

Sarah Hess, Director

The Retired and Senior Volunteer Program (RSVP) provides opportunities for people 55 and over to make a difference in their community through volunteer service. RSVP volunteers contribute anywhere from a few to over forty hours a week, serving thourgh schools, day care centers, police departments, hospitals and other nonprofit and public organizations to help meet critical community needs. RSVP offers maximum flexibility and choice to its volunteers. RSVP matches the personal interests and skills to older Americans with opportunities to help solve community problems and offer supplemental insurance while on duty, on-the-job training from the agency or organization where volunteers are placed.

1429 RSVP Kno-Ho-Co

2004 Campus Drive
Po Box 251
Mount Vernon, OH 43050
740-393-3633
Fax: 740-397-3306

Margaret Summers, Director

The Retired and Senior Volunteer Program (RSVP) provides opportunities for people 55 and over to make a difference in their community through volunteer service. RSVP volunteers contribute anywhere from a few to over forty hours a week, serving thourgh schools, day care centers, police departments, hospitals and other nonprofit and public organizations to help meet critical community needs. RSVP offers maximum flexibility and choice to its volunteers. RSVP matches the personal interests and skills to older Americans with opportunities to help solve community problems and offer supplemental insurance while on duty, on-the-job training from the agency or organization where volunteers are placed.

1430 RSVP Lake County
25 Public Square
Tech Center Room 109
Willoughby, OH 44094-7863
440-269-3015
Fax: 440-975-3741
kristen.kane@weschools.org
www.rsvplc.org

Cristen Kane, Director

The Retired and Senior Volunteer Program (RSVP) provides opportunities for people 55 and over to make a difference in their community through volunteer service. RSVP volunteers contribute anywhere from a few to over forty hours a week, serving thourgh schools, day care centers, police departments, hospitals and other nonprofit and public organizations to help meet critical community needs. RSVP offers maximum flexibility and choice to its volunteers. RSVP matches the personal interests and skills to older Americans with opportunities to help solve community problems and offer supplemental insurance while on duty, on-the-job training from the agency or organization where volunteers are placed.

1431 RSVP Mid-Ohio
35 N Park Street
Mansfield, OH 44902-1722
419-525-2816
Fax: 419-524-3467

Kathryn Mills, Director

The Retired and Senior Volunteer Program (RSVP) provides opportunities for people 55 and over to make a difference in their community through volunteer service. RSVP volunteers contribute anywhere from a few to over forty hours a week, serving thourgh schools, day care centers, police departments, hospitals and other nonprofit and public organizations to help meet critical community needs. RSVP offers maximum flexibility and choice to its volunteers. RSVP matches the personal interests and skills to older Americans with opportunities to help solve community problems and offer supplemental insurance while on duty, on-the-job training from the agency or organization where volunteers are placed.

1432 Railroad Retirement Board: Cincinnati Office
525 Vine Street
Suite 1940
Cincinnati, OH 45202-3125
513-684-3182
Fax: 513-684-3182; *Toll Free:* 877-772-5772
www.rrb.gov/field/do_cinc.asp

Jeffrey F Szabo, Representative

The Railroad Retirement Board (RRB) is an independent agency in the executive branck of the Federal Government. The RRB's primary function is to administer comprehensive retirement-survivor and unemployment-sickness benefit programs for the nation's railroad workers and their

families, under the Railroad Retirement and Railroad Unemployment Insurance Acts.

1433 Railroad Retirement Board: Cleveland District Office
AJC Federal Building, Room 907
1240 East 9th Street
Cleveland, OH 44199-2093
216-522-4053
Fax: 216-522-2320; *Toll Free:* 800-808-0772
www.rrb.gov/field/do_clev

Kevin B McCrone, Representative

The Railroad Retirement Board (RRB) is an independent agency in the executive branch of the Federal Government. The RRB's primary function is to administer comprehensive retirement-survivor and umemployment-sickenss benefit programs for the nation's railroad workers and their families, under the Railroad Retirement and Railroad Unemployment Insurance Acts.

1434 Retired Teachers Association
8050 N High Street
Suite 190
Columbus, OH 43235-6488
614-431-7002
Fax: 614-431-7003
mlauer@orta.org
www.oata.org

Ann Hanning, Executive Director
Tom Seamon, Publications Director
Mary Laurer, Administration/Tresurer

Represents members' interests;at STRS. Provides programs and networking opportunities for retirees.

1435 Senior Center of Sidney Shelby County
304 South West Avenue
Po Box 45365
Sidney, OH 45365-4362
937-492-5266
srcenter@ambarqmail.com
www.shelbysites.com/seniorcenter

Casey Beardslee, Director

Mission is to serve as a community focal point for programs and services promoting the well-being of older adults in the Sidney-Shelby County area.

1436 Western Reserve: Area Agency on Aging
11890 Fairhill Road
Suite 600
Cleveland, OH 44115-1405
216-621-8010
Fax: 216-621-9262; *Toll Free:* 800-626-7277
www.psa10a.org

Fatima Perkins, President
Marie Mirro Edmonds, Vice President
Robert Royer, Treasurer

Mission is to empower older adults to maintain wellness, independence, and dignity.

Oklahoma

1437 Aging Services Division
1900 Springlake Drive
Suite 40
Oklahoma City, OK 73107-2422

405-521-6734
Fax: 405-522-6739
www.okdhs.org

Lance Robertson, Director
Stacey Gholson, Operations

The division provides leadership in issues of concern to older Oklahomans, helps to develop communtiy-based systems which support independence and protect the quality of life of older persons and helps tp promote citizen involvement in planning and delivering those services.

1438 Central Oklahoma Economic Development District: Area Agency on Aging
PO Box 3398
Shawnee, OK 74802-3398
405-273-6410
Fax: 405-273-3213; *Toll Free:* 800-375-8255
jshea@sbcglobal.net
www.coedd.org
TDD 405-273-6410

Gregory Clifton, Executive Director
Floy K Alexander, Administrative Assistant
Theresa Beverage, Aging Specialist

Administers OAA programs in seven county rural area to Oklahomans 60 and older.

1439 Disability Determination Division
3535 NW 58th Street
Suite 500
Oklahoma City, OK 73124-0400
405-951-3400
Fax: 405-951-3529; *Toll Free:* 800-877-9977
info@okdrs.gov
www.okrehab.org
TTY: 405-951-3400

Dr Michael O'Brien, Executive Director

Expands opportunities for employment, independent life, and econmic self-sufficiency by helping Oklahomans with disabilities bridge barriers to success in workplace, school, and at home.

1440 Eastern Oklahoma Development District: Area: Agency on Aging
1012 North 38th Street
PO Box 1367
Muskogee, OK 74402-1367
918-682-7891
Fax: 918-682-5444
www.eoddok.org
TDD 918-684-5300

Ernie Moore, Executive irector
Kevin Wilson, Economic Director

EODD is a cooperative council of governments dedicated to improving the quality of life in eastern Oklahoma. EODD serves as an extension of the staffs of local governments which do not have adequate full-time staffs of their own or the state expertise required to meet the mandates of federal and state government.

1441 Kiamichi Economic Development: Area Agency on Aging
1002 Highway
2 North
Wilburton, OK 74578-0638

918-465-2367
Fax: 918-465-3873; *Toll Free:* 800-722-8180
kblaylock@keddo.org
www.keddo.org

Danny Baldwin, Executive Director

KEDDO is a legal trust authority set up to assist people in Southeast Oklahoma to plan and promote growth and development for the seven county area. The organization is directed by a Board of Trustees of person from each of the counties. The financing for KEDDO is a cooperative effort between Federal, State and Local Governments.

1442 Northern Oklahoma: Area Agency on Aging
2901 N Van Buren
Enid, OK 73703-2532
580-237-4810
Fax: 580-237-8230; *Toll Free:* 800-789-1149
noda.aaa.org

Brandi Atkinson, Director

1443 Oklahoma Association of Homes and Services for the Aging
Po Box 1383
El Reno, OK 73036
405-640-8040
Fax: 405-341-0976
info@leadingageok.org
www.leadingageok.org

Jessica Pfau, President
Lindsay Fick, Secretary
Jim O'Brien, Treasurer

A not-for-profit organization dedicated to establishing the highest standards of excellence for services in to the aging in Oklahoma.

1444 Oklahoma Association: Area Agencies on Gging
2400 N Lincoln Blvd
PO Box 25352
Oklahoma City, OK 73112-5911
405-942-8500
Fax: 405-943-4344
www.okdhs.org/aging

Helps to develop community-based systems which support independence and protect the quality of life of older persons and helps to promote itizen involvement in planning and delivering those services.

1445 Oklahoma Client Assistance Program
1111 N Lee
Suite 500
Oklahoma City, OK 73103
405-522-3702
cap@odc.ok.gov
www.odc.ok.gov

Provides accurate and timely information, referral and advocacy. We act as an intermediary to persons with disabilities and provide services for those with disabilities.

Year Founded: 1984

1446 Oklahoma Department of Human Services: Aging Services Division
1900 Springlake Drive
Suite 40
Oklahoma City, OK 73107-2422

405-521-2281
Fax: 405-521-2086
www.okdhs.org/divisionsoffices/visd/asd

Lance Robertson, Director

Provides leadership in issues of concern to older Oklahomans, helps to develop community-based systems which support independence and protect the quality of life of older persons and helps to promote citizen involvement in planning and delivering those services.

1447 Oklahoma Department of Veterans Affairs

2311 N Central Avenue
PO Box 53067
Oklahoma City, OK 73105-3200
405-521-3684
Fax: 405-521-6533; *Toll Free:* 888-655-2838
bwhite@odva.state.ok.us
www.ok.gov/ddva

Martha Spear, Executive Director
Vacant , Deputy Director
Rita Aragan, Cabinet Secretary

Provides a complete service to the State's veterans. This service includes nursing and domicilary care, financial assistance in emergencies, and field service counseling in the filing of claims for US Department of Veterans Affairs and state benefits.

1448 Oklahoma Developmental Disability Council

2401 NW 23rd Street
Suite 74
Oklahoma City, OK 73107-2431
405-521-4984
Fax: 405-521-4910; *Toll Free:* 800-836-4470
staff@okddc.ok.gov
www.okddc.ok.gov

Ann Trudgeon, Director

The mission of the Oklahoma Developmental Disabilities Council is to promote services and programs which enable persons with developmental disabilities to fully realize their maximum potential through increased independence and productivity, as well as through integration and inclusion in the community.

1449 Oklahoma Protection & Advocacy Agecny
Oklahoma Disability Law Center

2915 Classen Boulevard
300 Cameron Building
Oklahoma City, OK 73106
405-525-7755
Fax: 405-525-7759; *Toll Free:* 800-880-7755
odlcokc@flash.net
www.oklahomadisabilitylaw.org

Kayla Bower, Executive Director

The mission of the Oklahoma Disability Law Center is to protect, promote and expand the rights of people with disabilities. The ODLC mission reflects a belief that people with disabilities are entitled to be treated with dignity and respect; to be free from abuse, neglect, exploitation and discrimination. The ODLC mission also reflects the belief that people with disabilites are entitled to equal rights and to equally effective access to the same opportunities as are afforded to other members of society.

1450 Oklahoma Tax Commission

2501 N Lincoln Boulevard
Oklahoma City, OK 73194-1001
405-521-3160
www.oktax.state.ok.us

Thomas Kemp, Chairman
Jerry Johnson, Vice-Chairman
Dawn Cash, Secretary

The mission is to serve the people of Oklahoma by promoting tax compliance through quality service and fair administration.

1451 RSVP Altus

PO Box 1088
Altus, OK 73521
580-482-4141
Fax: 580-482-5433

Teresa Williams, Director

The Retired and Senior Volunteer Program (RSVP) provides opportunities for people 55 and over to make a difference in their community through volunteer service. RSVP volunteers contribute anywhere from a few to over forty hours a week, serving thourgh schools, day care centers, police departments, hospitals and other nonprofit and public organizations to help meet critical community needs. RSVP offers maximum flexibility and choice to its volunteers. RSVP matches the personal interests and skills to older Americans with opportunities to help solve community problems and offer supplemental insurance while on duty, on-the-job training from the agency or organization where volunteers are placed.

1452 RSVP Atoka

210 N Main Street
Coalgate, OK 74538-2872
580-927-2369
Fax: 580-927-3783

Phyllis Mixon, Director

The Retired and Senior Volunteer Program (RSVP) provides opportunities for people 55 and over to make a difference in their community through volunteer service. RSVP volunteers contribute anywhere from a few to over forty hours a week, serving thourgh schools, day care centers, police departments, hospitals and other nonprofit and public organizations to help meet critical community needs. RSVP offers maximum flexibility and choice to its volunteers. RSVP matches the personal interests and skills to older Americans with opportunities to help solve community problems and offer supplemental insurance while on duty, on-the-job training from the agency or organization where volunteers are placed.

1453 RSVP Bryan County

301 N 16th
PO Box 192
Durant, OK 74702
580-931-7147
Fax: 58-92- 258
bcrsvp@redriverok.com
bryancountyunitedway.org/

Robinson Pamela, Agency Director
Suman Pat, President
Clay Betty, Board Director of Secretary

People aged 55 or more in Bryan County, OK who participate and assist in various community programs. Volunteer program.

1454 RSVP Pottawatomie-Seminole Counties
400 North Bell
Shawnee, OK 74801
405-273-6410
Fax: 405-275-9442

Patricia Heer, Director

Provides opportunities for people 55 and over to make a difference in their community through volunteer service. RSVP volunteers contribute anywhere from a few to over forty hours a week, serving through schools, day care centers, police departments, hospitals and other nonprofit and public organizations to help meet critical community needs. RSVP matches the personal interests and skills of older Americans with opportunities to help solve community problems and offers supplemental insurance while on duty, on-the-job training from the agency or organization where volunteers are placed.

1455 RSVP Seven County
PO Box 569
117 W Russworm
Watonga, OK 73772-3817
580-623-7283
Fax: 580-623-7290
rsvp@opportunities-inc.org
opportunities-inc.org

Velda Wood, Director

Works with senior citizens age 55 and over who volunteer to work in their communities services such as hospital auxilaries, tutoring/mentoring and literacy programs with schools, assisting in nursing homes, clinics, libraries, museums, county offices, legal programs, senior centers and other related facilities.

1456 RSVP Tulsa
320 Southeast Delaware
Suite 4
Bartlesville, OK 74003
918-336-0330
Fax: 918-280-8659
rsvp@rsvptulsa.org
rsvptulsa.org

Ann Dougherty, Director

Matches the talents and interests of volunteers 55 and over with meaningful efforts that enhance the quality of our community.

1457 South Western Oklahoma Development Authority Area Agency on Aging
Clinton-Sherman Industrial Airpark
Building 420, Sooner Drive
PO Box 569
Burns Flat, OK 73624
580-562-4882
Fax: 580-562-4880; *Toll Free:* 800-627-4882
info@swoda.org
www.swoda.org

James Boyd, Director of Aging Services

Our mission is to strengthen local governments by providing services and technical assistance; promote orderly growth and development through job creation and the preservation of environmental integrity, and improve the quality of life by maximizing economic and social opportunities for the region and its population.

1458 Southern Oklahoma Development Association Area: Agency on Aging (SODA)
PO Box 709
224 W Evergreen Suite 202
Durant, OK 74702
580-920-1388
Fax: 580-920-1391; *Toll Free:* 800-211-2116
www.soda-aaa.org
TDD 405-226-2250

Kathy Weiner, Director

The Southern Oklahoma Development Association Area Agency on Aging strives to improve the quality of life of older Oklahomans by serving as their advocate; encourages older Oklahomans to fully and equally exercise their rights and benefits as citizens of this state and nation. The SODA/Area Agency on Aging administers programs providing nutrition services, outreach and information services, transportation, legal aid, ombudsman services, education/training, and other supportive services.

1459 Tulsa: Area Agency on Aging
111 S Greenwood Avenue
Suite 200
Tulsa, OK 74120-1410
918-596-7688
Fax: 918-596-7653; *Toll Free:* 800-211-2116
taaa@ci.tulsa.ok.us
www.cityoftulsa.org
TDD 918-582-8911

Clark Miller, Executive Director

Mission is to improve the quality of life by promoting independence, dignity, and health for senior citizens through advocacy, education and support of community-based services.

Oregon

1460 Access Technologies
2225 Lancaster Drive NE
Salem, OR 97305-1396
503-361-1201
Fax: 503-370-4530; *Toll Free:* 800-677-7512
www.accesstechnologiesinc.org

Laurie Brooks, President

A not-for-profit organization whose mission is to assure that persons with disabilities in Oregon will be able to secure and effectively use assistive technologies.

1461 Central Oregon Council on Aging
373 NE Greenwood Ave.
Bend, OR 97701
541-678-5483
Fax: 541-647-2689
admin@councilonaging.org
www.councilonaging.org

Carol Bro, Acting Executive Director
Michael Payne, Program Manager

The Council on Aging is the only agency in Central Oregon at the local level that is in business to provide leadership and guidance in developing and supporting an older person's ability to lead a dignified, safe, healthy and independent life.

1462 Douglas County: Area Agency on Aging
621 West Madrone
Roseburg, OR 97470
541-440-3500
Fax: 541-464-3901; *Toll Free:* 800-234-0985
vlnunenk@co.douglas.or.us
www.co.douglas.or.us

Peggy Madison, Administrator
Vanessa Becker, Deputy Adminstrator
Michelle Endicott, Administration

The AAA of Douglas County provides Older American Act and Medicaid services to those eligible among our county's 24,000 residents age 60 and older (23% of the total population) through its main office in Roseburg and eight community facilities throughout the County. We are committed to working together with our community partners to assist seniors and people with disabilities to enjoy independence, dignity, choice and quality of life.

1463 Gray Panthers of Portland
Gray Panthers
10 G Street NE
Suite 600
Washington, DC 20002
202-737-6637
Fax: 202-737-1160; *Toll Free:* 800-280-5362
info@graypanthers.org
www.graypanthers.org

Jan BenDor, National Chair
Brooke Hollister, Ph.D., Vice Chair
Jim Dawson, Treasurer

Gray Panthers of Portland is a gathering of mostly older activists who welcome people of all ages to join us in our work for human liberation and social justice.

Year Founded: 1970

1464 Harney County Senior Center
17 S Alder Avenue
PO Box 728
Burns, OR 97720
541-573-6024
Fax: 541-573-6025
angela.lamborn@co.harney.or.us
www.co.harney.or.us/seniorcenter.html

Angela Lamborn, Executive Director
Howard Weathers, Weatherization Manager
Vickie McLain, Nutrition Manager

Once known only as the senior center now the name reflects their value in our community. Senior and Community Services Center. The Harney County community is well served by a wide variety of services and programs offered by Senior and Community Services. These services are meant for everyone who qualify as well as senior citizens.

Year Founded: 1889

1465 Lane Council of Governments: Senior and Disabled Services Division
1015 Willamette Street
Eugene, OR 97401
541-682-4038
Fax: 541-682-3959
sds@lcog.org
www.sdslane.org
TTY: 541-682-4567

Brooke Emery, Program Manager
Brenda Wilson, Executive Director
Jody Cline, S&DS Director

The mission of S&DS is to advocacte for seniors and persons with disabilities and provide to them quality services and information that promote dignity, independence, and choice.

Year Founded: 1961

1466 Mid-Columbia Senior and Disabled Services
Mid-Columbia Center for Living
312 3rd Street
The Dalles, OR 97058
541-296-5452
Fax: 541-296-2731; *Toll Free:* 800-452-2333
info@mccfl.org
www.mccfl.org

Sally Zuck, Director

Mission is to provide comprehensive and culturally sensitive services in the least restrictive setting.

1467 Multnomah County Aging Services Division
421 SW Oak Street
Suite 510
Portland, OR 97219
503-988-3646
Fax: 503-248-3656
webmaster@multco.us
www.co.multnomah.or.us/ads
TTY: 503-988-3663

Marissa Madrigal, Chairman
Rod Underhill, District Attorney
Dan Staton, Multnomah County Sheriff

Mission is to assist older adults and persons with disabilities to live as independently as possible with a range of accessible, quality services that meet their diverse needs and preferences.

1468 Oregon Alliance of Senior & Health Services
7340 SW Hunziker
Suite 104
Tigard, OR 97223
503-684-3788
Fax: 503-624-0870
info@leadingageoregon.org
www.oashs.org

Bob Johnson, President
Dennis Whitted, Vice President/Housing
Lynn Szender, Vice President/Nursing

Mission is to represent and promote the common interests of its membership through leadership, advocacy, education and other services in order to enhance member's ability to serve their community.

1469 Oregon Cascades West Senior Services
Oregon Cascades West Council of Governments
1400 Queen Avenue SE
Suite 206
Albany, OR 97322
541-967-8630
Fax: 541-967-6423; *Toll Free:* 800-638-0510
www.ocwcog.org

Mary Abraham, Information & Referral Spclst.

The COG provides member governments and the people living within the region a broad range of programs and services.

1470 Oregon Commission on Disabilities
500 Summer Street NE
Salem, OR 97301
503-945-5944
Fax: 503-378-2897; *Toll Free:* 800-358-3117
www.oregon.dhs
TTY: 503-945-6214

Erin Kelly-Siehl, Director
Jim Scherzinger, Chief Operating Officer
Eric Moore, Chief Financial Officer

Year Founded: 1971

1471 Oregon Council on Developmental Disabilities
540 24th Place NE
Salem, OR 97301-4517
503-945-9941
Fax: 503-945-9947; *Toll Free:* 800-292-4154
ocdd@ocdd.org
www.ocdd.org

Jamie Daignault, Executive Director
Beth Kessler, Planning & Communications Coordi
Carol Loop, Office Specialist

Our mission is to join with Oregonians with developmental disabilities and their families to promote change, through self-determination, leading to a more accessible, inclusive and culturally responsive world.

1472 Oregon Department of Aging
500 Summer St NE 12
Salem, OR 97301-1073
503-945-5811; *Toll Free:* 800-282-8096
spd.web@state.or.us
www.oregon.gov/dhs
TTY: 800-282-8096

James Wilson, Administrator
Barry Donenfeld, Executive Director

Provides services and resources for the aging.

1473 Oregon Department of Revenue
955 Center Street NE
Salem, OR 97301-2555
503-378-4988
Fax: 503-945-8738; *Toll Free:* 800-356-4222
questions.dor@oregon.gov
www.oregon.gov/dor
TTY: 800-886-7204

Elizabeth Harchenko, Executive Director

Mission is to make tax systems work to fund the public service that preserve and enhance the quality of life for all citizens.

1474 Oregon Department of Veterans Affairs
700 Summer Street NE
Salem, OR 97301-1285
503-373-2000
Fax: 503-373-2362; *Toll Free:* 800-828-8801
www.oregon.gov/odva
TTY: 503-373-2217

Jim Willis, Director

Advocates for veterans, their dependents, and survivors. We are dedicated to providing quality programs and services to meet their current and future needs.

1475 Oregon Hearing Society
PO Box 30404
Portland, OR 97294
503-256-4233
Fax: 503-256-5367; *Toll Free:* 866-OHS-HEAR
www.ohsinc.org

Cheryl Blackman, President
Carol Sayre, Vice President
Scott Frink, Secretary

Representing and promoting the interests of hearing and professionals and the hearing aid consumers of the state of Oregon.

Year Founded: 1959

1476 Oregon Protection & Advocacy for Persons with Disabilities
620 SW Eth Avenue
5th Floor
Portland, OR 97204-1428
503-243-2081
Fax: 503-243-1738; *Toll Free:* 800-452-1694
www.oradvocacy.org

Elizabeth Arledge, Director Of Communications

An independent non-profit organization which provides legal advocacy services for people with disabilities anywhere in Oregon.

1477 Oregon Public Employees Retirement System
11410 SW 68th Parkway
Tigard, OR 97223
503-598-7377
Fax: 503-598-0561; *Toll Free:* 888-320-7377
www.oregon.gov/pers
TTY: 503-603-7766

John Thomas, Chairman
Pat West, Vice-Chair
Michael Jordan, Chief Operating Officer

We serve the people of Oregon by administering public employee benefit trusts to pay the right person the right benefit at the right time.

1478 Oregon Senior Services
500 Summer Street NE
Salem, OR 97301
503-945-5944
Fax: 503-378-2897
www.oregon.gov/dhs
TTY: 503-945-6214

Erin Kelly-Siehl, Director
Jim Scherzinger, Chief Operating Officer
Eric Moore, Chief Financial Officer

Mission is helping people become independent, healthy and safe.

Year Founded: 1971

1479 Pilot Rock Senior Center
144 North Alder Place
PO Box 130
Pilot Rock, OR 97868
541-443-2811
Fax: 541-443-2253

cityofpr@centurytel.net
www.cityofpilotorck.org

Teri Porter, City Recorder
Steve Draper, Public Works Supervisor
Wanda Young, Administrative Assistant

Senior center with activities for seniors.

1480 RSVP Clackamus

2051 Kaen Rd.
Oregon City, OR 97045
503-655-8581
Fax: 503-650-5752
bcc@clackamas.us
www.co.clackamas.or.us

John Ludlow, Chairman
Martha Schrader, Vice Chair
Tootie Smith, Commissioner

The Retired and Senior Volunteer Program (RSVP) provides opportunities for people 55 and over to make a difference in their community through volunteer service. RSVP volunteers contribute anywhere from a few to over forty hours a week, serving thourgh schools, day care centers, police departments, hospitals and other nonprofit and public organizations to help meet critical community needs. RSVP offers maximum flexibility and choice to its volunteers. RSVP matches the personal interests and skills to older Americans with opportunities to help solve community problems and offer supplemental insurance while on duty, on-the-job training from the agency or organization where volunteers are placed.

Year Founded: 1972

1481 RSVP Columbia County

375 S 18th Street
Suite C
Saint Helens, OR 97051
503-397-5655
Fax: 503-397-1183
rsvp@opusnet.com
www.columbiacountryrsvp.com/

Nancy Harwood, Director

1482 RSVP Coos County

1988 Newmark Avenue
Coos Bay, OR 97420
541-888-2525
Fax: 541-888-7120; *Toll Free:* 800-962-2838
rsvp@socc.edu
www.socc.edu/rsvp/

Tonya Schoonmaker, Director
Patty M. Scott, President

The Retired and Senior Volunteer Program (RSVP) provides opportunities for people 55 and over to make a difference in their community through volunteer service. RSVP volunteers contribute anywhere from a few to over forty hours a week, serving thourgh schools, day care centers, police departments, hospitals and other nonprofit and public organizations to help meet critical community needs. RSVP offers maximum flexibility and choice to its volunteers. RSVP matches the personal interests and skills to older Americans with opportunities to help solve community problems and offer supplemental insurance while on duty, on-the-job training from the agency or organization where volunteers are placed.

1483 RSVP Curry County

PO Box 746
94235 Moore Street
Gold Beach, OR 97444
541-247-3280
Fax: 541-247-2705
mcguinessv@co.curry.or.us
co.curry.or.us/rsvp/website/home_page.ht

Sharon Mather, Director

The Retired and Senior Volunteer Program (RSVP) provides opportunities for people 55 and over to make a difference in their community through volunteer service. RSVP volunteers contribute anywhere from a few to over forty hours a week, serving thourgh schools, day care centers, police departments, hospitals and other nonprofit and public organizations to help meet critical community needs. RSVP offers maximum flexibility and choice to its volunteers. RSVP matches the personal interests and skills to older Americans with opportunities to help solve community problems and offer supplemental insurance while on duty, on-the-job training from the agency or organization where volunteers are placed.

1484 RSVP Jackson County

1045 Ellendale Drive
Medford, OR 97504
541-857-7780
Fax: 541-857-7787
becky@retirement.org
www.retirement.org/rvmcs

Becky Snyder, Director

The Retired and Senior Volunteer Program (RSVP) provides opportunities for people 55 and over to make a difference in their community through volunteer service. RSVP volunteers contribute anywhere from a few to over forty hours a week, serving thourgh schools, day care centers, police departments, hospitals and other nonprofit and public organizations to help meet critical community needs. RSVP offers maximum flexibility and choice to its volunteers. RSVP matches the personal interests and skills to older Americans with opportunities to help solve community problems and offer supplemental insurance while on duty, on-the-job training from the agency or organization where volunteers are placed.

1485 RSVP Josephine County

201 NE 8th Street
Grants Pass, OR 97526
541-956-4050
Fax: 541-956-4056
www.ucancap.org/

Mike Fieldman, Executive Director
Dan McCue, Chief Financial Officer/ Chief O
Diana Smith, Executive Assistant

The Retired and Senior Volunteer Program (RSVP) provides opportunities for people 55 and over to make a difference in their community through volunteer service. RSVP volunteers contribute anywhere from a few to over forty hours a week, serving thourgh schools, day care centers, police departments, hospitals and other nonprofit and public organizations to help meet critical community needs. RSVP offers maximum flexibility and choice to its volunteers. RSVP matches the personal interests and skills to older Americans with opportunities to help solve community problems and offer supplemental insurance while on

duty, on-the-job training from the agency or organization where volunteers are placed.

1486 RSVP Lincoln County
203 North Main Street
Toldeo, OR 97391
541-574-2684
Fax: 541-336-1510
rsvp@ocwcog.org
rsvpoflbl.org/

Tamara Rosser, Director
Jennifer Grindy, Administrative Assistant
Holly Terlson, Volunteer Coordinator & Administ

Provides opportunities for people 55 and over to make a difference in their community through volunteer service. RSVP volunteers contribute anywhere from a few to over forty hours a week, serving through schools, day care centers, police departments, hospitals and other nonprofit and public organizations to help meet critical community needs. RSVP matches the personal interests and skills of older Americans with opportunities to help solve community problems and offers supplemental insurance while on duty, on-the-job training from the agency and organization where volunteers are placed.

1487 RSVP Linn Benton County
250 Broadalbin Street SW
Suite 2A
Albany, OR 97330-6312
541-753-9197
Fax: 541-812-0849
bfox@csc.gen.or.us
www.lbvision.org

Beth Fox, Director

The Retired and Senior Volunteer Program (RSVP) provides opportunities for people 55 and over to make a difference in their community through volunteer service. RSVP volunteers contribute anywhere from a few to over forty hours a week, serving thourgh schools, day care centers, police departments, hospitals and other nonprofit and public organizations to help meet critical community needs. RSVP offers maximum flexibility and choice to its volunteers. RSVP matches the personal interests and skills to older Americans with opportunities to help solve community problems and offer supplemental insurance while on duty, on-the-job training from the agency or organization where volunteers are placed.

1488 RSVP Washington County
18865 SW Johnson Street
Aloha, OR 97006
503-466-4749
Fax: 503-649-1530
www.lcsnw.org/

Roberta Nestaas, Presient & CEO

Mission is to connect volunteers 55 and older with volunteer opportunities that match their interes, experience and time commitment.

Year Founded: 1921

1489 Railroad Retirement Board: Oregon District Office
844 North Rush Street
Chicago, IL 60611-2092
312-751-4300
Fax: 503-326-2157; Toll Free: 877-772-5772

www.rrb.gov/field/do_port.asp
TTY: 312-751-4701

Judy Oxborrow, Representative

An independent agency in the executive branch of the Federal Government. The RRB's primary function is to administer comprehensive retirement-survivor and unemployment-sickness benefit programs for the nation's railroad workers and their families.

Year Founded: 1935

1490 Rogue Valley Council of Governments: Senior and Disability Services Division
155 North First Street
PO Box 3275
Central Point, OR 97502
541-664-6674
Fax: 541-664-7927
admin@rvcog.org
www.rvcog.org

Jim Lewis, President
Kay Harrison, 1st Vice President
Margie Moulin, Director

Assists seniors and adults with disabilities. Developed a network of services to help seniors and adults with disabilities live with dignity and independence.

Year Founded: 1968

1491 Vocational Rehabilitation Division
500 Summer Street NE
E-87
Salem, OR 97301
503-945-5880
Fax: 503-947-5010; Toll Free: 877-277-0513
vr.info@state.or.us
www.oregon.gov/dhs/vr

Stephanie Taylor, Administrator

OVRS is a state and federally funded program that works in partnership with the community and with businesses to develop employment opportunities for people who have disabilities

1492 Washington County: Area Agency on Aging
Washington County Deptartment of Aging Services
180 E Main St
Suite 226
Hillsboro, OR 97123-4026
503-846-3060
Fax: 503-846-3065; Toll Free: 855-673-2372
davsinfo@co.washington.or.us
www.co.washington.or.us/HHS/DAVS

Bob Davis, County Administrator
Don Bohn, Assistant County Administrator
Rob Masser

The mission is to create options for older persons to enable them to live independently in the appropriate care setting for as long as possible. This involves assessing need planning and coordinating services, developing services, advocating for their needs, and delivering and monitoring social and health services.

Pennsylvania

1493 Active Aging
1034 Park Avenue
Meadville, PA 16335
814-336-1792
Fax: 814-336-1705; *Toll Free:* 800-321-7705
aainc@activeaging.org
www.activeaging.org
TDD 814-333-3691

Pauline Mooney, Director

1494 Adams County Office for Aging
318 W Middle Street
Gettysburg, PA 17325
717-334-9296
Fax: 717-334-4715; *Toll Free:* 800-548-3240
inquiry@acofa.org
www.acofa.org

Vicki R Huffacker, Executive Director

A private non-profit agency dedicated to providing assistance to and for advocacy for older people within Adams County. Our mission is to assist older Adams Countians maintain their independence and their dignity within their own communities.

1495 Aging Services
1055 Oak Street
PO Box 519
Indiana, PA 15701-0519
724-349-4500
Fax: 724-349-9535; *Toll Free:* 800-442-8016
jmcquown@verizon.net
www.agingservicesinc.com

Jim McQuown, Executive Director

Aging Services, Inc. is a vital organization, comprised of a compassionate staff, dedicated to meeting the diverse needs of older adults in Indiana County by providing opportunities to enhance their social, physical and mental skills utilizing our various programs.

1496 Allegheny County Department of Aging
441 Smithfield Street
2nd Floor
Pittsburgh, PA 15222-2219
412-350-6905
Fax: 412-350-3091; *Toll Free:* 800-344-4319
SeniorLine@dhs.county.allegheny.pa.us
www.alleghenycounty.us/dhs/olderadults
TDD 412-350-2727

Mildred E Morrisson, Administrator

Provides and administers human services to county residents. Dedicated to meeting these human services needs, most particularly to the county's most vulnerable populations, through an extensive range of prevention, early intervention, crisis management and after-class services provided through its program offices.

1497 Area Agency on Aging: Luzerne & WyomingCounties
111 North Pennsylvania Boulevard
Wilkes Barre, PA 18701
570-822-1158
Fax: 570-823-9129; *Toll Free:* 800-252-1512

gdelivery@aginglw.org
www.aginglw.org

Mary Roselle, Admin. Services Director
Linda Kohut, Director of Community Services
Annette Grella, Director of Social Services

1498 Armstrong: Area Agency on Aging
450 East Market Street
Kittanning, PA 16201
724-548-3290
Fax: 724-548-3296; *Toll Free:* 800-368-1066
aaa@co.armstrong.pa.us
www.co.armstrong.pa.us

Janet D Talerico, Supervisor
Myra Miller, Controller
Scott Andreassi, District Attorney

A community service agency for older adults providing information and services to help seniors remain active and independent in the community.

1499 Beaver County Office on Aging
1020 8th Avenue
Beaver Falls, PA 15010
724-847-2262
Fax: 724-847-3490; *Toll Free:* 888-548-2262
Aging@BC0A.Us
www.bcoa.us

Tony Amadio, Chairman
Joe Spanik, Commissioner
Dennis Nichols, Commissioner

The Beaver County Office on Aging is committed to identifying the diverse needs of our aging population, providing quality services, preserving the dignity of the individual and advocating for the older persons rights.

Year Founded: 1802

1500 Blair Senior Services
1320 12th Avenue
Altoona, PA 16601
814-946-1235
Fax: 814-949-4857; *Toll Free:* 800-245-3282
www.blairsenior.org
TDD 814-949-4856

Dewey Adams, Chairman
Robert Scholl, Vice Chair
Patti Defibaugh, Secretary

A private, nonnon-profit organization dedicated to improving the health and welfare of older Blair County Residents. This is achieved through the coordination and implimention of programs designed to meet the needs of older persons in the community.

Year Founded: 1974

1501 Bucks County: Area Agency on Aging
55 East Court Street
Doylestown, PA 18901
215-348-6000
Fax: 215-348-9253; *Toll Free:* 888-942-8257
webmaster@co.bucks.pa.us
www.buckscounty.org
TDD 800-243-3767

Robert G. Loughery, Chairman
Charles H. Martin, Vice Chairman
William Penn, Founder

Services for older adults aged 60+.

Year Founded: 1682

1502 Bureau of Disability Determination
144 North Main Street
PO Box 2500
Greensburg, PA 15605
724-836-5100
Fax: 724-832-5284
www.state.pa.us

Robert P. Casey, Jr., Senator
Tommy Corbett, Governor
Jim Cawley, Lt. Governor

Determines what benefits a person is qualfied for regarding disability and SSA.

1503 Butler County: Area Agency on Aging
124 W. Diamond St.
Butler, PA 16001
724-285-4731
Fax: 724-282-1466; *Toll Free:* 888-367-2434
aaainfo@co.butler.pa.us
www.co.butler.pa.us
TDD 724-284-5473

James Eckstein, County Commissioner
William L. McCarrier, County Commissioner
A. Dale Pinkerton, County Commissioner

A wide range of senior services is available to Butler County residents over the age of 60. Most services are available on a donation basis.

1504 Centre County Office on Aging
420 Holmes Street
Room 245
Bellefonte, PA 16823-1488
814-355-6716
Fax: 814-355-6757; *Toll Free:* 800-494-2510
aging@co.centre.pa.us
www.co.centre.pa.us
TDD 814-355-6711

Steven G. Dershem, Chairman
C. Chris Exarchos, Vice Chair
Michael Pipe, Commissioner

Services include: information and referral, health insurance counseling, case work services, in-home services, protective services, home delivered meals, senior center programs, long term care ombudsman.

1505 Clearfield County: Area Agency on Aging
PO Box 550
103 North Front Street
Clearfield, PA 16830
814-765-2696
Fax: 814-765-2760; *Toll Free:* 800-225-8571
mail@ccaaa.net
www.ccaaa.net

John Kordish, Executive Director

Dedicated to providing a comprehensive array of the highest quality health and human services to resident of Clearfield County.

Year Founded: 1977

1506 Cumberland County Office of Aging
100 Claremont Road
Carlisle, PA 17015-8560

717-240-6110
Fax: 717-240-6118; *Toll Free:* 888-697-0371
aging@ccpa.net
www.ccpa.net/aging

Barbara Cross, Chairman
Jim Hertzler, Vice Chair
Terry Barley, Director

Provides coordinated services to county residents that are 60 years of age or older. Goal is to provide programs and services that allow the older adult to maintain their health, welfare and independence.

1507 Experience, Inc. : Area Agency on Aging
905 4th Avenue
Warren, PA 16365
814-723-3763
Fax: 814-723-6433; *Toll Free:* 800-281-6545
info@experienceinc.org
www.experienceinc.org

Danell Sowers, Executive Director
Beverly Mowrey, Long Term Care Director
Sue Himes, Director of Senior Centers

The mission is to provide or arrange for a comprehensive array of services to help offset the gradual loss of functional abilities typically experienced by the elderly. Our goal is to help a senior citizen maintain adequate functioning, and permit as independent a lifestyle as possible, preferably within their own home. Nutritious meals, activities and socialization are also provided at our local community senior centers.

Year Founded: 1968

1508 Franklin County: Area Agency on Aging
600 Norland Avenue
Suite 11
Chambersburg, PA 17201
717-264-4125
Fax: 717-261-3198; *Toll Free:* 800-528-3240
www.co.frankln.pa.us

David S. Keller, Chairman
Robert L Thomas, Commissioner
Robert G. Ziobrowski, Commissioner

Provides a planned program of supported services to those sixty years of age and older, intended to optimize independence, promote consumer choice and enhance quality of life.

1509 Greater Erie Community Action Committee
18 West 9th Street
Erie, PA 16501
814-459-4581
Fax: 814-456-0161; *Toll Free:* 800-769-2436
www.gecac.org

Gwendolyn White, Board Chairperson
Michael Butler, Vice Chair
Ronald A. Steele, Chief Executive Officer

A designated community action agency formed to provide advocacy and diverse services directed toward the elimination of poverty and the causes of poverty.

Year Founded: 1965

1510 Jefferson County: Area Agency on Aging
186 Main Street
Brookville, PA 15825

814-849-3096
Fax: 814-849-4655; *Toll Free:* 800-852-8036
www.jcaaa.org

Bill Sherman, Executive Director
Molly McNutt, HR/ Apprise Coordinator
Cheryl Muders, Long Term Care Director

Set up to administer and develop a program of comprehensive services for the elderly. to act as an advocate for the elderly, to provide various services to help the elderly remain in their homes for as long as possible and to assist the older person to remain a citizen in his or her community.

Year Founded: 1976

1511 Lackawanna County: Area Agency on Aging

135 Jefferson Avenue
Lower Level
Scranton, PA 18503
570-963-6740
Fax: 570-963-6401
www.lackawannacounty.org
TDD 717-299-7981

Timothy D. Rowland, Coroner
Gary A. DiBileo, Controller
Edward Karpovich, Treasurer

The AAA reflects a simple philosophy: to act as advocates for the aging and to serve, protect, enable, and empower older adults and persons with disabilities through the provision and continuous improvement of home and community based services.

1512 Lancaster County Office of Aging

150 North Queen Street
Lancaster, PA 17603
717-299-8000
Fax: 717-293-7234; *Toll Free:* 800-801-3070
aging@co.lancaster.pa.us
www.co.lancaster.pa.us/lanco_aging
TDD 717-299-7981

Dennis P. Stuckey, Chairman
Scott F. Martin, Vice Chairman
Jacqueline Burch, Executive Director

Supports the older person's right to decide his/her own destiny. Consumer self-determination, choice; supports the older person's right to risk; promote the independence and dignity; avoid aunnecessary/inappropriate institutionalization.

1513 Lawrence County: Area Agency on Aging

212 Ninth Street
Pittsburgh, PA 15222
412-456-6999
Fax: 724-658-7532
info@ccpgh.org
www.ccpgh.org/challenges

Susan Rauscher, Executive Director
Deacon Cliff Homer, Chief Operating Officer
Mary Bernhard, Director of Human Resources

Offers a wide range in programs and services for older persons ranging from job training and employment opportunities to in-home services for those who are seeking alternatives to nursing home care. Many social and recreational activities are available at community centers and satellite centers throughout Lawrence County. All services seek to enhance independence and to maintain the highest quality of life possible.

Year Founded: 1910

1514 Lebanon County: Area Agency on Aging

710 Maple Street
2nd Floor
Lebanon, PA 17046-3537
717-273-9262
Fax: 717-274-3882
lebcoaaa@lebcnty.org
www.lebcounty.org

Jamie A. Wolgemuth, County Administrator
Dr. Jeffrey Yocum, Coroner
Sallie A. Neuin, County Treasurer

Provide services to senior residents of Lebanon county.

Year Founded: 1723

1515 Life Insurance for Veterans: Veterans Benefits Administration
US Department of Veterans Affairs

810 Vermont Avenue NW
Washington, DC 20420
215-842-2000
Fax: 215-381-3084; *Toll Free:* 800-669-8477
www.va.gov

Jose D. Riojas, Chief of Staff
Will A. Gunn, General Counsel
Eric K. ShinSeki, Secretary of Veteran Affairs

Our insurance programs were developed to provide insurance benefits for veterans and service members who may not be able to get insurance from private companies because of the extra risks involved in military service, or a service connected disability.

Year Founded: 1636

1516 Luzerne-Wyoming Counties Area Agency onAging

111 N Pennsylvania Avenue
Wilkes Barre, PA 18701
570-822-1158
Fax: 570-823-9129; *Toll Free:* 800-252-1512
www.aginglw.org

Trula Hollywood, Executive Director
Linda Kohut, Community Services Director
Annette Grella, Social Services Director

Mission is to create a community environment that promotes the ability of all older persons to funtion with independence an dignity throughout their lives.

1517 Lycoming-Clinton Office of Aging

PO Box 3156
2138 Lincoln Street
Lock Haven, PA 17745
570-323-3096
Fax: 570-322-6869; *Toll Free:* 800-332-8555
flshrimp@stepcorp.org
www.state.pa.us

Tim Corbett, Governor
Jim Cawley, Lt. Governor
Robert P. Casey, Jr., Senator

Mission is to enhance the quality of life of all older Pennsylvanians by empowering diverse communities, the family and the individual.

1518 Mercer County: Area Agency on Aging
Mercer County Area Agency on Aging, Inc.
133 North Pitt Street
Mercer, PA 16137
724-662-6222
Fax: 724-662-0611
admin@mercercountyaging.org
www.mercercountyaging.org

Ann Marie Spiardi, Executive Director

Mission is to enrich the lives of older adults in Mercer County and enable them to maintain their independence through an array of programs and services.

1519 Mifflin-Juniata: Area Agency on Aging
Mifflin-Juniata Area Agency on Aging, Inc
249 West 3rd Street
Lewistown, PA 17044
717-242-0315
Fax: 717-242-1448; *Toll Free:* 800-348-2277
mifjunconf@mjaaa.com
www.mjaaa.com

Carlene S Hack, Director

Mission is to foster, promote, and provide fir the development of a comprehensive service system for persons over the age of 60, the enable aging with independence, dignity, and respect.

1520 Monroe County: Area Agency on Aging
Monroe County Vacation Bureau
724 Phillips Street
Suite B
Stroudsburg, PA 18360-2244
570-420-3735
Fax: 570-420-3734; *Toll Free:* 800-498-0330
monroeaging@co.monroe.pa.us
www.co.monroe.pa.us

John Moyer, Chairman
Charles Garris, Vice Chairman
Suzanne McCool, Commissioner

Mission is to improve the quality of life of older citizens through the coordination of exiting services and development of essential programs.
Year Founded: 1836

1521 Montgomery County Office on Aging and Adult Services
Montgomery County Office on Aging and Adult Servic
1430 DeKalb Pike
PO Box 311
Norristown, PA 19404
610-278-3601
Fax: 610-278-3769
www.mcaas.montcopa.org

Frank X. Custer, Director of Communications
Lauren M. Lambrugo, Chief Operating Officer/ Chief C
Uri Z. Monson, Chief Financial Officer

The Montgomery County Office of Aging and Adult Services is the agency responsible for planning, coordinating, and monitoring services for county residents, age 60 and older. As the area agency on aging, AAS is part of a state and national network of agencies established by the older persons through a wide range of service options.

1522 Northampton County: Area Agency on Aging
45 North 2nd Street
Easton, PA 18042
610-559-3000
Fax: 610-559-3297; *Toll Free:* 800-322-9269
NCInfo@northamptoncounty.org
www.northamptoncounty.org

Stacy Duke, Auditor
Stephen J. Barron Jr., CFE, County Controller
Frank S. Kedl, Audit Manager

Maintains and enhances the independence and dignity of older adults while providing protection as necessary.

1523 Northumberland County: Area Agency on Aging
Northumberland County Area Agency on Aging
322 North 2nd Street
Sunbury, PA 17801
570-495-2395
Fax: 570-644-4457; *Toll Free:* 877-622-2251
helpme@ncaging.org
www.ncaging.org/

Vinny Clausi, Chairman
Stephen Bridy, Vice Chairman
Richard J. Shoch, Commissioner

Mission is to serve as an advocate, and generally assist older citizens to remain active in their communities.

1524 Pennsylvania Association of Area Agencies on Aging Directors
Pennsylvania Association of Area Agencies on Aging
525 South 29th Street
Harrisburg, PA 17104
717-541-4214
Fax: 717-541-4217
www.p4a.org

Crystal Lowe, Executive Director
Arthur N. DiLoreto, Deputy Director
Eileen Carson, Project Specialist

Mission is to act as an advocate for the aging, promoting the continued wphysical, social, and economic self-sufficiency of seniors.
Year Founded: 1977

1525 Pennsylvania Association of Non-Profit Homes for the Aging
1100 Bent Creek Boulevard
Mechanicsburg, PA 17050
717-763-5724
Fax: 717-763-1057; *Toll Free:* 800-545-2270
info@leadingagepa.org
www.panpha.org

Ronald L Barth, Executive Director

Nursing homes, assisted living facilities, elderly housing, retirement communities.

1526 Pennsylvania Client Assistance Program
Client Assistance Program
1515 Market Street
Suite 1300
Philadelphia, PA 19102
215-557-7112
Fax: 215-557-7602; *Toll Free:* 888-745-2357
info@equalemployment.org

www.equalemployment.org
TDD 215-557-7112

Margaret Passio-McKenna, Senior Advocate
Stephen S. Pennington, Executive Director
Jamie C. Ray-Leonetti, Co-Director

Mission is to provide you with information and advice about rehabilitation programs.

1527 Pennsylvania Department of Revenue
Pennsylvania Department of Revenue
Strawberry Square Lobby
Harrisburg, PA 17128-0101
717-783-1405
Fax: 717-783-4447
www.revenue.state.pa.us

Tom Corbett, Governor
Mary McKee, Office Manager
Dan Meuser, Secretary

Mission is to administer the tax laws of the commonwealth in a fair and equitable manner.

1528 Pennsylvania Department on Aging
Commonwealth of Pennsylvania; Department of Aging
555 Walnut Street
5th Floor
Harrisburg, PA 17101-1919
717-783-1550
Fax: 717-783-6842; *Toll Free:* 800-225-7223
aging@pa.gov
www.aging.state.pa.us

Tom Corbett, Governor
Brian M. Duke, Secretary

Mission is to enhance the quality of life of all older Pennsylvanians by empowering diverse communities, the family, and the individual.

1529 Pennsylvania Developmental Disabilities Council
Pennslyvania Developmental Disabilities Council
Room 561 Forum Building
605 South Drive
Harrisburg, PA 17120
717-787-6057
Fax: 717-772-0738; *Toll Free:* 877-685-4452
www.paddc.org
TTY: 717-705-0819

Nancy Richey, Council Chairperson
Tom Corbett, Governor
Graham Mulholland, Executive Director

The Council engages in advocacy, systems change and capacity building for people with disabilities and their families in order to: Support people with disabilities in taking control of their own lives; Ensure access to goods, services, and supports; Build inclusive communities; Pursue a cross-disability agenda; Change negative societal attitudes towards people with disabilities.

Year Founded: 1970

1530 Pennsylvania Protection & Advocacy for Persons with Disabilities
Administration for Children & Families
901 D St. SW
Washington, DC 20447

202-401-9215
Fax: 202-205-9688; *Toll Free:* 800-692-7443
kenneth.wolfe@acf.hhs.gov
www.acf.hhs.gov

James Murray, Acting Director, Office of Regio
Jeannie Chaffin, Director, Office of Community Se
Mark Greenberg, Acting Assistant Secretary

Provide advocacy, information and referral for persons with disabilities and mental illness issues.

1531 Pennsylvania Public School Employees' Retirement System
Public School Employees' Retirement
5 North 5th Street
Harrisburg, PA 17101-1905
717-787-8540
Fax: 717-783-7275; *Toll Free:* 888-773-7748
ContactPSERS@pa.gov
www.psers.state.pa.us

Nathan G. Mains, Executive Director
Robert m. McCord, Treasurer
Carolyn C. Dumaresq, Acting Secretary

An agency of the Commonwealth of Pennsylvania who administers the pension plan for Pennsylvania's public school employees.

Year Founded: 1917

1532 Pennsylvania Society of Directors of Volunteer Services
Pennsylvania Society of Directors in Healthcare, I
PO Box 8600
Harrisburg, PA 17105-8600
717-564-9200
Fax: 717-561-5216

Mercedes Piesco, President
Carolyn Scanlan, CEO

1533 Perry County Office for Aging
Perry County Courthouse
2 East Main Street
PO Box 37
New Bloomfield, PA 17068
717-582-2131
Fax: 717-582-5162
rmeyer@perryco.org
www.perryco.org

Paul L. Rudy Jr., Commissioner
Brenda K. Benner, Commissioner
Stephen C. Naylor, Commissioner

Mission is to enhance the quality of life of all older Pennsylvanians by empowering diverse communities, the family, and the individual.

1534 Philadelphia Corporation for Aging
Philadelphia Corporation for Aging
642 North Broad Street
Philadelphia, PA 19130-3424
215-765-9000
Fax: 215-765-9066
info@pcaphl.org
www.pcacares.org/
TDD 215-765-9041

Holly Lange, President
Glenn D. Bryan, Vice Chair
sheri C. Gifford, Treasurer

Mission is to improve the quality of life for older persons and people with disabilities, and to assist them in achieving their maximum level of health, independence, and productivity.

Year Founded: 1965

1535 Pike County: Area Agency on Aging
Pike County Area Agency on Aging
150 Pike County Boulevard
Hawley, PA 18428-9107
570-775-5550
Fax: 570-775-5558; *Toll Free:* 800-233-8911
webmaster@pikepa.org
www.pikeaaa.org

Robin S. LoDolce, Executive Director
Ray Groll, Transportaion Manager
Barbara Paschell, Site Manager

1536 Potter County: Area Agency on Aging
PO Box 241
62 North Street
Roulette, PA 16746
814-544-7315
Fax: 814-544-9062; *Toll Free:* 800-800-2560
pottercountyhumansvcs.org
www.pottercountyhumansvcs.org
Sherry Hoffman, Aging Director
Jame Kockler, Administrator

Provides assessment, care management and services to eligible older adults, age 60 years and older.

Year Founded: 1987

1537 RSVP Allegheny County-Pittsburgh
225 Boulevard of the Allies
Pittsburgh, PA 15222-1615
412-263-3184
Fax: 412-263-5268
gueldnerm@usa.redcross.org
rsvp.pittsburghcares.org/

Linda Soldressen, Director

The Retired and Senior Volunteer Program (RSVP) provides opportunities for people 55 and over to make a difference in their community through volunteer service. RSVP volunteers contribute anywhere from a few to over forty hours a week, serving thourgh schools, day care centers, police departments, hospitals and other nonprofit and public organizations to help meet critical community needs. RSVP offers maximum flexibility and choice to its volunteers. RSVP matches the personal interests and skills to older Americans with opportunities to help solve community problems and offer supplemental insurance while on duty, on-the-job training from the agency or organization where volunteers are placed.

Year Founded: 1973

1538 RSVP Beaver County
Retired and Senior Volunteer Program of Beaver Cou
524 Franklin Avenue
Aliquippa, PA 15001-3728
724-378-7547
Fax: 724-378-9809
chaney@aaud.org
beavercountyrsvp.org/

Nathan Askins, Director

The Retired and Senior Volunteer Program (RSVP) provides opportunities for people 55 and over to make a difference in their community through volunteer service. RSVP volunteers contribute anywhere from a few to over forty hours a week, serving thourgh schools, day care centers, police departments, hospitals and other nonprofit and public organizations to help meet critical community needs. RSVP offers maximum flexibility and choice to its volunteers. RSVP matches the personal interests and skills to older Americans with opportunities to help solve community problems and offer supplemental insurance while on duty, on-the-job training from the agency or organization where volunteers are placed.

Year Founded: 1970

1539 RSVP Buck County
Retired and Senior Volunteer Program Bucks County
30 East Court Street
Doylestown, PA 18901
215-348-6000
Fax: 215-348-0356; *Toll Free:* 888-942-8257
webmaster@co.bucks.pa.us
www.buckscounty.org

Robert G. Loughery, Chairman
Charles H. Martin, Vice Chairman
Najja R. Orr, Director

The Retired and Senior Volunteer Program (RSVP) provides opportunities for people 55 and over to make a difference in their community through volunteer service. RSVP volunteers contribute anywhere from a few to over forty hours a week, serving thourgh schools, day care centers, police departments, hospitals and other nonprofit and public organizations to help meet critical community needs. RSVP offers maximum flexibility and choice to its volunteers. RSVP matches the personal interests and skills to older Americans with opportunities to help solve community problems and offer supplemental insurance while on duty, on-the-job training from the agency or organization where volunteers are placed.

1540 RSVP Capitol Region
RSVP of the Capitol Region, Inc.
50 Utley Drive
Suite 500
Camp Hill, PA 17011
717-541-9521
Fax: 717-541-8466; *Toll Free:* 800-870-2616
rsvp@rsvpcapreg.org
rsvpcapreg.org/

Carol A Oman, Director
Judy Bentz, Perry County Coordinator
Anne Meek

Volunteer recruitment and placement in Cumberland, Dauphin, Franklin and Perry counties.

1541 RSVP Centre County
420 Holmes Street
Room 245
Bellefonte, PA 16823-1488
814-355-6716
Fax: 814-355-6757; *Toll Free:* 800-479-0050
bquerry@co.centre.pa.us
www.co.centre.pa.us

Steven G. Dershem, Commissioner
Timothy T. Boyde, Director of Administrative Servi
Denise Elbell, Director of Financial Management

Retired and Senior Volunteer programs places adults ages 55+ in non-profit, government, and health care settings in Centre County PA.

1542 RSVP Chester County
Family Service of Chester County
310 North Matlack Street
West Chester, PA 19380
610-696-4900
Fax: 610-696-4476
www.familyservice.us/

Leslie Stauffer, Director
Vincent Pucher, Volunteer
Raman Patel, Volunteer

The Retired and Senior Volunteer Program (RSVP) provides opportunities for people 55 and over to make a difference in their community through volunteer service. RSVP volunteers contribute anywhere from a few to over forty hours a week, serving thourgh schools, day care centers, police departments, hospitals and other nonprofit and public organizations to help meet critical community needs. RSVP offers maximum flexibility and choice to its volunteers. RSVP matches the personal interests and skills to older Americans with opportunities to help solve community problems and offer supplemental insurance while on duty, on-the-job training from the agency or organization where volunteers are placed.

1543 RSVP Clearfield County
Clearfield County Area Agency on Aging, Inc.
103 North Front Street
PO Box 550
Clearfield, PA 16830
814-765-2696
Fax: 814-765-1730; *Toll Free:* 800-225-8571
www.ccaaa.net/

Donna English, Director

The Retired and Senior Volunteer Program (RSVP) provides opportunities for people 55 and over to make a difference in their community through volunteer service. RSVP volunteers contribute anywhere from a few to over forty hours a week, serving thourgh schools, day care centers, police departments, hospitals and other nonprofit and public organizations to help meet critical community needs. RSVP offers maximum flexibility and choice to its volunteers. RSVP matches the personal interests and skills to older Americans with opportunities to help solve community problems and offer supplemental insurance while on duty, on-the-job training from the agency or organization where volunteers are placed.

Year Founded: 1977

1544 RSVP Delaware County
Retired and Senior Volunteer Program of Delaware C
609 West State Street
Unit E
Media, PA 19063
610-565-5563
Fax: 610-565-5176
www.rsvpdelco.org/

Norma Testa, Executive Officer
Paul Graefe, RSVP Legends Band Director
Terry Mendenhall, RSVP Volunteer at Surrey Service

Provides volunteer assignments for persons age 55 or over with nonprofit public service agencies in Delaware County, PA. Volunteer oppurtuities are based on community need and are encouraged in areas where there is impact on the community.

Year Founded: 1972

1545 RSVP Greater Erie Community Action
Greater Erie Community Action Committee
18 West 9th Street
Erie, PA 16501
814-459-4581
Fax: 814-456-0161; *Toll Free:* 800-769-2436
www.gecac.org/

Gwendolyn White, Board Chairperson
Michael Michael, Vice Chair
Danny Jones, Treasurer

The Retired and Senior Volunteer Program (RSVP) provides opportunities for people 55 and over to make a difference in their community through volunteer service. RSVP volunteers contribute anywhere from a few to over forty hours a week, serving thourgh schools, day care centers, police departments, hospitals and other nonprofit and public organizations to help meet critical community needs. RSVP offers maximum flexibility and choice to its volunteers. RSVP matches the personal interests and skills to older Americans with opportunities to help solve community problems and offer supplemental insurance while on duty, on-the-job training from the agency or organization where volunteers are placed.

Year Founded: 1965

1546 RSVP Lackawanna County
Voluntary Action Center of Northeastern Pensylvani
538 Spruce Street
Suite 420
Scranton, PA 18503
570-347-5616
Fax: 570-341-5816
vac@vacnepa.org
www.vacnepa.org/

Nancy Post, Director

The Retired and Senior Volunteer Program (RSVP) provides opportunities for people 55 and over to make a difference in their community through volunteer service. RSVP volunteers contribute anywhere from a few to over forty hours a week, serving thourgh schools, day care centers, police departments, hospitals and other nonprofit and public organizations to help meet critical community needs. RSVP offers maximum flexibility and choice to its volunteers. RSVP matches the personal interests and skills to older Americans with opportunities to help solve community problems and offer supplemental insurance while on duty, on-the-job training from the agency or organization where volunteers are placed.

Year Founded: 1976

1547 RSVP Monroe County
Retired and Senior Volunteer Program Monroe County
411 Main Street
Suite 102-B
Stroudsburg, PA 18360
570-420-3747
Fax: 570-420-3732
www.co.monroe.pa.us/

Merle Turitz, RSVP Project Coordinator

The Retired and Senior Volunteer Program (RSVP) provides opportunities for people 55 and over to make a difference in their community through volunteer service. RSVP volunteers contribute anywhere from a few to over forty hours a week, serving thourgh schools, day care centers, police departments, hospitals and other nonprofit and public organizations to help meet critical community needs. RSVP offers maximum flexibility and choice to its volunteers. RSVP matches the personal interests and skills to older Americans with opportunities to help solve community problems and offer supplemental insurance while on duty, on-the-job training from the agency or organization where volunteers are placed.

1548 RSVP Westmoreland County
Westmoreland County Area Agency on Aging
Westmoreland CCC
145 Pavilion Lane
Youngwood, PA 15697
724-925-4213
Fax: 724-925-1150
www.co.westmoreland.pa.us/

Sylvia Detar, Director

The Retired and Senior Volunteer Program (RSVP) provides opportunities for people 55 and over to make a difference in their community through volunteer service. RSVP volunteers contribute anywhere from a few to over forty hours a week, serving thourgh schools, day care centers, police departments, hospitals and other nonprofit and public organizations to help meet critical community needs. RSVP offers maximum flexibility and choice to its volunteers. RSVP matches the personal interests and skills to older Americans with opportunities to help solve community problems and offer supplemental insurance while on duty, on-the-job training from the agency or organization where volunteers are placed.

Year Founded: 1967

1549 RSVP of Montgomery County
RSVP of Montgomery County, Inc.
925 Harvest Drive
Suite 100
Blue Bell, PA 19422
610-834-1040
Fax: 610-834-1087
tonyg@rsvpmc.org, rsvpwestern@rsvpmc.org, rsv
www.rsvpmc.org

Michele Spencer, Executive Director
Tony Giunta, Deputy Executive Director
Barbara Fitzgerald, Development Coordinator

The Retired and Senior Volunteer Program (RSVP) provides opportunities for people 55 and over to make a difference in their community through volunteer service. RSVP volunteers contribute anywhere from a few to over forty hours a week, serving thourgh schools, day care centers, police departments, hospitals and other nonprofit and pub-

lic organizations to help meet critical community needs. RSVP offers maximum flexibility and choice to its volunteers. RSVP matches the personal interests and skills to older Americans with opportunities to help solve community problems and offer supplemental insurance while on duty, on-the-job training from the agency or organization where volunteers are placed.

Frequency: Annual Year Founded: 1973; Number of Members: 3500

1550 RSVP of Venango County
One Dale Avenue
Franklin, PA 16323
814-432-9723
Fax: 814-432-9759
rsvp@co.venango.pa.us

Monica Vanderhoof, Director

Provides volunteer opportunities for peopled aged 55 and older.

Year Founded: 1972; Number of Members: 500

1551 Railroad Retirement Board: Altoona Pennslvania District Office
Railroad Retirement Board Office Altoona, PA
1514 11th Avenue
P.O. Box 990
Altoona, PA 16603-0990
877-772-5772
Fax: 814-946-3620
www.rrb.gov/field/do_alto.asp

William Lambert, Representative
Martin J. Dickman, Inspector General

Provides services to active and in active railroad employees regarding their benefits and retirement.

1552 Railroad Retirement Board: Harrisburg Pennsylvania District Office
Railroad Retirement Board Office Harrisburg, PA
Federal Building, Room 576
228 Walnut Street, P.O. Box 11697
Harrisburg, PA 17108-1697
877-772-5772
Fax: 717-221-3464
harrisburg@rrb.gov
www.rrb.gov/field/do_harr.asp

Karen E Keefer, District Manager
Martin J. Dickman, Inspector General

Provide services to active, inactive and retired rail employees filing for retirement or survivor benefits and also sickness and unemployment benefits.

1553 Railroad Retirement Board: Philadelphia Pennsylvania District Office
Railroad Retirement Board Office Piladelphia, PA
Nix Federal Building
900 Market Street, Room 301
Philadelphia, PA 19107-4293
877-772-5772
Fax: 215-597-2794
philadelphia@rrb.gov
www.rrb.gov/field/do_phil.asp

Edward M Chochek, Representative
Martin J. Dickman, Inspector General

Provides services to active and inactive railroad employees regarding retirement benefits.

1554 Railroad Retirement Board: Pittsburgh Pennsylvania District Office
Railroad Retirement Board Office Pittsburgh, PA
Moorhead Federal Building, Room 1511
1000 Liberty Avenue
Pittsburgh, PA 15222-4101
877-772-5772
Fax: 412-395-4711
www.rrb.gov/field/do_pitt.asp

Michael L Bauer, Representative
Martin J. Dickman, Inspector General

Provides services to both active and inactive railroad employees regarding retiremnt benefits.

1555 Railroad Retirement Board: Scranton Pennsylvania District Office
Railroad Retirement Board Office Scranton, PA
Siniawa Plaza II
717 Scranton Carbondale Highway
Scranton, PA 18508-1121
877-772-5772
Fax: 570-346-6042
scranton@rrb.gov
www.rrb.gov/field/do_scra.asp

Robert C Ralston, Representative
Martin J. Dickman, Inspector General

Provides services to active and inactive railroad employees regarding retirement benefits.

1556 Senior Adult Activities Center of Montgomery County
Senior Adult Activities Center of Montgomery Count
536 George Street
Norristown, PA 19401
610-275-1960
Fax: 610-275-0878
www.montcosaac.com

Linda Collins, Executive Director
Larry Reed, Site Manager
Kathy Phillips, Executive Secretary

Senior centers of Norristown, Ambler and Glenside, PA. Provides adult day care. Conducts educational, health, and recreational services for seniors at centers. Provides Meals on Wheels and congregate meals. Adult Day Care at Norristown site, as well. Publishes newsletter at no charge.

8 pages Frequency: Monthly

1557 Social Security for Public Employees
Pennsylvania Department of Labor & Industry
651 Boas Street
Room 1700
Harrisburg, PA 17121
717-787-5279
Fax: 717-783-4716
www.dli.state.pa.us

Stephen M Schmerin, Secretary

Our mission is to improve the quality of life and economic security for Pennsylvania workers and businesses, encourage labor-management cooperation, and prepare the Commonwealth's workforce for the jobs of the future.

Year Founded: 1913

1558 Somerset County: Area Agency on Aging
Area Agency on Aging of Somerset County
1338 South Edgewood Avenue
Somerset, PA 15501
814-443-2681
Fax: 814-445-4398; *Toll Free:* 800-452-0825
webmaster@somersetaaa.org
www.somersetaaa.org

Debbie Baker, Executive Director

Purpose is to help older and/or functionally challenged adults by working with individuals, families, and communities. Through the efforts of caring staff and volunteers, the Agency provides a wide variety of services to promote independence and quality of life.

1559 Southwestern Pennsylvania Partnership for Aging
Southwestern Pennsylvania Partnership for Aging (S
500 Commonwealth Drive
Warrendale, PA 15086
724-779-3200
Fax: 724-779-2131
info@swppa.org
www.swppa.org

Al Condeluci, Ph.D., President & CEO
Linda Doman, Vice President
JoAnne Andiorio, Secretary

The Southwestern Pennsylvania Partnership for Aging (SWPPA) is a regional coalition of individuals and groups who are committed to the well being of an aging population. Our mission is to serve as a catalyst to promote policies, programs and system change which will improve the quality of life of older adults.

Year Founded: 1990; Number of Members: 398

1560 Southwestern Pennsylvania: Area Agency on Aging
Southwestern Pennsylvania Partnership for Aging, I
305 Chamber Plaza
Charleroi, PA 15022-1607
724-489-8080
Fax: 724-489-1116; *Toll Free:* 888-300-2704
contact@swpa-aaa.org
www.swpa-aaa.org
TDD 724-483-5828
TTY: 724-483-5828

Leslie Grenfell, Executive Director
Timothy A. Landrin, Division Director, Long Term Car
Kathleen Gustine, Esq., Division Director, Legal Service

Mission is to promote the well-being of older adults through a planned, coordinated, and collaborative program of health and social services.

Year Founded: 1974

1561 Tioga, Bradford, Sullivan and Susquehanna Counties: Area Agency on Aging
220 Main Street
Towanda, PA 18848
570-265-6121
Fax: 570-265-5680; *Toll Free:* 800-982-4346

bfarley@bsstaaa.org
www.p4a.org/bsst.htm

William Farley, Director

Promotes independence, healthy lifestyles for Seniors and we provide support for family members who may serve as their caregivers.

Year Founded: 1981

1562 Union-Snyder: Area Agency on Aging
Union-Snyder Agency on Aging, Inc..
116 North 2nd Street
Lewisburg, PA 17837
570-524-2100
Fax: 570-524-0003; *Toll Free:* 800-533-1050
info@usaaa17.org
www.usaaa17.org

Peggy Chamberlain, President
Harry Adrian, Vice President
Carol Giesen, Secretary

Mission is to ensure the rights of older adults to live independent, menaingful, and dignified lives in their own homes and communities, make informed decisions concerning their care, and stay active and prductive for as long as possible.

Year Founded: 1999

1563 Voluntary Action Center of Northeastern Pennsylvania
Voluntary Action Center
Scranton Life Building
538 Spruce Street, Suite 420
Scranton, PA 18503
570-347-5616
Fax: 570-341-5816
vac@vacnepa.org
www.vacnepa.org

Ellen Stevens, Executive Director

Provides services to individuals and organizations in the areas of volunteerism, information and referral, and prevention.

Year Founded: 1976

1564 Wayne County: Area Agency on Aging
323 Tenth Street
Honesdale, PA 18431
570-253-4262
Fax: 570-253-9115; *Toll Free:* 800-648-9620
aging.co.wayne.pa.us/

Brian W. Smith, Chairman
Jacqueline Sturgis, Aging Administrator
Andrea Whyte, Human Services Administrator

Mission is to enhance their aging by promoting independence, choice and empowering our aging adults through partnerships and prgrams that improve and grow home and community based services.

1565 Westmoreland County: Area Agency on Aging
Westmoreland County Area Agency on Aging
2 North Main Street
Suite 101
Greensburg, PA 15601
724-830-3000
Fax: 724-830-4513; *Toll Free:* 800-442-8000
aaa@co.westmoreland.pa.us

www.co.westmoreland.pa.us/
TDD 412-830-4444

Sharon Casario, Production Assistant

Provides referrals and services for the aging.

Year Founded: 1773

Rhode Island

1566 Department of Mental Health, Retardation and Hospitals of Rhode Island
14 Harrington Road
Cranston, RI 02920-3080
401-462-3291
Fax: 401-462-3204
cstenning@bhddh.ri.gov
www.bhddh.ri.gov/
TDD 401-462-6087

Craig Stenning, Director

Committed to assuring access to quality services and supports for people with developmental disabilities, mental health and subsatnce abuse issues, and chronic long term medical conditions.

1567 Narragansett Senior Citizens Association
25 Fifth Avenue
Narragansett, RI 02882
401-789-1044
www.narragansettri.gov

Barbara E Wright, Senior Services Coordinator
Lisa Roy, Facility Coordinator

Serves Senior citizens. To help senior citizens fulfill and enjoy their leisure years with weekly group activities. Sponsors day trips, extended trips, chorus and senior stretch.

Year Founded: 1636

1568 RSVP Capital Region
RSVP of the Capital Region, Inc.
50 Utley Drive
Suite 500
Camp Hill, PA 17011
717-541-9521
Fax: 401-421-1079; *Toll Free:* 800-870-2616
rsvp@rsvpcapreg.org
rsvpcapreg.org/

Josh Hussey, Director

The Retired and Senior Volunteer Program (RSVP) provides opportunities for people 55 and over to make a difference in their community through volunteer service. RSVP volunteers contribute anywhere from a few to over forty hours a week, serving thourgh schools, day care centers, police departments, hospitals and other nonprofit and public organizations to help meet critical community needs. RSVP offers maximum flexibility and choice to its volunteers. RSVP matches the personal interests and skills to older Americans with opportunities to help solve community problems and offer supplemental insurance while on duty, on-the-job training from the agency or organization where volunteers are placed.

1569 RSVP Northern Rhode Island
Retired Senior Volunteer Program-Northern Rhode Is
PO Box 774
Woonsocket, RI 02895
401-766-2300
Fax: 401-769-6792
www.211ri.org/

Charles B Ryan, Director

The Retired and Senior Volunteer Program (RSVP) provides opportunities for people 55 and over to make a difference in their community through volunteer service. RSVP volunteers contribute anywhere from a few to over forty hours a week, serving thourgh schools, day care centers, police departments, hospitals and other nonprofit and public organizations to help meet critical community needs. RSVP offers maximum flexibility and choice to its volunteers. RSVP matches the personal interests and skills to older Americans with opportunities to help solve community problems and offer supplemental insurance while on duty, on-the-job training from the agency or organization where volunteers are placed.

1570 RSVP West Bay
224 Buttonwoods Avenue
Warwick, RI 02886-7506
401-732-4660
Fax: 401-739-2761
www.westbaycap.org/

Susan Lewis, Director

The Retired and Senior Volunteer Program (RSVP) provides opportunities for people 55 and over to make a difference in their community through volunteer service. RSVP volunteers contribute anywhere from a few to over forty hours a week, serving thourgh schools, day care centers, police departments, hospitals and other nonprofit and public organizations to help meet critical community needs. RSVP offers maximum flexibility and choice to its volunteers. RSVP matches the personal interests and skills to older Americans with opportunities to help solve community problems and offer supplemental insurance while on duty, on-the-job training from the agency or organization where volunteers are placed.

1571 Rhode Island Protection & Advocacy for Persons with Disabilities
Rhode Island Disability Law Center
275 Westminster Street
Suite 401
Providence, RI 02903-3434
401-831-3150
Fax: 401-274-5568; *Toll Free:* 800-733-5332
info@ridlc.org
www.ridlc.org
TTY: 401-831-5335

Raymond Bandusky, Director

Mission is to assist people with differing abilities in theor efforts to achieve full inclusion in society and to excercise their civil and humn rights through the provision of legal advocacy.

1572 Seniors Helping Others Volunteer Program of Washington County
Seniors Helping Others
25 Saint Dominic Road
Wakefield, RI 02879

401-789-2362
Fax: 401-789-1138
seniors@netsense.net
www.sho-ri.tripod.com

Fred Vanley, Volunteer Coordinator
Debra Tanner, Executive Director

South Carolina

1573 Aiken Area Council on Aging
Aiken Area Council on Aging, Inc.
159 Morgan Street NW
Aiken, SC 29801
803-648-5447
Fax: 803-649-1005; *Toll Free:* 866-228-5151
wwww.aacoa.net

Scott K Murphy, Executive Director
Charlotte McNichols, Finance Director
Sharon Cowden, Director of Services

Interested persons aged 60 and older. Provides focal point for information, advocacy, and other services for senior citizens. Promotes independence and quality of life.

1574 Catawba: Area Agency on Aging
Catawba Area Agency on Aging
2051 Ebenezer Road, Suite B
PO Box 4618
Rock Hill, SC 29732
803-329-9670
Fax: 803-329-6537; *Toll Free:* 800-662-8330
www.catawba-aging.com

Barbara Robinson, Executive Director
Deborah S. Lewis, Caregiver Advocate
Melissa R. Morrison, Long Term Care Ombudsman

Seeks to assist the entire population of the four county region, realizing that all generations have a stake in aging issues.

1575 Disability Determination Division
The South Carolina Vocational Rehabilitation Depar
1410 Boston Avenue
PO Box 15
West Columbia, SC 29171
803-896-6500
Fax: 803-896-6426; *Toll Free:* 800-832-7526
www.scvrd.net
TTY: 803-896-6553

Derle A. Lowder Sr., Agency Board Chairman
Dr. Roxanne Breland, Vice-Chair
Barbara G. Hollis, Executive Officer

Processes disabilikty claims

1576 Lancaster County Council on Aging
Lancaster County, SC
101 North Main Street
Lancaster, SC 29721
803-285-1565
Fax: 803-285-5691
www.mylancastersc.org

Lisa Robinson, Human Resources Director
Clay Catoe, Director
Debbie Horne, Administrator

Provides services for the elderly.

Year Founded: 1785

1577 Lowcountry Area Agency on Aging
634 Campground Road
P.O. Box 98
Yemassee, SC 29945
843-473-3991
Fax: 843-726-5165; *Toll Free:* 877-846-8148
office@lowcountrycog.org
www.lowcountrycog.org

Jordan Newman, Dir., Again/Disability Resources
Sabrena Graham, Executive Director
Sherry Smith, Finance Director

Plans, coordinates, and contracts with local providers for services to senior adults in the South Carolina service area of Beaufort, Colleton, Hampton & Jasper Counties.

1578 Lower Savannah: Area Agency on Aging
Lower Savannah Council of Governments
PO Box 850
Aiken, SC 29802
803-649-7981
Fax: 803-649-2248
info@lscog.org
www.lscog.org

Ronnie Young, Vice Chairman
Connie H. Shade, Executive Director
Nora D. Sanders, Assistant Executive Director

1579 Protection & Advocacy for People with Disabilities
Protection and Advocacy for People with Disabiliti
3710 Landmark Drive
Suite 208
Columbia, SC 29204
803-782-0639
Fax: 803-790-1946; *Toll Free:* 800-922-5225
info@pandasc.org
pandasc.org
TTY: 866-232-4525

J. Ashley Twombley, Chairman
Sherry Williams, Vice Chairman
Gloria M. Prevost, Executive Director

Mission is protecting and advancing disability rights.
Year Founded: 1973

1580 RSVP Carolina Low Country
8085 Rivers Avenue
Suite F
North Charleston, SC 29406
843-764-2323
Fax: 843-764-2318
dillonp@usa.redcross.org
www.lowcountryredcross.org

Pam Dillon, Director
Marlene Williamon, Area Coordintor

Engages persons 55 and older in volunteer service to meet critical community needs; and to provide a high quality experience that will enrich the lives of volunteers,

1581 RSVP Florence County
Senior Citizens Association (SCA)
600 Senior Way
Florence, SC 29505

843-669-6761
Fax: 843-665-2266; *Toll Free:* 877-856-5529
www.seniorcitizensassociation.com/

Julie Baxley, President
John Miller, Vice-President
Lisa Brown, Secretary

The Retired and Senior Volunteer Program (RSVP) provides opportunities for people 55 and over to make a difference in their community through volunteer service. RSVP volunteers contribute anywhere from a few to over forty hours a week, serving thourgh schools, day care centers, police departments, hospitals and other nonprofit and public organizations to help meet critical community needs. RSVP offers maximum flexibility and choice to its volunteers. RSVP matches the personal interests and skills to older Americans with opportunities to help solve community problems and offer supplemental insurance while on duty, on-the-job training from the agency or organization where volunteers are placed.
Year Founded: 1960

1582 RSVP Greenville
RSVP Greeneville
50 Directors Drive
Greenville, SC 29601-2935
864-467-3660
Fax: 864-467-3668
rsvpgreenville@gmail.com
www.rsvpgreenvillesc.com/

Mary Zachar, Director

The Retired and Senior Volunteer Program (RSVP) provides opportunities for people 55 and over to make a difference in their community through volunteer service. RSVP volunteers contribute anywhere from a few to over forty hours a week, serving thourgh schools, day care centers, police departments, hospitals and other nonprofit and public organizations to help meet critical community needs. RSVP offers maximum flexibility and choice to its volunteers. RSVP matches the personal interests and skills to older Americans with opportunities to help solve community problems and offer supplemental insurance while on duty, on-the-job training from the agency or organization where volunteers are placed.

1583 Santee-Lynches Council of Governments Area Agency on Aging
PO Box 1837
Sumter, SC 29151
803-775-7381
Fax: 803-773-9903
www.santeelynchescog.org/

Michael Mikota, Executive Director
Sharon Durden, Deputy & Finance Director
Shawn Keith, Aging Director

Mission is to help find a new way to find community assistance for seniors, adults with disabilities, and their caregivers.

1584 Social Security: West Columbia Disability Determination
The South Carolina Vocational Rehabilitation Depar
1410 Boston Avenue
PO Box 15
West Columbia, SC 29171

803-896-6500
Fax: 803-896-6553; Toll Free: 800-832-7526
info@scvrd.state.sc.us
www.scvrd.net

Derle A. Lowder Sr., Agency Board Chairman
Dr. Roxanne Breland, Vice-Chair
Barbara G. Hollis, Executive Officer

The South Carolina Vocational Rehabilitation Department's Disability Determination Services processes Social Security and Supplemental Security Income claims under the provisions of the Social Security Act.

1585 South Carolina Assistive Technology Projects
South Carolina Assistive Technology Program
USC School of Medicine
8301 Farrow Road
Columbia, SC 29203
803-935-5263
Fax: 803-935-5342; Toll Free: 800-915-4522
Janet.Jendron@uscmed.sc.edu
www.sc.edu/scatp
TDD 803-935-5263

Carol Page, Ph.D., Program Director
Mary Alice Bechtler, Program Coordinator
Leah Diggs, Research Assistant

A statewide program promoting assistive technology devices and services for persons of all ages with all disabilities.

1586 South Carolina Client Assistance Program
Office of the Governor of South Carolina
South Carolina Client Assistance Program
Edgar A. Brown Building
1205 Pendleton Street
Columbia, SC 29201
803-734-0285
Fax: 803-734-0546; Toll Free: 800-868-0040
cap@oepp.sc.gov
www.oepp.sc.gov/cap
TDD 803-734-1147

Denise Riley MSW, Director
Cindy Popenhagen, Program Administrator

The Client Assistance Program (CAP) helps citizens of the State by acting as advocates regarding services provided by the Vocational Rehabilitation Department (VR), Commission for the Blind, and all Independent Living programs and projects funded under the Rehabilitation Act of 1973. As advocates, CAP staff can investigate, negotiate, mediate, and pursue administrative, and other remedies to ensure that clients rights are protected.

1587 South Carolina Department of Aging
South Carolina Lieutenant Governor's Office on Agi
1301 Gervais Street
Suite 350
Columbia, SC 29201
803-734-9900
Fax: 803-734-9887; Toll Free: 800-868-9095
askus@aging.sc.gov
www.aging.sc.gov

Tony Kester, Executive Director
Catherine Angus, Volunteer Coordinator

Mission is to enhance the quality of life for seniors through advocating, planning, and developing resources in partner-

ship with state and local governements, non-profits and the private sector, individuals and advocates to meet the present and future aspirations of the growing senior population.

1588 South Carolina Department of Veterans Affairs
S.C. Governor's Office of Executive Policy and Pro
Edgar A. Brown Building
1205 Pendleton Street
Columbia, SC 29201
803-734-0200
Fax: 803-734-0421; Toll Free: 800-827-1000
va@oepp.sc.gov
www.govoepp.state.sc.us

Rhonda Walker, Director of Finance
Carol Smoak, Administrative Coordinator
Mary Smith, Director of Human Resources

Mission is to be the advocate for the state's 413,000 veterans in amatters that pertain to veterans.

Year Founded: 1776

1589 South Carolina Developmental Disability Council
South Carolina Developmental Disabilities Council
1205 Pendleton Street
Suite 461
Columbia, SC 29201
803-734-0465
Fax: 803-734-0241
javancleave@oepp.sc.gov
www.scddc.state.sc.us/
TTY: 803-734-1147

Valarie Bishop, Executive Director
Carol Niederhauser, Program Coordinator
Esther Williams, Administrative Specialist

Mission is to provide leadership in planning, funding, and implementing initiatives that lead to improved quality of life for people with developmental disabilities and their families.

1590 South Carolina Workers Compensation Commission
South Carolina Worker's Compensation Commission
PO Box 1715
1333 Main Street, Suite 500
Columbia, SC 29202-1715
803-737-5700
Fax: 803-737-1234
www.wcc.sc.gov

T. Scott Beck, Interim Chairman
Susan S. Barden, Vice Chairman
Amy Bracy, Administrative Assistant

Responsible for administering the workers' compensation law in South Carolina.

Year Founded: 1911

1591 Trident: Area Agency on Aging
Trident Area Agency on Aging

4450 Leeds Place West
Suite B
North Charleston, SC 29405

843-554-2275
Fax: 843-554-2284; *Toll Free:* 800-894-0415
info@tridentaaa.org
www.tridentaaa.net

Catherine O'Brien, President
Stephanie Blunt, Executive Director
Lisa Natividad, Finance Manager

Trident Area Agency on Aging plan, coordinate and offer services that help older adults remain in their home - if that is their preference - aided by services such as Meals-on-Wheels, homemaker assistance and whatever else it may take to make independent living a viable option.

South Dakota

1592 Division of Developmental Disabilities
South Dakota Department of Human Services
3800 East Highway 34, Hillsview Plaza
c/o 500 East Capital Avenue
Pierre, SD 57501
605-773-5990
Fax: 605-773-5483; *Toll Free:* 800-265-9684
www.state.sd.us/dhs
TTY: 605-773-6412

Lloyd Johnson, Assistant Director/ Accounts Pay
Dan Lusk, Division Director
Nick Cotton, Director of Budget & Finance

1593 RSVP Siouxland
Siouxland RSVP
1000 North West Avenue
Suite 260
Sioux Falls, SD 57104
605-362-2517
Fax: 605-271-5015
mnemec@good-sam.com
www.good-sam.com/rsvp/

Chellee Nemec, Project Director
Jackie Lukes, Volunteer Coordinator

RSVP is a national nonprofit organization that provides meaningful volunteer experiences for individuals 55+ within their local communities. Locally, the SIOUXLAND RSVP utilizes the time and talents of 600 volunteers in 200 local nonprofit organizations, health related facilities and public agencies in Minnehaha, Lincoln, and Union Counties in southeastern South Dakota.

1594 South Dakota Department of Aging
South Dakota Department of Social Services
700 Governors Drive
Pierre, SD 57501
605-773-3165
Fax: 605-773-6834
www.dss.sd.gov/elderlyservices

Kristin Kellar, Communications Director
Doug Dix, Deputy Financial Officer
Lynne Valenti, Deputy Secretary

1595 South Dakota Department of Military and Veterans Services
South Dakota Department of the Military
425 East Capitol Avenue
Pierre, SD 57501

605-773-3269
Fax: 605-773-5380; *Toll Free:* 877-579-0015
mva.sd.gov

Major Genera Reisch, Adjutant General
Connie Hohn, Budget & Finance Director
Steve Harding, Deputy Secretary

Mission is to provide highly trained and competent military units and individuals that will quickly respond to state emergencies and federal missions.

1596 South Dakota Department of Revenue
South Dakota Department of Revenue
425 East Capitol Avenue
Pierre, SD 57501-3185
605-773-3311
Fax: 605-773-6729; *Toll Free:* 800-829-9188
bustax@state.sd.us
dor.sd.gov/

Andy Gerlach, Secretary
Andy Gerlach, Secretary
David Wiest, Deputy Secretary

Focus is to serve and to support government services by collecting all taxes required by law.

1597 South Dakota Division of Rehabilitation
South Dakota Department of Human Services
3800 East Highway 34, Hillsview Plaza
c/o 500 East Capital Avenue
Pierre, SD 57501
605-773-5990
Fax: 605-773-5483; *Toll Free:* 800-265-9684
www.state.sd.us/dhs
TTY: 605-773-6412

Lloyd Johnson, Assistant Director/ Accounts Pay
Dan Lusk, Division Director
Nick Cotton, Director of Budget & Finance

Provides individualized services to assist people with significant disabilities to get and keep jobs that are compatible with their disability. Services can consist of: vocational rehabilitation counseling, assessment and diagnostic, work skills training, job site accommodations, job placement, and employer services.

1598 South Dakota Office of Adult Services
South Dakota Department of Social Services
700 Governors Drive
Pierre, SD 57501
605-773-3165
Fax: 605-773-4085; *Toll Free:* 866-854-5465
asa@state.sd.us
dss.sd.gov

Kristin Kellar, Communications Director
Doug Dix, Deputy Financial Officer
Lynne Valenti, Deputy Secretary

1599 South Dakota Protection Advocacy Services
Advocacy Services
221 South Central Avenue
Suite 38
Pierre, SD 57501
605-773-3181
Fax: 605-224-5125; *Toll Free:* 800-658-4782
sdas@sdadvocacy.com
www.sdadvocacy.com
TTY: 605-224-8294

Darlys Baum, Executive Director

1600 South Dakota Workers Compensation Board
South Dakota Department of Labor and Regulation
700 Governors Drive
Pierre, SD 57501-2291
605-773-3101
Fax: 605-773-6184
dlr.sd.gov

Lyle Harter, Director of Administrative Servi
Bret Afdahl, Division of Banking
Marcia Hultman, Secretary

Provides assistance for work related injuries and the benefits South Dakota Workers qualify for.

Tennessee

1601 East Tennessee: Area Agency on Aging
The East Tennessee Human Resource Agency
9111 Cross Park Drive
Suite D-100
Knoxville, TN 37923
865-691-2551
Fax: 865-531-7216
info@ethra.org
www.ethra.org
TDD 865-681-1990

William Baird, Chairman
Estelle Herron, Vice Chairman
Troy Beets, Secretary

Responsible for developing an advocacy and service delivery systems for persons 60and over and persons with disabilities.

1602 McMinn County Senior Citizens
McMinn County Senior Citizens, Inc.
PO Box 41
205 McMinn Avenue
Athens, TN 37371-0041
423-745-6830
Fax: 423-745-6803
mcminnsenior@comcast.net
www.mcminnseniors.com

Holly Currier, Executive Director & SHIP Counse
Tracey Davis, Assistant Director
Jane Wheeler, Activity/Program Coordinator & S

Year Founded: 1978; Number of Members: 625

1603 McMinn County Senior Citizens Inc.
PO Box 41
205 McMinn Avenue
Athens, TN 37371
423-745-6830
Fax: 423-745-6803
mcminnsenior@comcast.net
www.mcminnseniors.com

Holly Currier, Executive Director
Tracey Davis, Assistant Director
Jane Wheeler, Activity Coordinator

Extends senior citizen's quality of life by involving children and community in providing educational, physical, nutritional, intergenerational, recreational, and social programs including volunteer service opportunities. Serves ages 55+.

Year Founded: 1978; Number of Members: 665

1604 Midsouth: Area Agency on Aging
The Aging Commission of the Mid-South (ACMS)
2670 Union Avenue Extended
Suite 1000
Memphis, TN 38112
901-224-4100
Fax: 901-327-7755
www.agingcommission.org/

Dora Ivey, Executive Director
Gloria L. Collins, Chief Operating Officer/ Manager
Kathy Williams, Chief Financial Officer/ Manager

The Agency on Aging serves as the local point for aging services. The Agency on Aging also acts as the uniting link between senior citizens and agencies and programs that serve them.

1605 Northwest Tennessee: Area Agency on Aging and Disability
Northwest Tennessee Development District
124 Weldon Drive
PO Box 963
Martin, TN 38237-0963
731-587-4213
Fax: 731-588-5833; *Toll Free:* 800-750-6866
www.nwtddhra.org/

John A. Bucy, Executive Director
Betty Waggner, Assistant Financial Office/Offic
Melinda Goode, Special Projects/HR Director

Northwest Tennessee Area Agency on Aging strives to secure, promote and provide essential services to enhance the quality of life in a diverse and changing society. We meet this challenge through advocacy, coordination, building alliances, and promoting public awareness, guided by integrity, vision, and sustained commitment.

Year Founded: 1971

1606 RSVP Clarksville County
Clarksville-Montgomery County Community Action Age
PO Box 487
Clarksville, TN 37041-0487
931-896-1800
Fax: 931-648-5784
www.cmccaa.com/

Leslie Chiodini, Executive Director
Angie Lee, Fiscal Officer
Cindy Downing, Human Resources

The Retired and Senior Volunteer Program (RSVP) provides opportunities for people 55 and over to make a difference in their community through volunteer service. RSVP volunteers contribute anywhere from a few to over forty hours a week, serving thourgh schools, day care centers, police departments, hospitals and other nonprofit and public organizations to help meet critical community needs. RSVP offers maximum flexibility and choice to its volunteers. RSVP matches the personal interests and skills to older Americans with opportunities to help solve community problems and offer supplemental insurance while on duty, on-the-job training from the agency or organization where volunteers are placed.

Year Founded: 1978

1607 RSVP Knoxville-Knox County
Retired & Senior Volunteer Program
Knoxville-Knox
2247 Western Avenue
Knoxville, TN 37921-5756
865-524-2786
Fax: 865-546-0832
knoxooa@knoxseniors.org
www.knoxseniors.org/rsvp.html

Rebecca Hare, Director

The Retired and Senior Volunteer Program (RSVP) provides opportunities for people 55 and over to make a difference in their community through volunteer service. RSVP
volunteers contribute anywhere from a few to over forty
hours a week, serving thourgh schools, day care centers,
police departments, hospitals and other nonprofit and public organizations to help meet critical community needs.
RSVP offers maximum flexibility and choice to its volunteers. RSVP matches the personal interests and skills to
older Americans with opportunities to help solve community problems and offer supplemental insurance while on
duty, on-the-job training from the agency or organization
where volunteers are placed.

Year Founded: 1965

1608 Railroad Retirement Board: Tennessee District
Office
233 Cumberland Bend
Suite 104
Nashville, TN 37228-1806
877-772-5772
Fax: 615-736-7071
www.rrb.gov/field/do_nash.asp

Suzanna Givan, Representative

Administering retirement/survivor and unemployment/sick-
ness benefit programs for railroad workers and their
families.

1609 Tennessee Association of Homes and Services
for the Aging
LeadingAge of Tennessee
P. O. Box 41852
Nashville, TN 37204
615-970-7269
Fax: 615-726-3082
www.leadingagetennessee.org

David Glascoe, Chairman/President
Tom Sexton, Treasurer
Kirkland A. Mason, Secretary

Mission is expanding the world of possibilities for the aging.

1610 Tennessee Client Assistance Program
Department of Human Services
Citizens Plaza State Office Building , 14th Floor
400 Deaderick Street
Nashville, TN 37243-1403
615-313-5183
Fax: 615-741-6508; *Toll Free:* 800-732-5059
TN.TTAP@tn.gov
www.tennessee.gov/humanserv/rehab
TTY: 615-313-5695

Dr. Raquel Hatter, Commissioner

Mission is to help individuals with disabilities receive the
services for which they are eligible un the Rehabilitation
Act.

1611 Tennessee Commission on Aging and Disability
Tennessee Commission on Aging and Disability
502 Deaderick Street
9th Floor
Nashville, TN 37243-0860
615-741-2056
Fax: 615-741-3309
www.tn.gov/comaging

Jim Schulman, Executive Director
Kathy Zamata, Program Director

The Commission is the designated state agency on aging
and is mandated to provide leadrship relative to aging issues on behalf of older persons in the state.

1612 Tennessee Council on Developmental
Disabilities
Council on Developmental Disabilities
500 James Robertson Parkway
Davy Crockett Tower, First Floor
Nashville, TN 37243
615-532-6615
Fax: 615-532-6964
tnddc@tn.gov
www.state.tn.us/cdd
TTY: 615-741-4562

Wanda Willis, Executive Director
Errol Elshtain, Planning Coordinator

The Tennessee Council of Developmental Disabilities is a
State office that promotes public policies to increase and
support the inclusion of individuals with developmental
disabilities in their communities. The Council works with
public and private groups across the State to find necessary
supports for individuals with disabilities and their families,
so that they may have equal access to public education, employment, housing, health care, and all other aspects of
community life.

1613 Tennessee Department of Revenue
Department of Revenue
500 Deaderick Street
Andrew Jackson Building
Nashville, TN 37242
615-253-0600; *Toll Free: 800-342-1003*
TN.Revenue@tn.gov
www.state.tn.us/revenue

Richard H Roberts, Commissioner

Mission is to collect all the necessary taxes that are due by
law.

1614 Tennessee Department of Veterans Affairs
Department of Veteran Affairs
312 Rosa L Parks Avenue
Nashville, TN 37243
615-741-2931
Fax: 615-741-4785
TN.Veterans@tn.gov
www.state.tn.us/veteran/

Many-Bears Grinder, Commissioner
Noreen Henson, Executive Assistant to Commissio
Wendell Cheek, Deputy Commissioner

Mission is to serve veterans, their families and survivors with dignity and compassion.

1615 Tennessee Division of Rehabilitation Services
Department of Human Services
400 Deaderick Street
15th Floor
Nashville, TN 37243-1403
615-313-4700
Fax: 615-741-4165
www.tn.gov/humanserv

Raquel Hatter, Commissioner
Bill Russell, General Counsel
Shalonda Cawthon, Deputy Commissioner

The Division of Vocational Rehabilitation is the state's public program that helps people with physical and mental disabilities obtain or retain employment. Its mission is to provide opportunities and resources to eligible individuals with disabilities, leading to success in employment and independent living.

1616 Tennessee Technology Access Program
Department of Human Services
400 Deaderick Street
15th Floor
Nashville, TN 37243-1403
615-313-4700
Fax: 615-741-4165; *Toll Free:* 800-732-5059
tn.ttap@tn.gov
www.tn.gov/humanserv
TTY: 615-313-5695

Raquel Hatter, Commissioner
Bill Russell, General Counsel
Shalonda Cawthon, Deputy Commissioner

The Tennessee Technology Access Program (TTAP) is a statewide program designed to increase access to, and acquisition of, assistive technology devices and services.

1617 Upper Cumberland Area: Agency on Aging
The Upper Cumberland Development District
1225 South Willow Avenue
Cookeville, TN 38501
931-432-4111
Fax: 931-432-6010
www.ucdd.org

Mark Farley, Executive Director
Charlotte Burks, Senator
Charles Curtis, Representative

1618 Workers Compensation Division
Department of Labor and Workforce Development
220 French Landing Drive
Nashville, TN 37243
615-741-6642
Fax: 615-741-5078; *Toll Free:* 800-332-2667
wc.info@tn.gov
tn.gov/labor-wfd

Burns Phillips, Commissioner
Stephanie Mitchell, General Counsel
Marva Doremus, Administrator

Mission is to work as a team to promote workforce development and improve workplace safety and health throughout Tennessee.

Texas

1619 Administration for Community Living: Region VI
US Department of Health & Human Services
1301 Young Street
Room 736
Dallas, TX 75201
214-767-2971
Fax: 214-767-2951
www.aoa.gov

Percy Devine, Regional Administrator
Kathy Greenlee, Assistant Secretary AoA
Aviva Sufian, Deputy Assistant Secretary AoA

Region includes Arkansas, Louisiana, New Mexico, Oklahoma, and Texas. Provides supportive and nutrition services, including transportation, meals, and escorts, to individuals over the age of 60. Priority is given to those with the greatest economic and social need. Region VI: AR, LA, OK, NM, TX
Year Founded: 1965

1620 Alamo: Area Agency on Aging
Alamo Area Council of Governments
8700 Tesoro Drive
Suite 700
San Antonio, TX 78217-6228
210-362-5200
Fax: 210-225-5937
alamo.aging@aacog.com
www.aacog.com
TDD 800-456-5094
TTY: 800-735-2989

Dean Danos, Executive Director
Jeri Rainey, Chief Financial Officer
Anthony Jalomo, Senior Director of Disability Se

Supports older residents in 12 rural counties.

1621 Ark-Tex Council of Governments: Area Agency on Aging
Ark-Tex Council of Governments
4808 Elizabeth Street
Texarkana, TX 75503
903-832-8636
Fax: 903-832-3441; *Toll Free:* 800-372-4464
dmckinnon@atcog.org
www.atcog.org/areaAgencyAging.php

L D Williamson, Executive Director
Diane McKinnon, Manager

Serves seniors in 9 northeast Texas counties.

1622 Austin Disability Determination Services
Texas Department of Assistive and Rehabilitative S
PO Box 149198
Austin, TX 78714-9198
512-437-8000; *Toll Free:* 800-252-7009
www.dars.state.tx.us/

Terrell I Murphy, DARS Commissioner
Mary Elder, Deputy Commissioner
Alvin Miller

The DARS Division for Disability Determination Services (DDS), funded entirely through the Social Security Administration (SSA), makes disability determinations for Texans with severe disabilities who apply for benefits at their local Social Security Office and their applications are forwarded to DDS for a disability determination; however, SSA is responsbile for making final decisions as to whether or not a person is eligible to receive benefits.

1623 Bexar County: Area Agency on Aging
Alamo Area Council of Governments
8700 Tesoro Drive
Suite 700
San Antonio, TX 78217-6228
210-362-5200
Fax: 210-225-5937; *Toll Free:* 800-960-5201
mail@aacog.com
www.aacog.com
TDD 800-456-5094
TTY: 800-735-2989

Dean Danos, Executive Director
Jeri Rainey, Chief Financial Officer
Anthony Jalomo, Senior Director of Disability Se
Supports older residents of the Bexar Area.

1624 Bureau of Naval Personnel: Kingsville Retired Activities Office
Fleet and Family Support Center
Naval Air Station Kingsville Texas
746 Rosendahl Street
Kingsville, TX 78363
361-516-6333
Fax: 361-516-6927
www.navyfamily.com

The RAO serves as a link between local retired military and the active-duty community which provides assistance to retired military. It provides installation commanders with a means of providing more effective services and improving communication for the local retired community. The RAO is staffed and operated by volunteer retired military who assist other retired members, their families and survivors to receive entitled services and benefits. Through newsletters, seminars and appreciation days, the RAO supports quality of life issues throughout the retirement years to their fellow service members.

1625 Capital: Area Agency on Aging
Capital Area Council of Governments
6800 Burleson Road
Building 310, Ste. 165
Austin, TX 78744
512-916-6000
Fax: 512-916-6001
www.capcog.org

Judge Wayne Brascom, Chair
Mayor Marc Holm, 1st Vice-Chair
Jennifer Scott, Director
Services for 60+ individuals.
Year Founded: 1970

1626 Center for Lifelong Learning
The Osher Lifelong Learning Institute
UTEP 500 West University
Miners Hall Suite 209
El Paso, TX 79968
915-747-6280
Fax: 915-747-5538
contact@olliatutep.org
www.olliatutep.org

Winifred Dowling, Ph.D., Chair
Becky Duval Reese, Vice Chair
Peter A Rivera, Executive Director
Institute for learning in retirement.

1627 Coastal Bend: Area Agency on Aging
Area Agency on Aging of the Castal Bend
2910 Leopard Street
Corpus Christi, TX 78408-3614
361-883-3935
Fax: 361-883-5749; *Toll Free:* 800-817-5743
www.aaacoastalbend.org
TDD 800-456-5094
TTY: 800-735-2989

Mary Ganger, Director
Supports seniors in the Coastal Bend area.

1628 Concho Valle: Area Agency on Aging
Area Agency on Aging of the Concho Valley
2801 W Loop 306
Suite A
San Angelo, TX 76904
325-223-5704
Fax: 325-223-8233; *Toll Free:* 877-944-9666
toni.gutierrez@cvcog.org
www.cvcog.org/cvcog/aaa.html

Fred Deaton, Chair
Danny Neal, Vice Chairman
Jeffery Sutton, Executive Director
Our mission is to be the visible advocate and leader in the Concho Valley in providing for a comprehensive and coordinated continuum of services and opportunities so that older people can lead dignified, independent, and productive lives.

1629 Dallas Association of Directors of Volunteers - Brady Center Catholic Charities of Dallas
Dallas Association of Directors of Volunteers
P.O. Box 793763
Dallas, TX 75379
214-826-8330
Fax: 214-826-8579
www.dadv.org/

Lori Hudson, President
Elizabeth Bu Andrus, Vice President
Debra Polsky, Treasurer
Senior Centers provide nutritional meals at breakfast and lunch, social and recreational activities to seniors over the age of 60 years old. Bi-lingual staff coordinate a wide variety of activities, including health and safety classes.

1630 East Texas: Area Agency on Aging
East Texas Council of Governments
3800 Stone Road
Kilgore, TX 75662
903-218-6400
Fax: 903-983-1440; *Toll Free:* 800-442-8845
www.etcog.org

Mayor Angela Raiborn, Chair
Commissioner McKinney, 1st Vice-Chair
David Clveland, Executive Director
Provides support services to seniors in the East Texas area.
Year Founded: 1970

1631 Employees Retirement System of Texas
Employees Retirement System of Texas
PO Box 13207
Austin, TX 78711-3207
512-476-6431
Fax: 512-867-7438; *Toll Free:* 877-275-4377
www.ers.state.tx.us
TTY: 800-735-2989

Brian D. Ragland, Brian D. Ragland, Chair
Frederick E. Rowe, Jr., Vice-Chair
Ann S. Bishop, Executive Director

Serves seniors of Texas.

1632 Friends of Austin State Supported Living Center
Friends of Austin State Supported Living Center
2203 West 35th Street
Austin, TX 78703
512-374-6048
Fax: 512-374-6068
friends@ausslcfriends.org
www.ausslcfriends.org

Charles Bratcher, Center Director
Laura Murphy, Community Relations Director

Nonprofit advocacy group working for the benefit of residents of Austin State Supported Living Center.

Year Founded: 1956

1633 Golden Crescent: Area Agency on Aging
Golden Crescent Regional Planning Cimmission
120 South Main
Suite 210
Victoria, TX 77901
361-578-1587
Fax: 361-578-8865; *Toll Free:* 800-574-9745
cindyco@gcrpc.org
www.gcrpc.org
TDD 512-820-1262

Kenneth Finster, President
Joe E. Brannon, Executive Director
Wayne Dierlam, 1st Vice President

Supports seniors with funding provided by the Texas Department of Aging.

Year Founded: 1968

1634 Gray Panthers of Austin
Gray Panthers of Austin
8507 Lewis Mountain Drive
Austin, TX 78737
512-704-6675
Fax: 512-458-9727
ydugger@austin.rr.com
graypanthersaustin.org/

Leslie Aisenman, Convenor
Roland Scott, Treasurer
Maggie Kuhn, Founder

Promotes universal access to health care. Provides education on aging.

1635 Heart of Texas Council of Governments: Area Agency on Aging
Heart of Texas Council of Governments
1514 South New Road
Waco, TX 76711

254-292-1800
Fax: 254-756-0102
info@hot.cog.tx.us
www.hotcog.org

Honorable St Sharp, President
Hon Kay Taylor, Vice President
Hon. Bryan Ferguson, Secretary/ Treasurer

Provides access to needed social services, effective screening and assessment of individual needs, and advocacy for the older persons (age 60 and older) in the six-county region.

Year Founded: 1996

1636 Hill Country Community Action Association
Hill Country Community Action
2905 West Wallace
PO Box 846
San Saba, TX 76877
325-372-5167
Fax: 325-372-3526
hccaainc@centex.net
www.hccaa.com

Tama Shaw, Executive Director
Frances Little, Associate Director
Angela Miller, Human Resource Director

The purpose of the Agency is to promote the reduction of poverty, the revitalization of low-income communities, and the empowerment of familiies and individuals in the service area.

1637 Houston Harris County: Area Agency on Aging
Harris County: Area Agency on Aging
8000 N Stadium Drive
8th Floor
Houston, TX 77054-1823
832-393-4301
Fax: 713-794-9464; *Toll Free:* 800-213-8471
aging@houstontx.gov
www.houstontx.gov/health/Aging

Charlene Hunter James, Director

Strengthens services for the state's elderly population.

1638 Houston-Galveston: Area Agency on Aging
Houston-Galveston Area Council
PO Box 22777
Houston, TX 77227-2777
713-627-3200
Fax: 713-993-4578; *Toll Free:* 800-437-7396
Rick.Guerrero@h-gac.com
www.h-gac.com

William Bass, Chief GIS Specialist
Ronnie Barnes, Program Coordinator, Purchasing
Cynthia Aviles, Benefits Counselor

Manages Older Americans Act (OAA) and other state funded programs such as home-delivered meals and housekeeping services.

1639 Kings Manor Methodist Retirement System
King's Manor Methodist System
400 Ranger Street
P.O. Box 1999
Hereford, TX 79045
806-364-0661
Fax: 806-364-0675
www.kmmrs.com

Shelly Moss, Executive Director
Jim Layman, Chief Financial Officer
Yolanda Alaniz, Director of Nursing

The area's only not-for-profit, faith-based, community providing all levels of senior care in an affordable family atmosphere.

Year Founded: 1960

1640 Leading Age Texas
LeadingAge Texas
2205 Hancock Drive
Austin, TX 78756
512-467-2242
Fax: 512-467-2275
info@leadingagetexas.org
www.tahsa.org

George Linial, CAE, CASP

, President & CEO
Melanie Harrison, MPAff, Director of Education
Brandi Jimenez, Administrative Assistant/ Meetin

Association of non profit honest seniors for the aging in Texas.

Year Founded: 1959

1641 Lower Rio Grande Valley: Area Agency onAging
Lower Rio Grande Valley Development Council
301 West Railroad
Weslaco, TX 78596
956-682-3481
Fax: 956-631-4670; *Toll Free:* 800-365-6131
jgonzalez@lrgvdc.org
www.lrgvdc.org

Jose L Gonzalez, Director
Belinda Tyler, Program Administrator
Fina Martinez

Ensures that individuals aged 60 and over are treated with dignity, given independence, and provided with the opportunity to contribute to their communities.

Year Founded: 1984

1642 Middle Rio Grande: Area Agency on Aging
Middle Rio Grande Development Council
307 W Nopal
Carrizo Springs, TX 78834
830-876-3533
Fax: 830-876-9415; *Toll Free:* 800-224-4262
aaa.mrgdc.org
TDD 830-876-1260

Hon. Joel Rodriguez, Jr., President
Hon. Roberto Fernandez, 1st Vice President
Hon. Garry A Merritt, Secretary/ Treasurer

Dedicated to improving the lives of the elderly population of the Middle Rio Grande Area.

Year Founded: 1970

1643 North Central Texas: Area Agency on Aging
616 Six Flags Drive
PO Box 5888
Arlington, TX 76005-5888
817-695-9193
Fax: 817-695-9274; *Toll Free:* 800-272-3921
dgreen@nctcog.org
www.nctcog.org

Doni Green, Manager
Pat Borgfeldt, Volunteer Coordinator
Shannon Byrd

Serves seniors of North Central Texas.

1644 Panhandle: Area Agency on Aging
The Panhandle Regional Planning Commission
415 Southwest Eighth Avenue
PO Box 9257
Amarillo, TX 79105
806-372-3381
Fax: 806-373-3268; *Toll Free:* 800-642-6008
sleggett@theprpc.org
www.prpc.cog.tx.us

Brian Gillispie, Chair
Tom Velasquez, Vice Chair
Gary Pitne, Executive Director

Serves as the advocate for the Panhandle's elderly population.

Year Founded: 1969

1645 Permian Basin: Area Agency on Aging
Area Agency on Aging of the Permian Basin
2910 LaForce Boulevard
PO Box 60660
Midland, TX 79711
432-563-1061
Fax: 432-563-1728; *Toll Free:* 800-491-4636
plindsey@aaapb.com
www.aaapb.com

Jeannie Raglin, Director
Patti Lindsey, Operations Manager
Raynetta Williams, Benefits Counselor

Facilitates services for the elderly population of the Permian Basin.

1646 RSVP Big Spring
Big Spring Texas
1901 Simler Avenue
Big Spring, TX 79720-2732
432-267-1628
Fax: 432-264-2534
mmahaney@mybigspring.com
www.mybigspring.com

Larry McLellan, Mayor
Glen Carrigan, Council Member
Marcus M. Fernandez, Mayor Pro Tem

Provides opportunities for people 55 and over to make a difference in their community through volunteer service. RSVP volunteers contribute anywhere from a few to over forty hours a week, serving through schools, day care centers, police departments, hospitals and other nonprofit and public organizations to help meet critical community needs. RSVP matches the personal interests and skills of older Americans with opportunities to help solve community problems and offers supplemental insurance while on duty, on-the-job training from the agency or organization where volunteers are placed.

1647 RSVP Brazos Valley
The Brazos Valley Council of Governments
3991 East 29th Street
Bryan, TX 77803
979-595-2800
Fax: 979-595-2810

info@bvcog.org
www.bvcog.org

Mike Sutherland, 1st Vice Chair
Byron Ryder, President
Art Henson, Secretary

The Retired and Senior Volunteer Program (RSVP) provides opportunities for people 55 and over to make a difference in their community through volunteer service. RSVP volunteers contribute anywhere from a few to over forty hours a week, serving thourgh schools, day care centers, police departments, hospitals and other nonprofit and public organizations to help meet critical community needs. RSVP offers maximum flexibility and choice to its volunteers. RSVP matches the personal interests and skills to older Americans with opportunities to help solve community problems and offer supplemental insurance while on duty, on-the-job training from the agency or organization where volunteers are placed.

Year Founded: 1967

1648 RSVP Chisholm Trail County

1316 East McKinney Street
Denton, TX 76209
940-383-1508
Fax: 940-387-0862
info@rsvpserves.org
www.rsvpserves.org

Gloria Roberts, Chair
Betsy Haggard, Secretary
Melanie Vest, Treasurer

The Retired and Senior Volunteer Program (RSVP) provides opportunities for people 55 and over to make a difference in their community through volunteer service. RSVP volunteers contribute anywhere from a few to over forty hours a week, serving thourgh schools, day care centers, police departments, hospitals and other nonprofit and public organizations to help meet critical community needs. RSVP offers maximum flexibility and choice to its volunteers. RSVP matches the personal interests and skills to older Americans with opportunities to help solve community problems and offer supplemental insurance while on duty, on-the-job training from the agency or organization where volunteers are placed.

1649 RSVP Concho Valley

Concho Valley RSVP
618 South Chadbourne
San Angelo, TX 76903-6930
325-223-6388
Fax: 325-655-6294
dolores@cvrsvp.org
cvrsvp.org/contact.html

Dolores Schwertner, Director
Pam Klausner, RSVP Program Assistant
Denise Bloomquist, Executive Director

The Retired and Senior Volunteer Program (RSVP) provides opportunities for people 55 and over to make a difference in their community through volunteer service. RSVP volunteers contribute anywhere from a few to over forty hours a week, serving thourgh schools, day care centers, police departments, hospitals and other nonprofit and public organizations to help meet critical community needs. RSVP offers maximum flexibility and choice to its volunteers. RSVP matches the personal interests and skills to older Americans with opportunities to help solve community problems and offer supplemental insurance while on

duty, on-the-job training from the agency or organization where volunteers are placed.

Year Founded: 1981

1650 RSVP Concho Valley Texas

Concho Valley RSVP
618 South Chadbourne
San Angelo, TX 76903-6930
325-223-6388
Fax: 325-655-6294
dschwertner@wtrc.com
cvrsvp.org/contact.html

Dolores Schwertner, Director
Pam Klausner, RSVP Program Assistant
Denise Bloomquist, Executive Director

The Retired and Senior Volunteer Program (RSVP) provides opportunities for people 55 and over to make a difference in their community through volunteer service. RSVP volunteers contribute anywhere from a few to over forty hours a week, serving thourgh schools, day care centers, police departments, hospitals and other nonprofit and public organizations to help meet critical community needs. RSVP offers maximum flexibility and choice to its volunteers. RSVP matches the personal interests and skills to older Americans with opportunities to help solve community problems and offer supplemental insurance while on duty, on-the-job training from the agency or organization where volunteers are placed.

Year Founded: 1981

1651 RSVP Corpus Christi

City of Corpus Christi
1201 Leopard Street
Corpus Christi, TX 78401-2825
361-826-3105
Fax: 361-826-3113
www.cctexas.com

Ronald L. Olson, City Manager
Tamera Riley, Executive Assistant
Rebecca Huerta, City Secretary

The Retired and Senior Volunteer Program (RSVP) provides opportunities for people 55 and over to make a difference in their community through volunteer service. RSVP volunteers contribute anywhere from a few to over forty hours a week, serving thourgh schools, day care centers, police departments, hospitals and other nonprofit and public organizations to help meet critical community needs. RSVP offers maximum flexibility and choice to its volunteers. RSVP matches the personal interests and skills to older Americans with opportunities to help solve community problems and offer supplemental insurance while on duty, on-the-job training from the agency or organization where volunteers are placed.

Year Founded: 1852

1652 RSVP Dallas

3910 Harry Hines Boulevard
Dallas, TX 75219
214-823-5700
Fax: 214-826-2441
www.theseniorsource.org

J. Scott Wilson, Chairman
Molly H. Bogen, Executive Director
Matt Adams, Director

The Retired and Senior Volunteer Program (RSVP) provides opportunities for people 55 and over to make a difference in their community through volunteer service. RSVP volunteers contribute anywhere from a few to over forty hours a week, serving though schools, day care centers, police departments, hospitals and other nonprofit and public organizations to help meet critical community needs. RSVP offers maximum flexibility and choice to its volunteers. RSVP matches the personal interests and skills to older Americans with opportunities to help solve community problems and offer supplemental insurance while on duty, on-the-job training from the agency or organization where volunteers are placed.

Year Founded: 1961

1653 RSVP Deep East Texas
Deep East Texas Council of Governments
118 South First Street
Lufkin, TX 75901
936-634-2247
Fax: 936-634-2869; *Toll Free:* 800-256-7696
info@detcog.org
www.detcog.org
TDD 409-384-5975

Wes Suiter, President
Roy Boldon, 1st Vice President
Van Bush, Director

The Retired and Senior Volunteer Program (RSVP) provides opportunities for people 55 and over to make a difference in their community through volunteer service. RSVP volunteers contribute anywhere from a few to over forty hours a week, serving though schools, day care centers, police departments, hospitals and other nonprofit and public organizations to help meet critical community needs. RSVP offers maximum flexibility and choice to its volunteers. RSVP matches the personal interests and skills to older Americans with opportunities to help solve community problems and offer supplemental insurance while on duty, on-the-job training from the agency or organization where volunteers are placed.

1654 RSVP El Paso City
The Retired and Senior Volunteer Program (RSVP) E
300 North Campbell
El Paso, TX 79901
915-212-0000
Fax: 817-877-5807
home.elpasotexas.gov/

Adrian Duran, Executive Director
William L. Lilly, Director
Norma I. Corona, Volunteer Program Coordinator

The Retired and Senior Volunteer Program (RSVP) provides opportunities for people 55 and over to make a difference in their community through volunteer service. RSVP volunteers contribute anywhere from a few to over forty hours a week, serving though schools, day care centers, police departments, hospitals and other nonprofit and public organizations to help meet critical community needs. RSVP offers maximum flexibility and choice to its volunteers. RSVP matches the personal interests and skills to older Americans with opportunities to help solve community problems and offer supplemental insurance while on duty, on-the-job training from the agency or organization where volunteers are placed.

Year Founded: 1974

1655 RSVP Galveston County
The University of Texas Medical Branch at Galvesto
The University of Texas Medical Branch
301 University Boulevard
Galveston, TX 77555
409-772-5361
Fax: 409-747-2119
public.affairs@utmb.edu
www.utmb.edu
TDD 409-772-4200

David L. Callender, President
Carolee "Car King, Senior Vice President and Genera
Tom Riley, Vice President and Chief Health

The Retired and Senior Volunteer Program (RSVP) provides opportunities for people 55 and over to make a difference in their community through volunteer service. RSVP volunteers contribute anywhere from a few to over forty hours a week, serving though schools, day care centers, police departments, hospitals and other nonprofit and public organizations to help meet critical community needs. RSVP offers maximum flexibility and choice to its volunteers. RSVP matches the personal interests and skills to older Americans with opportunities to help solve community problems and offer supplemental insurance while on duty, on-the-job training from the agency or organization where volunteers are placed.

Year Founded: 1891

1656 RSVP Golden Triangle
South East Texas Regional Planning Commission
2210 Eastex Freeway
Beaumont, TX 77703
409-899-8444
Fax: 409-347-0138; *Toll Free:* 877-802-2200
setrpc@setrpc.org
www.setrpc.org

David Dubose, President
Glenn Johnson, 1st Vice President
Shaun P. Davis, Executive Director

The Retired and Senior Volunteer Program (RSVP) provides opportunities for people 55 and over to make a difference in their community through volunteer service. RSVP volunteers contribute anywhere from a few to over forty hours a week, serving though schools, day care centers, police departments, hospitals and other nonprofit and public organizations to help meet critical community needs. RSVP offers maximum flexibility and choice to its volunteers. RSVP matches the personal interests and skills to older Americans with opportunities to help solve community problems and offer supplemental insurance while on duty, on-the-job training from the agency or organization where volunteers are placed.

Year Founded: 1970

1657 RSVP Heart of Texas
Heart of Texas RSVP
1400 College Drive, CSC Room E108
McLennan Community College
Waco, TX 76708
254-299-8766
Fax: 254-299-8578
scopeland@mclennan.edu
www.hotrsvp.org

Susan Copeland, Executive Director
Rita Tejada, Volunteer Coordinator

The Retired and Senior Volunteer Program (RSVP) provides opportunities for people 55 and over to make a difference in their community through volunteer service. RSVP volunteers contribute anywhere from a few to over forty hours a week, serving thourgh schools, day care centers, police departments, hospitals and other nonprofit and public organizations to help meet critical community needs. RSVP offers maximum flexibility and choice to its volunteers. RSVP matches the personal interests and skills to older Americans with opportunities to help solve community problems and offer supplemental insurance while on duty, on-the-job training from the agency or organization where volunteers are placed.

Year Founded: 1990

1658 RSVP Houston County
**RSVP of the Texas Gulf Coast Community
Advisory Co**
5601 S Braeswood Boulevard
Houston, TX 77096-3907
713-729-3200
Fax: 713-551-7223
wmcfadden@jcchouston.org
www.rsvpvolunteers.com

Walt McFadden, Director

The Retired and Senior Volunteer Program (RSVP) provides opportunities for people 55 and over to make a difference in their community through volunteer service. RSVP volunteers contribute anywhere from a few to over forty hours a week, serving thourgh schools, day care centers, police departments, hospitals and other nonprofit and public organizations to help meet critical community needs. RSVP offers maximum flexibility and choice to its volunteers. RSVP matches the personal interests and skills to older Americans with opportunities to help solve community problems and offer supplemental insurance while on duty, on-the-job training from the agency or organization where volunteers are placed.

1659 RSVP Lubbock
Texas Tech University Health Sciences Center
3601 4th Street
Lubbock, TX 79430
806-743-3612
Fax: 806-743-3636
rsvp@ttu.edu
ttuhsc.edu/centers/aging/rsvp

Paula Grammas, Ph.D., Executive Director
Joan Blackmon, MBA, Program Coordinator
Carrie Crossland, Assistant Director, Finance & Ad

The Retired and Senior Volunteer Program (RSVP) provides opportunities for people 55 and over to make a difference in their community through volunteer service. RSVP volunteers contribute anywhere from a few to over forty hours a week, serving thourgh schools, day care centers, police departments, hospitals and other nonprofit and public organizations to help meet critical community needs. RSVP offers maximum flexibility and choice to its volunteers. RSVP matches the personal interests and skills to older Americans with opportunities to help solve community problems and offer supplemental insurance while on duty, on-the-job training from the agency or organization where volunteers are placed.

1660 RSVP Metro Tarrant
Senior Citizen Services of Greater Tarrant County
1400 Circle Drive
Fort Worth, TX 76119
817-413-4949
Fax: 817-877-5807
mlenton@scstc.org
www.scstc.org

Dr. Amy Moss, DO, President
Rev. Charles Graff, Vice President Programs
Linda Pugh, Vice President Resource Developm

The Retired and Senior Volunteer Program (RSVP) provides opportunities for people 55 and over to make a difference in their community through volunteer service. RSVP volunteers contribute anywhere from a few to over forty hours a week, serving thourgh schools, day care centers, police departments, hospitals and other nonprofit and public organizations to help meet critical community needs. RSVP offers maximum flexibility and choice to its volunteers. RSVP matches the personal interests and skills to older Americans with opportunities to help solve community problems and offer supplemental insurance while on duty, on-the-job training from the agency or organization where volunteers are placed.

Year Founded: 1967

1661 RSVP Midland
3301 Sinclair Avenue
Midland, TX 79707-6620
432-689-6693
Fax: 432-689-6699
director@cssmidland.org
www.cssmidland.org/rsvp

Saul Herrera, RSVP Director
Jody Sneed, Executive Director
Arleen Armstrong, Assistant Director

The Retired and Senior Volunteer Program (RSVP) provides opportunities for people 55 and over to make a difference in their community through volunteer service. RSVP volunteers contribute anywhere from a few to over forty hours a week, serving thourgh schools, day care centers, police departments, hospitals and other nonprofit and public organizations to help meet critical community needs. RSVP offers maximum flexibility and choice to its volunteers. RSVP matches the personal interests and skills to older Americans with opportunities to help solve community problems and offer supplemental insurance while on duty, on-the-job training from the agency or organization where volunteers are placed.

1662 RSVP North Texas
Texas Senior Corps
PO Box 5144
Wichita Falls, TX 76307
940-322-5281
Fax: 940-322-6743
dbooker@nortexrpc.org
texasseniorcorps.org

Dennis Wilde, Manager
Dee Anna Booker, Secretary

The Retired and Senior Volunteer Program (RSVP) provides opportunities for people 55 and over to make a difference in their community through volunteer service. RSVP volunteers contribute anywhere from a few to over forty hours a week, serving thourgh schools, day care centers, police departments, hospitals and other nonprofit and public organizations to help meet critical community needs. RSVP offers maximum flexibility and choice to its volunteers. RSVP matches the personal interests and skills to older Americans with opportunities to help solve community problems and offer supplemental insurance while on duty, on-the-job training from the agency or organization where volunteers are placed.

1663 RSVP Rio Grande Valley
Texas Senior Corps
5601 South Braeswood
Houston, TX 77096
713-595-8157
Fax: 713-551-7223
wmcfadden@erjcchouston.org
texasseniorcorps.org

Walter L. McFadden, President
Lidia Limas, Area Coordinator
Alvaro Herrera

Provides volunteer opportunities for persons 55 years of age or older. The purpose of the RSVP is to enrich retirement years for older adults through significant community service work. Encourages seniors to bring a lifetime of talent, experiences, skill, and hobbies to community projects and organization needing volunteer talent. A national program that is partially funded through the Corporation for national and Community Service, a federalagency.

Year Founded: 1983

1664 RSVP Runningwater Draw
Plainview, Texas
901 Broadway Street
Plainview, TX 79072
806-296-1100
Fax: 806-291-1979
rsvp@texasonline.net
www.plainviewtx.org

Greg Ingham, City Manager
Jeffrey Snyder, Assistant City Manager
Sarianne Beversdorf, CPA,, Director of Finance

The Retired and Senior Volunteer Program (RSVP) provides opportunities for people 55 and over to make a difference in their community through volunteer service. RSVP volunteers contribute anywhere from a few to over forty hours a week, serving thourgh schools, day care centers, police departments, hospitals and other nonprofit and public organizations to help meet critical community needs. RSVP offers maximum flexibility and choice to its volunteers. RSVP matches the personal interests and skills to older Americans with opportunities to help solve community problems and offer supplemental insurance while on duty, on-the-job training from the agency or organization where volunteers are placed.

1665 RSVP Swisher County
Texas Senior Corps
5601 South Braeswood
Houston, TX 77096
713-595-8157
Fax: 713-551-7223
rsvpswisher@cebridge.net
www.texasseniorcorps.org

Walter L. McFadden, President

The Retired and Senior Volunteer Program (RSVP) provides opportunities for people 55 and over to make a difference in their community through volunteer service. RSVP

volunteers contribute anywhere from a few to over forty hours a week, serving thourgh schools, day care centers, police departments, hospitals and other nonprofit and public organizations to help meet critical community needs. RSVP offers maximum flexibility and choice to its volunteers. RSVP matches the personal interests and skills to older Americans with opportunities to help solve community problems and offer supplemental insurance while on duty, on-the-job training from the agency or organization where volunteers are placed.

1666 RSVP Texas Panhandle
Texas Senior Corps, Texas Panhandle RSVP
321 West 7th Avenue
Amarillo, TX 79101
806-373-8389
Fax: 806-373-8380
larue.johnson@pcsvcs.org
texasseniorcorps.org/texaspanhandlersvp

LaRue Johnson, Director
Gloria Goyne, Coordinator

The Retired and Senior Volunteer Program (RSVP) provides opportunities for people 55 and over to make a difference in their community through volunteer service. RSVP volunteers contribute anywhere from a few to over forty hours a week, serving thourgh schools, day care centers, police departments, hospitals and other nonprofit and public organizations to help meet critical community needs. RSVP offers maximum flexibility and choice to its volunteers. RSVP matches the personal interests and skills to older Americans with opportunities to help solve community problems and offer supplemental insurance while on duty, on-the-job training from the agency or organization where volunteers are placed.

1667 RSVP Texoma
Texoma Council of Governments
1117 Gallagher Drive
Sherman, TX 75090
903-893-2161
Fax: 903-813-3511; *Toll Free:* 800-677-8264
lburleson@texoma.cog.tx.us
www.texoma.cog.tx

Honorable Cr Carter, II, President
Honorable Jo Roane, Vice President
Honorable Da Spindle, Secretary/Treasurer

Provides opportunities for people 55 and over to make a difference in their community through volunteer service. RSVP volunteers contribute anywhere form a few to over forty hours a week, serving through schools, day care centers, police departments, hospitals and other nonprofit and public organizations to help meet critical community needs. RSVP matches the personal interests and skills of older Americans with opportunities to help solve community problems and offers supplemental insurance while on duty, on-the-job trainng from the agency or organization where volunteers are placed.

1668 RSVP Travis County
Travis County, Texas
PO Box 1748
Austin, TX 78767
512-854-9020
Fax: 512-854-4131
fred.lugo@co.travis.tx.us
www.travis.tx.us

Fred Lugo, Director
Samuel T. Biscoe, County Judge
Dolores Ortega Carter, Treasurer

The Retired and Senior Volunteer Program (RSVP) provides opportunities for people 55 and over to make a difference in their community through volunteer service. RSVP volunteers contribute anywhere from a few to over forty hours a week, serving thourgh schools, day care centers, police departments, hospitals and other nonprofit and public organizations to help meet critical community needs. RSVP offers maximum flexibility and choice to its volunteers. RSVP matches the personal interests and skills to older Americans with opportunities to help solve community problems and offer supplemental insurance while on duty, on-the-job training from the agency or organization where volunteers are placed.

1669 Railroad Retirement Board: Fort Worth, Texas District Office
U.S. Railroad Retirement Board
819 Taylor Street, Room 10G02
PO Box 17420
Fort Worth, TX 76102-0420
817-978-2638
Fax: 817-978-2740; *Toll Free:* 877-772-5772
fortworth@rrb.gov
www.rrb.gov/field/do_fort.asp

Barbara Gettman, Representative
Martin J. Dickman, Inspector General

Administers retirement/survivor and unemployment/sickness benefit programs for railroad workers and their families.

1670 Railroad Retirement Board: Houston, Texas District Office
U.S. Railroad Retirement Board
1919 Smith Street
Suite 845
Houston, TX 77002-8098
713-209-3045
Fax: 713-759-0349; *Toll Free:* 877-772-5772
houston@rrb.gov
www.rrb.gov/field/do_hous.asp

Margie M Grimes, Representative
Martin J. Dickman, Inspector General

Administers retirement/survivor and unemployment/sickness benefit programs for railroad workers and their families.

1671 Rio Grande: Area Agency on Aging
The Rio Grande Council of Governments
8037 Lockheed Drive
Suite 100
El Paso, TX 79925
915-533-0998
Fax: 915-532-9385; *Toll Free:* 800-333-7082
www.riocog.org

Honorable Se Lewis, President
Honorable Je Calderon, 1st Vice President
Art Fierro, 2nd Vice President

Serves individuals 60 years of age and older and their families living in El Paso, Hudspeth, Culberson, Jeff Davis, Presidio and Brewster counties.

Year Founded: 1967

1672 Round Rock Volunteer Center
The Volunteer Center
1099 East Main Street
2nd Floor
Round Rock, TX 78683
512-733-7625
Fax: 512-733-7628
volrock@volrock.org
www.volrock.org

Heather Mich Riddle, Program Manager
Susan Dotson, Program Assistant

Connecting volunteers to nonprofit agencies.

1673 Shallowater Senior Citizens
The City of Shallowater
PO Box 246
Shallowater, TX 79363
806-832-4521
Fax: 806-832-4495
www.shallowatertx.us/

Robert Olmsted Jr., Mayor
Keny Arnold, Councilman
Rodney Cates, Councilman

Supports seniors in Shallowater.

Year Founded: 1913

1674 South Plains Association of Governments Area: Agency on Aging
The South Plains Association of Governments (SPAG)
1323 58th Street
Lubbock, TX 79412
806-762-8721
Fax: 806-765-9544; *Toll Free:* 800-858-1809
lrautis@spag.org
www.spag.org

Tim Pierce, Executive Director
Margo Boyd, Executive Assistant

Provides information and assistance to seniors on all aspects of all services including housing, employment and volunteer opportunities.

1675 South Texas: Area Agency on Aging
South Texas Development Council
PO Box 2187
Laredo, TX 78044-2187
956-722-3995
Fax: 512-722-2670; *Toll Free:* 800-292-5426
www.stdc.cog.tx.us

Jose Alfredo Guerra, Jr, Chairman
Cynthia Liendo-Espinoza, Vice Chairman
Amando Garza Jr., Executive Director

Promotes the improvement of the quality of life for the older population of South Texas.

1676 Southeast Texas: Area Agency on Aging
South East Texas Regional Planning Commission
2210 Eastex Freeway
Beaumont, TX 77703
409-899-8444
Fax: 409-347-0138; *Toll Free:* 800-395-5465
setrpc@setrpc.org
www.setrpc.org
TDD 409-347-2769

Glenn Johnson, President
Fred Williams, 1st Vice President
Shaun P. Davis, Executive Director

The Area Agency on Aging of Southeast Texas (AAASET) assists older individuals and their families in finding appropriate resources to further the independence and dignity of an older adult residing in Hardin, Jefferson or Orange County.

1677 Texas Association of Area Agencies on Aging
Texas Association of Area Agencies on Aging
1514 South New Road
Waco, TX 76711
254-772-9600
Fax: 254-756-0102; Toll Free: 866-772-9600
www.t4aging.org

Doni Van Ryswyk, President
Gary Luft, Vice President
Melissa Carter, Secretary

Carries out a program of advocacy and education for area agencies on aging.

1678 Texas Association of Directors of Volunteer Services
Texas Association of Directors of Volunteer Servic
PO Box 15587
Austin, TX 78761-5587
512-465-1000
Fax: 512-465-1090; Toll Free: 800-252-9403
tadvs.texas@gmail.com
www.tadvs.org

Christine Gonzalez, President
Ashleigh Jacobes, Vice President of Membership & W
Susie Tucker, Communications

Directors of volunteer services in hospitals and other health care settings.

1679 Texas Comptroller of Public Accountants
Texas Comptroller of Public Accountants
PO Box 13528
Capitol Station
Austin, TX 78711-3528
512-463-4000; *Toll Free: 800-531-5441*
susan.combs@cpa.state.tx.us
www.window.state.tx.us

Susan Combs, Texas Comptroller of Public Acco

Assists seniors with tax issues.

Year Founded: 1835

1680 Texas Council for Developmental Disabilities
6201 E Oltorf Street
Suite 600
Austin, TX 78741-7509
512-437-5432
Fax: 512-437-5434; Toll Free: 800-262-0334
tcdd@tcdd.texas.gov
www.tcdd.texas.gov

Mary Durheim, Chair
John W Thomas, Vice Chair
Beth Stalvey, Executive Director

The mission of the Texas Council for Developmental Disabilities (TCDD) is to create change so that all people with disabilities are fully included in their communities and exercise control over their own lives.

Number of Members: 27

1681 Texas Department of Aging and Disability Services
701 W 51st Street
PO Box 149030
Austin, TX 78751
512-438-3011
Fax: 512-438-4747; Toll Free: 800-458-9858
mail@dads.state.tx.us
www.dads.state.tx.us

Jon Weizenbaum, Interim Commissioner
Kristi Jordan, Assistant Commissioner
Gary Jessee

The Texas Department of Aging and Disability Services (DADS) mission is to provide a comprehensive array of aging and disability services, supports, and opportunities that are easily accessed in local communities.

1682 Texas Geriatrics Society
Texas Geriatrics Society
P. O. Box 130963
c/o Maggie Hayden
Dallas, TX 75313-0963
214-824-6027
haymags@sbcglobal.net
www.texasgeriatrics.org/

Yanping Ye, MD, President
Bassem Elsawy, MD, President Elect
Kim Higgins, DO, Secretary/ Treasurer

Represents members' interests; conducts lobbying activities. Provides assistance programs for retirees.

1683 Texas Governor's Committee for People With Disabilities
Office of the Governor
PO Box 12428
Austin, TX 78711-2428
512-463-2000
Fax: 512-463-5745; Toll Free: 800-843-5789
www.governor.state.tx.us
TDD 512-463-5764

Pat Pound, Executive Director
AnitaThigpen Perry, First Lady
Rick Perry, Governor

The Govenor's Committee on People with Disabilities envisions a state where people with disabilities have the opportunity to enjoy full and equal access to lives of independence, productivity and self determination.

1684 Texas Veterans Commission
Texas Veterans Commission
PO Box 12277
Austin, TX 78711-2277
512-463-5538
Fax: 512-463-3932; Toll Free: 800-252-VETS
info@tvc.texas.gov
www.tvc.state.tx.us

Eliseo Al Cantu, Jr., Chair
James H. Scott, Vice Chair
Thomas P Palladino, Executive Director

To assist veterans by informing them of their rights.

1685 Texas Workers Compensation Commission
Texas Department of Insurance Division of Workers'
7551 Metro Center Drive
Suite 100
Austin, TX 78744-1645
512-804-4000
Fax: 512-804-4101
www.tdi.texas.gov/wc/

Robert Shipe, Executive Director

1686 Texoma: Area Agency on Aging
Texoma Council of Governments
1117 Gallagher Drive
Sherman, TX 75090
903-893-2161
Fax: 903-813-3511; *Toll Free:* 800-677-8264
www.texoma.cog.tx.us/Aging/Aging.htm

Honorable Cr Carter, II, President
Honorable Jo Roane, Vice President
Honorable Da Spindle, Secretary/Treasurer

1687 West Central Texas Council of Governments-Area Agency on Aging
West Central Texas Council of Governments
3702 Loop 322
Abilene, TX 79602
325-672-8544
Fax: 325-675-5214; *Toll Free:* 800-928-2262
wctcog@wctcog.org
www.wctcog.org

Councilmembe Williams, President
Judge Gary Fuller, First Vice President
Tom K. Smith, Executive Director

Providing a bridge of coordinated services for persons over 60 to long-term services.

Utah

1688 Bear River: Area Agency on Aging
Bear River Association of Governments
170 North Main
Logan, UT 84321
435-752-7242
Fax: 435-752-6962; *Toll Free:* 877-772-7242
www.brag.utah.gov

Michelle Benson, Director
Rich Van Dyke, Commissioner

In conjunction with local Senior Centers, the Agency is a focal point for information available to Utah's older adults living in Box Elder, Cache, and Rich Counties.

Year Founded: 1971

1689 Disability Law Center at the Community Lal Center
Disability Law Center
205 North 400 West
Salt Lake City, UT 84103
801-363-1347
Fax: 801-363-1437; *Toll Free:* 800-662-9080
disabilitylawcenter.org

Adina Zahradnikova, Executive Director
Bryce Fifield Ph.D, Board Member
Barbara M. Campbell, Board Member

Enforces and strengthens laws that protect the opportunities, choices, and legal rights of people with disabilities in Utah.

1690 Division of Services for the People withDisabilities
Utah Division of Services for People with Disabili
195 North 1950 West
Salt Lake City, UT 84116
801-538-4200
Fax: 801-538-4279; *Toll Free:* 800-837-6811
dspd@utah.gov
www.dspd.utah.gov

Christine Nguyen, GRAMA Officer

Offers services for the totally blind, legally blind, visually impaired, mentally retarded blind and more with health, counseling, educational, recreational, rehabilitation, computer training and professional training services.

1691 Five County: Area Agency on Aging
Five County Association of Governments
1070 W 1600 S
St George, UT 84770
435-673-3548
Fax: 435-673-3540
cschonlaw@fivecounty.utah.gov
www.fivecounty.utah.gov

Bryan D. Thiriot., Executive Director
Jo Seegmiller, Human Resources Director

Plans, prepares and partners with federal, state and local governments to strengthen the role of southwestern Utah local officials in the execution of state and federal programs at the local level.

Year Founded: 1972

1692 Golden Age Center Uintah Health Care Special Service District
Uintah County Community Development
155 E 100 N
Vernal, UT 84078
435-781-5336
Fax: 435-781-5352
lmartin@co.uintah.ut.us
www.co.uintah.ut.us

Louise Martin, Director
Maxine Copley, Manager
Michael W. Wilkins, Clerk Auditor

We are here to serve the elderly population in our community. Available services include: nutrition, transportation, caregiver program, health insurance counseling.

Year Founded: 1973

1693 RSVP Cache County
Cache County Corp.
179 N Main Street
199 N Main Street
Logan, UT 84321
435-755-1850
Fax: 435-789-2171
lmartin@co.uintah.ut.us
www.cachecounty.org/rsvp/

Kathleen C. Howell, Assessor
Tamra Stones, Auditor
Karen A. Jeppesen, Treasurer

The Retired and Senior Volunteer Program (RSVP) provides opportunities for people 55 and over to make a difference in their community through volunteer service. RSVP volunteers contribute anywhere from a few to over forty hours a week, serving thourgh schools, day care centers, police departments, hospitals and other nonprofit and public organizations to help meet critical community needs. RSVP offers maximum flexibility and choice to its volunteers. RSVP matches the personal interests and skills to older Americans with opportunities to help solve community problems and offer supplemental insurance while on duty, on-the-job training from the agency or organization where volunteers are placed.

Year Founded: 1857

1694 RSVP Carbon County
Carbon County Utah
185 East Main Street
P.O. Box 893
Price, UT 84501
435-636-3183
Fax: 435-637-2905
www.carbon.utah.gov

Rebecca Mason, Contact

The Retired and Senior Volunteer Program (RSVP) provides opportunities for people 55 and over to make a difference in their community through volunteer service. RSVP volunteers contribute anywhere from a few to over forty hours a week, serving thourgh schools, day care centers, police departments, hospitals and other nonprofit and public organizations to help meet critical community needs. RSVP offers maximum flexibility and choice to its volunteers. RSVP matches the personal interests and skills to older Americans with opportunities to help solve community problems and offer supplemental insurance while on duty, on-the-job training from the agency or organization where volunteers are placed.

Year Founded: 1894

1695 RSVP Grand County
Grand County Utah
182 N 500 E
Moab, UT 84532
435-259-1302
Fax: 435-259-2601
jodyellis@frontiernet.net
www.grandcountyutah.net

Bill McCloskey, Operations Specialist
Orlinda Robertson, Human Resources Director
Terri Hines, Office Manager/Prosecutorial Ass

The Retired and Senior Volunteer Program (RSVP) provides opportunities for people 55 and over to make a difference in their community through volunteer service. RSVP volunteers contribute anywhere from a few to over forty hours a week, serving thourgh schools, day care centers, police departments, hospitals and other nonprofit and public organizations to help meet critical community needs. RSVP offers maximum flexibility and choice to its volunteers. RSVP matches the personal interests and skills to older Americans with opportunities to help solve community problems and offer supplemental insurance while on duty, on-the-job training from the agency or organization where volunteers are placed.

Year Founded: 1890

1696 RSVP Mountainland
Mountainland Association of Governments
586 East 800 North
Orem, UT 84097
801-229-3800
Fax: 801-229-3671
www.mountainland.org/aging

Jean Hatch, RSVP Program Manager
SueAnn Lawson, RSVP Volunteer Coordinator
Scott McBeth, Director, Aging and Family Servi

The Retired and Senior Volunteer Program (RSVP) provides opportunities for people 55 and over to make a difference in their community through volunteer service. RSVP volunteers contribute anywhere from a few to over forty hours a week, serving thourgh schools, day care centers, police departments, hospitals and other nonprofit and public organizations to help meet critical community needs. RSVP offers maximum flexibility and choice to its volunteers. RSVP matches the personal interests and skills to older Americans with opportunities to help solve community problems and offer supplemental insurance while on duty, on-the-job training from the agency or organization where volunteers are placed.

Year Founded: 1972

1697 RSVP Salt Lake County
Salt Lake County
2001 S State Street
Ste. S1500
Salt Lake City, UT 84190-4575
385-468-3200
Fax: 801-468-2989
vjhansen@slco.org
www.aging.slco.org

Barbara Drake, Program Manager

The Retired and Senior Volunteer Program (RSVP) provides opportunities for people 55 and over to make a difference in their community through volunteer service. RSVP volunteers contribute anywhere from a few to over forty hours a week, serving thourgh schools, day care centers, police departments, hospitals and other nonprofit and public organizations to help meet critical community needs. RSVP offers maximum flexibility and choice to its volunteers. RSVP matches the personal interests and skills to older Americans with opportunities to help solve community problems and offer supplemental insurance while on duty, on-the-job training from the agency or organization where volunteers are placed.

1698 RSVP Six County
RSVP and The Volunteer Connection
250 North Main
Suite B05
Richfield, UT 84701
435-893-0735
Fax: 435-893-0701
sbastian@sixcounty.com
www.volunteer-connection.com

Shara Bastian, Manager
Christy Nebeker, SMP Coordinator

The Retired and Senior Volunteer Program (RSVP) provides opportunities for people 55 and over to make a difference in their community through volunteer service. RSVP volunteers contribute anywhere from a few to over forty hours a week, serving thourgh schools, day care centers, police departments, hospitals and other nonprofit and public organizations to help meet critical community needs. RSVP offers maximum flexibility and choice to its volunteers. RSVP matches the personal interests and skills to older Americans with opportunities to help solve community problems and offer supplemental insurance while on duty, on-the-job training from the agency or organization where volunteers are placed.

Year Founded: 1998

1699 Railroad Retirement Board
US Railroad Retirement Board
125 S State Street
Suite 1205
Salt Lake City, UT 84138-1137
801-524-5725
Fax: 801-524-4313; *Toll Free:* 877-772-5772
saltlakecity@rrb.gov
www.rrb.gov/field/do-salt.asp

Frank Kurek, Representative
Martin J. Dickman, Inspector General

Assists retired railroad workers and their families with benefits.

1700 Salt Lake County Aging Services
Salt Lake County
2001 S State Street
Ste. S1500
Salt Lake City, UT 84190-4575
385-468-3200
Fax: 801-468-2852
slcoagingservices@slco.org
www.aging.slco.org
TDD 801-468-2480

Barbara Drake, Program Manager
Sharon Pierce, Manager

Promotes the independence of aging generations through advocacy, engagement and access to resources.

1701 San Juan: Area Agency on Aging
San Juan County Utah
PO Box 9
Monticello, UT 84535
435-587-3225
Fax: 435-587-2447
tgallegos@sanjuancounty.org
www.sanjuancounty.org

Bruce Adams, Chairman
Craig Halls, Attorney
Norman Johnson, Clerk/ Auditor

Promotes the dignity and well being of older persons - both as individuals within their families and in our communities.

1702 Six County: Area Agency on Aging
Six County Government
250 North Main Street
Richfield, UT 84701
435-893-0700
Fax: 435-893-0701; *Toll Free:* 888-899-4447
schristensen5@sixcounty.com
www.sixcounty.com

Russell Cowley, Executive Director
Lynnette Robinson, Chief Financial Officer
Jana Torgerson, Administrative Assist.

Serves seniors in Juab, Millard, Piute, Sanpete, Sevier, and Wayne counties.

1703 Tooele County Division of Aging and Adult Services
Tooele County
47 South Main Street
Tooele, UT 84074
435-843-3100
Fax: 435-882-6971; *Toll Free:* 866-704-3443
jmaher@co.tooele.ut.us
www.tooeleaging.org/

J.Bruce Clegg, Chairman

The mission of the Division of Aging and Adult Services is to provide leadership and advocacy in addressing issues that impact older Utahans, and serve elder and disabled adults needing protection from abuse, neglect or exploitation.

1704 Utah Center for Assistive Technology
The Utah Center for Assistive Technology
Judy Ann Buffmire Building
1595 West 500 South
Salt Lake City, UT 84104
801-887-9380
Fax: 801-887-9382
ucat.usor.utah.gov/

Starla Blackburn, Team administrator
Kent Remund, Director
Lynn Marcoux, Executive Secretary

A statewide program promoting assistive technology devices and services for persons of all ages with all disabilities.

Year Founded: 1988

1705 Utah Client Assistance Program
Disability Law Center
205 North 400 West
Salt Lake City, UT 84103
801-363-1347
Fax: 801-363-1437; *Toll Free:* 800-662-9080
nancyfriel@disabilitylawcenter.org
www.disabilitylawcenter.org
TTY: 800-550-4182

Adina Zahradnikova, Executive Director
Bryce Fifield Ph.D, Board Member
Barbara M. Campbell, Board Member

Protects the legal rights of people who apply for or are already clients of the state's Vocational Rehabilitation or Independent Living agencies.

1706 Utah Department of Aging
Aging Services Administrative Office
195 North 1950 West
Salt Lake City, UT 84116
801-538-3910
Fax: 801-538-4395; *Toll Free:* 877-4ag-ng0
debooth@utah.gov
www.hsdaas.utah.gov

Percy Devine III, Director

Administers a wide variety of home and community-based services for Utah residents who are 60 or older.

1707 Utah Department of Health
Utah Department of Health
P.O. Box 141010
Salt Lake City, UT 84114-1010

801-538-6003
Fax: 801-538-6036
www.health.utah.gov

W David Patton, Executive Director
Michael Hales, Director, Medicaid and Health Fi
Wu Xu, Ph.D, Director, Health Data and Inform

Protects the public's health through preventing avoidable illness, injury, disability and premature death.

1708 Utah Department of Human Services for People with Disabilities
Utah Division of Services for People with Disabili
195 North 1950 West?
Salt Lake City, UT 84116
801-538-4200
Fax: 801-538-4279; *Toll Free:* 800-837-6811
dspd@utah.gov
www.dspd.utah.gov

Christine Nguyen, GRAMA Officer

Provides services for people with disabilities in Utah.

1709 Utah Department of Human Services: Aging
Utah Department of Human Services
195 N 1950 W
Salt Lake City, UT 84116
801-538-4171
Fax: 801-538-4016; *Toll Free:* 877-424-4640
dirdhs@utah.gov
hsdaas.utah.gov

Ann Silverbe Williamson, Executive Director
Michael S Styles, Assistant Director
Nan Mendenhall

Oversees programs and services primarily delivered by a network of 12 Area Agencies on Aging (60 or older).

1710 Utah Office of Social Services: Department of Human Services
Utah Department of Human Services
195 North 1950 West
Salt Lake City, UT 84116
801-538-4171
Fax: 801-538-4016
www.dhs.utah.gov/

Ann Silverbe Williamson, Executive Director
Lisa-Michel Church, Executive Director

Information and referrals offering many different office locations for various counties in the state of Utah.

1711 Utah Retirement Systems
Utah Retirement Systems
560 E 200 S
Salt Lake City, UT 84102-2099
801-366-7700; *Toll Free:* 800-365-8772
www.urs.org

Brent Sonzini, Contact
Kyle Webb, Contact
Cory Wood

Provides comprehensive benefits to active and retired public employees in a courteous, timely, and professional manner.

1712 Utah State Association of Area Agencies on Aging
Bear River Association of Governments
170 North Main
Logan, UT 84321
435-752-7242
Fax: 435-752-6962; *Toll Free:* 877-772-7242
www.brag.utah.gov

Michelle Benson, Director
Rich Van Dyke, Commissioner

Supports seniors statewide.

Year Founded: 1971

1713 Utah State Tax Commission
Utah State Tax Commission
210 North 1950 West
Salt Lake City, UT 84134
801-297-2200
Fax: 801-297-7699; *Toll Free:* 800-662-4335
taxmaster@utah.gov
www.tax.utah.gov
TDD 801-297-2020

Pam Hendrickson, Manager

Oversees and enforces tax policy for Utah.

1714 Utah Workers Compensation Board
Labour Commission, State of Utah
160 East 300 South
3rd Floor
Salt Lake City, UT 84114-6600
801-530-6800
Fax: 801-530-6804; *Toll Free:* 800-530-5090
laborcom@utah.gov
www.laborcommission.utah.gov

Sherrie M. Hayashi, Commissioner & Department Direct
Jaceson Maughan, Deputy Commissioner General Coun
David Lamb, Administrative Services Division

Informs public about workers compensation.

1715 Weber-Morgan: Area Agency on Aging
Weber Human Services
237 26th Street
Ogden, UT 84401
801-625-3700
Fax: 801-778-6830
contactWHS@weberhs.org
www.weberhs.org
TDD 801-625-3638

Joe H. Ritchie, Chair
Matthew Bell, Weber County Commissioner
Jan M. Zogmaister, Weber County Commissioner

Provides support to seniors.

Vermont

1716 Central Vermont Council on Aging (CVCOA)
Central Vermont Council on Aging
59 North Main Street
Suite 200
Barre, VT 05641-4121
802-479-0531
Fax: 802-479-4235; *Toll Free:* 877-379-2600
cvcoa@cvcoa.org
www.cvcoa.org/

Dennis Minoli, President
Kay Charron, Vice President
John Castaldo, Directors

Supports independence, self-choice and security for all elders through a variety of programs.

1717 Champlain Valley: Area Agency on Aging
Champlain Valley Area Agency on Aging
76 Pearl Street
Suite 201
Essex Junction, VT 05452
802-865-0360
Fax: 802-865-0363
info@cvaa.org
www.cvaa.org
TDD 802-865-0360

Kathi Montieth, President
Glenn Jarrett, Vice President
Aaron Reynolds, Treasurer

A private, nonprofit United Way organization. We support people 60 and older in their efforts to remain active, healthy, financially, secure, and in control of their own lives. CVAA connects older people and the services thay need to live independently for as long as possible.

Year Founded: 1974

1718 Disability Determination Services
Department for Children and Families, DDS
93 Pilgrim Park Road
Suite 6
Waterbury, VT 05676
802-241-2463
Fax: 802-241-2492; *Toll Free:* 800-734-2463
vt.dd.waterbury@ssa.gov
www.dcf.state.vt.us

Trudy Lyon-Hart, Director
Dave Yacovone, DCF Commissioner

The Office of Disability Determination Services (DDS) serves Vermonters who apply for disability benefits under Social Security, Supplemental Security Income (SSI), and Medicaid programs. The mission of DDS is to provide applicants with accurate decisions as quickly as possible, as governed by Social Security federal statutes, regulations, and policy, with full and fair consideration of each applicant's situation and respect and concern for the individual's well-being and legal rights.

1719 Northeastern Vermont: Area Agency on Aging
Northeastern Vermont Area Agency on Aging
481 Summer Street
Suite 101
St Johnsbury, VT 05819
802-748-5182
Fax: 802-748-6622; *Toll Free:* 800-640-5119
info@nevaaa.org
www.nevaaa.org

Brenda B Smith, President
John Perry, Vice President
Rever Kennedy, Secretary

Supports older adults (age 60+) in the counties of Caledonia, Orleans and Essex.

Year Founded: 1979

1720 RSVP Chittenden County
United Way of Chittenden County
412 Farrell Street
Suite 200
South Burlington, VT 05403
802-864-7541
Fax: 802-864-7401
info@unitedwaycc.org
www.unitedwaycc.org

Charlotte Ancel, President
Michael Seaver, Vice President
Jeff McMahan, Secretary

The Retired and Senior Volunteer Program (RSVP) provides opportunities for people 55 and over to make a difference in their community through volunteer service. RSVP volunteers contribute anywhere from a few to over forty hours a week, serving thourgh schools, day care centers, police departments, hospitals and other nonprofit and public organizations to help meet critical community needs. RSVP offers maximum flexibility and choice to its volunteers. RSVP matches the personal interests and skills to older Americans with opportunities to help solve community problems and offer supplemental insurance while on duty, on-the-job training from the agency or organization where volunteers are placed.

1721 RSVP Green Mountain
Green Mountain Retired Senior Volunteer Program
215 Pleasant Street
Bennington, VT 05201
802-447-1545
Fax: 802-447-1868
rsvpvt.org/

Patricia Palencsar, Executive Director
Pam Meunier, Office Manager
Susan Armstrong, Program Manager

The Retired and Senior Volunteer Program (RSVP) provides opportunities for people 55 and over to make a difference in their community through volunteer service. RSVP volunteers contribute anywhere from a few to over forty hours a week, serving thourgh schools, day care centers, police departments, hospitals and other nonprofit and public organizations to help meet critical community needs. RSVP offers maximum flexibility and choice to its volunteers. RSVP matches the personal interests and skills to older Americans with opportunities to help solve community problems and offer supplemental insurance while on duty, on-the-job training from the agency or organization where volunteers are placed.

1722 RSVP Windham County
Green Mountain Retired Senior Volunteer Program
974 Western Avenue
Brattleboro, VT 05301
802-254-7515
Fax: 802-254-7519
pseares@greenmtncn.org
rsvpvt.org/

Patricia Palencsar, Executive Director
Pam Meunier, Office Manager
Peter Sears, Program Manager

RSVP is part of a nationwide program that offers people fifty-five and older the opportunity to have a positive impact on the quality of life in their communities, and on their own lives, by sharing their experience, abilities and skills through volunteer service.

1723 RSVP and The Volunteer Center
RSVP and The Volunteer Center
6 Court Street
Rutland, VT 05701-4134
802-775-8220
Fax: 802-775-8221
www.volunteersinvt.org/

Nan Hart, Executive Director

The Retired and Senior Volunteer Program (RSVP) provides opportunities for people 55 and over to make a difference in their community through volunteer service. RSVP volunteers contribute anywhere from a few to over forty hours a week, serving thourgh schools, day care centers, police departments, hospitals and other nonprofit and public organizations to help meet critical community needs. RSVP offers maximum flexibility and choice to its volunteers. RSVP matches the personal interests and skills to older Americans with opportunities to help solve community problems and offer supplemental insurance while on duty, on-the-job training from the agency or organization where volunteers are placed.

Year Founded: 1971

1724 RSVP of Central Vermont and the Northeast Kingdom-Barre
Volunteer Center of Central Vermont and the Northe
PO Box 433
Barre, VT 05641
802-828-4770
Fax: 802-828-5476
www.volunteervt.com/

J. Guy Isabelle, Director

The Retired and Senior Volunteer Program (RSVP) provides opportunities for people 55 and over to make a difference in their community through volunteer service. RSVP volunteers contribute anywhere from a few to over forty hours a week, serving thourgh schools, day care centers, police departments, hospitals and other nonprofit and public organizations to help meet critical community needs. RSVP offers maximum flexibility and choice to its volunteers. RSVP matches the personal interests and skills to older Americans with opportunities to help solve community problems and offer supplemental insurance while on duty, on-the-job training from the agency or organization where volunteers are placed.

1725 Southwestern Vermont Council on Aging
Southwestern Vermont Council on Aging
1085 US Route 4 East
Unit 2B
Rutland, VT 05701
802-786-5990
Fax: 802-786-5994; *Toll Free:* 800-642-5119
www.svcoa.org

Claire Granger, Bennington Manager

SVCOA helps individuals 60 plus meet the challenges of aging by providing meal support, case management, information and assistance and connection to other state benefits.

Year Founded: 1977

1726 Vermont Assistive Technology Projects
Vermont Assistive Technology Progarm
103 South Main Street
Weeks Building
Waterbury, VT 05671-2305
802-871-3353
Fax: 802-871-3048; *Toll Free:* 800-750-6355
atp.vermont.gov
TTY: 802-241-1464

Amber Fulcher, Program Director
Sharon Alderman, Assistive Technology Reuse Coord
Emma Cobb, Assistive Technology Services Co

Our mission is to increase awareness and change policies to ensure assistive technology (AT) is available to all Vermonters with disabilities.

1727 Vermont Client Assistance Program
Division for the Blind & Visually Impaired
57 North Main Street
Rutland, VT 05701
802-863-5620
Fax: 802-863-7152; *Toll Free:* 800-769-7459
www.dbvi.vermont.gov/cap

Eric Azildsen, Executive Director

Helps individuals who are applying for or receiving services from various Vermont agencies.

Year Founded: 1927

1728 Vermont Council on Aging
Central Vermont Council on Aging
59 North Main Street
Suite 200
Barre, VT 05641-4121
802-479-0531
Fax: 802-479-4235; *Toll Free:* 877-379-2600
cvcoa@cvcoa.org
www.cvcoa.org/

Dennis Minoli, President
Kay Charron, Vice President
John Castaldo, Directors

Provides support to seniors.

1729 Vermont Department of Disabilities, Aging and Independent Living
Department of Disabilities, Aging & Independent Li
103 South Main Street
Weeks Building
Waterbury, VT 05671-1601
802-241-2401
Fax: 802-241-2325
dail.vermont.gov
TTY: 802-241-3557

Susan Wehry, Commissioner
Douglas A. Racine, Secretary

The Department is part of the Agency of Human Services and provides a variety of services to Vermonters who are over the age of 60 or who have a disability.

1730 Vermont Department of Taxes
Vermont Department of Taxes
133 State Street
Montpelier, VT 05633-1401
802-828-2505
Fax: 802-828-5787; *Toll Free:* 866-828-2865

www.state.vt.us/tax
TDD 800-253-0191

Mary N Peterson, Commissioner

Assists with tax policies and problems.

1731 Vermont Developmental Disabilities Council
Vermont Developmental Disabilities Council
103 South Main Street
One North, Suite 117
Waterbury, VT 05671-0206
802-828-1310
Fax: 802-828-1321; *Toll Free:* 888-317-2006
vtddc@state.vt.us
www.ddc.vermont.gov

Karen Schwartz, Executive Director
Donna Bennett, Board Member
Jim Caffry

Helps build connections and supports that bring people with developmental disabilities and their families into the heart of Vermont communities.

1732 Vermont Protection and Advocacy Agency
Disability Rights Vermont
141 Main Street
Suite 7
Montpelier, VT 05602
802-229-1355
Fax: 802-229-1359; *Toll Free:* 800-834-7890
ed@DisabilityRightsVt.org
www.disabilityrightsvt.org/
TTY: 800-769-7459

Sarah Wendell-Launderville, President
David Gallagher, Vice President
Charlie Crocker, Treasurer

Legal services (protection and advocacy) for people with disabilities on legal issues arising from disability. Statewide. Adults and children. Employment, education, discrimination, housing, public benefits, health care.

Year Founded: 1970

1733 Vermont State Employees' Retirement System
Vermont Office of the State Treasurer
109 State Street
4th Floor
Montpelier, VT 05609-6200
802-828-2301
Fax: 802-828-5182; *Toll Free:* 800-642-3191
www.vermonttreasurer.gov/
TTY: 800-253-0191

Cynthia L Webster, Executive Secretary
Bert Pearce, State Treasurer

VSRS is the public pension plan provided by the State of Vermont for state employees.

1734 Vermont Veterans Affairs
Veteran Servics Directory
118 State Street
Montpelier, VT 05620-4401
802-828-3379
Fax: 802-828-5932; *Toll Free:* 888-666-9844
paul.perreault@state.vt.us
veterans.vermont.gov

Paul Perreault, Primary Contact

Consolidates the benefits and services available to veterans and their families in Vermont, regardless of the provider.

1735 Workers Compensation Board Vermont
Vermont Department of Labor
5 Green Mountain Drive
PO Box 488
Montpelier, VT 05601-0488
802-828-4000
Fax: 802-828-4022
labor-wccomp@state.vt.us
www.labor.vermont.gov
TDD 802-828-4203

Annie Noonan, Commissioner
Rose Lucenti, Director of Workforce Developmen
Steve Monahan, Director of Workers' Comp & Safe

Compensates and protects employees who suffer personal injury by accident arising out of and in the course of employement.

Virginia

1736 Alexandria Office of Aging and Adult Services
City of Alexandria
2525 Mount Vernon Avenue
Unit 5
Alexandria, VA 22301-1159
703-746-5999
Fax: 703-838-0886
maryann.griffin@alexandriava.gov
www.alexandriava.gov/Aging
TDD 703-836-1493

Michael Gilmore, Ph.D., Executive Director, Alexandria C
Suzanne T. Chris, Director of Social Services
Lisa Baker, Chief Staff Officer

Offers information, referral, outreach, home assessment, and assistance to Alexandria residents 60 years of age or older and their families.

1737 Arlington Area Agency on Aging
Department of Human Services
2100 Washington Blvd
Arlington, VA 22204
703-228-1300
Fax: 703-228-1174
dhs@arlingtonva.us
www.arlingtonva.us/
TDD 703-228-1788
TTY: 703-228-1788

Susanne Susanne, Director
Joan Planell, Deputy Director
Kurt Larrick, Communications Manager

The Arlington Agency on Aging serves Arlington residents aged 60 and older by providing to them and their families, friends and caregivers information on, assistance in accessing, and referrals to services and resources available for older residents of Arlington County.

1738 Crater District: Area Agency on Aging
Crater District Area Agency on Aging
23 Seyler Drive
Petersburg, VA 23805-9243
804-732-7020
Fax: 804-732-7232
cdaaa.org

David Sadowski, Director
Gladys Mason, Director of Programs

Helps Virginia's seniors to remain in their homes for as long as possible while helping to maintain their quality of life and independence.

1739 Disability Determination Services
Department for Aging & Rehabilitative Services
8004 Franklin Farms Drive
Henrico, VA 23229-5019
804-662-7000
Fax: 804-662-9532; *Toll Free:* 804-662-7000
dars@dars.virginia.gov
www.vadrs.org
TTY: 800-464-9950

Sharon Gottovi, Regional Director
Tamera Hargrove, Professional Relations Officer
Jim Rothrock, Commissioner

The Disability Determination Services (DDS), is a division within DRS, processes disability claims for benefits under the Social Security Disability Insurance and Supplemental Security Income Disability Programs. DDS is committed to making accurate, prompt decisions on disability claims under the Disability Insurance Benefits and Supplemental Security Income (SSI) Programs.

1740 Disability Determination Services: Roanoke
Disability Determination Services
111 Franklin Road SE
Suite 250
Roanoke, VA 24011
540-512-1880
Fax: 540-512-1990; *Toll Free:* 877-892-6871
www.vadrs.org/dds.htm

Betsy Stone, Regional Director
Europai Parker, Manager
Teresa Sizemore-Hernandez, Professional Relations Officer

Processes disability claims for benefits.

1741 District Three Governmental Cooperative
District Three Governmental Cooperative
4453 Lee Highway
Marion, VA 24354-2999
276-783-8157
Fax: 276-783-3003; *Toll Free:* 800-541-0933
district-three@smyth.net
www.district-three.org

Michael Guy, Executive Director

We are dedicated to improving the quality of life for our citizens, especially those who are elderly and those who need assistance with transportation. Our services are designed to help our citizens to live independently and productively as long as possible. We promote self-sufficiency and family care-giving.

1742 Eastern Shore Area: Agency on Aging,
Community Action Agency
Accomack County Virginia
5432-A Bayside Road
Exmore, VA 23350
757-442-9652
Fax: 757-442-9303; *Toll Free:* 800-452-5977
esaaa@aol.com
www.co.accomack.va.us/

Diane Musso, Executive Director
Todd E. Godwin, Sheriff

ESAAA/CAA is a community-based non-profit organization dedicated to providing comprehensive and high-quality human services. These services, for seniors and caregivers, include; outreach to the isolated, home-delivered meals, transportation services, inter-generational activities, legal services, long-term care ombudsman, and homemaker personal care.

Year Founded: 1634

1743 Fairfax Area: Agency on Aging
Fairfax County, Virginia
12000 Government Center Parkway
Fairfax, VA 22035
703-324-5411
Fax: 703-449-8689
www.fairfaxcounty.gov/service/aaa
TDD 703-803-7914

Grace Lynch, Director

Provides support to seniors in Fairfax County.

1744 Falls Church Senior Center
City Of Falls Church
223 Little Falls Street
Falls Church, VA 22046
703-248-5001
Fax: 703-536-8150
tbrowand@fallschurchva.gov
www.fallschurchva.gov
TTY: 703-248-5711

Tracy Browand, Senior Center Coordinator

Senior citizens in Arlington and Fairfax counties, and cities of Falls Church and Alexandria, VA. Provides health, education, recreation, and information services to area senior citizens. Sponsors lectures, classes, activities, and parties.

Year Founded: 1948

1745 Jefferson Area Board for Aging (JABA)
674 Hillsdale Drive
Suite 9
Charlottesville, VA 22901
434-817-5222
Fax: 434-817-5230
jabacares.org

Marta Keane, CEO

Area agency on aging.

Year Founded: 1975

1746 Lake County Area: Agency on Aging
Lake Country Area Agency on Aging
1105 W Danville Street
South Hill, VA 23970
434-447-7661
Fax: 434-447-4074; *Toll Free:* 800-252-4464
lakecaaa@lcaaa.org
lcaaa.org

Gwen Hinzman, President/CEO
Dean Lytle, Executive Vice President
Jo Ann Powell, Coordinator

Serving seniors in the South Central Virginia Counties of: Brunswick, Halifax, Mecklenburg

Year Founded: 1974

1747 League of Older Americans
Roanoke County, Virginia
PO Box 29800
Roanoke, VA 24018-0798
540-772-2006
Fax: 703-981-1487
www.roanokecountyva.gov

Joseph P. McNamara, Chairman
P. Jason Peters, Vice Chairman
Deborah C. Jacks, Clerk to the Board

The intent of the League is not to duplicate services delivered by other agencies for seniors but to ensure the delivery of existing and new services

Year Founded: 1838

1748 Loudoun County Area: Agency on Aging
Loudoun County Government
P.O. Box 7000
Leesburg, VA 20177
703-777-0100
Fax: 703-771-5161; *Toll Free:* 800-552-4464
aaa@loudoun.gov
www.loudoun.gov

Scott A. York, Chairman
Shawn M. Williams, Vice Chairman
Suzanne M. Volpe, Algonkian District

It is Loudoun County's central point of contact for seniors (55+) and their families. Fosters independence and healthy aging.

1749 Mercy Medical Airlift
Mercy Medical Airlift
PO Box 1940
Manassas, VA 20108-0804
703-361-1191
Fax: 703-257-1642; *Toll Free:* 800-296-1217
info@mercymedicalairlift.org
www.mercymedical.org

COL Norman E Johnson, Chairman
C.R. (Bud) Harper, Cice Chairman
Bill Edmunds, Director

Year Founded: 1972

1750 Mountain Empire Older Citizens
Mountain Empire Older Citizens, Inc.
PO Box 888
1501 Third Ave East
Big Stone Gap, VA 24219
276-523-4202
Fax: 276-523-4208; *Toll Free:* 800-252-6362
info@meoc.org
www.meoc.org

Marilyn Pace Maxwell, Executive Director
E Dennis Horton, Deputy Director
Linda Begley, Contact

MEOC is the designated area agency on aging and public transit provider for Lee, Scoot, and Wise counties, and the city of Norton, Va. Serves older persons with disabilities, caregivers, and the general public.

Year Founded: 1974

1751 NRCA RSVP (Retired and Senior VolunteerProgram) Floyd County
220 Parkway Lane South
Floyd, VA 24091-3083

540-745-2105
Fax: 540-745-2106
frsvp@nrcaa.org
www.swva.net/nrca/frsvp.htm

Valerie Mills, Program Director

Provides volunteer opportunities for persons age 55 or over to participate more fully in the life of their community. Lead with experience.

Year Founded: 1974; Number of Members: 267

1752 Northern Neck Middle Peninsula Area: Agency on Aging
Middle Peninsula-Northern Neck Community Services
5372B Old Virginia Street
Urbanna, VA 23175
804-758-5250
Fax: 804-758-5773; *Toll Free:* 800-305-BABY
www.mpnncsb.org/

Allyn W Gemerek, Director
Charles R. Walsh, Jr., LCSW, Executive Director

Provides support to senior area residents.

1753 Nutrition Services Incentive Program (NSIP)
Food & Nutrition Service
3101 Park Center Drive
Alexandria, VA 22302
703-305-2680
Fax: 703-305-2420
www.fns.usda.gov

Audrey Rowe, Administrator for Food & Nutriti
Kevin W. Concannon, Under Secretary for Food, Nutrit
Dr. Janey Thornton, Deputy Under Secretary for Food,

To improve diets of those people age 60 and older and their spouses (regardless of age) or disabled and handicapped persons, not yet 60, who reside in housing facilities occupied primarily by the elderly and at which congregate meals service for the elderly is provided. Also to increase the market for domestically produced foods acquired under surplus removal or price support operations.

Year Founded: 1969

1754 Prince William Area: Agency on Aging
Prince William Area County, Virginia
5 County Complex Court
Suite 240
Prince William, VA 22192
703-792-6439
Fax: 703-792-4734
SHenry@pwcgov.org.
www.pwcgov.org/aoa/
TDD 703-792-6444

Corey A. Stewart, Chairman At-Large
Michael C. May, Vice Chair
Sarah Henry, Analyst and Title VI Program Man

Serves older adults, their families and caregivers in the tri-jurisdictional area of Prince William County, the City of Manassas and the City of Manassas Park.

1755 RSVP Campbell County
Campbell County, Virginia
PO Box 100
Rustburg, VA 24588
434-332-9500
Fax: 804-332-9617

administration@campbellcountyva.gov
www.co.campbell.va.us/

Lynne Burnham, Program Manager
R. David Laurerell, County Administrator
Clifton M. Tweedy, Deputy County Administrator

Provides opportunities for people 55 and over to make a difference in their community through volunteer service. RSVP volunteers contribute anywhere from a few to over forty hours a week, serving through schools, day care centers, police departments, hospitals and other nonprofit and public organizations to help meet critical community needs. RSVP matches the personal interests and skills of older Americans with opportunities to help solve community problems and offers supplemental insurance while on duty, on-the-job training from the agency or organization where volunteers are placed.

Year Founded: 1781

1756 RSVP Clinch Valley
Clinch Valley Community Action, Inc.
The Donald E. Neal Building
200 E. Riverside Drive, PO Box 188
North Tazewell, VA 24630
276-988-5583
Fax: 276-988-4041; *Toll Free:* 800-273-9059
www.clinchvalleycaa.org

David T. Larimer, II, Chairperson
Brian Beck, Vice Chairperson
Joan Fugate, Secretary

The Retired and Senior Volunteer Program (RSVP) provides opportunities for people 55 and over to make a difference in their community through volunteer service. RSVP volunteers contribute anywhere from a few to over forty hours a week, serving through schools, day care centers, police departments, hospitals and other nonprofit and public organizations to help meet critical community needs. RSVP offers maximum flexibility and choice to its volunteers. RSVP matches the personal interests and skills to older Americans with opportunities to help solve community problems and offer supplemental insurance while on duty, on-the-job training from the agency or organization where volunteers are placed.

1757 RSVP Jefferson Area
674 Hillsdale Drive
Suite 9
Charlottesville, VA 22901
434-817-5245
Fax: 434-817-5230
mwilliams@jabacares.org
www.jabacares.org/

Martha Williams, Director
Donna Baker, Director of Operations
Jennifer Bivens, Human Resources Manager

1758 RSVP Loudoun
Loudoun County Government
P.O. Box 7000
Leesburg, VA 20177
703-777-0100
Fax: 703-771-5161; *Toll Free:* 800-552-4464
www.loudoun.gov/aaa

Scott A. York, Chairman
Shawn M. Williams, Vice Chairman
Suzanne M. Volpe, Algonkian District

The Retired and Senior Volunteer Program (RSVP) provides opportunities for people 55 and over to make a difference in their community through volunteer service. RSVP volunteers contribute anywhere from a few to over forty hours a week, serving though schools, day care centers, police departments, hospitals and other nonprofit and public organizations to help meet critical community needs. RSVP offers maximum flexibility and choice to its volunteers. RSVP matches the personal interests and skills to older Americans with opportunities to help solve community problems and offer supplemental insurance while on duty, on-the-job training from the agency or organization where volunteers are placed.

1759 RSVP Montgomery County
Health and Human Services Bldg.
210 S. Pepper Street
Ste. D
Christiansburg, VA 24073
540-382-5775
Fax: 540-381-6856
www.montgomerycountyva.gov/rsvp

Mary Critzer, Director Human Services
Angela Little, Director RSVP
Dawn Ramsey, Senior Program Assistant

The Retired and Senior Volunteer Program (RSVP) provides opportunities for people 55 and over to make a difference in their community through volunteer service. RSVP volunteers contribute anywhere from a few to over forty hours a week, serving though schools, day care centers, police departments, hospitals and other nonprofit and public organizations to help meet critical community needs. RSVP offers maximum flexibility and choice to its volunteers. RSVP matches the personal interests and skills to older Americans with opportunities to help solve community problems and offer supplemental insurance while on duty, on-the-job training from the agency or organization where volunteers are placed.

Year Founded: 1973

1760 RSVP Prince William
Volunteer Prince William
9248 Center Street
Manassas, VA 20110
703-369-5292
Fax: 703-369-5671
dragghianti@volunteerprincewilliam.org
www.volunteerprincewilliam.org

Mary E. Foley, Executive Director
Coleen Hersson, Retired & Senior Volunteer Progr
Bill Forquer, Adult Alternative Service Progra

Federally funded program designed to promote volunteerism in citizens 55 years of age and older. Program benefits included milelage reimbursment/cab service, supplemental accident insurance, volunteer training luncheons, volunteer get togethers, advisory board leadership roles, shirt and tote bags and more. Volunteer choose their volunteer site and set their own schedule.

Year Founded: 1981

1761 RSVP Pulaski County
New River Valley Agency on Aging
141 East Main Street
Suite 500
Pulaski, VA 24301

540-980-7720
Fax: 540-980-7724; *Toll Free:* 866-260-4417
nrvaoa@nrvaoa.org
www.nrvaoa.org

Tina King, M.S. Ed., Executive Director
Cassie Mills, Program Director/ Assistant to t
Jennifer Viers, Director of Finance & Administra

Provides opportunities for people 55 and over to make a difference in their community through volunteer service. RSVP volunteers contribute anywhere form a few to over forty hours a week, serving through schools, day care centers, police departments, hospitals and other nonprofit and public organizations to help meet critical community needs. RSVP matches the personal interests and skills of older Americans with opportunities to help solve community problems and offers supplemental insurance while on duty, on-the-job training from a agency or organization where volunteers are placed.

1762 RSVP Shenandoah Area
Shenandoah Area Agency on Aging
207 Mosby Lane
Front Royal, VA 22630
540-635-7141
Fax: 540-636-7810; *Toll Free:* 800-883-4122
information@shenandoahaaa.com
www.shenandoahaaa.com

Travis Clark, Chair
Tom Throckmorton, Vice Chair
Cathie Galvin, Executive Director

The Retired and Senior Volunteer Program (RSVP) provides opportunities for people 55 and over to make a difference in their community through volunteer service. RSVP volunteers contribute anywhere from a few to over forty hours a week, serving thourgh schools, day care centers, police departments, hospitals and other nonprofit and public organizations to help meet critical community needs. RSVP offers maximum flexibility and choice to its volunteers. RSVP matches the personal interests and skills to older Americans with opportunities to help solve community problems and offer supplemental insurance while on duty, on-the-job training from the agency or organization where volunteers are placed.

Year Founded: 1975

1763 Railroad Retirement Board: Richmond, Virginia District Office
US Railroad Retirement Board
400 N 8th Street
Ste. 470
Richmond, VA 23219-4819
877-772-5772
Fax: 804-771-8481
richmond@rrb.gov
www.rrb.gov/field/do_rich.asp

David P Griffith, Representative
Martin J. Dickman, Inspector General

Maintains information about retirement, survivor, and sickness benefits for railroad workers and their families.

1764 Railroad Retirement Board: Roanoke, Virginia District Office
US Railroad Retirement Board
First Campbell Square, Ste. 110
210 First Street SW, PO Box 270
Roanoke, VA 24002-0270
877-772-5772
Fax: 540-857-2769
roanoke@rrb.gov
www.rrb.gov/field/do_roan.asp

Martin J. Dickman, Inspector General

Maintains benefit and employment information for railroad workers and their families.

1765 Rappahannock Area: Agency on Aging
Rappahannock Area Agency on Aging
460 Landall Lane
Fredericksburg, VA 22405
540-371-3375
Fax: 540-371-3384; *Toll Free:* 800-262-4012
info@raaa16.org
www.raaa16.org

Joey Lambert, Chair
Leigh Wade, Executive Director
Pat Holland, Senior Services Coordinator

RAAA serves the needs and acts on behalf of persons aged 60 and older in the City of Fredericksburg and the surrounding counties of King George, Caroline, Spotsylvania and Stafford.

Year Founded: 1976

1766 Rappahannock-Rapidan Community Services Board and Area Agency on Aging
PO Box 1568
Culpeper, VA 22701
540-825-3100
Fax: 540-825-6245
rrcsb@rrcsb.org
www.rrcsb.org
TDD 540-825-7391
TTY: 540-825-7391

Elizabeth Blubaugh, Chair
Conway Porter, Vice Chair
Brian Buncan, Executive Director

Delivers services to the elderly within the region (Culpeper, Fauquier, Rappahannock, Orange, and Madison).

Year Founded: 1972

1767 Senior Connections The Capital Area: Agency
Senior Connections, The Capital Area Agency on Agi
24 East Cary Street
Richmond, VA 23219
804-343-3000
Fax: 804-649-2258; *Toll Free:* 800-989-2286
www.seniorconnections-va.org

John T. Robertson, Chairman
Felix Sarfo-Kantanka, Jr., Vice Chairman
Thelma B Watson, Executive Director

Serves persons age 60 and over in the City of Richmond and surrounding counties: Services provided: congregate meals, home-delivered meals, long-term care ombudsman, newsletter, volunteer program, foster grandparents, short-term home care, volunteer money management, partners in guardianship, Virginia insurance counseling and assistance project, senior employment, resource coordination, home equity conversion mortgage loan counseling, fan care.

Year Founded: 1973

1768 Virginia Association of Area Agencies on Aging
Virginia Association of Area Agencies on Aging
24 E Cary Street
Suite 100
Richmond, VA 23219
804-644-2804
Fax: 804-644-5640
info@thev4a.org
www.vaaaa.org

Betty Reams, Director
Thelma Watson, Executive Director

Advocates for the resources and policies that will allow older persons to lead meaningful lives. Making Virginia Elder Ready!

Year Founded: 1976

1769 Virginia Association of Nonprofit Homes for the Aging
Virginia Association of Nonprofit Homes for the Ag
4201 Dominion Boulevard
Suite 100
Glen Allen, VA 23060
804-965-5500
Fax: 804-965-9089
vanha@vanha.org
www.vanha.org

Sandee Levin, President
Dana Parsons, Legislative Affairs Legal Counsel
Sydney Thomas, Member Services Manager

Represents the interests of the not-for-profit facilities serving older adults in Virginia.

Year Founded: 1973

1770 Virginia Board for People with Disabilities
Virginia Board for People with Disabilities
1100 Bank Street
7th Floor
Richmond, VA 23219
804-786-0016
Fax: 804-783-1118; *Toll Free:* 800-846-4464
parsonbs@vbpd.state.va.us
www.vaboard.org/

John Kelly, Chair
Linda Broady-Myers, Vice Chair
Heidi Lawyer, Executive Director

The mission is to create a Commonwealth that advances opportunities for independence, personal decision-making and full participation in community life for individuals with developmental disabilities.

1771 Virginia Client Assistance Program
1910 Byrd Avenue
Suite 5
Richmond, VA 23230
804-225-2042
Fax: 804-662-7057; *Toll Free:* 800-552-3962
info@dLCV.org
www.vopa.state.va.us

Darrel T. Mason, Chair
Angela Thanyachareon, Vice Chair
Coleen Miller, Executive Director

Explains and protects the rights of and benefits to persons who are clients or or applicants for services provided by th Department of Rehabilitative Services, Department for the Blind, Centers for Independent Living, or programs funded under the Rehabilitation Act of 1973.

1772 Virginia Department for the Aging
Virginia Division for the Aging
1610 Forest Avenue
Suite 100
Richmond, VA 23229
804-662-9333
Fax: 804-662-9354; *Toll Free:* 800-552-3402
aging@vda.virginia.gov
www.vda.virginia.gov

Tim Catherman, M.H.A, Director, Aging Operations
AJ Hostetler, PR Director
Cecily Slasor, Customer Service Specialist

The Department's objective is to help Virginians find the information and services they need to lead healthy and independent lives as they grow older. Our mission is to foster the dignity, independence, and security of older Virginians by promoting partnerships with families and communities.

1773 Virginia Department of Taxation
Virginia Department of Taxation
PO Box 1115
Richmond, VA 23218-1115
804-367-8031
Fax: 804-254-6113
www.tax.virginia.gov

Kenneth W Thorson, Manager

Provides state income and business tax forms and information.

1774 Virginia Developmental Disability Council
Virginia Board for People with Disabilities
1100 Bank Street
7th Floor
Richmond, VA 23219
804-786-0016
Fax: 804-786-1118; *Toll Free:* 800-846-4464
www.vaboard.org

John Kelly, Chairman
Linda Broady-Myers, Vice Chair
Heidi Lawyer, Executive Director

Advances opportunities for individuals with developmental disabilities.

1775 Virginia Office for Protection and Advocacy
1910 Byrd Avenue
Suite 5
Richmond, VA 23230
804-225-2042
Fax: 804-662-7057; *Toll Free:* 800-552-3962
info@dLCV.org
www.vopa.state.va.us

Darrel T. Mason, Chair
Angela Thanyachareon, Vice Chair
Coleen Miller, Executive Director

Helps with disability-related problems like abuse, neglect and discrimination. Helps people with disabilities obtain services and treatment. Individuals with problems targeted in program priorities may receive advocacy services and/or legal representation.

Washington

1776 Abused Deaf Women's Advocacy Services

Abused Deaf Women's Advocacy Services (ADWAS)
8623 Roosevelt Way NE
Seattle, WA 98115
206-922-7088
Fax: 206-726-0017
adwas@adwas.org
www.adwas.org

Liz Gibson, Board Chair
Tiffany Williams, Executive Director
Nani Baran, Board Member

Advocacy group for deaf and deaf-blind women who have been mentally, physically, or sexually abused.

Year Founded: 1986

1777 Aging and Long Term Care of Eastern Washington

Aging and Long Term Care of Eastern Washington
1222 North Post
Spokane, WA 99201-2518
509-458-2509
Fax: 509-458-2003
action@altcew.org
www.altcew.org
TTY: 509-477-4442

Shelly O'Quinn, Spokane County Commissioner
Mike Fagan, Spokane City Council
Jerrie Allard, City of Spokane CD-Human Service

One of 13 area agencies on aging in Washington state. An administrative agency that funds programs and services that promote independence and keep older persons and individuals needing long term care living in their own homes for as long as possible.

Year Founded: 1978

1778 Bureau of Naval Personnel: Whidbey Island Retired Activities Office

Fleet & Family Support Center
Naval Air Station Whidbey Island
3675 W Lexington Street, Building 2256
Oak Harbor, WA 98278
360-257-8054
Fax: 360-257-8061
www.nioc-whidbeyisland.navy.mil

Commander Giangrasso, Commanding Officer
LCDR Dave Brown, Executive Officer
Albert John Ondo, Command Master Chief

The Fleet and Family Support Program throughout Navy Region Northwest is an on-base social service organization whose goal is to improve the quality of life for the Navy member and family through Counseling and Advocacy Prevention Services (CAPS) and Life Skills Programs.

1779 Disability Rights Washington

Disability Rights Washington
315 - 5th Avenue South
Suite 850
Seattle, WA 98104
206-324-1521
Fax: 206-957-0729; *Toll Free:* 800-562-2702
info@dr-wa.org
www.disabilityrightswa.org/
TTY: 206-957-0728

Mark Stroh, Executive Director
David Carlson, Director of Legal Advocacy
Andrea Kadlec, Director of Community Relations

DRW's mission is to advance the dignity, equality, and self-determination of people with disabilities.

Year Founded: 1975

1780 Gray Panthers of Seattle

Gray Panthers of Seattle
4649 Sunnyside Ave N
Seattle, WA 98103-6900
206-675-8859
Fax: 202-737-1160
graypanthers@qwest.net
www.scn.org/graypanthersofseattle/

Cynthia Adcock, Director

Work for social and economic justice and peace for all people.

1781 Kitsap County Area: Agency on Aging

Division of Aging and Long Term Care
614 Division Street
MS-5
Port Orchard, WA 98366
360-337-7129
Fax: 360-337-5746; *Toll Free:* 800-562-6418
www.agingkitsap.com/about.htm

Ade Ariwoola, Manager

Promote the health and well-being of senior Kitsap residents.

Year Founded: 1980

1782 Leading Age Wisconsin

LeadingAge Wisconsin
204 South Hamilton Street
Madison, WA 53703
608-255-7060
Fax: 608-255-7064
info@LeadingAgeWI.org
www.wahsa.org

Mike Christensen, Chair
Jim Williams, Vice Chair of Operations

Mari Beth Borek, Vice Chair of Member Services

Leading Age is the state association of not-for-profit organizations and other affiliated members dedicated to providing quality housing, health, community and related services to the elderly.

1783 Olympic Area: Agency on Aging

Olympic Area Agency on Aging
11700 Rhody Drive
Port Hadlock, WA 98339

360-379-5064
Fax: 360-379-4400; *Toll Free:* 866-720-4863
www.o3a.org

Roy B Walker, Executive Director
Barbie Rasmussen, Planning & Program Development D
Kim Younger, Chief Financial Officer

Provides services and programs to seniors.

1784 RSVP Clallam Jefferson County
Port Townsend Programs Office
823 Commerce Loop
Port Townsend, WA 98368
360-385-2571
Fax: 360-385-5185
action@olycap.org, info@olycap.org
www2.olycap.org/

Rich Ciccaro Rich Ciccarone, Board Chair
Robert Gray, Vice Chair
Dr. Ed Hopfner, Treasurer

The Retired and Senior Volunteer Program (RSVP) provides opportunities for people 55 and over to make a difference in their community through volunteer service. RSVP
volunteers contribute anywhere from a few to over forty
hours a week, serving thourgh schools, day care centers,
police departments, hospitals and other nonprofit and public organizations to help meet critical community needs.
RSVP offers maximum flexibility and choice to its volunteers. RSVP matches the personal interests and skills to
older Americans with opportunities to help solve community problems and offer supplemental insurance while on
duty, on-the-job training from the agency or organization
where volunteers are placed.

1785 RSVP Clark County
201 N.E. 73rd Street
Suite 101
Vancouver, WA 98665
360-694-6577
Fax: 360-694-6716
jeannep@hsc-wa.org
www.hsc-wa.org

Kris Olmstead, President
Cheryl Pfaff, Vice President
Jeanne Phipps, Director

Recruits volunteers 55 and older and matches their skills,
talents and time availability with the right
volunteerposition at one of 200 private and public non
profit organizations. Volunteers choose what, where and
how much time they give. Volunteers have the opportunity
to keep skills active, learn new ones and make new friends.
Provides supplemental insurance, limited mileage
reimbursment and recognition.

1786 RSVP Pierce County
United Way of Pierce County
PO Box 2215
1501 Pacific Ave., Suite 400
Tacoma, WA 98402
253-272-4263
Fax: 253-597-7481
web@uwpc.org
www.uwpc.org/

Debra Young, Board Chair
Jo Anne Coy, Secretary
Jennifer Nino, Treasurer

The Retired and Senior Volunteer Program (RSVP) provides opportunities for people 55 and over to make a difference in their community through volunteer service. RSVP
volunteers contribute anywhere from a few to over forty
hours a week, serving thourgh schools, day care centers,
police departments, hospitals and other nonprofit and public organizations to help meet critical community needs.
RSVP offers maximum flexibility and choice to its volunteers. RSVP matches the personal interests and skills to
older Americans with opportunities to help solve community problems and offer supplemental insurance while on
duty, on-the-job training from the agency or organization
where volunteers are placed.

1787 RSVP and Volunteer Center of Kittitas County
1206 N Dolarway Road
Suite 219
Ellensburg, WA 98926
509-962-4311
rsvp@fairpoint.net
rsvp-wa.org/ellensburg/

Carol Findley, RSVP Director

The Retired and Senior Volunteer Program (RSVP) provides opportunities for people 55 and over to make a difference in their community through volunteer service. RSVP
volunteers contribute anywhere from a few to over forty
hours a week, serving thourgh schools, day care centers,
police departments, hospitals and other nonprofit and public organizations to help meet critical community needs.
RSVP offers maximum flexibility and choice to its volunteers. RSVP matches the personal interests and skills to
older Americans with opportunities to help solve community problems and offer supplemental insurance while on
duty, on-the-job training from the agency or organization
where volunteers are placed.

Year Founded: 1974

1788 Railroad Retirement Board: Bellevue,
Washington District Office
US Railroad Retirement Board
155 108th Avenue NE
Bellevue, WA 98004
Fax: 425-450-5472; *Toll Free:* 877-772-5772
bellevue@rrb.gov
www.rrb.gov

Gregory Pesek, District Manager
Vonna Ward, Network Manager

Administers retirement/survivor and unemployment/sick-
ness benefit programs for railroad workers and their
families.

1789 Railroad Retirement Board: Spokane,
Washington District Office
US Railroad Retirement Board
920 W Riverside Avenue
Ste. 492 B
Spokane, WA 99201-1081
509-353-2795
Fax: 509-353-2741; *Toll Free:* 877-772-5772
www.rrb.gov/field/do_spok.asp

Nancy M Hand, Representative
Martin J. Dickman, Inspector General

Administers retirement/survivor and unemployment/sick-
ness benefit programs for railroad workers and their
families.

1790 Shoreline Lake Forest Park Senior Center
Shoreline Lake Forest Park Senior Center
18560 1st Avenue NE
Suite 1
Shoreline, WA 98155
206-365-1536
Fax: 206-364-8930
shorelinesc@seniorservices.org
www.shorelinelfpseniorcenter.org

Lee Fenton, President
David Chow, Vice President
Bob Lohmeyer, Director

Provides a wide range of activities and services for seniors 50 and over.

1791 Washington Association of Area Agencies on Aging
Washington Association of Area Agencies on Aging
4419 Harrison Avenue NW
Olympia, WA 98502
360-664-2168
Fax: 360-664-0791
mahardw@dshs.wa.gov
www.agingwashington.org/

Lori Brown, Chair
Dennis Mahar, Vice Chair
Jesse Eller, At-Large Member, Executive Commi

Provides a network of in-home and community services to older and diabled adults.

1792 Washington Client Assistance Program
Washington State Client Assistance Program
2531 Rainier Avenue S
5
Seattle, WA 98144
206-721-5999
Fax: 206-721-4537; Toll Free: 800-544-2121
jcap@qwestoffice.net
washingtoncap.org/
TTY: 206-721-6072

Jerry Johnsen, Director
Bob Huven, Rehabilitation Coordinator

Advocacy and information assistance for persons of disability seeking services through Vocational Rehabilitation or other program under the 1973 Rehabilitation Act as commented. We provide counseling.

1793 Washington Department of Retirement Systems
PO Box 48380
Olympia, WA 98504-8380
360-664-7000
Fax: 360-753-3166; Toll Free: 800-547-6657
www.drs.wa.gov
TTY: 360-586-5450

Maxine Hayes MD

Provides services to the retired.

1794 Washington Department of Revenue
Washington State Department of Revenue
PO Box 47450
Olympia, WA 98504-7450
360-236-4018; *Toll Free: 800-647-7706*
www.dor.wa.gov

Carol K. Nelson, Director

Provides tax payer assistance as the state's tax collection agency.

1795 Washington Department of Social and Health Services Aging and Adult Services
PO Box 47852
Olympia, WA 98504-7852
360-236-4018; *Toll Free: 800-422-3263*
wongma@dshs.wa.gov
www.aasa.dshs.wa.gov

Maxine Hayes MD

Provides support to family and other unpaid caregivers who care for an adult or senior with disabilities.

1796 Washington Department of Veterans Affairs
PO Box 41150
Olympia, WA 98504-1150
360-725-2200; *Toll Free: 800-562-0132*
webmaster@dva.wa.gov
www.dva.wa.gov
TDD 360-725-2199

Erwin Vidallon, Chief Financial Officer
Heidi Audette, Communications Director
Starleen Parsons, Human Resources Director

Provides information on benefits, services and programs for veterans.

1797 Washington State Aging & Disability Services Administration
640 Woodland Square Loop
Lacey, WA 98503
360-725-2300
Fax: 360-407-0369; Toll Free: 800-422-3263
www.aasa.dshs.wa.gov
TDD 800-737-7931

Kathy Leitch, Assistant Secretary

The Aging and Disability Services Administration assists children and adults with developmental delays or disabilities, cognitive impairment, chronic illness and related functional disabilities to gain access to needed services and supports by managing a system of long-term care and supportive services that are high quality, cost effective, and responsive to individual needs and preferences.

1798 Washington State Developmental Disabilities Council
2600 Martin Way, Suite F
PO Box 48314
Olympia, WA 98504-8314
425-753-3908
Fax: 360-586-6502; Toll Free: 800-634-4473
linda.west@ddc.wa.gov
www.wa.gov/ddc

Leslie Smith, Chair

The Washington State Developmental Disabilities Council is appointed by the Governor to promote a comprehensive system of services, and serve as an advocate and a planning body for Washington State's citizens with developmental disabilities.

1799 Washington Workers Compensation Board
Labour & Industries (L&I), Washington State
Department of Labor and Industries, 7273 Linderson Way SW

PO Box 44000
Olympia, WA 98504-4000
360-902-5800
Fax: 360-902-5798; *Toll Free:* 800-547-8367
www.lni.wa.gov

Gary Weeks, Director
Vickie Kennedy, Special Assistant to Director
Judy Schurke

Protecting workers wages and working conditions.

West Virginia

1800 Appalachian Area Agency on Aging
Appalachian Area Agency on Aging
1460 Main Street
PO Box 2
Princeton, WV 24740
304-425-1147
Fax: 304-487-3767; *Toll Free:* 800-473-1207
aaaa@citilink.net
www.aaaoa.org

Ramona Stanley, Executive Director
Mary Najar, Deputy Director
Myrna Wisman, Fiscal Officer

The AAAOA contracts with county aging programs to provide nutrition programs, transportation and other social services for seniors in thirteen counties in Southeastern West Virginia.

1801 Charleston Disability Determination Services
West Virginia Division of Rehabilitation Services
107 Capitol Street
Charleston, WV 25301-2609
304-343-5055
Fax: 304-353-4212
www.wvdrs.org

Jane Johnstone, Assistant Director

Under contract with the US Social Security Administration, the Disability Determination Services Section determines eligibility for Social Security Disability Insurance and Supplemental Security Income benefits.

1802 Clarksburg Disability Determination Services
West Virginia Division of Rehabilitation Services
Federal Center
320 West Pike Street, Suite 120
Clarksburg, WV 26301
304-624-0200
Fax: 304-624-0252
www.wvdrs.org

Janice A Holland, Interim Director

Under contract with the US Social Security Administration, the Disability Determination Services Section determines eligibility for Social Security Disability Insurance and Supplemental Security Income benefits.

1803 Northwestern Area: Agency on Aging
Belomar Regional Council
PO Box 2086
Wheeling, WV 26003
304-242-1800
Fax: 304-242-2437
lwilliams@belomar.org
www.belomar.org

Scott Hicks, Director
A. C. Wiethe, Assistant Director
Rick Healy, Housing Rehabilitation Specialis

The NWAAA maintains Older Americans Act programs through subgrants and contracts with senior centers within its 16 county PSA.

1804 Railroad Retirement Board: West Virginia District Office
US Railroad Retirement Board
New Federal Building, Room 145
640 4th Avenue, P.O. Box 2153
Huntington, WV 25721
304-529-5561
Fax: 304-529-5546; *Toll Free:* 877-772-5772
Janet.Terlop@rrb.gov
www.rrb.gov

Janet K Terlop, District Manager
Martin J. Dickman, Inspector General

The Railroad Retirement Board's mission is to administer retirement/survivor and unemployment/sickness insurance benefit programs for railroad workers and their families under the Railroad Retirement Act and the Railroad Unemployment Act.

1805 Upper Potomac Area Agency on Aging
Upper Potomac Area Agency on Aging, Inc.
Airport Road
PO Box 869
Petersburg, WV 26847
304-257-1221
Fax: 304-257-4958; *Toll Free:* 877-833-5084
upaaa@regioneight.org
www.upaaa.net/index

Scott Gossard, Executive Director
Janice Lantz, Fiscal Officer

Our mission is one of service, with emphasis on providing assistance to older West Virginians, with dignity and a caring spirit. The UPAAA believes its goal is to provide technical assistance, training, and counseling to county providers with the intent of enhancing the hapiness and standard of living of older West Virginians. In this way, we feel, elderly West Virginians will be able to retain their dignity and independence while remaining in their own households.

1806 West Virginia Advocates
West Virginia Advocates, Inc. (WVA)
1207 Quarrier Street
Ste. 400
Charleston, WV 25301
304-346-0847
Fax: 304-346-0867; *Toll Free:* 800-950-5250
www.wvadvocates.org
TDD 304-346-0847

Terry Dilcher, President
Clarice Hausch, Executive Director
Barbara Criner, Administrative Director

West Virginia Advocates protects and advocates for the human and legal rights of persons with disabilities. It is operated exclusively for charitable and educational purposes.

1807 West Virginia Bureau Of Senior Services
West Virginia Bureau of Senior Services
1900 Kanawha Boulevard E
Charleston, WV 25305

304-558-3317
Fax: 304-558-5609; *Toll Free:* 877-987-3646
www.wvseniorservices.gov/?

Robert E. Roswall, Commissioner
Lee Rodgers, Executive Secretary
Terry Hess, Finance Director

West Virginia Bureau of Senior Services lists senior programs from transportation to meals to exercise classes to in-home services throughout the state of West Virginia for seniors.

1808 West Virginia Department of Health
West Virginia Department of Health & Human Resourc
One Davis Square
Ste. 100 East
Charleston, WV 25301
304-558-0684
Fax: 304-558-1130
DHHRSecretary@wv.gov
dhhr.wv.gov

Karen L. Bowling, Cabinet Secretary

1809 West Virginia Developmental Disability Council
West Virginia Developmental Disabilities Council
110 Stockton Street
Charleston, WV 25387
304-558-0416
Fax: 304-558-0941
dhhrwvddc@wv.gov
www.ddc.wv.gov
TDD 304-558-2376

Jerri Stephens, Chair
Greg Bilonick, Council Member
Sarah Brown, Council Member

The Council's mission is to assure that West Virginians with developmental disabilities receive the services, supports and opportunities they need to achieve independence, productivity, integration and inclusion into the community.

Year Founded: 1972

1810 West Virginia Division of Tax and Revenue
West Virginia State Tax Department
PO Box 3784
Charleston, WV 25337-3784
304-558-3333; *Toll Free:* 800-982-8297
TaxWVTaxAid@wv.gov
www.state.wv.us/taxrev
TDD 800-282-9833

Urita Lanham, Executive Director
Mark W. Matkovich, Acting Commissioner

Provides tax support to the elderly.

1811 West Virginia Protection & Advocacy for Persons with Disabilities
West Virginia Advocates
1207 Quarrier Street
Suite 400
Charleston, WV 25301
304-346-0847
Fax: 304-346-0867; *Toll Free:* 800-950-5250
wvainfo@wvadvocates.org
www.wvadvocates.org
TDD 304-346-0847

Terry Dilcher, President
Barbara Criner, Administrative Director
Clarice Hausch, Executive Director

Provides potection for persons with disabilities.

1812 West Virginia State College University-Metro Area Agency on Aging
West Virginia State University
P.O. Box 1000
Dunbar, WV 25112-1000
304-766-3374
Fax: 304-766-4126; *Toll Free:* 800-987-2112
www.wvstateu.edu/

Thomas Susman, Chair
Ann Brothers Smith, Vice Chair
Brian O. Hemphill, Ph.D., President

Provides information and services on a range of assistance for older adults and those who care for them.

Year Founded: 1891

1813 West Virginia Workers Compensation Board of Review
West Virginia Offices of the Insurance Commissione
PO Box 2628
Charleston, WV 25329-2628
304-558-5230
Fax: 304-558-1322
www.wvinsurance.gov/boardofreview

W Jack Stevens, Member
Rita F. Hedrick-Helmick, Member
James D. Gray, Member

The Board of Review shall reverse, vacate or modify the order or decision of the administrative law judge if the substantial rights of the petitioner or petitioners have been prejudiced because the administrative law judge's findings.

Year Founded: 2003

Wisconsin

1814 Area Agency on Aging of Dane County
County of Dane, Winscon
2306 South Park St.
Madison, WI 53713
608-261-9930
Fax: 608-261-9787
aaa@countyofdane.com
www.co.dane.wi.us
TTY: 608-261-9905

Cheryl Batterman, Manager

The mission of the Dane County Commission on Aging is to advocate for older people in order to enable them to maintain their full potential and enhance their quality of life.

Year Founded: 1839

1815 Bay Area Managers of Volunteer Services
Bay Area Managers of Volunteer Services (BAMVS)
131 S Madison Street
Green Bay, WI 54301-4501
414-435-1101
Fax: 920-492-5965
bamvsgreenbay.wordpress.com/

Jody Weyers, President

Managers or coordinators of volunteer programs and volunteer supervisors in northeastern Wisconsin.

1816 Coalition of Wisconsin Aging Groups
Coalition of Wisconsin Aging Groups
2850 Dairy Drive
Suite 100
Madison, WI 53718
608-224-0606
Fax: 608-224-0607; *Toll Free:* 800-366-2990
cwag@cwag.org
www.cwag.org

Arlene Meyer, Board Chair / CEO
Leigh Roberts, Board Vice Chair
John Hendrick, Director, Legal and Program Serv

1817 Disability Rights Wisconsin
Disability Rights Wisconsin
131 W. Wilson St
Suite 700
Madison, WI 53703
608-267-0214
Fax: 608-267-0368; *Toll Free:* 800-928-8778
www.disabilityrightswi.org/
TTY: 888-758-6049

Frank Sterzen, President
Ted Skemp, Vice President
Dan Idzikowski, Executive Director

The protection and advocacy agency for people with disabilities in Wisconsin. DRW provides guidance, advice, investigation, negotiation, and in some cases legal representation to people with disabilities and their families. Local and state level systems advocacy and training are also provided.

Year Founded: 1977

1818 Governor's Committee for People with Disabilities
Winscon Department of Health Services
1 West Wilson Street
Madison, WI 53703
608-266-1865
Fax: 608-266-3386
DHSwebmaster@wisconsin.gov
www.dhfs.wisconsin.gov
TTY: 888-701-1251

A Governor's Committee was established with one goal: to improve employment opportunities for people with disabilities. The group's mission was broadened to cover many aspects of disability in Wisconsin, and the group became the Governor's Committee for People with Disabilites (GCPD).

1819 Leading Age Wisconsin
LeadingAge Wisconsin
204 S Hamilton Street
Madison, WI 53703
608-255-7060
Fax: 608-255-7064
info@LeadingAgeWI.org
www.leadingagewi.org/

Mike Christensen, Chair
Jim Williams, Vice Chair of Operations
Mari Bet Borek, Vice Chair of Member Services

1820 Milwaukee County Department on Aging
Department on Aging - Milwaukee County
1220 West Vliet St
Suite 302
Milwaukee, WI 53205
414-289-5950
Fax: 866-229-9695; *Toll Free:* 414-289-6874
county.milwaukee.gov/Aging
TDD 414-289-6874

Stephanie Su Stein, Director

The mission of the Milwaukee County Department on Aging is to affirm the dignity and value of older adults of Milwaukee County by supporting their choices for living in, and giving to, our community.

1821 RSVP Advocap
Advocap, Inc.
181 East North Water Street
Neenah, WI 54956
920-725-2791
Fax: 920-725-6337; *Toll Free:* 800-631-2791
mikeb@advocap.org
www.advocap.org/rsvp.html
TTY: 920-725-5035

Kara Klein, RSVP Director
Terri Stern, Manager
Michael Bone Michael Bonertz, Executive Director

The Retired and Senior Volunteer Program (RSVP) provides opportunities for people 55 and over to make a difference in their community through volunteer service. RSVP volunteers contribute anywhere from a few to over forty hours a week, serving thourgh schools, day care centers, police departments, hospitals and other nonprofit and public organizations to help meet critical community needs. RSVP offers maximum flexibility and choice to its volunteers. RSVP matches the personal interests and skills to older Americans with opportunities to help solve community problems and offer supplemental insurance while on duty, on-the-job training from the agency or organization where volunteers are placed.

Year Founded: 1966

1822 RSVP Brown County
Volunteer Center of Brown County
984 9th Street
Green Bay, WI 54304
920-429-9445
Fax: 920-429-9449
volunteercenter@volunteergb.org
www.volunteergb.org/rsvp.php

Christine Danielson, Executive Director

The Retired and Senior Volunteer Program (RSVP) provides opportunities for people 55 and over to make a difference in their community through volunteer service. RSVP volunteers contribute anywhere from a few to over forty hours a week, serving thourgh schools, day care centers, police departments, hospitals and other nonprofit and public organizations to help meet critical community needs. RSVP offers maximum flexibility and choice to its volunteers. RSVP matches the personal interests and skills to older Americans with opportunities to help solve community problems and offer supplemental insurance while on duty, on-the-job training from the agency or organization where volunteers are placed.

1823 RSVP Coulee Region
Coulee Region RSVP
2920 East Avenue South
Suite 104
La Crosse, WI 54601
608-785-0500
Fax: 608-785-2573; *Toll Free:* 888-822-1295
info@rsvplax.org
www.rsvplax.org/

Lynnetta P. Kopp, Executive Director
Heather M. Harpenau, Program Specialist
Amanda Tisch Buros, Assistant Director

The Retired and Senior Volunteer Program (RSVP) provides opportunities for people 55 and over to make a difference in their community through volunteer service. RSVP
volunteers contribute anywhere from a few to over forty
hours a week, serving thourgh schools, day care centers,
police departments, hospitals and other nonprofit and public organizations to help meet critical community needs.
RSVP offers maximum flexibility and choice to its volunteers. RSVP matches the personal interests and skills to
older Americans with opportunities to help solve community problems and offer supplemental insurance while on
duty, on-the-job training from the agency or organization
where volunteers are placed.

1824 RSVP Dane County
RSVP of Dane County
517 N Segoe Road
Suite 300
Madison, WI 53705
608-238-7787
Fax: 608-238-7931
info@rsvpdane.org
www.rsvpdane.org

Kelly Krein, President
Peg Davey, Vice President
Mike Foley, RSVP Board Member

The Retired and Senior Volunteer Program (RSVP) provides opportunities for people 55 and over to make a difference in their community through volunteer service. RSVP
volunteers contribute anywhere from a few to over forty
hours a week, serving thourgh schools, day care centers,
police departments, hospitals and other nonprofit and public organizations to help meet critical community needs.
RSVP offers maximum flexibility and choice to its volunteers. RSVP matches the personal interests and skills to
older Americans with opportunities to help solve community problems and offer supplemental insurance while on
duty, on-the-job training from the agency or organization
where volunteers are placed.

1825 RSVP Kenosha County Sponsored By Kenosha
Area Family And Aging Services, Inc.
Kenosha Area Family And Aging Services, Inc.
7730 Sheridan Road
Kenosha, WI 53143
262-658-0237
Fax: 262-658-2263; *Toll Free:* 866-658-0237
rsvp@kafasi.org
www.kafasi.org

Jayne Herring, President
David Schlichting, Vice President
Katie Oatsvall, Executive Director

RSVP(The Retired and Senior Volunteer Program) provides
adults 55+ with a wide variety of fulfilling and fun volun-

teer opportunities throughout Kenosha County. RSVP offers volunteers choice, flexibility, and the chance to make a
difference.
Year Founded: 1969

1826 RSVP Manitowoc County
Holy Family Memorial
2300 Western Avenue
PO Box 1450
Manitowoc, WI 54221-1450
920-320-2011
Fax: 920-686-7640; *Toll Free:* 800-994-3662
vc@hfmhealth.org
www.hfmhealth.org

William Casey, Chair
Jane Pfeffer, Vice Chair
Mark P. Herzog, President & CEO

The Retired and Senior Volunteer Program (RSVP) provides opportunities for people 55 and over to make a difference in their community through volunteer service. RSVP
volunteers contribute anywhere from a few to over forty
hours a week, serving thourgh schools, day care centers,
police departments, hospitals and other nonprofit and public organizations to help meet critical community needs.
RSVP offers maximum flexibility and choice to its volunteers. RSVP matches the personal interests and skills to
older Americans with opportunities to help solve community problems and offer supplemental insurance while on
duty, on-the-job training from the agency or organization
where volunteers are placed.
Year Founded: 1899

1827 RSVP Portage County
Portage County RSVP
Lincoln Center
1519 Water Street
Stevens Point, WI 54481
715-346-1401
Fax: 715-346-1418; *Toll Free:* 866-920-2525
adrc@co.portage.wi.us
www.co.portage.wi.us/adrc/rsvp.html
TTY: 715-346-1632

Cindy Piotrowski, Aging & Disability Resource Cent
Jeff Jester, RSVP Director
Donna Calhoun, Senior Center Director

The Retired and Senior Volunteer Program (RSVP) provides opportunities for people 55 and over to make a difference in their community through volunteer service. RSVP
volunteers contribute anywhere from a few to over forty
hours a week, serving thourgh schools, day care centers,
police departments, hospitals and other nonprofit and public organizations to help meet critical community needs.
RSVP offers maximum flexibility and choice to its volunteers. RSVP matches the personal interests and skills to
older Americans with opportunities to help solve community problems and offer supplemental insurance while on
duty, on-the-job training from the agency or organization
where volunteers are placed.

1828 RSVP Rock County
RSVP-Rock.org
2433 South Riverside Drive
Beloit, WI 53511
608-362-9593
Fax: 608-362-9820

rsvp@rsvp-rock.org
www.rsvp-rock.org/

Robert W Harlow, Executive Director
Linda Kleven, Assistant Director/Programs
Patty Hansberry, Seniors Volunteering for Seniors

The Retired and Senior Volunteer Program (RSVP) provides opportunities for people 55 and over to make a difference in their community through volunteer service. RSVP volunteers contribute anywhere from a few to over forty hours a week, serving though schools, day care centers, police departments, hospitals and other nonprofit and public organizations to help meet critical community needs. RSVP offers maximum flexibility and choice to its volunteers. RSVP matches the personal interests and skills to older Americans with opportunities to help solve community problems and offer supplemental insurance while on duty, on-the-job training from the agency or organization where volunteers are placed.

1829 RSVP Superior-Douglas
Catholic Charities Bureau
1416 Cumming Avenue
Superior, WI 54880
715-394-6617
Fax: 715-394-5951
ccbrecep@ccbsuperior.org
www.ccbsuperior.org

Matt Crowell, Chair
Kyle Torvinen, Vice Chair
Alan Rock, Charities Executive Director

RSVP develops and supports volunteer opportunities for adults 55 and over to share their talents and expertise in areas where needs are expressed in the community.

Year Founded: 1917

1830 RSVP Waukeesha County
210 NW Barstow Street
Suite 101
Waukesha, WI 53188
262-549-3348
Fax: 262-549-0436
www.rsvpwaukesha.org

Glen Choban, President
Kathy Gale, Executive Director
Sandi Ammerman, Associate Director

The Retired and Senior Volunteer Program (RSVP) provides opportunities for people 55 and over to make a difference in their community through volunteer service. RSVP volunteers contribute anywhere from a few to over forty hours a week, serving though schools, day care centers, police departments, hospitals and other nonprofit and public organizations to help meet critical community needs. RSVP offers maximum flexibility and choice to its volunteers. RSVP matches the personal interests and skills to older Americans with opportunities to help solve community problems and offer supplemental insurance while on duty, on-the-job training from the agency or organization where volunteers are placed.

Year Founded: 1981

1831 Railroad Retirement Board: Wisconsin District Office
Henry S. Reuss Plaza
310 W Wisconsin Avenue, Suite 1168
Milwaukee, WI 53203-2213

877-772-5772
Fax: 414-297-3833
www.rrb.gov/field/do_milw.asp

Thomas P Hammersley, Representative
Martin J. Dickman, Inspector General

1832 Retired Senior Volunteer Program of Western Dairyland
Western Dairyland Economic Opportunity Council, In
23122 Whitehall Road
PO Box 125
Independence, WI 54747
715-985-2391
Fax: 715-985-3239; *Toll Free:* 800-782-1063
info@WesternDairyland.org
www.westerndairyland.org/rsvp.phtml

Lyndon B. Johnson, President
James Schwartz, Manager

Year Founded: 1966

1833 Volunteer Center of Racine County
Volunteer Center of Racine County, Inc.
6216 Washington Avenue
Suite G
Racine, WI 53406
262-886-9612
Fax: 262-886-9632; *Toll Free:* 800-201-9490
info@volunteercenterofracine.org
www.volunteercenterofracine.org/

Marta Kultgen, President
Kurt Wahlen, Vice President
Marilyn Pelky, Executive Director

1834 Volunteer Services of Barron County
Volunteer Services of Barron County,Inc.
330 E. LaSalle Ave.
Room 112
Barron, WI 54812
715-236-2184
info@unitedwayricelake.org
www.unitedwayricelake.org/volunteer-serv

Rita Vanek, Manager

1835 WisTech Assistive Technology Program
Wisconsin Department of Health Services
1 West Wilson Street
Madison, WI 53703
608-266-1865
Fax: 608-266-3386
DHSwebmaster@wisconsin.gov
www.dhfs.wisconsin.gov
TTY: 888-701-1251

Sarah Lincoln, WisTech Support

A statewide program promoting assistive technology devices and services for persons of all ages with all disabilities.

1836 Wisconsin Aging and Long Term Care Board
Winscon Board on Aging and Long Term Care
1402 Pankratz Street
Suite 111
Madison, WI 53704-4001
608-246-7013
Fax: 608-246-7001; *Toll Free:* 800-242-1060

BOALTC@Wisconsin.Gov
longtermcare.wi.gov

Terry Lynch, Board Chair
Eva Arnold, Board Member
Tanya Meyer, Board Member

Year Founded: 1973

1837 Wisconsin Client Assistance Program
Wisconsin Client Assistance Program

PO Box 8911
2811 Agriculture Drive
Madison, WI 53708-8911
608-224-5070
Fax: 608-224-5069; Toll Free: 800-362-1290
linda.vegoe@datcp.state.wi.us
www.icdri.org/legal/WisconsinCAP.htm
TTY: 888-877-5939

Linda Vegoe, CAP Director
Deb Henderson-Guenther, Complaint Investigator

1838 Wisconsin Council on Developmental Disabilities
Wisconsin Council on Developmental Disabilities

201 West Washington Avenue
Suite 110
Madison, WI 53703
608-266-7826
Fax: 608-267-3906; Toll Free: 888-332-1677
help@wcdd.org
www.wcdd.org
TDD 608-266-6660
TTY: 608-266-6660

Jennifer Ondrejka, Executive Director
Helen Hartman, Office Manager

The Wisconsin Council on Developmental Disabilities was established to advocate on behalf of individuals with developmental disabilities, foster welcoming and inclusive communities, and improve the disability service system. The Council's mission is to help people with developmental disabilities become independent, productive, and included in all facets of community life.

1839 Wisconsin Department of Revenue
Wisconsin Department of Revenue

PO Box 8906
Madison, WI 53708-8906
608-266-2772
Fax: 608-267-0834
www.dor.state.wi.us

Richard G. Chandler, Secretary
Jack Jablonski, Deputy Secretary
Jennifer Western, Assistant Deputy Secretary

Wisconsin Department of Revenue's main goal is to implement good tax policy. The Department strives to lower the overall tax burden, ease the taxpaying process and wisely use tax dollars.

1840 Wisconsin Department of Veterans Affairs
The Wisconsin Department of Veterans Affairs (WDVA

PO Box 7843
201 West Washington Avenue
Madison, WI 53707-7843
608-266-1018
Fax: 608-264-7616; Toll Free: 800-947-8387

wisvets@dva.wisconsin.gov
www.wisvets.com

John A. Scocos, Secretary
Michael Trepanier, Deputy Secretary
Kathleen Marschman, Assistant Deputy Secretary

Offers an array of benefits and services to eligible Wisconsin veterans and their families.

Year Founded: 1945

1841 Wisconsin Retired Educators Association
Wisconsin Retired Educators' Association

6405 Century Avenue
Suite 201
Middleton, WI 53562
608-831-5115
Fax: 608-831-1694
wrea@wrea.net
www.wrea.net

Victor Bekkum, President
Annaliece Rynes, Assistant To Executive Director
David Bennett, Executive Director

WREA is the voice and choice of retired educators since 1951. WREA monitors and protects pension benefits, provides retirement information, and promotes volunteerism and community services.

Year Founded: 1969

1842 Wisconsin Workers Compensation Bureau
Wisconsin Compensation Rating Bureau

20700 Swenson Drive, #100
Waukesha, WI 53186
262-796-4540
Fax: 262-796-4400
donna.knepper@wcrb.org
www.wcrb.org

Bernard Rosa Bernard Rosauer, President
Nancy Kierzek, VP Vice President of Administrat
Beth Nickel, Vice President of Operations

The mission of the WCRB is to administer and enhance Wisconsin's system of worker's compensation classifications, rates, rating plans and forms.

Wyoming

1843 Wyoming Department of Aging
Aging Division Wyoming Department of Health

6101 Yellowstone Avenue
Cheyenne, WY 82002
307-777-7986
Fax: 307-777-5340; Toll Free: 800-442-2766
wyaging@wyo.gov
www.wyomingaging.org

Thomas O. Forslund, Director
Lee Clabots, Deputy Director
Bob Peck, Chief Financial Officer

1844 Wyoming Department of Health: Aging Division
Aging Division Wyoming Department of Health

6101 Yellowstone Avenue
Cheyenne, WY 82002
307-777-7986
Fax: 307-777-5340; Toll Free: 800-442-2766

wyaging@wyo.gov
health.wyo.gov/aging/

Thomas O. Forslund, Director
Lee Clabots, Deputy Director
Bob Peck, Chief Financial Officer

1845 Wyoming Department of Revenue
Wyoming Department of Revenue
122 W 25th Street
2nd Floor West
Cheyenne, WY 82002-0110
307-777-5200
Fax: 307-777-3632
dor@wyo.gov
www.revenue.state.wy.us

Dane Noble, Director
Christie Yurek, Manager of the Administrative Se
Brenda Arnold, Administrator of the Property Ta

1846 Wyoming Developmental Disability Council
122 West 25th Street, 1st Floor West
Herschler Bldg., Rm. 1608
Cheyenne, WY 82002
307-777-7230
Fax: 307-777-5690; *Toll Free:* 800-438-5791
http://ddcouncil.state.wy.us

Shannon Buller, Executive Director
Von Maul, Administrative Assistant
Samantha Janney, Public Information Officer

1847 Wyoming Division of Rehabilitation
Wyoming Department of Workforce Services
1510 East Pershing Blvd.
Cheyenne, WY 82002
307-777-3700
Fax: 307-777-5870
www.wyomingworkforce.org

Joan K. Evans, Director
Lisa M. Osvold, Deputy Director

Offers diagnostic, medical and surgical treatment, counseling, social work, professional training, employment services and computer training services for the disabled.

1848 Wyoming Workers Safety & Compensation Division
Wyoming Department Workforce Services
1510 E Pershing Boulevard
Cheyenne, WY 82002
307-777-3700
Fax: 307-777-5870
www.wyomingworkforce.org/

Joan K. Evans, Director
Lisa M. Osvold, Deputy Director

The Workers' Safety and Compensation Division administers the Workers' Compensation program in Wyoming. Benefit levels are based on the Statewide Average Monthly Wage at the time of injury. The Statewide Average Monthly Wage is established quarterly by Unemployment Insurance Commission information.

Awards, Honors & Prizes

National

1849 Clark Tibbitts Award
Association for Gerontology in Higher Education
1220 L Street North West
Suite 901
Washington, DC 20005-4018
202-289-9806
Fax: 202-289-9824
aghe@aghe.org
www.aghe.org

Janet C. Frank, President
M. Angela Baker, Director
Kelly Niles-Yokum, Secretary

For recognition of significant contributions to the advancement of gerontology as a field of study in institutions of higher learning. Selection is by nomination. A certificate is awarded each year at the annual meeting and the awardee presents a lecture at a plenary session. Established in 1980. Re-named in 1987 to honor Clark Tibbitts, a pioneer in the field of gerontological education who founded the US Administration on Aging and authored over 100 publications.

Year Founded: 1974

1850 Claude Pepper Award
Claude Pepper Foundation
636 West Call Street
Tallahassee, FL 32306-1122
850-644-9309
Fax: 850-644-9301
www.claudepepperfoundation.org

A not-for-profit corporation, established by Claude Pepper in 1986. Provides the resources to properly preserve, store, conserve, and make availiable the collection and to develop the curricula and public activities that would maximize its educational potential. Since its founding, the Foundation has not only fullfilled that purpose but developed programs to further the objectives of Senator Pepper.

Year Founded: 1986

1851 Community Outreach Awards
Hearing Loss Association of America
7910 Woodmont Avenue
Suite 1200
Bethesda, MD 20814
301-657-2248
Fax: 301-913-9413
www.hearingloss.org

Diana D. Bender, Ph.D., President
Dr. Margaret Wallhagen, Ph.D., Vice President
Anna Hall, Executive Director

To recognize chapters, groups, or individuals who have been involved in a project(s) which had a positive influence in the community on making hearing loss an issue of national concern. The recipients of these awards will have planted a seed of hope for hard of hearing people, followed through on the project, and have had the opportunity to watch the project grow to fruition. Any publicity generated by this activity will have had a positive impact on the goals of SHHH, as well as on the lives of hearing impaired persons in the community. Chapters, groups, or individual SHHH members may submit nominations of members for

these awards by completing an application for nomination. Members of the Executive Committee of the Board of Directors will select the recipients of the awards. The deadline for nominations is March 1. Awards are presented in two categories: Community Awareness; and Community Access. A plaque is awarded.

1852 Distinguished Mentorship in Gerontology Award
Gerontological Society of America
1220 L Street North West
Suite 901
Washington, DC 20005
202-842-1275
Fax: 202-842-1150
geron@geron.org
www.geron.org

James Appleby, Executive Director & CEO
Linda Krogh Harootyan, Deputy Executive Director
Chris Yoder, Senior Director, Finance and Adm

To recognize individuals who have fostered excellence and who have had a major impact on the field of gerontology by virtue of their mentoring, and whose inspiration is sought by students and colleagues. Membership in the BSS section is required.

Year Founded: 1939

1853 Distinguished Service in Aging Award
LeadingAge
2519 Connecticut Avenue North West
Washington, DC 20008-1520
202-783-2242
Fax: 202-783-2255
info@LeadingAge.org
www.aahsa.org

William L. (Minnix Jr., President/Chief Executive Office
Katrinka (Ka Smith Sloan, SVP /Chief Operating Officer
Cheryl Phillips, Senior Vice President of Public

To recognize a public figure who has performed extraordinary service to the aging that has had or could have an impact on the total field of care and service to the aging.

1854 Donald P. Kent Award
Gerontological Society of America
1220 L Street North West
Suite 901
Washington, DC 20005
202-842-1275
Fax: 202-842-1150
geron@geron.org
www.geron.org

James Appleby, Executive Director and CEO
Linda Krogh Harootyan, Deputy Executive Director
Chris Yoder, Senior Director, Finance and Adm

To recognize a member who exemplifies the highest standard of professional leadership through teaching, service, and the interpretation of gerontology to the larger society. Nominees must be fellows of the Society. The deadline for nominations is May 8. The award requires a lecture at the time of the annual scientific meeting. Established in 1973 to honor Donald P. Kent, a pioneer in the field of gerontology.

Year Founded: 1945

1855 Durward K. McDaniel Ambassador Award
American Council of the Blind
2200 Wilson Boulevard
Suite 650
Arlington, VA 22201-3354
202-467-5081
Fax: 703-465-5085; *Toll Free:* 800-424-8666
info@acb.org
www.acb.org

Kim Charlson, President
Jeff Thom, 1st Vice President

To recognize a blind or visually impaired person who has
performed distinguished service to the community or in the
state where he or she resides. A certificate is awarded annually at the Council's national convention. Established in
1964.

Year Founded: 1961

1856 Edward Henderson Memorial Student Award
American Geriatrics Society
40 Fulton Street
18th Floor
New York, NY 10038
212-308-1414
Fax: 212-832-8646
info.amger@americangeriatrics.org
www.americangeriatrics.org

James T. Pacala, MD, MS, AGSF, Chairman of the Board
Cathy Alessi, MD, AGSF, President
Jennie Chin Hansen, RN, MSN, FAAN, Chief Executive
Officer

For medical students demonstrating excellence and initiative in geriatrics.

Year Founded: 1942

1857 Employment Awards
Hearing Loss Association of America
7910 Woodmont Avenue
Suite 1200
Bethesda, MD 20814
301-657-2248
Fax: 301-913-9413
www.hearingloss.org

Diana D. Bender, Ph.D., President
Dr. Margaret Wallhagen, Ph.D., Vice President
Anna Hall, Executive Director

To recognize affiliates that have taken specific steps to initiate programs to provide support for senior, hard of hearing members.

1858 Excellence in Practice Award
LeadingAge
2519 Connecticut Avenue North West
Washington, DC 20008-1520
202-783-2242
Fax: 202-783-2255
info@LeadingAge.org
www.aahsa.org

William L. (Minnix Jr., President/Chief Executive Office
Katrinka (Ka Smith Sloan, SVP /Chief Operating Officer
Cheryl Phillips, Senior Vice President of Public

To recognize standards of excellence through programs that
address some of the most complex challenges in the field of
housing, care and services for the aging. By honoring
benchmark, best practices in AAHSA-member organizations, this award seeks to showcase programs that demonstrate superior achievement throughout the continuum of
aging services. An organization's total program of services
or an individual program may be nominated. Criteria for inclusion: demonstrates an overall level of excellence that far
exceeds what would be considered a merely good or even
commendable standard of care and service; emphasizes
quality of life for the individuals served, including the demonstrated capacity for change in response to their needs and
desires; provides tangible, quantifiable benefits to persons
being served; and in operation at least two years and
ongoing. Each receives a plaque.

1859 George Card Award
American Council of the Blind
2200 Wilson Boulevard
Suite 650
Arlington, VA 22201-3354
202-467-5081
Fax: 703-465-5085; *Toll Free:* 800-424-8666
info@acb.org
www.acb.org

Kim Charlson, President
Jeff Thom, 1st Vice President
Melanie Brunson, Executive Director

To honor an outstanding blind or visually impaired person
who has made noteworthy contributions to the welfare of
his fellow blind. A certificate is awarded occasionally. Established in 1968.

Year Founded: 1961

1860 Geriatric Oral Health Care Award
American Dental Association
211 East Chicago Avenue
Chicago, IL 60611-2678
312-440-2500
Fax: 312-440-4640
affiliates@ada.org
www.ada.org

Dr. Robert M Brandjord, President

To recognize and reward those individuals and organizations who have improved the oral health care of the elderly
through innovative health care delivery projects. The award
is open to any individual or organization responsible for developing research or projects that further the understanding
of dental caries, periodontal disease, denture stomatitis, or
other oral diseases in older Americans. The entry deadline
is May 15. The first prize consists of a monetary award of
$2,500 and a plaque. A meritorious award of $500 and a
plaque may also be awarded. Awarded annually at the ADA
annual session. The award is administered by the ADA.

Year Founded: 1859

1861 Glen Bollinger Humanitarian Award
HEAR Center
301 E Del Mar Boulevard
Pasadena, CA 91101
626-796-2016
Fax: 626-796-2320
info@hearcenter.org
www.hearcenter.org

Ellen S. Simon, Executive Director
Jennifer Ryen, Director of Development
Gayl Opatrny, Audiologist

To honor civic and service minded individuals for their efforts in behalf of hearing and speech impaired individuals, and for their loyalty and support of the HEAR Center. A plaque and/or trophy are awarded periodically. Established in 1979 for Glen H Bollinger, co-founder of HEAR (and founder of Sparkletts Drinking Water Corporation, Los Angeles) in memory of his generous contributions to the welfare of others.

Year Founded: 1954

1862 Glenn Foundation Award
Gerontological Society of America
1220 L Street North West
Suite 901
Washington, DC 20005
202-842-1275
Fax: 202-842-1150
geron@geron.org
www.geron.org

James Appleby, Executive Director and CEO
Linda Krogh Harootyan, Deputy Executive Director
Chris Yoder, Senior Director, Finance and Adm

For recognition of a significant research contribution in the biology of aging. Any scientist may be nominated for original research. A monetary prize of $2,500 is awarded annually at the annual meeting.

Year Founded: 1945

1863 Group Development Awards
Hearing Loss Association of America
7910 Woodmont Avenue
Suite 1200
Bethesda, MD 20814
301-657-2248
Fax: 301-913-9413
www.hearingloss.org

Diana D. Bender, Ph.D., President
Dr. Margaret Wallhagen, Ph.D., Vice President
Anna Hall, Executive Director

To honor SHHH groups that are developing successfully at a steady pace with a goal to prepare themselves to petition for chapter charter.

1864 Harold W. McGraw, Jr. Prize in Education
McGraw-Hill Financial
1221 Avenue of the Americas
New York, NY 10020-1095
212-512-2000
Fax: 212-512-4769
www.mcgraw-hill.com

Douglas L. Peterson, President & Chief Executive Offi
Jack F. Callahan, Jr., Executive Vice President , Chief
John Berisford, Executive Vice President , Human

To recognize individuals who have made significant contributions to the advancement of knowledge through education. The prize honors individuals whose accomplishments are making a difference today, and whose programs and ideas can serve as effective models for the education of future generations of Americans. Only individuals who are presently committed to the cause of education are eligible. Institutions, boards, organizations and other groups are not. Nominees need not be professional educators, nor is eligibility limited to traditional educational achievement. Individuals may be nominated in the areas of teaching, administration, policy planning, business, government,

publishing and adult education. Each year, a Nominating Committee, consisting of leaders in the educational community across the country, submit nominations to the Board of Judges. In addition, the Board of Judges considers nominations received directly, if they meet eligibility requirements, and include references from the educational community.

Year Founded: 1899

1865 Hobart Jackson Social Responsibility Award
LeadingAge
2519 Connecticut Avenue North West
Washington, DC 20008-1520
202-783-2242
Fax: 202-783-2255
info@LeadingAge.org
www.aahsa.org

William L. (Minnix Jr, President/Chief Executive Office
Katrinka (Ka Smith Sloan, SVP /Chief Operating Officer
Cheryl Phillips, Senior Vice President of Public

To recognize significant commitment to affirmative action goals. The nominees must show commitment to social justice and equal opportunity for minorities. Members, an agency of AAHSA, and/or individuals associated with an AAHSA agency are eligible.

1866 Innovation of the Year Awards
LeadingAge
2519 Connecticut Avenue North West
Washington, DC 20008-1520
202-783-2242
Fax: 202-783-2255
info@LeadingAge.org
www.aahsa.org

William L. (Minnix Jr., President/Chief Executive Office
Katrinka (Ka Smith Sloan, SVP /Chief Operating Officer
Cheryl Phillips, Senior Vice President of Public

To recognize creative problem solving within the AAHSA membership, to encourage professionals to document, display, and share their successes in the spirit of mutual helpfulness, and to motivate others to a higher level of development and professional practice. Three AAHSA members whose innovations in their own facilities have proven beneficial receive this award each year. An abstract of an innovation may be submitted in any of the following categories: care and services to residents or clients, management operations, and community or public relations. Recognition by AAHSA and peers at the annual meeting, publication of selected innovations, and presentation of selected papers at an education session during the annual meeting are awarded.

1867 Irving Diener Award
Blinded Veterans Association
477 H Street North West
Washington, DC 20001-2694
202-371-8880
Fax: 202-371-8258; *Toll Free:* 800-669-7079
bva@bva.org
www.bva.org

Mark Cornell, National President
Robert Dale Stamper, National Vice President
Al Avina, Executive Director

To recognize veterans for outstanding service to a regional group of the Association. Blinded veterans who are members or associate members are eligible for nomination. A scroll and a $50 stipend are awarded annually. Established in 1962 in honor of the late Irving Diener, a former member of the BVA National Advisory Committee.

Year Founded: 1945

1868 Irving S Wright Award of Distinction
American Federation for Aging Research (AFAR)
55 West 39th Street
16th Floor
New York, NY 10018
212-703-9977
Fax: 212-997-0330; *Toll Free:* 888-582-2327
info@afar.org, grants@afar.org
www.afar.org

William J. Lipton, JD, LLM, CPA, Chair, Board of Directors
Harvey Jay Cohen, M.D., President
Holly M. Brown-Borg, Ph.D., Vice President

To recognize exceptional accomplishments and contributions to the field of aging research. Nominations are by invitation only. A monetary award of $500 and a plaque are awarded annually. Established in 1981 to honor Dr Irving S Wright, founder of AFAR.

Year Founded: 1981

1869 Jack Weinberg Memorial Award for Geriatric Psychiatry
American Psychiatric Association
1000 Wilson Boulevard
Suite 1825
Arlington, VA 22209-3901
703-907-7300
Fax: 703-907-1085; *Toll Free:* 888-357-7924
apa@psych.org
www.psych.org

Jeffrey A. Lieberman, M.D., President
Saul Levin, M.D., M.P.A., APA Chief Executive Officer & Me
Paul Summergrad, M.D., President-Elect

For demonstrating leadership and exemplary work in geriatric psychiatry.

1870 Jacobus tenBroek Award
National Federation of the Blind
200 East Wells Street
at Jernigan Place
Baltimore, MD 21230
410-659-9314
Fax: 410-685-5653
nfb@nfb.org
nfb.org

Mark Riccobono, President

To honor the member of the Federation who has made an outstanding contribution to the welfare of the blind. A brass plate mounted on a walnut plaque is awarded as merited. Established in 1955.

Year Founded: 1940

1871 Jean Camper Cahn Award
The National Caucus and Center on Black Aged, Inc.
1220 L Street, North West
Suite 800
Washington, DC 20005

202-637-8400
Fax: 202-347-0895
info@ncba-aged.org
users.erols.com/ncba/

Karyne Jones, President/CEO
Elias Hussein, Executive Vice President
Angela Hughes

To recognize increasing minority participation in programs and services for the aging.

1872 John H. McAulay Award
Association for Education & Rehabilitation of the
1703 N. Beauregard Street
Suite 440
Alexandria, VA 22311
703-671-4500
Fax: 703-671-6391; *Toll Free:* 877-492-2708
aerbvi.org

Lou Tutt, Executive Director
Barbara James, Director, Membership & Office Op
Ginger Croce, Senior Director, Marketing & Off

For recognition of outstanding achievement in the placement of blind persons. Nominations must be accompanied by biographical material. Awarded biennially.

1873 Keystone Award
Hearing Loss Association of America
7910 Woodmont Avenue
Suite 1200
Bethesda, MD 20814
301-657-2248
Fax: 301-913-9413
www.hearingloss.org

Diana D. Bender, Ph.D., President
Dr. Margaret Wallhagen, Ph.D., Vice President
Anna Hall, Executive Director

To recognize individuals whose contributions to the formation and development of SHHH have been outstanding.

1874 Louise B Gerrard Award
National Association of States United for Aging an
1201 15th Street NW
Suite 350
Washington, DC 20005-2842
202-898-2578
Fax: 202-898-2583
info@nasua.org
www.nasuad.org/

Gloria Lawlah, President
James Bulot, Vice President
Lora Connolly, Secretary

To recognize the meritorious contributions of individuals committed to enhancing the quality of life of rural older Americans through improvements in policy, planning, advocacy or services. Practitioners, researchers, educators, service providers, administrators or public officials at the Federal, state or local levels whose exemplary efforts reflect improvement in the lives of the rural elderly are eligible.uise B. Gerrard, former Executive Director for the West Virginia Commission on Aging, whose pioneering efforts in the development of the Aging Network have impacted the lives of millions of older Americans, especially rural older persons.

Year Founded: 1964

1875 Major General Melvin J. Maas Achievement Award
Blinded Veterans Association
477 H Street North West
Washington, DC 20001-2694
202-371-8880
Fax: 202-371-8258; *Toll Free:* 800-669-7079
bva@bva.org
www.bva.org

Mark Cornell, National President
Robert Dale Stamper, National Vice President
Al Avina, Executive Director

To recognize the achievement of outstanding service-connected blinded veterans in their adjustment to blindness, participation in community affairs, and employment. From the beginning, presentation of this award has contributed to the enhancement of a positive image of blind people and to the elimination of the concept of helplessness. A monetary award and a scroll are awarded annually. Established in 1945 and renamed in 1973 to honor General Maas, a former president of BVA, Congressman, and Chairman of the President's Committee on the Handicapped.

Year Founded: 1945

1876 Marie Haug Student Award in Gerontology
University Center on Aging and Health
10900 Euclid Avenue
Cleveland, OH 44106
216-368-2000
Fax: 216-368-6389
pxc127@case.edu
fpb.case.edu/Centers/UCAH/

Teona Griggs, M.Ed., MA, Director of Student Services, Di
Donna Hassik, BA, Admissions Coordinator, Graduate
Dedra Hanna Adams, MPA, MA, Director of Financial Aid

To recognize excellence in aging studies. Awarded annually with a monetary prize and plaque. Established in 1990.

1877 Meritorious Service Award
LeadingAge
2519 Connecticut Avenue North West
Washington, DC 20008-1520
202-783-2242
Fax: 202-783-2255
info@LeadingAge.org
www.aahsa.org

William L. (Minnix Jr., President/Chief Executive Office
Katrinka (Ka Smith Sloan, SVP /Chief Operating Officer
Cheryl Phillips, Senior Vice President of Public

To recognize significant contributions to the field of long-term care, services, and housing for the elderly. Awarded to individuals whose organizations are full members of the association, or organizations that are full members. The nominee's accomplishments must show excellence, must have provided recognizable leadership in the aging services field, and must demonstrate a commitment to the nonprofit philosophy. The nominee's contribution must be of national importance.

1878 Migel Medal for Outstanding Service to Blind Persons
American Foundation for the Blind
2 Penn Plaza
Suite 1102
New York, NY 10121

212-502-7600
Fax: 888-545-8331; *Toll Free:* 800-232-5463
afbinfo@afb.net
www.afb.org

Carl Augusto, President & Chief Executive Offi
Rick Bozeman, Finance Director, Chief Financia
Kelly Bleach, Chief Administrative Officer

To honor professionals and volunteers whose dedication and achievements have significantly improved the lives of blind and visually-impaired people. Two medals are awarded annually: one to a professional; and one to a lay person. Presently it is awarded on Foundation Day, the fourth Thursday in October, following the annual meeting of the Board of Trustees. Established in 1937.

Year Founded: 1921

1879 Mildred M. Seltzer Distinguished Service Recognition
Association for Gerontology in Higher Education
1220 L Street North West
Suite 901
Washington, DC 20005-4018
202-289-9806
Fax: 202-289-9824
aghe@aghe.org
www.aghe.org

Janet C. Frank, President
M. Angela Baker, Director
Kelly Niles-Yokum, Secretary

For recognition and thanks to colleagues who are retired or near retirement and who have given significant service to the Association. A certificate of recognition and a lifetime subscription to the Association's newsletter, the AGHExchange, are awarded. Established in 1994, and renamed in 1995 to honor Mildred M. Seltzer, a nationally known gerontologist and senior faculty member at Miami's Scripps Gerontology Center.

Year Founded: 1974

1880 Milo D. Leavitt Memorial Lecture Award
American Geriatrics Society
40 Fulton Street
18th Floor
New York, NY
212-308-1414
Fax: 212-832-8646
info.amger@americangeriatrics.org
www.americangeriatrics.org

James T. Pacala, MD, MS, AGSF, Chairman of the Board
Cathy Alessi, MD, AGSF, President
Jennie Chin Hansen, RN, MSN, FAAN, Chief Executive
Officer

Recognizing a distinguished educator in the geriatric field.

Year Founded: 1942

1881 NCSC Community Service Award/Certificateof Merit
Senior Service America, Inc.
8403 Colesville Road
Suite 1200
Silver Spring, MD 20910
301-578-8900
Fax: 301-478-8947
contact@ssa-i.org
www.seniorserviceamerica.org/

Tony Sarmiento, Executive Director
Judy Alamprese, Director of Technical Assistance
Marta James, Deputy Director

Year Founded: 1961

1882 Nathan Shock New Investigator Award
Gerontological Society of America
1220 L Street North West
Suite 901
Washington, DC 20005
202-842-1275
Fax: 202-842-1150
geron@geron.org
www.geron.org

James Appleby, Executive Director and CEO
Linda Krogh Harootyan, Deputy Executive Director
Chris Yoder, Senior Director, Finance and Adm

To recognize outstanding original research in the field of gerontology. The deadline is May 8. A monetary award of $1,500 and a certificate are presented at the Biological Sciences Section annual business meeting at the Society's annual meeting. Established in 1986 by the Biological Sciences Section.

Year Founded: 1945

1883 National Federation of the Blind Scholarship Program
National Federation of the Blind
200 East Wells Street
at Jernigan Place
Baltimore, MD 21230
410-659-9314
Fax: 410-685-5653
nfb@nfb.org
nfb.org

Mark Riccobono, President

To recognize outstanding achievement by blind scholars. Applicants must be legally blind and be pursuing or planning to pursue a full-time post secondary course of study. Awarded on the basis of academic achievement, service to the community, and financial need. The deadline for applications is March 31.

Year Founded: 1940

1884 National Media Owl Awards
Retirement Research Foundation
8765 W Higgins Road
Suite 430
Chicago, IL 60631-4170
773-714-8080
Fax: 773-714-8089
info@rrf.org
www.rrf.org/

Nathaniel P. McParland, M.D, Chair
Irene Frye, Executive Director
Julie E. Kaufman, Ph.D.,, Senior Program Officer

Year Founded: 1950

1885 National Support Awards
Self Help for Hard of Hearing People
7910 Woodmont Avenue
Suite 1200
Bethesda, MD 20814-7022

301-657-2248
Fax: 301-913-9413
www.hearingloss.org

Anne Pope, President

To recognize the chapter or group that has made significant contributions to SHHH National by undertaking special projects or events that advance SHHH National programs. Chapters or groups may apply. A plaque is awarded. Formerly known as the Founders' Day Project Award.

1886 Ned E. Freeman Excellence in Writing Award
American Council of the Blind
2200 Wilson Boulevard
Suite 650
Arlington, VA 22201-3354
202-467-5081
Fax: 703-465-5085; *Toll Free:* 800-424-8666
info@acb.org
www.acb.org

Kim Charlson, President
Jeff Thom, 1st Vice President
Melanie Brunson, Executive Director

To recognize the author of the best article written specifically for the Braille Forum. A monetary prize and a certificate are awarded annually at the Council's national convention. Established in 1971.

Year Founded: 1961

1887 Nelson Cruikshank Award
Senior Service America, Inc.
8403 Colesville Road
Suite 1200
Silver Spring, MD 20910
301-578-8900
Fax: 301-478-8947
contact@ssa-i.org
www.seniorserviceamerica.org

Tony Sarmiento, Executive Director
Judy Alamprese, Director of Technical Assistance
Maarta Ames, Deputy Director

Year Founded: 1961

1888 New Investigator Awards
American Geriatrics Society
40 Fulton Street
18th Floor
New York, NY 10038
212-308-1414
Fax: 212-832-8646
info.amger@americangeriatrics.org
www.americangeriatrics.org

James T. Pacala, MD, MS, AGSF, Chairman of the Board
Cathy Alessi, MD, AGSF, President
Jennie Chin Hansen, RN, MSN, FAAN, Chief Executive Officer

Awarded for innovative research in geriatrics.

1889 Newel Perry Award
National Federation of the Blind
200 East Wells Street
at Jernigan Place
Baltimore, MD 21230
410-659-9314
Fax: 410-685-5653

nfb@nfb.org
nfb.org

Mark Riccobono, President

To honor an individual who has made an outstanding contribution to the welfare of the blind. Members of the Federation are not eligible. A brass plate mounted on a walnut plaque is awarded as merited. Established in 1973.

Year Founded: 1940

1890 Ollie Randall Award
National Council on Aging
251 18th Street S
Suite 500
Arlington, VA 22202
571-527-3900
info@ncoa.org
www.ncoa.org

James Firman, President & CEO

To recognize an individual who has made singular and outstanding contributions toward advancing the cause of the aging in accordance with the Council's philosophy of enabling the older person to live a dignified, healthy, and productive life. A Steuben glass trophy is awarded annually. Established in 1964 to honor Ollie A. Randall, an NCOA founder.

1891 Outstanding Continuing Education Student Awards
University Professional & Continuing Education Ass
1 Dupont Circle
Suite 615
Washington, DC 20036
202-659-3130
Fax: 202-785-0374
upcea.edu/

Karen Sibley, President
Robert J. Hansen, Chief Executive Officer
William McClure, Secretary/Treasurer

To recognize adult students over the age of 25 for their noteworthy achievements in the pursuit of excellence in continuing education. Two awards are presented. All award nominees must be attending institutions that are members of the University Professional and Continuing Education Association.

Year Founded: 1915

1892 Outstanding Newsletter Recognitions
Hearing Loss Association of America
7910 Woodmont Avenue
Suite 1200
Bethesda, MD 20814
301-657-2248
Fax: 301-913-9413
www.hearingloss.org

Diana D. Bender, Ph.D., President
Dr. Margaret Wallhagen, Ph.D., Vice President
Anna Hall, Executive Director

To recognize an outstanding editor of a chapter newsletter. Chapters publishing a regular newsletter are eligible for recognition. Recognizing that a newsletter is an excellent educational tool as well as a vehicle for basic information, judges look for the following: that the publication keeps members informed of Chapter activities; that it educates its readers about issues of concern that the data are accurate;

that the product is neat and easy to read; the size of its circulation; and how often it is issued. A plaque is awarded.

1893 Outstanding Service Medallion
American Association for Adult and Continuing Educ
10111 Martin Luther King, Jr. Highway
Suite 200C
Bowie, MD 20720
301-459-6261
Fax: 301-459-6241
office@aaace.org
www.aaace.org

Steven Schmidt, President
Jim Berger, Treasurer
Cle Anderson, Association Manager

To recognize a person who has an outstanding record of service to the profession of adult and continuing education at the state, national, or international level. The nominator and nominee must be AAACE members.

1894 Paul B Beeson Career Development Awardsin Aging Research Program
American Federation for Aging Research (AFAR)
55 West 39th Street
16th Floor
New York, NY 10018
212-703-9977
Fax: 212-997-0330; *Toll Free:* 888-582-2327
info@afar.org, grants@afar.org
www.afar.org/beeson

William J. Lipton, JD, LLM, CPA, Chair, Board of Directors
Harvey Jay Cohen, M.D., President
Holly M. Brown-Borg, Ph.D., Vice President

For outstanding research in the geriatric field.

Year Founded: 1981

1895 Peter J. Salmon Award - Blind Worker of the Year
National Industries for the Blind
1310 Braddock Place
Alexandria, VA 22314-1691
703-310-0500
Fax: 703-671-9053
services@nib.org
www.nib.org

The Honorabl Krump, Esq., Chairman
Louis J. Jablonski, Jr., Vice Chairman
Kevin A. Lynch, President and Chief Executive Of

To recognize an outstanding blind worker employed in an NIB Workshop below the administrative level. Each local Workshop selects a Blind Worker of the Year and the NIB selects the national winner for the Peter J. Salmon Award. A plaque is awarded at the Annual Meeting of the General Council of Workshops for the Blind. Established in 1968 in memory of Dr. Peter J. Salmon, who was instrumental in the establishment of NIB.

Year Founded: 1938

1896 Pfizer/AGS Postdoctoral Research Awards
American Geriatrics Society
40 Fulton Street
18th Floor
New York, NY 10038

212-308-1414
Fax: 212-832-8646
info.amger@americangeriatrics.org
www.americangeriatrics.org

James T. Pacala, MD, MS, AGSF, Chairman of the Board
Cathy Alessi, MD, AGSF, President
Jennie Chin Hansen, RN, MSN, FAAN, Chief Executive
Officer

Provides physicians interested in geriatrics with research and clinical training opportunities

Year Founded: 1942

1897 President's Award for Exceptional and Innovative Leadership in Adult and Continuing Education
American Association for Adult and Continuing Educ
10111 Martin Luther King, Jr. Highway
Suite 200C
Bowie, MD 20720
301-459-6261
Fax: 301-459-6241
office@aaace.org
www.aaace.org

Steven Schmidt, President
Jim Berger, Treasurer
Cle Anderson, Association Manager

To recognize exceptional leadership to, or in support of, adult and continuing education.need not be employed directly in the field of adult or continuing education.

1898 Professional Advisory Support Award
Hearing Loss Association of America
7910 Woodmont Avenue
Suite 1200
Bethesda, MD 20814
301-657-2248
Fax: 301-913-9413
www.hearingloss.org

Diana D. Bender, Ph.D., President
Dr. Margaret Wallhagen, Ph.D., Vice President
Anna Hall, Executive Director

To honor professionals in appreciation for what they are doing or have done to support the self help movement. To acknowledge how helpful these people can be with publicity, awareness, involvment in special events and in referring people with hearing loss to SHHH. The nominees must be current SHHH National members. Established in 1996.

1899 Purpose Prize
Civic Ventures
114 Sansome Street
Suite 850
Sanfrancisco, CA 94104
415-430-0141
Fax: 415-430-0144
info@civicventures.org
www.civicventures.org/nextchapter/

Ruth A. Wooden, Chairman
Michael A. Bailin, Vice Chair
Lewis M. Feldstein, Treasurer

Presented to people over 60 who are taking on society's biggest challenges. It's for those with the passion and experience to discover new opportunities, create new programs, and make lasting change.

1900 Rebuilding Together
Rebuilding Together
1899 L Street North West
Washington, DC 20036
973-971-0100
Fax: 973-971-0826; *Toll Free:* 800-473-4229
www.rebuildingtogether.org

Brad Segal, Chairman
Mell Meredith-Frazier, Vice Chairman
Sherry Chris, Director

Nonprofit organization dedicated to revitalizing communities by refurbising homes and community buildings. Honeywell is a leading national sponsor of Rebuilding Together and by combining the hard work of Honeywell volunteers, we are helping make life better for low-income homeowners — including elderly and disabled people and single-parent families in our hometowns all around the country.

1901 Retirement Research Foundation
8765 W Higgins Road
Suite 430
Chicago, IL 60630
773-714-8080
Fax: 773-714-8089
info@rrf.org
www.rrf.org

Jeane Frye, Executive Director
Downey R. Varey, Treasurer

The Retirement Research Foundation is devoted exclusively to improving the quality of life for our nation's older adults, especially those who are vulnerable due to advanced age, economic disadvantage, or disparity related to race and ethnicity. Since it was endowed in 1978, the Foundation has awarded grants totaling nearly $200 million to support innovative service, education, research, and advocacy projects that benefit older Americans nationwide.

1902 Richard Kalish Innovative Publication Award
Gerontological Society of America
1220 L Street North West
Washington, DC 20005
202-842-1275
Fax: 202-842-1150
geron@geron.org
www.geron.org

James Appleby, Executive Director and CEO
Linda Krogh Harootyan, Deputy Executive Director
Chris Yoder, Senior Director, Finance and Adm

To recognize insightful and innovative publications on aging and life course development in the behavioral and social sciences. Publications published in the past three years and written in English are eligible. A monetary prize of $500 is awarded annually at the annual meeting. Established in honor of Dr. Richard Kalish.

Year Founded: 1945

1903 Robert B. Irwin Award
National Industries for the Blind
1310 Braddock Place
Alexandria, VA 22314-1691
703-310-0500
Fax: 703-671-9053
services@nib.org
www.nib.org

The Honorabl Krump, Esq., Chairman
Louis J. Jablonski, Jr., Vice Chairman
Kevin A. Lynch, President and Chief Executive Of

To recognize an individual for significant contributions to an area related to sheltered workshop employment for blind persons. A plaque is awarded annually at the National Sales Meeting of The General Council of Workshops for the Blind. Established in 1953 in memory of Dr. Robert B. Irwin, who pioneered and led the way for creating employment opportunities for the blind.

Year Founded: 1938

1904 Robert S. Bray Award
American Council of the Blind
2200 Wilson Boulevard
Suite 650
Arlington, VA 22201-3354
202-467-5081
Fax: 703-465-5085; *Toll Free:* 800-424-8666
info@acb.org
www.acb.org

Kim Charlson, President
Jeff Thom, 1st Vice President
Melanie Brunson, Executive Director

To recognize outstanding achievement in extending library service, access to published materials, or the improvement of communication devices and techniques for the blind. Awarded occasionally. Established in 1975.

Year Founded: 1961

1905 Robert W. Kleemeier Award
Gerontological Society of America
1220 L Street North West
Washington, DC 20005
202-842-1275
Fax: 202-842-1150
geron@geron.org
www.geron.org

James Appleby, Executive Director and CEO
Linda Krogh Harootyan, Deputy Executive Director
Chris Yoder, Senior Director, Finance and Adm

To recognize a member for outstanding research in the field of gerontology. Nominees must be fellows of the Society. The award requires a lecture at the time of the annual scientific meeting. Established in 1965 in memory of Robert W. Kleemeier, the Society's twenty-first president.

Year Founded: 1945

1906 Rubens-Alcais Challenge
International Committee of Sports for the Deaf
PO Box #3441
Frederick, MD 21705-3441
Fax: 301-620-2990
office@ciss.org
www.deaflympics.com/

Rukhledev Valery, President
Chen Kang, Vice President - World Sports
Lanesman David, Vice President - World Youth Spo

To recognize countries that have promoted exceptionally well sports for the deaf. Member countries of the CISS are eligible. Awarded biennially. Established in 1967.

1907 Special Friend of Hearing Impaired People Award
Hearing Loss Association of America
7910 Woodmont Avenue
Suite 1200
Bethesda, MD 20814
301-657-2248
Fax: 301-913-9413
www.hearingloss.org

Diana D. Bender, Ph.D., President
Dr. Margaret Wallhagen, Ph.D., Vice President
Anna Hall, Executive Director

To recognize individuals who have worked diligently over a long period of time to improve the lives and circumstances of hearing-impaired people. Recipients are usually hearing people.

1908 Spirit of SHHH Award
Hearing Loss Association of America
7910 Woodmont Avenue
Suite 1200
Bethesda, MD 20814
301-657-2248
Fax: 301-913-9413
www.hearingloss.org

Diana D. Bender, Ph.D., President
Dr. Margaret Wallhagen, Ph.D., Vice President
Anna Hall, Executive Director

To recognize individuals whose continued selfless dedication to the development of SHHH has contributed to the success of the organization.

1909 State Public Official Award for Significant Legislative Achievement
AARP
601 East Street North West
Washington, DC 20049
202-434-2277
Fax: 202-434-3443; *Toll Free:* 888-687-2277
member@aarp.org
www.aarp.org
TTY: 877-434-7598

Gail E. Aldrich, Board Chair
Carol Raphael, Board Vice Chair
Robert G. Romasco, President

To recognize a public official, active or former, who has made a significant contribution, via legislative or administrative action, to the older citizens of the state and/or the field of aging. The award is based on the recipient's efforts on a specific issue. It is not given on a partisan basis or to imply, in any manner, AARP's endorsement of the candidacy of the recipients. The award is not issued during the election season. The award bears the logo of AARP and is presented by the State Legislative Committee.

Year Founded: 1958

1910 Trustee of the Year Award
LeadingAge
2519 Connecticut Avenue North West
Washington, DC 20008-1520
202-783-2242
Fax: 202-783-2255
info@LeadingAge.org
www.aahsa.org

William L. (Minnix Jr., President/Chief Executive Office
Katrinka (Ka Smith Sloan, SVP /Chief Operating Officer
Cheryl Phillips, Senior Vice President of Public

To recognize the outstanding achievements that a volunteer trustee or director has made to an AAHA member facility during his or her tenure on the member organization's board. The nominee must demonstrate a significant contribution to the well-being of the elderly and others the organization serves, must have displayed a personal commitment to the life of the organization, must have provided outstanding leadership to the organization and the community at large, and must have fostered growth and change through understanding the environment and the need for a continum of care for the elderly. Primary consideration is given to notable acts or unusual commitment to service. service. Each recipient will receive a plaque, one night's lodging to attend the annual meeting in New Orleans and complimentary registration to the annual meeting's Governance Assembly. Established in 1985.

1911 Vernon Henley Media Award
American Council of the Blind
2200 Wilson Boulevard
Suite 650
Arlington, VA 22201-3354
202-467-5081
Fax: 703-465-5085; *Toll Free:* 800-424-8666
info@acb.org
www.acb.org

Kim Charlson, President
Jeff Thom, 1st Vice President
Melanie Brunson, Executive Director

To recognize an individual, either sighted or blind, who has created a radio, television, or print media product conveying positive and useful information concerning blind people in general and the American Council of the Blind in particular. Nominations must be submitted by May 1. A plaque is awarded annually. Established in 1989 by the ACB Board of Publications to honor Vernon Henley.

Year Founded: 1961

1912 Walter T. Ridder Award
Hearing Loss Association of America
7910 Woodmont Avenue
Suite 1200
Bethesda, MD 20814
301-657-2248
Fax: 301-913-9413
www.hearingloss.org

Diana D. Bender, Ph.D., President
Dr. Margaret Wallhagen, Ph.D., Vice President
Anna Hall, Executive Director

To recognize an individual, an organization, or a corporation that has provided outstanding support (moral, financial, or both) to SHHH, enabling the organization to achieve goals that might otherwise not have been attained. Nominations of members are made by the SHHH Executive Committee, which includes the Executive Director, the group most familiar with the overall support given on the National level. Final selection of the recipient will be made by the Executive Commitee, or by a ballot among all members of the SHHH National Board of Directors. The deadline is March 1. A plaque is awarded.

1913 Widowed Persons Service Award
AARP
601 East Street North West
Washington, DC 20049
202-434-2277
Fax: 202-434-3443; *Toll Free:* 888-687-2277
member@aarp.org
www.aarp.org
TTY: 877-434-7598

Gail E. Aldrich, Board Chair
Carol Raphael, Board Vice Chair
Robert G. Romasco, President

To recognize Widowed Persons Service programs completing five years of successful operation. The Program Department presents a certificate.

Year Founded: 1958

Continuing Education

Alabama

1914 Shepherd's Center of America
5559 NW Barry Road
P.O. Box 333
Kansas City, MO 64154
816-960-2022
Fax: 205-933-7774
scheney@shepherdcenters.org
www.shepherdcenters.org

Ann McClung, Chair
Patrick Ryan, Pharm D, Vice Chair
Carl Nuzman, Treasurer

A pioneer in the field, the nationwide network of Shepherd's Centers offer endless possibilities to live life with meaning and purpose through educational programs, volunteer caregiving services and social programs that build community connections for all. Millions of lives have changed for the better as older adults are aging with dignity in the community.

Year Founded: 1974

1915 Shepherd's Center of Bluff Park
Shepherd's Centers of America
5559 NW Barry Road
#333
Kansas City, MO 64154
816-960-2022
Fax: 205-824-0228
scheney@shepherdcenters.org
www.shepherdscenter.org

Kay Wallick, Chair
William Kirby, Vice Chair
William Farrell, Treasurer/ Finance Committee

Individual centers partner with all faiths representing the diversity of their communities. The mission is to empower older adults to use their wisdom and skills for the good of their communities. Providing health enhancement, cultural enrichment and lifelong learning opportunities.

1916 UA College of Continuing Studies
University of Alabama
624 Paul W Bryant Drive
Tuscaloosa, AL 35401
205-348-6330
Fax: 205-348-9246; *Toll Free:* 866-307-3917
uadistance@ua.edu
continuingstudies.ua.edu

Craig Edelbrock, Dean
Dixie MacNeil, Senior Associate Dean
John Sikes, Executive Director

The College of Continuing Studies provides flexible and innovative educational opportunities, technical assistance and applied research that touches lives and creates opportunities in ways that make a difference and improve our world.

Alaska

1917 UAA Continuing Education Program
University of Alaska Anchorage
3211 Providence Drive
Anchorage, AK 99508
907-786-1800
bknygard@alaska.edu
www.uaa.alaska.edu

Bonnie Nygard, Administrator

The Continuing Educations Program at the University of Alaska Anchorage offers courses for personal enrichment, and professional development and training, from non-credit and Continuing Education Unit to Workforce Credentials, summer camps for kid, and college prep courses. Programs include business, computer skills, leadership development, education, engineering, fisheries, healthcare, and outdoor leadership.

1918 University of Alaska Southeast Campus: Adult Education Program
The Learning Center
1332 Seward Avenue
Sitka, AK 99835
907-747-7700
Fax: 907-747-7737; *Toll Free:* 800-478-6653
student.info@uas.alaska.edu
www.uas.alaska.edu/sitka/index.html

Jeff Johnston, Campus Director
Kathie Etulain, Assistant Campus Director
Bonnie Elsensohn

Full range of adult education services is available for all adults in Sitka at no charge through a contract with the Alaska Department of Labor and the Southeast Regional Resource Center.

Arizona

1919 ASU Continuing Education
Arizona State University
Tempe, AZ 85281
480-965-2100
darcy.richardson@asu.edu
ce.asu.edu

Darcy Richardson, Director
Adria Roode, Business Analyst
Phil Regier, Dean, Educational Initiatives

Offering opportunies for any individual adult who wants to expand their horizons and improve themselves by participating in noncredit courses, workshops or certificate programs. Programs include: art, architecture, childhood education, business, engineering, communication and media, English Immersion, history, healthcare, law, nonprofit management, lifelong learning, sciences, technologym sustainability, and writing.

1920 Custom Training and Education: Lifelong Learning Program
Phoenix College Downtown
640 North 1st Avenue
Phoenix, AZ 85003
602-223-4000
Fax: 602-223-4040
pc-cte@phoenixcollege.edu
www.phoenixcollege.edu

Anna Solley, Ed.D., President
Renee Perry, Administrative Assistant
Alfredo Herndanez

Formerly known as by the Senior Adult Program, promoting learning across the lifespan and adults of all ages. Courses are designed to provide informational and enriching learning opportunities without the pressure of tests and grades. Some classes are offered free of charge, while others are provided for minimal fees. Other features of the program include informal discussions with an emphasis on friendship and sharing.

1921 Lifelong Learning Program
Glendale Community College
Center for Learning Building
6000 West Olive Avenue
Glendale, AZ 85302
623-845-3812
Fax: 623-845-3818
cfl@gccaz.edu
www.gccaz.edu/cfl/

Dr. Irene Kovala, President
Dawn Meyer, Department Secretary/Reading-Eng
Carmela Arnoldt

Helps adults looking to improve their reading skills.

Year Founded: 1965

1922 Nursing Continuing Education
Gateway Community College
108 N 40th Street
Phoenix, AZ 85034
602-286-8544
rebecca.zagrodzky@gatewaycc.edu
www.gatewaycc.edu

Betty A Heying-Stanley, Interim Director
Rebecca Zagrodzky, Administrative Assistant
Brenda Laufer, Administrative/Marketing Ast.

The Nursing Continuing Education program is the largest of its kind in the state of Arizona, offering an exciting and comprehensive variety of classes for credit, ranging from one day workshops to full semester courses. NCE offers refresher classes during the fall semester for RNs who have not practiced nursing for more than five years, or who have inactive licenses.

1923 Pima Community College: Adult Education Programs
Pima Community College
4905 E. Broadway Blvd.
Tucson, AZ 85709-1010
520-206-4500
Fax: 520-884-8614; *Toll Free:* 800-860-PIMA
infocenter@pima.edu
www.pima.edu/pcae/
TTY: 520-206-4530

Lee. D Lambert, Chancellor
Deborah Yoklic, Assistant Vice Chancellor
Jeffery Silvyn, College General Counsel

Offering classes to adults for basic reading, writing and math, GED high-school equivalency preparation, English for speakers of other languages and citizenship preparation.

Year Founded: 1966

1924 Rio Salado Community College: Adult Basic Education Program
Rio Salado Community College
2323 W 14th Street
Tempe, AZ 85281
480-517-8000
Fax: 480-517-8030; *Toll Free:* 800-729-1197
www.riosalado.edu/programs/abe/Pages/Adu

Dr. Chris Bustamante, Ed.D., President
Kishia Brock, M.Ed., Vice President of Student Affair
Edward Kelty, M.Ed., Vice President of Information Se

Provides free instruction in basic skills, in the subjects required for the GED, English for speakers of other languages, and in citizenship, to students 16 years of age and older. Classes are offered at sites throughout Maricopa County, and meet during convenient daytime and evening hours. Books and materials are provided for students to use in the classroom.

Year Founded: 1979

1925 Senior Adult Educational Program
Scottsdale Community College
9000 E Chaparral Road
Scottsdale, AZ 85256-2626
480-423-6000
Fax: 480-423-6695
www.scottsdalecc.edu/senior

Jan L. Gehler, Ed.D, President
Carl Couch, VP of Administrative Services
Grant Gagnon, Chief Technology Officer

Providing courses and lecture series to adults; such as Health and Wellness, Language and Communications, Politics, History, Religion and Philosophy, and Arts and Humanities, Cinema.

Year Founded: 1969

1926 University of Arizona Continuing and Professional Education
University of Arizona
1955 E Sixth Street
Room 115
Tucson, AZ 85721
520-626-5091
rtc@email.arizona.edu
ce.arizona.edu

Rebecca Cook, Director
Ariel Gilbert-Knight, Program Manager
Melinda Davila, Program Coordinator

The University of Arizona office of Continuing & Professional Education provides innovative and engaging learning experiences that transform the lives of individuals, organizations and communities in Arizona and around the world. Programs include, but are not limited to: business, information technology, healthcare, law, web and graphic design, writing and communication, and accounting.

1927 University of Phoenix Continuing Education
University of Phoenix
1625 W Fountainhead Parkway
Tempe, AZ 85282-2371
Toll Free: 844-YES-UOPX
www.phoenix.edu

Peter Cohen, President
Byron Jones, Chief Financial Officer
Raghu Krishnaiah, Chief Operating Officer

Our programs make continuing education more accessible for the adult learner. Students can take online courses from anywhere, completing course work when it is convenient for them.

1928 YMCA Older Adult Programs
YMCA of Southern Arizona
PO Box 1111
Tucson, AZ 85702
520-623-5511
Fax: 520-624-1518
info@ywcatucson.org
www.tucsonymca.org/

Dane Woll, President and CEO
Kerry Dufour, V.P. Chief Development Officer
Cathy Scheirman, Chief Financial Officer

Programs for older adults include health and fitness, swimming classes, trips and programs, social clubs, and senior centers in addition to volunteer and service learning.

Arkansas

1929 Adult Education
Arkansas State University
7648 Victory Boulevard
Newport, AR 72112
870-512-7824; *Toll Free: 800-976-1676*
martha_taussig@asun.edu
www.asun.edu

Martha Taussig, Director

The classes are designed as General Education Development GED© prep classes and skills review classes for college or career advancement. The core areas offered are reading, math and language, with computer literacy and employability skills offered as an integrated part of the curriculum. All of the classes are free and open to adults aged 18 or older. Enrollment is open entry/open exit; students may start at any time.

1930 LifeQuest of Arkansas
LifeQuest of Arkansas
600 Pleasant Valley Dr
Little Rock, AR 72227
501-225-6073
Fax: 501-225-3759
info@LifeQuestOfArkansas.org
www.lifequestofarkansas.org/

Elaine Scott, Chair
Ronald H. Winters, Ph.D., Vice Chair
Ann Leek, Executive Director

Volunteer based, nonprofit established by and for active adults. We are dedicated to enhancing life's journey through the middle and later years through life long learning and meaningful volunteerism within a community of peers.

Year Founded: 1981

1931 Shepherd's Center of Beebe
Shepherd's Centers of America
5559 NW Barry Road
#333
Kansas City, MO 64154
816-960-2022
Fax: 205-824-0228

scheney@shepherdcenters.org
www.shepherdcenters.org

Kay Wallick, Chair
William Kirby, Vice Chair
William Farrell, Treasurer/ Finance Committee

Individual centers partner with all faiths representing the diversity of their communities. The mission is to empower older adults to use their wisdom and skills for the good of their communities. Providing health enhancement, cultural enrichment and lifelong learning opportunities.

1932 Shepherd's Center of Hot Springs
Shepherd's Centers of America
5559 NW Barry Road
#333
Kansas City, MO 64154
816-960-2022
Fax: 205-824-0228
scheney@shepherdcenters.org
www.shepherdcenters.org

Kay Wallick, Chair
William Kirby, Vice Chair
William Farrell, Treasurer/ Finance Committee

Individual centers partner with all faiths representing the diversity of their communities. The mission is to empower older adults to use their wisdom and skills for the good of their communities. Providing health enhancement, cultural enrichment and lifelong learning opportunities.

1933 Shepherd's Center of North Little Rock
Shepherd's Centers of America
5559 NW Barry Road
#333
Kansas City, MO 64154
816-960-2022
Fax: 205-824-0228
scheney@shepherdcenters.org
www.shepherdcenters.org

Kay Wallick, Chair
William Kirby, Vice Chair
William Farrell, Treasurer/ Finance Committee

Individual centers partner with all faiths representing the diversity of their communities. The mission is to empower older adults to use their wisdom and skills for the good of their communities. Providing health enhancement, cultural enrichment and lifelong learning opportunities.

1934 Shepherd's Center of SW Litte Rock
Shepherd's Centers of America
5559 NW Barry Road
#333
Kansas City, MO 64154
816-960-2022
Fax: 205-824-0228
scheney@shepherdcenters.org
www.shepherdcenters.org

Kay Wallick, Chair
William Kirby, Vice Chair
William Farrell, Treasurer/ Finance Committee

Individual centers partner with all faiths representing the diversity of their communities. The mission is to empower older adults to use their wisdom and skills for the good of their communities. Providing health enhancement, cultural enrichment and lifelong learning opportunities.

California

1935 California State University at Fullerton University Extended Education
California State University
2600 Nutwood Avenue
Suite 100
Fullerton, CA 92831
657-278-2611
Fax: 714-278-2088
ueeinfo@fullerton.edu
www.csufextension.org/

Carol Creighton, Director of Extension Programs
Christine Pircher Barnes, Asst Director Student Services
Dennis Robinson

University Extended Education provides quality learning experiences that extend access to the university into the community and around the globe. We offer a wide selection of educational programs that are accessible (online or in the classroom) and scheduled at convenient times. We have programs for working professionals and businesses, international students and groups, Open University and Intersession students, retirees and youth.

1936 College Avenue Adult Centers College Avenue Baptist Church Adult Ministries (CABC)
College Avenue Baptist Church
4747 College Avenue
San Diego, CA 92115
619-582-7222
Fax: 619-582-5346
suzannelederer@cabc.org
cabc.org/weconnect/adult.php

Sam Lloyd, Overseer Chairman
Mike Harris, Senior Pastor
Lara Blouin, CABC Preschool Director & Interi

The best place to begin forming relationships with others at CABC is in our varied communities. There are Sunday Communities and Mid-Week Communities, please check what is best for your schedule.

Year Founded: 1892

1937 Community Service Program of Van Nuys
Los Angeles Valley College
5800 Fulton Avenue
Valley Glen, CA 91401
818-947-2600
Fax: 818-947-2930
www.lavc.cc.ca.us/Calendar.html

Alma Johnson-Hawkins, President

Educational and recreational programs for children to senior adults, not for academic credit. Designed for those seeking enrichment, new skills. Also have extensive summer camps, sports oriented.

1938 Continuing Education Center at RB
Continuing Education Center at Rancho Bernardo
P. O. Box 28099
San Diego, CA 92198-0099
858-487-0464
Fax: 858-487-3740
www.cecrb.org/

Barbara Crouch, President Board of Directors
Jo Driscoll, VP/Secretary Board of Directors
Jim Reading

Continuing Education Center is a program of learning and sharing for adults in the North County area.

1939 Learning in Retirement Program (LIR)
University of California at Berkeley
101 Sproul Hall
UC Berkeley Campus
Berkeley, CA 94720-1550
510-642-6000
Fax: 510-643-1460
ucbrc@berkeley.edu
www.berkeley.edu/

Nicholas B. Dirks, Chancellor
George W. Breslauer, Executive Vice Chancellor
Gibor Basri, Vice Chancellor

1940 Modesto Institute for Continued Learning
Modesto Junior College
435 College Avenue
Modesto, CA 95350
209-575-6550
Fax: 209-575-6859
mjcadmissions@mjc.edu
www.mjc.edu/

Jill Stearns, President
Brenda Thames, VP of Student Services
Susan Kincade, VP of Instruction

MICL is an institute for mature learners, offering lectures, workshops, study and discussion groups, as well as trips and social events. All classes are not-for-credit and most have no tests, attendance requirements, homework or books to buy. They are a way to keep our brains exercised and stimulated as we age.

1941 Older Adult Program
Monterey Peninsula College
980 Fremont Street
Office/Administration Building
Monterey, CA 93940
831-646-4000
Fax: 831-655-2627
kkress@mpc.edu
www.mpc.edu/academics/olderadultprogram

Kathryn Kress, Coordinator
Bernadine C. Abbott, Technical Services Librarian, In
Nancy Harray, Instructor

The Older Adult Program, popularly know as the Learning is Living Program, offers special interest classes without charge to older adults at a variety of locations throughout the Monterey Peninsula. These non-credit courses meet at convenient senior citizen centers and other easily accessible places. A wide range of courses has been specially created to meet current growth patterns of senior citizens' education requirements.

1942 Osher Lifelong Learning Institute College of Extended Studies
SDSU College of Extended Studies
5250 Campanile Drive
Suite 2503
San Diego, CA 92182
619-594-2863
Fax: 619-594-5152
osher@mail.sdsu.edu
www.ces.sdsu.edu/osher/

Joe Shapiro, Dean
Francesca Ringland, Associate Dean of Programming
Wendy Evers, Executive Director of New Initia

Join us in an atmosphere of meaningful intellectual and social engagement without the burden of career preparation or emphasis on grades; students are given the opportunity to take academically rich courses that delve into topics that encourage discussion and intellectual stimulation.

1943 Peninsula Shepherd Senior Centers
Shepherd's Centers of America
5559 NW Barry Road
#333
Kansas City, MO 64154
816-960-2022
Fax: 205-824-0228
scheney@shepherdcenters.org
www.shepherdcenters.org/

Kay Wallick, Chair
William Kirby, Vice Chair
William Farrell, Treasurer/ Finance Committee

Our mission is to build and support a nationwide network of interfaith community-based centers that provide meaning and purpose for adults throughout their mature years.

1944 Plato Society of UCLA
University of California at Los Angeles
1083 Gayley Avenue
Los Angeles, CA 90024-3401
310-825-4321
Fax: 310-794-0672
www.ucla.edu/?

Gene Block, Chancellor
Scott Waugh, Executive vice Chancellor & Prov
Carole Golberg, Vice Chancellor, Academic Person

PLATO is a dynamic community of about 400 adults who have the time and commitment to continue a lifelong pursuit of knowledge. Each member researches, participates in - and periodically leads - weekly small group discussions of topics they've chosen. PLATO is not a passive experience. Like our namesake, we learn and teach through interactive dialogue - an educational opportunity like no other.

Year Founded: 1919

1945 Renaissance Society Center for Learning in Retirement
Renaissance Society CSU, Sacramento
Adams Building, Room 106
7750 College Town Dr.
Sacramento, CA 95819-6074
916-278-7834
rensoc@csus.edu
www.csus.edu/ORG/RENSOC/

Doris Keller, President
David Abelson, Vice President
Ivy Hendy, Secretary

The Renaissance Society is a participatory Center for Lifelong Learning in which members choose to study topics proposed by their peers who coordinate the seminar. These subjects constantly evolve from the interests of the members. The goals of the Society are to provide opportunities for continued learning and to foster creative expression for members.

Year Founded: 1986; Number of Members: 2,186

1946 Sage Society
California State University Northridge
18111 Nordhoff Street
Northridge, CA 91330
818-677-1200
Fax: 818-677-7863
elders@csun.edu
www.csun.edu/

Diane F. Harrison, President
Colin Donahue, VP & CFO

The SAGE Society is a learning-in-retirement organization for retired and semi-retired seniors interested in intellectual and cultural stimulation. SAGE offers a dynamic program for individuals who desire to share learning with like-minded people. SAGE operates under the auspices of the Roland Tseng College of Extended Learning at California State University Northridge.

1947 San Diego Community College District(SDCCD)
San Diego Community College District
3375 Camino Del Rio South
San Diego, CA 92108
619-388-6500; *Toll Free: 619-388-6913*
www.sdccd.edu

Constance M. Carroll, Ph.D., Chancellor
Richard Dittbenner, Government/Public Relations
John Nunes

Earn college credit online with courses developed and taught by professors from City, Mesa and Miramar colleges. SDCCD Online offers student support services designed to make your registration, educational planning and learning as efficient and user-friendly as possible.

1948 Sixty Plus Club
California State University of Bakersfield
9001 Stockdale Highway
Bakersfield, CA 93311-1022
661-654-CSUB
Fax: 661-664-3324
www.csub.edu/

Colleen Dillaway, CSUB Public Affairs & Communicat
Irma Cervantes, CSUB Public Affairs Coordinator

The Sixty-Plus Club (60+) at California State University, Bakersfield, offers a variety of seminars - past topics have included Retirement Planning, Positive Planning, Sex After 60, and Positive Psychology.

1949 UC Berkeley Retirement Center
University of California at Berkeley
1925 Walnut Street
#1550
Berkeley, CA 94720-1550
510-642-5461
Fax: 510-643-1460
ucbrc@berkeley.edu
thecenter.berkeley.edu

Patrick Cullinane MS, Director
Summer Scanlan, Project Manager

The University of California/UC Berkeley Retirement Center is dedicated to developing programs and services that contribute to the well being and creativity of retired faculty, staff and their families and that support the UC community.

Year Founded: 1997; Number of Members: 11,000

1950 UC San Diego Extension
University of California, San Diego
9500 Gilman Drive 0176
La Jolla, CA 92093-0176
858-534-3400
Fax: 858-534-7385
olli@ucsd.edu
extension.ucsd.edu/programs/osher

Mary Lindens Walshok, Associate Vice Chancellor, Publi
Vicki Krantz, Assistant Dean for Academic Plan
henry DeVries, Assistant Dean for External Affa

UC San Diego Extension was an early pioneer in the national movement of learning in retirement. Originally
named the Institute for Continued Learning, the program
began in 1974 in response to ideas offered by a group of retirees from New York who wished to replicate the learning
in retirement program they had participated in at the New
School for Social Research.

1951 University of San Francisco: Fromm Institute
for Lifelong Learning
The Fromm Institute for Lifelong Learning -
Univer
2130 Fulton Street
San Francisco, CA 94117-1080
415-422-6805
Fax: 415-422-6535
fromm@usfca.edu
usf.usfca.edu/fromm/?

Robert Fordham, Program Director
Hanna Fromm, Executive Director
Derek Leighnor

Educational program for retired persons at the University
of San Franscisco. Program offers day-time, non-credit,
college-level courses in a wide range of academic subjects
taught by retired professors. Three eight-week sessions per
year: fall, winter and spring. Call to be placed on our
mailing list.

Colorado

1952 Front Range Community College
Front Range Community College
3645 W 112th Avenue
Westminster, CO 80031
303-404-5000
Fax: 303-466-1623
www.frontrange.edu/

Andrew Dorsey, President
Joseph Harbouk, Ed.D., Vice President, Finance & Admini
Sandy Veltri, Ph.D., Vice President of Academic and S

Located near the crossroads of Adams, Boulder, Broom-
field, and Jefferson counties at the start of the U.S. 36 technology corridor, FRCC-Westminster blends up-to-date
technology with an old-fashioned commitment to personal
attention and small class size.

1953 University of Colorado Continuing Education
University of Colorado Boulder
1505 University Avenue
178 UCB
Boulder, CO 80309
303-492-5148
Fax: 303-492-5335; *Toll Free:* 800-331-2801
ceregistration@colorado.edu

www.ce.colorado.edu
TTY: 303-492-8905

Sara Thompson, Dean

The Division of Continuing Education is dedicated to providing quality, innovative lifelong learning opportunities to
a diverse student population by extending the educational
resources of the University of Colorado Boulder.

Connecticut

1954 Hartford Consortium for Higher Education
Adult Learning Program
Hartford Consortium for Higher Education
31 Pratt Street
4th Floor
Hartford, CT 06103
860-702-3801
Fax: 860-241-1130
mestey@metrohartford.com
www.hartfordconsortium.org/

Edward Klonoski, Chair
Pamela Trotm Reid, Vice Chair
Martin Estey, Ph.D., Executive Director

Founded in 1972, the Consortium is a vehicle for the development of joint programs that serve faculty, students and
the wider community. Its programs and initiatives include
Career Beginnings, Consortium Grant Program, Cross-reg-
istration, Fifth Graders Go To College and Regional
Roundtables.

1955 Learning for a Lifetime
Fairfield University
1073 N Benson Road
Fairfield, CT 06824
203-254-4000
Fax: 203-254-4119
webmaster@fairfield.edu
www.fairfield.edu/

Elizabeth Hastings, Director, Lifetime Education
Dr. Jocelyn Boryczka, Associate Professor of Politics

Membership is open to the intellectually curious. Explore
the world of arts and humanities by auditing one or two
courses each semester at Fairfield University on a space
available basis. Members attend monthly symposia led by
distinguished faculty members and also enjoy many free
lectures offered on campus, discounts at the Quick Center
for the Arts and access to the Di-Menna Nyselious Library
to name a few of the benefits offered.

1956 Taconic Learning Center (TLC)
Taconic Learning Center
PO Box 1752
Lakeville, CT 06039-1753
860-435-2922
www.taconiclearningcenter.org/uploads/Fa

Marion Haeberle, Manager

Non-credit, tuition-free, college-level courses in a wide
ariety of disciplines - art, literature, music, opera, the sciences, history, mathematics, current events, foreign affairs,
economics, the law, government, religion, foreign languages, health and welfare, and more!

1957 University of the Third Age of Asnuntuck
Asnunutck Community College
170 Elm Street
Enfield, CT 06082
860-253-3000
Fax: 860-253-3007; *Toll Free:* 800-501-3967
www.asnuntuck.edu/courses-programs/unive

James Lombella, President
Susan Beaudoin, Executive Assistant
Joseph Bleicher, Director of Human Resources

Programs are held at Asnuntuck Community College - past events have included trips to Radio City Christmas, Platzel Brauhaus Oktoberfest, and a Victorian Festival.

Year Founded: 1969

Delaware

1958 Academy of Lifelong Learning
University of Delaware
2700 Pennsylvania Avenue
115 Arsht Hall
Newark, DE 19716
302-831-2792
Fax: 302-573-4505
academy-ll@udel.edu
www.udel.edu/

Patrick T. Harker, President of the University
Lawrence White, Vice President and General Coun
Patricia Plu Wilson, Vice President and Chief of Staf

The Academy of Lifelong Learning provides opportunities for intellectual and cultural exploration and development for men and women of retirement age. It utilizes the members' wealth of experience and talent in planning and implementing college-level educational experiences.

Year Founded: 1743

1959 UD Professional & Continuing Studies
University of Delaware
ACCESS Center
501 S College Avenue
Newark, DE 19716
302-831-8843
Fax: 302-831-2789
continuing-ed@udel.edu
www.pcs.udel.edu

Dennis Assanis, President
Alan Brangman, Executive VP & Treasurer

The University of Delaware's Division of Professional and Continuing Studies (UD PCS) provides educational opportunities for anyone seeking to begin or complete their college career, enhance their professional skills or enrich their personal life. UD PCS also provides customized training and educational services to area businesses, organizations and professional associations.

District of Columbia

1960 Division of Continuing Education
University of the District of Columbia
4200 Connecticut Ave. NW
Washington, DC 20008

202-274-5000
mhailstock@udc.edu
www.udc.edu/ce/non_credit.htm

Dr. Elaine Crider, Chair
Christopher Bell, Esq, Vice Chair
Beverly Franklin, Executive Secretary

The Division of Continuing Education extends the resources of the University of the District of Columbia to the community by providing learning experiences in the form of short, non-credit activities, designed to provide opportunities for DC area residents to enrich and revitalize professional skills, expand career advancement opportunities, and promote personal growth and development.

Year Founded: 1851

1961 Osher Lifelong Learning Institute
Osher Lifelong Learning Institute
4400 Massachusetts Avenue NW
Washington, DC 20016
202-895-4860
Fax: 202-895-4865
olli@american.edu
www.olli-dc.org/contactus.html

Phil Schwartz, Chair
Dave Palmeter, Vice Chair
Linda B. Miller, Executive Committee

The Osher Lifelong Learning Institute is an association of, by, and for people who wish to continue to study and learn. OLLI is dedicated to the proposition that learning is a lifelong process, and curiosity never retires.

Florida

1962 Academy of Senior Professionals of Eckerd (ASPEC)
Eckerd College
4200 54th Avenue S
St Petersburg, FL 33711
727-864-8834
Fax: 727-864-2964; *Toll Free:* 800-456-9009
www.eckerd.edu/aspec/

Julia Lewis, President
Ken Wolfe, Director
Tom Alexander, Board Member

From the Visual arts to the Culinary Arts, Philosophy to Bicycling, Religions and Faiths to Science and Society, Literature to Laughing Matters, ASPEC Study Groups enrich the minds, hearts and souls of its 300 plus members. Weekly Social Hours at Lewis House and monthly events at local restaurants provide ASPEC members with the opportunity to socialize with each other and strengthen the ASPEC community.

1963 Institute of New Dimensions
Palm Beach State College
4200 Congress Avenue
Lake Worth, FL 33461
561-868-3350
Fax: 561-868-3379; *Toll Free:* 866-576-7222
www.palmbeachstate.edu/

Carolyn L. Williams, Chairperson
John W. Dowd III, Vice Chairperson
Dr. Dennis P Gallon, President

Year Founded: 1933

1964 Life Enrichment Center
Life Enrichment Center Tampa
9704 N Boulevard
Tampa, FL 33612
813-932-0241
Fax: 813-933-2256
info@LECTampa.org
www.lectampa.org/

T. J. Couch, Jr.,, Chairman
James Kallaher II, Vice Chair
Ronna J Metcalf, Executive Director

Year Founded: 1980

1965 Senior Summer School
Senior Summer School
PO Box 188
Madison, WI 53701
Toll Free: 800-847-2466
info@seniorsummerschool.com
www.seniorsummerschool.com

Offers adventurous senior citizens an affordable opportunity to enhance their summer through education, leisure, and discovery, at campus locations across the US and Canada.

Year Founded: 1985

1966 Shepherd's Center of Gainesville
Shepherd's Center of Gainesville
4000 NW 53rd Avenue
Gainesville, FL 32653
352-416-3050
Fax: 352-332-0400
bbannanna@hotmail.com
www.shepherdcenters.org/scamemberdetail.

Meg Malanaphy, Chair
Anna Langford, Director

Individual centers partner with all faiths representing the diversity of their communities. The mission is to empower older adults to use their wisdom and skills for the good of their communities. Providing health enhancement, cultural enrichment and lifelong learning opportunities.

Year Founded: 1998

1967 Shepherd's Center of Orange Park
Shepherd's Center of Orange Park
2105 Park Avenue
Suite 1
Orange Park, FL 32073
904-269-5315
Fax: 904-269-5315
scoop2105@att.net
tscoop.org/

Suzanne Tower, Chair
Arden Brey, Vice Chairman
Cindy Stewart, Executive Director

Individual centers partner with all faiths representing the diversity of their communities. The mission is to empower older adults to use their wisdom and skills for the good of their communities. Providing health enhancement, cultural enrichment and lifelong learning opportunities.

Georgia

1968 Northside Shepherd's Center
Shepherd's Center
2020 Peachtree Road NW
Atlanta, GA 30309-1465
404-352-2020
webmaster@shepherd.org.
www.shepherd.org/

Gary R. Ulicny, Ph.D., President and CEO
Bob Wiseman, Executive Director

Year Founded: 1975

1969 PACE II
Arthritis Foundation
1330 W. Peachtree Street
Suite 100
Atlanta, GA 30309
404-872-7100
Fax: 404-872-0457; *Toll Free:* 800-283-7800
www.arthritis.org

Daniel T. McGowan, Chair
Rowland W. Chang, Vice Chairman
Ann M. Palmer, President and CEO

1970 Perimeter Adult Learning and Services
Perimeter Adult Learning & Services (PALS), Inc.
1548 Mount Vernon Road
Dunwoody, GA 30338
770-698-0801
Fax: 770-617-7761
admin@plasonline.org
www.palsonline.org

Rev. Ron Gilreath, Chair
Bill Berger, President
Carla Masecar, Vice President

A nonprofit, interfaith organization for persons 50 and older in Dunwoody, Sandy Springs, Norcross and neighboring areas Metropolitan Atlanta. PALS is a volunteer organization sponsored by religious and civic groups, and by businesses. At present PALS' primary offerings are the quarterly sessions of the Lunch n' Learn program.

Year Founded: 1991

1971 Quality Living Services
Quality Living Services, Inc.
PO Box 311045
4001 Danforth Rd.
Atlanta, GA 30331
404-699-1686
Fax: 404-699-1687
www.qualitylivingservices.org/

Dr. Eula Cohen, Board of Directors President
Irene M. Richardson, Executive Director

1972 Senior University
Emory University
201 Dowman Drive
Atlanta, GA 30322
404-727-6123; *Fax:* 404-727-6001
www.emory.edu/

James W. Wagner, President
Stephen D. Sencer, Senior Vice President & General
Allison Dykes, Vice President & Secretary of th

Year Founded: 1836

Idaho

1973 Idaho State Continuing Education & Workforce Training
Idaho State University
921 S 8th Avenue
Pocatello, ID 83209
208-282-3372
cetrain.isu.edu

Arthur C Vailas, President

Offers noncredit courses, workshops, and certific programs for adults seeking to further their education, develop new business skills, and advance their careers.

Illinois

1974 Lifelong Learning Institute
Parkland College
2400 W Bradley Avenue
Champaign, IL 61821
217-351-2200
Fax: 217-356-7067; *Toll Free:* 800-346-8089
www.parkland.edu/

Thomas M. Bennett, Chairman
Dana Trimble, Vice-Chairman
Linden A. Warfel, Secretary

Educational enrichment programs for retirees or those nearly retired. Travelogues, lectures, classes in the arts, history, crafts, gardening, and a wide array of other topics.

Year Founded: 1967

1975 Older Adult Institute
College of DuPage
425 Fawell Boulevard
Glen Ellyn, IL 60137
630-942-2800
Fax: 630-858-3614
www.cod.edu/

Erin Birt, Board Chairman
Kathy Hamilton, Vice Chairman
Dr. Robert L Breuder, President

Offers mature adults an opportunity to engage in intellectual discovery through lifelong learning.

Year Founded: 1967

1976 Quality Care Conference
Alzheimer's Association
225 N. Michigan Ave.
Floor 17
Chicago, IL 60601-7633
312-335-8700
Fax: 866-699-1246; *Toll Free:* 800-272-3900
info@alz.org
www.alz.org
TDD 312-335-5886

Gerald Sampson, Chair
Harry Johns, President & CEO
Maria Carrillo, VP, Medical & Scientific Affairs

Selected educational sessions from the conference discussing topics such as special care units, drug therapies, behavior management, and care strategies.

Year Founded: 1980

1977 The Continuing Education Institute of Illinois
8770 W Bryn Mawr Avenue
Suite 1300
Chicago, IL 60631
773-930-3200
info@continuingeducationpartner.com
www.continuingeducationpartner.com

Cynthia Germain, Executive Director

The Continuing Education Institute of Illinois is a non-profit organization whose mission is to provide education and training services to professionals which are accessible, client driven, cost-effective and performance measured.

Indiana

1978 Forever Learning Institute
Forever Learning Institute
54191 Ironwood Road
South Bend, IN 46635
574-282-1901
Fax: 574-282-1901
jloranger2@netzero.net
www.foreverlearninginstitute.org

Elsie Nemeth, President
Carmen Piasecki, Vice President
Joseph Burt, Director

Forever Learning Institute's mission is to improve the quality and dignity of senior adult life through continuing intellectual challenge, spiritual reflection, and social interaction.

1979 High Street UMC Older Adult Ministry
Muncie High Street Church
219 S High Street
Muncie, IN 47305
765-747-8500
Fax: 765-741-5282
info@munciehighstreet.com
www.munciehighstreet.org/ministries/olde

Charlotte B Overmyer, Reverand, Director Older Adult Ministries
Jack Hartman, Religious Leader

High Street Methodist Church has an intention ministry by, for and with the older adults. Programs open to the community include Thursday Luncheon, Update Learning (continuing education), Senior Health Insurance Program, Elder-law Counseling, and various interest groups. High Street UMC is recognized as an advocate for the elderly in the community.

1980 Milestone Continuing Education
921 E Dupont Road
Suite 812
Fort Wayne, IN 46825
Fax: 800-886-1311; *Toll Free:* 800-709-8820
info@milestonece.com
www.milestonece.com

Offers online continuing education courses specializing in physical therapy, occupational therapy, athletic trainers, massage therapy, and chiropractics.

Iowa

1981 Chautauqua Program for Senior Adults
Cornell College
600 First Street SW
Mount Vernon, IA 52314-1098
319-895-4334
Fax: 319-895-5237
cstock@cornellcollege.edu
www.cornellcollege.edu/

Jonathan Brand, President
Year Founded: 1853

Kansas

1982 Cowley County Community College
Cowley College
125 S 2nd Street
PO Box 1147
Arkansas City, KS 67005
620-442-0430
Fax: 620-441-5350
admissions@cowley.edu
www.cowley.edu/

N. Clark Williams, President
Tony Crouch, Executive Vice President of Busi
Slade Griffiths, Vice President of Academic Affai
Year Founded: 1922

1983 Kansas Cosmosphere and Space Center
Kansas Cosmosphere and Space Center
1100 North Plum
Hutchinson, KS 67501-1499
620-662-2305
Fax: 620-662-3693; *Toll Free:* 800-397-0330
dianneb@cosmo.org
www.cosmo.org

Jim Remar, President & Chief Operating Offi
Richard Hollowell, Chief Executice Officer
Dianne (Wint Blick, Director of Development

The Kansas Cosmosphere and Space Center is home to one of the world's premier space museums, with a space artifact collection second only to the Smithsonian's National Air and Space Museum. The Cosmosphere's collections include such notable artifacts as the restored Apollo 13 command module 'Odyssey' and the largest collection of Russian space artifacts outside of Moscow. There is a week-long Elderhostel Astronaut Training Program for people 55+Space Museum, the Cosmosphere has an IMAX Dome Theater, a planetarium and Dr. Goddard's Lab, a live rocket science program. The Cosmosphere is also home to the Future Astronaut Training Program for students entering 7-10 and Space Camp for Seniors - The Elderhostel Astronaut Training Program for people 55 and older.

1984 Kansas Geriatric Education Center (KS-GEC)
Genetics Education Center
Center on Aging
Kansas City, KS 66160-7177
913-588-1549
Fax: 913-588-1201
www.kumc.edu/gec

Debra Collins, M.S. CGC, Genetic Counselor

KS-GEC provides information and support for developing community-based, long-term care for rural older people.

1985 Learning Resources Network (LERN)
PO Box 9
River Falls, WI 54022
715-426-9777
Fax: 785-539-7766; *Toll Free:* 800-678-5376
TammyP@lern.org
www.lern.org

Rebel Rush, Executive Director
Tammy Peterson, Contact

Aids in the development and growth of adult learning programs. Provides speakers, technical assistance and publications.

Year Founded: 1974

1986 Life Enrichment Program of El Dorado
Butler Community College
901 S Haverhill Road
El Dorado, KS 67042
316-321-2222
Fax: 316-322-3109
www.butlercc.edu/

Ron Engelbrecht, Chair Board of Trustees
Jim Wilson, Vice Chair Board of Trustees
Dr. Kimberly Krull, President

The Life Enrichment Service is an educational, entertaining and cultural program for citizens 60 years of age and above.

Year Founded: 1927

1987 Life Enrichment Program of North Newton
Bethel College
300 E 27th Street
North Newton, KS 67117
316-283-2500
Fax: 316-284-5286; *Toll Free:* 800-522-1887
www.bethelks.edu/

Perry D. White, President
Aaron Austin, Vice President for Student Life
Victoria Adame, Adjunct Instructor of Education

Educational weekly programs for adults age 60 and over.

Year Founded: 1887

1988 Shepherd's Center of Kansas City
Shepherd's Center of Kansas City, Kansas
757 Armstrong Avenue
Kansas City, KS 66101
913-281-8908
Fax: 913-281-8910
karenh@shepherdscenterkck.org
www.shepherdscenterkck.org/

Carol Levers, President
Sandy L. Scubelek, Vice President
Melissa Bynum, Executive Director

Individual centers partner with all faiths representing the diversity of their communities. The mission is to empower older adults to use their wisdom and skills for the good of their communities. Providing health enhancement, cultural enrichment and lifelong learning opportunities.

Year Founded: 1985

1989 Tabor College
Tabor College
400 S Jefferson
Hillsboro, KS 67063
620-947-3121
Fax: 620-947-2607
admissions@tabor.edu
www.tabor.edu

Dr. Jules Glanzer, President
Brenda Hamm, Campus Visit Coordinator/ Admiss
Michael Adamyk, Circulation Supervisor

Year Founded: 1908

1990 Washburn Walkers
Washburn University
1700 SW College Avenue
Topeka, KS 66621
785-670-1010
www.washburn.edu/

William Sneed, Chair
Jennifer McGivern, Vice Chair
Jerry B. Farley, President

Year Founded: 1865

Kentucky

1991 Donovan Scholars Program
University of Kentucky
Ligon House 658 Limestone
Lexington, KY 40506-0442
859-257-2658
Fax: 859-323-4940; *Toll Free:* 866-602-5862
Teresa.Hager@uky.edu
www.research.uky.edu/aging

Mike Smith, Executive Director
Diana S. Lockridge, Program Director
Teresa Hager, Registrar

Free education for seniors aged 65 and older.

1992 United Crescent Hill Ministries
United Crescent Hill Ministries
150 South State Street
Louisville, KY 40206
502-893-0346; *Fax:* 502-893-0352
www.uchmlouky.org/

Sue Gentry, Executive Director
Kim Michael, Coordinator of Senior Citizen Pr
Karen Tyler, Coordinator of Emergency Assista

Year Founded: 1974

Louisiana

1993 Centenary College of Louisiana
Centenary College of Louisiana
2911 Centenary Boulevard
Shreveport, LA 71104
318-869-5011
Fax: 318-869-5795; *Toll Free:* 800-234-4448
www.centenary.edu/

David Rowe, President
Connie Whittington, Executive Assistant to President
Michael Hemphill, Provost & Dean of the College

Year Founded: 1825

Maine

1994 Senior Adult Growth Exchange
University of Southern Maine
PO Box 9300
Portland, ME 04104
207-780-5900
Fax: 207-780-5954; *Toll Free:* 800-800-4USM
webmaster@usm.maine.edu
usm.maine.edu/

Theodora J. Kalikow, President
Michael R. Stevenson, Ph.D., Provost & VP for Academic Affair

Year Founded: 1878

Maryland

1995 Evergreen Society
Johns Hopkins University
237 Mergenthaler Hall
3400 N Charles Street
Baltimore, MD 21218
410-516-8000
Fax: 410-516-0864
www.jhu.edu/

Ronald J. Daniels, President
Kerry A. Ates, Vice President and Chief of Staf
Glenn M. Bieler, Vice President for Communication

Year Founded: 1876

1996 Institute for Retired Persons
Salisbury University
1101 Camden Avenue
Salisbury, MD 21801
410-543-6150
Fax: 410-543-6000; *Toll Free:* 888-543-0148
jmmaise@salisbury.edu
www.salisbury.edu/irp

Dr. Janet Dudley-Eshbach, Ph.D., President
Betty Crockett, Vice President of Administration
Dr. Diane Allen, SVP of Academic Affairs & Provos

The IRP offers continuing education designed for adults aged 50 and above. The IRP offers programs to enlighten, educate and offer better understanding of our world.

Year Founded: 1925

1997 Learning is for Everyone
Anne Arundel Community College
101 College Parkway
Arnold, MD 21012-1895
410-777-2222
Fax: 410-777-2822
helpdesk@aacc.edu
www.aacc.edu/

Martha Smith, President

1998 Prince George's Community College
Prince George's Community College
301 Largo Road
Largo, MD 20774-2199
301-336-6000
Fax: 301-386-7502
crawfoca@pgcc.edu
www.pgcc.edu/

Oretha Bridgwaters-Simms, Chair
E. Michael Walls, Vice President
Dr. Charlene Dukes, President

Educational programs designed for Maryland residents, age 60 and older. Explore art, music, health, history, and more in 13-15 week sessions. $50.00 trimester for unlimited classes.

Year Founded: 1958

1999 Renaissance Institue
Notre Dame of Maryland University
4701 N Charles Street
Baltimore, MD 21210
410-435-0100
Fax: 410-435-5937
www.ndm.edu/

Patricia J. Mitchel, Chair
Brenda Jews, Vice Chair
Joan Develin Coley, Ph.D., President

Year Founded: 1847

Massachusetts

2000 Five College Learning in Retirement
Five College Learning in Retirement
Smith College
Northampton, MA 01063
413-585-3756
5clir@smith.edu
5clir.org/

Carol T Christ, President
Liz Tiley, Office Manager

Year Founded: 1988

2001 Institute for Learning in Retirement
Harvard Institute for Learning in Retirement
51 Brattle Street
Cambridge, MA 02138-3701
617-495-4072
Fax: 617-495-9176
hilr@dcemail.harvard.edu
www.dce.harvard.edu/hilr/

Hunt Lambert, Dean of the Harvard Division of
Leonie Gordon, Assistant dean and director of t

Year Founded: 1977

2002 Learning in Later Life
Springfield College
263 Alden Street
Springfield, MA 01109-3797
413-748-3000
Fax: 413-748-3787
www.spfldcol.edu/resources/office-of.../

Tina Gorman, Director

Year Founded: 1885

2003 Seniors for Lifelong Learning
Curry College
1071 Blue Hill Avenue
Milton, MA 02186
617-333-0500
Fax: 617-333-2114
www.curry.edu/

Kenneth K. Quigley, Jr., President
Nathan Adkins, Assistant Director
Lynn Abrahams, Assistant Professor

Year Founded: 1879

2004 World Education
World Education, Inc.
44 Farnsworth Street
Boston, MA 02210
617-482-9485
Fax: 617-482-0617
wei@worlded.org
www.worlded.org/

Joel H. Lamstein, President
Shirley Burchfield, Ph.D., Vice President
Gill Garb, Executive Director

Assists in the development of adult education programs. Topics include literacy, health, nutrition, agriculture, income and family planning.

Year Founded: 1951

Michigan

2005 Emeritus College
Aquinas College
1607 Robinson Road SE
Grand Rapids, MI 49506-1799
616-632-8900
Fax: 616-732-4480
webmaster@aquinas.edu
www.aquinas.edu/

Year Founded: 1886

2006 University of Michigan: Learning in Retirement
Osher Lifelong Learning Institute
2401 Plymouth Road
Suite C
Ann Arbor, MI 48105-2193
734-998-9351
Fax: 734-998-9340
GerMedOll@umich.edu
www.umich.edu

Lisa Barton, Financial Coordinator
Abbie Lawrence-Jacobson, Program Coordinator
Abha S. Wiersba, Administrative Assistant

Year Founded: 1987

Missouri

2007 OASIS Institute
Oasis
11780 Borman Drive
Suite 400
Saint Louis, MO 63146
314-862-2933
Fax: 314-862-2149
mkerz@oasisnet.org
www.oasisnet.org/

Marcia Kerz, President
Dawn Anderson, Finance & Adminstration Director
Janice Branham, Communications & Technology Dire

OASIS is a national nonprofit educational organization designed to enhance the quality of life for mature adults. Offering challenging programs in the arts, humanities, wellness, technology and volunteer service, OASIS creates opportunities for older adults to continue their personal growth and provide meaningful service to the community.

Year Founded: 1982

2008 School of Metaphysics
School of Metaphysics
Hc 1
Box 15
Windyville, MO 65783
417-345-8411
Fax: 417-345-6668
som@som.org
www.som.org/

Dr. Daniel Condron, Chairperson
Dr. Laurel Clark, President
Ivy Norris, 1st Vice President

Conducts adult metaphysical education programs, sponsors social service, charity activities and children's services. Seeks to promote the creation of world peace and human spirituality.

Year Founded: 1973

2009 Shepherd's Center of Kansas City Central
Shepherd's Center Central
5200 Oak Street
Kansas City, MO 64112
816-444-1121
Fax: 916-444-1177; *Toll Free:* 800-547-7073
jwurth@sccentral.org
www.sccentral.org

Dale Walker, President
John McDonald, Vice President
Pamela Seymour, Executive Director

Individual centers partner with all faiths representing the diversity of their communities. The mission is to empower older adults to use their wisdom and skills for the good of their communities. Providing health enhancement, cultural enrichment and lifelong learning opportunities.

2010 Shepherd's Center of Raytown
Shepherd's Center of Raytown
7900 Blue Ridge Boulevard
Kansas City, MO 64138
816-356-9000
Fax: 816-356-6526
shepherdscenterr@sbcglobal.net
www.shepherdscenterraytown.org

Kim LeSage, President
Alice Wehmhoener, Vice President
Samantha Cummings, Board Member

Providing programs and supportive services to enable adults 55 and older to remain active and indpendent for as along as possible.

Year Founded: 1990

New Jersey

2011 Florham Institute for Lifelong Learning(FILL)
Farleigh Dickinson University
285 Madison Avenue
Madison, NJ 07940

973-443-8653
Fax: 973-443-8654
cuccini@fdu.edu
www.fdu.edu

Patrick J. Zenner, Chair
Sheldon Drucker, President
Anthony Ambrosio, Trustees

Program for people who are 62 years and older who wish to attend college for credit, credit towards a degree or simply audit, both Graduate and Undergraduate classes on available space for only $250 per class. We also offer Retired Persons Institute (RPI) classes, class day trips to museums, plays, parks, etc. We offer the program as many years as you want to participate.

New Mexico

2012 Amigos del Valle
Amigos Del Valle, Inc.
1116 N Conway Avenue
Mission, TX 78572
956-581-9494
Fax: 956-581-2210
www.advrgv.org/

Isaias Aguayo, Executive Director
Year Founded: 1974

New York

2013 American ORT
ORT America
75 Maiden Lane
Floor 10
New York, NY 10038
212-505-7700
Fax: 212-674-3057; *Toll Free:* 800-519-2678
info@ortamerica.org
www.aort.org

Larry Kadis, Chair
Linda Kirschbaum, National President
Alan Klugman, National Executive Director

Provides quality technical education and training to students in the international ORT network of schools in 60 countries around the world.

Year Founded: 1921

2014 College at Sixty
Fordham University at Lincoln Center
113 W 60th Street
Room 301
New York, NY 10023
212-636-6372
Fax: 212-636-6375
www.fordham.edu/collegeat60

Isabelle Frank, Ph.D., Dean, Fordham School of Professi
Cira T. Vernazza, Associate Dean and Director

For retired and pre-retirement men and women over 50 years of age, Fordham offers a variety of non-credit seminar courses, each of which meets two hours per week over a 13-week term. Subjects include fine and performing arts, literature, theology, psychology, history, philosophy, etc. Social events, topical lectures, and an annual trip to a destination of cultural or historical interest are also offered to College at Sixty students.

Year Founded: 1973

2015 Institute for Integrative Healthcare

2331 State Route 17K
Montgomery, NY 12549
845-361-3900
Fax: 845-361-1118; Toll Free: 800-364-5722
www.integrativehealthcare.org

Doug Alexander, Faculty Member
Shari Auth, Faculty Member
William E Baisley, Faculty Member

The Institute for Integrative Healthcare Studies was founded in 1996 to provide lifelong learning resources for healthcare professionals. In our mission of offering tools and ideas for professional growth, we serve our colleagues through educational opportunities that enhance their abilities and deepen their knowledge to practice safely and ethically.

Year Founded: 1996

2016 Institute for Retired Professionals at Syracuse
University College of Syracuse University

700 University Avenue
Syracuse, NY 13244-2530
315-443-4846
Fax: 315-443-4410; Toll Free: 866-498-9378
cps@uc.syr.edu
www.suce.syr.edu/IRP

Sandra Barrett, Senior Program Administrator
Stanley (Bud Buckhout, Administrator
Chris Cofer, Executive Director

Twice each month, members meet to hear speakers and share views. Topics include political and social issues, fine arts, science, environment, community organizations. September through May. Annual membership fee of $25.00.

Year Founded: 1972

2017 Institute for Senior Education
SUNY Rockland Community College

145 College Road
Suffern, NY 10901
845-574-4700
Fax: 845-574-4476
www.sunyrockland.edu/?

Cliff L. Wood, President
Ian Newman, 1st VP/ Grievance Chair
Saeed Safaie, 2nd VP/ Secretary & Negotiation

2018 Lifelong Learning Center
Rochester Institute of Technology

1 Lomb Memorial Drive
Rochester, NY 14623-5603
585-475-2411
Fax: 585-292-7697
www.rit.edu

Rose Marie Sepos, Program Director
Sara Connor, Staff Assistant
Julie Blowers

Lifelong learning center for adults over 50.

Year Founded: 1829

2019 Mainstream Westchester Community College
Westchester Community College

75 Grasslands Road
Valhalla, NY 10595
914-606-6600
Fax: 914-785-6526
www.sunywcc.edu/continuing_ed

Joseph N Hankin MD, President
Pat D'Imperio, Vice President and Dean of Admin
Eve Larner, Vice President of External Affai

Mainstream is an innovator in exciting educational programming and career change options for mature adults.

Year Founded: 1946

2020 My Turn Program
Kingsborough Community College

2001 Oriental Boulevard
Brooklyn, NY 11235-2398
718-368-5000
www.kbcc.cuny.edu/

Dr. Stuart Suss, Interim President
Dr. David Gomez, VP for Academic Administration
Bill Keller, VP for Finance & Administration

Year Founded: 1963

2021 OASIS Rochester
c/o Monroe Community Hospital

259 Monroe Avenue
Rochester, NY 14607
585-760-5440
Fax: 585-760-5439
prisminster@hotmail.com
www.oasisnet.org/Cities/East/RochesterNY

Priscilla Minster, Executive Director
Diane Boni, Contact
Diane Boni, Contact

OASIS is a national nonprofit educational organization designed to enhance the quality of life for mature adults. Offering challenging programs in the arts, humanities, wellness, technology and volunteer service, OASIS creates opportunities for older adults to continue their personal growth and provide meaningful service to the community. OASIS is nationally sponsored by Macy's Foundation.

2022 Pace Adult Resource Center
Pace University

1 Pace Plaza
New York, NY 10038
212-346-1200; *Toll Free: 800-874-PACE*
www.pace.edu

Mark M. Besca, Chair
Stephen J. Friedman, President
Barry M. Gosin, CEO

Year Founded: 1906

2023 Professionals and Executives in Retirement
Hofstra University

250 Hofstra University
Hempstead, NY 11549
516-463-6919
Fax: 516-463-4833
www.hofstra.edu/

Janis M. Meyer, Chair
James E. Quinn, Vice Chair
Stuart Rabinowitz, President

2024 Purchase College: School of Liberal Studies & Continuing Education
State University of New York
735 Anderson Hill Road
Purchase, NY 10577
914-251-6500
conted@purchase.edu
www.purchase.edu

Judith Lewis, Program Director

Offers a variety of noncredit certificate programs for adults to advance their professional careers or pursue a passion. Programs include: appraisal studies, art management, visual art, geographic information systems, home staging, interior design, museum studies, and social media marketing.

2025 Round Table at the School of Professional Development
Stony Brook University
N-201 Social and Behavioral Sciences
Stony Brook, NY 11794
631-632-7050
Fax: 631-632-9046
spd@stonybrook.edu
www.stonybrook.edu/spd/roundtable

Kevin Law, Chair
Samuel L. Stanley Jr., MD, President
Laura West, Secretary

The Round Table, a program within the School of Professional Development, is open to all retired and semi-retired individuals who are interested in expanding their intellectual horizons in a university setting.

2026 School of Education and Human Development Lyceum
Binghamton University, State University of New Yor
4400 Vestal Parkway East
Binghamton, NY 13902
607-777-2000
Fax: 607-777-6041
info@binghamton.edu
www.binghamton.edu/

Harvey G. Stenger, President
Terrence Kane, Chief of Staff
Margaret Kelly, Director of Special Events

Explore art, music, literature, science, history, current events, health, nature and more through lectures and slides, discussions, field trips and hands-on experience; all taught by volunteer course leaders from the Lyceum membership, the community, and current and retired faculty from Binghamton University and Broome Community College. Join with like-minded classmates to explore new areas without the pressure of assignments or exams. A wide variety of courses is offered each year with two terms in the Fall, a Winter term (Cabin Fever Break) and two in the Spring. Since its founding in 1988, Lyceum has grown to over 400 members. In lyceum's first ten years 650 courses were taught by more that 300 volunteer course leaders. Membership is open to all men and women over 50 years and older.

Year Founded: 1946

2027 Studies for Mature Adults
Skidmore College
815 North Broadway
Saratoga Springs, NY 12866
518-580-5000
Fax: 518-580-5749
info@skidmore.edu
www.skidmore.edu/

Philip A. Glotzbach, President
Elizabeth Bourque, Special Assistant to the Preside
Jeanne Sisson, Board Administrator

2028 Union College Academy for Lifelong Learning
Union College Academy for Lifelong Learning (UCALL
807 Union Street
Schenectady, NY 12308
518-388-6000; *Toll Free:* 888-843-6688
damariov@union.edu
www.union.edu/offices/ucall/

Stephen C. Ainlay, President
Valerie D'Amario, Director
Terri Mueller, Administrative Assistant

Year Founded: 1988

North Carolina

2029 Bennett College
Bennett College
900 E Washington Street
Greensboro, NC 27401
336-517-2100
Fax: 336-378-0511; *Toll Free:* 800-413-5323
www.bennett.edu

Dr. Rosalind Fuse-Hall, President
Latonya Flamer, Associate VP for Business and Fi
Dr. Rolanda Burney, Chief of Staff

Bennett College is a small, private, historically Black liberal arts college for women. The College offers women and education conducive in excellence in scholarly pursuits; preparation for leadership roles in the workplace, society, and the world; and life-long learning in technologically advanced, complex global society.

Year Founded: 1873

2030 Institute for Senior Scholars
Appalachian State University
PO Box 32042
Boone, NC 28608
828-262-2000
Fax: 828-262-4992
admissions@appstate.edu
www.appstate.edu/

Michael A. Steinback, Chair
Avery B. Hall, Sr., Vice Chair
Edwin Clark, Secretary

Year-round programs/activities in a lifelong learning program.

Year Founded: 1939

2031 LIFE
Mars Hill College
PO Box 370
100 Athletic Street
Mars Hill, NC 28754
828-689-1167
Fax: 828-689-1290; Toll Free: 866-642-4468
www.mhc.edu/

J. Dixon Free, Chair
Cheryl B. Pappas, Vice Chair
Dan Lunsford, President

Year Founded: 1856

2032 North Carolina Center for Creative Retirement
The University of North Carolina at Asheville
1 University Heights
Asheville, NC 28804-8511
828-251-6140
Fax: 828-251-6803
olli@unca.edu
olliasheville.com/

Catherine Frank, OLLI at UNC Asheville Executive
Jessika Carney, OLLI at UNC Asheville Administra
Ann Cadle, OLLI at UNC Asheville Budget Off

Has the threefold purpose of promoting lifelong learning, leadership, and community service opportunities for individuals 50 and over.

Year Founded: 1987

2033 Orange County Department on Aging:
Saturday School for Senior Citizens
Durham Tecnical Community College
1637 E Lawson Street
Durham, NC 27703
919-536-7200
Fax: 919-686-3346
www.durhamtech.edu/

Hon. MaryAnn Black, Chair
John Burness, Vice Chair
Dr. William Ingram, President

Year Founded: 1961

2034 Osher Lifelong Learning Institute
Duke University
PO Box 90700

Durham, NC 27708-0700

919-684-2703
Fax: 919-681-8235
learnmore@duke.edu
www.learnmore.duke.edu/olli

Jeanne Allen, Program Coordinator, Nonprofit M
Garry Crites, Director, Osher Lifelong Learnin
Mary Ende, Business Manager

An educational program offering noncredit liberal arts courses.

2035 Shepherd's Center of Greater Winston Salem
Shepherd's Center of Greater Winston Salem
1700 Ebert Street
Winston Salem, NC 27103
336-748-0217
Fax: 336-724-6545

shepcntr@bellsouth.net
www.shepherdscenter.org/

Ron Zambor, President
Judith Bailey, Ed.D., Vice President
Sam Matthews, Executive Director

The Shepherd's Center of Greater Winston-Salem is an interfaith ministry whose mission is to support and promote successful aging through educational, service, volunteer and support opportunities for older adults.

Year Founded: 1985

2036 Shepherd's Center of Kernersville
The Shepherd's Center of Kernersville
PO Box 2044
Kernersville, NC 27285-2044
336-996-6696
Fax: 336-996-7064
www.shepctrkville.com/

Bob Hicks, President
John Stone, Jr., 1st Vice President
Ruth Woosley, Executive Director

Individual centers partner with all faiths representing the diversity of their communities. The mission is to empower older adults to use their wisdom and skills for the good of their communities. Providing health enhancement, cultural enrichment and lifelong learning opportunities.

Year Founded: 1972

Ohio

2037 EHOVE Adult Career Center
EHOVE Career Center
316 West Mason Road
Milan, OH 44846
419-499-4663
Fax: 419-499-5391; Toll Free: 866-256-9707
AdultCareers@EHOVE.net
www.ehove.net

Dale VanLerberghe, Principal
Ben Chaffee, Executive Director of Adult Educ
David Jenkins, Operations Director

Individuals concerned w/public awareness and the quality of adult vocational education. Maintains an annual meeting, forums and publications.

Year Founded: 1968

2038 OASIS Akron
Oasis Outreach Opportunity, Inc.
847 Crouse Street
Akron, OH 44306
330-715-4477
Fax: 330-335-1468
lisa.arledge@gmail.com
www.oasisakron.org/

Lisa Arledge, Executive Director
Justin Edenhofer, Creative Arts Director
Jim Wright, Program Director

OASIS is a national nonprofit educational organization designed to enhance the quality of life for mature adults. Offering challenging programs in the arts, humanities, wellness, technology and volunteer service, OASIS creates opportunities for older adults to continue their personal growth and provide meaningful service to the community. OASIS is nationally sponsored by Macy's Foundation.

Year Founded: 2006

2039 Program Sixty
Ohio State University
Student Academic Services Building
281 W. Lane Ave.
Columbus, OH 43210
614-292-8860
Fax: 614-292-0492
www.osu.edu/

Anthony Basil, PhD, Director
Trey-Tyler Harte, Assistant PR/Communications

The Ohio State University of Continuing Education (CEd) is committed to offering diverse, quality programs and services that create a desire for lifelong learning. One of those programs is Program 60, which is adminstered by CEd. Program 60 (P60) is a unique opportunity for Ohio's older citizens to take courses at the Ohio State University for free. Individuals are welcome to participate in P60 if they are residents of the state of Ohio and 60 years of age or older.

2040 Senior Scholars
Case Western Reserve University
10900 Euclid Avenue
Cleveland, OH 44106
216-368-2000
Fax: 216-368-1861
www.case.edu/

Barbara R. Snyder, University President
W.A. Bud Baeslack III, Provost & Executive Vice Preside

Academic program for men and women age 50 and older. The program is designed for those who seek college-level work and intellectual stimulation but do not want or need academic credit. Offers an intersession and three 11-week seminars each semester. All programs are faculty led. Members may participate in all or part of each semester's program.

Year Founded: 1826

Oklahoma

2041 Oklahoma School for the Blind
Oklahoma School for the Blind
3300 Gibson Street
Muskogee, OK 74403
918-781-8200
Fax: 918-781-8300; *Toll Free:* 877-229-7136
www.osb.k12.ok.us

Steve Shelton, Chair
Lynda Collins, Vice Chair
James C. Adams, Superintendent

Our school's purpose is to meet the educational needs of blind and visually impaired students who are residents of the state by providing a program to help students reach their maximum potential.

Oregon

2042 OASIS Eugene
c/o Macy's
100 Valley River Center
Eugene, OR 97401

541-342-6611
Fax: 541-342-5187
www.oasisnet.org/Cities/West/EugeneOR.as

Meghan Weber, Contact
Shirley Kirkpatrick, Volunteer Program Manager

OASIS is a national nonprofit educational organization designed to enhance the quality of life for mature adults. Offering challenging programs in the arts, humanities, wellness, technology and volunteer service, OASIS creates opportunities for older adults to continue their personal growth and provide meaningful service to the community. OASIS is nationally sponsored by Macy's Foundation.

2043 OASIS Portland
c/o Macy's
621 SW Fifth Avenue
Fourth Floor
Portland, OR 97204
503-241-3059
Fax: 503-241-3068
www.oasisnet.org/Cities/West/PortlandOR

Jeanne Foster, Contact
Jane Griffin, Program Coordinator

OASIS is a national nonprofit educational organization designed to enhance the quality of life for mature adults. Offering challenging programs in the arts, humanities, wellness, technology and volunteer service, OASIS creates opportunities for older adults to continue their personal growth and provide meaningful service to the community. OASIS is nationally sponsored by Macy's Foundation.

2044 Senior Adult Learning Center
Portland State University
PO Box 751
Portland, OR 97207
503-725-3000
Fax: 503-725-4882
www.pdx.edu/ioa/senior-adult-learning-ce

Wim Wiewel, President
Dr Arezu Movahed, Director

Tuition free University, class adult program for Oregon Seniors 65 and over and a member shiporganization for anyone who is 50 years or older.

Year Founded: 1946

2045 Senior Venture
Southern Oregon University
1250 Siskiyou Boulevard
Ashland, OR 97520
541-552-6600
Fax: 541-552-6614; *Toll Free:* 800-257-0577
www.sou.edu/

Elisabeth Zinser, President
Earl Potter, EVP/Provost

Senior Ventures is a program of educational adventures combining lively classess with recreation and travel for active, life-long learners.

Pennsylvania

2046 Center for Learning in Retirement
Delaware Valley College
700 E Butler Avenue
Doylestown, PA 18901

215-345-1500
Fax: 215-345-5277; *Toll Free:* 800-2 D-lVal
www.delval.edu/

Dr. Bashar W Hanna, Vice President for Academic Affa

Wide variety of educational classes taught by peers, in-structors, and guest speakers

Year Founded: 1896

2047 Center for Lifelong Learning
Cedar Crest College
100 College Drive
Allentown, PA 18104
610-437-4471
Fax: 610-740-3786; *Toll Free:* 800-360-1222
lifelong@cedarcrest.edu
www.cedarcrest.edu

Carmen Twill Ambar, J.D, President
Elizabeth M. Meade, Ph.D., Provost

Basic educational courses for senior citizens

Year Founded: 1867

2048 Institute for Retired Persons
Wilson College
1015 Philadelphia Avenue
Chambersburg, PA 17201
717-264-4141
Fax: 717-264-1578
admissions@wilson.edu
www.wilson.edu/

John W. Gibb, Chair
Leslie L. Durgin '69, Vice Chair
Dr. Barbara Mistick, President

College level course for senior citizens

Year Founded: 1869

2049 Northampton County Area Community College
Northampton Community College
3835 Green Pond Road
Bethlehem, PA 18020
610-861-5300
Fax: 610-861-5070
www.northampton.edu

Karl A. Stackhouse, Chair
Robert R. Fehnel, Vice Chair
Bruce M. Browne, Secretary

Northampton Community College strives to prepare members of its community with the knowledge and critical skills they need to adapt to challenges in life and employment.

Year Founded: 1967

2050 OASIS Pittsburgh
Pittsburgh OASIS
Macys 10th Floor
400 Fifth Avenue
Pittsburgh, PA 15219-1713
412-232-2020
gweisberg@oasisnet.org
www.oasisnet.org/Cities/East/PittsburghP

Gail Weisberg, Director
John Spehar, Contact
Charity Leonette, Contact

A national nonprofit educational organization that enriches the quality of life for adults 50 and older by engaging them

in a lifelong learning and service programs so that they can learn, lead and contribute to their communities. Volunteers are the key to success of OASIS. Opportunities include tutors, mentors, office staff, instructors, entertainers and more. Membership is free.

2051 School of Living
School of Living
215 Julian Woods Lane
Julian, PA 16844
814-353-0130
Fax: 814-353-0130
office@schoolofliving.org
www.schoolofliving.org

David Harper, Chair
David Nuttall, President
Karen Stupski, Executive Director

Provides philosophy based adult education, focusing on homesteading, permaculture, and community land trusts

Year Founded: 1934

Rhode Island

2052 Brown Community for Learning in Retirement
Brown University
Alumnae Hall
Box 959
Providence, RI 02912
401-863-1000
Fax: 401-863-1121
admission@brown.edu
www.brown.edu/

Christina Paxson, President
Mark S. Schlissel, Provost
Elizabeth Huidekoper, Executive Vice President for Fin

Year Founded: 1764

South Carolina

2053 Shepherd's Center of Columbia
The Shepherd's Center of Columbia
3401 Trenholm Road
Columbia, SC 29204
803-779-4449
shepherdscent626@bellsouth.net
www.shepherdcentercolumbia.org/calendar.

Dottie Boatwright, Chair
Dorcas Giles, Director
Kay Wallick

Individual centers partner with all faiths representing the diversity of their communities. The mission is to empower older adults to use their wisdom and skills for the good of their communities. Providing health enhancement, cultural enrichment and lifelong learning opportunities.

2054 Shepherd's Center of Rock Hill
Shepherd's Center of Rock Hill, Inc.
PO Box 3046
Oakland Baptist Church 1067 Oakland Ave.
Rock Hill, SC 29730
803-328-1343
Fax: 803-328-3281
rhsc@comporium.net
www.shepherdscenterrh.org

Lisa Rumford, President
Jan Angel, Board Member
Kay Lee, Secretary

Individual centers partner with all faiths representing the diversity of their communities. The mission is to empower older adults to use their wisdom and skills for the good of their communities. Providing health enhancement, cultural enrichment and lifelong learning opportunities.

Year Founded: 1986

2055 Shepherd's Center of Spartanburg
Shepherd's Center of Spartanburg
393 East Main Street
Spartanburg, SC 29302
864-585-1999
Fax: 864-597-1711
info@spartanburgshepherdcenter.org
spartanburgshepherdcenter.org/

Rosa Lewis, Chair
Brigitte Wotier, Vice Chair
Cindy Tobias, Executive Director

Individual centers partner with all faiths representing the diversity of their communities. The mission is to empower older adults to use their wisdom and skills for the good of their communities. Providing health enhancement, cultural enrichment and lifelong learning opportunities.

Year Founded: 1978

Texas

2056 Learning Activities for Mature People
The University of Texas at Austin
One University Station
PO Box 7879
Austin, TX 78712-7879
512-471-3723
Fax: 512-471-1651
www.utexas.edu/

William Powers Jr., President
Gregory L. Fenves, Executive Vice President and Pro

Learning Activities for Mature People offers 36 large group lectures, one study seminar, one member-presented lecture per each six-week term; there are three time per year (fall, winter and spring). Membership is limited to 500, and members may attend any or all of the presentations; each presentation lasts an hour.

Year Founded: 1883

2057 OASIS Houston
Houston OASIS
9990 Richmond Avenue
Suite 102
Houston, TX 77042
713-957-2968
HoustonOasis@gmail.com
www.houstonoasis.org/

Marlene Matzner, Director
Jackie Brokenbourgh, Assistant
Kay Wallick

OASIS is a national nonprofit educational organization designed to enhance the quality of life for mature adults. Offering challenging programs in the arts, humanities, wellness, technology and volunteer service, OASIS creates opportunities for older adults to continue their personal

growth and provide meaningful service to the community. OASIS is nationally sponsored by Macy's Foundation.

Year Founded: 2012

2058 OASIS San Antonio
San Antonio OASIS
PO Box 291010
San Antonio, TX 78229
210-647-2546
Fax: 210-647-2432
bschmachtenberger@oasisnet.org
www.oasisnet.org/Cities/Central/SanAnton

Brenda Schmachtenberg, Executive Director
Mike Brown, Technology Coordinator
Greg Perkins, Administrative Assistant

OASIS is a national nonprofit educational organization designed to enhance the quality of life for mature adults. Offering challenging programs in the arts, humanities, wellness, technology and volunteer service, OASIS creates opportunities for older adults to continue their personal growth and provide meaningful service to the community. OASIS is nationally sponsored by Macy's Foundation.

2059 SAVE Senior Avocational/Vocational Education
Grayson County College
6101 Grayson Drive
Highway 691
Denison, TX 75020
903-463-6030
Fax: 903-463-5284
www.grayson.edu/

Alan Scheibmeir, President
Ron DeCento, Director Continuing Education
Shelle Cassell

SAVE representatives will be on-hand to answer questions and collect ideas for additional courses that may have broad interest for the 50+ year old citizens of the area.

Year Founded: 1992

2060 Senior Citizens Educational Program
Del Mar College
101 Baldwin Boulevard
Corpus Christi, TX 78404-3897
361-698-1200
Fax: 361-698-1092; *Toll Free:* 800-652-3357
www.delmar.edu/

Brenda Garcia, Intervention Specialist
Gary Rivera, Intervention Specialist

The Senior Citizens Educational Program encourages lifetime learning for older adults. The Del Mar College offers courses to seniors 65 or older, tuition free.

Year Founded: 1935

Virginia

2061 Elderscholar
Roanoke College
221 College Lane
Salem, VA 24153
540-375-2500
Fax: 540-375-2092
admissions@roanoke.edu

roanoke.edu/
TDD 800-388-2276

Morris M. Cregger, Jr.,, Chair
Kathryn S. Harkness, Vice Chair
Michael C. Maxey, President

Elderscholar is a educational program designed for seniors to allow them the opportunity to commute to campus on a regular basis for challenging academic programs. Offerings include six-week lecture series programs and book review programs.

Year Founded: 1842

2062 Environmental Alliance for Senior Involvement
Environmental Alliance for Senior Involvement
PO Box 250
Milford, CT 06460
203-779-0024
Fax: 203-779-0025
easi@easi.org
www.easi.org

Thomas P Benjamin, President

Is the largest senior enviromental action network in the world used to coordinate seniors as volunteers within their own communities, for enviromental and other good works.

Year Founded: 1991

2063 Shepherd's Center of Richmond
The Shepherd's Center of Richmond
3111 Northside Ave
Suite 400
Richmond, VA 23228
804-355-7282
Fax: 804-355-9856
info@TSCOR.org
www.tscor.org/

Linda Frank, Executive Director
Diana Rogers, Administrative Assistant
Julie Adams-Buchanan, Personal Services Coordinator

Individual centers partner with all faiths representing the diversity of their communities. The mission is to empower older adults to use their wisdom and skills for the good of their communities. Providing health enhancement, cultural enrichment and lifelong learning opportunities.

Washington

2064 Elderwise
900 University Street
Seattle, WA 98101
206-774-6606
Fax: 206-774-6607
info@elderwise.org
www.elderwise.org

Sandy Sabersky, Founding Director & Outreach Coo
Ann Koziol, Director of Communications
Tamara Keefe, Creative Programming Director

Cultural and artistic enrichment program designed to promote healthy aging for seniors through a multi-faceted venue based on respect for the wisdom of elders. Aims to improve the quality of life of seniors in Seattle, helpingto enhance and prolong the independence of this under-served population by providing healthy food, exercise, and intellectual and creative stimulation in a respectful, non-institutional environment.

Year Founded: 1997

2065 Focus on Mature Learning
Clark College
1933 Fort Vancouver Way
Vancouver, WA 98663
360-699-6398
Fax: 360-992-2868
www.clark.edu/

Royce Pollard, Chair
Rekah Strong, Vice Chair
Robert K. Knight, President

Year Founded: 1993

2066 Office of Continuing Education
Central Washington University
Barge Hall
400 E University Way
Ellensburg, WA 98926-7433
509-963-1504
Fax: 509-963-1690
www.cwuce.org

Richard Byham, Director
Doug Lonowski, Associate Director
Barbara Baines, Program Advisor

Provides liefelong learning opportunities for you, including a wide variety of credit and non-credit courses, certificates, and degree programs.

2067 Senior Adult Education
South Seattle Community College
6000 16th Avenue SW
Seattle, WA 98106
206-934-5300
Fax: 206-764-5807; *Toll Free:* 800-833-6388
www.southseattle.edu/

Albert Shen, Chair
Courtney Gregorie, Vice Chair
Charles Sims, Chief Human Resources Officer

2068 Seniors Program Institute for Extended Learning
Institute for Extended Learning
2917 W. Fort George Wright Drive
Spokane, WA 99224-5202
509-279-6000
Fax: 509-533-3226; *Toll Free:* 800-845-3324
www.iel.spokane.edu

S James Perez PhD, Executive Vice President
Dixie L Simmons EdD, VP Learning
Adrienne J Taber

The program offers a wide variety of non-credit courses designed specifically for seniors 55 years and older at senior centers, retirement housing, churches, other public locations, and community college campuses. Tuition ranges from $5 to $33 per course, depending on the total number of hours over the quarter (11 weeks). Explore art, history,w writing, computers, fitness, foreign language and more. Cost is $5 - $33 a quarter for courses.

Wisconsin

2069 Osher for Lifelong Learning Institute at UWM
UWM/School of Continuing Education
161 W Wisconsin Ave
Suite 6000
Milwaukee, WI 53203
414-227-3200
Fax: 414-227-3168; *Toll Free:* 800-222-3623
sce@uwm.edu
sce-osher.uwm.edu

Dr. Sammis White, Interim Dean
Tammy Benford, Business Office Manager
Oni Tate, HR Assistant

A program designed for older adults who share a love for learning throughout their lifetimes. Members enjoy innovative and enriching programs in a congenial setting with others who share their interests.

Wyoming

2070 Laramie Lyceum
University of Wyoming
1000 E. University Ave.
Laramie, WY 82071
307-766-1121
Fax: 307-766-3914
www.uwyo.edu/

Richard McGinity, Interim VP
Khaled Gasem, Associate Provost
Wilma Varga, Assistant to VP

Disability Aids & Assistive Devices

Automobile

2071 Adaptive Vans for the Physically Challenged
Mobility Works
810 Moe Drive
Akron, OH 44310
Fax: 330-633-0330; Toll Free: 800-638-8267
info@mobilityworks.com; www.mobilityworks.com/

Nathan Ahrens, Care Center Director
Todd Slates, Sales Maanger

Mobility Works builds adaptive vans for the disabled and their special needs. Adaptations include lowered floors, raised roofs, wheelchair lifts, custom interiors, custom exteriors, driving systems, power transfer seats, wheelchair tie downs, wheelchair ramps, remote entry systems, and rooftop wheelchair carriers for cars.

2072 Aeroquip Wheelchair Securement System
Kinedyne Corporation
3701 Greenway Circle
Lawrence, KS 66046-5442
785-841-4000
Fax: 785-841-3668; Toll Free: 800-848-6057
www.kinedyne.com

Hugh Lawrence, Plant Manager

Wheelchair users can have adaptable, safe, easily attached securement during transportation.

Year Founded: 1973

2073 Arcola Mobility
51 Kero Road
Carlstadt, NJ 07072-2601
201-507-8500
Fax: 201-507-5372; Toll Free: 800-272-6521
info@arcolasales.com; www.arcolamobility.com

Andrew Rolfe, President
John Akerlind, Controller
Linda Lemos, Advertising/ Marketing

Arcola sells new and used accessible vehicles and adaptive driving equipment including hand controls, wheelchair lifts and securement systems. Daily, weekly and monthly vehicle rentals available. Stairway lift, porch elevators and ramps for the home sold and rented.

2074 Braun Mobility Products
The Braun Corporation
631 West 11th Street
Winamac, IN 46996
Fax: 800-946-6305; Toll Free: 800-843-5438
www.braunlift.com
TDD 574-946-4670

Ralph W. Braun, Founder

Offers wheelchair lifts for vans and mobility products. The mission of The Braun Corporation is providing access to the world. We believe we provide a valuable service to wheelchair users, scooter users, and others who need extra help to get around. By producing and supporting a wide range of automotive mobility products, we aim to fill the needs of customers with a broad spectrum of abilities and challenges.

Year Founded: 1963

2075 Care Concepts
Concepts in Care
3233 W. Peoria Ave.
Suite 120
Phoenix, AZ 85029
602-942-9430
Fax: 602-942-1941; Toll Free: 800-322-1432
conceptsincare.org/

Cheri R Sanchez, Sales Manager

Lowered floor, wheelchair accessible Chrysler or Ford Windstar minivans, featuring in-floor or fold-down ramp system, cable operated power door, electro-mechanical kneel and a wide range of adaptive equipment.

2076 Classic
Ricon
7900 Nelson Road
Panorama City, CA 91402
818-267-3000
Fax: 818-267-3001; Toll Free: 800-322-2884
sales@RiconCorp.com
www.riconcorp.com

William Baldwin, CEO

Ricon has 36 years of experience in the design manufacture and installation of wheelchair lifts and ramps for commercial paratransit, transit motorcoach and passenger rail vehicles. As a part of our strategic plan to meet the growing needs of the transit industry, Ricon is rapidly becoming a leading supplier of anti-graffiti transit windows. Operating from a modern 225,000 square foot facility located in LA, Ricon is the largest manufacturer of its kind in the world.

Year Founded: 1971

2077 DW Auto & Home Mobility Specialties
DW Auto & Home Mobility
1208 N Garth Avenue
Columbia, MO 65203
573-449-3859
Fax: 573-449-4187; Toll Free: 800-568-2271
ContactUs@DWAuto.com
www.dwauto.com

Sheila Lynch, Business Manager
Darrell Whitmarsh, President
Shawn Bright

DW Auto is known throughout the industry as a leader in service and creativity. Darrell Whitmarsh's idea of catering to each individual person, and taking the time and extra effort to do so is what makes out company so successful.

Year Founded: 1967

2078 Dual Brakes Unit
Gresham Driving Aids
30800 Wixom Road
Wixom, MI 48393
248-624-1533
Fax: 248-624-6358; Toll Free: 800-521-8930
www.greshamdrivingaids.com

David Ohrt, General Manager
Dexter Jackson, Service Manager
Craig Wigginton, Sales Consultant

Manufacturers motor vehicle parts & accessories, manufactures industrial trucks & tractors and relays and industrial controls.

2079 Foot Steering
Drive Master Company
37 Daniel Road West
Fairfield, NJ 07004
973-808-9709
Fax: 973-808-9713
sales@drive-master.com
www.drive-master.com/

Peter B. Ruprecht, President
Christina Ruprecht, Vice President
Shelby Wells

For those customers without arms or the use of them, the foot steering system is usally combined with sensitzed steering and adaptations for other dash controlls. Drive-Master understands that most items concerning foot controlled steering need to be customized according to individual needs.

Year Founded: 1952

2080 General Motors Mobility Program for Persons with Disabilities
GM Mobility
PO Box 5053
Troy, MI 48807
Toll Free: 800-323-9935
www.gm.com/services/gm_mobility
TTY: 800-833-9935

Percy N Barnevik, Chairman
Erskine B Bowles, President
John H Bryan

General Motors is committed to helping persons with disabilities equip their vehicles for easier and safer travel. Through the GM Mobility Reimbursement Program, new vehicle purchasers/lessors who install or reinstall eligible adaptive mobility equipment can receive a combination of financial assistance and the protection and convenience of OnStar. (Valid through 09/30/08)

2081 Gresham Driving Aids
Gresham Driving Aids
30800 Wixom Road
Wixom, MI 48393
248-624-1533
Fax: 248-624-6358; *Toll Free:* 800-521-8930
www.greshamdrivingaids.com

David Ohrt, General Manager
Dexter Jackson, Service Manager
Craig Wigginton, Sales Consultant

Ofers a full-service package to physically challenged individuals including lowered floors, raised roofs and doors, and high-quad driver control systems. Dealer for Braun, Ricoh, Crow River and Bruno wheelchair lifts.

2082 Horizontal Steering
Drive Master Company
37 Daniel Road West
Fairfield, NJ 07004
973-808-9709
Fax: 973-808-9713
sales@drive-master.com
www.drive-master.com/

Peter B. Ruprecht, President
Christina Ruprecht, VP
Shelby Wells

Horizontal steering system is customized to meet the needs of the high-level spinally injured and all others who experience limited arm strength and range of motion.

Year Founded: 1952

2083 Joystick Driving Control
ACE MOBILITY, LLC
9850 E. 30th Street
Indianapolis, IN 46229
317-241-2444; *Toll Free:* 877-ACE-5301
info@acemobility.us
www.acemobility.us/

Jeff Ahnafield
Joe Kabat

Electronic microprocessor controlled hydraulic system specifically designed for persons with disabilities. It allows one-handed individuals and persons with impaired dexterity or limited and strength and range of motion to drive.

2084 Lazy Days RV Center
Lazy Days RV Center
6130 Lazy Days Boulevard
Seffner, FL 33584-2968
866-531-6820
Fax: 866-246-4408; *Toll Free:* 800-306-4002
www.lazydays.com

Jack Graham, Contact
Don Wallace, President

Customized recreational vehicles for people with disabilities. Specializing in wheelchair accessible bathrooms.

Year Founded: 1976

2085 Low Effort and No Effort Braking
Drive Master Company
37 Daniel Road West
Fairfield, NJ 07004
973-808-9709
Fax: 973-808-9713
sales@drive-master.com
www.drive-master.com/

Peter B Ruprecht, President
Christina Ruprecht, Vice President
Shelby Wells

Standard factory power breaks require 20 foot-pounds of pressure to operate. Drive-Master's low-effort modification reduces the required pressure to 11 foot-pounds. The no effort modification reduces the required pressure to 7 foot pounds (these statistics will vary slightly depending upon model of car or van.

Year Founded: 1952

2086 Low Effort and No Effort Steering
Drive Master Company
37 Daniel Road West
Fairfield, NJ 07004
973-808-9709
Fax: 973-808-9713
sales@drive-master.com
www.drive-master.com/

Peter B Ruprecht, President
Christina M Ruprecht, General Manager
J Shelby Wells

Drive-Master's Reduced Effort Steering modification boxes and steering racks are availiable for all American vans and most cars with factory power steering. All factory power steering units sent to Drive-Master will be modified to low or no effort and return shipped within 24 hours. Standard factory power steering requires approximately 40 ounces of effort to operate. Drive-Master's steering modifications can reduce the effort to 20-24 ounces (low effort) or 6-8 ounces (no effort) These statistics will vary depending on model of car and tire size.

Year Founded: 1952

2087 Mac's Lift Gate
Mac's Lift Gate Inc.
2801 South Street
Long Beach, CA 90805-3751
562-634-5962
Fax: 562-529-3466; *Toll Free:* 800-795-6227
sales@macsliftgate.com
www.macsliftgate.com

Lawrence MacDonald, Owner
Richard MacDonald, President

Vertical home lifts for cars and vans, new vans, conversions, scooters, and scooter lifts.

2088 Mini-Bus and Mini-Vans
Arcola Mobility
51 Kero Road
Carlstadt, NJ 07072-2601
201-507-8500
Fax: 201-507-5372; *Toll Free:* 800-272-6521
info@ArcolaSales.com
www.arcolamobility.com

Andrew Rolfe, President
John Akerlind, Controller
Linda Lemos, Advertising/ Marketing

Offers a virtually unlimited choice of chassis size, body style, floor plan and optional features. We provide transporters for almost every use, including school buses, vans, mini-coaches, medium-duty buses and personalized vans for the disabled.

2089 Mini-Rider
Ricon
7900 Nelson Road
Panorama City, CA 91402
818-267-3000
Fax: 818-267-3001; *Toll Free:* 800-322-2884
sales@RiconCorp.com
www.riconcorp.com

William Baldwin, CEO

Ricon has 36 years of experience in the design manufacture and installation of wheelchair lifts and ramps for commercial paratransit, transit motorcoach and passenger rail vehicles.

Year Founded: 1971

2090 Monmouth Vans-Access and Mobility Equipment
Mobility Works
5105 New Jersey
RT-33
Farmingdale, NJ 07727
732-919-1444
Fax: 732-919-0256; *Toll Free:* 877-275-4907
info@monmouthvans.com
www.mobilityworks.com/

Nathan Ahrens, Care Center Director
Christine, Client Care Center Team
Beth, Client Care Center Team

Vehicle modifications for driving by and/or transport of people with disabilities. Access equipment for buildings, e.g. ramps, stair lifts, pool lifts automatic door openers, and patient transfer lifts. Authorized dealer for Pride Jazzy and Scooters.

2091 Mr. Escort Manual Wheelchair Carrier
Worldwide Mobility
720 N Golden Key St.
Suite B6
Gilbert, AZ 85233
480-497-4692
Fax: 480-497-3834; *Toll Free:* 800-848-3433
service@worlwide-mobility.com
www.worldwide-mobility.com

A wheelchair carrier which is fitted with a padlock feature for safety and security.

Year Founded: 1987

2092 Power Seat Base (6-Way)
Ricon
7900 Nelson Road
Panorama City, CA 91402
818-267-3000
Fax: 818-267-3001; *Toll Free:* 800-322-2884
sales@RiconCorp.com
www.riconcorp.com

William Baldwin, CEO

Facilitates a driver's self-transfer from a wheelchair to the driving seat and allows optimal driving positioning.

Year Founded: 1971

2093 Rampvan
BraunAbility
4100 W Piedras Street
Farmington, NM 87401-3653
505-326-4538
Fax: 505-326-4846; *Toll Free:* 800-843-5438
www.braunability.com/

Ralph W. Braun, Founder

Accessible van offering automatic door and ramps.

Year Founded: 1963

2094 Rent-A-Van-Handicapped Driver Services
Mobility Works
1255 Kennestone Circle
Suite 100
Marietta, GA 30066
404-422-9674
Fax: 404-425-9535; *Toll Free:* 877-275-4907
www.mobilityworks.com/

Nathan Ahrens, Care Center Director
Christine, Client Care Center Team
Beth, Client Care Center Team

Handicapped Driver Services is a specialzed team of adaptive equipment professionals. Our compassionate and committed workforce is dedicated to providing increased vehicular mobility and independence to individuals not fully served by the traditional automotive market. Our team provides innovative solutions and superior products to assist each client in obtaining the highest quality of life possible.

2095 Special Access Vans
Explorer Van Company
2749 N. Fox Farm Road
Warsaw, IN 46581
574-267-7666
Fax: 574-267-7571
parts@explorervan.com
www.explorervan.com

Steve Kesler, President

Explorer Van Company is a leader in the van conversion business thanks to our very basic philosophy: We deliver more, not less, than we promise.

Year Founded: 1980

2096 Superarm Lift
Handicaps, Inc.
4335 S Santa Fe Drive
Englewood, CO 80110
303-782-2062
Fax: 303-761-6811; *Toll Free:* 800-782-4335
hereinfo@handicapsinc.com
www.handicapsinc.com

Made for vans and motorhomes. No platform is necessary and no doorways are blocked by lift that is simple and safe to use.

Year Founded: 1959

2097 Tim's Trim
Tim's Trim Inc
25 Bermar Park
Rochester, NY 14624-1541
585-429-6270; *Toll Free:* 888-468-6784
Info@TimsTrim.com, TimsTrimInc@yahoo.com
www.theoptionstore.com

Tim Miller, Owner

Offers vehicle modifications, drop floors, raised tops/doors, driving equipment, touch pads, and lifts.

Year Founded: 1978

2098 Transportation Equipment for People with Disabilities
Drive Master Company
37 Daniel Road West
Fairfield, NJ 07004
973-808-9709
Fax: 973-808-9713
sales@drive-master.com
www.drive-master.com/

Peter B Ruprecht, President
Christina Ruprecht, Vice President
Shelby Wells

Wheelchair lifts and ramps, hand and foot controls, steering and braking modifications, complete van conversions, home modifications, wheelchairs and scooters and wheelchair accessible van rentals.

Year Founded: 1952

2099 Transportation Made Easier
Drive Master Company
37 Daniel Road West
Fairfield, NJ 07004

973-808-9709
Fax: 973-808-9713
sales@drive-master.com
www.drive-master.com/

Peter B Ruprecht, President
Christina Ruprecht, Vice President
Shelby Wells

Our team has over fifty years of experience designing, installing, and servicing custom vehicle mobility solutions. Drive-Master has proven itself as an industry-leader in innovative solutions with unsurpassed quality. Our stat-of-the-art production facility allows us to quickly get you on the road. Drive-Master insalls and services all major brands of mobility products. We provide warranty repair, and tune-ups on all Drive-Master installed equip

Year Founded: 1952

2100 Ultra-Lite XL Hand Control
Drive Master Company
37 Daniel Road West
Fairfield, NJ 07004
973-808-9709
Fax: 973-808-9713
sales@drive-master.com
www.drive-master.com/

Peter B Ruprecht, President
Christina Ruprecht, Vice President
Shelby Wells

Allows the driver to operate a gas and brake by hand - push for brake - pull for gas. Can be installed in nearly every vehicle.

Year Founded: 1952

2101 Wheeler's Accessible Van Rentals
Wheelers Accessible Van Rentals
6614 W Sweetwater Avenue
Glendale, AZ 85304
623-776-8830
Fax: 623-878-0501; *Toll Free:* 800-456-1371
www.wheelersvanrentals.com

Judy Jordan, Reservations Manager
Gery King, Operations Developer

Offers customized van rentals to the disabled persons allowing them freedom and independence in their travel.

Year Founded: 1989

2102 Wright-Way
United Access
175 E. Interstate 30
Garland, TX 75043
972-240-8839
Fax: 972-240-0412; *Toll Free:* 877-669-0961
marketing@unitedaccess.com
www.wrightwayinc.com
TDD 877-659-1448

Tom Wright, President
Kathy Starnes, Inside Sales
Roy Jones

Various automobile control systems that use hand, foot and steering aids for the disabled, including complete vehicle modifications.

Year Founded: 1971

Bath

2103 Adjustable Raised Toilet Seat
Maxi-Aids, Inc.
42 Executive Boulevard
Farmingdale, NY 11735
631-752-0521
Fax: 631-752-0689; *Toll Free:* 800-522-6294
sales@maxiaids.com
www.maxiaids.com
TTY: 800-281-3555

Harold Zaretsky, President

Maxi-Aids has been an established special-needs provider for over two decades. In that time, we have evolved into the world's leading provider of adaptive products, products for independent living and products designed to enhance your lifestyle simply by making your every-day tasks easier.

2104 AirLift Toileting System from Mobility
Mobility Inc.- Mobility Products & Equipment
5726 La Jolla Boulevard
Suite 104
La Jolla, CA 92037-7342
714-730-0982
Fax: 858-456-8139; *Toll Free:* 866-456-8121
www.mobilityinc.net

Steve Winston, VP Sales
Eric Proffitt, VP Marketing

The Mobility AirLift toileting system makes it easy and painless to get on and off the toilet. With or without an assistant, the AirLift absorbs the user's weight, providing gentle lowering to a sitting position and smooth lifting to a standing position.

2105 Braun Corporation
The Braun Corporation
631 West 11th Street
Winamac, IN 46996
574-946-6153
Fax: 574-946-4670; *Toll Free:* 800-THE-LIFT
www.braunlift.com

William Roth, President
Ralph W. Braun, Founder

Offers a variety of assistive devices for the bath and surrounding environment.

Year Founded: 1963

2106 Clarke Health Care Products
Clarke Health Care Products
7830 Steubenville Pike
Oakdale, PA 15071
724-695-2122
Fax: 724-695-2922; *Toll Free:* 888-347-4537
info@clarkehealthcare.com
www.clarkehealthcare.com

Gerard Clarke, Owner

Clarke Health Care Products is located in Oakdale, Pennsylvania, just seven miles west of Pittsburgh. Our location contains the corporate office and eastern warehouse. Our focus is to search the world for unique products to make your daily activities easier.

Year Founded: 1989

2107 Commode Aluminum
Maxi-Aids, Inc.
42 Executive Boulevard
Farmingdale, NY 11735
631-752-0521
Fax: 631-752-0689; *Toll Free:* 800-522-6294
sales@maxiaids.com
www.maxiaids.com
TTY: 800-281-3555

Harold Zaretsky, President

Adjustable seat height for patient comfort.

2108 Crane Plumbing/Fiat Products
Crane Plumbing
41 Cairns Road
Mansfield, OH 44904
847-864-9777
Fax: 847-864-7652; *Toll Free:* 800-442-1902
www.craneplumbing.com

Carla Lindsey, Marketing Administrator
Reid L Beidler, CEO

Crane Plumbing LLC is one of the best-known manufacturers and distributors of plumbing fixtures and specialty plumbing products in North America. The Company offers various products and product lines that comprise all aspects of bathroom fixtures from a small porcelain sink to a luxury acrylic bath. Over 2,000 employees, many with decades of experience, distribute residential and commercial plumbing fixtures that blend modern design and efficiency with enduring beauty and style.

2109 Deluxe Bath Bench with Adjustable Legs
Maxi-Aids, Inc.
42 Executive Boulevard
Farmingdale, NY 11735
631-752-0521
Fax: 631-752-0689; *Toll Free:* 800-522-6294
sales@maxiaids.com
www.maxiaids.com
TTY: 800-281-3555

Harold Zaretsky, President

Features durable back support and adjustable legs with push-button adjustment that allows for wide range of height

2110 Driving Systems
Driving Systems, Inc
16139 Runnymede Street
Van Nuys, CA 91406
818-782-6485
Fax: 818-782-6485
info@drivingsystems.com
www.drivingsystems.com

Greg Paquin, Marketing Manager
Rudolf Schinz, President
William Butt

Designer grab bars with ergonomic grip. Available in colors and custom shapes. New fold down shower seat. Support grips extend out form the wall 24inches or 30 inches. Concealed fastener and modular components for many design possibilities. Price ranges from $30.00 to $280.00.

2111 Electric Leg Bag Emptier and Tub Slide Shower Chair
R.D. Equipment, Inc.
230 Percival Drive
West Barnstable, MA 02668
508-362-7498
Fax: 508-362-7498
info@rdequipment.com
www.rdequipment.com
TTY: 508-362-7498

Richard J Dagostino, Inventor/President
Diana M Pontieri, Sales Manager

Designed for independence, this small, lightweight battery-operated valve attaches to the bottom of the leg bag. A simple flip of the switch empties the leg bag, allowing the user to take in unlimited amounts of fluids. Tub Slide Shower Chair is a complete bathroom care system, with no need of costly renovations.

Year Founded: 1987

2112 Great Big Safety Tub Mat
Maxi-Aids, Inc.
42 Executive Boulevard
Farmingdale, NY 11735
631-752-0521
Fax: 631-752-0689; *Toll Free:* 800-522-6294
sales@maxiaids.com
www.maxiaids.com
TTY: 800-281-3555

Harold Zaretsky, President

Tub mat provides security against falls in the bath and shower.

2113 Long Handled Bath Sponges
Therapro, Inc.
225 Arlington Street
Framingham, MA 01702-8723
508-872-9494
Fax: 508-875-2062; *Toll Free:* 800-257-5376
info@therapro.com
www.theraproducts.com

Karen Conrad, Owner

Plastic-handled, 18-inch bath sponge. Handle may be heated and bent for easy reach.

Year Founded: 1986

2114 Modular Wall Grab Bars
Invacare Corporation
One Invacare Way
Elyria, OH 44035-4190
440-329-6000
Fax: 877-619-7996; *Toll Free:* 800-333-6900
info@invacare.com
www.invacare.com

A Malachi Mixon III, Chairman Of The Board
Gerald B Blouch, President/ Chief Executive Offic
Robert K. Gudbranson, Senior Vice President and Chief

Engineered for strength and beauty, these bars can be assembled in various combinations to fit any bath or shower.

Year Founded: 1885

2115 Roll-In Shower
BraunAbility
627 West 11th Street
Box 310
Winamac, IN 46996
574-946-6153
Fax: 800-946-6305; *Toll Free:* 800-843-5438
www.braunability.com/

Ralph W. Braun, Founder

Designed for easy access by wheelchair users as well as elderly people.

Year Founded: 1963

2116 Snug Seat
Snug Seat Inc.
12801 E. Independence Blvd.
P.O. Box 1739
Matthews, NC 28106
704-882-0666
Fax: 704-882-0751; *Toll Free:* 800-336-7684
information@snugseat.com
www.snugseat.com

Kirk MacKenzie, President
Scott Crosswhite, Vice President
Greg Tilley, Controller

Offers a wide range of products to meet the transportation, mobility, seating and bath aid needs for people of all ages. From car seats and standers for children with special needs to versatile and wheelchairs that offer adults customized options and the freedom to go anywhere with confidence.

Year Founded: 1987

2117 Suregrip Bathtub Rail
Invacare Corporation
One Invacare Way
Elyria, OH 44035-4190
440-329-6000
Fax: 877-619-7996; *Toll Free:* 800-333-6900
info@invacare.com
www.invacare.com

A Malachi Mixon III, Chairman Of The Board
Gerald B Blouch, President/ Chief Executive Offic
Robert K. Gudbranson, Senior Vice President and Chief

Compact and versatile, the bars have a soft-touch, contoured, white vinyl gripping area for added safety.

Year Founded: 1885

2118 Talking Bathroom Scale
Independent Living Aids, LLC
137 Rano Street
Buffalo, NY 14207
516-937-1848
Fax: 516-937-3906; *Toll Free:* 800-537-2118
techsupport@independentliving.com
www.independentliving.com

Marvin Sandler, President

Talking scale that will tell your weight.

2119 Terry-Wash Mitt
Therapro, Inc.
225 Arlington Street
Framingham, MA 01702-8723
508-872-9494
Fax: 508-875-2062; *Toll Free:* 800-257-5376

info@therapro.com
www.theraproducts.com

Karen Conrad, Owner

Includes a thumb socket and a palm pocket to hold a bar of soap.

Year Founded: 1986

2120 Terry-Wash Mitt - Medium Size
Therapro, Inc.
225 Arlington Street
Framingham, MA 01702-8723
508-872-9494
Fax: 508-875-2062; Toll Free: 800-257-5376
info@therapro.com
www.theraproducts.com

Karen Conrad, Owner

Includes a thumb socket and a palm pocket to hold a bar of soap.

Year Founded: 1986

2121 Toilet Guard Rail
Maxi-Aids, Inc.
42 Executive Boulevard
Farmingdale, NY 11735
631-752-0521
Fax: 631-752-0689; Toll Free: 800-522-6294
sales@maxiaids.com
www.maxiaids.com
TTY: 800-281-3555

Harold Zaretsky, President

Made of chrome-plated, heavy gauge steel. Fits securely to the toilet for maximum sturdiness.

2122 Tri-Grip Bathtub Rail
Maxi-Aids, Inc.
42 Executive Boulevard
Farmingdale, NY 11735
631-752-0521
Fax: 631-752-0689; Toll Free: 800-522-6294
sales@maxiaids.com
www.maxiaids.com
TTY: 800-281-3555

Harold Zaretsky, President

Two gripping heights for easy bathtub entrance or exit.

2123 Tub Slide Shower Chair
R.D. Equipment, Inc.
230 Percival Drive
West Barnstable, MA 02668
508-362-7498
Fax: 508-362-7498
info@rdequipment.com
www.rdequipment.com
TTY: 508-362-7498

Richard J Dagostino, Proprietor/Inventor
Diana M Pontieri, Sales Manager

The tub slide shower chair was designed for the elderly and disabled to make any bathroom (at home or when travelling) accessible with little or no renovations. Go from the bed, over the commode, and over the bathtub for a shower using one product. No transfers in the bathroom what so ever.

Year Founded: 1987

2124 Adjustable Bed
Golden Technologies
401 Bridge Street
Old Forge, PA 18518
570-451-7477
Fax: 800-628-5165; Toll Free: 800-624-6374
pobrien@goldentech.com
www.goldentech.com

Bob Golden, President

Trouble-free gear motor, safety features, dual massage variable speed timer and more, for the ultimate sleep experience.

2125 Bye-Bye Decubiti Air Mattress Overlay
Rand-Scot, Inc.
401 Linden Center Drive
Fort Collins, CO 80524
970-484-7967
Fax: 970-484-3800; Toll Free: 800-467-7967
info@randscot.com
randscot.com/

Joel Lerich, Founder
Barbara , Founder

Originally designed for hospital beds, converts any bed into an exceptionally therapeutic flotation unit when used between the conventional mattress and pad. The complete overlay is comprised of five individually inflatable, 100 percent natural rubber, ventilated sections enclosed within separate pockets of a soft velour cover. This sectional conformation to any configuration of electric or manual beds.

Year Founded: 1980

2126 DBC-1 DU-IT Bed Control
APT Technology
236A North Main Street
Shreve, OH 44676
330-567-2001
Fax: 330-567-3073; Toll Free: 888-549-2001
www.apt-technology.com

Controls a powered hospital bed via a single switch or it can control the bed as an accessory to an environmental control system. Controls head up, head down, feet up, feet down to increase patient comfort and independence.

2127 Foam Decubitus Bed Pads
Profex Medical Products
PO Box 140188
Memphis, TN 38114
314-727-0196
Fax: 901-454-9850; Toll Free: 800-325-0196
Customercare@profexmed.com
www.profexmed.com

Convoluted foam provides extra back support and comfort for wheelchair users.

Year Founded: 1938

2128 Hard Manufacturing Company
Hard Manufacturing Company, Inc.
230 Grider Street
Buffalo, NY 14215
716-893-1800
Fax: 716-896-2579; Toll Free: 800-873-4273

hardmfg@aol.com
www.hardmfg.com

Kevin Currier, Home Care Manager
William Godin, President

Manufactures metal cribs, hospital beds, mattresses and bedsprings and wood household furniture and furnishings.

Year Founded: 1876

2129 Priva Inc.
Fiber Links Textiles, Inc.
PO Box 448
Champlain, NY 12919-0448
514-356-8881
Fax: 514-356-0055; *Toll Free:* 800-761-8881
info@fiberlinktextiles.com
www.priva-inc.com

David Horowitz, President
Natasha Pietramala, Director, HHC Division

A leading manufacturer and distributor of branded and private label programs specialized in waterproof and absorbent textiles. Currently our channels of distribution are focused on Home Health Care, Home Furnishings, Infant & Juvenile, as well as the ever growing demand for environmentally safe multi-purpose reusable bags. These channels spread across North America into the UK, Spain & Australia.

Chairs

2130 Adjustable Rigid Chair
Graham-Field Health Products, Inc.
2935 Northeast Parkway
Atlanta, GA 30360
678-291-3207
Fax: 800-726-0601; *Toll Free:* 800-347-5678
cs@grahamfield.com
www.grahamfield.com

Kenneth Spett, President & Chief Executive Offi
Lori Kirschner, Senior Vice President, HR & Admi
Alan Spett, Senior Vice President, Operation

The Champion 3000 is a fully adjustable rigid frame chair weighing only 21 pounds with a new clamping system that adjusts seat height and angle without tools.

Year Founded: 1850

2131 Evac + Chair Emergency Wheelchair
Evac + Chair Corporation
3000 Marcus Avenue
Suite #3E6
Lake Success, NY 11042-1012
516-502-4240
Fax: 516-327-8220
sales@evac-chair.com
www.evac-chair.com

David Egen, Inventor of the EVAC+CHAIR

Gravity driven evaluation chair allows one non-disabled person to smoothly glide a seated passenger down fire stairs and across landings to exit on a combination of wheels and track belts. Pivots in own width for tight landing turns. Aluminum; weight 18 pounds. Compactly stores on wall mount, 38 by 20 by 9 inches. Maximum capacity 300 pounds. Self braking features. No installation, works on all fire exit stairs.

Year Founded: 1982

2132 Golden Power Lift Chair
Golden Technologies
401 Bridge Street
Old Forge, PA 18518
570-451-7477
Fax: 800-628-5165; *Toll Free:* 800-624-6374
pobrien@goldentech.com
www.goldentech.com

Diane Golden, Owner

Comes in different heights and widths to comfortably lift the user to a standing position.

2133 Lumex Recliner
Graham-Field Health Products, Inc.
2935 Northeast Parkway
Atlanta, GA 30360
678-291-3207
Fax: 800-726-0601; *Toll Free:* 800-347-5678
cs@grahamfield.com
www.grahamfield.com

Kenneth Spett, President & Chief Executive Offi
Lori Kirschner, Senior Vice President, HR & Admi
Alan Spett, Senior Vice President, Operation

Combines therapeutic benefits of position change with attractive appearance.

Year Founded: 1850

2134 Roll Chair
Bailey Manufacturing Company
PO Box 130
Lodi, OH 44254-0130
330-948-1080
Fax: 800-224-5390; *Toll Free:* 800-321-8372
www.baileymfg.com

Larry Strimple, President

The padded roll helps maintain proper hip abduction and prevents scissoring of the legs.

Year Founded: 1956

2135 Safari Tilt
Convaid Products
2830 California Street
Torrance, CA 90503
310-618-0111
Fax: 310-618-2166; *Toll Free:* 888-CON-AID
custservice@convaid.com
www.convaid.com

Merv Watkins, President/Owner

A semi-contour seat provides positioning with 5-45 degree tilt adjustment. One step design folds compactly into a lightweight chair.

Year Founded: 1976

2136 Spatial Tilt Custom Chair
Redman Power Chair
1601 S Pantano Road
Suite 107
Tucson, AZ 85710
Fax: 520-546-5530; *Toll Free:* 800-727-6684
www.redmanpowerchair.com

Don Redman, Chief Executive Officer
Paula Redman, Chief Financial Officer
Samuel Redman, General Manager

Custom chair designed for comfort with a solid seat and back with modifications available for seat depth, height or width.

2137 Special Needs III
Baby Jogger, LLC
8575 Magellan Parkway
Suite 1000
Richmond, VA 23227
804-726-1327
Fax: 804-262-6277; *Toll Free:* 800-241-1848
customerservice@babyjogger.com
www.babyjogger.com

Phil Baechler, Founder

A baby jogger offering wheels that are designed for smooth rides on all terrains, even sand and snow. The aluminum frame supports weight up to 150 pounds.

Year Founded: 1984

2138 Transfer Bench with Back
Invacare Corporation
One Invacare Way
Elyria, OH 44035-4190
440-329-6000
Fax: 877-619-7996; *Toll Free:* 800-333-6900
info@invacare.com
www.invacare.com

A Malachi Mixon III, Chairman Of The Board
Gerald B Blouch, President/ Chief Executive Offic
Robert K. Gudbranson, Senior Vice President and Chief

This bench with air-cushioned seat sections has a full, reversible backrest for safety and comfort.

Year Founded: 1885

Communication

2139 3M Brailler
Maxi-Aids, Inc.
42 Executive Boulevard
Farmingdale, NY 11735
631-752-0521
Fax: 631-752-0689; *Toll Free:* 800-522-6294
sales@maxiaids.com
www.maxiaids.com
TTY: 800-281-3555

Harold Zaretsky, President

For visually impaired, blind and sighted persons, produces braille on 3/8 and 1/2 inch vinyl tape. The dial has braille and regular characters.

2140 3M Large Printed Labeler
Maxi-Aids, Inc.
42 Executive Boulevard
Farmingdale, NY 11735
631-752-0521
Fax: 631-752-0689; *Toll Free:* 800-522-6294
sales@maxiaids.com
www.maxiaids.com
TTY: 800-281-3555

Harold Zaretsky, President

Ideal for persons with low vision. Can also be read tactually by blind persons with a knowledge of the print alphabet.

2141 ABLEDATA
AbleData
103 West Broad Street
Suite 400
Falls Church, VA 20910-3820
703-356-8035
Fax: 703-356-8314; *Toll Free:* 800-227-0216
abledata@neweditions.net
www.abledata.com
TTY: 703-992-8313

Katherine Belknap, Project Director
David Johnson, Publications Director
Carolyn Johnson

ABLEDATA is an electronic database of assistive technology and rehabilitation equipment products for children and adults with physical, cognitive and sensory disabilities. ABLEDATA staff can perform database searches or the database can be searched on the website.

2142 ACS Wireless
ACS Services,Inc.
10 Victor Square
Scotts Valley, CA 95066-3562
831-438-3883
Fax: 508-238-6365; *Toll Free:* 877-227-7773
sales@acs.com
www.acs.com

Phil Gattey, Chief Executive Officer
Gary Woerz, Chief Financial Officer
Beverly Robinson

Maker of several different types of telephone headsets depending on individual needs.

Year Founded: 1985

2143 AIPHONE Intercom Systems
Airphone Corporation
1700 130th Avenue NE
Bellevue, WA 98005-2262
425-455-0510
Fax: 425-455-0071; *Toll Free:* 800-692-0200
tech@aiphone.com, cs@aiphone.com
www.aiphone.com

Tak Kanie, President

AIPHONE manufactures audio and video intercom systems for home or business to help the physically disabled answer doors and communicate through physical barriers, also ADA-compliant emergency call intercom stations for use in public facilities.

Year Founded: 1970

2144 Ability Research
Ability Research, Inc.
PO Box 1721
Minnetonka, MN 55345-0721
952-939-0121
Fax: 952-890-8393
ability@skypoint.com
www.skypoint.com/~ability

John Severson, Manager

Manufacturers and marketers of assistive technology equipment.

2145 Able-Phone 100
Able-Phone
354 Chatfield Avenue
Biggs, CA 95917
530-846-7466
Fax: 530-846-7466; *Toll Free:* 800-456-4979
ablephone@juno.com
www.ablephone.com/

60 voice memories and enhanced voice recognition circuitry which provides accurate voice recognition.
Able-phone is the only company that manufactures a fully adapted cordless phone. The Able-Phone Model 100 gives you complete freedom from wires.

Year Founded: 1960

2146 Able-Phone 1900
Able-Phone
354 Chatfield Avenue
Biggs, CA 95917
530-846-7466
Fax: 530-846-7466; *Toll Free:* 800-456-4979
able-phone@juno.com
www.ablephone.com/

Totally hands free. No manipulation or operation or other mechanical devices required for complete controll of the Model 1900. The phone is operated by a puff or sip into the mouthpiece.

Year Founded: 1960

2147 Able-Switch SW-1
Able-Phone
354 Chatfield Avenue
Biggs, CA 95917
530-846-7466
Fax: 530-846-7466; *Toll Free:* 800-456-4979
able-phone@juno.com
www.ablephone.com/

Touch switch.

Year Founded: 1960

2148 AbleNet
AbleNet, Inc.
2625 Patton Road
Roseville, MN 55113
651-294-2200
Fax: 651-294-2259; *Toll Free:* 800-322-0956
customerservice@ablenetinc.com
www.ablenetinc.com

Bill Sproull, Chairman of the Board
Jennifer Thalhuber, President/ Chief Executive Offic
William Mills, Strategic Planning Chair

Designs, manufactures and markets simple technology devices for people with disabilities along with digitalized voice output communication aids for beginning communicators. Switches, environmental control units and mounting systems that allow electrical and battery operated toys and appliances to be accessed through a single switch.

Year Founded: 1985

2149 Access USA
Access-USA
242 James Street
PO Drawer 160
Clayton, NY 13624

800-623-2750
Fax: 800-563-1687; *Toll Free:* 800-263-2750
info@access-usa.com, deborah@access-usa.com
www.access-usa.com/

Deborah Webster, Contact

ACCESS USA provides all types of alternate media for people with blindness or visual impairments and/or hearing impairments. Documents (of all sizes) for transcription can be accepted as hard copy, disk copy or e-mail. Formats available include braille, large-type, simultaneous braille and print, audio recordings and electronic format. Video services include open and/or closed captioning and audio description. Specialties includes braille business cards, multipurpose braille labels and more.

2150 Adaptivation
Adaptivation, Inc
2225 W 50th Street
Suite 100
Sioux Falls, SD 57105
605-335-4445
Fax: 605-335-4446; *Toll Free:* 800-723-2783
info@adaptivation.com, sales@adaptivation.com
www.adaptivation.com

Jonathan Eckrich, President

Manfuacturer and retailer of speech generating devices, switches, and environmental control units.

Year Founded: 1992

2151 Adaptive Device Locator System
Academic Software, Inc.
3504 Tates Creek Road
Lexington, KY 40517-2601
859-552-1020
Fax: 253-799-4012
asistaff@acsw.com
www.acsw.com

Dr. Warren E Lacefield, President
Penelope D Ellis, COO/Sales & Marketing Director
Sylvia B Lacefield, Graphic Artist

Academic Software, Inc. (ASI) is a small Kentucky-based educational research, development, and consulting firm completing its 21st year as a corporation headquartered in Lexington. ASI specializes in the field of assistive technology and computer access for children and adults with disabilities and for health professionals who work with people with disabilities.

2152 Akron Resources
Akron Resources, Inc.
20 La Porte Street
Arcadia, CA 91006
626-254-9005
Fax: 626-254-9266; *Toll Free:* 800-841-0884
www.arkon.com

Paul Brassard, Owner
Aaron Roth, VP, Marketing and Sales
Benjamin Arana, Sr. Account Manager

Arkon seeks to provide innovative consumer solutions designed to enhance the function and experience of complimentary products for the car and home.

Year Founded: 1988

2153 Amplified Phones
HARC Mercantile Ltd.
5413 S. Westnedge Avenue
Suite A
Portage, MI 49002
269-324-1615
Fax: 269-324-2387; *Toll Free:* 800-445-9968
info@harc.com
www.harc.com
TTY: 269-324-1615

Mike Martinson, Managing Director

Low frequency ringer, indicator light, enhances or amplifies sound, some that automatically returns to normal dial tone when phone receiver is hung up, lighted easy to read dial pad and volume control boosts incoming sound.

Year Founded: 1960

2154 Amplified Portable Phone
HARC Mercantile Ltd.
5413 S. Westnedge Avenue
Suite A
Portage, MI 49002
269-324-1615
Fax: 269-324-2387; *Toll Free:* 800-445-9968
info@harc.com
www.harc.com
TTY: 269-324-1615

Mike Martinson, Managing Director

Portable amplified phones.

Year Founded: 1960

2155 Analog Switch Pad
Academic Software, Inc.
3504 Tates Creek Road
Lexington, KY 40517-2601
859-552-1020
Fax: 253-799-4012
asistaff@acsw.com
www.acsw.com

Dr. Warren E Lacefield, President
Penelope D Ellis, COO & Sales & Marketing Director
Sylvia B Lacefiled, Graphic Artist

Academic Software, Inc. (ASI) is a small Kentucky-based educational research, development, and consulting firm completing its 21st year as a corporation headquartered in Lexington. ASI specializes in the field of assistive technology and computer access for children and adults with disabilities and for health professionals who work with people with disabilities.

2156 Answerall 100
Able-Phone
354 Chatfield Avenue
Biggs, CA 95917
530-846-7466
Fax: 530-846-7466; *Toll Free:* 800-456-4979
ablephone@juno.com
www.ablephone.com/

A Panasonic answering machine which has been modified to accept both voice and TDD phone calls for individuals who are deaf or hearing impaired.

Year Founded: 1960

2157 Arkenstone
Freedom Scientific, Inc.
11800 31st Court North
St Petersburg, FL 33716-1805
727-803-8000
Fax: 727-803-8001; *Toll Free:* 800-444-4443
Info@FreedomScientific.com
www.freedomscientific.com

John Blake, President & Chief Executive Offi
Lee Hamilton, President/CEO

Offers various models of personal ready-to-read personal computers for the disabled.

2158 Artificial Larynx
HARC Mercantile Ltd.
5413 S. Westnedge Avenue
Suite A
Portage, MI 49002
269-324-1615
Fax: 269-324-2387; *Toll Free:* 800-445-9968
info@harc.com
www.harc.com
TTY: 269-324-1615

Mike Martinson, Managing Director

For people unable to use their larynx, a hand held speaking aid that simulates the natural vibrations on voice.

Year Founded: 1960

2159 Assistive Software Products
Innovation Management Group, Inc.
179 Niblick Road
Suite 454
Paso Robles, CA 93446
818-701-1579
Fax: 818-936-0200; *Toll Free:* 800-889-0987
cs@imgpresents.com, sales@imgpresents.com
www.imgpresents.com

Jerry Hussong, VP Sales/Marketing
Kermit Komm, Owner

IMG is the publisher of The Magnifier a 2x-10x Area Magnifier software program with Cursor Tracker; My-T-Soft AT Onscreen Keyboard software program with progrmmable Macro Panels and Word prediction Completion; and Joystick-To-Mouse software that lets any gamepad or joystick run Windows just like a mouse.

Year Founded: 1995

2160 Assistive Technology
Tobii ATI, North America
333 Elm Street
Dedham, MA 02026
781-461-8200
Fax: 617-461-8213; *Toll Free:* 800-793-9227
customercare@tobiiati.com, sales@tobiiati.com
www.tobiiati.com

James Lewis, President

A premiere developer of innovative technology solutions for people with physical and learning disabilities. Breakthrough products enable people of all ages and abilities to live and learn independently. Supportive material for teachers, clinicians, and those with disabilities.

Year Founded: 2007

2161 Augmentative Communication Systems (AAC)
ZYGO-USA
31805 Temecula Parkway
Suite 162
Temecula, CA 92592
510-493-0997
Fax: 951-303-9271; *Toll Free:* 888-321-6006
support@zygo-usa.com
www.zygo-usa.com

Lawrence Weiss, President

Full range of AAC systems and assistive technology including computer-based systems and computer access programs and devices.

Year Founded: 1974

2162 BIGmack Communication Aid
AbleNet, Inc.
2625 Patton Road
Roseville, MN 55113
651-294-2200
Fax: 651-294-2259; *Toll Free:* 800-322-0956
customerservice@ablenetinc.com
www.ablenetinc.com

Bill Sproull, Chairman of the Board
Jennifer Thalhuber, President/ Chief Executive Offic
William Mills, Strategic Planning Chair

A single message communication aid, BIGmack has 20 seconds of memory and has a 5 inches diameter switch surface.

Year Founded: 1985

2163 Big Number Pocket Sized Calculator
Independent Living Aids, LLC
137 Rano Street
Buffalo, NY 14207
516-937-1848
Fax: 516-937-3906; *Toll Free:* 800-537-2118
techsupport@independentliving.com
www.independentliving.com

Marvin Sandler, President

A handy pocket size calculator with big numbers that fits easily into purse or pocket.

2164 Big Red Switch
AbleNet, Inc.
2625 Patton Road
Roseville, MN 55113
651-294-2200
Fax: 651-294-2259; *Toll Free:* 800-322-0956
customerservice@ablenetinc.com
www.ablenetinc.com

Bill Sproull, Chairman of the Board
Jennifer Thalhuber, President/ Chief Executive Offic
William Mills, Strategic Planning Chair

Five inches across the top and activates no matter where on its surface it is touched. It is made of shatterproof plastic and contains a cord storage compartment. Also available in green, yellow and blue.

Year Founded: 1985

2165 Braille Blazer Printer
Freedom Scientific, Inc.
11800 31st Court North
St Petersburg, FL 33716-1805

727-803-8000
Fax: 727-803-8001; *Toll Free:* 800-444-4443
Info@FreedomScientific.com
www.freedomscientific.com

John Blake, President & Chief Executive Offi
Lee Hamilton, President/CEO

The Braille Blazer by Blazie Engineering is a portable, durable, and inexpensive Brailee embosser. Simply connect Braille Blazer to any personal computer to quickly produce high quality Braille text and graphics. It's small size and sturdy design make it perfect for the office, in school or at home. The Braille Blazer also features a built in speech synthesizer. It's TWO machines for the price of ONE.

2166 Braille Compass
Maxi-Aids, Inc.
42 Executive Boulevard
Farmingdale, NY 11735
631-752-0521
Fax: 631-752-0689; *Toll Free:* 800-522-6294
sales@maxiaids.com
www.maxiaids.com
TTY: 800-281-3555

Harold Zaretsky, President

For the visually impaired to find directions. Graduations raised for touch orientation, north arrow, East, South and West, by Braille letters, and inter-cardinal points by dots.

2167 Braille N' Speak
Blazie Engineering
272 Field End Road
Esatcote, MS HA4 9NA
020-858- 045
Fax: 020-858- 045
www.blazie.co.uk/

A compact, portable talking device with a seven-key Braille keyboard, may be used as a talking computer terminal, a braille to print transcriber and a word processor.

2168 Braille Touch-Time Watches
Independent Living Aids, LLC
137 Rano Street
Buffalo, NY 14207
516-937-1848
Fax: 516-937-3906; *Toll Free:* 800-537-2118
techsupport@independentliving.com
www.independentliving.com

Marvin Sandler, President

White dial with black numerals and hands makes telling time possible quickly and easily for the visually impaired. $44.95-$59.95.

2169 Braille/Print Protractor
American Printing House for the Blind
1839 Frankfort Avenue
PO Box 6085
Louisville, KY 40206-0085
502-895-2405
Fax: 502-899-2274; *Toll Free:* 800-223-1839
info@aph.org
www.aph.org

Tuck Tinsley, President
Bob Brasher, VP Advisory Services & Research
Gary Mudd

This cleverly designed Braille/Print Protractor allows visually impaired users to measure angles up to 180 degrees. Bold large type numbers and braille dots mark the degrees along the half circle of the protractor. Two braille dots mark 10 degree increments, while a single braille dot marks the 5 degree increments.

Year Founded: 1858

2170 Caleworthy
GW Micro, Inc.
725 Airport North Office Park
Fort Wayne, IN 46825
260-489-3671
Fax: 260-489-2608
sales@gwmicro.com, orders@gwmicro.com,support
www.gwmicro.com

Doug Geoffray, Vice President Development
Dan Weirich, VP Sales And Marketing
Lois Baich

A pop-up calculator that may be activated anytime. It includes support for ten memories and review of 50 entries.

Year Founded: 1990

2171 Captek/Science Products
CAPTEK Science Products
1043 Lincoln Highway
Berwyn, PA 19312
610-296-2111; *Toll Free:* 800-888-7400
info@captek.net
www.scienceproducts.org

Lee Benham, Owner

We adapt equipment to voice, mainly for the state Blind Vendors programs: cash registers, legal for trade scales, coin and currency sorters/counters, machine tools.

2172 Circline Illuminated Magnifier
Dazor Manufacturing Corporation
2079 Congressional
St. Louis, MO 63146
314-652-2400
Fax: 314-652-2069; *Toll Free:* 800-345-9103
info@dazor.com
www.dazor.com

Richard Kupferer, Marketing Coordinator
Mark Hogrebe, President
Henry Dazey, Founder

Provides even, shadow free light under the magnifying lens with a 22-watt circline fluorescent. The magnifier is mounted on a 'floating arm' that allows you to position the light source and lens with the touch of a finger.

Year Founded: 1938

2173 Clarity
4289 Bonny Oaks Drive
Suite 106
Chattanooga, TN 37406-1600
423-622-7793
Fax: 800-325-8871; *Toll Free:* 800-426-3738
claritysales@plantronics.com
www.clarityproducts.com

Carsten Trads, President
CJ Lindsey, Director of Finance
Jamie van den Bergh, VP- Sales & Marketing

Leading supplier of amplified telephones, notification systems, assistive listening devices and other communications devices for the hearing loss and Deaf markets. Clarity Power patented technology truly and positively impacts people's lives with every product created.

Year Founded: 1969

2174 Computer Paper for Brailling
Maxi-Aids, Inc.
42 Executive Boulevard
Farmingdale, NY 11735
631-752-0521
Fax: 631-752-0689; *Toll Free:* 800-522-6294
sales@maxiaids.com
www.maxiaids.com
TTY: 800-281-3555

Harold Zaretsky, President

Specially made paper for braille printing. 1,000 sheets/case, size 14 7/8 inches by 11 inches.

2175 Computer Switch Interface
AbleNet, Inc.
2625 Patton Road
Roseville, MN 55113
651-294-2200
Fax: 651-294-2259; *Toll Free:* 800-322-0956
customerservice@ablenetinc.com
www.ablenetinc.com

Bill Sproull, Chairman of the Board
Jennifer Thalhuber, President/ Chief Executive Offic
William Mills, Strategic Planning Chair

Allows single switch access to an Apple computer.

Year Founded: 1985

2176 Cordless Big Red Switch
AbleNet, Inc.
2625 Patton Road
Roseville, MN 55113
651-294-2200
Fax: 651-294-2259; *Toll Free:* 800-322-0956
customerservice@ablenetinc.com
www.ablenetinc.com

Bill Sproull, Chairman of the Board
Jennifer Thalhuber, President/ Chief Executive Offic
William Mills, Strategic Planning Chair

The Cordless Big Red Switch, when used in conjunction with either the Cordless Receiver or the Small Appliance Receiver, gives you cordless control of toys, games, and appliances in your environment.

Year Founded: 1985

2177 Cornell Communications
Cornell
7915 N 81st Street
Milwaukee, WI 53223
414-351-4660
Fax: 414-351-4657; *Toll Free:* 800-558-8957
sales@cornell.com
www.cornell.com

Pauline Haack, Inside Sales
Jerel Johnson, President

Cornell's Rescue Systems allow personnel to request emergency assistance. Applications include life safety emergency evacuation, parking garages and elevators. Voice and visual only systems are available. Call for our free Americans with Disabilities Act Accessibility Guideline.

Year Founded: 1970

2178 Darci Too
WesTest Engineering Corporation
810 Shepard Lane
Farmington, UT 84025
801-451-9191
Fax: 801-451-9393
webmail@westest.com
www.westest.com

A universal device which allows people with physical disabilities to replace the keyboard and mouse on a personal computer with a device that matches their physical capabilities. DARCI TOO works with almost any personal computer and provides access to all computer functions.

Year Founded: 1981

2179 DeltaTalker
Prentke Romich Company (PRC)
1022 Heyl Road
Wooster, OH 44691
330-262-1984
Fax: 330-263-4829; *Toll Free:* 800-262-1990
service@prentrom.com
www.prentrom.com

Dave Moffatt, President

A portable, electronic communication device that uses Minspeak so that symbols are used to represent words, sentences and phrases. The DT can be accessed by pressing keys scanning or optical pointing and can be configured with 8, 32 or 128 locations. It has both digitalized and synthesized speech. Optional infrared capabilities allow operation of remote controlled devices.

2180 Don Johnston
Don Johnston, Inc.
26799 W Commerce Drive
Volo, IL 60073
847-740-0749
Fax: 847-740-7326; *Toll Free:* 800-999-4660
info@donjohnston.com, support@donjohnston.com
www.donjohnston.com

Ruth Ziolkowski, President
Don Johnston, Founder

A provider of quality products and services that enable people with special needs to discover their potential and experience success. Products are developed for the areas of Physical Access, Augmentative Communication and for those who struggle with reading and writing.

Year Founded: 1980

2181 Doorbell Signalers
HARC Mercantile Ltd.
5413 S. Westnedge Avenue
Suite A
Portage, MI 49002
269-324-1615
Fax: 269-324-2387; *Toll Free:* 800-445-9968
info@harc.com
www.harc.com
TTY: 269-324-1615

Mike Martinson, Managing Director

Doorbell signalers to alert with either louder chime or flashing light.

Year Founded: 1960

2182 Duxbury Braille Translator
Duxbury Systems, Inc.
270 Littleton Road
Unit 6
Westford, MA 01886-3523
978-692-3000
Fax: 978-692-7912
info@duxsys.com, support@duxsys.com, orders@d
www.duxburysystems.com

Joe Sullivan, President
Peter Sullivan, VP of Software Development
Genevieve Sullivan, Treasurer

A complete line of braille easy to use word processing and translation software available for Windows (including NT), Macintosh, DOS, and UNIX. Applications for anyone wanting to produce or communicate with braille; signs, note cards, textbooks, business communications and forms, telephone bills, etc. Simple to use, FREE technical support. Free one year upgrades. DBT is for producing braille in English, Spanish, French, Portuguese, Italian, Latin

Year Founded: 1969

2183 Duxbury Systems
Duxbury Systems, Inc.
270 Littleton Road
Unit 6
Westford, MA 01886-3523
978-692-3000
Fax: 978-692-7912
info@duxsys.com, support@duxsys.com, orders@d
www.duxburysystems.com

Joe Sullivan, President
Peter Sullivan, VP of Software Development
Genevieve Sullivan, Treasurer

Software for the visually impaired.

Year Founded: 1969

2184 Enabling Technologies Company
Enabling Technologies
1601 NE Braille Place
Jensen Beach, FL 34957
772-225-3687
Fax: 772-225-3299; *Toll Free:* 800-777-3687
info@brailler.com
www.brailler.com

Greg Schenk, Marketing Executive

Manufactures the most complete line of American made braille embossers, including desk top or portable models capable of producing high quality single sided or interpoint braille. Also carry a complete line of adaptive technology aids for the blind community at affordable prices.

Year Founded: 1969

2185 Environment Control System
Airphone Corporation
1700 130th Avenue NE
Bellevue, WA 98005-2203
425-455-0510
Fax: 425-455-0071; *Toll Free:* 800-692-0200
tech@aiphone.com, cs@aiphone.com
www.aiphone.com

Chuck Watkins, Eastern Regional Sales Manager
Nancy McAlister, Western Regional Sales Manager
David McManamon

AIPHONE manufactures audio and video intercom systems for home or business to help the physically disabled answer doors and communicate through physical barriers; also ADA-compliant emergency call intercom stations for use in public facilities, and an Environmental Control System for persons with limited mobility.

Year Founded: 1970

2186 Extra Loud Alarm with Bed Shaker and ACPlug For Lamp
HARC Mercantile Ltd.
5413 S. Westnedge Avenue
Suite A
Portage, MI 49002
269-324-1615
Fax: 269-324-2387; *Toll Free:* 800-445-9968
info@harc.com
www.harc.com
TTY: 269-324-1615

Mike Martinson, Managing Director

Battery operated, easy to read, digital clock with extra loud alarm.

Year Founded: 1960

2187 Eyegaze Computer System
LC Technologies, Inc.
103636 Democracy Lane
Fairfax, VA 22030
703-385-8800
Fax: 703-385-7137; *Toll Free:* 800-393-4293
info309@eyegaze.com
www.eyegaze.com

John West, Sales & Information Contact
Nancy Cleveland, Contact, Eyegaze Edge, Schedulin
Erica Jeffery, Contact, Insurance, Medicare & M

Enables people with physical disabilities to do many things with their eyes that they would otherwise do with their hands.

Year Founded: 1986

2188 Flashing Lamp Telephone Ring Alerter
Independent Living Aids, LLC
137 Rano Street
Buffalo, NY 14207
516-937-1848
Fax: 516-937-3906; *Toll Free:* 800-537-2118
techsupport@independentliving.com
www.independentliving.com

Marvin Sandler, President

Once your phone is plugged into the Telephone Ring Alerter, the lamp light will flash with each ring, alerting you that there is a phone call.

2189 Font-Tools BIGFONT
Worthington Data Solutions
623 Swift St.
Santa Cruz, CA 95060
831-458-9938
Fax: 831-458-9964; *Toll Free:* 800-345-4220
wds@barcodehq.com
www.barcodehq.com

Steve Fent, Owner

Prints large text up to two inches tall on laser printers. It requires an IBM PC and runs from any MS-DOS language.

Year Founded: 1985

2190 GW Micro
GW Micro, Inc.
725 Airport North Office Park
Fort Wayne, IN 46825
260-489-3671
Fax: 260-489-2608
sales@gwmicro.com, orders@gwmicro.com,support
www.gwmicro.com

Doug Geoffray, Vice President Development
Dan Weirich, VP Sales & Marketing
Louis Biach

Computer hardware and software products for people with disabilities.

Year Founded: 1990

2191 Headmaster Plus
Prentke Romich Company (PRC)
1022 Heyl Road
Wooster, OH 44691
330-262-1984
Fax: 330-263-4829; *Toll Free:* 800-262-1984
info@prentrom.com
www.prentrom.com

Dave Moffatt, President

A headpointing system that takes the place of a mouse, and allows individuals who cannot use their hands but have good head control access to the computer. A transmitting unit sits atop the monitor and sends signals to the user's headset. The user puffs into a tube connected to the headset to make selections. Typing can be done with optional on-screen keyboards.

2192 Ideal-Phone
IDEAMATICS, Inc.
1364 Beverly Road
Suite 101
Mc Lean, VA 22101-3617
703-903-4972
Fax: 703-903-8949; *Toll Free:* 800-247-4332
ideamatics@ideamatics.net
www.ideamatics.com/

David L Danner, President, Founder
Michael A. Schwartz, VP
Mark Moore, VP of Operations

Integrates the personal computer and the telephone into a single, efficient workstation. It is ideal for mobility-impaired persons and others who need a hands-free operation of the phone. The Ideal-Phone includes one PC Board, a Plantronics headset, software for access and logging and complete documentation. It can be integrated into programs, or pops-up over any application. MS-DOS based, version 3.0 or higher are available.

Year Founded: 1975

2193 Induction Loop Receiver
HARC Mercantile Ltd.
5413 S. Westnedge Avenue
Suite A
Portage, MI 49002

269-324-1615
Fax: 269-324-2387; *Toll Free:* 800-445-9968
info@harc.com
www.harc.com
TTY: 269-324-1615

Mike Martinson, Managing Director

Sound induction receiver to be used with any loop system.

Year Founded: 1960

2194 Jelly Bean Switch
AbleNet, Inc.
2625 Patton Road
Roseville, MN 55113
651-294-2200
Fax: 651-294-2259; *Toll Free:* 800-322-0956
customerservice@ablenetinc.com
www.ablenetinc.com

Bill Sproull, Chairman of the Board
Jennifer Thalhuber, President/ Chief Executive Offic
William Mills, Strategic Planning Chair

A momentary touch switch made of shatterproof plastic, small and sensitive to 2-3 ounces of pressure, this switch is provided audible feedback when activated and is a compact version of the Big Red Switch.

Year Founded: 1985

2195 LT Switch
AbleNet, Inc.
2625 Patton Road
Roseville, MN 55113
651-294-2200
Fax: 651-294-2259; *Toll Free:* 800-322-0956
customerservice@ablenetinc.com
www.ablenetinc.com

Bill Sproull, Chairman of the Board
Jennifer Thalhuber, President/ Chief Executive Offic
William Mills, Strategic Planning Chair

A light touch version of the Plate Switch, beneficial to users with minimal strength.

Year Founded: 1985

2196 Laptops/Word Processors
Perfect Solutions Consulting, Inc
2685 Treanor Terrace
Wellington, FL 33414
561-790-1070
Fax: 561-790-0108; *Toll Free:* 800-726-7086
perfect@gate.net
www.perfectsolutions.com

Andrew Kramer, President

A computer for every student! Wireless talking laptop computers starting at $290.00 are ideal for all ages.

Year Founded: 1987

2197 Large Button Speaker Phone
HARC Mercantile Ltd.
5413 S. Westnedge Avenue
Suite A
Portage, MI 49002
269-324-1615
Fax: 269-324-2387; *Toll Free:* 800-445-9968
info@harc.com
www.harc.com
TTY: 269-324-1615

Mike Martinson, Managing Director

Speakerphone with or without remote control.

Year Founded: 1960

2198 Large Print Telephone Dial
Maxi-Aids, Inc.
42 Executive Boulevard
Farmingdale, NY 11735
631-752-0521
Fax: 631-752-0689; *Toll Free:* 800-522-6294
sales@maxiaids.com
www.maxiaids.com
TTY: 800-281-3555

Harold Zaretsky, President

Pressure sensitive dial with numbers that are easy to see for the disabled.

2199 Large Print Touch-Telephone Overlays
Maxi-Aids, Inc.
42 Executive Boulevard
Farmingdale, NY 11735
631-752-0521
Fax: 631-752-0689; *Toll Free:* 800-522-6294
sales@maxiaids.com
www.maxiaids.com
TTY: 800-281-3555

Harold Zaretsky, President

Pressure-sensitive and easy to apply overlays that make everyday phones accessible.

2200 Lighthouse Low Vision Products
Lighthouse International
111 E 59th Street
The Sol & Lillian Goldman Building
New York, NY 10022-1202
212-821-9200
Fax: 212-821-9707; *Toll Free:* 800-829-0500
info@lighthouse.org
www.lighthouse.org
TTY: 212-821-9713

Joseph A. Ripp, Chairman
Sarah E. Smith, Vice Chair & Treasurer
Mark G. Ackermann, President/CEO

Lighthouse International is the leading non-profit organization worldwide dedicated to preserving vision and to helping people of all ages overcome the challenges of vision loss.

Year Founded: 1905

2201 Line-A-Timers
Therapro, Inc.
225 Arlington Street
Framingham, MA 01702-8723
508-872-9494
Fax: 508-875-2062; *Toll Free:* 800-257-5376
info@theraproducts.com
www.theraproducts.com

Karen Conrad, Founder
Paul Weihrauch, Founder

Four flexible, translucent yellow plastic strips make reading easier for everyone. Static electricity holds strips against most types of reading material.

Year Founded: 1986

2202 Location Finder
Maxi-Aids, Inc.
42 Executive Boulevard
Farmingdale, NY 11735
631-752-0521
Fax: 631-752-0689; Toll Free: 800-522-6294
sales@maxiaids.com
www.maxiaids.com
TTY: 800-281-3555

Harold Zaretsky, President

Helps find house, apartment, car or office. Just press the transmitter and sound will be emitted indicating the location.

2203 Luminaud Inc.
8688 Tyler Boulevard
Mentor, OH 44060
440-255-9082
Fax: 440-255-2250; Toll Free: 800-255-3408
info@luminaud.com
www.luminaud.com

Thomas Lennox, President
Dorothy Lennox, VP

Catalog offers a line of artificial larynx, personal voice amplifiers, special switches, stoma covers and other communication, health and safety items.

50 pages Year Founded: 1972

2204 Magni-Cam
Innoventions, Inc.
10425 Bissonnet Street
Houston, TX 77099
281-879-6226
Fax: 281-879-6415; Toll Free: 800-854-6554
sales@innoventions.com
www.memorytesters.com/

David Feinstein, President & Founder
Charleen Freeman, Vice President Marketing

Magni-Cam is a hand-held, light weight, inexpensive, auto-focus electronic magnification system designed to meet the reading and writing needs of those with low vision. The system presents the image in black and white or in color with three different view modes. Connects to any TV monitor in minutes. System reads any surfact with no distortion. Two battery powered systems are availabe providing total portability and flexibility.

Year Founded: 1984

2205 Man's Low-Vision Quartz Watches
Independent Living Aids, LLC
137 Rano Street
Buffalo, NY 14207
516-937-1848
Fax: 516-937-3906; Toll Free: 800-537-2118
techsupport@independentliving.com
www.independentliving.com

Marvin Sandler, President

An inexpensive, easy-to-read watch with chrome case.

2206 MegaDots
Duxbury Systems, Inc.
270 Littleton Road
Unit 6
Westford, MA 01886-3523

978-692-3000
Fax: 978-692-7912
info@duxsys.com, support@duxsys.com, orders@d
www.duxburysystems.com

Joe Sullivan, President
Peter Sullivan, VP of Software Development
Genevieve Sullivan, Treasurer

A revolutionary new braille translator for the PC that lets you finish projects quickly and easily. Intelligent document importation recognizes what word processor your text is from and guesses that appropriate format for each paragraph, yielding high quality braille.

Year Founded: 1969

2207 Men's/Women's Low Vision Watches & Clocks
Maxi-Aids, Inc.
42 Executive Boulevard
Farmingdale, NY 11735
631-752-0521
Fax: 631-752-0689; Toll Free: 800-522-6294
sales@maxiaids.com
www.maxiaids.com
TTY: 800-281-3555

Harold Zaretsky, President

Choose from a wide range of watches from braille automatic to quartz pocket watches.

2208 MessageMate
Words+
42505 10th Street West
Lancaster, CA 93534-7059
661-723-6523
Fax: 888-298-9056; Toll Free: 800-869-8521
gaylon@words-plus.com
www.words-plus.com

Walt Wolosz, Manager

Lightweight, hand-held communicator providing high-quality analog recording capability using either direct select keyboards or 1 to 2 switch access.

Year Founded: 1981

2209 Metropolitan Washington Ear
The Metropolitan Washington Ear, Inc
12061 Tech Road
Silver Spring, MD 20904
301-681-6636
Fax: 301-625-1986
information@washear.org
www.washear.org

George Long, Chairman of the Board
Freddie L. Peaco, President Pro Tem
Neely Oplinger, Executive Director

This organization has pioneered audio description for blind audience members.

2210 Mini Teleloop
HARC Mercantile Ltd.
5413 S. Westnedge Avenue
Suite A
Portage, MI 49002
269-324-1615
Fax: 269-324-2387; Toll Free: 800-445-9968
info@harc.com
www.harc.com
TTY: 269-324-1615

Mike Martinson, Managing Director

Home induction loop amplifier for use with hearing aids equipped with T-Coil.

Year Founded: 1960

2211 Morse Code Equalizer
Words+
42505 10th Street West
Lancaster, CA 93534-7059
661-723-6523
Fax: 888-298-9056; *Toll Free:* 800-869-8521
gaylon@words-plus.com
www.words-plus.com

Walt Wolosz, Manager

Provides complete word processing and voice output communications with single or dual switch Morse code inputs. Originally designed for a blind user with only eyelid movement. The system can be used by both sighted and visually impaired persons.

Year Founded: 1981

2212 Multi-Scan Single Switch Activity Center
Academic Software, Inc.
3504 Tates Creek Road
Lexington, KY 40517-2601
859-552-1020
Fax: 253-799-4012
asistaff@acsw.com
www.acsw.com

Dr. Warren E Lacefield, President
Penelope D Ellis, COO & Sales & Marketing Director
Sylvia B. Lacefield, Graphic Artist

2213 Personal FM Systems
HARC Mercantile Ltd.
5413 S. Westnedge Avenue
Suite A
Portage, MI 49002
269-324-1615
Fax: 269-324-2387; *Toll Free:* 800-445-9968
info@harc.com
www.harc.com
TTY: 269-324-1615

Mike Martinson, Managing Director

Wireless FM systems transmits sound via a radio carrier wave.

Year Founded: 1960

2214 Personal Infrared Listening System
HARC Mercantile Ltd.
5413 S. Westnedge Avenue
Suite A
Portage, MI 49002
269-324-1615
Fax: 269-324-2387; *Toll Free:* 800-445-9968
info@harc.com
www.harc.com
TTY: 269-324-1615

Mike Martinson, Managing Director

Wireless method if listening to TV and radio with individually controlled amplification.

Year Founded: 1960

2215 Phillip Roy
Phillip Roy, Inc.
12651 Walsingham Road
Suite E
Largo, FL 33774
727-593-2700
Fax: 727-595-2685; *Toll Free:* 800-255-9085
info@philliproy.com
www.philliproy.com

Ruth Bralman PhD, President
Phillip Roy, Manager

Offers multimedia materials appropriate for use with individuals with disabilities. Programs range from preschool through the adult level. Many of the programs are high interest topics/low vocabulary, ideal for transition and employability skills. Materials are also available which focus on social and personal development. Call for a free catalog.

Year Founded: 1987

2216 Plantronics SP-04
Ablephone
354 Chatfield Avenue
Biggs, CA 95917
530-846-7466
Fax: 530-846-7466; *Toll Free:* 800-456-4979
ablephone@juno.com
www.ablephone.com/

Headset telephone for people who have a hard time grasping the telephone.

Year Founded: 1960

2217 PortaPower Plus
Words+
42505 10th Street West
Lancaster, CA 93534-7059
661-723-6523
Fax: 888-298-9056; *Toll Free:* 800-869-8521
gaylon@words-plus.com
www.words-plus.com

Walt Wolosz, Manager

Rechargeable battery pack designed to give longer life and remote usage time to laptop computers and other portable battery-operated devices and accessories. Requires a 12 volt auto adapter.

Year Founded: 1981

2218 Potomac Technology
Potomac Technology Services
77 S Washington Street
Suite 307
Rockville, MD 20850
301-637-8111
Fax: 301-637-8263; *Toll Free:* 800-433-2838
contact@pts-solutions.com
www.pts-solutions.com/

Patricia J Relihan, Manager

This catalog offers a variety of wake-up devices, alarm clocks, alerting systems, assistive listening devices, signalers, smoke detectors, TTY, telephones and telephone amplifiers.

24 pages

2219 Prentke Romich Company
Prentke Romich Company (PRC)
1022 Heyl Road
Wooster, OH 44691
330-262-1984
Fax: 330-263-4829; Toll Free: 800-262-1933
info@prentrom.com
www.prentrom.com

Barry Romich, Chairman
Joe Durbin, President
Dave Moffatt

The Prentke Romich Company is a full service company offering easy, yet powerful communication aids. The company believes in supporting customers before and after the sale by offering funding assistance, distance learning training, extended warranty, service assistance and much more. Visit our web-site to view our full-line catalogue, read about our success stories, and to sign up for our on-line newsletter.

2220 Prentke Romich Company Product Catalog
Prentke Romich Company (PRC)
1022 Heyl Road
Wooster, OH 44691
330-262-1984
Fax: 330-263-4829; Toll Free: 800-262-1933
info@prentrom.com
www.prentrom.com

Larry Gigax, Contact
Dave Moffatt, President

A full-line product catalog containing information on speech-output communication devices, environmental controls and computer access products.

2221 Remote Control Speakerphone
Clarity Products
4289 Bonny Oaks Drive
Suite 106
Chattanooga, TN 37406-1600
423-622-7793
Fax: 800-325-8871; Toll Free: 800-426-3738
claritycs@plantronics.com
www.clarityproducts.com

Carsten Trads, President
CJ Lindsey, Director of Finance
Jamie van den Bergh, VP- Sales & Marketing

A multi-functional speaker phone specially designed to meet the needs of motion-impaired persons who are unable to use a conventional phone without assistance.

Year Founded: 1969

2222 Resource Directory of Special Education and Rehabilitation Computer Products
Closing the Gap
PO Box 68
526 Main Street
Henderson, MN 56044
507-248-3294
Fax: 507-248-3810
info@closingthegap.com
www.closingthegap.com/

Dolores Hagen, President & Co-Founder
Connie Kneip, Vice President/ General Manager
Megan Turek, Managing Editor/ Advertising & E

About 300 suppliers of computer hardware and software designed for use by persons with disabilities. Entries include: Company or organization name, address, phone, description of products.

208 pages Frequency: Annual, Feb/Mar Year Founded: 1983

2223 Room Valet Visual-Tactile Alerting System
HARC Mercantile Ltd.
5413 S. Westnedge Avenue
Suite A
Portage, MI 49002
269-324-1615
Fax: 269-324-2387; Toll Free: 800-445-9968
info@harc.com
www.harc.com
TTY: 269-324-1615

Mike Martinson, Managing Director

ADA compliant built-in visual-tactile alerting system. The Room Valet is fully supervised and has power failure back up. Alerts to in-room smoke, building alarm, door, phone and alarm clock. Designed for permanent installation.

Year Founded: 1960

2224 SpeakEasy Communication Aid
AbleNet, Inc.
2625 Patton Road
Roseville, MN 55113
651-294-2200
Fax: 651-294-2259; Toll Free: 800-322-0956
customerservice@ablenetinc.com
www.ablenetinc.com

Bill Sproull, Chairman of the Board
Jennifer Thalhuber, President/ Chief Executive Offic
William Mills, Strategic Planning Chair

SpeakEasy is a digitalized Voice Output Communication Aid that is ideal for anyone who is beginning to develop communication skills such as making choices and identifying symbols. It holds 12 messages totaling four minutes and 20 seconds of recording time. It measures 7 1/2 inches by 1 3/4 inches and weighs only one pound. Activate messages using the built in keyboard or via external switch.

Year Founded: 1985

2225 Speech Discrimination Unit
HARC Mercantile Ltd.
5413 S. Westnedge Avenue
Suite A
Portage, MI 49002
269-324-1615
Fax: 269-324-2387; Toll Free: 800-445-9968
info@harc.com
www.harc.com
TTY: 269-324-1615

Mike Martinson, Managing Director

Speech Adjust-A-Tone improves speech discrimination for use with telephone and/or TV and radio.

Year Founded: 1960

2226 SpringBoard Plus
Prentke Romich Company (PRC)
1022 Heyl Road
Wooster, OH 44691
330-262-1984
Fax: 330-263-4829; Toll Free: 800-262-1933

info@prentrom.com
www.prentrom.com

Cherie Weaver, Marketing Coordinator

SpringBoard can be an excellent starting point for the child or adult just beginning the augmentative communication process. SpringBoard can also be the next step for someone who has demonstrated success with manual communication boards or static display devices with limited message capacity. SpringBoard is flexible, easy to customize and easy to support.

2227 Step-by-Step Communicator
AbleNet, Inc.
2625 Patton Road
Roseville, MN 55113
651-294-2200
Fax: 651-294-2259; *Toll Free:* 800-322-0956
customerservice@ablenetinc.com
www.ablenetinc.com

Bill Sproull, Chairman of the Board
Jennifer Thalhuber, President/ Chief Executive Offic
William Mills, Strategic Planning Chair

The Step-by-Step Communicator allows you to record a series of messages (as many as you want up to the 75 second limit). It has a 2 1/2 inch diameter switch surface and is 3 inches at its tallest point. Angled switch surface makes it easy to see and access.

Year Founded: 1985

2228 Stretch-View Wide-View Rectangular Illuminated Magnifier
Dazor Manufacturing Corporation
2079 Congressional
St. Louis, MO 63146
314-652-2400
Fax: 314-652-2069; *Toll Free:* 800-345-9103
info@dazor.com
www.dazor.com

Richard Kupferer, Marketing Coordinator
Mark Hogrebe, President
Harry Dazey, Founder

Provides shadow-free illumination or a highlighting effect under the magnifying lens with an 18-watt compact fluorescent light source. The magnifier is mounted on a floating arm that allows you to position the light source and lens with the touch of a finger.

Year Founded: 1938

2229 String Switch
AbleNet, Inc.
2625 Patton Road
Roseville, MN 55113
651-294-2200
Fax: 651-294-2259; *Toll Free:* 800-322-0956
customerservice@ablenetinc.com
www.ablenetinc.com

Bill Sproull, Chairman of the Board
Jennifer Thalhuber, President/ Chief Executive Offic
William Mills, Strategic Planning Chair

An activated switch beneficial for users with limited active movement or minimal strength.

Year Founded: 1985

2230 Strobe Light Signalers
HARC Mercantile Ltd.
5413 S. Westnedge Avenue
Suite A
Portage, MI 49002
269-324-1615
Fax: 269-324-2387; *Toll Free:* 800-445-9968
info@harc.com
www.harc.com
TTY: 269-324-1615

Mike Martinson, Managing Director

Strobe alerts. Plugs into receivers for signaling systems.

Year Founded: 1960

2231 Symbi-Key Computer Switch Interface
AbleNet, Inc.
2625 Patton Road
Roseville, MN 55113
651-294-2200
Fax: 651-294-2259; *Toll Free:* 800-322-0956
customerservice@ablenetinc.com
www.ablenetinc.com

Bill Sproull, Chairman of the Board
Jennifer Thalhuber, President/ Chief Executive Offic
William Mills, Strategic Planning Chair

The Symbi-Key can be programmed to simulate any key stroke or a series of keystrokes (up to 5 per key) for single switch access to software programs whether or not it was designed for switch access. Works well in DOS and all versions of Windows providing access to any IBM program.

Year Founded: 1985

2232 TAJ Braille Typewriter
Maxi-Aids, Inc.
42 Executive Boulevard
Farmingdale, NY 11735
631-752-0521
Fax: 631-752-0689; *Toll Free:* 800-522-6294
sales@maxiaids.com
www.maxiaids.com
TTY: 800-281-3555

Harold Zaretsky, President

Smooth edged, simple and sturdy construction. Creates braille on 8 1/2 x 11 paper.

2233 TTY's-Telephone Device for the Deaf
HARC Mercantile Ltd.
5413 S. Westnedge Avenue
Suite A
Portage, MI 49002
269-324-1615
Fax: 269-324-2387; *Toll Free:* 800-445-9968
info@harc.com
www.harc.com
TTY: 269-324-1615

Mike Martinson, Managing Director

With or without printer.

Year Founded: 1960

2234 TV & VCR Remote
AbleNet, Inc.
2625 Patton Road
Roseville, MN 55113

651-294-2200
Fax: 651-294-2259; *Toll Free:* 800-322-0956
customerservice@ablenetinc.com
www.ablenetinc.com

Bill Sproull, Chairman of the Board
Jennifer Thalhuber, President/ Chief Executive Offic
William Mills, Strategic Planning Chair

The TV and VCR Remote will control a TV, a VCR, or a TV that is connected through a VCR tuner. It may be programmed to control functions such as on and off, channel up, preprogrammed TV channels and if desired, other TV functions such as mute and pause.

Year Founded: 1985

2235 Talking Clocks
HARC Mercantile Ltd.
5413 S. Westnedge Avenue
Suite A
Portage, MI 49002
269-324-1615
Fax: 269-324-2387; *Toll Free:* 800-445-9968
info@harc.com
www.harc.com
TTY: 269-324-1615

Mike Martinson, Managing Director

Talking clocks with loud alarms, high and low volume control, choices of sound effects, hourly report options. Other languages are available.

Year Founded: 1960

2236 Talking Desktop Calculators
Maxi-Aids, Inc.
42 Executive Boulevard
Farmingdale, NY 11735
631-752-0521
Fax: 631-752-0689; *Toll Free:* 800-522-6294
sales@maxiaids.com
www.maxiaids.com
TTY: 800-281-3555

Harold Zaretsky, President

Unique voice synthesizers call out numerals and functions as they are keyed in, or read out data stored in memory.

2237 The Chatter Vox - Speech Amplifier
HARC Mercantile Ltd.
5413 S. Westnedge Avenue
Suite A
Portage, MI 49002
269-324-1615
Fax: 269-324-2387; *Toll Free:* 800-445-9968
info@harc.com
www.harc.com
TTY: 269-324-1615

Mike Martinson, Managing Director

Portable, body worn personal speech amplifier for people with a weak voice.

Year Founded: 1960

2238 Timex Easy Reader
Independent Living Aids, LLC
137 Rano Street
Buffalo, NY 14207
516-937-1848
Fax: 516-937-3906; *Toll Free:* 800-537-2118

techsupport@independentliving.com
www.independentliving.com

Marvin Sandler, President

An easy-to-read large face watch that's water resistant.

2239 U-Control II
Words+
42505 10th Street West
Lancaster, CA 93534-7059
661-723-6523
Fax: 888-298-9056; *Toll Free:* 800-869-8521
gaylon@words-plus.com
www.words-plus.com

Walt Wolosz, Manager

Works with the Words+ system (EX Keys, Morse WSKE, Scanning WSKE, Talking Screen) to provide wireless, portable control of items which are already infrared-controlled such as a TV, VCR, CD player, etc.

Year Founded: 1981

2240 Unisex Low Vision Watch
Independent Living Aids, LLC
137 Rano Street
Buffalo, NY 14207
516-937-1848
Fax: 516-937-3906; *Toll Free:* 800-537-2118
techsupport@independentliving.com
www.independentliving.com

Marvin Sandler, President

Unisex watch with large numbers and wide hands. Gold-toned case with either expansion or leather band. $10.95 to $49.95.

2241 Unity/128
Prentke Romich Company (PRC)
1022 Heyl Road
Wooster, OH 44691
330-262-1984
Fax: 330-263-4829; *Toll Free:* 800-262-1933
info@prentrom.com
www.prentrom.com

Dave Moffatt, President

A Minspeak application program available for the Liberator and Delta Talker communication devices. Provides single word vocabulary to people of all ages at varying stages of language development, who may be either cognitively intact or challenged.

2242 Universal Switch Mounting System
AbleNet, Inc.
2625 Patton Road
Roseville, MN 55113
651-294-2200
Fax: 651-294-2259; *Toll Free:* 800-322-0956
customerservice@ablenetinc.com
www.ablenetinc.com

Bill Sproull, Chairman of the Board
Jennifer Thalhuber, President/ Chief Executive Offic
William Mills, Strategic Planning Chair

Mounting system that allows switch placement in any position. A single lever locks all joints securely in place. Extends to 20 1/2 inches and holds up to five pounds. A mounting system for quick and easy positioning.

Year Founded: 1985

2243 Vantage Plus
Prentke Romich Company (PRC)
1022 Heyl Road
Wooster, OH 44691
330-262-1984
Fax: 330-263-4829; *Toll Free:* 800-262-1933
info@prentrom.com
www.prentrom.com

Dave Moffat, President

Vantage is the dynamic choice for powerful language and portable design. The enhanced operating system makes Vantage easy to customize and support. Vantage includes 4,8 and 15 location display options, plus the 45 and 84 location Unity Enhanced vocabulary.

2244 Vibrotactile Personal Alerting System
HARC Mercantile Ltd.
5413 S. Westnedge Avenue
Suite A
Portage, MI 49002
269-324-1615
Fax: 269-324-2387; *Toll Free:* 800-445-9968
info@harc.com
www.harc.com
TTY: 269-324-1615

Mike Martinson, Managing Director

Composed of a small wireless personal device that receives coded signals and a group of transmitters that send them.

Year Founded: 1960

2245 WINVISION
Artic Tech
1000 John R. Road
Suite 108
Troy, MI 48083-2724
248-588-7370
Fax: 313-588-2650
www.artictech.com

The premier access system for blind users of IBM personal computers.

2246 Weitbrecht Communications
Weitbrecht Communications, Inc.
1500 Olympic Boulevard
Santa Monica, CA 90404
310-656-4924
Fax: 310-450-9918; *Toll Free:* 800-233-9130
sales@weitbrecht.com
www.weitbrecht.com
TTY: 800-233-9130

Barbara Dreyfus, President

Catalog featuring a wide range of assistive devices for communication needs including telephones, amplifiers, signalers and more.

24 pages

2247 Whisper 2000
Ablephone
354 Chatfield Avenue
Biggs, CA 95917
530-846-7466
Fax: 530-846-7466; *Toll Free:* 800-456-4979
able-phone@juno.com
www.ablephone.com

Personal sound amplification system that features a transmitter, phone and relay system for the hard-of-hearing.

Year Founded: 1960

2248 WinSCAN-The Single Switch Interface for PCs with Windows
Academic Software, Inc.
3504 Tates Creek Road
Lexington, KY 40517-2601
859-552-1020
Fax: 253-799-4012
asistaff@acsw.com
www.acsw.com

Dr. Warren E Lacefield, President
Penelope D Ellis, COO & Sales & Marketing Director
Sylvia B Lacefield, Graphic Artist

2249 Words+ IST (Infrared, Sound, Touch)
Words+
42505 10th Street West
Lancaster, CA 93534-7059
661-723-6523
Fax: 888-298-9056; *Toll Free:* 800-869-8521
gaylon@words-plus.com
www.words-plus.com

Walt Wolosz, Manager

A unique switch that is activated by slight movement or faint sound. The switch provides user control when connected to a device driven by a single switch. Individuals are currently accessing a wide variety of communication and computer systems with movement using the IST switch.

Year Founded: 1981

Cushions and Wedges

2250 Action Products
Action Products, Inc.
954 Sweeny Drive
Hagerstown, MD 21740
301-797-1414
Fax: 301-733-2073; *Toll Free:* 800-228-7763
service@actionproducts.com
www.actionproducts.com

Nancy Eddington, Customer Service Manager
Fred Nelson, Seating/Positioning Specialist
Troy McKnigh

Wheelchair pads, mattress pads, positioning cushions and insoles that aids in the prevention and cure of pressure sores by reducing pressure. All products are made of Akton viscoelastic polymer that doesnot leak, flow or bottom out. Manufacturer of the Xact line of positioning cushions for patients with high risk of skin breakdown.

Year Founded: 1970

2251 Back-Huggar Pillow
Bodyline Comfort Systems
3730 Kori Road
Jacksonville, FL 32257
904-262-4068
Fax: 800-323-2225; *Toll Free:* 800-874-7715
info@bodyline.com
www.bodyline.com

Don Dodds, Office Manager
John Fiore, Owner

Exclusive design makes almost any seat more comfortable by exerting soothing pressure against back muscles and discs.

2252 Bye-Bye Decubiti (BBD)
Rand-Scot
401 Linden Center Drive
Fort Collins, CO 80524
970-484-7967
Fax: 970-484-3800; Toll Free: 800-467-7967
info@randscot.com
www.randscot.com

Joel Lerich, Founder
Barbara , Founder

The BBD therapeutic wheelchair cushions have been market-proven since 1951 - in the prevention and cure of pressure sores (decubiti). These natural rubber inflatable products have recently been expanded to include pediatric, sports and double-valve models. Moderately priced, they offer a viable and cost-effective alternative in the market. $84.00-$112.00

Year Founded: 1980

2253 Dynamic Systems
Dynamic Systems, Inc.
104 Morrow Branch Road
Leicester, NC 28748
828-683-3523
Fax: 828-683-3511; Toll Free: 855-SUN-ATE
www.sunmatecushions.com

Charles A Yost, CEO

SunMate orthopedic foam sheets and cushions, pudgee pads for pressure relief and skin breakdown prevention, laminar wheelchair cushions, and Foam-in-Place Seating for custom molding seat inserts. Sample packs and literature available upon request.

Year Founded: 1969

2254 ENHANCER Cushion
ROHO, Inc.
100 N Florida Avenue
Belleville, IL 62221-5429
618-277-9173
Fax: 618-277-9561; Toll Free: 800-851-3449
www.rohoinc.com

Tom Borcherding, President of the ROHO Group
Becky Pelton, VP of Human Resources
Bobby Graebe, Chief Executive Officer

Uses AIR IN PLACE progressive positioning for enhanced midline channeling of the femurs, lateral stability and tissue protection.

Year Founded: 1973

2255 Geo-Matt for High Risk Patients
Span-America Medical Systems, Inc.
70 Commerce Center
Greenville, SC 29615
864-288-8692
Fax: 864-288-8692; Toll Free: 800-888-6752
www.spanamerica.com

James D Ferguson, CEO

For over 30 years, Span America Medical Systems has offered the industry's most comprehensive line of specialty solutions for pressure management and patient positioning. Recognized in medical facilities throughout North America.

2256 HIGH PROFILE Dual Compartment Cushion
ROHO, Inc.
100 N Florida Avenue
Belleville, IL 62221-5429
618-277-9173
Fax: 618-277-9561; Toll Free: 800-851-3449
www.rohoinc.com

Tom Borcherding, President of the ROHO Group
Becky Pelton, VP of Human Resources
Bobby Graebe, Chief Executive Officer
Year Founded: 1973

2257 HIGH PROFILE Single Compartment Cushion
ROHO, Inc.
100 N Florida Avenue
Belleville, IL 62221-5429
618-277-9173
Fax: 618-277-9561; Toll Free: 800-851-3449
www.rohoinc.com

Tom Borcherding, President of the ROHO Group
Becky Pelton, VP of Human Resources
Bobby Graebe, Chief Executive Officer

With 4 inch cells, the HIGH PROFILE is the cushion of choice for individuals who suffer from ischemic ulcers (pressure sores) or who have a history of tissue breakdown.

Year Founded: 1973

2258 LOW PROFILE Dual Compartment Cushion
ROHO, Inc.
100 N Florida Avenue
Belleville, IL 62221-5429
618-227-9173
Fax: 618-277-9561; Toll Free: 800-851-3449
www.rohoinc.com

Tom Borcherding, President of the ROHO Group
Becky Pelton, VP of Human Resources
Bobby Graebe, Chief Executive Officer
Year Founded: 1973

2259 LOW PROFILE Single Compartment Cushion
ROHO, Inc.
100 N Florida Avenue
Belleville, IL 62221-5429
618-277-9173
Fax: 618-277-9561; Toll Free: 800-851-3449
www.rohoinc.com

Tom Borcherding, President of the ROHO Group
Becky Pelton, VP of Human Resources
Bobby Graebe, Chief Executive Officer

Offers 2 inch cells for active users protection against skin breakdown.

Year Founded: 1973

2260 Lumbo-Posture Back Support
Rand-Scot
401 Linden Center Drive
Fort Collins, CO 80524
970-484-7967
Fax: 970-484-3800; Toll Free: 800-467-7967

info@randscot.com
www.randscot.com

Joel Lerich, Founder
Barbara , Founder

Rubber inflatable back support that offers therapeutic relief to all who must sit for lengthy periods of time, whether used in a wheelchair, auto or bed.

Year Founded: 1980

2261 Lumex's Cushions and Mattresses
Graham-Field Health Products, Inc.
2935 Northeast Parkway
Atlanta, GA 30360
678-291-3207
Fax: 800-726-0601; *Toll Free:* 800-347-5678
cs@grahamfield.com, orders@grahamfield.com
www.grahamfield.com

Kenneth Spett, President/CEO
Lori Kirschner, Senior VP, Human Resources & Ami
Alan Spett, SVP, Operations

Line of cushions and pillows give comfort and independence to the physically challenged.

Year Founded: 1850

2262 Mini-Max Cushion
ROHO, Inc.
100 N Florida Avenue
Belleville, IL 62221-5429
618-277-9173
Fax: 618-277-9561; *Toll Free:* 800-851-3449
www.rohoinc.com

Tom Borcherding, President of the ROHO Group
Becky Pelton, VP of Human Resources
Bobby Graebe, Chief Executive Officer

Designed for the active individual with low risk of skin breakdown. The unique air cells of the MIN-MAX provide significant shock and impact absorption, skin protection and stability.

Year Founded: 1973

2263 NEXUS Wheelchair Cushioning System
ROHO, Inc.
100 N Florida Avenue
Belleville, IL 62221-5429
618-227-9173
Fax: 618-277-9561; *Toll Free:* 800-851-3449
www.rohoinc.com

Tom Borcherding, President of the ROHO Group
Becky Pelton, VP of Human Resources
Bobby Graebe, Chief Executive Officer

A unique modular cushion that mates a contoured polyurethane foam base with a DRY FLOTATION support pad. It is designed to give the user positioning and stability, while offering maximum protection to the ischia, sacrum and coccyx.

Year Founded: 1973

2264 Performance Gel Cushions
Spenco Medical Corporation
PO Box 2501
Waco, TX 76702
254-772-6000
Fax: 817-751-5799; *Toll Free:* 800-877-3626
www.spenco.com

Steven B Smith, Chairman/CEO
Dr. Wayman Spence, Founder

Spenco is an innovative healthcare company whose mission is to help people everywhere achieve more-more comfortably.

2265 QUADTRO Cushion
ROHO, Inc.
100 N Florida Avenue
Belleville, IL 62221-5429
618-277-9173
Fax: 618-277-9561; *Toll Free:* 800-851-3449
www.rohoinc.com

Tom Borcherding, President of the ROHO Group
Becky Pelton, VP of Human Resources
Bobby Graebe, Chief Executive Officer

For individuals who require special positioning of the pelvis or thighs and are at risk of skin breakdown, the QUADTRO, with 4 inch cell height and AIR IN PLACE, progressive positioning is the cushion of choice.

Year Founded: 1973

2266 Silicone Padding
Spenco Medical Corporation
PO Box 2501
Waco, TX 76702
817-772-6000
Fax: 817-751-5799; *Toll Free:* 800-877-3626
www.spenco.com

Steven B Smith, Chairman/CEO
Patty Smith, Controller
Dr. Wayman Spence, Founder

For the management of pressure sores, this padding provides a special support system which allows even distribution of pressure and cool, comfortable well-ventilated support.

2267 Spenco Medical Group
Spenco Medical Corporation
PO Box 2501
Waco, TX 76702
254-772-6000
Fax: 817-751-5799; *Toll Free:* 800-877-3626
spenco@spenco.com
www.spenco.com

Mark B Connors, VP Sales/Marketing
Patty Smith, Controller
Dr. Wayman Spence, Founder

Wheel chair cushions, Silicore mattress pads, wound dressings, second skin blister and burn pads, Polysorb insoles, elbow, knee, wrist supports, walking shoes.

Year Founded: 1967

2268 Sun-Mate Seat Cushions
Dynamic Systems, Inc.
104 Morrow Branch Road
Leicester, NC 28748
828-683-3523
Fax: 828-683-3511; *Toll Free:* 855-SUN-ATE
dsi@sunmatecushions.com
www.sunmatecushions.com

Charles A Yost, CEO
Ellie Brown, Operations Manager

Line of cushions, pads and accessory items for personal comfort of the disabled. SunMate Orthopedic foam cushions and sheets that contours slowly to give uniform pressure distribution and soft spring back. Liquid SunMate for Foam-in-Place Seating (FIPS) to make custom molded seat inserts.

Year Founded: 1969

2269 Wheelchair and Mattress Pads
Action Products, Inc.
954 Sweeney Drive
Hagerstown, MD 21740
301-797-1414
Fax: 301-733-2073; Toll Free: 800-228-7763
service@actionproducts.com
www.actionproducts.com

Troy McNight, President

Aids in the prevention and cure of pressure sores by reducing pressure.

Year Founded: 1970

Dressing Aids

2270 Button Aid
Maxi-Aids, Inc.
42 Executive Boulevard
Farmingdale, NY 11735
631-752-0521
Fax: 631-752-0689; Toll Free: 800-522-6294
sales@maxiaids.com
www.maxiaids.com
TTY: 800-281-3555

Harold Zaretsky, President

Makes buttoning possible with the use of only one hand.

2271 Deluxe Sock and Stocking Aid
Therapro, Inc.
225 Arlington Street
Framingham, MA 01702-8723
508-872-9494
Fax: 508-875-2062; Toll Free: 800-257-5376
info@theraproducts.com
www.theraproducts.com

Karen Conrad, Founder
Paul Weihrauch, Founder

Flexible plastic, lined with blue nylon to reduce friction and outside with beige terry cloth to hold sock firmly until it is on the foot.

Year Founded: 1986

2272 Dressing Stick
Maxi-Aids, Inc.
42 Executive Boulevard
Farmingdale, NY 11735
631-752-0521
Fax: 631-752-0689; Toll Free: 800-522-6294
sales@maxiaids.com
www.maxiaids.com
TTY: 800-281-3555

Harold Zaretsky, President

Helps put on coats, sweaters and garments even when arm and shoulder movement is limited.

2273 Elastic Shoelaces
Therapro, Inc.
225 Arlington Street
Framingham, MA 01702-8723
508-872-9494
Fax: 508-875-2062; Toll Free: 800-257-5376
info@theraproducts.com
www.theraproducts.com

Karen Conrad, Founder
Paul Weihrauch, Founder

The elastic laces allow the wearer to slip tied shoes on and off.

Year Founded: 1986

2274 Featherweight Reachers
Therapro, Inc.
225 Arlington Street
Framingham, MA 01702-8723
508-872-9494
Fax: 508-875-2062; Toll Free: 800-257-5376
info@theraproducts.com
www.theraproducts.com

Karen Conrad, Founder
Paul Weihrauch, Founder

Useful in dressing or retrieving objects.

Year Founded: 1986

2275 Folding Dressing Stick
EASE
3714 Copper Penny Lane
Auburn, CA 95602
928-636-9469
Fax: 530-888-6990; Toll Free: 800-327- 650
kmjc@northlink.com
www.accesswithease.com/

Helps the physically-challenged user put on shirts, coats and jackets easily. This dressing stick folds for easy storage.

2276 Mirror Go Lightly
AbleNet, Inc.
2625 Patton Road
Roseville, MN 55113
651-294-2200
Fax: 651-294-2259; Toll Free: 800-322-0956
customerservice@ablenetinc.com
www.ablenetinc.com

Bill Sproull, Chairman of the Board
Jennifer Thalhuber, President/ Chief Executive Offic
William Mills, Strategic Planning Chair

Framed in plastic, the mirror can be tilted to provide either a normal or magnified image, or to direct its lights at, or away from, the user.

Year Founded: 1985

2277 Molded Sock and Stocking Aid
Therapro, Inc.
225 Arlington Street
Framingham, MA 01702-8723
508-872-9494
Fax: 508-875-2062; Toll Free: 800-257-5376
info@theraproducts.com
www.theraproducts.com

Karen Conrad, Founder
Paul Weihrauch, Founder

Sock or stocking is pulled over the molded plastic and then can be put on more easily.

Year Founded: 1986

2278 Say What
Maxi-Aids, Inc.
42 Executive Boulevard
Farmingdale, NY 11735
631-752-0521
Fax: 631-752-0689; Toll Free: 800-522-6294
sales@maxiaids.com
www.maxiaids.com
TTY: 800-281-3555

Harold Zaretsky, President

Braille the tag with information that the wearer wants on the tag and place the tag on a hanger. The custom-identification program makes it easier for the user to remember and identify just the right clothes.

Health Aids

2279 AMI Aquamassage
AMI, Inc.
PO Box 808
Groton, CT 06340-0808
860-536-3735
Fax: 860-536-4362; Toll Free: 800-248-4031
sales@aquamassage.com
www.amiaqua.com

David M. Cote, President
Hilaire Cote, Sr. Vice President
Gerardo Aristi

The Aqua PT's 36 computer controlled water jets provide the effects of accupressure massage on three sides of the body in either two directions (pain management) or one direction (edema reduction). Concentrate on the full body, one area, or one specific problem point. The client remains clothed and dry. Aqua PT has adjustable water pressure and pulsating frequency, an automatic frequency, travel speed control and is easy to operate. $20,000-$24,000

Year Founded: 1988

2280 Digi-Flex
Therapro, Inc.
225 Arlington Street
Framingham, MA 01702-8723
508-872-9494
Fax: 508-875-2062; Toll Free: 800-257-5376
info@theraproducts.com
www.theraproducts.com

Karen Conrad, Founder
Paul Weihrauch, Founder

This is a unique hand and finger exercise unit. Recommended for use of individuation of fingers, web space and general strengthening of work hands.

Year Founded: 1986

2281 Digital and Audible Family Thermometer
Maxi-Aids, Inc.
42 Executive Boulevard
Farmingdale, NY 11735

631-752-0521
Fax: 631-752-0689; Toll Free: 800-522-6294
sales@maxiaids.com
www.maxiaids.com
TTY: 800-281-3555

Harold Zaretsky, President

Audible clinical thermometer.

2282 Electronic Stethoscopes
HARC Mercantile Ltd.
5413 S. Westnedge Avenue
Suite A
Portage, MI 49002
269-324-1615
Fax: 269-324-2387; Toll Free: 800-445-9968
info@harc.com
www.harc.com
TTY: 269-324-1615

Mike Martinson, Managing Director

High production fidelity with a number volume control wheel.

Year Founded: 1960

2283 Foot Inversion Tread
Bailey Manufacturing Company
Po Box 130
Lodi, OH 44254-0130
330-948-1080
Fax: 800-224-5390; Toll Free: 800-321-8372
www.baileymfg.com

Larry Strimple, President

Effective for correcting flat feet. These angled boards require the patient to walk on the outside of the foot instead of the arch.

Year Founded: 1956

2284 GA-SK
TDI
8630 Fenton Street
Suite 121
Silver Spring, MD 20910-3803
301-563-9112
Fax: 301-589-3797
info@TDIforAccess.org, advertising@TDIforAcce
www.tdiforaccess.org/
TTY: 301-589-3006

Claude Stout, Executive Director
John Skjeveland, Business Manager

A quarterly publication focusing on telecommunications and media access for people who are deaf, late-deafened, hard of hearing and deaf-blind.

40 pages Frequency: Quarterly Year Founded: 1968

2285 Hand/Nail Brush
EASE
3714 Copper Penny Lane
Auburn, CA 95602
928-636-9469
Fax: 530-888-6990; Toll Free: 800-327- 650
kmjc@northlink.com
www.accesswithease.com/

Suction cups hold this special brush in place.

2286 International Deaf/Tek, Inc.
Deaftek.USA
104 Catbriar Court
Summerville, SC 29485-8955
843-873-8444
Fax: 843-626-0270
deaftek@deaftek.org
www.deaftek.org
TTY: 843-851-6444

Brenda Monene RN, MEd, President

Provides the international electronic mail service, Deaftek, USA. This service is dedicated to communities that are deaf or hard of hearing; the service is used by individuals, organizations, agencies, schools, colleges and universities, service providers, and professionals in the field of deafness.

Year Founded: 1978

2287 Invacare Corporation
Invacare Corporation
1 Invacare Way
Elyria, OH 44035-4196
440-329-6000
Fax: 877-619-7996; *Toll Free:* 800-333-6900
www.invacare.com

A Malachi Mixon III, Chairman Of The Board
Gerald B Blouch, President/ Chief Executive Offic
Robert K. Gudbranson, Senior Vice President and Chief

The world's leading manufacturer and distributor of home health care products and mobility products for people with disabilities which are distributed worldwide through more than 10,000 provider locations in more than 80 countries.

Year Founded: 1885

2288 LS & S Products
LS & S
145 River Rock Drive
Buffalo, NY 14207
716-348-3500
Fax: 847-498-1482; *Toll Free:* 800-468-4789
info@lssproducts.com; www.lssproducts.com
TTY: 866-317-8533

Melissa T Balbach, President
John K Bace, Executive VP

LS&S has served the needs of the visually impaired and hard of hearing for over 20 years. We offer products that allow people to continue to live productive, independent lives. In order to find the right products, we constantly listen to customer feedback on products and ideas. In addition, we offer large print or cassette instructions for certain products upon request. Putting the customer first drives our mission at LS&S.

2289 MADAMIST 50/50 PSI Air Compressor
MADA, Inc.
625 Washington Ave
Carlstadt, NJ 07072
201-460-0454
Fax: 201-460-3509; *Toll Free:* 800-526-6370
www.madamedical.com

Jeffrey Adam, VP

The new compressor rated at 50 PSI is designed to drive humidifiers, nebulizers and mist tents, and ideal to administer pentamidine aerosol therapy.

Year Founded: 1969

2290 MedDev Corporation
MedDev Corporation
730 N Pastoria Avenue
Sunnyvale, CA 94085-3522
408-730-9702
Fax: 408-730-9732; *Toll Free:* 800-543-2789
info@meddev-corp.com
www.meddev-corp.com

Suzanne Gray, Owner

Aids to rehabilitate hands following injury or illness, including patented complementary FingerHelper, ThumbHelper and Iso HandHelper models. Med Dev also manufactures Soft Touch foam exercisers and the FiddlLink exerciser for digital dexterity. New for 2000, the Ultimate Hand Helper, an Ergonomically designed hand excerciser curved to confirm to the shape of the hand.

2291 Medi-Grip
Therapro, Inc.
225 Arlington Street
Framingham, MA 01702-8723
508-872-9494
Fax: 508-875-2062; *Toll Free:* 800-257-5376
info@theraproducts.com
www.theraproducts.com

Karen Conrad, Founder
Paul Weihrauch, Founder

Reasonably priced, non-skid material. This non-slip material is available in Marine Blue, Desert Sand and Burgundy, rolls 12 inches by 144 inches.

Year Founded: 1986

2292 Pill Splitter
EASE
3714 Copper Penny Lane
Auburn, CA 95602
928-636-9469
Fax: 530-888-6990; *Toll Free:* 800-327- 650
kmjc@northlink.com
www.accesswitease.com/

A mechanical device for opening pill bottles.

2293 Plum Enterprises
Plum Enterprises, Inc.
PO Box 85
Valley Forge, PA 19481
610-783-7377
Fax: 610-783-7577; *Toll Free:* 800-321-PLUM
info@plument.com
www.plument.com

Janice Carrington, CEO/ Founder

Patented Protective Wear made with material engineered specifically to absorb the energy of a fall. We exquisitley design each garment around its protective core with exacting detail and unmatched standards of quality.

Year Founded: 1983

2294 Plums Award Winning Protects Hip
Plum Enterprises, Inc.
Po Box 85
Valley Forge, PA 19481
610-783-7377
Fax: 610-783-7577; *Toll Free:* 800-321-PLUM
info@plument.com
www.plument.com

Janice Carrington, CEO/ Founder

Is engineered for safety, designed for exquiste simplicity.

Year Founded: 1983

2295 Protecta Capstet
Plum Enterprises, Inc.
Po Box 85
Valley Forge, PA 19481
610-783-7377
Fax: 610-783-7577; *Toll Free:* 800-321-PLUM
info@plument.com
www.plument.com

Janice Carrington, CEO/ Founder

Fits and works better than custom made helmets, lightest safest most comfortable. Prescribed post brain surgery, drop seizures, autism, hemophilia.

Year Founded: 1983

2296 ProtectaCap+PLUS, ProtectaHip
Plum Enterprises, Inc.
Po Box 85
Valley Forge, PA 19481
610-783-7377
Fax: 610-783-7577; *Toll Free:* 800-321-PLUM
info@plument.com
www.plument.com

Janice Carrington, CEO/ Founder

A distinctive dual core makes it the ultimate helmet for sports, hippo therapy and plagiocephaly.

Year Founded: 1983

2297 Talking Thermometers
Maxi-Aids, Inc.
42 Executive Boulevard
Farmingdale, NY 11735
631-752-0521
Fax: 631-752-0689; *Toll Free:* 800-522-6294
sales@maxiaids.com
www.maxiaids.com
TTY: 800-281-3555

Harold Zaretsky, President

Clearly announces temperature in Fahrenheit or Celcius.

2298 Therapy Putty
Therapro, Inc.
225 Arlington Street
Framingham, MA 01702-8723
508-872-9494
Fax: 508-875-2062; *Toll Free:* 800-257-5376
info@theraproducts.com
www.theraproducts.com

Karen Conrad, Founder
Paul Weihrauch, Founder

Designed to exercise and strengthen hands, ranging from soft to firm for developing a stronger grasp. Available in two, four and six ounce sizes. In unique clear fist shaped container.

Year Founded: 1986

2299 Battery Device Adapter
AbleNet, Inc.
2625 Patton Road
Roseville, MN 55113
651-294-2200
Fax: 651-294-2259; *Toll Free:* 800-322-0956
customerservice@ablenetinc.com
www.ablenetinc.com

Bill Sproull, Chairman of the Board
Jennifer Thalhuber, President/ Chief Executive Offic
William Mills, Strategic Planning Chair

A cable which connects to and adapts battery-operated devices for external switch control. Two sizes are available to adapt devices with AA or C and D size batteries.

Year Founded: 1985

2300 Custom Earmolds
Lloyds Hearing Aid
4435 Manchester Drive
Rockford, IL 61109
815-964-4191
Fax: 815-964-8378; *Toll Free:* 800-323-4212
www.lloydhearingaid.com

Andrew Palmquist, President
Marv Palmquist, Founder

Hearing aid molds, custom built to the exact fit of the customer.

2301 Duracell & Rayovac Hearing Aid Batteries
Lloyds Hearing Aid
4435 Manchester Drive
Rockford, IL 61109
815-964-4191
Fax: 815-964-8378; *Toll Free:* 800-323-4212
www.lloydhearingaid.com

Andrew Palmquist, President
Marv Palmquist, Founder

Batteries for hearing aids at discounted prices. As low as 70 cents each.

2302 HARC Mercantile-Division of HAC of America
HARC Mercantile Ltd.
5413 S. Westnedge Avenue
Suite A
Portage, MI 49002
269-324-1615
Fax: 269-324-2387; *Toll Free:* 800-445-9968
info@harc.com
www.harc.com
TTY: 269-324-1615

Mike Martinson, Managing Director

Specializes in products for the hard of hearing and deaf as required under ADA including visual alerting products for fire, phone, door, wake up, phone amplification, TTY, FM and infrared listening systems.

Year Founded: 1960

2303 Hearing Aid Batteries
HARC Mercantile Ltd.
5413 S. Westnedge Avenue
Suite A
Portage, MI 49002

269-324-1615
Fax: 269-324-2387; *Toll Free:* 800-445-9968
info@harc.com
www.harc.com
TTY: 269-324-1615

Mike Martinson, Managing Director

Hearing aid batteries in all popular sizes in mercury, zinc air, silver as well as Nicad and Varta, and batteries for electrolarynx and infrared systems.

Year Founded: 1960

2304 Hearing Aid Battery Testers
HARC Mercantile Ltd.
5413 S. Westnedge Avenue
Suite A
Portage, MI 49002
269-324-1615
Fax: 269-324-2387; *Toll Free:* 800-445-9968
info@harc.com
www.harc.com
TTY: 269-324-1615

Mike Martinson, Managing Director

From pocket size to professional type battery testers which test mercury, zinc air, silver, specialty and general usage batteries.

Year Founded: 1960

2305 Hearing Aid Dehumidifier
HARC Mercantile Ltd.
5413 S. Westnedge Avenue
Suite A
Portage, MI 49002
269-324-1615
Fax: 269-324-2387; *Toll Free:* 800-445-9968
info@harc.com
www.harc.com
TTY: 269-324-1615

Mike Martinson, Managing Director

Removes moisture from hearing aids and valuables. Contains desiccant pack and humidity guide, all in a rugged, vinyl case which provides protection and is water resistant.

Year Founded: 1960

2306 In the Ear Hearing Aid Battery Extractor
HARC Mercantile Ltd.
5413 S. Westnedge Avenue
Suite A
Portage, MI 49002
269-324-1615
Fax: 269-324-2387; *Toll Free:* 800-445-9968
info@harc.com
www.harc.com
TTY: 269-324-1615

Mike Martinson, Managing Director

Ideal tool to use when battery is stuck in battery compartment in ITE and canal hearing aids.

Year Founded: 1960

2307 Lloyd Hearing Aid Corporation
Lloyds Hearing Aid
4435 Manchester Drive
Rockford, IL 61109
815-964-4191
Fax: 815-964-8378; *Toll Free:* 800-323-4212

info@lloydhearingaid.com
www.lloydhearingaid.com

Marv Palmquist, Founder
Andrew Palmquist, President

Helps absorb any moisture that might damage the hearing aid.

2308 Mushroom Inserts
Lloyds Hearing Aid
4435 Manchester Drive
Rockford, IL 61109
815-964-4191
Fax: 815-964-8378; *Toll Free:* 800-323-4212
www.lloydhearingaid.com

Andrew Palmquist, President
Marv Palmquist, Founder

A universal earplug useful in wearing behind the ear type hearing instruments.

2309 Name Brand Hearing Aids
Lloyds Hearing Aid
4435 Manchester Drive
Rockford, IL 61109
815-964-4191
Fax: 815-964-8378; *Toll Free:* 800-323-4212
www.lloydhearingaid.com

Andrew Palmquist, President
Marv Palmquist, Founder

Hearing aids at discounts of up to 60%. Most makes and models with service to/from anywhere in the United States with a 30-day home trial.

2310 Oval Window Audio
Oval Window Audio
33 Wildflower Court
Nederland, CO 80466
303-447-3607
Fax: 303-447-3607
info@ovalwindowaudio.com
www.ovalwindowaudio.com
TDD 303-447-3607

Norman Lederman, Director of Research & Developme
Paula Hendricks, Educational Director

Manufacturer of induction loop hearing assistance technologies compatible with hearing aids already used by many hard of hearing people. Also multisensory sound systems for use in speech and music therapy and science classes.

Year Founded: 1984

Hobbies and Sports

2311 Score Card Set
American Printing House for the Blind
1839 Frankfort Avenue
PO Box 6085
Louisville, KY 40206-0085
502-895-2405
Fax: 502-899-2274; *Toll Free:* 800-223-1839
info@aph.org
www.aph.org

Tuck Tinsley, President
Bob Brasher, VP Advisory Services & Research
Gary Mudd

This handy card is made of durable plastic, has twenty buttons in two rows of ten and may be pushed up and down hundreds of times without wearing out. Can be used to keep count of the number of points scored by a sports team, or to count how many questions have been asked during '20 Questions.'

Year Founded: 1858

2312 Spectrum Aquatics
Spectrum Aquatics
7100 Spectrum Lane
Missoula, MO 59808
406-542-9781
Fax: 800-776-8057; Toll Free: 800-776-8056
info@spectrumaquatics.com
www.spectrumproducts.com/

Nabil Khaled, Director of Sales
Jon Mirkin, Business Development Specialist
Rob Nelson, Manager of Logistics & Customer

Leading manufacturers of assisted access lifts, stainless steel hydrotherapy tanks for the swimming pool and medical therapy markets.

Home Aids

2313 Abbey Home Healthcare
Abbey Home Healthcare Services, Inc.
3359 Belvedere Road
West Palm Beach, FL 33046
561-968-2425
Fax: 702-441-2632; Toll Free: 800-233-0098
www.abbeyhomehealth.com/

Ronald J Pion MD, Contact

Lifts, chairs, bathroom aids, bedroom aids, eating utensils and independent living aids for the physically challenged.

Year Founded: 1994

2314 Analog Clock Model
American Printing House for the Blind
1839 Frankfort Avenue
PO Box 6085
Louisville, KY 40206-0085
502-895-2405
Fax: 502-899-2274; Toll Free: 800-223-1839
info@aph.org
www.aph.org

Tuck Tinsley, President
Bob Brasher, VP/ Advisory Services & Research
Gary Mudd

The Analog Clock Model has hour and minute hands which are geared together and minute hands which are geared together and synchronized just like the hands on a functional clock. The hour hand is textured, while the minute hand is smooth and thin.

Year Founded: 1858

2315 Big Lamp Switch
Maxi-Aids, Inc.
42 Executive Boulevard
Farmingdale, NY 11735
631-752-0521
Fax: 631-752-0689; Toll Free: 800-522-6294
sales@maxiaids.com

www.maxiaids.com
TTY: 800-281-3555

Harold Zaretsky, President

This big, three-spoked knob replaces small rotating knobs which are a problem for those with arthritis or other limitations of the fingers.

2316 Cordless Receiver
AbleNet, Inc.
2625 Patton Road
Roseville, MN 55113
651-294-2200
Fax: 651-294-2259; Toll Free: 800-322-0956
customerservice@ablenetinc.com
www.ablenetinc.com

Bill Sproull, Chairman of the Board
Jennifer Thalhuber, President/ Chief Executive Offic
William Mills, Strategic Planning Chair

The Cordless Receiver in conjunction with the Cordless Big Red Switch, can be used anywhere a switch is currently used to control battery- or electrically - operated toys, games or appliances; augmentative communication systems; computers (through a computer switch interface).

Year Founded: 1985

2317 Dazor Manufacturing Corporation
Dazor Manufacturing Corporation
2079 Congressional
St. Louis, MO 63146
314-652-2400
Fax: 314-652-2069; Toll Free: 800-345-9103
info@dazor.com
www.dazor.com

Richard Kupferer, Marketing Coordinator
Morris Zuckerman, Inside Accounts Manager
Henry Dazey, Founder

Dazor is a US manufacturer of quality task lightning. Products include fluorescent, incandescent and halogen lighting fixtures to include illuminated magnifiers combine light and magnification to greatly enhance vision making activities such as reading as hobbies more enjoyable. All lamps come in a variety of mounting options to include desk bases, clamp on, floor stands and wall tracks. $95-$450.

Year Founded: 1938

2318 Dorma Architectural Hardware
DORMA
Dorma Drive Drawer AC
Reamstown, PA 17567
717-336-3881
Fax: 717-336-2106; Toll Free: 800-523-8483
jphillips@dorma-usa.com
www.dorma-usa.com

Larry O'Toole, CEO
John Bergstrom, Director Sales

DORMA provides a complete line of door controls including barrier-free units that comply with the Americans with Disabilities Act. A wide variety of surface applied and concealed closers and exit devices are available to address these requirements.

Year Founded: 1908

2319 Dual Switch Latch and Timer
AbleNet, Inc.
2625 Patton Road
Roseville, MN 55113
651-294-2200
Fax: 651-294-2259; Toll Free: 800-322-0956
customerservice@ablenetinc.com
www.ablenetinc.com

Bill Sproull, Chairman of the Board
Jennifer Thalhuber, President/ Chief Executive Offic
William Mills, Strategic Planning Chair

A Dual Switch Latch and Timer allows two users to activate two devices at a time in the latch, timed seconds or timed minutes mode of control.

Year Founded: 1985

2320 Emergency Response Telephone
HARC Mercantile Ltd.
5413 S. Westnedge Avenue
Suite A
Portage, MI 49002
269-324-1615
Fax: 269-324-2387; Toll Free: 800-445-9968
info@harc.com
www.harc.com
TTY: 269-324-1615

Mike Martinson, Managing Director

Press the emergency button and it dials up to 5 pre-programmed phone numbers of neighbors or family to get emergency help. Not monitored no monthly charge.

Year Founded: 1960

2321 Foot Placement Ladder
Bailey Manufacturing Company
PO Box 130
Lodi, OH 44254-0130
330-948-1080
Fax: 800-224-5390; Toll Free: 800-321-8372
www.baileymfg.com

Larry Strimple, President

Adjustable cross bars for different length steps. Reinforced metal crosses for easier climbing for the physically-disabled.

Year Founded: 1956

2322 Handy Reacher
EASE
3714 Copper Penny Lane
Auburn, CA 95602
928-636-9469
Fax: 530-888-6990; Toll Free: 800-327- 650
kmjc@northlink.com
www.accesswithease.com/

Long handled reacher retrieves items off high shelves.

2323 Knock Light
HARC Mercantile Ltd.
5413 S. Westnedge Avenue
Suite A
Portage, MI 49002
269-324-1615
Fax: 269-324-2387; Toll Free: 800-445-9968
info@harc.com
www.harc.com
TTY: 269-324-1615

Mike Martinson, Managing Director
Easily attaches to a door with velcro, portable.
Year Founded: 1960

2324 Longreach Reacher
Therapro, Inc.
225 Arlington Street
Framingham, MA 01702-8723
508-872-9494
Fax: 508-875-2062; Toll Free: 800-257-5376
info@theraproducts.com
www.theraproducts.com

Karen Conrad, Founder
Paul Weihrauch, Founder

Reacher is useful when reaching, sitting or when standing.
Year Founded: 1986

2325 Loop Scissors
Therapro, Inc.
225 Arlington Street
Framingham, MA 01702-8723
508-872-9494
Fax: 508-875-2062; Toll Free: 800-257-5376
info@theraproducts.com
www.theraproducts.com

Karen Conrad, Founder
Paul Weihrauch, Founder

Pliable, plastic handles that allow for easy and controlled cutting.
Year Founded: 1986

2326 Magnifier Highlights
Independent Living Aids, LLC
137 Rano Street
Buffalo, NY 14207
516-937-1848
Fax: 516-937-3906; Toll Free: 800-537-2118
techsupport@independentliving.com
www.independentliving.com

Marvin Sandler, President

Carries a full line of magnifiers, ranging from high-powered vision aids to hoppy instruments and accessories.

2327 Personal Amplifier
HARC Mercantile Ltd.
5413 S. Westnedge Avenue
Suite A
Portage, MI 49002
269-324-1615
Fax: 269-324-2387; Toll Free: 800-445-9968
info@harc.com
www.harc.com
TTY: 269-324-1615

Mike Martinson, Managing Director

Small personal amplifier with choice of headphones, earbuds or induction neckloop amplifies sounds for those who are hard of hearing.
Year Founded: 1960

2328 PowerLink 2 Control Unit
AbleNet, Inc.
2625 Patton Road
Roseville, MN 55113

651-294-2200
Fax: 651-294-2259; *Toll Free:* 800-322-0956
customerservice@ablenetinc.com
www.ablenetinc.com

Bill Sproull, Chairman of the Board
Jennifer Thalhuber, President/ Chief Executive Offic
William Mills, Strategic Planning Chair

The PowerLink 2 Control Unit allows switch operation of electrical appliances. It can be used to activate 1 or 2 appliances (up to 1700 watts combined). If 2 appliances are used, they will activate simultaneously. There are four modes of control on the PowerLink 2; direct mode, timed (seconds) mode, timed (minutes) mode and latch mode.

Year Founded: 1985

2329 Small Appliance Receiver
AbleNet, Inc.
2625 Patton Road
Roseville, MN 55113
651-294-2200
Fax: 651-294-2259; *Toll Free:* 800-322-0956
customerservice@ablenetinc.com
www.ablenetinc.com

Bill Sproull, Chairman of the Board
Jennifer Thalhuber, President/ Chief Executive Offic
William Mills, Strategic Planning Chair

The Small Appliance Receiver, in conjunction with the Cordless Big Red Switch, allows you to control small electrical appliances in the environment without a cord. It should only be used with low-wattage appliances (under 500 watts) which have two prong plugs (ie, radios, fans, lamps, blenders, etc.). It should not be used with heat generating appliances.

Year Founded: 1985

2330 Tactile Smoke Detector
HARC Mercantile Ltd.
5413 S. Westnedge Avenue
Suite A
Portage, MI 49002
269-324-1615
Fax: 269-324-2387; *Toll Free:* 800-445-9968
info@harc.com
www.harc.com
TTY: 269-324-1615

Mike Martinson, Managing Director

Battery powered smoke detector with transmitter signals to a receiver with a powerful bed shaker for night-time alerting.

Year Founded: 1960

2331 Telephone Signaler
HARC Mercantile Ltd.
5413 S. Westnedge Avenue
Suite A
Portage, MI 49002
269-324-1615
Fax: 269-324-2387; *Toll Free:* 800-445-9968
info@harc.com; www.harc.com
TTY: 269-324-1615

Mike Martinson, Managing Director

Plugs into phone jack to signal incoming calls with extra loud ring and flashing strobe light.

Year Founded: 1960

2332 Tinnitus Masker
HARC Mercantile Ltd.
5413 S. Westnedge Avenue
Suite A
Portage, MI 49002
269-324-1615
Fax: 269-324-2387; *Toll Free:* 800-445-9968
info@harc.com
www.harc.com
TTY: 269-324-1615

Mike Martinson, Managing Director

Bedside unit produces varied sounds to help mask tinnitus to let you sleep easy.

Year Founded: 1960

2333 Vibrating Personal Pager
HARC Mercantile Ltd.
5413 S. Westnedge Avenue
Suite A
Portage, MI 49002
269-324-1615
Fax: 269-324-2387; *Toll Free:* 800-445-9968
info@harc.com
www.harc.com
TTY: 269-324-1615

Mike Martinson, Managing Director

Small belt worn pager that vibrates when the call button is pressed. 100 foot range.

Year Founded: 1960

2334 Vibrating Watch
HARC Mercantile Ltd.
5413 S. Westnedge Avenue
Suite A
Portage, MI 49002
269-324-1615
Fax: 269-324-2387; *Toll Free:* 800-445-9968
info@harc.com
www.harc.com
TTY: 269-324-1615

Mike Martinson, Managing Director

Watches that vibrate on your wrist when the alarm goes off or as reminders for medication, etc. Automatically reset for specified period of time.

Year Founded: 1960

2335 Visual Smoke Detector
HARC Mercantile Ltd.
5413 S. Westnedge Avenue
Suite A
Portage, MI 49002
269-324-1615
Fax: 269-324-2387; *Toll Free:* 800-445-9968
info@harc.com
www.harc.com
TTY: 269-324-1615

Mike Martinson, Managing Director

Smoke detector with 177 candella strobe and 95 dB audible alarm. AC powered portable or hardwired models available.

Year Founded: 1960

2336 Weather Alert Systems
HARC Mercantile Ltd.
5413 S. Westnedge Avenue
Suite A
Portage, MI 49002
269-324-1615
Fax: 269-324-2387; *Toll Free:* 800-445-9968
info@harc.com
www.harc.com
TTY: 269-324-1615

Mike Martinson, Managing Director

Weather alert radio with choice of a flashing strobe or bedshaker to alert to any dangerous weather conditions.

Year Founded: 1960

Kitchen and Eating Aids

2337 Adjustable Clear Acrylic Tray
Bailey Manufacturing Company
PO Box 130
Lodi, OH 44254-0130
330-948-1080
Fax: 800-224-5390; *Toll Free:* 800-321-8372
www.baileymfg.com

Larry Strimple, President

Adjusts for height and depth and is equipped with a spill rim for easy to clean edges.

Year Founded: 1956

2338 Bagel Holder
Maxi-Aids, Inc.
42 Executive Boulevard
Farmingdale, NY 11735
631-752-0521
Fax: 631-752-0689; *Toll Free:* 800-522-6294
sales@maxiaids.com
www.maxiaids.com
TTY: 800-281-3555

Harold Zaretsky, President

Holds bagels in place for easy slicing.

2339 Big Bold Timer Low Vision
Maxi-Aids, Inc.
42 Executive Boulevard
Farmingdale, NY 11735
631-752-0521
Fax: 631-752-0689; *Toll Free:* 800-522-6294
sales@maxiaids.com
www.maxiaids.com
TTY: 800-281-3555

Harold Zaretsky, President

Sixty-minute mechanical timer with large, easy-to-read numbers for the vision impaired.

2340 Capscrew
EASE
3714 Copper Penny Lane
Auburn, CA 95602
928-636-9469
Fax: 530-888-6990; *Toll Free:* 800-327- 650
kmjc@northlink.com
www.accesswithease.com/

Remove lids and caps easily.

2341 Cordless Receiver
AbleNet, Inc.
2625 Patton Road
Roseville, MN 55113
651-294-2200
Fax: 651-294-2259; *Toll Free:* 800-322-0956
customerservice@ablenetinc.com
www.ablenetinc.com

Bill Sproull, Chairman of the Board
Jennifer Thalhuber, President/ Chief Executive Offic
William Mills, Strategic Planning Chair

The Cordless Receiver in conjunction with the Cordless Big Red Switch, can be used anywhere a switch is currently used to control battery- or electrically - operated toys, games or appliances; augmentative communication systems; computers (through a computer switch interface).

Year Founded: 1985

2342 Deluxe Long Ring Low Vision Timer Tactile
Maxi-Aids, Inc.
42 Executive Boulevard
Farmingdale, NY 11735
631-752-0521
Fax: 631-752-0689; *Toll Free:* 800-522-6294
sales@maxiaids.com
www.maxiaids.com
TTY: 800-281-3555

Harold Zaretsky, President

Bold black numerals on white background allows for easy reading at any distance.

2343 Easy Pour Locking Lid Pot
Maxi-Aids, Inc.
42 Executive Boulevard
Farmingdale, NY 11735
631-752-0521
Fax: 631-752-0689; *Toll Free:* 800-522-6294
sales@maxiaids.com
www.maxiaids.com
TTY: 800-281-3555

Harold Zaretsky, President

Baked enamel and dishwasher safe, the pot comes with an easy lid that locks in place for extra safety.

2344 Electric Can Opener & Knife Sharpener
Maxi-Aids, Inc.
42 Executive Boulevard
Farmingdale, NY 11735
631-752-0521
Fax: 631-752-0689; *Toll Free:* 800-522-6294
sales@maxiaids.com
www.maxiaids.com
TTY: 800-281-3555

Harold Zaretsky, President

Features include a powerful magnet lid holder, the ability to open odd-shaped cans, and easy operation for the physically challenged.

2345 Food Markers/Magnets
Maxi-Aids, Inc.
42 Executive Boulevard
Farmingdale, NY 11735
631-752-0521
Fax: 631-752-0689; *Toll Free:* 800-522-6294
sales@maxiaids.com

www.maxiaids.com
TTY: 800-281-3555

Harold Zaretsky, President

These are durable plastic markers, easily identified by touch, texture, shape and form which help the visually impaired orient themselves to food location on the plate.

2346 Food Markers/Rubberbands
Maxi-Aids, Inc.
42 Executive Boulevard
Farmingdale, NY 11735
631-752-0521
Fax: 631-752-0689; Toll Free: 800-522-6294
sales@maxiaids.com
www.maxiaids.com
TTY: 800-281-3555

Harold Zaretsky, President

These are durable plastic markers, easily identified by touch, texture, shape and form which help the visually impaired orient themselves to food location on the plate.

2347 Good Grips Cutlery
Therapro, Inc.
225 Arlington Street
Framingham, MA 01702-8723
508-872-9494
Fax: 508-875-2062; Toll Free: 800-257-5376
info@theraproducts.com
www.theraproducts.com

Karen Conrad, Owner

Stainless steel utensils have a special twist built into the metal to facilitate bending of a spoon or fork at any angle for right or left handed people.

2348 Guide A Knife
Maxi-Aids, Inc.
42 Executive Boulevard
Farmingdale, NY 11735
631-752-0521
Fax: 631-752-0689; Toll Free: 800-522-6294
sales@maxiaids.com
www.maxiaids.com
TTY: 800-281-3555

Harold Zaretsky, President

Adjustable food slicing system guides the knife for even, uniform slices while protecting the user.

2349 Handy-Helper Cutting Board
Maxi-Aids, Inc.
42 Executive Boulevard
Farmingdale, NY 11735
631-752-0521
Fax: 631-752-0689; Toll Free: 800-522-6294
sales@maxiaids.com
www.maxiaids.com
TTY: 800-281-3555

Harold Zaretsky, President

Laminated cutting board with unique features to hold food in place with corner ledge for cutting and spreading.

2350 Innerlip Plates
Therapro, Inc.
225 Arlington Street
Framingham, MA 01702-8723

508-872-9494
Fax: 508-875-2062; Toll Free: 800-257-5376
info@theraproducts.com
www.theraproducts.com

Karen Conrad, Founder
Paul Weihrauch, Founder

Food maybe pushed to the side of the plate, then scooped up with a fork and spoon. Available in beige or blue.

Year Founded: 1986

2351 Magnetic Card Reader
Maxi-Aids, Inc.
42 Executive Boulevard
Farmingdale, NY 11735
631-752-0521
Fax: 631-752-0689; Toll Free: 800-522-6294
sales@maxiaids.com
www.maxiaids.com
TTY: 800-281-3555

Harold Zaretsky, President

Produces audible labels so a recorded card could be taped on cans of food or a box of cake mix; even adding instructions for baking.

2352 Maxi Aid Braille Timer
Maxi-Aids, Inc.
42 Executive Boulevard
Farmingdale, NY 11735
631-752-0521
Fax: 631-752-0689; Toll Free: 800-522-6294
sales@maxiaids.com
www.maxiaids.com
TTY: 800-281-3555

Harold Zaretsky, President

Three raised dots at 15, 30 and 45, two raised dots at remaining five minute intervals and one raised dot at remaining two and a half minute intervals, offers ease of operation to make this a helpful aid for the visually impaired.

2353 Nosey Cup
Therapro, Inc.
225 Arlington Street
Framingham, MA 01702-8723
508-872-9494
Fax: 508-875-2062; Toll Free: 800-257-5376
info@theraproducts.com
www.theraproducts.com

Karen Conrad, Founder
Paul Weihrauch, Founder

For those with a stiff neck, or persons who can't tip their head back while drinking.

Year Founded: 1986

2354 Paring Boards
Therapro, Inc.
225 Arlington Street
Framingham, MA 01702-8723
508-872-9494
Fax: 508-875-2062; Toll Free: 800-257-5376
info@theraproducts.com
www.theraproducts.com

Karen Conrad, Founder
Paul Weihrauch, Founder

Suction feet stabilize board and stainless steel prongs hold food in place for easy one-handed cutting.

Year Founded: 1986

2355 PowerLink 2 Control Unit
AbleNet, Inc.
2625 Patton Road
Roseville, MN 55113
651-294-2200
Fax: 651-294-2259; Toll Free: 800-322-0956
customerservice@ablenetinc.com
www.ablenetinc.com

Bill Sproull, Chairman of the Board
Jennifer Thalhuber, President/ Chief Executive Offic
William Mills, Strategic Planning Chair

The PowerLink 2 Control Unit allows switch operation of electrical appliances. It can be used to activate 1 or 2 appliances (up to 1700 watts combined). If 2 appliances are used, they will activate simultaneously. There are four modes of control on the PowerLink 2; direct mode, timed (seconds) mode, timed (minutes) mode and latch mode. Meets safety standards from Underwriters Laboratory (UL) and Canadian Standards Association (CSA) for electrical

Year Founded: 1985

2356 Slicing Aid
Snug Seat Inc.
12801 E. Independence Blvd.
PO Box 1739
Matthews, NC 28106
704-882-0668
Fax: 704-882-0751; Toll Free: 800-336-7684
information@snugseat.com
www.snugseat.com

Kirk MacKenzie, President
Scott Crosswhite, VP
Greg Tiller, Controller

The design of these knives allows a better working posture and makes optimal use of strength in the arms and hands.

Year Founded: 1982

2357 Small Appliance Receiver
AbleNet, Inc.
2625 Patton Road
Roseville, MN 55113
651-294-2200
Fax: 651-294-2259; Toll Free: 800-322-0956
customerservice@ablenetinc.com
www.ablenetinc.com

Bill Sproull, Chairman of the Board
Jennifer Thalhuber, President/ Chief Executive Offic
William Mills, Strategic Planning Chair

The Small Appliance Receiver, in conjunction with the Cordless Big Red Switch, allows you to control small electrical appliances in the environment without a cord. It should only be used with low-wattage appliances (under 500 watts) which have two prong plugs (ie, radios, fans, lamps, blenders, etc.). It should not be used with heat generating appliances.

Year Founded: 1985

2358 Steel Food Guard
Maxi-Aids, Inc.
42 Executive Boulevard
Farmingdale, NY 11735

631-752-0521
Fax: 631-752-0689; Toll Free: 800-522-6294
sales@maxiaids.com
www.maxiaids.com
TTY: 800-281-3555

Harold Zaretsky, President

Provides stable area to push against while eating.

2359 Thick-n-Easy
Therapro, Inc.
225 Arlington Street
Framingham, MA 01702-8723
508-872-9494
Fax: 508-875-2062; Toll Free: 800-257-5376
info@theraproducts.com
www.theraproducts.com

Karen Conrad, Founder
Paul Weihrauch, Founder

Instant food thickener that sets in 30 seconds and will not become thicker even after refrigeration.

Year Founded: 1986

2360 Thumbs Up Cup
Therapro, Inc.
225 Arlington Street
Framingham, MA 01702-8723
508-872-9494
Fax: 508-875-2062; Toll Free: 800-257-5376
info@theraproducts.com
www.theraproducts.com

Karen Conrad, Founder
Paul Weihrauch, Founder

This cup is designed for those with limited strength or coordination or arthritis. The two backward-tilt handles and thumb rests allow finger joint to be used to their greatest mechanical advantage.

Year Founded: 1986

2361 Universal Hand Cuff
Therapro, Inc.
225 Arlington Street
Framingham, MA 01702-8723
508-872-9494
Fax: 508-875-2062; Toll Free: 800-257-5376
info@theraproducts.com
www.theraproducts.com

Karen Conrad, Founder
Paul Weihrauch, Founder

Comfortable cuff with Velcro strap holds utensils, toothbrushes, etc.

Year Founded: 1986

Lifts, Ramps, Elevators

2362 Access Industries/ThyssenKrupp Access
ThyssenKrupp Access Solutions
4001 E 138th Street
Grandview, MO 64030-2837
Fax: 816-763-4467; Toll Free: 800-829-9760
www.tkaccess.com

Thomas Hance, President
Ray Demes, VP Field Office Consumer Care
Chuck Herling

Committed to improving the quality of life. We are the world's most trusted name in accessibility solutions. Offers a full line of sairway lifts, wheelchair lifts, and elevators. Our nationwide network of certifies dealers ensures you will recieve a prompt, courteous, knowledge service from professional in your area.

Year Founded: 1811

2363 Accessibility Lift
Inclinator Company of America
601 Gibson Boulevard
Harrisburg, PA 17104
717-939-8420
Fax: 717-939-8075; Toll Free: 800-343-9007
www.inclinator.com

Paul R Krum, President

An economical lift for restricted usage that provides barrier-free access that can be used by churches, schools, lodging halls and meeting halls to meet compliance requirements, with the dignified convenience and freedom they deserve.

Year Founded: 1923

2364 AlumiRamp
AlumiRamp, Inc.
855 E Chicago Road
Quincy, MI 49082
Fax: 517-639-4314; Toll Free: 800-800-3864
sales@alumiramp.com
www.alumiramp.com

Linda Burke, President

Complete line of modular and portable ramps for both home and vehicle use. Welded construction and an wieght aluminum are featured on all our ramps.

Year Founded: 1986

2365 Amigo Mobility International
Amigo Mobility International
6693 Dixie Highway
Bridgeport, MI 48722-9725
989-777-0910
Fax: 800-334-7274; Toll Free: 800-692-6446
info@myamigo.com
myamigo.com

Beth Thieme, VP Commercial Sales
Alison Newkirk, West Region Account Manager
Sandy Roth

An industry leader in power-operated vehicles/motorized scooters. we provide innovative, durable and customized mobility solutions to mobility challenges facing the disabled, injured and seniors worldwide.

Year Founded: 1968

2366 Aquatic Access Pool Lifts for Pools and Spas
Aquatic Access Inc.
1921 Production Drive
Louisville, KY 40299
502-425-5817
Fax: 502-425-9607; Toll Free: 800-325-5438
info@aquaticaccess.com
www.aquaticaccess.com

Linda Nolan, President
Liz Waters, Marketing
John Nolan, Founder

Aquatic Access manufactures a variety of water-powered lifts that provide access to in-ground and above-ground pools, spas, therapy tubs, boats and docks. ADA compliant models available.

Year Founded: 1962

2367 Area Access
Area Access Inc.
7131 Gateway Court
Manassas, VA 20109
703-396-4949
Fax: 703-207-0446; Toll Free: 800-333-AREA
www.areaaccess.com

Scott Hobson, Owner

Serving the entire Mid-Atlantic with scooters, stairway lifts and elevators. Large inventory and fully stocked showrooms.

Year Founded: 1983

2368 Barrier Free Lifts
Barrier Free Lifts, Inc.
1620 SW 17th St
Ocala, FL 34471
703-361-6531
Fax: 866-378-3318; Toll Free: 800-582-8732
us-office@barrierfreelifts.com
www.barrierfreelifts.com/

Cecil K. Rider, Owner and President
Deborah Hensley, VP/Operations
Teresa Kirk, Administrative Assistant

Barrier Free ceiling and floor model lift systems are available in many models. Ceiling lifts can be portable, fully motorized and state-of-the-art to provide truly barrier-free equipment for lifting and transferring patients. Floor models include the premier LEXA with motorized spreader bar for patient positioning and the RAISA with motorized, adjustable knee pads for standing patients up and gait training. Ceiling lifts available with AIR TUBE

Year Founded: 2004

2369 Braille Plates for Elevator
Maxi-Aids, Inc.
42 Executive Boulevard
Farmingdale, NY 11735
631-752-0521
Fax: 631-752-0689; Toll Free: 800-522-6294
sales@maxiaids.com
www.maxiaids.com
TTY: 800-281-3555

Harold Zaretsky, President

The plates have curing type pressure sensitive material applied for metal to metal bonding.

2370 Bruno Independent Living Aids
Bruno Independent Living Aids
1780 Executive Drive
Po Box 84
Oconomowoc, WI 53066
262-567-4990
Fax: 262-953-5501; Toll Free: 800-882-8183
www.bruno.com

Michael R Bruno II, President/CEO
Patrick Foy, National Sales Manager
Anne Tyler

An ISO 9001 Certified Manufacturer of automotive lifts for scooter, wheelchairs, and powerchairs, three and four wheel scooters, and straight and custom curve stairlifts.

Year Founded: 1984

2371 Cheney's Liberty II
Handi-Lift, Inc.
730 Garden Street
Carlstadt, NJ 07072
201-933-0111
Fax: 201-933-0050; *Toll Free:* 800-432-LIFT
sales@handi-lift.com, drawings@handi-lift.com
www.handilift.com

Scott Darling, President

Economical lift for straight stairways.

Year Founded: 1975

2372 Classique
Handi-Lift, Inc.
730 Garden Street
Carlstadt, NJ 07072
201-933-0111
Fax: 201-933-0050; *Toll Free:* 800-432-LIFT
sales@handi-lift.com, drawings@handi-lift.com
www.handilift.com

Scott Darling, President

The Classique elevator answers access problems in churches, schools and small offices.

Year Founded: 1975

2373 Cub, SuperCub and Special Edition Scooters
Bruno Independent Living Aids
1780 Executive Drive
Po Box 84
Oconomowoc, WI 53066
262-567-4990
Fax: 262-953-5501; *Toll Free:* 800-882-8183
www.bruno.com

Michael R Bruno II, President/CEO
Patrick Foy, National Sales Manager
Anne Tyler

Bruno Independent Living Aids has over 12 different scooter models. Bruno Cub and SuperCub scooters, has front-or-rear wheel drive, in both 3-and-4 wheel versions and comes in four different colors plus a pediatric version. Each scooter can handle up to 300 pounds. Bruno Special Edition scooters resemble a fire engine, police car, Humvee and motorcycle.

Year Founded: 1984

2374 Custom Lift Residential Elevators
Waupaca Elevator Company
1726 N Ballard Road
Appleton, WI 54911
920-991-9082
Fax: 920-991-9087; *Toll Free:* 800-238-8739
info@waupacaelevator.com
www.waupacaelevator.com

Kari C Stumpf, Administration/Dealer Referrals

Waupac Elevator is an industry leader in the manufacturing of residential elevators and dumbwaiters. Our residential elevators can readily accommodate several people, a motorized wheelchair or scooter, or a wheelchair with a care-

giver. Consider Waupaca Elevator when you desire to add value, convenience, and reliability to today's homes.

Year Founded: 1957

2375 EZ-Access Portable Ramps
Homecare Products
1704 B St NW Ste 110
Auburn, WA 98001-1650
844-335-0816
Fax: 127-062-6604; *Toll Free:* 800-451-1903
www.homecaretechnology.co.uk/

Don Everard, VP Marketing
Deanne Sandvold, VP Sales

EZ-ACCESS Ramps bridge gaps over curbs and steps, allowing scooters and wheelchairs to continue on a smooth, safe course. Available in several different styles and sizes, ranging from a two-foot curb ramp to a 10-foot multi-purpose ramp. All ramps are made of anodized aluminum.

2376 Easy Pivot Transfer Machine
Rand-Scot, Inc.
401 Linden Center Drive
Fort Collins, CO 80524
970-484-7967
Fax: 970-484-3800; *Toll Free:* 800-467-7967
info@randscott.com
randscot.com/

Joel Lerich, Founder
Barbara , Founder

The Easy Pivot Patient Lifting System allows for strain-free, one-caregiver transfers of the disabled individual.

Year Founded: 1980

2377 Easy Stand
Altimate Medical, Inc.
262 W 1st. St.
Morton, MN 56270
507-697-6393
Fax: 507-697-6900; *Toll Free:* 800-342-8968
info@easystand.com
www.easystand.com

Alan Tholkes, President/CEO
Mark Schmitt, Sales & Marketing Director

Designed to make standing fast and simple. The easy to operate hydraulic lift system provides a controlled lifting and lowering. With the convenience of simply transferring to the chair and reaching a standing position in seconds with no straps to hassle with.

Year Founded: 1987

2378 EcoTraction Surface
Bike Track, Inc.
PO Box 235
Woodstock, VT 05091
802-457-3275
Fax: 802-457-3704; *Toll Free:* 888-663-8537
info@biketrack.com
www.biketrack.com

Nancy Hoblinest, Sales/Logistics
Barry McVey, President

2379 Economical Liberty
Handi-Lift, Inc.
730 Garden Street
Carlstadt, NJ 07072
201-933-0111
Fax: 201-933-0050; *Toll Free:* 800-432-LIFT
www.handilift.com

Doug Boydston, President/Co-Founder

Installs quickly and easily on most straight stairways. It
uses regular household current and mounts over the carpet
or directly to the stairs without marring.

2380 Elevette 2100
Inclinator Company of America
601 Gibson Boulevard
Harrisburg, PA 17104
717-939-8420
Fax: 717-939-8075; *Toll Free:* 800-343-9007
isales@inclinator.com
www.inclinator.com

Paul R Krum, President

A newly designed residential elevator which reduces
weight dramatically and permits the use of lower power
and less costly motors.

Year Founded: 1923

2381 Excel Stair Lift
ThyssenKrupp Access Solutions
4001 E 138th Street
Grandview, MO 64030-2837
800-925-3100
Fax: 816-763-4467; *Toll Free:* 800-925-3100
www.tkaccess.com

Thomas Hance, President
Ray Demes, VP Field Office Consumer Care
Chuck Herling

Installs easily on either side of a straight stairway for independent, step-free living. The lift fastens securely to the
stairs without marring walls and is adjustable to match any
stairway slope with an incline angle up to 45 degrees.
Available with battery back up.

Year Founded: 1811

2382 Ez International Inc./Ortho Kinetics
Electro Kinetic Technologies
W194 N11301 McCormick Drive
Germantown, WI 53022
262-250-7740
Fax: 262-250-7741; *Toll Free:* 800-824-1068
www.orthokinetics.com

William Grady, Sales Manager

Products to enhance people's lives through mobility. These
electric three and four wheel vehicles are designed to sur-
pass consumer expectations by providing total comfort,
convenience and performance features found nowhere else.
Ortho-Kinetics has a full line of vehicles for any
application.

2383 Handi Home Lift
Handi-Lift, Inc.
730 Garden Street
Carlstadt, NJ 07072
201-933-0111
Fax: 201-933-0050; *Toll Free:* 800-432-LIFT

sales@handi-lift.com
www.handilift.com

Douglas Boydston, Owner

An outdoor lift designed to provide access over porch stairs
or other steps that impede movement.

2384 Handi Prolift
Handi-Lift, Inc.
730 Garden Street
Carlstadt, NJ 07072
201-933-0111
Fax: 201-933-0050; *Toll Free:* 800-432-LIFT
sales@handi-lift.com
www.handilift.com

Douglas Boydston, Owner

Provides dependable vertical transportation for multi-level
buildings.

2385 Handi-Ramp
Handi-Ramp, Inc.
510 North Avenue
Libertyville, IL 60048
847-680-7700
Fax: 847-816-8866; *Toll Free:* 800-876-7267
info@handiramp.com
www.handi-ramp.com

Thom Disch, President and CEO
Ken Knapp, Contact

Provides a complete line of economical, ADA Compliant
access ramping products. Line includes Van attachable and
Wheelchair Tie Dows; Aluminum or Expanded Meal Folding Portables; aluminum channels; Portable, Sectional
Ramp Systems; Semi-Permanent Ramps, Platforms and
Systems. All ramp series are available in varied lengths and
widths in combination with platforms and optional hand
railing, single or double bar construction with return ends.
Specia

Year Founded: 1958

2386 Homewaiter
Inclinator Company of America
601 Gibson Boulevard
Harrisburg, PA 17104
717-939-8420
Fax: 717-939-8075; *Toll Free:* 800-343-9007
isales@inclinator.com
www.inclinator.com

Paul R Krum, President

With its roller truck riding in a specially formed monorail,
it is easy to install and highly adaptable to existing conditions. It can travel up to 35 feet, opening on any or all three
sides at different stations, whether at counter level or floor
level.

Year Founded: 1923

2387 Inclinette
Inclinator Company of America
601 Gibson Boulevard
Harrisburg, PA 17104
717-939-8420
Fax: 717-939-8075; *Toll Free:* 800-343-9007
isales@inclinator.com
www.inclinator.com

Paul Krum, President

Inclinette provides comfort and convenience in providing multi-floor access to persons who have difficulty climbing stairs.

Year Founded: 1923

2388 Leg Elevation Board
Bailey Manufacturing Company
PO Box 130
Lodi, OH 44254-0130
330-948-1080
Fax: 800-224-5390; *Toll Free:* 800-321-8372
www.baileymfg.com

Larry Strimple, President

Includes seven positions to a 30 degree incline, three pillows with Velcro, easy carry hand slot and a natural finish.

Year Founded: 1956

2389 Liberty LT
Handi-Lift, Inc.
730 Garden Street
Carlstadt, NJ 07072
201-933-0111
Fax: 201-933-0050; *Toll Free:* 800-432-LIFT
sales@handi-lift.com
www.handilift.com

Douglas Boydston, President/Co-Founder

Stair lift with dual armrests that lock into position. The comfortable, contoured seat is designed to swivel and move forward at the bottom or top landings to facilitate transfer.

2390 Minivator Residential Elevator
ThyssenKrupp Access Solutions
4001 E 138th Street
Grandview, MO 64030-2837
816-763-3100
Fax: 816-763-4467; *Toll Free:* 800-925-3100
www.tkaccess.com

Evelyn Johnson, Marketing Supervisor
Tom Hance, President

The perfect choice for a person who is contemplating moving from their multi-storied home because they cannot get up and down the stairs. The low cost, compact Minivator elevator can help these people live independently. The Minivator can be installed in the corner of a room without a shaft or hoistway, so the elevator doesn't have to disfigure the structure. The Minivator elevator can take a person or persons between floors in less than a minute

Year Founded: 1811

2391 Pool + Spa Lifts
Aquatic Access Inc.
1921 Production Drive
Louisville, KY 40299
502-425-5817
Fax: 502-425-9607; *Toll Free:* 800-325-5438
info@aquaticaccess.com
www.AquaticAccess.com

David Nolan, CEO
Linda Nolan, President

Provide independent or assisted access to in-ground pools. Lifts are powered with water pressure from a garden hose, and are portable. Some lifts have a three-hundred pound lift capacity and others have a four-hundred pound capacity,

perfect for commercial installations or home use. ADA compliant

Year Founded: 1987

2392 Pool Lifts for In-Ground Pools
Aquatic Access Inc.
1921 Production Drive
Louisville, KY 40299
502-425-5817
Fax: 502-425-9607; *Toll Free:* 800-325-5438
info@aquaticaccess.com
www.aquaticaccess.com

Kathy Nolan, Sales
Marie Worsham, Sales
John Nolan, Founder

Year Founded: 1962

2393 Porch-Lift Vertical Platform Lift
ThyssenKrupp Access Solutions
4001 E 138th Street
Grandview, MO 64030-2837
816-763-3100
Fax: 816-763-4467; *Toll Free:* 800-925-3100
www.tkaccess.com

Thomas Hance, President
Ray Demes, VP Field Office Consumer Affairs
Chuck Herling

Provide stairway access indoor and out for people who use wheelchairs. Lifting heights range from 1 to 144 feet and are available for both commercial and residential applications. Easy to install and operate, the units are space and cost efficient solutions to ADA compliance.

Year Founded: 1811

2394 RDL Supply
RDL Supply
11240 Gemini Lane
Dallas, TX 75229
214-630-3965
Fax: 214-560-0326; *Toll Free:* 800-688-1758
sales@rdlsupply.com
www.rdlsupply.com

Jim Goldthwaite, National Sales Manager
Sheri Martin, CEO

Power door, low energy door operators.

Year Founded: 1981

2395 Ricon Corporation
Ricon
7900 Nelson Road
Panorama City, CA 91402
818-267-3000
Fax: 818-267-3001; *Toll Free:* 800-322-2884
sales@RiconCorp.com
www.riconcorp.com

William Baldwin, CEO

Ricon corporation is a world leader in the manufacture of lifts and other mobility products for people with disabilities. The Ricon product line features the Activan(R) a lowered floor minivan conversion, wheelchair lifts power seat base and automatic door openers.

Year Founded: 1971

2396 Scooter, Power Chair and Wheelchair Lifts
Bruno Independent Living Aids
1780 Executive Drive
Po Box 84
Oconomowoc, WI 53066
262-567-4990
Fax: 262-953-5501; *Toll Free:* 800-882-8183
www.bruno.com

Michael R Bruno II, President/CEO
Patrick Foy, National Sales Manager
Anne Tyler

Over 18 different styles of automobile lifts for scooters,
wheelchairs, and powerchairs for nearly any car, van, truck,
or sport utility vehicle that can raise most scooters or
wheelchairs under 200 pounds and powerchairs up to 300
pounds. All Bruno lifts are eligible for reimbursement of up
to $1000.00 from GM, Saturn, Ford, and Chrysler under the
terms of their Mobility Programs.

Year Founded: 1984

2397 Silver Glide Stairway Lift
ThyssenKrupp Access Solutions
4001 E 138th Street
Grandview, MO 64030-2837
816-763-3100
Fax: 816-763-4467; *Toll Free:* 800-925-3100
www.tkaccess.com

Thomas Hance, President
Ray Demes, VP Field Office Consumer Care
Chuck Herling

The economical Silver-Glide easily installs on either side of
a straight stairway. The seat, armrest and footrest can be
folded to save stairway space when the unit is not in use.
The unit plugs into an outlet at the top or bottom of the
stairs and uses regular household current. Also available
with battery operated system. Heavy duty steel cable drive
system permits the rider to travel up to 20 feet.

Year Founded: 1811

2398 Sling Solutions
ArjoHuntleigh
2349 W. Lake Street
Addison, IL 60101
630-307-2756
Fax: 888-594-2756; *Toll Free:* 800-323-1245
usa.info@ArjoHuntleigh.com
www.arjohuntleigh.us/

Takes all the effort out of lifting while protecting the caregiver from the risk of backstrain.

Year Founded: 1975

2399 Smart Leg
Invacare Corporation
1 Invacare Way
Elyria, OH 44035-4190
440-329-6000
Fax: 877-619-7996; *Toll Free:* 800-333-6900
info@invacare.com; www.invacare.com

A Malachi Mixon III, Chairman Of The Board
Gerald B Blouch, President/ Chief Executive Offic
Robert K. Gudbranson, Senior Vice President and Chief

An ingenious elevating leg rest that automatically extends
to correctly fit every outstretched leg.

Year Founded: 1885

2400 Smooth Mover
Dixie Diners' Club
PO Box 1969
Tomball, TX 77377
832-616-3366
Fax: 832-201-0765; *Toll Free:* 800-233-3668
info@dixieusa.com
www.dixieusa.com

Bob Beeley, Chairman/ Founder
Brenda K. Oswalt, President
Jim Oswalt, Executive Vice President

Patient mover is a board designed to transfer patients from
bed to stretcher or table with one or two people.

Year Founded: 1975

2401 Stair & Glide Stairway Lift
ThyssenKrupp Access Solutions
4001 E 138th Street
Grandview, MO 64030-2837
816-763-3100
Fax: 816-763-4467; *Toll Free:* 800-925-3100
www.tkaccess.com

Thomas Hanceon, President
Gudrun Degenhart, Chief Operating Officer (COO)
Inge Delobelle, Chief Financial Officer (CFO)

Solves many multi-level accessibility problems in home.
Lifts easily to install on straight or curved stairways. The
rail attaches directly to steps without disturbing walls or
staircase. The heavy duty drive mechanism means reliable,
trouble-free operation. Public building and outdoor
packages available.

Year Founded: 1811

2402 StairLIFT SC & SL
Inclinator Company of America
601 Gibson Boulevard
Harrisburg, PA 17104
717-939-8420
Fax: 717-939-8075; *Toll Free:* 800-343-9007
isales@inclinator.com; www.inclinator.com

Paul R Krum, President

Simple, self-contained and efficient stair units.

Year Founded: 1923

2403 Stairway Elevators
Bruno Independent Living Aids
1780 Executive Drive
Po Box 84
Oconomowoc, WI 53066
262-567-4990
Fax: 262-953-5501; *Toll Free:* 800-882-8183
www.bruno.com

Michael R Bruno II, President/CEO
Patrick Foy, National Sales Manager
Anne Tyler

Bruno offers a full line of stairway elevators, including the
Electra-Ride II featuring access during power interruptions,
convenient installation, comfort and a powerful drive system. The Electra-Ride which features battery-powered
technology, a rail width of 25 inches and seat rotation for
easy transfers. The Comfort-Ride AC stair lift which is battery operated, has a rail width of 7.25 inches and folded
width of less than 14.5 inches.

Year Founded: 1984

2404 Stand Aid
Stand Aid of Iowa
1009 2nd Avenue
Po Box 386
Sheldon, IA 51201
712-324-2153
Fax: 712-324-5210; *Toll Free:* 800-831-8580
sales@stand-aid.com
www.stand-aid.com

Stand Aid can help you achieve independence and mobility safely and easily. Lifts you from a chair or bed with the flick of a switch, securing the user in an upright standing position.

2405 Straight and Custom Curved Stairlifts
Bruno Independent Living Aids
1780 Executive Drive
Po Box 84
Oconomowoc, WI 53066
262-567-4990
Fax: 262-953-5501; *Toll Free:* 800-882-8183
www.bruno.com

Michael R Bruno II, President/CEO
Patrick Foy, National Sales Manager
Anne Tyler

Bruno stairlifts can fit almost any curve or straight rail application and requires little or no structural modification to the stairway. Normal rail position for a Bruno inside turn is 7 inches to 8 inches from the wall or obstruction which is the tightest radius of any stairlift manufacturing company in the world. The Bruno inside turn is ideal for bi-level homes or staircases with mid-level doors.

Year Founded: 1984

2406 Sure Hands International
SureHandsr Lift & Care Systems
982 County Route 1
Pine Island, NY 10969-1205
845-258-6500
Fax: 845-258-6634; *Toll Free:* 800-724-5305
info@surehands.com
www.surehands.com

Thomas Herceg, President
Joyce Moraczewski, Marketing Coordinator
Ren, Van Raemdonck, Founder

SureHands lift and care systems are available in permanent and portable styles for homes and workplaces. The patented, self-adjusting body support with curve-around cups assures gentle, easy and secure transfers without the use of a sling. In many cases, transfers can be made independently. SureHands systems offers independence as a self-transfer tool. They provide assistance in bathing, hygiene care, positioning, standing, ambulation, exercising, and they are the back-saver for caregivers.

2407 SureHands Lift & Care Systems
SureHandsr Lift & Care Systems
982 County Route 1
Pine Island, NY 10969-1205
845-258-6500
Fax: 845-258-6634; *Toll Free:* 800-724-5305
info@surehands.com
www.surehands.com

Thomas Herceg, President
Joyce Moraczewski, Marketing Coordinator
Ren, Van Raemdonck, Founder

SureHands Lift & Care Systems offer a unique, patented and exlusive range of lift and transfer systems to meet private and institutional needs of individuals with motor disabilties. Includes permanent and portable models for homes, workplaces and recreation. The SureHands Body Support offers safe, easy and secure transfers for user and the opportunity for independent transfers for some. They are a back-save for caregivers. All lifts are easily ma

2408 Swing-A-Way
BraunAbility
627 West 11th Street
PO Box 310
Winamac, IN 46996
574-946-6153
Fax: 574-946-4670; *Toll Free:* 800-843-5438
www.braunability.com/

Ralph W. Braun, Founder

A swing lift for transporting patients from bed to bath and more. It features a gravity-down operation made possible by a newly designed pump module package. The new, quieter module features a built-in hand pump and a plastic reservoir for easy fluid checking. This is a vehicle lift not bath lift.

Year Founded: 1963

2409 Tilt 'n Tote, Roamer Riding Chair
WheelChair Carrier
7325 Douglas Road
Lambertville, MI 48144
734-568-6084
Fax: 734-568-6705; *Toll Free:* 800-541-3213
www.wheelchaircarrier.com

Christina Makulinski, Office Manager
Mike Siler, Engineering Manager
David Makulinski

Tilt 'n Tote is a wheelchair carrier that mounts to a Class 1 hitch on your vehicle. No lifting! Tilt the carrier to load your folding wheelchair. The Roamer Riding Chair is an electric powered mobility chair that folds to carry in trunk/backseat. weight of chair is only 35lbs without the battery.

Year Founded: 1977

2410 VPL Series Vertical Wheelchair Lift
ThyssenKrupp Access Solutions
4001 E 138th Street
Grandview, MO 64030-2837
816-763-3100
Fax: 816-763-4467; *Toll Free:* 800-925-3100
www.tkaccess.com

Thomas Hance, President
Gudrun Degenhart, Chief Operating Officer (COO)
Inge Delobelle, Chief Financial Officer (CFO)

Provide stairway access indoors and out for people who use wheelchairs. Lifting heights from 1 to 144 feet for loads up to 750 pounds are available for both commercial and residential applications. Easy to install and operate, the units are space and cost efficient solutions to ADA access compliance. Attendant operation, toe-guard enclosure and restricted access hoistway enclosure options are available.

Year Founded: 1811

2411 Vangater, Vangater II, Mini-Vangater
Braun Corporation
627 West 11th Street
PO Box 310
Winamac, IN 46996
574-946-6153
Fax: 574-946-4670; *Toll Free:* 800-THE-LIFT
www.braunlift.com

Jerry Sirjord, General Manager
Ralph W. Braun, Founder

Tri-fold and fold-in-half lifts represent a major innovation
in the field of adapted van transportation.

Year Founded: 1963

2412 Vertical Home Lift Sales
Mac's Lift Gate Inc.
2801 South Street
Long Beach, CA 90805-3751
562-634-5962
Fax: 562-529-3466; *Toll Free:* 800-795-6227
sales@macsliftgate.com
www.macsliftgate.com

Lawrence MacDonald, Owner

Sales and service of van and truck lifts. Sales and service of
wheel chair lifts for vans and automobiles. Sales, installation and service of vertical home lifts, scooter lifts and pool
lifts. Sales of scooters.

2413 Wecolator Stairway Lift
ThyssenKrupp Access Solutions
4001 E 138th Street
Grandview, MO 64030-2837
816-763-3100
Fax: 816-763-4467; *Toll Free:* 800-925-3100
www.tkaccess.com

Thomas Hance, President
Gudrun Degenhart, Chief Operating Officer (COO)
Inge Delobelle, Chief Financial Officer (CFO)

Solves many multi-level accessibility problems in home.
Lifts easily to install on straight or curved stairways. The
rail attaches directly to steps without disturbing walls or
staircase. The heavy duty drive mechanism means reliable,
trouble-free operation. Public building and outdoor
packages available.

Year Founded: 1811

2414 Wheelchair Carriers, Ramps, and Roamer
Riding Chair
WheelChair Carrier
7325 Douglas Road
Lambertville, MI 48144
734-568-6084
Fax: 734-568-6705; *Toll Free:* 800-541-3213
admin@wheelchaircarrier.com
www.wheelchaircarrier.com

Christina Makukinski, Office Manager
Mike Siler, Engineering Manager
David Makulinski

Wheelchair carriers for hitch mount on vehicles, portable
steel ramps, the Rider Roaming Chair, a lightweight,
foldable electric mobility aid. Carriers $199-$999, ramps
$189-429, the Roamer $1,995

Year Founded: 1977

2415 Ziggy Medi-Chair
LaszloChem
1805 Scherer Parkway
St. Charles, MO 63303
636-447-1312
Fax: 636-922-1698
suhaydal@yahoo.com, suhaydal@gmail.com
www.laszlochem.com/

Les Suhayda, President

A motorized lift and transfer system that maximizes time
and safety for disabled and bedridden patients. A
multifunctional product that benefits patients with disabilities and caregivers in a home or institutional enviroment. A
motorized system that lifts patients and saves caregivers
from injury and workman's compensation claims.

Scooters

2416 Amigo Centra
Amigo Mobility International
6693 Dixie Highway
Bridgeport, MI 48722-9725
989-777-0910
Fax: 800-334-7274; *Toll Free:* 800-692-6446
info@myamigo.com
myamigo.com

Allan Thiem, CEO

Features an adjustable handle that bends, making steering
comfortable and enjoyable. The rugged construction and
variable speed make it the perfect choice for indoor/out-
door mobility.

Year Founded: 1968

2417 Bravo! + Three-Wheel Scooter
Electro Kinetic Technologies
W194 N11301 McCormick Drive
Germantown, WI 53022
262-250-7740
Fax: 262-250-7741; *Toll Free:* 800-824-1068
www.ez-international.com

Designed to increase your mobility indoors. The Bravo!
plus has extendible rear wheels for outdoor use and comes
with easy to use finger tip controls and a maintenance free
gel-cell battery. Available in red, blue, green or light sand
gray with an optional power seat lift. Call for complete line
of 3 and 4-wheel electronic vehicles.

2418 Cruiser Bus Buggy 4MB
Convaid Products
2830 California Street
Torrance, CA 90503
310-618-0111
Fax: 310-618-2166; *Toll Free:* 888-CON-AID
www.convaid.com

Merv Watkins, Owner

In sizes from infant through young adult, this positioning
buggy is crash-tested.

Year Founded: 1976

2419 Explorer+ 4-Wheel Scooter
Electro Kinetic Technologies
W194 N11301 McCormick Drive
Germantown, WI 53022

262-250-7740
Fax: 262-250-7741; *Toll Free:* 800-824-1068
www.orthokinetics.com

William Grady, Sales Manager

A tough and rugged 4-wheel, rear-wheel drive, transaxle scooter designed to take you just about anywhere you want to go. Easy to use finger-tip controls and maintenance free gel-cell batteries and an extendible, take-apart frame, make the Explorer+ a perfect fit for people seeking greater mobility. Available in red, blue, green and gray, with an optional power seat lift.

2420 MVP+ 3-Wheel Scooter
Electro Kinetic Technologies
W194 N11301 McCormick Drive
Germantown, WI 53022
262-250-7740
Fax: 262-250-7741; *Toll Free:* 800-824-1068
www.ez-international.com

Thomas Dalums, Owner

The MVP+ is the rugged 3-wheel rear-wheel drive, tranaxle scooter with finger tip controls, and featuring an extendible, take-apart frame for a perfect fit. The MVP+ comes with maintenance free gel-cell batteries and is available in red, blue, green or light sand gray, with an optional power seat lift. $2,599-$3,099.

2421 Magni-Cam
American Printing House for the Blind
1839 Frankfort Avenue
PO Box 6085
Louisville, KY 40206-0085
502-895-2405
Fax: 502-899-2274; *Toll Free:* 800-223-1839
info@aph.org
www.aph.org

Tuck Tinsley, President
Bob Brasher, VP Advisory Services & Research
Gary Mudd

Magni-Cam is a light-weight, hand-held electronic magnifier that connects in minutes to any television set or computer monitor. It provides a crisp black and white image that enhances reading ability for people with low vision.

Year Founded: 1858

2422 Motorized Stander
Advanced Technology Corporation
115 Clemson Drive
Oak Ridge, TN 37830-7665
865-483-5756
Fax: 865-483-5860
info@atc-ssm.com
www.atc-ssm.com

Fahmy Haggag, Owner

Occupant-operated motorized vehicle that offers independence, increased mobility and ease of movement to disabled people.

2423 Outdoor Independence
Palmer Industries
PO Box 5707
Endicott, NY 13763
607-754-2957
Fax: 607-754-1954; *Toll Free:* 800-847-1304

palmer@palmerind.com
palmerind.com/

Jack Palmer, President

The futuristic electric three-wheeler designed to take you almost anywhere.

Year Founded: 1973

2424 Pace Saver Plus II
Leisure-Lift
1800 Merriam Lane
Kansas City, KS 66106
Fax: 913-722-2614; *Toll Free:* 800-255-0285
Leisure-Lift@Leisure-Lift.com
www.pacesaver.com

Bill Burke, Founder
Zella Burke, Founder

The scooter combines outdoor ruggedness with indoor maneuverability at a low price.

Year Founded: 1967

2425 Palmer Independence
Palmer Industries
PO Box 5707
Endicott, NY 13763
607-754-2957
Fax: 607-754-1954; *Toll Free:* 800-847-1304
palmer@palmerind.com
palmerind.com/

William C Brunner, CEO
Jack Palmer, President

Futuristic electric three wheeler designed to take the rider almost anywhere.

Year Founded: 1973

2426 Palmer Twosome
Palmer Industries
PO Box 5707
Endicott, NY 13763
607-754-2957
Fax: 607-754-1954; *Toll Free:* 800-847-1304
palmer@palmerind.com
palmerind.com/

All electric two seat vehicle for those who can't pedal.

Year Founded: 1973

2427 Quickie 2
Sunrise Medical (US) LLC
2842 Business Park Avenue
Fresno, CA 93727
760-930-1500
Fax: 800-300-7502; *Toll Free:* 800-333-4000
webmaster@sunmed.com
www.sunrisemedical.com

Michael Hammes, CEO

This custom, ultralight, folding, everyday scooter offers portability and performance plus modular flexibility.

2428 Ranger
Ranger All-Seasons
PO Box 132
George, IA 51237
712-475-2811
Fax: 712-475-2810; *Toll Free:* 800-225-3811

sales@rangerallseason.com
www.rangerallseason.com

Randy Rieeks, National Sales Manager
Larry Kruse, Owner

Makes 3 & 4 wheel electric scooters for physically challenged and elderly people. Ranger scooters feature two Patents. The first is for the easy disassembly of the scooter, which can be done in a matter of seconds. The second is for the easy to operate adjustable tiller. Ranger also manufactures an electric scooter and wheelchair lift for a car, van, pickup, or sport utility vehicle.

2429 Regal Scooters
Bruno Independent Living Aids
1780 Executive Drive
Po Box 84
Oconomowoc, WI 53066
262-567-4990
Fax: 262-953-5501; *Toll Free:* 800-882-8183
www.bruno.com

Michael R Bruno II, President/CEO
Patrick Foy, National Sales Manager
Anne Tyler

This line includes the Regal Standard, the regal large Adult, the Regal Small Adult, the Regal Pediatric, The Regal Ten models 65 and 75, and The Regal Four. These scooters offer adjustable flip-up armrests, pneumatic tires front and rear, and more.

Year Founded: 1984

2430 Regent
Golden Technologies
401 Bridge Street
Old Forge, PA 18518
574-517-477
Fax: 800-628-5165; *Toll Free:* 800-624-6374
pobrien@goldentech.com
www.goldentech.com

Top-rated performance scooter, with extra features and economically priced.

2431 Safari Scooter
Ranger All-Seasons
PO Box 132
George, IA 51237
712-475-2811
Fax: 712-475-2810; *Toll Free:* 800-225-3811
sales@rangerallseason.com
www.rangerallseason.com

Randy Rieeks, Sales Manager
Larry Kruse, Owner

Safari is Ranger's most popular scooter. Available in either a 40 inch or 43 inch frame length with an ultra-quiet, totally enclosed transacle drive. The Safari has some of the same features as the SOLO, the user-friendly take-apart and tiller adjustment, color impregnated - not painted- ABS plastic body. The most versatile Ranger Scooter, the Safari is an excellent choice for indoor use, and can take the place of most front wheel drive scooters.

Year Founded: 1986

2432 Scoota Bug
Golden Technologies
401 Bridge Street
Old Forge, PA 18518

570-451-7477
Fax: 800-628-5165; *Toll Free:* 800-624-6374
pobrien@goldentech.com
www.goldentech.com

Bob Golden, President

A lightweight, completely modular scooter, that disassembles and fits into most auto trunks.

2433 Sierra 3000/4000
Electro Kinetic Technologies
W194 N11301 McCormick Drive
Germantown, WI 53022
262-250-7740
Fax: 262-250-7741; *Toll Free:* 800-824-1068
www.ez-international.com

William Grady, Sales Manager

Look to the Sierra 3000/4000 series vehicles for comfort, convenience and performance. Increased leg and foot room, adjustable seat height and arm width, as well as adjustable tiller angle provide maximum comfort. For convenience, the Sierra is equipped with integrated cargo and cup holders and thumb/finger controls with built in wrist rest. Advanced safety features such as stall and free-wheeling situation identification and correction, anti rol

2434 Solo Scooter
Ranger All-Seasons
PO Box 132
George, IA 51237
712-475-2811
Fax: 712-475-2810; *Toll Free:* 800-225-3811
sales@rangerallseason.com
www.rangerallseason.com

Randy Rieeks, Sales Manager
Larry Kruse, Owner

The SOLO is Ranger's flagship model. Introduction of the SOLO 1991 set the standard for easy disassembly of a scooter. The SOLO has a long list of user friendly features including patented take-apart and tiller adjustment mechanisms, non-rusting aluminum frame, extra long, extra tall seats as standard, color impregnated-not painted-ABS plastic bodies, charger plug conveniently located on the Accelerator box and many more.

2435 Sterling
Golden Technologies
401 Bridge Street
Old Forge, PA 18518
570-451-7477
Fax: 800-628-5165; *Toll Free:* 800-624-6374
pobrien@goldentech.com
www.goldentech.com

Bob Golden, President

Rear-wheel-drive vehicle that represents the best in powered mobility.

2436 Super Scout Three Wheeler
Leisure-Lift
1800 Merriam Lane
Kansas City, KS 66106-4714
913-722-5658
Fax: 913-722-2614; *Toll Free:* 800-255-0285
Leisure-Lift@Leisure-Lift.com
www.pacesaver.com

Bill Burke, Founder
Zella Burke, Founder

Be free to be as active as you like with this three wheel scooter.

Year Founded: 1967

2437 Systems 2000
BioMedical Life Systems, Inc
PO Box 1360
Vista, CA 92085-1360
760-727-5600
Fax: 760-727-4220; *Toll Free:* 800-726-8367
information@bmls.com
www.bmls.com

This five-mode TENS device has four adjustable modulations, plus conventional settings and comes with a five-year warranty.

2438 TERRA-JET: Utility Vehicle
TERRA-JET USA
PO Box 918
Junction Hwy. 417 & 419
Innis, LA 70747
225-492-2249
Fax: 225-492-2226; *Toll Free:* 800-864-5000
Terra-Jet@Terra-Jet.com
www.members.tripod.com/~terrajet/

Larry Rabalais, General Manager
Dora Rabalais, Secretary/Treasurer

TERRA-JET utility vehicles are unique in its ability to traverse many different types of terrain in remote areas otherwise inaccessible. It has a multitude of uses for industry, sportsmen or the whole family. Uniquely designed, industrial duty construction of low maintenance and low fuel consumption. $7,000-$9,000.

Year Founded: 1973

2439 Tri-Wheelers
The Braun Corporation
627 West 11th Street
PO Box 310
Winamac, IN 46996
574-946-6153
Fax: 574-946-4670; *Toll Free:* 800-THE-LIFT
www.braunlift.com

Ralph W. Braun, Founder

Provides convenience features, producing a high efficiency performance with ultra-smooth operation.

Year Founded: 1963

2440 Triumph 3000/4000
Electro Kinetic Technologies
W194 N11301 McCormick Drive
Germantown, WI 53022
262-250-7740
Fax: 262-250-7741; *Toll Free:* 800-824-1068
www.ez-international.com

William Grady, Sales Manager

The Triumph 3000/4000 series vehicles provide unique comfort and convenience features found nowhere else. Digital Dash with soft touch keypad, deluxe seat with suspension and integral cargo and cup holders are just a few of these features. Equipped with TOPS 24 (Total Ortho Power System) ensures maximum power, performance and reli-

ability. Luxurious options such as velour or allante seat fabrics, stylized wheels, metallic or pearl color options an

2441 Triumph Scooter
Electro Kinetic Technologies
W194 N11301 McCormick Drive
Germantown, WI 53022
262-250-7740
Fax: 262-250-7741; *Toll Free:* 800-824-1068
www.ez-international.com

William Grady, Sales Manager

The sleek rugged three-wheel, rear-wheel drive, transaxle scooter with up-top controls, designed to help increase mobility and become more active. The Triumph is designed for both indoor and outdoor use. Available in red, blue, green or gray, with an optional power seat lift. $2,899-$3,399.

Stationery

2442 Address Book
The New Vision Store
919 Walnut Street
Philadelphia, PA 19107-5237
215-629-2990
webmaster@.thenewvisionstore.com
www.thenewvisionstore.com

The big print address book is the first personal book to provide enlarged writing spaces, making it easier to write down and retrieve information.

2443 Audio Book Contractors
Audio Book Contractors, LLC
PO Box 96
Riverdale, MD 20738-0096
301-439-5830
Fax: 301-439-5830
info@audiobookcontractors.com
www.audiobookcontractors.com

Flo Gibson, President/ Founder

Unabridged classic books on cassettes in sturdy vinyl covers with picture and spine windows.

Year Founded: 1983

2444 Audio Recordings
Access-USA
PO Box 160
242 James Street
Clayton, NY 13624
Fax: 800-563-1687; *Toll Free:* 800-263-2750
info@access-usa.com, deborah@access-usa.com
www.access-usa.com

Deborah Haight, EOA

Access-USA produces auctio recordings for businesses, organizations and entrepreneurs. Information such as brochures, reports, documents, etc. can be made accessible. Other formats available include braille, large print, braille business cards and video services.

2445 Beyond Sight
Beyond Sight, Inc.
5650 S Windermere Street
Littleton, CO 80120

303-795-6455
Fax: 303-795-6425
support@beyondsight.com
www.beyondsight.com

Scott Chaplick, President & Owner
Gina Wetzel, Sales & Merchandise Specialist

Products for the blind and visually impaired including talking clocks, watches, and calculators. They also carry a large selection of Braille products, magnifiers, reading machines, and computer equipment.

Year Founded: 1989

2446 Big Print Address Book
EASE
3714 Copper Penny Lane
Auburn, CA 95602
928-636-9469
Fax: 530-888-6990; *Toll Free:* 800-327- 650
kmjc@northlink.com
www.accesswithease.com/

Karen Clymer, President

Oversized organizer makes locating information easier for those with limited vision.

2447 Bold Line Paper
The New Vision Store
919 Walnut Street
1st Floor
Philadelphia, PA 19107-5237
215-629-2990
webmaster@.thenewvisionstore.com
www.thenewvisionstore.com

This pad consists of 100 sheets of paper with bold lines to help guide the writing of an individual with limited vision.

2448 Book Holder
EASE
3714 Copper Penny Lane
Auburn, CA 95602
928-636-9469
Fax: 530-888-6990; *Toll Free:* 800-327- 650
kmjc@northlink.com
www.accesswithease.com/

This hands free reading book holder enables the user to read hands free.

2449 Bookholder: Roberts
Therapro, Inc.
225 Arlington Street
Framingham, MA 01702-8723
508-872-9494
Fax: 508-875-2062; *Toll Free:* 800-257-5376
info@theraproducts.com
www.theraproducts.com

Karen Conrad, Founder
Paul Weihrauch, Founder

Gray plastic, ideal for hand free reading, adjusts to all sizes of books and prevents pages from flipping for the physically challenged.

Year Founded: 1986

2450 Braille Business Cards & More
Access-USA
242 James Street
PO Drawer 160
Clayton, NY 13624
315-686-0065
Fax: 800-563-1687; *Toll Free:* 800-263-2750
info@access-usa.com, deborah@access-usa.com
www.access-usa.com

Deborah Haight, EOA
Tim Baril, Owner

Braille on business cards, greeting cards, invitations, folders, plastic credit/ATM cards, advertising inserts, specialties and more.

2451 Braille Notebook
Maxi-Aids, Inc.
42 Executive Boulevard
Farmingdale, NY 11735
631-752-0521
Fax: 631-752-0689; *Toll Free:* 800-522-6294
sales@maxiaids.com
www.maxiaids.com
TTY: 800-281-3555

Harold Zaretsky, President

Made of heavy-duty board, covered with waterproof imitation leather and three rings for binding, including braille paper and titles.

2452 Brailled Desk Calendar
Maxi-Aids, Inc.
42 Executive Boulevard
Farmingdale, NY 11735
631-752-0521
Fax: 631-752-0689; *Toll Free:* 800-522-6294
sales@maxiaids.com
www.maxiaids.com
TTY: 800-281-3555

Harold Zaretsky, President

Schedule appointments, remember birthdays or write messages for a particular day.

2453 Bus and Taxi Sign
Maxi-Aids, Inc.
42 Executive Boulevard
Farmingdale, NY 11735
631-752-0521
Fax: 631-752-0689; *Toll Free:* 800-522-6294
sales@maxiaids.com
www.maxiaids.com
TTY: 800-281-3555

Harold Zaretsky, President

Signs that attract the attention of bus or taxi drivers.

2454 Calendars
American Printing House for the Blind
1839 Frankfort Avenue
PO Box 6085
Louisville, KY 40206-0085
502-895-2405
Fax: 502-899-2274; *Toll Free:* 800-223-1839
info@aph.org
www.aph.org

Tuck Tinsley, President
Bob Brasher, VP Advisory Services & Research
Gary Mudd

The American Printing House for the Blind offers three different styles of large type/braille calendars for learning and daily living. The Classroom Calendar Kit, The Individual Calendar Kit and the APH InSights Art Calendar.

Year Founded: 1858

2455 Card Chart
American Printing House for the Blind
1839 Frankfort Avenue
PO Box 6085
Louisville, KY 40206-0085
502-895-2405
Fax: 502-899-2274; Toll Free: 800-223-1839
info@aph.org
www.aph.org

Tuck Tinsley, President
Bob Brasher, VP Advisory Services & Research
Gary Mudd

The Card Chart is a handy device designed to hold the 3 1/2 x 2 inch braille/print cards sold by APH in a variety of products, such as the Expanded Dolch Word Cards.

Year Founded: 1858

2456 Deluxe Signature Guide
Maxi-Aids, Inc.
42 Executive Boulevard
Farmingdale, NY 11735
631-752-0521
Fax: 631-752-0689; Toll Free: 800-522-6294
sales@maxiaids.com
www.maxiaids.com
TTY: 800-281-3555

Harold Zaretsky, President

Rods supported by two rubber blocks facilitate writing.

2457 Finger Print Pen
Therapro, Inc.
225 Arlington Street
Framingham, MA 01702-8723
508-872-9494
Fax: 508-875-2062; Toll Free: 800-257-5376
info@theraproducts.com
www.theraproducts.com

Karen Conrad, Founder
Paul Weihrauch, Founder

This pen was designed for those with limited digital mobility and decreased ability to grasp a conventional writing tool.

Year Founded: 1986

2458 Highlighter and Note Tape
Therapro, Inc.
225 Arlington Street
Framingham, MA 01702-8723
508-872-9494
Fax: 508-875-2062; Toll Free: 800-257-5376
info@theraproducts.com
www.theraproducts.com

Karen Conrad, Founder
Paul Weihrauch, Founder

A great way to highlight and draw attention to words without damaging original. Price ranges from $4.00-$7.00.

Year Founded: 1986

2459 Letter Writing Guide
Independent Living Aids, LLC
137 Rano Street
Buffalo, NY 14207
516-937-1848
Fax: 516-937-3906; Toll Free: 800-537-2118
techsupport@independentliving.com
www.independentliving.com

Marvin Sandler, President

Sturdy plastic sheet with 13 apertures corresponding to standard line spacing.

2460 Lettering Guide Value Pack
Independent Living Aids, LLC
137 Rano Street
Buffalo, NY 14207
516-937-1848
Fax: 516-937-3906; Toll Free: 800-537-2118
techsupport@independentliving.com
www.independentliving.com

Marvin Sandler, President

Included in this useful pack are four durable plastic lettering and number guides for tracing letters when the individual is unable to write letters unassisted.

2461 Maxi Marks
Maxi-Aids, Inc.
42 Executive Boulevard
Farmingdale, NY 11735
631-752-0521
Fax: 631-752-0689; Toll Free: 800-522-6294
sales@maxiaids.com
www.maxiaids.com
TTY: 800-281-3555

Harold Zaretsky, President

Braille writing and identification products.

2462 Plastic Card Holder
Therapro, Inc.
225 Arlington Street
Framingham, MA 01702-8723
508-872-9494
Fax: 508-875-2062; Toll Free: 800-257-5376
info@theraproducts.com
www.theraproducts.com

Karen Conrad, Founder
Paul Weihrauch, Founder

For those with reduced finger control.

Year Founded: 1986

2463 Raised Line Drawing Kit
Maxi-Aids, Inc.
42 Executive Boulevard
Farmingdale, NY 11735
631-752-0521
Fax: 631-752-0689; Toll Free: 800-522-6294
sales@maxiaids.com
www.maxiaids.com
TTY: 800-281-3555

Harold Zaretsky, President

For writing script or drawing graphs by the use of special plastic paper.

2464 Signature and Address Self-Inking Stamps
Independent Living Aids, LLC
137 Rano Street
Buffalo, NY 14207
516-937-1848
Fax: 516-937-3906; *Toll Free:* 800-537-2118
techsupport@independentliving.com
www.independentliving.com

Marvin Sandler, President

Gives thousands of impressions before requiring re-inking.

2465 Steady Write
Maxi-Aids, Inc.
42 Executive Boulevard
Farmingdale, NY 11735
631-752-0521
Fax: 631-752-0689; *Toll Free:* 800-522-6294
sales@maxiaids.com
www.maxiaids.com
TTY: 800-281-3555

Harold Zaretsky, President

Furnishes the writer with increased holding capacity and stabilizes the hand.

2466 Weighted Holders
Therapro, Inc.
225 Arlington Street
Framingham, MA 01702-8723
508-872-9494
Fax: 508-875-2062; *Toll Free:* 800-257-5376
info@theraproducts.com
www.theraproducts.com

Karen Conrad, Founder
Paul Weihrauch, Founder

These weighted holders allow for more control along with proprioceptive feedback to encourage better writing skills.

Year Founded: 1986

2467 Wings & Wheels Greeting Cards
Wings & Wheels, Inc.
10700 Jersey Blvd.
Suite 400B
Rancho Cucamonga, CA 07801-5603
716-763-3213
Fax: 909-989-9103; *Toll Free:* 800-422-5309
sales@wingsandwheels.com
www.wingsandwheels.com/

Nanette Courtine, Owner
Garret Willat, Founder
Sean Franke, Founder

Offer inclusive greeting cards. Depicts people with disabilities on the cards.

Walking Aids

2468 Adjustable Incline Board
Bailey Manufacturing Company
PO Box 130
Lodi, OH 44254-0130
330-948-1080
Fax: 800-244-5390; *Toll Free:* 800-321-8372

baileymfg@baileymfg.com
www.baileymfg.com

Larry Strimple, President

Bailey manufactures more than 500 rehabilitation and therepeutic products for physical/occupations therapists, work hardening and sports medicine to use with their patients and clients in facilities or at home.

Year Founded: 1956

2469 Aluminum Adjustable Support Canes for the Blind
Maxi-Aids, Inc.
42 Executive Boulevard
Farmingdale, NY 11735
631-752-0521
Fax: 631-752-0689; *Toll Free:* 800-522-6294
sales@maxiaids.com
www.maxiaids.com
TTY: 800-281-3555

Harold Zaretsky, President

Adjustable canes for the visually impaired.

2470 Aluminum Crutches
Arista Homes
600 Applewood Crescent
Vaughan, ON L4K 4B4
905-660-5000
Fax: 905-660-8805; *Toll Free:* 800-223-1984
clientcare@aristahomes.com, sales@aristahomes
www.aristahomes.com/

Stephen Howard, Manager

Lightweight aluminum crutches with wood underarms and handgrips.

2471 Aluminum Walking Canes
Maxi-Aids, Inc.
42 Executive Boulevard
Farmingdale, NY 11735
631-752-0521
Fax: 631-752-0689; *Toll Free:* 800-522-6294
sales@maxiaids.com
www.maxiaids.com
TTY: 800-281-3555

Harold Zaretsky, President

Lightweight but strong, these walking canes are made of a heavy gauge aluminum tube with safety locknuts and heavy-duty rubber tips.

2472 Deluxe Standard Wood Cane
Arista Homes
600 Applewood Crescent
Vaughan, ON L4K 4B4
905-660-5000
Fax: 905-660-8805; *Toll Free:* 800-223-1984
clientcare@aristahomes.com, sales@aristahomes
www.aristahomes.com/

Stephen Howard, Manager

A standard old-fashioned wooden cane for the physically challenged.

2473 Dolomite Walkers
Clarke Health Care Products
7830 Steubenville Pike
Oakdale, PA 15071

724-695-2122
Fax: 724-695-2922; *Toll Free:* 888-347-4537
info@clarkehealthcare.com
www.clarkehealthcare.com

Gerard Clarke, Owner

Dolomite walkers are available in 3 models and 8 sizes. All
come with back supports, baskets, curb climbers.

Year Founded: 1989

2474 Maxi Superior Cane
Maxi-Aids, Inc.
42 Executive Boulevard
Farmingdale, NY 11735
631-752-0521
Fax: 631-752-0689; *Toll Free:* 800-522-6294
sales@maxiaids.com
www.maxiaids.com
TTY: 800-281-3555

Harold Zaretsky, President

Convenient folding cane designed for optimum balance.
Tapered joints provide rigidity when open, and are made of
heavy gauge aluminum.

2475 Push-Button Quad Cane
Arista Homes
600 Applewood Crescent
Vaughan, ON L4K 4B4
905-660-5000
Fax: 905-660-8805; *Toll Free:* 800-223-1984
clientcare@aristahomes.com, sales@aristahomes
www.aristahomes.com/

Stephen Howard, Manager

A reliable walking cane offering independence to the physically challenged user.

2476 Rand-Scot
Rand-Scot, Inc.
401 Linden Center Drive
Fort Collins, CO 80524
970-484-7967
Fax: 970-484-3800; *Toll Free:* 800-467-7967
info@randscot.com
randscot.com/

Joel Lerich, Founder
Darcy Thor, Business Manager
Barbara , Founder

Offers a line of patient lifts and standers for the disabled.
Manufactures the EasyPivot patient lift for 1 person transfers. A video is available plus, no charge for potential users.
$800.-$3,000.

Year Founded: 1980

2477 Rigid Aluminum Cane with Golf Grip
Maxi-Aids, Inc.
42 Executive Boulevard
Farmingdale, NY 11735
631-752-0521
Fax: 631-752-0689; *Toll Free:* 800-522-6294
sales@maxiaids.com
www.maxiaids.com
TTY: 800-281-3555

Harold Zaretsky, President

A straight, tubular, heavy gauge aluminum rigid cane for
blind and visually impaired persons.

2478 WCIB Heavy-Duty Folding Cane
Maxi-Aids, Inc.
42 Executive Boulevard
Farmingdale, NY 11735
631-752-0521
Fax: 631-752-0689; *Toll Free:* 800-522-6294
sales@maxiaids.com
www.maxiaids.com
TTY: 800-281-3555

Harold Saretsky, President

A four section aluminum folding cane with a golf-type grip
handle and flexible wrist loop. #1749015, 34-60"

2479 Walker Leg Support
Sammons Preston
1000 Remington Blvd
Suite 210
Bolingbrook, IL 60440-5177
630-378-6000
Fax: 630-378-6010; *Toll Free:* 800-323-5547
customersupport@patterson-medical.com
www.sammonspreston.com

For lower externity trauma. An alternative to crutches that
allows safe, stable ambulation and frees hands and arms for
daily tasks.

Wheelchairs

2480 Bariatric Wheelchairs Regency
Gendron, Inc.
520 W. Mulberry St.
Suite 100
Bryan, OH 43506
Fax: 419-636-9261; *Toll Free:* 800-537-2521
sales@gendroninc.com
www.gendroninc.com

Steven Cotter, President/CEO
Roberta Jacobs, National Sales Manager
Robin Robin, Customer Service

Bariatric wheelchairs, for users weighing up to seven hundred pounds. Manual and power styles built to order for
specific needs.

Year Founded: 1871

2481 Big Bounder Power Wheelchair
21st Century Scientific, Inc.
4931 N. Manufacturing Way
Coeur d'Alene, ID 83815
208-667-8800
Fax: 208-667-6600; *Toll Free:* 800-448-3680
21st@wheelchairs.com
www.wheelchairs.com

Ronald E Prior Ph.D., CEO
Susan Harris, CFO/Webmaster

Manufactured for the obese in virtually any dimension. Its
powerful motors and rugged frame can accommodate users
up to 1000 lb. 21st Century Scientific unique construction
option can reduce the overall width of the chair by as much
as 3 inches. This may make the difference between using
normal doorways or remodeling a home. $10,695.

2482 Bil Jax Construction/Rental
Gendron, Inc.
520 W. Mulberry St.
Suite 100
Bryan, OH 43506
Fax: 419-636-9261; *Toll Free:* 800-537-2521
sales@gendroninc.com; www.gendroninc.com

Steven Cotter, President/CEO
Roberta Jacobs, National Sales Manager
Robin Robin, Customer Service

Manufacturers of wheelchairs for a variety of other applications, specializing in obese patient products.

Year Founded: 1871

2483 Bounder Plus Power Wheelchair
21st Century Scientific, Inc.
4931 N. Manufacturing Way
Coeur d'Alene, ID 83815
208-667-8800
Fax: 208-667-6600; *Toll Free:* 800-448-3680
21st@wheelchairs.com
www.21stcenturyscientific.com

Dr. Ronald E Prior Ph.D, President & Founder
Susan Harris, CFO/Webmaster

Available in widths of 16 to 20 feet for users up to 500 pounds with a 2 year warranty on the entire chair. It offers all the standard features of a BOUNDER, plus reinforced rear wheel mounts, reinforced caster barrels, and super duty upholstery (with double liner and web straps under every screw). The BOUNDER Plus also features tandem cross struts, middle vertical support strut, seat rails supported at five points, and back upholstery attached wwith machine screws.

Year Founded: 1979

2484 Bounder Power Wheelchair
21st Century Scientific, Inc.
4931 N. Manufacturing Way
Coeur d'Alene, ID 83815
208-667-8800
Fax: 208-667-6600; *Toll Free:* 800-448-3680
21st@wheelchairs.com
www.21stcenturyscientific.com

Dr. Ronald E Prior Ph.D, President & Founder
Susan Harris, CFO/Webmaster

Available in a variety of widths from 16"-20" to 18 feet for users up to 500 pounds. Its powerful 1/3 HP motors can achieve top speeds of over 10 mph. The rugged frame is constructed with steel tubing. The standard 12 position Adjustable Front Forks, made of 1/4 inch thick steel, provides impact dampening and seat tilt adjustment. A Dual Group 27 Sliding Battery Box provides extended range and easy battery maintenance.

Year Founded: 1979

2485 Breezy
Sunrise Medical (US) LLC
2842 Business Park Avenue
Fresno, CA 93727
760-930-1500
Fax: 800-300-7502; *Toll Free:* 800-333-4000
webmaster@sunmed.com; www.sunrisemedical.com

Michael Hammes, CEO

This lightweight chair is durable, comfortable and flexible enough to meet the needs of a wide range of wheelchair users.

2486 Champion 1000
Graham-Field Health Products, Inc.
2935 Northeast Parkway
Atlanta, GA 30360
678-291-3207
Fax: 800-726-0601; *Toll Free:* 800-347-5678
cs@grahamfield.com
www.grahamfield.com

Kenneth Spett, President & Chief Executive Offi
Lori Kirschner, Senior Vice President, HR & Admi
Alan Spett, Senior Vice President, Operation

Ultralight wheelchair designed to improve mobility. $1,689

Year Founded: 1850

2487 Champion 2000
Graham-Field Health Products, Inc.
2935 Northeast Parkway
Atlanta, GA 30360
678-291-3207
Fax: 800-726-0601; *Toll Free:* 800-347-5678
cs@grahamfield.com; www.grahamfield.com

Kenneth Spett, President & Chief Executive Offi
Lori Kirschner, Senior Vice President, HR & Admi
Alan Spett, Senior Vice President, Operation

Rigid chair that folds side-to-side. $1,765

Year Founded: 1850

2488 Champion 3000
Graham-Field Health Products, Inc.
2935 Northeast Parkway
Atlanta, GA 30360
678-291-3207
Fax: 800-726-0601; *Toll Free:* 800-347-5678
cs@grahamfield.com; www.grahamfield.com

Kenneth Spett, President & Chief Executive Offi
Lori Kirschner, Senior Vice President, HR & Admi
Alan Spett, Senior Vice President, Operation

The high-performance chair built for perfectionists. $1,695

Year Founded: 1850

2489 Compax 12
Convaid Products
2830 California Street
Torrance, CA 90503
310-618-0111
Fax: 310-618-2166; *Toll Free:* 888-CON-AID
www.convaid.com

Merv Watkins, Owner

This wheelchair folds to the size of a small golf bag and weighs 19 pounds.

Year Founded: 1976

2490 Convaid Products
Convaid Products
2830 California Street
Torrance, CA 90503
310-618-0111
Fax: 310-618-2166; *Toll Free:* 888-CON-AID
www.convaid.com

Mervyn Watkins, Owner

Five different styles of wheelchairs. COnvaid's mission is to be sensitive to the broad needs of physically challenged children, and just as important, sensitive to the needs of the caregivers.

Year Founded: 1976

2491 Eagle Sportschairs
Eagle Sportschairs, LLC
2351 Parkwood Road
Snellville, GA 30039
770-972-0763
Fax: 770-985-4885; *Toll Free:* 800-932-9380
eaglesportschairs@gmail.com
www.eaglesportschairs.com

Barry Ewing, Owner
Bernice Marston, Customer Service

The Eagle line of custom lightweight performance chairs includes a range of options to fit all racing and sport needs including; track, baseball, quad-rugby, tennis, field events and waterski. Also popular for daily use. We are able to customize any chair to accommodate size and disability, and all frames have a full five year warranty.

Year Founded: 1980

2492 Evacu-Trac
Garaventa Emergency Evacuation Chairs
PO Box L-1
Blaine, WA 98230
360-332-2231; *Toll Free:* 866-824-8314
productinfo@evacutrac.com
www.evacutrac.com

This emergency evacuation chair is designed for safety and fast operation.

2493 Gem Wheelchair and Scooter Service
Gem Wheelchair and Scooter Service
176-39 Union Turnpike
Flushing, NY 11366
718-969-8600
Fax: 718-969-8300; *Toll Free:* 800-943-3578
help@gemwheelchairservice.com
www.gemwheelchairsservice.com/

Jeff Bochner, President

GEM repairs and sells all makes and models of manual and motorized wheelchairs and power scooters. Clients are in all five New York City Boroughs and Nassau County. Workers Compensatation, Medicare and Medicaid accepted, pick-up and delivery and loaner equipment services available. Huge replacement parts inventory.

2494 Gendron
Gendron, Inc.
520 W. Mulberry St.
Suite 100
Bryan, OH 43506
Fax: 419-636-9261; *Toll Free:* 800-537-2521
sales@gendroninc.com; www.gendroninc.com

Steven Cotter, President/CEO
Roberta Jacobs, National Sales Manager
Robin Robin, Customer Service

Manufacturer of wheelchairs for a variety of other applications, specializing in bariatric mobility products.

Year Founded: 1871

2495 Geronimo
Redman Power Chair
1601 S Pantano Road
Suite 107
Tucson, AZ 85710
Fax: 520-546-5530; *Toll Free:* 800-727-6684
info@redmanpowerchair.com
www.redmanpowerchair.com

Paula Redman, Chief Financial Officer
Don Redman, Chief Executive Officer
Samuel Redman, General Manager

Wheelchair offering direct drive, two year electronic guarantee and micro controls.

2496 HiRider
Gaymar Industries
10 Centre Drive
Orchard Park, NY 14127-2295
716-662-2551
Fax: 716-662-0748; *Toll Free:* 800-828-7341
websalescontact@gaymar.com
www.gaymar.com

Frank Lumbar, CEO
Dr. Thomas P Stewart, President

A wheelchair that provides mobility in both sitting and standing positions.

2497 Innovative Products Unlimited
Innovative Products Unlimited
2120 Industrial Drive
Niles, MI 49120
269-684-5050
Fax: 888-757-4734; *Toll Free:* 800-833-2826
ipu@ipu.com
www.ipu.com

Wheelchairs and accessories.

Year Founded: 1985

2498 Klassic-Plus
KareCo International, Inc.
21530 Gledhill Street
Chatsworth, CA 91311
732-752-9292
Fax: 818-717-0651; *Toll Free:* 877-495-7921
info@kareco.com; www.kareco.com/

Kevin O'Neil, Owner

Stainless steel lightweight wheelchair offers standard features.

2499 LEVO Standing Wheelchairs
LEVO USA
7105 Northland Terrace
Brooklyn Park, MN 55428
763-544-7779
Fax: 763-582-0442; *Toll Free:* 888-538-6872
request@levousa.com
www.levousa.com

Daniel Johnson, CEO, Founder

LEVO will be the leader in stand-up wheelchairs. We will provide our clients with innovative solutions and products, delivering the greatest value, supported with exceptional service.

Year Founded: 1975

2500 Lightweight Breezy
Motion Design
249 Muriwai Valley Road
RDI Waimauku
Auckland, NZ 0881
649-411-8230; *Fax:* 649-411-8237
info@motiondesign.co.nz
www.motiondesign.co.nz/

Gary Anderson, General Manager
Tim Brown, Business Development Manager
Loma Page, Admistration Manager

A lightweight wheelchair.

2501 Permobil Max 90
Permobil Inc.
300 Duke Drive
Lebanon, TN 37090
Fax: 800-231-3256; *Toll Free:* 800-736-0925
info@permobil.com, techsupport@permobil.com
www.permobilusa.com

Larry Jackson, President & Chief Executive Offi
Tom Rolick, Vice President Sales
Darin Lowery, Vice President of Operations

The power wheelchair for those needing an easily maneuverable and quiet indoor chair but who also need to use their chair outdoors.

Year Founded: 1960

2502 Permobil Super 90
Permobil Inc.
300 Duke Drive
Lebanon, TN 37090
Fax: 800-231-3256; *Toll Free:* 800-736-0925
info@permobil.com, techsupport@permobil.com
www.permobilusa.com

Larry Jackson, President & Chief Executive Offi
Tom Rolick, Vice President Sales
Darin Lowery, Vice President of Operations

The power wheelchair is designed for travel over uneven and hilly terrain outdoors and indoors.

Year Founded: 1960

2503 Posture-Glide Lounger
Graham-Field Health Products, Inc.
2935 Northeast Parkway
Atlanta, GA 30360
678-291-3207
Fax: 800-726-0601; *Toll Free:* 800-347-5678
cs@grahamfield.com
www.grahamfield.com

Kenneth Spett, President & Chief Executive Offi
Lori Kirschner, Senior Vice President, HR & Admi
Alan Spett, Senior Vice President, Operation

Provides all day comfort and safe, independent mobilization with feet or hands. The ergonomically engineered seat back provides correct support.

Year Founded: 1850

2504 Power Chairs
Bruno Independent Living Aids
1780 Executive Drive
PO Box 84
Oconomowoc, WI 53066

262-567-4990
Fax: 262-953-5501; *Toll Free:* 800-882-8183
www.bruno.com

Michael R Bruno II, President/CEO
Patrick Foy, National Sales Manager
Anne Tyler

Products available in front and rear wheel drive. Our power chairs have excellent directional stability, rock solid construction and durability.

Year Founded: 1984

2505 Power for Off-Pavement
Redman Power Chair
1601 S Pantano Road
Suite 107
Tucson, AZ 85710
Fax: 520-546-5530; *Toll Free:* 800-727-6684
info@redmanpowerchair.com
www.redmanpowerchair.com

Don Redman, Chief Executive Officer
Paula Redman, Chief Financial Officer
Samuel Redman, General Manager

Power-drive wheelchair has a solid seat and safely and securely handle knolls and off-pavement terrain.

2506 Redman Apache
Redman Power Chair
1601 S Pantano Road
Suite 107
Tucson, AZ 85710
Fax: 520-546-5530; *Toll Free:* 800-727-6684
info@redmanpowerchair.com
www.redmanpowerchair.com

Don Redman, Chief Executive Officer
Paula Redman, Chief Financial Officer
Samuel Redman, General Manager

These ultralight, active use wheelchairs offer quick release rear wheels, adjustable arm height and detachable arm swing-away.

2507 Redman Crow Line
Redman Power Chair
1601 S Pantano Road
Suite 107
Tucson, AZ 85710
Fax: 520-546-5530; *Toll Free:* 800-727-6684
info@redmanpowerchair.com
www.redmanpowerchair.com

Don Redman, Chief Executive Officer
Paula Redman, Chief Financial Officer
Samuel Redman, General Manager

Reclining wheelchair that reclines a full 90 degrees to flat and can be stopped anywhere on the axis.

2508 Roll-Aid
Stand Aid of Iowa
1009 2nd Ave
PO Box 386
Sheldon, IA 51201
712-324-2153
Fax: 712-324-5210; *Toll Free:* 800-831-8580
sales@stand-aid.com
www.stand-aid.com

Mike Kleinwolterink, Owner

Adapts to fit all standard collapsible wheelchairs. It is convenient, portable and provides electric rollator mobility instantly.

2509 Rolls 2000 Series
Invacare Corporation
One Invacare Way
Elyria, OH 44035-4190
440-329-6000
Fax: 877-619-7996; Toll Free: 800-333-6900
info@invacare.com
www.invacare.com

A Malachi Mixon III, Chairman Of The Board
Gerald B Blouch, President/ Chief Executive Offic
Robert K. Gudbranson, Senior Vice President and Chief

These wheelchairs are the first light-weight wheelchairs designed for rental use.

Year Founded: 1885

2510 Sidekick Walk & Ride Power Wheelchair
21st Century Scientific, Inc.
4931 N. Manufacturing Way
Coeur d'Alene, ID 83815
208-667-8800
Fax: 208-667-6600; Toll Free: 800-448-3680
21st@wheelchairs.com
www.21stcenturyscientific.com

Dr. Ronald E Prior Ph.D., President & Founder
Susan Harris, CFO/Webmaster

Manufactured for people up to 200 pounds with walking disabilities. It is lightweight, easy to use and transport, and competitively priced. The patent pending Walk and Ride feature allows the user to drive the SIDEKICK as a normal power wheelchair or walk behind it as a power walker using controls located on the push-handles.

Year Founded: 1979

2511 Sport Lite 4000
Gendron, Inc.
520 W. Mulberry St.
Suite 100
Bryan, OH 43506
Fax: 419-636-9261; Toll Free: 800-537-2521
sales@gendroninc.com
www.gendroninc.com

Steven Cotter, VP Sales
Roberta Jacobs, National Sales Manager
Robin Robin, Customer Service

Swing-away armrests made of durable stainless steel and detachable anti-tippers.

Year Founded: 1871

2512 Sportaid
2462 Centerville Rosebud Road
Loganville, GA 30052
770-554-5130
Fax: 770-554-5944; Toll Free: 800-743-7203
stuff@sportaid.com
www.sportaid.com

Jimmy Green, Contact
Norma Carden, Office Manager
Stacy Green, Sportaid

Offers an assortment of wheelchairs (everyday and racing), wheelchair sports equipment, replacement tires, hubs, spokes, pushrims, cushions and more. Call for free catalog.
Year Founded: 1987

2513 Wizz-ard
Wheelchairs of Kansas
204 W 2nd St.
PO Box 320
Ellis, KS 67637
785-726-4885
Fax: 800-337-2447; Toll Free: 800-537-6454
wokinfo@go2wok.com
www.wheelchairsofkansas.com

A large-frame wheelchair constructed of high quality, stress tested stainless steel to insure durability and peak performance.

2514 YM 9000 Ride-Lite Series
Invacare Corporation
1 Invacare Way
Elyria, OH 44035-4190
440-329-6000
Fax: 877-619-7996; Toll Free: 800-333-6900
info@invacare.com
www.invacare.com

A Malachi Mixon III, Chairman Of The Board
Gerald B Blouch, President/ Chief Executive Offic
Robert K. Gudbranson, Senior Vice President and Chief

This wheelchair has adjustable toggle wheel locks with brackets that bolt through the frame, composite pneumatic wheels and casters, and foam-padded back upholstery.

Year Founded: 1885

Wheelchair Accessories

2515 Air Liftunlimited
Air Lift Unlimited Inc.
1212 Kerr Gulch
Evergreen, CO 80439
303-526-4700
Fax: 303-526-4774; Toll Free: 800-776-6771
info@airlift.com
www.airlift.com/contact.html

Phyllis King, Sales Associate

Conveniently attaches liquid oxygen or cylinder unit to any size wheelchair or walker.

2516 Convert-Able Table
Rehab and Educational Aids for Living (R.E.A.L Inc
187 S Main Street
Dolgeville, NY 13329-1455
315-429-3071
Fax: 315-429-3071; Toll Free: 800-696-7041
rdesign@twcny.rr.com
www.realdesigninc.com

Specially designed for use with wheelchairs, this table has push button height adjustment and interchangeable tops so it can become a desk, art easel, etc.

2517 Curtis Instruments
Curtis Instruments, Inc.
200 Kisco Avenue
Mount Kisco, NY 10549
914-666-2971; *Fax:* 914-666-2188
www.curtisinst.com

Stuart Marwell, President & CEO
John Kenneally, Application Engineer
Nancy A Korman, National Sales Manager

Provides a readable, accurate indication of battery, in easy to read type of display. Innovative, efficient motor speed controllers for single or dual PM motor vehicles.

Year Founded: 1960

2518 East Penn Manufacturing Company
East Penn Manufacturing Company, Inc.
Deka Road
Lyon Station, PA 19536
610-682-6361
Fax: 610-682-4781
eastpenn@eastpenn-deka.com
www.dekabatteries.com

DeLight Breidegam, Chairman
Daniel R Langdon, President
Harold Eberly, VP Sales

Specially engineered for demanding deep-cycle applica-tions Gelled electrolyte Deka Dominator Batteries provides maintenance-free operation, longer battery life and hours of reliable performance. Their excellent recharge characteris-tics provide quick turn-a-round time.

Year Founded: 1946

2519 Lester Dual-Mode Battery Charger
Lester Electrical
625 W A Street
Lincoln, NE 68522-1794
402-477-8988; *Fax:* 402-474-1769
sales@lesterelectrical.com, service@lesterele
www.lesterelectrical.com

Edith Earnest, Sales Service Coordinator
James L Carrier, President

Replaceable electrolyte batteries require an entirely differ-ent charge cycle than do sealed batteries.

Year Founded: 1963

2520 Lestronic II
Lester Electrical
625 West A Street
Lincoln, NE 68522-1794
402-477-8988; *Fax:* 402-474-1769
sales@lesterelectrical.com, service@lesterele
www.lesterelectrical.com

James Carrier, President

Fully automatic battery charger.

Year Founded: 1963

2521 Mat Factory
Mat Factory Inc.
6726 N. Figueroa Street
Los Angeles, CA 90042
949-645-3122
Fax: 323-254-4545; *Toll Free:* 800-628-7626
www.matfactoryinc.com

Roger Maloney, President
Peggy Maloney, Owner

The safety deck II is an interlocking grid system made from recycled rubber tires. The tiles are set directly on top of the ground and permit grass to grow through the holes and cover the surface. It provides barrier free access for wheelchairs.

2522 Skyway
Skyway Machine, Inc.
4451 Caterpillar Road
Redding, CA 96003
530-243-5151
Fax: 530-243-5104; *Toll Free:* 800-332-3357
sales@skywaywheels.com
www.skywaytuffwheels.com

Parrey Cremeans, Sales Department
Rein Stolz, Engineering Department
Patrick McEachen, Customer Service

For over 20 years Skyway has been the world leader in composite wheels. Supplying over 650 different wheel combinations for wheelchairs, lawn and garden products, bicycles, and a large assortment of wheeled devices. Wheel sizes range from 5 to 24 inch diameter.

Year Founded: 1974

2523 Wheelchair Aide
Graham-Field Health Products, Inc.
2935 Northeast Parkway
Atlanta, GA 30360
678-291-3207
Fax: 800-726-0601; *Toll Free:* 800-347-5678
cs@grahamfield.com
www.grahamfield.com

Kenneth Spett, President & Chief Executive Offi
Lori Kirschner, Senior Vice President, HR & Admi
Alan Spett, Senior Vice President, Operation

This is a heavy-duty wheelchair comfort tray which sur-rounds the wheelchair user and provides a large, smooth surface for dining, writing, hobbies or work. The heavy gauge plastic tray is easy to clean and attaches with two Velcro straps.

Year Founded: 1850

2524 Wheelchair Work Table
Bailey Manufacturing Company
PO Box 130
Lodi, OH 44254-0130
330-948-1080
Fax: 800-224-5390; *Toll Free:* 800-321-8372
www.baileymfg.com

Larry Strimple, President

An adjustable height, functional, individual cut-out work table featuring a wood-grain laminate, scratch resistant top with chrome plated steel legs.

Year Founded: 1956

Aging

Associations & Organizations

2525 AARP
601 E Street NW
Washington, DC 20049
Toll Free: 888-687-2277
member@aarp.org
www.aarp.org
TTY: 877-434-7598

Jo Ann Jenkins, CEO

Formerly the American Association of Retired Persons. AARP is a collection of diverse individuals and ideas working as one to influence positive change and improve the lives of those 50 and over. AARP reflects a wide range of attitudes, cultures, lifestyles, and beliefs.

Year Founded: 1958; Number of Members: 37,000,000+

2526 AARP Alabama
201 Monroe Street
Suite 1880
Montgomery, AB 36104
Toll Free: 866-542-8167
alaarp@aarp.org
states.aarp.org

Candi Williams, Interim State Director

Year Founded: 2001; Number of Members: 450,000

2527 AARP Arizona
16165 N 83rd Avenue
Suite 201
Peoria, AZ 85382
Toll Free: 866-389-5649
aarpaz@aarp.org
states.aarp.org

Cynthia Fagyas, Contact

2528 AARP Arkansas
1701 Centerview Drive
Suite 205
Little Rock, AR 72211
Fax: 501-227-7710; *Toll Free:* 866-554-5379
araarp@aarp.org
states.aarp.org

2529 AARP California: Pasadena
200 S Los Robles Avenue
Suite 400
Pasadena, CA 91101-2422
Fax: 626-583-8500; *Toll Free:* 866-448-3614
caaarp@aarp.org
states.aarp.org/contact-aarp-california

Resources for online classes, training and more. Topics include Computers/Technology, Health/Wellbeing, Personal Finance. AARP Membership open to individuals age 50+, benefits include access to insurance services, travel discounts, advice on healthy living, financial planning, consumer protection. AARP represents members on issues like Medicare, Social Security, and consumer safety. Publications include the AARP Magazine and AARP Bulletin.

2530 AARP California: Sacramento
1415 L Street
Suite 960
Sacramento, CA 95814
Fax: 916-446-2223; *Toll Free:* 866-448-3614
caaarp@aarp.org
states.aarp.org/contact-aarp-california

Resources for online classes, training and more. Topics include Computers/Technology, Health/Wellbeing, Personal Finance. AARP Membership open to individuals age 50+, benefits include access to insurance services, travel discounts, advice on healthy living, financial planning, consumer protection. AARP represents members on issues like Medicare, Social Security, and consumer safety. Publications include the AARP Magazine and AARP Bulletin.

2531 AARP California: San Francisco
150 Post Street
Suite 450
San Francisco, CA 94108
Fax: 415-986-3467; *Toll Free:* 866-448-3614
caaarp@aarp.org
states.aarp.org/contact-aarp-california

2532 AARP Colorado
303 E 17th Avenue
Denver, CO 80203
Fax: 303-764-5999; *Toll Free:* 866-554-5376
coaarp@aarp.org
states.aarp.org

Resources for online classes, training and more. Topics include Computers/Technology, Health/Wellbeing, Personal Finance. AARP Membership open to individuals age 50+, benefits include access to insurance services, travel discounts, advice on healthy living, financial planning, consumer protection. AARP represents members on issues like Medicare, Social Security, and consumer safety. Publications include the AARP Magazine and AARP Bulletin.

2533 AARP Connecticut
21 Oak Street
Suite 104
Hartford, CT 06106
Toll Free: 866-295-7279
ctaarp@aarp.org
states.aarp.org/aarp-connecticut

Resources for online classes, training and more. Topics include Computers/Technology, Health/Wellbeing, Personal Finance. AARP Membership open to individuals age 50+, benefits include access to insurance services, travel discounts, advice on healthy living, financial planning, consumer protection. AARP represents members on issues like Medicare, Social Security, and consumer safety. Publications include the AARP Magazine and AARP Bulletin.

Number of Members: 600,000

2534 AARP Delaware
1100 North Market Street
Suite 1201
Wilmington, DE 19801
Toll Free: 866-227-7441
www.aarp.org/de

Resources for online classes, training and more. Topics include Computers/Technology, Health/Wellbeing, Personal Finance. AARP Membership open to individuals age 50+, benefits include access to insurance services, travel discounts, advice on healthy living, financial planning, consumer protection. AARP represents members on issues like Medicare, Social Security, and consumer safety. Publications include the AARP Magazine and AARP Bulletin.

2535 AARP Florida: Doral
3750 NW 87th Avenue
Suite 650
Doral, FL 33178
Fax: 786-804-4544; *Toll Free:* 866-595-7678
flaarp@aarp.org
states.aarp.org

Resources for online classes, training and more. Topics include Computers/Technology, Health/Wellbeing, Personal Finance. AARP Membership open to individuals age 50+, benefits include access to insurance services, travel discounts, advice on healthy living, financial planning, consumer protection. AARP represents members on issues like Medicare, Social Security, and consumer safety. Publications include the AARP Magazine and AARP Bulletin.

2536 AARP Florida: St. Petersburg
400 Carillon Parkway
Suite 100
St. Petersburg, FL 33716
Fax: 727-369-5191; *Toll Free:* 866-595-7678
flaarp@aarp.org
states.aarp.org

Resources for online classes, training and more. Topics include Computers/Technology, Health/Wellbeing, Personal Finance. AARP Membership open to individuals age 50+, benefits include access to insurance services, travel discounts, advice on healthy living, financial planning, consumer protection. AARP represents members on issues like Medicare, Social Security, and consumer safety. Publications include the AARP Magazine and AARP Bulletin.
Number of Members: 2.7 million

2537 AARP Florida: Tallahassee
200 West College Avenue
Suite 304
Tallahassee, FL 32301
Fax: 850-222-8968; *Toll Free:* 866-595-7678
flaarp@aarp.org
states.aarp.org

Resources for online classes, training and more. Topics include Computers/Technology, Health/Wellbeing, Personal Finance. AARP Membership open to individuals age 50+, benefits include access to insurance services, travel discounts, advice on healthy living, financial planning, consumer protection. AARP represents members on issues like Medicare, Social Security, and consumer safety. Publications include the AARP Magazine and AARP Bulletin.

2538 AARP Georgia
999 Peachtree Street NE
Suite 1100
Atlanta, GA 30309
Fax: 404-815-7940; *Toll Free:* 866-295-7281
gaaarp@aarp.org
states.aarp.org
Serena Garcia, Media Contact

Resources for online classes, training and more. Topics include Computers/Technology, Health/Wellbeing, Personal Finance. AARP Membership open to individuals age 50+, benefits include access to insurance services, travel dis-

counts, advice on healthy living, financial planning, consumer protection. AARP represents members on issues like Medicare, Social Security, and consumer safety. Publications include the AARP Magazine and AARP Bulletin.

2539 AARP Hawaii
1132 Bishop Street
Suite 1920
Honolulu, HI 96813
Fax: 808-537-2288; *Toll Free:* 866-295-7282
hiaarp@aarp.org
states.aarp.org/aarp-hawaii

Resources for online classes, training and more. Topics include Computers/Technology, Health/Wellbeing, Personal Finance. AARP Membership open to individuals age 50+, benefits include access to insurance services, travel discounts, advice on healthy living, financial planning, consumer protection. AARP represents members on issues like Medicare, Social Security, and consumer safety. Publications include the AARP Magazine and AARP Bulletin.
Number of Members: 150,000

2540 AARP Idaho
250 S 5th Street
Suite 800
Boise, ID 83702
Fax: 202-288-4424; *Toll Free:* 866-295-7284
aarpid@aarp.org
states.aarp.org/contact-aarp-idaho
Randy Simon, Media Contact

Resources for online classes, training and more. Topics include Computers/Technology, Health/Wellbeing, Personal Finance. AARP Membership open to individuals age 50+, benefits include access to insurance services, travel discounts, advice on healthy living, financial planning, consumer protection. AARP represents members on issues like Medicare, Social Security, and consumer safety. Publications include the AARP Magazine and AARP Bulletin.

2541 AARP Illinois
222 N LaSalle Street
Suite 710
Chicago, IL 60601
Fax: 312-372-2204; *Toll Free:* 866-448-3613
aarpil@aarp.org
states.aarp.org/aarp-illinois-contact-us
Gerardo Cardenas, Media Contact

Resources for online classes, training and more. Topics include Computers/Technology, Health/Wellbeing, Personal Finance. AARP Membership open to individuals age 50+, benefits include access to insurance services, travel discounts, advice on healthy living, financial planning, consumer protection. AARP represents members on issues like Medicare, Social Security, and consumer safety. Publications include the AARP Magazine and AARP Bulletin.

2542 AARP Indiana
One North Capitol Avenue
Suite 1275
Indianapolis, IN 46204-2025
Fax: 317-423-2211; *Toll Free:* 866-448-3618
inaarp@aarp.org
states.aarp.org/aarp-indiana
Katie Moreau, Media Contact

Resources for online classes, training and more. Topics include Computers/Technology, Health/Wellbeing, Personal

Finance. AARP Membership open to individuals age 50+, benefits include access to insurance services, travel discounts, advice on healthy living, financial planning, consumer protection. AARP represents members on issues like Medicare, Social Security, and consumer safety. Publications include the AARP Magazine and AARP Bulletin.

2543 AARP Iowa
600 E Court Avenue
Suite 100
Des Moines, IA 50309
Fax: 515-244-7767; *Toll Free:* 866-554-5378
ia@aarp.org
states.aarp.org/contact-us-2

Ann Black, Media Contact

Resources for online classes, training and more. Topics include Computers/Technology, Health/Wellbeing, Personal Finance. AARP Membership open to individuals age 50+, benefits include access to insurance services, travel discounts, advice on healthy living, financial planning, consumer protection. AARP represents members on issues like Medicare, Social Security, and consumer safety. Publications include the AARP Magazine and AARP Bulletin.

2544 AARP Kansas
6220 SW 29th Street
Suite 300
Topeka, KS 66614
Fax: 785-232-1465; *Toll Free:* 866-448-3619
ksaarp@aarp.org
states.aarp.org/contact-us-4

Mary Tritsch, Media Contact

Resources for online classes, training and more. Topics include Computers/Technology, Health/Wellbeing, Personal Finance. AARP Membership open to individuals age 50+, benefits include access to insurance services, travel discounts, advice on healthy living, financial planning, consumer protection. AARP represents members on issues like Medicare, Social Security, and consumer safety. Publications include the AARP Magazine and AARP Bulletin.

2545 AARP Kentucky
10401 Linn Station Road
Suite 121
Louisville, KY 40223
Toll Free: 866-295-7275
kyaarp@aarp.org
states.aarp.org/contact-aarp-kentucky

Scott Wegenast, Contact

Resources for online classes, training and more. Topics include Computers/Technology, Health/Wellbeing, Personal Finance. AARP Membership open to individuals age 50+, benefits include access to insurance services, travel discounts, advice on healthy living, financial planning, consumer protection. AARP represents members on issues like Medicare, Social Security, and consumer safety. Publications include the AARP Magazine and AARP Bulletin.

2546 AARP Louisiana
301 Main Street
Suite 1012
Baton Rouge, LA 70825
Toll Free: 866-448-3620
la@aarp.org
states.aarp.org/contact-aarp-louisiana
Denise Bottcher, Communications Director

Resources for online classes, training and more. Topics include Computers/Technology, Health/Wellbeing, Personal Finance. AARP Membership open to individuals age 50+, benefits include access to insurance services, travel discounts, advice on healthy living, financial planning, consumer protection. AARP represents members on issues like Medicare, Social Security, and consumer safety. Publications include the AARP Magazine and AARP Bulletin.

2547 AARP Maine
53 Baxter Boulevard
Portland, ME 04101
Toll Free: 866-554-5380
me@aarp.org
states.aarp.org/about-aarp-maine-3

Lori Parham, State Director
Amy Gallant, Director, Advocacy & Outreach
Jane Margesson, Director, Comms. & Media Relats.

Resources for online classes, training and more. Topics include Computers/Technology, Health/Wellbeing, Personal Finance. AARP Membership open to individuals age 50+, benefits include access to insurance services, travel discounts, advice on healthy living, financial planning, consumer protection. AARP represents members on issues like Medicare, Social Security, and consumer safety. Publications include the AARP Magazine and AARP Bulletin.

2548 AARP Maryland
200 St. Paul Place
Suite 2510
Baltimore, MD 21202
Fax: 410-837-0269; *Toll Free:* 866-542-8163
mdaarp@aarp.org
states.aarp.org

Nancy Carr, Comms. Representative

Resources for online classes, training and more. Topics include Computers/Technology, Health/Wellbeing, Personal Finance. AARP Membership open to individuals age 50+, benefits include access to insurance services, travel discounts, advice on healthy living, financial planning, consumer protection. AARP represents members on issues like Medicare, Social Security, and consumer safety. Publications include the AARP Magazine and AARP Bulletin.

2549 AARP Massachusetts
1 Beacon Street
Suite 2301
Boston, MA 02108
Fax: 617-723-4224; *Toll Free:* 866-448-3621
ma@aarp.org
states.aarp.org

Cindy Campbell, Comms. Director

2550 AARP Michigan
309 N Washington Square
Suite 110
Lansing, MI 48933
Fax: 517-482-2794; *Toll Free:* 866-227-7448
miaarp@aarp.org
states.aarp.org/welcome-to-aarp-michigan

Resources for online classes, training and more. Topics include Computers/Technology, Health/Wellbeing, Personal Finance. AARP Membership open to individuals age 50+, benefits include access to insurance services, travel discounts, advice on healthy living, financial planning, consumer protection. AARP represents members on issues like

Medicare, Social Security, and consumer safety. Publications include the AARP Magazine and AARP Bulletin.

2551 AARP Minnesota

30 E 7th Street
Suite 1200
St. Paul, MN 55101
Toll Free: 866-554-5381
aarpmn@aarp.org
states.aarp.org/contact-aarp-minnesota

Will Phillips, State Director
Seth Boffeli, Comms. Director
Jay Haapala, Outreach Director

Resources for online classes, training and more. Topics include Computers/Technology, Health/Wellbeing, Personal Finance. AARP Membership open to individuals age 50+, benefits include access to insurance services, travel discounts, advice on healthy living, financial planning, consumer protection. AARP represents members on issues like Medicare, Social Security, and consumer safety. Publications include the AARP Magazine and AARP Bulletin.

2552 AARP Mississippi

141 Township Avenue
Suite 302
Ridgeland, MS 39157
Fax: 601-898-5429; *Toll Free:* 866-554-5382
msaarp@aarp.org
states.aarp.org

Ronda Gooden, Media Contact

Resources for online classes, training and more. Topics include Computers/Technology, Health/Wellbeing, Personal Finance. AARP Membership open to individuals age 50+, benefits include access to insurance services, travel discounts, advice on healthy living, financial planning, consumer protection. AARP represents members on issues like Medicare, Social Security, and consumer safety. Publications include the AARP Magazine and AARP Bulletin.

2553 AARP Missouri

9200 Ward Parkway
Suite 350
Kansas City, MO 64114
Fax: 816-561-3107; *Toll Free:* 866-389-5627
aarpmo@aarp.org
states.aarp.org/contact-aarp-missouri-2

Anita Parran, Media Contact

Resources for online classes, training and more. Topics include Computers/Technology, Health/Wellbeing, Personal Finance. AARP Membership open to individuals age 50+, benefits include access to insurance services, travel discounts, advice on healthy living, financial planning, consumer protection. AARP represents members on issues like Medicare, Social Security, and consumer safety. Publications include the AARP Magazine and AARP Bulletin.

2554 AARP Montana

30 W 14th Street
Suite 301
Helena, MT 59601
Toll Free: 866-295-7278
sdahl@aarp.org
states.aarp.org/about-aarp-montana

Stacia Dahl, Media Contact

Resources for online classes, training and more. Topics include Computers/Technology, Health/Wellbeing, Personal

Finance. AARP Membership open to individuals age 50+, benefits include access to insurance services, travel discounts, advice on healthy living, financial planning, consumer protection. AARP represents members on issues like Medicare, Social Security, and consumer safety. Publications include the AARP Magazine and AARP Bulletin.

Number of Members: 150,000

2555 AARP Nebraska

301 S 13th Street
Suite 201
Lincoln, NE 68508
Fax: 402-323-6908; *Toll Free:* 866-389-5651
neaarp@aarp.org
states.aarp.org

Devorah Lanner, Media Contact

Resources for online classes, training and more. Topics include Computers/Technology, Health/Wellbeing, Personal Finance. AARP Membership open to individuals age 50+, benefits include access to insurance services, travel discounts, advice on healthy living, financial planning, consumer protection. AARP represents members on issues like Medicare, Social Security, and consumer safety. Publications include the AARP Magazine and AARP Bulletin.

Number of Members: 200,000

2556 AARP Nevada

5820 S Eastern Avenue
Suite 190
Las Vegas, NV 89119
Toll Free: 866-389-5652
aarpnv@aarp.org
states.aarp.org/contact-aarp-nevada

Hilarie Grey, Media Contact

2557 AARP New Hampshire

45 South Main Street
Suite 202
Concord, NH 03301
Fax: 603-224-6211; *Toll Free:* 866-542-8168
nh@aarp.org
states.aarp.org

Resources for online classes, training and more. Topics include Computers/Technology, Health/Wellbeing, Personal Finance. AARP Membership open to individuals age 50+, benefits include access to insurance services, travel discounts, advice on healthy living, financial planning, consumer protection. AARP represents members on issues like Medicare, Social Security, and consumer safety. Publications include the AARP Magazine and AARP Bulletin.

2558 AARP New Jersey

101 Rockingham Row
Princeton, NJ 08540
Fax: 609-987-4634; *Toll Free:* 866-542-8165
aarpnj@aarp.org
states.aarp.org/contactaarpnj

Jeff Abramo, Media Contact

Resources for online classes, training and more. Topics include Computers/Technology, Health/Wellbeing, Personal Finance. AARP Membership open to individuals age 50+, benefits include access to insurance services, travel discounts, advice on healthy living, financial planning, consumer protection. AARP represents members on issues like Medicare, Social Security, and consumer safety. Publications include the AARP Magazine and AARP Bulletin.

2559 AARP New Mexico
535 Cerrillos Road
Santa Fe, NM 87501
Toll Free: 866-389-5636
nmaarp@aarp.org
states.aarp.org/tag/aarp-new-mexico

Resources for online classes, training and more. Topics include Computers/Technology, Health/Wellbeing, Personal Finance. AARP Membership open to individuals age 50+, benefits include access to insurance services, travel discounts, advice on healthy living, financial planning, consumer protection. AARP represents members on issues like Medicare, Social Security, and consumer safety. Publications include the AARP Magazine and AARP Bulletin.

2560 AARP New York: Albany
One Commerce Plaza
Suite 706
Albany, NY 12260
Fax: 212-644-6390; *Toll Free:* 866-227-7442
nyaarp@aarp.org
states.aarp.org

Stacey Kratz, Media Contact

Resources for online classes, training and more. Topics include Computers/Technology, Health/Wellbeing, Personal Finance. AARP Membership open to individuals age 50+, benefits include access to insurance services, travel discounts, advice on healthy living, financial planning, consumer protection. AARP represents members on issues like Medicare, Social Security, and consumer safety. Publications include the AARP Magazine and AARP Bulletin.

2561 AARP New York: New York
780 Third Avenue
33rd Floor
New York, NY 12260
Fax: 212-644-6390; *Toll Free:* 866-227-7442
nyaarp@aarp.org
states.aarp.org

Stacey Kratz, Media Contact

Resources for online classes, training and more. Topics include Computers/Technology, Health/Wellbeing, Personal Finance. AARP Membership open to individuals age 50+, benefits include access to insurance services, travel discounts, advice on healthy living, financial planning, consumer protection. AARP represents members on issues like Medicare, Social Security, and consumer safety. Publications include the AARP Magazine and AARP Bulletin.

2562 AARP New York: Rochester
Monroe Community Hospital
435 E Henrietta Road
Rochester, NY 14620
Fax: 212-644-6390; *Toll Free:* 866-227-7442
nyaarp@aarg.org
states.aarp.org

Stacey Kratz, Media Contact

2563 AARP North Carolina
1511 Sunday Drive
Suite 312
Raleigh, NC 27607
Toll Free: 866-389-5650
ncaarp@aarp.org
www.aarp.org/nc

Resources for online classes, training and more. Topics include Computers/Technology, Health/Wellbeing, Personal Finance. AARP Membership open to individuals age 50+, benefits include access to insurance services, travel discounts, advice on healthy living, financial planning, consumer protection. AARP represents members on issues like Medicare, Social Security, and consumer safety. Publications include the AARP Magazine and AARP Bulletin.

Number of Members: 1.1 million

2564 AARP North Dakota
107 W Main Avenue
Bismarck, ND 58501
Fax: 701-255-2242; *Toll Free:* 866-554-5383
aarpnd@aarp.org
states.aarp.org/aarp-north-dakota

Resources for online classes, training and more. Topics include Computers/Technology, Health/Wellbeing, Personal Finance. AARP Membership open to individuals age 50+, benefits include access to insurance services, travel discounts, advice on healthy living, financial planning, consumer protection. AARP represents members on issues like Medicare, Social Security, and consumer safety. Publications include the AARP Magazine and AARP Bulletin.

2565 AARP Ohio
17 S High Street
Suite 800
Columbus, OH 43215
Fax: 614-224-9801; *Toll Free:* 866-389-5653
ohaarp@aarp.org
states.aarp.org

Resources for online classes, training and more. Topics include Computers/Technology, Health/Wellbeing, Personal Finance. AARP Membership open to individuals age 50+, benefits include access to insurance services, travel discounts, advice on healthy living, financial planning, consumer protection. AARP represents members on issues like Medicare, Social Security, and consumer safety. Publications include the AARP Magazine and AARP Bulletin.

Number of Members: 1.5 million

2566 AARP Oklahoma
126 N Bryant Avenue
Edmond, OK 73034
Fax: 405-340-9776; *Toll Free:* 866-295-7277
ok@aarp.org
states.aarp.org/contact-aarp-oklahoma

Sean Voskuhl, State Director

Resources for online classes, training and more. Topics include Computers/Technology, Health/Wellbeing, Personal Finance. AARP Membership open to individuals age 50+, benefits include access to insurance services, travel discounts, advice on healthy living, financial planning, consumer protection. AARP represents members on issues like Medicare, Social Security, and consumer safety. Publications include the AARP Magazine and AARP Bulletin.

2567 AARP Oregon
9200 SE Sunnybrook Boulevard
Suite 410
Clackamas, OR 97015
Toll Free: 866-554-5360
oraarp@aarp.org
states.aarp.org/about-aarp-oregon

Jerry Cohen, State Director

Resources for online classes, training and more. Topics include Computers/Technology, Health/Wellbeing, Personal Finance. AARP Membership open to individuals age 50+, benefits include access to insurance services, travel discounts, advice on healthy living, financial planning, consumer protection. AARP represents members on issues like Medicare, Social Security, and consumer safety. Publications include the AARP Magazine and AARP Bulletin.

Number of Members: 500,000

2568 AARP Pennsylvania: Harrisburg

30 North 3rd Street
Suite 750
Harrisburg, PA 17101
Fax: 717-236-4078; *Toll Free:* 866-389-5654
aarppa@aarp.org
states.aarp.org/your-local-aarp-office

Steve Gardner, Media Contact
Jacklyn Isasi, Media Contact

Resources for online classes, training and more. Topics include Computers/Technology, Health/Wellbeing, Personal Finance. AARP Membership open to individuals age 50+, benefits include access to insurance services, travel discounts, advice on healthy living, financial planning, consumer protection. AARP represents members on issues like Medicare, Social Security, and consumer safety. Publications include the AARP Magazine and AARP Bulletin.

Year Founded: 1987; Number of Members: 1.8 million

2569 AARP Pennsylvania: Philadelphia

1650 Market Street
Suite 675
Philadelphia, PA 19103
Fax: 215-665-8529; *Toll Free:* 866-389-5654
aarppa@aarp.org
states.aarp.org/your-local-aarp-office

Steve Gardner, Media Contact
Jacklyn Isasi, Media Contact

Resources for online classes, training and more. Topics include Computers/Technology, Health/Wellbeing, Personal Finance. AARP Membership open to individuals age 50+, benefits include access to insurance services, travel discounts, advice on healthy living, financial planning, consumer protection. AARP represents members on issues like Medicare, Social Security, and consumer safety. Publications include the AARP Magazine and AARP Bulletin.

Year Founded: 1987; Number of Members: 1.8 million

2570 AARP Rhode Island

10 Orms Street
Suite 200
Providence, RI 02904
401-248-2663
Fax: 401-272-0596; *Toll Free:* 866-542-8170
ri@aarp.org
states.aarp.org/contact

John Martin, Comms. Director

Resources for online classes, training and more. Topics include Computers/Technology, Health/Wellbeing, Personal Finance. AARP Membership open to individuals age 50+, benefits include access to insurance services, travel discounts, advice on healthy living, financial planning, consumer protection. AARP represents members on issues like Medicare, Social Security, and consumer safety. Publications include the AARP Magazine and AARP Bulletin.

2571 AARP South Carolina

1201 Main Street
Suite 1720
Columbia, SC 29201
Toll Free: 866-389-5655
scaarp@aarp.org
states.aarp.org/weve-moved

Resources for online classes, training and more. Topics include Computers/Technology, Health/Wellbeing, Personal Finance. AARP Membership open to individuals age 50+, benefits include access to insurance services, travel discounts, advice on healthy living, financial planning, consumer protection. AARP represents members on issues like Medicare, Social Security, and consumer safety. Publications include the AARP Magazine and AARP Bulletin.

2572 AARP South Dakota

5101 S Nevada Avenue
Suite 150
Sioux Falls, SD 57108
Toll Free: 866-542-8172
sdaarp@aarp.org
states.aarp.org

Resources for online classes, training and more. Topics include Computers/Technology, Health/Wellbeing, Personal Finance. AARP Membership open to individuals age 50+, benefits include access to insurance services, travel discounts, advice on healthy living, financial planning, consumer protection. AARP represents members on issues like Medicare, Social Security, and consumer safety. Publications include the AARP Magazine and AARP Bulletin.

2573 AARP Tennessee

150 4th Avenue N
Suite 180
Nashville, TN 37219
Toll Free: 866-295-7274
tnaarp@aarp.org
states.aarp.org/about-aarp-tennessee

Rebecca Kelly, State Director
Rob Naylor, Comms. Director

Resources for online classes, training and more. Topics include Computers/Technology, Health/Wellbeing, Personal Finance. AARP Membership open to individuals age 50+, benefits include access to insurance services, travel discounts, advice on healthy living, financial planning, consumer protection. AARP represents members on issues like Medicare, Social Security, and consumer safety. Publications include the AARP Magazine and AARP Bulletin.

Number of Members: 645,000

2574 AARP Texas: Austin

98 San Jacinto
Suite 750
Austin, TX 78701
Toll Free: 866-227-7443
txaarp@aarp.org
states.aarp.org/contact-aarp-texas

Resources for online classes, training and more. Topics include Computers/Technology, Health/Wellbeing, Personal Finance. AARP Membership open to individuals age 50+, benefits include access to insurance services, travel discounts, advice on healthy living, financial planning, consumer protection. AARP represents members on issues like Medicare, Social Security, and consumer safety. Publications include the AARP Magazine and AARP Bulletin.

2575 AARP Texas: Dallas
8140 Walnut Hill Lane
Suite 108
Dallas, TX 75231
Toll Free: 866-227-7443
txaarp@aarp.org
states.aarp.org/contact-aarp-texas

Resources for online classes, training and more. Topics include Computers/Technology, Health/Wellbeing, Personal Finance. AARP Membership open to individuals age 50+, benefits include access to insurance services, travel discounts, advice on healthy living, financial planning, consumer protection. AARP represents members on issues like Medicare, Social Security, and consumer safety. Publications include the AARP Magazine and AARP Bulletin.

2576 AARP Texas: Houston
2323 S Shepherd
Suite 1100
Houston, TX 77019
Toll Free: 866-227-7443
txaarp@aarp.org
states.aarp.org/contact-aarp-texas

Resources for online classes, training and more. Topics include Computers/Technology, Health/Wellbeing, Personal Finance. AARP Membership open to individuals age 50+, benefits include access to insurance services, travel discounts, advice on healthy living, financial planning, consumer protection. AARP represents members on issues like Medicare, Social Security, and consumer safety. Publications include the AARP Magazine and AARP Bulletin.

2577 AARP Utah
6975 Union Park Center
Suite 320
Midvale, UT 84047
e-mail: utaarp@aarp.org
states.aarp.org/contact-us-3

Alan Ormsby, State Director

Resources for online classes, training and more. Topics include Computers/Technology, Health/Wellbeing, Personal Finance. AARP Membership open to individuals age 50+, benefits include access to insurance services, travel discounts, advice on healthy living, financial planning, consumer protection. AARP represents members on issues like Medicare, Social Security, and consumer safety. Publications include the AARP Magazine and AARP Bulletin.

Number of Members: 211,000

2578 AARP Vermont
199 Main Street
Suite 225
Burlington, VT 05401
Fax: 802-651-9805; *Toll Free:* 866-227-7451
vtaarp@aarp.org
states.aarp.org/contact-info

Resources for online classes, training and more. Topics include Computers/Technology, Health/Wellbeing, Personal Finance. AARP Membership open to individuals age 50+, benefits include access to insurance services, travel discounts, advice on healthy living, financial planning, consumer protection. AARP represents members on issues like Medicare, Social Security, and consumer safety. Publications include the AARP Magazine and AARP Bulletin.

2579 AARP Virgin Islands
4093 Diamond Ruby
Suite 6
Christiansted, VI 00820
340-713-2002
Fax: 340-692-2544
viaarp@aarp.org
states.aarp.org/aarp-virgin-islands

Denyce E. Singleton, State Director

Number of Members: 20,000

2580 AARP Virginia
707 E Main Street
Suite 910
Richmond, VA 23219
Fax: 804-819-1923; *Toll Free:* 866-542-8164
vaaarp@aarp.org
states.aarp.org/contact-aarp-virginia

Resources for online classes, training and more. Topics include Computers/Technology, Health/Wellbeing, Personal Finance. AARP Membership open to individuals age 50+, benefits include access to insurance services, travel discounts, advice on healthy living, financial planning, consumer protection. AARP represents members on issues like Medicare, Social Security, and consumer safety. Publications include the AARP Magazine and AARP Bulletin.

2581 AARP Washington
18000 International Boulevard
Suite 1020
SeaTac, WA 98188
Fax: 206-517-9350; *Toll Free:* 866-227-7457
aarpwa@aarp.org
www.aarp.org/wa

Resources for online classes, training and more. Topics include Health/Wellbeing, Caregiving Resources, Computers/Technology, and more. AARP Membership open to individuals age 50+, benefits include access to insurance services, travel discounts, advice on healthy living, financial planning, consumer protection. AARP represents members on issues like Medicare, Social Security, and consumer safety. Publications include the AARP Magazine and AARP Bulletin.

Number of Members: 960,000

2582 AARP Washington, DC
601 E Street NW
Washington, DC 20049
202-434-7700
Fax: 202-434-7710; *Toll Free:* 866-554-5384
dcaarp@aarp.org
states.aarp.org

Louis Davis Jr., State Director

Number of Members: 88,500

2583 AARP West Virginia
300 Summers Street
Suite 400
Charleston, WV 25301
Fax: 304-344-4633; *Toll Free:* 866-227-7458
wvaarp@aarp.org
states.aarp.org/about-aarp-west-virginia

Resources for online classes, training and more. Topics include Computers/Technology, Health/Wellbeing, Personal Finance. AARP Membership open to individuals age 50+, benefits include access to insurance services, travel discounts, advice on healthy living, financial planning, consumer protection. AARP represents members on issues like Medicare, Social Security, and consumer safety. Publications include the AARP Magazine and AARP Bulletin.

2584 AARP Wisconsin
222 W Washington Avenue
Suite 600
Madison, WI 53703
Fax: 608-251-7612; *Toll Free:* 866-448-3611
wistate@aarp.org
states.aarp.org

Jim Flaherty, Media Contact

Resources for online classes, training and more. Topics include Computers/Technology, Health/Wellbeing, Personal Finance. AARP Membership open to individuals age 50+, benefits include access to insurance services, travel discounts, advice on healthy living, financial planning, consumer protection. AARP represents members on issues like Medicare, Social Security, and consumer safety. Publications include the AARP Magazine and AARP Bulletin.

Number of Members: 800,000

2585 AARP Wyoming
2020 Carey Avenue
Mezzanine
Cheyenne, WY 82009
Toll Free: 866-663-3290
wyaarp@aarp.org
states.aarp.org/aarp-wyoming

Tim Summers, State Director

Resources for online classes, training and more. Topics include Computers/Technology, Health/Wellbeing, Personal Finance. AARP Membership open to individuals age 50+, benefits include access to insurance services, travel discounts, advice on healthy living, financial planning, consumer protection. AARP represents members on issues like Medicare, Social Security, and consumer safety. Publications include the AARP Magazine and AARP Bulletin.

2586 ACL Regional Support Center: Region I
Administration for Community Living
John F. Kennedy Building
Room 2075
Boston, MA 02203
617-565-1158
Fax: 617-565-4511
www.acl.gov

Kathleen Otte, Regional Administrator

Region includes CT, MA, ME, NH, RI, VT

2587 ACL Regional Support Center: Region II
Administration for Community Living
26 Federal Plaza
Room 38-102
New York, NY 10278
212-264-2976
Fax: 212-264-0114
www.acl.gov

Kathleen Otte, Regional Administrator

Region includes NY, NJ, PR, VI

2588 ACL Regional Support Center: Region III
Administration for Community Living
Atlanta Federal Center
61 Forsyth Street SW, Suite 5M69
Atlanta, GA 30303-8909
215-356-1683
Fax: 215-861-4625
www.acl.gov

Costas Miskis, Regional Administrator

Region includes DC, DE, MD, PA, VA, WV

2589 ACL Regional Support Center: Region IV
Administration for Community Living
Atlanta Federal Center
61 Forsyth Street, Suite 5M69
Atlanta, GA 30303-8909
404-562-7600
Fax: 404-562-7598
www.acl.gov

Costas Miskis, Regional Administrator

Region includes AL, FL, GA, KY, MS, NC, SC, TN

2590 ACL Regional Support Center: Region IX
Administration for Community Living
90 7th Street
T-1800
San Francisco, CA 94103
415-437-8780
Fax: 415-437-8782
www.acl.gov

David Ishida, Regional Administrator

Region includes CA, NV, AZ, HI, GU, CNMI, AS

2591 ACL Regional Support Center: Region V
Administration for Community Living
233 N Michigan Avenue
Suite 790
Chicago, IL 60601-5519
312-938-9855
Fax: 312-886-8533
www.acl.gov

Jim Varpness, Regional Administrator

Region includes IL, IN, MI, MN, OH, WI

2592 ACL Regional Support Center: Region VI
Administration for Community Living
1301 Young Street
Room 736
Dallas, TX 75201
214-767-2971
Fax: 214-767-2951
www.acl.gov

Percy Devine, Regional Administrator

Region includes AR, LA, OK, NM, TX

2593 ACL Regional Support Center: Region VII
Administration for Community Living
233 N Michigan Avenue
Suite 790
Chicago, IL 60601-5519
312-938-9855
Fax: 312-886-8533
www.acl.gov

Jim Varpness, Regional Administrator

Region includes IA, KS, MO, NE

2594 ACL Regional Support Center: Region VIII
Administration for Community Living
999 18th Street, South Terrace
Suite 496
Denver, CO 80202
303-844-2951
Fax: 303-844-2943
www.acl.gov

Percy Devine, Regional Administrator

Region includes CO, MT, UT, WY, ND, SD

2595 ACL Regional Support Center: Region X
Administration for Community Living
Blanchard Plaza, RX-33, Room 859
2201 Sixth Avenue
Seattle, WA 98121
206-615-2298
Fax: 206-615-2305
www.acl.gov

David Ishida, Regional Administrator

Regions include AK, ID, OR, WA

2596 ADAPT
1640-A E 2nd Street
Suite 200
Austin, TX 78702
303-744-0717
Fax: 303-733-6211
adapt@adapt.org
www.adapt.org

Babs Johnson, Contact

ADAPT is a national grass-roots community that organizes
disability rights activists to engage in nonviolent direct action, including civil disobedience, to assure the civil and
human rights of people with disabilities to live in freedom.

2597 AMDA - The Society for Post-Acute and
Long-Term Care Medicine
10500 Little Patuxent Parkway
Suite 210
Columbia, MD 21044
410-740-9743
Fax: 410-740-4572; *Toll Free:* 800-876-2632
info@paltc.org
paltc.org

Heidi K White, MD, MHS, MEd, President
Arif Nazir, MD, FACP, CMD, Vice President
Chritoper E Laxton, CAE, Executive Director

The only medical specialty society representing the community of over 50,000 medical directors, physicians, nurse
practitioners, physician assistants, and other practitioners
working in the various post-acute and long-term care
(PA/LTC) settings.

Year Founded: 1978

2598 Administration on Aging
Administration for Community Living
330 C Street SW
Washington, DC 20201
202-401-4634
www.aoa.gov

Created to administer the Older Americans Act of 1965.

2599 Advancing Excellence in America's Nursing
Homes
www.nhqualitycampaign.org

Jay Sackman, Chair
Donna Adair, Secretary
Dheeraj Mahajan, Treasurer

Coalition of 28 organizations working to make nursing
homes better places to live, work and visit.

Year Founded: 2006

2600 AgainCare.org
9015 Strada Stell Court
Suite 203
Naples, FL 34109
239-594-3222
www.agingcare.com

Joe Buckheit, President
Christina Hardy, Vice President
Ashley Huntsberry-Lett, Editor-In-Chief

An online resource for aiding family caregivers.
AgingCare.com covers questions on assisted living,
long-term and home care, veterans benefits, Alzheimer's
disease, financial aid, funeral planning, and more.

2601 Alliance for Aging Research
1700 K Street NW
Suite 740
Washington, DC 20006
202-293-2856
Fax: 202-955-8394
info@agingresearch.org
www.agingresearch.org

Sue Peschin, President & CEO

Non-profit organization dedicated to supporting and accel-
erating the pace of medical discoveries to vastly improve
the universal human experience of aging and health.

2602 Alliance for Retired Americans
815 16th Street NW
4th Floor
Washington, DC 20006
202-637-5399
retiredamericans.org

Robert Roach Jr., President
Joe Peters Jr., Secretary & Treasurer

National grassroots organization advocates for a progressive political and social agenda that improves the lives of
retirees and older Americans.

Year Founded: 2001; Number of Members: 4.3 million

2603 American Association for Geriatric Psychiatry
6728 Old McLean Village Drive
McLean, VA 22101
703-556-9222
Fax: 703-556-8729
main@aagponline.org
www.aagponline.org

Christopher Wood, Executive Director

Information and resources for physician members and affiliates on improving quality of life for older persons with
mental disorders. Provides news, facts, tools and expert information for adults coping with mental health issues and
aging.

Year Founded: 1978; Number of Members: 2000

2604 American Geriatrics Society

40 Fulton Street
18th Fl.
New York, NY 10038
212-308-1414
Fax: 212-832-8646; *Toll Free:* 800-247-4779
info.amger@americangeriatrics.org
www.americangeriatrics.org

Nancy E. Lundebjerg, CEO

The premier professional organization of healthcare providers dedicated to improving the health and well-being of older adults. With an active membership of over 6,000 health care professionals, the AGS has a long history of affecting change in the provision of healthcare in older adults. The AGS Foundation for Health in Aging (FHA) aims to build a bridge between the research and practice of geriatrics health care professionals and the public. The FHA advocates on behalf of older adults and their special needs through public education, clinical research and public policy.

Year Founded: 1942; Number of Members: 5,000+

2605 American Public Health Association

800 I Street NW
Washington, DC 20001
202-777-2742
Fax: 202-777-2534
www.apha.org
TTY: 202-777-2500

Georges C. Benjamin, Executive Director

Public health awareness association.

2606 American Society on Aging

575 Market Street
Suite 2100
San Francisco, CA 94105-2869
415-974-9600
Fax: 415-974-0300; *Toll Free:* 800-537-9728
info@asaging.org
www.asaging.org

Robert Stein, President & CEO
Robert R. Lowe, COO

Health care and social service professionals, educators, researchers, administrators, businesspersons, students, and senior citizens. Works to enhance the well-being of older individuals and to foster unity among those working with and for the elderly. Offers 25 continuing education programs for professionals in aging-related fields. Publishes 'Aging Today,' a bi-monthly newspaper, and 'Generations,' a quarterly journal.

Year Founded: 1954; Number of Members: 5,000

2607 American Urogynecologic Society

2025 M Street NW
Suite 800
Washington, DC 20036
202-367-1167
Fax: 202-367-2167
info@augs.org
www.augs.org

Michelle Zinnert, Executive Director
Colleen Hughes, Associate Executive Director

The leader in female pelvic medicine and reconstructive surgery.

Year Founded: 1979

2608 Argentum

1650 King Street
Suite 602
Alexandria, VA 22314
703-894-1805
www.alfa.org

James Balda, President/CEO
Maribeth Bersani, Chief Operating Officer
Gina Mamone, Chief Financial Officer

Argentum is the leading national association exclusively dedicated to supporting companies operating professionally managed, resident-centered senior living communities and the older adults and families they serve.

Year Founded: 1990

2609 Arizona Center on Aging

Arizona Center on Aging
1807 E Elm Street
Tucson, AZ 85719
520-626-5800
Fax: 520-626-5801
info@aging.arizona.edu
www.aging.arizona.edu

Mindy Fain, MD, Co-Director
Janko Nikolich-Zugish, MD, Co-Director

The mission at Arizona Center of Aging (ACOA) is to promote healthy and functional lives for older adults through comprehensive programs in research, education and training, and clinical care.

2610 Association for Adult Development and Aging

5999 Stevenson Avenue
Alexandria, VA 22304-3300
703-823-9800 Toll free: 800-347-6647
www.aadaweb.org

Wendy Killam, President

A division of the American Counseling Association. Individuals holding a master's degree or its equivalent in adult counseling or a related field. Seeks to: improve the competence and skills of ACA and AADA members; expand professional work opportunities in adult development and aging counseling; promote the development of guidelines for professional preparation of counselors. Provides leadership and information to families, legislators, communitty service agencies, counselors, and other service providers in professions related to adult development and aging. Serves as forum for the discussion of ethical, social, and technical issues related to counseling adults across the life span.

Year Founded: 1986

2611 BrightFocus Foundation

22512 Gateway Center Drive
Clarksburg, MD 20871-2005
301-948-3244
Fax: 301-258-9454; *Toll Free:* 800-437-2423
jphilabaum@brightfocus.org
www.brightfocus.org

Dave Marks, VP, Finance & Administration
Diane Bovenkamp, VP, Scientific Affairs
Michael Buckley, VP, Public Affairs

Offers updated and trustworthy information on research, treatments, and resources. Free publications and newsletters.

Year Founded: 1973

2612 Brookdale Center for Healthy Aging and Longevity of Hunter College
2180 3rd Avenue
8th Floor
New York, NY 10035
212-396-7835
Fax: 212-396-7852
info@brookdale.org
www.brookdale.org

Ruth Finkelstein, PhD, Executive Director
Jerry Antonatos, MPA, Director, Finance/Administration
Geoff Rogers, Director, Learning Development

The Brookdale Center for Healthy Aging is a leader and innovator in public policy, research, and education related to aging and elder justice. We are a part of Hunter College, the City University of New York. We work in partnership with a wide range of agencies and non-governmental organizations to promote ethical treatment of older adults and other vulnerable populations in social service and healthcare systems and to develop educational curricula and training for professionals who work with older adults.

Year Founded: 1974

2613 Center for Benefits Access
National Council on Aging
251 18th Street S
Suite 500
Arlington, VA 22202
571-527-3900
centerforbenefits@ncoa.org
www.ncoa.org/centerforbenefits

Leslie Fried, Director

Benefits outreach and enrollment for seniors and younger adults with disabilities.

Year Founded: 1950

2614 Center for Healthy Aging
National Council on Aging
251 18th Street S
Suite 500
Arlington, VA 22202
571-527-3900
cha@ncoa.org
www.ncoa.org

Binod Suwal, Senior Program Manager

Helping older adults live longer and healthier lives through evidence-based health promotion and disease prevention programs.

Year Founded: 1950

2615 Center for Medicare Advocacy
PO Box 350
Willimantic, CT 06226
860-456-7790
Fax: 860-456-2614
mshepard@medicareadvocacy.org
www.medicareadvocacy.org

Judith A. Stein, Executive Director

Offers consultation, training, presentation, and materials on wide array of topics pertaining to aging.

Year Founded: 1986

2616 Center for Positive Aging
1440 Dutch Valley Place NE
Suite 120
Atlanta, GA 30324-5367
404-872-9191
Fax: 404-872-1737
www.centerforpositiveaging.org

Katie Jones, Chair
Ellen Miller, Treasurer
Carolyn Roper, Secretary

The Center for Positive Aging is a partnership of individuals, community organizations and congregations working together to provide health, educational and recreational opportunities for older persons and their families. Through our programs, services, and affiliations, we educate people of all ages and walks of life about living independent and creative lives. Programs and services availacle from the Center include: Computers Made Easy classes, Educational classes, Eldercare Forums, Exercise videos, 'Focus on Fitness' exercise classes, Health Care Information, Information and Referral, Meals on Wheels, Support Groups, Trips and Special Events, and Workshops for Exercise Leaders.

Year Founded: 1982

2617 Center for Social Gerontology
2307 Shelby Avenue
Ann Arbor, MI 48103
734-665-1126
Fax: 734-665-2071
tcsg@tcsg.org
www.tcsg.org

Penelope Hommel, Co-director
James A. Bergman, Co-director

Purpose is to advance the well-being of older people in the US through research, education, technical assistance, and training. Focuses primarily on legal rights, guardianship and alternative protective services, and delivery of legal services. Provides consulting services. Develops and researches standards for the provision of guardianship services for older people; works to improve the court processes for determining the need for guardianship through development and evaluation of a new model. Conducts periodic training on legal rights and legal resources, for legal advocates, nonlawyers who work with the elderly, and older consumers.

Year Founded: 1972

2618 Easter Seals
One Concorde Gate
Suite 700
Toronto, ON M3C 3N6
416-421-8377
Fax: 416-696-1035; *Toll Free:* 800-668-6252
info@easterseals.org
www.easterseals.org

Duncan Hawthorne, Chair

Provides services to those with physical disabilities to help them achieve greater independence, accessibility, and integration.

Year Founded: 1922

2619 Experience Works
4401 Wilson Boulevard
Suite 1100
Arlington, VA 22203

703-522-7272
Fax: 703-522-0141; *Toll Free:* 866-397-9757
www.experienceworks.org

Roger Noonan, Chairman
Sally A. Boofer, President & CEO
Richard Schorr, CFO

Helps low income seniors with multiple barriers to employment, get the training they need to find good jobs in their local community.

Year Founded: 1965

2620 Harvey A. Friedman Center for Aging
Washington University
St. Louis, Campus Box 8217
660 S. Euclid
St. Louis, MO 63110
314-747-9212
centerforaging@wustl.edu
publichealth.wustl.edu/aging

Nancy Morrow-Howell, PhD, Director
Stephanie Herbers, Center Manager
Jeanie Bryant, Administrative Coordinator

The Center promotes research, education, policy and service initiatives that enable older adults to remain healthy, active, empowered, contributing and independent for as long as possible.

Year Founded: 1998

2621 International Network for the Preventionof
Elder Abuse
The Somers Law Firm
PO Box 368
Nassau, NY 12123
518-281-2777
www.inpea.net

Susan B. Somers, President
Pamela Teastor, Secretary
Cynthia Thomas, Treasurer

Organization for the prevention of elder abuse.

Year Founded: 1997

2622 Jewish Council for the Aging of
GreaterWashington
12320 Parklawn Drive
Rockville, MD 20852-1726
301-255-4200
jodie.rasch@AccessJCA.org
www.accessjca.org
TDD 301-881-5263

Jodie Rasch, Administrator

Seeks to assist the elderly of all faiths lead independent lives. Provides transportation, job search assistance, fitness training, computer training and information and referrals. Conducts educational programs and presents an annual productive aging award. Maintains speakers' bureau.

Year Founded: 1973

2623 Leadership Council of Aging Organizations
202-216-8387
lcao@ncpssm.org
www.lcao.org

Coalition of national non-profit organizations concerned with the well-being of older Americans.

Number of Members: 72

2624 LeadingAge
2519 Connecticut Avenue NW
Washington, DC 20008-1520
202-783-2242
Fax: 202-783-2255
info@leadingage.org
www.leadingage.org

Katrinka Smith Sloan, President & CEO

The work of LeadingAge is focused on advocacy, leadership development, and applied research and promotion of effective services, home health, hospice, community services, senior housing, continuing care communities, nursing homes, as well as technology solutions to seniors and thers with special needs.

Year Founded: 1961

2625 Medicare Rights Center: New York
266 West 37th Street
3rd Floor
New York, NY 10018
212-869-3850
Fax: 212-869-3532
info@medicarerights.org
www.medicarerights.org

Joe Baker, President

Seeks to ensure the rights of senior citizens and people with disabilities to quality, affordable health care. Provides counseling services to Medicare beneficiaries with health insurance problems and questions; compiles information on inquiries to detect issues and systemic problems in Medicare claims administration. Educates beneficiaries, advocates, providers, and social workers about developments in Medicare law and how to handle problems. Monitors trends and changes in Medicare laws, regulations, and guidelines.

Year Founded: 1989; Number of Members: 49 million

2626 Medicare Rights Center: Washington, DC
1825 K Street NW
Suite 400
Washington, DC 20006
202-637-0961
Fax: 202-637-0962
info@medicarerights.org
www.medicarerights.org

Joe Baker, President

A consumer service organization that works to ensure access to affordable health care for older adults and peoplw tih disabilities through counseling and advocacy, educational programs, and public policy intiatives.

Year Founded: 1989; Number of Members: 49 million

2627 National Alliance for Caregiving
4720 Montgomery Lane
Suite 205
Bethesda, MD 20814
301-718-8444
Fax: 301-951-9067
info@caregiving.org
www.caregiving.org

Gail Gibson Hunt, President & CEO

Coalition of organizations focused on improving the lives of family caregivers.

Year Founded: 1996

2628 National Asian Pacific Center on Aging

napca.org

Wesley Lum, President & CEO
Donavan Lam, CFO

Advocating for the specific needs of aging Asian Americans and Pacific Islanders.

Year Founded: 1979

2629 National Center for Creative Aging

4125 Albemarle Street NW
Washington, DC 20016-2105
202-895-9456
Fax: 202-895-9483
info@creativeaging.org
www.creativeaging.org

Developing programs based on the understanding that creative expression is vital to healthy aging.

2630 National Center on Elder Abuse

Administration on Aging

c/o USC Keck School of Medicine, Dept. of Family
Medicine & Geriatrics
1000 South Fremont Avenue, Unit 22 Bld. A-6
Alhambra, CA 91803
855-500-3537
Fax: 626-457-4090
www.ncea.aoa.gov

The NCEA is an Administration on Aging Resource Center that provides up-to-date information on elder abuse, neglect and exploitation to policy makers and the public.

Year Founded: 1988

2631 National Chronic Disease Self-Management Resource Center

Center for Healthy Aging

251 18th Street S
Suite 500
Arlington, VA 22202
571-527-3900
www.ncoa.org

Supporting the expansion and sustainability of evidence-based health promotion and disease prevention programs in the community and online.

2632 National Clearinghouse on Abuse in Later Life

1245 E Washington Avenue
Suite 150
Madison, WI 53703
608-255-0539
Fax: 608-255-3560
ncall@wcadv.org
www.ncall.us

Bonnie Brandl, Director

Working to end abuse in later life.

2633 National Committee to Preserve Social Security & Medicare

10 G Street NE
Suite 600
Washington, DC 20002
202-216-0420
Fax: 202-216-0446; Toll Free: 800-966-1935

Max Richtman, President & CEO

Leading advocates for the protection of Social Security and Medicare.

Year Founded: 1982

2634 National Council on Aging

251 18th Street S
Suite 500
Arlington, VA 22202
571-527-3900
www.ncoa.org

James Firman, President & CEO

Emphasizes the needs for in-home and community-based health care and social services designed to help older persons remain in or return to their homes and live independently, works to educate and assist voluntary organizations to help develop such services.

Year Founded: 1950

2635 National Falls Prevention Resource Center

Center for Healthy Aging

251 18th Street S
Suite 500
Arlington, VA 22202
571-527-3900
www.ncoa.org

Supporting the implementation and dissemination of evidence-based falls prevention programs and strategies across the nation.

2636 National Institute of Senior Centers

National Council on Aging

251 18th Street S
Suite 500
Arlington, VA 22202
571-527-3900
www.ncoa.org

Supporting the nation's senior centers.

Year Founded: 1950

2637 National Institutes of Health

9000 Rockville Pike
Bethesda, MD 20892
301-496-4000
nihinfo@od.nih.gov
www.nih.gov
TTY: 301-402-9612

Francis S. Collins, Director

The nation's medical research agency.

Year Founded: 1887

2638 National Older Worker Career Center

3811 N Fairfax Drive
Suite 900
Arlington, VA 22203
703-558-4200
gmerrill@nowcc.org
www.nowcc.org

Gregory A. Merrill, President & CEO

National non-profit promoting experienced workers as staffing options to government agencies.

2639 National Resource Center on Nutrition, Physical Activity & Aging
Florida International University
OE 200
Miami, FL 33199
305-348-1517
Fax: 305-348-1518
nutritionandaging@fiu.edu
nutritionandaging.fiu.edu

Nancy S. Wellman, Director

Promoting better nutrition and active healthy aging.

2640 National Senior Citizens Law Center: Los Angeles
3660 Wilshire Boulevard
Suite 718
Los Angeles, CA 90010
213-639-0930
www.justiceinaging.org

Vanessa Barrington, Comms. Director

Legal services support center specializing in the legal problems of the elderly poor. Acts as advocate on behalf of elderly, poor clients in litigation and administrative affairs. Sponsors conferences and workshops on areas of the law affecting the elderly. See Legal Resources chapter for specific state resorces.

2641 National Senior Citizens Law Center: Oakland
1330 Broadway
Suite 525
Oakland, CA 94612
510-663-1055
www.justiceinaging.org

Vanessa Barrington, Comms. Director

Advocates nationwide to promote the independence and well-being of low-income elderly individuals, as well as persons with disabilities, with particular emphais on women and racial and ethnic minorities. Advocates through litigation and agency representation and assistance to attotneys and paralegals in field programs.

2642 National Senior Citizens Law Center: Washington, DC
1444 Eye Street NW
Suite 1100
Washington, DC 20005
202-289-6976
www.justiceinaging.org

Vanessa Barrington, Comms. Director

Advocates nationwide to promote the independence and well-being of low-income elderly individuals, as well as persons with disabilities, with particular emphasis on women and racial and ethnic minorities. Advocates through litigation, legistlative and agency representation and assistance to attorneys and paralegals in field programs.

2643 National Senior Corps Association
1316 E McKinney
Denton, TX 76209
940-383-1508
Fax: 940-383-1509
info@nscatogether.org
www.nscatogether.org

Gary Goosman, President
Lynnetta Kopp, Vice President
Diana Corona, Treasurer

Provides service for aging adults.

Year Founded: 2007; Number of Members: 500+

2644 Office for American Indian, Alaskan Native and Native Hawaiian Elders
Administration for Community Living
330 C Street SW
Washington, DC 20201
202-401-4634Toll free: 800-677-1116
olderindians@acl.hhs.gov
olderindians.acl.gov/about

Lance Robertson, Asst. Secretary for Aging
Mary Lazare, Principal Deputy Administrator

The Office for American Indians, Alaskan Natives, and Native Hawaiians advises the Secretary, through the Assistant Secretary for Children and Families, on matters relating to Native Americans. It represents the concerns of Native Americans and serves as the focal point in the Department on the full range of developmental, social, and economic strategies that support Native American self-determination and self-sufficiency. Under Title VI of the Older Americans Act, the AoA awards grants directly to tribes and tribal organizations and native organizations for nutrition services, information, and assistance, transportation, and at-home support services.

2645 Points of Light: Atlanta
600 Means Street
Suite 210
Atlanta, GA 30318
404-979-2900
Fax: 404-979-2901
www.pointsoflight.org

Tracy Hoover, CEO
Alison Doerfler, Executive Director

Mobilizing people to take action on the causes they care about.

2646 Points of Light: Washington, DC
1625 K Street NW
Suite 500
Washington, DC 20006
404-979-2900
Fax: 404-979-2901
www.pointsoflight.org

Tracy Hoover, CEO
Alison Doerfler, Executive Director

Mobilizing people to take action on the causes they care about.

2647 SeniorGuidance.org
www.seniorguidance.org

SeniorGuidance.org provides comprehensive resources on various senior living options, including: assisted living facilities, senior living communities, nursing homes, independent living communities, continuing care retirement communities (CCRC) and all other long term senior care options.

2648 Unbound
1 Elmwood Avenue
Kansas City, KS 66103

913-384-6500Toll free: 800-875-6564
mail@unbound.org
www.unbound.org

Scott Wasserman, President & CEO
Paul Pearce, Director of Global Strategy
Martin Kraus, Director of Finance

Seeks to advance the physical, mental, spiritual, and social welfare of the economically disadvantaged, especially children and aging persons in developing countries. US sponsors provide financial support and correspond with individuals in need; volunteers help provide social services, including medical, educational, and nutritional programs. Provides Christian education and guidance. Conducts orientation program for volunteers and Mission Awareness trips to Mexico and Central America.

Year Founded: 1981

2649 Virginia Center on Aging
Virginia Commonwealth University, Virginia Center
730 East Broad Street
2nd Floor
Richmond, VA 23298
804-828-1525
Fax: 804-828-7905
vcoa@vcu.edu
sahp.vcu.edu/departments/vcoa

Edward F Ansello, PhD, Director
Rachel Ramierez, Executive Director
Constance L Coogle, PhD, Associate Director of Research

The Virginia Center on Aging is a statewide agency created by the Virginia General Assembly, with our home at Virginia Commonwealth University. For 40 years, VCoA has worked diligently to protect and improve the quality of life of older Virginians, so that they may remain independent and contributing members in their communities. Our four program areas include, elder abuse prevention, dementia research, geriatrics training, and lifelong learning.

Year Founded: 1978

Books

2650 36 Hour Day: A Family Guide to Caring for Persons with Alzheimer Disease
Hachette Book Group
237 Park Avenue
New York, NY 10017
www.hachettebookgroup.com/

Michael Pietsch, Chief Executive Officer
Joe Mangan, EVP, Chief Operating Officer
Sophie Cottrell, VP, Communications Director

The trusted bible for families affected by dementia disorders. Provides all the practical and specific advice you need to make care easier, improve quality of life, and lift the whole family's spirit. Features the latest medical research and news on current delivery of care, with new appendices including Web site and association listings.

512 pages Year Founded: 1837

2651 Activities for the Elderly: Volume 1-A Guide to Quality Programming
Idyll Arbor, Inc.
39129 264th Ave SE
Enumclaw, WA 98022

360-825-7797
Fax: 360-825-5670
sales@IdyllArbor.com
www.IdyllArbor.com

Sandra D Parker, Author
Carol Will, Author
Cheryl L Burke

A collection of 75 practical activities and programs for therapists working with older adults. In addition to the instruction and helpful hints for each activity, the authors have also included the therapeutic benefits of each activity. Paperback.

171 pages

2652 Activities for the Elderly: Volume 2-Working with Residents with Significant Physical and Cognitive Diseases
Idyll Arbor, Inc.
39129 264th Ave SE
Enumclaw, WA 98022
360-825-7797
Fax: 360-825-5670
sales@IdyllArbor.com
www.IdyllArbor.com

A collection of 86 practical activities for residents who are very impaired because of dementia or other severe disabilities. This book provides the therapist with instructions and helpful hints, as well as the therapeutic benefits for each activity. Spiral bound.

135 pages

2653 Adult Children & Aging Parents
American Counseling Association
5999 Stevenson Avenue
Alexandria, VA 22304
703-823-9800
Fax: 703-823-0252; *Toll Free:* 800-347-6647
www.counseling.org

Cirecie A. West-Olatunji, President
Richard Yep, Executive Director
Thelma Daley, Treasurer

Provides effective intervention strategies and suggestions for counselors who work with older persons, individually and with the family. Offers information on many vital topics such as Alzheimer's Disease, retirement, elder abuse and suicide.

216 pages Year Founded: 1952

2654 Aging Children & Aging Parents
American Counseling Association
5999 Stevenson Avenue
Alexandria, VA 22304
703-823-9800
Fax: 703-823-0252; *Toll Free:* 800-347-6647
www.counseling.org

Cirecie A. West-Olatunji, President
Richard Yep, Executive Director
Thelma Daley, Treasurer

Full of facts and statistics about aging, as well as emotional issues that face the elderly and their families.

216 pages Year Founded: 1952

2655 Aging Comes of Age
Westminster John Knox Press
100 Witherspoon Street
Louisville, KY 40202-1396
502-569-8308
Fax: 800-541-5113; *Toll Free:* 800-523-1631
customer_service@wjkbooks.com
www.wjkbooks.com/

Marc Lewis, President & Publisher
Monty Anderson, VP & Chief Operations Officer, T
Robert Ratcliff, Executive Director

Following retirement, older people today are starting new
businesses, returning to universities, becoming world travelers, and setting new patterns of divorce and remarriage.
In this 'why to' book, eighty year old Frank Hutchison
gives encouragement to mature persons who wish to have
satisfying personal lives while contributing to society. He
states that an expanded life can be yours if you become
aware of it and if you genuinely want it.

120 pages

2656 Aging in Stride: A Practical Guide for Older
Adults & Their Families
CareSource
PO Box 8738
Dayton, OH 45401-8738
Fax: 206-682-2901; *Toll Free:* 800-488-0134
service@caresource.com
www.caresource.com
TTY: 800-750-0750

Michael E. Ervin, MD, Chairperson
Pamela B. Morris, President & CEO
Terry Rapoch, Director

A guide to the full range of aging and caregiver issues, including arranging in home services, maintaining health and
independence; selecting and moving to retirement housing;
addressing legal and financial issues; and doing advance
health care planning. Contains a variety of user friendly
forms and checklists, an extensive glossary, links to other
resources, and index.

368 pages

2657 Aging, Physical Activity, and Health
Human Kinetics
PO Box 5076
1607 N Market Street
Champaign, IL 61820
217-351-5076
Fax: 217-351-1549; *Toll Free:* 800-747-4457
info@hkusa.com
www.humankinetics.com

Brian Holding, CEO
Rainer Martens, Founder
Marilyn Martens, Founder

Reference for exercise scientists, gerontologists, geriatric
medicine specialists, physiologists, and other professionals
who work with older populations.

496 pages 1997 Year Founded: 1974

2658 Aging, Rights and Quality of Life: Prospects for
Older People with Developmental Disabilities
Paul H. Brookes Publishing Co., Inc.
PO Box 10624
Baltimore, MD 21285-0624

410-337-9580
Fax: 410-337-8539; *Toll Free:* 800-638-3775
www.brookespublishing.com/

Paul H. Brookes, Chairman of the Board
Jeffrey D. Brookes, President
Melissa A. Behm, Executive Vice President

In this groundbreaking new book, the leading authorities in
the fields of aging and developmental disabilities provide
you with an interdisciplinary analysis of the critical issues
in the lives of older adults with developmental disabilities.
Hardcover.

416 pages Year Founded: 1978

2659 Aging, Spirituality and Well-Being
Jessica Kingsley Publishers Inc.
400 Market Street
Suite 400
Philadelphia, PA 19106
215-922-1161
Fax: 215-922-1474; *Toll Free:* 866-416-1078
hello.usa@jkp.com
www.jkp.com

Jessica Kingsley, Chairman, Founder
Jemima Kingsley, Director
Laurie Kingsley, Vice President of Sales and Mark

Explores how well-being is not about physical health alone
(having purpose in life and continual spiritual growth are
vital elements for older people) and guides as to how the
particular needs of this age group can be addresses, and
how meaningful care and support can be given.

224 pages 1904 Year Founded: 1987

2660 Art of Getting Well
Hunter House
PO Box 2914
Alameda, CA 94501
510-865-5282
Fax: 510-865-4295; *Toll Free:* 800-266-5592
ordering@hunterhouse.com
www.hunterhouse.com

Christina Sverdrup, Customer Service Manager
David Spero RN, Author

A five step plan for maximazing health when you have a
chronic illness.

224 pages

2661 Beat the Nursing Home Trap: A Consumer's
Guide to Assisted Living and Long Term Care
NOLO
950 Parker Street
Berkeley, CA 94710
510-549-1976
Fax: 510-548-5902; *Toll Free:* 800-955-4775
www.nolo.com

Chris Braun, President, General Manager
Jonathan Rochez, Vice President, Engineering
Mary Randolph, Editor-in-Chief

Don't guess. Use this book to figure out how to choose a
nursing home, or find a viable alternative. Covers how to
get the most out of Medicare and other benefit programs.

336 pages Year Founded: 1971

2662 Caregiver Survival Series: Positive Caregiver Attitudes
National Stroke Association
9707 E Easter Lane
Suite B
Centennial, CO 80112
303-649-9299
Fax: 303-649-1328; *Toll Free:* 800-787-6537
info@stroke.org
www.stroke.org/

Michael D. Walker, MD, Chairman
George Davis, Jr., Vice Chairman
James Baranski, CEO

Down-to-earth strategies for developing positive attitudes toward care receivers, caregivers and life in general.

Year Founded: 1984

2663 Caregivers' Roller Coaster
Loyola Press, A Jesuit Ministry
3441 N Ashland Avenue
Chicago, IL 60657
Fax: 773-281-0555; *Toll Free:* 800-621-1008
customerservice@loyolapress.com
www.loyolapress.com/

A simply written self-help guide for caregivers of the frail elderly. Offers support for men and women, not trained professionals, who find themselves caring for aging family members in their own homes. Offers practical advice and information on Alzheimer's, Medicare, insurance and community services for the elderly.

150 pages

2664 Caring for Those You Love: A Guide to Compassionate Care for the Aged
Horizon Publishers
191 N 650 East
Bountiful, UT 84010-3628
801-292-7102
LDSHorizonPublishers@gmail.com
ldshorizonpublishers.com/

Duane S. Crowther, Owner
Jean D. Crowther, Chief Executive Officer

This book is a practical guide to coping with special problems of the aged and infirm, and examines the many challenges of caring for the elderly on a personal and family level.

Year Founded: 1971

2665 Caring for Your Parents: The Complete AARP Guide
Sterling Publishing Company, Inc.
387 Park Avenue South
New York, NY 10016
212-532-7160 Toll free: 800-367-9692
custservice@sterlingpublishing.com
www.sterlingpublishing.com

Amir Aczel, Author
Caroline Ada Miller, Author
Jonathan Adler, Author

Offers both sensitive counsel and a practical road map through the complex emotional terrain many of us face as our parents age. This eye-opening book guides readers through a new, creative approach to caregiving that turns familial duty into a journey of emotional development and resolution.

256 pages

2666 Caring for the Disabled Elderly
The Brookings Institution
1775 Massachusetts Avenue NW
Washington, DC 20036
202-797-6000
Fax: 202-797-6004
www.brookings.edu/

John L. Thornton, Chairman
Strobe Talbott, President
Steven Bennett, Vice President and Chief Operati

Financial information for the elderly.

318 pages Year Founded: 1916

2667 Change for the Better
AARP
601 E Street NW
Washington, DC 20049
202-434-3525
Fax: 202-434-3443; *Toll Free:* 888-687-2277
member@aarp.org
www.aarp.org
TTY: 877-434-7598

Gail E. Aldrich, Board Chair
Robert G. Romasco, President
Dr. Ethel Pe Andrus, Founder

Overview of the ways in which older people can provide leadership and create environmental and housing changes that will make their communities better places to live.

Year Founded: 1958

2668 Chiropractor's Self-Help Back and Body Book
Hunter House
PO Box 2914
Alameda, CA 94501
510-865-5282
Fax: 510-865-4295; *Toll Free:* 800-266-5592
ordering@hunterhouse.com
www.hunterhouse.com

Christina Sverdrup, Customer Service Manager
Samuel Homola DC, Author

How to relieve common aches and pains at home and on the job.

320 pages

2669 Communicating with Older Adults: A Guide for Health Care & Senior Service Professionals & Staff
CareSource
PO Box 8738
Dayton, OH 45401-8738
Fax: 206-682-2901; *Toll Free:* 800-488-0134
service@caresource.com
www.caresource.com
TTY: 800-750-0750

Diane Kenny, Contact

A handbook for health care senior care professionals and workers on how to communicate more effectively with older patients and consumers. This book reports on findings of research funded by the Retirement Research, SPRY, and Robert Wood Johnson Foundations. Contains research based recommendations for clinical care workers, senior living workers, and senior information and referral staff.

124 pages

2670 Community Recreation and People with Disabilities for Inclusion
Paul H. Brookes Publishing Co., Inc.
PO Box 10624
Baltimore, MD 21285-0624
410-337-9580
Fax: 410-337-8539; *Toll Free:* 800-638-3775
www.brookespublishing.com/

Paul H. Brookes, Chairman of the Board
Jeffrey D. Brookes, President
Melissa A. Behm, Executive Vice President

Updates abound in the second edition of this respected manual for professionals designing community recreation programs to include people with disabilities. Paperback.

368 pages Year Founded: 1978

2671 Community Supports for Aging Adults with Lifelong Disabilities
Paul H. Brookes Publishing Co., Inc.
PO Box 10624
Baltimore, MD 21285-0624
410-337-9580
Fax: 410-337-8539; *Toll Free:* 800-638-3775
www.brookespublishing.com/

Paul H. Brookes, Chairman of the Board
Jeffrey D. Brookes, President
Melissa A. Behm, Executive Vice President

Drawing on field-tested experiences and situations that can be applied to almost any setting, this text gives you practical approaches to real-life challenges facing people with disabilities as they grow older. An essential resource for anyone working with older adults. Hardcover.

560 pages Year Founded: 1978

2672 Cycling Past 50
Human Kinetics
PO Box 5076
1607 N Market Street
Champaign, IL 61820
217-351-5076
Fax: 217-351-1549; *Toll Free:* 800-747-4457
info@hkusa.com
www.humankinetics.com

Brian Holding, CEO
Rainer Martens, Founder
Marilyn Martens, Founder

The author shows cyclists that with proper training and the right attitude, the years after 50 can be their best ever. Written for cyclists of all types this book provides basic and advanced training programs, racing strategies, and injury prevention tips for middle-aged cyclists.

264 pages 1998 Year Founded: 1974

2673 Elder Care
Center for Public Representation
22 Green Street
Northampton, MA 1060
413-586-6024
Fax: 413-586-5711
info@cpr-ma.org

www.centerforpublicrep.org/
TTY: 413-586-6024

Bob Agoglia, President
Cathy Costanzo, Executive Director
Steven J. Schwartz, Litigation Director

A compendium of alternatives for providing and financing long-term care. This practical guide provides the most comprehensive and comforting information to help navigate a number of consumer mine fields.

224 pages Year Founded: 1972

2674 Elder Fit: A Health and Fitness Guide
American Alliance for Health, Physical Education,
1900 Association Drive
Reston, VA 20191-1598
703-476-3400
Fax: 703-476-9527; *Toll Free:* 800-213-7193
aaalf@aahperd.org
www.aahperd.org

Gale Wiedow, President
E. Paul Roetert, Chief Executive Officer
Frances E. Cleland, Director

Senior citizens need planned fitness activities! This book gives instructors a comprehensive exercise and fitness program designed for older adults.

2675 Exercise for Older Adults
Human Kinetics
PO Box 5076
1607 N Market Street
Champaign, IL 61820
217-351-5076
Fax: 217-351-1549; *Toll Free:* 800-747-4457
info@hkusa.com
www.humankinetics.com

Brian Holding, CEO
Rainer Martens, Founder
Marilyn Martens, Founder

Reference for health and fitness instructors, strength and conditioning professionals, personal trainers, athletic trainers, physical therapists, and kinesiotherapists.

244 pages 1998 Year Founded: 1974

2676 Falling in Old Age
Springer Publishing Company
11 West 42nd Street
15th Floor
New York, NY 10036
212-431-4370
Fax: 212-941-7842; *Toll Free:* 877-687-7476
cs@springerpub.com, journals@springerpub.com
www.springerpub.com

James C. Costello, Vice President, Journal Publishi
Theodore C. Nardin, Chief Executive Officer & Publis
Diana Osborne, Production Manager

Presented are practical techniques for the prevention of falls and for determining and correcting the causes.

Year Founded: 1950

2677 Feil Method, VALIDATION
Validation
21987 Byron Road
Cleveland, OH 44122

216-921-6606
Fax: 216-751-6434
naomi@vfvalidation.org
vfvalidation.org/

Frances Bulloff, J.D., President
Naomi Feil, LCSW, Founder and Director in Chief

G. Michael Leader, Honorary Member

A method of communicating with very old people.

135 pages Year Founded: 1982

2678 Financial Power of Attorney Workbook: Who Will Finance If You Can't?
NOLO
950 Parker Street
Berkeley, CA 94710
510-549-1976
Fax: 510-548-5902; *Toll Free:* 800-955-4775
www.nolo.com

Chris Braun, President, General Manager
Jonathan Rochez, Vice President, Engineering
Mary Randolph, Editor-in-Chief

To help people create their own durable power of attorney with step-by-step instructions.

160 pages Year Founded: 1971

2679 Fitness for the Aged, Disabled and Industrial Worker
Human Kinetics
PO Box 5076
1607 N Market Street
Champaign, IL 61820
217-351-5076
Fax: 217-351-1549; *Toll Free:* 800-747-4457
info@hkusa.com
www.humankinetics.com

Brian Holding, CEO
Rainer Martens, Founder
Marilyn Martens, Founder

The proportion of elderly and disabled citizens in Western countries is on the rise. And industrial workers are increasingly exposed to various health risks. These two factors are resulting in health problems that cannot be ignored.

304 pages Year Founded: 1974

2680 Functional Fitness Assessment for Adults
American Alliance for Health, Physical Education,
1900 Association Drive
Reston, VA 20191-1598
703-476-3400
Fax: 703-746-9527; *Toll Free:* 800-213-7193
aaalf@aahperd.org
www.aahperd.org

Gale Wiedow, President
E. Paul Roetert, Chief Executive Officer
Frances E. Cleland, Director

This field test assesses the functional fitness of adults over 60 years of age. It is designed to serve the larger population through field based measurement techniques that can be used in a facility where older persons live and can be conducted by personnel not necessarily trained for clinical responsibilities.

24 pages

2681 Gerontology: Responding to an Aging Society
Jessica Kingsley Publishers
73 Collier Street
London, England, N1 9BE
207-833-2307
Fax: 207-837-2917
hello@jkp.com
www.jkp.com

Jessica Kingsley, Chairman & Managing Director, Fo
Jemima Kingsley, Director
Laurie Schlesinger, Vice President of Sales and Mark

This book aims specifically to recent developments in gerontology, and includes expert contributions from the disciplines of geography, economics, sociology and social policy.

200 pages Year Founded: 1987

2682 Get Fit While You Sit
Hunter House
PO Box 2914
Alameda, CA 94501
510-865-5282
Fax: 510-865-4295; *Toll Free:* 800-266-5592
ordering@hunterhouse.com
www.hunterhouse.com

Christina Sverdrup, Customer Service Manager
Charlene Torkelson, Author

Easy workouts from your chair, three total body workout programs that can be done from your chair-anywhere. $17.95 for Spiral Bound.

160 pages

2683 Grandparenting with Love and Logic
Alexander Graham Bell Association for the Deaf
3417 Volta Place, NW
Washington, DC 20007
202-337-5220
Fax: 202-337-8314
info@agbell.org
www.agbell.org
TTY: 202-337-5220

Donald M. Goldberg, Ph.D., President
Alexander T. Graham, Executive Director & CEO
John Alberg, Ph.D, Director

This book offers easy-to-use techniques to show grandparents how to develop and nurture fulfilling relationships with both their children and grandchildren based on the love and logic philosophy.

276 pages

2684 I Can't Chew Cookbook
Hunter House Publisher
PO Box 2914
Alameda, CA 94501
510-865-5282
Fax: 510-865-4295; *Toll Free:* 800-266-5592
ordering@hunterhouse.com
www.hunterhouse.com

Christina Sverdrup, Customer Service Manager
J Randy Wilson, Author

Delicious soft-diet recipes for people with chewing, swallowing and Dry-Mouth Disorders. $22.95 Spiral Bound.

224 pages

2685 Journey to Pain Relief
Hunter House
PO Box 2914
Alameda, CA 94501
510-865-5282
Fax: 510-865-4295; *Toll Free:* 800-266-5592
ordering@hunterhouse.com
www.hunterhouse.com

Christina Sverdrup, Customer Service Manager
Phyllis Berger, Author

Hands-on guide to breakthroughs in pain treatment.

288 pages

2686 Joy of Laziness
Hunter House
PO Box 2914
Alameda, CA 94501
510-865-5282
Fax: 510-865-4295; *Toll Free:* 800-266-5592
ordering@hunterhouse.com
www.hunterhouse.com

Christina Sverdrup, Customer Service Manager
Peter Axt PhD, Author
Michaela Axt Gadermann MD

Why life is better slower-and how to get there.

160 pages

2687 Knowing Your Rights
AARP
601 E Street NW
Washington, DC 20049
202-434-3525
Fax: 202-434-3443; *Toll Free:* 888-687-2277
member@aarp.org
www.aarp.org
TTY: 877-434-7598

Gail E. Aldrich, Board Chair
Robert G. Romasco, President
Dr. Ethel Pe Andrus, Founder

Describes how changes in Medicare's reimbursement policies are designed to reduce health care costs and suggests
steps that Medicare beneficiaries, their families and friends
can take to assure that they continue to receive quality care
under the Prospective Payment System.

19 pages Year Founded: 1958

2688 Living Well in a Nursing Home
Hunter House
PO Box 2914
Alameda, CA 94501
510-865-5282
Fax: 510-865-4295; *Toll Free:* 800-266-5592
ordering@hunterhouse.com
www.hunterhouse.com

Christina Sverdrup, Customer Service Manager
Lynn Dickinson MA, Author
Xenia Vosen PhD

Positive aspects of nursing homes. How to recognize signs
that a family member needs extra support. How to identify
and select the best facility.

288 pages

2689 Long-Term Care: How to Plan and Pay for It
NOLO
950 Parker Street
Berkeley, CA 94710
510-549-1976
Fax: 510-548-5902; *Toll Free:* 800-955-4775
www.nolo.com

Chris Braun, President, General Manager
James Rochez, Vice President, Engineering
Mary Randolph, Editor-in-Chief

Allows you to evaluate long-term care insurance, arrange
home care, explore options beyond nursing homes, choose
a nursing facility, get the most out of Medicare, Medicaid
and other benefit programs, protect your assets, and recognize and prevent elder fraud. Also contains a chapter on
hospice care, and up-to-date benefit numbers, laws and
taxes, as well as the latest resources and websites.

384 pages 1906 Year Founded: 1971

2690 Managing Aging and Human Services Agencies
Springer Publishing Company
11 West 42nd Street
15th Floor
New York, NY 10036
212-431-4370
Fax: 212-941-7842; *Toll Free:* 877-687-7476
cs@springerpub.com, journals@springerpub.com
www.springerpub.com

James C. Costello, Vice President, Journal Publishi
Theodore C. Nardin, Chief Executive Officer & Publis
Diana Osborne, Production Manager

Offers specialized information for the human resources
professional who works with the elderly.

160 pages Year Founded: 1950

2691 Menopause Without Medicine
Hunter House
PO Box 2914
Alameda, CA 94501
510-865-5282
Fax: 510-865-4295; *Toll Free:* 800-266-5592
ordering@hunterhouse.com
www.hunterhouse.com

Christina Sverdrup, Customer Service Manager
Linda Ojeda PhD, Author

Menopause Without Medicine, 5th Editon. Non medical
approach to menopause. Covers Heart Disease, mood
swings, cognitive decline, osteoporosis, weight control,
insomnia.

400 pages

2692 Night Light: A Book of Nighttime Meditations
Hazelden
15251 Pleasant Valley Road
PO Box 11
Center City, MN 55012-0011
651-213-4200
Fax: 651-213-4426; *Toll Free:* 800-257-7810
info@hazelden.org
www.hazelden.org

Mark Mishek, President & CEO
James A. Blaha, VP Finance & Administration/ CFO
Ann Bray, General Counsel & VP of Startegi

366 meditations designed to help relax and encourage prayer. Reminds readers to look to their Higher Power for strength, reassurance, comfort and guidance.

400- pages Year Founded: 1949

2693 Nolo's Guide to Social Security Disability: Getting and Keeping Your Benefits
NOLO
950 Parker Street
Berkeley, CA 94710
510-549-1976
Fax: 510-548-5902; *Toll Free:* 800-955-4775
www.nolo.com

Chris Braun, President, General Manager
Jonathan Rochez, Vice President, Engineering
Mary Randolph, Editor-in-Chief

Not many bureaucratic programs are as large- and as con-fusing- as Social Security disability. This book shows you the ins and outs of the system.

350 pages Year Founded: 1971

2694 Older & Wiser: A Workbook for Coping with Aging
New Harbinger Publications
5674 Shattuck Avenue
Oakland, CA 94609
510-652-0215
Fax: 800-652-1613; *Toll Free:* 800-748-6273
customerservice@newharbinger.com
www.newharbinger.com

Matthew McKay, Owner
Patrick Fanning, Founder

This compassion guide teaches the practical skills and elic-its personal insight necessary to meet the demands of aging in our society.

300 pages Year Founded: 1973

2695 Older Americans, Vital Communities
Johns Hopkins University Press
2715 North Charles Street
Baltimore, MD 21218-4363
410-516-6900
Fax: 410-516-6998
webmaster@jhupress.jhu.edu
www.press.jhu.edu

Erik A. Smist, Director, Finance and Administra
Timothy D. Fuller, Chief Information Officer
Jack Holmes, Development and Publicity Office

This thought-provoking work grapples with the vast range of issues associated with the aging population and chal-lenges people of all ages to think more boldly and more creatively about the relationship between older Americans and their communities.

224 pages Year Founded: 1878

2696 Part of the Community: Strategies for Including Everyone
Paul H. Brookes Publishing Co., Inc.
PO Box 10624
Baltimore, MD 21285-0624
410-337-9580
Fax: 410-337-8539; *Toll Free:* 800-638-3775
www.brookespublishing.com/

Paul H. Brookes, Chairman of the Board
Jeffrey D. Brookes, President
Melissa A. Behm, Executive Vice President

Full of models and strategies on designing natural commu-nity supports rather than separate programs, this book shows you how to help individuals with disabilities achieve their goals and benefit from inclusion. Emphasizing inclu-sion as a lifelong process and offering creative prob-lem-solving techniques, this cutting edge bookk enables you to improve the lives of individuals with disabilities in your community. Paperback.

288 pages Year Founded: 1978

2697 Power of Attorney for Health Care
Center for Public Representation
22 Green Street
Northampton, MA 1060
413-586-6024
Fax: 413-586-5711; *Toll Free:* 800-369-0388
info@cpr-ma.org
www.centerforpublicrep.org/
TTY: 413-586-6024

Bob Agoglia, President
Cathy Costanzo, Executive Director
Steven J. Schwartz, Litigation Director

Discusses Wisconsin law regarding medical decisions, the Cruzan case and ethical considerations in addition to legal implications and advantages of this document. Book tells how to create a personalized Power of Attorney document, including language for the 'Special Provisions' portion.

132 pages Year Founded: 1972

2698 Prostate Health Workbook
Hunter House
PO Box 2914
Alameda, CA 94501
510-865-5282
Fax: 510-865-4295; *Toll Free:* 800-266-5592
ordering@hunterhouse.com
www.hunterhouse.com

Christina Sverdrup, Customer Service Manager
Newton Malerman, Author

A practical guide for the prostate cancer patients.

160 pages

2699 Racial and Ethnic Differences in the Health of Older Americans
The National Academies Press
500 Fifth Street NW
Washington, DC 20001
202-334-3313
Fax: 202-334-2451; *Toll Free:* 888-624-8373
customerservice@nap.edu
www.nap.edu

Ann Merchant, Deputy Executive Director for Co
Barbara Klin Popo, Director
Stephen Mautner, Executive Editor

Examines trends in mortality rates and selected causes of disability (cardiovascular disease, dementia) for older peo-ple of different racial and ethnic groups.

312 pages

2700 Running Past 50
Human Kinetics
PO Box 5076
1607 N Market Street
Champaign, IL 61820
217-351-5076
Fax: 217-351-1549; *Toll Free:* 800-747-4457
info@hkusa.com
www.humankinetics.com

Brian Holding, CEO
Rainer Martens, Founder
Marilyn Martens, Founder

The author shows how to make adjustments to running programs so that training becomes more effective and satisfying. He also discusses physical adjustments and pacing in workouts, getting proper rest, and incorporating walking into workouts.

256 pages 1998 Year Founded: 1974

2701 Social Security, Medicare and Pensions
NOLO
950 Parker Street
Berkeley, CA 94710
510-549-1976
Fax: 510-548-5902; *Toll Free:* 800-955-4775
www.nolo.com

Chris Braun, President, General Manager
Jonathan Rochez, Vice President, Engineering
Mary Randolph, Editor-in-Chief

A plain-English guide explaining the ins and outs of the Social Security system: retirement, disability and benefits for dependents and survivors.

320 pages Year Founded: 1971

2702 Strength Training Past 50
Human Kinetics
PO Box 5076
1607 N Market Street
Champaign, IL 61820
217-351-5076
Fax: 217-351-1549; *Toll Free:* 800-747-4457
info@hkusa.com
www.humankinetics.com

Brian Holding, CEO
Rainer Martens, Founder
Marilyn Martens, Founder

Provides research based guidelines and tools to help anyone over 50 develop and perform a sound, safe strength training program.

240 pages 1998 Year Founded: 1974

2703 Strength Training for Seniors
Human Kinetics
PO Box 5076
1607 N Market Street
Champaign, IL 61820
217-351-5076
Fax: 217-351-1549; *Toll Free:* 800-747-4457
info@hkusa.com
www.humankinetics.com

Brian Holding, CEO
Rainer Martens, Founder
Marilyn Martens, Founder

Reference for health and fitness instructors, strength and conditioning professionals, personal trainers, athletic trainers, physical therapists, and kinesiotherapists.

232 pages 1999 Year Founded: 1974

2704 The Elder Care Sourcebook
McGraw-Hill Financial
1221 Avenue of the Americas
New York, NY 10020-1095
212-512-2000
Fax: 212-512-4769
www.mcgraw-hill.com

Douglas L. Peterson, President & Chief Executive Offi
Jack F. Callahan, Jr., Executive Vice President , Chief
John Berisford, Executive Vice President , Human

Presents a wealth of information on concerns of elderly people, from nutrition to physical and mental health to sexuality to pharmaceuticals to bereavement and more. A comprehensive overview of the demographics of the aging population is also featured, along with actual case histories.

304 pages 1902 Year Founded: 1899

2705 What Are Old People For? How Elders Will
Save the World
VanderWyk & Burnham
1610 Long Leaf Circle
St. Louis, MO 63146
314-432-3435
Fax: 314-993-4485
quickpublishing@sbcglobal.net
www.vandb.com

William H Thomas, Author

Nodding to popular culture, history, science, and literature, a passionate and persuasive case is made for removing our ageist blinders and seeing old age as a developmental stage of life.

370 pages 1904

2706 Work Options for Older Americas
University of Notre Dame Press
310 Flanner Hall
Notre Dame, IN 46556
574-631-6346
Fax: 574-631-8148
undpress@nd.edu
undpress.nd.edu/

Diane Schaut, Business Manager
Rebecca DeBoer, Managing Editor
Charles Von Hof, Sr. Acquisitons Editor

Brings together discussion of these issues by well-known economists and scholars in other fields, from the Government Accountability Office, the AARPÆPublic Policy Institute, the U.S. Department of Labor, and academia.

392 pages Year Founded: 1949

2707 Work, Health and Income Among the Elderly
The Brookings Institution
1775 Massachusetts Avenue NW
Washington, DC 20036
202-797-6000
Fax: 202-797-6004
www.brookings.edu/

John L. Thornton, Chairman
Strobe Talbott, President
Steven Bennett, Vice President and Chief Operati

Employment, health and financial information for the elderly.

276 pages Year Founded: 1916

2708 Writing from Within
Hunter House
PO Box 2914
Alameda, CA 94501
510-865-5282
Fax: 510-865-4295; *Toll Free:* 800-266-5592
ordering@hunterhouse.com
www.hunterhouse.com

Christina Sverdrup, Customer Service Manager
Bernard Selling, Author

Writing from Within, 3rd Edition. A guide to creativity and life story writing.

320 pages

Directories

2709 A Place to Live: Housing Alternatives for the Elderly in Arizona
Division of Aging And Adult Services
1789 W Jefferson Street
Suite 950A
Phoenix, AZ 85007
602-542-4446
Fax: 602-542-6655; *Toll Free:* 877-767-2385
www.azdes.gov/aging/

Joe Slattery, Mailing Contact
Rex Critchfield, Manager

Alternative senior citizen housing in Arizona.

45 pages

2710 A World of Options: A Guide to International, Educational, Exchange, Community Service...for Persons with Disabilities
Mobility International USA
132 E. Broadway
Suite 343
Eugene, OR 97401
541-343-1284
Fax: 541-343-6812
info@miusa.org
www.miusa.org
TTY: 541-343-1284

Susan Sygall, CEO
Cindy Lewis, Editor
Christa Bucks, Editor

Hundreds of educational programs, workcamps, transportation and travel advisory services for persons with disabilities. Entries include: Name, address, phone, geographical area served, financial data, eligibility requirements, descriptions of projects. Personal stories included. Paperback.ith TDD.

400 pages Year Founded: 1981

2711 AAAS Resource Directory of Scientists and Engineers with Disabilities
American Assoc for the Advancement of Science (AAA
1200 New York Avenue NW
Washington, DC 20005-3928
202-326-6400
Fax: 202-289-4950
www.aaas.org/

William Press, Chair
Phillip A. Sharp, President
Alan I. Leshner, Chief Executive Officer

Approximately 1,000 disabled scientists and engineers offering their services as consultants, speakers, role models, and peer reviewers. Entries include: Scientist's and engineer's name, address, degree(s), position, disability, age of onset, consulting interest.

158 pages Year Founded: 1848

2712 AHA Guide to the Health Care Field
American Hospital Association (AHA)
155 N. Wacker Dr.
Chicago, IL 60606
312-422-3000
Fax: 312-422-4506; *Toll Free:* 800-424-4301
www.aha.org/

James H. Hinton, Chairman
Ricahrd J. Umbdenstock, President & CEO
Alan D. Aviles, Director

Hospitals, networks, multi-health care systems, freestanding ambulatory surgery centers, psychiatric facilities, long-term care facilities, substance abuse programs, hospices, Health Maintenance Organizations (HMOs), and other health-related organizations. Entries include: For hospitals—Facility name, address, phone, administrator's name, number of beds, facilities and services, number of employees, expenses, other statistics. For other. organizations—Name, address, phone, fax, name and title of contact.

963 pages Frequency: Annual Year Founded: 1899

2713 Age Care Sourcebook: A Resource Guide for the Aging and Their Families
Simon & Schuster Consumer Group
1230 Avenue of the Americas
New York, NY 10020-1513
212-698-7000
Fax: 212-767-2993; *Toll Free:* 800-223-1360
www.simonandschuster.com

Carolyn Reidy, President & CEO
Richard L. Simon, Founder
M. Lincoln Schuster, Senior Vice President of Public

Publication includes: List of more than 600 state and local agencies that provide information or assistance for the care of the elderly. Entries include: Agency name, address, phone, branch office locations. Principal content is a resource guide for adult children having to care for their aging parents, including information on financial planning, retirement housing, medical care, and wills.

Year Founded: 1924

2714 American Association of Homes and Services for the Aging: Directory of Members
LeadingAge
2519 Connecticut Avenue North West
Washington, DC 20008-1520
202-661-5700
Fax: 202-783-2255
info@LeadingAge.org
www.aahsa.org

William L. (Minnix Jr., President/Chief Executive Office
Katrinka (Ka Smith Sloan, SVP /Chief Operating Officer
Cheryl Phillips, Senior Vice President of Public

Over 5,200 nonprofit member homes and health facilities; over 800 business firm suppliers, individuals, and other associate members. Entries include: Name of home, address, phone, names of administrative staff, sponsorship, levels of care, services.

500 pages Frequency: Annual

2715 American Blue Book of Funeral Directors
Kates-Boylston Publications
3349 Route 138
Building D, Suite D
Wall, NJ 07719
732-767-9300
Fax: 732-730-2515; *Toll Free:* 800-500-4585
www.kates-boylston.com

Thomas A. Parmalee, Executive Director
Amy Fidalgo, Marketing & Production Manager
Patti Martin-Bartsche, Editor

Listing of manufactures and suppliers of funeral equipment, as well as funeral homes primarily found in the USA and Canada.

908 pages Frequency: Annual Year Founded: 1877

2716 Association for Continuing Higher Education Directory
Association for Continuing Higher Education (ACHE)
OCCE Administration Building, Room 233
1700 Asp Avenue
Norman, OK 73072-6400
843-574-6658
Fax: 405-325-4888; *Toll Free:* 800-807-2243
admin@acheinc.org
www.acheinc.org/

Ynez C. Henningsen, Operations Manager & Executive S
V. Stan Khrapak, Operations Associate & Graduate

Directory of institutions and individual professionals that assist in continuing education.

102 pages Frequency: Annual, March

2717 Bailey
Bailey Manufacturing Company
PO Box 130
Lodi, OH 44254-0130
330-948-1080
Fax: 800-224-5390; *Toll Free:* 800-321-8372
www.baileymfg.com

Dave Bailey, Owner

Catalog of ambulation aids, balance aids, benches, chairs, exercise devices, tables, stools, rehabilitation and physical therapy equipment for the physically challenged.

51 pages Year Founded: 1956

2718 Best 25 Catalog Resources for Making Life Easier
Making Life Easier
9042 Aspen Grove Lane
Madison, WI 53717-2700
608-824-0401
Fax: 608-274-6993
shelly@makinglifeeasier.com
www.makinglifeeasier.com

Shelley Peterman Schwarz, Author
Deborah , Director of Marketing & Developm

Unique reference guide to locate thousands of useful and hard-to-find adaptive devices to make dressing, eating, cooking, grooming, communicating, playing, exercising, etc. easier, safer and less frustrating for people of all ages and disabilities. A comprehensive reference for people with disabilities, caregivers and healthcare professionals.

30 pages

2719 CARF Directory of Organizations with Accredited Programs
CARF International
6951 East Southpoint Road
Tucson, AZ 85756-9407
520-325-1044
Fax: 520-318-1129; *Toll Free:* 888-281-6531
postmaster@carf.org
www.carf.org/
TTY: 888-281-6531

Brian J Boon, Ph.D., President & CEO
Amanda E. Birch, Administrator of Operations
Leslie Ellis-Lang, Managing Director of Child & You

About 2,500 organizations in 5,000 locations offering more than 11,000 medical rehabilitation, behavioral health, and employment and community support services that have been accredited by CARF. Entries include: Organization name, address, phone, name and title of chief executive, accredited programs offered, accreditation outcome.

358 pages Frequency: Annual Year Founded: 1966

2720 Cardiac Rehabilitation Directory
infoUSA
1020 E 1st Street
Papillion, NE 68046
402-593-4600
Fax: 402-331-5481; *Toll Free:* 800-835-5856
internet@infousa.com
www.infousa.com/

Bill Hippen, Vice President

Listings of cardiac rehabilitation programs

Frequency: Annual

2721 Complete Directory for People with Chronic Illness
Grey House Publishing
4919 Route 22
PO Box 56
Amenia, NY 12501-0056
518-789-8700
Fax: 518-789-0556; *Toll Free:* 800-562-2139
books@greyhouse.com
www.greyhouse.com

Richard Gottlieb, President & Co-Founder
Laura Mars, Editoral Director
Leslie Mackenzie, Publisher & Co-Founder

The Complete Directory for People with Chronic Illness provides a comprehensive overview of 80 chronic illnesses and information on condition-specific support services and resources. Each new edition has been designed to offer assistance to all those involved in the chronic illness community, with resources for patients, families, healthcare professionals, and other caregivers.

1200 pages

2722 Complete Directory for People with Disabilities
Grey House Publishing
4919 Route 22
PO Box 56
Amenia, NY 12501-0056
518-789-8700
Fax: 518-789-0556; *Toll Free:* 800-562-2139
books@greyhouse.com
www.greyhouse.com

Richard Gottlieb, President & Co-Founder
Laura Mars, Editoral Director
Leslie Mackenzie, Publisher & Co-Founder

This resource details independent living centers, rehabilitation facilities, state and federal agencies, associations and support groups, and provides immediate access to the latest products and services for people with disabilities, such as periodicals, books, assistive devices, employment, education, camps and travel.

1000 pages

2723 Complete Directory of Large Print Books and Serials
Bowker
630 Central Ave
New Providence, NJ 07974
908-286-1090
Fax: 908-771-7704; *Toll Free:* 888-269-5372
info@bowker.com
www.bowker.com

D Gravesande, Editor
R Crego, Editor

Publication includes: List of over 340 publishers and distributors of more than 12,000 books, 200 periodicals, and paperbacks printed in at least 14-point type. Entries include: For publishers—Company name, address. Principal content of publication is bibliography of large type books, newspapers, periodicals, and paperback bestsellers.

350 pages Frequency: Annual, January Year Founded: 1872

2724 Complete Listing of Nursing Facilities and Home for the Aged Beds when Licensed as a Part of a Nursing Facility
North Carolina Dept of Human Resources
2711 Sullivan Drive
Raleigh, NC 27695
919-515-2135
Fax: 919-515-7543
www.ncsu.edu/human_resources/

Barbara Carroll, Associate Vice Chancellor
Jessie Sova, Director, EPA Administration
Joanna Carter, Administrative Assistant

About 400 nursing facilities. Entries include: Name, address, phone, name of administrator, whether certified for Medicare and/or Medicaid, number of beds for nursing care.

25 pages Frequency: Monthly

2725 Complete Mental Health Directory
Grey House Publishing
4919 Route 22
PO Box 56
Amenia, NY 12501-0056
518-789-8700
Fax: 518-789-0556; *Toll Free:* 800-562-2139
books@greyhouse.com
www.greyhouse.com

Richard Gottlieb, President & Co-Founder
Laura Mars, Editoral Director
Leslie Mackenzie, Publisher & Co-Founder

The first comprehensive resource covering the field of behavioral health, with critical information for both the layman and the health professional. For the layman, this directory offers understandable descriptions of 21 mental health disorders as well as detailed information on associations, support groups and mental health facilities. For the professional, it offers information on managed care, government agencies and provider organizations.

800 pages

2726 Consumer's Directory of Continuing Care Retirement Communities
LeadingAge
2519 Connecticut Avenue North West
Washington, DC 20008-1520
202-661-5700
Fax: 202-783-2255
info@LeadingAge.org
www.aahsa.org

William L. (Minnix Jr., President/Chief Executive Office
Katrinka (Ka Smith Sloan, SVP /Chief Operating Officer
Cheryl Phillips, Senior Vice President of Public

500 retirement communities providing an integrated continuum of short-term and long-term care, including health care, housing, and home and community-based services. Entries include: Community name, address, phone, size fee, services, agreement and refund options.

610 pages

2727 Continuing Care Retirement Community Directory
LeadingAge
2519 Connecticut Avenue North West
Washington, DC 20008-1520
202-661-5700
Fax: 301-206-9789
info@LeadingAge.org
www.aahsa.org

William L. (Minnix Jr., President/Chief Executive Office
Katrinka (Ka Smith Sloan, SVP /Chief Operating Officer
Cheryl Phillips, Senior Vice President of Public

A national consumer's directory of continuing care retirement communities. This directory is a vital tool for individuals searching and evaluating a community for themselves or a loved one.

2728 **Council for Health and Human Service Ministries: Directory of Services**
Council for Health and Human Service Ministries
700 Prospect Avenue
Cleveland, OH 44115
866-822-8224
Fax: 216-736-2251
sickberb@chhsm.org
www.chhsm.org/

Margaret M. Mullan, Chair
Hugh Meyers, Vice Chair
Bryan Sickbert, President and CEO

About 300 social welfare agencies, retirement homes, children's residential homes, hospitals, and other health and human service facilities affiliated with the United Church of Christ. Entries include: Agency name, type of institution and summary of services offered, certifications and memberships, name of chief administrator, mailing address, phone, and conference assignment.

90 pages Frequency: Annual Year Founded: 1961

2729 **Data Resources in Gerontology: A Directory of Selected Information Vendors, Databases, and Archives**
Gerontological Society of America
1220 L Street North West
Washington, DC 20005
202-842-1275
Fax: 202-842-1150
geron@geron.org
www.geron.org

James Appleby, Executive Director and CEO
Linda Krogh Harootyan, Deputy Executive Director
Chris Yoder, Senior Director, Finance and Adm

Approximately 55 vendors of database access/information sources, bibliographic or reference databases, and data archives related to aging; regional census offices; state agencies, universities, libraries, and regional and local governments that provide census information. Entries include: For vendors—Company name, address, phone, description of product/service. For regional census offices—Name, address, phone, geographical area servedFor others—Name, address, phone, name and title of contact, geographical area served.

45 pages Year Founded: 1945

2730 **Directory of Aging Resources**
Business Publishers, Inc.
2222 Sedwick Drive
Durham, NC 27713
301-589-5103
Fax: 800-508-2592; *Toll Free:* 800-223-8720
www.bpinews.com/

Kimberly Gilbert, Managing Editor
Alexa Chew, Contributing Editor
Mary Compton, Publisher

Organizations, professionals, universities, and federal, state, and local government agencies in the US involved with aging issues. Entries include: Organization, company or agency name, names of programs or divisions, address, phone, fax, e-mail address, TTY/TTD numbers, names and titles of key personnel, number of members or constituents, mission or goals, jurisdiction, activities and services, publications, funding sources.

500 pages Frequency: Annual Year Founded: 1963

2731 **Directory of American Baptist Retirement Homes, Nursing Homes, Children's Homes & Special Services**
American Baptist Churches USA
PO Box 851
Valley Forge, PA 19482-0851
610-768-2000
Fax: 610-768-2309; *Toll Free:* 800-ABC-3USA
webmaster@abc-usa.org
www.abc-usa.org

Victoria Buff, Mailing Contact
Thomas Helwys, Founder

125 member American Baptist related retirement, nursing, and children's homes and special services. Entries include: Institution name, address, phone, facilities available.

14 pages Frequency: Annual Year Founded: 1612

2732 **Directory of Community Care Facilities**
California Department of Social Services
744 P Street
Ms 19-50
Sacramento, CA 95814-6413
916-324-4031
Fax: 916-323-8352
www.cdss.ca.gov/

Will Lightbourne, Director
Pat Leary, Chief Deputy Director
Pete Cervinka, Program Deputy Director for Bene

Adoption and home finding agencies, residential care facilities for adults and children, preschool care centers, and day care centers located in California and licensed by the California Department of Social Services. Health facilities are not listed. Entries include: Facility name, address, phone; name of director or administrator; capacity; license limitations (age, sex, hours of care, etc.).

2,400 pages Frequency: Quarterly Year Founded: 1903

2733 **Directory of Department of Veterans Affairs Facilities**
U.S. Department of Veterans Affairs
810 Vermont Avenue NW
Washington, DC 20420
202-273-5803
Fax: 202-273-6891; *Toll Free:* 800-827-1000
www.va.gov/

Eric K. Shinseki, Secretary of Veterans Affairs
Jose D. Riojas, Chief of Staff
Will A. Gunn, General Counsel

About 345 facilities, including medical centers and regional offices with associated outpatient clinics, veterans outreach centers, and other offices; national cemeteries, and data processing centers. Entries include: Location (state, county, city), congressional district, congressional representative, station numbers, code for facility type.

40 pages Frequency: Biennial Year Founded: 1636

2734 **Directory of Health Education Programs for Elders**
Center on Aging Studies\Univ Missouri-Kansas City
5100 Rockhill Road
Kansas City, MO 64110
816-235-1000
Fax: 816-235-5193
cas.umkc.edu/agingstudies/

Murray Blackwelder, President
Curt Crespino, Vice Chancellor
Lee Morton, Chancellor

Lists 36 health education programs for the elderly in rural areas. Entries include: Name, address, phone of program, bibliography and abstracts of relevant publications and reviews.

219 pages Year Founded: 1929

2735 Directory of Health, Medical, and Disability Sites on the World Wide Web and Internet
Twin Peaks Press
PO Box 8
Vancouver, WA 98666-0088
360-694-2462
Fax: 360-696-3210; *Toll Free:* 800-637-2256
twinpeak@pacifier.com
home.pacifier.com/~twinpeak/

Helen Hecker RN, Editor, Founder

Internet and World Wide Web sites related to health and disabilities in categories such as alternative medicine, disorders, genetics, nutrition, women's health, and many others. Entries include: Name, contact information.

Year Founded: 1982

2736 Directory of Jewish Homes and Housing for the Aged in the United States and Canada
Association of Jewish Aging Services
2519 Connecticut Ave NW
Washington, DC 20008
202-543-7500
Fax: 202-543-4090
info@ajas.org
www.ajas.org

Donald J Shulman, President & CEO

Nonprofit Jewish homes and housing for the aged in the United States and Canada. Entries include: Facility name, address, number of beds or units, admission requirements and procedures, name of administrator and description of residents' characteristics, financial data, services offered.

300 pages Frequency: Biennial Year Founded: 1960

2737 Directory of Long Term Care Facilities
Illinois Department of Public Health
525 W Jefferson Street
Springfield, IL 62761
217-782-5180
Fax: 217-785-4200
www.idph.state.il.us/

Wendy Fry, Editor

Long term care facilities licensed by the state, including skilled care, skilled intermediate care, sheltered community living facilities, and persons under age 22. Entries include: Facility name, address, phone, level of care, number of beds, type of ownership, approvals, provider association, name of administrator.

141 pages Frequency: Bi-annual

2738 Directory of Services for the Widowed in the United States and Canada
AARP
601 E Street NW
Washington, DC 20049

202-434-3525
Fax: 202-434-6474; *Toll Free:* 888-687-2277
member@aarp.org
www.aarp.org
TTY: 877-434-7598

Gail E. Aldrich, Board Chair
Robert G. Romasco, President
Dr. Ethel Pe Andrus, Founder

Forms of assistance as well as counseling offered for widows and widowers. Directory of nearly 500 associations, services and agencies nationwide.

65 pages Frequency: Biennial Year Founded: 1958

2739 Directory of Suicide Prevention/Crisis Intervention Agencies in the United States
American Association of Suicidology
5221 Wisconsin Avenue, NW
Washington, DC 20015
202-237-2280
Fax: 202-237-2282; *Toll Free:* 800-273-TALK
aikule@ix.netcom.com
www.suicidology.org

Julie Cerel, Ph.D., Board Chair
William Schmitz, Jr., Psy.D., President
Amy Boland, CPA, Treasurer

About 600 suicide prevention and crisis intervention centers. Entries include: Center name, sponsoring organization name (if different), address, phone, emergency phone number, hours of service.

60 pages Frequency: Annual Year Founded: 1968

2740 Directory of Survivors of Suicide Support Groups
American Association of Suicidology
5221 Wisconsin Avenue, NW
Washington, DC 20015
202-237-2280
Fax: 202-237-2282; *Toll Free:* 800-273-TALK
amyjomc@ix.netcom.com
www.suicidology.org

Julie Cerel, Ph.D., Board Chair
William Schmitz, Jr., Psy.D., President
Amy Boland, CPA, Treasurer

220 support groups in the US and Canada for family, friends, and other survivors of people who commit suicide. Entries include: Name, address, phone.

28 pages Frequency: Annual Year Founded: 1968

2741 Directory of Travel Agencies for the Disabled
Twin Peaks Press
PO Box 8
Vancouver, WA 98666-0088
360-694-2462
Fax: 360-696-3210; *Toll Free:* 800-637-2256
twinpeak@pacifier.com
home.pacifier.com/~twinpeak/

Helen Hecker, Editor, Founder

Number of listings: 370. Entries include: Company name, address, phone, fax, names and titles of key personnel, subsidiary and branch names and locations, description of services.

80 pages Frequency: Quarterly Year Founded: 1982

2742 Elderhostel Catalog
Road Scholar
11 Avenue de Lafayette
Boston, MA 02111
978-323-4141
Fax: 617-426-0701; *Toll Free:* 800-454-5768
www.elderhostel.org
TTY: 877-426-2167

Michael Zoob, Editor
James Moses, CEO

Short-course educational, residential programs on about 1,900 campuses in North America, South America, Asia, and Europe which are available to persons 55 years of age or older and their adult companions. Programs include noncredit courses taught by regular faculty (and sometimes based on local resources or culture). Campus living accommodations and meals are provided. In United States and Canada cost is an average of $325.00 per week; Alaska, Hawaii, and overseas programs are more. Entries include: Institution name, location, description of setting, programs available, dates, brief travel information.

100 pages Frequency: 8x Year Year Founded: 1975

2743 Federal Benefits for Veterans and Dependents
US Department of Veterans Affairs
810 Vermont Avenue NW
Washington, DC 20420
202-273-6763Toll free: 800-273-8255
www.va.gov

Eric K. Shinseki, Secretary of Veterans Affairs
Sloan D. Gibson, Deputy Secretary of Veterans Aff
Jose D. Riojas, Chief of Staff

Publication includes: List of VA offices, assistance centers, insurance claims offices, medical facilities, and national cemeteries. Entries include: For offices—Name, address, phone, type of office or facility. For cemeteries—Name, address, phone. Principal content of publication is description of veterans' benefits.

100 pages Frequency: Annual Year Founded: 1636

2744 Financial Aid for Veterans, Military Personnel and Their Dependents
Reference Service Press
5000 Windplay Drive
Suite 4
El Dorado Hills, CA 95762-9319
916-939-9620
Fax: 916-939-9626
info@rspfunding.com
www.rspfunding.com/

Gail A. Schlachter, President & Founder
R David Weber, Editor-in-Chief
Mike Fields, Database & Website Manager

Organizations that offer approximately 1,100 scholarships, fellowships, loans, grants, awards, and internships to veterans, military personnel, and their families. Entries include: Organization name, address, phone, financial data, requirements for eligibility, duration, special features and limitations, deadline, number of awards.

350 pages Frequency: Biennial Year Founded: 1977

2745 Financial Aid for the Disabled and Their Families
Reference Service Press
5000 Windplay Drive
Suite 4
El Dorado Hills, CA 95762-9319
916-939-9620
Fax: 916-939-9626
info@rspfunding.com
www.rspfunding.com/

Gail A. Schlachter, President & Founder
R David Weber, Editor-in-Chief
Mike Fields, Database & Website Manager

Over 900 scholarships, fellowships, grants, loans, and awards to disabled persons or their family members. Entries include: Program name, sponsor name, address, phone, description of program including purpose, financial data, and eligibility requirements.

370 pages Frequency: Biennial Year Founded: 1977

2746 Funding in Aging
Foundation Center
79 5th Avenue/ 16th Street
New York, NY 10003-3076
212-620-4230
Fax: 212-807-3677; *Toll Free:* 800-424-9836
foundationcenter.org/

P. Russell Hardin, Chairman
Barron M. Tenny, Vice Chairman
Bradford K. Smith, President

1,000 foundations and private organizations that offer funding for programs about aging. Entries include: For federal government agencies—Agency name, address, phone; regional office name, address, phone; description of program, types of assistance awarded, eligibility requirements, description of past programs funded by the agency, application procedure. For state government agencies—Agency name, address, phone. For private organizations—Organization name, address, phone, description of funding program, types of financial assistance available, description of publications. For foundations—Foundation name, address, phone, names of key personnel, description of program, assets, amount of money awarded, deadline date for application, description of publications.

294 pages Year Founded: 1956

2747 Golden Opportunities
Peterson's
PO Box 2123
Princeton, NJ 08544-1019
609-258-3060
Fax: 609-258-6743; *Toll Free:* 800-338-3282
uaoffice@princeton.edu
www.petersons.com/

Andrew Carroll, Editor
Rick Pinto, Partner

Organizations that need and welcome senior volunteers. Principal content of publication is selecting the right volunteer activity.

384 pages Year Founded: 1746

2748 Grants for Literacy, Reading &
Adult/Continuing Education
Foundation Center
79 5th Avenue/ 16th Street
New York, NY 10003-3076
212-620-4230
Fax: 212-807-3677; *Toll Free:* 800-424-9836
foundationcenter.org/

P. Russell Hardin, Chairman
Barron M. Tenny, Vice Chairman
Bradford K. Smith, President

In past years this organization has awarded grants to foundations that support reading, adult basic education, continuing education programs, and literacy. This directory contains the recipient foundations general information as well as the grant limitations, amount and spending patterns.

Year Founded: 1956

2749 Grants of Aging
Foundation Center
79 5th Avenue/ 16th Street
New York, NY 10003-3076
212-620-4230
Fax: 212-807-3677; *Toll Free:* 800-424-9836
foundationcenter.org/

P. Russell Hardin, Chairman
Barron M. Tenny, Vice Chairman
Bradford K. Smith, President

114 pages Year Founded: 1956

2750 Great Buys for People over 50
Penguin Group (USA)
375 Hudson Street
New York, NY 10014-3657
212-366-2372
Fax: 212-366-2933; *Toll Free:* 800-526-0275
academic@penguin.com
www.us.penguingroup.com/

John Makinson, Chairman and Chief Executive
Susan Peters Kennedy, President
James C. Clark, Senior Vice President for Distri

Mail order firms, bargain retail outlets, and other sources of bargain apparel, food, appliances, home furnishings, crafts kits, and other items appropriate for persons over 50; firms offering discounted fees for their services; and special services. Entries include: Name, address, phone, description, credit cards accepted, price of catalog.

420 pages Year Founded: 1936

2751 Greatest of Ease Company Catalog
3022 Buchanan Street
San Francisco, CA 94123
415-606-4416
Fax: 415-441-4319; *Toll Free:* 800-845-1208
dpuri@yahoo.com
personalpagers.tripod.com/go/

Offers 127 products designed to enable and enhance your independence and make everyday tasks a little easier.

2752 Guide to the Nation's Hospices
National Hospice and Palliative Care Organization
1731 King Street
Suite 100
Alexandria, VA 22314

703-837-1500
Fax: 703-837-1233; *Toll Free:* 800-646-6460
nhpco_info@nhpco.org
www.nhpco.org/

Ronald Fried, Chair
Linda Rock, Vice Chair
J. Donald Schumacher, President/CEO

About 3,000 hospices, palliative care centers, and other programs serving terminally ill persons. Entries include: Name of hospice program, address, and phone, fax, e-mail address, website, name and title of principal executive, service area, scope of services, budget and patient size.

350 pages Frequency: Annual

2753 Home Care Agencies, Hospices and Nursing
Pools
NC Dept of Human Resources
116 West Jones Street
Raleigh, NC 27603
919-807-4800
Fax: 919-733-0653
askhr@nc.gov
www.oshr.nc.gov/

C. Neal Alexander, Jr., State Human Resources Director
Paula Woodhouse, Deputy Director
PJ Warren, Executive Assistant to Director

Computer printout. Covers more than 725 home care agencies, nursing pools, and hospice programs in North Carolina. Entries include: Agency name, address, phone; agency director; Medicare/Medicaid certification.

131 pages

2754 Home Health Service Directory
infoUSA
1020 E 1st Street
Papillion, NE 68046
402-593-4600
Fax: 402-331-5481; *Toll Free:* 800-835-5856
internet@infousa.com
www.infousa.com/

Bill Hippen, Vice President

A health care directory for patients restricted to thier homes.

Frequency: Annual

2755 Homes Nursing Directory
infoUSA
1020 E 1st Street
Papillion, NE 68046
402-593-4600
Fax: 402-331-5481; *Toll Free:* 800-835-5856
internet@infousa.com
www.infousa.com/

Bill Hippen, Vice President

Over 23,000 listings of programs related to home nursing care.

Frequency: Annual

2756 Hospices Directory
infoUSA
1020 E 1st Street
Papillion, NE 68046
402-593-4600
Fax: 402-331-5481; *Toll Free:* 800-835-5856

internet@infousa.com
www.infousa.com/

Bill Hippin, Vice President

Number of listings: 2,639. Entries include: Name, address, phone, size of advertisement, name of owner or manager, number of employees, year first in 'Yellow Pages.' Compiled from telephone company 'Yellow Pages,' nationwide.

2757 ILRU Directory of Centers, SILCs, and Related Organizations (Independent Living Research Utilization)
Independent Living Research Utilization Program
TIRR Memorial Hermann Research Center
1333 Moursund Street
Houston, TX 77030-3405
713-520-0232
Fax: 713-520-5785
ilru@ilru.org
www.ilru.org
TTY: 713-520-0232

Lex Frieden, Director, ILRU
Vinh Nguyen, Program Director
Sharon Finney, Information & Communication Spec

List of independent living programs for disabled people.

80 pages Frequency: Annual, January Year Founded: 1977

2758 In-Home Care Services Directory
infoUSA
1020 E 1st Street
Papillion, NE 68046
402-593-4600
Fax: 402-331-5481; *Toll Free:* 800-835-5856
internet@infousa.com
www.infousa.com/

Bill Hippin, Vice President

Directory of in-home care related listings.

Frequency: Annual

2759 Information & Referral Services Directory
Nursing Home
infoUSA
1020 E 1st Street
Papillion, NE 68046
402-593-4600
Fax: 402-331-5481; *Toll Free:* 800-835-5856
internet@infousa.com
www.infousa.com/

Bill Hippin, Vice President

Directory with over 350 listings of nursing homes. Available online.

Frequency: Annual

2760 International Directory of Research and Researchers in Comparative Gerontology
University of South Florida
4202 E. Fowler Avenue
Tampa, FL 33620
813-974-2011
Fax: 727-553-1126
www.usf.edu/

Dr. Judy Genshaft, President & Chief Executive Offi
Dr. Ralph Wilcox, Provost and Executive Vice Presi

Over 300 research projects in comparative gerontology conducted since 1984; international coverage. Entries include: Project title; sponsoring institution, organization, or individual name, address, phone; biographical data for researchers, description of study.

380 pages Frequency: Quadrennial Year Founded: 1956

2761 International Telephone Directory for TDD Users
Gallaudet University
800 Florida Avenue, NE
Washington, DC 20002-3695
202-651-5000
Fax: 800-621-8476; *Toll Free:* 800-621-2736
clerc.center@gallaudet.edu
www.gallaudet.edu
TTY: 888-630-9347

Dr. T. Alan Hurwitz, President
Paul Kelly, Vice President for Administratio
Catherine Murphy, Executive Director, Communicatio

Offers 12,000 TDD members and organizations serving deaf people.

190 pages Year Founded: 1864

2762 Large Print Loan Library Catalog
Lighthouse International
111 East 59th Street
The Sol and Lillian Goldman Building
New York, NY 10022-1202
212-821-9200
Fax: 212-821-9707; *Toll Free:* 800-829-0500
info@lighthouse.org
www.navh.org
TTY: 212-821-9713

Ann Illuzzi, Manager
Winifred Holt, Co-Founder
Edith Holt, Co-Founder

Listing of over 6500 commercially published and NAVH large print books avaiable through NAVH on a loan basis. Includes a limited selection of titles available for purchase.

Year Founded: 1905

2763 Legal Rights of Persons with Disabilities: An Analysis of Federal Law
LRP Publications
747 Dresher Road
Suite 500
Horsham, PA 19044
215-784-0941
Fax: 215-784-9639; *Toll Free:* 800-341-7874
custserve@lrp.com
www.lrp.com
TTY: 215-658-0938

Kenneth F. Kahn, President
Gary Bagin, Director Communications

A comprehensive analysis of the rights accorded individuals with disabilities under federal law covering such issues as: Definitions of individuals with disabilities, reasonable accomidations, architectural barriers, access to transportation and communication services, education, and newborns.

1536 pages Year Founded: 1977

2764 Meals on Wheels Assoiation of America Directory
Meals on Wheels Association of America
413 N. Lee Street
Alexandria, VA 22314
703-548-5558
Fax: 703-548-5274; *Toll Free:* 888-998-6325
mowaa@mowaa.org
www.mowaa.org/

Vinsen Faris, CFRE, Chair
Liz Seman, Vice Chair
Jeffrey Smythe, MPA, Secretary/Treasurer

Online Directory of companies and organizations serving the needs of the elderly. Meals on Wheels home-delivers food to older citizens who are homebound.

130 pages Frequency: Annual Year Founded: 1940

2765 Medical Device Market Place
Grey House Publishing
4919 Route 22
PO Box 56
Amenia, NY 12501-0056
518-789-8700
Fax: 518-789-0556; *Toll Free:* 800-562-2139
books@greyhouse.com
www.greyhouse.com

Richard Gottlieb, President & Co-Founder
Laura Mars, Editoral Director
Leslie Mackenzie, Publisher & Co-Founder

The two-volume Medical Device Market Place provides data on the 13,000 Medical Device companies licensed to sell medical devices in the United States, and the 67,000 products they represent.

1900 pages

2766 Mental Retardation & Developmentally Disabled Services Directory
infoUSA
1020 E 1st Street
Papillion, NE 68046
402-593-4600
Fax: 402-331-5481; *Toll Free:* 800-835-5856
internet@infousa.com
www.infousa.com/

Bill Hippen, Vice President

Number of listings: 2,759. Entries include: Name, address, phone, size of advertisement, name of owner or manager, number of employees, year first in 'Yellow Pages.' Compiled from telephone company 'Yellow Pages,' nationwide.

2767 Mentally Disabled and the Law
William S Hein & Company
2350 North Forest Rd.
Getzville, NY 14068
716-882-2600
Fax: 716-883-8100; *Toll Free:* 800-828-7571
mail@wshein.com
www.wshein.com

William Hein, Chairman of the Board
Kevin Marmion, President
Shannon Hein, Vice President, Sales

Offers information on treatment rights, the provider-patient relationship, and the rights of the mentally disabled persons in the community.

867 pages Year Founded: 1980

2768 NARIC Guide to Disability and Rehabilitation Periodicals
National Rehabilitation Information Center
8400 Corporate Drive
Suite 500
Landover, MD 20785
301-459-5984
Fax: 301-459-4263; *Toll Free:* 800-346-2742
naricinfo@kra.com
www.naric.com
TTY: 301-459-5984

Mark X. Odum, Project Director
Jessica H. Chaiken, Media and Information Services M
Natalie J. Collier, Library and Acquisitions Manager

Listing of more than 400 national, local and international rehabiliatation newsletters and journals.

170 pages Year Founded: 1982

2769 NIDRR Program Directory
National Rehabilitation Information Center
8400 Corporate Drive
Suite 500
Landover, MD 20785
301-459-5984
Fax: 301-459-4263; *Toll Free:* 800-346-2742
naricinfo@kra.com
www.naric.com
TTY: 301-459-5984

Mark X. Odum, Project Director
Jessica H. Chaiken, Media and Information Services M
Natalie J. Collier, Library and Acquisitions Manager

A directory of NIDRR funded demonstrations and research projects.

318 pages Frequency: Annual Year Founded: 1982

2770 NLADA Directory of Legal Aid and Defender Offices in the United States and Territories
National Legal Aid & Defender Association
1140 Connecticut Avenue NW
Suite 900
Washington, DC 20036
202-452-0620
Fax: 202-872-1031
linfo@nlada.org
www.nlada100years.org/

Lillian Johnson, Chairperson
Rosita Stanley, Vice-Chairperson
Jo-Ann Wallace, President and CEO

Approximately 3,600 civil legal aid and indigent defense organizations in the United States; includes programs for specific groups such as prisoners, senior citizens, the disabled, etc. Entries include: Agency name, address, phone, director's name.

265 pages Frequency: Biennial-Spring Year Founded: 1911

2771 National Directory of Educational Programs in Gerontology and Geriatrics
Association for Gerontology in Higher Education
1220 L Street, NW
Suite 901
Washington, DC 20005-4018
202-289-9806
Fax: 202-289-9824

aghe@aghe.org
www.aghe.org/

Janet C. Frank, President
M. Angela Baker, Director
Kelly Niles-Yokum, Secretary

Over 1,000 degree and certificate programs and concentrations in the field of gerontology available at 507 institutions of higher education. Entries include: Institution name, name and title of contact, address, phone, fax, e-mail address, overview of campus gerontology instruction/activity, description of gerontology programs(s), year program began, number of credit courses offered, number of faculty teaching aging, and special resources. available.

Year Founded: 1972

2772 National Directory of Healthcare and Human Service Ministries
United Methodist Association
2800 W. Main Street
Tupelo, MS 38801-3027
662-269-2955
Fax: 662-269-2956; Toll Free: 800-411-9901
umassociation.org/

Rev. Nancy S Hull, Board Chair
Rev. Stephen Vinson, President/ CEO
Shelly L. Ward, Secretary

95 hospitals, 62 child care facilities, 345 long-term care facilities, 67 annual conferences, and 115 community centers connected with a connectional unit of The United Methodist Church. Entries include: Institution name, address, phone, name of executive, list of services.

137 pages Frequency: Annual

2773 National Home Care and Hospice Directory
National Association for Home Care & Hospice
228 7th Street SE
Washington, DC 20003
202-547-7424
Fax: 202-547-3540
ads@nahc.org, exec@nahc.org
www.nahc.org

Andrea Devoti, Chair
Lucy Andrews, Vice Chair
Val J. Halamandaris, President

Approximately 17,000 home care and hospice providers in the US & Puerto Rico. Entries include: Agency name, address, phone, fax, director's name, product/service provided, area served.

960 pages Frequency: Annual, January

2774 National Yellow Book of Funeral Directors
Nomis Publications, Inc.
PO Box 5159
Youngstown, OH 44514
330-965-2380
Fax: 330-965-2381; Toll Free: 800-321-7479
info@nomispublications.com
www.nomispublications.com/

Lucille A. (McGuire, President
Kimberly McGuire-Graham, Vice President
Margaret (Pe Rouzzo, Secretary/Treasurer

20,000 United States and Canadian funeral homes; Veteran's Administration hospitals and regional offices; major hospitals; foreign consulates and branch offices; daily papers; mortuary colleges. Entries include: Name of home, address, phone, code for shipping points, city code for daily papers available for obituaries.

1,000 pages Frequency: Annual Year Founded: 1974

2775 Nursing & Convalescent Homes Directory
infoUSA
1020 E 1st Street
Papillion, NE 68046
402-593-4600
Fax: 402-331-5481; Toll Free: 800-835-5856
internet@infousa.com
www.infousa.com/

Bill Hippen, Vice President

Number of listings: 20,736. Entries include: Name, address, phone (including area code), size of advertisement, year first in 'Yellow Pages,' name of owner or manager, number of employees. Compiled from telephone company 'Yellow Pages,' nationwide.

Frequency: Annual

2776 Options: A Directory of Child and Senior Services
Five Star Publications, Inc.
PO Box 6698
Chandler, AZ 85246
480-940-8182
Fax: 480-940-8787; Toll Free: 866-471-0777
infor@fivestarsupport.com
www.fivestarsupport.com

Linda F Radke, President

Over 350 care services for children and senior citizens; primary coverage of Arizona with some national listings. Entries include: Facility/service name, address, phone, hours and days of week open, year established, commission or regulatory agency granting the operating license, ownership, available discounts, available handicapped facilities/services, and a description of services written by the listee.

90 pages Year Founded: 1985

2777 Over 50 Directory & Handbook
Area 10 Agency on Aging
631 West Edgewood Drive
Ellettsville, IN 47429
812-876-3383
Fax: 812-876-9922; Toll Free: 800-844-1010
www.area10agency.org/

Jewel Echelbarger, Exeuctive Director
Jason Carnes, Director
Marsha Keith, Director

A free guide of local services and business who support local seniors, offer quality merchandise and services and many offer a senior discount.

Year Founded: 1981

2778 Pension & Profit Sharing Plan Companies Directory
infoUSA
1020 E 1st Street
Papillion, NE 68046
402-593-4600
Fax: 402-331-5481; Toll Free: 800-835-5856
internet@infousa.com
www.infousa.com/

Bill Hippen, Vice President

Number of listings: 5,428. Entries include: Name, address, phone (including area code), size of advertisement, year first in 'Yellow Pages,' name of owner or manager, number of employees. Compiled from telephone company 'Yellow Pages,' nationwide.

Frequency: Annual

2779 Pensions & Investments: 1,000 Largest Retirement Funds
Crain Communications, Inc.
150 N. Michigan Ave.
Chicago, IL 60601
312-649-5200
Fax: 312-649-5228
jmurphy@crain.com
www.pionline.com

Chris J. Battaglia, Publisher
William A. Morrow, Executive Vice President/Operati
Nancy K. Webman, Editor

The nations largest retirement plans compiled into a directory.

Frequency: Annual, January Year Founded: 1916

2780 Products for People With Disabilities
LS&S Group
145 River Rock Drive
Buffalo, NY 14207
716-348-3500
Fax: 847-498-1482; *Toll Free:* 800-468-4789
info@lssproducts.com
www.lssproducts.com
TDD 866-317-8533

Melissa Balbach, President
John K Bace, Executive VP

2781 Publicist's Guide to Senior Media
Promoworks
300 North Martingale Road
Schaumburg, IL 60173
888-310-3555
Fax: 805-379-1029
www.promoworks.com/

Pete Tarnapoli, CEO
Julie Beck, General Manager
Karen Carlborg, Senior Director Client Services

Directory of newspapers, media and syndicated columnists that are senior oriented.

130 pages Frequency: Biennial Year Founded: 1999

2782 Purple Directory: National Listing of African-American Funeral Firms
SHUGAR'S
PO Box 38665
Detroit, MI 48238-0665
313-836-8600
Fax: 313-836-8600; *Toll Free:* 800-377-9129
purfuneral@aol.com
www.purpledirectory.com

Miriam E Pipes, Editor-in-Chief, President, Foun

Approximately 2,700 Afircan American funeral firms, in the US Entries include: Firm name, address, phone; some listings include fax and name and title of contact.

248 pages Frequency: Bi Annually Year Founded: 1979

2783 Rehabilitation Services Directory
infoUSA
1020 E 1st Street
Papillion, NE 68046
402-593-4600
Fax: 402-331-5481; *Toll Free:* 800-835-5856
internet@infousa.com
www.infousa.com/

Bill Hippen, Vice President

Directory of rehabilitation programs.

Frequency: Annual

2784 Retirement Planning Service Directory
infoUSA
1020 E 1st Street
Papillion, NE 68046
402-593-4600
Fax: 402-331-5481; *Toll Free:* 800-835-5856
internet@infousa.com
www.infousa.com/

Bill Hippen, Vice President

Number of listings: 2,396. Entries include: Name, address, phone, size of advertisement, name of owner or manager, number of employees, year first in 'Yellow Pages.' Compiled from telephone company 'Yellow Pages,' nationwide.

2785 Senior Citizens Service Organizations Directory
infoUSA
1020 E 1st Street
Papillion, NE 68046
402-593-4600
Fax: 402-331-5481; *Toll Free:* 800-835-5856
internet@infousa.com
www.infousa.com/

Bill Hippen, Vice President

Number of listings: 7,212. Entries include: Name, address, phone (including area code), size of advertisement, year first in 'Yellow Pages,' name of owner or manager, number of employees. Compiled from telephone company 'Yellow Pages,' nationwide.

Frequency: Annual

2786 Senior Citizens Services
Gale
27500 Drake Road
Farmington Hills, MI 48331-3535
248-699-4253
Fax: 248-699-8069; *Toll Free:* 800-877-GALE
galeord@gale.com
www.gale.cengage.com/

Alexander Broich, President, International
Dean D. Durbin, Chief Financial Officer
Michael E. Hansen, Chief Executive Officer

15,000 organizations from the private sector that provide senior services, 57 State Agencies on Aging, 670 Area Agencies on Aging. Separated into four volumes each available separately: Northeastern States, Southern and Mid-Atlantic States, Midwestern States, and Western States. Entries include: Contact information and description of services.

1,852 pages

2787 Senior Media Directory
Creative Ink, Inc.
PO Box 22383
Beaverton, OR 55122-0383
503-690-5693
Fax: 877-245-9904
info@creativeink.com
www.creativeink.com/

Pat Picard, Sales Manager

Approximately 1,250 radio and television programs, newspapers, periodicals, other publications, and marketing and mailing programs that have targeted the senior citizen audience. Entries include: Name, address, phone, fax, e-mail, website, names and titles, circulation, PR contacts, etc. Paperback.

200 pages Frequency: Annual, Februa.

2788 State Vocational Rehabilitation Agencies
US Office Special Educ and Rehabilitative Serv.
400 Maryland Avenue, SW
Washington, DC 20202
202-205-8358
Fax: 202-205-9163; *Toll Free:* 800-USA-LEAR
www2.ed.gov/about/offices/list/osers/rsa

Arne Duncan, Secretary of Education
Jim Shelton, Acting Deputy Secretary
Martha Kanter, Under Secretary

State government agencies responsible for vocational rehabilitation activities, including those for the blind. Entries include: Agency name, address, phone, name and title of director, federal Rehabilitation Services Administration region number.

11 pages Frequency: Triannually Year Founded: 1980

2789 Travelin' Talk Directory
Travelin' Talk
PO Box 3534
Clarksville, TN 37043-3534
931-552-6670
Fax: 931-552-1182
www.travelintalk.net/

Rick Crowder, Founder

Over 1,000 resources for travelers with disabilities; international coverage. Entries include: Company, organization, or personal name, address, phone, biographical data for individuals, geographical area served, descriptions of services, projects, etc. $35.00

550 pages Year Founded: 1987

2790 US Aging Policy Interest Groups
Greenwood Publishing Group, Inc.
88 Post Road W
PO Box 5007
Westport, CT 06881-5007
203-226-3571
Fax: 203-226-1502; *Toll Free:* 800-225-5800
www.harcourt.com/bu_info/greenwood.html

David Van Tassel, Editor
Elaine Meyer, Editor
Wayne Smith

83 organizations interested in aging and aging policies. Entries include: Organization name, address, phone, fax, purpose and background, funding, primary concerns, activities, publications.

288 pages

2791 USTA Adult and Senior National Championships Booklet
Florentine Press
160 Varick Street
Floor 6
New York, NY 10013-1220
212-633-1110
Fax: 212-633-8831
info@theflorentinepress.com
www.theflorentinepress.com/

Anne Humes, Editor
Susan Shaffer, Editor
Steve Fromkes

Directory of associations that promote senior activities and over 250 listings of clubs and organizations that offer tennis for seniors.

65 pages

2792 United States Naval Academy Alumni Association: Register of Alumni
United States Naval Academy Alumni Association
247 King George Street
Annapolis, MD 21402
410-295-4000
Fax: 410-269-0151
SAAC@usna.com, membership@usna.com, events@us
www.usna.com/

ADM Robert J Natter, USN (Ret.), Chair
Ltgen Jack W Klimp, USMC (Ret.), Vice Chair
Byron F. Marchant, President & CEO

About 88,000 graduates and former naval cadets and midshipmen, living and deceased. Entries include: Name, date of birth, state appointed from, address (including duty address, if still on active duty), decorations, date of resignation or retirement, date and place of death and widow's name, where applicable.

700 pages Frequency: Annual, Aug. Year Founded: 1931

2793 University of Continuing Education Association: Membership Directory
University Continuing Education Association
1 Dupont Circle
Suite 615
Washington, DC 20036
202-659-3130
Fax: 202-785-0374
upcea.edu/

Robert Hansen, CEO
Lori Derkay, COO
Robert Colburn, Finance & Administration Coordin

Almost 400 college and University departments which offer continuing educations programs

175 pages Frequency: Annual, Sept. Year Founded: 1915

2794 Veterans & Military Organizations Directory
infoUSA
1020 E 1st Street
Papillion, NE 68046
402-593-4600
Fax: 402-331-5481; *Toll Free:* 800-835-5856
internet@infousa.com
www.infousa.com/

Bill Hippen, Vice President

Number of listings: 8,849. Entries include: Name, address, phone (including area code), size of advertisement, year first in 'Yellow Pages,' name of owner or manager, number of employees. Compiled from telephone company 'Yellow Pages,' nationwide.

Frequency: Annual

2795 Volunteer Vacations
Chicago Review Press
814 N Franklin Street
Chicago, IL 60610
312-337-0747
Fax: 312-337-5110; *Toll Free:* 800-888-4741
www.chicagoreviewpress.com/

Allison Felus, Managing Editor
Cynthia Sherry, Publisher
Michelle Williams, Developmental Editor

Directory of more than 280 foundations and organizations that sponsor volunteer expeditions in environmental and wild life preservation.

480 pages Frequency: Biennial, March Year Founded: 1973

2796 Wheel Chairs & Scooters Directory
infoUSA
1020 E 1st Street
Papillion, NE 68046
402-593-4600
Fax: 402-331-5481; *Toll Free:* 800-835-5856
internet@infousa.com
www.infousa.com/

Bill Hippen, Vice President

Number of listings: 3,857. Entries include: Name, address, phone (including area code), size of advertisement, year first in Yellow Pages, name of owner or manager, number of employees. Compiled from telephone company Yellow Pages, nationwide.

Frequency: Annual

2797 Wheel Chairs Renting Directory
infoUSA
1020 E 1st Street
Papillion, NE 68046
402-593-4600
Fax: 402-331-5481; *Toll Free:* 800-835-5856
internet@infousa.com
www.infousa.com/

Bill Hippen, Vice President

Number of listings: 594. Entries include: Name, address, phone, size of advertisement, name of owner or manager, number of employees, year first in Yellow Pages. Compiled from telephone company Yellow Pages, nationwide.

Journals, Magazines

2798 A Better Tomorrow
Thomas Nelson
5301 Wisconsin Avenue NW
Suite 620
Washington, DC 20015-2015
202-364-8000
Fax: 202-364-8910
www.thomasnelson.com/

Bruce Barbour, Publisher
Dale Hanson, Editor

Magazine focusing on issues and concerns of senior citizens.

Frequency: Quarterly Year Founded: 1798

2799 AARP Bulletin
AARP
601 E Street NW
Washington, DC 20049
Toll Free: 888-687-2277
www.aarp.org

Resources for online classes, training and more. Topics include Computers/Technology, Health/Wellbeing, Personal Finance. AARP Membership open to individuals age 50+, benefits include access to insurance services, travel discounts, advice on healthy living, financial planning, consumer protection. AARP represents members on issues like Medicare, Social Security, and consumer safety. Publications include the AARP Magazine and AARP Bulletin.

2800 AARP The Magazine
AARP
601 E Street NW
Washington, DC 20049
Toll Free: 888-687-2277
member@aarp.org
www.aarp.org/magazine
TTY: 877-434-7598

Mary C. Hickey, Editor in Chief

AARP The Magazine is the world's largest circulation magazine and the definitive lifestyle publication for AARP's nearly 40 million members and Americans 50 and over.

Frequency: Monthly

2801 ACE Fitness Matters
American Council on Exercise (ACE)
4851 Paramount Drive
San Diego, CA 92123
858-576-6500
Fax: 858-576-6564; *Toll Free:* 888-825-3636
support@acefitness.org
www.acefitness.org/

Herb Flentye, Chair
Scott Murdoch, PhD., RD, Vice Chair
Scott Goudeseune, President & CEO

Consumer magazine covering health and fitness news.

Frequency: Bimonthly Year Founded: 1985

2802 AER Report
Association for Education & Rehabilitation of the
1703 N. Beauregard Street
Suite 440
Alexandria, VA 22311
703-671-4500
Fax: 703-671-6391
www.aerbvi.org/

Jim Adams, President
Lou Tutt, Executive Director
Deborah Gold, Director

Contains organizational news, conference dates and information concerning services to visually impaired people.

Year Founded: 1984

2803 Adapted Physical Activity Quarterly
Human Kinetics
PO Box 5076
1607 N Market Street
Champaign, IL 61820
217-351-5076
Fax: 217-351-1549; *Toll Free:* 800-747-4457
info@hkusa.com
www.humankinetics.com

Brian Holding, CEO
Rainer Martens, Founder
Marilyn Martens, Founder

Journal on the study of physical activity for special populations.

Frequency: Quarterly Year Founded: 1974

2804 Aging International
Transaction Publishers
35 Berrue
New Brunswick, NJ 08901
732-445-1245
Fax: 732-445-3138; *Toll Free:* 888-999-6778
orders@transactionpub.com
www.transactionpub.com/

Mary E. Curtis, Chair
Irving Louis Horowitz, Co-Founder
Michael Celletto, Secretary

Journal dedicated to the well-being of older persons worldwide. Explores productive aging, empowerment, life-long learning, health promotion, and services for the elderly, with an emphasis on sharing both common concerns and practical applications. Focuses on social and economic issues, public policies, and use of resources. Published in cooperation with the International Federation on Aging.

Frequency: Quarterly Year Founded: 1962

2805 Aging News Alert
CD Publications
2222 Sedwick Drive
Durham, NC 27713
301-588-6380
Fax: 800-508-2592; *Toll Free:* 855-237-1396
info@cdpublications.com
www.cdpublications.com

Michael Gerecht, President

Twice-monthly newsletter reporting on senior programs, funding opportunities and federal actions affecting the elderly.

Year Founded: 1961

2806 Aging Research & Training News
Business Publishers, Inc.
2222 Sedwick Drive
Durham, NC 27713
Fax: 800-508-2592; *Toll Free:* 800-223-8720
www.bpinews.com

Kimberly Gilbert, Managing Editor
Alexa Chew, Contributing Editor
Mary Compton, Publisher

Compilation of studies of aging populations; reports on innovative programs with aging community; federal funding and laws.

8 pages Year Founded: 1963

2807 Aging and Society
Cambridge University Press
32 Avenue of the Americas
New York, NY 10013-2473
212-924-3900
Fax: 212-691-3239; *Toll Free:* 800-221-4512
info@cup.org
www.cambridge.org/us/information/contact

Ken Blakemore, Editor
Bill Bythwway, Editor
Richard Ziemacki

International journal publishing on topics which further the understanding of human aging. The journal of the Centre for policy on aging and the British Socie for Gerontology.

Frequency: Bimonthly

2808 American Journal of Speech-Language Pathology
American Speech-Language-Hearing Association (ASHA
2200 Research Boulevard
Rockville, MD 20850-3289
301-296-5700
Fax: 301-296-8580; *Toll Free:* 800-638-8255
nsslha@asha.org, productsales@asha.org
www.asha.org/
TTY: 301-296-5650

Elizabeth S. McCrea, PhD, CCC-SLP, President
Barbara K. Cone, PhD, CCC-A, Vice President for Academic Affa
Carolyn W. Higdon, EdD, CCC-SLP, Vice President for Finance

2809 American Legion Magazine
American Legion National Headquarters
PO Box 1055
700 N. Pennsylvania St.
Indianapolis, IN 46206
317-630-1200
Fax: 317-630-1223; *Toll Free:* 800-433-3318
www.legion.org/

Daniel S. Wheeler, National Adjutant
Philip B. Onderdonk Jr., National Judge Advocate
George A. Buskirk Jr., National Treasurer

General interest magazine for veterans.

Frequency: Monthly Year Founded: 1919

2810 American Rehabilitation Services Administration (RSA)
American Rehabilitation Services Administration (R
400 Maryland Avenue, SW
Washington, DC 20202
202-205-8296
Fax: 202-205-9874; *Toll Free:* 800-USA-LEAR
www2.ed.gov/about/offices/list/osers/rsa

Arne Duncan, Secretary of Education
Jim Shelton,. Acting Deputy Secretary
Martha Kanter, Under Secretary

Magazine on rehabilitation of the handicapped.

Frequency: Quarterly Year Founded: 1980

2811 Assistive Technology
RESNA
1700 N Moore Street
Suite 1540
Arlington, VA 22209
703-524-6686
Fax: 202-524-6630
www.resna.org

Alex Mihailidis, PhD, P.Eng, President
Jamie Arasz Prioli, ATP, Secretary
Paul J. Schwartz, MSIE, ATP, R, Treasurer

Journal focusing on assistive technology for persons with disabilities.

2812 Audecibel
International Hearing Society
16880 Middlebelt Road
Suite 4
Livonia, MI 48154
734-522-7200
Fax: 734-522-0200; *Toll Free:* 800-521-5247
www.ihsinfo.org/

Amanda Ciccantelli, Administrative Assistant
Bernadette " Demicoli, Member Services Coordinator
Sandra den Boer, Communications Specialist

Magazine publishing technical articles and product announcements on hearing aids and hearing.

Frequency: Quarterly

2813 Buena Vida
Casiano Communications
1700 Fern ndez Juncos Avenue
San Juan, PR 00909
787-728-3000
Fax: 787-268-1001; *Toll Free:* 800-468-8167
nationalsales@casiano.com
www.casiano.com/

Manuel A. Casiano, Chairman & CEO
Carlos Rom, Executive Vice President
Nora Casiano, Vice President & Business Manage

Health and fitness magazine.

Frequency: Monthly Year Founded: 1973

2814 Challenge Magazine
Disabled Sports, USA
451 Hungerford Drive
Suite 100
Rockville, MD 20850
301-217-0960
Fax: 301-217-0968
dsusa@dsusa.org
www.disabledsportsusa.org/

Robert Meserve, President
Steven Goodwin, Vice President
Kirk Bauer, Executive Director

Magazine providing information on sports for people with physical disabilities.

Frequency: Quarterly Year Founded: 1967

2815 Closing the Gap, Inc.
P.O. Box 68
Henderson, MN 56044
507-248-3294
Fax: 507-248-3810

info@closingthegap.com
www.closingthegap.com

Megan Turek, President
Marc Hagen, Vice President

Online membership that includes access to the Solutions on-line magazine and archives, archived webinars and the Resource Directory, a guide to over 2,000 products for children and adults with disabilities

Year Founded: 1983

2816 Communication Outlook: Artificial Language Laboratory
Artificial Language Laboratory
405 Computer Center
Michigan State University
Lansing, MI 48824-1042
517-353-0870
Fax: 517-353-4766
artlang@pilot.msu.edu
www.msu.edu/~artlang/CommOut.html

Dr. John B. Eulenberg, Ph.D., Director
Stephen R. Blosser, B.S.M.E., Technical Director
Rebecca Ann Baird, Editor, Communication Outlook

Magazine reporting on the newest developments in the application of technology for neurologically impaired persons.

Frequency: Quarterly Year Founded: 1972

2817 Computer-Disability News
Easter Seals
233 South Wacker Drive
Suite 2400
Chicago, IL 60606
312-726-6200
Fax: 312-726-1494; *Toll Free:* 800-221-6827
www.easterseals.com/

Richard W. Davidson, Chairman
Sandra L. Bouwman, 1st Vice Chairman
Joseph G. Kern, 2nd Vice Chairman

Magazine highlighting news for persons with disabilities.

Frequency: Quarterly Year Founded: 1934

2818 Conscious Choice
Conscious Communications
920 N Franklin Street
Suite 202
Chicago, IL 60610-3473
312-440-4373
Fax: 312-751-3973
www.consciouscomms.com/

Ross Thompson, Managing Editor
Jim Slama, Publisher

Consumer magazine covering health, nutrition and environmental issues.

Frequency: Bimonthly

2819 Contemporary Gerontology
Springer Publishing Company
11 West 42nd Street
15th Floor
New York, NY 10036
212-431-4370
Fax: 212-941-7842; *Toll Free:* 877-687-7476

cs@springerpub.com, journals@springerpub.com
www.springerpub.com

James C. Costello, Vice President, Journal Publishi
Theodore C. Nardin, Chief Executive Officer & Publis
Diana Osborne, Production Manager

Scholarly journal covering gerontology.

Frequency: Quarterly Year Founded: 1950

2820 Disability Rag's Ragged Edge Magazine
Advocado Press
PO Box 145
Louisville, KY 40201
502-894-9492
Fax: 502-899-9562
www.advocadopress.org/

Mary Johnson, Mailing Contact/Editor

Magazine of debate on disability rights issues. ISSN#
1095-3949

35 pages Frequency: Bimonthly

2821 Disability Rights Now
Disability Rights Education and Defense Fund
3075 Adeline Street
Suite 210
Berkeley, CA 94703
510-644-2555
Fax: 510-841-8645; *Toll Free:* 800-466-4232
info@dredf.org
dredf.org/
TTY: 510-841-8645

Claudia Center, President and Chair
Susan Henderson, Executive Director
Ingrid Tischer, Director of Development

Free quarterly publication describing the activities of the
Disability Rights Education and Defense Fund, available in
alternative formats.

Year Founded: 1979

2822 Disability Statistics Report
Institute for Health & Aging
2 Koret Way, #N-319X
UCSF Box 0602
San Francisco, CA 94143-0602
415-476-1435
Fax: 415-476-9707
info@nursing.ucsf.edu
nursing.ucsf.edu/iha

David Vlahov, RN, PhD, Dean and Professor
Yolanda Abrea, Fiscal Analyst
Phoebe Byers, Communications Coordinator

Magazine providing statistical data on disability in the US
as collected by the Disability Statistics Program.

Year Founded: 1907

2823 Disability Studies Quarterly
University of Hawaii at Manoa
2500 Campus Road
Honolulu, HI 96822
808-956-8111
Fax: 808-956-3162
manoa.hawaii.edu/

M.R.C. Greenwood, President
Tom Apple, Chief Executive Officer

Scholarly journal containing articles on all aspects of disability.

Frequency: Quarterly

2824 Disabled American Veterans Magazines
Disabled American Veterans National
Headquarters
PO Box 14301
Cincinnati, OH 45250-0301
859-441-7300
Fax: 859-441-8056
www.dav.org/

Thomas K Keller, Editor
James Chaney, Mailing Contact

Veterans magazine on disability issues.

Frequency: Bimonthly

2825 Disabled People as Second Class Citizens
Springer Publishing Company
11 West 42nd Street
15th Floor
New York, NY 10036
212-431-4370
Fax: 212-941-7842; *Toll Free:* 877-687-7476
cs@springerpub.com, journals@springerpub.com
www.springerpub.com

James C. Costello, Vice President, Journal Publishi
Theodore C. Nardin, Chief Executive Officer & Publis
Diana Osborne, Production Manager

Disability and legal practice.

320 pages Year Founded: 1950

2826 Domestic Mistreatment of the Elderly: Towards
Prevention
AARP
601 E Street NW
Washington, DC 20049
202-434-3525
Fax: 202-434-3443; *Toll Free:* 888-687-2277
member@aarp.org
www.aarp.org
TTY: 877-434-7598

Gail E. Aldrich, Board Chair
Robert G. Romasco, President
Dr. Ethel Pe Andrus, Founder

This comprehensive publication addresses the problem of
mistreatment or neglect in the home.

39 pages Year Founded: 1958

2827 Duplex Planet
Duplex Planet
PO Box 1230
Saratoga Springs, NY 12866
518-692-7410
Fax: 518-692-8208
info@duplexplanet.com, booking@duplexplanet.c
www.duplexplanet.com/

David Greenberger, Editor/ Founder

Consumer journal covering issues of aging and popular culture.

Frequency: Bimonthly Year Founded: 1979

2828 Eating Well Magazine
Eating Well
6221 Shelburne Road
Suite 100
Charlotte, VT 05482
802-985-4500
Fax: 802-425-3675; *Toll Free:* 800-344-3350
www.eatingwell.com

Thomas Witschi, President
Brierley Wright, Managing Editor
Jessie Price, Editor-in-Chief

Food magazine with emphasis on delicious low-fat cooking and sensible nutrition.

Year Founded: 1990

2829 Educational Gerontology
Taylor & Francis
711 3rd Avenue
8th Floor
New York, NY 10017
212-216-7800
Fax: 212-564-7854; *Toll Free:* 800-634-7064
www.taylorandfrancis.com/

D Barry Lumsden, Editor
Kevin Bradley, CEO

Journal publishing original research in the fields of gerontology, adult education, and the social and behavioral sciences.

Year Founded: 1936

2830 Elderly Health Services Letter
Health Resources Online
P.O. Box 456
Allenwood, NJ 08720
800-516-4343
Fax: 732-292-1111
info@healthresourcesonline.com
www.healthresourcesonline.com

Robert K Jenkins, Publisher

An essential tool for senior services professionals. Stays on top of the most current challenges facing senior services professionals, including financing and funding senior services, marketing, positioning senior services for managed care, getting administrative support and more.

Year Founded: 1978

2831 Experimental Aging Research
Taylor & Francis
711 3rd Avenue
8th Floor
New York, NY 10017
212-216-7800
Fax: 212-564-7854; *Toll Free:* 800-634-7064
www.taylorandfrancis.com/

Jeffrey Elias, Editor
Kevin Bradley, CEO

International journal devoted to the scientific study of the aging process.

Frequency: Quarterly Year Founded: 1936

2832 Fitness Diet and Exercise Guide
Family Circle
110 5th Avenue
New York, NY 10011-5614
212-463-1673
Fax: 212-463-1906; *Toll Free:* 800-627-4444
fcfeedback@familycircle.com
www.familycircle.com/

Darcy Jacobs, Executive Editor
Linda Fears, Vice President/Editor in Chief
Robb Riedel, Managing Editor

Magazine suggesting ways to eat healthier and exercise better.

2833 Focus on Geriatric Care and Rehabilitation
Aspen Publishers
7201 McKinney Circle
Frederick, MD 21704
301-644-3599
Fax: 800-901-9075; *Toll Free:* 800-234-1660
www.aspenpublishers.com/

Bob Lemmond, President & CEO
Gustavo Dobles, Vice President & Chief Content O
Susan Pikitch, Vice President & Chief Financial

Monthly journal written for nurses, occupational therapists and administrators in geriatric settings.

2834 Generations
American Society on Aging
575 Market Street
Suite 2100
San Francisco, CA 94105-2869
415-974-9600
Fax: 415-974-0300; *Toll Free:* 800-537-9728
www.asaging.org

Louis Colbert, Chairperson
Tobi Abramson, Director
Patricia J. Volland, Treasurer

Peer-review quarterly journal featuring guest editor.

Year Founded: 1954

2835 Generations, Journal of the American Society on Aging
American Society on Aging
575 Market Street
Suite 2100
San Francisco, CA 94105-2869
415-974-9600
Fax: 415-974-0300; *Toll Free:* 800-537-9728
www.asaging.org

Louis Colbert, Chairperson
Tobi Abramson, Director
Patricia J. Volland, Treasurer

Magazine for health, social service, and other professionals who work with older people; presenting in-depth view of a specific topic in aging emphasizing research and practice.

Frequency: Quarterly Year Founded: 1954

2836 Geriatrics
ModernMedicine
7500 Old Oak Boulevard
Cleveland, OH 44130-3343
440-891-2769
Fax: 440-891-2635
www.geri.com

Don Berman, Director, Business Development
Terry Tetzlaff, Digital Traffic Coordinator
Laura Mcelwee, Digital Design Manager

Peer-reviewed, clinical journal for physicians and laypersons relating to medical care of middle-aged and older adults.

Frequency: Monthly

2837 Gerontologist
Gerontological Society of America
1220 L Street North West
Washington, DC 20005
202-842-1275
Fax: 202-842-1150
geron@geron.org
www.geron.org

James Appleby, Executive Director and CEO
Linda Krogh Harootyan, Deputy Executive Director
Chris Yoder, Senior Director, Finance and Adm

Multidisciplinary peer-reviewed journal presenting new concepts, clinical ideas, and applied research in gerontology. Includes book and audiovisual reviews.

Frequency: Bimonthly Year Founded: 1945

2838 Gerontology
S. Karger Publishers, Inc.
PO Box 529
26 West Avon Road
Unionville, CT 06085
860-675-7834
Fax: 860-675-7302; *Toll Free:* 800-828-5479
karger@snet.net
www.karger.com/

W Meier-Rage, Managing Editor
Monica Brendel, President
Samuel Karger, Founder

Medical journal.

Frequency: Bimonthly Year Founded: 1890

2839 Get Up and Go
Liberty Media Corporation
11551 Forest Central Drive
Suite 305
Dallas, TX 75243-3920
214-341-9429
Fax: 214-341-9779; *Toll Free:* 877-772-1518
www.libertymedia.com/

John C. Malone, Chairman
Gregory B. Maffei, President & CEO
Richard N. Baer, Senior Vice President and Genera

Magazine (tabloid) for people age 50 and over.

Frequency: Monthly Year Founded: 1991

2840 Impact!
World Institute on Disability (WID)
3075 Adeline Street
Suite 280
Berkeley, CA 94703
510-225-6400
Fax: 510-225-0477
wid@wid.org
www.wid.org/
TTY: 510-225-0478

Paul W. Schroeder, Chair
Linda M. Dardarian, Vice Chair
Anita Shafer Aaron, Executive Director

Magazine reporting on the activities of the World Institute on Disability.

Frequency: Semiannual Year Founded: 1983

2841 Independent Living Provider
Equal Opportunity Publications
1160 E Jericho Turnpike
Suite 200
Huntington, NY 11743-5405
516-421-9421
Fax: 516-421-0359
info@eop.com
www.eop.com/

Tamara Flaum-Dreyfuss, President and Publisher
Maureen Gladstone, Account Executive
Denise Mas, Account Executive

Business magazine for home health care.

Frequency: Quarterly Year Founded: 1968

2842 Informer
The Simon Foundation for Continence
PO Box 815
Wilmette, IL 60091
847-864-3913
Fax: 847-864-9758; *Toll Free:* 800-23S-mon
info@simonfoundation.org
www.simonfoundation.org

Cheryle Gartley, President and Founder
Elizabeth Tr LaGro, Vice President, Communications a
Twila Yednock, Director of Special Events

Magazine for persons with bladder or bowel incontinence.

Frequency: Quarterly Year Founded: 1985

2843 Inside MS
National Multiple Sclerosis Society
733 3rd Avenue
3rd Floor
New York, NY 10017
212-986-3240
Fax: 212-986-7981; *Toll Free:* 800-FIG-HTMS
editor@nmss.org
www.nationalmssociety.org/

Eli Rubenstein, Chairman of the Board
Cynthia Zagieboylo, President & CEO
Mindy B. Alpert, Director

Magazine for people with multiple sclerosis, their families, attending professionals, and interested donors. Provides information on coping, research, legislation, medical advances and disability rights advocacy.

80 pages Frequency: Quarterly

2844 International Journal of Aging and Human Development
Baywood Publishing Company, Inc.
PO Box 337
26 Austin Avenue
Amityville, NY 11701
631-691-1270
Fax: 631-691-1770; *Toll Free:* 800-638-7819
info@baywood.com
www.baywood.com/

Adult development and aging featuring original research theory, critial reviews.

2845 International Psychogeriatrics
Springer Publishing Company
11 West 42nd Street
15th Floor
New York, NY 10036
212-431-4370
Fax: 212-941-7842; *Toll Free:* 877-687-7476
cs@springerpub.com, journals@springerpub.com
www.springerpub.com

James C. Costello, Vice President, Journal Publishi
Theodore C. Nardin, Chief Executive Officer & Publis
Diana Osborne, Production Manager

Scholarly journal covering psychogeriatric practice, research, and education worldwide.

Frequency: Quarterly Year Founded: 1950

2846 International Rehabilitation Review
Rehabilitation International
125 E 21st Street
4th Floor
New York, NY 10010
212-420-1500
Fax: 212-505-0871
ri@riglobal.org
www.riglobal.org/

Jan A. Monsbakken, President
Patrick Fougeyrollas, Vice President
Martin Grabois, Deputy Vice President

Magazine overviewing the activities programs in the disability and rehabilitation fields.

Year Founded: 1972

2847 Journal of AAA
American Academy of Audiology
11480 Commerce Park Drive
Suite 220
Reston, VA 20191
703-790-8466
Fax: 703-790-8631; *Toll Free:* 800-222-2336
www.audiology.org/

Deborah Carlson, PhD, Chair
Bettie Borton, AuD, President
Lisa Christensen, Members-at-Large

Year Founded: 1990

2848 Journal of Aging and Ethnicity
Springer Publishing Company
11 West 42nd Street
15th Floor
New York, NY 10036
212-431-4370
Fax: 212-941-7842; *Toll Free:* 877-687-7476
cs@springerpub.com, journals@springerpub.com
www.springerpub.com

James C. Costello, Vice President, Journal Publishi
Theodore C. Nardin, Chief Executive Officer & Publis
Diana Osborne, Production Manager

Scholarly journal for researchers and professionals in gerontology and geriatrics, emphasizing the ethnic population of North America.

Year Founded: 1950

2849 Journal of Aging and Health
Sage Publications
2455 Teller Road
Thousand Oaks, CA 91320
805-499-0721
Fax: 805-499-0871
linfo@sagepub.com
www.sagepub.in/

Kyriakos S Markides, Editor
C Anderson, Circulation Manager
Sara Miller McCurne, Founder

Journal presenting research relative to the social and behavioral factors related to aging and health.

Frequency: Quarterly Year Founded: 1965

2850 Journal of Aging and Physical Activity
Human Kinetics
PO Box 5076
1607 N Market Street
Champaign, IL 61820
217-351-5076
Fax: 217-351-1549; *Toll Free:* 800-747-4457
info@hkusa.com
www.humankinetics.com

Brian Holding, CEO
Rainer Martens, Founder
Marilyn Martens, Founder

Journal examining the relationship between physical activity and the aging process.

Frequency: Quarterly Year Founded: 1974

2851 Journal of American Aging Association
American Aging Association
52373 Tyndall Falls Drive
Olmstead Falls, OH 44138
440-793-6565
Fax: 440-793-6598
ameraging@gmail.com
www.americanaging.org

Mitch Harman, Chairperson
LaDora Thompson, President
Peggy Harris, Business Manager, Vice President

Year Founded: 1970

2852 Journal of Developmental and Physical Disabilities
Kluwer Academic Publishers
101 Philip Drive
Norwell, MA 02061
212-620-8000
Fax: 212-463-0742
vlib.ustu.ru/storon/kluwer/

Vincent B Hassett, Editor
V Hersen, Advertising Manager
Rudiger Gebauer

Professional journal.

Frequency: Quarterly

2853 Journal of Ethics, Law, and Aging
Springer Publishing Company
11 West 42nd Street
15th Floor
New York, NY 10036

212-431-4370
Fax: 212-941-7842; *Toll Free:* 877-687-7476
cs@springerpub.com, journals@springerpub.com
www.springerpub.com

James C. Costello, Vice President, Journal Publishi
Theodore C. Nardin, Chief Executive Officer & Publis
Diana Osborne, Production Manager

Scholarly journal covering ethical and legal issues regarding aging for professionals who plan, administer, and provide and finance services to the elderly.

Frequency: Semiannual Year Founded: 1950

2854 Journal of Mental Health and Aging
Springer Publishing Company
11 West 42nd Street
15th Floor
New York, NY 10036
212-431-4370
Fax: 212-941-7842; *Toll Free:* 877-687-7476
cs@springerpub.com, journals@springerpub.com
www.springerpub.com

James C. Costello, Vice President, Journal Publishi
Theodore C. Nardin, Chief Executive Officer & Publis
Diana Osborne, Production Manager

Scholarly journal covering aging population for mental health professionals.

Year Founded: 1950

2855 Journal of Rehabilitation
National Rehabilitation Association
P.O. Box 150235
Alexandria, VA 22315
703-836-0850
Fax: 703-836-0848; *Toll Free:* 888-258-4295
www.nationalrehab.org/
TDD 703-836-0849

David Beach David Beach, President
Patricia Leahy, Interim Executive Director
Sandra Mulliner, Administrative Assistant

Rehabilitation journal.

Frequency: Quarterly Year Founded: 1923

2856 Journal of Religion, Spirituality & Aging
www.tandfonline.com

James W. Ellor, Editor

Features articles, research reports and reviews of new books and audiovisual resources on religion and aging.

Frequency: Quarterly

2857 Journal of Therapeutic Horticulture
American Horticultural Therapy Association
610 Freedom Business Center
Suite 110
King of Prussia, PA 19406
610-992-0020
Fax: 301-869-2397
ahta.org/

MaryAnne Millan, HTR, President
Leigh Anne Starling, MS, CRC, HTR, Vice President
Rene Malone, MS, CTRS, HTR, Treasurer

Journal containing articles on the therapeutic aspects of gardening and agriculture for persons with disabilities.

Frequency: Annual Year Founded: 1973

2858 Journal of the Association for Persons with Severe Handicaps
TASH
1001 Connecticut Avenue, NW
Suite 235
Washington, DC 20036
202-540-9020
Fax: 202-540-9019; *Toll Free:* 800-482-TASH
info@tash.org
tash.org/

David Westling, President
Jean Trainor, Vice President
Barbara Trader, Executive Director

Special education journal presenting articles that report original research, authoritative and comprehensive reviews, and conceptual and practical position papers offering new directions for people with disabilities.

Frequency: Quarterly Year Founded: 1970

2859 Kaleidoscope: Exploring the Expirence of Disability through Literature & Fine Arts
United Disability Services
701 S Main Street
Akron, OH 44311-1019
330-762-9755
Fax: 330-762-0912
www.udsakron.org

Karen A. Bozzelli, Chairperson
Bill Choler, Vice Chairperson
Gary Knuth, President/CEO

Magazine featuring articles on literature and the arts. Disabilitiy related.

64 pages Frequency: Bi-Annually

2860 Macrobiotics Today
George Ohsawa Macrobiotic Foundation
PO Box 3998
Chico, CA 95927-3998
530-566-9765
Fax: 530-566-9768; *Toll Free:* 800-232-2372
gomf@earthlink.net, gomf@ohsawamacrobiotics.c
www.ohsawamacrobiotics.com/

Carl Ferr,, President
Peter Milbury, Director
Tim Galanek, Director

Magazine covering macrobiotics, health, and nutrition.

Frequency: Bimonthly Year Founded: 1978

2861 Magazines in Special Media for the Handicapped
National Library Service for the Blind and Physic
1291 Taylor Street NW
Washington, DC 20011
202-707-5100
Fax: 202-707-0712; *Toll Free:* 800-424-8567
nls@loc.gov, nlsref@loc.gov
www.loc.gov/nls
TDD 202-707-0744

Karen Keninger, Director
Isabella Marqu,s de Castilla, Deputy Director
Erica Vaughns, Executive Assistant to the Direc

Publication includes: List of over 100 public and private organizations that publish magazines in Braille, on cassette, on disc and computer diskette, or in large print or moon type for visually impaired and physically disabled individuals. Entries include: Name of publisher, address, price. Principal content is a bibliography of periodicals, with brief description, frequency, format, and price of each.

Frequency: Biennial

2862 Massage Therapy Journal
American Massage Therapy Association
500 Davis Street
Suite 900
Evanston, IL 60201-4695
847-864-0123
Fax: 847-864-5196; *Toll Free:* 877-905-0577
info@amtamassage.org
www.amtamassage.org/

Winona Bontrager, President
Rachel Mann, Vice President
Bill Brown, Executive Director

Magazine focusing on professional massage therapy benefits, techniques, research, news, and practitioners.

Frequency: Quarterly

2863 Mature Health
New York - Haymarket
114 West 26th Street
4th Floor
New York, NY 10001
646-638-6000
www.haymarket.com/office/usa/new_york/de

Michael Heseltine, Chairman
Kevin Costello, Chief Group Executive
Brian Freeman, Chief Operating Officer

Magazine featuring articles on health aspects of aging, as well as articles on recreation and leisure.

Year Founded: 1964

2864 Mature Years
United Methodist Publishing House
201 8th Avenue S
PO Box 801
Nashville, TN 37202-0801
615-749-6000
Fax: 615-749-6079
newscope_office@econet.org
umph.org/

Neil Alexander, President/Publisher
Jeff Barnes, Executive Director
Steve Cashion, Executive Director of Applicatio

Magazine promoting the physical and spiritual well-being of older adults.

Frequency: Quarterly Year Founded: 1789

2865 Men's Health
Rodale Inc
400 South 10th Street
Emmaus, PA 18098
610-967-5171
Fax: 610-967-7725; *Toll Free:* 800-848-4735
RodaleBooks@cdsfulfillment.com
www.rodaleinc.com/working-at-rodale

Maria Rodale, CEO and Chairman
Scott D. Schulman, President
Heather Rodale, Vice President, Leadership Devel

Magazine offering health advice for men.

Year Founded: 1930

2866 Mental Health Report
Business Publishers, Inc.
2222 Sedwick Drive
Durham, NC 27713
301-495-5570
Fax: 800-508-2592; *Toll Free:* 800-223-8720
custserv@bpinews.com
www.bpinews.com

Kimberly Gilbert, Managing Editor
Alexa Chew, Contributing Editor
Mary Compton, Publisher

Magazine reporting on legislation affecting the mentally ill and their families.

Year Founded: 1963

2867 Modern Maturity
AARP
601 E Street NW
Washington, DC 20049
202-434-2277
Fax: 888-687-2277; *Toll Free:* 202-434-3525
member@aarp.org
www.aarp.org
TTY: 877-434-7598

Gail E. Aldrich, Board Chair
Robert G. Romasco, President
Dr. Ethel Pe Andrus, Founder

Offers news and information of concern to those 50 and older. Features articles on current events, health, recreation, housing, family life, legislation and other issues.

Year Founded: 1958

2868 National Easter Seal Communicator
Easter Seals
233 South Wacker Drive
Suite 2400
Chicago, IL 60606
312-726-6200
Fax: 312-726-1494; *Toll Free:* 800-221-6827
www.easterseals.com/

Richard W. Davidson, Chairman
Sandra L. Bouwman, 1st Vice Chairman
Joseph G. Kern, 2nd Vice Chairman

Magazine for persons with any type of disability.

Year Founded: 1934

2869 New Living
New Living Magazine
PO Box 1001
Patchogue, NY 11772
631-751-8819
Fax: 631-751-8910; *Toll Free:* 800-NEW-LIVI
www.newliving.com

Christine Ly Harvey, Publisher and Editor-in-Chief

Features and articles about holistic health and fitness;herbal remedies, preventive medicine, nutrition, mind/body health, spirituality, fitness, recipes, book reviews and more!

Frequency: Monthly

2870 PN
PVA Publications
2111 E Highland Avenue
Suite 180
Phoenix, AZ 85016-4702
602-224-0500
Fax: 602-224-0507; *Toll Free:* 888-888-2201
www.pn-magazine.com

Richard Hoover, Editor
Sherri Shea, Marketing & Circulation Director
Suzi Hubbard, Ciculation Coordinator

Magazine spotlighting independent living for paraplegics and quadriplegics.

Frequency: Monthly

2871 Physical Disabilities—Education & Related Services
Council for Exceptional Children
2900 Crystal Drive
Suite 1000
Arlington, VA 22202-3557
703-620-3660
Fax: 703-264-1637; *Toll Free:* 888-232-7733
www.cec.sped.org/
TTY: 866-915-5000

Robin D. Brewer, President
Joni L. Baldwin, Member-at-Large
James P. Heiden, Treasurer

Professional magazine covering research, instructional innovations and issues regarding education and physical disabilities.

Frequency: Semiannual

2872 Polio Network News
Post-Polio Health International (PHI)
4207 Lindell Boulevard
Suite 110
Saint Louis, MO 63108-2930
314-534-0475
Fax: 314-534-5070
info@post-polio.org
www.post-polio.org

William G. Stothers, President/Chairperson
Saul J. Morse, Vice President
Joan L. Headley, MS, Executive Director

Quarterly newsletter for polio survivors. Contains current information about the late efects of polio, encourages research and promotes networking among the post-polio community worldwide. Publish an annual Post-Polio Directory.

12 pages Frequency: Quarterly Year Founded: 1958

2873 Post-Polio Health International
Post-Polio Health International (PHI)
4207 Lindell Boulevard
Suite 110
St Louis, MO 63108-2930
314-534-0475
Fax: 314-534-5070
info@post-polio.org
www.post-polio.org

William G Stothers, President/Chairperson
Saul J Morse, Vice President
Brian Tiburzi, Executive Director

International organization concerning advocacy and research for polio survivors and ventilator-dependent individuals. Newsletters are called Post-Polio Health and Ventilator Assisted Living.

8 pages Frequency: Biannual Year Founded: 1958

2874 Prevention
Rodale Inc
400 South 10th Street
Emmaus, PA 18098
610-967-5171
Fax: 910-967-8963; *Toll Free:* 800-848-4735
RodaleBooks@cdsfulfillment.com
rodaleinc.com/

Maria Rodale, CEO and Chairman
Scott D. Schulman, President
Paul A. McGinley, EVP/General Counsel and Chief Ad

Magazine containing articles on wellness, preventive medicine, self-care, and fitness.

Frequency: Monthly

2875 Remedy
Rx Remedies
500 Highway 51 North
Suite Q
Ridgeland, MS 39157
601-981-0070
Fax: 800-729-0167; *Toll Free:* 800-826-1197
www.rxremediesms.com/

Joan Montgomery, Publisher

Consumer magazine covering health and wellness for individuals over 50 years in the US.

Frequency: Bimonthly

2876 Research on Aging
Sage Publications
2455 Teller Road
Thousand Oaks, CA 91320
805-499-0721
Fax: 805-499-0871
info@sagepub.com
www.sagepub.in/

Angela M O'Rand, Editor
Blaise R Simqu, CEO
Sara Miller McCurne, Founder

Social gerontology journal.

Frequency: Bimonthly Year Founded: 1965

2877 SELF Magazine
Cond, Nast
4 Times Square
New York, NY 10036
212-286-2860
Fax: 212-880-8248; *Toll Free:* 800-223-0780
communications@condenast.com
www.condenast.com/

Rochelle Udell, Editor-in-Chief
Larry Burstein, Publisher

Magazine serving as a health sourcebook for contemporary women.

Frequency: Monthly

2878 Secure Retirement, The Newsmagazine for Mature Americans
The National Committee to Preserve Social Security
10 G Street, NE
Suite 600
Washington, DC 20002-4215
202-822-9459
Fax: 202-822-9612
www.ncpssm.org/

Carroll L. Estes, Ph.D, Chair
Maya Rockeymoore, Ph.D., Vice Chair
Max Richtman, J.D., President & CEO

Magazine for senior citizens and others interested in politics and government and how they affect senior concerns and issues.

Year Founded: 1982

2879 Senior Times Magazine
Senior Times Magazine
4400 NW 36th Avenue
Gainesville, FL 32601
352-372-5468
Fax: 352-373-9178
www.seniortimesmagazine.com/

Charlie Delatorre, Publisher
Albert Issac, Editor-in-Chief
Hank McAfee, Creative Director

Magazine devoted to educating senior citizens on recreational, political, health and financial issues.

Frequency: Monthly

2880 Serenity
Little Sisters of The Poor
601 Maiden Choice Lane
Baltimore, MD 21228
410-744-9367
Fax: 410-788-5614
serenitys@littlesistersofthepoor.org
www.littlesistersofthepoor.org/

S R Marguerite, Publications Coordinator
Saint Jeanne Jugan, Founder

Magazine making known the apostolate of Little Sisters of the Poor and providing a positive view of the elderly and the respect due them.

32 pages Frequency: Quarterly Year Founded: 1839

2881 Spirit of Change Magazine
Spirit of Change Magazine
PO Box 405
Uxbridge, MA 01569
508-278-9640
Fax: 508-278-9641
info@spiritofchange.org
www.spiritofchange.org/

Carol Bedrosian, Publisher/Editor
Michella Bedrosian, Advertising Director
Gail Lord, Book Reviewer

Consumer magazine covering holistic health and New Age issues.

Frequency: Bimonthly Year Founded: 1987

2882 The American Wanderer
American Volkssport Association (AVA)
1001 Pat Booker Road
Suite 101
Universal City, TX 78148
210-659-2112
Fax: 210-659-1212
AVAHQ@ava.org
www.ava.org

Henry Rosales, Executive Director, AVA

Consumer magazine covering sports and health news.

Frequency: Bimonthly

2883 VANTAGE
Signature Group Inc.
15-598 Falconbridge Rd.
Sudbury, ON P3A 5K6
877-688-1989
Fax: 877-688-0808
www.signaturegroupinc.com/

Paul Misniak, Publisher
Joanie Davies, Mailing Contact

Magazine for active consumers over 55 years of age.

Frequency: Bimonthly

2884 VFW Auxiliary
Ladies Auxiliary to the VFW
406 W 34th Street
10th Floor
Kansas City, MO 64111
816-561-8655
Fax: 816-931-4753
info@ladiesauxvfw.org
www.ladiesauxvfw.org/

Armithea "Si Borel, National President
Marilyn Ebersole, Mailing Contact/Editor
Jan Owens, National Secretary

VFW auxiliary patriotic services magazine.

Year Founded: 1914

2885 Vegetarian Voice
North American Vegetarian Society
PO Box 72
Dolgeville, NY 13329
518-568-7970
Fax: 518-568-7979
navs@telenet.net
www.navs-online.org

Maribeth Abrams, Managing Editor
Brian Graff, Executive Manager

Consumer magazine covering vegetarianism, health, cooking, environmental and animal protection issues.

40 pages Frequency: Quarterly Year Founded: 1974

2886 Veggie Life
EGW.com
4075 Papazian Way
208
Fremont, CA 94538
925-671-9852
Fax: 925-671-0692
www.egw.com/

Shanna Masters, Editor
Rickie Wilson, Advertising Manager

Consumer magazine covering health, nutrition, and vegetarian cooking.

68 pages Frequency: Quarterly

2887 Vim & Vigor Magazine
McMurry
1010 E. Missouri Ave.
Phoenix, AZ 85014
602-395-5850
Fax: 602-395-5853; Toll Free: 800-282-5850
mcmurrytmg.com/

Matthew Peterson, CEO
Fred Petrovsky, COO
Kim Caviness, Chief Content Officer

Magazine offering articles on health, fitness, and medical research.

Frequency: Quarterly Year Founded: 1984

2888 WebMD Magazine
WebMD, LLC
395 Hudson Street
New York, NY 10014
www.webmd.com/magazine

Vanessa Cognard, Publisher
Kristy Hammam, Editor in Chief

2889 Whole Life
Whole Life Enterprises
PO Box 2058
New York, NY 10159-2058

Marc Medoff, Publisher/Editor

Magazine focusing on the mind-body-spirit connection, with emphasis on dietary awareness and personal health.

Frequency: Bimonthly

Newspapers

2890 Aging Today
American Society on Aging
575 Market Street
Suite 2100
San Francisco, CA 94105-2869
415-974-9600
Fax: 415-974-0300; Toll Free: 800-537-9728
www.asaging.org

Louis Colbert, Chairperson
Tobi Abramson, Director
Patricia J. Volland, Treasurer

Newspaper (tabloid) for health, social service, and other professionals who work with older people.

Year Founded: 1954

2891 Bulletin
AARP
601 E Street NW
Washington, DC 20049
202-434-2277
Fax: 888-687-2277; Toll Free: 202-434-3525
member@aarp.org
www.aarp.org
TTY: 877-434-7598

Gail E. Aldrich, Board Chair
Robert G. Romasco, President
Dr. Ethel Pe Andrus, Founder

Frequency: 11x/year Year Founded: 1958

2892 Fifty Plus Advocate
Fifty Plus Advocates
131 Lincoln Street
Worcester, MA 01605-2408
508-752-2512
Fax: 508-752-9057
ddavis@fiftyplusadvocate.com
www.fiftyplusadvocate.com/

Reva Capellan, Office Manager
Karen Higgins, Editor
Donna Davis, Contact

Newspaper for senior citizens.

Year Founded: 1975

2893 Health Perspective
Clayton-Davis & Associates, Inc.
230 S. Bemiston
Clayton, MO 63105
314-862-7800
Fax: 314-721-5171
info@claytondavis.com
www.claytondavis.com/

Irvin Davis, Chair
Jennifer Davis, President
Ruth Sirko, Editor

Consumer health tabloid.

Frequency: Monthly Year Founded: 1953

2894 Jewish Veteran
Jewish War Veterans of the United States of Americ
1811 R Street NW
Washington, DC 20009
202-265-6280
Fax: 202-234-5662
jwv@jwv.org
www.jwv.org/

Herb Rosenbleeth, National Executive Director
Larry Richardson, Director of Operations
Christy Turner, Executive Assistant/ Desktop Pub

2895 Lovin' Life After 50
Lovin' Life After 50
EOS Publishing, LLC
3200 N. Hayden, Suite 210
Scottsdale, AZ 85251
480-348-0343
Fax: 480-348-2109
info@lovinlifeafter50.com, advertising@lovinl
www.lovinlife.com

Debbie Close, Account Executive

Newspaper for senior citizens.

Frequency: Monthly Year Founded: 1979

2896 New York Times Large Type Weekly
New York Times Company
229 W 43rd Street
New York, NY 10036-3913
212-556-1234
www.nytco.com/

Abbe Serphos, Executive Director Corporate Com
Eileen M. Murphy, Vice President, Corporate Commun
Stephanie Serino, Executive Director Content Licen

Newspaper for persons with impaired vision.

Newsletters, Pamphlets

2897 A Lifetime of Freedom from Smoking
American Lung Association
55 W. Wacker Drive
Suite 1150
Chicago, IL 60601
212-315-8700
Fax: 202-452-1805; *Toll Free:* 800-LUN-USA
www.lung.org/

Ross P. Lanzafame, Esq., Chair
Kathryn A. Forbes, CPA, Vice Chair
Harold Wimmer, President and Chief Executive Of

Companion manual helps persons stay quit once they have
stopped smoking.

28 pages Year Founded: 1904

2898 A Profile of Older Americans
AARP
601 E Street NW
Washington, DC 20049
202-434-2277
Fax: 888-687-2277; *Toll Free:* 202-434-3525
member@aarp.org
www.aarp.org
TTY: 877-434-7598

Gail E. Aldrich, Board Chair
Robert G. Romasco, President
Dr. Ethel Pe Andrus, Founder

Offers information on aging, retirement, illnesses and more
for the elderly population.

Year Founded: 1958

2899 AARP Newsletter
AARP
601 E Street NW
Washington, DC 20049
202-434-2277
Fax: 888-687-2277; *Toll Free:* 202-434-3525
www.aarp.org
TTY: 877-434-7598

Gail E. Aldrich, Board Chair
Robert G. Romasco, President
Dr. Ethel Pe Andrus, Founder

4 pages Frequency: Bimonthly Year Founded: 1958

2900 AARP Pharmacy Service
AARP
601 E Street NW
Washington, DC 20049
202-434-2277
Fax: 888-687-2277; *Toll Free:* 202-434-3525
www.aarp.org
TTY: 877-434-7598

Gail E. Aldrich, Board Chair
Robert G. Romasco, President
Dr. Ethel Pe Andrus, Founder

4 pages Frequency: Bimonthly Year Founded: 1958

2901 ADARA Updated
ADARA
PO Box 480
Myersville, MD 21773
501-868-8850
Fax: 501-868-8812
www.adara.org/

Michelle Niehaus, LCSW, President
Steve Hmaerdinger, Vice President
Jean Baker, Secretary

Updates readers on events, resources, legislation, information of national interest, conferences, workshops and employment opportunities. Information from and about local
chapters, special interest sections, and national organizations is included in this publication.

Year Founded: 1961

2902 AGHE Exchange Newsletter
Association for Gerontology in Higher Education
1220 L Street, NW
Suite 901
Washington, DC 20005-4018
202-289-9806
Fax: 202-289-9824
aghe@aghe.org
www.aghe.org/

JanetC. Frank, President
M. Angela Baker, Director
Leland Bret Waters, Treasurer

16-20 pages Frequency: Quarterly Year Founded: 1974

2903 AUL Forum
Americans United for Life
655 15th St NW
Suite 410
Washington, DC 20005
202-289-1478
Fax: 312-786-2131
info@aul.org, press@aul.org
www.aul.org/

Jay Cunningham, CFP, Chairman
Eileen J. O'Connor, Vice Chairman
Charmaine Yoest, Ph.D., President

Frequency: Quarterly Year Founded: 1971

2904 Abstracts in Social Gerontology
Sage Publications
2455 Teller Road
Thousand Oaks, CA 91320
805-499-0721
Fax: 805-499-0871
info@sagepub.com
www.sagepub.in/

Julie L Moore, Editor
Jane Saquet, Publisher
Sara Miller McCurne, Founder

Annotated bibliography of books, journal articles, and documents relevant to social gerontology.

Frequency: Quarterly Year Founded: 1965

2905 Aging Research and Training News
Business Publishers, Inc.
2222 Sedwick Drive
Durham, NC 27713

301-495-5570
Fax: 800-508-2592; *Toll Free:* 800-223-8720
custserv@bpinews.com
www.bpinews.com

Kimberly Gilbert, Managing Editor
Alexa Chew, Contributing Editor
Mary Compton, Publisher

Reports on sources of government and private sector grant and contract opportunities.

10 pages Frequency: Monthly Year Founded: 1963

2906 American Geriatrics Society Newsletter
American Geriatrics Society
40 Fulton Street
18th Floor
New York, NY 10038
212-308-1414
Fax: 212-832-8646
info.amger@americangeriatrics.org
www.americangeriatrics.org

James T. Pacala, MD, MS, AGSF, Chairman of the Board
Cathy Alessi, MD, AGSF, President
Jennie Chin Hansen, RN, MSN, FAAN, Chief Executive
Officer

16-20 pages Frequency: Quarterly Year Founded: 1942

2907 American Health Care Association
American Health Care Association
1201 L Street NW
Washington, DC 20005
202-842-4444
Fax: 202-842-3860
support@ahca.org
www.ahcancal.org/

Leonard Russ, Chairman
Dave Kyllo, Vice President

8 pages

2908 American Senior Newsletter
Butler County Department on Aging
2101 Dearborn
Suite 302
Augusta, KS 67010
316-775-0500
Fax: 316-775-0555; *Toll Free:* 800-279-3655
www.bucoks.com

Crysatl Noles, Director
Brenda Louthan, Assistant Director/ Program Mana
Melody Gault, RSVP Program Manager

Subscription is free, but donations to help offset postage are appreciated.

Year Founded: 1989

2909 Americans with Disabilities Act Resource Manual
Arthritis Foundation
1330 W. Peachtree Street
Suite 100
Atlanta, GA 30309
404-872-7100
Fax: 404-872-0457; *Toll Free:* 800-283-7800
www.arthritis.org/georgia/

Daniel T. McGowan, Chairman
Michael V. Ortman, Co-Vice Chair
Ann M. Palmer, President & CEO

2910 An Ounce of Prevention is Worth a Poundof Cure
Alliance for Aging Research
1700 K Street NW
Suite 740
Washington, DC 20006
202-293-2856
Fax: 202-955-8394
info@agingresearch.org
www.agingresearch.org

Daniel Perry, President/CEO
Cynthia Bens, Public Policy Director
Michael Maroni

Federal funding, health, medical innovation, policy, and quality of care.

2911 Audiology Express
American Academy of Audiology
11480 Commerce Park Drive
Suite 220
Reston, VA 20191
703-790-8466
Fax: 703-790-8631; *Toll Free:* 800-222-2336
www.audiology.org/

Deborah Carlson, PhD, Chair
Bettie Borton, AuD, President
M. Samantha Lewis PhD, Members-at-Large

Year Founded: 1990

2912 Between Classes
Road Scholar
11 Avenue de Lafayette
Boston, MA 02111
978-323-4141
Fax: 617-426-0701; *Toll Free:* 800-454-5768
www.elderhostel.org
TTY: 877-426-2167

Michael Zoob, Editor
James Moses, CEO

Year Founded: 1975

2913 Bulletin on Long-Term Care Law
Health Resources
Post Office Box 3623
Hueytown, AL 35023
817-785-4656
Fax: 800-941-6920; *Toll Free:* 800-471-4007
service@healthresources.net
www.healthresources.net/

Robert K Jenkins, Publisher

Covers federal and state laws and regulations governing long-term care facilities, compliance problems, changes to the Medicare and Medicaid programs, litigation and coverage of news of importance to long-term care providers.

Year Founded: 1995

2914 Center for Aging Newsletter
University of Alabama at Birmingham
1720 2nd Ave South
Birmingham, AL 35294

205-934-4011
Fax: 205-975-5930
www.uab.edu/
TDD 205-934-4642

Tim L. Pennycuff, University Archivist, Assistant
Jennifer L. Beck, Library Assistant III
Michael A. Flannery, Associate Director for Historica

8 pages Frequency: Monthly Year Founded: 1831

2915 Cigarette Smoking
American Lung Association
55 W. Wacker Drive
Suite 1150
Chicago, IL 60601
212-315-8700
Fax: 202-452-1805; *Toll Free:* 800-LUN-USA
www.lung.org/

Ross P. Lanzafame, Esq., Chair
Kathryn A. Forbes, CPA, Vice Chair
Harold Wimmer, President and Chief Executive Of

Leaflet presenting the facts about how cigarette smoke is related to lung disease.

Year Founded: 1904

2916 Conscious Aging: Through Their Art, a Couple Finds Beauty and Peace in Aging
Alliance for Aging Research
1700 K Street NW
Suite 740
Washington, DC 20006
202-293-2856
Fax: 202-955-8394
info@agingresearch.org
www.agingresearch.org

Daniel Perry, President/CEO
Cynthia Bens, Public Policy Director
Michael Maroni

Newletter on how not to focus on what you have a chieved but what you are accomplishing now as you age.

2917 Council for Disability Rights
The Council for Disability Rights
20 N Wacker Drive
Suite 1540
Chicago, IL 60606-2903
312-444-9484
Fax: 312-444-1977
www.disabilityrights.org/

Josephine E Holzer, Executive Director/Editor
Dorie Stewart, Information Specialist

Promotes human rights of persons with disabilities and their families. Offers a job placement service, legal referrals, information services, a website and monthly newsletter (CDR Reports).

Year Founded: 1981

2918 Disability Compliance Bulletin
LRP Publications
747 Dresher Road
Suite 500
Horsham, PA 19044
215-784-0941
Fax: 215-784-9639; *Toll Free:* 800-341-7874
custserve@lrp.com

www.lrp.com
TTY: 215-658-0938

Kenneth F. Kahn, President
Honora O'Connell, Product Group Manager

This biweekly newsletter gives you timely coverage and insightful analyses of the latest developments in disability law. You'll learn the most recent case law dealing with the Americans with Disabilities Act, the Family and Medical Leave Act, and more. Disability Compliance Bulletin will help you understand the laws' obligations and show you emerging legal trends.

24 pages Frequency: Biweekly Year Founded: 1977

2919 Disability Notes
Social Security Admin Office of Disability
Windsor Park Building
6401 Security Blvd.
Baltimore, MD 21235
410-965-3987
Fax: 410-965-6503
www.socialsecurity.gov/

Newsletter focusing on disability programs offered by Social Security and other agencies.

Frequency: Quarterly

2920 Disability Rights Now
Disability Rights Education and Defense Fund
3075 Adeline Street
Suite 210
Berkeley, CA 94703
510-644-2555
Fax: 510-841-8645; *Toll Free:* 800-466-4232
info@dredf.org
dredf.org/
TTY: 510-841-8645

Claudia Center, President & Chair
Susan Henderson, Executive Director
Ingrid Tischer, Directo of Development

Free quarterly publication describing the activities of the Disability Rights Education and Defense Fund, available in alternative formats.

Frequency: Quarterly Year Founded: 1979

2921 Don't Let Your Dreams Go Up in Smoke
American Lung Association
55 W. Wacker Drive
Suite 1150
Chicago, IL 60601
212-315-8700
Fax: 202-452-1805; *Toll Free:* 800-LUN-USA
www.lung.org/

Ross P. Lanzafame, Esq., Chair
Kathryn A. Forbes, CPA, Vice Chair
Harold Wimmer, President and Chief Executive Of

Photos, testimonials and clear language to deliver the message that everyone can and should stop smoking.

Year Founded: 1904

2922 Federal Laws of the Mentally Handicapped: Laws, Legislative Histories and Admin. Documents
William S. Hein & Co., Inc.
2350 North Forest Road
Getzville, NY 14068

716-882-2600
Fax: 716-883-8100; *Toll Free:* 800-828-7571
mail@wshein.com
www.wshein.com/

William Hein, Chair
Kevin Marmion, President
Shannon Hein, Vice President, Sales

Chronological compilation of all relevant federal laws dealing with the mentally handicapped along with supporting documentation necessary to create a complete legislative history.

Frequency: 42 Volumes Year Founded: 1980

2923 Freedom From Smoking Flyer
American Lung Association
55 W. Wacker Drive
Suite 1150
Chicago, IL 60601
212-614-2800
Fax: 202-452-1805; *Toll Free:* 800-LUN-USA
www.lung.org/

Ross P. Lanzafame, Esq., Chair
Kathryn A. Forbes, CPA, Vice Chair
Harold Wimmer, President and Chief Executive Of

4 color flyer describing all FFS programs.

Year Founded: 1904

2924 Gerontology News
Gerontological Society of America
1220 L Street North West
Washington, DC 20005
202-842-1275
Fax: 202-842-1150
geron@geron.org
www.geron.org

James Appleby, Executive Director and CEO
Linda Krogh Harootyan, Deputy Executive Director
Chris Yoder, Senior Director, Finance and Adm

12 pages Frequency: Monthly Year Founded: 1945

2925 Gerontology Special Interest Section Quarterly
American Occupational Therapy Association
4720 Montgomery Ln
Suite 200
Bethesda, MD 20814-3449
301-652-6611
Fax: 301-652-7711; *Toll Free:* 800-SAY-AOTA
ajotsis@asta.org
www.aota.org/
TDD 800-377-8555

Barbara Scanlon, Managing Editor

Quarterly newsletter for occupational therapy practitioners, focusing on issues relating to gerontology practice.

4 pages Frequency: Quarterly Year Founded: 1917

2926 Have Fun! Figure Out the Smoking Puzzle
American Lung Association
55 W. Wacker Drive
Suite 1150
Chicago, IL 60601
212-315-8700
Fax: 202-452-1805; *Toll Free:* 800-LUN-USA
www.lung.org/

Ross P. Lanzafame, Esq., Chair
Kathryn A. Forbes, CPA, Vice Chair
Harold Wimmer, President and Chief Executive Of

Crossword puzzles make stimulating points on the effects of smoking.

Year Founded: 1904

2927 Healing Choices
Healing Choices
144 Saint Johns Place
Brooklyn, NY 11217-3402
718-636-4433
Fax: 718-616-0186
www.ralphmoss.com

A unique series of in-depth reports on nearly every cancer diagnosis. Choose the report that corresponds to the exact type of cancer you are concered with, and within days you will receeive Dr. Moss's report on the most successful alternative and complementary treatment approches relevant to the condition.

2928 Home Health Line
United Communications Group (UCG)
9737 Washingtonian Blvd
Suite 200
Gaithersburg, MD 20878-7364
301-287-2700
Fax: 301-287-2039; *Toll Free:* 800-929-4824
info@ucg.com
www.ucg.com/

Nancy Becker, Partner-President
Todd Foreman, Partner-CEO
Jon Slabaugh, Managing Director, Business Deve

8-16 pages Frequency: Weekly Year Founded: 1977

2929 Hospice Letter
Health Resources
Post Office Box 3623
Hueytown, AL 35023
817-785-4656
Fax: 800-941-6920; *Toll Free:* 800-471-4007
service@healthresources.net
www.healthresources.net/

Robert K Jenkins, Publisher

Year Founded: 1995

2930 Housing for Seniors Report
CD Publications
2222 Sedwick Drive
Durham, NC 27713
301-588-6380
Fax: 800-508-2592; *Toll Free:* 855-237-1396
info@cdpublications.com
www.cdpublications.com

Michael Gerecht, President

Monthly newsletter with practical advice for senior housing managers on marketing, financing and management issues.

Year Founded: 1961

2931 IDF Patient and Family Handbook
Immune Deficiency Foundation
40 W Chesapeake Avenue
Suite 308
Towson, MD 21204

410-321-6647
Fax: 410-321-9165; *Toll Free:* 800-296-4433
info@primaryimmune.org
primaryimmune.org/

John Seymour, PhD, LMFT, Chair
Steve Fietek, Vice Chair
Marcia Boyle, President & Founder

Year Founded: 1980

2932 ILRU Insights
ILRU Research/Training Center Independent Living
TIRR Memorial Hermann Research Center
1333 Moursund Street
Houston, TX 77030-3405
713-520-0232
Fax: 713-520-5785
ilru@ilru.org
www.ilru.org/
TTY: 713-520-0232

Lex Frieden, Director
Vinh Nguyen, Program Director
Roxy Funchess, Administrative Secretary

The national newsletter for independent living offers the reader information on laws, social issues, medicine and more for the disabled person.

10 pages Year Founded: 1977

2933 Impotence Causes and Treatments
American Medical Systems (AMS)
10700 Bren Road West
Minnetonka, MN 55343
952-933-4666
Fax: 952-930-6373; *Toll Free:* 800-328-3881
americanmedicalsystems.com/

Camille Farhat, Group President
Pam Balthazor, VP Commercial Excellence
Steve Blum, General Manager Women's Health

Offers information on what impotence is, physical and emotional causes, treatments, questions and answers.

Year Founded: 1972

2934 Informer
Simon Foundation for Continence
PO Box 815
Wilmette, IL 60091
847-864-3913
Fax: 847-864-9758; *Toll Free:* 800-237-4666
www.simonfoundation.org/

Cheryle B Gartley, President and Founder
Elizabeth Tr Lagrow, Vice President, Communications a
Twila Yednock, Director of Special Events

Seeks to bring the topic of incontinence out of the closet and remove the associated stigma; provides information to patients, their families, and the health care professionals who provide patient care.

Year Founded: 1983

2935 International Ventilator Users Network (IVUN) News
Post-Polio Health International (PHI)
4207 Lindell Boulevard
Suite 110
Saint Louis, MO 63108-2930

314-534-0475
Fax: 314-534-5070
info@post-polio.org
www.post-polio.org

William G. Stothers, President/Chairperson
Saul J. Morse, Vice President
Joan L. Headley, MS, Executive Director

IVUN is a worldwide network of ventilator users and health professionals experienced in and committed to home care and long term mechanical ventilation. IVUN News, a quarterly newsletter, offers articles on family adjustments, equipment, techniques, travel, ethical issues, medical topics, and resources. ISSN# 1066-534x. We also publish the annual IVUN Resource Directory. ($5.00)

8 pages Frequency: Quarterly Year Founded: 1958

2936 Is There a Safe Tobacco?
American Lung Association
55 W. Wacker Drive
Suite 1150
Chicago, IL 60601
212-315-8700
Fax: 202-452-1805; *Toll Free:* 800-LUN-USA
www.lung.org/

Ross P. Lanzafame, Esq., Chair
Kathryn A. Forbes, CPA, Vice Chair
Harold Wimmer, President and Chief Executive Of

Offers information on the health risks of cigarette smoking, pipes and cigars.

Year Founded: 1904

2937 Knowing Your Rights
AARP
601 E Street NW
Washington, DC 20049
202-434-2277
Fax: 888-687-2277; *Toll Free:* 202-434-3525
member@aarp.org
www.aarp.org
TTY: 877-434-7598

Gail E. Aldrich, Board Chair
Robert G. Romasco, President
Dr. Ethel Pe Andrus, Founder

Describes how changes in Medicare's reimbursement policies are designed to reduce health care costs and suggests steps that Medicare beneficiaries, their families and friends can take to assure that they continue to receive quality care under the Prospective Payment System.

19 pages Year Founded: 1958

2938 Legal Action Center
Legal Action Center (LAC)
236 Massachusetts Avenue NE
Suite 505
Washington, DC 20002-4980
202-544-5478
Fax: 202-544-5712
lacdc@lac.org
www.lac.org/

Daniel K. Mayers, Esq, Chair
Anita R. Marton, Vice President
Robert B. Levy, Director of Development

Provides technical assistance and education programs for employers and employees on ADA issues related to individuals with drug and alcohol abuse and HIV disease.

Year Founded: 1973

2939 Let's Solve the Smokeword Puzzle
American Lung Association
55 W. Wacker Drive
Suite 1150
Chicago, IL 60601
212-315-8700
Fax: 202-452-1805; *Toll Free:* 800-LUN-USA
www.lung.org/

Ross P. Lanzafame, Esq., Chair
Kathryn A. Forbes, CPA, Vice Chair
Harold Wimmer, President and Chief Executive Of

Fifth graders will love getting an antismoking message through solving a crossword puzzle.

Year Founded: 1904

2940 Lifetime of Freedom from Smoking
Maintenance Manual
American Lung Association
55 W. Wacker Drive
Suite 1150
Chicago, IL 60601
212-315-8700
Fax: 202-452-1805; *Toll Free:* 800-LUN-USA
www.lung.org/

Ross P. Lanzafame, Esq., Chair
Kathryn A. Forbes, CPA, Vice Chair
Harold Wimmer, President and Chief Executive Of

Companion manual helps persons stay quit once they have stopped smoking.

28 pages Year Founded: 1904

2941 NAHC Report
National Association for Home Care & Hospice
228 7th Street SE
Washington, DC 20003
202-547-7424
Fax: 202-547-3540
ads@nahc.org, exec@nahc.org
www.nahc.org

Andrea Devoti, Chair
Lucy Andrews, Vice Chair
Val J. Halamandaris, President

6-16 pages Frequency: Weekly

2942 NAPCA Voices
National Asian Pacific Center on Aging
1511 Third Avenue
Suite 914
Seattle, WA 98101-1626
206-624-1221
Fax: 206-624-1023
napca.org

Debbie Louie, Editor & Designer

Quarterly newsletter of the National Asian Pacific Center on Aging.

8 pages Frequency: 3-4

2943 NARIC Quarterly
National Rehabilitation Information Center
8400 Corporate Drive
Suite 500
Landover, MD 20785
301-459-5984
Fax: 301-459-4263; *Toll Free:* 800-346-2742
www.naric.com
TTY: 301-459-5984

Mark X. Odum, Project Director
Jessica H. Chaiken, Media and Information Services M
Natalie J. Collier, Library and Acquisitions Manager

18 pages Frequency: Quarterly Year Founded: 1982

2944 NCD Bulletin
National Council on Disability
1331 F Street NW
Suite 850
Washington, DC 20004
202-272-2004
Fax: 202-272-2022
www.ncd.gov/
TTY: 202-272-2074

Jeff Rosen, Chairperson
Kamilah Oni Martin-Proctor, Co-Vice Chair
Lynnae Ruttledge, Co-Vice Chair

Reports on the latest issues and news affecting people with disabilities.

2 pages Frequency: Monthly Year Founded: 1978

2945 NHO NewsLine
National Hospice and Palliative Care Organization
1731 King Street
Suite 100
Alexandria, VA 22314
703-837-1500
Fax: 703-837-1233; *Toll Free:* 800-646-6460
www.nhpco.org/

Ronald Fried, Chair
Linda Rock, Vice Chair
J. Donald Schumacher, PsyD, President & CEO

6-8 pages Frequency: Semimonthly Year Founded: 1992

2946 NSCLC Washington Weekly
National Senior Citizens Law Center
1444 Eye Street, NW
Suite 1100
Washington, DC 20005
202-289-6976
Fax: 202-289-7224
nsclc@nsclc.org
www.nsclc.org/

Robert K. Johnson, Esq., Chair
Barrett S. Litt, Esq., Vice Chair
Kevin Prindiville, Executive Director

4 pages Year Founded: 1972

2947 National Veterans Legal Services Program
Newsletter
National Veterans Legal Services Program
(NVLSP)
P. O. Box 65762
Washington, DC 20035
202-265-8305
Fax: 202-328-0063

info@nvlsp.org
www.nvlsp.ORG

Ronald S. Flagg, Chair
Ronald Abrams, Joint Executive Director
Evelyn Anderson, Chief Financial Officer

Non-profit veterans law firm. Recruits volunteer lawyers to handle cases before the US Court of Veterans Claims. Engages in many activities around Agent Orange and VA reform.

Frequency: Quarterly Year Founded: 1970

2948 News from the Points of Light Foundation
Points of Light Foundation
1625 K Street NW
Suite 500
Washington, DC 20006
404-979-2900
Fax: 404-979-2901
www.pointsoflight.org

Tracy Hoover, President
Richard Dubose, Chief Development Officer
Scott Geller, Chief Technology Officer

Frequency: Monthly Year Founded: 1987

2949 Newsline
Sertoma Foundation
1912 E Meyer Boulevard
Kansas City, MO 64132
816-333-8300
Fax: 816-333-4320
Infosertoma@sertomahq.org
www.sertoma.org/

Tim Hazel, President
Debby Larsen, Senior Vice President
Don Bartelmay, Junior Vice President

Reports on activities of the Sertoma Foundation in the field of speech and hearing impairments.

Year Founded: 1912

2950 Nicotine Addiction and Cigarettes
American Lung Association
55 W. Wacker Drive
Suite 1150
Chicago, IL 60601
212-315-8700
Fax: 202-452-1805; *Toll Free:* 800-LUN-USA
www.lung.org/

Ross P. Lanzafame, Esq., Chair
Kathryn A. Forbes, CPA, Vice Chair
Harold Wimmer, President and Chief Executive Of

Offers information on nicotine and cigarette smoking.

Year Founded: 1904

2951 No Smoking: Lungs at Work
American Lung Association
55 W. Wacker Drive
Suite 1150
Chicago, IL 60601
212-315-8700
Fax: 202-452-1805; *Toll Free:* 800-LUN-USA
www.lung.org/

Ross P. Lanzafame, Esq., Chair
Kathryn A. Forbes, CPA, Vice Chair
Harold Wimmer, President and Chief Executive Of

Describes how lungs work and how they are affected by smoking.

Year Founded: 1904

2952 Noticias
National Hispanic Council on Aging
734 15th Street NW
Suite 1050
Washington, DC 20005
202-347-9733
Fax: 202-347-9735
www.nhcoa.org

6 pages Frequency: Quarterly Year Founded: 1980

2953 Now Where Did I Put My Keys?
AARP
601 E Street NW
Washington, DC 20049
202-434-3525
Fax: 202-434-3443; *Toll Free:* 888-687-2277
member@aarp.org
www.aarp.org
TTY: 877-434-7598

Gail E. Aldrich, Board Chair
Robert G. Romasco, President
Dr. Ethel Pe Andrus, Founder

Your copies of this brochure won't last long on your information counter.

Year Founded: 1958

2954 Nursing Home Law Letter
National Senior Citizens Law Center
1444 Eye Street, NW
Suite 1100
Washington, DC 20005
202-289-7224
Fax: 202-289-7224
nsclc@nsclc.org
www.nsclc.org/

Robert K. Johnson, Esq., Chair
Barrett S. Litt, Esq., Vice Chair
Kevin Prindiville, Executive Director

6-10 pages Frequency: Quarterly Year Founded: 1972

2955 Nutrition Action Healthletter
Center for Science in the Public Interest
1220 L St. N.W.
Suite 300
Washington, DC 20005
202-332-9110
Fax: 202-265-4954
cspi@cspinet.org, cspinews@cspinet.org
www.cspinet.org

Tom Gegax, Chair
Sushma Palmer, Director
Don Allen, Director of Finance

The nation's leading consumer group concerned with food and nutrition issues. Focuses on diseases that result from consuming too many calories, too much fat, sodium and sugar such as cancer and heart disease.

16 pages Year Founded: 1970

2956 Older Americans Report
Business Publishers, Inc.
2222 Sedwick Drive
Durham, NC 27713
301-495-5570
Fax: 800-508-2592; *Toll Free:* 800-223-8720
custserv@bpinews.com
www.bpinews.com

Kimberly Gilbert, Managing Editor
Alexa Chew, Contributing Editor
Mary Compton, Publisher

Handles issues like long term care, Social Security, nutrition, retirement and other programs that effect older Americans.

8-10 pages Frequency: Weekly Year Founded: 1963

2957 Plain Talk About Depression
Superintendent of Documents
PO Box 371954
Pittsburgh, PA 15250-7954
202-512-1800
Fax: 202-512-2250
history.nasa.gov/gpo/order.html

A flyer discussing types of depression, major depression, symptoms and causes.

2958 Positive Living
APLA
611 South Kingsley Drive
Los Angeles, CA 90005
213-201-1600
Fax: 213-201-1500
info@apla.org
www.apla.org/

Rodney Gould, Chair
Mark Perrin, Vice Chair
Dean Hale, Treasurer

Year Founded: 1983

2959 Positively Aware
Test Positive Aware Network
5050 N Broadway Street
Suite 300
Chicago, IL 60640
773-989-9400
Fax: 773-989-9494
www.tpan.com/

Joel Bosch, Chair
Scott Cook, Ph.D., Vice Chair
Jeff Berry, Interim CEO

Chicago area HIV related services directory, that includes HIV news items, events and clinical trials in the Chicago area.

2960 Program Booklet
Women For Sobriety, Inc.
PO Box 618
Quakertown, PA 18951
215-536-8026
Fax: 215-536-9026; *Toll Free:* 800-333-1606
WFSobriety@aol.com
www.womenfor sobriety.org

Dr. Jean Kirkpatrick, Founder

Purse size booklet that explains the Thirteen Statements of Dr. Kirkpatrick's New Life program, statement by statement.

Year Founded: 1976

2961 Q&A About Smoking and Health
American Lung Association
55 W. Wacker Drive
Suite 1150
Chicago, IL 60601
212-315-8700
Fax: 202-452-1805; *Toll Free:* 800-LUN-USA
www.lung.org/

Ross P. Lanzafame, Esq., Chair
Kathryn A. Forbes, CPA, Vice Chair
Harold Wimmer, President and Chief Executive Of

Gives fact-crammed answers to questions on smoking and health.

Year Founded: 1904

2962 Quality Care
National Association for Continence (NAFC)
P.O. Box 1019
Charleston, SC 29402-1019
843-377-0900
Fax: 843-377-0905; *Toll Free:* 800-BLA-DER
memberservices@nafc.org
www.nafc.org

Donna Deng, MD, Chairperson
Nancy Hicks, Vice-Chairperson
Steven Gregg, Executive Director

Committed to alleviating the social stigma associated with bladder control problems. A source of education, advocacy, and support to the public and to the health profession about the causes, prevention, diagnosis, treatments, and management alternatives for incontinence.

Year Founded: 1980

2963 Quality Care Advocate
The National Consumer Voice for Quality Long-Term
1001 Connecticut Avenue, NW
Suite 425
Washington, DC 20036
202-332-2275
Fax: 866-230-9789
info@theconsumerservice.org
www.nccnhr.org

Lisa Tripp, Chair
Bill Lamb, President
Afsoon Namini, Vice President

News, views, and inspiration to help you be a better advocate. Covers Congressional action, regulatory developments, state and local advocacy campaigns, important research, and more.

8 pages Frequency: 8 issues Year Founded: 1975

2964 Report on Disability Programs
Business Publishers, Inc.
2222 Sedwick Drive
Durham, NC 27713
301-495-5570
Fax: 800-508-2592; *Toll Free:* 800-223-8720
custserv@bpinews.com
www.bpinews.com

Kimberly Gilbert, Managing Editor
Alexa Chew, Contributing Editor
Mary Compton, Publisher

Follows all programs and funding sources in education, housing, job training, therapy, Social Security Supplemental Security Income, Medicare, Medicaid and more. Also covers the latest on the Americans with Disabilities Act.

Frequency: BiWeekly Year Founded: 1963

2965 Retired Enlisted Association: Voice
Retired Enlisted Association
1111 S Abilene Court
Aurora, CO 80012
303-752-0660
Fax: 303-752-0835; *Toll Free:* 800-338-9337
treahq@trea.org
www.trea.org/

Richard Delaney, President
John Adams, 1st Vice President
Paul Ott, 2nd Vice President

48 pages Frequency: Monthly Year Founded: 1963

2966 SAGE Newsletter
Senior Action in A Gay Environment (SAGE)
305 7th Avenue
15th Floor
New York, NY 10001
212-741-2247
Fax: 212-366-1947
info@sageusa.org
www.sageusa.org/

Rosalyn Richter, Co-Chair
Michael Adams, Executive Director
Patricia Wil Patricia Wiley, Secretary

4 pages Frequency: Monthly Year Founded: 1978

2967 Secondhand Smoke
American Lung Association
55 W. Wacker Drive
Suite 1150
Chicago, IL 60601
212-315-8700
Fax: 202-452-1805; *Toll Free:* 800-LUN-USA
www.lung.org/

Ross P. Lanzafame, Esq., Chair
Kathryn A. Forbes, CPA, Vice Chair
Harold Wimmer, President and Chief Executive Of

Documents the effects of tobacco smoke on nonsmokers.

Year Founded: 1904

2968 Selling to Seniors
CD Publications
2222 Sedwick Drive
Durham, NC 27713
301-588-6380
Fax: 800-508-2592; *Toll Free:* 855-237-1396
info@cdpublications.com
www.cdpublications.com

Michael Gerecht, President

Monthly newsletter reporting on innovative ways businesses can better reach the over-50 market.

Year Founded: 1961

2969 Should Tobacco Advertising and Promotion Be Banned
American Lung Association
55 W. Wacker Drive
Suite 1150
Chicago, IL 60601
212-431-7489
Fax: 202-452-1805; *Toll Free:* 800-LUN-USA
www.lung.org/

Ross P. Lanzafame, Esq., Chair
Kathryn A. Forbes, CPA, Vice Chair
Harold Wimmer, President and Chief Executive Of

Answers many questions about tobacco advertising and promotion, and explains how ads are targeted to vulnerable populations.

Year Founded: 1904

2970 Simon Foundation for Continence
Simon Foundation for Continence
PO Box 815
Wilmette, IL 60091
847-864-3913
Fax: 847-864-9758; *Toll Free:* 800-237-4666
www.simonfoundation.org/

Cheryle B Gartley, President and Founder
Elizabeth Tr Lagrow, Vice President, Communications a
Twila Yednock, Director of Special Events

Publishes items of interest to people with bladder or bowel incontinence, including medical articles, helpful devices, publications and a pen pal list.

Year Founded: 1983

2971 Sobering Thoughts
Women For Sobriety, Inc.
PO Box 618
Quakertown, PA 18951
215-536-8026
Fax: 215-536-9026; *Toll Free:* 800-333-1606
www.womenforsobriety.org

Rebecca Fenner, Director
Dr. Jean Kirkpatrick, Founder

A monthly membership newsletter for women with an addiction problem who wish for recovery and start a new life.

16 pages Year Founded: 1976

2972 Social Security Bulletin
US Social Security Administration
4301 Connecticut Avenue NW
Room 209
Washington, DC 20008-2304
202-282-7138
Fax: 202-282-7219
www.ssa.gov/

Reports on results of research and analysis pertinent to the Social Security and SSI programs.

Frequency: Monthly

2973 Sounding Board
Sanders-Brown Center on Aging
101 Sanders Brown Building
800 S. Limestone Street
Lexington, KY 40536-0230

859-323-6040
Fax: 859-323-2866
www.uky.edu/coa/

Deborah D Danner, Editor
Linda J. Van Eldik, Ph.D., Director

8 pages Frequency: Semiannual Year Founded: 1979

2974 Stop Smoking: A Guide to Your Options
American Lung Association
55 W. Wacker Drive
Suite 1150
Chicago, IL 60601
212-315-8700
Fax: 202-452-1805; *Toll Free:* 800-LUN-USA
www.lung.org/

Ross P. Lanzafame, Esq., Chair
Kathryn A. Forbes, CPA, Vice Chair
Harold Wimmer, President and Chief Executive Of

Describes a variety of approaches to smoking cessation. Offers guidance on how to choose a program.

Year Founded: 1904

2975 Telephone Pioneer
Pioneers
1801 California Street
Suite 225
Denver, CO 80202
303-571-1200
Fax: 303-572-0520; *Toll Free:* 800-872-5995
info@pioneersvolunteer.org
www.telecompioneers.org/

Michael Sears, Chair
Charlene Hill, Executive Director
Cheri Jones, Director

Year Founded: 1911

2976 The Common Denominator: The Key to
Extending Healthspan
Alliance for Aging Research
750 17th Street NW
Suite 740
Washington, DC 20006
202-293-2856
Fax: 202-955-8394
info@agingresearch.org
www.agingresearch.org

Daniel Perry, President/CEO
Cynthia Bens, Public Policy Director
Michael Maroni

Newletter on how responses to stress can accelerate aging and the risks of disease.

2977 Topics in Geriatric Rehabilitation
Aspen Publishers
7201 McKinney Circle
Frederick, MD 21704
301-644-3599
Fax: 800-901-9075; *Toll Free:* 800-234-1660
www.aspenpublishers.com/

Bob Lemmond, President & CEO
Gustavo Dobles, Vice President & Chief Content O
Susan Pikitch, Vice President & Chief Financial

Peer-review journal presenting clinical, basic and applied research as well as theoretical information.

Frequency: Quarterly

2978 United States Department of the Interior:
National Park Service
Department of the Interior
1849 C Street, N.W.
Washington, DC 20240
202-208-3100
feedback@ios.doi.gov
www.doi.gov/

Jon Jarvis, Director
Maureen Foster, Chief of Staff
Peggy O'Dell, Deputy Director, Operations

Offers an informational packet containing books, guides and tours for the disabled and elderly.

2979 University Center on Aging and Health
Newsletter
Case Western Reserve University
10900 Euclid Avenue
Cleveland, OH 44106
216-368-2000
Fax: 216-368-6389
mlw4@po.cwru.edu
www.case.edu/

Barbara R. Snyder, University President
W. A. Bud Baeslack III, Provost and Executive Vice Presi

16 pages Frequency: Semiannual Year Founded: 1826

2980 Unpuffables Promotional Brochure
American Lung Association
55 W. Wacker Drive
Suite 1150
Chicago, IL 60601
212-315-8700
Fax: 202-452-1805; *Toll Free:* 800-LUN-USA
www.lung.org/

Ross P. Lanzafame, Esq., Chair
Kathryn A. Forbes, CPA, Vice Chair
Harold Wimmer, President and Chief Executive Of

Describes the ALA Unpuffables program.

Year Founded: 1904

2981 Volunteer Committees of Art Museums of
Canada and the United States News
Council of the Virginia Museum of the Fine Arts
200 N. Boulevard
Richmond, VA 23220-4007
804-340-1400
Fax: 804-340-1548
www.vmfa.state.va.us/council/

Benjamin W. Rawles III, President and Director
Kelly B. Armstrong, Vice President and Director
H. Hiter Harris III, Treasurer and Director

4-8 pages Year Founded: 1955

2982 Volunteers of America
1660 Duke Street
Alexandria, VA 22314
703-548-2288
Fax: 703-684-1972; *Toll Free:* 800-899-0089
ams@voa.org
www.voa.org/

Dawn Batts, Chair
Richard Cavanagh, Vice Chair
Mike King, President/CEO

24 pages Year Founded: 1896

2983 Washington Watch
United Cerebral Palsy Associations
1825 K Street NW
Suite 600
Washington, DC 20006
202-776-0406
Fax: 202-785-3508; *Toll Free:* 800-872-5827
ucp.org/
TDD 202-973-7197

Woody Connette, Chair
Ian Ridlon, Vice Chair
Stephen Bennett, President and Chief Executive Of

Dependable, timely information on national legislative and regulatory issues affecting people with disabilities and their families.

4 pages Frequency: Bi-weekly Year Founded: 1948

2984 What's Your Cigarette Smoking IQ?
American Lung Association
55 W. Wacker Drive
Suite 1150
Chicago, IL 60601
212-315-8700
Fax: 202-452-1805; *Toll Free:* 800-LUN-USA
www.lung.org/

Ross P. Lanzafame, Esq., Chair
Kathryn A. Forbes, CPA, Vice Chair
Harold Wimmer, President and Chief Executive Of

Brief true-or-false quiz that tests a persons knowledge of the effects of smoking.

Year Founded: 1904

2985 Working Age
AARP
601 E Street NW
Washington, DC 20049
202-434-3525
Fax: 202-434-3443; *Toll Free:* 888-687-2277
member@aarp.org
www.aarp.org
TTY: 877-434-7598

Gail E. Aldrich, Board Chair
Robert G. Romasco, President
Dr. Ethel Pe Andrus, Founder

8 pages Year Founded: 1958

Videos, Audio Tapes

2986 A Safer Place
Fanlight Productions
c/o Icarus Films
32 Court Street, 21st Floor
Brooklyn, NY 11201
718-488-8900
Fax: 718-488-8642; *Toll Free:* 800-876-1710
info@fanlight.com, sales@icarusfilms.com
www.fanlight.com

Sandy St Louis, Distribution Director
Kelli English, Publicity Coordinator
Ben Achtenberg, Founder

Profiles two elderly adults who were helped by social service agencies to recognize and get help for the abusive situations they were living in. 20-minute video.

2987 Age Base
Brookdale Foundation Group
300 Frank W. Burr Blvd.
Suite 13
Teaneck, NJ 07666
201-836-4602
Fax: 201-836-4342
vcb@brookdalefoundation.org
www.brookdalefoundation.org/

Stephen L. Schwartz, President
Mary Ann Van Clief, Vice President
Maria Asenjo, Secretary

Over 800 direct service programs for the elderly, including programs for the home-bound, health promotions, and senior citizen classes. Database includes: Program name, address, phone, contact, date established, description, group of elderly served, funding level and source.

Frequency: Continuous Year Founded: 1950

2988 As Times Goes By
Fanlight Productions
c/o Icarus Films
32 Court Street, 21st Floor
Brooklyn, NY 11201
718-488-8900
Fax: 718-488-8642; *Toll Free:* 800-876-1710
info@fanlight.com, sales@icarusfilms.com
www.fanlight.com

Canadian Broadcasting Corp., Contact
Ben Achtenberg, Founder

Humans are sexual until the very end. The seniors profiled in this video open share their experiences with love, romance and growing old. 23 minutes.

2989 Assistive Devices Information Network
The University of Iowa
University of Iowa
Iowa City, IA 52242
319-335-3500
Fax: 319-384-9273; *Toll Free:* 800-331-3027
webmaster@uiowa.edu
www.uiowa.edu/

Sally Mason, President

Provides information on assistive devices, the vendors who make them, and suggestions on how to order.

2990 Choice & Challenge: Caring for Aggressive Older Adults Across Levels of Care
Fanlight Productions
c/o Icarus Films
32 Court Street, 21st Floor
Brooklyn, NY 11201
718-488-8900
Fax: 718-488-8642; *Toll Free:* 800-876-1710
info@fanlight.com, sales@icarusfilms.com
www.fanlight.com

Ben Achtenberg, Founder

Presents a series of real-life situations in which health care providersmust cope with behaviorally impaired and aggressive elders. 22-minute video.

2991 Depression in Older Adults
Fanlight Productions
c/o Icarus Films
32 Court Street, 21st Floor
Brooklyn, NY 11201
718-488-8900
Fax: 718-488-8642; *Toll Free:* 800-876-1710
info@fanlight.com, sales@icarusfilms.com
www.fanlight.com

Ben Achtenberg, Founder

Depression in later life is common and very treatable. This video explores its causes and current approaches. 30-minute video.

2992 Elder Abuse: 5 Case Studies
Fanlight Productions
c/o Icarus Films
32 Court Street, 21st Floor
Brooklyn, NY 11201
718-488-8900
Fax: 718-488-8642; *Toll Free:* 800-876-1710
info@fanlight.com, sales@icarusfilms.com
www.fanlight.com

Ben Achtenberg, Founder

Illuminates the fear and ambivalence experienced by elderly people abused by family members and their struggles to find help. 40-minute video.

2993 ElderNet
ElderNet, Inc.
246 Walnut Street
Suite B
Newton, MA 02460-1639
617-244-1774
Fax: 617-558-5504
www.eldernet.com

A seniors' guide to health, housing, legal, financial, retirement, lifestyles, news, and entertainment information on the World Wide Web. Click on the front door.

2994 Emergency Care for the Elderly
Alzheimer's Disease Education & Referral Center
National Institute on Aging, Building 31, Room 5C27
31 Center Drive, MSC 2292
Bethesda, MD 20892
Fax: 301-495-3334; *Toll Free:* 800-222-2225
niaic@nia.nih.gov
www.nia.nih.gov/alzheimers
TTY: 800-222-4225

Richard J. Hodes, M.D., Director
Marie A. Bernard. M.D., Deputy Director
Patrick Shirdon, Director of Management

Designed to teach paramedics, EMTs and first responders to address issues presented by geriatric patients. One videotape, manual and two student booklets. Produced by University of Pittsburgh.

Year Founded: 1974

2995 Golden Years?
Fanlight Productions
c/o Icarus Films
32 Court Street, 21st Floor
Brooklyn, NY 11201
718-488-8900
Fax: 718-488-8642; *Toll Free:* 800-876-1710
info@fanlight.com, sales@icarusfilms.com
www.fanlight.com

Ben Achtenberg, Founder

A graphic and disturbing look at the growing incidence of domestic abuse against those over sixty-five. 60-minute vide.

2996 Grandparents Raising Grandchildren
Fanlight Productions
c/o Icarus Films
32 Court Street, 21st Floor
Brooklyn, NY 11201
718-488-8900
Fax: 718-488-8642; *Toll Free:* 800-876-1710
info@fanlight.com, sales@icarusfilms.com
www.fanlight.com

Ben Achtenberg, Founder

It was supposed to be their golden years, a time to relax and spoil the grandchildren. For nearly 4 million grandparents, a new reality is taking shape as they are taking on sole responsiblity for raising their children's children. This hard-hitting investigation exploses some of the difficulties surrounding this growing phenomenon and explores the emotional and financial difficulties that these families face. 37-minute video.

2997 Guide to Helping Elderly Relatives Near and Far
National Stroke Association
96 Inverness Drive E
Suite I
Englewood, CO 80112-5311
303-649-9299
Fax: 303-649-1328; *Toll Free:* 800-787-6537
info@stroke.org
www.stroke.org

James Baranski, CEO

Suggestions on how to deal with the fear and frustration of coping with long-distance caregiving, family communication, care alternatives, and much more. 92 minute video.

2998 I'm Pretty Old
Fanlight Productions
c/o Icarus Films
32 Court Street, 21st Floor
Brooklyn, NY 11201
718-488-8900
Fax: 718-488-8642; *Toll Free:* 800-876-1710
info@fanlight.com, sales@icarusfilms.com
www.fanlight.com

Ben Achtenberg, Founder

An engaging look at several elderly men and woman as they adapt to the realities of living in a nursing home. 20-minute video.

2999 Label Reading and Shopping
American Diabetes Association
1701 North Beauregard Street
Alexandria, VA 22311
203-639-0385
Fax: 203-639-0292; *Toll Free:* 800-342-2383
www.diabetes.org/adact

Dwight Holing, Chair
Larry Hausner, MBA, CEO
Debbie Johnson, CPA, CFO

Provides practical information on how to shop and what to look for on labels.

3000 Line Dancing Video
Center for Positive Aging
1440 Dutch Valley Place NE
Suite 120
Atlanta, GA 30324-5367
404-872-9191
Fax: 404-872-1737
positiveaging@mindspring.com
www.centerforpositiveaging.org/

Walter Coffey, President & CEO
Jacque Thornton, Sr. Vice President
Susan Watkins, Dir. Of Member Services

A unique and exciting new line dancing video designed especially for adults over 50. Executed at a safe, easy pace that lets you learn the steps while achieving the mobility, timing, flexibility, stamina, and muscle control that helps insure lasting fitness. 45-minute video.

Year Founded: 1982

3001 My Mother, My Father
Fanlight Productions
c/o Icarus Films
32 Court Street, 21st Floor
Brooklyn, NY 11201
718-488-8900
Fax: 718-488-8642; *Toll Free:* 800-876-1710
info@fanlight.com, sales@icarusfilms.com
www.fanlight.com

Ben Achtenberg, Founder

Portraits of four families caring for aging parents; their choices include care at home, use of a variety of support services, and nursing home placement. 33-minute video.

3002 My Mother, My Father: Seven Years Later
Fanlight Productions
c/o Icarus Films
32 Court Street, 21st Floor
Brooklyn, NY 11201
718-488-8900
Fax: 718-488-8642; *Toll Free:* 800-876-1710
info@fanlight.com, sales@icarusfilms.com
www.fanlight.com

Ben Achtenberg, Founder

Revisits each family seven years from the first study, to explore changes in family dynamics and the caregivers' thoughts about their own aging. 33-minute video.

3003 Not My Home
Fanlight Productions
c/o Icarus Films
32 Court Street, 21st Floor
Brooklyn, NY 11201

718-488-8900
Fax: 718-488-8642; *Toll Free:* 800-876-1710
info@fanlight.com, sales@icarusfilms.com
www.fanlight.com

Suzanne Babin, Author
Tynette Deveaux, Author
Ben Achtenberg, Founder

A compelling look at life inside a nursing home, as residents, families, and staff discuss their problems and rewards. 45-minute video.

3004 Personals
Fanlight Productions
c/o Icarus Films
32 Court Street, 21st Floor
Brooklyn, NY 11201
718-488-8900
Fax: 718-488-8642; *Toll Free:* 800-876-1710
info@fanlight.com, sales@icarusfilms.com
www.fanlight.com

Ben Achtenberg, Founder

A group of senior citizens reveal their longing for love and perform it on stage with energy and laughter. 37-minute video.

3005 Quality Care Conference
Alzheimer's Association
225 N Michigan Avenue
Floor 17
Chicago, IL 60601-7633
312-335-8700
Fax: 866-699-1246; *Toll Free:* 800-272-3900
info@alz.org
www.alz.org
TDD 312-335-5886

Gerald Sampson, Chair
Electa Anderson, Director
Deborah Jones, Secretary

Selected educational sessions from the conference discussing topics such as special care units, drug therapies, behavior management, and care strategies.

3006 Right to Decide
Fanlight Productions
c/o Icarus Films
32 Court Street, 21st Floor
Brooklyn, NY 11201
718-488-8900
Fax: 718-488-8642; *Toll Free:* 800-876-1710
info@fanlight.com, sales@icarusfilms.com
www.fanlight.com

Ben Achtenberg, Founder

Informed by the Patient Self-Determination Act, these outstanding physician-patient interviews explore patients' hopes, fears, and golas regarding end-of-life care. 43-minute video.

3007 Sexuality & Aging
Fanlight Productions
c/o Icarus Films
32 Court Street, 21st Floor
Brooklyn, NY 11201
718-488-8900
Fax: 718-488-8642; *Toll Free:* 800-876-1710

info@fanlight.com, sales@icarusfilms.com
www.fanlight.com

Ben Achtenberg, Founder

Explores society's attitudes and myths about sexuality in later life, while several elders contribute their perspectives on the importance of continued intimacy. 60-minute video.

3008 Signs for Computing Terminology
National Association of the Deaf
8630 Fenton Street
Suite 820
Silver Spring, MD 20910
301-587-1788
Fax: 301-587-1791
www.nad.org
TTY: 301-587-1789

Christopher Wagner, President
Melissa S. Draganac-Hawk, Vice President
Kirsten Poston, Secretary

Three videotapes designed to accompany the text, Signs for Computing Terminology (separately listed). Videotape #1 covers prefixes, suffixes, and vocabulary A-D. Videotape #2 covers vocabulary E-O. Videotape #3 cover vocabulary P-W.

Year Founded: 1880

3009 Solution Starts with You
Simon Foundation for Continence
PO Box 815
Wilmette, IL 60091
847-864-3913
Fax: 847-864-9758; *Toll Free:* 800-237-4666
www.simonfoundation.org/

Cheryle B Gartley, President and Founder
Elizabeth Tr Lagrow, Vice President, Communications a
Twila Yednock, Director of Special Events

Video that seeks to bring the topic of incontinence out of the closet and remove the associated stigma; provides information to patients, their families, and the health care professionals who provide patient care.

Year Founded: 1983

3010 Stay Fit Video
Center for Positive Aging
1440 Dutch Valley Place NE
Suite 120
Atlanta, GA 30324-5367
404-872-9191
Fax: 404-872-1737
positiveaging@mindspring.com
www.centerforpositiveaging.org/

Walter Coffey, President & CEO
Jacque Thornton, Sr. Vice President
Susan Watkins, Dir. Of Member Services

Designed especially for the older adults, STAY FIT FOR LIFE offers stretching exercises that are safe, effective and motivating with easy-to-follow routines. With this video, you can quickly acquire increased flexibility and muscle strength, and improve your posture, balance, and cordination. This 45-minute video features ten minutes of limbering movements and static stretches while seated, 20 minutes of muscle-strengthening and free-standing floor moevments, 10 minutes of cool-down stretches, and five minutes of relaxation exercises. Also includes modifica-

tions for standing and sitting exercises for those with different levels of physical fitness.

Year Founded: 1982

3011 Tonight's the Night
Fanlight Productions
c/o Icarus Films
32 Court Street, 21st Floor
Brooklyn, NY 11201
718-488-8900
Fax: 718-488-8642; *Toll Free:* 800-876-1710
info@fanlight.com, sales@icarusfilms.com
www.fanlight.com

Canadian Broadcasting Corp., Contact
Ben Achtenberg, Founder

Three senior couples describe the evolution of their sexual relationnships, while experts stress the importance of more accepting social attitudes about sexuality and aging. 25-minute video.

3012 Way We Die
Fanlight Productions
c/o Icarus Films
32 Court Street, 21st Floor
Brooklyn, NY 11201
718-488-8900
Fax: 718-488-8642; *Toll Free:* 800-876-1710
info@fanlight.com, sales@icarusfilms.com
www.fanlight.com

Ben Achtenberg, Founder

Intimately filmed interviews between caregivers and terminally ill patients encourage professionals to attend more closely to their patients' values, needs, and wishes. 24-minute video.

3013 We Will Remember
Compassion Books
7036 State Hwy 80 South
Burnsville, NC 28714
828-675-5909
Fax: 828-675-9687; *Toll Free:* 828-675-5909
orders@compassionbooks.com
www.compassionbooks.com

Bruce Greene, Vice President
Donna O'Toole, Founder

A video meditation that uses the beauty of natural photography, soothing music and gentle words to give permission and encouragement in using the memories of the past for healing in the present.

Frequency: 10 Minutes Year Founded: 1981

Websites

3014 60 Plus Association
60 Plus Association
515 King Street
Suite 315
Alexandria, VA 22314
703-807-2070
Fax: 703-807-2073
info@60plus.org
www.60plus.org

James L. Martin, Chairman
Amy Noore Frederick, President
Pat Boone, National Spokesman

A non-partisan seniors advocacy group with a free enterprise, less government, less taxes approach to seniors issues.

Year Founded: 1992

3015 AARP

601 E Street NW
Washington, DC 20049
Toll Free: 888-687-2277
member@aarp.org
www.aarp.org

Jo Ann Jenkins, CEO

AARP is a nonprofit membership organization of persons 50 and older dedicated to addressing their needs and interests. AARP is dedicated to enhancing quality of life for all as we age. We lead positive social change and deliver value to members through information, advocacy and service.

Year Founded: 1958

3016 AARP-Consumer Protection
AARP

601 E Street NW
Washington, DC 20049
202-434-3525
Fax: 202-434-3443; *Toll Free:* 888-687-2277
member@aarp.org
www.aarp.org
TTY: 877-434-7598

Gail E. Aldrich, Board Chair
Robert G. Romasco, President
Dr. Ethel Pe Andrus, Founder

AARP is a nonprofit membership organization of persons 50 and older dedicated to addressing their needs and interests. AARP is dedicated to enhancing quality of life for all as we age. We lead positive social change and deliver value to members through information, advocacy and service.

Year Founded: 1958

3017 Age in place
National Aging In Place Council

1400 16th Street NW
Suite 420
Washington, DC 20036
202-939-1770
Fax: 202-265-4435
jhoefer@dworbell.com
naipc.org

Peter Bell, President
Marty Bell, Executive Director

Web site with resources for planning for housing and care needs.

3018 Age of Reason
Weird Seniors

www.ageofreason.com

Over 5,000 Links to sites of interest to the over 50 age group.

3019 American Academy of Dermatology
American Academy of Dermatology

PO Box 4014
Schaumburg, IL 60168
847-240-1280
Fax: 847-240-1859; *Toll Free:* 866-503-SKIN
www.aad.org

Dirk M. Elston, MD, President
Lisa A. Garner, MD, Vice President
Robert T. Brodell,MD, Director

An organization of doctors who specialize in diagnosing and treating skin problems.

Year Founded: 1938

3020 American Academy of Otolaryngology-Head& Neck Surgery
American Academy of Otolaryngology

1650 Diagonal Road
Alexandria, VA 22314-2857
703-836-4444
www.entnet.org

Richard Waguespack, MD, President
David R. Nielsen, MD, EVP & CEO
Paul T. Fass, MD, Director- Private Practice

Advance the art and science of otalaryngology-head and neck surgury through state-of-the-art education, research, and learning; and to unite, serve, and represent the interests of its members and their patients to the public.

3021 American Association of Homes and Services for the Aging
LeadingAge

2519 Connecticut Avenue North West
Washington, DC 20008-1520
202-661-5700
Fax: 301-206-9789
info@LeadingAge.org
www.aahsa.org

William L. (Minnix Jr., President/Chief Executive Office
Katrinka (Ka Smith Sloan, SVP /Chief Operating Officer
Cheryl Phillips, Senior Vice President of Public

Organizations dedicated to providin high-quality health care, housing and services to the nation's elderly.

3022 American Association of Retired Persons(AARP)
AARP

601 E Street NW
Washington, DC 20049
202-434-3525
Fax: 202-434-3443; *Toll Free:* 888-687-2277
member@aarp.org
www.aarp.org
TTY: 877-434-7598

Gail E. Aldrich, Board Chair
Robert G. Romasco, President
Dr. Ethel Pe Andrus, Founder

AARP is the nation's leading organization for people age 50 and older. Information and education, advocacy, and community services provided by a network of local chapters and experienced volunteers throughout the country.

Year Founded: 1958

3023 American Lung Association
55 W Wacker Drive
Suite 1150
Chicago, IL 60601
Toll Free: 800-548-8252
info@lung.org
www.lung.org

Harold P. Wimmer, President & CEO

A voluntary organization interested in the prevention and control of lung disease.

Year Founded: 1904

3024 American Prostate Society
American Prostate Society
www.americanprostatesociety.com/

Organization dedicated exclusively to using existing medical capabilities to reduce death due to prostate cancer and to reduce unnecessary or ineffective prostate surgery.

3025 American Society of Colon and Rectal Surgeons
American Society of Colon and Rectal Surgeons
85 W. Algonquin Rd
Suite 550
Arlington Heights, IL 60005
847-290-9184
Fax: 847-290-9203
ascrs@fascrs.org
www.fascrs.org

Michael J. Stamos, MD, President
Martin A. Luchtefeld, MD, Vice President
Charles E. Littlejohn, MD, Secretary

Represents more than 1000 board certified colon and rectal surgeons and other surgeons dedicated to advancing and promoting the science and practice of the treatment of patients with diseases and disorders affecting the colon, rectum and anus.

Year Founded: 1899

3026 Caresource Healthcare Communications
CareSource
P.O. Box 8738
Dayton, OH 45401-8738
Toll Free: 800-488-0134
www.caresource.com/
TTY: 800-750-0750

Pamela B. Morris, President & CEO
Bobby Jones, Chief Operating Officer
Dan Mccabe, Chief Administrative Officer

This web site is a free information and resource pool for senior services community. It includes a community bulletin board for coming events, a database of senior and caregiver opportunities, directories of services and service providers, and extensive forms library.

Year Founded: 1989

3027 Centers for Medicare and Medicaid Services (CMS)
Centers for Medicare and Medicaid Services
7500 Security Blvd.
Baltimore, MD 21244
410-786-3000 Toll free: 877-267-2323
www.cms.hhs.gov
TTY: 410-786-0727

Jonathan Blum, Principal Deputy Administrator
Tim Love, Chief Operating Officer
Marilyn Tavenner, Administrator

CMS, part of the Federal Government, administers health insurance through Medicare and Medicaid. CMS regulates hospitals, nursing homes, and home health agencies.

Year Founded: 1965

3028 Consultation and Education Unlimited
www.staug.com

Complete catalog on line of items to help those in pain or with physical disabilities with tasks of daily living.

3029 Council of Better Business Bureau
Council of Better Business Bureau
3033 Wilson Blvd.
Suite 600
Arlington, VA 22201
703-276-0100
www.bbb.org/

Sharon Abrams, Chair
Mary E. Power,CAE, President & CEO
Beverly Baskin, SVP, Chief Mission Officer

BBBOnLine's mission is to promote trust and confidence on the Internet through the BBBOnLine Reliability and Privacy Seal Programs. BBBOnLine's web site seal programs allows companies with web sites to display the seals once they have been evaluated and confirmed to meet the program requirements.

3030 ElderCareMatters.com
561-406-5293
www.eldercarematters.com

National directory of elder and senior care resources.

3031 ElderConnect
Elder Connect
107 North Main Street
Anderson, SC 29621
864-934-5600
jean@elderconnect.net
elderconnect.net/

Becky Morlok, President
Jean Mahaffey, Ph.D., Executive Director

Information of over 33,000 acute rehabilitation providers, retirement communities, and providers specializing in all levels of long-term nursing care as well as home health agencies.

Year Founded: 1984

3032 Eldercare Locator
Department of Health and Human Services
Toll Free: 800-677-1116
eldercarelocator@n4a.org
www.eldercare.gov

Eldercare Locator links those who need assistance with state and local area agencies on aging and community-based organizations that serve older adults and their caregivers.

3033 Elderhostel
Road Scholar
11 Avenue de Lafayette
Boston, MA 02111

978-323-4141
Fax: 617-426-0701; *Toll Free:* 800-454-5768
www.elderhostel.org
TTY: 877-426-2167

Michael Zoob, Editor
James Moses, CEO

Elderhostel.

Year Founded: 1975

3034 Family Meds
Family Meds
461 Cooke Street
Farmington, CT 6032
Fax: 877-471-6008; *Toll Free:* 888-787-2800
customersupport@familymeds.com
www.familymeds.com

Jeff P. D'Alessandro, RPh, Pharmacist

A site providing information on impotence and its various
treatments, including over the counter, natural, and prescription medication choices.

3035 Federal Trade Commission
Federal Trade Commission
600 Pennsylvania Avenue
Washington, DC 20580
www.ftc.gov

Randolph W. Tritell, Director
David B. Robbins, Executive Director
Bajinder Paul, Chief Information Officer & Dirc

The FTC site includes news and alerts, consumer protection
and anti-trust information.

3036 Fidelco Guide Dog Foundation
Fidelco Guide Dog Foundation
103 Vision Way
Bloomfield, CT 6002
860-243-5200
Fax: 860-769-0567
admissions@fidelco.org, Info@fidelco.org
www.fidelco.org

Eliot D. Russman, CEO and Executive Director

Fidelco breeds, raises, trains, and places German shepherd
guide dogs with men and women who are visually impaired, primarily in the Northeast.

Year Founded: 1960

3037 Food Allergy Network
Food Allergy Research & Education, Inc. (FARE)
7925 Jones Branch Dr.
Suite 1100
Mclean, VA 22102
Fax: 703-691-2713; *Toll Free:* 800-929-4040
www.foodallergy.org

Todd J. Slotkin, Chair
Janet Atwater, Vice Chair & Secretary
Veronica LaFemina, Vice President of Communications

Information to help families living with food allergies, and
to increase public awareness about food allergies and
anaphylaxis.

3038 Friends-In-Art
The American Council of the Blind
2220 Wilson Boulevard
Suite 650
Arlingtonn, VA 22201-3354
202-467-5081
Fax: 703-465-5085; *Toll Free:* 800-424-8666
info@acb.org
www.acb.org

Kim Charlson, President
Jeff Thom, 1st Vice President
Marlaina Lieberg, 2nd Vice President

Offers consultation to program planners in establishing accessible art and museum exhibits and presents Performing
Arts Showcases.

Year Founded: 1961

3039 General Fitness
General Fitness
425 Pleasant St
Fall River, MA 2724
508-677-4933
www.generalfitness.net/

Important reasons why senior citizens should exercise regardless of age.

3040 Generations Online
Generations on Line
3637 Chestnut Street
Philadelphia, PA 19104
215-222-6400
www.generationsonline.com

Tobby Dichter, CEO
VJ Pappas, COO
Katie Burke, Administrator

3041 Gerontological Society of America
Gerontological Society of America
1220 L Street North West
Washington, DC 20005
202-842-1275
Fax: 202-842-1150
geron@geron.org
www.geron.org

James Appleby, Executive Director and CEO
Linda Krogh Harootyan, Deputy Executive Director
Chris Yoder, Senior Director, Finance and Adm

Provides researchers, educators, practitioners, and policy
makers with opportunities to understand, advance, integrate, and use basic and applied research on aging to improve the quality of life as one ages.

Year Founded: 1945

3042 Grand Times
Grand Times
403 Village Drive
El Cerrito, CA 94530
510-527-4337
mail3@grandtimes.com
www.grandtimes.com

Reece R. Halpern, Publisher

A weekly Internet magazine foe seniors. Controversial, entertaining and informative, Grand Times celebrates life's
opportunities and examines life's challanges.

Year Founded: 1995

3043 HMOs4seniors.com
HealthMetrix Research
PO Box 30041
Columbus, OH 43230
614-236-8345
info@medicarenewswatch.com
www.hmos4seniors.com

Alan Mittermaier, President

Dedicated to assisting seniors and caregivers with making informed choices regarding Medicare and Choice options.

Year Founded: 1999

3044 Hazelden
Hazelden
15251 Pleasant Valley Rd.
Center city, MN 55012
651-213-4200Toll free: 800-257-7810
info@hazelden.org
www.hazelden.com

Mark Mishek, President & CEO
James A. Blaha, VP Finance & Administration/ CFO
Nick Motu, VP, Marketing & Communications

Organization dedicated to providing quality rehabilitation, education and professional services for chemical dependency and related addictive behaviors.

Year Founded: 1949

3045 Healing Well
HealingWell.com LLC
e-mail: admin@healingwell.com
www.healingwell.com

Peter Waite, Founder& CEO

An online health resource guide to medical news, chat, information and articles, newsgroups and message boards, books, disease-related web sites, medical directories, and more for patients, friends, and family coping with disabling diseases, disorders, or chronic illnesses.

Year Founded: 1996

3046 Immune Deficiency Foundation
Immune Deficiency Foundation
40 W Chesapeake Avenue
Suite 308
Towson, MD 21204
410-321-6647
Fax: 410-321-9165; *Toll Free:* 800-296-4433
info@primaryimmune.org
primaryimmune.org/

John Seymour, PhD, LMFT, Chair
Steve Fietek, Vice Chair
Marcia Boyle, President & Founder

Offers information and referral services to immune deficient patients and their families.

Year Founded: 1980

3047 International Association of Eating Disorder Professionals
The International Association of Eating Disorders
PO Box 1295
Pekin, Il 61555-1295

Fax: 800-800-8126; *Toll Free:* 800-800-8126
iaedpmembers@earthlink.net
www.iaedp.com

Bonnie Harken, Managing Director
Blanche Williams, Assistant Managing Director & Me
Tammy Beasley, Certification Director

Supplies printed information and sponsors meetings and other activities. Publishes a directory of speech instructors and maintains a list of sources for supplies for laryngectomee.

Year Founded: 1985

3048 Internet Health Coalition
iHealthCoalition.org
www.ihealthcoalition.org

The mission of the Internet Healthcare Coalition is quality healthcare resources on the Internet.

Year Founded: 1997

3049 Living Will Form
Easy Legal Form/Paralegal Services
33309 1st Way South
Suite 203
Federal Way, WA 98003
523-874-0649
kda31952@gmail.com
www.easylegalforms.net/

Kristen D. Alcoba, Paralegal-Owner

These are easy-to-use law documents that you individually customize for your specific needs.

Year Founded: 1992

3050 Medical Library Association
Medical Library Association
65 East Wacker Place
Suite 1900
Chicago, IL 60601-7246
312-419-9094
Fax: 312-419-8950
info@mlahq.org
www.mlanet.org

Dixie Jones, President
Kristine M. Alpi, Director
Angela Dixon, Director

A nonprofit, educational organization of more than 1,100 institutions and 3,600 individual members in the health sciences information field, committed to educating health information professionals, supporting health information research, promoting access to the world's health sciences information, and working to ensure that the best health information is available to all.

Year Founded: 1898

3051 Medicare
Medicare.gov
7500 Security Boulevard
Baltimore, MD 21244
Toll Free: 800-MED-CARE
www.medicare.gov
TTY: 877-486-2048

Official US Government website for people with Medicare.

3052 Mediconsult
Mediconsult Planning & Consulting Services Sdn. Bh
A13/5/5 One Ampang Business Avenue
Jalan Ampang Utama 2/2, 68000 Ampang
Selangor, Ma
60 - 42-3 32
Fax: 60 - 42-3 31
info@mediconsult.com.my
www.mediconsult.com.my/

Dieter Nassler, Mediconsult Director
Sharif Lough Abdullah, Mediconsult Director
Nguyen Thi Dung, Mediconsult Director

Provides links to information on disease, illness, and disorders, including such content areas as conference highlights, educational material, journal articles, research, news, and support.

3053 MedlinePlus
U.S. National Library of Medicine
8600 Rockville Pike
Bethesda, MD 20894
e-mail: custserv@nlm.nih.gov
medlineplus.gov

Produced by the National Library of Medicine - the world's largest medical library - MedlinePlus is the National Institutes of Health's Web site for patients and their families and friends.

3054 Merck & Company
Merck & Co.
One Merck Drive
P.O. Box 100
Whitehouse Station, NJ 08889-0100
908-423-1000Toll free: 800-444-2080
www.merck.com

Kenneth C. Frazier, Chaairman &CEO
Richard R. Deluca Jr., EVP, Merck Animal Health
Cuong Viet Do, EVP & Chief Strategy Officer

This site features several sections from the on-line version of the doctors' bible, the recently updated Merck Manual of Medical Information-Home Edition, the definitive guide to disease, diagnosis, prevention and treatment. Click on Publications.

Year Founded: 1654

3055 NIA Publishers
National Institute on Aging
31 Center Drive, MSC 2292
Bethesda, MD 20892
Toll Free: 800-222-2225
niaic@nia.nih.gov
www.niapublications.org
TTY: 800-222-4225

Robin Barr, Director
Vicky Autrey, Branch Chief
Catherine Amores, Information Systems Security Off

Free publications online.

Year Founded: 1974

3056 NIH Senior Health
National Institutes of Health
e-mail: custserv@nlm.nih.gov
nihseniorhealth.gov

Reliable, easy to understand aging-related health information for older adults. This site was developed by the National Institute on Aging (NIA), and the National Library of Medicine (NLM) both parts of the National Institutes of Health (NIH).

3057 National Academy on Aging
Gerontological Society of America
1220 L Street North West
Washington, DC 20005
202-842-1275
Fax: 202-842-1150
geron@geron.org
www.geron.org

James Appleby, Executive Director and CEO
Linda Krogh Harootyan, Deputy Executive Director
Chris Yoder, Senior Director, Finance and Adm

Promotes the scientific study of aging.
Year Founded: 1945

3058 National Association for Continence
National Association for Continence (NAFC)
P.O. Box 1019
Charleston, SC 29402-1019
843-377-0900
Fax: 843-377-0905; *Toll Free:* 800-BLA-DER
memberservices@nafc.org
www.nafc.org

Donna Deng, MD, Chairperson
Nancy Hicks, Vice-Chairperson
Steven Gregg, Executive Director

Committed to alleviating the social stigma associated with bladder control problems. Information to consumers and health professionals and advocating on their behalf to increase public awareness about incontinence.

Year Founded: 1980

3059 National Association for Home Care and Hospice (NAHC)
National Association for Home Care & Hospice
228 7th Street SE
Washington, DC 20003
202-547-7424
Fax: 202-547-3540
ads@nahc.org, exec@nahc.org
www.nahc.org

Andrea Devoti, Chair
Lucy Andrews, Vice Chair
Val J. Halamandaris, President

Providers of home health care, hospice, and homemaker-home health aide services; interested individuals and organizations. Develops and promotes high standards of patient care in home care services. Seeks to affect legislative and regulatory processes concerning home care services; gathers and disseminates home care industry data; develops public relations strategies; works to increase political visibility of home care services. Interprets home care services to governmental and private sector bodies affecting the delivery and financing of such services. Provides legal and accounting consulting services; conducts market research and compiles statistics. Offers members insurance discounts. Sponsors educational programs for organizations and individuals concerned with home care services.

3060 National Association of Professional Geriatric Care Managers (PGCM)
National Association of Professional Geriatric Car
3275 West Ina Road
Suite 130
Tuscon, AZ 85741
520-881-8008
Fax: 520-325-7925
www.caremanager.org

Emily Saltz, MSW, LICSW, CMC, President
Amy Abrams, MPH, MSW, CMC, Director
Jeffrey S. Pine, MS, MSPH, CMC, Treasurer

Information resource for those interested in the field of geriatriccare while supporting quality care and services for the elderly.

Year Founded: 1985

3061 National Association of State Units on Aging
National Association of State Units on Aging & Dis
1201 15th Street, NW
Suite 350
Wsahington, DC 20005
202-898-2578
Fax: 202-898-2583
info@nasuad.org
www.nasuad.org/

Gloria Lawlah, President
James Bulot, Vice President
Lora Connolly, Secretary

Offers support, information and technical assistance to state units on aging.

Year Founded: 1964

3062 National Center on Elder Abuse
www.elderabusecenter.org

3063 National Crime Prevention Council
1201 Connecticut Avenue
Suite 200
Washington, DC 20036
202-466-6272
www.ncpc.org

Ann M. Harkins, President & CEO

This organization works to prevent crime and drug use in many ways, including developing materials for parents and children.

Year Founded: 1982

3064 National Domestic Violence Hotline
The National Domestic Violence Hotline
P.O. Box 161810
Austin, TX 78716
512-794-1133 Toll free: 800-799-SAFE
hotline.media@ndvh.org
www.thehotline.org/
TTY: 800-787-3224

Maury Lane, Chair
Catrina Steinocher Wilson, Vice-Chair
Sheila Casey, Board Member

At the National Domestic Violence Hotline (NDVH), we continue our commitment to answering this call for help by creating the NDVH Advisory Board, consisting of eleven prominent national leaders who are committed to raising

awareness and the resources necessary to ensure that the Hotline's lifesaving work continues.

Year Founded: 1994

3065 National Heart, Lung, & Blood Institute
NHLBI Health Information Center
PO Box 30105
Bethesda, MD 20824-0105
301-592-8573
nhlbiinfo@nhlbi.nih.gov
www.nhlbi.nih.gov

Gary H. Gibbons, Director

The mission is to improve meaning of one American people by supporting and understanding research to prevent, detect, diagnose and treat diseases of heart, lungs, blood vessels, and sleep disorders.

Year Founded: 1887

3066 National Institute of Dental and Craniofacial Research
National Institute of Dental and Craniofacial Rese
National Institutes of Health
Bethesda, MD 20892-2190
301-496-4261
Fax: 301-480-4098; *Toll Free:* 866-232-4528
nidcrinfo@mail.nih.gov
www.nidcr.nih.gov

Our mission is to improve oral, dental and craniofacial health through research, research training, and the dissemination of health information.

3067 National Institute of Neurological Disorders and Stroke
National Institute of Neurological Disorders &Stro
P.O. Box 5801
Bethesda, MD 20824
301-496-5751 Toll free: 800-352-9424
www.ninds.nih.gov

Story C. Landis, Ph.D., Director
Caroline Lewis, Executive Officer
Ken Frushour, Budget Officer

Offers a brochure on stroke. The leading supporter of research on brain and nervous system disorders, including stroke.

3068 National Institute on Aging
National Institute on Aging
31 Center Drive, MSC 2292
Bethesda, MD 20892
Toll Free: 800-222-2225
niaic@nia.nih.gov
www.nih.gov/nia
TTY: 800-222-4225

Robin Barr, Director
Vicky Autrey, Branch Chief
Catherine Amores, Information Systems Security Off

The NIA promotes healthy aging by conducting and supporting biomedical, social, and behavioral research and public education.

Year Founded: 1974

3069 National Institutes of Health
9000 Rockville Pike
Bethesda, MD 20892

301-496-4000
nihinfo@od.nih.gov
www.nih.gov
TTY: 301-402-9612

Francis S. Collins, Director

The nation's medical research agency.

Year Founded: 1887

3070 National Meditation Center
National Meditation Center (NMC)
936-445-0095
www.nationalmeditation.org/

Master Hughes, Director

A humanitarian agency with volunteer camps to the Philippines. We need seniors for our volunteer projects overseas and here in America.

3071 National Organization for Victim Assistance
National Organization for Victim Assistance
510 King Street
Suite 424
Alexandria, VA 22314
703-535-6682
Fax: 703-535-5500; *Toll Free:* 800-879-6682
www.trynova.org

Hon. Tim Jeffries, President
Andrew Yurick, VP for Administration
Dr. Will Marling, Executive Director

NOVA's mission is to promote rights and services for victims of crime and crisis everywhere.

Year Founded: 1975

3072 Office on Smoking and Health
Centers for Disease Control and Prevention
1600 Clifton Rd.
Atlanta, GA 30333
Toll Free: 800-CDC-INFO
www.cdc.gov
TTY: 888-232-6348

Offers reference services to researchers through the Technical Information Center. Publishes and distributes a number of titles in the field of smoking and health.

3073 Onhealth
MedicineNet, Inc.
www.onhealth.com

A search engine providing links to websites with information on illnesses, diseases, and disorders.

3074 Partnership for Prescription Assistance
Partnership for Prescription Assistance (PPA)
Toll Free: 888-4PP- NOW
www.pparx.org

Our mission is to increase awareness of patient assistance programs and boost enrollment of those who are eligible. The Partnership for Prescription Assistance offers a single point of access to more than 475 public and private patient assistance programs, including more than 150 programs offered by pharmaceutical companies.

Year Founded: 2005

3075 QuackWatch
QuackWatch
Chatham Crossing, Suite 107/208
11312 U.S. 15-501 North
Chapel Hill, NC 27517
www.quackwatch.org

Dr. Stephen Barrett, Founder

A nonprofit corporation whose purpose is to combat health-related frauds, myths, fads, fallacies, and misconduct. Its primary focus is on quackery-related information that is difficult or impossible to get elsewhere.

Year Founded: 1969

3076 Randolph-Sheppard Vendors of America
American Council of the Blind
2200 Wilson Boulevard
Suite 650
Arlington, VA 22201-3354
202-467-5081
Fax: 703-465-5085; *Toll Free:* 800-424-8666
info@acb.org
www.acb.org

Kim Charlson, President
Jeff Thom, 1st Vice President
Melanie Brunson, Executive Director

Protects the interests of blind vendors, seeks proper implementation of the Randolph-Sheppard Act and encourages facility locations in more visible and profitable areas.

Year Founded: 1961

3077 Retirement Planning
www.vanguard.com/

F. William McNabb III, Chairman and CEO
John C. Bogle, Founder
Mortimer J. Buckley, Managing Director

Helps you create a personal financial plan based on information you enter.

Year Founded: 1970

3078 Senior Housing Net
10 Almaden Blvd.
Suite 800
San Jose, CA 95113
www.seniorhousing.net

Michele Conn, VP, Corporate Development
Alison Schwartz, VP of Communications

Comprehensive guide to retirement communities, assisted living residences, Alzheimer's facilities, and nursing homes nationwide.

3079 Senior Job Bank
Senior Job Bank
P.O. Box 508
Marlborough, MA 1752
Toll Free: 888-501-0804
publisher@seniorjobbank.org
www.seniorjobbank.com

Year Founded: 1975

3080 Senior Law Home Page
Senior Law Home Page
350 Fifth Avenue
Suite 4310
New York, NY 10118

212-387-8400
goldfarb@seniorlaw.com
www.seniorlaw.com

Ira Salzman, Attorney
Michael Kutzin, Publisher
David Goldfarb, Education Reporter

Information about Elder Law, Medicare, Medicaid, estate planning, trusts and the rights of the elderly and disabled.

3081 Senior Summer School
Senior Summer School
P.O. Box 188
Madison, WI 53701
Toll Free: 800-847-2466
info@seniorsummerschool.com
www.seniorsummerschool.com

The Education Vacation for seniors. Visit college campuses across the US and Canada from 2 to 10 weeks during the summer.

Year Founded: 1985

3082 Senior Times
The Senior Times
4077 Decarie Boulevard
Montreal, QC H4A 3J8
514-484-5033
Fax: 514-484-8254
editor@theseniortimes.com
www.theseniortimes.com

Barbara Moser, Publisher & Managing Editor
Kristine Berey, Assistant Editor
Thelma Gearey, Office Manager

By, for, and about exraordinary seniors.

Year Founded: 1986

3083 Senior Women's Travel
20 Van Winkle Road
Hudson, NY 12534
917-880-6732
maryann@poshnosh.com
www.poshnosh.com

Mary Ann Zimmerman, President and Founder

Senior Women's Travel brings a new dimension to senior travel and eliminates many of the annoyances of single travel. It's for 50+ women, with a large cultural appetite, who love to shop and eat.

3084 United Ostomy Association
United Ostomy Associations of America, Inc. (UOAA)
P.O. Box 512
Northfield, MN 55057-0512
Toll Free: 800-826-0826
info@ostomy.org, ostomyvisitor@ostomy.org
www.uoa.org

Ken Aukett, Chair
George Salamy, Vice Chair
Susan Burns, President

Produces and distributes materials about ostomy care and management; through trained UOA members, offers practical assistance and emotional support to ostomy patients; sponsors annual youth rally and state and regional conferences for local affiliates; has 500 chapters to serve people locally.

Year Founded: 1943

3085 WebMD
WebMD, LLC
www.webmd.com

Kristy Hammam, SVP, Content & Programming
Michael Smith, Chief Medical Editor

Credible information, in-depth reference material, health management tools and supportive communities.

3086 Webhelp
Webhelp
161, Rue de Courcelles
Paris, 75 1 44 40 33
e-mail: contact@fr.webhelp.com
www.webhelp.com

J,r,my C"me, Communication Director

Provides links to information, including research, treatment, prevention, support, and more.

3087 Women's Health
The New York Times Company
212-556-7194Toll free: 800-NYT-MES
kerrie@nytimes.com, inytsubs@nytimes.com
www.nytimes.com

Click on Web Specials-women's health to reach this site operated by *The New York Times*. Consult Resources for a guide to more than 100 women-related Web sites.

Year Founded: 1851

Research Centers

3088 Ackerman Institute for the Family
Ackerman Institute for the Family
936 Broadway
New York, NY 10010
212-879-4900
Fax: 212-744-0206
ackerman@ackerman.org
www.ackerman.org

John R. O'Neill, Chair
Lois Braverman, LCSW, President
Nathan W. Ackerman, Founder

Provides mental health care professionals with new skills, and brings innovative perspectives to community service agencies and other health care facilities.

Year Founded: 1960

3089 Aging Research Institute
LeadingAge Kansas
217 SE 8th Avenue
Topeka, KS 66603-3906
785-233-7443
Fax: 785-233-9471; *Toll Free:* 800-264-5242
jgrace@kahsa.org
www.kahsa.org

Kevin Reimer, Chair
Debra Harmon Zehr, President and CEO
Dana Weaver, COO

Managed care and nursing facilities staff recruitment and retention.

3090 Aging Research: National Institute on Aging, Public Health Service
US Department of Health and Human Services
200 Independence Avenue, S.W.
Washington, DC 20201
301-496-4996
Fax: 301-402-0010; *Toll Free:* 800-422-6237
www.hhs.gov/

To encourage biomedical, social, and behavioral research, and research training directed toward greater understanding of the aging process and the diseases, special problems, and needs of people as they age.

Year Founded: 1798

3091 Aging in America
Morningside House Aging in America
1000 Pelham Parkway S
Bronx, NY 10461
718-824-4004
Fax: 413-586-1121; *Toll Free:* 877-AGI-GNY
admissiondept@aiamsh.org
www.aiamsh.org/

Dr. William Smith, President/Chief Executive Office
Julie Dalton, VP

Research and services organization for professionals in gerontology. Objectives are: to produce, implement and share effective and affordable programs and services that improve the quality of life for the elderly community; to better prepare professionals and students interested in, or currently involved with, aging and the aged.

Year Founded: 1977

3092 Alliance for Aging Research
Alliance for Aging Research
1700 K Street NW
Suite 740
Washington, DC 20006
202-293-2856
Fax: 202-955-8394; *Toll Free:* 800-497-0360
info@agingresearch.org
www.agingresearch.org

Daniel Perry, Executive Director

Gerontologists and other medical professionals, executives and members of Congress are participants. Works to increase private and public research into aging. Supports policies concerning: productive aging; independence for older Americans; successful aging. Public and professional educational literature, newsletter web site.

3093 American Aging Association
American Aging Association (AGE)
25373 Tyndall Falls Drive
Olmsted Falls, OH 44138
440-793-6565
Fax: 440-793-6598
americanaging@gmail.com
www.americanaging.org

Mitch Harman, MD, PhD, Chair
LaDora Thompson, PhD, President
Peggy Harris, Vice President

Laymen and scientists primarily in the biomedical field. Dedicated to helping people live better, longer by promoting biomedical aging studies directed toward slowing down the aging process, informing the public of the progress of aging research and of practical means of achieving a long

and healthy life and increasing knowledge of gerontology among physicians and other health workers.

Year Founded: 1970

3094 American Federation for Aging Research
American Federation for Aging Research (AFAR)
55 West 39th Street
16th Floor
New York, NY 10018
212-703-9977
Fax: 212-997-0330; *Toll Free:* 888-582-2327
info@afar.org, grants@afar.org
www.afar.org

William J. Lipton, JD, LLM, CPA, Chair
Harvey Jay Cohen, M.D., President
Holly M. Brown-Borg, Ph.D., Vice President

Year Founded: 1981

3095 Arthur M Fishberg Research Center in Neurobiology
Mt. Sinai Medical Center
PO Box 1065
New York, NY 10029
212-659-5992
Fax: 212-996-9785
www.mssm.edu.neurobio/home-page.html

Neurobiological systems in humans and mammals, emphasizing aging research. Specific interests include the neuroendocrinology of stress, reproduction and metabolism, the molecular biology of Alzheimer's disease, schizophrenia, and other neurological/psychiatric diseases, and growth factors and growth factor receptor gene expression in the central nervous system.

3096 Baylor College of Medicine: Roy M and Phyllis Gough Center on Aging
Huffington Center on Aging (HCOA)
Baylor College of Medicine
One Baylor Plaza, MS230
Houston, TX 77030
713-798-5804
Fax: 713-798-6688
pa-webteam@bcm.edu, askemployment@bcm.edu
www.hcoa.org

James T. Hackett, Chair
Carolyn Dine King, Vice Chair and Board Secretary
Paul Klotman, M.D., President & CEO

Internal unit of Baylor College representing research into the biology of aging.

Year Founded: 1943

3097 Baylor University Institute for Gerontological Studies
PO Box 97320
One Bear Place
Waco, TX 76798-7320
254-710-6400
Fax: 254-710-6455
First name_last name@baylor.edu
www.baylor.edu/gerontology

Krista Barrett, Field Education Program Manager/
Jeanie Fitzpatrick, Assistant to the Dean
Angela Pool Funai, Research and Grants Coordinator

Physical, emotional, social, and spiritual needs of older persons, including family solidarity in later life, geriatric dentistry, problems of the older offender, and life-long learning.

3098 Boston University Gerontology Center
Boston University Institute for Geriatric Social W
264 Bay State Road
Boston, MA 02215
617-358-2626
Fax: 617-358-2636
cader@bu.edu
www.bu.edu/cader/

Scott Miyake Geron, M.S.W., Ph.D, Director and Principal Investiga
Bronwyn Keefe, M.S.W., M.P.H.,, Associate Director and Academic
Kathy Kuhn, M.S.W., L.I.C.S., Director of Workforce Developmen

Gerontology, including biological, psychological, social, medical, and humanistic concerns relating to aging and the elderly. Identifies socially relevant problems in the fields of gerontology and human development, socioeconomic factors impinging upon the lives and well-being of older adults, historical context in which values and attitudes toward the aging have been defined and redefined, and the medical and social services developed to serve the older person in American society.

3099 Brain Research Institute University of California, Los Angeles
The Brain Research Institute (BRI)
1506 Gonda (Goldschmied) Neuroscience and Genetics Research Center
Los Angeles, CA 90095-1761
310-825-5061
Fax: 310-206-5855
lmaninger@mednet.ucla.edu
www.bri.ucla.edu

Christopher Evans, PhD., Director
J. David Jentsch, PhD., Associate Director for Research
Michael S. Levine, PhD., Associate Director for Education

Brain and central nervous system, including interdisciplinary studies in developmental neurobiology, molecular neurobiology, neuroanatomy, neurobiophysics, neurochemistry, neurocytology, neuroendocrinology, neuroimaging, neuromuscular physiology, neuropathology, neuropharmacology, neurophysiology, behavior, neuroimmunology, and experimental epilepsy.

Year Founded: 1959

3100 Brandeis University Institute for Health Policy
The Heller School for Social Policy and Management
415 South Street (MS 035)
Waltham, MA 02254-9110
781-736-3820
Fax: 781-736-3865
www.brandeis.edu/heller/ihp/ihp

Lisa M. Lynch, PhD., Dean
Ron Etlinger, Chief Administrative Officer
Kristen Stevens, Sr. Executive Administrator & As

Health services research and policy analysis, focusing on the design, development, implementation, and evaluation of innovative financing and delivery systems. Specific areas of research include establishing and implementing national health care expenditure limits, all-payer payment systems, an Alcohol and Drug Services Survey, the changing trends of substance abuse, financing and reimbursement of drug abuse treatment programs, and long-term care for the elderly, including home care services for the disabled elderly and cost effective models and standards for assisted living. Operates the [Center for Substance Abuse Services Research], [Center for Drug Abuse Policy Analysis], [Center on Vulnerable Populations], and the [National Resource Center].

3101 Brandeis University Policy Center on Aging
The Heller School for Social Policy and Management
415 South Street (MS 035)
Waltham, MA 02254-9110
781-736-3820
Fax: 781-736-3865
NATWONCTR@brandeis.edu
www.brandeis.edu/heller/ihp/ihp

Lisa M. Lynch, PhD., Dean
Ron Etlinger, Chief Administrative Officer
Kristen Stevens, Sr. Executive Administrator & As

Retirement income adequacy and policy, long term care and health service delivery, aging and mental health, supportive service in senior housing and resource allocation for the elderly. Generates, synthesizes, and disseminates knowledge on policy alternatives affecting the economic security of the aging; analyzes the economic, legal, administrative, and political consequences and feasibility of alternative policies; participates in the formulation and implementation of policy; and trains professionals for careers focused in the area of policy analysis.

3102 Brookdale Center for Healthy Aging and Longevity
2180 3rd Avenue
8th Floor
New York, NY 10035
212-396-7835
Fax: 212-396-7852
info@brookdale.org
www.brookdale.org

Jerry Antonatos, MPA, Dir., Finance & Administration
Ruth Finkelstein, PhD, Executive Director
Goeff Rogers, Director, Learning & Development

The Brookdale Center for Healthy Aging is a leader and innovator in public policy, research, and education related to aging and elder justice. We are a part of Hunter College, the City University of New York. We work in partnership with a wide range of agencies and non-governmental organizations to promote ethical treatment of older adults and other vulnerable populations in social service and healthcare systems and to develop educational curricula and training for professionals who work with older adults.

Year Founded: 1974

3103 Brown University Center for Gerontologyand Health Care Research
121 South Main Street
6th Floor
Providence, RI 02912
401-863-3211
Fax: 401-863-3489
CGCHR@brown.edu
www.chcr.brown.edu/

Christina Paxson, President
Elizabeth Huidekoper, Executive Vice President for Fin
Beverly Ledbetter, Vice President and General Couns

Fundamental and applied research relating to aging, chronic disease, and long-term care with particular emphasis on the assessment of function and health status and its application to diagnosis, prognosis and monitoring of long-term care. Offers data collection and teaching and training services.

Year Founded: 1764

3104 Brown University Population Studies and Training Center
Population Studies & Training Center, Brown Univer
PO Box 1836
68 Waterman St.
Providence, RI 02912
401-863-2668
Fax: 401-863-3351
Population_Studies@brown.edu
www.pstc.brown.edu/

Anna Aizer, Associate Professor of Economics
Susan M. Allen, Professor of Health Services Pol
Melani Cammett, Associate Professor of Political

Family and household demography, health and fertility transitions in developing nations, infant mortality, child health, social and economic development, migration/immigration and population distribution, aging and health in developed societies and developing nations. Develops new methods for assessing the dynamics of population change, evaluates the causes and consequences of these changes assessment of policies to influence population change. Focuses on quantitative and qualitative methods in the collection and analysis of demographic data, uses econometric and biostatistical methods in demographic analysis. Promotes the knowledge of the patterns, factors, and consequences of population change, and makes this knowledge available for formulating and evaluating population policy.

3105 Case Western Reserve University Center for Biomedical Ethics
Case Western Reserve University
10900 Euclid Avenue
Cleveland, OH 44106
216-368-2000
Fax: 216-368-8713; *Toll Free:* 800-773-2633
xx245@po.cwru.edu
www.cwru.edu/cwru/dept/med/bioethics/bio

Thomas Murray PhD, Director
Edward M Hundert, President

Bioethics, including human genetics, decisions to end life, aging, and reproductive alternatives.

Year Founded: 1826

3106 Case Western Reserve University Elderly Care Research Center
Case Western Reserve University
10900 Euclid Avenue
Cleveland, OH 44106
216-368-2000
Fax: 216-368-8713
exk@po.cwru.edu
www.cwru.edu/

Edward Hundert, President

Aging, health, and mental health, including public policy issues, predictors of wellness and vulnerability, environmental and social influences on well-being of the elderly, cross-national and cross-cultural comparisons, and health and mental health outcomes of stress, coping, and adaptation.

Year Founded: 1826

3107 Case Western Reserve University School of Medicine
Case Western Reserve University
2103 Cornell Rd.
5129 WRB
Cleveland, OH 44106-7288
216-368-3611
Fax: 216-368-0494
pathology@case.edu, pathwebmaster@case.edu
www.case.edu/med/pathology

John B Lowe MD, Chair Department of Pathology

Immunology, immunopathology, aging, cell biology, neurobiology, Alzheimer disease, oncology, and drug delivery.

Year Founded: 1826

3108 Case Western Reserve University: University Center on Aging and Health
Case Western Reserve University
10900 Euclid Avenue
Cleveland, OH 44106
216-368-2000
Fax: 216-368-6389
pxc127@case.edu
www.cwru.edu/

Diane Lynn Morris PhD RN, Director
May L Wykle PhD RN, Dean
Barbara R Snyder

Conducts, supports, and facilitates research at the University Center on Aging and Health, including the effects of stress and strains, and elderly physical health on persons over 65 years of age. Emphasizes prevention, diagnosis, treatment, management of illness or disability, and service utilization of care giver.

Year Founded: 1826

3109 Center for Human Services
University Research Co., LLC.
7200 Wisconsin Avenue
Suite 600
Bethesda, MD 20814
301-654-8338
Fax: 301-941-8427
dnicholas@urc-chs.com
www.urc-chs.com

Barbara N. Turner, President
Dr. David Nicholas, Director

Quality healthcare research
Year Founded: 1968

3110 Center for Neural Recovery and Rehabilitation Research
Helen Hayes Hospital
51-55 Route 9W North
West Haverstraw, NY 10993

845-786-4000
Fax: 845-947-3097; *Toll Free:* 888-70 -EHAB
info@helenhayeshospital.org, webmaster@helenh
www.helenhayeshospital.org/cnrrcnt.htm
TTY: 845-947-3187

Ann C. O'Sullivan, Chair
Dr. Newton Shaffer, Founder
Kathleen Sweeney, Director

Epilepsy, brain injury, and neuroendocrinology. Degenerative neurological disorders such as Huntington's and Alzheimer's diseases are also investigated.

Year Founded: 1900

3111 Center for the Study of Pharmacy and Therapeutics for the Elderly
University of Maryland School of Pharmacy
20 North Pine Street
Baltimore, MD 21201
410-706-7650
Fax: 410-706-4012; *Toll Free:* 877-706-2434
lamycenter@rx.umaryland.edu
www.pharmacy.umaryland.edu

Natalie D. Eddington, PhD, FAAPS,, Dean and Professor
William J. Cooper, Senior Associate Dean for Admini
Richard Dalby, PhD, Associate Dean for Academic Affa

Provides educational programs, researches gerontology and geriatrics. Also compiles statistics and maintains a speaker's bureau.

Year Founded: 1841

3112 Central Michigan University: Center for Adult Longitudinal Studies
Central Michigan University
1200 S. Franklin St
Mount Pleasant, MI 48859
989-774-4000
Fax: 517-794-7406
www.cmich.edu/ACA-CIC

William R. Kanine, Chair
George E. Ross, President
Michael A. Gealt, Executive Vice President/Provost

Measurement of psychological and consumer behavior dimensions of the aging process for adults over the entire lifespan.

Year Founded: 1892

3113 Columbia University Irving Center for Clinical Research
Columbia University
116th Street and Broadway,
Ph 10
New York, NY 10027
212-854-1754
Fax: 212-305-3213
www.columbia.edu/

Lee C. Bollinger, President
Robert Kasdin, Senior EVP
John H. Coatsworth, Provost

Multidisciplinary studies of human disease and clinical pharmacology. Areas include arrhythmia control, heart failure, atherosclerosis, nutrition, metabolism, clinical pharmacology, dermatology, endocrinology, hypertension, immunology, mineral metabolism and skeletal disease, neuromuscular disease, physiology, pulmonary disease, pulmonary physiology, reproductive research studies, neurology (including dementia, stroke, and seizure disorders), oncology, AIDS/infectious disease, geriatrics, epidemiology, and substance abuse.

Year Founded: 1954

3114 Coriell Institute for Medical Research
403 Haddon Avenue
Camden, NJ 08103-1505
856-966-7377
Fax: 856-964-0254
webmaster@coriell.org
www.coriell.org

Joseph L Mintzer, Executive VP/COO
Josefina J Nash, Director Information Systems

Cell and molecular biology, microbiology, genetics, aging, cancer and cancer immunology, tumor virology, antibodies, genetic disorders, vascular disorders, infectious diseases and virus/chromosome relationships, environmental mutagenesis, and genetic probes. Studies utilization of cells grown in tissue culture for isolation and characterization of tumor cell antigens, viruses, genetic abnormalities, tumor viruses, and chromosomes.

3115 Creighton University Center for Health Policy and Ethics
Creighton University
2500 California Plaza
Omaha, NE 68178
402-280-2700
Fax: 402-280-5735
info@creighton.edu
www.creighton.edu/

Steven Friedriche, Manager

Cross-cultural ethics, ethical issues involving the elderly and neonates, health care reform, legal ethics, medical economics, nursing ethics, pharmacy ethics, racial and ethnic health concerns, religious ethics, rural health policy, and women's issues.

Year Founded: 1878

3116 Creighton University Center for Healthy Aging
Creighton University
2500 California Plaza
Omaha, NE 68178
402-280-2700
Fax: 402-280-5735
info@creighton.edu
www.creighton.edu/

Timothy R. Lannon, S.J., President
Colette O'Meara-McKinney, Associate Vice President
Shirley Spain, Senior Manager

Focuses on human development, aging and health care for the elderly.

Year Founded: 1878

3117 Dartmouth College Center for Evaluative Clinical Sciences
Geisel School of Medicine
1 Rope Ferry Rd.
Hanover, NH 03755-1404
603-650-1200
Fax: 603-650-1202; *Toll Free:* 877-367-1797
Geisel.Administration@dartmouth.edu
www.dartmouth.edu/dms/cecs

Chip Souba, MD, ScD, MBA, VP & Dean
Jeff Robbins, Executive Director

Evaluative clinical science and health care delivery, including medical care epidemiology, health policy, health behavior, efficacy of medical procedures, quality of medical and surgical care, distribution of health care resources, medical interventions and consequences for patients, care at the end of life, distribution of health care resources across hospital market areas, geriatric health, and sociology of medical organizations.

Year Founded: 1797

3118 Duke University Center for the Study of Aging and Human Development
Duke University
Box 3003 DUMC
Room 3502 Busse Building, Blue Zone, Duke South
Durham, NC 27710
919-660-7500
Fax: 919-668-0453
www.geri.duke.edu

Harvey J Cohen MD, Director
Linda K. George, PhD, Associate Director
Kenneth E. Schmader, Associate Director and Director

Human and animal physiology, immunology, neuroendocrinology, pharmacology, carcinogenesis, enzyme biochemistry, free radical effects, membrane and receptor function, bone metabolism and osteoporosis, central nervous system structure and function, Alzheimer's disease, dementia, cognitive processes, psychometrics, human personality and behavior, family structure and intergenerational relationships, social factors and illness, epidemiology of agingand chronic illness, stress and coping, cell growth and differentiation, signal transduction, and the demographics and economics of aging populations. The Aging Center coordinates research, training, and clinical services in aging for the University. The Division of Geriatrics focuses research on the basic and clinical aspects of aging, emphasizing neoplasia, bone and musculoskeletal disorders and rehabilitation involved, immunology, cardiovascular diseases, cerebrovascular disease/dementia, enzymatic and cellular basis for aging, and health services delivery for the aged.

Year Founded: 1955

3119 Duke University General Clinical Research Center
Duke University
PO Box 3854
Durham, NC 27708
919-684-8111
Fax: 919-681-8829
www.duke.edu/rankincru

Harvey J Cohen MD, Director
Linda K. George, PhD, Associate Director
Kenneth E. Schmader, Associate Director and Director

Multidisciplinary, clinical research into the cause, progression, prevention, control, and cure of human disease. Sample projects have studied immunodeficiency diseases, Alzheimer's disease, food allergy, X-linked hypophosphatemic rickets, and cardiovascular disease.

Year Founded: 1955

3120 Economic and Social Research Institute
The Economic and Social Research Institute (ESRI)
Whitaker Square
Sir John Rogerson's Quay
Dublin 2, DC 20037-1235
353-1 8-3200
Fax: 353-1 8-3210
www.esri.ie/

Frances Ruane, Director

Year Founded: 1960

3121 Edmund S. Muskie School of Public Service
University of Southern Maine
PO Box 9300
Portland, ME 04104
207-780-4430
Fax: 207-780-4417; *Toll Free:* 800-800-4USM
webmaster@usm.maine.edu
usm.maine.edu/

Theodora J. Kalikow, President
Michael R. Stevenson, PhD., Provost & VP of Academic Affairs

Health, rehabilitation and special education, aging, mental health, developmental disabilities, children, youth, and families, and alcoholism. Projects include program evaluations, policy/planning analysis and research, training systems, training and curriculum materials, policy forums, and communication technologies.

Year Founded: 1988

3122 Ethel Percy Andrus Gerontology Center
USC Davis School of Gerontology
3715 McClintock Avenue
Los Angeles, CA 90089-0191
213-740-5156
Fax: 213-740-8241
ldsgero@usc.edu
www.usc.edu/gero

Pinchas Cohen, M.D.,, Dean
Jen Brewer, Administrative Assistant
Maria Henke, M.A., Associate Dean

Gerontology, including interdisciplinary studies on biological, behavioral, social, and environmental aspects of aging process. Develops and evaluates curricula for training scientific and professional personnel specializing in study of aging processes and for improving associated personal, medical and social disorders, cognitive behavior, employment and retirement, state politics of aging, Alzheimer's disease, income maintenance and more.nd reproductive aspects of aging. Also responsible for coordination of graduate and postgraduate instruction and research training in gerontology conducted within academic disciplines of architecture, biology, economics, education, linguistics, pharmacy, political science, psychology, psychiatry, public administration, urban and regional planning, social work, and sociology at the University.

Year Founded: 1975

3123 Families and Work Institute
Families and Work Institute
267 5th Avenue
Floor 2
New York, NY 10016-7503

212-465-2044
Fax: 212-465-8637
www.familiesandwork.org

Ellen Galinsky, President and Co-Founder
Anne Weisberg, Vice President - Strategy
John Boose, Art Director

Child care, elder care, family and work issues, men and families, diversity, flexibility, community planning, organizational change, and public policy.

Year Founded: 1989

3124 Florida Policy Exchange Center on Aging
Florida Policy Exchange Center on Aging (FPECA)
13301 Bruce B. Downs Blvd.
MHC 1300
Tampa, FL 33612
813-974-2414
Fax: 813-974-5766
fpeca.cbcs.usf.edu/

Larry Polivka, Director
Kathryn Hyer, Ph.D., MPP, Associate Professor and Director

Aging and aging related issues and policies, particularly effective, innovative programs for elderly in other countries. Activities include studies on crime, housing, health care, aging, service delivery issues, and other issues regarding the elderly.

Year Founded: 1992

3125 Florida State University: Pepper Institute on Aging and Public Policy
Florida State University
600 W. College Avenue
Tallahassee, FL 32306
850-644-2525
Fax: 850-644-2304
mhardy@garnet.acns.fsu.edu
www.fsu.edu/pia

Melissa Hardy, Contact

Public policy issues affecting the elderly, including health care, income security, and social welfare. Research programs have included historical and comparative studies of income security programs for the elderly, the elderly in the work force, the elderly and the political system, gender and racial dimensions of poverty in old age, retirement decisions, elder abuse in Florida health care facilities, and alternatives to nursing home care and health care financing.

3126 Fordham University Third Age Center
Fordham University
Rose Hill Campus
Bronx, NY 10458
718-817-1000
Fax: 718-817-4769
www.fordham.edu

Concentrates on the intellectual, emotional, economic, spiritual, and cultural opportunities that confront the elderly. Programs include studies on the interface of informal and formal support systems, long-term care and service delivery, alternative forms of housing, older persons in families, neighborhood ethnography, life styles of the suburban elderly, employment and the older worker, religion and aging.

3127 Georgia Consortium on the Psychology of Aging
Institute of Gerontology
255 E. Hancock Avenue
University of Georgia
Athens, GA 30602-5775
706-425-3222
Fax: 706-425-3221
gerontology@uga.edu
www.geron.uga.edu

Toni P. Miles, Director
Anne P. Glass, Associate Director and Graduate
Kerstin Gers Emerson, Assistant Professor

Psychology of aging, including basic studies in cognition, and clinical diagnosis and treatment of behavioral dysfunctions most often found with the aged. The Consortium was formed to share training and research resources and to foster interaction between psychologists and other scientists.

Year Founded: 1785

3128 Georgia State University Center for Mature Consumer Studies
Georgia State University
P.O. Box 3965
Atlanta, GA 30302-3965
404-880-9595
Fax: 404-651-4198
gmoschis@gsu.edu
www.gsu.edu/mkteer/cmcs

Mark Becker, President
Jimmy George, Manager

Mature consumer marketing, with emphasis on industries of special importance to the older consumer, including financial services, health care, housing, leisure, insurance, technology, mass media, and telecommunications industries. Studies include analysis of older consumer needs, lifestyles, purchasing habits and consumption patterns. Serves as an information resource, assisting in strategy development for reaching the mature consumer market.

3129 Geriatrics Education and Research Institute
University of North Texas Health
3500 Camp Bowie Blvd.
Fort Worth, TX 76107
817-735-2600
Fax: 817-735-2486
tfairchi@hsc.unt.edu
unthsc.edu/

Michael R Williams, DO, MD, MBA, President
Jennifer M Treviño, MBA, Vice President of Administration
Thomas Yorio, PhD, Provost and EVP Academic Affairs

Biology of aging, including fundamental chemical and molecular biological changes that may cause aging; health promotion in older adults including health programs promoting physical, psychological, and social well being; geriatric care and practice including evaluation of new clinical programs, physical/mental functions, long term care system development focusing on case management, and in-home health screen/assessment of home-bound elderly.

Year Founded: 1970

3130 Gerontological Society of America
Gerontological Society of America
1220 L Street North West
Washington, DC 20005
202-842-1275
Fax: 202-842-1150
geron@geron.org
www.geron.org

James Appleby, Executive Director and CEO
Linda Krogh Harootyan, Deputy Executive Director
Chris Yoder, Senior Director, Finance and Adm

The society was formed in 1945 to promote the scientific study of aging, to encourage exchanges among researchers and practitioners from the various disciplines related to gerontology and to foster the use of gerontological research in forming public policy. Publishes five scientific journals.

Year Founded: 1945

3131 Harvard Brain Tissue Resource Center
Harvard Brain Tissue Resource Center
115 Mill Street
Belmont, MA 02478-1041
Toll Free: 800-272-4622
hbtrc@mclean.harvard.edu
www.brainbank.mclean.org

Francine M. Benes, M.D., Ph.D., Director
John C. Hedreen, MD, Associate Director, Chief of Neu
T. Wilson Woo, MD, PhD, Associate Director

Provides tissues to the neuroscience community for studies of movement disorders, major psychoses, and dementia.

3132 Harvard University Division of Health Policy Research and Education
Harvard School of Public Health
Office of Admissions
158 Longwood Avenue
Boston, MA 02115-5810
617-432-1031
Fax: 617-432-7080
newhouse@hcp.med.harvard.edu
www.hsph.harvard.edu/

Julio Frenk, Dean
David Hunter, Dean for Academic Affairs
Michael Grusby, Sr. Associate Dean Academic Affa

Coordinates health policy resources throughout the University, including suggestion of new research initiatives, stimulation of educational activities, coordination of research and educational efforts, promotion of multidisciplinary analysis of complex health policy issues, and dissemination of health policy findings.

Year Founded: 1913

3133 Harvey A. Friedman Center for Aging
Washington University in St. Louis
Campus Box 8217
660 S. Euclid
Saint Louis, MO 63110
314-747-9212
Fax: 888-617-4513
publichealth@wustl.edu
wucfa.wustl.edu

Lenise Cummings-Vaughn, MD, Assistant Professor

The Center promotes research, education, policy and service initiatives that enable older adults to remain healthy, active, empowered, contributing and independent for as long as possible.

Year Founded: 1998

3134 Huffington Center on Aging
Baylor College of Medicine
1 Baylor Plaza
Houston, TX 77030
713-798-4951
Fax: 713-798-6688
askemployment@bcm.edu, pa-webteam@bcm.edu
www.bcm.edu/

Paul Klotman, M.D, President and CEO
Steve Sigworth, MD, VP & Chief Medical Officer
Lorie Tabak, Chief of Staff

Cell and molecular biology of aging, cardiovascular disease, and ethics in long-term care.

Year Founded: 1900

3135 Hunter College of City University of New York: Brookdale Center on Aging
Hunter College
695 Park Ave
New York, NY 10065
212-772-4000
Fax: 646-366-1041
www.hunter.cuny.edu

Jennifer J. Raab, President
Vita Rabinowitz, Provost and Vice President
Eija Ayravainen, Vice President

Legal support program for social workers, paralegals, attorneys and other professionals engaged in providing advocacy assistance to the elderly poor.

Year Founded: 1870

3136 Indiana Family Institute
Indiana Family Institute
140 North First Street
Zionsville, IN 46077
317-423-9178
Fax: 317-423-9421; *Toll Free:* 800-269-2959
www.hoosierfamily.org

Ryan McCann, Director of Operations and Publi
Curt Smith, Journalist
John Brockma Crane, Author

Family issues research.

3137 Indiana University Bloomington Center on Aging and Aged
Indiana University Bloomington
107 S. Indiana Ave.
Bloomington, IN 47405-7000
812-855-4848
Fax: 812-855-6194
AskIU@iu.edu
www.indiana.edu/rugs/ctrdir/caa

Suzanne Thorin, Manager

Gerontology, including developmentally disabled, handicapped, minorities, rural-isolated, and mainstream aging populations.

3138 Indiana University: Purdue University at Indianapolis Hackney Dermatopathology Research Laboratory

Indiana University Indianapolis
420 University Blvd.
Indianapolis, IN 46202
317-274-5555
AskIU@iu.edu
www.indiana.edu/rugs/ctrdir/hdrl

Daniel F Spandau, Director
Charles Bantz, Manager

Skin diseases, including skin cancer and psoriasis and the genetic changes that occur with these conditions. Wound healing and the aging of skin are also studied.

3139 Institute for Community Inclusion

Institute for Community Inclusion
100 Morrissey Boulevard
Boston, MA 02125
617-287-4300
Fax: 617-287-4352
ici@umb.edu
www.communityinclusion.org
TTY: 617-287-4350

William Kiernan, Director
Quinn Barbour, Contact

Research in health issues and the community.
Year Founded: 1967

3140 International Center for the Disabled

340 E 24th Street
New York, NY 10010
212-585-6020
Fax: 212-585-6002
jkirk@icdnyc.org
www.icdnyc.org

Justin B. Wender, Chair
Dr. Richard Weber, Vice Chair
Christopher Wu, Vice Chair

Promising techniques designed to prevent, reduce, and control disabilities arising from persistent physical disorders. Studies focus on the control of deterioration and disability associated with recurring ear infections in children, symptom magnification in those with disabling conditions, and factors associated with gainful employment. Other projects examine the parameters of post-laryngectomy speech, nerve conduction patterns in overuse syndromes, relapse factors in alcoholism, and methods used in the management of individuals with Alzheimer's disease. Techniques that prove effective are transferred to ICD clinical programs and communicated to professionals nationally and internationally.

3141 Johns Hopkins University Institute for Policy Studies

Wyman Building
3400 N Charles Street
Baltimore, MD 21218-2608
410-516-7174
Fax: 410-516-8233
ips.jhu.edu

William R Brody, CEO
Donald Steinwachs,Ph.D., Interim Director
Carey Borkoski, Ph.D., Assistant Director

Economic development, at risk youth, economic structural change, problems of the elderly, future of the welfare state, the role of nonprofit organizations, youth employment, human resource investment, crime and delinquency, public finance, housing, regional capital flows.

3142 Johns Hopkins University: Center for Immunization Research

Johns Hopkins University School of Hygiene
624 North Broadway
Room 117
Baltimore, MD 21295
410-955-1622
Fax: 410-955-2791
www.jhsph.edu/research/centers-and-insti

Dr. Ruth Karron, Director
Florence C. George, Finance Manager
Frederick San Mateo, BA, Senior Programmer/Analyst

Research in vaccine immunization

3143 Kent State University Exercise Physiology Lab

162 Gym Annex
Kent, OH 44242-0001
330-672-2930
Fax: 330-672-2250
eglickma@kent.edu
www.kent.edu/ehhs/exph/index.cfm

Ellen L Glickman, PhD FACSM, Professor, Exercise Physiology &

Exercise physiology, body composition, and physical fitness, including studies of protein metabolism and exercise, cardiovascular/respiratory responses during exercise in heat and cold, an neuromuscular integration/biomechanics, and psychosocial reactivity to behavioral stressors.

3144 Lion's Club International

300 W 22nd Street
Oak Brook, IL 60523-8842
630-571-5466
Fax: 630-571-8890
lions@lionsclubs.org
www.lionsclubs.org

Barry J. Palmer, International President
Joseph Preston, First Vice President
Dr. Jitsuhir Yamada, Second Vice President

International organization with over 1.4 million members dedicated to the largest blindness prevention program ('SightFirst').

3145 Maharishi International University: Lab for Health & Aging Studies

1000 N 4th Street
Fairfield, IA 52557
641-472-7000
www.mum.edu

DR. Craig Pearson, Executive Vice president

3146 Mankind Research Foundation

1315 Apple Avenue
Silver Spring, MD 20910-3307
301-587-8686
Fax: 301-587-8688
www.uvbi.com

Dr. Carl Schneider, President
Nader A Dakak MD

General health research

Year Founded: 1973

3147 Massachusetts Institute of Technology General Clinical Research Center

77 Massachusetts Ave
Cambridge, MA 2139-4307
617-253-1000
dick@mit.edu
TTY: 61- 25- 934

Dr. Richard J Wartman, Program Director
Joe Graham, Manager

Normal human metabolism, physiology, and behavior, including studies on hormones (melatonin and sleep), fates of deuterated amino acids, behavioral and neuroendocrine effect of foods (carbohydrate, protein, and caffeine), effects of drugs on memory and other behaviors, and endocrine and metabolic effects on aging. Also studies human diseases such as obesity, Alzheimer's disease, brain injury, Parkinson's disease, seasonal depression, use of brain imaging techniques to follow metabolic events, and facilitation of smoking withdrawal by psychopharmacologic agents.

3148 Mayo Clinic and Foundation-General Clinical Research Center

St. Mary's Hospital
200 First Street SW
Rochester, MN 55905
507-284-2511
Fax: 507-538-7802
andersen@mayo.edu
www.mayoclinic.org

Jeffrey Rome, Manager

Researches inpatient and outpatient sleep pattern, cardiac telemetry monitoring, endocrinology and many other medical issues.

Year Founded: 1971

3149 Minneapolis Medical Research Foundation

701 Park Avenue
Suite PP7.700
Minneapolis, MN 55415
612- 87- 53
www.mmrf.org

Paul Pentel, President
Carla Erickson, Director

General health research

Year Founded: 1952

3150 Mount Sinai School of Medicine of City University of New York

Department of Geriatrics & Adult Development
PO Box 1070
New York, NY 10029
212-241-5561
Fax: 212-860-9737
www.icahn.mssm.edu

Siu Albert, Chair

Health, long-term care, and productive aging, emphasizing policy implications for future generations and institutions.

3151 National Institute on Aging

US Department of Health & Human Services
31 Center Drive
Room 5c27
Bethesda, MD 2292
301-496-1752
Fax: 301-496-1072
www.nia.nih.gov

The Institute conducts and supports biomedical and behavioral research to increase the knowledge of the aging process and associated physical, psychological, and social factors resulting from advanced age. Incontinence, menopause, susceptibility to disease, and memory loss are among the areas of special concern.

3152 National Institute on Aging Gerontology Research Center

251 Bayview Boulevard
Suite 100
Baltimore, MD 21224-6825
410-558-8110
longod@grc.nia.nih.gov
www.grc.nia.nih.gov/

Robin Barr, Director

Gerontology research, including molecular genetics, human physiology, personality, behavioral research, and Alzheimer's disease studies.

3153 National Institute on Aging: Information Center

31 Center Drive
Room 5c27
Bethesda, MD 20892
301-496-1752Toll free: 800-222-2225
www.nia.nih.gov

Richard J. Hodes, M.D., Director
Marie A. Bernard, M.D., Deputy Director
Patrick Shirdon, Director of Management

Concerned with the health problems of older Americans. The Center offers free printed materials, including fact sheets about going to the hospital and about prostate problems.

3154 Neuropsychiatric Research Institute

700 1st Avenue S
Fargo, ND 58103
701-293-1335
Fax: 701-293-3226
mail@nrifargo.com
www.narifargo.com

James Mitchell, President

Basic and clinical studies of the central nervous system. Specific applications include eating disorders, studies of Alzheimer's disease, Parkinson's disease, Huntington's disease, and schizophrenia.

3155 New York State Institute for Basic Research in Developmental Disabilities

1050 Forest Hill Road
Staten Island, NY 10314-6399
718-494-0600
Fax: 718-494-0833
www.omr.state.ny.us/

Dr Piotr B Kozlowski, Director
William T Brown MD

3156 Nisonger Center for Mental Retardation and Developmental Disabilities
Ohio State University
281 W. Lane Avenue
Columbus, OH 43210
614-292-8365
Fax: 614-292-3727
reiss.7@osu.edu
www.osu.edu

Steven Reiss, Executive Director

Developmental disabilities, psychometric assessment, rehabilitation engineering, psychopathology, psychopharmacology, adults and aging, and family studies. Special attention given to applied research related to mental retardation and development and implementation of training programs to prepare professional personnel to work with the developmentally disabled. Provides early childhood classes for developmentally disabled preschoolers and offers information services to clients, students, staff, and faculty.

3157 Noll Physiological Research Center
Pennsylvania State University
129 Noll Laboratory Building
University Park, PA 16802
814-865-3453
Fax: 814-865-4602
www.noll.psu.edu

Metabolic adaptations to stress, biology of aging, and environmental and exercise physiology. Studies the effects of aging, physical activity, nutritional status, and heat, cold, and altitude stress on muscle metabolism and function, thermoregulation and cardiovascular control, immune function, and carbohydrate, insulin, and protein metabolism.

3158 Northwestern University: Buehler Center on Aging
750 N Lake Shore Drive
Suite 601
Chicago, IL 60611
312-503-3087
Fax: 312-503-5868
www.nwu.edu/aging/index.htm

Dr. James R Webster, Director
Linda Emmanuel, Executive Director

Aging research

Year Founded: 1982

3159 Northwestern University: General Clinical Research Center
303 E Chicago Avenue
Chicago, IL 60611-3072
312-503-8649
www.northwestern.edu

Ennio C Rossi MD

Year Founded: 1961

3160 Ohio State University Neuroscience Program
333 W 10th Avenue
Columbus, OH 43210
614-292-2379
ngsp@osu.edu
www.ngsp.osu.edu

Spinal cord injury, tumor biology, neuromuscular disease, epilepsy, Parkinson Disease, multiple sclerosis, stroke, neu-

ral development, regeneration, plasticity, regeneration, molecular neurobiology, and neuroimmunology.

3161 Olive View: UCLA Education and Researchnstitute
14445 Olive View Drive
Sylmar, CA 91342
818-364-3205
ovinfo@earthlink.net
www.uclaoliveview.org

Soma Wali, MD, FACP, Program Director
Michael Rotblatt, MD, PharmD, Sr. Associate Program Director
Richard Tennant, MD, Associate Program Director

Researches head injury, neurology, perinatal issues, genetic counseling and other health related studies.

Year Founded: 1986

3162 Oregon Research Institute
1776 Millrace Drive
Eugene, OR 97403
541-484-2123
Fax: 541-484-1108
www.ori.org

Amy Greenwold, Manager

Behavioral sciences, including studies in tobacco prevention and cessation, compliance with diabetic regimens, children's social skills, personality structure, drug abuse prevention, depression and family interaction, special education technology, adolescent depression, and community child-rearing practices. Provides behavioral research and consultation services to other public and private agencies in fields of education, health, and mental health.

3163 Orentreich Foundation for the Advancement of Science
855 Route 301
Cold Spring, NY 10516
845-265-4200
www.orentreich.org

Norman Orentreich, President

Dermatology, aging, endocrinology, and serum markers for human diseases.

3164 Pennsylvania State University Center for Developmental and Health Genetics
101 Amy Gardner House
University Park, PA 16802
814-865-5471
Fax: 814-863-4768
www.psu.edu

Gerald McCleam, Director
Randy Deike, Manager

Role of genetics in infant, child, and adolescent behavioral development, in aging, and in common drug and health problems. Also studies molecular, nutritional and immunological genetics. Uses human and animal model research projects to study personality, cognition, functional capacity, immune system functioning, and use and effects of alcohol and tobacco.

3165 Pennsylvania State University Gerontology Center
312 Old Main
University Park, PA 16802

814-865-7517
arh1@psu.edu
www.hhdev.psu.edu/CENTERS

Broad interdisciplinary approach to questions on aging. Major areas of research are cognition in aging, developmental methodology, family and informal supports, and animal models of aging. Specific topics include reversing cognitive decline, human services for the elderly, caregiving, urinary incontinence, and the use of pharmaceutical products.

3166 Pennsylvania State University: Noll Physiological Research Center
129 Noll Laboratory Building
University Park, PA 16802
814-865-3453
Fax: 814-865-4602
www.noll.psu.edu

Researches metabolic adaptations to stress, the effects of physical activities, nutritional status and other related topics.

Year Founded: 1963

3167 Peter Lamy Center for Drug Therapy and Aging
University of Maryland School Pharmacy
20 North Pine Street
Baltimore, MD 21201
410-706-7650
Fax: 410-706-4012
lamycenter@rx.umaryland.edu
www.pharmacy.umaryland.edu

Natalie D. Eddington, PhD, FAAPS,, Dean

The Lamy Center is dedicated to improving drug therapy for aging adults through innovative research, education and clinical initiatives.

3168 Population Reference Bureau
1875 Connecticut Avenue NW
Suite 520
Washington, DC 20009
202-328-3937
Fax: 202-328-3937; *Toll Free:* 800-877-9881
popref@prb.org
www.prb.org

James Scott, President, CEO

Demography, particularly national and international population trends as they relate to education, aging, employment, minority populations, health and welfare, and the environment.

3169 Portland State University Institute on Aging
PO Box 751
Portland, OR 97207-0751
503-725-4043
www.upa.pdx.edu/ioa

Alba Scholz, Manager

Adult development and aging, including health and social care systems, social and economic life maintenance, political behavior, age status, economic behavior, social and psychological phenomena, and communication.

3170 Purdue University: Center for Research on Aging
1202 W. State Street
West Lafayette, IN 47907-2055
765-494-9692
Fax: 765-494-2180
www.purdue.edu/aging

Kenneth F. Ferraro, Ph.D., Director

Social science research on aging, health and health care delivery.

3171 Rehabilitation Research and Training Center on Aging With a Disability
Rancho Los Amigos Medical Center
7601 Imperial Highway
Downey, CA 90242
562-401-7111
www.agingwithdisability.org
TDD 562-401-
TTY: 562-401-8450

Jorge Orozco, PT, CEO

Aging research

3172 Research Institute of the Hebrew Home of Greater Washington
6121 Montrose Road
Rockville, MD 20852
301-881-0300
Fax: 301-770-8309
cohen-mansfield@hebrew-home.org
www.hebrew.org

Warren R. Slavin, CEO/President
Douglas W. Sherman, Secretary

Gerontology, aging, and issues concerning the elderly, focusing on nursing home residents, their families, and staff. Areas include: agitated behaviors among the elderly; stress in families caring for elderly relatives; staff stress; back injuries among staff caretakers; the preferences of nursing home residents regarding life-sustaining treatments; standardized assessment procedures of the physical and emotional states of nursing home residents; sleep patterns of nursing home residents; the use of physical restraints in the nursing home; and the use of psychotropic medication in the nursing home.

3173 Retirement Research Foundation
8765 W Higgins Road
Suite 430
Chicago, IL 60631-4170
773-714-8080
Fax: 773-714-8089
info@rrf.org
www.fdncenter.org/grantmaker/rrf/new

Patrick McCarthy, President/CEO

Supports research to improve the well-being of elderly persons in the US Also provides support for model demonstration projects.

3174 Rockefeller University Laboratory of Neuroendocrinology
1230 York Avenue
New York, NY 10065
e-mail: Bruce.McEwen@rockefeller.edu
www.rockefeller.edu

Seeks to locate brain sites and understand the mechanisms by which hormones promote neural plasticity and thereby alter endocrine function, behavior, neurological states, and mood. Also studies the influence of gonadal and adrenal hormones on aging in the brain.

3175 Rush University Neuroscience Institute
Rush-Presbyterian-St. Luke's Medical Center
1653 W Congress Pkwy
Chicago, IL 60612
312-942-5000
www.rush.edu

Dr. Jacob H Fox, Chairperson
Larry J. Goodman, CEO

Alzheimer's disease, Parkinson's disease, and stroke, including community-based studies, clinical investigations, and laboratory investigations using brain tissue and animal experimentation. Studies also focus on development of new drugs to improve symptoms of multiple sclerosis.

3176 Rush University: Rush Institute for Healthy Aging
1645 W Jackson Boulevard
Suite 675
Chicago, IL 60612-3276
312-421-8940
Fax: 312-942-2861
devans2@rush.edu
www.rush.edu

Dennis A Evans PhD, Contact

Epidemiology of Alzheimer's disease, community-based studies of Alzheimer's disease and other common problems of older persons, physical functions among older persons, and statistical methods in aging research.

3177 Rutgers University Institute for Health, Health Care Policy: and Aging Research
112 Paterson Street
New Brunswick, NJ 08901-1293
848- 93- 841
caboyer@rci.rutgers.edu
www.ihhcpar.rutgers.edu

Joel C. Cantor, Sc.D., Director

Research divisions include and focus on the impact of stress on emotional states and health and risk behaviors and how these latter factors influence the immune system and morbidity and mortality.ms.

3178 San Jose State University Gerontology Education and Training Center
1 Washington Square
San Jose, CA 95112
408-924-1000
www.sjsu.edu/

Gerontology and the social aspects of aging, focusing on personal autonomy of elderly persons in long-term care and ethnogerontology.

3179 SeniorNet
5237 Summerlin Commons Boulevard
Suite 314
Fort Myers, FL 33907
239-275-2202
Fax: 239- 27- 250

seniornet@aol.com
www.seniornet.org

Interaction between computers and older individuals through online telecomputer system. Studies include psychological effects of the computer on the individual at the introduction, learning, and user levels.

3180 Southwest Foundation for Biomedical Research
PO Box 760549
San Antonio, TX 78245-0549
210- 25- 940
fledford@sfbr.org
www.txbiomed.org/

Richard Schlosberg, Chairman
Lewis J. Moorman III, Vice Chairman

Aging research
Year Founded: 1941

3181 Syracuse University Biological Research Laboratories
Syracuse University
114 Life Sciences Complex
Syracuse, NY 13244
315-443-3186
Fax: 314-443-2012
hrlevy@mailbox.syr.edu
www.biology.syr.edu

Aging and aging conditions research.

3182 Syracuse University Center for Policy Research
426 Eggers Hall
Syracuse, NY 13244-1020
315-443-3114
Fax: 314-443-1081
ctrpol@syr.edu
www-cpr.maxwell.syr.edu

Leonard M. Lopoo, Director

Economics and demography of aging, income security policy, long-term care, gender and minority aging, and cross-national aging comparisons.

3183 Tampa Bay Research Institute
10900 Roosevelt Boulevard N
St Petersburg, FL 33716
727-576-6675
Fax: 727-577-9862
www.tbri.org

Akiko Tanaka, CEO

3184 Temple University: General Clinical Research Center
Medical education and research Building
Room 1040
Philadelphia, PA 19140
215-707-4045
Fax: 215-707-0170
www.temple.edu

Bryant Tabb, Director

3185 Thomas Jefferson University: Center for Research in Medical Education
Jefferson Medical College
1025 Walnut Street
Room 119
Philadelphia, PA 19107

215-955-8907
Fax: 215-923-6939
www.jefferson.edu

Joseph Gonnella MD, Director

3186 Tulane University Occupational Lung Disease Center
School of Medicine
1430 Tulane Avenue
New Orleans, LA 70112
504-988-5187
www.tulane.edu

Dr. Hans Weill, Director
James V Talano MD

3187 UCSF Memory and Aging Center
Sandler Neurosciences Center
675 Nelson Rising Lane, Suite 190
San Francisco, CA 94143
415-353-2057
www.memory.ucsf.edu

Dr. Bruce Miller, Director

The UCSF Memory and Aging Center provides the highest quality of care for individuals with cognitive problems, to conduct research for degenerative brain diseases, and to educate health professionals, patients, and their families. The Memory and Aging Center also publishes a biannual newsletter, as well as other publications.

Year Founded: 1998

3188 USDA Human Nutrition Research Center on Aging
711 Washington Street
Boston, MA 02111
617- 55- 300
www.hnrca.tufts.edu

Simin Nibkin Meydani, D.V.M., Director

Investigates the relationship of nutrition to aging, including research programs in nutrient metabolism, nutrient requirements, nutritional epidemiology, functional systems, and drug-nutrient interactions.

3189 University at Albany: State University of New York Ringel Institute of Gerontology
State University of New York
135 West Avenue
Albany, NY 12222
518-442-5346
Fax: 518-442-3823
iog@albany.edu
www.albany.edu/iog

Frank D Andraia, Executive Director

Applied research on aging, primarily in the social sciences, and services for the elderly, including studies on institutional and noninstitutional care of the elderly, nursing homes, day care, foster home care, the church as service provider, retirement and preretirement, and other social aspects of aging. Collaborates in the development of community programs and their evaluation.

3190 University of Akron Institute for Life Span Development and Gerontology
University of Akron
340 Arts and Sciences Building
Akron, OH 44325-4307

330-972-6724
Fax: 330-972-5174
hsterns@uakron.edu
www3.uakron.edu/ilsdg

Harvey L Sterns, Director

Improving older adult cognitive functioning, aging and work, mental retardation and aging, training and retraining adult older workers, gender identity, human development, health and aging, and family and aging. Programs concentrate on aging changes in perception, perceptual style, selective attention, and learning and memory. Other studies focus on performance appraisal and selection of older adult workers.

3191 University of California, San Francisco Center for Social and Behavioral Sciences
3333 California Street
San Francisco, CA 94143-0612
415- 47- 304
Fax: 415-826-3381
www.nursing.ucsf.edu

Morris Schambelan, MD

Sponsors pre- and postdoctoral research and training activities in the areas of stress and illness, cognitive factors in health behavior, mental health and aging, adult development, gerontology, Alzheimer's Disease, and AIDS.

3192 University of California: Center for Health & Community
3333 California Street
Suite 465
San Francisco, CA 94143-0844
415-476-7408
Fax: 415-502-1010
chc@chc.ucsf.edu
www.chc.ucsf.edu

Nancy E Adler PhD, Director
Dina Dudum MPA, Manager

Facilitate multidisciplinary research that will provide comprehensive understanding of problems of health, illness and health care.

Year Founded: 1984

3193 University of California: San Diego Center for Population Research
06339500 Gilman Drive
La Jolla, CA 92093
858-534-3703
repromed@ucsd.edu
www.repromed.ucsd.edu

Homer G Chin, Chief, Obstetrics & Gynecology
Steven C Plaxe, Chief, Gynecologic Oncology
Thomas R Moore, Director, Perinatal Medicine

Hypothalamic control of the pituitary and gonadal function in human and animal models, focusing on issues related to neuroendicrine metabolic dysfunction in the aging population.

3194 University of California: San Francisco Institute for Health and Aging
Laurel Hights Campus 3333
Suite 340
San Francisco, CA 94143

415-502-5200
Fax: 415-502-5208
www.nurseweb.ucsf.edu/iha
Wendy Max, Director
Lena Borodina, Manager

Aging health policy issues and policy alternatives; state discretionary policies in long-term care, social services, and income maintenance; private sector involvement in supporting health and social services for the elderly; effects of intergovernmental relations and state and federal fiscal conditions on services to the elderly; coordination between state and local aging programs and health planning, financing, and regulatory programs; specialhealth and social service needs of the low-income, isolated elderly; enrollment of the elderly in health maintenance and social/health organizations; gender issues; Alzheimers' disease resources and program evaluation; AIDS; international alcohol; health promotion and injury and disease prevention; disability statistics; and health status of the elderly, with special emphasis on selected acute and chronic health conditions.

3195 University of Chicago Brain Research Institute
5801 South Ellis Avenue
Chicago, IL 60637
773-702-1234
infocenter@uchicago.edu
www.uchicago.edu

Bryce Wier MD, Director
Sue Curtis, Manager

Alzheimer's disease, amyotrophic lateral sclerosis, myasthenia gravis, AIDS, sleep and sleep disorders, dyslexia, hyperkinesia, epilepsy and epileptoid disorders, mental retardation, mental illness, and brain and nervous system disorders such as multiple sclerosis, muscular dystrophy, cerebral palsy, encephalitis, Parkinson's disease, stroke, cerebral hemorrhage, aneurysm tumor, head injury, and intractable pain. Conducts basic research in neurophysiology, neuropharmacology, neuroanatomy, molecular biology, neuroimmunology, and virology.

3196 University of Chicago Committee on Human Development
5736 S Woodlawn Avenue
Chicago, IL 60637
773-702-3971
www.humdev.uchicago.edu

Susan Cohen, Manager

Conducts research and graduate study in life course development (including child and adolescent development, adult development and aging, and philosophy of development), mental health research (including personality psychology), and cross-cultural studies (including psychological anthropology and cultural psychology). Seeks to provide education for innovative careers in research and teaching, and to contribute to the interdisciplinary understanding of human behavior.

3197 University of Connecticut Health Center: Biomolecular Structure Analysis Center
263 Farmington Avenue
Farmington, CT 06030
860-679-2000

Dr. Leo G Herbette, Director
Lee Ann Maximowicz, Administrator

Drug-membrane interaction, drug-receptor interaction, membrane drug design, pulmonary surfactant research, and collagen structure research as it relates to cardiology, alcoholism, Alzheimer's disease, CNS disorders, skeletal and smooth muscle disorders, and atherosclerosis.

3198 University of Florida Brain Institute
JHMHC
PO Box 100015
Gainesville, FL 32610-0015
352-273-8500
Fax: 352-846-0185
www.ufbi.ufl.edu

William G Luttge PhD, Director

Peripheral Nerve Trauma Research Program, including biomaterials research, peripheral nerve regeneration, and mechanisms and control of pain associated with peripheral nerve trauma; Head Injury Research Program, including injury- and/or stroke-induced problems with memory, language, attention, emotion, motor skills, and epilepsy; molecular, cellular, and immunological mechanisms involved in nerve cell death and injury following stroke or closed head injury; Neurodegenerative Diseases Program, including molecular biologic studies of genetic bases of a variety of neurologic dysfunctions, including neurodegenerative movement disorders, cell biological studies on Batten's disease, and cell biological and MRI studies of laboratory animal models of multiple sclerosis. Additional studies include the underlying causes of Alzheimer's disease; the neurobiological consequences of alcohol and cocaine abuse in both adults and fetuses; and the molecular and cellular mechanisms and the behavioral and neurologic consequences of such viral-induced neurodegenerative diseases as AIDS, polio, and measles.

3199 University of Florida Health Policy and Epidemiology
2004 Mowry Road
PO Box 100231
Gainesville, FL 32610
352-273-5468
www.hpe.ufl.edu

Dr. Thomas A. Pearson, Executice VP

Policy research and evaluations of long-term care and aging, hospital cost controls, regulatory and administrative methods in the health sector, health economics and financing, maternal and child health, HIV/AIDS, community epidemiology, outcomes research.

3200 University of Florida: Claude D Pepper Center for Research on Oral Health in Aging
PO Box 100405
Gainesville, FL 32610
352-273-5800
mheft@dental.ufl.edu
www.dental.ufl.edu

Health services research and basic oral-health functions of the elderly, including the development of periodontal disease, the effects of medications on saliva production, and the effects of aging on the senses.

3201 University of Florida: Institute for Gerontology
PO Box 117335
Gainesville, FL 32611

352-392-3261
rwest@geron.ufl.edu
www.gerou.ufl.edu

Robin Lea West, Contact

Faculty associates conduct interdisciplinary studies on family economic status, labor force participation and survivorship in life course perspective, alternative living environments for older people, political attitudes and policy issues in aging, preventive health self-care learning for intergenerational groups, nutritional status of elderly, memory fitness and intelligence in adulthood and old age, training needs of counselors and physician assistants, age-sensitive counseling and self-help resource development, geriatric dentistry, older driver fitness and transportation safety, ambulatory health care case mix management for older persons, caregiving, and demography.

3202 University of Georgia: Gerontology Center

255 E. Hancock Avenue
Athens, GA 30602-5775
706-425-3222
Fax: 706-425-3221
gerontology@uga.edu
www.geron.uga.edu

Leonard W Poon PhD, Director

Aging, focusing on applied gerontology, demography as it relates to the aged, mental and physical health of the oldest-old, Alzheimer's disease and other dementia in the aged, and cognitive aging, especially memory for pictures.

3203 University of Illinois Health Systems Research
College of Medicine

1601 Parkview Avenue
Rockford, IL 61107
815-395-5630
Fax: 815-395-5602; *Toll Free:* 800-854-4461
www.rockford.uic.edu/hsr.htm

Joel B Cowen, Assistant Dean

Community health, including primary care, public health, geriatrics, substance abuse, evaluation of delivery of health services, survey research, focus groups, demographic studies, health care planning, program evaluation, and feasibility studies.

3204 University of Iowa Center for Health Services
Research

200 Hawkins Drive
Iowa City, IA 52242
319-384-3830
www.public-health.uiowa.edu/hmp/

Delivery, organization, and financing of health care. Studies the health practices and needs of specific populations such as individuals in rural areas. Develops multidisciplinary research teams from the University's ten colleges and facilitates interaction between researchers, policy makers, and providers to address regional health care problems.

3205 University of Kansas Laboratory of Biological
Anthropology
Department of Anthropology

622 Fraiser Hall
Lawrence, KS 66045
785-864-4172
crawford@ku.edu
www.ukans.edu

Michael H Crawford PhD, Director

Cancer etiology, twin research, aging and longevity, genetic epidemiology, anthropological genetics in Saint Vincent, Hungary, Mexico, Siberia, Belize, rural and urban US ethnic enclaves, dental anthropology, forensic medicine, and skeletal identification.

3206 University of Kansas Neurobiology Research
Laboratory

4801 E Linwood Boulevard
Kansas City, MO 64128-2226
816-861-4700
Fax: 816-922-3375
www.kumc.edu/kcbamc/research/nbrl

Barry W Festoff, Director
Kent Hill, Executive Director

Development, plasticity, and diseases of the nervous system. Studies focus on synaptic formation and metabolism; roles of serine proteases and inhibitors (serpins); regulation of amyloid precursor protein processing in Alzheimer's disease; and biological markers in head injuries.

3207 University of Kansas: Center on Aging
Kansas University Medical Center

3901 Rainbow Boulevard
Kansas City, KS 66160
913-588-5000
Fax: 913-588-1201
www2.kumc.edu/coa

Linda J Redford, RN, PhD, Director

Provides support for interdisciplinary research on issues of age and aging.

3208 University of Kansas: Gerontology Center

1000 Sunnyside Avenue
Room 3090
Lawrence, KS 66045-7555
785-864-4130
Fax: 785-864-5063
www.gerontology.ku.edu

David J. Ekerdt, Director

Aging and the problems of the aged, including applied and social gerontology, family caregiving, minority aging, service to the aging, cognitive aging, and housing options for elders.

3209 University of Kentucky: Sanders-Brown Center
on Aging

800 S Limestone Street
Lexington, KY 40536-0230
859-323-6040
Fax: 859-323-2866
www.mc.uky.edu/coa

Linda J. Van Eldik, PhD, Director

Biology of aging, including studies on the aging nervous systems, Alzheimer's disease, stroke, immunology.

3210 University of Maryland Division of Infectious
Diseases

10 S Pine Street
Room 900
Baltimore, MD 21201-1116
410-706-7560Toll free: 800-492-5538
www.umm.edu

Infections in the elderly, including infection from urinary catheterization, epidemiology of nursing home patients, tests of antimicrobial agents, and pharmacokinetics and microbiology using animal models and clinical techniques.

3211 University of Maryland: Center for the Study of Pharmacy and Therapeutics for the Elderly
School of Pharmacy
20 N Pine Street
Baltimore, MD 21201
410-706-7650
Fax: 410-706-4012
www.pharmacy.unmaryland.edu

Natalie D Eddington, PhD, FAAPS,, Dean

Geriatrics and gerontology, focusing on drug use in the elderly and the development of artificial intelligence programs in support of optimal drug use. Also responsible for three elder care programs, the Parke-Davis Center for the Education of the Elderly, the Elder-Health Program, and the Maryland Caregiver Program.

3212 University of Maryland: Center on Aging
2367 SPH Building
College Park, MD 20742-2611
301-405-2469
Fax: 301-405-2542
lwilson@umd.edu
www.sph.umd.edu/hlsa/aging

Laura B Wilson, Contact
Sue Anne Schwartz, Coordinator

Gerontology, including senior service and volunteerism, long-term care financing, service credit banking, informal caregiving, aging and disabilities, productive aging, health care delivery systems and cost containment. Conducts health assessment and longitudinal data base projects on aging in the Interdisciplinary Health Research Laboratory.

Year Founded: 1974

3213 University of Massachusetts at Boston: Gerontology Institute and Center
100 Morrissey Boulevard
Dorchester, MA 02125
617-287-7300
Fax: 617-287-7080
geronto@umb.edu
www.geront.umb.edu

Robert P Gerary, Managing Editor

Aging Journal of Aging social policy, including health care, economics, security, long-term care, productive aging, systems delivery, older women's issues, and minority issues.

110 pages Frequency: Quarterly

3214 University of Miami Center for Neurological Diseases
PO Box 16960
Miami, FL 33101-6960
305-243-6732
Fax: 305-243-1632; Toll Free: 800-707-5589
www.neurologu.med.miami.edu

Adams David MD, Contact
Matilde Camjel, Manager

Neuroscience, including physiological, neurochemical, anatomical, metabolic, neuropharmacological and vascular mechanisms that account for normal brain function, and the changes in these which underlie neurological diseases such

as stroke, senile dementia, epilepsy, Parkinson's syndrome, Alzheimer's disease, multiple sclerosis, amyotrophic lateral sclerosis (ALS), and other neurological dysfunctions.

3215 University of Miami Touch Research Institute
PO Box 16820
Miami, FL 33101-6820
305-585-5160
Fax: 305-243-6488
www.miami.edu/touch-research

Tiffany M Field PhD, Contact
Noris Reyes, Manager

Sense of touch, including the biology of touch in health and development, and the role of touch therapy in medicine and the treatment of disease. Specific research areas include the use of massage in enhancing immune function in AIDS and cancer patients, massage effects on growth in premature infants, underlying mechanism responsible for the relationship between touch and physical growth and emotional development in infants and children, the role of massage in sports medicine and wound healing, the effects of touch therapy on addictive personalities, pain reduction during invasive medical procedures, and alleviation of skin disorders such as eczema and psoriasis. Studies the effects of touch on persons of all ages.

3216 University of Miami: Center on Adult Development and Aging
1695 N.W. 9th Avenue
Suite 3204
Miami, FL 33136
305-355-9080
Fax: 305-355-9076
centeronaging.med.miami.edu

Chaerles B. Nemeroff, M.D., Ph.D, Director

Biochemistry, neuropsychiatry, and clinical treatment of Alzheimer's disease and related disorders, including brain reactive antibodies and autoimmune responses. Also studies ethnicity and aging, human factors and aging, aging and developmental disabilities, biology of aging, osteoporosis, social and behavioral patterns of older persons and families, stress and aging, nutrition and aging, and demographics of elderly population in Florida and specific areas in Florida, including studies relating to the migration of elderly persons around the U.S., and the improvement of the quality of life for the elderly. Recently, awarded 11-year contract for the Women's Health Intiative, a 45-site national longitudinal clinical trial which follows the health of post-menopausal women.

3217 University of Michigan Center for Human Growth and Development
500 S. State Street
Ann Arbor, MI 48109
734-764-1817
blozoff@umich.edu
www.umich.edu/tld/chgd

Betsy Lozoff PhD, Director

Human growth and development through childhood and adolescence, including interdisciplinary studies on normal and abnormal behavioral, physical, and mental development, focusing especially on the challenges to children who grow up in adverse conditions.

3218 University of Michigan: Antiviral Laboratory
4222 School of Dentistry
1500 E. Medical Center Drive
Ann Arbor, MI 48109
734-615-0863 Toll free: 855-855-0863
jcdrach@umich.edu
www.umich.edu

Dr. John C Drach Hd, Contact

Antiviral research

Year Founded: 1970

3219 University of Michigan: Institute of Gerontology
300 N Ingalls Street
Ann Arbor, MI 48109-2007
734-764-3493
Fax: 734-936-2116
www.med.umich.edu

Joan A Faulkner PhD, Director

Gerontological research studies in the behavioral, biological, clinical, and social sciences and the humanities.

3220 University of Minnesota: Center on Aging
School of Public Health
PO Box 197
Minneapolis, MN 55455
612-624-1185
www.coa.umn.edu
Aging.

3221 University of Missouri Kansas City: Center for Aging Studies
5100 Rockhill Road
Kansas City, MO 64110
816-235-1000
breytspraak@umkc.edu
www.iml.umkc.edu/cas

Stephen W Lehmkuhle, Manager

Caregiving to the elderly, health care systems and costs, health promotion/disease prevention, public perceptions of Social Security, voluntarism among the elderly, the care of Chinese elderly, and rural elderly. Rural studies include program assessment and testing in areas of health promotion/disease prevention, caregiving intergenerational relationships and the elderly, transportation, and housing.

3222 University of North Dakota: UND Centerfor Rural Health
501 North Columbia Road Stop 9037
Grand Forks, ND 58202-9307
701- 77- 384
Fax: 701-777-6779
bgibbens@medicine.nodak.edu
medicine.nodak.edu/crh

Gary Hart, PhD, Director

Rural health care delivery, especially in the areas of health professional shortage areas, the viability of rural health facilities, aging population, Native American health care, and uncompensated care. Collaborates with other research organizations throughout the nation.

3223 University of North Texas Health Science Center at Forth Worth: Geriatrics Education and Research Institute
3500 Camp Bowie Boulevard
Fort Worth, TX 76107
817-735-2000
tfairchi@hsc.unt.edu
www.hsc.unt.edu/research.aging.htm

Michael R Williams, DO, MD, MBA, President
Jennifer M Treviño, MBA, VP

Geriatric research.

Year Founded: 1991

3224 University of North Texas: Center for Studies in Aging
Department of Applied Gerontology
PO Box 310919
Denton, TX 76203
940-565-2411
Fax: 940-565-4370
lusky@scs.cmm.unt.edu
www.unt.edu/aging

Donald Grose, Manager

Social gerontology, including employee job performance in nursing homes, impact of leadership on culture of nursing homes and retirement communities, the Native American elderly, development of databases and models for community services planning, geriatric programs in community health centers, mediation and aging, and the low-income minority elderly. Conducts demographic, social-psychological, and evaluation studies and surveys for cities, labor unions, churches, and other client groups.

3225 University of Northern Iowa: Center for Social and Behavioral Research
College of Social & Behaviora
Cedar Falls, IA 50614
319-273-2311
GENE.LUTZ@UNI.EDU
www.csbs.csbs.uni.edu/college/centers/cs

Robert D Koob, CEO

Geography, history, home economics, political science, psychology, sociology, anthropology, criminology, social work, and public policy, including studies on adolescents, adult education, airline passengers, airports, educational needs assessment, elderly, environmental impact assessment, highways, human services needs assessment, outdoor recreation, radio listening habits, substance abuse, and television viewing habits. Performs feasbility studies on proposed projects such as sports complexes and auditoriums. Conducts special surveys for groups, organizations, localities, regions, and social aggregates.

3226 University of Pennsylvania Institute on Aging
3615 Chestnut Street
Philadelphia, PA 19104-2676
215-662-2746
Fax: 215-573-8684
www.med.upenn.edu/aging

John Q. Trojanowski, MD, PhD, Director
Laura Trean, Manager

Biomedical and social science research on aging, including cellular mechanisms of aging, Alzheimer's disease, sleep disturbances, arthritis, osteoporosis, population demographics of aging, nursing home quality, organization and structure of life care communities, social security, and social support systems for the aged.

3227 University of Pennsylvania: Center for Clinical Epidemiology and Biostatistics
School of Medicine
423 Guardian Drive
Philadelphia, PA 19104-6021
215-898-0901
strom@cceb.upenn.edu
www.cceb.med.upenn.edu

Harold I. Feldman, MD, MSCE, Director

Epidemiology of disease and risk factors of clinical importance, especially pharamacoepidemiology, molecular epidemiology, cancer, cardiovascular disease, renal disease, women's health, reproductive epidemiology, emergency medicine, injury, and aging.

3228 University of Pittsburgh University Center for Social and Urban Research
121 University Place
Pittsburgh, PA 15260-2600
412-624-4141
Fax: 412-624-4810
www.pitt.edu/ucsur

Urban and regional analysis, child and family development, gerontology, intergenerational studies, and environmental policy. Conducts survey research, sampling, and data processing and analysis. Research findings are used for policy making at the international, national, regional, and local levels.

3229 University of South Dakota Social Science Research Institute
414 E Clark Street
Vermillion, SD 5706
605-677-6240
www.usd.edu

James W. Abbott, President

Research includes studies on organizations, economic and social development, criminology, juvenile delinquency, child abuse, aged population, communications, social work and welfare, court administration, jury selection and community surveys for litigation, prison education, alcoholism, medical and educational problems on American Indian reservations, and follow-up on juvenile offenders. Conducts anthropological studies, including site preservation.

3230 University of Southern California: Institute for Health Promotion and Disease Prevention Research
Health sciences campus
Los Angeles, CA 90033
323- 44- 110
carljohn@hsc.usc.edu
www.usc.edu/go/ipr

C Anderson Johnson PhD, Director

Disease prevention

Year Founded: 1980

3231 University of Tennessee: Knoxville Society for the Study of Social Problems
906 McClung Tower
Knoxville, TN 37996

865-974-3620
Fax: 865-974-7013
tomhood@utk.edu
www.it.utk.edu/sssp

Dr. Thomas C Hood, Executive Officer

Community research and development; crime and juvenile delinquency; drinking and drugs; racial and ethnic minorities; conflict, social action, and change; the family; poverty, class, and inequality; psychiatric sociology; social problems theory; sociology and social welfare; youth, aging, and the life course; educational problems; environment and technology; labor studies; sexual behavior; politics and communities; law and society; and health and health policy and services.

3232 University of Texas-Houston Health Science Center Mental Sciences Institute
University of Texas
7000 Fannin Street
Houston, TX 77030
713-500-3130
www.uth.tmc.edu/med/msi/index

Giuseppe N. Colasurdo, M.D., President

Biochemical and behavioral aspects of psychiatric diseases, particularly physiopathology and pharmacology of alcohol and drug addiction, and affective and anxiety disorders. Performs basic and clinical studies in neuroendocrinology, metabolism, behavioral science, disorders, mental retardation, neurochemistry, psychophysiology, biochemistry, crime and delinquency, and gerontology.

3233 University of Utah Human Performance Research Laboratory
250 S 1850 E
Room 200
Salt Lake City, UT 84112
801-581-8379
www.health.utah.edu

Kerry Jacques, Director

Effects of exercise and environment on muscular, cardiovascular, respiratory, nervous, and thermoregulatory systems of the human body. Programs are conducted on exercise and multiple sclerosis patients, women at risk for osteoporosis, exercise and functional abilities and health benefits.

3234 University of Utah: Gerontology Center
10 South 2000 East
Salt Lake City, UT 84112
801-581-3414
nursing.utah.edu/

Health and social sciences as they relate to the aged, including long-term care, gerontology curriculum and standards, bereavement of the elderly, in-home and respite care services, the family as a support system, family caregiving, and intergenerational families.

3235 University of Washington Northwest: Geriatric Education Center
PO Box 357262
Seattle, WA 98195-7262
206-616-4276
Fax: 206-616-3064
sgural@u.washington.edu
nwgec.org/

Provides education and training in geriatrics to health professionals, educators, and practitioners in Washington, Alaska, Montana, and Idaho.

3236 University of West Florida: Center on Aging
Department of Social Work
11000 University Parkway
Pensacola, FL 32514
850- 47- 329
beechems@prodigy.net
www.uwf.edu/coa

John Cavanaugh, President

Gerontology, including rural elderly, housing, and death. Develops and evaluates training material for aging services.

3237 University of Wisconsin-Madison
Neuropsychology Laboratory
600 Highland Avenue
Madison, WI 53792
608-262-1818
Fax: 608-263-6211
www.uwhealth.org

Clinical neuropsychology in neuropsychological correlates of epilepsy, cognitive and affective changes in aging, and differential diagnosis of dementia with a view toward cognitive and memory remediation.

3238 University of Wisconsin: Madison Institute on Aging
1300 University Avenue
Madison, WI 53706
608-262-1818
Fax: 608-263-6211
aging@ssc.wisc.edu
www.aging.wisc.edu

Carol Ryff, Director

Aging, including life course studies, biogerontology, social geroltology, and clinical geriatrics. Specific areas of study include, but are not limited to, Alzheimer's disease, caloric intake, coping with later life stress, demography, falls after hospital discharge, free radicals, housing and environment for older adults, muscle loss, osteoporosis, resilience in adulthood, primates, psychological well-being, swallowing disorders, and visual systems.

3239 University of Wisconsin: Milwaukee Institute on Aging and Environment
School of Architecture and Urban Planning
PO Box 413
Milwaukee, WI 53201
414-229-2991
Fax: 414-229-6976
aging@uwm.edu
www.uwm.edu/dept/iae

Uriel Cohen, Director

Interaction betweeen the aged and the environment, with emphasis on environments for people with dementia. Specific issues include innovative environmental planning, programming, and design practice for enhancement of the quality of life of older persons; behavioral and social impacts of institutional settings; constraints of zoning in the creation of innovative forms of community housing; optimal thermal and luminous conditions for older persons; and the social history of the nursing home as a building type.

3240 Veterans Affairs Medical Center: Geriatric Research, Education and Clinical Center
1601 SW Archer Road
Gainesville, FL 32608-1135
352-374-6051
Fax: 352-371-6142
dlowenth@pharmacology.ufl.edu
www.med.ufl.edu/pharm/facdata/GRECC

Luann Cox, Manager

Geropharmacology, including mechanisms of drug action, pharmacokinetics, therapeutic uses, drug abuse, polypharmacy and drug compliance as it applies to geriatric patients. Clinical research is conducted in the areas of exercise in the healthy, frail, and elderly, cardiovascular function, and cognitive disorders in the elderly. Basic research is conducted in pharmacologic mechanisms of temperature regulation, obesity, febril response to infections, immunology, and muscle strength.

3241 Virginia Center on Aging
Virginia Commonwealth University
730 East Broad Street
Richmond, VA 23298-0239
804-828-1525
Fax: 804-828-7905
lhwaters@hsc.vcu.edu
www.sahp.vcu.edu/vcoa/
Edward F Ansello, Director
Connie Coogle PhD, Assoc. Director of Research

Mental and physical health of the elderly, focusing on community-living and health-related factors of aging. Studies include: eldercare responsibilities of employed family caregivers, staffing requirements in residential care facilities, impact of aging of adults with developmental disabilities, minority healthcare utilization, caregiving of demented elders, research and documentation project on rural geropharmacy.

3242 Wayne State University Center for Health Research
5557 Cass Avenue
Detroit, MI 48202
313-577-4135
Fax: 313-577-5777
www.nursing.wayne.edu/

Nursing, urban health, pain reduction in hospitalized children, adolescent health, teen pregnancy, aging, chronicity, health education and promotion (e.g. smoking cessation), community health, psychosocial oncology, health behavior, self care, stress and coping, parent/child health, family health, caregivers of aged individuals, drug use, violence and abuse, sleep patterns, risk-taking with respect to teen pregnancy and sexually transmitted diseases (including HIV), and transcultural nursing. Multidisciplinary studies involve health professionals and faculty members from disciplines such as nursing, psychology, sociology, anthropology, medicine, and epidemiology.

3243 Wayne State University: Institute of Gerontology
87 E Ferry Street
Detroit, MI 48202
313- 66- 260
Fax: 313-664-2666
ioginfo@wayne.edu
www.iog.wayne.edu

Tina Abbott, Chair

Gerontology, including studies on public policy, acute and long-term health care, service delivery, aging process, family relations, and work and retirement.

3244 Wichita State University: Gerontology Center

1845 Fairmount Street
Wichita, KS 67260
316-978-3456
www.webs.wichita.edu

Dr. Teresa Radebaugh, Director

Gerontology.

3245 Woodrow Wilson School of Public and International Affairs: Center for Health Care Strategies
Princeton University

353 Nassau Street
Princeton, NJ 08540-1013
609-258-4800
mail@chcs.org
www.chcs.org

Christopher Eisgruber, CEO

Development and implementation of effective health and social policy for all Americans.

3246 Yeshiva University: Resnick Gerontology Center
Albert Einstein College of Medicine

1300 Morris Park Avenue
Bronx, NY 10461
718-430-2000
crystal@aecom.yu.edu
www.einstein.yu.edu/

Joe Verghese, Chief

Alzheimer's disease and other dementia. Conducts the [Bronx Aging Study], a ten-year longitudinal study of the Bronx elderly. Also conducts a teaching nursing project, a biochemical research assessment program, and drug studies.

3247 AIDS Community Resources
ACR Health
627 West Genesee Street
Syracuse, NY 13204
315-475-2430
Fax: 315-472-6515; *Toll Free:* 800-475-2430
information@ACRhealth.org
acrhealth.org

Shannon O'Connor, Chair
Anthony Adornato, Vice Chair
Franchesca Clemente, Secretary

ACR Health is a not-for-profit, community-based organization providing a range of support services to individuals with chronic diseases, including HIV/AIDS, diabetes, heart disease, obesity, asthma, substance use disorders, and serious mental illnesses, with the goal of positive health outcomes. ACR Health provides a wide variety of targeted prevention and sexual health services to individuals, from youth through adulthood, as well as to communit y groups and organizations, with the goal of informed and responsible decision making.

Year Founded: 1983

3248 AIDSinfo
P.O. Box 4780
Rockville, MD 20849-6303
Fax: 301-315-2818; *Toll Free:* 800-448-0440
contactus@aidsinfo.nih.gov
www.aidsinfo.nih.gov
TTY: 888-480-3739

A call-in service where trained staff offers quick access to federally approved HIV/AIDS treatment and prevention guidelines, clinical trials, and other research-related information. AIDSinfo is a U.S. Department of Health and Human Services (DHHS) project that offers the latest federally approved information on HIV/AIDS clinical research, treatment and prevention, and medical practice guidelines for people living with HIV/AIDS, their families and friends, health care providers, scientists, and researchers.

Year Founded: 2002

3249 American Civil Liberties Union: HIV
125 Broad Street
18th Floor
New York, NY 10004
212-549-2500
www.aclu.org

Susan N. Herman, President
Anthony D. Romero, Executive Director
Dorothy M. Ehrlich, Deputy Executive Director

Offers legislative and employment information, public awareness materials and support for persons with HIV/AIDS and their families.

Year Founded: 1920; Number of Members: 500,000+

3250 CDC National Prevention Information Network
800-232-4636
npin-info@cdc.gov
npin.cdc.gov
TTY: 888-232-6348

CDCNPIN is the US reference, referral and distribution service for informtion on HIV/AIDS, STOs and TB.

3251 Committee of Ten Thousand
202-681-2351
info@cott1.org
www.cott1.org

Carl Weixler, President
Mary Lou Murphy, Co-Vice President
Terry MacNeill, Co-Vice President

The Committee of Ten Thousand is an education, advocacy and support organization for persons with hemophilia who contracted HIV/AIDS from tainted blood products.

Year Founded: 1989

3252 HIV Wisdom for Older Women
340 Southwest Blvd
Kansas City, KS 66103-2150
913-722-3100
Fax: 913-722-2542
jane@hivwisdom.org
www.hivwisdom.org

Jane P. Fowler, Director

HIV prevention in older women and support for those who are infected.

Year Founded: 2002

3253 Health Education AIDS Liaison (HEAL)
347-867-4497
michaelellner2@gmail.com
www.healaids.com

Michael Ellner, President
Roberto Giraldo, MD, Board Member
Barnett J Weiss, Board Member

Alternative and holistic support groups and resources for people with HIV.

Year Founded: 1982

3254 Health Information Network
7211 Greenwood Avenue N
Seattle, WA 98103
206-784-5655
Fax: 206-784-3240
information@healthinfonetwork.org
www.healthinfonetwork.org

Offers information, public awareness and support for women with HIV/AIDS and the public in general.

Year Founded: 1981

3255 Immune Deficiency Foundation
110 West Road
Suite 300
Towson, MD 21204
Fax: 410-321-9165; *Toll Free:* 800-296-4433
primaryimmune.org

John G Boyle, President & CEO
Sarah Rose, CFO
Christoper Scalchunes, VP, Research

The only national charitable organization aimed at fighting the primary immune deficiency diseases. The founders included parents of children with primary immune deficiency, immunologists who treat immune deficient patients and other individuals with an interest in helping others. The Foundation's main goal is to improve the care and treatment of adults and children with primary immune deficiency diseases and to promote public education and awareness about the diseases.

Year Founded: 1980

3256 Life Force: Women Fighting AIDS
NYC Service
175 Remsen Street
Suite 1100
Brooklyn, NY 11201
718-797-0937
Fax: 718-797-4011
www.nycservice.org/organizations/138

Nur Ibrahim, Treasurer

A support network offering legislative information, educational awareness and support for women with HIV/AIDS.

Year Founded: 1989

3257 NAMES Project Foundation: AIDS MemorialQuilt
204 14th Street NW
Atlanta, GA 30318-5304
404-688-5500
Fax: 404-688-5552
info@aidsquilt.org
www.aidsquilt.org

Julie Rhoad, Executive Director

To preserve, care for, and use the AIDS Memorial Quilt to foster healing, heighten awareness, and inspire action in the struggle against HIV and AIDS.

Year Founded: 1987

3258 National AIDS Housing Coalition
727 15th Street NW
11th Floor
Washington, DC 20005
202-347-0333
Fax: 202-347-3411
rbennett@nationalaidshousing.org
nationalaidshousing.org

Arturo Bendixen, President
Jeff Allen, Secretary
Charlie Frew, Treasurer

Works to end the HIV/AIDS epidemic by ensuring that persons living with the condition have quality, affordable, and appropriate housing.

3259 National Association on HIV over Fifty
38 Chauncy Street
Suite 500
Boston, MA 02111
617-233-7107
Fax: 617-262-5667
hivoverfifty.org

NAHOF is a membership organization promoting the availability of a full range of education, prevention, service, and health care programs for people over age 50 and affected by HIV.

3260 National Hospice and Palliative Care Organization
1731 King Street
Suite 100
Alexandria, VA 22314
703-837-1500
Fax: 703-837-1233; *Toll Free:* 800-646-6460
nhpco_info@nhpco.org
www.nhpco.org

Edo Banach, President & CEO
John Mastrojoin III, Chief Operating Officer
Cathy Gibney, Chief Financial Officer

The organization is committed to improving end of life care and expanding access to hospice care with the goal of profoundly enhancing quality of life for people dying in America, and their loved ones.

Year Founded: 1978

3261 National Minority AIDS Council
1000 Vermont Avenue NW
Suite 200
Washington, DC 20005
202-483-6622
Fax: 202-483-1135
communications@nmac.org
nmac.org

Paul Kawata, Executive Director

Mission is to develop leadership in communitites of color to end the HIV/AIDS epidemic.

3262 National Native American AIDS Prevention Center
1031 33rd Street
Suite 270
Denver, CO 80205
720-382-2244
Fax: 720-382-2248
www.nnaapc.org

Alexander White Tail Feather, Executive Director

Sole mission of this organization is to promote AIDS education, prevention and cures for Native Americans suffering from the illness.

Year Founded: 1987

3263 Project Inform
273 Ninth Street
San Francisco, CA 94103
415-558-8669
Fax: 415-558-0684; *Toll Free:* 877-435-7443
www.projectinform.org

Dana Van Gorder, Executive Director

Project Inform encourages the development of better treatments and cures for both HIV and hepatitis C.

3264 URSA Institute
390 4th Street
San Francisco, CA 94107
415-777-1922
info@ursa-institute.org
www.ursa-institute.org

Social policies, including AIDS prevention and education, crime and justice, aging, economic development, health care, housing, mental health, substance abuse, public education, public media, and public advertising.

3265 Whitman-Walker Health
Washington, DC
202-745-7000
www.whitman-walker.org

Mark Edward, Chair

Community health centers in Washington with expertise in LGBT & HIV care.

Year Founded: 1973

Books

3266 100 Questions and Answers About AIDS and HIV
Jones and Bartlett Publishers
5 Wall Street
Burlington, MA 01803
978-443-5000
Fax: 978-443-8000; *Toll Free:* 800-832-0034
info@jbpub.com
www.jbpub.com

Joel E Gallant MD/MPH, Author

Provides answers to the most common questions asked by patients with HIV and AIDS, their partners, and their family members. An invaluable resource for people with HIV infection or for those who care about them. Also includes useful information on prevention and testing for HIV-negative readers.

209 pages 1907

3267 AIDS: Distinguishing Between Fact and Opinion
Greenhaven Press
PO Box 9187
Farmington Hills, MI 48333-9187
www.gale.cengage.com/

Bruce Glassman, Owner

For beginning debaters, reports and classroom use this book offers three debates: Can AIDS be spread by casual contact? Should the Food and Drug Administration make AIDS drugs more available? Is AIDS a moral issue?.

3268 About AIDS
New Readers Press
104 Marcellus Street
Syracuse, NY 13204
800-448-8878Toll free: 866-894-2100
www.newreaderspress.com

3269 An Annotated Bibliography of Recent Empirical Research in Methadone
National Clearinghouse for Alcohol and Drug Info.
PO Box 2345
Rockville, MD 20847-2345
301-468-2600
Fax: 301-468-2600; *Toll Free:* 800-729-6686
healthliteracy.worlded.org/

Provides guidelines and suggestions to investigators engaged in the demanding and essential task of followup research on intravenous drug users who have contracted AIDS.

97 pages

3270 Color of Light
Hazelden
PO Box 11
Center City, MN 55012-0011
651-213-4200
Fax: 651-213-4793; *Toll Free:* 800-328-9000
customersupport@hazelden.org
www.hazelden.org

Ellen Breyer, President

These 366 meditations speak to both the practical and spiritual journey of living with HIV/AIDS, and demonstrate how to integrate personal values with those offered in chemical dependency recovery and the Twelve Steps.

400 pages

3271 Guide to Living With HIV Infection
Johns Hopkins University Press
2715 N Charles Street
Baltimore, MD 21218-4319
410-516-6900
Fax: 410-516-6998; *Toll Free:* 800-537-5487
www.jhu.edu/press/index.html

William Brody, President

This guidebook includes detailed discussions of new drugs; special considerations of the stages of infection; facts about opportunistic infection; and new information on prevention.

440 pages

3272 HIV/AIDS and Older Adults: Challenges for Individuals, Families, and Communities
Springer Publishing Company
11 West 42nd Street
15th Floor
New York, NY 10036
Fax: 212-941-7842; *Toll Free:* 877-687-7476
www.springerpub.com

Charles A Emlet MSW/PhD, Editor

Focuses on the ways in which HIV/AIDS can affect older adults. The chapters in this book discuss the variety of HIV/AIDS problems that we face at the individual, family and community levels.

216 pages 1904

3273 HIV: Third Edition
American College of Physicians
190 North Independence Mall West
Philadelphia, PA 19106-1572
215-351-2400Toll free: 800-523-1546
www.acponline.org

Susan Thompson Hingle, Chair

This comprehensively revised and updated new edition features all the practical guidance physicians need to care for HIV-infected patients. Details antiretroviral therapy; opportunistic infections, common clinical syndromes, long-term treatment complications; and the mangement of HIV in women, pregnant women, minorities, IV-drug users, and other special populations.

446 pages

3274 Learning AIDS
American Foundation for AIDS Research
120 Wall Street
Floor 13
New York, NY 10005-3908
212-806-1600
Fax: 212-806-1601; *Toll Free:* 800-392-6327
www.amfar.org

Kenneth Cole, Chairman

Lists organizations that distribute materials and information.

3275 Longitudinal Studies of HIV Infection in Intravenous Drug Users
National Clearinghouse for Alcohol and Drug Info.
PO Box 2345
Rockville, MD 20847-2345
301-468-2600
Fax: 301-468-2600; *Toll Free:* 800-729-6686
www.health.org

This monograph is based upon papers and discussions from a NIDA technical review concerned with the methodological problems encountered in natural history studies of drug-related AIDS.

3276 Lving Well with HIV & AIDS
Bull Publishing Company
PO Box 1377
Boulder, CO 80306
800-676-2855
Fax: 303-545-6354
www.bullpub.com

Allen L Gifford MD, Author
Kate Lorig RN, Author
Diana Laurent MPH, Author

Offers the latest information based on the HIV care guidelines from the Department of Health & Human Services and the Center for Disease Control. Discusses a shift in treatments emphasis to the ways of managing side effects such as lypodystrophy, redistribution of body fat, cardiac risks, and concerns with vulnerability to other aliments called comorbidities.

295 pages

3277 No Longer Immune: A Counselor's Guide to AIDS
American Counseling Association
5999 Stevenson Avenue
Alexandria, VA 22304-3304
800-347-6647
Fax: 800-473-2329; *Toll Free:* 800-347-6647
www.counseling.org

Covers a broad range of issues such as working with specific populations, handling pre- and posttesting situations, coping with fear, grief and survivor guilt, preventing caregiver burnout and dealing with countertransference.

295 pages

3278 Psychosocial Interventions in HIV Illness
Jason Aronson
PO Box 15100
York, PA 17405-7100
Fax: 201-840-7242; *Toll Free:* 800-782-0015
www.aronson.com

240 pages

3279 The First Year: HIV: An Essential Guide for the Newly Diagnosed
Perseus Books Group
250 West 57th Street
15th Floor
New York, NY 10016
212-340-8100
www.perseusbooksgroup.com

Brett Grodeck

Guides readers through their first seven days following diagnosis, then the next three weeks of their first month, and finally the next eleven months of their first year-to provide answers and advice that will help everyone newly diagnosed with HIV come to terms with their condition and the lifestyle changes that accompany it.

1903

3280 The Guide to Living with HIV Infection
Johns Hopkins University Press
2715 North Charles Street
Baltimore, MD 21218-4363
410-516-6900
Fax: 410-516-6968
www.press.jhu.edu

John G Bartlett MD, Author
Ann K Finkbeiner, Author

Developed at the Johns Hopkins AIDS Clinic is the most complete source of medical, emotional, social, and practical advice available for those infected with HIV and their loved ones. Provides essential information for making decisions about treatment and testing in a world transformed by new research and pharamcotherapy.

408 pages 1906

Directories

3281 AIDS Action Bulletin
AIDS Action Baltimore
10 E Eager Street
Apartment 1
Baltimore, MD 21202
410-837-2437
Fax: 410-837-2438
www.aidsactionbaltimore.org/

A directory of clinical research in AIDS for Baltimore and Washington.

3282 AIDS Crisis in America
ABC-CLIO
PO Box 1911
Santa Barbara, CA 93116-1911
805-968-1911
Fax: 805-685-9685; *Toll Free:* 800-368-6868
www.abc-clio.com/

Mary Ellen Hombs, Editor

Directory of organizations in the U.S that deal with AIDS issues.

268 pages

3283 AIDS Directory
LRP Publications
747 Dresher Road, Suite 500
P.O. Box 980
Horsham, PA 19044

215-784-0860
Fax: 215-784-9639; *Toll Free:* 800-341-7874
www.lrp.com
TDD 215-658-0938

William Feldman, Editor

Directory of over 1,5000 educational, prevention, research and treatment organizations and government agencies working at national and state awareness.

808 pages

3284 AIDS Funding: A Guide to Giving by Foundations & Charitable Organizations
Foundation Center
79 5th Avenue
New York, NY 10003-3034
212-620-4230
Fax: 212- 80- 367; *Toll Free:* 800-424-9836
foundationcenter.org/

Sara Engelhardt, President

Includes current information on the grantmaking programs of foundations and corparate giving programs as well as public charities.

206 pages Frequency: 1997

3285 AIDS and Deafness: Resource Directory
CDC National Aids Clearinghouse
PO Box 6003
Rockville, MD 20849-6003
800-458-5231
Fax: 301-562-1050; *Toll Free:* 800-243-7012
www.cdcnpin.org/

Computer printout. Lists national, state, and local organizations that offer AIDS (Acquired Immune Deficiency Syndrome)-related services to deaf and hard-of-hearing people; coverage includes Canada and the United Kingdom. Entries include: Organization name, address, phone, hotline numbers, hours of operation, access procedures, TTY/TDD numbers, names and titles of key personnel, geographic area served, description, product/service.
Databasecompiled in cooperation with Gallaudet Research Institute at Gallaudet University.

3286 AIDS/HIV Treatment Directory
American Foundation for AIDS Research
120 Wall Street
Floor 13
New York, NY 10005-3908
212-806-1600
Fax: 212-806-1601; *Toll Free:* 800-392-6327
www.amfar.org

Jerome Radwin, Manager

Directory has resources and assistance as well as lists active recruiting clinical tests on approved and experimental treatments for HIV, AIDS and opportunitistic infections.

Frequency: Biennial

3287 Local AIDS Services: The National Directory
US Conference of Mayors
1620 I Street NW
Washington, DC 20006-4005
202-293-7330
Fax: 202-293-2352
info@usmayors.org
usmayors.org/

2,500 organizations that provide various information and services for AIDS coordinators and other health-related professionals.

3288 New York State Directory of AIDS/HIV Clinical Trials
Treatment Information Services - AmFAR
120 Wall Street
Floor 13
New York, NY 10005-3908
212-806-1600
Fax: 212-806-1601
giving.amfar.org

Jerome Radwin, Manager

Provides the reader with easy to read, accurate information on clinical trials which are enrolling patients at sites throughout New York State and the surrounding area.

3289 Resources and Services Database
Centers for Disease Control
1600 Clifton Road NE
Atlanta, GA 30333
Toll Free: 800-232-4636
www.cdc.gov/

Describes more than 16,000 organizations that provide HIV and AIDS prevention, education and social services. These include public health departments, community and social service organizations, hospitals and clinics.

Journals, Magazines

3290 Critical Path AIDS Project/AIDS Library
1233 Locust Street
5th Floor
Philadelphia, PA 19107
215- 98- 444
fight.org/

Articles and reprints on experimental treatments and alternative therapies, and a listing of Philadelphia-area resources.

Frequency: Monthly

Newsletters, Pamphlets

3291 AIDS Health Pamphlets
Greenhaven Press
P.O. Box 9187
Farminton Hills, MI 48333-9187
www.gale.cengage.com/

Bruce Glassman, Owner

Offers informational pamphlets on How serious is AIDS? Is AIDS a moral issue? Is AIDS testing effective? and How can the spread of AIDS be prevented?.

3292 AIDS Medicines in Development
Pharmaceutical Research & Manufacturers of America
950 F Street
NW? Suite 300
Washington, DC 20004
202-835-3400
Fax: 202- 83- 341
www.phrma.org/

An annual chart of antivirals, as well as information on diagnostics and vaccines.

3293 AIDS News
Northern California Chapter of the NHF
7700 Edgewater Drive
Suite 710
Oakland, CA 94621
510-568-6243
Fax: 510-568-6111
www.hemophilia.org/

Robin Brratton, Manager

Provides current information for people who need to cope mentally and physically with the issues of virus infection and transmission. Provides answers to questions about AIDS, ARC, HIV infection and transmission prevention.

3294 AIDS and Hemophilia: Protecting Yourself and Others
Northern California Chapter, NHF
Nhf 7700 Edgewater Drive
Suite 710
Oakland, CA 94621
510-568-6243
Fax: 510-568-6111
www.hemophilia.org

Robin Brratton, Manager

Explains HIV transmission via sex, needle sticks and blood spills.

12 pages

3295 AIDS: What We Need to Know
March of Dimes Resource Center
1275 Mamaroneck Avenue
White Plains, NY 10605
914- 99- 448
resourcecenter@modimes.org
www.modimes.org
TTY: 914-997-4764

One to two page review and color brochure written for the general public.

3296 APLA Update
AIDS Project Los Angeles
611 South Kingsley Drive
Los Angeles, CA 90005
213-201-1600
www.apla.org/

Rodney Gould, Chair

Presents news about AIDS and programs of AIDS Project Los Angeles to people affected by the disease.

20 pages

3297 Americans with Disabilities Act: What It Means for People with AIDS
American Civil Liberties Union AIDS Project
125 Broad Street
New York, NY 10004
212-549-2500
www.aclu.org

3298 Basics of HIV Disease: Questions and Answers
National Hemophilia Foundation
116 W 32nd Street
Floor 11
New York, NY 10001
212- 32- 370
Fax: 212-328-3777
www.hemophilia.org/

This publication contains basic information about hemophilia and HIV disease.

28 pages

3299 Be Smart About HIV
American Red Cross
1616 Fort Myer Drive
17th Floor
Arlington, VA 22209-3110
703-312-8724
Fax: 703-312-8738

Sandra L Mertz, Product Manager

This brochure offers very simple and informative information on the HIV virus. Half of this brochure is in English and the other half is in Spanish.

3300 Clinical Focus
Immune Deficiency Foundation
40 West Chesapeake Avenue
Suite 308
Towson, MD 21204
Toll Free: 800-296-4433
idf@primaryimmune.org
www.primaryimmune.org

John Seymour, PhD, LMFT, Chair

Bi-annual publication for medical professionals covering current issues and information regarding clinical approaches to primary immune deficiencies.

3301 Clinical Presentation of the Primary Immunodeficiency Diseases
Immune Deficiency Foundation
40 West Chesapeake Avenue
Suite 308
Towson, MD 21204
Toll Free: 800-296-4433

John Seymour, PhD, LMFT, Chair

A primer for physicians.

3302 Clinical Update
Immune Deficiency Foundation
40 West Chesapeake Avenue
Suite 308
Towson, MD 21204
Toll Free: 800-296-4433

John Seymour, PhD, LMFT, Chair

3303 Employee Attitudes About AIDS
National Leadership Coalition on AIDS
1730 M Street NW
Suite 905
Washington, DC 20036
202-429-0930
Fax: 202-872-1977
www.hrtips.org/

A national survey of what working Americans think. Includes information on background surveys of AIDS in the workplace, key findings, conlusions, executive summaries and methodology.

3304 HIV Disease in People with Hemophilia: Your Questions Answered
National Hemophilia Foundation
116 W 32nd Street
Floor 11
New York, NY 10001
212- 32- 370
Fax: 212-328-3777
www.hemophilia.org/

Discusses hemophilia and HIV disease, AIDS, management of HIV disease, risks to sexual partners, and issues for children with hemophilia.

48 pages

3305 HIV Frontline
Center for AIDS Prevention Studies
50 Beale Street
Suite 1300
San Francisco, CA 94105
415-597-9100
caps.ucsf.edu/

Dr. Leon McKusick, Contact
Cynthia Gomez, Manager

Monthly newsletter aimed at mental health and healthcare professionals who counsel people living with HIV/AIDS.

3306 HIV Infection and AIDS
NIAID Office of Communications and Public Liason
6610 Rockledge Drive,MSC 6612
Bethesda, MD 20892-6612
301-496-5717
Fax: 301-402-3573
www.niaid.nih.gov

Offers information on transmission, treatment, early symptoms, diagnosis, prevention and research.

3307 HIV Treatment Information Exchange (HTIE)
National Hemophilia Foundation
116 W 32nd Street
Floor 11
New York, NY 10001
212- 32- 370
Fax: 212-328-3777
www.hemophilia.org/

Indexes and reprints articles from leading consumer-oriented HIV treatment newsletters. Areas covered include antiviral/retroviral treatments, opportunistic infections, immunotherapies, nutritional therapies, alternative therapies, and women's issues. Also highlights recent news stories involving HIV/AIDS treatments.

3308 Infections Linked to AIDS
NIAID Office of Communications and Public Liason
6610 Rockledge Drive,MSC 6612
Bethesda, MD 20892-6612
301-496-5717
Fax: 301-402-3573
www.niaid.nih.gov

Offers information on infections related to HIV/AIDS and referral numbers of where to receive help.

3309 Managing Tuberculosis and HIV Infection in Today's General Workplace
National Leadership Coalition on AIDS
1730 M Street NW
Suite 905
Washington, DC 20036
202-429-0930
Fax: 202-872-1977

Offers information on tuberculosis, HIV and AIDS in the workplace. How employers can protect themselves, special precautions to be taken, and the ADA and other legal information on this issue.

3310 NMAC Update
National Minority AIDS Council
1931 13th Street NW
Washington, DC 20009-4432
202-483-6622
Fax: 202-483-1135
communications@nmac.org
nmac.org/

A newsletter reporting on public policy issues and information on subjects in organizational management.

3311 Our Immune System
Immune Deficiency Foundation
40 West Chesapeake Avenue
Suite 308
Towson, MD 21204
Toll Free: 800-296-4433

John Seymour, PhD, LMFT, Chair

A booklet, in comic book form offering information and descriptions on the body's immune system.

22 pages

3312 Primary Immune Deficiency Diseases: A Guide for Nurses
Immune Deficiency Foundation
40 West Chesapeake Avenue
Suite 308
Towson, MD 21204
Toll Free: 800-296-4433
idf@primaryimmune.org

John Seymour, PhD, LMFT, Chair

Offers information on primary immune deficiency diseases to nurses working with patients suffering from these illnesses.

3313 Report to Members
National Leadership Coalition on AIDS
1730 M Street NW
Suite 905
Washington, DC 20036
202-429-0930
Fax: 202-872-1977

Offers information on new medical research and breakthroughs, legal information and more to management personnel concerned with HIV/AIDS in the workplace.

3314 Small Business and AIDS: How AIDS can Affect Your Business
National Leadership Coalition on AIDS
1730 M Street NW
Suite 905
Washington, DC 20036

202-289-0930
Fax: 202-872-1977

Offers the employer information on legal issues surrounding HIV in the workplace, educational programs, what employees need to know, health insurance and facts about AIDS.

3315 Taking the HIV (AIDS) Test: How to Help Yourself
NIAID Office of Communications and Public Liason
6610 Rockledge Drive,MSC 6612
Bethesda, MD 20892-6612
301-496-5717
Fax: 301-402-3573
www.niaid.nih.gov

Offers information on the AIDS test, how it works, how it can help and should it be taken.

3316 Testing Positive for HIV
NIAID Office of Communications and Public Liason
6610 Rockledge Drive,MSC 6612
Bethesda, MD 20892-6612
301-496-5717
Fax: 301-402-3573
www.niaid.nih.gov

Information on what a positive HIV test means, how not to spread the disease to others, and various health and dieting tips.

3317 Testing for HIV Infection
American Red Cross
1616 Fort Myer Drive
17th Floor
Arlington, VA 22209-3110
703-312-8724
Fax: 703-312-8738

Sandra L Mertz, Product Manager

Videos, Audio Tapes

3318 AIDS
Rosen Publishing Group
29 E 21st Street
New York, NY 10010
212-777-3017
Fax: 888-436-4643; *Toll Free:* 800-237-9932
www.rosenpublishing.com

Roger Rosen, President

This video presents moving portraits of people living with AIDS who generously share their experience with AIDS. Includes views on sex, condoms, and life.

3319 Our Immune System
Immune Deficiency Foundation
40 W Chesapeake Avenue
Suite 308
Towson, MD 21204
Toll Free: 800-296-4433
primaryimmune.org/contact-us

Marcia Boyle, CEO

Slide set.

Websites

3320 AIDS Info
P.O. Box 4780
Rockville, MD 20849-6303
Fax: 301-315-2818; *Toll Free:* 800-448-0440
ContactUs@aidsinfo.nih.gov
www.aidsinfo.nih.gov

A call in service where trained staff offers quick access to federally approved HIV/AIDS treatment and prevention guidelines, clinical trials, and other research-related information.

3321 Arkansas Department of Health
4815 W Markham Street
Little Rock, AR 72205
501-661-2000
www.healthy.state.ar

Provides educational materials such as pamphlets and films, conducts HIV and AIDS research and operates a speakers bureau.

3322 National AIDS Information Clearinghouse
www.cdcnac.org

Provides information and materials for employers on national, state and local resources related to HIV/AIDS in the workplace.

3323 Pennsylvania Department of Health: Bureau of HIV/AIDS
625 Forster Street
8th Floor
Harrisburg, PA 17120
877-724-3258
www.state.pa.com

Tom Corbett, Governor
Michael Wolf, Secretary

Offers various community health education presentations, counseling and testing sites. Also offers practical support services, counseling, HIV testing, a hotline and referrals.

3324 Project Inform Hotline
273 Ninth Street
San Francisco, CA 94103
415-558-8669
Fax: 415-558-0684; *Toll Free:* 877-435-7443
www.projectinform.org

Christopher Esposito, President
Ferdinand Garcia, Vice President
Fred Dillon, Secretary

HIV/AIDS treatment information.

3325 The Body: The Complete HIV/AIDS Resource
Remedy Health Media
750 3rd Avenue
6th Floor
New York, NY 10017
www.thebody.com

Myles Helfand, Editorial Director
J.D. Davids, Managing Editor

3326 Vermont Department of Healt: HIV/AIDS Program
www.state.vt.us

We provide riask reduction and health education services, Anonymous HIV counseling and testing sites through Vermont, HIV/AIDS educational materials.

3327 Virginia Department of Health: Division HIV/STD

www.vdh.state.va.us/std

The division provides a toll free hotline for HIV/STD and viral Hepatitis information, education, confidentiality and anonymous testing. Tghe division provides referrals for AIDS medication assistance and outpatient care services for income eligible persons with HIV.

Research Centers

3328 Aaron Diamond AIDS Research Center

455 1st Avenue
7th Floor
New York, NY 10016
212-448-5000
Fax: 212-725-1126
www.adarc.org

David D Ho MD, Director

AIDS research.

3329 Agency for Health Care Research and Quality

540 Gaither Road
Suite 2000
Rockville, MD 20850
301- 42- 136
www.ahcpr.gov

Operated by a branch of the US Department of Health and Human Services, this site provides recommendations (in layman's lingo) on the prevention and treatment of common illnesses and conditions. Just click on Clinical Information, then on Clinical Practice Guidelines Online, then on Consumer's Guides.

3330 American Foundation for AIDS Research

120 Wall Street
Floor 13
New York, NY 10005-3908
212-806-1600
Fax: 212-806-1601
www.amfar.org

Kenneth Cole, Chairman of the Board
Kevin Robert Frost, Chief Executive Officer
Bradley Jensen, Chief Financial Officer

Supports research in basic, clinical, prevention and public policy and publishes the AIDS/HIV Experimental Treatment Directory.

3331 Arizona State University: School of Health Administration & Policy

300 E. University Drive
Suite 345
Tempe, AZ 85287-7305
480-965-7774
www.asu.edu

Eugene S Schneller PhD, Director

Offers research into healthcare delivery issues in the US including program evaluation, rural health and swing beds, new systems and AIDS in managed care systems.

3332 Asian AIDS Project

730 Polk Street
Floor 4
San Francisco, CA 94109-7813
415-292-3400
Fax: 415-292-3404
www.apiwellness.org

Lance Toma, LCSW, Executive Director
Yvonne Watson, CPA, Director of Finance & Administra
Lina Sheth, MPH, Director of Programs

Offers support and information for Asian Americans with HIV/AIDS.

3333 Cascade AIDS Project: Women's Phone Network

208 SW 5th Avenue
#800
Portland, OR 97204
503-223-5907
Fax: 503-223-6437
info@cascadeaids.org
cascadeaids.org

Charles Washington, President
Warren Jimenez, Vice President
Amanda Hurley, Director of Housing

3334 Center for Blood Research

800 Huntington Avenue
Boston, MA 02115-6399
617-731-6470
Fax: 617-278-3493
lanner@cbr.med.harvard.edu
www.wellness.com

Fred Rosen, Managing Director

Offers research into blood disorders including multidisciplinary studies on AIDS and hemophilia, cancer and diabetes research as well.

3335 Center for Disease Control

1600 Clifton Road NE
Stop E47
Atlanta, GA 30333
404-639-3311
www.cdc.gov

Elizabeth R Unger PhD

Offers reprints, reports, public awareness and educational materials, research grants, and support for persons with HIV/AIDS.

3336 City of Hope National Medical Center: Beckman Research
Virology & Infectious Diseases

1500 Duarte Road
Duarte, CA 91010
626-256-4673
www.cityofhope.org

Dr. John A Zaia, Chair and Professor
Michael Barish, Chair and Professor, Neuroscienc
Ashley Baker Lee, Senior Vice President of Researc

Developmental research into the treatment of AIDS.

3337 Clinical Research Center
Northwestern Center for Clinical Research
680 N Lake Shore Drive
Suite 1220
Chicago, IL 60611-8708
312-503-6227
www.ocrt@northwestern.edu

Dr. Tom Schnitzer, Program Director

Offers research into complications and effects of AIDS and
HIV infection on the human body.

**3338 Dana-Farber Cancer Institute: National Drug
Discovery Group for AIDS Treatment**
450 Brookline Avenue
Boston, MA 02115
617-632-3000Toll free: 86- 40- 332
www.dana-farber.org/contact-us.aspx

Harvey Cantor, MD,Chair

3339 Developmental Evaluation Center
Children's Hospital
300 Longwood Avenue
Boston, MA 02115
617-355-6000Toll free: 800-355-7944
www.childrenshospital.org

Sandra L. Fenwick, President , CEO

Studies developmental effects of infants at risk and development effects of congenital HIV infection.

**3340 Dwight David Eisenhower Army Medical
Center**
Department of Clinical Investigation
300 E Hospital Road
Fort Gordon, GA 30905
706-787-5811
www.ddeamc.amedd.army.mil

Col. Kent M Plowman MC, Chief

Focuses research on cardiac disorders, immune deficiencies
and AIDS.

**3341 Emory University: National Cooperative Drug
Discovery for AIDS Treatment**
Department of Pediatrics
2015 Uppergrate Road
Room 504
Atlanta, GA 30322
404-712-8356
www.pedsresearch.org

Dr. Raymond F Schanzi, Principal
Thomas Abshire, MD

**3342 Emory University: Yerkes Regional Primate
Research Center**
201 Dowman Drive
Atlanta, GA 30322
404-727-6123
insel@rmy.emory.edu
www.emory.edu

Dr. Thomas R Insel MD, Director
Thomas Emory, Owner

Immune research.

**3343 George Washington National Cooperative Drug
Discovery/AIDS Treatment**
2300 Eye Street NW
Washington, DC 20037
202- 99- 35
Fax: 202-994-1753
smhs.gwu.edu

Studies and researches natural products and synthetic
anti-AIDS agents.

**3344 Indiana University Bloomington: Rural Center
for the Study and Promotion of AIDS/STD
Prevention (RCAP)**
801 E 7th Street
Bloomington, IN 47405-3085
812- 85- 797
Fax: 812-855-3936
aids@indiana.edu
www.indiana.edu/~aids

William L Yarber, Director
Suzanne Thorin, Manager

AIDS research.

**3345 Johns Hopkins University: Center for
Communication Programs**
111 Market Place
Suite 310
Baltimore, MD 21202
410-659-6300
Fax: 410-659-6266
info@jhuccp.org
www.jhuccp.org

Susan Krenn, Director

Health communications, family planning and AIDS prevention research.

3346 Kaiser Foundation Research Institute
3505 Broadway
Suite 112
Oakland, CA 94611-5714
510-450-2000
Fax: 510-873-5130

Paul Lairson MD, Director

3347 Mariposa Education and Research Foundation
3123 Schweitzer Drive
Topanga, CA 90290
www.wysk.com

Bruce Voeller PhD, President

Research involving the prevention of AIDS.

**3348 Medical University of South Carolina: Health
Services Administration**
College of Health
Charleston, SC 29425
843-792-2300
academicdepartments.musc.edu

Mark S. Sothmann, President

Devoted to public health policy and health care management including AIDS research.

3349 National Hemophilia Foundation: Hemophillia and AIDS/HIV Network (HANDI)
110 Greene Street
Suite 406
New York, NY 10012-3838
212-328-3700
Fax: 212-328-3777
handi@hemophilia.org
www.hemophilia.org

Alan Kinniburgh, CEO

Dedicated to the treatment and the cure of hemophilia, AIDS and other blood related disorders. This foundation wishes to improve the quality of life of all those affected through promotion and support of research, education and other services.

3350 Northwestern Connecticut AIDS Project
100 Migeon Avenue
Torrington, CT 06790
860-482-1596
Fax: 860-482-3606
www.nwctaids.org

Patricia Lafayette, Executive Director

A nonprofit organization offering support and a variety of services to people with AIDS and their loved ones. Provides education to all segments of the public about AIDS prevention and treatment.

3351 SUNY at Buffalo: National Cooperative Drug Discovery Group for AIDS Treatment
Department of Biochemistry
131 Biomedical Education Building
Buffalo, NY 14214
716-829-3466
medicine.buffalo.edu

Michael E. Cain MD., Vice President

3352 Sansum Diabetes Research Institute
2219 Bath Street
Santa Barbara, CA 93105-4321
805-682-7638
Fax: 805-682-3332
info@sansum.org
www.sansum.org

Rem Laan, Executive Director

3353 Stanford University: General Clinical Research Center
300 Pasteur Drive
Unit 1
Palo Alto, CA 94305-2200
650-723-6073
Fax: 650-725-6698
www.leland.stanford.edu/dept/gcrc

Dr. David Stevenson, Director
Howard Sussman, MD

3354 Stanford University:National Cooperative Drug Discover /AIDS Group
Department of Pathology
800 Welch Road
Palo Alto, CA 94304
650- 49- 649
Fax: 650- 72- 855
spectrum.stanford.edu

3355 UCLA AIDS Clinical Research Center
10940 Wilshire Blvd.
Los Angeles, CA 90024-1678
310-794-4419
Fax: 310- 79- 395
aidsinstitute.ucla.edu

Irvin S.Y. Chen, PhD, Director
Ora Yadin, MD

3356 University of Alabama at Birmingham: National Cooperative Drug/AIDS
Department of Pediatrics
1600 7th Avenue South
Birmingham, AL 35233
205-638-9100
www.uab.edu

Sergio Stagno, Department Chairman

3357 University of California: Institute of Health Policy Studies
333 California Street
Suite 625
San Francisco, CA 94104-2600
415-476-4921
Fax: 415-476-0705
healthpolicy.ucsf.edu

Philip R Lee, Director
Harold Luft, Executive Director

Health policy and AIDS research.

3358 University of California: Los Angeles Clinical AIDS Research & Education
10833 Le Conte Avenue
Room Bh-412
Los Angeles, CA 90095-1793
310-794-1456
Fax: 310-206-3311
www.med.ucla.edu/carectr/carehome.htm

Alan Fogelman, M.D., Executive Chair

AIDS research

Year Founded: 1983

3359 University of California: San Diego Center for AIDS Research
9500 Gilman Drive
La Jolla, CA 92093-5004
858-534-8805
Fax: 619-822-1934
csussman@ucsd.edu
ari.ucsd.edu

Flossie Wong-Staal PhD, Director
Gerry R Boss, MD

AIDS research

Year Founded: 1994

3360 University of California: San Francisco Center for AIDS Prevention Studies
Prevention Science Group
50 Beale Street
Suite 1300
San Francisco, CA 94105
415-597-9100
fcoates@psg.ucsf.edu
www.caps.ucsf.edu/capsweb

3361 University of Hawaii: Hawaii AIDS Clinical Research Program

3675 Kilauea Avenue
6th Floor
Honolulu, HI 96816
808-441-1573
Fax: 808-735-7047
gerschen@hawaii.edu
www.hawaii.edu/hacrp/gerschenson.html

AIDS research

Year Founded: 1990

3362 University of Maryland: Center for Research, Grants & Contracts

655 W Lombard Street
Baltimore, MD 21201
410-706-3100
www.nursing.umaryland.edu

Focuses research on public and health policy laws, including AIDS research.

3363 University of Maryland: Division of Infectious Diseases

10 S Pine Street
Baltimore, MD 21201-1192
410-706-7070
Fax: 410-706-8414
medschool.umaryland.edu

Focuses research on elderly studies including drug use, treatments and infectious diseases of the aged.

3364 University of Michigan: National Cooperative Drug/AIDS Group
School of Dentistry, Dept. of Biologic Sciences

1011 N University Avenue
Ann Arbor, MI 48109-1012
734-763-6933
dent.umich.edu

Joseph I. Helman, DMD, Chair

Focuses on the design of new drugs to fight AIDS.

3365 University of North Carolina: General Clinical Research Center

Cb 7600
Chapel Hill, NC 27599
919-962-2211
www.med.unc.edu

William L. Roper MD, MPH, Dean

Focuses on public policy and health research pertaining to the AIDS community and sexually transmitted disease studies.

3366 University of South Florida: Center for HIV Education & Research

13301 Bruce B Downs Boulevard
Tampa, FL 33612
813-974-4430
Fax: 831-974-8451
contact@usfcenter.org
usfcenter.org

Jeffrey Beal, MD, AAHIVS, Director

Treatment of persons affected and infected with HIV, provides current AIDS information to physicians and operates

a resource center to provide educational materials as well as consultations.

3367 University of Vermont: Office of Health Promotion Research

1 S Prospect Street
Burlington, VT 05401
802-656-4187
Fax: 802-656-8826
www.uvm.edu/~ohpr

Thomas Sullivan, President

Research done into public policy and human health including AIDS information and evaluation.

3368 Utah Department of Health: Division of Community Health Services

PO Box 141010
Salt Lake City, UT 84114-1010
801-538-6003
health.utah.gov/

W. David Patton PhD, Executive Director

Secures and distributes funds for AIDS prevention services, provides educational programs and counseling to the general public, AIDS service organizations, health workers and groups at risk.

3369 Wayne State University: Center for Health Research
College of Nursing

5557 Cass Avenue
Detroit, MI 48202-3615
313-577-4082
Fax: 313-577-5777
www.comm.wayne.edu/nursing/nursing.html

Dr. Ada Jacox, Associate Dean
Janet Harden, Executive Director

AIDS and HIV infection research and studies.

3370 Whitehead Institute for Biomedical Research

9 Cambridge Center
Cambridge, MA 02142
617-258-5000
info@wi.mit.edu
www.wi.mit.edu/home.html

David C. Page, Director

AIDS information and research.

3371 Worcester Foundation for Biomedical Research: Biology/Drug Discovery/AIDS Group
University of Massachusetts Medical School

55 Lake Avenue North
Worcester, MA 01655
508-856-2000
www.umassmed.edu/

Developmental research on new advances and drug therapies for HIV infection and the prevention of AIDS.

Allergies

Associations & Organizations

3372 Allergy & Asthma Network
8229 Boone Boulevard
Suite 260
Vienna, VA 22182
Fax: 703-288-5271; Toll Free: 800-878-4403
www.allergyasthmanetwork.org

Nonprofit seeks to end needless death and suffering due to asthma, allergies and related conditions through outreach, education, advocacy and research.

Year Founded: 1985

3373 American Academy of Allergy Asthma & Immunology
555 East Wells Street
Suite 1100
Milwaukee, WI 53202-3823
414-272-6071
Fax: 414-272-6070; Toll Free: 800-822-2762
info@aaaai.org
www.aaaai.org

Membership organization for allergists and immunologists and patient's resource for allergies, asthma and immune deficiency disorders.

Number of Members: 6,800+

3374 American Academy of Environmental Medicine
6505 E Central Avenue
Suite 296
Wichita, KS 67206
316-684-5500
defox@aaemonline.org
aaemonline.org

De Rodgers-Fox, Executive Director

Promoting health and serving the public through education about the interaction between humans and the environment.

Year Founded: 1965

3375 American College of Allergy, Asthma & Immunology
85 West Algonquin Road
Suite 550
Arlington Heights, IL 60005
847-427-1200
Fax: 847-427-1294
college.acaai.org

Rick Slawny, Executive Director

Promoting excellence in patient care through research, education and advocacy.

Year Founded: 1942

3376 American Lung Association
55 W Wacker Drive
Suite 1150
Chicago, IL 60601
Toll Free: 800-548-8252
info@lung.org
www.lung.org

Harold P. Wimmer, President & CEO

A voluntary organization interested in the prevention and control of lung disease. Promotes and distributes public awareness information on a variety of lung disorders, including allergies.

Year Founded: 1904

3377 American Lung Association: Alabama
1678 Montgomery Highway
Suite 104-355
Birmingham, AL 35216
205-258-5367
alaal@lungse.org
www.lung.org

Working to save lives by improving lung health and preventing lung disease.

3378 American Lung Association: Alaska
1075 S Check Street
Suite 205
Wasilla, AK 99654
907-357-3110
kt.mckee@lung.org
www.lung.org

Working to save lives by improving lung health and preventing lung disease.

3379 American Lung Association: Arizona
2819 E Broadway Boulevard
Tucson, AZ 85716
520-323-1812
azinfo@lungs.org
www.lung.org

Working to save lives by improving lung health and preventing lung disease.

3380 American Lung Association: Arkansas
14524 Cantrell Road
Suite 140, Box 214
Little Rock, AR 72223
e-mail: alaar@lungse.org
www.lung.org

Working to save lives by improving lung health and preventing lung disease.

3381 American Lung Association: California
2020 Camino Del Rio North
Suite 200
San Diego, CA 92108
619-297-3901
ellen.sherwood@lung.org
www.lung.org

Working to save lives by improving lung health and preventing lung disease.

3382 American Lung Association: Colorado
5600 Greenwood Plaza Boulevard
Suite 100
Greenwood Village, CO 80111
303-388-4327
coinfo@lungs.org
www.lung.org

Working to save lives by improving lung health and preventing lung disease.

3383 American Lung Association: Connecticut
45 Ash Street
East Hartford, CT 06108
860-289-5401
info@lungne.org
www.lung.org

Working to save lives by improving lung health and preventing lung disease.

3384 American Lung Association: Delaware
630 Churchmans Road
Suite 202
Newark, DE 19702
302-737-6414
llyons@lunginfo.org
www.lung.org

Working to save lives by improving lung health and preventing lung disease.

3385 American Lung Association: District of Columbia
1301 Pennsylvania Avenue NW
Washington, DC 20004
202-747-5541
lungdc@lunginfo.org
www.lung.org

Working to save lives by improving lung health and preventing lung disease.

3386 American Lung Association: Florida
2701 N Australian Avenue
Suite 100
West Palm Beach, FL 33407
561-659-7644
alafse@lungse.org
www.lung.org

Working to save lives by improving lung health and preventing lung disease.

3387 American Lung Association: Georgia
2452 Spring Road
Smyrna, GA 30080
770-434-5864
alaga@lungse.org
www.lung.org

Working to save lives by improving lung health and preventing lung disease.

3388 American Lung Association: Hawaii
810 Richards Street
Suite 750
Honolulu, HI 96813
808-537-5966
kim.nguyen@lung.org
www.lung.org

Working to save lives by improving lung health and preventing lung disease.

3389 American Lung Association: Idaho
1412 W Idaho Street
Suite 100
Boise, ID 83702
208-345-5864
heather.kimmel@lung.org
www.lung.org

Working to save lives by improving lung health and preventing lung disease.

3390 American Lung Association: Illinois
3000 Kelly Lane
Springfield, IL 62711
217-787-5864
info@lungil.org
www.lung.org

Working to save lives by improving lung health and preventing lung disease.

3391 American Lung Association: Indiana
115 West Washington Street
Suite 1180-South
Indianapolis, IN 46204
317-819-1181
info@lungin.org
www.lung.org

Working to save lives by improving lung health and preventing lung disease.

3392 American Lung Association: Iowa
2530 73rd Street
Des Moines, IA 50322
515-309-9507
info@lungia.org
www.lung.org

Working to save lives by improving lung health and preventing lung disease.

3393 American Lung Association: Kansas
8400 W 110th Street
Suite 130
Overland Park, KS 66210
913-353-9165
info@lungks.org
www.lung.org

Working to save lives by improving lung health and preventing lung disease.

3394 American Lung Association: Kentucky
4100 Churchman Avenue
Louisville, KY 40215
502-363-2652
barry.gottschalk@lung.org
www.lung.org

Working to save lives by improving lung health and preventing lung disease.

3395 American Lung Association: Louisiana
2325 Severn Avenue
Suite 8
Metairie, LA 70001
504-828-5864
alala@lungse.org
www.lung.org

Working to save lives by improving lung health and preventing lung disease.

3396 American Lung Association: Maine
122 State Street
Augusta, ME 04330
207-622-6394
info@lungne.org
www.lung.org

Working to save lives by improving lung health and preventing lung disease.

3397 American Lung Association: Maryland
211 E Lombard Street
Suite 260
Baltimore, MD 21202
202-747-5541
lungmd@lunginfo.org
www.lung.org

Working to save lives by improving lung health and preventing lung disease.

3398 American Lung Association: Massachusetts
393 Maple Street
Springfield, MA 01105
413-737-3506
info@lungne.org
www.lung.org

Working to save lives by improving lung health and preventing lung disease.

3399 American Lung Association: Michigan
1475 E 12 Mile Road
Madison Heights, MI 48071
248-784-2000
midland@lung.org
www.lung.org

Working to save lives by improving lung health and preventing lung disease.

3400 American Lung Association: Minnesota
490 Concordia Avenue
St. Paul, MN 55103
651-227-8014
info@lungmn.org
www.lung.org

Working to save lives by improving lung health and preventing lung disease.

3401 American Lung Association: Mississippi
1599 Bienville Boulevard
Suite D
Ocean Springs, MS 39564
678-478-0314
alams@lungse.org
www.lung.org

Working to save lives by improving lung health and preventing lung disease.

3402 American Lung Association: Missouri
7745 Carondelet Avenue
Suite 305
Clayton, MO 63105
314-627-5505
missouri@lung.org
www.lung.org

Working to save lives by improving lung health and preventing lung disease.

3403 American Lung Association: Montana
c/o American Lung Association
822 John Street
Seattle, WA 98109

206-441-5100
infomtp@lung.org
www.lung.org

Working to save lives by improving lung health and preventing lung disease.

3404 American Lung Association: Nebraska
8990 West Dodge
Suite 226
Omaha, NE 68114
402-502-4950
info@lungnb.org
www.lung.org

Working to save lives by improving lung health and preventing lung disease.

3405 American Lung Association: Nevada
10615 Double R Boulevard
Reno, NV 89521
775-829-5864
nvinfo@lungs.org
www.lung.org

Working to save lives by improving lung health and preventing lung disease.

3406 American Lung Association: New Hampshire
51 Islington Street
Cloudport Unit 1
Portsmouth, NH 03801
603-369-3977
info@lungne.org
www.lung.org

Working to save lives by improving lung health and preventing lung disease.

3407 American Lung Association: New Jersey
PO Box 10188
Newark, NJ 07101
908-685-8040
jgrinwald@lunginfo.org
www.lung.org

Working to save lives by improving lung health and preventing lung disease.

3408 American Lung Association: New Mexico
5911 Jefferson Street NE
Albuquerque, NM 87109
Toll Free: 800-586-4872
nminfo@lungs.org
www.lung.org

Working to save lives by improving lung health and preventing lung disease.

3409 American Lung Association: New York
237 Mamaroneck Avenue
Suite 205
White Plains, NY 10605
914-347-2094
info@lungne.org
www.lung.org

Working to save lives by improving lung health and preventing lung disease.

3410 American Lung Association: North Carolina
514 Daniels Street
Suite 109
Raleigh, NC 27605
919-792-1641
alanc-r@lungse.org
www.lung.org

Working to save lives by improving lung health and preventing lung disease.

3411 American Lung Association: North Dakota
212 N Second Street
Bismarck, ND 58501
701-223-5613
info@lungnd.org
www.lung.org

Working to save lives by improving lung health and preventing lung disease.

3412 American Lung Association: Ohio
PO Box 415
Sandusky, OH 44871
419-663-5864
pat.volz@lung.org
www.lung.org

Working to save lives by improving lung health and preventing lung disease.

3413 American Lung Association: Oklahoma
730 W Wilshire Boulevard
Suite 105
Oklahoma City, OK 73116
405-748-4674
okinfo@lungs.org
www.lung.org

Working to save lives by improving lung health and preventing lung disease.

3414 American Lung Association: Oregon
16037 SW Upper Boones Ferry Road
Suite 165
Tigard, OR 97224
503-924-4094
infomtp@lung.org
www.lung.org

Working to save lives by improving lung health and preventing lung disease.

3415 American Lung Association: Pennsylvania
Marywood University
2300 Adams Avenue
Scranton, PA 18509
570-346-1784
adelonti@lunginfo.org
www.lung.org

Working to save lives by improving lung health and preventing lung disease.

3416 American Lung Association: Rhode Island
260 West Exchange Street
Suite 102 B
Providence, RI 02903
401-421-6487
info@lungne.org
www.lung.org

Working to save lives by improving lung health and preventing lung disease.

3417 American Lung Association: South Carolina
2030 North Church Place
Spartanburg, SC 29303
864-764-1777
upstate@lungse.org
www.lung.org

Working to save lives by improving lung health and preventing lung disease.

3418 American Lung Association: South Dakota
490 Concordia Avenue
St. Paul, MN 55103
651-227-8014
info@lungsd.org
www.lung.org

Working to save lives by improving lung health and preventing lung disease.

3419 American Lung Association: Tennessee
One Vantage Way
Suite C120
Nashville, TN 37228
615-329-1151
gail.bost@lung.org
www.lung.org

Working to save lives by improving lung health and preventing lung disease.

3420 American Lung Association: Texas
8207 Callaghan Road
Suite 140
San Antonio, TX 78230
210-308-8978
txinfo@lungs.org
www.lung.org

Working to save lives by improving lung health and preventing lung disease.

3421 American Lung Association: Utah
3920 South 1100 East
Suite 240
Salt Lake City, UT 84124
801-484-4456
utinfo@lungs.org
www.lung.org

Working to save lives by improving lung health and preventing lung disease.

3422 American Lung Association: Vermont
372 Hurricane Lane
Suite 101
Williston, VT 05495
802-876-6500
info@lungne.org
www.lung.org

Working to save lives by improving lung health and preventing lung disease.

3423 American Lung Association: Virginia
9702 Gayton Road
Suite 110
Richmond, VA 23238

804-302-5740
lungva@lunginfo.org
www.lung.org

Working to save lives by improving lung health and preventing lung disease.

3424 American Lung Association: Washington
822 John Street
Seattle, WA 98109
206-441-5100
infomtp@lung.org
www.lung.org

Working to save lives by improving lung health and preventing lung disease.

3425 American Lung Association: West Virginia
2102 Kanawha Boulevard E
Charleston, WV 25311
304-342-6600
cfields@lunginfo.org
www.lung.org

Working to save lives by improving lung health and preventing lung disease.

3426 American Lung Association: Wisconsin
13100 W Lisbon Road
Suite 700
Brookfield, WI 53005
262-703-4200
info@lungwi.org
www.lung.org

Working to save lives by improving lung health and preventing lung disease.

3427 American Lung Association: Wyoming
c/o American Lung Association
822 John Street
Seattle, WA 98109
206-441-5100
infomtp@lung.org
www.lung.org

Working to save lives by improving lung health and preventing lung disease.

3428 Asthma and Allergy Foundation of America
8201 Corporate Drive
Suite 1000
Landover, MD 20785
Toll Free: 800-727-8462
info@aafa.org
www.aafa.org

Cary Sennett, President & CEO

The Foundation was formed to alleviate suffering and loss from asthma and allergy disorders. The Foundation offers a nationwide network of chapters and support groups and provides education and emotional support for patients and their families.

Year Founded: 1953

3429 Food Allergy Research & Education (FARE)
7925 Jones Branch Drive
Suite 1100
McLean, VA 22102
703-691-3179
Fax: 703-691-2713; *Toll Free:* 800-929-4040
www.foodallergy.org

James R. Baker, CEO & Chief Medical Officer

A nonprofit organization established to help families living with food allergies, and to increase public awareness about food allergies and anaphylaxis. Also provides emotional support and educational information.

3430 Immune Deficiency Foundation
110 West Road
Suite 300
Towson, MD 21204
Fax: 410-321-9165; *Toll Free:* 800-296-4433
info@primaryimmune.org
primaryimmune.org

Marcia Boyle, President and Founder

National non-profit patient organization dedicated to improving the diagnosis, treatment and quality of life of persons with primary immunodeficiency diseases (PI) through advocacy, education and research.

Year Founded: 1980

3431 National Association of School Nurses
1100 Wayne Avenue
Suite 925
Silver Spring, MD 20910
240-821-1130
Fax: 301-585-1791; *Toll Free:* 866-627-6767
nasn@nasn.org
www.nasn.org

Donna J. Mazyck, Executive Director

Optimizing student health.

3432 National Eczema Association
4460 Redwood Highway
Suite 16D
San Rafael, CA 94903
415-499-3474
Fax: 415-472-5345; *Toll Free:* 800-818-7546
info@nationaleczema.org
nationaleczema.org

Julie Block, President & CEO

Improving quality of life for individuals with eczema through research, support and education.

3433 World Allergy Organization
555 East Wells Street
Suite 1100
Milwaukee, WI 53202-3823
414-276-1791
Fax: 414-276-3349
info@worldallergy.org
www.worldallergy.org

Justin Dodge, Executive Director

International organization building global alliance of allergy societies to advance excellence in care, research, education and training.

Year Founded: 1951

Books

3434 Allergies A to Z
Facts on File
11 Penn Plaza
Floor 15
New York, NY 10001

212-967-8090Toll free: 800-322-8755
medinformer.org/

This vital resource for the one in five Americans who suffer from allenes provides reliable, up-to-date information on every aspect of this condition.

368 pages

3435 Allergy Plants That Cause Sneezing and Wheezing
Asthma and Allergy Foundation of America
8201 Corporate Drive
Suite 1000
Landover, MD 20785
Toll Free: 800-727-8462
Info@aafa.org
www.aafa.org

Lynn Hanessian, Chair

Destined to be displayed on coffee tables, the spectacular photographs in this book actually show allergy sufferers what causes their sneezing and wheezing.

64 pages

3436 Allergy Practice Worlwide
World Allergy Organization
555 East Wells Street
Suite 1100
Milwaukee, WI 53202
414-276-1791
Fax: 414-276-3349
info@worldallergy.org
www.worldallergy.org

Ruby Pawankar, President
Jennie Smazik, Executive Director
Amanda Hegg, Program Manager

Book with references towards allergic diseases, asthma, and possible immunities.

3437 Allergy Prevalence Survey
World Allergy Organization
555 East Wells Street
Suite 1100
Milwaukee, WI 53202
414-276-1791
Fax: 414-276-3349
info@worldallergy.org
www.worldallergy.org

Ruby Pawankar, President
Jennie Smazik, Executive Director
Amanda Hegg, Program Manager

Book with references towards allergic diseases, asthma, and possible immunities.

3438 Allergy-Free Garening: The Revolutionary Guide to Healthy Landscaping
Ten Speed Press
PO Box 7123
Berkely, CA 94707-0123
510-559-1600
www.tenspeed.com

Thomas Leo Ogren, Author

This extensively researched, comprehensive, plant-by-plant reference alerts gardeners and helps them make landscaping choices that can drastically reduce their exposure to harmful allergens.

256 pages

3439 Best Guide to Allergy
Humana Press
999 Riverview Drive
Suite 208
Totowa, NJ 07512-1165
973-256-1699
Fax: 973-256-8341
www.superpages.com/

Thomas Lanigan, Owner

Practical everyday approaches to your allergy and asthma problems, including food allergies, environmental control, skin conditions, allergy testing and shots, and more.

232 pages

3440 Essential Allergy
Blackwell Science
350 Main Street
Malden, MA 02148-5089
781-388-8250
Fax: 781-388-8255; *Toll Free:* 800-215-1000
csbooks@blacksci.com
www.blackwellscience.com

Gordan Tibbitts III, President

3441 Food Allergies for Dummies
For Dummies
10475 Crosspoint Boulevard
Indianapolis, IN 46256
877-762-2974
Fax: 800-597-3299
www.dummies.com

Robert A Wood MD, Author

This concise guide shows you how to identify and avoid food that triggers reactions. Covers how to care for a child with food allergies, such as getting involved with his/her school's allergy policies, packing safe lunches, and empowering him/her to take responsibility for his allergy.

384 pages

3442 Food Allergy: A Primer for People
Asthma and Allergy Foundation of America
8201 Corporate Drive
Suite 1000
Landover, MD 20785
Toll Free: 800-727-8462
www.aafa.org

Bill McLin, Executive Director

Food allergies demystified.

66 pages

3443 Indoor Allergens: Assessing & Controlling Adverse Health Effects
National Academy Press
500 5th Street NW
Washington, DC 20001
Toll Free: 800-624-6242
zjones@nas.edu
www.nap.edu

This unique volume summarizes what is known about indoor allergens and how they affect human health and how they can be controlled.

320 pages 1993

3444 International Collaboration in Asthma, Allergy, And Immunology
World Allergy Organization
555 East Wells Street
Suite 1100
Milwaukee, WI 53202-3823
414-276-1791
Fax: 414-276-3349
info@worldallergy.org
www.worldallergy.org

Ruby Pawankar, President
Jennie Smazik, Executive Director
Amanda Hegg, Program Manager

Book with references towards allergic diseases, asthma, and possible immunities.

3445 Prevention of Allergy and Allergic Asthma
World Allergy Organization
555 East Wells Street
Suite 1100
Milwaukee, WI 53202
414-276-1791
Fax: 414-276-3349
info@worldallergy.org
www.worldallergy.org

Ruby Pawankar, President
Jennie Smazik, Executive Director
Amanda Hegg, Program Manager

Book with references towards asthma and a possible cure for it.

3446 Taming Asthma and Allergy by Controlling Your Environment
Allergy Control Products
1620-D Satellite Road
Duluth, GA 30097
www.allergycontrol.com

Tells how to avoid allergens in simple, straight forward directions and also explains the reasons through interesting case examples.

170 pages

3447 WAO White Book on Allergy
World Allergy Organization
555 East Wells Street
Suite 1100
Milwaukee, WI 53202
414-276-1791
Fax: 414-276-3349
info@worldallergy.org
www.worldallergy.org

Ruby Pawankar, President
Jennie Smazik, Executive Director
Amanda Hegg, Program Manager

Book with references towards allergic diseases and asthma.

Newsletters, Pamphlets

3448 Allergies and You
American Lung Association
1740 Broadway
New York, NY 10019-4315

212-315-8700
Fax: 212-315-8870
american-lung-association

Answers basic questions about allergy, particularly as it relates to asthma.

3449 FAN Flashbacks
Food Allergy Network
7925 Jones Branch Drive
Suite 1100
McLean, VA 22102
703-691-3179
Fax: 703-691-2713; *Toll Free:* 800-929-4040
www.foodallergy.org

Todd J. Slotkin, Chairman
John L. Lehr, CEO
Irvin Andr, Alexander, Chief Financial Officer

Series of reprints on specific topics of Food Allergy News. Specific pamphlets offer information on wheat, milk, soy, peanuts and special occasion tips.

3450 Food Allergy News
Food Allergy Network
7925 Jones Branch Drive
Suite 1100
McLean, VA 22102
703-691-3179
Fax: 703-691-2713; *Toll Free:* 800-929-4040
www.foodallergy.org

Todd J. Slotkin, Chairman
John L. Lehr, CEO
Irvin Andr, Alexander, Chief Financial Officer

Contains allergy-free recipes, practical tips such as birthday party, trick-or-treating and travel tips, a dietitian's column, medical information and product information.

8 pages

3451 Food Allergy and Atopic Dermatitis
Food Allergy Network
7925 Jones Branch Drive
Suite 1100
McLean, VA 22102
703-691-3179
Fax: 703-691-2713; *Toll Free:* 800-929-4040
www.foodallergy.org

Todd J. Slotkin, Chairman
John L. Lehr, CEO
Irvin Andr, Alexander, Chief Financial Officer

The purpose of this booklet is to provide tips and other sources of information to help parents raise a child who is afflicted with Atopic Dermatitis.

12 pages

3452 Just One Little Bite Can Hurt! Important Facts About Anaphylaxis
Food Allergy Network
7925 Jones Branch Drive
Suite 1100
McLean, VA 22102
703-691-3179
Fax: 703-691-2713; *Toll Free:* 800-929-4040
www.foodallergy.org

Todd J. Slotkin, Chairman
John L. Lehr, CEO
Irvin Andr, Alexander, Chief Financial Officer

Offers information on what Anaphylaxis is, what the patient should do if they have a reaction and important medical safety tips regarding the illness.

8 pages

3453 MA Report
Allergy and Asthma Network/Mothers of Asthmatics
8229 Boone Boulevard
Suite 260
Vienna, VA 22182
Fax: 703-288-5271; *Toll Free:* 800-878-4403
www.aanma.org

Michael Amato, Chair

Monthly newsletter providing members with insider information on medical research, new products, practical how-to tips and helpful hints, updates on legislation, product recalls, prevention and coping techniques and much more.

Frequency: 12

3454 Nutrition Guide to Food Allergies
Food Allergy Network
7925 Jones Branch Drive
Suite 1100
McLean, VA 22102
703-691-3179
Fax: 703-691-2713; *Toll Free:* 800-929-4040
www.foodallergy.org

Todd J. Slotkin, Chairman
John L. Lehr, CEO
Irvin Andr, Alexander, Chief Financial Officer

Offers answers to the most commonly asked questions about food allergies, common allergy-causing foods and resources for the patient.

24 pages

3455 Something in the Air: Airborne Allergens
National Institute of Allergy & Infectious Disease
6610 Rockledge Drive
MSC 6612
Bethesda, MD 20892-6612
301-496-5717
Fax: 301-402-0120
www.niaid.nih.gov

Offers information on the symptoms to airborne substances, pollen, mold, dust, animal, chemical allergies and treatments for them.

3456 Tips to Remember
American Academy of Allergy & Immunology
611 E Wells Street
Suite 4a
Milwaukee, WI 53202-3816
414-272-6071
Fax: 414-272-6070; *Toll Free:* 800-822-2762
latexallergyresources.org/

A set of 23 informational pamphlets offering information on various aspects of allergies and asthma from allergies in the elderly to what is an allergic reaction.

3457 Allergy and Asthma Network Mothers of Asthmatics
8229 Boone Boulevard
Suite 260
Vienna, VA 22182
Fax: 703-288-5271; *Toll Free:* 800-878-4403
www.aanma.org

Michael Amato, Chair

A nonprofit association dedicated to educating families with asthma and allergies. Facilitates communication of accurate information among patients, parents, physicians and industry. Provides an important communication link among the home, school, physician and pharmaceutical industry in an effort to help families create a management program for those with asthma and allergies.

3458 American Academy of Allergy and Immunology
www.aaaai.org

Strives to serve the public through information on asthma and allergies, as well as referrals to allergists. Also offers pollen and mold statistics from the Committee on Pollen & Molds.

3459 American Lung Association
www.lung.org

A voluntary organization interested in the prevention and control of lung disease. Promotes and distributes public awareness information on a variety of lung disorders, including allergies.

Year Founded: 1904

3460 Asthma and Allergy Foundation of America
www.aafa.org

Voluntary health organization dedicated to improving the quality of life for people with asthma and allergies and their caregivers through education, research and advocacy. The network of affiliated chapters and educational support groups.

3461 Food Allergy Anaphylaxis Network
www.foodallergy.org

A nonprofit organization established to help families living with food allergies, and to increase public awareness about food allergies and anaphylaxis. Also provides emotional support and educational information.

Research Centers

3462 Allergy Research Foundation
PO Box 18
Aylesbury, Bu HP22 4XJ
296-655-818
Fax: 310-575-9292
philip_goddard@tiscali.co.uk
www.allergyresearchfoundation.org

Billy Loftus, Manager
Professor Jo Brostoff, Chairman

Non-profit, independent organization that deals with allergy related issues.

Year Founded: 1988

3463 John Hopkins Asthma & Allergy Center
5501 Hopkins Bayview Circle
Baltimore, MD 21224-6801
410-550-2101
Fax: 410-550-3256
jhuellergy@jhmi.edu
www.hopkinsmedicine.org/allergy

Bruce S Bochner MD, Director
Peter S Creticos MD, Clinical Director

Treatment of allergies, asthma and other lung disorders.

Year Founded: 1976

3464 La Jolla Institute for Allergy and Immunology
9420 Athena Circle
La Jolla, CA 92037
858-752-6500
www.liai.org

Tai Nguyen, CFO

A nonprofit public benefit corporation dedicated to basic biomedical research and training. The essential purpose of the Institute is to use innovative approaches to advance our knowledge of how the immune system works, to study the regulatory mechanisms involved in the onset and mainte-nance of immune response, and to develop new, more so-phisticated and precise strategies and/or therapies for managing various immunological and allergic disorders.

3465 Mayo Clinic and Foundation: Allergy Disease Research Laboratory
200 1st Street SW
Rochester, MN 55905
507-284-2511
gleich@mayo.edu
www.mayoclinic.org/

Provides a focus for research into the causes, prevention and management of allergic diseases.

3466 National Institute of Allergy and Infectious Diseases
6610 Rockledge Drive
MSC 6612
Bethesda, MD 20892-6612
301-496-5717
Fax: 301-402-3573; *Toll Free:* 866-284-4107
www.niaid.nih.gov
TDD 800-877-8339

Conducts and supports research on allergies; focused on understanding what happens to the body during the aller-gic process. Educates patients and health care workers in con-trolling allergic disease; offers various research centers that conduct and evaluate educational programs focused on methods to control allergic diseases.

3467 National Jewish Center for Medical and Research Center
1400 Jackson Street
Denver, CO 80206-2762
303-388-4461
Fax: 303-290-2165; *Toll Free:* 800-222-5864
www.nationaljewish.org/

Basic and clinical research into the causes and treatments of asthmatic disorders.

3468 Research Institute of Palo Alto Medical Foundation
795 El Camino Real
Palo Alto, CA 94301
650-326-8120
Fax: 650-329-9114
www.pamf.org/research/?

Harold Hal Luft PhD., Director

Clinical and general medical sciences research including allergy and immunology disorders.

3469 Scripps Clinic and Research Foundation: Autoimmune Disease Center
4275 Campus Point Court
Cp10
San Diego, CA 92121
Toll Free: 800-727-4777
www.scrippsclinic.com

Susan Taylor, Executive Director

Immunologic studies on the development of allergic disor-ders.

3470 State University of New York Health Science Center at Stony Brook: Asthma and Allergic Diseases Center
HSC Level T16-040
State University of New York
Level 2,Room 271
Stony Brook, NY 11794-8276
631-444-2111
Fax: 631-444-6035
www.stonybrook.edu/

Allergy research.

Year Founded: 1979

3471 Tufts University: Asthma and Allergic Diseases Cooperative Research Center
School of Medicine
750 Washington Street
Boston, MA 02111-1526
617-636-9700
start.cortera.com/

Allergy research.

3472 University of Colorado: Immunology Center
1250 14th street
Denver, CO 80262
303-556-2400
www.ucdenver.edu/

Allergy research.

3473 University of Florida: General Clinical Research Center
PO Box 100219
Gainesville, FL 32610-0219
352-273-8700
Fax: 352-273-8703
www.ctsi.ufl.edu

Micheal Good, Dean
David Guzick, Vice President

Studies on allergies and immunology.

3474 University of Michigan: Montgomery Allergy Research Laboratory
500 South State Street
Ann Arbor, MI 48109
734-764-1817
www.umich.edu/

3475 University of Texas: Southwestern Medical Center
5323 Harry Hines Boulevard
Dallas, TX 75390
214-648-3111
www.utsouthwestern.edu/

Daniel K. Podolsky MD, President

Immunodermatology department researching allergies and immune disorders.

3476 University of Wisconsin: Allergy/Asthma Clinical Research Unit
Medical School, H6/367 CSC
600 Highland Avenue
Madison, WI 53792
608-263-6400Toll free: 800-323-8942
mjb@medicine.wisc.edu
www.medicine.wisc.edu/sections/allergy

Allergy research.

Year Founded: 1972

Alzheimer's Disease

Associations & Organizations

3477 Alzheimer's & Dementia Resource Center
1506 Lake Highland Drive
Orlando, FL 32803
407-843-1910
adrccares.org

Nancy Squillacioti, Executive Director

A non profit organization, has been athe forerunner in Central Florida bringing Alzheimer specific education and support to family caregivers as well as professional care providers.

Year Founded: 1984

3478 Alzheimer's Aid Society of Northern California
2641 Cottage Way
Suite 4
Sacramento, CA 95825
916-483-2002Toll free: 800-540-3340
info@alzaid.org
alzaid.org

Sheryl Ashby, President

Family support: provide needed support and advice for victims and their families. Counseling and emotional support are a major need. Education and information for lay and professional people. To aid and support research into the causes, treatment, prevention and cure for Alzheimer's disease. To advocate the social needs of the afflicted population, provide information to increase public awareness. Bimonthly newsletters and a multitute of direct services, including distribution of free information packets, in-service training, workshops, home visits and 24-hour one-on-on phone call availability are supported through donations.

Year Founded: 1981; Number of Members: 15,000

3479 Alzheimer's Association
225 N Michigan Avenue
17th Floor
Chicago, IL 60601
312-335-8700
Fax: 866-699-1246; *Toll Free:* 800-272-3900
info@alz.org
www.alz.org

Harry Johns, President & CEO
Richard Hovland, COO

Combats Alzheimer's disease and related disorders. Seeks to destroy the myth that what were once called 'senile behaviors' are a natural part of aging. Works to develop family support systems for relatives of victims of the disease.

Year Founded: 1980

3480 Alzheimer's Association Autopsy Assistance Network
Alz. Assoc. Western & Central Washington State
12721 30th Avenue NE
Suite 101
Seattle, WA 98125-1696
206-363-5500Toll free: 800-848-7097
alz.org

Provides families with information regarding autopsy, assists in obtaining a confirmed diagnosis, provides tissue for Alzheimer's disease research and establishes diagnosis for the purpose of clinical and epidemiological studies.

3481 Alzheimer's Association: Alabama-FloridaPanhandle
2151 Highland Avenue
Suite 210
Birmingham, AL 35205
Toll Free: 800-272-3900
info@alz.org
www.alz.org

Year Founded: 1980

3482 Alzheimer's Association: Alaska
225 N Michigan Avenue
Suite 1700
Chicago, IL 60601
312-335-8700
Fax: 866-699-1246; *Toll Free:* 800-272-3900
www.alz.org/alaska
TDD 312-335-5886

Year Founded: 1980

3483 Alzheimer's Association: Aloha
1050 Ala Moana Boulevard
Suite 2610
Honolulu, HI 96814-4906
808-591-2771
Fax: 808-591-9071; *Toll Free:* 800-272-3900
alohainfo@alz.org
www.alz.org/hawaii

Christine Payne, Executive Director

Year Founded: 1980

3484 Alzheimer's Association: Arkansas
210 N Walton Avenue
Suite 25
Bentonville, AR 72712
479-273-5559Toll free: 800-272-3900
www.alz.org/arkansas

Susan Neyman, Executive Director

Year Founded: 1980

3485 Alzheimer's Association: California Central
1528 Chapala Street
Suite 204
Santa Barbara, CA 93101
805-892-4259
Fax: 805-892-4250; *Toll Free:* 800-272-3900
cacentral-info@alz.org
www.alz.org/cacentral

Rhonda Spiegel, Executive Director
Donna Beal, VP, Programs & Advocacy
Mitchel Sloan, VP, Development & Communications

The Alzheimer's Association is the world's leading voluntary health organization in Alzheimer's care, support and research. Our mission is to eliminate Alzheimer's disease through the advancement of research, to provide and enhance care and support for all affected, and to reduce the risk of dementia through the promotion of brain health. The California Central Chapter provides services in Santa Barbara, Ventura and San Luis Obispo counties.

Year Founded: 1980; Number of Members: 11-50

3486 Alzheimer's Association: California Southland
5670 Wilshire Boulevard
Suite 1800
Los Angeles, CA 90036
323-309-8821Toll free: 800-272-3900
www.alz.org/socal

To eliminate Alzheimer's disease through the advancement of research; to provide and enhance care and support for all affected; and to reduce the risk of dementia through the promotion of brain health.

Year Founded: 1980

3487 Alzheimer's Association: Capital of Texas
106 E 6th Street
Suite 900
Austin, TX 78701
512-592-0990Toll free: 800-272-3900
www.alz.org/texascapital

Year Founded: 1980

3488 Alzheimer's Association: Central & NorthFlorida
2180 West State Road 434
Suite 1100
Longwood, FL 32779
Toll Free: 800-272-3900
www.alz.org/cnfl

The Central and North Florida Chapter provides services and programs in 31 counties. Our mission is to eliminate Alzheimer's disease through the advancement of research, to provide and enhance care and support for individuals, their families and caregivers.

Year Founded: 1980

3489 Alzheimer's Association: Central & Western Virginia
1160 Pepsi Place
Suite 306
Charlottesville, VA 22901
434-973-6122Toll free: 800-272-3900
www.alz.org/cwva

Year Founded: 1980

3490 Alzheimer's Association: Central Illinois
612 W Glen Avenue
Peoria, IL 61614
309-681-1100
Fax: 309-681-1101; *Toll Free:* 800-272-3900
infocentralil@alz.org
www.alz.org/illinoiscentral

Chris Nauman, Office Manager

To help optimize the quality of life for people with Alzheimer's Disease and their families through advocacy, education, suport and service delivery, while actively promoting research to eliminate the disease.

Year Founded: 1980

3491 Alzheimer's Association: Central New York
441 W Kirkpatrick Street
Syracuse, NY 13204-1361
315-472-4201
Fax: 315-472-4202; *Toll Free:* 800-272-3900
cny-info@alz.org
www.alz.org/centralnewyork

Year Founded: 1980

3492 Alzheimer's Association: Central Ohio
1379 Dublin Road
Columbus, OH 43215
614-457-6003Toll free: 800-272-3900
www.alz.org/centralohio

Vince McGrail, Executive Director & CEO
Year Founded: 1980

3493 Alzheimer's Association: Central and Western Kansas
1820 E Douglas Avenue
Wichita, KS 67214
316-267-7333
Fax: 316-267-6369; *Toll Free:* 800-272-3900
cwkshelpline@alz.org
www.alz.org/cwkansas

Information, resources and services for patients and families. Education and Training fro family and professional caregivers. Directed Training for medical emergency and law enforcement personnel. Public awarness, Advocacy and Public Policy.

Year Founded: 1980

3494 Alzheimer's Association: Cleveland Area
23215 Commerce Park Drive
Suite 300
Beachwood, OH 44122
216-342-5565Toll free: 800-272-3900
info@alz.org
www.alz.org/cleveland

Year Founded: 1980

3495 Alzheimer's Association: Colorado
455 Sherman Street
Suite 500
Denver, CO 80203
303-813-1669
Fax: 303-813-1670; *Toll Free:* 800-272-3900
info@alz.org
www.alz.org/co

The primary provider of local information services to Alzheimer patients and families in Colorado, the leading funder of AD research and the leading voice representing those dealing with dementia on public policy issues.

Year Founded: 1980

3496 Alzheimer's Association: Connecticut
200 Executive Boulevard
Suite 4B
Southington, CT 06489
860-828-2828
Fax: 860-571-8613; *Toll Free:* 800-272-3900
info@alz.org
www.alz.org/ct

Eleonora Tornatore-Mikesh, President & CEO
James Vumbaco, CFO & COO
Year Founded: 1980

3497 Alzheimer's Association: Delaware Valley
399 Market Street
Suite 102
Philadelphia, PA 19106
Toll Free: 800-272-3900
info@alz.org
www.alz.org/delval

Wendy Campbell, President & CEO
Linda Coppinger, Executive Director
Year Founded: 1980

3498 Alzheimer's Association: Desert Southwest

1028 E McDowell Road
Phoenix, AZ 85006-2622
602-528-0545
Fax: 602-528-0546; *Toll Free:* 800-272-3900
deborah.schaus@alz.org
www.alz.org/dsw

Serves the state of Arizona and Southern Nevada.

Year Founded: 1980

3499 Alzheimer's Association: East Central Iowa

317 7th Avenue SE
Suite 402
Cedar Rapids, IA 52401
Toll Free: 800-272-3900
www.alz.org/eci

Year Founded: 1980

3500 Alzheimer's Association: Eastern North Carolina

3739 National Drive
Suite 110
Raleigh, NC 27612
Toll Free: 800-272-3900
www.alz.org/nc

Year Founded: 1980

3501 Alzheimer's Association: Eastern Tennessee

1545 Western Avenue
Suite 110A
Knoxville, TN 37921
Fax: 865-544-6249; *Toll Free:* 800-272-3900
info@alz.org
www.alz.org/tn

Angelia Jones, Executive Director

Year Founded: 1980

3502 Alzheimer's Association: Florida Gulf Coast

14010 Roosevelt Boulevard
Suite 709
Clearwater, FL 33762
727-578-2558Toll free: 800-272-3900
www.alz.org/flgulfcoast

Gloria Smith, President & CEO
Chuck Albrecht, COO

Serving 17 Florida Counties. Care Consultations, 24/7
Helpline, Support Groups, Caregiver Education, Library,
Information and Referral.

Year Founded: 1984

3503 Alzheimer's Association: Georgia

41 Perimeter Center East
Suite 550
Atlanta, GA 30346
404-728-1181
Fax: 404-636-9768; *Toll Free:* 800-272-3900
www.alz.org/georgia

Leslie Gregory, President & CEO

Year Founded: 1980

3504 Alzheimer's Association: Greater Cincinnati

644 Linn Street
Suite 1026
Cincinnati, OH 45203
513-721-4284
Fax: 513-345-8446; *Toll Free:* 800-272-3900
www.alz.org/cincinnati

Paula Kollstedt, Executive Director

Year Founded: 1980

3505 Alzheimer's Association: Greater Dallas

3001 Knox Street
Suite 200
Dallas, TX 75025
214-540-2400
Fax: 214-827-2064; *Toll Free:* 800-272-3900
helpline@alzdallas.org
www.alz.org/greaterdallas

Mark Denzin, Executive Director

The Alzheimer's Association is dedicated to providing support and assistance to persons affected by Alzheimer's disease and to their families and other caregivers through the Chapter's core services. The Dallas Chapter currently provides service for a thirty-four county area including: Anderson, Bowie, Camp, Cass, Cherokee, Collin, Cooke, Dallas, Delta, Denton, Ellis, Fannin, Franklin, Grayson, Gregg, Harrison, Henderson, Hopkins, Hunt, Kaufman, Lamar, Marion, Morris, Navarro, Panola, Rains, Red River, Rockwall, Rusk, Smith, Titus, Upshur, Van Zandt and Wood Counties.

Year Founded: 1980

3506 Alzheimer's Association: Greater East Ohio Area

70 W Streetsboro Street
Suite 201
Hudson, OH 44236
Fax: 330-650-0568; *Toll Free:* 800-272-3900
info@alz.org
www.alz.org/akroncantonyoungstown

Pam Schuellerman, Executive Director
Liz Mulroy, Program Director

Year Founded: 1980

3507 Alzheimer's Association: Greater Idaho

6126 W State Street
Suite 305
Boise, ID 83703
208-206-0041
Fax: 866-201-5957; *Toll Free:* 800-272-3900
www.alz.org/idaho

MacKenzie Rodgers, Executive Director

The Alzheimer's Association Greater Idaho serves the citizens of Idaho and South Eastern Oregon. We are a part of the National Alzheimer's Association. Our mission is to eliminate Alzheimer's disease through the advancement of research; to provide and enhance care and support for all affected, and to reduce the risk of dementia through the promotion of brain health.

Year Founded: 1980

3508 Alzheimer's Association: Greater Illinios

8430 W Bryn Mawr
Chicago, IL 60631

847-933-2413
Fax: 847-933-2417; *Toll Free:* 800-272-3900
gi.chapter@alz.org
www.alz.org/illinois

Erna Colborn, President & CEO
Janet Devlin, CFO

A national voluntary health agency dedicated to researching the prevention, cure and treatment of Alzheimer's disease and related disorders and to providing support and assistance to individuals with alzheimer's disease, their families and caregivers.

Year Founded: 1980

3509 Alzheimer's Association: Greater Indiana
50 E 91st Street
Suite 100
Indianapolis, IN 46240
Toll Free: 800-272-3900
www.alz.org/indiana

Year Founded: 1980

3510 Alzheimer's Association: Greater Iowa
1730 28th Street
West Des Moines, IA 50266
515-440-2722Toll free: 800-272-3900
greateriowa@alz.org
www.alz.org/greateriowa

Michelle Kelman, Snr. Program & Event Coordinator
Year Founded: 1980

3511 Alzheimer's Association: Greater Kentucky & Southern Indiana
Kaden Tower
6100 Dutchmans Lane
Suite 401
Louisville, KY 40205
502-451-4266
Fax: 502-456-2701; *Toll Free:* 800-272-3900
infoky-in@alz.org
www.alz.org/kyin

Year Founded: 1980

3512 Alzheimer's Association: Greater Maryland
1850 York Road
Suite D
Timonium, MD 21093
Toll Free: 800-272-3900
www.alz.org/maryland

Year Founded: 1980

3513 Alzheimer's Association: Greater Michigan
25200 Telegraph Road
Suite 100
Southfield, MI 48033
248-351-0280
Fax: 248-351-0419; *Toll Free:* 800-272-3900
helplinegmc@alz.org
www.alz.org/gmc

The Chapter's mission is to enhance the quality of life for all persons affected by Alzheimer's disease and related disorders through comprehensive educational programs, compassionate services, access to resources and support for research.

Year Founded: 1980

3514 Alzheimer's Association: Greater Missouri
2400 Bluff Creek Drive
Columbia, MO 65201
Toll Free: 800-272-3900
www.alz.org/greatermissouri

Year Founded: 1980

3515 Alzheimer's Association: Greater New Jersey
3 Eves Drive
Suite 310
Marlton, NJ 08053
973-866-8143Toll free: 800-272-3900
www.alz.org/nj

Year Founded: 1980

3516 Alzheimer's Association: Greater Pennsylvania
2595 Interstate Drive
Suite 100
Harrisburg, PA 17110
Toll Free: 800-272-3900
www.alz.org/pa

Year Founded: 1980

3517 Alzheimer's Association: Greater Richmond
4600 Cox Road
Suite 130
Glen Allen, VA 23060
804-967-2580
Fax: 804-967-2588; *Toll Free:* 800-272-3900
www.alz.org/grva

Marie D. Kolendo, CEO

The Chapter provides educational and support services to individuals with Alzheimer's disease, their families, and caregivers. Services include a telephone helpline, support groups, educational programs, case manager services, a respite scholarship program, a lending library, the National Safe Return Program, and a quarterly newsletter with caregiving tips. In addition, the Chapter offers in-service training to professional caregivers.

Year Founded: 1980

3518 Alzheimer's Association: Greater Wisconsin
2900 Curry Lane
Suite A
Green Bay, WI 54311
920-469-2110Toll free: 800-272-3900
info@alz.org
www.alz.org/gwwi

Year Founded: 1980

3519 Alzheimer's Association: Heart of America
3846 W 75th Street
Prairie Village, KS 66208
913-831-3888
Fax: 913-831-1916; *Toll Free:* 800-272-3900
jan.horn@alz.org
www.alz.org/kansascity

Year Founded: 1980

3520 Alzheimer's Association: Houston & Southeast Texas
6055 S Loop East
Houston, TX 77087

713-314-1313
Fax: 713-314-1315; *Toll Free:* 800-272-3900
www.alz.org/texas

Richard Elbein, CEO

Alzheimer's Association of Houston and Southeast Texas consits or families, caregivers, scientists, health professionals, and concerned citizens commited to finding a cure for Alzheimer's disease and to easing the burden of Alzheimer's and related disorders on patients and their familes and loved ones.

Year Founded: 1980

3521 Alzheimer's Association: Hudson Valley
2 Jefferson Plaza
Suite 103
Poughkeepsie, NY 12601
845-471-2655Toll free: 800-272-3900
info@alzhudsonvalley.org
www.alz.org/hudsonvalley

Year Founded: 1980

3522 Alzheimer's Association: Long Island
425 Broadhollow Road
Suite 307
Melville, NY 11747
631-629-6950Toll free: 800-272-3900
www.alz.org/longisland

Doug Davidson, Executive Director
Kate Anastasia, Program Director

Year Founded: 1980

3523 Alzheimer's Association: Louisiana
3445 N Causeway Boulevard
Suite 902
Metairie, LA 70002
504-613-6505Toll free: 800-272-3900
www.alz.org/louisiana

Brian Berrigan, Exeutive Director

Year Founded: 1980

3524 Alzheimer's Association: Maine
383 U.S. Route 1
Suite 2C
Scarborough, ME 04074
207-772-0115
Fax: 207-289-3705; *Toll Free:* 800-272-3900
www.alz.org/maine

Laura Trenholm, Executive Director

Year Founded: 1980

3525 Alzheimer's Association: Massachusetts - New Hampshire
480 Pleasant Street
Watertown, MA 02472
617-868-6718
Fax: 617-868-6720; *Toll Free:* 800-272-3900
info@alz.org
www.alz.org/manh

Year Founded: 1980

3526 Alzheimer's Association: Miami Valley
31 W Whipp Road
Dayton, OH 45459

937-291-3332
Fax: 937-291-0463; *Toll Free:* 800-272-3900
www.alz.org/dayton

Eric VanVlymen, Executive Director

Year Founded: 1980

3527 Alzheimer's Association: Michigan GreatLakes
564 South Main Street
Suite 200
Ann Arbor, MI 48104
734-369-2716Toll free: 800-272-3900
www.alz.org/mglc

Year Founded: 1980

3528 Alzheimer's Association: Mid South
4825 Trousdale Drive
Suite 220
Nashville, TN 37220
615-315-5880Toll free: 800-272-3900
www.alz.org/altn

Jim Ward, President & CEO

Year Founded: 1980

3529 Alzheimer's Association: Minnesota-North Dakota
7900 West 78th Street
Suite 100
Minneapolis, MN 55439
952-830-0512
Fax: 952-830-0513; *Toll Free:* 800-272-3900
info@alz.org
www.alz.org/mnnd

Susan Spalding, CEO

Year Founded: 1980

3530 Alzheimer's Association: Mississippi Chapter
207 W Jackson Street
Suite 1
Ridgeland, MS 39157
769-230-0611Toll free: 800-272-3900
ms-info@alz.org
www.alz.org/ms

Mary Kim Smith, Executive Director
Rachel Corkern, Director of Development
Cindy Widdig, Dir., Community Outreach

Mission is to eliminate Alzheimer's disease through the advancement of research; to provide and enhance care and support for all affected; and to reduce the risk of dementia through the promotion of brain health.

Year Founded: 1980

3531 Alzheimer's Association: Montana
3010 11th Avenue North
Billings, MT 59101
406-252-3053Toll free: 800-272-3900
www.alz.org/montana

Lynn Mullowney, Executive Director

Year Founded: 1980

3532 Alzheimer's Association: National Capital Area
3701 Pender Drive
Suite 400
Fairfax, VA 22030

703-359-4440
Fax: 703-359-4441; *Toll Free:* 800-272-3900
info@alz.org
www.alz.org/nca

Chris Broullire, President & CEO

Year Founded: 1980

3533 Alzheimer's Association: Nebraska

11711 Arbor Street
Suite 110
Omaha, NE 68144
402-502-4301
Fax: 402-502-7001; *Toll Free:* 800-272-3900
www.alz.org/nebraska

Viv Ewing, Executive Director

Serves persons with Alzheimer's disease and their families
in 80 counties across Nebraska and the entire state of Wyoming. The mission is to enhance the quality of life for all
persons affected by Alzheimer's disease and related disorders through comprehansive educational programs, compassionate services, access to resources and support for
research.

Year Founded: 1980

3534 Alzheimer's Association: New Mexico

9500 Montgomery Boulevard NE
Suite 121
Albuquerque, NM 87111
505-266-4473
Fax: 505-266-0108; *Toll Free:* 800-272-3900
www.alz.org/newmexico

Gary Giron, Executive Director
Lorey Esquibel, Director of Operations

Year Founded: 1980

3535 Alzheimer's Association: New York City

600 3rd Avenue
2nd Floor
New York, NY 10016
646-418-4466Toll free: 800-272-3900
www.alz.org/nyc

3536 Alzheimer's Association: North Central Texas

2630 West Freeway
Suite 100
Fort Worth, TX 76102
817-336-4949Toll free: 800-272-3900
www.alz.org/northcentraltexas

Theresa Hocker, President & CEO

Year Founded: 1980

3537 Alzheimer's Association: Northeastern New York

4 Pine West Plaza
Suite 405
Albany, NY 12205
518-867-4999
Fax: 518-867-4997; *Toll Free:* 800-272-3900
infoeny@alz.org
www.alz.org/northeasternny

Elizabeth Smith Boivin, Executive Director & CEO

Year Founded: 1980

3538 Alzheimer's Association: Northern California & Northern Nevada

2290 North First Street
Suite 101
San Jose, CA 95131
323-309-8821Toll free: 800-272-3900
www.alz.org/norcal

Year Founded: 1980

3539 Alzheimer's Association: Northwest Ohio

2500 North Reynolds Road
Toledo, OH 43615-2820
419-537-1999
Fax: 419-536-5591; *Toll Free:* 800-272-3900
www.alz.org/nwohio

Salli Bollin, Executive Director
Cheryl Conley, Program Director

Mission is to enhance quality Of life of all persons affected
by Alzheimer's disease and related memory loss disorders.

Year Founded: 1980

3540 Alzheimer's Association: Oklahoma

2448 E 81st Street
Suite 3000
Tulsa, OK 74137
918-392-5000Toll free: 800-272-3900
oksocial@alz.org
www.alz.org/oklahoma

Year Founded: 1980

3541 Alzheimer's Association: Orange County

600 Anton Boulevard
11th Floor
Costa Mesa, CA 92626
Toll Free: 800-272-3900
www.alz.org/oc

Year Founded: 1980

3542 Alzheimer's Association: Oregon

1650 Northwest Naito Parkway
Suite 190
Portland, OR 97209
Toll Free: 800-272-3900
www.alz.org/oregon

Alzheimer's information and resources.

Year Founded: 1980

3543 Alzheimer's Association: Rhode Island

245 Waterman Street
Suite 306
Providence, RI 02906
Toll Free: 800-272-3900
www.alz.org/ri

Donna McGowan, Executive Director

The mission is to help support Alzheimers families in
Rhode Island.

Year Founded: 1980

3544 Alzheimer's Association: Rochester & Finger Lakes

435 East Henrietta Road
Rochester, NY 14620
Toll Free: 800-272-3900
www.alz.org/rochesterny

Year Founded: 1980

3545 Alzheimer's Association: San Antonio & South Texas
10223 McAllister Freeway
Suite 100
San Antonio, TX 78216
Toll Free: 800-272-3900
www.alz.org/sanantonio

Year Founded: 1980

3546 Alzheimer's Association: San Diego/Imperial
2305 Historic Decatur Road
Suite 100
San Diego, CA 92106
Toll Free: 800-272-3900
www.alz.org/sandiego

Year Founded: 1980

3547 Alzheimer's Association: South Carolina
4124 Clemson Boulevard
Suite L
Anderson, SC 29621
Toll Free: 800-272-3900
info@alz.org
www.alz.org/sc

Year Founded: 1980

3548 Alzheimer's Association: South Central Wisconsin
2820 Walton Commons
Suite 132
Madison, WI 53718
Toll Free: 800-272-3900
www.alz.org/scwisc

Year Founded: 1980

3549 Alzheimer's Association: South Dakota
1000 North West Avenue
Suite 250
Sioux Falls, SD 57104
Toll Free: 800-272-3900
www.alz.org/sd

Year Founded: 1980

3550 Alzheimer's Association: Southeast Florida
3333 Forest Hill Boulevard
West Palm Beach, FL 33406
Toll Free: 800-272-3900
www.alz.org/seflorida

Year Founded: 1980

3551 Alzheimer's Association: Southeastern Virginia
6350 Center Drive
Suite 102
Norfolk, VA 23502
757-459-2405
Fax: 757-461-7902; *Toll Free:* 800-272-3900
infoseva@alz.org
www.alz.org/seva

Year Founded: 1980

3552 Alzheimer's Association: Southeastern Wisconsin
620 South 76th Street
Suite 160
Milwaukee, WI 53214
414-479-8800Toll free: 800-272-3900
www.alz.org/sewi

Tom Hlavacek, Executive Director
Krista Scheel, Program Director

Year Founded: 1980

3553 Alzheimer's Association: St. Louis
9370 Olive Boulevard
St. Louis, MO 63132-3214
Toll Free: 800-272-3900
www.alz.org

Year Founded: 1980

3554 Alzheimer's Association: Utah
855 East 4800 South
Suite 100
Salt Lake City, UT 84107
801-265-1944Toll free: 800-272-3900
www.alz.org/utah

Ronnie Daniel, Executive Director
Kate Nederostek, Program Director

Year Founded: 1980

3555 Alzheimer's Association: Vermont
300 Cornerstone Drive
Suite 130
Williston, VT 05495
802-316-3839Toll free: 800-272-3900
www.alz.org/vermont

Martha Richardson, Executive Director
Jane Mitchell, Development Director

The Alzheimer's Association is the only voluntary health organization dedicated to research aimed at the prevention, care, and treatment of Alzheimer's disease and related disorders, while providing support and assistance to those affected with the disease and their families.

Year Founded: 1980

3556 Alzheimer's Association: Washington State
North Tower, 100 W Harrison Street
Suite N200
Seattle, WA 98119
Toll Free: 800-272-3900
www.alz.org/alzwa

Year Founded: 1980

3557 Alzheimer's Association: West Texas
110 Mesa Park
Suite 250
El Paso, TX 79912
915-544-1799
Fax: 915-544-8746; *Toll Free:* 800-272-3900
vlosoya@alz.org
www.alz.org/westtexas

Year Founded: 1980

3558 Alzheimer's Association: West Virginia
1601 Second Avenue
Charleston, WV 25387

304-343-2717Toll free: 800-272-3900
info@alz.org
www.alz.org/wv

Laurel Walker, Executive Director

Year Founded: 1980

3559 Alzheimer's Association: Western Carolina

4600 Park Road
Suite 250
Charlotte, NC 28209
980-498-7760
Fax: 980-939-1306; *Toll Free:* 800-272-3900
infonc@alz.org
www.alz.org/northcarolina

Dedicated to improving life for those with Alzheimer's and related disorders and their families and caregivers. Provides patient and family services designed to support an estimated 77,000 persons with the disease in North Carolina's 49 western counties. Services include a 24-hour toll-free helpline, family support groups, and a national Safe Return Program, as well as family, caregiver, professional and community education.

Year Founded: 1980

3560 Alzheimer's Association: Western New York

2805 Wehrle Drive
Suite 6
Williamsville, NY 14221
Fax: 716-626-2255; *Toll Free:* 800-272-3900
www.alz.org/wny

Leilani Joven Pelletier, Executive Director

Year Founded: 1980

3561 Alzheimer's Association: Wyoming

2232 Dell Range Boulevard
Suite 220
Cheyenne, WY 82009
307-316-2892Toll free: 800-272-3900
www.alz.org/wyoming

Janet Lewis, Executive Director

Year Founded: 1980

3562 Alzheimer's Disease Education and Referral Center (ADEAR)

National Institute on Aging
Building 31, 31 Center Drive
Room 5C27
Bethesda, MD MSC 2292
Toll Free: 800-438-4380
adear@nia.nih.gov
www.nia.nih.gov/alzheimers

A service of the National Institute on Aging, the ADEAR Center distributes information on Alzheimer's disease, on current research activities and on services available to patients and family members. Offers free publications. List available upon request.

Year Founded: 1990

3563 Alzheimer's Drug Discovery Foundation

57 W 57th Street
Suite 904
New York, NY 10019
212-901-8000
info@alzdiscovery.org
www.alzdiscovery.org

Howard Fillit, Executive Director

Funds the most promising Alzheimer's drug research worldwide.

Year Founded: 1998

3564 Alzheimer's Foundation of America

322 Eighth Avenue
7th Floor
New York, NY 10001
646-638-1542
Fax: 646-638-1546; *Toll Free:* 866-232-8484
www.alzfdn.org

Charles J. Fuschillo Jr., President & CEO
Josie Di Chiara, SVP, External Relations

Number of Members: 1,600

3565 American Academy of Neurology

201 Chicago Avenue
Minneapolis, MN 55415
612-928-6000
Fax: 612-454-2746; *Toll Free:* 800-879-1960
memberservices@aan.com
www.aan.com

Professional society of medical doctors specializing in brain and nervous system diseases. Maintains placement service. Sponsors research and educational programs. Compiles statistics. Publishes scientific journal.

Year Founded: 1948

3566 American Board of Psychiatry and Neurology

2150 E Lake Cook Road
Suite 900
Buffalo Grove, IL 60089
847-229-6500
Fax: 847-229-6600
questions@abpn.com
www.abpn.com

Larry R. Faulkner, President & CEO

The mission of the ABPN is to develop and provide valid and reliable procedures for certification and maintenance of certification in psychiatry and neurology.

Year Founded: 1934

3567 BrightFocus Foundation

22512 Gateway Center Drive
Clarksburg, MD 20871-2005
301-948-3244
Fax: 301-258-9454; *Toll Free:* 800-437-2423
jphilabaum@brightfocus.org
www.brightfocus.org

Dave Marks, VP, Finance & Administration
Diane Bovenkamp, VP, Scientific Affairs
Michael Buckley, VP, Public Affairs

Offers updated and trustworthy information on research, treatments, and resources. Free publications and newsletters.

Year Founded: 1973

3568 CareScout

60 Hickory Drive
4th Floor
Waltham, MA 02451
Fax: 800-513-8860; *Toll Free:* 800-571-1918
www.carescout.com

Robert N. Bua, President

Care advocates help thousands of families each year find the most appropriate home health aids, assisted living facilities, and nursing homes.

Year Founded: 1997

3569 Clayton County Alzheimer's Services Center
7251 Mt. Zion Circle
Morrow, GA 30260
770-603-4090
Fax: 770-603-4092
info@asc-ga.org
www.asc-ga.org

The mission of ASC is to enhance and prolong the highest quality of life for person's with Alzheimer's Disease and other related disorders and for their families.

3570 John Douglas French Alzheimer's Foundation
11620 Wilshire Boulevard
Suite 270
Los Angeles, CA 90025-1768
310-445-4650
www.jdfaf.org

Mike Minchin, President & CEO

Funds scientific and medical research into the cause, cure and prevention of Alzheimer's disease.

3571 The Tender
4501 Church Road
Mt. Laurel, NJ 08054
856-234-5999
Fax: 856-234-9074
tenderadc@aol.com
www.thetender.org

Barbara Fetty, Executive Director

Caring for frail seniors and people with Alzheimer's in Burlington County, NJ since 1977.

Year Founded: 1977

Books

3572 36-Hour Day
Alzheimer's Association
919 N Michigan Avenue
Suite 1000
Chicago, IL 60611-1696
773-342-4722
Fax: 312-335-1110; *Toll Free:* 800-272-3900
info@alz.org
www.alz.org

Gerald Sampson, Chair
Deborah Jones, Secretary
Thomas J. Winkel, Treasurer

A family guide to caring for persons with Alzheimer's disease, related dementing illnesses, and memory loss later in life. Spanish version available.

422 pages

3573 A Handbook of Activities for Persons With Dementia
Johns Hopkins University Press
2715 N Charles Street
Baltimore, MD 21218-4319

301-338-6900
Fax: 301-338-6998
www.press.jhu.edu
192 pages

3574 ABC's of Dementia
Canyonlands Publishing
10320 W Indian School Road
Phoenix, AZ 85037-5822
602-224-9796
Fax: 623-877-9887

Jim Moritz, Owner

Provides basic information about the syndrome of Alzheimer's dementia. The topics include definition of the dementia syndrome, general characteristics, diagnosis, informational resources and treatment.

3575 Activity Programming for Persons with Dementia: A Sourcebook
Alzheimer's Association
919 N Michigan Avenue
Suite 1000
Chicago, IL 60611-1696
312-335-8700
Fax: 312-335-1110; *Toll Free:* 800-272-3900
info@alz.org
www.alz.org

Gerald Sampson, Chair
Deborah Jones, Secretary
Thomas J. Winkel, Treasurer

Provides direction and suggestions for designing activities for people with Alzheimer's disease and other related dementias. Each activity is described and illustrated. Includes a list of reference materials and organizations.

138 pages

3576 Alzheimer Early Stages
Hunter House Publisher
PO Box 2914
Alameda, CA 94501
510-865-5282
Fax: 510-865-4295; *Toll Free:* 800-266-5592
ordering@hunterhouse.com
www.hunterhouse.com

Christina Sverdrup, Customer Service Manager
Daniel Kuhn MSW, Author

First steps in caring and treatments. This book is for family memebrs and friends of those recently diagnosed with Alzheimer's Disease.

320 pages

3577 Alzheimer's Disease Orientation Kit
Alzheimer's Association
919 N Michigan Avenue
Suite 1000
Chicago, IL 60611-1696
312-335-8700
Fax: 312-335-1110; *Toll Free:* 800-272-3900
info@alz.org
www.alz.org

Gerald Sampson, Chair
Deborah Jones, Secretary
Thomas J. Winkel, Treasurer

A collection of materials developed to familiarize the audience with Alzheimer's disease and its effects on the patient and family. Includes the Orientation to Alzheimer's Disease videotape, Learning Guide and Caregiver Packet.

3578 Alzheimer's Disease Treatment and Family Stress: Directions for Research
Superintendent of Documents
PO Box 371954
Pittsburgh, PA 15250-7954
202-512-2250
Fax: 202-512-2250

Presents a collection of papers giving current information on research investigations that increase the understanding of the nature and consequences of family caregiving.

486 pages

3579 Alzheimer's Disease: A Guide to Federal Programs
Alzheimer's Disease Education & Referral Center
PO Box 8250
Silver Spring, MD 20907-8250
Fax: 301-495-3334; *Toll Free:* 800-438-4380

Directory of Alzheimer's disease programs sponsored by federal agencies. Listed agency by agency, it provides locations and telephone numbers for multi-site activities and demonstration programs, and lists information resources.

113 pages

3580 Alzheimer's Disease: A Handbook for Caregivers
Mosby-Year Book
11830 Westline Industrial Drive
Saint Louis, MO 63146-3313
314-872-8370
Fax: 432-432-1380; *Toll Free:* 800-426-4545
www.mosby.com

For nurses and caregivers without nursing degrees. Discusses the structure and functioning of the human brain, clinical aspects of Alzheimer's, management of dementia, issues of ethics, law, stress and abuse of elders, community support, and optimistic research areas.

451 pages

3581 Alzheimer's Disease: Activity-Focused Care
Butterworth-Heinemann
225 Wildwood Avenue
Woburn, MA 01801-2025
781-904-2500
Fax: 800-446-6520; *Toll Free:* 800-366-2665
www.bh.com

Information for professional and family caregivers on activity-focused care for Alzheimer's patients.

436 pages

3582 Alzheimer's Handbook
Branden Publishing Company
17 Station Street
Box 843
Brookline, MA 02445-7995
617-734-2045
Fax: 617-734-2046
www.branden.com

3583 Alzheimer's, Stroke and 29 Other Neurological Disorders Sourcebook
Omnigraphics
155 West Congress
Suite 200
Detroit, MI 48226
313-961-1340
Fax: 313-961-1383; *Toll Free:* 800-234-1340
www.omnigraphics.com

Georgiann Lavginiger, Customer Service Manager
Peter E Ruffner, President

Provides vital information for the nontechnical reader focusing on Alzheimer's Disease, stroke and various neurological disorders. Answers thousands of questions related to afflications of the central nervous system with each chapter reviwing a particular disorder and offers in-depth discussions.

3584 Alzheimer's: The Answers You Need
Elder Books
PO Box 490
Forest Knolls, CA 94933
415-488-9002
Fax: 415-488-4720; *Toll Free:* 800-909-2673
www.elderbooks.com

Designed for people in the early stages of Alzheimer's. Question-and-answer format provides information about the nature and causes of AD.

138 pages

3585 Complete Guide to Alzheimer's Proofing Your Home
Purdue University Press
504 West State Street
West Lafayette, IN 47907-2058
Fax: 419-281-6883; *Toll Free:* 800-247-6553
www.thepress.purdue.edu/

Guide to modify homes of Alzheimer's patients to facilitate caregiving.

496 pages

3586 Confronting Alzheimer's Disease
American Assn. of Homes & Services for the Aging
901 E Street NW
Suite 500
Washington, DC 20004-2037
202-661-5700
Fax: 202-783-2255

Daniel Smith, Vice President

A resource for administrators, professional caregivers and families dealing with Alzheimer's Disease and related disorders.

225 pages

3587 Coping and Caring: Living with Alzheimer's Disease
AARP Fulfillment
601 E Street NW
Washington, DC 20049
202-434-2277
Fax: 202-434-3443; *Toll Free:* 800-424-3410
member@aarp.org
www.aarp.org

William D Novelli, CEO

Addresses the questions: What is Alzheimer's? How does the disease progress? How long does it last? How can families cope?.

24 pages

3588 Designing for Alzheimer's Disease: Strategies for Creating Better Care Environment
John Wiley & Sons
111 River Street
Hoboken, NJ 07030-5774
201-748-6000
Fax: 201-748-6088
info@wiley.com
www.wiley.com

Elizabeth C Brawley, Author

A practical, thorough approach to the development of therapeutic special care settings. Equips designers and care providers with the information they need to plan environments that can greatly enhance the lives of those with alzheimer's.

340 pages

3589 From Theory to Therapy: The Development of Drugs for Alzheimer's Disease
Alzheimer's Association
919 N Michigan Avenue
Suite 1000
Chicago, IL 60611-1696
312-335-8700
Fax: 312-335-1110; *Toll Free:* 800-272-3900
info@alz.org
www.alz.org

Gerald Sampson, Chair
Deborah Jones, Secretary
Thomas J. Winkel, Treasurer

Provides a layman's explanation of how experimental drugs are being developed and tested for Alzheimer's disease, and information about patient participation in clinical drug trials.

44+ pages

3590 Guidelines for Dignity
Alzheimer's Association
919 N Michigan Avenue
Suite 1000
Chicago, IL 60611-1696
312-335-8700
Fax: 312-335-1110; *Toll Free:* 800-272-3900
info@alz.org
www.alz.org

Gerald Sampson, Chair
Deborah Jones, Secretary
Thomas J. Winkel, Treasurer

A resource for providers who are offerng Alzheimer/dementia care in residential settings. Eight goals target specific issues to be addressed and present practical ideas and advice. This resource for facility professionals corresponds to the Family Guide for Alzheimer Care in Residential Settings, which can be used as a companion resource.

40 pages

3591 Handbook of Activities for Persons with Dementia
Johns Hopkins University Press
2715 N Charles Street
Baltimore, MD 21218-4319
410-516-6900
Fax: 410-516-6998; *Toll Free:* 800-537-5487
www.jhu.edu/press/index.html

William Brody, President

192 pages

3592 Hospice Care for Patients with Advanced Progressive Dementia
Springer Publishing Company
11 West 42nd Street
15th Floor
New York, NY 10036
212-431-4370
Fax: 212-941-7842
www.springerpub.com

Ursula Springer, President

Discusses adpating hospice care for terminally ill patients with dementia. Topics include infections, eating difficulties, and providing palliative care.

305 pages

3593 Interventions for Alzheimer's Disease: A Caregiver's Complete Reference
Health Professions Press
PO Box 10624
Baltimore, MD 21285
410-337-9585
Fax: 410-337-8539; *Toll Free:* 888-337-8808

Melissa Behm, President

For professionals who plan, administer or provide services to Alzheimer's patients.

239 pages

3594 Just the Facts & More Kit
Alzheimer's Association
919 N Michigan Avenue
Suite 1000
Chicago, IL 60611-1676
312-335-8700
Fax: 312-335-1110; *Toll Free:* 800-272-3900
info@alz.org
www.alz.org

Gerald Sampson, Chair
Deborah Jones, Secretary
Thomas J. Winkel, Treasurer

Two-sided, easy-to-read fact sheets on a variety of topics of interest to caregivers of Alzheimer's patients.

3595 Key Elements of Dementia Care
Alzheimer's Association
919 N Michigan Avenue
Suite 1000
Chicago, IL 60611-1676
312-335-8700
Fax: 312-335-1110; *Toll Free:* 800-272-3900
info@alz.org
www.alz.org

Gerald Sampson, Chair
Deborah Jones, Secretary
Thomas J. Winkel, Treasurer

Defines, describes, and illustrates dementia-capable care throughout the range of residential care settings.

90 pages

3596 Learning to Speak Alzheimer's A Groundbreaking Approach for Everyone Dealing with the Disease
Houghton Mifflin
222 Berkeley Street
Boston, MA 02116
617-351-5000
www.houghtonmifflinbooks.com

Joanne Koenig Coste, Author

Offers a practical appraoch to the emotional well-being of both patients and caregivers that emphasizes relating to patients in their own reality.

256 pages

3597 Living in the Labyrinth: A Personal Journey Through the Maze of Alzheimers
Dell Publishing
1745 Broadway
New York, NY 10019
212-782-9000
Fax: 800-659-2436; *Toll Free:* 800-726-0600
www.randomhouse.com

Peter Olsen, CEO

3598 Safe Return Home: An Inspirational Book for Caregivers of Alzheimer's
Andrews McMeel Publishing Company
PO Box 419263
Kansas City, MO 64193
816-932-6700
Fax: 800-437-8683; *Toll Free:* 800-826-4216
www.uclick.com

Kathleen W Andrews, CEO

Impact of Alzheimer's on patients and their families by using the Crankshaft cartoon and personal reminiscences.

112 pages

3599 Speaking Our Minds: Personal Reflections from Individuals with Alzheimer's
WH Freeman and Company
41 Madison Avenue
New York, NY 10010-2202
212-576-9400
Fax: 212-689-2383

Elizabeth Widdicombe, President

Personal reflections of people with Alzheimer's disease.

161 pages

3600 Therapeutic Activity for Persons with Alzheimer
Pro-Ed
8700 Shoal Creek Boulevard
Austin, TX 78757-6816
Fax: 800-897-3202; *Toll Free:* 800-397-7633

A program of functional skills for activities of daily living. Hardcover.

3601 Understanding Alzheimer's Disease
University Press of Mississippi
3825 Ridgewood Road
Jackson, MS 39211
601-432-6205
Fax: 601-432-6217
press@ihl.state.ms.us
www.upress.state.ms.us

A guide to understanding a devastating illness that affects a significant segment of the elderly population.

150 pages

3602 Useful Information on Alzheimer's Disease
National Clearinghouse for Alcohol and Drug Abuse
PO Box 2345
Rockville, MD 20847-2345
301-468-2600
Fax: 301-468-2600; *Toll Free:* 800-729-6686
www.health.org

24 pages

3603 When Memory Fails: Helping the Alzheimer's & Dementia Patient
Plenum Press
233 Spring Street
Floor 7
New York, NY 10013-1522
212-620-8000
Fax: 212-463-0742

Rudiger Gebauer, Owner

296 pages

Directories

3604 Alzheimer's Disease
Franklin Watts
PO Box 1796
Danbury, CT 06816-1796
Fax: 800-374-4329; *Toll Free:* 800-621-1115
www.publishing.grolier.com

Elaine Landau, Editor

Support organizations for family members of Alzheimer's patients. Entries include: Organization name, address, phone. Principal content of publication is true stories of patients, treatments currently used, and research concerning the cause of the illness.

3605 Alzheimer's Disease: A Guide for Families
Addison-Wesley Publishing Company
Jacob Way
Reading, MA 01867
617-944-3700
Fax: 617-942-1117; *Toll Free:* 800-552-2259

Katie Courtice, Contact
Lenore S Powell, Contact

Publication includes: List of about 60 chapters of the Alzheimer's Disease and Related Disorders Association. Entries include: Chapter name, address, phone, name of contact person.

Journals, Magazines

3606 Early Stage Alzheimer's Care: A Guide for Community Based Programs
Springer Publishing Company
11 West 42nd Street
15th Floor
New York, NY 10036
212-431-4370
Fax: 212-941-7842
www.springerpub.com

Ursula Springer, President

3607 Research & Practice
Alzheimer's Association
919 N Michigan Avenue
Suite 1000
Chicago, IL 60611-1676
312-335-8700
Fax: 312-335-1110; *Toll Free:* 800-272-3900
info@alz.org
www.alz.org

Gerald Sampson, Chair
Deborah Jones, Secretary
Thomas J. Winkel, Treasurer

Provides practical information for healthcare professionals on the current status of prominent areas of Alzheimer research.

Newsletters, Pamphlets

3608 Advances
Alzheimer's Association
919 N Michigan Avenue
Suite 1000
Chicago, IL 60611-1676
312-335-8700
Fax: 312-335-1110; *Toll Free:* 800-272-3900
info@alz.org
www.alz.org

Gerald Sampson, Chair
Deborah Jones, Secretary
Thomas J. Winkel, Treasurer

Provides information related to research and caregiving.

3609 Alzheimer's Advocates Handbook
Alzheimer's Association
919 N Michigan Avenue
Suite 1000
Chicago, IL 60611-1676
312-335-8700
Fax: 312-335-1110; *Toll Free:* 800-272-3900
info@alz.org
www.alz.org

Gerald Sampson, Chair
Deborah Jones, Secretary
Thomas J. Winkel, Treasurer

Guide for the individual advocate, offering tips in letter writing, meeting with public officials and getting results.

20 pages

3610 Alzheimer's Association National Brochure
Alzheimer's Association
919 N Michigan Avenue
Suite 1000
Chicago, IL 60611-1676
312-335-8700
Fax: 312-335-1110; *Toll Free:* 800-272-3900
info@alz.org
www.alz.org

Gerald Sampson, Chair
Deborah Jones, Secretary
Thomas J. Winkel, Treasurer

Describes the Alzheimer's Association and its services.

3611 Alzheimer's Association Newsletter
Lexington\Bluegrass Chapter
801 S Limestone
Suite E
Lexington, KY 40508-3222
859-266-5283
Fax: 859-268-4764

Pat McCray, Editor
Marcey Ansley, Executive Director

8 pages Frequency: Quarterly

3612 Alzheimer's Association Tarrant County Chapter
PO Box 9709
Fort Worth, TX 76147-2709
817-336-4949
Fax: 817-336-4966; *Toll Free:* 800-471-
theresa.hocker@alz.org
www.alz.org

David Burr, President
Meharvan Singh PhD, Vice President
Susan J. Wilcox, Treasurer

Newsletter for those afflicted with Alzheimer's Disease. Includes education, support groups, case management, telephone helpline, and referral to services (i.e. long-term care, adult daycare, medical assistance, legal assistance, etc.).

8 pages

3613 Alzheimer's Disease: A Guide to Federal Programs
Alzheimer's Disease Education & Referral Center
PO Box 8250
Silver Spring, MD 20907-8250
Fax: 301-495-3334; *Toll Free:* 800-438-4380

R. Jordon Smyth , Jr., CFA, Chair
Eric Steinmiller, Vice Chair
Jodi Lyons, Secretary

Directory of Alzheimer's disease programs sponsored by federal agencies. Listed agency by agency, it provides locations and telephone numbers for multi-site activities and demonstration programs, and lists information resources.

113 pages

3614 Alzheimer's Disease: An Overview
Alzheimer's Association
919 N Michigan Avenue
Suite 1000
Chicago, IL 60611-1676
312-335-8700
Fax: 312-335-1110; *Toll Free:* 800-272-3900

info@alz.org
www.alz.org

Gerald Sampson, Chair
Deborah Jones, Secretary
Thomas J. Winkel, Treasurer

Basic facts on Alzheimer's disease, including a glossary.

3615 Alzheimer's Disease: Services You May Need
Alzheimer's Association
919 N Michigan Avenue
Suite 1000
Chicago, IL 60611-1696
312-335-8700
Fax: 312-335-1110; *Toll Free:* 800-272-3900
info@alz.org
www.alz.org

Gerald Sampson, Chair
Deborah Jones, Secretary
Thomas J. Winkel, Treasurer

Guide to services available to Alzheimer's disease caregivers.

3616 Alzheimer's Disease: Statistics
Alzheimer's Association
919 N Michigan Avenue
Suite 1000
Chicago, IL 60611-1696
312-335-8700
Fax: 312-335-1110; *Toll Free:* 800-272-3900
info@alz.org
www.alz.org

Gerald Sampson, Chair
Deborah Jones, Secretary
Thomas J. Winkel, Treasurer

Indicates basic information on incidence, prevalence, cost of care, etc.

3617 Alzheimer's Research Review
American Health Assistance Foundation
15825 Shady Grove Road
Suite 140
Rockville, MD 20850-4015
301-948-3244
Fax: 301-258-9451; *Toll Free:* 800-437-2423
www.brightfocus.org/

Gerald Sampson, Chair
Deborah Jones, Secretary
Thomas J. Winkel, Treasurer

4-6 pages

3618 Care for Advanced Alzheimer's Disease
Alzheimer's Association
919 N Michigan Avenue
Suite 1200
Chicago, IL 60611-1694
312-335-8700
Fax: 312-335-1110; *Toll Free:* 800-272-3900
info@alz.org
www.alz.org

Gerald Sampson, Chair
Deborah Jones, Secretary
Thomas J. Winkel, Treasurer

Suggestions for coping with caregiving problems that commonly occur late in the progression of Alzheimer's disease.

3619 Caregiver Stress: Signs to Watch for... Steps to Take
Alzheimer's Association
919 N Michigan Avenue
Suite 1200
Chicago, IL 60611-1694
312-335-8700
Fax: 312-335-1110; *Toll Free:* 800-272-3900
info@alz.org
www.alz.org

Gerald Sampson, Chair
Deborah Jones, Secretary
Thomas J. Winkel, Treasurer

Learn to recognize the warning signs and discover techniques for reducing stress.

3620 Caregiving at Home
Alzheimer's Association
919 N Michigan Avenue
Suite 1000
Chicago, IL 60611-1696
312-335-8700
Fax: 312-335-1110; *Toll Free:* 800-272-3900
info@alz.org
www.alz.org

Gerald Sampson, Chair
Deborah Jones, Secretary
Thomas J. Winkel, Treasurer

Suggestions for considering and planning home care for the person with dementia.

3621 Caring for Alzheimer's Patients
Perseus Books
233 Spring Street
New York, NY 10013-1522
212-368-0770
Fax: 800-324-3791; *Toll Free:* 800-221-8002

Gerald Sampson, Chair
Deborah Jones, Secretary
Thomas J. Winkel, Treasurer

This handbook is designed for families, friends, and health-care professionals coping with the myriad of problems encountered by those afflicted with Alzheimer's disease.

308 pages

3622 Charitable Trusts
Alzheimer's Association
919 N Michigan Avenue
Suite 1000
Chicago, IL 60611-1696
312-335-8700
Fax: 312-335-1110; *Toll Free:* 800-272-3900
info@alz.org
www.alz.org

Gerald Sampson, Chair
Deborah Jones, Secretary
Thomas J. Winkel, Treasurer

Explains the benefits of several types of charitable trusts, including Unitrusts, Charitable Remainder Annuity Trusts, and Charitable Lead Trusts.

3623 Drug Fact Sheets
Alzheimer's Association
919 N Michigan Avenue
Suite 1000
Chicago, IL 60611-1696
312-335-8700
Fax: 312-335-1110; *Toll Free:* 800-272-3900
info@alz.org
www.alz.org

Gerald Sampson, Chair
Deborah Jones, Secretary
Thomas J. Winkel, Treasurer

Concerns experimental drugs currently being tested.

3624 Especially for the Alzheimer Caregiver
Alzheimer's Association
919 N Michigan Avenue
Suite 1000
Chicago, IL 60611-1696
312-335-8700
Fax: 312-335-1110; *Toll Free:* 800-272-3900
info@alz.org
www.alz.org

Gerald Sampson, Chair
Deborah Jones, Secretary
Thomas J. Winkel, Treasurer

Offers suggestions for the Alzheimer caregiver on how to
cope with caregiving.

3625 Ethical Considerations: Issues in Diagnostic
Disclosure
Alzheimer's Association
919 N Michigan Avenue
Suite 1000
Chicago, IL 60611-1696
312-335-8700
Fax: 312-335-1110; *Toll Free:* 800-272-3900
info@alz.org
www.alz.org

Gerald Sampson, Chair
Deborah Jones, Secretary
Thomas J. Winkel, Treasurer

Discusses the individual's right to know the Alzheimer's
diagnosis. Provides tips on disclosing the diagnosis and
communicating with family members.

2 pages

3626 Exploring Care Options for a Relative with
Alzheimer's Disease
American Assn. of Homes & Services for the Aging
901 E Street NW
Suite 500
Washington, DC 20004-2037
202-661-5700

3627 Family Guide for Alzheimer's Care in
Residential Settings
Alzheimer's Association
919 N Michigan Avenue
Suite 1000
Chicago, IL 60611-1676
312-335-8700
Fax: 312-335-1110; *Toll Free:* 800-272-3900
info@alz.org
www.alz.org

Gerald Sampson, Chair
Deborah Jones, Secretary
Thomas J. Winkel, Treasurer

This guide for families corresponds to Guidelines for Dignity which can be used as a companion resource. It provides 50 checkpoints for families to consider as they plan
for long-term residential care for their Alzheimer/dementia
patient. A checklist to use in evaluating residential settings
is included.

40 pages

3628 Guidelines for Dignity
Alzheimer's Association
919 N Michigan Avenue
Suite 1000
Chicago, IL 60611-1676
312-335-8700
Fax: 312-335-1110; *Toll Free:* 800-272-3900
info@alz.org
www.alz.org

Gerald Sampson, Chair
Deborah Jones, Secretary
Thomas J. Winkel, Treasurer

A resource for providers who are offerring Alzheimer/de-
mentia care in residential settings. Eight goals target specific issues to be addressed and present practical ideas and
advice.

40 pages

3629 Home Safety for the Alzheimer's Patient
Alzheimer's Disease Education & Referral Center
PO Box 8250
Silver Spring, MD 20907-8250
Fax: 301-495-3334; *Toll Free:* 800-438-4380

Gerald Sampson, Chair
Deborah Jones, Secretary
Thomas J. Winkel, Treasurer

Practical guide for those who provide in-home care to people with Alzheimer's disease or related disorders. Designed
to improve home safety and identify problems and solutions to prevent increase accieents. Increases the patient's
security and freedom.

32 pages

3630 If You Have Alzheimer's Disease: What You
Should Know, What You Can Do
Alzheimer's Association
919 N Michigan Avenue
Suite 1000
Chicago, IL 60611-1676
312-335-8700
Fax: 312-335-1110; *Toll Free:* 800-272-3900
info@alz.org
www.alz.org

Gerald Sampson, Chair
Deborah Jones, Secretary
Thomas J. Winkel, Treasurer

Guide for the person with Alzheimer's disease. Includes
suggestions of things to do that will help the person cope.

3631 Is it Alzheimer's? Warning Signs You Should Know
Alzheimer's Association
919 N Michigan Avenue
Suite 1000
Chicago, IL 60611-1676
312-335-8700
Fax: 312-335-1110; *Toll Free:* 800-272-3900
info@alz.org
www.alz.org

Gerald Sampson, Chair
Deborah Jones, Secretary
Thomas J. Winkel, Treasurer

Contains a list of symptoms and answers to the most frequently asked questions.

3632 Memory and Aging
Alzheimer's Association
919 N Michigan Avenue
Suite 1000
Chicago, IL 60611-1676
312-335-8700
Fax: 312-335-1110; *Toll Free:* 800-272-3900
info@alz.org
www.alz.org

Gerald Sampson, Chair
Deborah Jones, Secretary
Thomas J. Winkel, Treasurer

Compares age-associated memory impairment with disease-caused memory impairment.

3633 National Public Policy Program to Conquer Alzheimer's Disease
Alzheimer's Association
919 N Michigan Avenue
Suite 1000
Chicago, IL 60611-1676
312-335-8700
Fax: 312-335-1110; *Toll Free:* 800-272-3900
info@alz.org
www.alz.org

Gerald Sampson, Chair
Deborah Jones, Secretary
Thomas J. Winkel, Treasurer

Summary of the Association's public policy goals, objectives and policies.

12 pages

3634 Private Long-Term Care Insurance: To Buy or Not to Buy?
Alzheimer's Association
919 N Michigan Avenue
Suite 1000
Chicago, IL 60611-1676
773-298-9988
Fax: 312-335-1110; *Toll Free:* 800-272-3900
info@alz.org
www.alz.org

Chai Leung, Owner

Consumer guide to making decisions about purchasing a long-term care insurance policy, including affordability, key points to look for, and alternatives to long-term care insurance.

4 pages

3635 Respite Care Guide: How to Find What's Right for You
Alzheimer's Association
919 N Michigan Avenue
Suite 1000
Chicago, IL 60611-1676
312-335-8700
Fax: 312-335-1110; *Toll Free:* 800-272-3900
info@alz.org
www.alz.org

Gerald Sampson, Chair
Deborah Jones, Secretary
Thomas J. Winkel, Treasurer

Designed to help caregivers and persons with dementia recognize the benefits of respite care as well as identify which respite care services will best meet their needs.

18 pages

3636 Ronald & Nancy Reagan Research Institute: To Treat and Prevent Alzheimer's Disease
Alzheimer's Association
919 N Michigan Avenue
Suite 1000
Chicago, IL 60611-1676
312-335-8700
Fax: 312-335-1110; *Toll Free:* 800-272-3900
info@alz.org
www.alz.org

Gerald Sampson, Chair
Deborah Jones, Secretary
Thomas J. Winkel, Treasurer

Describes the goals of the Alzheimer's Association Ronald & Nancy Reagan Research Institute.

3637 Safe Return Brochure
Alzheimer's Association
919 N Michigan Avenue
Suite 1000
Chicago, IL 60611-1676
312-335-8700
Fax: 312-335-1110; *Toll Free:* 800-272-3900
info@alz.org
www.alz.org

Gerald Sampson, Chair
Deborah Jones, Secretary
Thomas J. Winkel, Treasurer

General information on the Safe Return program. Includes the registration form.

3638 Standing By You: Family Support Groups
Alzheimer's Association
919 N Michigan Avenue
Suite 1000
Chicago, IL 60611-1676
312-335-8700
Fax: 312-335-1110; *Toll Free:* 800-272-3900
info@alz.org
www.alz.org

Gerald Sampson, Chair
Deborah Jones, Secretary
Thomas J. Winkel, Treasurer

Explains how family members, particularly the caregiver of the person with Alzheimer's, can benefit from family support groups.

3639 Steps to Enhancing Communication
Alzheimer's Association
919 N Michigan Avenue
Suite 1000
Chicago, IL 60611-1676
312-335-8700
Fax: 312-335-1110; *Toll Free:* 800-272-3900
info@alz.org
www.alz.org

Gerald Sampson, Chair
Deborah Jones, Secretary
Thomas J. Winkel, Treasurer

Offers caregivers techniques for improving their approach to listening to and communication with the individual with Alzheimer's disease.

12 pages

3640 Steps to Enhancing Your Home: Modifying the Environment
Alzheimer's Association
919 N Michigan Avenue
Suite 1000
Chicago, IL 60611-1676
312-335-8700
Fax: 312-335-1110; *Toll Free:* 800-272-3900
info@alz.org
www.alz.org

Gerald Sampson, Chair
Deborah Jones, Secretary
Thomas J. Winkel, Treasurer

Offers caregivers tips for reducing accidents in the home and creating an environment that supports the changing needs of the individual with Alzheimer's disease.

12 pages

3641 Steps to Finding Home Health Care
Alzheimer's Association
919 N Michigan Avenue
Suite 1000
Chicago, IL 60611-1676
312-335-8700
Fax: 312-335-1110; *Toll Free:* 800-272-3900
info@alz.org
www.alz.org

Gerald Sampson, Chair
Deborah Jones, Secretary
Thomas J. Winkel, Treasurer

Provides practical strategies for finding in-home care for the person with Alzheimer's disease.

15 pages

3642 Steps to Getting a Diagnosis: Finding Out if It's Alzheimer's Disease
Alzheimer's Association
919 N Michigan Avenue
Suite 1000
Chicago, IL 60611-1676
312-335-8700
Fax: 312-335-1110; *Toll Free:* 800-272-3900
info@alz.org
www.alz.org

Gerald Sampson, Chair
Deborah Jones, Secretary
Thomas J. Winkel, Treasurer

Educates individuals and their families on the importance of seeking a diagnosis, and the various test completed to obtain an accurate diagnosis.

12 pages

3643 Steps to Planning Activities: Structuring the Day at Home
Alzheimer's Association
919 N Michigan Avenue
Suite 1000
Chicago, IL 60611-1676
312-335-8700
Fax: 312-335-1110; *Toll Free:* 800-272-3900
info@alz.org
www.alz.org

Gerald Sampson, Chair
Deborah Jones, Secretary
Thomas J. Winkel, Treasurer

Guides the caregiver in planning meaningful activities for the person with Alzheimer's disease.

12 pages

3644 Steps to Understanding Challenging Behaviors
Alzheimer's Association
919 N Michigan Avenue
Suite 1000
Chicago, IL 60611-1676
312-335-8700
Fax: 312-335-1110; *Toll Free:* 800-272-3900
info@alz.org
www.alz.org

Gerald Sampson, Chair
Deborah Jones, Secretary
Thomas J. Winkel, Treasurer

Offers caregivers ways to respond to the changing behaviors, including anxiety, agitation, and aggression that the individual with Alzheimer's disease is experiencing.

12 pages

3645 Steps to Understanding Legal Issues: Planning for the Future
Alzheimer's Association
919 N Michigan Avenue
Suite 1000
Chicago, IL 60611-1676
312-335-8700
Fax: 312-335-1110; *Toll Free:* 800-272-3900
info@alz.org
www.alz.org

Gerald Sampson, Chair
Deborah Jones, Secretary
Thomas J. Winkel, Treasurer

Provides information on legal issues such as legal capacity, powers of attorney, wills and living wills, and guardianship.

12 pages

3646 Taxes and Alzheimer's Disease
Alzheimer's Association
919 N Michigan Avenue
Suite 1000
Chicago, IL 60611-1676
312-335-8700
Fax: 312-335-1110; *Toll Free:* 800-272-3900

info@alz.org
www.alz.org

Gerald Sampson, Chair
Deborah Jones, Secretary
Thomas J. Winkel, Treasurer

A series of three consumer education brochures about tax issues that may affect people with Alzheimer's and their families. Address the household and dependent care credit, federal employment texes, and the itemized deduction for medical expenses. Also includes a preliminary explanation of the medical deduction for long-term care expenses clarified by the Kassebaum-Kennedy health insurance law.

3647 Terms & Tips: An Alzheimer Care Handbook
Alzheimer's Association
919 N Michigan Avenue
Suite 1000
Chicago, IL 60611-1676
312-335-8700
Fax: 312-335-1110; *Toll Free:* 800-272-3900
info@alz.org
www.alz.org

Gerald Sampson, Chair
Deborah Jones, Secretary
Thomas J. Winkel, Treasurer

Offers an explanation for over 250 terms and offers practical caregiver ideas and tips. Primarily for people with dementia and their caregivers, family members, and all providers of hands-on assistance.

84 pages

3648 Time Out!
Alzheimer's Association
919 N Michigan Avenue
Suite 1000
Chicago, IL 60611-1676
312-335-8700
Fax: 312-335-1110; *Toll Free:* 800-272-3900
info@alz.org
www.alz.org

Gerald Sampson, Chair
Deborah Jones, Secretary
Thomas J. Winkel, Treasurer

Details the Association's position supporting a national respite care policy and recommends actions for federal and state policy makers.

14 pages

3649 Understanding Medicaid Long Term Care: A Primer for Alzheimer Advocates
Alzheimer's Association
919 N Michigan Avenue
Suite 1000
Chicago, IL 60611-1676
312-335-8700
Fax: 312-335-1110; *Toll Free:* 800-272-3900
info@alz.org
www.alz.org

Gerald Sampson, Chair
Deborah Jones, Secretary
Thomas J. Winkel, Treasurer

Provides current information about the Medicaid program, including eligibility rules.

30 pages

3650 Wills and Bequests
Alzheimer's Association
919 N Michigan Avenue
Suite 1000
Chicago, IL 60611-1676
773-651-1369
Fax: 312-335-1110; *Toll Free:* 800-272-3900
info@alz.org
www.alz.org

Bill Walls, Owner

How to make a bequest to fight Alzheimer's disease through a will.

3651 World Without Alzheimer's: A Dream Within Reach
Alzheimer's Association
919 N Michigan Avenue
Suite 1000
Chicago, IL 60611-1676
312-335-8700
Fax: 312-335-1110; *Toll Free:* 800-272-3900
info@alz.org
www.alz.org

Gerald Sampson, Chair
Deborah Jones, Secretary
Thomas J. Winkel, Treasurer

Covers the major trends and promising developments in conquering Alzheimer's disease.

10 pages

3652 You Can Make a Difference: 10 Ways to Help an Alzheimer Family
Alzheimer's Association
919 N Michigan Avenue
Suite 1000
Chicago, IL 60611-1676
773-777-4567
Fax: 312-335-1110; *Toll Free:* 800-272-3900
info@alz.org
www.alz.org

Kwang Yoo, Owner

Information specifically for friends, explaining how Alzheimer's disease affects the entire family and suggesting practical ways to assist.

Videos, Audio Tapes

3653 A Thousand Tomorrows
Fanlight Productions
32 Court Street
21st Floor
Brooklyn, NY 11201
Fax: 718-488-8642; *Toll Free:* 800-876-1710
info@fanlight.com
www.fanlight.com

Spouses of people with Alzheimer's talk candidly about the impact of the illness on intimacy and sexuality. 30-minute video.

3654 Agitation... It's a Sign
Fanlight Productions
32 Court Street
21st Floor
Brooklyn, NY 11201

Fax: 718-488-8642; *Toll Free:* 800-876-1710
info@fanlight.com
www.fanlight.com

A variety of caregivers share their experiences and thoughts on providing for residents with Alzheimer's while providing vivid examples of the techniques and concepts that have worked in their facilities. 14-minute videotape.

3655 Alzheimer's Disease
Fanlight Productions
32 Court Street
21st Floor
Brooklyn, NY 11201
Fax: 718-488-8642; *Toll Free:* 800-876-1710
info@fanlight.com
www.fanlight.com

Dartmouth Hitchcock Medical, Center

From 'The Dr. Is In' series. The stories of three families offer caregivers thechance to share experiences and learn practical strategies for keeping people with Alzheimer's engaged in life. 29-minute videotape.

3656 Alzheimer's Disease: an Educational Training Program for Social Workers
Alzheimer's Disease Education & Referral Center
PO Box 8250
Silver Spring, MD 20907-8250
Fax: 301-495-3334; *Toll Free:* 800-438-4380

Gerald Sampson, Chair
Deborah Jones, Secretary
Thomas J. Winkel, Treasurer

For training social workers who are not familiar working with Alzheimer's patients and families. Four videotapes and one manual. Produced by the University of Pittsburgh.

3657 Another Home for Mom
Fanlight Productions
32 Court Street
21st Floor
Brooklyn, NY 11201
Fax: 718-488-8642; *Toll Free:* 800-876-1710
info@fanlight.com
www.fanlight.com

A couple confront the difficult decision of whether to place the husband's mother, who has Alzheimer's Disease, in a nursing home. 28-minute video.

3658 Caring... Sharing: The Alzheimer's Caregiver
Fanlight Productions
32 Court Street
21st Floor
Brooklyn, NY 11201
Fax: 718-488-8642; *Toll Free:* 800-876-1710
info@fanlight.com
www.fanlight.com

Explores the frustrations, fears, loneliness, anger and guilt - as well as moment of joy - experienced by those who care for lvoed ones with Alzheimer's Disease. 38-minute video

3659 In and Out of Time
Fanlight Productions
32 Court Street
21st Floor
Brooklyn, NY 11201

Fax: 718-488-8642; *Toll Free:* 800-876-1710
info@fanlight.com
www.fanlight.com

A tender personal chronicle of the filmmaker's grandmother's loss of memory due to Alzheimer's disease. 14-minute video.

3660 Memories of Love: Caring for the Caregiver
Alzheimer's Disease Education & Referral Center
PO Box 8250
Silver Spring, MD 20907-8250
Fax: 301-495-3334; *Toll Free:* 800-438-4380

Gerald Sampson, Chair
Deborah Jones, Secretary
Thomas J. Winkel, Treasurer

Produced by the University of Pittsburgh, this video features African-American members of a lay support group sharing personal perspectives of Alzheimer's and coping strategies.

3661 Resisting Care... Putting Yourself in Their Shoes
Fanlight Productions
32 Court Street
21st Floor
Brooklyn, NY 11201
Fax: 718-488-8642; *Toll Free:* 800-876-1710
info@fanlight.com
www.fanlight.com

Assisted Living Federation of, America

A variety of caregivers share their experiences and thoughtso n providing for residents with Alzheimer's while providing vivid examples of the techniques and concepts that have worked in their facilities. 14-minute video.

3662 Something Should be Done About Grandma Ruthie
Fanlight Productions
32 Court Street
21st Floor
Brooklyn, NY 11201
Fax: 718-488-8642; *Toll Free:* 800-876-1710
info@fanlight.com
www.fanlight.com

A moving and unsettling portrait of the filmmaker's family as they struggle to deal with her grandmother's deteriorating mental condition. 54-minute video.

3663 Speaking for Them: Identifying Psychiatric Complications in Alzheimer's Patients
Alzheimer's Disease Education & Referral Center
PO Box 8250
Silver Spring, MD 20907-8250
Fax: 301-495-3334; *Toll Free:* 800-438-4380

Gerald Sampson, Chair
Deborah Jones, Secretary
Thomas J. Winkel, Treasurer

Shows nursing staff in long-term care facilities to differentiate and describe psychiatric complications of Alzheimer's disease. Includes one video and syllabus. Produced by the University of California.

3664 Wandering: It Is a Problem?
Fanlight Productions
32 Court Street
21st Floor
Brooklyn, NY 11201
Fax: 718-488-8642; *Toll Free:* 800-876-1710
info@fanlight.com
www.fanlight.com

Assisted Living Federation of, America

A variety of caretivers share their experiences and thoughts on providing for residents with Alzheimer's while providing vivid examples of the techniques and concepts that have worked in their facilities. 14-minute video.

3665 Waves of Stone
Alzheimer's Association
919 N Michigan Avenue
Suite 1000
Chicago, IL 60611-1676
312-335-8700
Fax: 312-335-1110; *Toll Free:* 800-272-3900
info@alz.org
www.alz.org

Gerald Sampson, Chair
Deborah Jones, Secretary
Thomas J. Winkel, Treasurer

PBS documentary on Alzheimer's disease that discusses both scientific research and caregiver issues.

Websites

3666 Alzheimer Research Forum
1 Main Street
13th Floor
Cambridge, MA 2142
www.alzforum.org

Dedicated to understanding Alzheimer's disease and related disorders.

3667 Alzheimer Support
www.alzheimersupport.com

Serves Alzheimer's sufferers and their loved ones by reporting the latest news in research and treatment, making hard-to-find, recommended nutritional supplements available at manufacturer-direct low prices, and, most importantly, donating profits from each purchase to fund Alzheimer's medical research.

3668 Alzheimer's Association Hotline
www.alz.org

A 24-hour telephone information line offering information on Alzheimer's and local chapters across the country to Alzheimer's patients, families and caregivers.

3669 Alzheimer's Disease Center
1660 S Columbian Way
Seattle, WA 98108
206-764-2609Toll free: 800-317-5382
www.depts.washington.edu/adrcweb

Researchers work to translate advances into improved care and diagnosis for Alzheimer's patients.

3670 Alzheimer's Disease International
64 Great Sufflok Street
London, UK

442-798- 088
Fax: 442-792- 235
www.alz.co.uk

We aim to help establish and strengthen Alzheimer associations throughout the world, and to raise global awareness about Alzheimer's disease and all other causes of dementia.

3671 Alzheimer's Foundation of America
322 Eighth Avenue
7th Floor
New York, NY 10001
646-638-1542
Fax: 646-638-1546; *Toll Free:* 866-232-8484
www.alzfdn.org

Charles J. Fuschillo Jr., President & CEO
Josie Di Chiara, SVP, External Relations

3672 American Academy of Neurology
201 Chicago Avenue
Minneapolis, MN 55415
Fax: 612-454-2746; *Toll Free:* 800-879-1960
www.aan.com

Professional society of medical doctors specializing in brain and nervous system diseases. Maintains placement service. Sponsors research and educational programs. Compiles statistics. Publishes scientific journal.

3673 American Board of Psychiatry and Neurology
2150 East Lake Cook Road
Suite 900
Buffalo Grove, IL 60089
847-229-6500
Fax: 847-299-6600
www.abpn.com

Physicians with specialized training in psychiatry, neurology, child neurology, child adolescent psychiatry, clinical neurophysiology, and geriatric psychiatry. Determines eligibility requirements, administers examinations, and certifies physicians.

3674 American Health Assistance Foundation
25512 Gateway Center Drive
Clarksburg, MD 20871
800-437-2423
Fax: 301-258-9454
www.ahaf.org

Funds research programs for heart disease, glaucoma, and Alzheimer's disease. Provides financial assistance through Alzheimer's Family Relief Program. Public education materials on programs, brochures, and applications are provided. Hours: 9am to 5pm Monday-Friday.

3675 Steps for Caregivers: Caring for Persons with Alzheimer's Disease
www.alz.org

Provides guidance and support for caregivers of those with Alzheimer's.

Research Centers

3676 Arizona Alzheimer's Consortium
4745 N 7th Street
Suite 105
Phoenix, AZ 85014-3666

602-839-6525
azalz.org

A leader in statewide collaboration in Alzheimer's Disease research.

Year Founded: 1998

3677 Arthritis Foundation: Michigan

1050 Wilshire Drive
Suite 302
Troy, MI 48084
248-649-2891
Fax: 248-649-2895
www.arthritis.org/michigan

Mary Sue Lanigan, Development Director

Offers information and referral services, catalog of publications, physician referral list, speakers bureau, public forums and more for the arthritis community of Michigan.

Year Founded: 1948

3678 Arthur M Fishberg Research Center in Neurobiology
Mt. Sinai Medical Center

1 Gustave L Levy Place
New York, NY 10029
212-241-6500
Fax: 212-590-3300
www.mountsinai.org/

Kenneth L. Davis MD, CEO

Studies and research done in neurobiological systems and the molecular biology of Alzheimer's disease, schizophrenia and growth factors.

3679 Banner Alzheimer's Institute

2901 N Central Avenue
Suite 160
Phoenix, AZ 85012
602-747-4483
Fax: 602-839-6906
baiinfo@bannerhealth.com
banneralz.org

Eric M. Reiman, Executive Director

3680 Baylor College of Medicine Center for Allergy & Immunological Disorders

1 Baylor Plaza
Houston, TX 77030
713-798-7313
Fax: 713-798-5780
wshearer@bcm.tmc.edu
https://www.bcm.edu

William T Shearer MD, PhD, Director
Mark M Udden, MD

3681 Boston University Alzheimer's Disease Center
Boston University School of Medicine

72 E Concord Street
B-7800
Boston, MA 02118
617-414-1077
Fax: 617-414-1197; Toll Free: 888-458-2823
buad@bu.edu
www.bu.edu/alzresearch

One of 29 Alzheimer's Disease Centers funded by the National Institutes of Health.

Year Founded: 1996

3682 Center for Senility Studies: Alzheimer's Disease Treatment Research

161 N Dithridge Street
Pittsburgh, PA 15213-2646
412-621-4132

Arthur C Walsh MD, President
Cathy Painter, Manager

Nonprofit organization dealing in research of Alzheimer's disease, senility and elderly/aging disorders.

3683 Columbia University Alzheimer's Disease Research Center
Department of Pathology

630 W 168th Street
New York, NY 10032
212-305-6719
Fax: 212-305-2301
pathology.columbia.edu/

Michael L Shelanski, Director

Alzheimer's disease and elderly care. Serves as a resource for tissue, cells, and DNA from Alzheimer's disease and control patients. Areas of research include epidemiology, cell biology, molecular biology, and care-giving.

3684 Duke University General Clinical Research Center
Medical Center

PO Box 3854
Durham, NC 27710
919-477-9292
Fax: 252-684-5041
marke001@mc.duke.edu
www.duke.edu/rankincru

Dr. M Louis Markert, Program Director
Michael Duke, Owner

Multidisciplinary, clinical research into the cause and prevention of human diseases such as Alzheimer's.

3685 Emory University Alzheimer's Disease Center

201 Dowman Drive
Atlanta, GA 30322
404-727-6123
www.alzheimers.emory.edu

Allan Levey, Director

3686 Fisher Center for Alzheimer's Research Foundation

110 E 42nd Street
16th Floor
New York, NY 10017
Fax: 212-915-1319; Toll Free: 800-259-4636
info@alzinfo.org
www.alzinfo.org

Kent L. Karosen, President & CEO

Provides a broad range of information on research, treatment, legal and financial planning.

3687 Georgetown University: International Center for Interdiciplinary Studies of Immunology

3800 Reservoir Road NW
Washington, DC 20007
202-444-2000
www.georgetown.edu/

John J. DeGioia, President
Thomas Banchoff, Vice President

Studies of immunology and allergic disorders.

3688 Gerontology Research Institute

4940 Eastern Avenue
Baltimore, MD 21224-2735
410-558-8185

Dr. George Martin, Director

Nonprofit organization focusing on gerontology research including Alzheimer's disease studies.

3689 Indiana University-Purdue University at Indianapolis: Center for Alzheimer's Disease & Related Neuropsychiatric Disorder

420 University Boulevard
Indianapolis, IN 46202
317-274-5555
www.iupui.edu/

Alzheimer's Disease and related neuropsychiatric disorders characterized by memory loss and mood disorders in the elderly.

3690 Institute of the Neurosciences Research Program

Smith Hall Annex

1230 York Avenue
New York, NY 10021-6307
212-570-8975
Fax: 212-570-7628
www.rockefeller.edu/

David Rockefeller, Honorary Chair
Russell L. Carson, Chair
David I. Hirsh, Vice Chair

Nonprofit organization focusing on Alzheimer's and related disorders.

3691 Johns Hopkins University: Alzheimer's Disease Research Center

720 Rutland Avenue
Baltimore, MD 21205
410-502-5164
Fax: 410-955-9777
edelman1@jhmi.edu
www.alzresearch.org/

Dr. Donald L Price, Director
Elaine Delman, Administrator

Alzheimer's disease, including basic and applied studies of symptoms and psychiatric problems.

3692 Knight Alzheimer's Disease Research Center

4488 Forest Park
Suite 101
St. Louis, MO 63112
314-286-2881
alzheimer.wustl.edu

3693 Massachusetts Alzheimer's Disease Research Center

16th Street
Charlestown, MA 02129
617-726-3987
Fax: 617-724-1480
madrc.mgh.harvard.edu/

John H Growdon MD, Director

Coordinates research on Alzheimer's disease, including memory loss, dementia, neuropathology, neuropsychology, neurochemistry, and investigational drug studies. Projects focus on biochemical studies on the abnormal proteins that accumulate in the brains of Alzheimer's patients, possible genetic markers or familial traits, anatomical and neuro-transmitter abnormalities, and clinical studies of behavior and neuropharmacology.

3694 Mount Sinai School of Medicine of City University of New York: Alzheimer's Disease Research Center

University of New York

1428 Madison Avenue
New York, NY 10029
212-241-6500
icahn.mssm.edu/

Dr. Kenneth L Davis, Chairman
Donnie Sauls, Manager

Etiology, diagnosis, and treatment of Alzheimer's disease and related dementias. Clinical studies include trials of new drugs and biological markers and longitudinal follow-up studies. An active autopsy network obtains brain material from Alzheimer patients.

3695 NHI Clinical Center

9000 Rockville Pike
Bethesda, MD 20892
301-496-2563
Fax: 301-402-2984
www.cc.nih.gov

Established in 1953 as the research hospital of the National Institutes of Health. Designed so that patient care facilities are close to research laboratories so new findings of basic and clinical scientists can be quickly applied to the treatment of patients. Upon referral by physicians or self-referral, qualifying patients are admitted to NIH clinical studies.

3696 Nathan Kline Institute for Psychiatric Research: Center for Alzheimer's Disease

140 Old Orangeburg Road
Orangeburg, NY 10962
845-398-5500
Fax: 914-398-5510
nixon@nki.rfmh.org
www.rfmh.org/

Donald C. Goff M.D., Director
Antonio Convit M.D., Deputy Director

Molecular neuroscience and aging, including molecular neurobiology of proteases, signal transduction, neurodegenerative disease, protein/peptide analytical techniques, molecular genetics, vesicle biology, transgenic modeling.

3697 National Alzheimer's Coordinating Center

4311 11th Avenue NE
Suite 300
Seattle, WA 98105
206-543-8637
Fax: 206-616-5927
naccmail@uw.edu
www.alz.washington.edu

Coordinating data collection and fostering collaborative research among Alzheimer's Disease centers.

Year Founded: 1999

3698 National Cell Repository for Alzheimer's
Toll Free: 800-526-2839
alzstudy@iu.edu
ncrad.iu.edu

Tatiana Foroud, Principal Investigator

Providing biological samples and data to researchers to
help them find genetic factors in Alzheimer's Disease and
dementia.

Year Founded: 1990

3699 Ohio State University Neuroscience Program
333 W 10th Avenue
Columbus, OH 43210-1239
614-292-6192
Fax: 614-292-1544
www.osu.edu/

John Oberdick, Chiar Co Director
Dana McTigue, Co-Director

Specializes in brain disorders such as Alzheimer's disease.

**3700 Rockefeller University: Zachary and Elizabeth
M Fisher Center for Research on Alzheimer's
Disease**
1230 York Avenue
New York, NY 10065
212-327-8000
Fax: 212-327-7974
www.rockefeller.edu/graduate/cenzach

David Rockefeller, Honorary Chair
Russell L. Carson, Chair
David I. Hirsh, Vice Chair

Alzheimer's disease, including how brain cells process the
amyloid precursor phosphoprotein (APP) leading to the
production of b-amlyoid, a major component of the plaques
that are a hallmark of Alzheimer's disease.

3701 Rush University Alzheimer's Disease Center
1653 W. Congress Parkway
Chicago, IL 60612
312-942-4463
Fax: 312-942-4154
www.rush.edu

Dr. Jacob H Fox, Co-Director

Alzheimer's disease, including causes, treatment, and cure.
Conducts clinical trials of new drug treatments and analyzes potential risk factors in the development of Alzheimer's disease.

**3702 State University College at Plattsburgh:
Biochemisrty/Biophysics Program**
101 Broad Street
Plattsburgh, NY 12901
518-564-2000
www.plattsburgh.edu/

Offers research services into genetic engineering relating to
physiology and molecular aspects of Alzheimer's Disease.

**3703 State University of New York at Stony Brook:
Cognitive and Behavioral Neuroscience**
Nicholis Road
Stony Brook, NY 11790
631-632-6000
www.stonybrook.edu/

Mary Ann Short, Department Administrator

Alzheimer's disease research.
Year Founded: 1993

**3704 Sun Health Research Institute: Alzheimers
Center**
PO Box 6030
Sun City, AZ 85376
623-832-5350
Fax: 623-832-5498
www.sunhealth.org

Alzheimer's disease, Parkinson's disease, rheumatoid arthritis, and other age-related diseases. Research focuses on
molecular genetics molecular/cell biology, protein chemistry, and immunology of degenerative disorders affecting
the elderly.

**3705 UC Irvine Alzheimer's Disease Research Center
UCI MIND**
2642 Biological Sciences III
Irvine, CA 92697-4545
www.mind.uci.edu

Andrea J. Tenner, Director
David Cribbs, Associate Director

Internationally recognized research into age-related disorders of the brain.

**3706 UT Southwestern Medical Center Alzheimer's
Disease Center**
UT Southwestern Medical Center
5323 Harry Hines Boulevard
Dallas, TX 75390
214-648-3111
www.utsouthwestern.edu

Roger N. Rosenberg, Director
Perrie M. Adams, Deputy Director

**3707 University of California, Los Angeles
Alzheimer's Disease Center**
710 Westwood Plaza
Los Angeles, CA 90095-1769
310-825-0703
Fax: 310-825-6956
jcummings@mednet.ucla.edu
www.neurology.ucla.edu/

Diagnosis, pathophysiology, and treatment of dementing
illnesses such as Alzheimer's disease.

**3708 University of Chicago: Brain Research Institute
Department of Neurology**
5841 S Maryland Avenue
Chicago, IL 60637
773-702-6390
neurology.uchicago.edu/
Studies brain disorders including Alzheimer's disease.

**3709 University of Iowa: Alzheimer's Disease
Research Center
College of Medicine**
200 Hawkins Drive
Iowa City, IA 52242-1009
319-356-4296
Fax: 319-356-4505; *Toll Free:* 800-854-4461
www.medicine.uiowa.edu/

Alzheimer's disease and related conditions. Departments with participating specialists include anatomy, radiology, pathology, ophthalmology, psychology.

3710 University of Kentucky: Alzheimer's Disease Research Center

800 S Limestone
Lexington, KY 40536-0230
859-323-6040
Fax: 859-323-2866
www.uky.edu/

Alzheimer's disease, focusing on the cause, treatment, and eventual cure.

3711 University of Miami: Center for Neurological Diseases

1501 NW 9th Avenue
Miami, FL 33136-1407
305-547-6946
uhealthsystem.com

Noble David MD, Vice Chairperson

Focuses on aged disorders such as Alzheimer's research.

3712 University of Michigan: Alzheimer's Disease Research Center
Department of Neurology

1500 E Medical Drive Center
Ann Arbor, MI 48109-5316
734-936-9070
sgilman@umich.edu
www.med.umich.edu/

Sid Gilman MD, Chairman

Alzheimer's disease and other neurodegenerative diseases associated with dementia, including Parkinson's disease, multiple system atrophy, progressive supranuclear palsy, and olivopontocerebellar atrophy. Studies involve positron emission tomography (PET) scanning of patients with neurological disorders, neuropathological studies of patients with neurodegenerative illnesses, animal models, and a statewide public opinion survey on Alzheimer's disease.

3713 University of Texas Southwestern Medical Center at Dallas: Alzheimer's Disease Center
Department of Psychiatry

5323 Harry Hines Boulevard
Dallas, TX 75235
214-648-3111
Fax: 214-648-2450
mcullu@mednet.swmed.edu
www.utsouthwestern.edu/

Daniel K. Podolsky, President

Alzheimer's diseaese and aging in the brain, focusing on loss of cognitive functions and test measurements including IQ, problem solving, abstract thinking, spatial and dexterity skills, attention and concentration, language function, and memory.

3714 University of Washington: Alzheimer's Disease Research Center

1660 S Columbian Way
Seattle, WA 98108
206-764-2069 Toll free: 800-317-5382
www.depts.washington.edu/adrcweb/

Sydeny Lewis, Education Coordinator

Basic mechanisms underlying the development of adult dementing disorders, with particular attention to heritable susceptibility factors underlying Alzheimer's disease.

3715 Winifred Masterson Burke Medical Research Institute
Cornell University

785 Mamaroneck Avenue
White Plains, NY 10605
914-597-2500
web@burke.org
www.burke.org/

Clinical and basic studies in metabolic and nutritional aspects of degenerative diseases of the nervous system, especially Alzheimer's disease.

3716 Wisconsin Alzheimer's Disease Research Center
Univ. of Wisconsin Sch. of Medicine & Publ. Health

600 Highland Avenue
J5/1 Mezzanine
Madison, WI 53792-2420
608-263-2582
adrc@medicine.wisc.edu
www.adrc.wisc.edu

Investigators conduct basic, clinical and behavioral research.

3717 Yeshiva University: Resnick Gerontology Center
Albert Einstein College of Medicine

1300 Morris Park Avenue
Bronx, NY 10461
718-430-2000
www.einstein.yu.edu/

Amy Ehrlich, MD

Alzheimer's disease and other dementia studies.

Arthritis

Associations & Organizations

3718 American College of Rheumatology
2200 Lake Boulevard NE
Atlanta, GA 30319
404-633-3777
Fax: 404-633-1870
www.rheumatology.org
Joan M. Von Feldt, President

3719 American Orthopaedic Association
9400 W Higgins Road
Suite 205
Rosemont, IL 60018-4975
847-318-7330
Fax: 847-318-7339
info@aoassn.org
www.aoassn.org
Kevin P. Black, President
William N. Levine, Secretary
Rick W. Wright, Treasurer

Professional society of bone and joint surgeons. Seeks to further knowledge in the diagnosis and treatment of crippling diseases.
Year Founded: 1887

3720 Arthritis Consulting Services
2787 E Oakland Park Boulevard
Suite 204
Ft Lauderdale, FL 33306
954-739-3202
Fax: 206-350-1884; *Toll Free:* 800-327-3027
www.stoparthritis.com

Provides information on holistic approaches to the treatment of arthritis.

3721 Arthritis Foundation
1355 Peachtree Street NE
6th Floor
Atlanta, GA 30309
404-872-7100
www.arthritis.org
Ann M. Palmer, President & CEO
Karen Larson, CFO
David McLoughlin, COO

A nonprofit organization that depends on volunteers to provide services to help people with arthritis. Supports research to find ways to cure and prevent arthritis and provides services to improve the quality of life for those affected by arthritis. Provides help through information, referrals, speakers bureaus, forums, self-help courses, and various support groups and programs nationwide.
Year Founded: 1948

3722 Arthritis Foundation: Alabama
500 Office Park Drive
Suite 200
Birmingham, AL 35223
205-979-5700
Fax: 205-979-4172; *Toll Free:* 800-879-7896
www.arthritis.org/alabama
Kayla Smeraglia, Development Director

Founded in 1948, this chapter affects thousands of lives through programs, services, information and referrals, public and professional education and more for residents of Alabama. Research is a great priority of the chapter which supports the advancements that are made by local researchers at the University of Alabama at Birmingham. In addition to research, the Alabama Chapter seeks to improve the quality of life for those affected by arthritiis.
Year Founded: 1948

3723 Arthritis Foundation: Alaska
615 East 82nd Avenue
Suite 104
Anchorage, AK 99518
907-277-2784
Fax: 907-277-2783; *Toll Free:* 888-391-9389
www.arthritis.org/alaska
Anna Campione, Development Manager

3724 Arthritis Foundation: Arizona
5009 E Washington Street
Suite 125
Phoenix, AZ 85034
602-212-9900
Fax: 602-264-0563
www.arthritis.org/arizona
Laura Rolfe, Executive Director

Offers information and referral hotlines, support groups, public forums, summer camps, speakers bureau, self-help courses, self-help devices, aquatics programs and a lending library for persons living with arthritis.
Year Founded: 1948

3725 Arthritis Foundation: Arkansas
10 Corporate Hill Drive
Suite 220
Little Rock, AR 72205
501-664-7242
Fax: 501-664-6588; *Toll Free:* 800-482-8858
www.arthritis.org/arkansas
Angela Harris, Executive Director
Year Founded: 1948

3726 Arthritis Foundation: California
800 West 6th Street
Suite 1250
Los Angeles, CA 90017
Fax: 323-954-5790; *Toll Free:* 800-954-2873
www.arthritis.org/california
Asher Garfinkel, Exec. Director, LA & Ctrl. Coast
Teresa Dinh, Exec. Director, Orange County
Nancy Coate, Exec. Director, San Diego
Year Founded: 1948

3727 Arthritis Foundation: Central & WesternPennsylvania
790 Holiday Drive
Suite 11
Pittsburgh, PA 15220
412-566-1645
www.arthritis.org/pennsylvania

Serves 28 counties in the central Pennsylvania area. More than 441,233 persons in the chapter area are affected with one of the forms of arthritis seriously enough to require medical care. The chapter offers research services, professional education and training, parent and community services and public health education.

Year Founded: 1948

3728 Arthritis Foundation: Colorado

2280 S Albion Street
Denver, CO 80222-4906
303-756-8622
Fax: 303-759-4349; *Toll Free:* 888-391-9389
www.arthritis.org/colorado

Laura Rosseisen, President

Serves Colorado and Wyoming and is dedicated to finding solutions to over 100 forms of arthritis which affect millions of people nationwide.

Year Founded: 1948

3729 Arthritis Foundation: Connecticut

35 Cold Spring Road
Suite 411
Rocky Hill, CT 06067
860-563-1177
Fax: 860-563-6018; *Toll Free:* 800-541-8350
www.arthritis.org/connecticut

Luellen Perkins, Senior Development Director

3730 Arthritis Foundation: Delaware

4720 Montgomery Lane
Suite 300
Bethesda, MD 20814
202-787-5333Toll free: 800-365-3811
www.arthritis.org/delaware

Lisa Boccia, Executive Director

Offers services to residents in Delaware who are affected by arthritis and related diseases. Also raises funds for research toward the national effort to seek a cure.

Year Founded: 1948

3731 Arthritis Foundation: Eastern Pennsylvania

111 S Independence Mall East
Suite 500
Philadelphia, PA 19106
215-574-3060
Fax: 215-574-3070
www.arthritis.org/eastern-pennsylvania

Sheila Brown, Operations Manager
Sullanie Mertus, Program Manager

3732 Arthritis Foundation: Florida

14499 N Dale Mabry Highway
Suite 139
Tampa, FL 33618
813-968-7000
Fax: 813-968-1119
www.arthritis.org/florida

Judy Dorn, Regional Vice President

3733 Arthritis Foundation: Georgia

PO Box 78423
Atlanta, GA 30357
404-237-8771Toll free: 800-933-7023
www.arthritis.org/georgia

Jamie Johnson, Senior Executive Director
Ayana Charleston, Program and Services Director

Offers people with arthritis and their families information and support, as well as activities designed to help manage the disease, improve daily functioning and lead to independence.

Year Founded: 1948

3734 Arthritis Foundation: Hawaii

2752 Woodlawn Drive
Suite 5-204B
Honolulu, HI 96822
808-596-2900
Fax: 808-596-2904; *Toll Free:* 800-462-0743
www.arthritis.org/hawaii

Maile Kawamura, Executive Director
Shanelle Ganiron, Development Manager

Year Founded: 1948

3735 Arthritis Foundation: Idaho

4424 South 700 East
Suite 180
Salt Lake City, UT 84107
801-536-0990
Fax: 801-536-0991; *Toll Free:* 888-391-9389
www.arthritis.org/idaho

Scott Weaver, CEO
Lisa B. Fall, President

3736 Arthritis Foundation: Illinois

35 E Wacker Drive
Suite 2260
Chicago, IL 60601
312-372-2080
Fax: 312-372-2081; *Toll Free:* 800-735-0096
www.arthritis.org/illinois

Tom Fite, Heartland Region CEO
Chris Crowley, Area VP, Chicago
Jenny Conder, Area VP, Central Illinois

Year Founded: 1948

3737 Arthritis Foundation: Indiana

615 N Alabama Street
Suite 430
Indianapolis, IN 46204
317-879-0321
Fax: 317-876-5608; *Toll Free:* 800-783-2342
www.arthritis.org/indiana

Tom Fite, Heartland Region CEO
Jenny Conder, Area Vice President

Offers programs and services for the arthritis community of Indiana.

Year Founded: 1948

3738 Arthritis Foundation: Iowa

4949 Pleasant Street
Suite 202
West Des Moines, IA 50266
515-278-0636
Fax: 515-278-2603; *Toll Free:* 866-378-0636
www.arthritis.org/iowa

Tom Fite, Heartland Region CEO

Year Founded: 1948

3739 Arthritis Foundation: Kansas
1900 West 75th Street
Suite 200
Prairie Village, KS 66208
913-262-2233
Fax: 913-262-2288; *Toll Free:* 888-719-5670
www.arthritis.org/kansas

Tom Fite, Heartland Region CEO
Steve Rock, Area Vice President

The only organization in the area representing the National Office in support of its international research program and in providing services throughout the bi-state area. Offers a wide range of services and programs to deal with the needs of persons with arthritis and their family members such as speakers bureaus, aquatic programs, self-help courses, physician referrals and the American Juvenile Arthritis Organization.

Year Founded: 1948

3740 Arthritis Foundation: Kentucky
2908 Brownsboro Road
Suite 117
Louisville, KY 40206
502-585-1866
Fax: 502-585-1657
www.arthritis.org/kentucky

Molly Young, Kentucky Branch Director

Active with ongoing support and exercise programs, educational programs, and special events for individuals with arthritis or a related disease, and others interested in finding out more about arthritis and helping to find a cure.

Year Founded: 1948

3741 Arthritis Foundation: Louisiana
10 Corporate Hill Drive
Suite 220
Little Rock, AR 72205
501-664-7242
Fax: 501-664-6588; *Toll Free:* 800-482-8858
www.arthritis.org/louisiana

Angela Harris, Executive Director
Emily Pearce, Programs & Services Director

Develops funds for medical research programs, enhances public awareness of arthritis, and provides service programs for those with arthritis.

Year Founded: 1948

3742 Arthritis Foundation: Maine
6 Chenell Drive
Suite 260
Concord, NH 03301
603-224-9322
Fax: 603-224-3778; *Toll Free:* 800-639-2113
www.arthritis.org/maine

Margaret Duffy, Community Engagement Director
Thomas Bringle, Development Manager

3743 Arthritis Foundation: Maryland
9891 Broken Land Parkway
Suite 101
Columbia, MD 21046
202-787-5333Toll free: 800-365-3811
www.arthritis.org/maryland

Lisa Boccia, Executive Director
Lauren Yankolonis, Development Director

This chapter supports research both locally and nationally to help find causes, better treatments and ways to prevent the many forms of arthritis. Offers various educational booklets and brochures, a physician referral service a speakers bureau, self-help courses land and water excersises and activities for children.

Year Founded: 1948

3744 Arthritis Foundation: Massachusetts
29 Crafts Street
Suite 450
Newton, MA 02458
617-244-1800
Fax: 617-558-7686; *Toll Free:* 800-766-9449
www.arthritis.org/massachusetts

Erica D'Agostino, Executive Director

Offers essential information, research programs and services for the close-to-one-million Massachusetts residents with arthritis.

Year Founded: 1948

3745 Arthritis Foundation: Metropolitan Washington
4720 Montgomery Lane
Suite 300
Bethesda, MD 28209
202-787-5333Toll free: 800-365-3811
arthritis.org/metropolitan-washington

Lisa Boccia, Executive Director
Jody Haltenhof, Development Manager

Year Founded: 1948

3746 Arthritis Foundation: Minnesota
1876 Minnehaha Avenue W
Saint Paul, MN 55104
651-644-4108
Fax: 651-644-4219; *Toll Free:* 800-333-1380
www.arthritis.org/minnesota

Tiffany Layden, Area Director
Lindsey Kumlien, Executive Director

Nonprofit organization providing programs and services North Dakota and South Dakota areas, to anyone affected by arthritis in the Minnesota area. Offers aquatic programs, support groups, juvenile arthritis support groups, research, grants program and information and referrals.

Year Founded: 1948

3747 Arthritis Foundation: Mississippi
500 Office Park Drive
Suite 200
Birmingham, AL 35223
205-979-5700
Fax: 205-979-4172; *Toll Free:* 800-879-7896
www.arthritis.org/mississippi

Over 6,800 Mississippians volunteer their services to help the chapter with fund raising and program support. Programs include land and water based exercise classes, and support groups, direct assistance to needy individuals to purchase arthritis medications and special equipment.

Year Founded: 1948

3748 Arthritis Foundation: Missouri
9433 Olive Street
Suite 100
St. Louis, MO 63132

314-991-9333
Fax: 314-991-4020; *Toll Free:* 800-406-2491
www.arthritis.org/missouri

Jan Bignall, Area Vice President
Year Founded: 1948

3749 Arthritis Foundation: Montana
PO Box 8113
Missoula, MT 59807
406-203-3019Toll free: 888-391-9389
www.arthritis.org/montana

Scott Weaver, CEO

3750 Arthritis Foundation: Nebraska
600 N 93rd Street
Suite 206
Omaha, NE 68114
402-330-6130
Fax: 402-330-6167; *Toll Free:* 800-642-5292
www.arthritis.org/nebraska

Tom Fite, Heartland Region CEO
Sally Stalnaker, Director of Special Events

For close to 40 years the Arthritis Foundation has been the source for help and hope to the 253,000 Nebraskans and residents of Pottawattamie County, Iowa, with arthritis. Provides a wide variety of services designed to help people better cope with arthritis and live happier, fuller lives.

Year Founded: 1948

3751 Arthritis Foundation: Nevada
PO Box 778213
Henderson, NV 89077
702-367-6381Toll free: 800-477-7679
www.arthritis.org/nevada

Valerie Jones, Executive Director
Crystal Schulz, Community Development Manager

3752 Arthritis Foundation: New Hampshire
6 Chenell Drive
Suite 260
Concord, NH 03301
603-224-9322
Fax: 603-224-3778; *Toll Free:* 800-639-2113
www.arthritis.org/new-hampshire

Margaret Duffy, Community Engagement Director
Thomas Bringle, Development Manager

3753 Arthritis Foundation: New Jersey
555 Route 1 South
Suite 220
Iselin, NJ 08830
732-283-4300
Fax: 732-283-4633
www.arthritis.org/new-jersey

Amy Boright Siperstein, Regional Director
Peggy Lotkowictz, Program Director

Offers various programs for the residents of New Jersey including support groups, self-help courses, water exercise and arthritis fitness classes and informational public forums.

Year Founded: 1948

3754 Arthritis Foundation: New Mexico
8100 Wyoming Boulevard NE
Suite M4
Albuquerque, NM 87113
505-200-1924
www.arthritis.org/new-mexico

Offers public education information, referrals, educational materials, chapter lending library, professional education resources and support groups for the residents of New Mexico.

Year Founded: 1948

3755 Arthritis Foundation: New York
122 E 42nd Street
18th Floor
New York, NY 10168
212-984-8700
Fax: 212-984-8728
www.arthritis.org/new-york

Ingrid Montecino, President & CEO
Year Founded: 1948

3756 Arthritis Foundation: North Carolina
4530 Park Road
Suite 230
Charlotte, NC 28209
704-705-1808
Fax: 704-529-0626; *Toll Free:* 800-365-3811
www.arthritis.org/north-carolina

Judy Dorn, Executive Director, Charlotte
Candy Fuller, Executive Director, Raleigh
Year Founded: 1948

3757 Arthritis Foundation: North Dakota
PO Box 1208
Fargo, ND 58107
701-388-1988Toll free: 800-333-1380
www.arthritis.org/north-dakota

Darci Hustrulid, Executive Director

3758 Arthritis Foundation: Northern California
657 Mission Street
Suite 603
San Francisco, CA 94105
415-356-1230
Fax: 415-356-1240; *Toll Free:* 888-391-9389
www.arthritis.org/northern-california

Scott Weaver, CEO
Deborah Jackson, President

Offers information and referral services, hotlines, resources, booklets, physician referral lists and more for the Nevada arthritis community.

Year Founded: 1948

3759 Arthritis Foundation: Ohio
4630 Richmond Road
Suite 240
Cleveland, OH 44128
216-831-7000Toll free: 800-245-2275
www.arthritis.org/ohio

Offers information and referral services, self-help courses, aquatics program, equipment loans, clinics, home assessment and continuing education to help more than 300,000 people in Central Ohio, including over 5,000 children affected with the 100 types of arthritis.

Year Founded: 1948

3760 Arthritis Foundation: Oklahoma
710 W Wilshire Creek
Suite 101
Oklahoma City, OK 73116
405-936-3366
Fax: 405-936-0617; *Toll Free:* 800-627-5486
www.arthritis.org/oklahoma
Year Founded: 1948

3761 Arthritis Foundation: Oregon
9700 SW Capitol Highway
Suite 160
Portland, OR 97219
503-245-5695
Fax: 503-245-5691; *Toll Free:* 888-391-9389
www.arthritis.org/oregon

Scott Weaver, CEO
Cindy Bishop, Development Manager

Offers public education, information and referrals, self-help courses, exercise programs, fund raising activities and more for the residents of Oregon and Clark County, Washington, that are managing with arthritis.

Year Founded: 1948

3762 Arthritis Foundation: Rhode Island
2348 Post Road
Suite 104
Warwick, RI 02886
401-739-3773
Fax: 401-739-8990
www.arthritis.org/rhode-island

Rebecca Farnlof, Community Engagement Director
Melissa Behm, Development Manager
Offers programs and services for persons in the Rhode Island area that are living with arthritis.

Year Founded: 1948

3763 Arthritis Foundation: South Carolina
4530 Park Road
Suite 230
Charlotte, NC 28209
704-705-1808Toll free: 800-365-3811
www.arthritis.org/south-carolina

Lisa Shultz, Executive Director

3764 Arthritis Foundation: South Dakota
PO Box 90445
Sioux Falls, SD 57109
605-201-7973Toll free: 800-333-1380
www.arthritis.org/south-dakota

Darci Hustrulid, Executive Director

3765 Arthritis Foundation: Tennessee
209 10th Avenue South
Suite 123
Nashville, TN 37203
615-806-8538
Fax: 615-261-9184; *Toll Free:* 866-227-3850
www.arthritis.org/tennessee

Melissa LaBonge, Executive Director

This chapter serves the residents of Tennessee by offering research and fellowship grants, self-help courses, aquatics program, educational programs, pharmacy services, loan

closet, information and referrals, public forums and seminars, support groups and a telethon for persons living with arthritis.

Year Founded: 1948

3766 Arthritis Foundation: Texas
4300 MacArthur Avenue
Suite 245
Dallas, TX 75209
214-826-4361
Fax: 214-824-5842; *Toll Free:* 800-442-6653
www.arthritis.org/texas

Aims to improve lives in Northern Texas through leadership in the prevention, control, and cure of arthritis and related diseases.

Year Founded: 1948

3767 Arthritis Foundation: Utah
4424 South 700 East
Suite 180
Salt Lake City, UT 84107
801-536-0990
Fax: 801-536-0991; *Toll Free:* 888-391-9389
www.arthritis.org/utah

Scott Weaver, CEO
Lisa B. Miller, President

3768 Arthritis Foundation: Vermont
6 Chenell Drive
Suite 260
Concord, NH 03301
603-224-9322
Fax: 603-224-3778; *Toll Free:* 800-639-2113
www.arthritis.org/vermont

Margaret Duffy, Community Engagement Director
Thomas Bringle, Development Manager

3769 Arthritis Foundation: Virginia
7202 Glen Forest Drive
Suite 305
Richmond, VA 23226
804-665-9950
Fax: 804-359-4900; *Toll Free:* 800-365-3811
www.arthritis.org/virginia

Laura Boone, Executive Director

Serves as a source of health and hope to the over 1 million Virginians living with arthritis. Provides the opportunity to learn about self-care through services such as land and aquatic exercise programs. Committed to information and education services, community programs, research support and fundraising.

Year Founded: 1948

3770 Arthritis Foundation: Washington
115 NE 100th St.
Suite 350
Seattle, WA 98125
206-547-2707
Fax: 206-547-2805; *Toll Free:* 888-391-9389
www.arthritis.org/washington

Scott Weaver, CEO

Offers arthritis helplines and information lines for residents of Washington state. Provides self-help courses, arthritis aquatic programs and resources for persons living with various forms of arthritis.

3771 Arthritis Foundation: West Virginia
1116 Smith Street
Charleston, WV 25301
304-205-1510
www.arthritis.org/west-virginia

3772 Arthritis Foundation: Wisconsin
10427 W Lincoln Avenue
Suite 1300
West Allis, WI 53227
414-321-3933
Fax: 414-321-0365; *Toll Free:* 800-333-1380
www.arthritis.org/wisconsin

Tiffany Layden, Area Director
Megan Cooley, Executive Director

Programs offered include aquatics and land exercise programs, self-help courses, professional public education and information and refferal.

Year Founded: 1948

3773 Arthritis Foundation: Wyoming
2280 South Albion Street
Denver, CO 80222
303-756-8622
Fax: 303-759-4349; *Toll Free:* 888-391-9389
www.arthritis.org/wyoming

Scott Weaver, CEO

3774 Association of Rheumatology Health Professionals
2200 Lake Boulevard NE
Atlanta, GA 30319
404-633-3777
Fax: 404-633-1870
www.rheumatology.org

Elizabeth A. Schlenk, President

Nurses, occupational and physical therapists, social workers, psychologists, vocational counselors, physicians, pharmacists, and other health professionals concerned with the practice, education, and research of rheumatic diseases. Seeks to establish a scientific base of knowledge to improve the quality and provision of health services to individuals with rheumatic diseases. Disseminates information regarding the study and treatment of rheumaticdiseases. Develops and implements medical and scientific programs in the field of rheumatology. A section of the Arthritis Foundation.

3775 Hahnemann University Hospital Orthopaedic Institute
Feinstein Building
216 N Broad Street
2nd Floor
Philadelphia, PA 19102
215-762-2663
www.hahnemannhospital.com/our-services
Year Founded: 1993

3776 Kuzell Institute for Arthritis and Infectious Diseases
2200 Webster Street
San Francisco, CA 94115
415-561-1734

One of seven units comprising the Medical Research Institute of San Francisco that offers basic and applied research in arthritis and related diseases.
Year Founded: 1980

3777 Warren Grant Magnuson Clinical Center
National Institutes of Health Clinical Center
9000 Rockville Pike
Bethesda, MD 20892
301-496-4000
www.cc.nih.gov

Established in 1953, the NIH Clinical Center is the nation's largest hospital totally dedicated to clinical research. Designed so that patient care facilities are close to research laboratories so new findings of basic and clinical scientists can be quickly applied to the treatment of patients. Upon referral by physicians, patients are admitted to NIH clinical studies.

Year Founded: 1953

Books

3778 250 Tips for Making Life with Arthritis Easier
Professional Book Distributing
PO Box 6996
Alpharetta, GA 30023-6996
770-442-8633
Fax: 770-442-9742; *Toll Free:* 800-207-8633
julie.katz@pbd.com
www.arthritis.org

Scott A Dockter, CEO

What do aerosol cooking spray and snow-shoveling have in common? Learn the answer to this question, and other clever and handy tips to make your life with-or without-arthritis easier. Plus learn about helpful serviced you didn't know were available through you bank, post office, phone company, grocery store, and other businesses you frequent.
88 pages

3779 Arthritic's Cookbook
Zebra Books
119 West 40th Street
New York, NY 10018
212-407-1500
www.kensingtonbooks.com/

Steven Zacharius, Chairman, President & CEO

3780 Arthritis Helpbook: A Tested Self-Management Program for Coping
Addison-Wesley
Rr 128
Reading, MA 01867
781-944-3700
Fax: 781-944-9338; *Toll Free:* 800-552-2259
288 pages

3781 Arthritis Rx: A Cutting-Edge Program for a Pain-Free Life
American Book Company
10267 Kingston Pike
Knoxville, TN 37922

865-966-7454
Fax: 865-675-0557
www.americanbookco.com

Nutrition and other supplements for managing arthritis; The Arthritis RX diet, including an anti-inflammatory nutrition plan and a sample week of meals, recipes, and exercises; The Arthritis RX exercises: three step-by-step exercise series, ranging from a gentle motion regimen to a strenuous core body workout, all demonstrated through over 100 precise photographs.

3782 Arthritis Self-Help Book
Addison-Wesley
Rr 128
Reading, MA 01867
781-944-3700
Fax: 781-944-9338; *Toll Free:* 800-552-2259

A useful and informative book used in conjunction with the Arthritis Foundation's Self-Help Course.

3783 Arthritis Sourcebook: Everything You Need to Know
Lowell House
220 Avenue of the Stars
Suite 300
Los Angeles, CA 90067
310-552-7555
Fax: 310-552-7573

252 pages

3784 Arthritis and Common Sense
1230 Avenue of the Americas
New York, NY 10020
212-698-7000
Fax: 212-698-7099
www.simonsays.com

The arthritis sufferer will find a simple dietary plan that may help to alleviate the pains and symptoms of this disease, without the use of drugs of any kind.

3785 Arthritis, What Exercises Work: Breakthrough Even after Drugs & Surgery Have Failed
MacMillan
175 Fifth Avenue
New York, NY 10010
646-307-5151Toll free: 888-330-8477
customerservice@mpsvirginia.com
us.macmillan.com

Arthritis/exercise therapy.

3786 Arthritis: A Comprehensive Guide
Addison-Wesley
Rr 128
Reading, MA 01867
781-944-3700
Fax: 781-944-9338; *Toll Free:* 800-552-2259

Reviews types of arthritis, different aspects of treatment including exercise, medications, surgery, the role of diet and an extensive section on challenges of daily living.

3787 Arthritis: Taking Care of Yourself Health Guide for Understanding Your Arthritis
Addison-Wesley
Rr 128
Reading, MA 01867

781-944-3700
Fax: 781-944-9338; *Toll Free:* 800-552-2259

3788 Bone Up on Arthritis
Arthritis Foundation
1330 W Peachtree Street
Suite 100
Atlanta, GA 30309
404-872-7100
Fax: 404-872-0457; *Toll Free:* 800-283-7800
help@arthritis.org
www.arthritis.org

Daniel T. McGowan, Chair
Rowland W. (Chang, Vice Chair
Ann M. Palmer, President and CEO

A self-help education packet designed for home-study use, this program can improve your pain and function levels by teaching proven self-help techniques.

3789 Clinical Care in the Rheumatic Disease
Professional Book Distributing
PO Box 6996
Alpharetta, GA 30023-6996
770-442-8633
Fax: 770-442-9742; *Toll Free:* 800-207-8633
julie.katz@pbd.com
www.arthritis.org

Scott A Dockter, CEO

This book was written for all health professionals caring for people with rheumatic diseases and for students in these disciplines.

224 pages

3790 Exercise Beats Arthritis
Bull Publishing
PO Box 208
Palo Alto, CA 94302
650-322-2855
Fax: 650-327-3300; *Toll Free:* 800-676-2855
bullpublishing@msn.com
www.bullpub.com

Easy-to-follow program will help arthritis sufferers of all ages manage the problems of living with this condition. In depth look at minimizing the pain and limitations of arthritis, keep their joints mobile, increase muscle strength, strengthen bones and ligaments, perform daily tasks more easily.

144 pages

3791 In Control
Arthritis Foundation
1330 W Peachtree Street
Suite 100
Atlanta, GA 30309
404-872-7100
Fax: 404-872-0457; *Toll Free:* 800-283-7800
help@arthritis.org
www.arthritis.org

Daniel T. McGowan, Chair
Rowland W. (Chang, Vice Chair
Ann M. Palmer, President and CEO

An excellent at-home program which includes video, audio cassettes and the Arthritis Helpbook. Provides tools to help meet the challenges of arthritis.

3792 Living With Rheumatoid Arthritis
Johns Hopkins University Press
2715 N Charles Street
Baltimore, MD 21218-4363
410-516-6900
Fax: 410-516-6998; *Toll Free:* 800-537-5487
www.jhu.edu/press/index.html

Kathleen Keane, Director

This book offers practical and usable answers to the questions of everyday life. The authors provide clear explanations of the causes, diagnosis, and treatment of the disease, and why medication, joint protection, physical activity, and good nutrition are essential components of care.

280 pages

3793 Preventing & Reversing Arthritis Naturally
Bear & Company
PO Box 388
Rochester, VT 05767-0388
800-246-8648
Fax: 802-767-3726
info@innertraditions.com
www.innertraditions.com/

A comprehensive self-help program designed to prevent and reverse degenerative inflammatory diseases without drugs and their unwelcome side effects.

272 pages Year Founded: 1995

3794 Toward Healthy Living - A Wellness Journal,
Arthritis Foundation Distribution Center
Professional Book Distributing
PO Box 6996
Alpharetta, GA 30023-6996
770-442-8633
Fax: 770-442-9742; *Toll Free:* 800-207-8633
julie.katz@pbd.com
www.arthritis.org

Scott A Dockter, CEO

This spiral-bound journal has ample pages where you can unleash you thoughts, plus scales to monitor your mook and pain. Throught the book you will also find wisdom from a variety of famous and ordinary people - those who live with chronic ilness, and those whose life lessons can help you gain a more positive outlook on daily living.

144 pages

3795 Yoga for Arthritis: The Complete Guide
WW Norton & Company
500 Fifth Avenue
New York, NY 10110
212-354-5500
Fax: 212-869-0856
www.wwnorton.com

A comprehensive, user-friendly medical yoga program designed for management and prevention of arthritis, with over 400 illustrations..

Directories

3796 Aids for Arthritis
35 Wakefield Drive
Medford, NJ 08055

609-654-6918
Fax: 609-654-8631; *Toll Free:* 800-654-0707
www.aidsforarthritis.com

Offers hundreds of arthritis self-help devices at low costs. Shop on website or call for catalog.

3797 Maxi Aids
42 Executive Boulevard
Farmingdale, NY 11735
631-752-0521
Fax: 631-752-0689; *Toll Free:* 800-522-6294
sales@maxiaids.com
www.maxiaids.com

Catalog of aids and appliances for the arthritic, visually impaired, hearing impaired, physically challenged, mature adult and for the needs of home health care.

131 pages

Journals, Magazines

3798 Arthritis Today
Arthritis Foundation
1330 W Peachtree Street NW
Atlanta, GA 30309-2922
404-872-7100
Fax: 404-872-9559; *Toll Free:* 800-933-7800

Daniel T. McGowan, Chair
Ann M. Palmer, President and CEO

The authoritative and respected source of information for persons with arthritis, their families and health professionals who manage their care. As the official magazine of the Arthritis Foundation, it is backed by the Foundation's experience of 44 years and leadership in the fight against arthritis. This magazine gives its readers the advice, information and inspiration they need to live better with arthritis.

Newsletters, Pamphlets

3799 Alerter
San Diego Area Chapter of the Arthritis
Foundation
9089 Clairemont Mesa Boulevard
Suite 300
San Diego, CA 92123-1225
858-492-1090
Fax: 619-492-9248; *Toll Free:* 800-422-

Daniel T. McGowan, Chair
Ann M. Palmer, President and CEO

Offers chapter updates, information on activities and events, resources and medical research for members.

3800 Ankylosing Spondylitis
Arthritis Foundation
1330 W Peachtree Street
Suite 100
Atlanta, GA 30309
404-872-7100
Fax: 404-872-0457; *Toll Free:* 800-283-7800
help@arthritis.org
www.arthritis.org

Daniel T. McGowan, Chair
Rowland W. (Chang, Vice Chair
Ann M. Palmer, President and CEO

3801 Arthritis Accent
Arthritis Foundation Southern N.E. Chapter
35 Cold Spring Road
Suite 411
Rocky Hill, CT 06067-3164
860-563-1177
Fax: 860-563-6018; *Toll Free:* 800-541-8350
www.arthritis.org

Stephen Evangelista, CEO
Sue Nesci, Vice President
Luellen Perkins, Senior Director of Develpoment

Newsletter that contains information on chapter events and activities.

3802 Arthritis Answers: Basic Information About Arthritis
Arthritis Foundation
1330 W Peachtree Street
Suite 100
Atlanta, GA 30309
404-872-7100
Fax: 404-872-0457; *Toll Free:* 800-283-7800
help@arthritis.org
www.arthritis.org

Daniel T. McGowan, Chair
Rowland W. (Chang, Vice Chair
Ann M. Palmer, President and CEO

3803 Arthritis Arizona Southwest
Chapter - Arthritis Foundation Greater Southwest
777 E Missouri Avenue
Suite 119
Phoenix, AZ 85014-2831
602-264-7679
Fax: 602-264-0563; *Toll Free:* 800-477-7679
info.caz@arthritis.org
www.arthritis.org

Michele Gama, Editor
Vikki Scarafiotti, President

A chapter newsletter offering updated information and resources pertaining to persons affected by arthritis.

3804 Arthritis Foundation Services
Arthritis Foundation
1330 W Peachtree Street
Suite 100
Atlanta, GA 30309
404-872-7100
Fax: 404-872-0457; *Toll Free:* 800-283-7800
help@arthritis.org
www.arthritis.org

Daniel T. McGowan, Chair
Rowland W. (Chang, Vice Chair
Ann M. Palmer, President and CEO

3805 Arthritis Information: Advocacy and Government Affairs
Arthritis Foundation
1330 W Peachtree Street
Suite 100
Atlanta, GA 30309
404-872-7100
Fax: 404-872-0457; *Toll Free:* 800-283-7800
help@arthritis.org
www.arthritis.org

Daniel T. McGowan, Chair
Rowland W. (Chang, Vice Chair
Ann M. Palmer, President and CEO

3806 Arthritis News
Wisconsin Chapter of the Arthritis Foundation
10427 W Lincoln Avenue
Suite 1300
West Allis, WI 53227
414-321-3933
Fax: 414-321-0365; *Toll Free:* 800-333-1380
www.arthritis.org

Maureen Blattner, Health Promotion Coordinator
Kim Wilbur, Administrator

Offers information on activities, events, medical research, information and referrals to persons living in the Wisconsin area that are afflicted with arthritis.

3807 Arthritis Observer
Rocky Mountain Chapter of the Arthritis Foundation
2280 S Albion Street
Denver, CO 80222-4906
303-756-8622
Fax: 303-759-0359; *Toll Free:* 800-475-6447

Daniel T. McGowan, Chair
Rowland W. (Bing) Chang, Vice Chair
Patricia Novak Nelson, Vice Chair

Offers chapter information and updates on fund-raising events and activities, resources and publications and medical updates for the arthritis community.

3808 Arthritis Reporter
New York Chapter of the Arthritis Foundation
122 E 42nd Street
Floor 18
New York, NY 10168-1899
212-984-8700
Fax: 212-878-5960

Daniel T. McGowan, Chair
Rowland W. (Bing) Chang, Vice Chair
Patricia Novak Nelson, Vice Chair

Chapter newsletter offering information on upcoming events, activities and groups for the arthritis community.

3809 Arthritis Update of Rhode Island
Southern NE Chapter of the Arthritis Foundation
37 N Blossom Street
East Providence, RI 02914-2728
401-434-5792
Fax: 401-434-5779

Offers information, activities, events and updates on the chapter.

3810 Arthritis Volunteer
Tennessee Chapter of the Arthritis Foundation
1719 W End Avenue
Suite 303w
Nashville, TN 37203-5123
615-320-7626
Fax: 615-329-3982

Keeps members up-to-date on arthritis developments and on programs, services and special events in Tennessee.

3811 Arthritis and Diet
NAMSIC, National Institutes of Health
1 Ams Circle
Bethesda, MD 20892-0001
301-495-4484
Fax: 301-718-6366; *Toll Free:* 877-226-4267
www.nih.gov/niams/
TTY: 301-565-2966

Offers information on nutrition and diet pertaining to the arthritis community.

16 pages

3812 Arthritis and Employment: You Can Get the Job You Want
Arthritis Foundation
1330 W Peachtree Street
Suite 100
Atlanta, GA 30309
404-872-7100
Fax: 404-872-0457; *Toll Free:* 800-283-7800
help@arthritis.org
www.arthritis.org

Daniel T. McGowan, Chair
Rowland W. (Chang, Vice Chair
Ann M. Palmer, President and CEO

3813 Arthritis and Inflammatory Bowel Disease
Arthritis Foundation
1330 W Peachtree Street
Suite 100
Atlanta, GA 30309
404-872-7100
Fax: 404-872-0457; *Toll Free:* 800-283-7800
help@arthritis.org
www.arthritis.org

Daniel T. McGowan, Chair
Rowland W. (Chang, Vice Chair
Ann M. Palmer, President and CEO

3814 Arthritis and Vocational Rehabilitation
Arthritis Foundation
1330 W Peachtree Street
Suite 100
Atlanta, GA 30309
404-872-7100
Fax: 404-872-0457; *Toll Free:* 800-283-7800
help@arthritis.org
www.arthritis.org

Daniel T. McGowan, Chair
Rowland W. (Chang, Vice Chair
Ann M. Palmer, President and CEO

3815 Arthritis on the Job: You Can Work With It
Arthritis Foundation
1330 W Peachtree Street
Suite 100
Atlanta, GA 30309
404-872-7100
Fax: 404-872-0457; *Toll Free:* 800-283-7800
help@arthritis.org
www.arthritis.org

Daniel T. McGowan, Chair
Rowland W. (Chang, Vice Chair
Ann M. Palmer, President and CEO

3816 Arthritis, Rheumatic Diseases and Related Disorders
Nat'l Arthritis/Skin Diseases Info. Clearinghouse
9000 Rockville Pike
Bethesda, MD 20892
301-496-4000
NIHinfo@od.nih.gov
www.nih.gov/
TTY: 301-402-9612

Francis S. Collins M.D, PhD, Director

This pamphlet offers information, technical articles and research on arthritis and related disorders. Also included are referral organizations to help patients uncover more information.

3817 Arthritis: Do You Know?
Arthritis Foundation
1330 W Peachtree Street
Suite 100
Atlanta, GA 30309
404-872-7100
Fax: 404-872-0457; *Toll Free:* 800-283-7800
help@arthritis.org
www.arthritis.org

Daniel T. McGowan, Chair
Rowland W. (Chang, Vice Chair
Ann M. Palmer, President and CEO

A brief overview of arthritis and the services of the Arthritis Foundation.

3818 Aspirin and Other Nonsteroidal Anti-Inflammatory Drugs
Arthritis Foundation
1330 W Peachtree Street
Suite 100
Atlanta, GA 30309
404-872-7100
Fax: 404-872-0457; *Toll Free:* 800-283-7800
help@arthritis.org
www.arthritis.org

Daniel T. McGowan, Chair
Rowland W. (Chang, Vice Chair
Ann M. Palmer, President and CEO

3819 Back Pain
Arthritis Foundation
1330 W Peachtree Street
Suite 100
Atlanta, GA 30309
404-872-7100
Fax: 404-872-0457; *Toll Free:* 800-283-7800
help@arthritis.org
www.arthritis.org

Daniel T. McGowan, Chair
Rowland W. (Chang, Vice Chair
Ann M. Palmer, President and CEO

3820 Behcet's Disease
Arthritis Foundation
1330 W Peachtree Street
Suite 100
Atlanta, GA 30309
404-872-7100
Fax: 404-872-0457; *Toll Free:* 800-283-7800
help@arthritis.org
www.arthritis.org

Daniel T. McGowan, Chair
Rowland W. (Chang, Vice Chair
Ann M. Palmer, President and CEO

3821 Bursitis, Tendonitis and other Soft Tissue
Arthritis Foundation
1330 W Peachtree Street
Suite 100
Atlanta, GA 30309
404-872-7100
Fax: 404-872-0457; Toll Free: 800-283-7800
help@arthritis.org
www.arthritis.org

Daniel T. McGowan, Chair
Rowland W. (Chang, Vice Chair
Ann M. Palmer, President and CEO

3822 CPPD Crystal Deposition Disease
Arthritis Foundation
1330 W Peachtree Street
Suite 100
Atlanta, GA 30309
404-872-7100
Fax: 404-872-0457; Toll Free: 800-283-7800
help@arthritis.org
www.arthritis.org

Daniel T. McGowan, Chair
Rowland W. (Chang, Vice Chair
Ann M. Palmer, President and CEO

3823 Carpal Tunnel Syndrome
Arthritis Foundation
1330 W Peachtree Street
Suite 100
Atlanta, GA 30309
404-872-7100
Fax: 404-872-0457; Toll Free: 800-283-7800
help@arthritis.org
www.arthritis.org

Daniel T. McGowan, Chair
Rowland W. (Chang, Vice Chair
Ann M. Palmer, President and CEO

Offers an introduction to Carpal Tunnel, causes, symptoms, diagnosis and resources.

3824 Corticosteriod Medications
Arthritis Foundation
1330 W Peachtree Street
Suite 100
Atlanta, GA 30309
404-872-7100
Fax: 404-872-0457; Toll Free: 800-283-7800
help@arthritis.org
www.arthritis.org

Daniel T. McGowan, Chair
Rowland W. (Chang, Vice Chair
Ann M. Palmer, President and CEO

3825 Diet and Arthritis
Arthritis Foundation
1330 W Peachtree Street
Suite 100
Atlanta, GA 30309
404-872-7100
Fax: 404-872-0457; Toll Free: 800-283-7800

help@arthritis.org
www.arthritis.org

Daniel T. McGowan, Chair
Rowland W. (Chang, Vice Chair
Ann M. Palmer, President and CEO

3826 Ehlers-Danlos Syndrome
Arthritis Foundation
1330 W Peachtree Street
Suite 100
Atlanta, GA 30309
404-872-7100
Fax: 404-872-0457; Toll Free: 800-283-7800
help@arthritis.org
www.arthritis.org

Daniel T. McGowan, Chair
Rowland W. (Chang, Vice Chair
Ann M. Palmer, President and CEO

3827 Exercise and Your Arthritis
Arthritis Foundation
1330 W Peachtree Street
Suite 100
Atlanta, GA 30309
404-872-7100
Fax: 404-872-0457; Toll Free: 800-283-7800
help@arthritis.org
www.arthritis.org

Daniel T. McGowan, Chair
Rowland W. (Chang, Vice Chair
Ann M. Palmer, President and CEO

Types of exercise for people with arthritis and how to do them.

3828 Factor Fax
NE California Chapter - Arthritis Foundation
3040 Explorer Drive
Suite 1
Sacramento, CA 95827-2729
916-368-5599
Fax: 916-368-5596; Toll Free: 800-571-3456
arthritisinsight.com/

Offers information on all of the chapter's activites, events and resources for the arthritis community of central California.

3829 Family
Arthritis Foundation
1330 W Peachtree Street
Suite 100
Atlanta, GA 30309
404-872-7100
Fax: 404-872-0457; Toll Free: 800-283-7800
help@arthritis.org
www.arthritis.org

Daniel T. McGowan, Chair
Rowland W. (Chang, Vice Chair
Ann M. Palmer, President and CEO

Effects of arthritis on family life and ways to cope.

3830 Family: Making the Difference
Arthritis Foundation
1330 W Peachtree Street
Suite 100
Atlanta, GA 30309

404-872-7100
Fax: 404-872-0457; *Toll Free:* 800-283-7800
help@arthritis.org
www.arthritis.org

Daniel T. McGowan, Chair
Rowland W. (Chang, Vice Chair
Ann M. Palmer, President and CEO

3831 Gold Treatment
Arthritis Foundation
1330 W Peachtree Street
Suite 100
Atlanta, GA 30309
404-872-7100
Fax: 404-872-0457; *Toll Free:* 800-283-7800
help@arthritis.org
www.arthritis.org

Daniel T. McGowan, Chair
Rowland W. (Chang, Vice Chair
Ann M. Palmer, President and CEO

3832 Gout
Arthritis Foundation
1330 W Peachtree Street
Suite 100
Atlanta, GA 30309
404-872-7100
Fax: 404-872-0457; *Toll Free:* 800-283-7800
help@arthritis.org
www.arthritis.org

Daniel T. McGowan, Chair
Rowland W. (Chang, Vice Chair
Ann M. Palmer, President and CEO

3833 Guide to Effective Volunteer Lobbying
Arthritis Foundation
1330 W Peachtree Street
Suite 100
Atlanta, GA 30309
404-872-7100
Fax: 404-872-0457; *Toll Free:* 800-283-7800
help@arthritis.org
www.arthritis.org

Daniel T. McGowan, Chair
Rowland W. (Chang, Vice Chair
Ann M. Palmer, President and CEO

3834 Health, Life and Disability Insurance for People with Arthritis
Arthritis Foundation
1330 W Peachtree Street
Suite 100
Atlanta, GA 30309
404-872-7100
Fax: 404-872-0457; *Toll Free:* 800-283-7800
help@arthritis.org
www.arthritis.org

Daniel T. McGowan, Chair
Rowland W. (Chang, Vice Chair
Ann M. Palmer, President and CEO

Information about these three types of insurance.

3835 Hydroxychloroquine
Arthritis Foundation
1330 W Peachtree Street
Suite 100
Atlanta, GA 30309
404-872-7100
Fax: 404-872-0457; *Toll Free:* 800-283-7800
help@arthritis.org
www.arthritis.org

Daniel T. McGowan, Chair
Rowland W. (Chang, Vice Chair
Ann M. Palmer, President and CEO

3836 Living and Loving: Information About Sexuality and Intimacy
Arthritis Foundation
1330 W Peachtree Street
Suite 100
Atlanta, GA 30309
404-872-7100
Fax: 404-872-0457; *Toll Free:* 800-283-7800
help@arthritis.org
www.arthritis.org

Daniel T. McGowan, Chair
Rowland W. (Chang, Vice Chair
Ann M. Palmer, President and CEO

3837 Managing Your Activities
Arthritis Foundation
1330 W Peachtree Street
Suite 100
Atlanta, GA 30309
404-872-7100
Fax: 404-872-0457; *Toll Free:* 800-283-7800
help@arthritis.org
www.arthritis.org

Daniel T. McGowan, Chair
Rowland W. (Chang, Vice Chair
Ann M. Palmer, President and CEO

3838 Managing Your Fatigue
Arthritis Foundation
1330 W Peachtree Street
Suite 100
Atlanta, GA 30309
404-872-7100
Fax: 404-872-0457; *Toll Free:* 800-283-7800
help@arthritis.org
www.arthritis.org

Daniel T. McGowan, Chair
Rowland W. (Chang, Vice Chair
Ann M. Palmer, President and CEO

3839 Managing Your Health Care
Arthritis Foundation
1330 W Peachtree Street
Suite 100
Atlanta, GA 30309
404-872-7100
Fax: 404-872-0457; *Toll Free:* 800-283-7800
help@arthritis.org
www.arthritis.org

Daniel T. McGowan, Chair
Rowland W. (Chang, Vice Chair
Ann M. Palmer, President and CEO

3840 Managing Your Pain
Arthritis Foundation
1330 W Peachtree Street
Suite 100
Atlanta, GA 30309
404-872-7100
Fax: 404-872-0457; *Toll Free:* 800-283-7800
help@arthritis.org
www.arthritis.org

Daniel T. McGowan, Chair
Rowland W. (Chang, Vice Chair
Ann M. Palmer, President and CEO

3841 Managing Your Stress
Arthritis Foundation
1330 W Peachtree Street
Suite 100
Atlanta, GA 30309
404-872-7100
Fax: 404-872-0457; *Toll Free:* 800-283-7800
help@arthritis.org
www.arthritis.org

Daniel T. McGowan, Chair
Rowland W. (Chang, Vice Chair
Ann M. Palmer, President and CEO

3842 Methotrexate
Arthritis Foundation
1330 W Peachtree Street
Suite 100
Atlanta, GA 30309
404-872-7100
Fax: 404-872-0457; *Toll Free:* 800-283-7800
help@arthritis.org
www.arthritis.org

Daniel T. McGowan, Chair
Rowland W. (Chang, Vice Chair
Ann M. Palmer, President and CEO

3843 Myositis
Arthritis Foundation
1330 W Peachtree Street
Suite 100
Atlanta, GA 30309
404-872-7100
Fax: 404-872-0457; *Toll Free:* 800-283-7800
help@arthritis.org
www.arthritis.org

Daniel T. McGowan, Chair
Rowland W. (Chang, Vice Chair
Ann M. Palmer, President and CEO

3844 Osteoarthritis
Arthritis Foundation
1330 W Peachtree Street
Suite 100
Atlanta, GA 30309
404-872-7100
Fax: 404-872-0457; *Toll Free:* 800-283-7800
help@arthritis.org
www.arthritis.org

Daniel T. McGowan, Chair
Rowland W. (Chang, Vice Chair
Ann M. Palmer, President and CEO

Offers introductions, examples, explanations and research
pertaining to this type of arthritis.

3845 Osteonecrosis
Arthritis Foundation
1330 W Peachtree Street
Suite 100
Atlanta, GA 30309
404-872-7100
Fax: 404-872-0457; *Toll Free:* 800-283-7800
help@arthritis.org
www.arthritis.org

Daniel T. McGowan, Chair
Rowland W. (Chang, Vice Chair
Ann M. Palmer, President and CEO

3846 Overcoming Rheumatoid Arthritis
Michigan Chapter of the Arthritis Foundation
23999 Northwestern Highway
210
Southfield, MI 48075-2528
810-350-3030

Provides extensive information about the disease and treatment, with an emphasis on what you can do for yourself.

3847 Penicillamine
Arthritis Foundation
1330 W Peachtree Street
Suite 100
Atlanta, GA 30309
404-872-7100
Fax: 404-872-0457; *Toll Free:* 800-283-7800
help@arthritis.org
www.arthritis.org

Daniel T. McGowan, Chair
Rowland W. (Chang, Vice Chair
Ann M. Palmer, President and CEO

3848 Polyarteritis Nodosa and Wegener's
Granulomatosis
Arthritis Foundation
1330 W Peachtree Street
Suite 100
Atlanta, GA 30309
404-872-7100
Fax: 404-872-0457; *Toll Free:* 800-283-7800
help@arthritis.org
www.arthritis.org

Daniel T. McGowan, Chair
Rowland W. (Chang, Vice Chair
Ann M. Palmer, President and CEO

3849 Polymyalgia Rheumatica and Giant Cell
Arthritis
Arthritis Foundation
1330 W Peachtree Street
Suite 100
Atlanta, GA 30309
404-872-7100
Fax: 404-872-0457; *Toll Free:* 800-283-7800
help@arthritis.org
www.arthritis.org

Daniel T. McGowan, Chair
Rowland W. (Chang, Vice Chair
Ann M. Palmer, President and CEO

3850 Pseudoxanthoma Elasticum Fact Sheet
Arthritis Foundation
1330 W Peachtree Street
Suite 100
Atlanta, GA 30309
404-872-7100
Fax: 404-872-0457; *Toll Free:* 800-283-7800
help@arthritis.org
www.arthritis.org

Daniel T. McGowan, Chair
Rowland W. (Chang, Vice Chair
Ann M. Palmer, President and CEO

3851 Psoriatic Arthritis
NAMSIC, National Institutes of Health
1 Ams Circle
Bethesda, MD 20892-0001
301-495-4484
Fax: 301-718-6366; *Toll Free:* 877-226-4267
www.nih.gov/niams/
TTY: 301-565-2966

3852 Raynaud's Phenomenon
Arthritis Foundation
1330 W Peachtree Street
Suite 100
Atlanta, GA 30309
404-872-7100
Fax: 404-872-0457; *Toll Free:* 800-283-7800
help@arthritis.org
www.arthritis.org

Daniel T. McGowan, Chair
Rowland W. (Chang, Vice Chair
Ann M. Palmer, President and CEO

3853 Reflex Sympathetic Dystrophy Syndrome Fact Sheet
Arthritis Foundation
1330 W Peachtree Street
Suite 100
Atlanta, GA 30309
404-872-7100
Fax: 404-872-0457; *Toll Free:* 800-283-7800
help@arthritis.org
www.arthritis.org

Daniel T. McGowan, Chair
Rowland W. (Chang, Vice Chair
Ann M. Palmer, President and CEO

3854 Reiter's Syndrome
Arthritis Foundation
1330 W Peachtree Street
Suite 100
Atlanta, GA 30309
404-872-7100
Fax: 404-872-0457; *Toll Free:* 800-283-7800
help@arthritis.org
www.arthritis.org

Daniel T. McGowan, Chair
Rowland W. (Chang, Vice Chair
Ann M. Palmer, President and CEO

3855 Rheumatoid Arthritis
NAMSIC, National Institutes of Health
1 Ams Circle
Bethesda, MD 20892-0001

301-495-4484
Fax: 301-718-6366; *Toll Free:* 877-226-4267
www.nih.gov/niams/
TTY: 301-565-2966

Offers an introduction and definition of Rheumatoid Arthritis, treatments, causes, objectives, daily living, resources and medical information.

3856 Spectrum
Michigan Chapter of the Arthritis Foundation
17117 W 9 Mile Road
Suite 950
Southfield, MI 48075-4516
248-424-9001
Fax: 248-424-9005; *Toll Free:* 800-968-3030
info.mi.semr@arthritis.org
arthritisinsight.com/

Promotes various activities and programs and provides current information about arthritis.

3857 Surgery: Information to Consider
Arthritis Foundation
1330 W Peachtree Street
Suite 100
Atlanta, GA 30309
404-872-7100
Fax: 404-872-0457; *Toll Free:* 800-283-7800
help@arthritis.org
www.arthritis.org

Daniel T. McGowan, Chair
Rowland W. (Chang, Vice Chair
Ann M. Palmer, President and CEO

3858 Volunteer Voice
Kentucky Chapter of the Arthritis Foundation
410 W Chestnut Street
Suite 750
Louisville, KY 40202-2368
Toll Free: 800-633-5335

Newsletter offering information and updates on chapter activities, events, camps, juvenile programs and government/legislative information.

Videos, Audio Tapes

3859 Arthritis Foundation Distribution Center: Pool Exercise Program
PO Box 6996
Alpharetta, GA 30023-6996
770-442-8633
Fax: 770-442-9742; *Toll Free:* 800-207-8633
julie.katz@pbd.com
www.arthritis.org

Scott A Dockter, CEO

This video features water exercises that will help you increase and maintain joint flexibility, strengthen and tone muscles, and increase endurance. All exercises are performed in water at chest level. No swimming skills are necessary.

3860 FIT Video
Arthritis Foundation
PO Box 6996
Alpharetta, GA 30023-6996
Fax: 770-442-9742; *Toll Free:* 800-207-8633

Research Centers

3861 Arthritis, Musculoskeletal & Skin Diseases Research: Public Health Service
US Department of Health and Human Services
9000 Rockville Pike
Room 4c32
Bethesda, MD 20892
301-496-4000
NIHinfo@od.nih.gov
www.nih.gov/
TTY: 301-402-9612

Francis S. Collins M.D, PhD, Director

To extramurally support basic laboratory research and clinical investigations, and to provide post-doctoral biomedical research training for individuals interested in careers in health sciences and fields related to these programs.

3862 Boston University: Arthritis Center
Conte Building
5th Floor
Boston, MA 02118
617-638-8000
Fax: 617-534-3573

Dr. Joseph Korn MD, Director
Syed S Ahmed, MD

3863 Boston University: Robert Dawson Evans Memorial Department of Clinical Research
75 E Newton Street
Boston, MA 02118-2657
617-638-7250
Fax: 617-638-7931
profiles.bu.edu/

David Center , MD

Integral unit of the University Hospital specializing in arthritis and connective tissue studies.

3864 Brigham and Women's Hospital: Robert B Brigham Arthritis Center
75 Francis Street
Boston, MA 02115-6106
617-732-6816
Fax: 617-732-5766

Dr. Matthew Liang, Director
Judith Kennedy, Manager

Research studies into arthritis and rheumatic diseases.

3865 Bucknell University Immunobiology Research Laboratory
Department of Biology
Lewisburg, PA 17837
570-577-2000
www.bucknell.edu

John C. Bravman, President

Studies into autoimmune diseases, particularly the causes of rheumatoid arthritis.

3866 Harrington Arthritis Research Center
300 N 18th Street
Phoenix, AZ 85006
602-254-0377
www.newswise.com/

Research into the various areas of arthritis, including assistive devices, joint repair and replacement, medical treatment and early detection and prevention.

3867 Medical University of South Carolina: Arthritis Clinical Research Center
171 Ashley Avenue
Charleston, SC 29425
843-792-8999
Fax: 843-792-7121

E Carwile LeRoy, Director
Fred Crawford, Manager

Offers basic and clinical research on various types of arthritis.

3868 Multipurpose Arthritis & Musculoskeletal Center
1720 2nd Avenue
Birmingham, AL 35294
205-934-4011
www.uab.edu/

Arthritis and related rheumatic disorders are studied.

3869 Multipurpose Arthritis and Musculoskeletal Disease Center
University of California, San Diego
9500 Gilman Drive
La Jolla, CA 92093
858-534-2230
ucsd.edu/

Causes and treatment of arthritis.

3870 National Arthritis and Musculoskeletal and Skin Diseases Information Clearinghouse
1 Ams Circle
Bethesda, MD 20892-0001
301-495-4484
Fax: 301-718-6366; Toll Free: 877-226-4267
www.nih.gov/niams
TTY: 301-565-2966

Supports and provides clinical and public information and research to increase understanding of the many rheumatic diseases and related disorders. Also provides lists and order forms for their resources and materials.

3871 National Institute of Arthritis and Musculoskeletal and Skin Disease
1 Ams Circle
Bethesda, MD 20892-0001
301-495-4484
Fax: 301-718-6366; Toll Free: 877-226-4267
www.niams.nih.gov
TTY: 301-565-2966

The Institute is a public service that provides health information and information sources. Supports research into the causes, treatment and prevention of arthritis and musculokeletal and skin diseases, the training of basic and clinical scientists to carry out this research, and dissemination of information on research progress in these diseases. Provides health information and resources.

3872 Northwestern University: Multipurpose Arhritis & Musculoskeletal Center
303 E Chicago Avenue
Chicago, IL 60611

312-503-1687
offices.northwestern.edu/

Conducts biomedical, educational and health services research into musculoskeletal diseases.

3873 Oklahoma Medical Research Foundation

825 NE 13th Street
Oklahoma City, OK 73104
405-271-6673
Fax: 405-271-3980; *Toll Free:* 800-522-0211
omrf.org/

Scott A. Armstrong MD, Phd

Focuses on arthritis and muscoloskeletal disease research.

3874 Oklahoma Medical Research Foundation: Arthritis Immunology Research

825 NE 13th Street
Oklahoma City, OK 73104
405-271-6673
Fax: 405-271-3980; *Toll Free:* 800-522-0211

Scott A. Armstrong MD, Phd

3875 Pearlman Biomedical Research Institute

Mt. Sinani Medical Center
4300 Alton Road
Miami Beach, FL 33140
305-674-2121
www.msmc.com/

Pulmonary medicine, arthritis, sleep disorders and gynecology departments of research.

3876 Rehabilitation Institute of Chicago

345 E Superior Street
Chicago, IL 60611
312-238-2883
Fax: 312-238-2900
www.ric.org/

Joanne C. Smith MD, President & CEO
Edward B. Case, Executive VP &CFO
Laura L. Ferrio, Vice President

3877 Rosalind Russell Medical Research Center for Arthritis

350 Parnassus Avenue
Suite 600
San Francisco, CA 94117
415-476-1192
www.rosalindrussellcenter.ucsf.edu/

Paula R. Gambs, Chair

Arthritis research and its probable causes.

3878 University of Michigan: Orthopaedic Research Laboratories

109 Zina Pitcher Place
Room 2003
Ann Arbor, MI 48109-2200
734-936-7417
Fax: 734-747-0003

Andrea Alford Phd
Ann De Mare, Executive Director

Develops and studies the causes and treatments for arthritis including new devices and assistive aids.

3879 University of Missouri: Columbia Arthritis Center

MA427 Health Sciences Center
1 Hospital Drive
Columbia, MO 65212
573-882-4677
Fax: 573-884-3996

Gordon C Sharp MD, Director

Research into arthritis and rheumatic diseases.

Cancer

Associations & Organizations

3880 ACS Cancer Action Network
American Cancer Society
555 11th Street NW
Suite 300
Washington, DC 20004
202-661-5700
www.acscan.org

Gary M. Reedy, CEO
Christopher Hansen, President

Advocacy organization of the American Cancer Society.

3881 AMC Cancer Fund
University of Colorado
13001 East 17th Place
MS F-500
Aurora, CO 80045
303-724-7824
Fax: 303-724-7828
contactus@amc.org
www.amc.org

Gary Kortz, Chair
Steven D Toltz, Treasurer
Cherryl Kisling, Secretary

AMC aims to create hope through science by raising funds through engaging corporations, civic organizations and individuals in special events, education and outreach efforts.

3882 American Cancer Society
250 Williams Street NW
Atlanta, GA 30303
Toll Free: 800-227-2345
www.cancer.org

Gary M. Reedy, CEO
Otis W. Brawley, Chief Medical & Scientific Ofc.
Sharon Byers, Chief Development Officer

The American Cancer Society is the nationwide community-based voluntary health organization dedicated to eliminating cancer as a major health problem by preventing cancer, saving lives, and diminishing suffering from cancer, through research, education, advocacy and service.

Year Founded: 1913

3883 American Cancer Society: Acton
American Cancer Society
43 Nagog Park
Suite 110
Acton, MA 01720-3426
781-894-6633 Toll free: 800-227-2345
www.cancer.org
TTY: 866-228-4327

Gary M Reedy, CEO
Otis W Brawley, MD, Chief Medical/Scientific Officer
Catherine Mickle, CFO

Nationwide, community-based voluntary health organization dedicated to eliminating cancer as a major health problem by preventing cancer, saving lives, and diminishing suffering from cancer through research, education, advocacy, and service.

Year Founded: 1913

3884 American Cancer Society: Alameda
American Cancer Society
1001 Marina Village Parkway
Suite 300
Alameda, CA 94501
510-893-7900 Toll free: 800-227-2345
www.cancer.org
TTY: 866-228-4327

Gary M Reedy, CEO
Otis W Brawley, MD, Chief Medical/Scientific Officer
Catherine Mickle, CFO

Nationwide, community-based voluntary health organization dedicated to eliminating cancer as a major health problem by preventing cancer, saving lives, and diminishing suffering from cancer through research, education, advocacy, and service.

Year Founded: 1913

3885 American Cancer Society: Alaska
3851 Piper Street
Suite U240
Anchorage, AK 99508
907-277-8696 Toll free: 800-227-2345
www.cancer.org
TTY: 866-228-4327

Gary M Reedy, CEO
Otis W Brawley, MD, Chief Medical/Scientific Officer
Catherine Mickle, CFO

Nationwide, community-based voluntary health organization dedicated to eliminating cancer as a major health problem by preventing cancer, saving lives, and diminishing suffering from cancer through research, education, advocacy, and service.

Year Founded: 1913

3886 American Cancer Society: Albuquerque
8500 Menaul Boulevard NE
Suite A500
Albuquerque, NM 87112
505-260-2105 Toll free: 800-227-2345
www.cancer.org
TTY: 866-228-4327

Gary M Reedy, Chief Executive Officer
Otis W Brawley, MD, Chief Medical/Scientific Officer
Catherine Mickle, Chief Financial Officer

Nationwide, community-based voluntary health organization dedicated to eliminating cancer as a major health problem by preventing cancer, saving lives, and diminishing suffering from cancer through research, education, advocacy, and service.

Year Founded: 1913

3887 American Cancer Society: Amarillo
3915 Bell Street
Amarillo, TX 79109
806-353-4306 Toll free: 800-227-2345
www.cancer.org
TTY: 866-228-4327

Gary M Reedy, Chief Executive Officer
Otis W Brawley, MD, Chief Medical/Scientific Officer
Catherine Mickle, Chief Financial Officer

Nationwide, community-based voluntary health organization dedicated to eliminating cancer as a major health problem by preventing cancer, saving lives, and diminishing

suffering from cancer through research, education, advocacy, and service.

Year Founded: 1913

3888 American Cancer Society: Amherst

101 John James Audubon Parkway
Amherst, NY 14228
716-689-6981Toll free: 800-227-2345
www.cancer.org
TTY: 866-228-4327

Gary M Reedy, CEO
Otis W Brawley, MD, Chief Medical/Scientific Officer
Catherine Mickle, CFO

Nationwide, community-based voluntary health organization dedicated to eliminating cancer as a major health problem by preventing cancer, saving lives, and diminishing suffering from cancer through research, education, advocacy, and service.

Year Founded: 1913

3889 American Cancer Society: Athens

105 Westpark Drive
Suite C
Athens, GA 30606
706-549-4893Toll free: 800-227-2345
www.cancer.org
TTY: 866-228-4327

Gary M Reedy, Chief Executive Officer
Otis W Brawley, MD, Chief Medical/Scientific Officer
Catherine Mickle, Chief Financial Officer

Nationwide, community-based voluntary health organization dedicated to eliminating cancer as a major health problem by preventing cancer, saving lives, and diminishing suffering from cancer through research, education, advocacy, and service.

Year Founded: 1913

3890 American Cancer Society: Atlanta

250 Williams Street NW
Atlanta, GA 30303
404-816-7800Toll free: 800-227-2345
www.cancer.org
TTY: 866-228-4327

Gary M Reedy, Chief Executive Officer
Otis W Brawley, MD, Chief Medical/Scientific Officer
Catherine Mickle, Chief Financial Officer

Nationwide, community-based voluntary health organization dedicated to eliminating cancer as a major health problem by preventing cancer, saving lives, and diminishing suffering from cancer through research, education, advocacy, and service.

Year Founded: 1913

3891 American Cancer Society: Augusta

2607 Commons Boulevard
Augusta, GA 30909
706-731-9900Toll free: 800-227-2345
www.cancer.org
TTY: 866-228-4327

Gary M Reedy, Chief Executive Officer
Otis W Brawley, MD, Chief Medical/Scientific Officer
Catherine Mickle, Chief Financial Officer

Nationwide, community-based voluntary health organization dedicated to eliminating cancer as a major health prob-

lem by preventing cancer, saving lives, and diminishing suffering from cancer through research, education, advocacy, and service.

Year Founded: 1913

3892 American Cancer Society: Austin

11000 N Mopac Expressway
Suite 100
Austin, TX 78759
512-919-1800Toll free: 800-227-2345
www.cancer.org
TTY: 866-228-4327

Gary M Reedy, Chief Executive Officer
Otis W Brawley, MD, Chief Medical/Scientific Officer
Catherine Mickle, Chief Financial Officer

Nationwide, community-based voluntary health organization dedicated to eliminating cancer as a major health problem by preventing cancer, saving lives, and diminishing suffering from cancer through research, education, advocacy, and service.

Year Founded: 1913

3893 American Cancer Society: Bakersfield

1831 Truxtun Avenue
Suite 150
Bakersfield, CA 93301
661-327-2424Toll free: 800-227-2345
www.cancer.org
TTY: 866-228-4327

Gary M Reedy, Chief Executive Officer
Otis W Brawley, MD, Chief Medical/Scientific Officer
Catherine Mickle, Chief Financial Officer

Nationwide, community-based voluntary health organization dedicated to eliminating cancer as a major health problem by preventing cancer, saving lives, and diminishing suffering from cancer through research, education, advocacy, and service.

Year Founded: 1913

3894 American Cancer Society: Baltimore

405 Williams Court
Suite 120
Baltimore, MD 21220
410-931-6850Toll free: 800-227-2345
www.cancer.org
TTY: 866-228-4327

Gary M Reedy, CEO
Otis W Brawley, MD, Chief Medical/Scientific Officer
Catherine Mickle, CFO

Nationwide, community-based voluntary health organization dedicated to eliminating cancer as a major health problem by preventing cancer, saving lives, and diminishing suffering from cancer through research, education, advocacy, and service.

Year Founded: 1913

3895 American Cancer Society: Barry County

129 Jefferson Avenue SE
Grand Rapids, MI 49503
616-364-6121Toll free: 800-227-2345
www.cancer.org
TTY: 866-228-4327

Gary M Reedy, Chief Executive Officer
Otis W Brawley, MD, Chief Medical/Scientific Officer
Catherine Mickle, Chief Financial Officer

Nationwide, community-based voluntary health organization dedicated to eliminating cancer as a major health problem by preventing cancer, saving lives, and diminishing suffering from cancer through research, education, advocacy, and service.

Year Founded: 1913

3896 American Cancer Society: Baton Rouge
10528 Kentshire Court
Baton Rouge, LA 70810
225-927-0782Toll free: 800-227-2345
www.cancer.org
TTY: 866-228-4327

Gary M Reedy, Chief Executive Officer
Otis W Brawley, MD, Chief Medical/Scientific Officer
Catherine Mickle, Chief Financial Officer

Nationwide, community-based voluntary health organization dedicated to eliminating cancer as a major health problem by preventing cancer, saving lives, and diminishing suffering from cancer through research, education, advocacy, and service.

Year Founded: 1913

3897 American Cancer Society: Beaumont
American Cancer Society
4 Bayou Brandt Drive
Suite B
Beaumont, TX 77706
409-924-0576Toll free: 800-227-2345
www.cancer.org
TTY: 866-228-4327

Gary M Reedy, CEO
Otis W Brawley, MD, Chief Medical/Scientific Officer
Catherine Mickle, CFO

Nationwide, community-based voluntary health organization dedicated to eliminating cancer as a major health problem by preventing cancer, saving lives, and diminishing suffering from cancer through research, education, advocacy, and service.

Year Founded: 1913

3898 American Cancer Society: Bethlehem
American Cancer Society
3893 Adler Place
Suite 170
Bethlehem, PA 18017
610-882-5774Toll free: 800-227-2345
www.cancer.org
TTY: 866-228-4327

Gary M Reedy, CEO
Otis W Brawley, MD, Chief Medical/Scientific Officer
Catherine Mickle, CFO

Nationwide, community-based voluntary health organization dedicated to eliminating cancer as a major health problem by preventing cancer, saving lives, and diminishing suffering from cancer through research, education, advocacy, and service.

Year Founded: 1913

3899 American Cancer Society: Billings
1903 Central Avenue
Billings, MT 59102
406-256-7150Toll free: 800-227-2345
www.cancer.org
TTY: 866-228-4327

Gary M Reedy, Chief Executive Officer
Otis W Brawley, MD, Chief Medical/Scientific Officer
Catherine Mickle, Chief Financial Officer

Nationwide, community-based voluntary health organization dedicated to eliminating cancer as a major health problem by preventing cancer, saving lives, and diminishing suffering from cancer through research, education, advocacy, and service.

Year Founded: 1913

3900 American Cancer Society: Birmingham
1100 Ireland Way
Suite 300
Birmingham, AL 35205-7014
205-879-2242Toll free: 800-227-2345
www.cancer.org
TTY: 866-228-4327

Gary M Reedy, Chief Executive Officer
Otis W Brawley, MD, Chief Medical/Scientific Officer
Catherine Mickle, Chief Financial Officer

Nationwide, community-based voluntary health organization dedicated to eliminating cancer as a major health problem by preventing cancer, saving lives, and diminishing suffering from cancer through research, education, advocacy, and service.

Year Founded: 1913

3901 American Cancer Society: Blue Bell
American Cancer Society
480 Norristown Road
Suite 150
Blue Bell, PA 19422
Toll Free: 888-202-1487
www.cancer.org
TTY: 866-228-4327

Gary M Reedy, CEO
Otis W Brawley, MD, Chief Medical/Scientific Officer
Catherine Mickle, CFO

Nationwide, community-based voluntary health organization dedicated to eliminating cancer as a major health problem by preventing cancer, saving lives, and diminishing suffering from cancer through research, education, advocacy, and service.

Year Founded: 1913

3902 American Cancer Society: Boise
2676 Vista Avenue
Boise, ID 83705
208-343-4609Toll free: 800-227-2345
www.cancer.org
TTY: 866-228-4327

Gary M Reedy, Chief Executive Officer
Otis W Brawley, MD, Chief Medical/Scientific Officer
Catherine Mickle, Chief Financial Officer

Nationwide, community-based voluntary health organization dedicated to eliminating cancer as a major health problem by preventing cancer, saving lives, and diminishing suffering from cancer through research, education, advocacy, and service.

Year Founded: 1913

3903 American Cancer Society: Bowling Green
952 Fairview Avenue
Suite 4
Bowling Green, KY 42101

270-782-3654Toll free: 800-227-2345
www.cancer.org
TTY: 866-228-4327

Gary M Reedy, Chief Executive Officer
Otis W Brawley, MD, Chief Medical/Scientific Officer
Catherine Mickle, Chief Financial Officer

Nationwide, community-based voluntary health organization dedicated to eliminating cancer as a major health problem by preventing cancer, saving lives, and diminishing suffering from cancer through research, education, advocacy, and service.

Year Founded: 1913

3904 American Cancer Society: Brockton
1324 Belmont Street
Suite 204-101
Brockton, MA 02301
508-584-9600Toll free: 800-227-2345
www.cancer.org
TTY: 866-228-4327

Gary M Reedy, CEO
Otis W Brawley, MD, Chief Medical/Scientific Officer
Catherine Mickle, CFO

Nationwide, community-based voluntary health organization dedicated to eliminating cancer as a major health problem by preventing cancer, saving lives, and diminishing suffering from cancer through research, education, advocacy, and service.

Year Founded: 1913

3905 American Cancer Society: Bronx
American Cancer Society
2426 Eastchester Road
Suite 211
Bronx, NY 10469
718-991-4576Toll free: 800-227-2345
www.cancer.org
TTY: 866-228-4327

Gary M Reedy, CEO
Otis W Brawley, MD, Chief Medical/Scientific Officer
Catherine Mickle, CFO

Nationwide, community-based voluntary health organization dedicated to eliminating cancer as a major health problem by preventing cancer, saving lives, and diminishing suffering from cancer through research, education, advocacy, and service.

Year Founded: 1913

3906 American Cancer Society: Brooklyn
503 Fifth Avenue
Suite 2A
Brooklyn, NY 11215
718-237-7850Toll free: 800-227-2345
www.cancer.org
TTY: 866-228-4327

Gary M Reedy, Chief Executive Officer
Otis W Brawley, MD, Chief Medical/Scientific Officer
Catherine Mickle, Chief Financial Officer

Nationwide, community-based voluntary health organization dedicated to eliminating cancer as a major health problem by preventing cancer, saving lives, and diminishing suffering from cancer through research, education, advocacy, and service.

Year Founded: 1913

3907 American Cancer Society: Burbank
American Cancer Society
500 N Victory Boulevard
Burbank, CA 91502
818-841-3800Toll free: 800-227-2345
www.cancer.org
TTY: 866-228-4327

Gary M Reedy, CEO
Otis W Brawley, MD, Chief Medical/Scientific Officer
Catherine Mickle, CFO

Nationwide, community-based voluntary health organization dedicated to eliminating cancer as a major health problem by preventing cancer, saving lives, and diminishing suffering from cancer through research, education, advocacy, and service.

Year Founded: 1913

3908 American Cancer Society: Campbell
747 Camden Avenue
Suite B
Campbell, CA 95008
408-871-1062Toll free: 800-227-2345
www.cancer.org
TTY: 866-228-4327

Gary M Reedy, CEO
Otis W Brawley, MD, Chief Medical/Scientific Officer
Catherine Mickle, CFO

Year Founded: 1913

3909 American Cancer Society: Canfield
525 N Broad Street
Canfield, OH 44406-9274
888-227-6446Toll free: 800-227-2345
www.cancer.org
TTY: 866-228-4327

Gary M Reedy, CEO
Otis W Brawley, MD, Chief Medical/Scientific Officer
Catherine Mickle, CFO

Nationwide, community-based voluntary health organization dedicated to eliminating cancer as a major health problem by preventing cancer, saving lives, and diminishing suffering from cancer through research, education, advocacy, and service.

Year Founded: 1913

3910 American Cancer Society: Cedar Knolls
American Cancer Society
7 Ridgedale Avenue
Suite 103
Cedar Knolls, NJ 07927
973-285-8010Toll free: 800-227-2345
www.cancer.org
TTY: 866-228-4327

Gary M Reedy, CEO
Otis W Brawley, MD, Chief Medical/Scientific Officer
Catherine Mickle, CFO

Nationwide, community-based voluntary health organization dedicated to eliminating cancer as a major health problem by preventing cancer, saving lives, and diminishing suffering from cancer through research, education, advocacy, and service.

Year Founded: 1913

3911 American Cancer Society: Cedar Rapids
4080 First Avenue NE
Suite 101
Cedar Rapids, IA 52402
319-365-5241 Toll free: 800-227-2345
www.cancer.org
TTY: 866-228-4327

Gary M Reedy, Chief Executive Officer
Otis W Brawley, MD, Chief Medical/Scientific Officer
Catherine Mickle, Chief Financial Officer

Nationwide, community-based voluntary health organization dedicated to eliminating cancer as a major health problem by preventing cancer, saving lives, and diminishing suffering from cancer through research, education, advocacy, and service.

Year Founded: 1913

3912 American Cancer Society: Charleston
American Cancer Society
3508 Staunton Avenue
Third Floor
Charleston, WV 25314
304-347-5850 Toll free: 800-227-2345
www.cancer.org
TTY: 866-228-4327

Gary M Reedy, CEO
Otis W Brawley, MD, Chief Medical/Scientific Officer
Catherine Mickle, CFO

Nationwide, community-based voluntary health organization dedicated to eliminating cancer as a major health problem by preventing cancer, saving lives, and diminishing suffering from cancer through research, education, advocacy, and service.

Year Founded: 1913

3913 American Cancer Society: Charlotte
1901 Brunswick Avenue
Suite 100
Charlotte, NC 28207
704-552-6147 Toll free: 800-227-2345
www.cancer.org
TTY: 866-228-4327

Gary M Reedy, Chief Executive Officer
Otis W Brawley, MD, Chief Medical/Scientific Officer
Catherine Mickle, Chief Financial Officer

Nationwide, community-based voluntary health organization dedicated to eliminating cancer as a major health problem by preventing cancer, saving lives, and diminishing suffering from cancer through research, education, advocacy, and service.

Year Founded: 1913

3914 American Cancer Society: Charlottesville
American Cancer Society
1445 E Rio Road
Suite 104
Charlottesville, VA 22901
434-978-7423 Toll free: 800-227-2345
www.cancer.org
TTY: 866-228-4327

Gary M Reedy, CEO
Otis W Brawley, MD, Chief Medical/Scientific Officer
Catherine Mickle, CFO

Nationwide, community-based voluntary health organization dedicated to eliminating cancer as a major health prob-

lem by preventing cancer, saving lives, and diminishing suffering from cancer through research, education, advocacy, and service.

Year Founded: 1913

3915 American Cancer Society: Chattanooga
6221 Shalloword Road
Suite 102
Chattanooga, TN 37421
423-267-8613 Toll free: 800-227-2345
www.cancer.org
TTY: 866-228-4327

Gary M Reedy, Chief Executive Officer
Otis W Brawley, MD, Chief Medical/Scientific Officer
Catherine Mickle, Chief Financial Officer

Nationwide, community-based voluntary health organization dedicated to eliminating cancer as a major health problem by preventing cancer, saving lives, and diminishing suffering from cancer through research, education, advocacy, and service.

Year Founded: 1913

3916 American Cancer Society: Cherry Hill
American Cancer Society
1851 Old Cuthbert Road
Cherry Hill, NJ 08034
856-616-1650 Toll free: 800-227-2345
www.cancer.org
TTY: 866-228-4327

Gary M Reedy, CEO
Otis W Brawley, MD, Chief Medical/Scientific Officer
Catherine Mickle, CFO

Nationwide, community-based voluntary health organization dedicated to eliminating cancer as a major health problem by preventing cancer, saving lives, and diminishing suffering from cancer through research, education, advocacy, and service.

Year Founded: 1913

3917 American Cancer Society: Chicago
225 N Michigan Ave
Suite 1200
Chicago, IL 60601
312-372-0471 Toll free: 800-227-2345
www.cancer.org
TTY: 866-228-4327

Gary M Reedy, Chief Executive Officer
Otis W Brawley, MD, Chief Medical/Scientific Officer
Catherine Mickle, Chief Financial Officer

Nationwide, community-based voluntary health organization dedicated to eliminating cancer as a major health problem by preventing cancer, saving lives, and diminishing suffering from cancer through research, education, advocacy, and service.

Year Founded: 1913

3918 American Cancer Society: Chico
1165 East Avenue
Suite 100
Chico, CA 95926
530-342-4567 Toll free: 800-227-2345
www.cancer.org
TTY: 866-228-4327

Gary M Reedy, CEO
Otis W Brawley, MD, Chief Medical/Scientific Officer
Catherine Mickle, CFO

Nationwide, community-based voluntary health organization dedicated to eliminating cancer as a major health problem by preventing cancer, saving lives, and diminishing suffering from cancer through research, education, advocacy, and service.

Year Founded: 1913

3919 American Cancer Society: Cincinnati
2808 Reading Road
Cincinnati, OH 45206
888-227-6446 Toll free: 800-227-2345
www.cancer.org
TTY: 866-228-4327

Gary M Reedy, Chief Executive Officer
Otis W Brawley, MD, Chief Medical/Scientific Officer
Catherine Mickle, Chief Financial Officer

Nationwide, community-based voluntary health organization dedicated to eliminating cancer as a major health problem by preventing cancer, saving lives, and diminishing suffering from cancer through research, education, advocacy, and service.

Year Founded: 1913

3920 American Cancer Society: Clearfield
American Cancer Society
26 S 2nd Street
Suite 102
Clearfield, PA 16830
814-765-1315 Toll free: 800-227-2345
www.cancer.org
TTY: 866-228-4327

Gary M Reedy, CEO
Otis W Brawley, MD, Chief Medical/Scientific Officer
Catherine Mickle, CFO

Nationwide, community-based voluntary health organization dedicated to eliminating cancer as a major health problem by preventing cancer, saving lives, and diminishing suffering from cancer through research, education, advocacy, and service.

Year Founded: 1913

3921 American Cancer Society: Cleveland
American Cancer Society
10501 Euclid Avenue
Cleveland, OH 44102-2204
Toll Free: 888-227-6446
www.cancer.org
TTY: 866-228-4327

Gary M Reedy, CEO
Otis W Brawley, MD, Chief Medical/Scientific Officer
Catherine Mickle, CFO

Nationwide, community-based voluntary health organization dedicated to eliminating cancer as a major health problem by preventing cancer, saving lives, and diminishing suffering from cancer through research, education, advocacy, and service.

Year Founded: 1913

3922 American Cancer Society: Colorado Springs
1445 N Union Boulevard
Suite B100
Colorado Springs, CO 80909

719-636-5101 Toll free: 800-227-2345
www.cancer.org
TTY: 866-228-4327

Gary M Reedy, Chief Executive Officer
Otis W Brawley, MD, Chief Medical/Scientific Officer
Catherine Mickle, Chief Financial Officer

Nationwide, community-based voluntary health organization dedicated to eliminating cancer as a major health problem by preventing cancer, saving lives, and diminishing suffering from cancer through research, education, advocacy, and service.

Year Founded: 1913

3923 American Cancer Society: Columbia
200 Center Point Circle
Suite 100
Columbia, SC 29210-1790
803-750-1693 Toll free: 800-227-2345
www.cancer.org
TTY: 866-228-4327

Gary M Reedy, Chief Executive Officer
Otis W Brawley, MD, Chief Medical/Scientific Officer
Catherine Mickle, Chief Financial Officer

Nationwide, community-based voluntary health organization dedicated to eliminating cancer as a major health problem by preventing cancer, saving lives, and diminishing suffering from cancer through research, education, advocacy, and service.

Year Founded: 1913

3924 American Cancer Society: Columbus
233 12th Street
Suite 710
Columbus, GA 31901
706-324-4573 Toll free: 800-227-2345
www.cancer.org
TTY: 866-228-4327

Gary M Reedy, Chief Executive Officer
Otis W Brawley, MD, Chief Medical/Scientific Officer
Catherine Mickle, Chief Financial Officer

Nationwide, community-based voluntary health organization dedicated to eliminating cancer as a major health problem by preventing cancer, saving lives, and diminishing suffering from cancer through research, education, advocacy, and service.

Year Founded: 1913

3925 American Cancer Society: Corpus Christi
210 S Carancachua
Suite 301
Corpus Christi, TX 78401
361-857-0134 Toll free: 800-227-2345
www.cancer.org
TTY: 866-228-4327

Gary M Reedy, Chief Executive Officer
Otis W Brawley, MD, Chief Medical/Scientific Officer
Catherine Mickle, Chief Financial Officer

Nationwide, community-based voluntary health organization dedicated to eliminating cancer as a major health problem by preventing cancer, saving lives, and diminishing suffering from cancer through research, education, advocacy, and service.

Year Founded: 1913

3926 American Cancer Society: Culver City
5731 W Slauson Avenue
Suite 200
Culver City, CA 90230
310-348-0356Toll free: 800-227-2345
www.cancer.org
TTY: 866-228-4327

Gary M Reedy, CEO
Otis W Brawley, MD, Chief Medical/Scientific Officer
Catherine Mickle, CFO

Nationwide, community-based voluntary health organization dedicated to eliminating cancer as a major health problem by preventing cancer, saving lives, and diminishing suffering from cancer through research, education, advocacy, and service.

Year Founded: 1913

3927 American Cancer Society: Cumberland
1050 East Industrial Boulevard
Unit 3
Cumberland, MD 21502
301-722-2145Toll free: 800-227-2345
www.cancer.org
TTY: 866-228-4327

Gary M Reedy, Chief Executive Officer
Otis W Brawley, MD, Chief Medical/Scientific Officer
Catherine Mickle, Chief Financial Officer

Nationwide, community-based voluntary health organization dedicated to eliminating cancer as a major health problem by preventing cancer, saving lives, and diminishing suffering from cancer through research, education, advocacy, and service.

Year Founded: 1913

3928 American Cancer Society: Dallas
8900 John W Carpenter Fwy
Dallas, TX 75247
214-819-1200Toll free: 800-227-2345
www.cancer.org
TTY: 866-228-4327

Gary M Reedy, Chief Executive Officer
Otis W Brawley, MD, Chief Medical/Scientific Officer
Catherine Mickle, Chief Financial Officer

Nationwide, community-based voluntary health organization dedicated to eliminating cancer as a major health problem by preventing cancer, saving lives, and diminishing suffering from cancer through research, education, advocacy, and service.

Year Founded: 1913

3929 American Cancer Society: Daytona Beach
LakeSide North Executive Center
1737 North Clyde Morris Boulevard, Suite 140
Daytona Beach, FL 32117
386-274-3274Toll free: 800-227-2345
www.cancer.org
TTY: 866-228-4327

Gary M Reedy, Chief Executive Officer
Otis W Brawley, MD, Chief Medical/Scientific Officer
Catherine Mickle, Chief Financial Officer

Nationwide, community-based voluntary health organization dedicated to eliminating cancer as a major health problem by preventing cancer, saving lives, and diminishing suffering from cancer through research, education, advocacy, and service.

Year Founded: 1913

3930 American Cancer Society: Denver
2255 S Oneida Street
Denver, CO 80224
303-758-2030Toll free: 800-227-2345
www.cancer.org
TTY: 866-228-4327

Gary M Reedy, Chief Executive Officer
Otis W Brawley, MD, Chief Medical/Scientific Officer
Catherine Mickle, Chief Financial Officer

Nationwide, community-based voluntary health organization dedicated to eliminating cancer as a major health problem by preventing cancer, saving lives, and diminishing suffering from cancer through research, education, advocacy, and service.

Year Founded: 1913

3931 American Cancer Society: Des Moines
1717 Ingersoll Avenue
Suite 111
Des Moines, IA 50309
515-253-0147Toll free: 800-227-2345
www.cancer.org
TTY: 866-228-4327

Gary M Reedy, Chief Executive Officer
Otis W Brawley, MD, Chief Medical/Scientific Officer
Catherine Mickle, Chief Financial Officer

Nationwide, community-based voluntary health organization dedicated to eliminating cancer as a major health problem by preventing cancer, saving lives, and diminishing suffering from cancer through research, education, advocacy, and service.

Year Founded: 1913

3932 American Cancer Society: Dublin
5555 Frantz Road
Dublin, OH 43017
888-227-6446Toll free: 800-227-2345
www.cancer.org
TTY: 866-228-4327

Gary M Reedy, Chief Financial Officer
Otis W Brawley, MD, Chief Medical/Scientific Officer
Catherine Mickle, Chief Financial Officer

Nationwide, community-based voluntary health organization dedicated to eliminating cancer as a major health problem by preventing cancer, saving lives, and diminishing suffering from cancer through research, education, advocacy, and service.

Year Founded: 1913

3933 American Cancer Society: Duluth
6500 Sugarloaf Parkway
Suite 260
Duluth, GA 30097
770-814-0211Toll free: 800-227-2345
www.cancer.org
TTY: 866-228-4327

Gary M Reedy, Cheif Executive Officer
Otis W Brawley, MD, Chief Medical/Scientific Officer
Catherine Mickle, Chief Financial Officer

Nationwide, community-based voluntary health organization dedicated to eliminating cancer as a major health problem by preventing cancer, saving lives, and diminishing

suffering from cancer through research, education, advocacy, and service.

Year Founded: 1913

3934 American Cancer Society: Eagan
American Cancer Society
950 Blue Gentian Road
Suite 100
Eagan, MN 55121
651-255-8100Toll free: 800-227-2345
www.cancer.org
TTY: 866-228-4327

Gary M Reedy, CEO
Otis W Brawley, MD, Chief Medical/Scientific Officer
Catherine Mickle, CFO

Nationwide, community-based voluntary health organization dedicated to eliminating cancer as a major health problem by preventing cancer, saving lives, and diminishing suffering from cancer through research, education, advocacy, and service.

Year Founded: 1913

3935 American Cancer Society: East Lansing
1755 Abbey Road
East Lansing, MI 48823
517-332-3300Toll free: 800-227-2345
www.cancer.org
TTY: 866-228-4327

Gary M Reedy, Chief Executive Officer
Otis W Brawley, MD, Chief Medical/Scientific Officer
Catherine Mickle, Chief Financial Officer

Nationwide, community-based voluntary health organization dedicated to eliminating cancer as a major health problem by preventing cancer, saving lives, and diminishing suffering from cancer through research, education, advocacy, and service.

Year Founded: 1913

3936 American Cancer Society: East Syracuse
6725 Lyons Street
P.O. Box 7
East Syracuse, NY 13057
315-437-7025Toll free: 800-227-2345
www.cancer.org
TTY: 866-228-4327

Gary M Reedy, Chief Executive Officer
Otis W Brawley, MD, Chief Medical/Scientific Officer
Catherine Mickle, Chief Financial Officer

Nationwide, community-based voluntary health organization dedicated to eliminating cancer as a major health problem by preventing cancer, saving lives, and diminishing suffering from cancer through research, education, advocacy, and service.

Year Founded: 1913

3937 American Cancer Society: El Centro
400 S Eighth Street
El Centro, CA 92243
760-352-6656Toll free: 800-227-2345
www.cancer.org
TTY: 866-228-4327

Gary M Reedy, CEO
Otis W Brawley, MD, Chief Medical/Scientific Officer
Catherine Mickle, CFO

Nationwide, community-based voluntary health organization dedicated to eliminating cancer as a major health problem by preventing cancer, saving lives, and diminishing suffering from cancer through research, education, advocacy, and service.

Year Founded: 1913

3938 American Cancer Society: El Paso
10801 Gateway West
Suite 500
El Paso, TX 79935
915-633-1231Toll free: 800-227-2345
www.cancer.org
TTY: 866-228-4327

Gary M Reedy, Chief Executive Officer
Otis W Brawley, MD, Chief Medical/Scientific Officer
Catherine Mickle, Chief Financial Officer

Nationwide, community-based voluntary health organization dedicated to eliminating cancer as a major health problem by preventing cancer, saving lives, and diminishing suffering from cancer through research, education, advocacy, and service.

Year Founded: 1913

3939 American Cancer Society: Eldersburg
1393 Progress Way
Suite 908
Eldersburg, MD 21784
410-781-4316Toll free: 800-227-2345
www.cancer.org
TTY: 866-228-4327

Gary M Reedy, Chief Executive Officer
Otis W Brawley, MD, Chief Medical/Scientific Officer
Catherine Mickle, Chief Financial Officer

Nationwide, community-based voluntary health organization dedicated to eliminating cancer as a major health problem by preventing cancer, saving lives, and diminishing suffering from cancer through research, education, advocacy, and service.

Year Founded: 1913

3940 American Cancer Society: Erie
2115 W 38th Street
Erie, PA 16508
814-866-5174Toll free: 800-227-2345
www.cancer.org
TTY: 866-228-4327

Gary M Reedy, Chief Executive Officer
Otis W Brawley, MD, Chief Medical/Scientific Officer
Catherine Mickle, Chief Financial Officer

Nationwide, community-based voluntary health organization dedicated to eliminating cancer as a major health problem by preventing cancer, saving lives, and diminishing suffering from cancer through research, education, advocacy, and service.

Year Founded: 1913

3941 American Cancer Society: Eugene
2350 Oakmont Way
Suite 200
Eugene, OR 97401
541-484-2211Toll free: 800-227-2345
www.cancer.org
TTY: 866-228-4327

Gary M Reedy, Chief Executive Officer
Otis W Brawley, MD, Chief Medical/Scientific Officer
Catherine Mickle, Chief Financial Officer

Nationwide, community-based voluntary health organization dedicated to eliminating cancer as a major health problem by preventing cancer, saving lives, and diminishing suffering from cancer through research, education, advocacy, and service.

Year Founded: 1913

3942 American Cancer Society: Eureka
611 Harris Street
Eureka, CA 95503
707-442-1436Toll free: 800-227-2345
www.cancer.org
TTY: 866-228-4327

Gary M Reedy, CEO
Otis W Brawley, MD, Chief Medical/Scientific Officer
Catherine Mickle, CFO

Nationwide, community-based voluntary health organization dedicated to eliminating cancer as a major health problem by preventing cancer, saving lives, and diminishing suffering from cancer through research, education, advocacy, and service.

Year Founded: 1913

3943 American Cancer Society: Evansville
5250 Vogel Road
Main Level
Evansville, IN 47715
812-475-9244Toll free: 800-227-2345
www.cancer.org
TTY: 866-228-4327

Gary M Reedy, CEO
Otis W Brawley, MD, Chief Medical/Scientific Officer
Cahterine Mickle, CFO

Nationwide, community-based voluntary health organization dedicated to eliminating cancer as a major health problem by preventing cancer, saving lives, and diminishing suffering from cancer through research, education, advocacy, and service.

Year Founded: 1913

3944 American Cancer Society: Everett
3120 McDougall Avenue
Suite 100
Everett, WA 98201
425-340-4293Toll free: 800-227-2345
www.cancer.org
TTY: 866-228-4327

Gary M Reedy, Chief Executive Officer
Otis W Brawley, MD, Chief Medical/Scientific Officer
Catherine Mickle, Chief Financial Officer

Nationwide, community-based voluntary health organization dedicated to eliminating cancer as a major health problem by preventing cancer, saving lives, and diminishing suffering from cancer through research, education, advocacy, and service.

Year Founded: 1913

3945 American Cancer Society: Fairlawn
American Cancer Society
3500 Embassy Parkway
Suite 150
Fairlawn, OH 44333

330-517-2060Toll free: 800-227-2345
www.cancer.org
TTY: 866-228-4327

Gary M Reedy, CEO
Otis W Brawley, MD, Chief Medical/Scientific Officer
Catherine Mickle, CFO

Nationwide, community-based voluntary health organization dedicated to eliminating cancer as a major health problem by preventing cancer, saving lives, and diminishing suffering from cancer through research, education, advocacy, and service.

Year Founded: 1913

3946 American Cancer Society: Fargo
4646 Amber Valley Parkway
Fargo, ND 58104
701-433-7580Toll free: 800-227-2345
www.cancer.org
TTY: 866-228-4327

Gary M Reedy, Chief Executive Officer
Otis W Brawley, MD, Chief Medical/Scientific Officer
Catherine Mickle, Chief Financial Officer

Nationwide, community-based voluntary health organization dedicated to eliminating cancer as a major health problem by preventing cancer, saving lives, and diminishing suffering from cancer through research, education, advocacy, and service.

Year Founded: 1913

3947 American Cancer Society: Flint
2413 S Linden
Suite A
Flint, MI 48532
810-733-3702Toll free: 800-227-2345
www.cancer.org
TTY: 866-228-4327

Gary M Reedy, Chief Executive Officer
Otis W Brawley, MD, Chief Medical/Scientific Officer
Catherine Mickle, Chief Financial Officer

Nationwide, community-based voluntary health organization dedicated to eliminating cancer as a major health problem by preventing cancer, saving lives, and diminishing suffering from cancer through research, education, advocacy, and service.

Year Founded: 1913

3948 American Cancer Society: Flushing
131-07 40th Road
Suite E28
Flushing, NY 11354
718-263-2224Toll free: 800-227-2345
www.cancer.org
TTY: 866-228-4327

Gary M Reedy, Chief Executive Officer
Otis W Brawley, MD, Chief Medical/Scientific Officer
Catherine Mickle, Chief Financial Officer

Nationwide, community-based voluntary health organization dedicated to eliminating cancer as a major health problem by preventing cancer, saving lives, and diminishing suffering from cancer through research, education, advocacy, and service.

Year Founded: 1913

3949 American Cancer Society: Fort Lauderdale
American Cancer Society
3363 W Commercial Boulevard
Suite 100
Fort Lauderdale, FL 33309
954-564-0880 Toll free: 800-227-2345
www.cancer.org
TTY: 866-228-4327

Gary M Reedy, CEO
Otis W Brawley, MD, Chief Medical/Scientific Officer
Catherine Mickle, CFO

Nationwide, community-based voluntary health organization dedicated to eliminating cancer as a major health problem by preventing cancer, saving lives, and diminishing suffering from cancer through research, education, advocacy, and service.

Year Founded: 1913

3950 American Cancer Society: Fort Myers
4575 Via Royale
Suite 110
Fort Myers, FL 33919
239-936-1113 Toll free: 800-227-2345
www.cancer.org
TTY: 866-228-4327

Gary M Reedy, Chief Executive Officer
Otis W Brawley, MD, Chief Medical/Scientific Officer
Catherine Mickle, Chief Financial Officer

Nationwide, community-based voluntary health organization dedicated to eliminating cancer as a major health problem by preventing cancer, saving lives, and diminishing suffering from cancer through research, education, advocacy, and service.

Year Founded: 1913

3951 American Cancer Society: Fort Walton Beach
99 Elgin Parkway NE
Suite 37
Fort Walton Beach, FL 32548
850-244-3813 Toll free: 800-227-2345
www.cancer.org
TTY: 866-228-4327

Gary M Reedy, Chief Executive Officer
Otis W Brawley, MD, Chief Medical/Scientific Officer
Catherine Mickle, Chief Financial Officer

Nationwide, community-based voluntary health organization dedicated to eliminating cancer as a major health problem by preventing cancer, saving lives, and diminishing suffering from cancer through research, education, advocacy, and service.

Year Founded: 1913

3952 American Cancer Society: Fort Wayne
111 E Ludwig Road
Suite 105
Fort Wayne, IN 46825
260-471-3911 Toll free: 800-227-2345
www.cancer.org
TTY: 866-228-4327

Gary M Reedy, CEO
Otis W Brawley, MD, Chief Medical/Scientific Officer
Catherine Mickle, CFO

Nationwide, community-based voluntary health organization dedicated to eliminating cancer as a major health problem by preventing cancer, saving lives, and diminishing

suffering from cancer through research, education, advocacy, and service.

Year Founded: 1913

3953 American Cancer Society: Fort Worth
3301 West Fwy
Fort Worth, TX 76107
817-737-9990 Toll free: 800-227-2345
www.cancer.org
TTY: 866-228-4327

Gary M Reedy, Chief Executive Officer
Otis W Brawley, MD, Chief Medical/Scientific Officer
Catherine Mickle, Chief Financial Officer

Nationwide, community-based voluntary health organization dedicated to eliminating cancer as a major health problem by preventing cancer, saving lives, and diminishing suffering from cancer through research, education, advocacy, and service.

Year Founded: 1913

3954 American Cancer Society: Frackville
American Cancer Society
101 W Frack Street
Frackville, PA 17931
570-874-1413 Toll free: 800-227-2345
www.cancer.org
TTY: 866-228-4327

Gary M Reedy, CEO
Otis W Brawley, MD, Chief Medical/Scientific Officer
Catherine Mickle, CFO

Nationwide, community-based voluntary health organization dedicated to eliminating cancer as a major health problem by preventing cancer, saving lives, and diminishing suffering from cancer through research, education, advocacy, and service.

Year Founded: 1913

3955 American Cancer Society: Framingham
American Cancer Society
30 Speen Street
Framingham, MA 01701
508-270-4600 Toll free: 800-227-2345
www.cancer.org
TTY: 866-228-4327

Gary M Reedy, CEO
Otis W Brawley, MD, Chief Medical/Scientific Officer
Catherine Mickle, CFO

Nationwide, community-based voluntary health organization dedicated to eliminating cancer as a major health problem by preventing cancer, saving lives, and diminishing suffering from cancer through research, education, advocacy, and service.

Year Founded: 1913

3956 American Cancer Society: Fresno
2222 W Shaw Avenue
Suite 201
Fresno, CA 93711
559-451-0722 Toll free: 800-227-2345
www.cancer.org
TTY: 866-228-4327

Gary M Reedy, Chief Executive Officer
Otis W Brawley, MD, Chief Medical/Scientific Officer
Catherine Mickle, Chief Financial Officer

Nationwide, community-based voluntary health organization dedicated to eliminating cancer as a major health problem by preventing cancer, saving lives, and diminishing suffering from cancer through research, education, advocacy, and service.

Year Founded: 1913

3957 American Cancer Society: Gainesville
2565 Thompson Bridge Road
Suite 114
Gainesville, GA 30501
770-297-1176 Toll free: 800-227-2345
www.cancer.org
TTY: 866-228-4327

Gary M Reedy, Chief Executive Officer
Otis W Brawley, MD, Chief Medical/Scientific Officer
Catherine Mickle, Chief Financial Officer

Nationwide, community-based voluntary health organization dedicated to eliminating cancer as a major health problem by preventing cancer, saving lives, and diminishing suffering from cancer through research, education, advocacy, and service.

Year Founded: 1913

3958 American Cancer Society: Gainesville, FL
American Cancer Society
2119 SW 16th Street
Gainesville, FL 32608
352-376-6866 Toll free: 800-227-2345
www.cancer.org
TTY: 866-228-4327

Gary M Reedy, CEO
Otis W Brawley, MD, Chief Medical/Scientific Officer
Catherine Mickle, CFO

Nationwide, community-based voluntary health organization dedicated to eliminating cancer as a major health problem by preventing cancer, saving lives, and diminishing suffering from cancer through research, education, advocacy, and service.

Year Founded: 1913

3959 American Cancer Society: Glen Allen
4240 Park Place Court
Glen Allen, VA 23060
804-527-3700 Toll free: 800-227-2345
www.cancer.org
TTY: 866-228-4327

Gary M Reedy, Chief Executive Officer
Otis W Brawley, MD, Chief Medical/Scientific Officer
Catherine Mickle, Chief Financial Officer

Nationwide, community-based voluntary health organization dedicated to eliminating cancer as a major health problem by preventing cancer, saving lives, and diminishing suffering from cancer through research, education, advocacy, and service.

Year Founded: 1913

3960 American Cancer Society: Grand Junction
2754 Compass Drive
Suite 100
Grand Junction, CO 81506
970-242-9593 Toll free: 800-227-2345
www.cancer.org
TTY: 866-228-4327

Gary M Reedy, Chief Executive Officer
Otis W Brawley, MD, Chief Medical/Scientific Officer
Catherine Mickle, Chief Financial Officer

Nationwide, community-based voluntary health organization dedicated to eliminating cancer as a major health problem by preventing cancer, saving lives, and diminishing suffering from cancer through research, education, advocacy, and service.

Year Founded: 1913

3961 American Cancer Society: Greater Tampa
3709 W Jetton Avenue
Tampa, FL 33629-5146
813-253-0541 Toll free: 800-227-2345
www.cancer.org
TTY: 866-228-4327

Gary M Reedy, Chief Executive Officer
Otis W Brawley, MD, Chief Medical/Scientific Officer
Catherine Mickle, Chief Financial Officer

Nationwide, community-based voluntary health organization dedicated to eliminating cancer as a major health problem by preventing cancer, saving lives, and diminishing suffering from cancer through research, education, advocacy, and service.

Year Founded: 1913

3962 American Cancer Society: Greater Ventura
2186 Knoll Drive
Suite A
Ventura, CA 93003
805-644-4237 Toll free: 800-227-2345
www.cancer.org
TTY: 866-228-4327

Gary M Reedy, Chief Executive Officer
Otis W Brawley, MD, Chief Medical/Scientific Officer
Catherine Mickle, Chief Financial Officer

Nationwide, community-based voluntary health organization dedicated to eliminating cancer as a major health problem by preventing cancer, saving lives, and diminishing suffering from cancer through research, education, advocacy, and service.

Year Founded: 1913

3963 American Cancer Society: Greeley
8221 W 20th Street
Suite A
Greeley, CO 80634
970-356-9727 Toll free: 800-227-2345
www.cancer.org
TTY: 866-228-4327

Gary M Reedy, Chief Executive Officer
Otis W Brawley, MD, Chief Medical/Scientific Officer
Catherine Mickle, Chief Financial Officer

Nationwide, community-based voluntary health organization dedicated to eliminating cancer as a major health problem by preventing cancer, saving lives, and diminishing suffering from cancer through research, education, advocacy, and service.

Year Founded: 1913

3964 American Cancer Society: Green Bay
2100 Riverside Drive
Suite 201
Green Bay, WI 54301

920-338-1541Toll free: 800-227-2345
www.cancer.org
TTY: 866-228-4327

Gary M Reedy, Chief Executive Officer
Otis W Brawley, MD, Chief Medical/Scientific Officer
Catherine Mickle, Chief Financial Officer

Nationwide, community-based voluntary health organization dedicated to eliminating cancer as a major health problem by preventing cancer, saving lives, and diminishing suffering from cancer through research, education, advocacy, and service.

Year Founded: 1913

3965 American Cancer Society: Greenbelt
American Cancer Society
7500 Greenway Center Drive
Suite 300
Greenbelt, MD 20770
301-982-2161Toll free: 800-227-2345
www.cancer.org
TTY: 866-228-4327

Gary M Reedy, CEO
Otis W Brawley, MD, Chief Medical/Scientific Officer
Catherine Mickle, CFO

Nationwide, community-based voluntary health organization dedicated to eliminating cancer as a major health problem by preventing cancer, saving lives, and diminishing suffering from cancer through research, education, advocacy, and service.

Year Founded: 1913

3966 American Cancer Society: Greensboro
American Cancer Society
7027 Albert Pick Road
Suite 104
Greensboro, NC 27409
336-834-0844Toll free: 800-227-2345
www.cancer.org
TTY: 866-228-4327

Gary M Reedy, CEO
Otis W Brawley, MD, Chief Medical/Scientific Officer
Catherine Mickle, CFO

Nationwide, community-based voluntary health organization dedicated to eliminating cancer as a major health problem by preventing cancer, saving lives, and diminishing suffering from cancer through research, education, advocacy, and service.

Year Founded: 1913

3967 American Cancer Society: Greensburg
American Cancer Society
510 Pellis Road
Suite 203
Greensburg, PA 15601
724-834-9081Toll free: 800-227-2345
www.cancer.org
TTY: 866-228-4327

Gary M Reedy, CEO
Otis W Brawley, MD, Chief Medical/Scientific Officer
Catherine Mickle, CFO

Nationwide, community-based voluntary health organization dedicated to eliminating cancer as a major health problem by preventing cancer, saving lives, and diminishing

suffering from cancer through research, education, advocacy, and service.

Year Founded: 1913

3968 American Cancer Society: Greenville
154 Milestone Way
Greenville, SC 29615
864-627-1903Toll free: 800-227-2345
www.cancer.org
TTY: 866-228-4327

Gary M Reedy, Chief Executive Officer
Otis W Brawley, MD, Chief Medical/Scientific Officer
Catherine Mickle, Chief Financial Officer

Nationwide, community-based voluntary health organization dedicated to eliminating cancer as a major health problem by preventing cancer, saving lives, and diminishing suffering from cancer through research, education, advocacy, and service.

Year Founded: 1913

3969 American Cancer Society: Greenville, NC
American Cancer Society
930 Wellness Drive
Suite B
Greenville, NC 27834
252-695-9028Toll free: 800-227-2345
www.cancer.org
TTY: 866-228-4327

Gary M Reedy, CEO
Otis W Brawley, MD, Chief Medical/Scientific Officer
Catherine Mickle, CFO

Nationwide, community-based voluntary health organization dedicated to eliminating cancer as a major health problem by preventing cancer, saving lives, and diminishing suffering from cancer through research, education, advocacy, and service.

Year Founded: 1913

3970 American Cancer Society: Greenwood
P.O. Box 1741
Greenwood, SC 29648
864-321-1166Toll free: 800-227-2345
www.cancer.org
TTY: 866-228-4327

Gary M Reedy, Chief Executive Officer
Otis W Brawley, MD, Chief Medical/Scientific Officer
Catherine Mickle, Chief Financial Officer

Nationwide, community-based voluntary health organization dedicated to eliminating cancer as a major health problem by preventing cancer, saving lives, and diminishing suffering from cancer through research, education, advocacy, and service.

Year Founded: 1913

3971 American Cancer Society: Harrisonburg
American Cancer Society
420 Neff Avenue
Suite 210
Harrisonburg, VA 22801
540-434-3360Toll free: 800-227-2345
www.cancer.org
TTY: 866-228-4327

Gary M Reedy, CEO
Otis W Brawley, MD, Chief Medical/Scientific Officer
Catherine Mickle, CFO

Nationwide, community-based voluntary health organization dedicated to eliminating cancer as a major health problem by preventing cancer, saving lives, and diminishing suffering from cancer through research, education, advocacy, and service.

Year Founded: 1913

3972 American Cancer Society: Hershey
American Cancer Society
Route 422 & Sipe Avenue
Hershey, PA 17033
717-533-6144Toll free: 800-227-2345
www.cancer.org
TTY: 866-228-4327

Gary M Reedy, CEO
Otis W Brawley, MD, Chief Medical/Scientific Officer
Catherine Mickle, CFO

Nationwide, community-based voluntary health organization dedicated to eliminating cancer as a major health problem by preventing cancer, saving lives, and diminishing suffering from cancer through research, education, advocacy, and service.

Year Founded: 1913

3973 American Cancer Society: Hilo
58 Kinoole Street
Suite 104
Hilo, HI 96720
808-935-9763Toll free: 800-227-2345
www.cancer.org
TTY: 866-228-4327

Gary M Reedy, Chief Executive Officer
Otis W Brawley, MD, Chief Medical/Scientific Officer
Catherine Mickle, Chief Financial Officer

Nationwide, community-based voluntary health organization dedicated to eliminating cancer as a major health problem by preventing cancer, saving lives, and diminishing suffering from cancer through research, education, advocacy, and service.

Year Founded: 1913

3974 American Cancer Society: Hollidaysburg
American Cancer Society
1004 N Juniata Street
Hollidaysburg, PA 16648
814-695-9232Toll free: 800-227-2345
www.cancer.org
TTY: 866-228-4327

Gary M Reedy, CEO
Otis W Brawley, MD, Chief Medical/Scientific Officer
Catherine Mickle, CFO

Nationwide, community-based voluntary health organization dedicated to eliminating cancer as a major health problem by preventing cancer, saving lives, and diminishing suffering from cancer through research, education, advocacy, and service.

Year Founded: 1913

3975 American Cancer Society: Holyoke
59 Bobala Road
Holyoke, MA 01040
413-734-6000Toll free: 800-227-2345
www.cancer.org
TTY: 866-228-4327

Gary M Reedy, CEO
Otis W Brawley, MD, Chief Medical/Scientific Officer
Catherine Mickle, CFO

Nationwide, community-based voluntary health organization dedicated to eliminating cancer as a major health problem by preventing cancer, saving lives, and diminishing suffering from cancer through research, education, advocacy, and service.

Year Founded: 1913

3976 American Cancer Society: Honolulu
2370 Nuuanu Avenue
Honolulu, HI 96817
808-595-7544Toll free: 800-227-2345
www.cancer.org
TTY: 866-228-4327

Gary M Reedy, CEO
Otis W Brawley, MD, Chief Medical/Scientific Officer
Catherine Mickle, CFO

Nationwide, community-based voluntary health organization dedicated to eliminating cancer as a major health problem by preventing cancer, saving lives, and diminishing suffering from cancer through research, education, advocacy, and service.

Year Founded: 1913

3977 American Cancer Society: Houston
2500 Forden Road
Suite 100
Houston, TX 77063
713-706-5690Toll free: 800-227-2345
www.cancer.org
TTY: 866-228-4327

Gary M Reedy, CEO
Otis W Brawley, MD, Chief Medical/Scientific Officer
Catherine Mickle, CFO

Nationwide, community-based voluntary health organization dedicated to eliminating cancer as a major health problem by preventing cancer, saving lives, and diminishing suffering from cancer through research, education, advocacy, and service.

Year Founded: 1913

3978 American Cancer Society: Huntsville
2745 Bob Wallace Avenue
Suite A
Huntsville, AL 35805
256-536-1855Toll free: 800-227-2345
www.cancer.org
TTY: 866-228-4327

Gary M Reedy, CEO
Otis W Brawley, MD, Chief Medical/Scientific Officer
Catherine Mickle, CFO

Nationwide, community-based voluntary health organization dedicated to eliminating cancer as a major health problem by preventing cancer, saving lives, and diminishing suffering from cancer through research, education, advocacy, and service.

Year Founded: 1913

3979 American Cancer Society: Indianapolis
5635 W 96th Street
Suite 100
Indianapolis, IN 46278

317-344-7800Toll free: 800-227-2345
www.cancer.org
TTY: 866-228-4327

Gary M Reedy, CEO
Otis W Brawley, MD, Chief Medical/Scientific Officer
Catherine Mickle, CFO

Nationwide, community-based voluntary health organization dedicated to eliminating cancer as a major health problem by preventing cancer, saving lives, and diminishing suffering from cancer through research, education, advocacy, and service.

Year Founded: 1913

3980 American Cancer Society: Jackson

1380 Livingston Lane
Jackson, MS 39213
601-362-8874Toll free: 800-227-2345
www.cancer.org
TTY: 866-228-4327

Gary M Reedy, CEO
Otis W Brawley, MD, Chief Medical/Scientific Officer
Catherine Mickle, CFO

Nationwide, community-based voluntary health organization dedicated to eliminating cancer as a major health problem by preventing cancer, saving lives, and diminishing suffering from cancer through research, education, advocacy, and service.

Year Founded: 1913

3981 American Cancer Society: Jackson, TN

2935 US Highway 45 Bypass
Jackson, TN 38305
731-664-4663Toll free: 800-227-2345
www.cancer.org
TTY: 866-228-4327

Gary M Reedy, CEO
Otis W Brawley, MD, Chief Medical/Scientific Officer
Catherine Mickle, CFO

Nationwide, community-based voluntary health organization dedicated to eliminating cancer as a major health problem by preventing cancer, saving lives, and diminishing suffering from cancer through research, education, advocacy, and service.

Year Founded: 1913

3982 American Cancer Society: Jacksonville

1430 Prudential Drive
Jacksonville, FL 32207
904-398-0537Toll free: 800-227-2345
www.cancer.org
TTY: 866-228-4327

Gary M Reedy, CEO
Otis W Brawley, MD, Chief Medical/Scientific Officer
Catherine Mickle, CFO

Nationwide, community-based voluntary health organization dedicated to eliminating cancer as a major health problem by preventing cancer, saving lives, and diminishing suffering from cancer through research, education, advocacy, and service.

Year Founded: 1913

3983 American Cancer Society: Jefferson City

2409 Hyde Park Road
Jefferson City, MO 65109

573-635-4821Toll free: 800-227-2345
www.cancer.org
TTY: 866-228-4327

Gary M Reedy, CEO
Otis W Brawley, MD, Chief Medical/Scientific Officer
Catherine Mickle, CFO

Nationwide, community-based voluntary health organization dedicated to eliminating cancer as a major health problem by preventing cancer, saving lives, and diminishing suffering from cancer through research, education, advocacy, and service.

Year Founded: 1913

3984 American Cancer Society: Johnson City

American Cancer Society
13 Beech Street
Johnson City, NY 13790
607-766-6900Toll free: 800-227-2345
www.cancer.org
TTY: 866-228-4327

Gary M Reedy, CEO
Otis W Brawley, MD, Chief Medical/Scientific Officer
Catherine Mickle, CFO

Nationwide, community-based voluntary health organization dedicated to eliminating cancer as a major health problem by preventing cancer, saving lives, and diminishing suffering from cancer through research, education, advocacy, and service.

Year Founded: 1913

3985 American Cancer Society: Kansas City

American Cancer Society
1100 Pennsylvania Avenue
Kansas City, MO 64105
913-432-3277Toll free: 800-227-2345
www.cancer.org
TTY: 866-228-4327

Gary M Reedy, CEO
Otis W Brawley, MD, Chief Medical/Scientific Officer
Catherine Mickle, CFO

Nationwide, community-based voluntary health organization dedicated to eliminating cancer as a major health problem by preventing cancer, saving lives, and diminishing suffering from cancer through research, education, advocacy, and service.

Year Founded: 1913

3986 American Cancer Society: Kearney

3808 28th Avenue
Suite E
Kearney, NE 68845
308-237-7481Toll free: 800-227-2345
www.cancer.org
TTY: 866-228-4327

Gary M Reedy, CEO
Otis W Brawley, MD, Chief Medical/Scientific Officer
Catherine Mickle, CFO

Nationwide, community-based voluntary health organization dedicated to eliminating cancer as a major health problem by preventing cancer, saving lives, and diminishing suffering from cancer through research, education, advocacy, and service.

Year Founded: 1913

3987 American Cancer Society: Kennesaw

3380 Chastain Meadows Parkway NW
Suite 200
Kennesaw, GA 30144
770-429-0089Toll free: 800-227-2345
www.cancer.org
TTY: 866-228-4327

Gary M Reedy, CEO
Otis W Brawley, MD, Chief Medical/Scientific Officer
Catherine Mickle, CFO

Nationwide, community-based voluntary health organization dedicated to eliminating cancer as a major health problem by preventing cancer, saving lives, and diminishing suffering from cancer through research, education, advocacy, and service.

Year Founded: 1913

3988 American Cancer Society: Knoxville

871 N Weisgarber Road
Knoxville, TN 37909
865-584-1668Toll free: 800-227-2345
www.cancer.org
TTY: 866-228-4327

Gary M Reedy, CEO
Otis W Brawley, MD, Chief Medical/Scientific Officer
Catherine Mickle, CFO

Nationwide, community-based voluntary health organization dedicated to eliminating cancer as a major health problem by preventing cancer, saving lives, and diminishing suffering from cancer through research, education, advocacy, and service.

Year Founded: 1913

3989 American Cancer Society: Lafayette

1604 W Pinhook Road
Suite 203
Lafayette, LA 70508
337-237-3736Toll free: 800-227-2345
www.cancer.org
TTY: 866-228-4327

Gary M Reedy, CEO
Otis W Brawley, MD, Chief Medical/Scientific Officer
Catherine Mickle, CFO

Nationwide, community-based voluntary health organization dedicated to eliminating cancer as a major health problem by preventing cancer, saving lives, and diminishing suffering from cancer through research, education, advocacy, and service.

Year Founded: 1913

3990 American Cancer Society: Lake County

100 Tri-State International
Suite 125
Lincolnshire, IL 60069
847-317-0025Toll free: 800-227-2345
www.cancer.org
TTY: 866-228-4327

Gary M Reedy, CEO
Otis W Brawley, MD, Chief Medical/Scientific Officer
Catherine Mickle, CFO

Nationwide, community-based voluntary health organization dedicated to eliminating cancer as a major health problem by preventing cancer, saving lives, and diminishing suffering from cancer through research, education, advocacy, and service.

Year Founded: 1913

3991 American Cancer Society: Lakeland

122 East Main Street
Suite 215
Lakeland, FL 33801
863-688-2326Toll free: 800-227-2345
www.cancer.org
TTY: 866-228-4327

Gary M Reedy, Chief Executive Officer
Otis W Brawley, MD, Chief Medical/Scientific Officer
Catherine Mickle, Chief Financial Officer

Nationwide, community-based voluntary health organization dedicated to eliminating cancer as a major health problem by preventing cancer, saving lives, and diminishing suffering from cancer through research, education, advocacy, and service.

Year Founded: 1913

3992 American Cancer Society: Lakes Region

1120 S Gooddman Street
Rochester, NY 14620
585-288-1950Toll free: 800-227-2345
www.cancer.org
TTY: 866-228-4327

Gary M Reedy, CEO
Otis W Brawley, MD, Chief Medical/Scientific Officer
Catherine Mickle, CFO

Nationwide, community-based voluntary health organization dedicated to eliminating cancer as a major health problem by preventing cancer, saving lives, and diminishing suffering from cancer through research, education, advocacy, and service.

Year Founded: 1913

3993 American Cancer Society: Lancaster

314 Good Drive
Lancaster, PA 17603
717-397-3745Toll free: 800-227-2345
www.cancer.org
TTY: 866-228-4327

Gary M Reedy, CEO
Otis W Brawley, MD, Chief Medica/Scientific Officer
Catherine Mickle, CFO

Nationwide, community-based voluntary health organization dedicated to eliminating cancer as a major health problem by preventing cancer, saving lives, and diminishing suffering from cancer through research, education, advocacy, and service.

Year Founded: 1913

3994 American Cancer Society: Las Vegas

6165 S Rainbow Boulevard
Suite 12
Las Vegas, NV 89118
702-798-5938Toll free: 800-227-2345
www.cancer.org
TTY: 866-228-4327

Gary M Reedy, CEO
Otis W Brawley, MD, Chief Medical/Scientific Officer
Catherine Mickle, CFO

Nationwide, community-based voluntary health organization dedicated to eliminating cancer as a major health problem by preventing cancer, saving lives, and diminishing

suffering from cancer through research, education, advocacy, and service.

Year Founded: 1913

3995 American Cancer Society: Latham
American Cancer Society
1 Penny Lane
Latham, NY 12110
518-220-6901 Toll free: 800-227-2345
www.cancer.org
TTY: 866-228-4327

Gary M Reedy, CEO
Otis W Brawley, MD, Chief Medical/Scientific Officer
Catherine Mickle, CFO

Nationwide, community-based voluntary health organization dedicated to eliminating cancer as a major health problem by preventing cancer, saving lives, and diminishing suffering from cancer through research, education, advocacy, and service.

Year Founded: 1913

3996 American Cancer Society: Lawton
1320 NW Homestead Drive
Suite D
Lawton, OK 73505
580-353-5001
www.cancer.org

Gary M Reedy, CEO
Otis W Brawley, MD, Chief Medical/Scientific Officer
Catherine Mickle, CFO

Nationwide, community-based voluntary health organization dedicated to eliminating cancer as a major health problem by preventing cancer, saving lives, and diminishing suffering from cancer through research, education, advocacy, and service.

Year Founded: 1913

3997 American Cancer Society: Lexington
1504 College Way
Lexington, KY 40502
859-276-3223 Toll free: 800-227-2345
www.cancer.org
TTY: 866-228-4327

Gary M Reedy, CEO
Otis W Brawley, MD, Chief Medical/Scientific Officer
Catherine Mickle, CFO

Nationwide, community-based voluntary health organization dedicated to eliminating cancer as a major health problem by preventing cancer, saving lives, and diminishing suffering from cancer through research, education, advocacy, and service.

Year Founded: 1913

3998 American Cancer Society: Lihue
3343 Kanakolu Street
Lihue, HI 96766
808-245-2942 Toll free: 800-227-2345
www.cancer.org
TTY: 866-228-4327

Gary M Reedy, CEO
Otis W Brawley, MD, Chief Medical/Scientific Officer
Catherine Mickle, CFO

Nationwide, community-based voluntary health organization dedicated to eliminating cancer as a major health prob-

lem by preventing cancer, saving lives, and diminishing suffering from cancer through research, education, advocacy, and service.

Year Founded: 1913

3999 American Cancer Society: Lincoln
5733 S 34th Street
Suite 500
Lincoln, NE 68516
402-423-4888 Toll free: 800-227-2345
www.cancer.org
TTY: 866-228-4327

Gary M Reedy, CEO
Otis W Brawley, MD, Chief Medical/Scientific Officer
Catherine Mickle, CFO

Nationwide, community-based voluntary health organization dedicated to eliminating cancer as a major health problem by preventing cancer, saving lives, and diminishing suffering from cancer through research, education, advocacy, and service.

Year Founded: 1913

4000 American Cancer Society: Little Rock
901 N University Avenue
Little Rock, AR 72207
501-664-3480 Toll free: 800-227-2345
www.cancer.org
TTY: 866-228-4327

Gary M Reedy, CEO
Otis W Brawley, MD, Chief Medical/Scientific Officer
Catherine Mickle, CFO

Nationwide, community-based voluntary health organization dedicated to eliminating cancer as a major health problem by preventing cancer, saving lives, and diminishing suffering from cancer through research, education, advocacy, and service.

Year Founded: 1913

4001 American Cancer Society: Long Beach
444 W Ocean Boulevard
Suite 1070
Long Beach, CA 90802
562-437-0791 Toll free: 800-227-2345
www.cancer.org
TTY: 866-228-4327

Gary M Reedy, CEO
Otis W Brawley, MD, Chief Medical/Scientific Officer
Catherine Mickle, CFO

Nationwide, community-based voluntary health organization dedicated to eliminating cancer as a major health problem by preventing cancer, saving lives, and diminishing suffering from cancer through research, education, advocacy, and service.

Year Founded: 1913

4002 American Cancer Society: Louisville
1640 Lyndon Farm Court
Suite 104
Louisville, KY 40223
502-584-6782 Toll free: 800-227-2345
www.cancer.org
TTY: 866-228-4327

Gary M Reedy, CEO
Otis W Brawley, MD, Chief Medical/Scientific Officer
Catherine Mickle, CFO

Nationwide, community-based voluntary health organization dedicated to eliminating cancer as a major health problem by preventing cancer, saving lives, and diminishing suffering from cancer through research, education, advocacy, and service.

Year Founded: 1913

4003 American Cancer Society: Lubbock
American Cancer Society
3513 10th Street
Lubbock, TX 79415
806-792-7126Toll free: 800-227-2345
www.cancer.org
TTY: 866-228-4327

Gary M Reedy, CEO
Otis W Brawley, MD, Chief Medical/Scientific Officer
Catherine Mickle, CFO

Nationwide, community-based voluntary health organization dedicated to eliminating cancer as a major health problem by preventing cancer, saving lives, and diminishing suffering from cancer through research, education, advocacy, and service.

Year Founded: 1913

4004 American Cancer Society: Lufkin
American Cancer Society
212 Gene Samford Drive
Lufkin, TX 75904
936-634-2940Toll free: 800-227-2345
www.cancer.org
TTY: 866-228-4327

Gary M Reedy, CEO
Otis W Brawley, MD, Chief Medical/Scientific Officer
Catherine Mickle, CFO

Nationwide, community-based voluntary health organization dedicated to eliminating cancer as a major health problem by preventing cancer, saving lives, and diminishing suffering from cancer through research, education, advocacy, and service.

Year Founded: 1913

4005 American Cancer Society: Lynchburg
2050 Langhorne Road
Suite 201
Lynchburg, VA 24501
434-845-0973Toll free: 800-227-2345
www.cancer.org
TTY: 866-228-4327

Gary M Reedy, CEO
Otis W Brawley, MD, Chief Medical/Scientific Officer
Catherine Mickle, CFO

Nationwide, community-based voluntary health organization dedicated to eliminating cancer as a major health problem by preventing cancer, saving lives, and diminishing suffering from cancer through research, education, advocacy, and service.

Year Founded: 1913

4006 American Cancer Society: Macon
804 Cherry Street
Suite A
Macon, GA 31201
478-743-6391Toll free: 800-227-2345
www.cancer.org
TTY: 866-228-4327

Gary M Reedy, CEO
Otis W Brawley, MD, Chief Medical/Scientific Officer
Catherine Mickle, CFO

Nationwide, community-based voluntary health organization dedicated to eliminating cancer as a major health problem by preventing cancer, saving lives, and diminishing suffering from cancer through research, education, advocacy, and service.

Year Founded: 1913

4007 American Cancer Society: Madison
8317 Elderberry Road
Madison, WI 53717
608-833-4555Toll free: 800-227-2345
www.cancer.org
TTY: 866-228-4327

Gary M Reedy, CEO
Otis W Brawley, MD, Chief Medical/Scientific Officer
Catherine Mickle, CFO

Nationwide, community-based voluntary health organization dedicated to eliminating cancer as a major health problem by preventing cancer, saving lives, and diminishing suffering from cancer through research, education, advocacy, and service.

Year Founded: 1913

4008 American Cancer Society: Manasquan
American Cancer Society
2310 Route 34
Suite 1D
Manasquan, NJ 08736
732-292-3112Toll free: 800-227-2345
www.cancer.org
TTY: 866-228-4327

Gary M Reedy, CEO
Otis W Brawley, MD, Chief Medical/Scientific Officer
Catherine Mickle, CFO

Nationwide, community-based voluntary health organization dedicated to eliminating cancer as a major health problem by preventing cancer, saving lives, and diminishing suffering from cancer through research, education, advocacy, and service.

Year Founded: 1913

4009 American Cancer Society: Manhattan
American Cancer Society
132 W 32nd Street
New York, NY 10001
212-565-8700Toll free: 800-227-2345
www.cancer.org
TTY: 866-228-4327

Gary M Reedy, CEO
Otis W Brawley, MD, Chief Medical/Scientific Officer
Catherine Mickle, CFO

Nationwide, community-based voluntary health organization dedicated to eliminating cancer as a major health problem by preventing cancer, saving lives, and diminishing suffering from cancer through research, education, advocacy, and service.

Year Founded: 1913

4010 American Cancer Society: Marco Island
583 Tallwood Court
Suite 101
Marco Island, FL 34145

239-642-6216Toll free: 800-227-2345
www.cancer.org
TTY: 866-228-4327

Gary M Reedy, CEO
Otis W Brawley, MD, Chief Medical/Scientific Officer
Catherine Mickle, CFO

Nationwide, community-based voluntary health organization dedicated to eliminating cancer as a major health problem by preventing cancer, saving lives, and diminishing suffering from cancer through research, education, advocacy, and service.

Year Founded: 1913

4011 American Cancer Society: Marion
American Cancer Society
4503 W DeYoung Street
Suite 200 C
Marion, IL 62959
618-998-9898Toll free: 800-227-2345
www.cancer.org
TTY: 866-228-4327

Gary M Reedy, CEO
Otis W Brawley, MD, Chief Medical/Scientific Officer
Catherine Mickle, CFO

Nationwide, community-based voluntary health organization dedicated to eliminating cancer as a major health problem by preventing cancer, saving lives, and diminishing suffering from cancer through research, education, advocacy, and service.

Year Founded: 1913

4012 American Cancer Society: Martinsville
American Cancer Society
1079 Spruce Street
Martinsville, VA 24112
276-638-8944Toll free: 800-227-2345
www.cancer.org
TTY: 866-228-4327

Gary M Reedy, CEO
Otis W Brawley, MD, Chief Medical/Scientific Officer
Catherine Mickle, CFO

Nationwide, community-based voluntary health organization dedicated to eliminating cancer as a major health problem by preventing cancer, saving lives, and diminishing suffering from cancer through research, education, advocacy, and service.

Year Founded: 1913

4013 American Cancer Society: Maryville
American Cancer Society
5 Schiber Court
Building A
Maryville, IL 62062
618-288-2320Toll free: 800-227-2345
www.cancer.org
TTY: 866-228-4327

Gary M Reedy, CEO
Otis W Brawley, MD, Chief Medical/Scientific Officer
Catherine Mickle, CFO

Nationwide, community-based voluntary health organization dedicated to eliminating cancer as a major health problem by preventing cancer, saving lives, and diminishing suffering from cancer through research, education, advocacy, and service.

4014 American Cancer Society: McAllen
American Cancer Society
1200 E Ridge Road
Suite 1
McAllen, TX 78503
956-682-8320Toll free: 800-227-2345
www.cancer.org
TTY: 866-228-4327

Gary M Reedy, CEO
Otis W Brawley, MD, Chief Medical/Scientific Officer
Catherine Mickle, CFO

Nationwide, community-based voluntary health organization dedicated to eliminating cancer as a major health problem by preventing cancer, saving lives, and diminishing suffering from cancer through research, education, advocacy, and service.

Year Founded: 1913

4015 American Cancer Society: Medford
31 W 6th Street
Medford, OR 97501
541-779-6091Toll free: 800-227-2345
www.cancer.org
TTY: 866-228-4327

Gary M Reedy, CEO
Otis W Brawley, MD, Chief Medical/Scientific Officer
Catherine Mickle, CFO

Nationwide, community-based voluntary health organization dedicated to eliminating cancer as a major health problem by preventing cancer, saving lives, and diminishing suffering from cancer through research, education, advocacy, and service.

Year Founded: 1913

4016 American Cancer Society: Melbourne
American Cancer Society
5545 N Wickham Road
Suite 107
Melbourne, FL 32940
321-253-0361Toll free: 800-227-2345
www.cancer.org
TTY: 866-228-4327

Gary M Reedy, CEO
Otis W Brawley, MD, Chief Medical/Scientific Officer
Catherine Mickle, CFO

Nationwide, community-based voluntary health organization dedicated to eliminating cancer as a major health problem by preventing cancer, saving lives, and diminishing suffering from cancer through research, education, advocacy, and service.

Year Founded: 1913

4017 American Cancer Society: Memphis
1378 Union Avenue
Memphis, TN 38104
901-278-2000Toll free: 800-227-2345
www.cancer.org
TTY: 866-228-4327

Gary M Reedy, CEO
Otis W Brawley, MD, Chief Medical/Scientific Officer
Catherine Mickle, CFO

Nationwide, community-based voluntary health organization dedicated to eliminating cancer as a major health problem by preventing cancer, saving lives, and diminishing suffering from cancer through research, education, advocacy, and service.

Year Founded: 1913

4018 American Cancer Society: Miami
American Cancer Society
8095 NW 12th Street
Suite 200
Doral, FL 33126
305-594-4363 Toll free: 800-227-2345
www.cancer.org
TTY: 866-228-4327

Gary M Reedy, CEO
Otis W Brawley, MD, Chief Medical/Scientific Officer
Catherine Mickle, CFO

Nationwide, community-based voluntary health organization dedicated to eliminating cancer as a major health problem by preventing cancer, saving lives, and diminishing suffering from cancer through research, education, advocacy, and service.

Year Founded: 1913

4019 American Cancer Society: Midland
American Cancer Society
2304 W Wadley
Midland, TX 79705
432-683-6374 Toll free: 800-227-2345
www.cancer.org
TTY: 866-228-4327

Gary M Reedy, CEO
Otis W Brawley, MD, Chief Medical/Scientific Officer
Catherine Mickle, CFO

Nationwide, community-based voluntary health organization dedicated to eliminating cancer as a major health problem by preventing cancer, saving lives, and diminishing suffering from cancer through research, education, advocacy, and service.

Year Founded: 1913

4020 American Cancer Society: Mishawaka
130 Red Coach Drive
Mishawaka, IN 47715
574-257-9789 Toll free: 800-227-2345
www.cancer.org
TTY: 866-228-4327

Gary M Reedy, CEO
Otis W Brawley, MD, Chief Medical/Scientific Officer
Catherine Mickle, CFO

Nationwide, community-based voluntary health organization dedicated to eliminating cancer as a major health problem by preventing cancer, saving lives, and diminishing suffering from cancer through research, education, advocacy, and service.

Year Founded: 1913

4021 American Cancer Society: Missoula
3550 Mullan Road
Suite 103
Missoula, MT 59808
406-542-2191 Toll free: 800-227-2345
www.cancer.org
TTY: 866-228-4327

Gary M Reedy, Chief Executive Officer
Otis W Brawley, MD, Chief Medical/Scientific Officer
Catherine Mickle, Chief Financial Officer

Nationwide, community-based voluntary health organization dedicated to eliminating cancer as a major health problem by preventing cancer, saving lives, and diminishing suffering from cancer through research, education, advocacy, and service.

Year Founded: 1913

4022 American Cancer Society: Mobile
1110 Montlimar Drive
Suite 420
Mobile, AL 36609
251-344-9856 Toll free: 800-227-2345
www.cancer.org
TTY: 866-228-4327

Gary M Reedy, CEO
Otis W Brawley, MD, Chief Medical/Scientific Officer
Catherine Mickle, CFO

Nationwide, community-based voluntary health organization dedicated to eliminating cancer as a major health problem by preventing cancer, saving lives, and diminishing suffering from cancer through research, education, advocacy, and service.

Year Founded: 1913

4023 American Cancer Society: Modesto
1101 Sylvan Avenue
Suite C-150
Modesto, CA 95350
209-524-7242 Toll free: 800-227-2345
www.cancer.org
TTY: 866-228-4327

Gary M Reedy, CEO
Otis W Brawley, MD, Chief Medical/Scientific Officer
Catherine Mickle, CFO

Nationwide, community-based voluntary health organization dedicated to eliminating cancer as a major health problem by preventing cancer, saving lives, and diminishing suffering from cancer through research, education, advocacy, and service.

Year Founded: 1913

4024 American Cancer Society: Montgomery
3054 McGehee Road
Montgomery, AL 36111
334-288-3432 Toll free: 800-227-2345
www.cancer.org
TTY: 866-228-4327

Gary M Reedy, CEO
Otis W Brawley, MD, Chief Medical/Scientific Officer
Catherine Mickle, CFO

Nationwide, community-based voluntary health organization dedicated to eliminating cancer as a major health problem by preventing cancer, saving lives, and diminishing suffering from cancer through research, education, advocacy, and service.

Year Founded: 1913

4025 American Cancer Society: Morgantown
122 S High Street
Morgantown, WV 26501

304-296-8155Toll free: 800-227-2345
www.cancer.org
TTY: 866-228-4327

Gary M Reedy, CEO
Otis W Brawley,, Chief Medical/Scientific Officer
Catherine Mickle, CFO

Nationwide, community-based voluntary health organization dedicated to eliminating cancer as a major health problem by preventing cancer, saving lives, and diminishing suffering from cancer through research, education, advocacy, and service.
Year Founded: 1913

4026 American Cancer Society: Myrtle Beach
950 48th Avenue N
Suite 101
Myrtle Beach, SC 29577
843-213-0333Toll free: 800-227-2345
www.cancer.org
TTY: 866-228-4327

Gary M Reedy, CEO
Otis W Brawley, MD, Chief Medical/Scientific Officer
Catherine Mickle, CFO

Nationwide, community-based voluntary health organization dedicated to eliminating cancer as a major health problem by preventing cancer, saving lives, and diminishing suffering from cancer through research, education, advocacy, and service.
Year Founded: 1913

4027 American Cancer Society: Naples
American Cancer Society
5020 Tamiami Trail N
Suite 108
Naples, FL 34103
239-261-0337Toll free: 800-227-2345
www.cancer.org
TTY: 866-228-4327

Gary M Reedy, CEO
Otis W Brawley, MD, Chief Medical/Scientific Officer
Catherine Mickle, CFO

Nationwide, community-based voluntary health organization dedicated to eliminating cancer as a major health problem by preventing cancer, saving lives, and diminishing suffering from cancer through research, education, advocacy, and service.
Year Founded: 1913

4028 American Cancer Society: Nashville
2000 Charlotte Avenue
Nashville, TN 37203
615-327-0991Toll free: 800-227-2345
www.cancer.org
TTY: 866-228-4327

Gary M Reedy, CEO
Otis W Brawley, MD, Chief Medical/Scientific Officer
Catherine Mickle, CFO

Nationwide, community-based voluntary health organization dedicated to eliminating cancer as a major health problem by preventing cancer, saving lives, and diminishing suffering from cancer through research, education, advocacy, and service.
Year Founded: 1913

4029 American Cancer Society: New Castle
92 Reads Way
Suite 205
New Castle, DE 19720
302-324-4227Toll free: 800-227-2345
www.cancer.org
TTY: 866-228-4327

Gary M Reedy, CEO
Otis W Brawley, MD, Chief Medical/Scientific Officer
Catherine Mickle, CFO

Nationwide, community-based voluntary health organization dedicated to eliminating cancer as a major health problem by preventing cancer, saving lives, and diminishing suffering from cancer through research, education, advocacy, and service.
Year Founded: 1913

4030 American Cancer Society: New Hampshire
American Cancer Society
2 Commerce Drive
Suite 110
Bedford, NH 03110
603-472-8899Toll free: 800-227-2345
www.cancer.org
TTY: 866-228-4327

Gary M Reedy, CEO
Otis W Brawley, MD, Chief Medical/Scientific Officer
Catherine Mickle, CFO

Nationwide, community-based voluntary health organization dedicated to eliminating cancer as a major health problem by preventing cancer, saving lives, and diminishing suffering from cancer through research, education, advocacy, and service.
Year Founded: 1913

4031 American Cancer Society: New Orleans
2605 River Road
New Orleans, LA 70121
504-469-0021Toll free: 800-227-2345
www.cancer.org
TTY: 866-228-4327

Gary M Reedy, CEO
Otis W Brawley, MD, Chief Medical/Scientific Officer
Catherine Mickle, CFO

Nationwide, community-based voluntary health organization dedicated to eliminating cancer as a major health problem by preventing cancer, saving lives, and diminishing suffering from cancer through research, education, advocacy, and service.
Year Founded: 1913

4032 American Cancer Society: New Windsor
121 Executive Drive
New Windsor, NY 12533
845-440-2549Toll free: 800-227-2345
www.cancer.org
TTY: 866-228-4327

Gary M Reedy, CEO
Otis W Mickle, Chief Medical/Scientific Officer
Catherine Mickle, CFO

Nationwide, community-based voluntary health organization dedicated to eliminating cancer as a major health problem by preventing cancer, saving lives, and diminishing suffering from cancer through research, education, advocacy, and service.

Year Founded: 1913

4033 American Cancer Society: Newport News
11835 Canon Boulevard
Suite A102
Newport News, VA 23606
757-591-8330Toll free: 800-227-2345
www.cancer.org
TTY: 866-228-4327

Gary M Reedy, CEO
Otis W Brawley, MD, Chief Medical/Scientific Officer
Catherine Mickle, CFO

Nationwide, community-based voluntary health organization dedicated to eliminating cancer as a major health problem by preventing cancer, saving lives, and diminishing suffering from cancer through research, education, advocacy, and service.

Year Founded: 1913

4034 American Cancer Society: North Charleston
5900 Core Avenue
Suite 504
North Charleston, SC 29406
843-744-1922Toll free: 800-227-2345
www.cancer.org
TTY: 866-228-4327

Gary M Reedy, CEO
Otis W Brawley, MD, Chief Medical/Scientific Officer
Catherine Mickle, CFO

Nationwide, community-based voluntary health organization dedicated to eliminating cancer as a major health problem by preventing cancer, saving lives, and diminishing suffering from cancer through research, education, advocacy, and service.

Year Founded: 1913

4035 American Cancer Society: Norwalk
38 Richards Avenue
Norwalk, CT 06854-2318
203-563-0740Toll free: 800-227-2345
www.cancer.org
TTY: 866-228-4327

Gary M Reedy, CEO
Otis W Brawley, MD, Chief Medical/Scientific Officer
Catherine Mickle, CFO

Nationwide, community-based voluntary health organization dedicated to eliminating cancer as a major health problem by preventing cancer, saving lives, and diminishing suffering from cancer through research, education, advocacy, and service.

Year Founded: 1913

4036 American Cancer Society: Oak Brook Terrace
1801 Meyers Road
Ste 100
Oak Brook Terrace, IL 60181
630-932-1141Toll free: 800-227-2345
www.cancer.org
TTY: 866-228-4327

Gary M Reedy, Chief Executive Officer
Otis W Brawley, MD, Chief Medical/Scientific Officer
Catherine Mickle, Chief Financial Officer

Nationwide, community-based voluntary health organization dedicated to eliminating cancer as a major health problem by preventing cancer, saving lives, and diminishing

suffering from cancer through research, education, advocacy, and service.

Year Founded: 1913

4037 American Cancer Society: Oklahoma City
6525 N Meridian Avenue
Suite 110
Oklahoma City, OK 73116
405-843-9888Toll free: 800-227-2345
www.cancer.org
TTY: 866-228-4327

Gary M Reedy, CEO
Otis W Brawley, MD, Chief Medical/Scientific Officer
Catherine Mickle, CFO

Nationwide, community-based voluntary health organization dedicated to eliminating cancer as a major health problem by preventing cancer, saving lives, and diminishing suffering from cancer through research, education, advocacy, and service.

Year Founded: 1913

4038 American Cancer Society: Omaha
9850 Nicholas Street
Suite 200
Omaha, NE 68114
402-393-5800Toll free: 800-227-2345
www.cancer.org
TTY: 866-228-4327

Gary M Reedy, CEO
Otis W Brawley, MD, Chief Medical/Scientific Officer
Catherine Mickle, CFO

Nationwide, community-based voluntary health organization dedicated to eliminating cancer as a major health problem by preventing cancer, saving lives, and diminishing suffering from cancer through research, education, advocacy, and service.

Year Founded: 1913

4039 American Cancer Society: Onalaska
American Cancer Society
1285 Ruby Street
Suite 103
Onalaska, WI 54650
608-783-5000Toll free: 800-227-2345
www.cancer.org
TTY: 866-228-4327

Gary M Reedy, CEO
Otis W Brawley, MD, Chief Medical/Scientific Officer
Catherine Mickle, CFO

Nationwide, community-based voluntary health organization dedicated to eliminating cancer as a major health problem by preventing cancer, saving lives, and diminishing suffering from cancer through research, education, advocacy, and service.

Year Founded: 1913

4040 American Cancer Society: Orange County Region
1940 E Deere Avenue
Suite 100
Santa Ana, CA 92705
949-261-9446Toll free: 800-227-2345
www.cancer.org
TTY: 866-228-4327

Gary M Reedy, CEO
Otis W Brawley, MD, Chief Medical/Scientific Officer
Catherine Mickle, CFO

Nationwide, community-based voluntary health organization dedicated to eliminating cancer as a major health problem by preventing cancer, saving lives, and diminishing suffering from cancer through research, education, advocacy, and service.

Year Founded: 1913

4041 American Cancer Society: Osage Beach

2926 E Battlefield
Springfield, MO 65804
417-881-4668Toll free: 800-227-2345
www.cancer.org
TTY: 866-228-4327

Gary M Reedy, CEO
Otis W Brawley, MD, Chief Medical/Scientific Officer
Catherine Mickle, CFO

Nationwide, community-based voluntary health organization dedicated to eliminating cancer as a major health problem by preventing cancer, saving lives, and diminishing suffering from cancer through research, education, advocacy, and service.

Year Founded: 1913

4042 American Cancer Society: Paducah

3140 Parisa Drive
Paducah, KY 42003
270-444-0375Toll free: 800-227-2345
www.cancer.org
TTY: 866-228-4327

Gary M Reedy, CEO
Otis W Brawley, MD, Chief Medical/Scientific Officer
Catherine Mickle, CFO

Nationwide, community-based voluntary health organization dedicated to eliminating cancer as a major health problem by preventing cancer, saving lives, and diminishing suffering from cancer through research, education, advocacy, and service.

Year Founded: 1913

4043 American Cancer Society: Palm Beach

235 S County Road 2
Palm Beach, FL 33480
561-655-3449Toll free: 800-227-2345
www.cancer.org
TTY: 866-228-4327

Gary M Reedy, CEO
Otis W Brawley, MD, Chief Medical/Scientific Officer
Catherine Mickle, CFO

Nationwide, community-based voluntary health organization dedicated to eliminating cancer as a major health problem by preventing cancer, saving lives, and diminishing suffering from cancer through research, education, advocacy, and service.

Year Founded: 1913

4044 American Cancer Society: Palm Desert

73-161 Fred Waring Drive
Suite 100
Palm Desert, CA 92260
760-568-2691Toll free: 800-227-2345
www.cancer.org
TTY: 866-228-4327

Gary M Reedy, CEO
Otis W Brawley, MD, Chief Medical/Scientific Officer
Catherine Mickle, CFO

Nationwide, community-based voluntary health organization dedicated to eliminating cancer as a major health problem by preventing cancer, saving lives, and diminishing suffering from cancer through research, education, advocacy, and service.

Year Founded: 1913

4045 American Cancer Society: Panama City

4001 W 23rd Street
Suite C
Panama City, FL 32405
850-785-9205Toll free: 800-227-2345
www.cancer.org
TTY: 866-228-4327

Gary M Reedy, CEO
Otis W Brawley, MD, Chief Medical/Scientific Officer
Catherine Mickle, CFO

Nationwide, community-based voluntary health organization dedicated to eliminating cancer as a major health problem by preventing cancer, saving lives, and diminishing suffering from cancer through research, education, advocacy, and service.

Year Founded: 1913

4046 American Cancer Society: Pasadena
American Cancer Society

99 S Lake Avenue
Suite 400
Pasadena, CA 91101
626-795-7774Toll free: 800-227-2345
www.cancer.org
TTY: 866-228-4327

Gary M Reedy, CEO
Otis W Brawley, MD, Chief Medical/Scientific Officer
Catherine Mickle, CFO

Nationwide, community-based voluntary health organization dedicated to eliminating cancer as a major health problem by preventing cancer, saving lives, and diminishing suffering from cancer through research, education, advocacy, and service.

Year Founded: 1913

4047 American Cancer Society: Pensacola

5401 Corporate Woods Drive
Suite 100
Pensacola, FL 32504
850-475-0850Toll free: 800-227-2345
www.cancer.org
TTY: 866-228-4327

Gary M Reedy, CEO
Otis W Brawley, MD, Chief Medical/Scientific Officer
Catherine Mickle, CFO

Nationwide, community-based voluntary health organization dedicated to eliminating cancer as a major health problem by preventing cancer, saving lives, and diminishing suffering from cancer through research, education, advocacy, and service.

Year Founded: 1913

4048 American Cancer Society: Peoria
4234 N Knoxville Avenue
Suite B
Peoria, IL 61614
309-688-3488Toll free: 800-227-2345
www.cancer.org
TTY: 866-228-4327

Gary M Reedy, CEO
Otis W Brawley, MD, Chief Medical/Scientific Officer
Catherine Mickle, CFO

Nationwide, community-based voluntary health organization dedicated to eliminating cancer as a major health problem by preventing cancer, saving lives, and diminishing suffering from cancer through research, education, advocacy, and service.

Year Founded: 1913

4049 American Cancer Society: Perrysburg
American Cancer Society
740 Commerce Drive
Suite B
Perrysburg, OH 43551
Toll Free: 888-227-6446
www.cancer.org
TTY: 866-228-4327

Gary M Reedy, CEO
Otis W Brawley, MD, Chief Medical/Scientific Officer
Catherine Mickle, CFO

Nationwide, community-based voluntary health organization dedicated to eliminating cancer as a major health problem by preventing cancer, saving lives, and diminishing suffering from cancer through research, education, advocacy, and service.

Year Founded: 1913

4050 American Cancer Society: Philadelphia
American Cancer Society
1626 Locust Street
Philadelphia, PA 19103
215-985-5400Toll free: 800-227-2345
www.cancer.org
TTY: 866-228-4327

Gary M Reedy, CEO
Otis W Brawley, MD, Chief Medical/Scientific Officer
Catherine Mickle, CFO

Nationwide, community-based voluntary health organization dedicated to eliminating cancer as a major health problem by preventing cancer, saving lives, and diminishing suffering from cancer through research, education, advocacy, and service.

Year Founded: 1913

4051 American Cancer Society: Phoenix
4550 E Bell Road
Suite 126
Phoenix, AZ 85032
602-224-0524Toll free: 800-227-2345
www.cancer.org
TTY: 866-228-4327

Gary M Reedy, CEO
Otis W Brawley, MD, Chief Medical/Scientific Officer
Catherine Mickle, CFO

Nationwide, community-based voluntary health organization dedicated to eliminating cancer as a major health problem by preventing cancer, saving lives, and diminishing

suffering from cancer through research, education, advocacy, and service.

Year Founded: 1913

4052 American Cancer Society: Pittsburgh
320 Bilmar Drive
Pittsburgh, PA 15205
412-919-1100Toll free: 800-227-2345
www.cancer.org
TTY: 866-228-4327

Gary M Reedy, CEO
Otis W Brawley, MD, Chief Medical/Scientific Officer
Catherine Mickle, CFO

Nationwide, community-based voluntary health organization dedicated to eliminating cancer as a major health problem by preventing cancer, saving lives, and diminishing suffering from cancer through research, education, advocacy, and service.

Year Founded: 1913

4053 American Cancer Society: Portland
0330 SW Curry Street
Portland, OR 97239
503-295-6422Toll free: 800-227-2345
www.cancer.org
TTY: 866-228-4327

Gary M Reedy, CEO
Otis W Brawley, MD, Chief Medical/Scientific Officer
Catherine Mickle, CFO

Nationwide, community-based voluntary health organization dedicated to eliminating cancer as a major health problem by preventing cancer, saving lives, and diminishing suffering from cancer through research, education, advocacy, and service.

Year Founded: 1913

4054 American Cancer Society: Raleigh
8300 Health Park
Suite 10
Raleigh, NC 27615
919-334-5218Toll free: 800-227-2345
www.cancer.org
TTY: 866-228-4327

Gary M Reedy, CEO
Otis W Brawley, MD, Chief Medical/Scientific Officer
Catherine Mickle, CFO

Nationwide, community-based voluntary health organization dedicated to eliminating cancer as a major health problem by preventing cancer, saving lives, and diminishing suffering from cancer through research, education, advocacy, and service.

Year Founded: 1913

4055 American Cancer Society: Reno
691 Sierra Rose Drive
Suite A
Reno, NV 89511
775-329-0609Toll free: 800-227-2345
www.cancer.org
TTY: 866-228-4327

Gary M Reedy, CEO
Otis W Brawley, MD, Chief Medical/Scientific Officer
Catherine Mickle, CFO

Nationwide, community-based voluntary health organization dedicated to eliminating cancer as a major health problem by preventing cancer, saving lives, and diminishing suffering from cancer through research, education, advocacy, and service.

Year Founded: 1913

4056 American Cancer Society: Rhode Island
931 Jefferson Boulevard
Suite 3004
Warwick, RI 02886
401-243-2600Toll free: 800-227-2345
www.cancer.org
TTY: 866-228-4327

Gary M Reedy, CEO
Otis W Brawley, MD, Chief Medical/Scientific Officer
Catherine Mickle, CFO

Nationwide, community-based voluntary health organization dedicated to eliminating cancer as a major health problem by preventing cancer, saving lives, and diminishing suffering from cancer through research, education, advocacy, and service.

Year Founded: 1913

4057 American Cancer Society: Riverside
6355 Riverside Avenue
Riverside, CA 92506
951-683-6415Toll free: 800-227-2345
www.cancer.org
TTY: 866-228-4327

Gary M Reedy, CEO
Otis W Brawley, MD, Chief Medical/Scientific Officer
Catherine Mickle, CFO

Nationwide, community-based voluntary health organization dedicated to eliminating cancer as a major health problem by preventing cancer, saving lives, and diminishing suffering from cancer through research, education, advocacy, and service.

Year Founded: 1913

4058 American Cancer Society: Roanoke
2840 Electric Road
Suite 106A
Roanoke, VA 24018
540-774-2716Toll free: 800-227-2345
www.cancer.org
TTY: 866-228-4327

Gary M Reedy, CEO
Otis W Brawley, MD, Chief Medical/Scientific Officer
Catherine Mickle, CFO

Nationwide, community-based voluntary health organization dedicated to eliminating cancer as a major health problem by preventing cancer, saving lives, and diminishing suffering from cancer through research, education, advocacy, and service.

Year Founded: 1913

4059 American Cancer Society: Rochester
2900 43 Street NW
Suite 350
Rochester, MN 55901
507-287-2044Toll free: 800-227-2345
www.cancer.org
TTY: 866-228-4327

Gary M Reedy, CEO
Otis W Brawley, MD, Chief Medical/Scientific Officer
Catherine Mickle, CFO

Nationwide, community-based voluntary health organization dedicated to eliminating cancer as a major health problem by preventing cancer, saving lives, and diminishing suffering from cancer through research, education, advocacy, and service.

Year Founded: 1913

4060 American Cancer Society: Rocky Hill
American Cancer Society
825 Brook Street
1-91 Tech Court
Rocky Hill, CT 06067
203-379-4700Toll free: 800-227-2345
www.cancer.org
TTY: 866-228-4327

Gary M Reedy, CEO
Otis W Brawley, MD, Chief Medical/Scientific Officer
Catherine Mickle, CFO

Nationwide, community-based voluntary health organization dedicated to eliminating cancer as a major health problem by preventing cancer, saving lives, and diminishing suffering from cancer through research, education, advocacy, and service.

Year Founded: 1913

4061 American Cancer Society: Rogers
5434 Walsh Lane
Suite 100
Rogers, AR 72758
479-273-3906Toll free: 800-227-2345
www.cancer.org
TTY: 866-228-4327

Gary M Reedy, CEO
Otis W Brawley, MD, Chief Medical/Scientific Officer
Catherine Mickle, CFO

Nationwide, community-based voluntary health organization dedicated to eliminating cancer as a major health problem by preventing cancer, saving lives, and diminishing suffering from cancer through research, education, advocacy, and service.

Year Founded: 1913

4062 American Cancer Society: Sacramento
1545 River Park Drive
Suite 100
Sacramento, CA 95815
916-446-7933Toll free: 800-227-2345
www.cancer.org
TTY: 866-228-4327

Gary M Reedy, Chief Executive Officer
Otis W Brawley, MD, Chief Medical/Scientific Officer
Catherine Mickle, Chief Financial Officer

Nationwide, community-based voluntary health organization dedicated to eliminating cancer as a major health problem by preventing cancer, saving lives, and diminishing suffering from cancer through research, education, advocacy, and service.

Year Founded: 1913

4063 American Cancer Society: Saint Cloud
3721 23rd Street S
Suite 102
Saint Cloud, MN 56301
320-255-0220Toll free: 800-227-2345
www.cancer.org
TTY: 866-228-4327

Gary M Reedy, Chief Executive Officer
Otis W Brawley, Chief Medical/Scientific Officer
Catherine Mickle, Chief Financial Officer

Nationwide, community-based voluntary health organization dedicated to eliminating cancer as a major health problem by preventing cancer, saving lives, and diminishing suffering from cancer through research, education, advocacy, and service.

Year Founded: 1913

4064 American Cancer Society: Saint Louis
4207 Lindell Boulevard
Saint Louis, MO 63108
314-286-8100Toll free: 800-227-2345
www.cancer.org
TTY: 866-228-4327

Gary M Reedy, CEO
Otis W Brawley, MD, Chief Medical/Scientific Officer
Catherine Mickle, CFO

Nationwide, community-based voluntary health organization dedicated to eliminating cancer as a major health problem by preventing cancer, saving lives, and diminishing suffering from cancer through research, education, advocacy, and service.

Year Founded: 1913

4065 American Cancer Society: Salinas
945 S Main Street
Suite 201
Salinas, CA 93901
831-442-2992Toll free: 800-227-2345
www.cancer.org
TTY: 866-228-4327

Gary M Reedy, CEO
Otis W Brawley, MD, Chief Medical/Scientific Officer
Catherine Mickle, CFO

Nationwide, community-based voluntary health organization dedicated to eliminating cancer as a major health problem by preventing cancer, saving lives, and diminishing suffering from cancer through research, education, advocacy, and service.

Year Founded: 1913

4066 American Cancer Society: Salisbury
1315 Mt Hermon Road
Suite D
Salisbury, MD 21804
410-749-1624Toll free: 800-227-2345
www.cancer.org
TTY: 866-228-4327

Gary M Reedy, CEO
Otis W Brawley, MD, Chief Medical/Scientific Officer
Catherine Mickle, CFO

Nationwide, community-based voluntary health organization dedicated to eliminating cancer as a major health problem by preventing cancer, saving lives, and diminishing suffering from cancer through research, education, advocacy, and service.

Year Founded: 1913

4067 American Cancer Society: Salt Lake City
375 E 100 S
1st Floor
Salt Lake City, UT 84111
801-493-4700Toll free: 800-227-2345
www.cancer.org
TTY: 866-228-4327

Gary M Reedy, Chief Executive Officer
Otis W Brawley, MD, Chief Medical/Scientific Officer
Catherine Mickle, Chief Financial Officer

Nationwide, community-based voluntary health organization dedicated to eliminating cancer as a major health problem by preventing cancer, saving lives, and diminishing suffering from cancer through research, education, advocacy, and service.

Year Founded: 1913

4068 American Cancer Society: San Antonio
8115 Datapoint Drive
2nd Floor
San Antonio, TX 78229-3266
210-614-4211Toll free: 800-227-2345
www.cancer.org
TTY: 866-228-4327

Gary M Reedy, CEO
Otis W Brawley, MD, Chief Medical/Scientific Officer
Catherine Mickle, CFO

Nationwide, community-based voluntary health organization dedicated to eliminating cancer as a major health problem by preventing cancer, saving lives, and diminishing suffering from cancer through research, education, advocacy, and service.

Year Founded: 1913

4069 American Cancer Society: San Diego
5333 Mission Center Road
Suite 105
San Diego, CA 92108
619-299-4200Toll free: 800-227-2345
www.cancer.org
TTY: 866-228-4327

Gary M Reedy, CEO
Otis W Brawley, MD, Chief Medical/Scientific Officer
Catherine Mickle, CFO

Nationwide, community-based voluntary health organization dedicated to eliminating cancer as a major health problem by preventing cancer, saving lives, and diminishing suffering from cancer through research, education, advocacy, and service.

Year Founded: 1913

4070 American Cancer Society: Santa Barbara
1432 Chapala Street
Santa Barbara, CA 93101
805-963-1576Toll free: 800-227-2345
www.cancer.org
TTY: 866-228-4327

Gary M Reedy, CEO
Otis W Brawley, MD, Chief Medical/Scientific Officer
Catherine Mickle, CFO

Nationwide, community-based voluntary health organization dedicated to eliminating cancer as a major health problem by preventing cancer, saving lives, and diminishing

suffering from cancer through research, education, advocacy, and service.

Year Founded: 1913

4071 American Cancer Society: Santa Rosa

1451 Guerneville Road
Suite 220
Santa Rosa, CA 95403
707-545-6720Toll free: 800-227-2345
www.cancer.org
TTY: 866-228-4327

Gary M Reedy, CEO
Otis W Brawley, MD, Chief Medical/Scientific Officer
Catherine Mickle, CFO

Nationwide, community-based voluntary health organization dedicated to eliminating cancer as a major health problem by preventing cancer, saving lives, and diminishing suffering from cancer through research, education, advocacy, and service.

Year Founded: 1913

4072 American Cancer Society: Sarasota

2970 University Parkway
Suite 104
Sarasota, FL 34243
941-365-2858Toll free: 800-227-2345
www.cancer.org
TTY: 866-228-4327

Gary M Reedy, Chief Executive Officer
Otis W Brawley, MD, Chief Medical/Scientific Officer
Catherine Mickle, Chief Financial Officer

Nationwide, community-based voluntary health organization dedicated to eliminating cancer as a major health problem by preventing cancer, saving lives, and diminishing suffering from cancer through research, education, advocacy, and service.

Year Founded: 1913

4073 American Cancer Society: Savannah

4849 Paulsen Street
Suite 102
Savannah, GA 31405
912-355-5196Toll free: 800-227-2345
www.cancer.org
TTY: 866-228-4327

Gary M Reedy, CEO
Otis W Brawley, MD, Chief Medical/Scientific Officer
Catherine Mickle, CFO

Nationwide, community-based voluntary health organization dedicated to eliminating cancer as a major health problem by preventing cancer, saving lives, and diminishing suffering from cancer through research, education, advocacy, and service.

Year Founded: 1913

4074 American Cancer Society: Seattle

2120 First Avenue N
Seattle, WA 98109
206-283-1153Toll free: 800-227-2345
www.cancer.org
TTY: 866-228-4327

Gary M Reedy, CEO
Otis W Brawley, MD, Chief Medical/Scientific Officer
Catherine Mickle, CFO

Nationwide, community-based voluntary health organization dedicated to eliminating cancer as a major health problem by preventing cancer, saving lives, and diminishing suffering from cancer through research, education, advocacy, and service.

Year Founded: 1913

4075 American Cancer Society: Sioux Falls

4904 S Technopolis Drive
Sioux Falls, SD 57106-4230
605-361-8277Toll free: 800-227-2345
www.cancer.org
TTY: 866-228-4327

Gary M Reedy, CEO
Otis W Brawley, MD, Chief Medical/Scientific Officer
Catherine Mickle, CFO

Nationwide, community-based voluntary health organization dedicated to eliminating cancer as a major health problem by preventing cancer, saving lives, and diminishing suffering from cancer through research, education, advocacy, and service.

Year Founded: 1913

4076 American Cancer Society: Southfield

20450 Civic Center Drive
Southfield, MI 48076
248-663-3400Toll free: 800-227-2345
www.cancer.org
TTY: 866-228-4327

Gary M Reedy, CEO
Otis W Brawley, MD, Chief Medical/Scientific Officer
Catherine Mickle, CFO

Nationwide, community-based voluntary health organization dedicated to eliminating cancer as a major health problem by preventing cancer, saving lives, and diminishing suffering from cancer through research, education, advocacy, and service.

Year Founded: 1913

4077 American Cancer Society: Spokane

920 N Washington Street
Suite 200
Spokane, WA 99201
509-455-3440Toll free: 800-227-2345
www.cancer.org
TTY: 866-228-4327

Gary M Reedy, CEO
Otis W Brawley, MD, Chief Medical/Scientific Officer
Catherine Mickle, CFO

Nationwide, community-based voluntary health organization dedicated to eliminating cancer as a major health problem by preventing cancer, saving lives, and diminishing suffering from cancer through research, education, advocacy, and service.

Year Founded: 1913

4078 American Cancer Society: Springfield

675 E Linton Avenue
Springfield, IL 62703-5902
217-523-4503Toll free: 800-227-2345
www.cancer.org
TTY: 866-228-4327

Gary M Reedy, CEO
Otis W Brawley, MD, Chief Medical/Scientific Officer
Catherine Mickle, CFO

Nationwide, community-based voluntary health organization dedicated to eliminating cancer as a major health problem by preventing cancer, saving lives, and diminishing suffering from cancer through research, education, advocacy, and service.

Year Founded: 1913

4079 American Cancer Society: State College
1375 Martin Street
Suite 206
State College, PA 16803
814-234-1023Toll free: 800-227-2345
www.cancer.org
TTY: 866-228-4327

Gary M Reedy, CEO
Otis W Brawley, MD, Chief Medical/Scientific Officer
Catherine Mickle, CFO

Nationwide, community-based voluntary health organization dedicated to eliminating cancer as a major health problem by preventing cancer, saving lives, and diminishing suffering from cancer through research, education, advocacy, and service.

Year Founded: 1913

4080 American Cancer Society: Staten Island
1200 South Avenue
Suite 305
Staten Island, NY 10314
718-987-8871Toll free: 800-227-2345
www.cancer.org
TTY: 866-228-4327

Gary M Reedy, CEO
Otis W Brawley, MD, Chief Medical/Scientific Officer
Catherine Mickle, CFO

Nationwide, community-based voluntary health organization dedicated to eliminating cancer as a major health problem by preventing cancer, saving lives, and diminishing suffering from cancer through research, education, advocacy, and service.

Year Founded: 1913

4081 American Cancer Society: Statesboro
201 S Main Street
Suite A
Statesboro, GA 30458
912-764-7410Toll free: 800-227-2345
www.cancer.org
TTY: 866-228-4327

Gary M Reedy, CEO
Otis W Brawley, MD, Chief Medical/Scientific Officer
Catherine Mickle, CFO

Nationwide, community-based voluntary health organization dedicated to eliminating cancer as a major health problem by preventing cancer, saving lives, and diminishing suffering from cancer through research, education, advocacy, and service.

Year Founded: 1913

4082 American Cancer Society: Stockton
207 E Alpine Avenue
Stockton, CA 95204
209-941-2676Toll free: 800-227-2345
www.cancer.org
TTY: 866-228-4327

Gary M Reedy, CEO
Otis W Brawley, MD, Chief Medical/Scientific Officer
Catherine Mickle, CFO

Nationwide, community-based voluntary health organization dedicated to eliminating cancer as a major health problem by preventing cancer, saving lives, and diminishing suffering from cancer through research, education, advocacy, and service.

Year Founded: 1913

4083 American Cancer Society: Stroudsburg
American Cancer Society
2158 W Main Street
Stroudsburg, PA 18360
570-420-1685Toll free: 800-227-2345
www.cancer.org
TTY: 866-228-4327

Gary M Reedy, CEO
Otis W Brawley, MD, Chief Medical/Scientific Officer
Catherine Mickle, CFO

Nationwide, community-based voluntary health organization dedicated to eliminating cancer as a major health problem by preventing cancer, saving lives, and diminishing suffering from cancer through research, education, advocacy, and service.

Year Founded: 1913

4084 American Cancer Society: Suffolk Region
75 Davids Drive
Hauppauge, NY 11788
631-436-7070Toll free: 800-227-2345
www.cancer.org
TTY: 866-228-4327

Gary M Reedy, CEO
Otis W Brawley, MD, Chief Medical/Scientific Officer
Catherine Mickle, CFO

Nationwide, community-based voluntary health organization dedicated to eliminating cancer as a major health problem by preventing cancer, saving lives, and diminishing suffering from cancer through research, education, advocacy, and service.

Year Founded: 1913

4085 American Cancer Society: Suisun City
American Cancer Society
700 Main Street
Suite 102
Suisun City, CA 94585
707-425-5006Toll free: 800-227-2345
www.cancer.org
TTY: 866-228-4327

Gary M Reedy, CEO
Otis W Brawley, MD, Chief Medical/Scientific Officer
Catherine Mickle, CFO

Nationwide, community-based voluntary health organization dedicated to eliminating cancer as a major health problem by preventing cancer, saving lives, and diminishing suffering from cancer through research, education, advocacy, and service.

Year Founded: 1913

4086 American Cancer Society: Tacoma
1313 Broadway
Suite 100
Tacoma, WA 98402

253-272-5767Toll free: 800-227-2345
www.cancer.org
TTY: 866-228-4327

Gary M Reedy, CEO
Otis W Brawley, MD, Chief Medical/Scientific Officer
Catherine Mickle, CFO

Nationwide, community-based voluntary health organization dedicated to eliminating cancer as a major health problem by preventing cancer, saving lives, and diminishing suffering from cancer through research, education, advocacy, and service.

Year Founded: 1913

4087 American Cancer Society: Tallahassee

2619 Centennial Boulevard
Suite 101
Tallahassee, FL 32308
850-297-0588Toll free: 800-227-2345
www.cancer.org
TTY: 866-228-4327

Gary M Reedy, CEO
Otis W Brawley, MD, Chief Medical/Scientific Officer
Catherine Mickle, CFO

Nationwide, community-based voluntary health organization dedicated to eliminating cancer as a major health problem by preventing cancer, saving lives, and diminishing suffering from cancer through research, education, advocacy, and service.

Year Founded: 1913

4088 American Cancer Society: Taylor
American Cancer Society

712 S Keyser Avenue
Taylor, PA 18517
570-562-9749Toll free: 800-227-2345
www.cancer.org
TTY: 866-228-4327

Gary M Reedy, CEO
Otis W Brawley, MD, Chief Medical/Scientific Officer
Cathrine Mickle, CFO

Nationwide, community-based voluntary health organization dedicated to eliminating cancer as a major health problem by preventing cancer, saving lives, and diminishing suffering from cancer through research, education, advocacy, and service.

Year Founded: 1913

4089 American Cancer Society: Tinley Park

17060 Oak Park Avenue
Tinley Park, IL 60477
708-633-7770Toll free: 800-227-2345
www.cancer.org
TTY: 866-228-4327

Gary M Reedy, CEO
Otis W Brawley, MD, Chief Medical/Scientific Officer
Catherine Mickle, CFO

Nationwide, community-based voluntary health organization dedicated to eliminating cancer as a major health problem by preventing cancer, saving lives, and diminishing suffering from cancer through research, education, advocacy, and service.

Year Founded: 1913

4090 American Cancer Society: Topeka

1315 SW Arrowhead Road
Topeka, KS 66604-4020
785-273-4422Toll free: 800-227-2345
www.cancer.org
TTY: 866-228-4327

Gary M Reedy, CEO
Otis W Brawley, MD, Chief Medical/Scientific Officer
Catherine Mickle, CFO

Nationwide, community-based voluntary health organization dedicated to eliminating cancer as a major health problem by preventing cancer, saving lives, and diminishing suffering from cancer through research, education, advocacy, and service.

Year Founded: 1913

4091 American Cancer Society: Topsham

1 Bowdoin Mill Island
Suite 300
Topsham, ME 04086-1240
207-373-3700Toll free: 800-227-2345
www.cancer.org
TTY: 866-228-4327

Gary M Reedy, CEO
Otis W Brawley, MD, Chief Medical/Scientific Officer
Catherine Mickle, CFO

Nationwide, community-based voluntary health organization dedicated to eliminating cancer as a major health problem by preventing cancer, saving lives, and diminishing suffering from cancer through research, education, advocacy, and service.

Year Founded: 1913

4092 American Cancer Society: Tucson
American Cancer Society

2015 W River Road
Tucson, AZ 85704
520-222-8607Toll free: 800-227-2345
www.cancer.org
TTY: 866-228-4327

Gary M Reedy, CEO
Otis W Brawley, MD, Chief Medical/Scientific Officer
Catherine Mickle, CFO

Nationwide, community-based voluntary health organization dedicated to eliminating cancer as a major health problem by preventing cancer, saving lives, and diminishing suffering from cancer through research, education, advocacy, and service.

Year Founded: 1913

4093 American Cancer Society: Tulsa

4110 S 100th E Ave, Grant Building
Suite 101
Tulsa, OK 74146
918-743-6767Toll free: 800-227-2345
www.cancer.org
TTY: 866-228-4327

Gary M Reedy, CEO
Otis W Brawley, MD, Chief Medical/Scientific Officer
Catherine Mickle, CFO

Nationwide, community-based voluntary health organization dedicated to eliminating cancer as a major health problem by preventing cancer, saving lives, and diminishing suffering from cancer through research, education, advocacy, and service.

Year Founded: 1913

4094 American Cancer Society: Tuscon

2015 W River Road
Tucson, AZ 85704
520-222-8607Toll free: 800-227-2345
www.cancer.org
TTY: 866-228-4327

Gary M Reedy, CEO
Otis W Brawley, MD, Chief Medical/Scientific Officer
Catherine Mickle, CFO

Nationwide, community-based voluntary health organization dedicated to eliminating cancer as a major health problem by preventing cancer, saving lives, and diminishing suffering from cancer through research, education, advocacy, and service.

Year Founded: 1913

4095 American Cancer Society: Tyler

American Cancer Society
1301 S Broadway
Tyler, TX 75701
903-597-1348Toll free: 800-227-2345
www.cancer.org
TTY: 866-228-4327

Gary M Reedy, CEO
Otis W Brawley, MD, Chief Medical/Scientific Officer
Catherine Mickle, CFO

Nationwide, community-based voluntary health organization dedicated to eliminating cancer as a major health problem by preventing cancer, saving lives, and diminishing suffering from cancer through research, education, advocacy, and service.

Year Founded: 1913

4096 American Cancer Society: Utica

American Cancer Society
110 Lomond Court
Utica, NY 13502
315-724-8125Toll free: 800-227-2345
www.cancer.org
TTY: 866-228-4327

Gary M Reedy, CEO
Otis W Brawley, MD, Chief Medical/Scientific Officer
Catherine Mickle, CFO

Nationwide, community-based voluntary health organization dedicated to eliminating cancer as a major health problem by preventing cancer, saving lives, and diminishing suffering from cancer through research, education, advocacy, and service.

Year Founded: 1913

4097 American Cancer Society: Valencia

25020 W Avenue
Stanford Unit 170
Valencia, CA 91355
661-298-0886Toll free: 800-227-2345
www.cancer.org
TTY: 866-228-4327

Gary M Reedy, CEO
Otis W Brawley, MD, Chief Medical/Scientific Officer
Catherine Mickle, CFO

Nationwide, community-based voluntary health organization dedicated to eliminating cancer as a major health problem by preventing cancer, saving lives, and diminishing

suffering from cancer through research, education, advocacy, and service.

Year Founded: 1913

4098 American Cancer Society: Vermont

55 Day Lane
Williston, VT 05495-4420
802-872-6300Toll free: 800-227-2345
www.cancer.org
TTY: 866-228-4327

Gary M Reedy, CEO
Otis W Brawley, MD, Chief Medical/Scientific Officer
Catherine Mickle, CFO

Nationwide, community-based voluntary health organization dedicated to eliminating cancer as a major health problem by preventing cancer, saving lives, and diminishing suffering from cancer through research, education, advocacy, and service.

Year Founded: 1913

4099 American Cancer Society: Vero Beach

3375 20th Street
Suite 100
Vero Beach, FL 32960
772-562-2272Toll free: 800-227-2345
www.cancer.org
TTY: 866-228-4327

Gary M Reedy, CEO
Otis W Brawley, MD, Chief Medical/Scientific Officer
Catherine Mickle, CFO

Nationwide, community-based voluntary health organization dedicated to eliminating cancer as a major health problem by preventing cancer, saving lives, and diminishing suffering from cancer through research, education, advocacy, and service.

Year Founded: 1913

4100 American Cancer Society: Vienna

American Cancer Society
124 Park Street SE
Suite 100
Vienna, VA 22180-0699
703-938-5550Toll free: 800-227-2345
www.cancer.org
TTY: 866-228-4327

Gary M Reedy, CEO
Otis W Brawley, MD, Chief Medical/Scientific Officer
Catherine Mickle, CFO

Nationwide, community-based voluntary health organization dedicated to eliminating cancer as a major health problem by preventing cancer, saving lives, and diminishing suffering from cancer through research, education, advocacy, and service.

Year Founded: 1913

4101 American Cancer Society: Villages

American Cancer Society
Highway 441, Building 200
Suite 205
Lady Lake, FL 32159
352-350-2273Toll free: 800-227-2345
www.cancer.org
TTY: 866-228-4327

Gary M Reedy, CEO
Otis W Brawley, MD, Chief Medical/Scientific Officer
Catherine Mickle, CFO

Nationwide, community-based voluntary health organization dedicated to eliminating cancer as a major health problem by preventing cancer, saving lives, and diminishing suffering from cancer through research, education, advocacy, and service.

Year Founded: 1913

4102 American Cancer Society: Virginia Beach

4416 Expressway Drive
Virginia Beach, VA 23452
757-493-7940 Toll free: 800-227-2345
www.cancer.org
TTY: 866-228-4327

Gary M Reedy, CEO
Otis W Brawley, MD, Chief Medical/Scientific Officer
Catherine Mickle, CFO

Nationwide, community-based voluntary health organization dedicated to eliminating cancer as a major health problem by preventing cancer, saving lives, and diminishing suffering from cancer through research, education, advocacy, and service.

Year Founded: 1913

4103 American Cancer Society: Waco

1700 Lake Success Drive
Waco, TX 76710
254-753-0806 Toll free: 800-227-2345
www.cancer.org
TTY: 866-228-4327

Gary M Reedy, CEO
Otis W Brawley, MD, Chief Medical/Scientific Officer
Catherine Mickle, CFO

Nationwide, community-based voluntary health organization dedicated to eliminating cancer as a major health problem by preventing cancer, saving lives, and diminishing suffering from cancer through research, education, advocacy, and service.

Year Founded: 1913

4104 American Cancer Society: Wailuku

95 Mahalani Street
Cameron Center, Suite 27
Wailuku, HI 96793
808-244-5553 Toll free: 800-227-2345
www.cancer.org
TTY: 866-228-4327

Gary M Reedy, CEO
Otis W Brawley, MD, Chief Medical/Scientific Officer
Catherine Mickle, CFO

Nationwide, community-based voluntary health organization dedicated to eliminating cancer as a major health problem by preventing cancer, saving lives, and diminishing suffering from cancer through research, education, advocacy, and service.

Year Founded: 1913

4105 American Cancer Society: Walnut Creek

2185 N California Boulevard
Suite 290
Walnut Creek, CA 94596

925-934-7640 Toll free: 800-227-2345
www.cancer.org
TTY: 866-228-4327

Gary M Reedy, CEO
Otis W Brawley, MD, Chief Medical/Scientific Officer
Catherine Mickle, CFO

Nationwide, community-based voluntary health organization dedicated to eliminating cancer as a major health problem by preventing cancer, saving lives, and diminishing suffering from cancer through research, education, advocacy, and service.

Year Founded: 1913

4106 American Cancer Society: Waukesha

N19 W24350 Riverwood Drive
Waukesha, WI 53188
262-523-5500 Toll free: 800-227-2345
www.cancer.org
TTY: 866-228-4327

Gary M Reedy, CEO
Otis W Brawley, MD, Chief Medical/Scientific Officer
Catherine Mickle, CFO

Nationwide, community-based voluntary health organization dedicated to eliminating cancer as a major health problem by preventing cancer, saving lives, and diminishing suffering from cancer through research, education, advocacy, and service.

Year Founded: 1913

4107 American Cancer Society: West Palm Beach

621 Clearwater Park Road
West Palm Beach, FL 33401
561-366-0013 Toll free: 800-227-2345
www.cancer.org
TTY: 866-228-4327

Gary M Reedy, CEO
Otis W Brawley, MD, Chief Medical/Scientific Officer
Catherine Mickle, CFO

Nationwide, community-based voluntary health organization dedicated to eliminating cancer as a major health problem by preventing cancer, saving lives, and diminishing suffering from cancer through research, education, advocacy, and service.

Year Founded: 1913

4108 American Cancer Society: White Pines

2 Lyon Place
White Plains, NY 10601
914-949-4800 Toll free: 800-227-2345
www.cancer.org
TTY: 866-228-4327

Gary M Reedy, CEO
Otis W Brawley, MD, Chief Medical/Scientific Officer
Catherine Mickle, CFO

Nationwide, community-based voluntary health organization dedicated to eliminating cancer as a major health problem by preventing cancer, saving lives, and diminishing suffering from cancer through research, education, advocacy, and service.

Year Founded: 1913

4109 American Cancer Society: Wichita
330 South Main
Suite 100
Wichita, KS 67202
316-265-3400 Toll free: 800-227-2345
www.cancer.org
TTY: 866-228-4327

Gary M Reedy, CEO
Otis W Brawley, ME, Chief Medical/Scientific Officer
Catherine Mickle, CFO

Nationwide, community-based voluntary health organization dedicated to eliminating cancer as a major health problem by preventing cancer, saving lives, and diminishing suffering from cancer through research, education, advocacy, and service.

Year Founded: 1913

4110 American Cancer Society: Williamsport
American Cancer Society
1948 E 3rd Street
Williamsport, PA 17701
570-326-4149 Toll free: 800-227-2345
www.cancer.org
TTY: 866-228-4327

Gary M Reedy, CEO
Otis W Brawley, MD, Chief Medical/Scientific Officer
Catherine Mickle, CFO

Nationwide, community-based voluntary health organization dedicated to eliminating cancer as a major health problem by preventing cancer, saving lives, and diminishing suffering from cancer through research, education, advocacy, and service.

Year Founded: 1913

4111 American Cancer Society: Wilmington
American Cancer Society
2202 Wrightsville Avenue
Suite 111
Wilmington, NC 28403
910-254-4870 Toll free: 800-227-2345
www.cancer.org
TTY: 866-228-4327

Gary M Reedy, CEO
Otis W Brawley, MD, Chief Medical/Scienific Officer
Catherine Mickle, CFO

Nationwide, community-based voluntary health organization dedicated to eliminating cancer as a major health problem by preventing cancer, saving lives, and diminishing suffering from cancer through research, education, advocacy, and service.

Year Founded: 1913

4112 American Cancer Society: Winter Park
American Cancer Society
507 N New York Avenue
Suite 100
Winter Park, FL 32789
407-843-8680 Toll free: 800-228-2345
www.cancer.org
TTY: 866-228-4327

Gary M Reedy, CEO
Otis W Brawley, MD, Chief Medical/Scientific Officer
Catherine Mickle, CFO

Nationwide, community-based voluntary health organization dedicated to eliminating cancer as a major health problem by preventing cancer, saving lives, and diminishing suffering from cancer through research, education, advocacy, and service.

Year Founded: 1913

4113 American Cancer Society: Wyoming
333 S Beech Street
Casper, WY 82601
307-577-4892 Toll free: 800-227-2345
www.cancer.org
TTY: 866-228-4327

Gary M Reedy, Chief Executive Officer
Otis W Brawley, MD, Chief Medical/Scientific Officer
Catherine Mickle, Chief Financial Officer

Nationwide, community-based voluntary health organization dedicated to eliminating cancer as a major health problem by preventing cancer, saving lives, and diminishing suffering from cancer through research, education, advocacy, and service.

Year Founded: 1913

4114 American Lung Association
55 W Wacker Drive
Suite 1150
Chicago, IL 60601
Toll Free: 800-548-8252
info@lung.org
www.lung.org

Harold P. Wimmer, President & CEO

Working to save lives by improving lung health and preventing lung disease.

4115 American Lung Association: Alabama
1678 Montgomery Highway
Suite 104-355
Birmingham, AL 35216
205-258-5367
alaal@lungse.org
www.lung.org

Working to save lives by improving lung health and preventing lung disease.

4116 American Lung Association: Alaska
1075 S Check Street
Suite 205
Wasilla, AK 99654
907-357-3110
kt.mckee@lung.org
www.lung.org

Working to save lives by improving lung health and preventing lung disease.

4117 American Lung Association: Arizona
2819 E Broadway Boulevard
Tucson, AZ 85716
520-323-1812
azinfo@lungs.org
www.lung.org

Working to save lives by improving lung health and preventing lung disease.

4118 American Lung Association: Arkansas
14524 Cantrell Road
Suite 140, Box 214
Little Rock, AR 72223
e-mail: alaar@lungse.org
www.lung.org

Working to save lives by improving lung health and preventing lung disease.

4119 American Lung Association: California
2020 Camino Del Rio North
Suite 200
San Diego, CA 92108
619-297-3901
ellen.sherwood@lung.org
www.lung.org

Working to save lives by improving lung health and preventing lung disease.

4120 American Lung Association: Colorado
5600 Greenwood Plaza Boulevard
Suite 100
Greenwood Village, CO 80111
303-388-4327
coinfo@lungs.org
www.lung.org

Working to save lives by improving lung health and preventing lung disease.

4121 American Lung Association: Connecticut
45 Ash Street
East Hartford, CT 06108
860-289-5401
info@lungne.org
www.lung.org

Working to save lives by improving lung health and preventing lung disease.

4122 American Lung Association: Delaware
630 Churchmans Road
Suite 202
Newark, DE 19702
302-737-6414
llyons@lunginfo.org
www.lung.org

Working to save lives by improving lung health and preventing lung disease.

4123 American Lung Association: District of Columbia
1301 Pennsylvania Avenue NW
Washington, DC 20004
202-747-5541
lungdc@lunginfo.org
www.lung.org

Working to save lives by improving lung health and preventing lung disease.

4124 American Lung Association: Florida
2701 N Australian Avenue
Suite 100
West Palm Beach, FL 33407
561-659-7644
alafse@lungse.org
www.lung.org

Working to save lives by improving lung health and preventing lung disease.

4125 American Lung Association: Georgia
2452 Spring Road
Smyrna, GA 30080
770-434-5864
alaga@lungse.org
www.lung.org

Working to save lives by improving lung health and preventing lung disease.

4126 American Lung Association: Hawaii
810 Richards Street
Suite 750
Honolulu, HI 96813
808-537-5966
kim.nguyen@lung.org
www.lung.org

Working to save lives by improving lung health and preventing lung disease.

4127 American Lung Association: Idaho
1412 W Idaho Street
Suite 100
Boise, ID 83702
208-345-5864
heather.kimmel@lung.org
www.lung.org

Working to save lives by improving lung health and preventing lung disease.

4128 American Lung Association: Illinois
3000 Kelly Lane
Springfield, IL 62711
217-787-5864
info@lungil.org

Working to save lives by improving lung health and preventing lung disease.

4129 American Lung Association: Indiana
115 West Washington Street
Suite 1180-South
Indianapolis, IN 46204
317-819-1181
info@lungin.org
www.lung.org

Working to save lives by improving lung health and preventing lung disease.

4130 American Lung Association: Iowa
2530 73rd Street
Des Moines, IA 50322
515-309-9507
info@lungia.org
www.lung.org

Working to save lives by improving lung health and preventing lung disease.

4131 American Lung Association: Kansas
8400 W 110th Street
Suite 130
Overland Park, KS 66210
913-353-9165
info@lungks.org
www.lung.org

Working to save lives by improving lung health and preventing lung disease.

4132 American Lung Association: Kentucky
4100 Churchman Avenue
Louisville, KY 40215
502-363-2652
barry.gottschalk@lung.org
www.lung.org

Working to save lives by improving lung health and preventing lung disease.

4133 American Lung Association: Louisiana
2325 Severn Avenue
Suite 8
Metairie, LA 70001
504-828-5864
alala@lungse.org
www.lung.org

Working to save lives by improving lung health and preventing lung disease.

4134 American Lung Association: Maine
122 State Street
Augusta, ME 04330
207-622-6394
info@lungne.org
www.lung.org

Working to save lives by improving lung health and preventing lung disease.

4135 American Lung Association: Maryland
211 E Lombard Street
Suite 260
Baltimore, MD 21202
202-747-5541
lungmd@lunginfo.org
www.lung.org

Working to save lives by improving lung health and preventing lung disease.

4136 American Lung Association: Massachusetts
393 Maple Street
Springfield, MA 01105
413-737-3506
info@lungne.org
www.lung.org

Working to save lives by improving lung health and preventing lung disease.

4137 American Lung Association: Michigan
1475 E 12 Mile Road
Madison Heights, MI 48071
248-784-2000
midland@lung.org
www.lung.org

Working to save lives by improving lung health and preventing lung disease.

4138 American Lung Association: Minnesota
490 Concordia Avenue
St. Paul, MN 55103
651-227-8014
info@lungmn.org
www.lung.org

Working to save lives by improving lung health and preventing lung disease.

4139 American Lung Association: Mississippi
1599 Bienville Boulevard
Suite D
Ocean Springs, MS 39564
678-478-0314
alams@lungse.org
www.lung.org

Working to save lives by improving lung health and preventing lung disease.

4140 American Lung Association: Missouri
7745 Carondelet Avenue
Suite 305
Clayton, MO 63105
314-627-5505
missouri@lung.org
www.lung.org

Working to save lives by improving lung health and preventing lung disease.

4141 American Lung Association: Montana
c/o American Lung Association
822 John Street
Seattle, WA 98109
206-441-5100
infomtp@lung.org
www.lung.org

Working to save lives by improving lung health and preventing lung disease.

4142 American Lung Association: Nebraska
8990 West Dodge
Suite 226
Omaha, NE 68114
402-502-4950
info@lungnb.org
www.lung.org

Working to save lives by improving lung health and preventing lung disease.

4143 American Lung Association: Nevada
10615 Double R Boulevard
Reno, NV 89521
775-829-5864
nvinfo@lungs.org
www.lung.org

Working to save lives by improving lung health and preventing lung disease.

4144 American Lung Association: New Hampshire
51 Islington Street
Cloudport Unit 1
Portsmouth, NH 03801
603-369-3977
info@lungne.org
www.lung.org

Working to save lives by improving lung health and preventing lung disease.

4145 American Lung Association: New Jersey
PO Box 10188
Newark, NJ 07101

908-685-8040
jgrinwald@lunginfo.org
www.lung.org

Working to save lives by improving lung health and preventing lung disease.

4146 American Lung Association: New Mexico
5911 Jefferson Street NE
Albuquerque, NM 87109
Toll Free: 800-586-4872
nminfo@lungs.org
www.lung.org

Working to save lives by improving lung health and preventing lung disease.

4147 American Lung Association: New York
237 Mamaroneck Avenue
Suite 205
White Plains, NY 10605
914-347-2094
info@lungne.org
www.lung.org

Working to save lives by improving lung health and preventing lung disease.

4148 American Lung Association: North Carolina
514 Daniels Street
Suite 109
Raleigh, NC 27605
919-792-1641
alanc-r@lungse.org
www.lung.org

Working to save lives by improving lung health and preventing lung disease.

4149 American Lung Association: North Dakota
212 N Second Street
Bismarck, ND 58501
701-223-5613
info@lungnd.org
www.lung.org

Working to save lives by improving lung health and preventing lung disease.

4150 American Lung Association: Ohio
PO Box 415
Sandusky, OH 44871
419-663-5864
pat.volz@lung.org
www.lung.org

Working to save lives by improving lung health and preventing lung disease.

4151 American Lung Association: Oklahoma
730 W Wilshire Boulevard
Suite 105
Oklahoma City, OK 73116
405-748-4674
okinfo@lungs.org
www.lung.org

Working to save lives by improving lung health and preventing lung disease.

4152 American Lung Association: Oregon
16037 SW Upper Boones Ferry Road
Suite 165
Tigard, OR 97224
503-924-4094
infomtp@lung.org
www.lung.org

Working to save lives by improving lung health and preventing lung disease.

4153 American Lung Association: Pennsylvania
Marywood University
2300 Adams Avenue
Scranton, PA 18509
570-346-1784
adelonti@lunginfo.org
www.lung.org

Working to save lives by improving lung health and preventing lung disease.

4154 American Lung Association: Rhode Island
260 West Exchange Street
Suite 102 B
Providence, RI 02903
401-421-6487
info@lungne.org
www.lung.org

Working to save lives by improving lung health and preventing lung disease.

4155 American Lung Association: South Carolina
2030 North Church Place
Spartanburg, SC 29303
864-764-1777
upstate@lungse.org
www.lung.org

Working to save lives by improving lung health and preventing lung disease.

4156 American Lung Association: South Dakota
490 Concordia Avenue
St. Paul, MN 55103
651-227-8014
info@lungsd.org
www.lung.org

Working to save lives by improving lung health and preventing lung disease.

4157 American Lung Association: Tennessee
One Vantage Way
Suite C120
Nashville, TN 37228
615-329-1151
gail.bost@lung.org
www.lung.org

Working to save lives by improving lung health and preventing lung disease.

4158 American Lung Association: Texas
8207 Callaghan Road
Suite 140
San Antonio, TX 78230
210-308-8978
txinfo@lungs.org
www.lung.org

Working to save lives by improving lung health and preventing lung disease.

4159 American Lung Association: Utah

3920 South 1100 East
Suite 240
Salt Lake City, UT 84124
801-484-4456
utinfo@lungs.org
www.lung.org

Working to save lives by improving lung health and preventing lung disease.

4160 American Lung Association: Vermont

372 Hurricane Lane
Suite 101
Williston, VT 05495
802-876-6500
info@lungne.org
www.lung.org

Working to save lives by improving lung health and preventing lung disease.

4161 American Lung Association: Virginia

9702 Gayton Road
Suite 110
Richmond, VA 23238
804-302-5740
lungva@lunginfo.org
www.lung.org

Working to save lives by improving lung health and preventing lung disease.

4162 American Lung Association: Washington

822 John Street
Seattle, WA 98109
206-441-5100
infomtp@lung.org
www.lung.org

Working to save lives by improving lung health and preventing lung disease.

4163 American Lung Association: West Virginia

2102 Kanawha Boulevard E
Charleston, WV 25311
304-342-6600
cfields@lunginfo.org
www.lung.org

Working to save lives by improving lung health and preventing lung disease.

4164 American Lung Association: Wisconsin

13100 W Lisbon Road
Suite 700
Brookfield, WI 53005
262-703-4200
info@lungwi.org
www.lung.org

Working to save lives by improving lung health and preventing lung disease.

4165 American Lung Association: Wyoming

c/o American Lung Association
822 John Street
Seattle, WA 98109

206-441-5100
infomtp@lung.org
www.lung.org

Working to save lives by improving lung health and preventing lung disease.

4166 American Thoracic Society

25 Broadway
New York, NY 10004
212-315-8600
Fax: 212-315-6498
atsinfo@thoracic.org
www.thoracic.org

Atul Malhotra, President

To improve health worldwide by advancing research, clinical care, and public health in respiratory disease, critical illness, and sleep disorders.

Year Founded: 1905

4167 Aptium Oncology

4607 Lakeview Canyon Road
Suite 260
Westlake Village, CA 91361
818-851-9455
wscruggs@aptiumoncology.com
www.aptiumoncology.com

Wesley L Scruggs, Chief Information Officer
Suzanne Bledsoe, Vice President
Nicole C Valdez, IT Manager

Provider of diagnostic and therapeutic services to patients with catastrophic illnesses requiring sophisticated long-term care, principally in the areas of cancer, kidney disease, organ transplantation and immunodeficiency diseases.

4168 Association for the Cure of Cancer of the Prostate
Prostrate Cancer Foundation

1250 4th Street
Santa Monica, CA 90401
310-570-4700
Fax: 310-570-4701; *Toll Free:* 800-757-2873
info@pcf.org
www.pcf.org

Mike Milken, Founder and Chairman
Jonathan W Simons, MD, President and CEO
Ralph Finerman, Chief Financial Officer

The Prostate Cancer Foundation is dedicated to ending death and suffering from prostate cancer through research.

Year Founded: 1993

4169 Association of Community Cancer Centers

11600 Nebel Street
Suite 201
Rockville, MD 20852
301-984-9496
Fax: 301-770-1949
accc-cancer.org

Christian G. Downs, Executive Director

Institutions (517), individuals (300), and 14 state oncology societies involved in the provision of community cancer care. Fosters communication among providers of community cancer care; seeks to improve the quality of care available to cancer patients in community settings; encourages clinical research utilizing the community as a setting.

Year Founded: 1974

4170 CanHelp
P.O. Box 1678
Livingston, NJ 07039
Fax: 888-800-0201; *Toll Free:* 800-364-2341
joan@canhelp.com
www.canhelp.com

Joan Runfola, Director & Owner

Offers reports for cancer patients on orthodox and alternative therapies.

Year Founded: 1983

4171 Cancer Care
Public Information Associates
275 Seventh Avenue
22nd Floor
New York, NY 10001
212-712-8400
Fax: 212-712-8495; *Toll Free:* 800-813-4673
info@cancercare.org
www.cancercare.org

Patricia J Goldsmith, CEO
Brian Tomlinson, Chief Program/Comm. Officer
John Rutigliano, COO

Voluntary social service agency that functions as the service arm of the National Cancer Care Foundation. Provides professional social work counseling and guidance to help patients and families cope with the emotional, psychological, and financial consequences of cancer. In conjunction with professional counseling and where appropriate to the individual casework plan, supplementary financial aid may be given to self-supporting families to share the cost of home care services such as nursing care, home health aides, housekeepers, child care, and transportation.

Year Founded: 1944; Number of Members: 100

4172 Cancer Caring Center
4117 Liberty Avenue (Bloomfield)
Pittsburgh, PA 15224
412-622-1212
Fax: 412-622-1216
info@cancercaring.org
cancercaring.org

Rebecca Whitlinger, Executive Director
Stephanie Samolovitch, Director of Support Services
Wendy A. Myers, Support Care Coordinator

Provides a wide variety of support services to cancer patients, their families and friends, including support groups, education classes, personal counseling, telephone helpline.

Year Founded: 1988

4173 Cancer Control Society and Cancer Book House
2043 N Berendo Street
Los Angeles, CA 90027
323-663-7801
Fax: 323-663-7757
www.cancercontrolsociety.com

Lorraine Rosenthal, Co-Founder
Frank Cousineau, President
Charles Wintner, Vice President

An informational organization offering books, films, videos, clinic tours and lists of patients with cancer.

Year Founded: 1973

4174 Cancer Federation
711 W Ramsey Street
P.O. Box 1298
Banning, CA 92220
951-849-4325
Fax: 951-849-0156; *Toll Free:* 866-804-4325
info@cancerfed.org
www.cancerfed.org

Jules Vautrot, EdD, President
Ralph Carlton, Treasurer

Offers a quarterly magazine, holds free meetings, counsels cancer patients and their families, maintains a lending library of materials on cancer and more.

Year Founded: 1977

4175 Cancer Prevention Institute of California
2201 Walnut Avenue
Suite 300
Fremont, CA 94538
510-608-5000
Fax: 510-608-5095; *Toll Free:* 888-315-5988
education@cpic.org
www.cpic.org

Donna Randall, CEO

Year Founded: 1971

4176 Cancer Victors and Friends
PO Box 745
Lakeport, CA 95453
310-822-5032
contact@cancervictors.net
www.cancervictors.net

Offers referrals to recovered patients and provides information packets.

Year Founded: 1963

4177 Cancer and Leukemia Group B
Cancer and Leukemia Group B
230 West Monroe
Suite 2050
Chicago, IL 60606
773-702-9171
Fax: 312-345-0117
marciak@uchicago.edu
www.calgb.org

Michael Kelly, Director, Protocol Operations
Marcia Kelly, Administrative Coordinator
Denise Collins Brennan, Interim Chief Financial Officer

a cancer research cooperative group focused on seven major disease areas: leukemia, lymphoma, breast cancer, lung cancer, gastrointestinal malignancies, genito-urinary malignancies, and melanoma.

Year Founded: 1956

4178 Chemocare
Toll Free: 844-268-3901
chemocare@ccf.org
www.chemocare.com

CHEMOcare is a telephone support network for chemotherapy and/or radiation patients. They have a newsletter, a tollfree information line, and offer peer counseling and advocacy.

Year Founded: 2002

4179 Chemotherapy Foundation

183 Madison Avenue
Suite 403
New York, NY 10016
212-213-9292
Fax: 212-213-3831
info@chemotherapyfoundation.org
www.chemotherapyfoundation.org

Franco M Muggia, Chairman and Medical Director
Craig Effron, Secretary/Treasurer
Edward Ambinder, MD, Director of Medical Symposia

The Chemotherapy Foundation is dedicated to developing more effective methods of treatment for the control and cure of cancer. They provide educational materials and provide funds for innovative chemotherapy research, and sponsor professional and public educational symposia.

Year Founded: 1968

4180 Corporate Angel Network

Westchester County Airport
One Loop Road
White Plains, NY 10604-1215
914-328-1313
Fax: 914-328-3938
info@corpangelnetwork.org
www.corpangelnetwork.org

Gina Russo, Executive Director
Astrid Reynolds, Program Development Director
Randall Greene, Chairman

A service which fills available space on corporate airplanes with cancer patients in need of transportation to treatment centers.

Year Founded: 1981

4181 Duke Cancer Institute
Duke University

10 Bryan Searle Drive
Seeley Mudd Building, 2nd floor
Durham, NC 27710
919-419-4621
Fax: 919-681-7385
www.cancer.duke.edu

Michael B Kastan, MD, PhD, Executive Director
Steven Patierno, PhD, Deputy Director
Karen E Butler, Director of Communications

Duke Cancer Institute is home to more than 300 researchers and physicians dedicated to assembling each patient's entire clinical team and treatment resources in a single building. Duke Cancer Institute integrates patient care, research and education.

Year Founded: 1973

4182 Exceptional Cancer Patients

Woodbridge, CT
203-288-2839
bugsyssiegel@sbcglobal.net
berniesiegelmd.com

Bernie Siegel, MD, Founder

Support groups for those suffering from cancer.

Year Founded: 1978

4183 Gilda's Club

195 W Houston Street
New York, NY 10014
212-647-9700
Fax: 212-647-1151
info@gildasclubnyc.org
www.gildasclubnyc.org

Lily Safani, Chief Executive Officer
Migdalia Torres, Executive Director
Michelle Ramlochan, Executive Assistant to the CEO

To support, educate, and empower cancer patients and their families through programs such as support groups, educational lectures, and healthy lifestyle workshops for anyone impacted by cancer.

Year Founded: 1995; Number of Members: 5000

4184 Gilda's Club: Metro Detroit

3517 Rochester Road,
Royal Oak, MI 48073
248-577-0800
info@gildasclubdetroit.org
gildasdetroit.wpengine.com

Ronald K Weiner, Chair
Todd Sinclair, Vice Chair
Tina Wheeler, Secretary

To support, educate, and empower cancer patients and their families through programs such as support groups, educational lectures, and healthy lifestyle workshops for anyone impacted by cancer.

Year Founded: 1998

4185 Gilda's Club: Quad Cities

1234 East River Drive
Davenport, IA 52803
563-326-7504
Fax: 563-323-1658
www.gildasclubqc.org

Joy McMeekan, Interim Executive Director
Melissa Wright, Program Director
Anita Shaft, Program Manager

To support, educate, and empower cancer patients and their families through programs such as support groups, educational lectures, and healthy lifestyle workshops for anyone impacted by cancer.

Year Founded: 1995

4186 Gilda's Club: South Florida

119 Rose Drive
Fort Lauderdale, FL 33316
954-763-6776
Fax: 954-763-6779
info@gildasclubsouthflorida.org
www.gildasclubsouthflorida.org

Heather Miller, Chair
Leonard Goldberg, Vice Chair
Sean Pleus, Treasurer

To support, educate, and empower cancer patients and their families through programs such as support groups, educational lectures, and healthy lifestyle workshops for anyone impacted by cancer.

Year Founded: 1989

4187 International Cancer Information Service Group (ICISG)
www.icisg.org

Kevin Babb, President
Anna Boltong, Vice President

Provides information on cancer causes, prevention, detection, diagnosis, and rehabilitation. Offers referrals to doctors, cancer centers, and support groups.

4188 International Holistic Center
4640 N Federal Highway
Suite F
Ft. Lauderdale, FL 33308
954-903-9426
Fax: 954-533-8616
ihchealthfusion.com

Elizabeth King, CEO
Year Founded: 1989

4189 Kidney Cancer Association
9450 SW Gemini Drive
Unit 38269
Beaverton, OR 97008-7105
Fax: 847-332-1051; *Toll Free:* 800-850-9132
office@kidneycancer.org
www.kidneycancer.org

William Bro, VP & Executive Secretary
Jennifer Fitzgerald, Accounts Payable & Receivale
Stephanie Shirley, Donations & Fundraising Events

A nationwade charity dedicated specifically to eradication of death and suffering from renal cancers.

Year Founded: 1990

4190 Leukemia & Lymphoma Society
3 International Drive
Suite 200
Rye Brook, NY 10573
914-949-5213
Fax: 914-949-6691
www.lls.org

Louis J. DeGennaro, President & CEO
Rosemarie Loffredo, Chief Financial Officer
Mark Roithmayr, Chief Development Officer

A national voluntary health agency dedicated to finding cures for leukemia and blood related illnesses and improving the quality of life for patients and their families.

4191 Leukemia & Lymphoma Society: Alabama Chapter
3500 Blue Lake Drive
Suite 225
Birmingham, AL 35243
205-989-0098
regan.goldberg@lls.org
www.lls.org

Regan Goldberg, Executive Director
Julie Moon, Office Manager
Maggie Rountree, Campaign Manager

Dedicated to finding cures for leukemia and related cancers and to improving the quality of life for patients and their families.

4192 Leukemia & Lymphoma Society: California Southland Chapter
4929 Wilshire Boulevard
Suite 800
Los Angeles, CA 90010
310-342-5800
shannon.sullivan@lls.org
www.lls.org

Shannon Sullivan, Executive Director
Lauren Plichta, Sr Director, Special Events
Nancy Rink, Operations Director

Dedicated to finding cures for leukemia and related cancers and to improving the quality of life for patients and their families.

Year Founded: 1949

4193 Leukemia & Lymphoma Society: Central Ohio Chapter
2225 Citygate Drive
Suite A
Columbus, OH 43219
614-476-7194
breana.shawver@lls.org
www.lls.org

Breana Shawyer, Executive Director

Dedicated to finding cures for leukemia and related cancers and to improving the quality of life for patients and their families.

4194 Leukemia & Lymphoma Society: Central Pennsylvania Chapter
101 Erford Road
Suite 201
Camp Hill, PA 17011
717-652-6520
laura.macneill@lls.org
www.lls.org

Laura MacNeill, Executive Director
Tara Reyka, Sr Development Director

Dedicated to finding cures for leukemia and blood related illnesses and improving the quality of life for patients and their families.

4195 Leukemia & Lymphoma Society: Central Valley Branch
340 W Fallbrook Avenue
Suite 101
Fresno, CA 93711
559-435-1482
debbie.truhett@lls.org
www.lls.org

Debbie Truhett, Executive Director
Casey Fitzpatrick, Director, Donor Development
Douglas Macnab, Operations Director

Dedicated to finding cures for leukemia and blood related illnesses and improving the quality of life for patients and their families.

4196 Leukemia & Lymphoma Society: Connecticut Chapter
3 Landmark Square
Suite 330
Stamford, CT 06901

203-388-9160
deborah.barker@lls.org
www.lls.org

Deborah Barker, Executive Director
Roger Drake, Senior Campaign Director
Diana Rukaj, Special Events Director

Dedicated to finding cures for leukemia and related cancers and to improving the quality of life for patients and their families. Serves residents of the counties: Hartford, Litchfield, Middlesex, New Haven, Tolland, and Windham.

4197 Leukemia & Lymphoma Society: Delaware Chapter

1300 Grant Avenue
Suite 100
Wilmington, DE 19806
302-661-7300
brook.rowe@lls.org
www.lls.org

Brook Patterson Rowe, Executive Director

Dedicated to finding cures for leukemia and blood related illnesses and improving the quality of life for patients and their families.

Year Founded: 1949

4198 Leukemia & Lymphoma Society: Eastern Pennsylvania Chapter

100 N 20th Street
Suite 405
Philadelphia, PA 19103
610-238-0360
ellen.rubesin@lls.org
www.lls.org

Ellen Rubesin, Executive Director
Laurent Iannucci, Sr Dir., Corporate Development
Janet Butley, Field Operations Director

Dedicated to finding cures for leukemia and related cancers and to improving the quality of life for patients and their families.

4199 Leukemia & Lymphoma Society: Gateway Chapter

1972 Innerbelt Business Center
St. Louis, MO 63114
314-590-2230
debbie.kersting@lls.org
www.lls.org

Debbie Kersting, Executive Director

Dedicated to finding cures for leukemia, lymphoma, Hodgkin's disease and myeloma and to improving the quality of life for patients and thier families.

Year Founded: 1949

4200 Leukemia & Lymphoma Society: Georgia Chapter

2859 Paces Ferry Road SE
Suite 725
Atlanta, GA 30339
404-720-7900
piper.medcalf@lls.org
www.lls.org

Piper Medcalf, Executive Director
Audrey Skopitz, Development Director

Dedicated to finding cures for leukemia and related cancers and to improving the quality of life for patients and their families.

Year Founded: 1949

4201 Leukemia & Lymphoma Society: Greater Sacramento Area

7750 College Town Drive
Suite 210
Sacramento, CA 95826
916-929-4720
jenaye.shepherd@lls.org
www.lls.org

Jenaye Sheperd, Executive Director
Cherrie Caballero, Operations Director

Dedicated to finding cures for leukemia and related cancers and to improving the quality of life for patients and their families.

Year Founded: 1949

4202 Leukemia & Lymphoma Society: Illinois Chapter

954 W Washington Boulevard
Suite 305
Chicago, IL 60607
312-651-7350
pam.swenk@lls.org
www.lls.org

Pamela Swenk, Executive Director
Jan Rohacik, Sr Dir., Donor Development
Ashley Bloom, Sr Dir., Special Events

Dedicated to finding cures for leukemia and related cancers and to improving the quality of life for patients and their families.

Year Founded: 1949

4203 Leukemia & Lymphoma Society: Indiana Chapter

9075 North Meridian
Suite 150
Indianapolis, IN 46260
317-860-3840
patricia.clark@lls.org
www.lls.org

Trish Clark, Executive Director

Dedicated to finding cures for leukemia and blood related illnesses and improving the quality of life for patients and their families.

Year Founded: 1949

4204 Leukemia & Lymphoma Society: Iowa Chapter

Century 1 Building
2700 Westown Parkway, Suite 260
West Des Moines, IA 50266
515-270-6169
melanie.brown@lls.org
www.lls.org

Melanie Brown, Executive Director

Dedicated to finding cures for leukemia, lymphoma, and related cancers, and to improving the quality of life for patients and thier families.

Year Founded: 1949

4205 Leukemia & Lymphoma Society: Kentucky and Southern Indiana Chapter
301 East Main Street
Suite 100
Louisville, KY 40202-1077
502-584-8490
helen.overfield@lls.org
www.lls.org

Helen Overfield, Executive Director
Meredith Johnson, Operations Manager

Dedicated to finding cures for leukemia and blood related illnesses and improving the quality of life for patients and their families.

Year Founded: 1949

4206 Leukemia & Lymphoma Society: Long Island Chapter
3 Huntington Quadrangle
Suite 202S
Melville, NY 11747
631-370-7530
sara.lipsky@lls.org
www.lls.org

Sara Lipsky, Executive Director
Meghana Golden, Development Director

Dedicated to finding cures for leukemia and blood related illnesses and improving the quality of life for patients and their families.

Year Founded: 1949

4207 Leukemia & Lymphoma Society: Maryland Chapter
100 Painters Mill Road
Suite 800
Owings Mills, MD 21117
443-471-1600
jonathan.v.wilson@lls.org
www.lls.org

Jonathan V Wilson, Executive Director
Sheronda Booker, Director, Donor Development

Dedicated to finding cures for leukemia and related cancers and to improving the quality of life for patients and their families.

Year Founded: 1949

4208 Leukemia & Lymphoma Society: Massachusetts Chapter
9 Erie Drive
Suite 101
Natick, MA 01760
508-810-1300
laura.macneill@lls.org
www.lls.org

Laura MacNeill, Executive Director

Dedicated to finding cures for leukemia and blood related illnesses and improving the quality of life for patients and their families.

Year Founded: 1949

4209 Leukemia & Lymphoma Society: Michigan Chapter
1471 E Twelve Mile Road
Madison Heights, MI 48071

248-581-3900
doug.glazier@lls.org
www.lls.org

Doug Glazier, Executive Director
Healther Tull, Officer Manager
Jo Belz, Administrative Asssistant

Dedicated to finding cures for leukemia and blood related illnesses and improving the quality of life for patients and their families.

Year Founded: 1949

4210 Leukemia & Lymphoma Society: Mid-America Chapter
6811 Shawnee Mission Parkway
Suite 202
Shawnee Mission, KS 66202-4001
913-262-1515
carli.good@lls.org
www.lls.org

Carli Howard Good, Executive Director
Megan Clemens, Deputy Executive Director

Dedicated to finding cures for leukemia and related cancers and to improving the quality of life for patients and their families.

Year Founded: 1949

4211 Leukemia & Lymphoma Society: Minnesota Chapter
1711 Broadway Street NE
Minneapolis, MN 55413
612-259-4600
teri.cannon@lls.org
www.lls.org

Teri Cannon, Executive Director

Dedicated to finding cures for leukemia and blood related illnesses and improving the quality of life for patients and their families.

Year Founded: 1949

4212 Leukemia & Lymphoma Society: Mississippi and Louisiana Chapter
3636 S I-10 Service Road
Suite 304
Metairie, LA 70001
504-837-0945
katie.triplett@lls.org
www.lls.org

Katie Triplett, Executive Director

Dedicated to finding cures for leukemia and related cancers and to improving the quality of life for patients and their families.

Year Founded: 1949

4213 Leukemia & Lymphoma Society: Nebraska Chapter
12100 W Center Road
Suite 1, Suite 202
Omaha, NE 68144
402-344-2242
jenna.sager@lls.org
www.lls.org

Jenna Sager, Area Director

Dedicated to finding cures for leukemia and blood related illnesses and improving the quality of life for patients and their families.

Year Founded: 1949

4214 Leukemia & Lymphoma Society: New Jersey Chapter
14 Commerce Drive
Suite 301
Cranford, N 07016
908-956-6644
jana.boyer@lls.org
www.lls.org

Jana Boyer, Executive Director

Dedicated to finding cures for leukemia and related cancers and to improving the quality of life for patients and their families.

Year Founded: 1949

4215 Leukemia & Lymphoma Society: New Mexico Chapter
6100 Indian School Road NE
Suite 225
Albuquerque, NM 87110
505-872-0141
kristja.falvo@lls.org
www.lls.org

Kris Falvo, Managing Director

Dedicated to finding cures for leukemia and blood related illnesses and improving the quality of life for patients and their families.

Year Founded: 1949

4216 Leukemia & Lymphoma Society: New York City Chapter
61 Broadway
Suite 400
New York, NY 10006
212-376-7100
jim.roberts@lls.org
www.lls.org

Jim Roberts, Executive Director
Kyle Hale, Sr Dir., Corporate Development

Dedicated to finding cures for leukemia and blood related illnesses and improving the quality of life for patients and their families.

Year Founded: 1949

4217 Leukemia & Lymphoma Society: North Carolina Chapter
401 Harrison Oaks Boulevard
Suite 200
Cary, NC 27513
919-367-4100
emily.blust@lls.org
www.lls.org

Emily Blust, Executive Director

Dedicated to finding cures for leukemia and related cancers and to improving the quality of life for patients and their families.

Year Founded: 1949

4218 Leukemia & Lymphoma Society: North Texas Chapter
8111 Lyndon B Johnson Fwy
Suite 425
Dallas, TX 75251
972-996-5900
patricia.thomson@lls.org
www.lls.org

Patricia Thomson, Executive Director
Stacey Russell, Deputy Executive Director
Kacy Lowe, Sr Dir., Donor Development

Dedicated to finding cures for leukemia and blood related illnesses and improving the quality of life for patients and their families.

Year Founded: 1949

4219 Leukemia & Lymphoma Society: Northern Ohio Chapter
5700 Brecksville Road
3rd Floor
Independence, OH 44131
216-264-5680
lindsay.silverstein@lls.org
www.lls.org

Lindsay Silverstain, Executive Director
Jessica Whittimore, Director, Special Events
Kerri Peterson-Davis, Director, Donor Development

Dedicated to finding cures for leukemia and related cancers and to improving the quality of life for patients and their families.

Year Founded: 1949

4220 Leukemia & Lymphoma Society: Northern and Central Florida Chapter
341 N Maitland Avenue
Suite 100
Maitland, FL 32751
407-898-0733
alison.thompson@lls.org
www.lls.org

David Wiggins, Interim Executive Director
Alison Thompson, Operations Director
Jill Nugent, Senior Campaign Director

Dedicated to finding cures for leukemia and related cancers and to improving the quality of life for patients and their families.

4221 Leukemia & Lymphoma Society: Oklahoma Chapter
500 N Broadway Avenue
Suite 250
Oklahoma City, OK 73102
405-943-8888
patricia.thomson@lls.org
www.lls.org

Patricia Thompson, Executive Director

Dedicated to finding cures for leukemia and related cancers and to improving the quality of life for patients and their families.

Year Founded: 1949

4222 Leukemia & Lymphoma Society: Oregon SW Washington Idaho Montana Chapter
9320 SW Barbur Boulevard
Suite 350
Portland, OR 97219
503-245-9866
stephanie.carlson@lls.org
www.lls.org

Stephanie Carlson, Executive Director
Jeffry Reaume, Revenue Director
Shannon Gianola, Donor Development Director

Dedicated to finding cures for leukemia,lymphoma and myeloma quality of life for patients and their families.
Year Founded: 1949

4223 Leukemia & Lymphoma Society: Palm Beach Chapter
3230 Commerce Place
Suite B
West Palm Beach, FL 33407
561-616-8682
pam.payne@lls.org
www.lls.org

Pamela Payne, Executive Director

Dedicated to finding cures for leukemia and related cancers and to improving the quality of life for patients and their families.
Year Founded: 1949

4224 Leukemia & Lymphoma Society: Rhode Island Chapter
2348 Post Road
Suite 114
Warwick, RI 02886
401-943-8888
laura.macneill@lls.org
www.lls.org

Laura MacNeill, Executive Director
Emily Morash, Area Director, MWOY

Dedicated to finding cures for leukemia and blood related illnesses and improving the quality of life for patients and their families.
Year Founded: 1949

4225 Leukemia & Lymphoma Society: Rocky Mountain Chapter
720 S Colorado Boulevard
Suite 500-S
Denver, CO 80246
720-440-8620
rebecca.russell@lls.org
www.lls.org

Rebecca Russell, Executive Director
Jessica Milnes, Development Director
Alexandra Zaranka, Operations Manager

Dedicated to finding cures for Leukemia, and related cancers, and to improving the quality of life for patients and their families.
Year Founded: 1949

4226 Leukemia & Lymphoma Society: San Diego & Hawaii Chapter
3890 Murphy Canyon Road
Suite 150
San Diego, CA 92123
858-277-1800
Fax: 858-277-1748
kathlene.seymour@lls.org
www.lls.org

Kathlene Seymour, Executive Director
Nayana Sangani, Operations Manager
Sherrie Rosenberger, Front Officer Coordinator

Dedicated to finding cures for leukemia and related cancers and to improving the quality of life for patients and their families.
Year Founded: 1949

4227 Leukemia & Lymphoma Society: South Carolina Chapter
107 Westpark Boulevard
Suite 150
Columbia, SC 29210
803-731-4060
paul.jeter@lls.org
www.lls.org

Paul Jeter, Executive Director
Robin Rolin, Campaign Manager
Shanna Banks, Office Manager

Dedicated to finding cures for leukemia and blood related illnesses and improving the quality of life for patients and their families.
Year Founded: 1949

4228 Leukemia & Lymphoma Society: South Central Texas Chapter
1218 Arion Parkway
Suite 102
San Antonio, TX 78216
210-998-5400
clarissa.flores@lls.org
www.lls.org

Clarissa Flores, Executive Director
Alana Seger, Area Director
Linda Juarez, Director of Operations

Dedicated to finding cures for leukemia and related cancers and to improving the quality of life for patients and their families.
Year Founded: 1949

4229 Leukemia & Lymphoma Society: Southern Florida Chapter
200 S Park Road
Suite 140
Hollywood, FL 33021
954-744-5300
deann.hazey@lls.org
www.lls.org

DeAnn Hazey, Executive Director
Tatiana Marquez Mendez, Officer Manager/Bookkeeper

Dedicated to finding cures for leukemia and blood related illnesses and improving the quality of life for patients and their families.
Year Founded: 1949

4230 Leukemia & Lymphoma Society: Southern Nevada Chapter

6280 S Valley View Boulevard
Suite 342
Las Vegas, NV 89118
702-436-4220
elizabeth.hunterton@lls.org
www.lls.org

Elizabeth Hunterton, Executive Director

Dedicated to finding cures for leukemia and blood related illnesses and improving the quality of life for patients and their families.

Year Founded: 1949

4231 Leukemia & Lymphoma Society: Southern Ohio Chapter

4370 Glendale Milford Road
Cincinnati, OH 45242
513-698-2828
tom.carleton@lls.org
www.lls.org

Tom Carleton, Executive Director
Dawn Berryman, Sr Campaign Director
Roseann Hayes, Campaign Director

Dedicated to finding cures for leukemia and blood related illnesses and improving the quality of life for patients and their families.

Year Founded: 1949

4232 Leukemia & Lymphoma Society: Suncoast Chapter

3505 East Frontage Road
Suite 145
Tampa, FL 33607
813-963-6461
sherri.stitt@lls.org
www.lls.org

Sherri Stitt, Executive Director

Dedicated to finding cures for leukemia and blood related illnesses and improving the quality of life for patients and their families.

Year Founded: 1949

4233 Leukemia & Lymphoma Society: Tennessee Chapter

404 BNA Drive
Suite 102
Nashville, TN 37217
615-331-2980
jeff.parsley@lls.org
www.lls.org

Jeff Parsley, Executive Director

Dedicated to finding cures for leukemia and blood related illnesses and improving the quality of life for patients and their families.

Year Founded: 1949

4234 Leukemia & Lymphoma Society: Texas Gulf Coast

5433 Westheimer
Suite 300
Houston, TX 77056

713-840-0483
billiesue.parris@lls.org
www.lls.org

Billie Sue Parris, Executive Director
Charley Tauer, Development Director
Nunzi Pritchett, Operations Manager

Dedicated to finding cures for leukemia and related cancers and to improving the quality of life for patients and their families.

Year Founded: 1949

4235 Leukemia & Lymphoma Society: Upstate New York & Vermont Chapter

1 Marcus Boulevard
Suite 104
Albany, NY 12205
518-438-3583
maureen.thornton@lls.org
www.lls.org

Maureen O'Brien-Thornton, Executive Director
Karla Pagan, Office Manager

Dedicated to finding cures for leukemia and related cancers and to improving the quality of life for patients and their families.

Year Founded: 1949

4236 Leukemia & Lymphoma Society: Utah Chapter

310 E 4500 S
Suite 240
Murray, UT 84107
801-281-6618
stacie.kulp@lls.org
www.lls.org

Stacie Kulp, Executive Director
Susan Henson, Sr Campaign Manager

Dedicated to finding a cure for leukemia, lymphoma, and realted diseases, and to improving the quality of life for patients and their families.

Year Founded: 1949

4237 Leukemia & Lymphoma Society: Virginia Chapter

5540 Falmouth Street
Suite 101
Richmond, VA 23230
804-673-5690
nicholas.faraone@lls.org
www.lls.org

Nick Farone, Executive Director
Julia Schranck, Operations Manager

Dedicated to finding a cure for leukemia and related cancers and to improving the quality of life for patients and thier families.

Year Founded: 1949

4238 Leukemia & Lymphoma Society: Washington & Alaska Chapter

5601 6th Avenue S
Suite 182
Seattle, WA 98108
206-628-0777
Fax: 206-292-9791; Toll Free: 800-955-4572
anne.gillingham@lls.org
www.lls.org

Anne Gillingham, Executive Director
Julia Carter, Senier Director
Erin Paschall, Patient Access Manager

Dedicated to finding cures for blood cancers, such as leukemia, lymphoma and myeloma, while also providing education and support services to patients, their caregivers and health care professionals.

Year Founded: 1949

4239 Leukemia & Lymphoma Society: Western Pennsylvania/West Virginia Chapter

River Walk Corporate Centre 333 E Carson Street
Suite 441
Pittsburgh, PA 15219
412-395-2873
christina.massari@lls.org
www.lls.org

Tina Massari-Thompson, Executive Director
Robert Stout, Operations Director
Jeanne Caliguiri, Director of Development

Dedicated to finding cures for leukemia and realted cancers and to improving the quality of life for patients and thier families.

Year Founded: 1949

4240 Leukemia & Lymphoma Society: Western and Central New York Chapter

4043 Maple Road
Suite 105
Amherst, NY 14226
716-834-2578
nancy.hails@lls.org
www.lls.org

Nancy Hails, Executive Director
Luann Burgio, Deputy Director

Dedicated to finding cures for leukemia and related cancers and to improving the quality of life for patients and their families.

4241 Leukemia & Lymphoma Society: Wisconsin Chapter

200 S Executive Drive
Suite 203
Brookfield, WI 53005
262-790-4701
liz.klug@lls.org
www.lls.org

Liz Klug, Executive Director
Kortney Hamm, Sr Campaign Director

Dedicated to finding cures for leukemia and blood related illnesses and improving the quality of life for patients and their families.

Year Founded: 1949

4242 Look Good... Feel Better

American Cancer Society
250 Williams Street NW
Atlanta, GA 30303
Toll Free: 800-395-5665
lookgoodfeelbetter.org

Program developed with the help of the Cosmetic, Toiletry and Fragrance Association Foundation in cooperation with the American Cancer Society. Focuses on techniques that can help people undergoing cancer treatment.

Year Founded: 1989

4243 Lung Cancer Alliance

1700 K Street NW
Suite 660
Washington, DC 20006
202-463-2080Toll free: 800-298-2436
info@lungcanceralliance.org
lungcanceralliance.org

Laurie Fenton Ambrose, President & CEO
Emily Eyres, Chief Operating Officer
Edythe Whidden, Chief Administrative Officer

Non-profit organization solely dedicated to help people with lung cancer improve their quality of life through increased advocacy, support and education.

Year Founded: 1995

4244 Mary Bird Perkins Cancer Center

4950 Essen Lane
Baton Rouge, LA 70809
225-767-0847
Fax: 225-215-1215
feedback@marybird.com
www.marybird.org

Todd D Stevens, President & CEO
Jonas Fontenot, PhD, COO, Chief of Physics
Dana Neucere, CFO & CAO

Mary Bird Perkins Cancer Center is Louisiana's leading cancer care organization, dedicated to improve survivorship and lessen the burden of cancer.

Year Founded: 1960

4245 National Coalition for Cancer Survivorship

1010 Wayne Avenue
Suite 315
Silver Spring, MD 20910
Toll Free: 877-622-7937
info@canceradvocacy.org
www.canceradvocacy.org

Shelley Fuld Nasso, CEO

Founded in 1986 by and for people with cancer and those who care for them, the National Coalition for Cancer Survivorship (NCCS) is the only patient-led organization advocating on behalf of survivors of all types of cancer. NCCS's mission is to ensure quality cancer care for all americans by leading and strenghtening the survivorship movement, empowering cancer survivors and advocating on issues that affect cancer survivors' quality of life.

Year Founded: 1986

4246 National Health Federation

PO Box 688
Monrovia, CA 91017
626-357-2181
Fax: 626-303-0642
contact-us@thenhf.com
www.thenhf.com

4247 National Marrow Donor Program

500 N 5th Street
Minneapolis, MN 55401-1206
Toll Free: 800-627-7692
foundation@nmdp.org
bethematch.org

Jeffrey W. Chell, CEO

The program helps patients find marrow donors and supports them through the transplant process.

4248 Norris Cotton Cancer Center
Dartmouth-Hitchcock Medical Center
One Medical Center Drive
Lebanon, NH 03756
603-653-9000Toll free: 800-639-6918
cancerhelp@dartmouth.edu
cancer.dartmouth.edu

Mark A. Israel, Director

Norris Cotton Cancer Center is dedicated to reducing the burden of cancer among the people of New England, and playing a significant part in the world effort to eliminate cancer.

Year Founded: 1970

4249 Oncology Nursing Society
125 Enterprise Drive
Pittsburgh, PA 15275
412-859-6100
Fax: 412-859-6162; Toll Free: 866-257-4667
help@ons.org
www.ons.org

Susan Schneider, President
Brenda Nevidjon, Chief Executive Officer
Barbara Holmes Gobel, Secretary

Registered nurses interested in oncology. Seeks to: promote high professional standards in oncology nursing; provide a network for the exchange of information, resources, and peer support; encourage nurses to specialize in oncology; promote and develop educational programs in oncology nursing extending through the graduate level; identify, encourage, and foster nursing research in improving the quality of patient care. Conducts instructional and abstract sessions.

Year Founded: 1975; Number of Members: 39,000

4250 Patient Advocates for Advanced Cancer Treatments
11555 Jadon Court NE
P.O. Box 45
Sparta, MI 49345
616-453-1477
Fax: 616-453-1846
paact@paact.help
www.paactusa.org

Richard H Profit Jr, President & CEO
Molly Meyers, Manager of Business Operations
Janet Ney, Co-Founder

Offers state-of-the-art detection, diagnostics, evaluations and treatments for all stages of prostate cancer and related problems.

Year Founded: 1985

4251 People Against Cancer
604 East Street
P.O. Box 10
Otho, IA 50569
515-972-4444
Fax: 515-972-4415; Toll Free: 800-662-2623
info@peopleagainstcancer.net
www.peopleagainstcancer.net

Frank D Wiewel, Founder

People Against Cancer is a grassroots, non-profit, member-supported, public benefit organization dedicated to finding members the most effective treatment for their type of cancer.

Year Founded: 1964

4252 Physicians Committee for Responsible Medicine
5100 Wisconsin Avenue NW
Suite 400
Washington, DC 20016
202-686-2210
Fax: 202-686-2216
pcrm@pcrm.org
www.pcrm.org

Neal Barnard, MD, President
Stacey Glaeser, Director of Human Resources
Doug Hall, Publications Director

The Physicians Committee is leading a revolution in medicine, publishing educational literature on nutrion, health, and ethics and effectiveness in research.

Year Founded: 1985

4253 Prostate Cancer Foundation
1250 Fourth Street
Santa Monica, CA 90401
310-570-4700
Fax: 310-570-4701; Toll Free: 800-757-2873
info@pcf.org
www.pcf.org

Jonathan W. Simons, President & CEO
Ralph Finerman, CFO, Treasurer & Secretary

PCF's mission is to accelerate the world's most promising prostate cancer research for better treatments and cures.

4254 Reach to Recovery
American Cancer Society
250 Williams Street NW
Atlanta, GA 30303
Toll Free: 800-227-2345
info@canceradvocacy.org
www.cancer.org

A rehabilitation program for women who have or have had breast cancer. The program helps breast cancer patients meet the physical, emotional and cosmetic needs related to their disease and its treatment. The American Cancer Society Reach To Recovery program matches trained volunteer breast cancer survivors to people living with breast cancer. Through face-to-face visits or by phone, Reach To Recovery volunteer visitors provide understanding and hope to individuals who need support during their breast cancer experience.

Year Founded: 1913

4255 Support for People with Oral and Head and Neck Cancer
P.O. Box 53
Locust Valley, NY 11560-0053
Fax: 516-671-8794; Toll Free: 800-377-0928
info@spohnc.org
www.spohnc.org

Nancy E Leupold, President and founder
James J Sciubba, PhD, Vice President
Gail Fass, Secretary

Non-profit organization founded in 1991 to address the broad emotional, physical and humanistic needs of oral and head and neck cancer patients.

Year Founded: 1991

4256 Sylvester Comprehensive Cancer Center
University of Miami Health System
1475 NW 12th Avenue
Miami, FL 33136
305-243-1000Toll free: 800-545-2292
sylvester.org
TTY: 305-243-3170

Richard Ballard, CEO
Lazara Pagan, COO
Year Founded: 1976

4257 The Second Opinion
1200 Gough Street
Suite 500
San Francisco, CA 94109
415-775-9956
mail@thesecondopinion.org
www.thesecondopinion.org

Robert Ignoffo, Pharm D, Interim President
Ann Lanzerotti, MD, Secretary
Linus So, Treasurer

This foundation offers, at no charge, a second opinion consultation to individuals diagnosed with cancer. The patient and a family member or friend meet with an interdisciplinary panel of local cancer specialists with expertise in radiation therapy, chemotherapy, surgery, radiology, and pathology.

Year Founded: 1974

4258 United Ostomy Association of America
P.O. Box 525
Kennebunk, ME 04043-0525
Toll Free: 800-826-0826
www.ostomy.org

Susan Burns, President
Jim Murray, Vice President
George Salamy, Treasurer

The United Ostomy Associations of America, Inc. (UOAA) is a nonprofit organization that supports, empowers, and advocates for people who have had or who will have ostomy or continent diversion surgery.

Year Founded: 2005

Books

4259 3rd Opinion: International Directory to Complementary Therapy Centers
Avery Publishing Group
120 Old Broadway
New Hyde Park, NY 11040-5015
516-741-2155
Fax: 516-742-1892; *Toll Free:* 800-548-5757

Discusses over 300 alternative treatment cancer centers, educational centers, support groups and other research services.

4260 ACS Bookstore
American Cancer Society
e-mail: acsbooks@cancer.org
www.cancer.org/cancer/bookstore

4261 Alternative Medicine Magazine's Definitive Guide to Cancer
The Crown Publishing Group
1745 Broadway
New York, NY 10019
212-782-9000
Fax: 510-559-1629; *Toll Free:* 800-841-2665
www.crownpublishing.com

Comprehensive guide to cancer helps patients and their caregivers learn about causes and prevention of cancer; offset the side effects of conventional medicine; evaluate effective alternative treatments; utilize natural therapies involving diet, lifestyle, and nutritional supplements; and achieve deep healing through a mind-body-spirit approach.

4262 Ask the Doctor: Breast Cancer
Andrews McMeel Publishing
PO Box 419263
Kansas City, MO 64193
816-932-6700
Fax: 800-437-8683; *Toll Free:* 800-826-4216
www.uclick.com

Kathleen W Andrews, CEO
128 pages Year Founded: 1970

4263 Cancer Dictionary
Facts on File
11 Penn Plaza
Floor 15
New York, NY 10001-2006
212-766-9152
Fax: 212-967-8107; *Toll Free:* 800-322-8755

Maggie Kok, Owner
352 pages

4264 Cancer Facts and Figures
American Cancer Society
1599 Clifton Road NE
Atlanta, GA 30329-4250
404-320-3333Toll free: 800-ACS-2345
claire.greenwell@cancer.org
www.cancer.org

John Seffrin PhD, CEO
Publishes over 57 treatment centers.

4265 Cancer Rates and Risks
National Cancer Institute
6116 Executive Boulevard
Suite 3036a
Bethesda, MD 20892
301-929-1779

This book is a compact guide to statistics, risk factors, and risks for major cancer sites.

136 pages

4266 Cancer Sourcebook
Omnigraphics
155 W.Congress
Suite 200
Detroit, MI 48226

313-961-1340
Fax: 800-875-1340; *Toll Free:* 800-234-
contact@omnigraphics.com
www.omnigraphics.com

Peter E Ruffner, President

Offers basic information on cancer types, symptoms, diagnostic methods, and treatments. Includes statistics on cancer occurrences worldwide and the risks associated with known carcinogens and activities.

Year Founded: 1940

4267 Cancer Therapy: The Independant Consumer's Guide to Non-Toxic Treatment & Prevention
Equinox Press
144 Saint Johns Place
Brooklyn, NY 11217-3402
718-636-4433
Fax: 718-636-0186
www.ralphmoss.com

A must for cancer patients and their families who want: Practical information on the most promising non-toxic treatments; Scientific evidence in readable language; Well-documented resource lists and medical references.

528 pages

4268 Cancer-Free: Your Guide to Gentle
AuthorHouse
1663 Liberty Drive
Suite 200
Bloomington, IN 47403
888-519-5121
www.authorhouse.com

This book tells you how to work with the medical system anywhere in the world to save the life of those you care about.

4269 Everyone's Guide To Cancer Therapy
Andrews McMeel Publishing
PO Box 419263
Kansas City, MO 64193
816-932-6700
Fax: 800-437-8683; *Toll Free:* 800-826-4216

Kathleen W Andrews, CEO

848 pages

4270 Everyone's Guide to Cancer Therapy
Andrews McMeel Publishing LLC
100 Front Street
Riverside, NJ 08075
800-943-9839
Fax: 800-943-9831
www.andrewsmcmeel.com

Inside Everyone's Guide to Cancer, the world's top cancer specialists-141 to be exact-provide the latest medical breakthroughs, treatments, and accessible information on the more than 200 forms of cancer, highlighting the 54 most common types of the disease.

4271 Home Care Guide for Cancer
Johns Hopkins University Press
2715 N Charles Street
Baltimore, MD 21218-4319
410-516-6900
Fax: 410-516-6998; *Toll Free:* 800-537-5487
www.jhu.edu/press/index.html

William Brody, President

This easy to use workbook was designed for home cargivers, patients, support groups, and education programs; it features easy to read type, and index for quick reference, and advice on twenty common cancer caregiving problems.

260 pages

4272 No Less a Woman
Simon & Schuster
1819 L Street NW
Washington, DC 20036-3807
202-293-0202
Fax: 202-293-0202

Offers intimate interviews that explore the major issues of coping and surviving breast cancer, from diagnosis and treatment to physical and psychological recovery. In their own words, ten women describe how they successfully adjusted to the changes in their bodies and their feelings about themselves.

288 pages

4273 Older Than My Mother: A Nurse's Life & Triumph
Ananse Press
PO Box 22565
Seattle, WA 98122-0565
206-325-8205

This book describes childhood as a young African-American woman in the rural Louisiana, struggles to become a nurse, and the development of a strong self-advocacy that has led to her longevity as a breast cancer survivor..

4274 Prostate Health Workbook
Hunter House Publisher
PO Box 2914
Alameda, CA 94501
510-865-5282
Fax: 510-865-4295; *Toll Free:* 888-519-5121
ordering@hunterhouse.com
www.hunterhouse.com

Christina Sverdrup, Customer Service Manager
Newton Malerman, Author

A practical guide for the prostate cancer patients.

160 pages

4275 Teratologies: A Cultural Study of Cancer
Routledge
29 W 35th Street
Floor 10
New York, NY 10001-2299
212-244-3336
Fax: 212-248-4724; *Toll Free:* 800-634-7064
www.routledge.com

A distinctively feminist look at how cancer is perceived, experienced and theorized in contemprary society. Beginning with powerful personal accounts of her own illness, as well as self-help manuals and patients' personal stories, Jackie Stacey explores changing beliefs about the causes and treatments of cancer in both biomedecine and its increasingly popular alternative counterparts.

4276 What to Eat if you Have Cancer
McGraw-Hill Companies
7500 Chavenelle Road
Dubuque, IA 52002
877-833-5524
Fax: 614-759-3749
pbg.ecommerce_custserv@mcgraw-hill.com
www.mhprofessional.com

Improved dietary habits can support cancer treatment programs; yet too few cancer guides provide much information on just what kind of diet should be followed. Enter this title, written by two licensed nutritionists and focusing on foods which reduce toxicity from chemotherapy and increase the body's recovery process. From supplement dos and don'ts to insights on natural foods, this covers many topics.

Journals, Magazines

4277 Coping: Living with Cancer
Media America
4 New York Plaza
New York, NY 10004
212-545-4800
Fax: 615-794-0179
www.americanmediainc.com

David J. Pecker, Chair
Chris Polimeni, Executive VP
Eric S. Klee, Secretary

Consumer magazine for people whose lives have been touched by cancer.

Frequency: Bimonthly Year Founded: 1940

4278 Diseases of the Colon and Rectum
American Society of Colon and Rectal Surgeons
85 W Algonquin Road
Suite 550
Arlington Heights, IL 60005-4460
847-290-9184
Fax: 847-290-9273
www.fascrs.org

Information for professionals specializing in the diagnosis and treatment of colorectal disorders.

4279 Journal of Cancer Education
Hanley & Belfus
210 S 13th Street
Philadelphia, PA 19107-5467
215-546-4995
Fax: 215-790-9330; *Toll Free:* 800-962-

A peer-reviewed quarterly journal that addresses varied aspects of cancer education for physicians, dentists, nurses, students, social workers, and other allied health professionals. Articles include reports of original results of educational research and discussions of current problems and techniques in cancer education.

4280 Skin Cancer Foundation Journal
Skin Cancer Foundation
85 W.Algonquin Rd
Suite 550
Arlington Heights, IL 60005
847-290-9184
Fax: 847-290-9203

ascrs@fascrs.org
www.skincancer.org

Michael J. Stamos, President
Terry C. Hicks, President-Elect
Martin A. Luchtefeld, VP

A collection of articles by physicians, scientists and lay writers on the subject.

Frequency: Once a year

Newsletters, Pamphlets

4281 Advanced Cancer: Living Each Day
National Cancer Institute
Building 31
Bethesda, MD 20892
301-496-7406
Fax: 301-480-8105
www.cancer.gov

Harold E. Varmus, Director

Booklet delving into all aspects of everyday living with cancer. Offers information on coping, how children react, facing the unknown, living wills, additional resources and making treatment decisions.

30 pages

4282 Breast Cancer: Understanding Treatment Options
National Cancer Institute
Building 31
Bethesda, MD 20892
301-496-7406
Fax: 301-480-8105
www.cancer.gov

Harold E. Varmus, Director

Summarizes the biopsy procedure and examines the pros and cons of various types of breast surgery. It discusses lumpectomy and radiation therapy as primary treatment.

19 pages

4283 Cancer of the Bladder: Research Report
National Cancer Institute
Building 31
Bethesda, MD 20892
301-496-7406
Fax: 301-480-8105
www.cancer.gov

Harold E. Varmus, Director

Offers information on the types of bladder cancer, mortality rates, diagnosis, symptoms, therapies, rehabilitation, clinical trials, and selected references.

4284 Cancer of the Colon and Rectum: Research Report
National Cancer Institute
Building 31
Bethesda, MD 20892
301-496-7406
Fax: 301-480-8105
www.cancer.gov

Harold E. Varmus, Director

Informative pamphlet offering factual statistics on causes and prevention, detection, diagnosis, staging, treatment, followup, clinical trials and selected references.

4285 Cancer of the Ovary: Research Report
National Cancer Institute
Building 31
Bethesda, MD 20892
301-496-7406
Fax: 301-480-8105
www.cancer.gov

Harold E. Varmus, Director

4286 Cancer of the Pancreas: Research Report
National Cancer Institute
Building 31
Bethesda, MD 20892
301-496-7406
Fax: 301-480-8105
www.cancer.gov

Harold E. Varmus, Director

Offers information on the various types of pancreatic cancer, treatments, surgical procedures, chemotherapy, biological therapy, hormone therapy, clinical trials and selected references.

4287 Cancer of the Uterus: Research Report
National Cancer Institute
Building 31
Bethesda, MD 20892
301-496-7406
Fax: 301-480-8105
www.cancer.gov

Harold E. Varmus, Director

4288 Chemotherapy and You: A Guide to Self-Help During Treatment
National Cancer Institute
Building 31
Bethesda, MD 20892
301-496-7406
Fax: 301-480-8105
www.cancer.gov

Harold E. Varmus, Director

Explains chemotherapy and addresses problems and concerns of patients undergoing this treatment.

4289 Clearing the Air: A Guide to Quitting Smoking
National Cancer Institute
Building 31
Bethesda, MD 20892
301-496-7406
Fax: 301-480-8105
www.cancer.gov

Harold E. Varmus, Director

Offers hints on quitting smoking and cancer prevention.

24 pages

4290 Diet, Nutrition and Cancer Prevention: A Guide to Food Choices
National Cancer Institute
Building 31
Bethesda, MD 20892

301-496-7406
Fax: 301-480-8105
www.cancer.gov

Harold E. Varmus, Director

Describes what is known about diet, nutrition and cancer prevention. Provides information about foods that contain components like fiber, fat and vitamins that may affect a person's risk of getting certain cancers.

4291 Diet, Nutrition and Cancer Prevention: The Good News
National Cancer Institute
Building 31
Bethesda, MD 20892
301-496-7406
Fax: 301-480-8105
www.cancer.gov

Harold E. Varmus, Director

Provides an overview of dietary guidelines that may assist individuals in reducing their risks for some cancers.

16 pages

4292 Do the Right Thing: Get a Mammogram
National Cancer Institute
Building 31
Bethesda, MD 20892
301-496-7406
Fax: 301-480-8105
www.cancer.gov

Harold E. Varmus, Director

Targets black women age 40 and older. Describes the importance of regular mammograms in the early detection of breast cancer.

4293 Eating Hints: Recipes and Tips for Better Nutrition During Cancer Treatment
National Cancer Institute
Building 31
Bethesda, MD 20892
301-496-7406
Fax: 301-480-8105
www.cancer.gov

Harold E. Varmus, Director

Provides recipes that help patients meet their needs for good nutrition during treatment.

4294 Facing Forward: A Guide for Cancer Survivors
National Cancer Institute
Building 31
Bethesda, MD 20892
301-496-7406
Fax: 301-480-8105
www.cancer.gov

Harold E. Varmus, Director

Presents a concise overview of important survivor issues, including ongoing health needs, psychosocial concerns, insurance and employment.

43 pages

4295 Facts About Lung Cancer
American Lung Association
55 W. Wacker Drive
Suite 1150
Chicago, IL 60601

800-LUN-GUSA
Fax: 202-452-1805
www.lung.org

Ross P. Lanzafame, Chair
Kathryn A. Forbes, Vice Chair
John F. Emanuel, Treasurer/Secretary

4296 Immune System: How it Works
National Cancer Institute
Building 31
Bethesda, MD 20892
301-496-7406
Fax: 301-480-8105
www.cancer.gov

Harold E. Varmus, Director

Written for the high school level, this booklet explains the human immune system for the general public. It describes the sophistication of the body's immune responses, the impact of immune disorders and the relation of the immune system to cancer therapies.

28 pages

4297 Mastectomy: A Treatment for Breast Cancer
National Cancer Institute
Building 31
Bethesda, MD 20892
301-496-7406
Fax: 301-480-8105
www.cancer.gov

Harold E. Varmus, Director

Presents information about the different types of breast surgery, explains what to expect at the hospital and during the recovery period.

25 pages

4298 Melanoma Newsletter
Skin Cancer Foundation
85 W.Algonquin Rd
Suite 550
Arlington Heights, IL 60005
847-290-9184
Fax: 847-290-9203
ascrs@fascrs.org
www.skincancer.org

Michael J. Stamos, President
Terry C. Hicks, President-Elect
Martin A. Luchtefeld, VP

For medical investigators and practitioners.

Frequency: Quarterly

4299 Melanoma: Research Report
National Cancer Institute
Building 31
Bethesda, MD 20892
301-496-7406
Fax: 301-480-8105
www.cancer.gov

Harold E. Varmus, Director

Offers information on types of skin cancer, detection, diagnosis, staging, treatment, clinical trials, selected references and additional information for patients with skin cancer.

4300 Nutrition for Patients Receiving Chemotherapy/Radiation Treatment
National Cancer Institute
Building 31
Bethesda, MD 20892
301-496-7406
Fax: 301-480-8105
www.cancer.gov

Harold E. Varmus, Director

Describes the importance of maintaining nutritional intake while receiving chemotherapy and radiation.

4301 Once a Year for a Lifetime
National Cancer Institute
Building 31
Bethesda, MD 20892
301-496-7406
Fax: 301-480-8105
www.cancer.gov

Harold E. Varmus, Director

Targets all women age 40 and older describing the importance of regular mammograms in the early detection of breast cancer.

4302 Oral Cancers: Research Report
National Cancer Institute
Building 31
Bethesda, MD 20892
301-496-7406
Fax: 301-480-8105
www.cancer.gov

Harold E. Varmus, Director

Describes types of oral cancer, causes and risk factors, symptoms, prevention, detection, diagnosis, treatment, staging, methods of treatments, followup care, clinical trials and selected references for more information.

4303 Pap Test: It Can Save Your Life
National Cancer Institute
Building 31
Bethesda, MD 20892
301-496-7406
Fax: 301-480-8105
www.cancer.gov

Harold E. Varmus, Director

Easy-to-read pamphlet tells women of the importance of getting a Pap test, how often to get it done and where to go to get it.

4304 Questions and Answers About Breast Lumps
National Cancer Institute
Building 31
Bethesda, MD 20892
301-496-7406
Fax: 301-480-8105
www.cancer.gov

Harold E. Varmus, Director

Describes some of the most common noncancerous breast lumps and what can be done about them.

22 pages

4305 Questions and Answers About Choosing a Mammography Facility
National Cancer Institute
Building 31
Bethesda, MD 20892
301-496-7406
Fax: 301-480-8105
www.cancer.gov

Harold E. Varmus, Director

Lists questions to ask in selecting a quality mammography facility.

4306 Questions and Answers About Metastatic Cancer
National Cancer Institute
Building 31
Bethesda, MD 20892
301-496-7406
Fax: 301-480-8105
www.cancer.gov

Harold E. Varmus, Director

Presents information on detection, treatment methods and common areas of reoccurrence.

4307 Questions and Answers About Pain Control
National Cancer Institute
Building 31
Bethesda, MD 20892
301-496-7406
Fax: 301-480-8105
www.cancer.gov

Harold E. Varmus, Director

Discusses pain control using both medical and nonmedical methods.

4308 Radiation Therapy and You: A Guide To Self-Help During Treatment
National Cancer Institute
BUILDING 31
Bethesda, MD 20892
301-496-7406
Fax: 301-480-8105
www.cancer.gov

Harold E. Varmus, Director

Explains radiation therapy and addresses concerns of patients receiving radiation treatment.

4309 Research Report: Adult Kidney Cancer and Wilms' Tumor
National Cancer Institute
Building 31
Bethesda, MD 20892
301-496-7406
Fax: 301-480-8105
www.cancer.gov

Harold E. Varmus, Director

4310 Skin Cancer: Preventable and Curable
Skin Cancer Foundation
85 W.Algonquin Rd
Suite 550
Arlington Heights, IL 60005
847-290-9184
Fax: 847-290-9203

ascrs@fascrs.org
www.skincancer.org

Michael J. Stamos, President
Terry C. Hicks, President-Elect
Martin A. Luchtefeld, VP

Brochure on preventing and curing skin cancer

4311 Skin Cancers: Basal Cell and Squamous Cell Carcinomas: Research Report
National Cancer Institute
Building 31
Bethesda, MD 20892
301-496-7406
Fax: 301-480-8105
www.cancer.gov

Harold E. Varmus, Director

Offers information on types of skin cancer, incidence and mortality, risk factors, prevention, symptoms, detection, diagnosis, staging, treatment, followup care and clinical trials.

4312 Students with Cancer: A Resource for the Educator
National Cancer Institute
Building 31
Bethesda, MD 20892
301-496-7406
Fax: 301-480-8105
www.cancer.gov

Harold E. Varmus, Director

Designed for teachers who have students with cancer in their classrooms or schools.

22 pages

4313 Sun and Skin News
Skin Cancer Foundation
85 W.Algonquin Rd
Suite 550
Arlington Heights, IL 60005
847-290-9184
Fax: 847-290-9203
ascrs@fascrs.org
www.skincancer.org

Michael J. Stamos, President
Terry C. Hicks, President-Elect
Martin A. Luchtefeld, VP

Deals with skin cancer and related subjects in non-technical terms.

4314 Sunlight, Ultraviolet Radiation and the Skin
National Cancer Institute
Building 31
Bethesda, MD 20892
301-496-7406
Fax: 301-480-8105
www.cancer.gov

Harold E. Varmus, Director

4315 Support for People with Oral, Head and Neck Cancer
PO Box 53
Locust Valley, NY 11560
516-759-5333
Fax: 516-671-8794; *Toll Free:* 800-377-0928

www.spohnc.org
TDD inf- sp-hnc

Nancy Leupold, President
James J. Sciubba, VP
Gail Fass, Secretary

This a patient-run support program. Other services include patient networking oportunities, a national newsletter, a resource library, and insurance information and assistance.

4316 Taking Time: Support for People with Cancer & People Who Care for Them
National Cancer Institute
Building 31
Bethesda, MD 20892
301-496-7406
Fax: 301-480-8105
www.cancer.gov

Harold E. Varmus, Director

Discusses the emotional sides of cancer. how to deal with the disease and learn to talk with friends, family members and others about cancer.

4317 Testicular Cancer: Research Report
National Cancer Institute
Building 31
Bethesda, MD 20892
301-496-7406
Fax: 301-480-8105
www.cancer.gov

Harold E. Varmus, Director

4318 Testicular Self-Examination
National Cancer Institute
Building 31
Bethesda, MD 20892
301-496-7406
Fax: 301-480-8105
www.cancer.gov

Harold E. Varmus, Director

Contains information about risks and symptoms of testicular cancer and provides instructions on how to perform testicular self-examination.

4319 What Are Clinical Trials All About?
National Cancer Institute
Building 31
Bethesda, MD 20892
301-496-7406
Fax: 301-480-8105
www.cancer.gov

Harold E. Varmus, Director

Explains clinical trials (studies of new cancer treatments) to help patients decide if they want to take part in a trial.

4320 What You Need to Know About Bladder Cancer
National Cancer Institute
Building 31
Bethesda, MD 20892
301-496-7406
Fax: 301-480-8105
www.cancer.gov

Harold E. Varmus, Director

Offers information on the history, symptoms, diagnosis, treatment, followup care, support groups, medical terms and resources for more information.

4321 What You Need to Know About Cancer
National Cancer Institute
Building 31
Bethesda, MD 20892
301-496-7406
Fax: 301-480-8105
www.cancer.gov

Harold E. Varmus, Director

Offers information on signs and symptoms, diagnosis, treatment, early detection and advances in medical technology.

4322 What You Need to Know About Cancer of the Colon and Rectum
National Cancer Institute
Building 31
Bethesda, MD 20892
301-496-7406
Fax: 301-480-8105
www.cancer.gov

Harold E. Varmus, Director

Offers information on symptoms, diagnosis, treatments, and support for cancer patients.

4323 What You Need to Know About Cervical Cancer
National Cancer Institute
Building 31
Bethesda, MD 20892
301-496-7406
Fax: 301-480-8105
www.cancer.gov

Harold E. Varmus, Director

Areas covered include early detection, symptoms, treatments, diagnosis, followup care, support, medical terms and resources.

4324 What You Need to Know About Esophagus Cancer
National Cancer Institute
Building 31
Bethesda, MD 20892
301-496-7406
Fax: 301-480-8105
www.cancer.gov

Harold E. Varmus, Director

Offers information on symptoms, causes, preventions, diagnosis, support, medical terms and available resources.

4325 What You Need to Know About Kidney Cancer
National Cancer Institute
Building 31
Bethesda, MD 20892
301-496-7406
Fax: 301-480-8105
www.cancer.gov

Harold E. Varmus, Director

Offers factual information on diagnosis, symptoms, prevention, treatment and referral sources.

4326 What You Need to Know About Larynx Cancer
National Cancer Institute
Building 31
Bethesda, MD 20892
301-496-7406
Fax: 301-480-8105
www.cancer.gov

Harold E. Varmus, Director

Offers information on what cancer is, symptoms, diagnosis, treatment options, side effects of medication, rehabilitation, learning to speak again, living with cancer, causes and preventions, medical terms and resources.

4327 What You Need to Know About Lung Cancer
National Cancer Institute
Building 31
Bethesda, MD 20892
301-496-7406
Fax: 301-480-8105
www.cancer.gov

Harold E. Varmus, Director

Offers information on types of lung cancer, symptoms, diagnosis, treatments, support, medical terms and resources.

4328 What You Need to Know About Oral Cancers
National Cancer Institute
Building 31
Bethesda, MD 20892
301-496-7406
Fax: 301-480-8105
www.cancer.gov

Harold E. Varmus, Director

Offers information on symptoms, diagnosis, treatments, rehabilitation, followup care, support, medical terms and resources for cancer patients.

4329 What You Need to Know About Ovarian Cancer
National Cancer Institute
Building 31
Bethesda, MD 20892
301-496-7406
Fax: 301-480-8105
www.cancer.gov

Harold E. Varmus, Director

Early detection, symptoms, diagnosis, treatments, medical terms and resources for further information.

4330 What You Need to Know About Pancreatic Cancer
National Cancer Institute
Building 31
Bethesda, MD 20892
301-496-7406
Fax: 301-480-8105
www.cancer.gov

Harold E. Varmus, Director

Offers information on symptoms, diagnosis, treatment, support, medical terms and resources.

4331 What You Need to Know About Prostate Cancer
National Cancer Institute
Building 31
Bethesda, MD 20892
301-496-7406
Fax: 301-480-8105
www.cancer.gov

Harold E. Varmus, Director

Offers information on symptoms, diagnosis, treatment options, side effects of medications, followup care, living with cancer and support resources for patients.

4332 What You Need to Know About Skin Cancer
National Cancer Institute
Building 31
Bethesda, MD 20892
301-496-7406
Fax: 301-480-8105
www.cancer.gov

Harold E. Varmus, Director

Offers information on types of skin cancer, symptoms, causes, prevention, treatment planning, treating skin cancer, research and medical terms.

4333 What You Need to Know About Testicular Cancer
National Cancer Institute
Building 31
Bethesda, MD 20892
301-496-7406
Fax: 301-480-8105
www.cancer.gov

Harold E. Varmus, Director

Offers information on the symptoms, diagnosing of testicular cancer, side effects of treatments, followup care, support for patients, cancer research, medical terms and resources.

4334 What You Need to Know About Uterine Cancer
National Cancer Institute
Building 31
Bethesda, MD 20892
301-496-7406
Fax: 301-480-8105
www.cancer.gov

Harold E. Varmus, Director

Offers information on symptoms, diagnosing cancer of the uterus, treatments, followup care, support for patients, medical terms and resources.

4335 What You Need to Know About...
National Cancer Institute
Building 31
Bethesda, MD 20892
301-496-7406
Fax: 301-480-8105
www.cancer.gov

Harold E. Varmus, Director

This is a series of booklets, broken down in this directory. Each provides information about a specific type of cancer. These booklets discuss emotional issues, treatment, diagnosis, symptoms and questions to ask the doctor about cancer.

4336 When Cancer Recurs: Meeting the Challenge Again
National Cancer Institute
Building 31
Bethesda, MD 20892
301-496-7406
Fax: 301-480-8105
www.cancer.gov

Harold E. Varmus, Director

Offers information on why cancer can recur, where cancers can recur, diagnosing recurrent cancer, treatment methods and resources that offer more help.

4337 When Someone in Your Family Has Cancer
National Cancer Institute
Building 31
Bethesda, MD 20892
301-496-7406
Fax: 301-480-8105
www.cancer.gov

Harold E. Varmus, Director

Written for young people whose parent or sibling has cancer.

28 pages

4338 Who Is This Person Who Helped Save My Life?
Bone Marrow Foundation
515 Madison Avenue
Suite 1130
New York, NY 10022-5102
212-838-3029
Fax: 212-223-0081; *Toll Free:* 800-365-1336
thebmf@bonemarrow.org
www.bonemarrow.org

Robert Fishman, President
Elaine Textor, VP
Andrew Robin, Treasurer/Secretary

Discusses the wide range of emotions for a patient in the process of searching for and identifying a donor.

4339 Why Do You Smoke?
National Cancer Institute
Building 31
Bethesda, MD 20892
301-496-7406
Fax: 301-480-8105
www.cancer.gov

Contains a self-test to determine why people smoke and suggest alternatives that can help them stop and prevent cancer.

Videos, Audio Tapes

4340 Living with Ovarian Cancer
National Ovarian Cancer Coalition
2501 Oak Lawn Avenue
Suite 435
Dallas, TX 75219
949-385-6170
Fax: 214-273-4201; *Toll Free:* 888-682-7426
jmonaco@ovarian.org
www.ovarian.org

Elizabeth Isham Cory, President
Dr. Allison Garrett, Co-Chair
April Donahue, Treasurer

Videotape for women who have been recently diagnosed with ovarian cancer. Created to orient and inform patients and their families; describes the experiences of individuals intimately connected with the disease.

Websites

4341 American Cancer Society
318 Main Street
Vincennes, IN 47591
812-886-9007
Fax: 812-886-9008; *Toll Free:* 800-227-2345
claire.greenwell@cancer.org
www.cancer.org
TTY: 866-228-4327

W. Phil Evans, MD, FACR, President
Tim E. Byers, MD, MPH, First Vice President
Douglas K. Kelsey, MD, PhD, FAAP, Second Vice President

Provides free printed materials, offers a range of services to patients and their families.

Year Founded: 1913

4342 Bone Marrow Foundation
Bone Marrow Foundation
515 Madison Avenue
Suite 1130
New York, NY 10022-5102
212-838-3029
Fax: 212-223-0081; *Toll Free:* 800-365-1336
thebmf@bonemarrow.org
www.bonemarrow.org

Robert Fishman, President
Elaine Textor, VP
Andrew Robin, Treasurer/Secretary

4343 National Ovarian Cancer Coalition
National Ovarian Cancer Coalition
2501 Oak Lawn Avenue
Suite 435
Dallas, TX 75219
949-385-6170
Fax: 214-273-4201; *Toll Free:* 888-682-7426
jmonaco@ovarian.org
www.ovarian.org

Elizabeth Isham Cory, President
Dr. Allison Garrett, Co-Chair
April Donahue, Treasurer

Research Centers

4344 AMC Cancer Research Center
1600 Pierce Street
Lakewood, CO 80214-1897
303-239-3422
Fax: 303-233-9562

David Silberberg, President

Offers research activities, publications, meetings, educational activities, public services, testing services, community-based cancer control programs and knowledge of cancer mortality rates.

4345 Albany Medical College: Joint Center for Cancer and Blood Disorders
43 New Scotland Avenue
Albany, NY 12208
518-262-3125
Fax: 518-445-5011
www.amc.edu

Gregory R Harper, Acting Head
James J Barba, CEO
Greg McGarry, Former VP

Offers research in the fields of cancer and blood disorders, focusing on radiotherapy, pathology and surgery.

4346 American Institute for Cancer Research
1759 R Street NW
Washington, DC 20009-2585
202-328-7744
Fax: 202-328-7226; *Toll Free:* 800-843-8114
aicrweb@aicr.org
www.aicr.org

Marilyn Gentry, President
Melvin Hutson, Chairman
Lawrence Pratt, VC

Fosters research on diet, nutrition and cancer. Call toll free to request educational materials, information on specific cancers, and personalized answers to your nutrition questions.

Year Founded: 1982

4347 Arizona State University: Cancer Research Institute
University Drive
Tempe, AZ 85287
480-965-3351

George R Pettit, Director

Offers research into new cancer drugs and treatments.

4348 Baylor University: Bone Marrow Transplantation Research Center
3409 Worth Street
Suite 410
Dallas, TX 75246-2053
214-820-3361
Fax: 214-820-6890

Joseph W Fay MD, Director
Rebecca Robbins, Manager

Offers bone marrow transplantation research in leukemia studies.

4349 Bone Marrow Foundation
Bone Marrow Foundation
515 Madison Avenue
Suite 1130
New York, NY 10022-5102
212-838-3029
Fax: 212-223-0081; *Toll Free:* 800-365-1336
thebmf@bonemarrow.org
www.bonemarrow.org

Robert Fishman, President
Elaine Textor, VP
Andrew Robin, Treasurer/Secretary

4350 Boston University Cancer Research Center
72 E Concord Street
Boston, MA 02118-2307

617-638-4173
Fax: 617-638-4176
www.bumc.bu.edu

Douglas V Faller, PhD, MD
Glenn St Marie, Manager
Deborah Lowe, Administrative

4351 Brigham Young University: Cancer Research Center
S125 Esc
Provo, UT 84602
801-378-4636
www.cancerresearch.byu.edu

Daniel L Simmons, Director
Kim L O'Neill, Associate Director
Merrill J Bateman, President

Year Founded: 1977

4352 Brown University: Division of Biology and Medicine
PO Box G-A1
Providence, RI 02912
401-274-3990
Fax: 401-863-2660
www.biomed.brown.edu

Dr. Pierre Gallleti, VP
Ted Brown, President
Jabbar R. Bennett, PhD, Associate Dean

Interdisciplinary studies in biological and medical sciences including studies in health care problems and fields of research such as cancer and diabetes.

4353 Cancer Center of Wake Forest University: Bowman Gray School of Medicine
300 S Hawthorne Road
Winston Salem, NC 27157
336-758-5000
Fax: 336-758-4324
www.wakehealth.edu

William C Gordon, CEO

4354 Cancer Research Center
3501 Berrywood Drive
Columbia, MO 65201-6570
573-875-2255

Dr. Abraham Eisenstark, Director
Marnie Tutt, Executive Director

4355 Cancer Research Center: Albert Einstein College of Medicine
1300 Morris Park Avenue
Bronx, NY 10461-1900
718-430-2302
Fax: 718-822-6538
aecc@aecom.yu.edu
www.einstein.yu.edu

4356 Cancer Research Foundation of America
1600 Duke Street
Alexandria, VA 22314-3466
703-836-4412
Fax: 703-836-4413
mmcleod@crfa.org
www.preventcancer.or

521

Scott McIntyre, Chairperson
Carolyn Aldige, President and Founder
Gary Lytle, VC

4357 Cancer Research Institute
New England Deaconess Hospital
330 Brookline Ave
Boston, MA 02215-5324
617-667-7000
Fax: 212-832-9376; *Toll Free:* 800-439-0183
www.bidmc.org

Allan Bufferd, Treasurer
Daniel Jick, Chair
Carol Anderson, VC

4358 Cancer Research Institute of New York
29 Broadway
4th Floor
New York, NY 10006
212-688-7515
Fax: 212-832-9376; *Toll Free:* 800-99C-ANCE
info@cancerresearch.org
www.cancerresearch.org

Jill O'Donne Tormey, PhD, CEO/Dir., Scientific Affairs
Brian M Brewer, Dir., Marketing/Communications

Cancer Research Institute (CRI) is the world's leading non-profit organization dedicated exclusively to harnessing the immune system's power to conquer all cancers.

Year Founded: 1953

4359 Cancer Therapy and Research Center
7979 Wurzbach Rd
San Antonio, TX 78229-3779
210-450-1000
Fax: 210-692-9823; *Toll Free:* 800-340-2872
www.ctrc.net

Thompson Ian M, MD, Executive Director
Ortiz Sheri, Relationship Manager
Jackson Mary, Director

Year Founded: 1974

4360 City of Hope Clinical Cancer Research Center
1450 E Duarte Road
Duarte, CA 91010
626-359-8111
Fax: 626-301-8111
www.cityofhope.org

Paul A Chervenick, Director
Argelia J Sandoval, MD

4361 College of Physicians & Surgeons: Columbia University Cancer Center
College of Physicians and Surgeons
630 W 168th Street
New York, NY 10032-3795
212-305-2575
www.ps.columbia.edu

William L Young, MD

4362 Colorado Cancer Research Program
Presbyterian-St. Luke's Medical Center
1719 E 19th Avenue
Denver, CO 80218-1235

303-839-6000
Fax: 303-839-7294
www.pslmc.com

Ester Hayden, Executive Director
Mimi Roberson, CEO

4363 Colorectal Center at St Elizabeth's Medical Center of Boston
736 Cambridge Street
5th Floor
Boston, MA 02135-2907
617-789-3000
Fax: 617-789-3204
www.semc.org

Robert Haddad, CEO

Multidisplinary service for the diagnosis and management of medical and surgical disorders of the colon and rectum.

4364 Columbia University Comprehensive Cancer Center
701 W 168th Street
New York, NY 10032-2704
212-851-4680
Fax: 212-305-6889
www.hiccc.columbia.edu

I Bernard Weinstein, Director
Stephen Emerson,PhD, MD
Sadie Maloof, MBA, Director

Year Founded: 1911

4365 Dana-Farber Institute: Division of Biostistics & Epidemiology
450 Brookline Ave
Boston, MA 02215
617-632-3000
Fax: 617-737-8614
bcb@jimmy.harvard.edu
www.bcb.dfci.harvard.edu

Dr. Marvin Zelen, Chief
Edward Benz, President
Karen Abbet, Administration

Integral unit of the Institute organized into laboratories of biostatistics, computing and epidemiology.

4366 Eastern Cooperative Oncology Group
420 N Charter Street
Room 4765
Madison, WI 53706
608-263-6650
Fax: 608-262-4403
www.ecog.dfci.harvard.edu

Dr. Tormey, Chairperson

Studies into cancer, including biological response modifiers and cancer studies.

4367 Emory University: Georgia Center for Cancer Statistics
201 Dowman Drive
Atlanta, GA 30322-1013
404-727-6069
Fax: 404-727-8737
www.emory.edu

Raymond S Greenberg MD, PhD, Director
William T Branch Jr, MD

Serves as a cancer registry for five counties of metropolitan Atlanta and ten rural counties of central Georgia.

4368 Emory University: Winship Cancer Center
1365 Clifton Road NE
Atlanta, GA 30322-1013
404-778-1900
Fax: 404-248-5016; *Toll Free:* 888-946-7447
www.winshipcancer.emory.edu

Kenneth W Sell MD, Director
Thomas Emory, Owner

A clinical cancer center coordinating basic and clinical cancer research.

Year Founded: 1937

4369 Fox Chase Cancer Center: Institute for Cancer Research
333 Cottman Ave
Philadelphia, PA 19111-2497
215-728-6900
Fax: 215-728-3574
www.fccc.edu

Minhhuyen Nguyen, MD
Comprehensive cancer center

4370 Fred Hutchinson Cancer Research Center
1100 Fairview Avenue N
Seattle, WA 98109-4433
206-288-1024
www.fhcrc.org

Lee Hartwell, CEO

4371 Georgetown University: Vincent T Lombardi Cancer Research Center
3800 Reservoir Road NW
Washington, DC 20007-2113
202-342-2400
Fax: 202-687-6402
www.lombardi.georgetown.edu

Marc Lippman MD, Director
Joy Drass, CEO

4372 Geraldine Brush Cancer Research Institute
Medical Research Institute
2330 Clay Street
San Francisco, CA 94115-1932
415-561-1728
Fax: 415-561-1390

Dr. Helene S Smith, Director

4373 Goodwin Institute for Cancer Research
1850 NW 69th Avenue
Plantation, FL 33313-4569
954-587-9020
Fax: 954-587-6378
www.rgicr.nova.edu

Claire Thuning-Robinson, Director
Richard Dix, Executive Director

4374 Hauptman-Woodward Medical ResearchInstitute
700 Ellicott Street
Buffalo, NY 14203-1102

716-898-8600
Fax: 716-898-8660
www.hwi.buffalo.edu

Richard Aubrecht, Ph.D., Chairman of the Board
Eaton E. Lattman, Ph.D., Executive Director & CEO
Robert H. Blessing, Ph.D., Vice President and Interim Chair

Nonprofit organization devoted to cancer research.

4375 Heimlich University
2368 Victory Parkway
Suite 410
Cincinnati, OH 45206-2810
513-221-0002
Fax: 513-221-0003

Henry J Heimlich MD, President

Malaria therapy for cancer and Lyme Disease.

4376 Henry Vogt Cancer Research Institute
James Graham Brown Cancer Center
529 S Jackson Street
Louisville, KY 40292
502-562-0082
Fax: 502-588-7799
www.browncancercenter.org

Roger H Herzig MD, Director

4377 Hereditary Cancer Institute
Creighton University
Omaha, NE 68178
402-280-2700
Fax: 402-280-1734
www.creighton.edu

Henry T Lynch MD, President

Offers research into hereditary cancer including studies of its incidence and patterns.

4378 Hipple Cancer Research Center
601 W Riverview Avenue
Dayton, OH 45406-5543
937-293-8508
Fax: 937-293-7652
www.ohiocancer.org

Dr. Martin Murphy Jr, President

Nonprofit organization focusing research activities primarily on cancer, studies on human tumor cloning, hormone purification and human tumor marker identification.

4379 Howard University Cancer Center
2041 Georgia Avenue NW
Washington, DC 20060
202-865-6711
Fax: 202-667-1686
www.cancer.howard.edu

Dr. Alfred Goldson, Interim Director
Sandra Holt, Administrator

4380 Illinois Cancer Center
200 S Michigan Avenue
Chicago, IL 60604-2402
312-739-0600
Fax: 312-986-0404
www.illinoiscancercare.com

Shirley Lansky MD, President

Serves as a consortium cancer research center for the state of Illinois in National Cancer Institute's nationwide program for coordinating basic and clinical cancer research.

4381 Illinois Oncology Research Association

900 Main Street
Suite 780
Peoria, IL 61602-1067
309-672-5681
Fax: 312-986-0404
www.illinoiscancercare.com

Robert Cooper, Director
James Knost, MD

Research into cancer treatments.

4382 Indiana University Laboratory for Experimental Oncology
School of Medicine

702 Barnhill Drive
Indianapolis, IN 46202-5128
317-274-7921
Fax: 317-274-3939
www.med.stanford.edu

Prof. George Weber MD, Director

4383 Institute for Cancer and Blood Research

150 N Robertson Boulevard
Beverly Hills, CA 90211-2142
310-657-4706
Fax: 310-657-2185
www.cincinnatichildrens.org

Dr. Howard Bierman, Scientific Director
Susan Kane, Administrator

4384 Iowa Oncology Research Association

300 E Locust St
Des Moines, IA 50309
515-244-7586
Fax: 515-244-7757
www.iora.org

Roscoe F Morton MD, Principal Investigator
Sherri Rickabaugh, Administrator

Clinical cancer studies and research.

Year Founded: 1878

4385 Ireland Cancer Center at Case Western Reserve University

2074 Abington Road
Cleveland, OH 44106
216-844-5432
Fax: 216-844-1129

Patty Balas, Manager

4386 JL and Helen Kellogg Cancer Care Center
Evanston Hospital

2650 Ridge Avenue
Evanston, IL 60201-1718
847-570-2000
Fax: 847-570-2918

Dr. JD Khandekar, Director
Raymond Grady, CEO

Integral unit of the Evanston Hospital, this center researches treatment and diagnosis of cancer, including phase 1 and phase 2 studies.

4387 John P Caulfield Technology Extension Center for Cancer Treatment

1 Bruce Street
Newark, NJ 07103-2709
973-456-4600
Fax: 973-456-7047

David M Goldenberg, Director

Develops and provides new and more effective technologies for the early detection, diagnosis and treatment of cancer.

4388 Johns Hopkins Oncology Center

401 N Broadway
Room B156
Baltimore, MD 21287
410-955-5222
www.hopkinskimmelcancercenter.org

Edward Chambers, Administrator

4389 Jonsson Comprehensive Cancer Center
University of California at Los Angeles

100 Ucla Medical Plaza
Suite 255
Los Angeles, CA 90024-6900
310-443-8999
Fax: 310-825-5268; *Toll Free:* 800-825-2631
www.cancer.ucla.edu

Robert Mohr DPM, Owner

4390 Kansas State University: Center for Basic Cancer Research
Division of Biology

1 Chalmers Hall
Kansas State University
Manhattan, KS 66506
785-532-6705
Fax: 785-532-6707
cancerresearch@k-state.edu
www.kso.edu/cancer.center

Dr. Rob Denell, Director
Terry C. Johnson, Founder
Dr. Keith Chapes, Associate Director

4391 Kaplan Cancer Center
New York University Medical Center

550 1st Avenue
New York, NY 10016-6402
212-964-1800
Fax: 212-263-2150
www.myelomabeacon.com

Mitchell Kaplan CPA, Owner

The mission of NYU Cancer Institute is to decrease and eliminate cancer as a significant helth problem throughout New York, the nation, and the world, by developing and maintaining excellent programs in patient care, research, education and prevention.

4392 Kentucky Cancer Program

800 Rose Street
Lexington, KY 40536
859-219-0772
Fax: 859-258-1902
www.kycancerprogram.org

Gilbert H Friedell, Director
Candace Robbinnette, Manager

4393 Koch Institute for Integrated CancerResearch at MIT
77 Massachusetts Avenue
Cambridge, MA 02139-4307
617-253-6403
Fax: 617-324-2238
cancer@mit.edu
ki.mit.edu/

Tyler Jacks, Director
Anne E. Deconinck, Executive Director
Jacqueline Lees, Associate Director

4394 La Jolla Cancer Research Foundation
10901 N Torrey Pines Road
La Jolla, CA 92037-1005
858-646-3100
Fax: 858-455-0181

Erkki Rudslahti MD, President

4395 Leukemia Research Foundation
4761 W Touhy Avenue
Suite 211
Lincolnwood, IL 60712-1622
312-982-1480
Fax: 312-982-1485
www.nfcr.org

Janie Weisenberg, Executive Director
Judith P. Barnhard, Chairman
Robert T. Bosserman, Founder

Founded to conquer leukemia by funding research into the causes and cures of the disease and to enrich the quality of life by those touched by leukemia.

4396 Mayo Comprehensive Cancer Center
200 First Street SW
Rochester, MN 55905
507-284-2511
www.mayo.edu

Denis Cortese, President

4397 Melanoma Research Foundation
1411 K Street, NW
Suite 800
Washington, DC 20005
202-347-9675
Fax: 202-347-9678; *Toll Free:* 800-MRF-1290
info@melanoma.org
www.melanoma.org

Timothy Turnham, Ph.D., Executive Director

Founded in October 1996 by melanoma patients and their families to support research which will lead to a cure for melanoma. Strictly a volunteer organization - not one person will receive compensation for his or her efforts.

4398 Natalie Warren Bryant Cancer Center
St. Francis Hospital
5151 S Yale Avenue
Tulsa, OK 74135-7404
918-494-2273
Fax: 918-494-1886
www.saintfrancis.com

Dr. Alan M Keller, Principal Investor

Year Founded: 1975

4399 National Cancer Institute
US Department of Health & Human Services
9609 Medical Center Drive
Bethesda, MD 20892-9760
301-496-2481
Fax: 301-402-2594; *Toll Free:* 800-422-6237
www.nci.nih.gov

Harold Varmus, M.D., Director

NCI grants and contracts support cancer research in most of the Nation's university medical centers and many other non-Federal institutions. NCI also coordinates the cancer research programs of Federal and private institutions in accordance with a constantly updated National Cancer Program, which encompasses the lines of research effort considered to be most important in solving the major problems of cancer.

4400 National Foundation for Cancer Research
4600 E West Highway
Suite 525
Bethesda, MD 20814
301-654-1250
Fax: 301-654-5824; *Toll Free:* 800-321-2873
info@nfcr.org
www.nfcr.org

Franklin C. Salisbury Jr., CEO
Sujuan Ba, President & COO

Year Founded: 1973

4401 New York University: Kaplan Comprehensive Cancer Center
550 1st Avenue
New York, NY 10016-6402
212-263-5349
Fax: 212-263-8211
www.nyu.edu/kccc/homepage.html

Franco Muggia MD, Director

4402 Ohio State University Comprehensive Cancer Center
Arthur G James Cancer Hospital
300 W. 10th Ave.
Columbus, OH 43210-1240
614-293-3810Toll free: 800-293-5066
jamesline@osumc.edu
cancer.osu.edu

Michael A. Caligiuri, MD, Director
Jeff Walker, MBA, Senior Executive Director
Peter Shields, MD, Deputy Director

4403 Ohio State University: Clinical Research Center
2115 Davis Medical Research Center
480 Medical Center Drive
Columbus, OH 43210-1240
614-293-6140
Fax: 614-293-6140
www.osu.edu

William B. Malarkey, Program Director
David Phillips, Administrative Manager
Diane Habash, Bionutrition Manager

Provides facilities and financial support for inpatient and outpatient cancer research.

4404 Oklahoma Medical Research Foundation: Immunology & Cancer Research
825 NE 13th Street, MS 23
Oklahoma City, OK 73104-5097
405-271-7905
Fax: 405-271-8568
paul-kincade@omrf.org
omrf.org

Dr. Stephen Prescott, President
Mike D. Morgan, Executive Vice Presidnet & COO
Adam Cohen, Senior VP & General Counsel

4405 Purdue University Cancer Center
Hansen Life Sciences Research Building, Room 141
201 S. University Street
West Lafayette, IN 47907-2064
765-494-9129
Fax: 765-494-9193
cancerresearch@purdue.edu
www.cancerresearch.purdue.edu

Dr. Timothy Ratliff, Director
Tim Bobillo, Director of Development
Doug Cuttell, Managing Director

4406 Robert H. Lurie Comprehensive Cancer Center of Northwestern University
303 E Chicago Avenue
L3 - 125
Chicago, IL 60611-3072
312-908-5250
Fax: 312-908-1372
cancer.northwestern.edu

Leonidas Platanias, MD, PhD, Interim Director
Al Benson III, MD, FACP, Associate Director
David Cella, PhD, Associate Director

4407 Roger Williams Cancer Research
Roger Williams Medical Center
825 Chalkstone Avenue
Providence, RI 02908
401-456-2000
Fax: 401-456-6793
www.rwmc.org/

Sheri L. Smith, Ph.D.,, Chair
Rev. Kenneth Sicard, Vice Chairman
Kenneth H. Belcher, President

4408 Roswell Park Cancer Institute
Roswell Park Cancer Institute (RPCI)
Elm and Carlton Streets
Buffalo, NY 14263
716-845-2300Toll free: 877-275-7724
askrpci@roswellpark.org
www.roswellpark.org/

Donna Gioia, Chair
Donald L. Trump, MD, President and CEO
Sylvia M. Tokasz, Consultant

Year Founded: 1898

4409 Salk Institute for Biological Studies Library
Salk Institute for Biological Studies
10010 N Torrey Pines Rd
La Jolla, CA 92037
858-453-4100
Fax: 858-453-8534
webrequest@salk.edu, communications@salk.edu

www.salk.edu/

Irwin Mark Jacobs, Sc.D., Chair
Darlene Marcos Shiley, Co-Vice Chair
Theodore W. Waitt, Co-Vice Chair

Basic science research in the areas of molecular biology, genetics, neuroscience, AIDS, Alzheimer's disease, biochemistry, cancer, neurobiology, plant biology, structural biology, virology.

Year Founded: 1960

4410 Skin Cancer Foundation
The Skin Cancer Foundation
149 Madison Avenue
Suite 901
New York, NY 10016
212-725-5176
Fax: 212-725-5751
www.skincancer.org/

Perry Robins, MD, President
Mary Stine, Executive Director
Carla Barry-Austin, Director, Marketing Communicatio

Conducts public and medical education programs to help reduce skin cancer. Major goals are to increase public awareness of the importance of taking protective measures against the damaging rays of the sun and to teach people how to recognize the early signs of skin cancer.

Year Founded: 1979

4411 University of Alabama at Birmingham: Comprehensive Cancer Center
University of Alabama at Birmingham
1720 2nd Ave South
Birmingham, AL 35294
205-934-4011
Fax: 205-975-7428
www.uab.edu/
TDD 205-934-4642

Ray L. Watts, M.D., President
Richard L. Margison, VP, Financial Affairs, Administr
Louis Dale,Ph.D., VP, Equity & Diversity

Year Founded: 1831

4412 University of Arizona Cancer Center
The University of Arizona Cancer Center
3838 North Campbell Avenue
Tucson, AZ 85719-1454
520-694-CURE
Fax: 520-626-2032
azcc.arizona.edu/

Anne E. Cress, PhD, Interim Cancer Center Director
Jesse D. Martinez, PhD, Chief Scientific Officer
M. Peter Lance, MD, Chief Cancer Control Officer

Year Founded: 1976

4413 University of California: Berkeley Cancer Research Laboratories
University of California at Berkeley
447 Life Science Addition
Berkeley, CA 94720-2751
510-642-0411
Fax: 510-642-5741
crl.berkeley.edu/

Russell Vance, Director
Judith Yee, Manager
Holly Aaron, Imaging Center Specialist

Research with a special emphasis on mammary and hepatic cancers.

Year Founded: 1951

4414 University of California: Irvine Cancer Research Institute
UC Irvine Department of Molecular Biology & Bioche
Irvine, CA 92717
949-824-4915
Fax: 714-886-4023
cchughes@uci.edu, bvarela@uci.edu
mbb.bio.uci.edu/

Christopher Hughes, Professor & Chair
Bessy J. Varela, Department Administrator
Vanessa Lopez, Director of Finance
Year Founded: 1858

4415 University of California: San Diego Cancer Center
UC San Diego Moores Cancer Center
3855 Health Sciences Drive
La Jolla, CA 92093
858-534-7000
Fax: 858-534-7628
cancer.ucsd.edu/

William (Bil Koman Jr., Chairman
Scott M. Lippman, MD, Director
Sandy T. Liarakos, CFRE, Executive Director of Developmen
Year Founded: 1978

4416 University of California: San Francisco Cancer Research Institute
UCSF Helen Diller Family Comprehensive Cancer Cent
PO Box 0981
San Francisco, CA 94143-0981
415-476-2557
Fax: 415-476-3541; Toll Free: 888-689-8273
communications@cc.ucsf.edu
cancer.ucsf.edu/

Frank McCormick, PhD, FRS, Director
Martin McMahon, PhD, Asst. Director
Rena J. Pasick, DrPH, Asst. Director

4417 University of Chicago: Cancer Research Center
University of Chicago Cancer Research Foundation
5841 S Maryland Avenue
MC 1140
Chicago, IL 60637
773-702-6180
Fax: 773-702-0666; Toll Free: 855-702-8222
feedback@bsd.uchicago.edu
cancer.uchicago.edu/

Mary Ellen Connellan, MA, Executive Director
Michelle M. Le Beau, PhD, Director
Marcy A. List, PhD, Associate Director for Administr
Year Founded: 1972

4418 University of Chicago: Clinical Nutrition Research Unit
University of Chicago Cancer Research Foundation
5841 S Maryland Avenue
MC 1140
Chicago, IL 60637
773-702-6180Toll free: 855-702-8222
feedback@bsd.uchicago.edu
cancer.uchicago.edu/

Mary Ellen Connellan, MA, Executive Director
Michelle M. Le Beau, PhD, Director
Marcy A. List, PhD, Associate Director for Administr
Year Founded: 1972

4419 University of Kansas Cancer Center
The University of Kansas Cancer Center
3901 Rainbow Boulevard
Kansas City, KS 66160-7220
913-588-1227
Fax: 913-588-4701; Toll Free: 800-332-6048
www.kucancercenter.org/

Roy Jensen, MD, Director
Shrikant Anant, PhD, Associate Director, Cancer Preve
Teresa Christenson, Associate Director, Administrati

4420 University of Michigan Cancer Center
University of Michigan Comprehensive Cancer Center
1500 East Medical Center Drive
CCGC 6-303
Ann Arbor, MI 48109-0944
734-936-4000
Fax: 734-936-9582
mcancer.org/

Max S. Wicha, M.D., Director
Kathleen Cooney, M.D., Deputy Director for Clinical Ser
Maha H. Hussain, M.D., Associate Director of Clinical R
Year Founded: 1986

4421 University of Minnesota: Coordinating Centers for Biometric Research
University of Minnesota University Office Plaza
2221 University Avenue SE
Minneapolis, MN 55414
612-626-8887
Fax: 612-626-9054
www1.umn.edu/twincities/maps/UOffPl/

Thomas A Louis, Division Head
Cancer research
Year Founded: 1972

4422 University of Minnesota: Masonic Cancer Center
University of Minnesota Masonic Cancer Center
425 East River Road
Minneapolis, MN 55455
612-625-5411
Fax: 612-625-8966; Toll Free: 888-CAN-ER M
www.cancer.umn.edu/

Ruth Bachman, Chair
Douglas Yee, M.D., Director
Susan Collins, Finance and Operations Director
Year Founded: 1991

4423 University of Nebraska at Omaha: Eppley Institute for Research in Cancer
Eppley Institute for Research in Cancer and Allied
985950 Nebraska Medical Center
Omaha, NE 68198-5950
402-559-4090
Fax: 402-559-4651
www.unmc.edu/eppley/

Jeffery P. Gold, M.D., Director
Dr. Jennifer Larsen, MD, Vice-Chancellor for Research
Don Leuenberger, Vice-Chancellor for Business & F

Focuses on the causes, prevention and early detection of cancer.

Year Founded: 1960

4424 University of New Mexico Cancer Center
University of New Mexico Cancer Center
900 Camino De Salud NE
Albuquerque, NM 87131
505-277-0111
Fax: 505-277-2841; *Toll Free:* 800-225-5866
cancer.unm.edu/

Cheryl L. Willman, MD, Director
Wadih Arap, MD, PhD, Deputy Chair

4425 University of New Mexico: Center for Non-Invasive Diagnosis
The University of New Mexico
1 University of New Mexico
Albuquerque, NM 87131
505-277-2631
Fax: 505-277-3173
uac@unm.edu
uac.unm.edu/non-degree/

Dr. Nicholas Matwiyoff, Director

Cardiology and cancer research.

4426 University of Pennsylvania Cancer Center
Abramson Cancer Center of the University of Pennsy
3535 Market Street
Suite 750
Philadelphia, PA 19104-3309
215-898-0578
Fax: 215-573-2800; *Toll Free:* 800-789-PENN
holly.auer@uphs.upenn.edu
www.penncancer.org/

Chi Dang, MD, PhD, Director
Robert F. Wynne, Executive Director for Administr
Joseph R. Carver, MD, Chief of Staff

4427 University of Pennsylvania: Comparative Leukemia Unit
University of Pennsylvania, School of Veterinary M
382 W Street Road
Kennett Square, PA 19348
610-444-5800
Fax: 610-925-8123
www.vet.upenn.edu/about/campuses/new-bol

Joan Hendricks, VMD, PhD, Dean
Malcolm J. Keiter, Associate Dean, Admissions
Robert Schieri, MBA, CPA, Vice Dean and Chief Financial Of

Year Founded: 1952

4428 University of Southern California's Hematology, Hematologic Malignancy and Retroviral Research Program
USC Norris Comprehensive Cancer Center
1441 Eastlake Avenue
Los Angeles, CA 90033
323-865-3000
Fax: 323-865-0060; *Toll Free:* 800-USC-CARE
horner@hsc.usc.edu
ccnt.hsc.usc.edu/hamatology/index.html

Stephen Gruber, M.D., Ph.D., M, Director
John Baker, Senior Executive Director for De
Amy S. Lee, Ph.D., Associate Director for Basic Res

Cancer research.

Year Founded: 1973

4429 University of Southern California: Comprehensive Cancer Center
USC Norris Comprehensive Cancer Center
1441 Eastlake Avenue
Los Angeles, CA 90033
323-865-3000Toll free: 800-USC-CARE
ccnt.hsc.usc.edu/hamatology/index.html

Stephen Gruber, M.D., Ph.D., M, Director
John Baker, Senior Executive Director for De
Amy S. Lee, Ph.D., Associate Director for Basic Res

Year Founded: 1973

4430 University of Southern California: Kenneth T Norris Jr Comprehensive Cancer Center
USC Norris Comprehensive Cancer Center
1441 Eastlake Avenue
Los Angeles, CA 90033
323-865-3000Toll free: 800-USC-CARE
ccnt.hsc.usc.edu/hamatology/index.html

Stephen Gruber, M.D., Ph.D., M, Director
John Baker, Senior Executive Director for De
Amy S. Lee, Ph.D., Associate Director for Basic Res

Year Founded: 1973

4431 University of Tennessee: Memphis Cancer Center
The University of Tennessee Health Science Center
920 Madison Ave.
Memphis, TN 38163
901-448-5500
Fax: 901-528-5033
www.uthsc.edu/cancer/
TDD 901-448-7382

Dr. Joe DiPietro, President
Keith Carver, Executive Assistant
Jane Pullum, Administrative Assistant

Year Founded: 1911

4432 University of Texas: MD Anderson Cancer Center
The University of Texas MD Anderson Cancer Center
1515 Holcombe Boulevard
Houston, TX 77030
713-792-2121
www.mdanderson.org/

Ronald A. DePinho, M.D., President
Tom Buchholz, M.D., Executive Vice President and Phy
Leon J. Leach, Ph.D., Executive Vice President and Chi

Year Founded: 1941

4433 University of Texas: Medical Branch at Galveston Cancer Center
UTMB Public Affairs
301 University Boulevard
Galveston, TX 77555-0144
409-772-1011
Fax: 409-772-4865
public.affairs@utmb.edu
www.utmb.edu/cancer/

David L. Callender, MD, MBA, FA, President
Carolee "Car King, JD, Senior Vice President and Genera
Sheila Lidstone, Chief of Staff, Office of the Pr

Year Founded: 1891

4434 University of Vermont Cancer Center
University of Vermont College of Medicine
The Courtyard at Given
4th Floor North, 89 Beaumont Avenue

Burlington, VT 5405

802-656-4414
Fax: 802-656-8788; Toll Free: 877-540-HOPE
www.vermontcancer.org/

Gary Stein, Ph.D., Co-Director Professor, Chair, Bi
Kimberly Luebbers, MSHS, R.N.,, Deputy Director for Administrati

Year Founded: 1974

4435 Utah Cancer Center
University of Utah School of Medicine
30 N. 1900 E.
Salt Lake City, UT 84132
801-581-7201
Fax: 801-585-2300
medicine.utah.edu/

Vivian S. Lee, MD, Ph.D, MBA, Dean, School of Medicine
Carrie L. Byington, MD, Vice Dean, Academic Affairs & Fa
Wayne M. Samuelson, MD, Vice Dean, Education

Year Founded: 1905

4436 Virginia Commonwealth University: Massey Cancer Center
VCU Massey Cancer Center
401 College St.
PO Box 980037
Richmond, VA 23298-0037
804-828-0450
Fax: 804-828-8453
AskMassey@vcu.edu
www.massey.vcu.edu/

I David Goldman MD, Director

Gene regulation and prevention of cancer.

4437 Warren Grant Magnuson Clinical Center
10 Center Drive
Bethesda, MD 20892
301-496-2563
Fax: 301-402-2984; Toll Free: 800-411-1222

prpl@mail.cc.nih.gov
www.cc.nih.gov
TTY: 866-411-1010

John I. Gallin, MD, Clinical Center Director
Maureen E. Gormley, MPH, MA, RN, COO
Maria D. Joyce, MBA, CPA, CFO

Established in 1953 as the research hospital of the National Institutes of Health. Designed so that patient care facilities are close to research laboratories so new findings of basic and clinical scientists can be quickly applied to the treatment of patients. Upon referral by physicians, patients are admitted to NIH clinical studies.

4438 Wayne State University Center for Molecular Biology
Center for Molecular Medicine and Genetics
Wayne
3127 Scott Hall
540 East Canfield
Detroit, MI 48201
313-577-5323
Fax: 313-577-5218
sshaw@wayne.edu
genetics.wayne.edu/

Lawrence I. Grossman, Ph.D., fessor and Director
John Kamholz, M.D.,Ph.D., Professor of Neurology & of Mole
Gerald L. Feldman, M.D., Ph.D, Professor of Molecular Medicine

Research focusing on human conditions such as cancer and neuromuscular disorders.

4439 West Virginia University: Mary Babb Randolph Cencer Center
1 Medical Center Dr
Morgantown, WV 26506
304-598-4500
Fax: 304-293-4667; Toll Free: 877-427-2894
www.wvucancer.org

Laura F Gibson, Deputy Director
Scot Remick, Director
Pamela J Foley, Office Manager

4440 Yale University: Comprehensive Cancer Center
333 Cedar Street
New Haven, CT 06510
203-785-4095
Fax: 203-785-4116
yalecancercenter.org

Thomas J Lynch, Jr., MD, Director
Kevin Vest, MBA, FACHE, Deputy Director, Administration
Chad Ellis, PhD, Deputy Director, Research

Death & Bereavement

Associations & Organizations

4441 A Little Hope - The National Foundationfor Grieving Children Teens and Families
20 Sterling Road S
Armonk, NY 10504
e-mail: info@alittlehope.org
www.alittlehope.org

Richard H. Schimel, President
Tanhya Vancho Schimel, Vice President & Secretary
Sanford Weintraub, Treasurer

The foundation's mission is to help provide bereavement support services and grief counseling for children, teens and young adults who have experienced the loss of a parent, sibling, or a loved one, regardless of the circumstances of the death.

Year Founded: 2002

4442 Association for Death Education and Counseling
One Parkview Plaza
Suite 800
Oakbrook Terrace, IL 60181
847-686-2240
Fax: 847-686-2251
adec@adec.org
www.adec.org

Christopher Hall, President
Heidi L. Parker, Secretary
William G. Hoy, Treasurer

Professional organization dedicated to promoting excellence and recognizing diversity in death education, care of the dying, grief counseling, and research in thantology. Based on quality research, theory and practice, the association provides information, support, and resources to the public.

4443 Compassion Books
7036 State Highway 80 South
Burnsville, NC 28714
828-675-5909
Fax: 828-675-9687; *Toll Free:* 800-970-4220
orders@compassionbooks.com
www.compassionbooks.com

A resource organization providing networking, training and resources related to loss and grief, death and dying, comfort and hope. The organization's primary concern is to help people of all ages transform the despair and hopelessness that often accompanies death and loss into healing awareness and a deeper spiritual connectedness to all life.

Year Founded: 1981

4444 Compassion and Choices
PO Box 101810
Denver, CO 80250
Fax: 866-312-2690; *Toll Free:* 800-247-7421
www.compassionandchoices.org

Barbara Coombs Lee, President
Marcia Campbell, CFO
Trish Bernstein, COO

Provides information, counseling, and emotional support to terminally ill patients who are deciding how life should come to an end. This includes counseling patients and families about intensive pain management, comfort or hospice care, and safe, effective methods for hastening death.

Year Founded: 1993

4445 Compassionate Friends
PO Box 3696
Oak Brook, IL 60522
630-990-0010
Fax: 630-990-0246; *Toll Free:* 877-969-0010
nationaloffice@compassionatefriends.org
www.compassionatefriends.org

Alan Pedersen, Executive Director
Lisa Corrao, COO

A national organization that offers 470 local chapters that give support to people who have experienced the death of a child. Offers monthly support meetings to get through the difficult times and learn how to cope.

Year Founded: 1969

4446 Gundersen Health System
1900 South Avenue
La Crosse, WI 54601
608-782-7300Toll free: 800-362-9567
www.gundersenhealth.org

Scott Rathgaber, CEO

Seeks to promote bereavement care by developing and continually improving bereavement training and support materials and by providing respectful, compassionate care for those experiencing a loss.

Year Founded: 1981

4447 Hospice Foundation of America
1710 Rhode Island Avenue NW
Suite 400
Washington, DC 20036
202-457-5811Toll free: 800-854-3402
hospicefoundation.org

Amy Tucci, President & CEO

Provides leadership in the development and application of hospice and its philosophy of care with the goal of enhancing the U.S. health care system and the role of hospice within it.

4448 International Cemetery, Cremation and Funeral Association
107 Carpenter Drive
Suite 100
Sterling, VA 20164
703-391-8400
Fax: 703-391-8416; *Toll Free:* 800-645-7700
www.iccfa.com

Robert M. Fells, Executive Director
Nadira E. Baddeliyanage, Director, Operations
Robert Treadway, Director, Communications

Serves the needs of the cemetery, funeral service, cremation and memorialization professions with a number of services and products.

Year Founded: 1887

4449 National Association for Home Care & Hospice
Hospice Association of America
228 7th Street SE
Washington, DC 20003

202-546-4759
Fax: 202-547-9559
www.nahc.org/haa
Denise Schrader, Chair

Promotes the concepts of hospice, a philosophy of health care which is expressed through the provision of a variety of medical and nonmedical services to terminally ill patients and their families.

Year Founded: 1982

4450 National Hospice and Palliative Care Organization
1731 King Street
Suite 100
Alexandria, VA 22314
703-837-1500
Fax: 703-837-1233
www.nhpco.org

J. Donald Schumacher, President & CEO
John Mastrojohn, EVP & COO

To lead and mobilize social change for improved care at the end of life.

4451 National Institute for Jewish Hospice
732 University Street
North Woodmere, NY 11581
516-791-9888Toll free: 800-446-4448
nijh.org

Shirley Lamm, Executive Director

Serves as a resource center that seeks to help terminal patients and their families deal with their grief by providing information on traditional Jewish views on death, dying and managing the loss of a loved one.

Year Founded: 1985

4452 Rainbows for all Children
1007 Church Street
Suite 408
Evanston, IL 60201
847-952-1770
Fax: 847-952-1774
rainbows.org

A support program operating in 7 countries for individuals who have suffered a significant loss in their lives due to death, divorce or any other painful transition.

Year Founded: 1983

4453 Right to Life League of Southern California
1028 N Lake Avenue
Suite 207
Pasadena, CA 91104
626-398-6100
Fax: 626-398-6101
media@rtllsc.org
www.rtllsc.org

The Right to Life League of Southern California is an education and service organization dedicated to the support and protection of innocent human life from conception to natural death. We exist to defend the God-given gift of life. We are dedicated to exerting every effort to produce a universal change of heart, resulting in the cessation of the deliberate termination of innocent human life.

Year Founded: 1967

4454 Anatomy of Bereavement
Jason Aronson Publishers
400 Keystone Industrial Park
Dunmore, PA 18512-1507
Fax: 201-840-7242; *Toll Free:* 800-782-0015
www.aronson.com

In this comprehensive book, Dr. Raphael describes all the stages of mourning and healing.

454 pages

4455 Compassion Book Service
Mail Order Division
7036 State Hwy 80 South
Burnsville, NC 28714-7569
828-675-5909
Fax: 828-675-9687
orders@compassionbooks.com
www.compassionbooks.com

Bruce Greene, Vice President

The country's largest mail-order collection of carefully selected books, audios and videos on death and dying, bereavement and change, comfort, healing and hope, collected from hundreds of publishers in the United States.

4456 Grief, Dying and Death
Research Press
PO Box 9177
Champaign, IL 61826-9177
217-352-3273
Fax: 217-352-1221; *Toll Free:* 800-519-2707
rp@researchpress.com
www.researchpress.com

Russell Pence, President

A comprehensive manual providing theoretical background and practical treatment interventions necessary for working with those who are bereaved or dying.

488 pages

4457 Love You Forever
Compassion Books
477 Hannah Branch Road
Burnsville, NC 28714-7569
828-675-5950
Fax: 828-675-9687
www.compassionbooks.com

This endearing and heart-warming story shows how love can survive death and is passed down for generations to come.

4458 On Death and Dying
MacMillan
175 Fifth Avenue
New York, NY 10010
646-307-5151
us.macmillan.com

A wonderful book offering information on how to deal and cope with death and dying.

4459 Recovery from Bereavement
Jason Aronson Publishers
400 Keystone Industrial Park
Dunmore, PA 18512-1507

Fax: 201-840-7242; *Toll Free:* 800-782-0015
www.aronson.com

Outstanding authorities on loss and bereavement discuss the factors that play a role in successful recovery.

344 pages

4460 So Many of My Friends Have Moved Away or Died
AARP Fulfillment
601 E Street NW
Washington, DC 20049
202-434-2277
Fax: 202-434-3443; *Toll Free:* 800-424-3410
member@aarp.org
www.aarp.org

Willilam D Novelli, CEO

A typical problem faced by older persons, discussion focuses on coping with the loss of old friends and finding new ones.

4461 Talking About Death
Beacon Press
25 Beacon Street
Boston, MA 02108-2824
617-742-2110
Fax: 617-723-3097
www.beacon.org

Helen Atwan, Executive Director

4462 The Tender Scar: Life After the Death of a Spouse
Kregel Publications
PO Box 2607
Grand Rapids, MI 49501-2607
616-451-4775
Fax: 616-451-9330
www.kregel.gospelcom.net

Written by a former physician and recent widower, this warmly practical book guides the bereaved through the grief process and explains how to live after the death of a spouse.

4463 The Wisdom of Death: Six Paths to Understanding Loss and Grief
AuthorHouse
1663 Liberty Drive
Suite 200
Bloomington, IN 47403
888-519-5121
www.authorhouse.com

4464 Treatment of Complicated Mourning
Research Press
PO Box 9177
Champaign, IL 61826-9177
217-352-3273
Fax: 217-352-1221; *Toll Free:* 800-519-2707
rp@researchpress.com
www.researchpress.com

Russell Pence, President

The first book to specifically focus on complicated mourning, often referred to as unresolved or abnormal grief. It provides caregivers with practical therapeutic strategies that are necessary when traditional grief counseling is insufficient.

768 pages

4465 Understanding Dying, Death and Bereavement
Cengage Learning
10 Davis Drive
Belmont, CA 94002
650-595-2350
academic.cengage.com

Coverage encompasses the study of death and dying, the American experience, growing up with death, cultural perspectives including life after death, the dying process, and living with a terminal illness.

Directories

4466 National Directory of Bereavement Support Groups and Services
ADM Publishing
PO Box 608606
Orlando, FL 32860-8606
407-774-5260
Fax: 407-774-5260; *Toll Free:* 800-299-7716
www.admpublishing.com

Mary M Wong, Editor

More than 2,500 bereavement support groups and resources in 12 categories: AIDS, death of a child, death of an infant, general bereavement, grieving children, homicide/murder, organ/tissue donation, pet loss, suicide, vehicular homicide, the widowed, 24-hour crisis hotlines. Entries include: Name, address, phone, fax, geographical area served, requirements for eligibility, description of services offered.

130 pages Frequency: Biennial, June

Websites

4467 Grief and Loss
AARP
601 E Street NW
Washington, DC 20049
Toll Free: 888-687-2277
www.aarp.org/relationships/grief-loss
TTY: 877-434-7598

Jo Ann Jenkins, CEO
Lawrence Flanagan, President

Offers information and resources pertaining to grief and loss. Assists communities in coping and bereavement programs.

Year Founded: 1958; Number of Members: 37,000,000+

4468 ProCon.org
233 Wilshire Boulevard
Suite 200
Santa Monica, CA 90401
310-451-9596
info@procon.org
euthanasia.procon.org

Jay Rakow, CEO
Kambiz Akhavan, President & Managing Editor

Pros and cons of controversial issues.

Research Centers

4469 Center for Thanatology Research
391 Atlantic Avenue
Brooklyn, NY 11217-1701
718-858-3026
Fax: 718-858-3026
rhalporn@pipeline.com
www.thanatology.org

Roberta Halporn, Director

Aging, dying, death, bereavement, and gravestone studies.

4470 University of Minnesota: Center for Bioethics
410 Church Street SE
Suite N504
Minneapolis, MN 55455
612-624-9440
Fax: 612-624-9108
www.med.umn.edu/bioethics

Jeffrey Kahn, Executive Director

Biomedical ethics and ethical issues in health care and
health policy, including the use of fetal tissue in medicine,
human genetics and genetic counseling, ethical issues in
long-term care, humane care of dying people, ethics and
cost-containment, health care reform, and ethics of managed care. Sets up task forces on related issues.

Depression/Mental Health

Associations & Organizations

4471 Alabama Department of Mental Health
PO Box 301410
Montgomery, AL 36130-1410
334-242-3454
Fax: 334-242-0725
alabama.dmh@mh.alabama.gov
www.mh.alabama.gov

James V. Perdue, Commissioner

4472 Alaska Department of Health and Social Services Division of Behavioral Health
3601 C Street
Suite 878
Anchorage, AK 99503
907-269-3600Toll free: 907-269-3623
dhss.alaska.gov/dbh

Randall Burns, Acting Director

4473 American Board of Psychiatry and Neurology
2150 E Lake Cook Road
Suite 900
Buffalo Grove, IL 60089
847-229-6500
Fax: 847-229-6600
www.abpn.com

Larry R. Faulkner, President & CEO
Paul Whittington, CIO
Robin Callen, CFO

Physicians with specialized training in psychiatry, neurology, child neurology, child adolescent psychiatry, clinical neurophysiology, and geriatric psychiatry. Determines eligibility requirements, administers examinations, and certifies physicians.

Year Founded: 1934

4474 Anxiety and Depression Association of America
8701 Georgia Avenue
Suite 412
Silver Spring, MD 20910
240-485-1001
www.adaa.org

Susan K. Gurley, Interim Executive Director
Mary E.L. Gies, Program Director

Offers help, support and information for persons with anxiety disorders, manic and depressive disorders and mental illness.

Year Founded: 1980

4475 Arizona Department of Health Services Division of Behavioral Health Services
150 N 18th Avenue
2nd Floor
Phoenix, AZ 85007
602-364-4558
Fax: 602-364-4570; *Toll Free:* 800-867-5808
dbhsinfo@azdhs.gov
www.azdhs.gov/bhs

4476 Arkansas Department of Human Services Division of Behavioral Health Services
305 South Palm Street
Little Rock, AR 72205
501-686-9164
Fax: 501-686-9182
humanservices.arkansas.gov
TDD 501-686-9176

Charlie Green, Director
Paula Stone, Assistant Clinical Director
Pam Dodson, Assistant Clinical Director

4477 California Department of Health Care Services
1501 Capitol Avenue
PO Box 997413
Sacramento, CA 95899-7413
www.dhcs.ca.gov

Jennifer Kent, Director

4478 Colorado Department of Health Care Behavioral Health Services Programs
1570 Grant Street
Denver, CO 80203-1818
303-866-2993
Fax: 303-866-4411
www.colorado.gov

Susan E. Birch, Executive Director

4479 Connecticut Department of Health & Addiction Services
410 Capitol Avenue
PO Box 341431
Hartford, CT 06134
860-418-7000
www.ct.gov/dmhas

Miriam E. Delphin-Rittmon, Commissioner
Nancy Navarretta, Deputy Commissioner

4480 Delaware Health & Social Services Division of Substance Abuse & Mental Health
1901 N Du Pont Highway
Main Building
New Castle, DE 19720
302-255-9399
Fax: 302-255-4427
www.dhss.delaware.gov/dhss/dsamh

Michael Barbieri, Director

4481 Depression and Bipolar Support Alliance
55 E Jackson Boulevard
Suite 490
Chicago, IL 60604
Fax: 312-642-7243; *Toll Free:* 800-826-3632
www.dbsalliance.org

Allen Doerderlein, President
Cindy Specht, Executive Vice President

Consists of 250 patient groups providing support and direct services to persons with clinical depression.

4482 District of Columbia Department of Behavioral Health
64 New York Avenue NE
3rd Floor
Washington, DC 20002

202-673-2200
Fax: 202-673-3433
dbh@dc.gov
dbh.dc.gov
TTY: 202-673-7500

Tanya A. Royster, Director

4483 Georgia Department of Behavioral Health & Developmental Disabilities

Two Peachtree Street NW
24th Floor
Atlanta, GA 30303
404-657-2252
Fax: 404-463-7149
terri.timberlake@dbhdd.ga.gov
dbhdd.georgia.gov

Terri Timberlake, Dir, Off. of Adult Mental Health

4484 Hawaii Department of Health Adult Mental Health Division

1250 Punchbowl Street
Suite 256
Honolulu, HI 96813
808-586-4686
Fax: 808-586-4745
health.hawaii.gov/amhd

4485 Idaho Mental Health Services

healthandwelfare.idaho.gov

Richard Armstrong, Director

4486 Indiana Family & Social Services Administration Division of Mental Health & Addiction

Toll Free: 800-901-1133
www.in.gov/fssa/dmha

4487 Iowa Department of Human Services

Toll Free: 800-972-2017
dhs.iowa.gov

4488 Kansas Department of Health & Environment

Curtis State Office Building
1000 SW Jackson
Topeka, KS 66612
www.kdheks.gov

4489 Kentucky Department of Behavioral Health, Developmental & Intellectual Disabilities

275 E Main Street 4WG
Frankfort, KY 40621
502-564-4456
Fax: 502-564-9010
dbhdid.ky.gov/dbh

Natalie Kelly, Director

4490 Lewy Body Dementia Association

912 Killian Hill Road SW
Lilburn, GA 30047
404-935-6444
Fax: 480-422-5434
www.lbda.org

Mike Koehler, CEO
Mark Wall, Vice President
Angela Taylor, Director of Programs

Raising awareness of Lewy body dementias and supporting sufferers, their families and caregivers.

4491 Louis de la Parte Florida Mental Health Institute

University of South Florida
13301 Bruce B. Downs Boulevard
MHC 1100
Tampa, FL 33612
813-974-1992
Fax: 813-974-4699
home.fmhi.usf.edu

Dean Serovich, Executive Director

Mental health care, including aging and mental health, child and family studies, community mental health, and mental health law and policy.

Year Founded: 1967

4492 Louisiana Department of Health & Hospitals Office of Behavioral Health

PO Box 629
Baton Rouge, LA 70821-0629
225-342-9500
Fax: 225-342-5568
dhh.louisiana.gov

Rochelle Head-Dunham, Medical Director

4493 Maine Department of Health & Human Services

State House Station 11
41 Anthony Avenue
Augusta, ME 04333-0011
207-287-2595
Fax: 207-287-4334
www.maine.gov/dhhs/samhs/mentalhealth

Sheldon Wheeler, Director

4494 Maryland Department of Health & Mental Hygiene

201 W Preston Street
Baltimore, MD 21201-2399
410-402-8198
Fax: 410-402-8056; *Toll Free:* 877-402-8221
dhmh.maryland.gov/ohcq/mh

4495 Massachusetts Health & Human Services Department of Mental Health

25 Staniford Street
Boston, MA 02114
617-626-8000 Toll free: 800-221-0053
dmhinfo@dmh.state.ma.us
www.mass.gov/dmh
TTY: 617-727-9842

Joan Mikula, Commissioner

Most mental health services, including medication and therapy are provided through health insurance - MassHealth (Medicaid), the Massachusetts Health Connector (health insurance marketplace) or through private insurance (employer-based). The Department of Mental Health (DMH) has a specialized role in the healthcare delivery system as DMH provides supplemental services for people with the most serious needs.

4496 Mental Health America
2000 N Beauregard Street
6th Floor
Alexandria, VA 22311
703-684-7722
Fax: 703-684-5968; *Toll Free:* 800-969-6642
www.nmha.org

Paul Gionfriddo, President & CEO

Serves over 700 affiliates nationally providing information,
publications and other services.

Year Founded: 1909

**4497 Mental Health, Developmental Disabilities, and
Substance Abuse Services**
NC Department of Health and Human Services
2001 Mail Service Center
Raleigh, NC 27699-2001
919-855-4800
www.ncdhhs.gov/divisions/mhddsas

Courtney Cantrell, Contact

Community-based mental health, developmental disabilities and substance abuse services are managed through a
network of local management entities that cover the state's
100 counties. These programs oversee and manage local
services.

**4498 Michigan Department of Health & Human
Services**
Capitol View Building
201 Townsend Street
Lansing, MI 48913
www.michigan.gov/mdhhs

4499 Minnesota Department of Human Services
651-431-2225
mn.gov/dhs/people-we-serve

4500 Mississippi Department of Mental Health
1101 Robert E. Lee Building
230 N Lamar Street
Jackson, MS 39201
601-359-1288
Fax: 601-359-6295; *Toll Free:* 877-210-8513
www.dmh.ms.gov
TDD 601-359-6230

4501 Missouri Department of Mental Health
1706 East Elm Street
Jefferson City, MO 65101
573-751-4122
Fax: 573-751-8224; *Toll Free:* 800-364-9687
dmh.mo.gov

Mark Stringer, Director

**4502 Montana Department of Public Health &
Human Services Mental Health Services
Bureau**
PO Box 4210
Helena, MT 59604-4210
www.dphhs.mt.gov

Richard Opper, Director

4503 National Institute of Mental Health
Fax: 301-443-4279; *Toll Free:* 866-615-6464
nimhinfo@nih.gov

www.nimh.nih.gov
TTY: 866-415-8051

Bruce Cuthbert, Acting Director

Lead federal agency for research on mental disorders.

**4504 Nebraska Department of Health & Human
Services Division of Behavioral Health**
PO Box 95026
Lincoln, NE 68509-5026
402-471-3121
dhhs.ne.gov

Sheri Dawson, Director

4505 Nevada Division of Public & Behavioral Health
775-684-4200
Fax: 775-684-4211
dpbh@health.nv.gov
dpbh.nv.gov

4506 New Hampshire Bureau of Behavioral Health
105 Pleasant Street
Concord, NH 03301
603-271-5000Toll free: 800-852-3345
www.dhhs.nh.gov/dcbcs/bbh/index.htm

**4507 New Jersey Department of Human
ServicesDivision of Mental Health & Addiction
Services**
Capital Place One
PO Box 700
Trenton, NJ 08625
Toll Free: 800-382-6717
www.state.nj.us/humanservices/dmhas/home

**4508 New Mexico Human Services Department
Behavioral Health Services Division**
PO Box 2348
Santa Fe, NM 87504
505-476-9266
Fax: 505-476-9277
www.hsd.state.nm.us

Wayne Lindstrom, Director

4509 New York State Office of Mental Health
44 Holland Avenue
Albany, NY 12229
Toll Free: 800-597-8481
www.omh.ny.gov

**4510 North Carolina Mental Health, Developmental
Disabilities, & Substance Abuse Services**
2001 Mail Service Center
Raleigh, NC 27699-2001
919-855-4800
www.ncdhhs.gov/divisions/mhddsas

Courtney Cantrell, Contact

4511 North Dakota Behavioral Health Services
1237 W Divide Avenue
Suite 1C
Bismarck, ND 58501-1208
701-328-8920
Fax: 701-328-8969; *Toll Free:* 800-755-2719
dhsbhdiv@nd.gov
www.nd.gov/dhs/services/mentalhealth

Pamela Sagness, Director

4512 Ohio Mental Health & Addiction Services
30 E Broad Street
8th Floor
Columbus, OH 43215-3430
614-466-2596 Toll free: 877-275-6364
mha.ohio.gov
TTY: 614-752-9696

Tracy J. Plouck, Director

4513 Oklahoma Department of Mental Health & Substance Abuse Services
PO Box 53277
Oklahoma City, OK 73152-3277
405-522-3908
Fax: 405-522-3650; Toll Free: 800-522-9054
ok.gov/odmhsas
TDD 405-522-3851

Terri White, Commissioner
Durand Crosby, COO

4514 Oregon Addictions and Mental Health Services
500 Summer Street NE
Salem, OR 97301-1079
503-945-5763
Fax: 503-378-8467
amh.web@state.or.us
www.oregon.gov/oha/amh
TTY: 800-375-2863

The AMH division of the Oregon Health Authority provides Oregonians access to mental health and addiction services and supports meeting the needs of adults and children to live, be educated, work and participate in their communities and to help them achieve optimum physical, mental and social well being.

4515 Pennsylvania Department of Human Services
PO Box 2675
Harrisburg, PA 17105-2675
www.dhs.pa.gov

4516 Rhode Island Department of Behavioral Healthcare, Developmental Disabilities & Hospitals
14 Harrington Road
Cranston, RI 02920
401-462-2339
Fax: 401-462-3204
www.bhddh.ri.gov

Maria Montanaro, Director

4517 South Carolina Department of Mental Health
2414 Bull Street
Columbia, SC 29202
803-898-8581
www.state.sc.us/dmh

4518 South Dakota Department of Social Services Division of Behavioral Health
811 E 10th
Dept. 9
Sioux Falls, SD 57103
605-367-5236
Fax: 605-367-5239
dss.sd.gov/behavioralhealth

Tiffany Wolfgang, Contact

4519 Tennessee Department of Mental Health &Substance Abuse Services
500 Deaderick Street
Nashville, TN 37243
615-532-6500
tn.gov/behavioral-health

E. Douglas Varney, Commissioner

The Department is the state's mental health and developmental disabilities authority and is responsible for system planning, setting policy and quality standards, system monitoring and evaluation, disseminating public information and advocating for persons of all ages who have mental illness, serious emotional disturbance or developmental disability.

4520 Texas Department of State Health Services
PO Box 149347
Austin, TX 78714-9347
512-776-7111 Toll free: 888-963-7111
www.dshs.state.tx.us/MHSA
TDD 800-735-2989

Offers information and referrals.

4521 Utah Department of Human Services Division of Substance Abuse & Mental Health
195 N 1950 W
Salt Lake City, UT 84116
801-538-3939
Fax: 801-538-9892
dsamh@utah.gov
dsamh.utah.gov

4522 Vermont Department of Mental Health
Redstone Building
26 Terrace Street
Montpelier, VT 05609-1101
802-828-3867
Fax: 802-828-1717
mentalhealth.vermont.gov

Frank Reed, Commissioner

4523 Virginia Department of Behavioral Health and Developmental Services
PO Box 1797
Richmond, VA 23218-1797
804-786-3921
Fax: 804-371-6638
www.dbhds.virginia.gov
TDD 804-371-8977

Jack Barber, Interim Commissioner

4524 Washington State Department of Social and Health Services - Mental Health & Addiction Services
PO Box 11699
Tacoma, WA 98411-9905
www.dshs.wa.gov

Kevin W. Quigley, Secretary
Carla Reyes, Ass. Sec., Behav. Health & Rcvry
Year Founded: 2009

4525 West Virginia Bureau for Behavioral Health & Health Facilities
350 Capitol Street
Room 350
Charleston, WV 25301
304-356-4811
Fax: 304-558-1008
www.dhhr.wv.gov/bhhf

4526 Wisconsin Department of Health Services-Division of Mental Health & Substance Abuse Services
PO Box 7851
Madison, WI 53707-7851
608-266-2717
www.dhs.wisconsin.gov/mh/index.htm

Joyce Allen, Director

4527 Wyoming Department of Health - Behavioral Health Division
6101 Yellowstone Road
Suite 220
Cheyenne, WY 82002
307-777-6494
Fax: 307-777-5849; *Toll Free:* 800-535-4006
www.health.wyo.gov/mhsa/index.htm

Thomas O. Forslund, Director
Korin Schmidt, Deputy Director
Eric McVicker, Chief Financial Officer

The Mental Health Division of the Wyoming Department of Health exists to be a leader in providing high-quality behavioral services that anticipate and respond to the changing needs of persons served. Our strategic plan is to advocate for and participate in the development and maintenance of a comprehensive system of mental health services and supports throughout Wyoming, which stresses independence, dignity, security, and recovery.

Books

4528 Anxiety & Depression in Adults & Children
Sage Publications
2455 Teller Road
Thousand Oaks, CA 91320-2218
805-499-0721
Fax: 805-499-0871
www.adaa.org/living-with-anxiety

Blaise R Simqu, CEO

304 pages

4529 Depression & Antidepressants: A Guide
Lithium Information Center
7617 Mineral Point Road
Suite 300
Madison, WI 53717-1623
608-827-2470
Fax: 608-827-2479
www.miminc.org

Margaret Baudhuin, Manager

48 pages 1999

4530 Depression and Its Treatment
Warner Books
1271 Avenue of the Americas
New York, NY 10020-1300
212-522-7200
www.abebooks.com

Laurence J Kirshbaum, CEO

A layman's guide to help one understand and cope with America's #1 mental health problem.

157 pages

4531 Depression, the Mood Disease
Johns Hopkins University Press
2715 N Charles Street
Baltimore, MD 21218-4319
410-516-6900
Fax: 410-516-6998; *Toll Free:* 800-537-5487
www.jhu.edu/press/index.html

William Brody, President

This book explores the many faces of an illness that will affect as many as 36 million Americans at some point in their lives. Updated to reflect state-of-the-art treatment.

240 pages

4532 Listening to Depression: How Understanding Your Pain Can Heal Your Life
New Harbinger
5674 Shattuck Avenue
Oakland, CA 94609
800-748-6273
Fax: 510-652-5472
www.newharbinger.com

Depression For Dummies is to present you with the facts on depression and explain the options for dealing with it..

4533 Mood Apart
Basic Books
10 E 53rd Street
New York, NY 10022-5244
212-832-5550
Fax: 212-207-7203
www.goodreads.com

C Propopulon, Owner

An overview of the depression and manic depression and the available treatments for them.

363 pages

4534 National Institute of Mental Health
Science Writing, Press, and Dissemination Branch
6001 Executive Boulevard, Room 6200, MSC 9663
Bethesda, MD 20892-9663
Fax: 301-443-4279; *Toll Free:* 866-615-6464
nimhinfo@nih.gov
www.nimh.nih.gov
TTY: 866-415-8051

Alissa Gallagher, Branch Chief

A variety of publications is available from this Federal research Institute that conducts and supports research that focuses on the causes, diagnosis, prevention and treatment of severe mental illnesses. The Institute Office of Communications provides a public inquiries line that is staffed with trained information specialists who respond to information requests from the lay public, clinicians, and the scientific community.

4535 Overcoming Depression
Harper & Row
10 E 53rd Street
New York, NY 10022-5244
212-207-7000
Fax: 212-207-7203
www.abebooks.com/Overcoming-Depression-P

Jane Friedman, CEO

318 pages

4536 Questions & Answers About Depression & Its Treatment
Charles Press Publishers
PO Box 15715
Philadelphia, PA 19103
215-496-9616
Fax: 215-496-9637
www.charlespresspub.com

Lauren Meltzer, Owner

All the questions you'd like to ask, asked and answered.

136 pages

4537 The Mindful Way through Depression: Freeing Yourself from Chronic Unhappiness
Guilford Press
72 Spring Street
New York, NY 10012
800-365-7006
Fax: 212-966-6708
info@guilford.com
www.guilford.com

The Mindful Way through Depression draws on the collective wisdom of four internationally renowned mindfulness experts, including bestselling author Jon Kabat-Zinn, to provide effective relief from the most prevalent psychological disorder.

Directories

4538 Depression in the Elderly: Multimedia Sourcebook
Greenwood Publishing Group
88 Post Road W
5007
Westport, CT 06880-4208
203-226-3571
Fax: 203-226-6009; *Toll Free:* 800-225-5800
www.greenwood.com

John J Miletich, Editor
Wayne Smith, President

Information providers, associations, and television programs related to depression in the elderly. Entries include: Contact information. Principal content of publication is annotated entries for a variety of alternate formats covering material from 1970-96.

Journals, Magazines

4539 Journal of Mental Health and Aging
Springer Publishing Company
536 Broadway
New York, NY 10012-3915

212-431-4370
Fax: 212-941-7842
www.springerpub.com

Donna Cohen, Editor
Rafael Ortiz, Advertising Manager
Ursula Springer, President

Scholarly journal covering aging population for mental health professionals.

4540 Journal of the American Psychoanalytic Association
American Psychoanalytic Association
309 E 49th Street
New York, NY 10017-1601
212-752-0450
Fax: 212-593-0571
central.office@apsa.org
www.apsa.org

Dean K Stine, Executive Director
Dottie Jeffries, Director Public Affairs
Steven T Levy, Editor

Quarterly journal.

250 pages 1911 Frequency: 4

4541 Journals of Gerontology; Psychological Sciences & Social Sciences
Gerontological Society of America
1030 15th Street NW
Suite 250
Washington, DC 20005-1526
202-842-1275
Fax: 202-842-1150
geron@geron.org
www.geron.org

Elizabeth Borgen, Contact
Carol Schutz, Executive Director

Two journals under one cover presenting scientific articles and research in the fields of biology and medicine, as they relate to aging.

Frequency: Bimonthly

4542 Rehabilitation Counseling Bulletin
American Counseling Association
5999 Stevenson Avenue
Alexandria, VA 22304-3304
703-823-9800
Fax: 703-823-0252; *Toll Free:* 800-347-6647
www.counseling.org

Stephren Brooks, Editor
Richard Yep, Executive Director

Journal including new information on the rehabilitation field, career development, and job placement of persons with special needs.

Frequency: Quarterly

Newsletters, Pamphlets

4543 Adjustment, Adaptation and Accomodation: Psychological Approaches
National Parkinson Foundation
1501 NW 9th Avenue
Miami, FL 33136-1407

305-547-6666
Fax: 305-548-4403; *Toll Free:* 800-327-4545
www.parkinson.org

Jose Garcia-Pedrosa, Executive Director

Coping strategies for Parkinson's disease.

4544 Bell
National Mental Health Association
1021 Prince Street
Alexandria, VA 22314-2979
703-684-7722
Fax: 703-684-5968
www.nmha.org
TDD 800-433-5959

Sandy Alexander, Publications Manager
Patrick Cody, Senior Director Media Relations
Micheal Faenze, CEO

Targets public and private mental health organizations as well as interested corporations, agencies and individuals. The Bell contains information about a variety of issues pertaining to mental health, including: the effects of managed care on mental health care; the implications of Congressional decisions for mental health; prevention efforts on the local, state and national levels; national anti-stigma efforts and national public education camppaigns.

Frequency: Monthly

4545 Depression and Recovery From Chemical Dependency
Hazelden
15251 Pleasant Valley Road
Center City, MN 55012-9640
651-257-4010
Fax: 651-213-4426; *Toll Free:* 800-328-9000
www.hazelden.org

Ellen Breyer, President

Outlines depression's warning signs.

4546 Mental Health Law Reporter
Business Publishers
951 Pershing Drive
Silver Spring, MD 20910-4400
301-587-6300
Fax: 301-584-4530; *Toll Free:* 800-274-6737
www.bpinews.com

Leonard A Eiserer, Publisher
Bonnie Becker, Editor
Adam Goldstein, President

Brings you the most timely, focused and thorough information on the legal issues that concern mental health practitioners in mental health litigation. Topics include: malpractice litigation, patient-therapist confidentiality, sexual victimization of patients, the insanity defense, social security administrative case law and much more.

8 pages

4547 NFDI Newsletter
National Foundation for Depressive Illness
PO Box 2257
New York, NY 10116-2257
212-268-4260
Fax: 212-268-4434; *Toll Free:* 800-248-4344
pross@att.net
www.depression.org

Amy C Russell, Administrator

To correct the myths and misconceptions surrounding the illness and help reverse the devastating effects depression has on the individual and our society and to inform the public, primary health care providers, other healthcare professionals and corporations about depression and manic depression and to provide the information about correct diagnosis and treatment and the availability of qualified doctors and support groups.

4 pages

4548 National Council News
Nat'l Council of Community Mental Health Center
12300 Twinbrook Parkway
Suite 320
Rockville, MD 20852-1606
301-984-6200
Fax: 301-881-7159
www.thenationalcouncil.org

Linda Rosenberg, CEO

Gives you news about legislative and regulatory developments, public policy and mental health issues, editorials, perspectives, new publications and seminars.

4549 Public Policy Report
National Council of Community Mental
Health Center 12300 Twinbrook Parkway
Suite 320
Rockville, MD 20852
301-984-6200
Fax: 301-881-7159
www.thenationalcouncil.org

Linda Rosenberg, CEO

Information on promoting advocacy, action and association for people with mental disabilities.

Frequency: Monthly

Research Centers

4550 National Alliance for Research on Schizophrenia and Depression
60 Cuttermill Road
Suite 404
Great Neck, NY 11021-3104
516-829-0091
Fax: 516-487-6930
info@narsad.org

Steve Doochin, Executive Director

Raises and distributes funds for scientific research into the causes, cures and treatments, and prevention of severe mental illness, primarily schizophrenia and depression.

4551 St. Louis University: Department of Psychiatry
1221 S Grand Boulevard
Saint Louis, MO 63104-1016
314-577-8742
Fax: 314-664-7248
waldmans@wpogate.slu.edu
www.slucare.edu/clinical/psychiatry

Adult and child psychiatry, geriatric psychiatry, psychopharmacology, psychology, and behavioral medicine, including psychophysiologic reactions in pyschotherapeutic relationships, personality profiles in a general hospital population, emotional response to cardiovascular surgery, emotional responses of children to chronic illness, factors influencing career choice in medicine, and impact of direct entry into psychiatric training on residents and their training programs.

4552 University of Minnesota: Division of Health Services Research and Policy

420 Delaware Street SE
Minneapolis, MN 55455
612-624-6151
Fax: 612-624-2196
krale001@maroon.tc.umn.edu
www.hsr.umn.edu

Long-term care, health insurance, managed health care, patient care outcomes, rural health services, and health policy analysis.

4553 University of Pennsylvania: Depression Research Unit
School of Medicine, Department of Psychiatry

3600 Spruce Street
Philadelphia, PA 19104-4211
215-662-3462
Fax: 215-662-6443
DRU@mail.med.upenn.edu
www.med.upenn.edu/dru/

Jay D Amsterdam MD, Director
Maryanne Giampapa, Manager

Focuses on mental health and depression.

4554 University of Pittsburgh Medical Center: Clinic Western Psychiatric Institute and Clinic

3811 Ohara Street
Pittsburgh, PA 15213-2593
412-624-9167
www.wpic.pitt.edu

Oscar G Bukstein MD

Advancement of basic and clinical knowledge in psychological, biological, environmental, and social interactions related to mental health and psychiatric care. Conducts research on psychiatric disorders, including depression, schizophrenia, anorexia nervosa, Alzheimer's disease, autism, anxiety, obsessive-compulsive disorders, and borderline disorders.adolescent and young adult disorders, affective disorders, psychogeriatrics, schizophrenia, and children's services. Clinical laboratory investigations include studies in clinical pharmacology, neuroendocrinology, psychophysiology, neuropharmacology, neurophysics, molecular neurobiology and genetics, and EEG sleep. Also researches health habits and precursors of medical disease states such as hypertension, diabetes, obesity, effects of drug abuse, and epidemiology of psychiatric disorders.

4555 Yale University: Behavioral Medicine Clinic
Yale School of Medicine

333 Cedar Street
New Haven, CT 06510-3206
203-785-4095
www.psychiatry.yale.edu

Hoyle Leigh MD, Director
Margaret Wylie, Manager

Focuses on mental disorders including schizophrenia and depression.

4556 Yale University: Ribicoff Research Facilities

34 Park Street
New Haven, CT 06510
203-432-0828
Fax: 203-562-7079
www.psychiatry.yale.edu

George Heninger MD, Director
Terri Boustad, Administrator

Clinical research in the areas of schizophrenia, depression and mental disorders.

Diabetes

Associations & Organizations

4557 Academy of Nutrition & Dietetics
120 South Riverside Plaza
Suite 2000
Chicago, IL 60606-6995
312-899-0040 Toll free: 800-877-1600
www.eatrightpro.org

Mary Beth Whalen, Executive Director

Offers information and support to those with special diet needs due to a variety of health issues, includiung diabetes and allergies.

Year Founded: 1917; Number of Members: 75,000+

4558 American Association of Diabetes Educators
200 W Madison Street
Suite 800
Chicago, IL 60606
Toll Free: 800-338-3633
www.diabeteseducator.org

Charles Macfarlane, CEO
Brad Neal, CFO
Ken Widelka, COO

An independent, multidisciplinary organization of health professionals involved in teaching persons with diabetes. The mission is to enhance the competence of health professionals who teach persons with diabetes, advance the specialty practice of diabetes education, and to improve the quality of diabetes education and care for all those affected by diabetes.

4559 American Diabetes Association
1701 North Beauregard Street
Alexandria, VA 22311
Toll Free: 800-342-2383
www.diabetes.org

Robin Richardson, Chair
Kevin L. Hagan, CEO

Offers a network of 52 affiliates with over 55,000 volunteers, including a professional membership of more than 10,000 physicians, social workers, nutritionists, educators and nurses.

Year Founded: 1940

4560 American Diabetes Association: Alabama
3918 Montclair Rd
Suite 218
Birmingham, AL 35213
205-870-5172
Fax: 205-879-2903; Toll Free: 800-342-2383
www.diabetes.org

Stephanie Willis, Market Director
Year Founded: 1940

4561 American Diabetes Association: Alaska
801 W Fireweed Lane
Suite 103
Anchorage, AK 99503
907-272-1424
Fax: 907-272-1428; Toll Free: 800-342-2383
www.diabetes.org

Michelle Cassano, Executive Director
Cyrese Gorrin, Manager, Development
Year Founded: 1940

4562 American Diabetes Association: Arizona
5333 N 7th St
Suite B-212
Phoenix, AZ 85014
602-861-4731
Fax: 602-995-1344; Toll Free: 800-342-2383
www.diabetes.org

Anne Dennis, Area Director
Thomas Donohue, Regional Director, Proj. Mngmnt.
Year Founded: 1940

4563 American Diabetes Association: Arkansas
320 Executive Court
Suite 104
Little Rock, AR 72205
501-221-7444
Fax: 501-221-3138; Toll Free: 800-342-2383
www.diabetes.org

Rick Selig, Director
Becki Swindell, Manager
Year Founded: 1940

4564 American Diabetes Association: Central Florida
2290 Lucien Way
Suite 230
Maitland, FL 32751
407-660-1926
Fax: 407-660-1080; Toll Free: 800-342-2383
www.diabetes.org

Carly Zampiceni, Regional Director, Florida
Nicole Donelson, Area Director, Ctrl & SW Florida
Year Founded: 1940

4565 American Diabetes Association: Central Ohio
1900 Crown Park Court
Suite H
Columbus, OH 43235
614-436-1917
Fax: 614-221-0348; Toll Free: 800-342-2383
www.diabetes.org

Lori Butterfield, Executive Director, Greater Ohio
William Hesse, Campaign Manager, Tour de Cure
Year Founded: 1940

4566 American Diabetes Association: Central Texas
Building 2
9430 Research Boulevard, Suite 150
Austin, TX 78759
512-472-9838
Fax: 512-472-9672; Toll Free: 800-342-2383
ctxinfo@diabetes.org
www.diabetes.org

Michelle Peacock, Executive Director, Ctrl. Texas
Year Founded: 1940

4567 American Diabetes Association: Colorado
2460 W 26th Avenue
Suite 500C
Denver, CO 80211

720-855-1102
Fax: 720-855-1302; *Toll Free:* 800-342-2383
www.diabetes.org

Sue Glass, Vice President, Western Division
Jennifer Klass, Area Director, CO/MT/WY
Kristin Barry, Regional Associate Director
Year Founded: 1940

4568 American Diabetes Association: Connecticut & Western Massachusetts
2080 Silas Deane Highway
2nd Floor
Rocky Hill, CT 06067
203-639-0385
Fax: 860-257-4320; *Toll Free:* 800-342-2383
www.diabetes.org

Patti Clair, Associate Director
Hope Jays, Manager, Special Events
Year Founded: 1940

4569 American Diabetes Association: Districtof Columbia
1400 16th Street NW
Suite 410
Washington, DC 20036
202-331-8303
Fax: 202-331-1402; *Toll Free:* 800-342-2383
www.diabetes.org

Mary Merritt, Executive Director
Kim Cameron, Associate Director, Tour de Cure
Year Founded: 1940

4570 American Diabetes Association: Eastern Pennsylvania & Delaware
150 Monument Road
Suite 100
Philadelphia, PA 19004
610-828-5003
Fax: 610-667-1761; *Toll Free:* 800-342-2383
bala_office@diabetes.org
www.diabetes.org

Denise Andersen, Regional Director
Year Founded: 1940

4571 American Diabetes Association: Georgia
Harris Tower
233 Peachtree Street
Suite 2225
Atlanta, GA 30303
404-320-7100
Fax: 404-581-1904; *Toll Free:* 800-342-2383
www.diabetes.org

Rena Cozart, Regional Director, South
Tiffany Kirkland, Area Director, Georgia
Year Founded: 1940

4572 American Diabetes Association: Hawaii
Pioneer Plaza
900 Fort Street Mall, Suite 940
Honolulu, HI 96813
808-947-5979
Fax: 808-546-7502; *Toll Free:* 800-342-2383
www.diabetes.org

Leslie Lam, Executive Director
Danielle Tuata, Events Director
Year Founded: 1940

4573 American Diabetes Association: Iowa
317 7th Avenue SE
Suite 202B
Cedar Rapids, IA 52401
319-247-5124
Fax: 319-247-5125; *Toll Free:* 800-342-2383
www.diabetes.org
Year Founded: 1940

4574 American Diabetes Association: Kansas
608 W Douglas Avenue
Suite 100
Wichita, KS 67203
316-684-6091Toll free: 800-342-2383
www.diabetes.org
Year Founded: 1940

4575 American Diabetes Association: Kentucky
161 St. Matthews Avenue
Suite 3
Louisville, KY 40207
502-452-6072
Fax: 502-893-2698; *Toll Free:* 800-342-2383
www.diabetes.org
Year Founded: 1940

4576 American Diabetes Association: Louisiana & Mississippi
2424 Edenborn Avenue
Suite 660
Metairie, LA 70001
Fax: 504-834-2797; *Toll Free:* 888-342-2383
www.diabetes.org

John Guzzardo, Executive Director
Year Founded: 1940

4577 American Diabetes Association: Maryland
2002 Clipper Park Road
Suite 110
Baltimore, MD 21211
410-265-0075
Fax: 410-235-4048; *Toll Free:* 800-342-2383
www.diabetes.org

Kathy Rogers, Executive Director
Year Founded: 1940

4578 American Diabetes Association: Massachusetts, Maine, Rhode Island, New Hampshire, Vermont & Connecticut
10 Speen Street
2nd Floor
Framingham, MA 01701
617-482-4580
Fax: 508-626-4260; *Toll Free:* 800-342-2383
www.diabetes.org

Chris Boynton, Executive Director, New England
Year Founded: 1940

4579 American Diabetes Association: Michigan
300 Galleria Officentre
Suite 111
Southfield, MI 48034
248-433-3830
Fax: 248-352-0261; *Toll Free:* 800-342-2383
www.diabetes.org

Debbie O'Leary, Sr. Executive Director
Year Founded: 1940

4580 American Diabetes Association: Minnesota & North Dakota
8000 W 78th Street
Suite 175
Edina, MN 55439
763-593-5333
Fax: 952-582-9000; *Toll Free:* 800-342-2383
www.diabetes.org

David Becker, Executive Director
Year Founded: 1940

4581 American Diabetes Association: Missouri
2833-B East Battlefield Road
Suite 100
Springfield, MO 65804
417-890-8400
Fax: 417-890-8484; *Toll Free:* 800-342-2383
www.diabetes.org

Renee Steele-Paulsell, Regional Director
Year Founded: 1940

4582 American Diabetes Association: Montana
112 S First Avenue
Suite 5 #323
Laurel, MT 59044
406-256-0616
Fax: 877-684-7059; *Toll Free:* 800-342-2383
www.diabetes.org
Year Founded: 1940

4583 American Diabetes Association: Nebraska& South Dakota
14216 Dayton Circle
Suite 6
Omaha, NE 68137
402-571-1101
Fax: 402-572-8141; *Toll Free:* 800-342-2383
www.diabetes.org

Doug Bickford, Executive Director
Ellen Myer, Manager, Tour de Cure (Nebraska)
Year Founded: 1940

4584 American Diabetes Association: New Jersey
CenterPointe II
1160 U.S. 22, Suite 103
Bridgewater, NJ 08807
732-469-7979
Fax: 908-722-4887; *Toll Free:* 800-342-2383
www.diabetes.org

Denise Andersen, Regional Director
Year Founded: 1940

4585 American Diabetes Association: New York
333 7th Avenue
10th Floor
New York, NY 10001
212-725-4925
Fax: 212-725-8916; *Toll Free:* 800-342-2383
www.diabetes.org

Elaine Curran, VP, Development
Gina Ihne, Director, Corp. Development
Robin Hahn, Assoc. Director, Corp. Devel.
Year Founded: 1940

4586 American Diabetes Association: No. California
1970 Broadway
Suite 425
Oakland, CA 94612
510-654-4499
Fax: 510-893-2376; *Toll Free:* 800-342-2383
www.diabetes.org

Michael Chae, Executive Director
Tom Hall, Director, Tour de Cure
Year Founded: 1940

4587 American Diabetes Association: North Carolina
1300 Baxter Street
Suite 150
Charlotte, NC 28204
704-373-9111
Fax: 704-373-9113; *Toll Free:* 800-342-2383
www.diabetes.org

Dianne Roth, Executive Director
Year Founded: 1940

4588 American Diabetes Association: North Texas
4100 Alpha Road
Suite 100
Dallas, TX 75244
972-392-1181
Fax: 972-392-1366; *Toll Free:* 800-342-2383
www.diabetes.org

Quin Neal, Sr. Exec. Director, North Texas
Year Founded: 1940

4589 American Diabetes Association: Northeast Ohio
4500 Rockside Road
Suite 440
Independence, OH 44131
216-328-9989
Fax: 216-328-0007; *Toll Free:* 800-342-2383
www.diabetes.org

Lori Butterfield, Executive Director, Greater Ohio
Year Founded: 1940

4590 American Diabetes Association: Oklahoma
4334 NW Expressway
Suite 265
Oklahoma City, OK 73116
405-840-3881
Fax: 405-810-8427; *Toll Free:* 800-342-2383
www.diabetes.org
Year Founded: 1940

4591 American Diabetes Association: Oregon
4380 SW Macadam Avenue
Suite 210
Portland, OR 97239
503-736-2770
Fax: 503-227-2090; *Toll Free:* 800-342-2383
www.diabetes.org

Andrea Bruno, Regional Director, Northwest
Alison Bruun, Market Director

4592 American Diabetes Association: So. California
611 Wilshire Boulevard
Suite 900
Los Angeles, CA 90017
323-966-2890
Fax: 213-489-4375; *Toll Free:* 800-342-2383
www.diabetes.org

Cassie Shafer, Regional Director, So. Calif.
Jennifer Campbell, Area Director

4593 American Diabetes Association: Tennessee
220 Great Circle Road
Suite 134
Nashville, TN 37228
615-298-3066
Fax: 615-271-2151; *Toll Free:* 800-342-2383
www.diabetes.org
Year Founded: 1940

4594 American Diabetes Association: Utah & Nevada
4424 South 700 East
#100
Salt Lake City, UT 84107
801-363-3024
Fax: 801-261-3005; *Toll Free:* 800-342-2383
www.diabetes.org

Jeff Bird, Market Director, UT/NV
Year Founded: 1940

4595 American Diabetes Association: Virginia
Greenbrier Tower II
870 Greenbrier Circle, Suite 404
Chesapeake, VA 23320
757-424-6662
Fax: 757-420-0490; *Toll Free:* 800-342-2383
www.diabetes.org

Deanie Eldridge, Executive Director
Amie Holman, Associate Director, Tour de Cure
Year Founded: 1940

4596 American Diabetes Association: Washington
2815 Eastlake Avenue E
Suite 240
Seattle, WA 98102
206-282-4616
Fax: 206-282-4732; *Toll Free:* 800-342-2383
www.diabetes.org

Paul Tobin, Market Director
Year Founded: 1940

4597 American Diabetes Association: West Texas & New Mexico
8008 Slide Road
Suite 12-A
Lubbock, TX 79424

806-794-0691
Fax: 806-794-1394; *Toll Free:* 800-342-2383
www.diabetes.org
Year Founded: 1940

4598 American Diabetes Association: West Virginia
PO Box 21903
Lexington, KY 40522
859-268-9129
Fax: 502-714-7313; *Toll Free:* 800-342-2383
www.diabetes.org

4599 American Diabetes Association: Western Pennsylvania
100 W Station Square Drive
Suite 1900
Pittsburgh, PA 15219
412-824-1181
Fax: 412-471-1315; *Toll Free:* 800-342-2383
pittsburgh@diabetes.org
www.diabetes.org

Julie Keller Heverly, Executive Director
Year Founded: 1940

4600 American Diabetes Association: Wisconsin
375 Bishop's Way
Suite 220
Brookfield, WI 53005
414-778-5500
Fax: 262-797-9270; *Toll Free:* 800-342-2383
www.diabetes.org
Year Founded: 1940

4601 American Diabetes Association: Wyoming
2460 W 26th Avenue
Suite 500C
Denver, CO 80211
720-855-1102
Fax: 720-855-1302; *Toll Free:* 800-342-2383
www.diabetes.org

Sue Glass, Vice President, Western Division
Jennifer Klass, Area Director, CO/MT/WY
Kristin Barry, Regional Associate Director
Year Founded: 1940

4602 American Gastroenterological Association
4930 Del Ray Avenue
Bethesda, MD 20814
301-654-2055
Fax: 301-654-5920
member@gastro.org
www.gastro.org

Michael Camilleri, President

Physicians of internal medicine certified in gastroenterology; radiologists, pathologists, surgeons, and physiologists with special interest and competency in gastroenterology. Studies normal and abnormal conditions of the digestive organs and problems connected with their metabolism; conducts scientific research; offers placement services.

Year Founded: 1897; Number of Members: 16,000+

4603 Diabetes Care and Education
Academy of Nutrition & Dietetics
120 South Riverside Plaza
Suite 2000
Chicago, IL 60606
www.dce.org

Betty Krauss, Chair
Claudia Shwide-Slavin, Secretary
Paula Kellogg Leibovitz, Treasurer

Responds to the needs of diabetes organizations and industry with regard to diabetes nutrition issues, promotes clinical and educational research to imrpove diabetes management, develop guideleines for the nutritional management of diabetes and maintain a network of practicing dieticians available for consultation services to health professionals and people with diabetes.

4604 Diabetes Hands Foundation
1962 University Avenue
Suite One
Berkeley, CA 94704
510-898-1301
Fax: 510-295-2519
diabeteshandsfoundation.org

Gene Kunde, CEO

Mission is to connect, engage, and empower people touched with diabetes.

Year Founded: 1962

4605 Endocrine Society
2055 L Street NW
Suite 600
Washington, DC 20036
202-971-3636Toll free: 888-363-6274
societyservices@endocrine.org
www.endocrine.org

Lisa H. Fish, President
Kenneth H. Hupart, Secretary Treasurer

Mission is to promote excellence in research, education, and the clinical practice endocrinology.

Year Founded: 1916

4606 Joslin Diabetes Center
One Joslin Place
Boston, MA 02215
617-309-2400
diabetes@joslin.harvard.edu
www.joslin.org

Peter Amenta, President & CEO

Mission is to prevent, treat, and cure diabetes.

4607 National Certification Board for Diabetes Educators
330 East Algonquin Road
Suite 4
Arlington Heights, IL 60005
847-228-9795Toll free: 877-239-3233
info@ncbde.org
www.ncbde.org

John Johnson, Chair

The Board for Diabetes Educators is dedicated to promoting excellence in the field of diabetes education through the development, maintenance, and protection of the certified Diabetes Educator credential and the certification process.

Year Founded: 1986

4608 National Eye Institute
31 Center Drive
MSC 2510
Bethesda, MD 20892-2510
301-496-3583
2020@nei.nih.gov
nei.nih.gov

Mission is to promote public and professional awareness of the importance of diagnosis and treatment of diabetic eye disease. NEHEP is a partnership with various public and private organizations that plan and implemtn eye health education programs targeted to a variety of high-risk audiences.

4609 National Kidney Disease Program
Nat Inst of Diabetes & Digestive & Kidney Diseases
Bethesda, MD 20892-2560
301-496-3583
www.niddk.nih.gov

Griffin P. Rodgers, Director

Mission is to reduce the morbidity and mortality caused ny kidney disease and its complications.

Year Founded: 2000

Books

4610 101 Tips for Improving Your Blood Sugar
American Diabetes Association
1701 N Beauregard Street
Alexandria, VA 22311-1742
Fax: 703-549-6995; *Toll Free:* 800-232-3472
www.diabetes.org

Lee Barona, National Call Center Director
Jacqueline Amaya, Operations Manager

Tips for 101 common situations and questions to reduce the risk of complications from blood sugar at the wrong level.

122 pages

4611 50 Secrets of the Longest Living People with Diabetes
Perseus Books Group
250 West 57th St.
15th Floor
New York, NY 10107
212-340-8100
www.perseusbooksgroup.com

David Steinberger, President & CEO
Sheri R Colberg MD, Author
Steven V Edelman MD, Author

From interviews with more than fifty people who have thrived with the condition for as many as 84 years, the authors distill their lifelong habits into fifty user-friendly, easy-to-adopt secrets.

Year Founded: 1999

4612 Balance Your Act: A Book for Adults with Diabetes
Pritchett & Hull
3440 Oakcliff Road, NE
Suite 110
Atlanta, GA 30340-3006

770-451-0602Toll free: 800-241-4925
www.p-h.com
Betty Westmoreland, President
96 pages

4613 Caring for the Diabetic Soul
American Diabetes Association
1660 Duke Street
Suite 100
Alexandria, VA 22314-3427
Fax: 703-549-6995; *Toll Free:* 800-232-3472
www.diabetes.org

Restoring emotional balance for yourself and your family.

213 pages

4614 Clinical Practice Recommendations
American Diabetes Association
1660 Duke Street
Suite 100
Alexandria, VA 22314-3427
Fax: 703-549-6995; *Toll Free:* 800-232-3472
www.diabetes.org

Features all current position and consensus statements of
the American Diabetes Association.

4615 Control Diabetes the Easy Way
Random House Trade Books
400 Hahn Road
Westminster, MD 21157-4627
410-848-1900
Fax: 800-659-2436; *Toll Free:* 800-733-3000
www.randomhouse.com
Year Founded: 1998

4616 Diabetes A to Z
American Diabetes Association
1660 Duke Street
Alexandria, VA 22314-3473
Fax: 703-549-6995; *Toll Free:* 800-232-3472
www.diabetes.org

Dictionary-style guidebook discussing basic terms and issues concerning diabetes. Third edition.

202 pages

**4617 Diabetes Burnout: What To Do When You
Can't Take It Anymore**
American Diabetes Association
1701 North Beauregard Street
Alexandria, VA 22311
Toll Free: 800-342-2383
www.diabetes.org
William H Polonsky PhD/CDE, Author

Provides the tools you need to keep from being over-
whelmed, addressing such issues as dealing with friends
and family, and how you can better handle the stress for
better health.

348 pages

4618 Diabetes Education Goals
American Diabetes Association
1660 Duke Street
Suite 100
Alexandria, VA 22314-3427

Fax: 703-549-6995; *Toll Free:* 800-232-3472
www.diabetes.org

Features advice on how to assess, plan, and evaluate patient
education and counseling programs. Covers both short-term
and in-depth goals. Focuses on the education process and
assessing the unique needs of each patient.

64 pages

4619 Diabetes Medical Nutrition Therapy
American Diabetes Association
1660 Duke Street
Suite 100
Alexandria, VA 22314-3427
Fax: 703-549-6995; *Toll Free:* 800-232-3472
www.diabetes.org

A professional guide to management and nutrition education resources. Provides in-depth coverage of nutrition assessment, goal setting, intervention, and outcome
evaluation. Information is provided on specific resources
and case studies are cited for practical examples.

4620 Diabetes Mellitus: A Practical Handbook
Bull Publishing
P.O. Box 1377
Boulder, CO 80306
303-545-6350
Fax: 303-545-6354; *Toll Free:* 800-676-2855
bullpublishing@msn.com
www.bullpub.com
Jim Bull, Owner
Emily Sewell, Vice President of Operations
Claire Cameron, Director of Marketing

Helpful and user-friendly, the guide teaches readers how to
balance diet, medication, and exercise for optimal health,
7th edition.

212 pages

4621 Diabetes Self-Management
RA Rapaport Publishing
150 W 22nd Street
Suite 800
New York, NY 10011-2421
212-989-0200
Fax: 212-989-4786; *Toll Free:* 800-234-0923
editor@diabetes-self-mgmt.com
www.diabetesselfmanagement.com
Ingrid Strauch, Managing Editor
Diane Fennell, Web Editor
Alwa Cooper, Associate Editor

Publishes practical, how-to information, focusing on the
day-to-day and long-term aspects of diabetes in a positive
and upbeat style. Gives subscribers up-to-date news, facts,
and advice to help them maintain their wellness and make
informed decisions regarding their health.

56 pages Year Founded: 1983

4622 Diabetes Sourcebook - Vol. 3
Omnigraphics
155 West Congress
Suite 200
Detroit, MI 48226
313-961-1340
Fax: 800-875-1340; *Toll Free:* 800-234-1340
contact@omnigraphics.com
omnigraphics.com

Peter E Ruffner, President
Year Founded: 1956

4623 Diabetes Teaching Guide for People Who Use Insulin
Joslin Diabetes Center
1 Joslin Place
Boston, MA 02215-5306
617-732-2400
Fax: 617-732-2487
diabetes@joslin.harvard.edu
www.joslin.org

Ralph M. James, Chairman
Barry D. Libert, Chief Executive Officer
Geoffery S. Rehnert, Founder and Co-CEO

Discusses the causes of diabetes, the role of diet and exercise, meal planning and complications. Also provide information on drawing blood, mixing and injecting insulin.

4624 Diabetes: Your Complete Exercise Guide
Human Kinetics Publishers
1607 N Market Street
PO Box 5076
Champaign, IL 61820
217-351-5076
Fax: 217-351-1549; *Toll Free:* 800-747-4457
info@hkusa.com
www.humankinetics.com

Part of the Cooper Clinic and Research Institute Fitness Series providing exercise rehabilitation for persons with diabetes.

144 pages

4625 Diabetic's Guide to Health and Fitness
Human Kinetics Publishers
1607 N Market Street
PO Box 5076
Champaign, IL 61820
217-351-5076
Fax: 217-351-1549; *Toll Free:* 800-747-4457
info@hkusa.com
www.humankinetics.com

Information about achieving and maintaining physical fitness and proper health living with diabetes.

272 pages

4626 Fitness Book: For People with Diabetes
American Diabetes Association
1660 Duke Street
Suite 100
Alexandria, VA 22314-3427
Fax: 703-549-6995; *Toll Free:* 800-232-3472
www.diabetes.org

Advice on learning to exercise to lose weight, exercise safely, increase your competitive edge, get your mind and body ready to exercise, and more.

149 pages

4627 How To Cook for People with Diabetes
American Diabetes Association
1660 Duke Street
Suite 100
Alexandria, VA 22314-3427
Fax: 703-549-6995; *Toll Free:* 800-232-3472
www.diabetes.org

150 recipes featuring unusual techniques.

205 pages

4628 Intensive Diabetes Management
American Diabetes Association
1660 Duke Street
Suite 100
Alexandria, VA 22314-3427
Fax: 703-549-6995; *Toll Free:* 800-232-3472
www.diabetes.org

Delivers practical advice on how to help your patients achieve better glucose control through intensified management.

128 pages

4629 Maximizing the Role of Nutrition in Diabetes Management
American Diabetes Association
1660 Duke Street
Suite 100
Alexandria, VA 22314-3427
Fax: 703-549-6995; *Toll Free:* 800-232-3472
www.diabetes.org

Integrates medical, nutritional, and behavioral sciences and recognizes the importance of each in total diabetes care.

64 pages

4630 Medical Management of Type II Diabetes
American Diabetes Association
1660 Duke Street
Suite 100
Alexandria, VA 22314-3427
Fax: 703-549-6995; *Toll Free:* 800-232-3472
www.diabetes.org

Complete overview of Type II diabetes, including diagnosis and classification, pathogenesis, and prevention/treatment of complications.

112 pages

4631 Prediabetes: What You Need to Know to Keep Diabetes Away
Perseus Books Group
250 West 57th St.
15th Floor
New York, NY 10107
212-340-8100
www.perseusbooksgroup.com

David Steinberger, President & CEO
Sheri R Colberg MD, Author
Steven V Edelman MD, Author

This first-ever practical guide offers fifty essential, informative ideas and simple steps to help this vast and rapidly growing constituency manager their condition and thereby reduce their chances of developing full-blown diabetes.

Year Founded: 1999

4632 Stop Prediabetes Now: The Ultimate Planto Lose Weight and Prevent Diabetes
Wiley
10475 Crosspoint Boulevard
Indianapolis, IN 46256
Fax: 800-597-3299; *Toll Free:* 877-762-2974
www.wiley.com

Stephen M. Smith, President and Chief Executive Of
Ellis E. Cousens, Executive Vice President, Chief
John Kritzmacher, Executive Vice President, Chief

Offers a practical step-by-step program for improving eating habots and using nutritional supplements to reverse prediabetes and related weight problems. Also includes shopping instructions, meal plans, and easy-to-prepare recipes.

304 pages Year Founded: 1807

4633 The First Year: Type 2 Diabetes: An Essential Guide for the Newly Diagnosed
Perseus Books Group
250 West 57th St.
15th Floor
New York, NY 10107
212-340-8100
www.perseusbooksgroup.com

David Steinberger, President & CEO
Sheri R Colberg MD, Author
Steven V Edelman MD, Author

Uniquely guides you step-by-step through your first year with diabetes, walking you through everything you need to learn and do each day of your first week after diagnosis, each subsequent week of the first month, and each subsequent month of the crucial first year.

Year Founded: 1999

4634 The New Glucose Revolution for Diabetes
Perseus Books Group
250 West 57th St.
15th Floor
New York, NY 10107
212-340-8100
www.perseusbooksgroup.com

David Steinberger, President & CEO
Sheri R Colberg MD, Author
Steven V Edelman MD, Author

The first comprehensive guide to using the glycemic index to control type 1 diabetes, type 2 diabetes, and more. Includes GI-based recipes and menus for type 1, type 2, prediabetes, gestational diabetes, and juvenile diabetes, as well as related conditions like obesity and celiac disease, plus practical dietary guidance on sugar, sweeteners, alcohol, snacking, and eating out.

Year Founded: 1999

4635 The Official Pocket Guide for Diabetic Exchanges
American Diabetes Association
1701 North Beauregard Street
Alexandria, VA 22311
Toll Free: 800-342-2383
www.diabetes.org

Dwight Holing, Chairman
Larry Hausner, Chief Executive Officer
Shreen Arent, Executive Vice President, Govern

Newly updated with expanded food lists and carbohydrate for every food. ADA's official guide that goes anywhere you go-to the grocery store, out to eat, on vacation. Use it to be sure you are chosing the right foods and portion sizes.

64 pages

4636 Therapy for Diabetes Mellitus and Related Disorders
American Diabetes Association
1701 North Beauregard Street
Suite 100
Alexandria, VA 22311
Fax: 703-549-6995; *Toll Free:* 800-342-2383
www.diabetes.org

Dwight Holing, Chairman
Larry Hausner, Chief Executive Officer
Shreen Arent, Executive Vice President, Govern

Guides through the treatment of specific problems of persons with diabetes. Represents the views and experience of leading clinicians in a concise, practical approach to treatment.

384 pages

4637 Type 2 Diabetes: Your Healthy Living Guide
American Diabetes Association
1701 North Beauregard Street
Alexandria, VA 22311
Fax: 703-549-6995; *Toll Free:* 800-342-2383
www.diabetes.org

A thorough guide to staying healthy with Type 2. Includes everything from choosing a health care team and eating and exercising properly to self-monitoring, insulin, dealing with complications, and keep mentally fit.

180 pages

4638 Voice of the Diabetic
6520 North Western Avenue
Suite 100
Oklahoma City, OK 73116-7334
573-875-8911
Fax: 573-875-8902
www.voiceofdiabetes.org

J. Robertt Dark, Executive Producer
Anastasia Chehak, Host

Personal stories and practical guidelines by blind diabetics and medical professionals, medical news, resource column and a recipe corner.

28 pages Frequency: Quarterly

Directories

4639 Buyer's Guide
American Diabetes Association
PO Box 186
Villanova, PA 19085
Fax: 703-549-6995; *Toll Free:* 800-232-3472
www.buyersguide.com

John Deneen, Founder & CEO

A catalog listing all manufacturers of insulin, syringes, pumps, test strips, monitors and more.

4640 Diabetes Dictionary
National Diabetes Information Clearinghouse
1 Information Way
Bethesda, MD 20892-2560
301-496-3583
Fax: 301-907-8906
www.niddk.nih.gov

Griffin P. Rodger, Director

Illustrated glossary of more than 300 deabetes-related terms.

64 pages

Journals, Magazines

4641 Clinical Diabetes
American Diabetes Association
1701 N Beauregard Street
Alexandria, VA 22311
clinical.diabetesjournals.org

Davida F. Kruger, Editor in Chief

Providing all diabetes care providers with information on advances and state-of-the-art care.

Frequency: Quarterly

4642 Diabetes
American Diabetes Association
1701 N Beauregard Street
Alexandria, VA 22311
Fax: 703-549-6995; *Toll Free:* 800-232-3472
editorialoffice@diabetes.org
diabetes.diabetesjournals.org

Michael Eisenstein, Publisher
K.S. Nair, Editor in Chief

Diabetes publishes original research about the physiology and pathophysiology of diabetes mellitus.

Frequency: Monthly

4643 Diabetes Care
American Diabetes Association
1701 N Beauregard Street
Alexandria, VA 22311
Fax: 703-549-6995; *Toll Free:* 800-232-3472
diabetescare@diabetes.org
care.diabetesjournals.org

Michael Eisenstein, Publisher
William T. Cefalu, Editor in Chief

The journal promotes better patient care by serving the needs of all health professionals caring for patients with diabetes.

Frequency: Monthly

4644 Diabetes Forecast
American Diabetes Association
1701 N Beauregard Street
Alexandria, VA 22311
Toll Free: 800-806-7801
www.diabetesforecast.org

Lois A. Witkop, Publisher
Paris Roach, Editor in Chief

The monthly lifestyle magazine for people with diabetes, featuring complete, in-depth coverage of all aspects of living with diabetes.

Frequency: Bimonthly

4645 Diabetes Spectrum
American Diabetes Association
1701 N Beauregard Street
Alexandria, VA 22311
spectrum.diabetes.org

Joshua J. Neumiller, Editor in Chief

Peer-reviewed original research and review articles on topics in diabetes prevention and medical management.

Frequency: Quarterly

Newsletters, Pamphlets

4646 Clinical Diabetes
American Diabetes Association
1701 North Beauregard Street
Alexandria, VA 22311
Fax: 703-549-6995; *Toll Free:* 800-342-2383
www.diabetes.org

A bi-monthly newsletter providing practical treatment information for primary care physicians.

4647 Dental Tips for Diabetics
National Diabetes Information Clearinghouse
1 Information Way
Bethesda, MD 20892-2560
301-496-3583
Fax: 301-907-8906
www.niddk.nih.gov

Griffin P. Rodger, Director

Discusses the relationship between diabetes and periodontal disease. Describes the symptoms of periodontal problems and preventive measures.

4648 Diabetes Advisor
American Diabetes Association
1701 North Beauregard Street
Alexandria, VA 22311
Fax: 703-549-6995; *Toll Free:* 800-342-2383
www.diabetes.org

Lynn Nicholas, CEO

Offers informative articles and research in the area of diabetes for professionals and patients. Offers facts and research on diagnosis, symptoms, technology and the newest devices for persons with diabetes, as well as referral and hotline numbers.

4649 Diabetes Dateline
National Diabetes Information Clearinghouse
1 Information Way
Bethesda, MD 20892-2560
301-654-3583
Fax: 301-907-8906
www.niddk.nih.gov

Griffin P. Rodger, Director

This bulletin features news about current issues in diabetes research and control, special events, patient and professional meeting, and new publications available from NDIC and other organizations.

4650 Diabetes Educator
American Association of Diabetes Educators
200 W. Madison Street
Suite 800
Chicago, IL 60606
312-644-2233
Fax: 312-644-4411; *Toll Free:* 800-338-3633
www.diabeteseducator.org

James J Balija, Executive Director

Offers information to health professionals working with persons with diabetes.

4651 Diabetes Self-Management
RA Rapaport Publishing
150 W 22nd Street
Suite 800
New York, NY 10011-2421
212-989-0200
Fax: 212-989-4786; *Toll Free:* 800-989-0200
www.diabetesselfmanagement.com

James Hazlett, Editor
Melissa Glim, Associate Editor
Jim Moorehead, Manager

Publishes practical, how-to information, focusing on the day-to-day and long-term aspects of diabetes in a positive and upbeat style. Gives subscribers up-to-date news, facts, and advice to help them maintain their wellness and make informed decisions regarding their health.

56 pages Frequency: BiMonthly

4652 Diabetic Foot Care
American Diabetes Association
1701 North Beauregard Street
Alexandria, VA 22311
Fax: 703-549-6995; *Toll Free:* 800-342-2383
www.diabetes.org

Booklet discussing early detection and prompt treatment of diabetic foot problems.

12 pages

4653 Diabetic Traveler
1701 N Beauregard Street
Alexandria, VA 22311-1742
Toll Free: 800-342-2383

Maury E Rosenbaum, Contact

Provides information to assist individuals with diabetes to plan safe travel. Includes information like adjusting insulin doses on air flights, reviews of storage cases for insulin and diabetes supplies, emergency medical contacts in designated destinations, information on carrying medical history. Written by a diabetic and reviewed by a medical advisory panel of experts.

6 pages Frequency: Quarterly

4654 Do Your Level Best: Start Controlling Your Blood Sugar Today
National Diabetes Information Clearinghouse
1 Information Way
Bethesda, MD 20892-2560
301-496-3583
Fax: 301-907-8906
www.niddk.nih.gov

Griffin P. Rodger, Director

Provides comprehensive information in an easy to read format for people with Type I and Type II diabetes.

4655 End-Stage Renal Disease: Choosing A Treatment That's Right for You
National Diabetes Information Clearinghouse
1 Information Way
Bethesda, MD 20892-2560
301-496-3583
Fax: 301-907-8906
www.niddk.nih.gov

Griffin P. Rodger, Director

Patient education booklet reviews three main treatment modalities for end-stage renal disease.

4656 Healthy Food Choices
American Diabetes Association
1701 North Beauregard Street
Alexandria, VA 22311
Fax: 703-549-6995; *Toll Free:* 800-342-2383
www.diabetes.org

Pamphlet containing the basics of good nutrition.

4657 Type II Diabetes
Chronimed Publishing
1701 N Beauregard Street
Alexandria, VA 22311-1742
612-513-6475
Fax: 952-443-2806; *Toll Free:* 800-848-2793
www.diabetes.org/diabetes-basics/type-2/

Explains the basics of what diabetes is and how it is treated.

4658 Type II Diabetes Prevention Pyramids
Chronimed Publishing
1701 N Beauregard Street
Alexandria, VA 22311-1742
612-513-6475
Fax: 952-443-2806; *Toll Free:* 800-848-2793

Teaches ways to decrease risks by improving nutrition, increasing physical activity, and balancing stress.

21 pages

4659 Understanding Gestational Diabetes
National Diabetes Information Clearinghouse
1 Information Way
Bethesda, MD 20892
301-654-3327
Fax: 301-907-8906
www.niddk.nih.gov

A guide for women who develop diabetes during pregnancy. It discusses symptoms and diagnosis of gestational diabetes, risk factors, tests during pregnancy and daily management including the use of insulin and blood glucose monitoring.

44 pages

Videos, Audio Tapes

4660 ADA Clinical Education Series on CD-Rom
American Diabetes Association
1701 North Beauregard Street
Alexandria, VA 22311
Fax: 703-549-6995; *Toll Free:* 800-342-2383
www.diabetes.org

Features complete texts of Medical Management of Type 1 Diabetes, Medical Management of Type 2 Diabetes, Therapy for Diabetes Mellitus and Related Disorders, and Medical Management of Pregnancy Complicated by Diabetes.

4661 Black Experience
American Diabetes Association/Conn. Affiliate
1701 North Beauregard Street
Alexandria, VA 22311

Fax: 703-549-6995; *Toll Free:* 800-342-2383
www.diabetes.org

Designed to increase awareness of diabetes in the black community.

4662 Diabetes & Exercise Video
American Diabetes Association
1701 North Beauregard Street
Alexandria, VA 22311
Fax: 703-549-6995; *Toll Free:* 800-342-2383
www.diabetes.org

Lynn Nichols, CEO

A video offering information on how to maintain good health and exercise in controlling diabetes.

4663 Diabetes Update - Glucose Toxicity: The Need for 24-Hour Control
American Diabetes Association/Conn. Affiliate
1701 North Beauregard Street
Alexandria, VA 22311
Fax: 703-549-6995; *Toll Free:* 800-342-2383
www.diabetes.org

Explores the two new issues in understanding Type II Diabetes: the important role of hepatic glucose overproduction and the concept of glucose toxicity.

4664 Diabetes and You
American Diabetes Association/Conn. Affiliate
1701 North Beauregard Street
Alexandria, VA 22311
Fax: 703-549-6995; *Toll Free:* 800-342-2383
www.diabetes.org

A 4-part series that emphasizes the important role patients play in their diabetes management.

4665 Diabetes: What You Need to Know
American Diabetes Association/Conn. Affiliate
1701 North Beauregard Street
Alexandria, VA 22311
Fax: 703-549-6995; *Toll Free:* 800-342-2383
www.diabetes.org

Created to increase patient awareness of the classic signs of diabetes and emphasizes the importance to reduce risks of serious complications.

4666 Diabetic Foot
American Diabetes Association/Conn. Affiliate
1701 North Beauregard Street
Alexandria, VA 22311
Fax: 703-549-6995; *Toll Free:* 800-342-2383
www.diabetes.org

Explains what to look for and what to do when a problem is suspected or detected in the diabetic foot.

4667 Guidelines for Managing Diabetes During Brief Illness
Chronimed Publishing
PO Box 59032
Minneapolis, MN 55459
612-513-6475
Fax: 612-443-2806; *Toll Free:* 800-848-2793

Offers instructions and food suggestions to help prevent the development of ketoacidosis in persons with diabetes during common brief illnesses that interrupt regular food intake. 50 slides/cassette. Item No. 4101.

4668 How to Measure and Inject Insulin
Chronimed Publishing
PO Box 59032
Minneapolis, MN 55459
612-513-6475
Fax: 952-443-2806; *Toll Free:* 800-848-2793

Provides step-by-step instructions on how to draw up, measure, and inject insulin. Also reviews types of insulin and syringes, storage of insulin, and injection sites. 12 minutes. Item No. 4125. Also available as 62 slides/cassette (Item No. 4150).

4669 Living Well with Diabetes
American Diabetes Association/Conn. Affiliate
1701 North Beauregard Street
Alexandria, VA 22311
Fax: 703-549-6995; *Toll Free:* 800-342-2383
www.diabetes.org

Presents two patient role models who are successfully following a treatment plan for noninsulin dependent diabetes.

4670 On Top of My Game: Living with Diabetes
American Diabetes Association/Conn. Affiliate
1701 North Beauregard Street
Alexandria, VA 22311
Fax: 703-549-6995; *Toll Free:* 800-342-2383
www.diabetes.org

Six patients and their families share their day-to-day frustrations and successes in managing diabetes.

Websites

4671 Diabetes Forecast
American Diabetes Association
1701 N Beauregard Street
Alexandria, VA 22311
www.diabetesforecast.org

Kelly Rawlings, Editorial Director

4672 National Diabetes Information Clearinghouse
Nat Inst of Diabetes & Digestive & Kidney Diseases
Bethesda, MD 20892-2560
301-496-3583
www.niddk.nih.gov

Offers various materials, resources, books, pamphlets and more for persons and families in the area of diabetes.

4673 National Digestive Diseases InformationClearinghouse
Nat Inst of Diabetes & Digestive & Kidney Diseases
Bethesda, MD 20892-2560
301-496-3583
www.niddk.nih.gov

Mission is to serve as a digestive disease informational, educational, and referral resource for health professionals and the public.

Research Centers

4674 Diabetes Education and Research Center
Franklin Medical Building
829 Spruce Street
Suite 302
Philadelphia, PA 19107-5752

215-925-1481
Fax: 215-928-9150
www.libertynet.org/~diabetes
Ronald Morgan, Manager

4675 Diabetes Research Center
University of Virginia Diabetes Center
200 S. Park Road, Suite 100
Charlottesville, VA 22908
434-295-1551
Fax: 434-982-3796
jts@virginia.edu
www.diabetesresearch.org

Eugene J Barrett, Director
Richard De Butts, Owner

The mission of this center is to improve the quality and quanity of health care available to persons with diabetes in Virginia through the provision of professional education, assistance in program planning and development, and of educational resources realting to diabetes

4676 Diabetes Research and Training Center: University of Alabama at Birmingham
Department of Medicine
University Station
Birmingham, AL 35294
205-934-4116
Fax: 205-934-4389

Dr. Jeffrey Kudlow, Director

4677 Endocrinology Research Laboratory
Cabrini Medical Center
247 3rd Avenue
New York, NY 10010-7457
212-995-6000
www.endocrinology.ucsd.edu/research.html

Dr. Leonid Poretsky, Director
Robert Chaloner, CEO

Focuses on the effects of insulin and insulin-like growth factors on human body functions.

4678 International Diabetes Center: Institute for Research & Education Health System
3800 Park Nicollet Boulevard
Minneapolis, MN 55416-2533
952-993-3393
Fax: 952-993-0501; *Toll Free:* 888-637-2675
idccustsvc@parknicollet.com
www.idcpublishing.com

Kathy Reynolds, Manager

Research center which improves the quality of life of individuals with diabetes and those at rick of developing diabetes by undertaking ckinical car, education, research, and outreach activities that stimulate and support health.

4679 Joslin Diabetes Center
1 Joslin Place
Boston, MA 02215-5394
617-732-2400
Fax: 617-732-2487; *Toll Free:* 800-JOS-LIN1
diabetes@joslin.harvard.edu
www.joslin.org

Kenneth E Quickle Jr, MD, President

Offers research into diabetes mellitus, including investigations on chemical composition.

4680 Multiple District 22: Lions Vision Research Foundation
PO Box 1714
Baltimore, MD 21203-1714
410-955-1883
Fax: 41- 78- 395
www.lionsvision.org

Heather Mays, Administrative Manager

Promotes eye research in eye diseases of all types, particularly those related to diabetes, such as diabetic retinopathy, cataracts, glaucoma, and low vision impairment. Works directly with the Wilmer Eye Institute of the Johns Hopkins Medical Institutes, Baltimore, MD in support of its research into eye diseases and cures. Sponsors Lions Vision Days each October. Currently running Lions Vision 2000 campaign to raise a 4 million dollar endowmentfor the Low Vision department at Wilmer.

4681 National Institute of Diabetes & Digestive & Kidney Disease
US Department of Health and Human Services
9000 Rockville Pike
Bldg 31
Bethesda, MD 20892
301-496-3583
Fax: 301-496-7422; *Toll Free:* 800-422-6237

Elizabeth Singer, Executive Director

The Institute conducts, fosters, and supports basic and clinical research into the causes, prevention, diagnosis, and treatment of the various metabolic and digestive diseases. It covers the broad areas of diabetes, blood, endocrine, and metabolic diseases; digestive diseases and nutrition; and kidney and urologic diseases.

4682 Omaha Department of Veteran Affairs Medical Center Research Service
4101 Woolworth Avenue
Omaha, NE 68105-1850
402-346-8800
Fax: 402-449-0604

Lynell W Klassen MD, Associate Chief

4683 University of California, Irvine: UCI Diabetes Research Program
Department of Medicine, Med Sci I C264
Irvine, CA 92697
949-824-5011
www.uci.edu/

M Arthur Charles MD, PhD, Head Master

Basic and clinical diabetes research.

4684 University of Chicago: Diabetes Research & Training Center
5801 South Ellis
Chicago, IL 60637
773-702-1234
Fax: 773-702-4427

Dr. Arthur Rubenstein, Director
Sue Curtis, Manager

4685 University of Miami: Diabetes Research Institute
1450 NW 10th Avenue
Miami, FL 33136-1011

305-243-6504
Fax: 305-243-4404

Daniel H Mintz MD, Scientific Director

4686 University of Pittsburgh: Nutrition and Biochemistry Laboratory
Graduate School of Public Health
505 Parran Hall
Pittsburgh, PA 15261
412-624-4141
Fax: 412-624-7397
rwe2@pitt.edu

Rhobert Evans MD, Director

Focuses on, diabetes and obesity research. AIDS, cardio-vascular disease, wide range of analytical techniques to analyse cytokines, hormones, vitamins and fatty acids.

4687 University of Texas: General Clinical Research Center
7703 Floyd Curl Drive
San Antonio, TX 78229-3901
210-567-8400
Fax: 210-567-6693

Gregory Mundy MD, Program Director

Focuses on diabetes and infectious disease research.

4688 University of Washington: Diabetes Endocrinology Research Center
1660 S Columbian Way
Seattle, WA 98108-1532
206-764-2222
Fax: 206-764-2598

Daniel Porte Jr, Director
Jodie K Haselkorn, MD

4689 Vanderbilt University: Diabetes Research and Training Center
B3307 Medical Center N
Nashville, TN 37232
615-322-2571
Fax: 615-322-2198

Dr. Oscar B Crofford, Director
Rhonda Venable, PhD

4690 Veterans Affairs Medical Center: Research Service
500 Foothill Drive
Salt Lake City, UT 84148
801-582-1565
Fax: 801-583-9624

Andrew Deiss MD, Associate Chief
James Floyd, Executive Director

Diabetes and cancer research.

4691 Virginia Mason Research Center
1000 Seneca Street
Seattle, WA 98101-2744
206-583-6525
Fax: 206-223-7543

Dwight Sutton PhD, Director
Jerry Nepom, Executive Director

Immunology and diabetes research.

4692 Warren Grant Magnuson Clinical Center
6100 Executive Boulevard
Suite 3c01
Bethesda, MD 20892
301-496-2563
Fax: 301-402-2984
www.cc.nih.gov

Established in 1953 as the research hospital of the National Institutes of Health. Designed so that patient care facilities are close to research laboratories so new findings of basic and clinical scientists can be quickly applied to the treatment of patients. Upon referral by physicians, patients are admitted to NIH clinical studies.

4693 Washington University: Diabetes Research and Training Center
660 S Euclid Avenue
Campus Box 8086
Saint Louis, MO 63110-1093
314-362-7080
Fax: 314-454-6225
www.diabetesresearchcenter.dom.wustl.edu

Jean E. Schaffer, Director
Clay F. Semenkovich, Executive Director
Philip E. Cryer, Associate Director

Hearing Impaired

Associations & Organizations

4694 ADARA
1204 Queen Street NE
Washington, DC 20002
www.adara.org

John Gournaris, President
Deb Guthmann, Secretary
Della Thomas, Treasurer

Professional networking for excellence in service delivery with individuals who are deaf or hard of hearing. A partnership of national organizations, local affiliates, professional sections, and individual members working together to support social services and rehabilitation delivery for deaf and hard of hearing people.

Year Founded: 1960

4695 Abledata
103 W Broad Street
Suite 400
Falls Church, VA 22046
Fax: 703-356-8314; Toll Free: 800-227-0216
abledata@neweditions.net
www.abledata.com
TTY: 703-992-8313

An information and referral project that maintains a database of 20,000-plus assistive technology products. The project also produces fact sheets on types of devices and other aspects of assistive technology.

4696 Abused Deaf Women's Advocacy Services
8623 Roosevelt Way NE
Seattle, WA 98115
206-922-7088
Fax: 206-726-0017
adwas@adwas.org
www.adwas.org

Libby Stanley, Executive Director
Karent Carlson, Finance Chair
Liz Gibson, Chair

Advocacy group for deaf and deaf-blind women who have been mentally, physically, or sexually abused.

Year Founded: 1986

4697 Academy of Dispensing Audiologists
446 E High Street
Suite 10
Lexington, KY 40507
866-493-5544
Fax: 859-271-0607
info@audiologist.org
www.audiologist.org

Alicia Spoor, President
Larry Schmidbauer, Secretary
Patricia Dabrowski, Treasurer

ADA is focused on helping audiologists succeed in all aspects of practice, with a particular emphasis on the business of audiology.

Year Founded: 1977

4698 Academy of Rehabilitative Audiology
e-mail: ara@audrehab.org
www.audrehab.org

Claire Bernstein, PhD, President
Sherri Smith, PhD, Treasurer
Laura Ann Wilber, PhD, Parliamentarian

Provides professional education, research, and interest in programs for hearing impaired persons.

Year Founded: 1966

4699 Alexander Graham Bell Association for the Deaf and Hard of Hearing
3417 Volta Place NW
Washington, DC 20007
202-337-5220
Fax: 202-337-8314
info@agbell.org
www.agbell.org

Emilio Alonso-Mendoza, CEO

Nonprofit working to ensure that every child and adult with hearing loss has the opportunity to thrive in mainstream society.

4700 American Academy of Audiology
11480 Commerce Park Drive
Suite 220
Reston, VA 20191
703-790-8466
Fax: 703-790-8631; Toll Free: 802-222-3366
infoaud@audiology.org
www.audiology.org

Erin Miller, Chair

A professional organization of individuals dedicated to providing high quality hearing care to the public. Provides professional development, education and research and provides increased public awareness of hearing disorders and audiologic services.

Year Founded: 1988

4701 American Academy of Otolaryngology - Head & Neck Surgery
1650 Diagonal Road
Alexandria, VA 22314-2857
703-836-4444
Fax: 703-683-5100
www.entnet.org

Sujana S. Chandrasekhar, President
Scott P. Stringer, Secretary/Treasurer
James C. Denneny III, Executive Vice President and CEO

Professional society of medical doctors specializing in otolaryngology (diseases of the ear, nose and throat) and head and neck surgery. Represents otolaryngology in governmental and socioeconomic areas and provides high-quality medical education for otolaryngologists. Coordinates Combined Otolaryngological Spring Meetings for ten national otolaryngological societies. Operates job information exchange service and museum.

4702 American Auditory Society
PO Box 779
Pennsville, NJ 08070
Fax: 650-763-9185; Toll Free: 877-746-8315
amaudsoc@comcast.net
www.amauditorysoc.org

Harvey Abrams, President
Anil Lalwani, Treasurer

Year Founded: 1960

4703 American Cochlear Implant Alliance

PO Box 103
McLean, VA 22101-0103
703-534-6146
info@acialliance.org
www.acialliance.org

Donna L. Sorkin, Executive Director

Nonprofit advocating for improved access to cochlear implants for patients of all ages.

Year Founded: 2010

4704 American Neurotology Society

4960 Dover Street NE
St. Petersburg, FL 33703
217-638-0801
Fax: 727-800-9428
administrator@americanneurotologysociety.com
www.americanneurotologysociety.com

Physicians and audiologists interested in the diagnosis and treatment of hearing and balance disorders. Promotes education and research in the field of neurotology.

4705 American Speech-Language-Hearing Association

2200 Research Boulevard
Rockville, MD 20850-3289
301-296-5700
Fax: 301-296-8580; *Toll Free:* 800-638-8255
www.asha.org
TTY: 301-296-5650

Andrea Falzarano, Director

A professional and scientific organization for speech-language pathologists; audiologists and speech, language and hearing scientists concerned with commutation disabilities. Provides information and referral and a toll-free HELPLINE number for consumers to inquire about speech, language or hearing disabilities.

Year Founded: 1925; Number of Members: 150,000

4706 American Tinnitus Association

503-248-9985
tinnitus@ata.org
www.ata.org

Membership organization that carries out and supports research and education on tinnitus. Provides resources to both professionals and patients about seeking help and information. Publishes quarterly journal, Tinnitus Today. $25 annual membership includes subscription to Tinnitus Today.

Year Founded: 1971

4707 Arizona Commission for the Deaf & Hard of Hearing

100 N. 15th Avenue
Suite 104
Phoenix, AZ 85007
602-542-3323
Fax: 602-542-3380; *Toll Free:* 800-352-8161
info@acdhh.az.gov
www.acdhh.org
TTY: 800-352-8161

Sherri Collins, Executive Director
Carmen M Green, Deputy Director
Curtis Humphries, Business Manager

The purpose of the Arizona Commission for the Deaf and the Hard of Hearing is to ensure, in partnership with the public and private sector, accessibility for the Deaf and the Hard of Hearing to improve the quality of life.

Year Founded: 1977

4708 Association of Late-Deafened Adults

8038 Macintosh Lane
Suite 2
Rockford, IL 61107
815-332-1515
info@alda.org
www.alda.org
TTY: 815-332-1515

Steve Larew, President

ALDA reaches out to deafened individuals regardless of age of onset who are seeking their place as a deafened person.

4709 Berks Deaf and Hard of Hearing Service

2045 Centre Avenue
Reading, PA 19605
610-685-4523
Fax: 610-685-4526
www.bdhhs.org
TTY: 484-388-4086

Kandy Reyes, President
Sarah Cline Foltz, Executive Secretary
Michelle Gromlich, Administrative Assistant

BDHHS offers services for Deaf and Hard of Hearing individuals and their families in Berks County, Pennsylvania, the surrounding counties, as well as in New Jersey, Delaware, and Baltimore, Maryland.

4710 Better Hearing Institute

1444 I Street, NW
Suite 700
Washington, DC 20005
www.betterhearing.org
TDD 800-327-9355

A nonprofit educational organization that implements national public information programs on hearing loss and available medical, surgical, hearing aid and rehabilitation assistance for millions with uncorrected hearing problems. Its award-winning series of television, radio and print media public service messages include many celebrities who overcame hearing loss. BHI maintains a toll-free Hearing HelpLine telephone service that provides information.

Year Founded: 1973

4711 Betty and Leonard Phillips Deaf Action Center

601 Jordan Street
Shreveport, LA 71101-4748
318-425-7781
Fax: 318-226-1299
raydra@deafactioncenter.org
www.deafactioncenter.org

David W Hylan, Jr, Executive Director

The center provides comprehensive services through one central agency 'to bridge the gap' between the hearing and deaf worlds. Since its inception, the Center has made every effort to identify those deaf individuals who have specific needs and to provide adequate services for them.

Year Founded: 1982

4712 Canine Assistance for the Disabled

3160 Francis Road
Milton, GA 30004
770-664-7178
Fax: 770-664-7820; *Toll Free:* 800-771-7221
info@canineassistants.org
www.canineassistants.org

Jennifer Arnold, Executive Director
Melissa Payton, Director of Operations
Grace Murphy, Director of Development

Provides individuals with physical or hearing impairments with a dog trained to assist in meeting daily needs. Offers Service Dogs for the physically disabled that can open doors, turn off and on lights, pull wheelchairs up ramps, etc. Signal Dogs for the deaf and hard of hearing person become 'ears' for their masters and Social Dogs that help disabled persons build their self-esteem and confidence.

4713 Carl & Ruth Shapiro Family National Center for Accessible Media

WGBH Media Access Group
One Guest Street
Boston, MA 02135
617-300-3400
Fax: 617-300-1035
ncam@wgbh.org
ncam.wgbh.org
TTY: 617-300-2489

Donna Danielewski, Director

Year Founded: 1836

4714 Center for Community and Professional Services

Pennsylvania School for the Deaf
100 W School House Lane
Philadelphia, PA 19144-3403
215-951-4700
Fax: 215-951-4708
ccps@psd.org
www.psd.org
TTY: 215-754-4770

Classes and assistance for the deaf and hard of hearing. Involved in operation of George W. Nevil Home for aged and infirm deaf and blind-deaf persons. Operates camping facility. Bestows awards.

Year Founded: 1820

4715 Center for Hearing & Communication - Florida

2900 W Cypress Creek Road
Fort Lauderdale, FL 33309
954-601-1930
chchearing.org
TTY: 954-601-1938

Laurie Hanin, Executive Director
Margaret Brown, Regional Executive Director

Improving the quality of life for children and adults with all degrees of hearing loss and auditory challenges.

Year Founded: 1910

4716 Center for Hearing & Communication - NewYork

50 Broadway
6th Floor
New York, NY 10004
917-305-7766
chchearing.org
TTY: 917-305-7999

Laurie Hanin, Executive Director

Improving the quality of life for children and adults with all degrees of hearing loss and auditory challenges.

Year Founded: 1910

4717 Central Institute for the Deaf

825 S Taylor Avenue
St Louis, MO 63110
314-977-0132
Fax: 314-977-0023; *Toll Free:* 877-444-4574
cid@cid.edu
cid.edu

Carrue L Johnson, President
Robin M Feder, Executive Director
Dennis M Reagan, Treasurer

Central Institute for the Deaf is a nonprofit institute dedicated to teaching children who are deaf and hard of hearing to listen, talk, read and succeed. CID partners with universities, educators, and other professionals worldwide to help children communicate to achieve their fullest potential.

Year Founded: 1916

4718 Cleveland Hearing & Speech Center

11635 Euclid Avenue
Cleveland, OH 44106-4319
216-231-8787
Fax: 216-231-7141
info@chsc.org
www.chsc.org

Jennell C. Vicki, Executive Director

Offers research and studies into speech, language and hearing disorders.

Year Founded: 1921

4719 Committee for Purchase from People who are Blind or Severely Disabled

U.S. AbilityOne Commission
1401 S Clark Street
Suite 715
Arlington, VA 22202-3259
703-603-2100 Toll free: 800-999-5963
info@abilityone.gov
www.abilityone.gov

James M Kesteloot, Chair
Tina Ballard, Executive Director

A federal agency that administers the Javits-Wagner-O'Day Program, directing federal agencies to purchase products and services from nonprofit agencies that employ people who are blind or have other severe disabilities. Provides a wide range of vocational options to individuals with severe disabilities.

4720 Communication Service for the Deaf

2028 E Ben White Boulevard
Suite 240-5250
Austin, TX 78741

www.csd.org

Chris Soukup, Chief Executive Officer
Brad Hermes, Chief Financial Officer
Dominic Lacy, Chief Innovation Officer

Offers peer counseling, information and referrals and advocacy services.

Year Founded: 1975

4721 Communications Services for the Deaf and Hard of Hearing

1175 Revolution Mill Drive
Suite 15
Greensboro, NC 27405
336-275-8878
Fax: 336-273-0015
info@csdhh.org
www.csdhh.org
TTY: 336-542-3981

Kelle Owens, Executive Director
Paige Sprinkle, Program Coordinator

Provides services to the deaf and hearing impaired.

Year Founded: 1975; Number of Members: 9

4722 Conference of Educational Administrators Serving the Deaf

P.O. Box 116
Washington Grove, MD 20880
202-999-2204
ceasd@ceasd.org
www.ceasd.org
TTY: 202-866-6248

Sandra Edwards, President
Mindi Failing, Treasurer
Stacey Katz Shapiro, Secretary

Focuses on improvements in the education of deaf and hard of hearing people through research, personnel development, advocacy and training.

Year Founded: 1868

4723 Connecticut Deaf and Hard of Hearing Services
Connecticut Department of Rehabilitation Services

184 Windsor Avenue
Windsor, CT 06095
860-424-5055
DORS.Interpreting@ct.gov
www.dhoh.ct.gov
TTY: 800-671-0737

The Deaf and Hard of Hearing Counseling Unit primarily provides adjustment counseling for individuals, couples and family specific to Deaf, Hard of Hearing, and children of Deaf adults. Some examples of counseling may include: managing stress related to communication barriers; issues related to hearing loss; understanding Deaf, Hard of Hearing or Kid of Deaf Adult/Children of Deaf Adult (KODA/CODA) identity; enhancing daily skills and other daily challenges that may be encountered daily with being Deaf, Hard of Hearing or KODA/CODA.

Year Founded: 1974

4724 Convention of American Instructors of the Deaf

PO Box 377
Bedford, TX 76095-0377

817-354-8414
caid@swbell.net
www.caid.org

Christina Yuknis, President

The professional organization for teachers, administrators, educational interpreters, residential personnel, and other professionals involved in education of the deaf. CAID provides biennial conventions, networking of professionals with shared interests through Special Interest Groups, and advocacy for national and state legislation concerning the deaf.

4725 Deaf & Hard of Hearing Service Center

5340 N Fresno Street
Fresno, CA 93710
559-225-3323
Fax: 559-225-0116
info@dhhsc.org
www.dhhsc.org

Michelle L. Bronson, Executive Director

4726 Deaf & Hard of Hearing Service Center Inc.

5340 N Fresno Street
Fresno, CA 93710
559-225-3323
Fax: 559-225-0116
info@dhhsc.org
www.dhhsc.org
TTY: 559-225-3323

Janice Smith-Warshaw, President
Tim Spires, Treasurer
Peter Crume, Secretary

dHHSC offers classes in ASL, basic English, and citizenship preparation for Deaf and Hard of Hearing Immigrants in the Chicagoland area.

Year Founded: 1984

4727 Deaf Counseling, Advocacy & Referral Agency

14895 E 14th Street
Suite 200
San Leandro, CA 94578
510-343-6670
info@dcara.org
www.dcara.org

Raymond Rodgers, Executive Director
David Kerr, Deputy Director
Debby Buchan, Program Developer

Promotes self-determination, independence and celebration of American Sign Language.

Year Founded: 1962

4728 Deaf REACH

3722 12th Street NE
Washington, DC 20017
202-832-6681
maym@deaf-reach.org
www.deaf-reach.org

Michele May, Executive Director

Offers referral, education, advocacy, counseling, and housing services for deaf mentally ill, multihandicapped and/or low income deaf people in the metro District of Columbia area.

Year Founded: 1972

4729 Deaf Seniors of Georgia
Georgia Association of the Deaf
P.O. Box 7023
Columbus, GA 31908
e-mail: gadsocialmedia@gmail.com
gadeaf.org/deaf-seniors

Robert Jones, President
Debra Barnick, Vice President
Duwayne Dukes, Secretary

Division of Georgia Association of the Deaf dedicated to
deaf seniors.

Year Founded: 1910

4730 Described and Captioned Media Program
1447 E Main Street
Spartanburg, SC 29307
864-585-1778
Fax: 800-538-5636; Toll Free: 800-237-6213
info@dcmp.org
dcmp.org
TDD 800-237-6819
TTY: 864-585-2617

Howard A Rosenblum, CEO

Distributes described and captioned educational media to
deaf and hard of hearing individuals, schools and organizations serving deaf and hard of hearing person, families of
deaf and hard of hearing children to promote and provide
equal access to communication and learning.

4731 Dogs for Better Lives
10175 Wheeler Road
Central Point, OR 97502
541-826-9220Toll free: 800-990-3647
info@dogsforbetterlives.org
www.dogsforbetterlives.org

Blake Matray, President & CEO
John Drach, Training Director
Harvey Potts, Devlopment Director

Trains hearing dogs to alert deaf persons to certain sounds.
Dogs are chosen from pet adoption shelters and assigned on
the basis of a prioritized waiting list. Four to five months of
training teaches them to alert their masters to the sounds of
alarm clocks, smoke alarms, doorbells, oven timers, telephones, etc.

Year Founded: 1977

4732 Eaton-Peabody Laboratory of Auditory
Physiology
243 Charles Street
Boston, MA 02114
617-523-7900
www.masseyeandear.org

Ken Holmes, Chief Financial Officer
John Fernandez, President and CEO
Jeff Pikeiams, Chief Operating Officer

Auditory system and auditory information processing, including ear-brain interactions in normal and pathologic
hearing.

4733 Florida Dog Guides for the Deaf
2016 27th Street E
Bradenton, FL 34208
941-748-8245
floridadogguides@gmail.com
www.floridadogguidesftd.org

Brandy Decker, Office Manager

Florida Dog Guides FTD is a certified Service Dog, Therapy Dog and Dog Obedience Training Center specializing
in personalized dog training for Service Dogs, Therapy
Dogs and Veteran Dogs for over 30 years.

Year Founded: 1984

4734 Gallaudet University
800 Florida Avenue NE
Washington, DC 20002
202-651-5000
usherla.deberry@gallaudet.edu
www.gallaudet.edu

Roberta Cordano, President

A comprehensive multipurpose educational institution serving deaf and hard of hearing individuals through education,
research and public service. Disseminates information
through such units as the Gallaudet University Press; Research Institute; Pre-College Outreach; College for Continuing Education; Media Distribution Center and the
National Information Center on Deafness.

4735 Georgia Center of the Dead and Hard of
Hearing
4151 Memorial Drive
Suite 103-B
Decatur, GA 30032
404-292-5312
Fax: 404-299-3642; Toll Free: 800-541-0710
www.gcdhh.org
TTY: 404-381-8447

Jimmy Peterson, Executive Director
LaQuanda Jackson, Executive Assistant
DeAnna Swope, Case Manager

Dedicated to helping Georgians who are deaf, hard of hearing, late deafened or deaf-blind improve their quality of
life.

4736 HEAR Center
301 E Del Mar Boulevard
Pasadena, CA 91101
626-796-2016
Fax: 626-796-2320
info@hearcenter.org
www.hearcenter.org

Ellen Simon, Executive Director
Deborah Lorino, Office Manager
Berenice Castro, COO

Auditory and verbal program designed to help hearing impaired children, infants and adults lead normal and productive lives. Seeks to develop auditory techniques to aid
people who have communication problems due to deafness.
Offers diagnostic evaluations for hearing. And hearing aid
dispensing. Aural rehabilitation program.

Year Founded: 1954

4737 Hands Organization for the Deaf and Hard of
Hearing
Ridge Academy
2501 W 103rd Street
Chicago, IL 60655-1003
773-233-0033
www.ridgeacademy.org

Kenneth Koll, Principal

A nonprofit organization of both deaf and hearing persons working together to address the needs and concerns of the deaf community. The organization is working to raise the consciousness of the hearing world to the realities of deafness, and to bridge the gap between services already in place for the deaf and the large number of deaf people who have never been reached by those services.

Year Founded: 2000

4738 Hear Now
Starkey Hearing Foundation
6700 Washington Avenue
South Eden Prairie, MN 55344
866-354-3254
Fax: 952-828-6900; Toll Free: 800-328-8602
info@starkeyfoundation.org
www.starkeyhearingfoundation.org

Richard Brown, President
Elizabeth Tulach, Vice President
Jeff Papineau, Treasurer

Hear Now is an application-based program that provides hearing help to low-income Americans, funded and organized by the Starkey Hearing Foundation.

Year Founded: 1984

4739 Hearing Education and Awareness for Rockers
H.E.A.R.
1405 Lyon Street
San Francisco, CA 94115
415-409-3277
help@hearnet.com
www.hearnet.com
TTY: 415-476-7600

Kathy Peck, Executive Director

Educates the public about the real dangers of hearing loss resulting from repeated exposure to excessive noise levels.

Year Founded: 1988

4740 Hearing Industries Association
1444 I Street, NW
Suite 700
Washington, DC 20005
202-449-1090
info@hearing.org
www.hearing.org

Carole M Rogin, President

The association for hearing aid manufacturers and suppliers of component parts.

4741 Hearing Loss Association of America
7910 Woodmont Avenue
Suite 1200
Bethesda, MD 20814
301-657-2248
Fax: 301-913-9413
www.hearingloss.org

Barbara Kelley, Acting Executive Director

Assistance, resources and advocacy for people with hearing loss and their families.

Year Founded: 1979

4742 Helen Keller National Center for Deaf-Blind Youths & Adults
141 Middle Neck Road
Sands Point, NY 11050
516-944-8900
hkncinfo@hknc.org
www.helenkeller.org

Joseph F. Bruno, President & CEO
Marc Feldman, CFO

A team of experts tailors action plans with deaf-blind individuals using cutting-edge technology and hands-on learning.

Year Founded: 1967

4743 House Ear Institute
2100 W 3rd Street
Suite 111
Los Angeles, CA 90057
213-989-6701
Fax: 213-989-7473
saugustine@hei.org
www.hei.org

Jennifer Derebery, MD, Board of Directors
Gregory Lekovic, MD, Board of Directors
Marc Schwartz, MD, Board of Directors

Studies the causes of hearing impairments and trains professionals in diagnosis, treatment and rehabilitation.

Year Founded: 1946; Number of Members: 180

4744 International Catholic Deaf Association
e-mail: icdaus1989@gmail.com
www.icda-us.org

Jean Cox, President
Kate Slosar, Vice President
Aline Shaw, Secretary

Promotes ministry for Catholic deaf people with chapters encouraging to arrange Sunday masses for deaf people in their local areas with the liturgy presented in sign language.
Year Founded: 1987

4745 International Deaftek.USA
Aurora, CO
303-366-1970
www.deaftek.org

Provides an international electronic mail service; dedicated to communities that are deaf or hard of hearing; the service is used by individuals, organizations, agencies, schools, colleges and universities, service providers, and professionals in the field of deafness.

Year Founded: 1978

4746 International Hearing Dog
International Hearing Dog
5901 E 89th Avenue
Henderson, CO 80640
303-287-3277
Fax: 303-287-3425
info@hearingdog.org
www.hearingdog.org

Samuel Cheris, Chairman
Anne Musial, Vice Chair
Matt Bailey, Treasurer

Trains dogs to assist persons who are deaf or hard-of-hearing, with and without multiple disabilities, at no cost to the recipient.

Year Founded: 1979

4747 International Hearing Society

16880 Middlebelt Road
Suite 4
Livonia, MI 48154
734-522-7200
Fax: 734-522-0200
kburch@ihsinfo.org
www.ihsinfo.org

Kathleen Mennillo, Executive Director
Richard Giles, President
Antonio F Calderon, MD, Treasurer

The society recognizes the need for promoting and maintaining the highest possible standards for its members in the best interest of the consumer. As the membership organization for thousands of independent specialists, IHS conducts programs in competency accreditation, education and training, and promotes specialty-level certification for its members.

Year Founded: 1951

4748 International Lutheran Deaf Association
Lutheran Deaf Mission Society

9907 Sappington Road
St Louis, MO 63128
e-mail: DeafLutheran@q.com
www.deafjesus.org

Rev. Tim Eckert, Executive Director

Promotes ministry for deaf people throughout the Lutheran Church-Missouri.

Year Founded: 1894

4749 Iowa Hearing Association

1001 Office Park Road
Suite 105
West Des Moines, IA 50265
515-440-6057
Fax: 515-440-6057
apmsthomas@aol.com
www.iowahearingassociation.org

Cory Popelka, President
Steve Harrison, Treasurer
Bev Thomas, Executive Director

The mission of the Iowa Hearing Association is to promote and encourage an effective program of public education as to the benefits of the use of hearing aids.

4750 Kansas Hearing Society

2812 E Menlo
Wichita, KS 67211
316-209-6697
kansashearingsociety.org

Irene Wagner, Executive Director
Haris Zafar, PhD, President
Brad Hilderman, Vice President

The Kansas Hearing Society, Inc. exists to meet the educational and advocacy needs of both Audiologists and Hearing Instrument Specialists in the State of Kansas. The Society also retains a lobbying firm to keep track of state legislative issues that impact members.

4751 Lexington School for the Deaf

25-26 75th Street
East Elmhurst, NY 11370
718-350-3300
Fax: 718-899-9846
www.lexnyc.org
TTY: 917-832-1676

Cindy Casson, Development Director
Russell Rosen, President
Ralph Reiser, Vice President

Offers a comprehensive range of services to deaf, hard of hearing and speech impaired persons from infancy to elderly through its affiliate agencies: The Center for Mental Health Services; The Lexington Hearing and Speech Center, Lexington Vocational Services, and the Lexington School for the Deaf. Also provides services through its research division which houses the only federally funded Rehabilitation Engineering Center.

Year Founded: 1865

4752 Michigan Speech Language Hearing Association

790 W Lake Lansing Road
Suite 400
East Lansing, MI 48823
517-332-5691
msha@att.net
www.michiganspeechhearing.org

Natalie Douglas, President
Katherine Elder, Secretary
Sherry Riedel, Treasurer

Speech pathologists, audiologists, and teachers of the hearing-impaired. Promotes professional development among those working in the speech, language, and hearing field.

Year Founded: 2006

4753 NTID Center on Employment
National Technical Institute for the Deaf

52 Lomb Memorial Drive
Rochester, NY 14623
585-475-6400
www.ntid.rit.edu/nce

Gerard Buckley, President

Operated by the National Technical Institute for the Deaf at Rochester Institute of Technology, the National Center was established to promote successful employment of RIT's deaf graduates. NCED offers training and consultations to employers and professionals working with deaf persons.

Year Founded: 1829

4754 National Association for Hearing & Speech Action
American Speech-Language-Hearing Association

2200 Research Boulevard
Rockville, MD 20850-3289
301-296-5700
Fax: 301-296-8580; *Toll Free:* 800-498-2071
www.asha.org/NAHSA
TTY: 301-296-5650

Arlene A. Pietranton, President
Joseph Cerquone, Executive Director

Professional membership association for speech pathologists and audiologists. Offers referrals to doctors. Free information packets are available.

Year Founded: 1972; Number of Members: 13,000

4755 National Association of the Deaf

8630 Fenton Street
Suite 820
Silver Spring, MD 20910
301-587-1788
Fax: 301-587-1791
nad.org
TTY: 301-587-1789

Howard A. Rosenblum, CEO

Nation's largest organization safeguarding the accessability and civil rights of 28 million deaf and hard of hearing Americans in eduaction, employment, health care, and tele-communications. Focuses on grassroots advocate and empowermet, captioned media deafness-related information and publications, legal assistance, and policy development.

Year Founded: 1880

4756 National Association of the Deaf Law & Advocacy Center

National Association of the Deaf
8630 Fenton Street
Suite 820
Silver Spring, MD 20910
301-587-1788
Fax: 301-587-1791
nad.org
TTY: 301-587-1789

Howard A. Rosenblum, CEO

The NAD Law and Advocacy Center educates, advocates, and litigates on behalf of and to empower deaf and hard of hearing people.

Year Founded: 1880

4757 National Black Deaf Advocates

P.O. Box 564
Secane, PA 19018
e-mail: info@nbda.org
www.nbda.org

Evon Black, President
Samuel Holden, Vice President
Anquinette Kimble, Secretary

NBDA is the leading advocacy organization of black deaf and hard of hearing people in the United States.

Year Founded: 1082; Number of Members: 700

4758 National Captioning Institute

3725 Concorde Parkway
Suite 100
Chantilly, VA 20151
703-917-7600
Fax: 703-917-9853
www.ncicap.org

Gene Chao, Chairman & CEO
Jill Toschi, President & COO

Formed in 1979, the nonprofit National Captioning Institute is the global captioning leader, supplying the highest quality closed-captioning services to the television, cable, and home video industries.

Year Founded: 1979

4759 National Catholic Office for the Deaf

7202 Buchanan Street
Landover Hills, MD 20784
Fax: 301-577-1684
info@ncod.org
www.ncod.org

Assists in the coordination of the efforts of people and organizations involved in the church's ministry with deaf and hard of hearing people; serves as a resource center for information concerning spirtual needs and religious educational materials; and assists bishops and pastors with their pastoral duties to people who are deaf or hard of hearing.

4760 National Center on Deafness

California State University, Northridge
18111 Nordhoff Street
Northridge, CA 91330
818-677-1200
www.csun.edu/ncod

Cathy McLeod, Director

Taking full advantage of the educational, social, and cultural opportunities a large public university has to offer poses a challenge to the most gifted student. For students who are deaf or hard of hearing, the obsacles are multiplied.

Year Founded: 1964

4761 National Congress of Jewish Deaf

jewishdeafcongress.org

Jacob Salem, President
Andrew St. Cyr, Vice President
Simon Roffe, Treasurer

Publishes a quarterly newsletter and holds a conference every two years. The group has a listing of deaf synagogues and deaf Jewish groups in major metropolitan areas around the country. Also publishes a book on Jewish signs.

Year Founded: 1956

4762 National Cued Speech Association

National Cued Speech Association
1300 Pennsylvania Avenue, NW
Suite 190-713
Washington, DC 20004
Toll Free: 800-459-3529
www.cuedspeech.org
TTY: 800-459-3529

Anne Huffman, President
Suhad Keblawi, Treasurer
Claire Klossner, Secretary

Provides instruction, support services and information pertaining to deafness and the application of Cued Speech. The center provides classes and workshops in Cued Speech, maintains a speakers bureau and provides counseling and support for hearing-impaired adults and their families.

Year Founded: 1966

4763 National Family Association for Deaf-Blind

141 Middle Neck Road
Sands Point, NY 11050
Fax: 516-883-9060; *Toll Free:* 800-255-0411
nfadbinfo@gmail.com
nfadb.org

Clara Berg, President
Julie McGuire, Treasurer
Patti McGowan, Secretary

NFADB advocates for all persons who are deaf-blind of any chronological age and cognitive ability, supports national policy to benifit people who are deaf-blind, encourages the founding and strengthening of family organizations in each state, shares information related to deaf-blindness, provides resources and referrals, collaborates with professionals, and assists in the develpment of materials and training seminars which benefit family members.

4764 National Institute on Deafness and Other Communication Disorders
31 Center Drive
MSC 2320
Bethesda, MD 20892-2320
301-496-7243
Fax: 301-402-0018
nidcdinfo@nidcd.nih.gov
www.nidcd.nih.gov

James F. Battey Jr., Director

Part of the National Institutes of Health, the NIDCD conducts and supports research in hearing, balance, taste, smell, voice, speech and language.

Year Founded: 1988

4765 National Organization for Hearing Research Foundation
PO Box 421
Narberth, PA 19072
610-649-6114
info@nohrfoundation.org
nohrfoundation.org

The Foundation was established in order to fund and support medical research into the causes, preventions, treatments and cures for hearing loss and deafness.

Year Founded: 1990

4766 National Rehabilitation Information Center
8400 Corporate Drive
Suite 500
Landover, MD 20785
Toll Free: 800-346-2742
www.naric.com

Mark X. Odum, Project Director

4767 National Technical Institute for the Deaf
Rochester Institute of Technology
52 Lomb Memorial Drive
Rochester, NY 14623
585-475-6400
www.ntid.rit.edu

Gerard Buckley, President

Provides technological postsecondary education to deaf and hard-of-hearing students. One of seven colleges of Rochester Institute of Technology.

Year Founded: 1829

4768 National Theatre of the Deaf
Monte Cristo Cottage
325 Pequot Avenue
New London, CT 06320

860-574-9063
Fax: 860-574-9107
info@ntd.org
www.ntd.org

Betty Beekman, Executive Director

Concentrates on artistic and theatrical professional development of deaf actors.

Year Founded: 1967

4769 Nebraska Commission for the Deaf & Hard of Hearing
4600 Valley Road
Suite 420
Lincoln, NE 68510-4844
402-471-3593
Fax: 402-742-2357; *Toll Free:* 800-545-6244
ncdhh@nebraska.gov
ncdhh.nebraska.gov

John C Wyvill, Executive Director
Natasha Olsen, Business Manager

The mission of the Nebraska Commission for the Deaf and Hard of Hearing is to promote and advocate for Nebraskans who are Deaf, Deaf-Blind or Hard of Hearing; to achieve equality and opportunity in social, educational, vocational, and legal aspects impacting their daily lives; and to enhance and monitor access to effective communication and telecommunication technology.

Year Founded: 1993

4770 New Jersey Academy of Audiology
American Academy of Audiology
11480 Commerce Park Drive
Suite 220
Reston, VA 20191
703-790-8466
Fax: 703-790-8631; *Toll Free:* 800-222-2336
ttolpegin@audiology.org
www.audiology.org

Promotes audiology to consumers, physicians, and schools through outreach and continuing educational programs.

Number of Members: 12000

4771 North Carolina Department of Human Resources: Deaf & Hard of Hearing Division
2301 Mail Service Center
Raleigh, NC 27699-2301
919-874-2212Toll free: 800-851-6099
dsdhh.information@dhhs.nc.gov
www.ncdhhs.gov/divisions/dsdhh
TTY: 919-890-0859

Bill Rabon, President

The North Carolina Council for the Deaf and the Hard of Hearing was established to advise the Department of Health and Human Services and the Department of Public Instruction on matters pertaining to services provided to deaf and hard of hearing individuals and their families.

Year Founded: 1970

4772 Pittsburgh Hearing, Speech and Deaf Services
Center for Hearing & Deaf Services
1945 5th Avenue
Pittsburgh, PA 15219-5547
412-281-1375
ahart@hdscenter.org

www.hdscenter.org
TTY: 412-281-1375

Amy Hart, President & CEO
Deborah DeFazio, Chief Financial Officer
Patricia Maurer, Director, Development

Provides diagnostic, rehabilitative, and support services for persons who are deaf, hard of hearing, or speech impaired. Offers hearing tests, hearing aid sales and repair, and assistive listening/signaling devices. Offers speech/language evaluation and therapy; provides sign language interpreting, psychological, mental health counseling and social rehabilitation services.

Year Founded: 1920

4773 Providence Speech and Hearing Center

1301 Providence Avenue
Orange, CA 92868
714-923-1521
Fax: 714-639-2593
pshc@pshc.org
pshc.org

Lewis Jaffe, President
Casey Immel, Treasurer
Marlene Woodworth, Secretary

Providence speech and hearing center's mission is to provide the highest quality services available in the identification, diagnosis, treatment and prevention of speech, language and hearing disorders for persons of all ages.

Year Founded: 1965

4774 Regional Resource Center on Deafness
Western Oregon University

345 Monmouth Avenue N
Monmouth, OR 97361
503-838-8000Toll free: 877-877-1593
rrcd@wou.edu
www.wou.edu

Cheryl Davis, Director

The mission is to prepare professionals in the Northwest who are qualified to serve the unique communication, rehabilitation, and educational needs of deaf and hard of hearing children and adults. The center offers graduate and undergraduate degree programs for professionals entering various fields that serve this population, continuing education opportunities for currently particing professionals; and consultation and community service activities designed to enhance the quality of life for all citizens who are hard of hearing or deaf.

Year Founded: 1856

4775 Registry of Interpreters for the Deaf

333 Commerce Street
Alexandria, VA 22314
703-838-0030
Fax: 703-838-0454
ridinfo@rid.org
www.rid.org
TTY: 571-257-3957

Melvin Walker, President
Josh Pennise, Secretary
Sandra Maloney, Vice President

The Registry of Interpreters for the Deaf strives to advocate for the best practices in interpreting, professional development for practitioners and for the highest standards in the

provisions of interpreting services for diverse users of languages that are signed or spoken.

Year Founded: 2011; Number of Members: 7,000

4776 Rochester Institute of Technology: National Technical Institute for the Deaf
NTID at College of Rochester Technology

52 Lomb Memorial Drive
Rochester, NY 14623
585-475-6400
ntidmc@rit.edu
www.ntid.rit.edu
TTY: 585-743-1366

Dr. Gerard Buckley, President

Provides technical and professional education and training for deaf students.

Year Founded: 1829

4777 South Carolina Association of the Deaf

437 Center Street
West Columbia, SC 29169
803-794-3175
Fax: 803-794-4420
www.scadservices.org
TTY: 803-794-7059

Sherry Williams, President
Anita M. Steichen-McDaniel, Executive Director
Joy Hill, Administrative Assistant

Advocates for hearing impaired persons. Acts as an information clearinghouse. Provides interpreter information, does statewide interpreter assessments, sells assistive devices for the deaf and hard of hearing.

Year Founded: 1911

4778 The Betty & Leonard Phillips Deaf ActionCenter of Louisiana

601 Jordan Street
Shreveport, LA 71101
318-425-7781
www.deafactioncenter.org

Angie Evans, Office Manager

Supports and promotes the non-hearing population of Central Louisiana.

Year Founded: 1982

4779 Travis County Services for the Deaf and Hard of Hearing

2201 Post Road
Suite 100
Austin, TX 78704
512-410-1598
Fax: 512-854-9289
angeline.champagne@traviscountytx.gov
www.traviscountytx.gov

Stacy Landry, Program Manager
Julie Erickson, Case Manager
Tom Turner, Case Manager

Promotes participation in recreational activities by the deaf. Provides social services, advocacy, and communications access by people who are deaf. Makes available interpreter services to facilitate communication between deaf people and agencies and corporations.

4780 Treasure Valley Hearing and Balance Clinics
1084 N Cole Road
Boise, ID 83704
208-549-5431
www.treasurevalleyhearing.com

Jacquie Elcox, Chief Executive Officer
Denice Sawin, Audiologist Assistant

Provides hearing assesments, treatment to hearing loss, and healthcare otions to hard of hearing individuals.

Year Founded: 1990

4781 USA Deaf Sports Federation
PO Box 22011
Santa Fe, NM 87502
e-mail: support@usdeafsports.org
usdeafsports.org

Governing body for all deaf sports and recreation in the United States. Seventeen different sports organizations and 200 member clubs are affiliates. Publishes a newsletter three times a year and an annual magazine.

4782 Virginia Department of Deaf and Hard ofHearing
1602 Rolling Hills Drive
Suite 203
Henrico, VA 23229-5012
804-662-9502Toll free: 800-552-7917
www.vddhh.org
TTY: 800-552-7917

Ronald Lanier, Director
Eric Raff, Deputy Director
Leslie Hutcheson, Administration/Policy Manager

Works to reduce the communication barriers between persons who are deaf or hard of hearing and their families and the professionals who serve them. Operates with the full understanding that communication is the most critical issue facing persons who are deaf or hard of hearing.

4783 Washington Hearing and Speech
Sibley Center for Rehabilitation Medicine
5255 Loughboro Road NW
Washington, DC 20016
202-537-4010
www.hopkinsmedicine.org

Lauren K. Dickstein, Senior Audiologist
Daniel Weinstein, Snr. Speech-Language Pathologist

Offers individuals with hearing or speech impairments, in the DC area, speech reading classes, audiological services and new aids.

Year Founded: 1890

4784 Wisconsin Alliance of Hearing Professionals
P.O. Box 161
Evansville, WI 53536
608-882-6571
dqj@jjaassociates.com
wahpinfo.org

Todd Beyer, President
Peter Zellmer, Vice President
Michelle Krier, Secretary-Treasurer

The Alliance is the statewide association of the hearing instrument specialists and audiologists. Its purpose is to foster, promote and protect the professional interests and general welfare of its members and the hearing impaired.

Year Founded: 1901

Books

4785 Advanced Sign Language Vocabulary
Charles C Thomas Publisher
2600 S 1st Street
P.O. Box 19265
Springfield, IL 62704-4730
217-789-8980
Fax: 217-789-9130
books@ccthomas.com
www.ccthomas.com
TDD 217-789-8980
TTY: 217-789-8980

Michael P Thomas, President

A resource text for educators, interpreters, parents and sign language instructors.

202 pages Year Founded: 1927

4786 American Deaf Culture
Gallaudet University
800 Florida Avenue
NE
Washington, DC 20002-3695
202-651-5000
Fax: 800-621-8476; Toll Free: 800-621-2736
visitors.center@gallaudet.edu
www.gallaudet.edu
TTY: 888-630-9347

Dr. T. Alan Hurwitz, President
Edward Bosso, Vice President for the Laurent C
Charity Reedy, Chief Enrollment Management Offi

This book presents a collection of classic articles which have been selected to provide a variety of perspectives on language and culture of deaf people in America.

132 pages Year Founded: 1864

4787 American Deaf Culture: An Anthology
Sign Media
4020 Blackburn Lane
Burtonsville, MD 20866-1167
301-421-0268
Fax: 301-421-0270; Toll Free: 800-475-4756
www.signmedia.com
TTY: 301-421-4460

Verden Ness, President
Barbara Olmert, Director Marketing
Sherman Wilcox, Editor

Features Deaf and hearing authors offering their experience and perspectives on cultural values, ASL, social interaction in the Deaf community, education, folklore, and more.

Year Founded: 1979

4788 American Sign Language: A Beginning Course
National Association of the Deaf
814 Thayer Avenue
Silver Spring, MD 20910-4504
301-587-6282
Fax: 301-587-4873
www.nad.org
TTY: 301-587-1789

Howard A. Rosenblum, CEO
Shane H. Feldman, COO
Andrew S. Phillips, Staff Attorney

An interactive approach to teaching and learning American Sign Language, with 700 sign illustrations, each accompanied by an object drawing.

199 pages Year Founded: 1880

4789 Basic Course in Manual Communication
Gallaudet University
800 Florida Avenue
NE
Washington, DC 20002-3695
202-651-5000
Fax: 800-621-8476; *Toll Free:* 800-621-2736
visitors.center@gallaudet.edu
www.gallaudet.edu
TTY: 888-630-9347

Dr. T. Alan Hurwitz, President
Edward Bosso, Vice President for the Laurent C
Charity Reedy, Chief Enrollment Management Offi

Teach your students manual communication - that living, changing, growing language of signs.

158 pages Year Founded: 1864

4790 Basic Sign Communication: Vocabulary
National Association of the Deaf
814 Thayer Avenue
Silver Spring, MD 20910-4504
301-587-6282
Fax: 301-587-4873
www.nad.org
TTY: 301-587-1789

Howard A. Rosenblum, CEO
Shane H. Feldman, COO
Andrew S. Phillips, Staff Attorney

Features sections on Sign Vocabulary, Numbers, and Classifiers. Contains 1000 illustrated signs, organized alphabetically by gloss for quick reference.

162 pages Year Founded: 1880

4791 Book of Name Signs
Gallaudet University
800 Florida Avenue
NE
Washington, DC 20002-3695
202-651-5000
Fax: 800-621-8476; *Toll Free:* 800-621-2736
visitors.center@gallaudet.edu
www.gallaudet.edu
TTY: 888-630-9347

Dr. T. Alan Hurwitz, President
Edward Bosso, Vice President for the Laurent C
Charity Reedy, Chief Enrollment Management Offi

Discusses the rules for American Sign Language name sign formation and their appropriate use.

112 pages Year Founded: 1864

4792 Bridges Beyond Sound
Brookes Publishing
PO Box 10624
Baltimore, MD 21285-0624
410-337-9580
Fax: 410-337-8539; *Toll Free:* 800-638-3775

submit@brookespublishing.com
www.brookespublishing.com

Paul Brooks, Owner

An instructional workbook on understanding and including students with a hearing loss. Supplement to the Bridges Beyond Sound videotape. Besides the videotape script, background information on hearing loss, discussion questions, activities, and reproducible worksheets are included.

176 pages

4793 Chelsea: The Story of a Signal Dog
Gallaudet University
800 Florida Avenue
NE
Washington, DC 20002-3695
202-651-5000
Fax: 800-621-8476; *Toll Free:* 800-621-2736
visitors.center@gallaudet.edu
www.gallaudet.edu
TTY: 888-630-9347

Dr. T. Alan Hurwitz, President
Edward Bosso, Vice President for the Laurent C
Charity Reedy, Chief Enrollment Management Offi

This is a story of a young deaf couple and their Belgian sheepdog, who acts as their 'ears'. It explains how these dogs are trained and paired with their new owners.

169 pages Year Founded: 1864

4794 Choices in Deafness
Woodbine House
6510 Bells Mill Road
Bethesda, MD 20817-1636
301-897-3570
Fax: 301-897-5838; *Toll Free:* 800-843-7323
info@woodbinehouse.com
www.woodbinehouse.com

Irv Shapell, Owner

A useful aid in choosing the appropriate communication option for a child with a hearing loss. Experts present the following communication options: Auditory-Verbal Approach, Bilingual-Bicultural Approach, Cued Speech, Oral Approach, and Total Communication. This new edition explains medical causes of hearing loss, the diagnostic process, audiological assessment, and cochlear implants. Children and parents also offer their personal experiences.

275 pages

4795 Cognition, Education and Deafness
Gallaudet University
800 Florida Avenue
NE
Washington, DC 20002-3695
202-651-5000
Fax: 800-621-8476; *Toll Free:* 800-621-2736
visitors.center@gallaudet.edu
www.gallaudet.edu
TTY: 888-630-9347

Dr. T. Alan Hurwitz, President
Edward Bosso, Vice President for the Laurent C
Charity Reedy, Chief Enrollment Management Offi

The work of 54 authors is gathered in this definitive collection of current research on deafness and cognition. The articles are grouped into seven sections: cognition, problem solving, thinking processes, language development, reading methodologies, measurement of potential, and intervention programs.

260 pages Year Founded: 1864

4796 Come Sign with Us
Gallaudet University
800 Florida Avenue
NE
Washington, DC 20002-3695
202-651-5000
Fax: 800-621-8476; *Toll Free:* 800-621-2736
visitors.center@gallaudet.edu
www.gallaudet.edu
TTY: 888-630-9347

Dr. T. Alan Hurwitz, President
Edward Bosso, Vice President for the Laurent C
Charity Reedy, Chief Enrollment Management Offi

Lessons including fingerspelling and signing are overviewed.

Year Founded: 1864

4797 Communicating with Deaf People: An Introduction
Gallaudet University
800 Florida Avenue
NE
Washington, DC 20002-3695
202-651-5000
Fax: 800-621-8476; *Toll Free:* 800-621-2736
visitors.center@gallaudet.edu
www.gallaudet.edu
TTY: 888-630-9347

Dr. T. Alan Hurwitz, President
Edward Bosso, Vice President for the Laurent C
Charity Reedy, Chief Enrollment Management Offi

This illustrated publication introduces the various ways deaf people can communicate, including gesture and facial expression, speech-reading, fingerspelling and other manual communication systems.

20 pages Year Founded: 1864

4798 Communication Access for Persons with Hearing Loss
Alexander Graham Bell Association for the Deaf
3417 Volta Place, NW
Washington, DC 20007-2753
202-337-5220
Fax: 202-337-8314
info@agbell.org
listeningandspokenlanguage.org
TTY: 202-337-5220

Alexander T. Graham, Executive Director
Judy Harrison, Director of Programs
June Martin, Development and Outreach Manager

Filled with information about available technologies, this book explores equipment and options available uner the ADA. The book stresses that technology is a tool, not a solution, for combination hearing loss and for improving communication.

306 pages

4799 Communication Disorders in Aging
Gallaudet University
800 Florida Avenue
NE
Washington, DC 20002-3695
202-651-5000
Fax: 800-621-8476; *Toll Free:* 800-621-2736
visitors.center@gallaudet.edu
www.gallaudet.edu
TTY: 888-630-9347

Dr. T. Alan Hurwitz, President
Edward Bosso, Vice President for the Laurent C
Charity Reedy, Chief Enrollment Management Offi

This text presents contemporary practices in the medical and clinical assessment of the aged, reviews clinical evaluation techniques, and provides a comprehensive discussion of neurological imaging techniques.

528 pages Year Founded: 1864

4800 Communication Issues Among Deaf People
Gallaudet University
800 Florida Avenue
NE
Washington, DC 20002-3695
202-651-5000
Fax: 800-621-8476; *Toll Free:* 800-621-2736
visitors.center@gallaudet.edu
www.gallaudet.edu
TTY: 888-630-9347

Dr. T. Alan Hurwitz, President
Edward Bosso, Vice President for the Laurent C
Charity Reedy, Chief Enrollment Management Offi

Monograph discussing important aspects of communication including total communication and the value of ASL.

138 pages Year Founded: 1864

4801 Communication Issues Among Deaf People - Eyes, Hands, and Voices
National Association of the Deaf
814 Thayer Avenue
Silver Spring, MD 20910-4504
301-587-6282
Fax: 301-587-4873
www.nad.org
TTY: 301-587-1789

Howard A. Rosenblum, CEO
Shane H. Feldman, COO
Andrew S. Phillips, Staff Attorney

Includes over thirty relevant articles reflecting a wide range of perceptions and attitutes on communication among deaf people.

145 pages Year Founded: 1880

4802 Communication Issues Related to Hearing Loss
Self Help for Hard of Hearing People
7910 Woodmont Avenue
Suite 1200
Bethesda, MD 20814-7022
301-657-2248
Fax: 301-913-9413
national@shhh.org
www.hearingloss.org
TTY: 301-657-2249

Anna Gilmore Hall, Executive Director
Barbara Kelly, Deputy Executive Director and Ed
Lise Hamlin, Director of Public Policy

An overview of causes and effects of hearing loss on those who experience it - both people with hearing loss and their families. Helpful also to professionals who provide services to people with hearing loss.

Year Founded: 1979

4803 Communication Therapy for Hearing Impaired Adults

Alexander Graham Bell Association for the Deaf
3417 Volta Place, NW
Washington, DC 20007-2753
202-337-5220
Fax: 202-337-8314
info@agbell.org
listeningandspokenlanguage.org
TTY: 202-337-5220

Alexander T. Graham, Executive Director
Judy Harrison, Director of Programs
June Martin, Development and Outreach Manager

A conversation-based aural habilitation approach offers assessment materials and relevant therapy procedures for hearing impaired adults in daily conversation.

228 pages

4804 Communication and Adult Hearing Loss

Alexander Graham Bell Association for the Deaf
3417 Volta Place, NW
Washington, DC 20007-2753
202-337-5220
Fax: 202-337-8314
info@agbell.org
listeningandspokenlanguage.org
TTY: 202-337-5220

Alexander T. Graham, Executive Director
Judy Harrison, Director of Programs
June Martin, Development and Outreach Manager

This informative book was written for anyone who wants to communicate more effectively with a person with adult hearing loss.

136 pages

4805 Communication-Based Learning Communities

Alexander Graham Bell Association for the Deaf
3417 Volta Place, NW
Washington, DC 20007-2753
202-337-5220
Fax: 202-337-8314
info@agbell.org
listeningandspokenlanguage.org
TTY: 202-337-5220

Alexander T. Graham, Executive Director
Judy Harrison, Director of Programs
June Martin, Development and Outreach Manager

This 1995 monograph of The Volta Review examines how teachers work with students who are deaf or hard of hearing to construct knowledge rather than to transmit information to students and to create meaningful context.

169 pages

4806 Comprehensive Reference Manual for Signers and Interpreters 4th Edition

Charles C Thomas Publisher
2600 S 1st Street
P.O. Box 19265
Springfield, IL 62704-4730
217-789-8980
Fax: 217-789-9130; Toll Free: 800-258-8980
books@ccthomas.com
www.ccthomas.com
TDD 217-789-8980
TTY: 217-789-8980

Michael P Thomas, President

Manual for signers. Paperback only.

314 pages 1994 Year Founded: 1927

4807 Comprehensive Signed English Dictionary

Harris Communications
15155 Technology Drive
Eden Prairie, MN 55344-2273
952-906-1180
Fax: 952-906-1099; Toll Free: 800-825-6758
www.harriscomm.com
TTY: 800-825-9187

Robert Harris, President
Karen L Saulnier, Author
Bill Williams, National Sales Manager

Complete dictionary offers 3,100 signs, including signs reflecting contemporary vocabulary.

457 pages Year Founded: 1982

4808 Conversational Sign Language II

Harris Communications
15155 Technology Drive
Eden Prairie, MN 55344-2273
952-906-1180
Fax: 952-906-1099; Toll Free: 800-825-6758
www.harriscomm.com
TTY: 800-825-9187

Robert Harris, President
Bill Williams, National Sales Manager

This book presents English words and their American Sign Language equivalents.

218 pages Year Founded: 1982

4809 Coping with the Multi-Handicapped Hearing Impaired: A Practical Approach

Charles C Thomas Publisher
2600 S 1st Street
P.O. Box 19265
Springfield, IL 62704-4730
217-789-8980
Fax: 217-789-9130; Toll Free: 800-258-8980
books@ccthomas.com
www.ccthomas.com
TDD 217-789-8980
TTY: 217-789-8980

Michael P Thomas, President

Professional text offers suggestions on how to deal with the multi-handicapped deaf person. Available in cloth, paperback and hardcover.

90 pages Year Founded: 1927

4810 Dancing Without Music
Gallaudet University
800 Florida Avenue
NE
Washington, DC 20002-3695
202-651-5000
Fax: 800-621-8476; *Toll Free:* 800-621-2736
visitors.center@gallaudet.edu
www.gallaudet.edu
TTY: 888-630-9347

Dr. T. Alan Hurwitz, President
Edward Bosso, Vice President for the Laurent C
Charity Reedy, Chief Enrollment Management Offi

Investigates being deaf and its ramifications in society.

320 pages Year Founded: 1864

4811 Deafness 1993-2013
National Association of the Deaf
814 Thayer Avenue
Silver Spring, MD 20910-4504
301-587-1788
Fax: 301-587-4873
www.nad.org
TTY: 301-587-1789

Howard A. Rosenblum, CEO
Shane H. Feldman, COO
Andrew S. Phillips, Staff Attorney

Over 30 articles cover such topics as magnet schools, deaf
identity, technology, multicultural education, communication, leadership, and sign language research.

Year Founded: 1880

4812 Discovering Sign Language
Gallaudet University
800 Florida Avenue
NE
Washington, DC 20002-3695
202-651-5000
Fax: 800-621-8476; *Toll Free:* 800-621-2736
visitors.center@gallaudet.edu
www.gallaudet.edu
TTY: 888-630-9347

Dr. T. Alan Hurwitz, President
Edward Bosso, Vice President for the Laurent C
Charity Reedy, Chief Enrollment Management Offi

Here is a book of information about deaf people and sign
communication.

104 pages Year Founded: 1864

4813 Do You Hear Me?
Alexander Graham Bell Association for the Deaf
3417 Volta Place, NW
Washington, DC 20007-2753
202-337-5220
Fax: 202-337-8270
info@agbell.org
listeningandspokenlanguage.org
TTY: 202-337-5220

Alexander T. Graham, Executive Director
Judy Harrison, Director of Programs
June Martin, Development and Outreach Manager

This little book is a collection of all the jokes and cartoons
that help the author cope with his hearing impairment. He
believes strongly that family members and friends who offer encouragement and understanding play and extremely
important role in whether people with hearing losses decide
to seek professional help to overcome the problems that
their hearing loss causes.

138 pages

4814 Ear Book
Gallaudet University
800 Florida Avenue
NE
Washington, DC 20002-3695
202-651-5000
Fax: 800-621-8476; *Toll Free:* 800-621-2736
visitors.center@gallaudet.edu
www.gallaudet.edu
TTY: 888-630-9347

Dr. T. Alan Hurwitz, President
Edward Bosso, Vice President for the Laurent C
Charity Reedy, Chief Enrollment Management Offi

A how-to book on obtaining and using an otoscope, recognizing and managing common ear disorders, when to call
the doctor and when your child needs ear tubes.

136 pages Year Founded: 1864

4815 Educating the Deaf: Psychology, Principles and
Practices
Gallaudet University
800 Florida Avenue
NE
Washington, DC 20002-3695
202-651-5000
Fax: 800-621-8476; *Toll Free:* 800-621-2736
visitors.center@gallaudet.edu
www.gallaudet.edu
TTY: 888-630-9347

Dr. T. Alan Hurwitz, President
Edward Bosso, Vice President for the Laurent C
Charity Reedy, Chief Enrollment Management Offi

Offers extensive coverage of the background and history of
the education of the deaf, as well as specific information on
working with multihandicapped students.

383 pages Year Founded: 1864

4816 Encyclopedia of Deafness and Hearing
Disorders
Gallaudet University
800 Florida Avenue
NE
Washington, DC 20002-3695
202-651-5000
Fax: 800-621-8476; *Toll Free:* 800-621-2736
visitors.center@gallaudet.edu
www.gallaudet.edu
TTY: 888-630-9347

Dr. T. Alan Hurwitz, President
Edward Bosso, Vice President for the Laurent C
Charity Reedy, Chief Enrollment Management Offi

Presents the most current information on deafness and
hearing disorders in an authoritative A-to-Z compendium.

278 pages Year Founded: 1864

4817 FM Auditory Training Systems
Alexander Graham Bell Association for the Deaf
3417 Volta Place, NW
Washington, DC 20007-2753

202-337-5220
Fax: 202-337-8270
info@agbell.org
listeningandspokenlanguage.org
TTY: 202-337-5220

Alexander T. Graham, Executive Director
Judy Harrison, Director of Programs
June Martin, Development and Outreach Manager

This brand new text is a collection of papers written by notable experts in the field of FM auditory training systems and speech development.

254 pages

4818 GA and SK Etiquette
Gallaudet University
800 Florida Avenue
NE
Washington, DC 20002-3695
202-651-5000
Fax: 800-621-8476; *Toll Free:* 800-621-2736
visitors.center@gallaudet.edu
www.gallaudet.edu
TTY: 888-630-9347

Dr. T. Alan Hurwitz, President
Edward Bosso, Vice President for the Laurent C
Charity Reedy, Chief Enrollment Management Offi

This booklet presents guidelines for proper usage of the TDD. It includes everything you wanted to know about sending and receiving TDD calls.

53 pages Year Founded: 1864

4819 Gallaudet Encyclopedia of Deaf People and Deafness
Gallaudet University
800 Florida Avenue
NE
Washington, DC 20002-3695
202-651-5000
Fax: 800-621-8476; *Toll Free:* 800-621-2736
visitors.center@gallaudet.edu
www.gallaudet.edu
TTY: 888-630-9347

Dr. T. Alan Hurwitz, President
Edward Bosso, Vice President for the Laurent C
Charity Reedy, Chief Enrollment Management Offi

Three-volume set of research and information on deaf people and deafness.

1400 pages Year Founded: 1864

4820 HEAR: Solutions, Skills, and Sources for People with Hearing Loss
DK Publishing
375 Hudson Street
New York, NY 10014
646-674-4000
Fax: 201-256-0000; *Toll Free:* 806-318-571
ecommerce@us.penguingroup.com
us.dk.com

4821 Hear: Solutions, Skills, and Sources for People with Hearing Loss
Alexander Graham Bell Association for the Deaf
3417 Volta Place, NW
Washington, DC 20007-2753

202-408-7901
Fax: 202-337-8270
info@agbell.org
listeningandspokenlanguage.org
TTY: 202-337-5220

Alexander T. Graham, Executive Director
Judy Harrison, Director of Programs
June Martin, Development and Outreach Manager

This practical, well-designed self-help guide is a valuable resource for people who are hard of hearing and their families and friends. HEAR features real-life case studies and interviews with people who have become hard of hearing. The reader will learn about sound and how we hear; tips for making changes, finding self-help groups, and knowing your rights; about types of hearing loss and hearing tests.ing loss, from hearing aids to cochlear implant.

128 pages

4822 Hearing Rehabilitation for Deafened Adults: A Psychosocial Approach
Wiley
10475 Crosspoint Boulevard
Indianapolis, IN 46256
317-572-3000
Fax: 317-572-4000; *Toll Free:* 877-762-2974
www.wiley.com

Peter B. Wiley, Chairman of the Board
Stephen M. Smith, President and Chief Executive Of
Jesse C. Wiley, Editor and Member of the Board

Provides the reader with a psycho-social framework for understanding practice, while offering a range of practical strategies,tools and counseling ideas for use in the clinic.

200 pages Year Founded: 1807

4823 Hearing in Aging
Alexander Graham Bell Association for the Deaf
3417 Volta Place, NW
Washington, DC 20007-2753
202-337-5220
Fax: 202-337-8270
info@agbell.org
listeningandspokenlanguage.org
TTY: 202-337-5220

Alexander T. Graham, Executive Director
Judy Harrison, Director of Programs
June Martin, Development and Outreach Manager

A useful title for hearing professionals that discusses rehabilitative services and delivery for adults with age-related hearing loss.

302 pages

4824 How to Survive a Hearing Loss
Gallaudet University
800 Florida Avenue
NE
Washington, DC 20002-3695
202-651-5000
Fax: 800-621-8476; *Toll Free:* 800-621-2736
visitors.center@gallaudet.edu
www.gallaudet.edu
TTY: 888-630-9347

Dr. T. Alan Hurwitz, President
Edward Bosso, Vice President for the Laurent C
Charity Reedy, Chief Enrollment Management Offi

This book presents the results of the author's intensive research about hearing and the ear.

241 pages Year Founded: 1864

4825 I Didn't Hear the Dragon Roar
Gallaudet University
800 Florida Avenue
NE
Washington, DC 20002-3695
202-651-5000
Fax: 800-621-8476; *Toll Free:* 800-621-2736
visitors.center@gallaudet.edu
www.gallaudet.edu
TTY: 888-630-9347

Dr. T. Alan Hurwitz, President
Edward Bosso, Vice President for the Laurent C
Charity Reedy, Chief Enrollment Management Offi

The remarkable true story of a deaf woman's journey from Hong Kong to Katmandu.

251 pages Year Founded: 1864

4826 I Think I Have a Hearing Problem! What Should I Do?
Self Help for Hard of Hearing People
7910 Woodmont Avenue
Suite 1200
Bethesda, MD 20814-7022
301-657-2248
Fax: 301-913-9413
national@shhh.org
www.hearingloss.org
TTY: 301-657-2249

Anna Gilmore Hall, Executive Director
Barbara Kelly, Deputy Executive Director and Ed
Lise Hamlin, Director of Public Policy

A basic introduction to hearing loss and where to go for help.

Year Founded: 1979

4827 In All Our Affairs: Making Crises Work for You
Al-Anon Family Group Headquarters
1600 Corporate Landing Parkway
Virginia Beach, VA 23454-5617
757-563-1600
Fax: 757-563-1655; *Toll Free:* 800-356-9996
afgwso@al-anon.org
www.al-anon.alateen.org

Shatters the silence surrounding crises that go hand in hand with alcoholism.

256 pages

4828 Interpretation: A Sociolinguistic Model
Gallaudet University
800 Florida Avenue
NE
Washington, DC 20002-3695
202-651-5000
Fax: 800-621-8476; *Toll Free:* 800-621-2736
visitors.center@gallaudet.edu
www.gallaudet.edu
TTY: 888-630-9347

Dr. T. Alan Hurwitz, President
Edward Bosso, Vice President for the Laurent C
Charity Reedy, Chief Enrollment Management Offi

This text presents a sociolinguistically sensitive model of the interpretation process. The model applies to interpretation in any two languages although this one focuses on ASL and English.

199 pages Year Founded: 1864

4829 Introduction to Communication
Gallaudet University
800 Florida Avenue
NE
Washington, DC 20002-3695
202-651-5000
Fax: 800-621-8476; *Toll Free:* 800-621-2736
visitors.center@gallaudet.edu
www.gallaudet.edu
TTY: 888-630-9347

Dr. T. Alan Hurwitz, President
Edward Bosso, Vice President for the Laurent C
Charity Reedy, Chief Enrollment Management Offi

Curriculum materials exploring the areas of sound, hearing and interpersonal communication.

100 pages Year Founded: 1864

4830 Invisible Condition: The Human Side of Hearing Loss
Self Help for Hard of Hearing People
7910 Woodmont Avenue
Suite 1200
Bethesda, MD 20814-7022
301-657-2248
Fax: 301-913-9413
national@shhh.org
www.hearingloss.org
TTY: 301-657-2249

Anna Gilmore Hall, Executive Director
Barbara Kelly, Deputy Executive Director and Ed
Lise Hamlin, Director of Public Policy

A collection of 14 years of editorials by the author from the SHHH Journal.

Year Founded: 1979

4831 Journey Into the DEAF-WORLD
DawnSignPress
6130 Nancy Ridge Drive
San Diego, CA 92121-3223
858-625-0600
Fax: 858-625-2336; *Toll Free:* 800-549-5350
www.dawnsign.com

Barry Howland, Marketing Director
Joe Dannis, President

Provides explanation about the nature and meaning of the DEAF-WORLD. Comprehensive work discusses latest findings and theories for Deaf Studies students and professionals working with Deaf people.

528 pages Year Founded: 1700

4832 Joy of Listening: An Auditory Training Program
Alexander Graham Bell Association for the Deaf
3417 Volta Place, NW
Washington, DC 20007-2753
202-337-5220
Fax: 202-337-8270
info@agbell.org

listeningandspokenlanguage.org
TTY: 202-337-5220

Alexander T. Graham, Executive Director
Judy Harrison, Director of Programs
June Martin, Development and Outreach Manager

This manual contains lessons to improve listening skills, auditory discrimination, attention span, memory , and sequencing in children with hearing losses. The lessons can be used when working with children alone, or in small groups.

160 pages

4833 Joy of Signing
Gallaudet University
800 Florida Avenue
NE
Washington, DC 20002-3695
202-651-5000
Fax: 800-621-8476; *Toll Free:* 800-621-2736
visitors.center@gallaudet.edu
www.gallaudet.edu
TTY: 888-630-9347

Dr. T. Alan Hurwitz, President
Edward Bosso, Vice President for the Laurent C
Charity Reedy, Chief Enrollment Management Offi

This manual on signing includes illustrations, information on sign origins, practice sentences, and step-by-step descriptions of hand positions and movements.

336 pages Year Founded: 1864

4834 Keys to Living with Hearing Loss
Self Help for Hard of Hearing People
7910 Woodmont Avenue
Suite 1200
Bethesda, MD 20814-7022
301-657-2248
Fax: 301-913-9413
national@shhh.org
www.hearingloss.org
TTY: 301-657-2249

Anna Gilmore Hall, Executive Director
Barbara Kelly, Deputy Executive Director and Ed
Lise Hamlin, Director of Public Policy

Guidebook that provides helpful advice on a wide range of topics, from living alone with a hearing loss, to going to the hospital, to legal rights.

Year Founded: 1979

4835 Learning To Hear Again
Alexander Graham Bell Association for the Deaf
3417 Volta Place, NW
Washington, DC 20007-2753
202-337-5220
Fax: 202-337-8270
info@agbell.org
listeningandspokenlanguage.org
TTY: 202-337-5220

Alexander T. Graham, Executive Director
Judy Harrison, Director of Programs
June Martin, Development and Outreach Manager

This audiologic rehabilitation curriculum guide is designed to help audiologists and speech language pathologist provide rehabilitation and education for adults with hearing losses. The authors are practicing audiologists and have

used these methods successfully in individual and group sessions. This comprehensive manual comprises lesson plans, activities, and materials ready to be duplicated and distributed to clients. Three-ring binder.

224 pages

4836 Learning to See: American Sign Language as a Second Language
Alexander Graham Bell Association for the Deaf
3417 Volta Place, NW
Washington, DC 20007-2753
202-337-5220
Fax: 202-337-8270
info@agbell.org
listeningandspokenlanguage.org
TTY: 202-337-5220

Alexander T. Graham, Executive Director
Judy Harrison, Director of Programs
June Martin, Development and Outreach Manager

Provides a comprehensive introduction to the history and structure of ASL to the deaf community.

134 pages

4837 Legal Rights of Hearing-Impaired People
Gallaudet University
800 Florida Avenue
NE
Washington, DC 20002-3695
202-651-5000
Fax: 800-621-8476; *Toll Free:* 800-621-2736
visitors.center@gallaudet.edu
www.gallaudet.edu
TTY: 888-630-9347

Dr. T. Alan Hurwitz, President
Edward Bosso, Vice President for the Laurent C
Charity Reedy, Chief Enrollment Management Offi

Includes updated interpretations of legislation affecting hearing-impaired people, including chapters dealing with the ADA.

297 pages Year Founded: 1864

4838 Lessons in Laughter: The Autobiography of a Deaf Actor
Gallaudet University
800 Florida Avenue
NE
Washington, DC 20002-3695
202-651-5000
Fax: 800-621-8476; *Toll Free:* 800-621-2736
visitors.center@gallaudet.edu
www.gallaudet.edu
TTY: 888-630-9347

Dr. T. Alan Hurwitz, President
Edward Bosso, Vice President for the Laurent C
Charity Reedy, Chief Enrollment Management Offi

Born deaf of deaf parents, Bernard Bragg dreamed of using sign language to act. This book recounts how he starred in his own television show.

237 pages Year Founded: 1864

4839 Lipreading Made Easy Book and Video Tape
Alexander Graham Bell Association for the Deaf
3417 Volta Place, NW
Washington, DC 20007-2753

202-337-5220
Fax: 202-337-8270
info@agbell.org
listeningandspokenlanguage.org
TTY: 202-337-5220

Alexander T. Graham, Executive Director
Judy Harrison, Director of Programs
June Martin, Development and Outreach Manager

This photo primer was written to satisfy the need for easy practice-at-home material for people who want to learn the basics of lipreading. 120 minute videotape that gives one hour lessons.

32 pages

4840 Lisa and Her Soundless World
Resources for Rehabilitation
22 Bonad Road
Winchester, MA 01890-1302
781-368-9094
Fax: 781-368-9096
info@rfr.org
www.rfr.org

Describes the impact deafness has on communication and functioning in a hearing world. Lisa, born with a severe hearing loss, was not diagnosed as hearing impaired until her parents were worried about her lack of speech and other children had rejected her.

30 pages

4841 Look Now, Hear This: Combined Auditory Training and Speechreading Instruction
Charles C Thomas Publisher
2600 S 1st Street
P.O. Box 19265
Springfield, IL 62704-4730
217-789-8980
Fax: 217-789-9130; *Toll Free:* 800-258-8980
books@ccthomas.com
www.ccthomas.com
TDD 217-789-8980
TTY: 217-789-8980

Michael P Thomas, President

230 pages Year Founded: 1927

4842 Looking Back: A Reader on the History of Deaf Communities & Sign Language
Gallaudet University
800 Florida Avenue
NE
Washington, DC 20002-3695
202-651-5000
Fax: 800-621-8476; *Toll Free:* 800-621-2736
visitors.center@gallaudet.edu
www.gallaudet.edu
TTY: 888-630-9347

Dr. T. Alan Hurwitz, President
Edward Bosso, Vice President for the Laurent C
Charity Reedy, Chief Enrollment Management Offi

Renowned researchers from around the world present provocative findings in six areas relating to the deaf culture.

558 pages Year Founded: 1864

4843 Meeting Halfway in ASL
DeafLife
PO Box 23380
Rochester, NY 14692-3380
585-442-6370
Fax: 585-442-6371
www.deaflife.com
TTY: 716-442-6370

Matthew S. Moore, Publisher

Illustrated photographic sign-language book containing 1,300 photos.

Year Founded: 1986

4844 Mental Health Services for Deaf People
Gallaudet University
800 Florida Avenue
NE
Washington, DC 20002-3695
202-651-5000
Fax: 800-621-8476; *Toll Free:* 800-621-2736
visitors.center@gallaudet.edu
www.gallaudet.edu
TTY: 888-630-9347

Dr. T. Alan Hurwitz, President
Edward Bosso, Vice President for the Laurent C
Charity Reedy, Chief Enrollment Management Offi

Contains information on over 350 mental health programs and services for deaf people across the United States.

210 pages Year Founded: 1864

4845 Missing Words: The Family Handbook on Adult Hearing Loss
Gallaudet University
800 Florida Avenue
NE
Washington, DC 20002-3695
202-651-5000
Fax: 800-621-8476; *Toll Free:* 800-621-2736
visitors.center@gallaudet.edu
www.gallaudet.edu
TTY: 888-630-9347

Dr. T. Alan Hurwitz, President
Edward Bosso, Vice President for the Laurent C
Charity Reedy, Chief Enrollment Management Offi

Written by a mother who lost her hearing and her daughter, learning to cope.

304 pages Year Founded: 1864

4846 NAD Deaf Awareness Kit
National Association of the Deaf
814 Thayer Avenue
Silver Spring, MD 20910-4504
301-587-1788
Fax: 301-587-4873
www.nad.org
TTY: 301-587-1789

Howard A. Rosenblum, CEO
Shane H. Feldman, COO
Andrew S. Phillips, Staff Attorney

Includes information that can be used both during Deaf Awareness Week and year-round to recognize the accomplishments and heritage of the deaf community.

Year Founded: 1880

4847 On My Own
Gallaudet University
800 Florida Avenue
NE
Washington, DC 20002-3695
202-651-5000
Fax: 800-621-8476; *Toll Free:* 800-621-2736
visitors.center@gallaudet.edu
www.gallaudet.edu
TTY: 888-630-9347

Dr. T. Alan Hurwitz, President
Edward Bosso, Vice President for the Laurent C
Charity Reedy, Chief Enrollment Management Offi

Book examining doorbell devices, alarm clocks, telephone amplifiers and other assistive devices for the deaf.

50 pages Year Founded: 1864

4848 Other Side of Silence
Gallaudet University
800 Florida Avenue
NE
Washington, DC 20002-3695
202-651-5000
Fax: 800-621-8476; *Toll Free:* 800-621-2736
visitors.center@gallaudet.edu
www.gallaudet.edu
TTY: 888-630-9347

Dr. T. Alan Hurwitz, President
Edward Bosso, Vice President for the Laurent C
Charity Reedy, Chief Enrollment Management Offi

Explores the deaf community through interviews from across the country.

256 pages Year Founded: 1864

4849 Outsiders in a Hearing World
Gallaudet University
800 Florida Avenue
NE
Washington, DC 20002-3695
202-651-5000
Fax: 800-621-8476; *Toll Free:* 800-621-2736
visitors.center@gallaudet.edu
www.gallaudet.edu
TTY: 888-630-9347

Dr. T. Alan Hurwitz, President
Edward Bosso, Vice President for the Laurent C
Charity Reedy, Chief Enrollment Management Offi

An introduction to the social world of deaf people. The author gives a sociologists view of what it's like to be deaf.

240 pages Year Founded: 1864

4850 Senior Citizen Program Packet
Self Help for Hard of Hearing People
7910 Woodmont Avenue
Suite 1200
Bethesda, MD 20814-7022
301-657-2248
Fax: 301-913-9413
national@shhh.org
www.hearingloss.org
TTY: 301-657-2249

Anna Gilmore Hall, Executive Director
Barbara Kelly, Deputy Executive Director and Ed
Lise Hamlin, Director of Public Policy

Information and ideas for anyone working with groups of older adults with hearing loss. Materials include a model program of one senior center, information on communication access and assistive devices, coping strategies, publications, programs, and resources.

Year Founded: 1979

4851 Signing Exact English
Modern Signs Press
PO Box 1181
Los Alamitos, CA 90720-1181
562-596-8548
Fax: 562-795-6614; *Toll Free:* 800-572-7332
modsigns@modernsignspress.com
www.modernsignspress.com
TTY: 310-493-4168

Esther Zawolkow, President
Gerilee Gustason, Executive Director

A reference manual containing manual signs representing nearly 4,000 words, plus signs for letters, numbers, prefixes and suffixes.

479 pages

4852 Signing Illustrated
Gallaudet University
800 Florida Avenue
NE
Washington, DC 20002-3695
202-651-5000
Fax: 800-621-8476; *Toll Free:* 800-621-2736
visitors.center@gallaudet.edu
www.gallaudet.edu
TTY: 888-630-9347

Dr. T. Alan Hurwitz, President
Edward Bosso, Vice President for the Laurent C
Charity Reedy, Chief Enrollment Management Offi

A guide presenting illustrations of over 1,350 signs.

85 pages Year Founded: 1864

4853 Signs for Computing Terminology
Gallaudet University
800 Florida Avenue
NE
Washington, DC 20002-3695
202-651-5000
Fax: 800-621-8476; *Toll Free:* 800-621-2736
visitors.center@gallaudet.edu
www.gallaudet.edu
TTY: 888-630-9347

Dr. T. Alan Hurwitz, President
Edward Bosso, Vice President for the Laurent C
Charity Reedy, Chief Enrollment Management Offi

This sign reference will facilitate communication among deaf persons involved with computers by providing a significant vocabulary base for the computing field of today and tomorrow.

182 pages Year Founded: 1864

4854 Silent Alarm: On the Edge with a Deaf EMT
Gallaudet University
800 Florida Avenue
NE
Washington, DC 20002-3695
202-651-5000
Fax: 800-621-8476; *Toll Free:* 800-621-2736

visitors.center@gallaudet.edu
www.gallaudet.edu
TTY: 888-630-9347

Dr. T. Alan Hurwitz, President
Edward Bosso, Vice President for the Laurent C
Charity Reedy, Chief Enrollment Management Offi

Silent Alarm tells the gripping story of survival and the good that the author did as a topnotch EMT.

160 pages Year Founded: 1864

4855 Software to Go
Gallaudet University
800 Florida Avenue
NE
Washington, DC 20002-3695
202-651-5000
Fax: 800-621-8476; *Toll Free:* 800-621-2736
visitors.center@gallaudet.edu
www.gallaudet.edu
TTY: 888-630-9347

Dr. T. Alan Hurwitz, President
Edward Bosso, Vice President for the Laurent C
Charity Reedy, Chief Enrollment Management Offi

Lists and describes commercial software that may be borrowed by educators of hearing impaired students.

100 pages Year Founded: 1864

4856 Speak Out! Tips on Speaking in Public for Individuals with a Hearing Loss
Self Help for Hard of Hearing People
7910 Woodmont Avenue
Suite 1200
Bethesda, MD 20814-7022
301-657-2248
Fax: 301-913-9413
national@shhh.org
www.hearingloss.org
TTY: 301-657-2249

Anna Gilmore Hall, Executive Director
Barbara Kelly, Deputy Executive Director and Ed
Lise Hamlin, Director of Public Policy

Learn how to be an effective speaker.

Year Founded: 1979

4857 Speech & Lip Reading
Charles C Thomas Publisher
2600 S 1st Street
P.O. Box 19265
Springfield, IL 62704-4730
217-789-8980
Fax: 217-789-9130; *Toll Free:* 800-258-8980
books@ccthomas.com
www.ccthomas.com
TDD 217-789-8980
TTY: 217-789-8980

Michael P Thomas, President
Year Founded: 1927

4858 Understanding Deafness Socially
Charles C Thomas Publisher
2600 S 1st Street
P.O. Box 19265
Springfield, IL 62704-4730

217-789-8980
Fax: 217-789-9130; *Toll Free:* 800-258-8980
books@ccthomas.com
www.ccthomas.com
TDD 217-789-8980
TTY: 217-789-8980

Michael P Thomas, President

A look at the social difficulties of being hearing impaired in a 'hearing' society.

168 pages Year Founded: 1927

4859 VISION
National Catholic Office for the Deaf
7202 Buchanan Street
Landover Hills, MD 20784-2236
301-577-1684
Fax: 301-577-1690
www.ncod.org

Kevin C. Rhoades, Episcopal Represenative
Fr. Paul Zirimenya, Region I - West
Arthine Vicks Powers, Region II -The South

Published as a pastoral service for the deaf and hard of hearing.

16 pages Frequency: Quarterly

4860 When the Mind Hears
Gallaudet University
800 Florida Avenue
NE
Washington, DC 20002-3695
202-651-5000
Fax: 800-621-8476; *Toll Free:* 800-621-2736
visitors.center@gallaudet.edu
www.gallaudet.edu
TTY: 888-630-9347

Dr. T. Alan Hurwitz, President
Edward Bosso, Vice President for the Laurent C
Charity Reedy, Chief Enrollment Management Offi

Comprehensive history of the deaf and their relationship with hearing academic communities.

414 pages Year Founded: 1864

4861 Working With Deaf People: Accessibility and Accommodation in the Workplace
Charles C Thomas Publisher
2600 S 1st Street
P.O. Box 19265
Springfield, IL 62704-4730
217-789-8980
Fax: 217-789-9130; *Toll Free:* 800-258-8980
books@ccthomas.com
www.ccthomas.com
TDD 217-789-8980
TTY: 217-789-8980

Michael P Thomas, President

Reveals the kinds of patterns of work adjustment problems that can surface among deaf employees, including the points of view of both supervisors and deaf people.

250 pages Year Founded: 1927

Directories

4862 AIDS and Deafness: Resource Directory
CDC National Aids Clearinghouse
PO Box 6003
Rockville, MD 20849-6003
800-458-5231
Fax: 301-562-1050; *Toll Free:* 800-243-7012
www.cdcnac.org

Computer printout. Lists national, state, and local organizations that offer AIDS (Acquired Immune Deficiency Syndrome)-related services to deaf and hard-of-hearing people; coverage includes Canada and the United Kingdom. Entries include: Organization name, address, phone, hotline numbers, hours of operation, access procedures, TTY/TDD numbers, names and titles of key personnel, geographic area served, description, product/service.
Databasecompiled in cooperation with Gallaudet Research Institute at Gallaudet University.

4863 American Annals of the Deaf: Reference Issue
Gallaudet University
800 Florida Avenue
NE
Washington, DC 20002-3695
202-651-5000
Fax: 800-621-8476; *Toll Free:* 800-621-2736
visitors.center@gallaudet.edu
www.gallaudet.edu
TTY: 888-630-9347

Dr. T. Alan Hurwitz, President
Edward Bosso, Vice President for the Laurent C
Charity Reedy, Chief Enrollment Management Offi

Publication includes: Lists of educational programs and services, supportive and rehabilitation programs and services, and research and information programs and services focusing on the deaf and aurally handicapped. Entries include: Generally, name of sponsoring organization, address, and description of programs offered. School listings include staff and enrollment data.

208 pages Frequency: Annual Year Founded: 1864

4864 Assistive Devices Demonstration Centers
Gallaudet University
800 Florida Avenue
NE
Washington, DC 20002-3695
202-651-5000
Fax: 800-621-8476; *Toll Free:* 800-621-2736
visitors.center@gallaudet.edu
www.gallaudet.edu
TTY: 888-630-9347

Dr. T. Alan Hurwitz, President
Edward Bosso, Vice President for the Laurent C
Charity Reedy, Chief Enrollment Management Offi

A resource list identifying demonstration centers across the United States.

Year Founded: 1864

4865 Audiologists Directory
InfoUSA
PO Box 27347
Omaha, NE 68127
402-593-4600
Fax: 402-331-5481; *Toll Free:* 800-555-6124

admin@abii.com.au
www.abii.com.au
Bill Hippin, Vice President

Number of listings: 3,617. Entries include: Name, address, phone (including area code), size of advertisement, year first in 'Yellow Pages,' name of owner or manager, number of employees. Compiled from telephone company 'Yellow Pages,' nationwide.

4866 Directory of Auditory-Oral Programs
Alexander Graham Bell Association for the Deaf
3417 Volta Place, NW
Washington, DC 20007-2753
202-337-5220
Fax: 202-337-8270
info@agbell.org
listeningandspokenlanguage.org
TTY: 202-337-5220

Alexander T. Graham, Executive Director
Judy Harrison, Director of Programs
June Martin, Development and Outreach Manager

This directory lists auditory-oral programs in public and private schools, auditory-oral programs in speech and hearing centers, and therapists who offer private tutoring and auditory-oral therapy.

204 pages

4867 Directory of National Organizations of and for Deaf and Hard of Hearing People
Gallaudet University
800 Florida Avenue
NE
Washington, DC 20002-3695
202-651-5000
Fax: 800-621-8476; *Toll Free:* 800-621-2736
visitors.center@gallaudet.edu
www.gallaudet.edu
TTY: 888-630-9347

Dr. T. Alan Hurwitz, President
Edward Bosso, Vice President for the Laurent C
Charity Reedy, Chief Enrollment Management Offi

National focus and nonprofit organizations who serve the deaf and hard of hearing. Entries include: Name, address, phone, names and titles of key personnel, name and title of contact, publications and description of available services.

8 pages Frequency: Annual Year Founded: 1864

4868 Greater Los Angeles Agency on Deafness, Inc. (GLAD)
2222 Laverna Avenue
Los Angeles, CA 90041-2625
323-478-8000
Fax: 323-550-4205; *Toll Free:* 323-892-2225
info@gladinc.org
www.gladinc.org

Robert Sidansky, President
Dr. Patricia Hughes, Chief Executive Officer

Resources and information on several programs and organizations that provide accessibility for deaf and hard of hearing community in addition to our services of advocacy, peer counseling, communication assistance, job development, and community education.

Year Founded: 1969

4869 Leading National Publications of and for Deaf People
Gallaudet University
800 Florida Avenue
NE
Washington, DC 20002-3695
202-651-5000
Fax: 800-621-8476; *Toll Free:* 800-621-2736
visitors.center@gallaudet.edu
www.gallaudet.edu
TTY: 888-630-9347

Dr. T. Alan Hurwitz, President
Edward Bosso, Vice President for the Laurent C
Charity Reedy, Chief Enrollment Management Offi

Identifies publications with national circulations to deaf audiences.

Year Founded: 1864

4870 National Directory of Hearing Assistance Technology Assistive Device Demo Centers
Self Help for Hard of Hearing People
7910 Woodmont Avenue
Suite 1200
Bethesda, MD 20814-7022
301-657-2248
Fax: 301-913-9413
national@shhh.org
www.hearingloss.org
TTY: 301-657-2249

Anna Gilmore Hall, Executive Director
Barbara Kelly, Deputy Executive Director and Ed
Lise Hamlin, Director of Public Policy

Year Founded: 1979

Journals, Magazines

4871 ASHA Magazine: ASHA Leader
American Speech-Language-Hearing Association
10801 Rockville Pike
Rockville, MD 20852-3226
301-897-5700
Fax: 301-571-0457; *Toll Free:* 800-638-8255
www.betterhearing.org
TTY: 301-897-5700

Nancy A. Creaghead, President
Arlene Pietranton, Executive Director
Joanne K. Jessen, Editor-In-Chief

Association publication containing news, notices of events and activities and information for members on issues facing the profession.

16 pages Year Founded: 1973

4872 American Annals of the Deaf
Gallaudet University
800 Florida Avenue
NE
Washington, DC 20002-3695
202-651-5000
Fax: 800-621-8476; *Toll Free:* 800-621-2736
visitors.center@gallaudet.edu
www.gallaudet.edu
TTY: 888-630-9347

Dr. T. Alan Hurwitz, President
Edward Bosso, Vice President for the Laurent C
Charity Reedy, Chief Enrollment Management Offi

Scholarly journal at the forefront of research related to the education of deaf people. Annual reference Issue identifies programs and services for deaf people nationwide.

Year Founded: 1864

4873 American Journal of Audiology
American Speech-Language-Hearing Association
10801 Rockville Pike
Rockville, MD 20852-3226
301-897-5700
Fax: 301-571-0457; *Toll Free:* 800-638-8255
www.betterhearing.org
TTY: 301-897-5700

Nancy A. Creaghead, President
Arlene Pietranton, Executive Director
Joanne K. Jessen, Editor-In-Chief

Year Founded: 1973

4874 Auricle
Auditory-Verbal International
2121 Eisenhower Avenue
Suite 402
Alexandria, VA 22314-4688
703-739-1049
Fax: 703-739-0395
audiverb@aol.com
www.auditory-verbal.org
TTY: 703-739-0874

Peter L. Saltonstall, President & CEO
Pamela Gavin, Chief Operating Officer
Russell Teagarden, Senior Vice President of Medical

To provide the choice of listening and speaking as the way of life for children and adults who are deaf on hard of hearing.

Year Founded: 1987

4875 Deaf Life
DeafLife
PO Box 23380
Rochester, NY 14692-3380
585-442-6370
Fax: 585-442-6371
www.deaflife.com

Matthew S. Moore, Publisher

This magazine focuses on profiles, news, controversial issues, cultural topics and more relating to the Deaf community.

50 pages Year Founded: 1986

4876 Deaf-Blind American
National Association of the Deaf
8630 Fenton Street
Suite 820
Silver Spring, MD 20910-4504
301-587-1788
Fax: 310-587-1791
www.nad.org
TTY: 301-587-1789

Howard A. Rosenblum, CEO
Shane H. Feldman, COO
Andrew S. Phillips, Staff Attorney

A journal of the American Association of the Deaf-Blind with articles on new technology, legislation news affecting deaf-blind Americans, success storeis on deaf-blind, conference news, and many other topics of interest to deaf-blind people.

Year Founded: 1880

4877 Hearing Loss Magazine
Hearing Loss Association of America
7910 Woodmount Avenue
Suite 1200
Bethesda, MD 20814
301-657-2248
Fax: 301-913-9413
www.hearingloss.org

Barbara Kelley, Editor in Chief

Award-winning magazine featuring the stories of people with hearing loss and the latest information on products, services, research and technology in the hearing health care field. Available to HLAA members.

Frequency: Bimonthly Year Founded: 1980

4878 Journal of Speech and Hearing Disorders
American Speech-Language-Hearing Association
10801 Rockville Pike
Rockville, MD 20852-3226
301-897-5700
Fax: 301-571-0457; *Toll Free:* 800-638-8255
www.betterhearing.org
TTY: 301-897-5700

Nancy A. Creaghead, President
Arlene Pietranton, Executive Director
Joanne K. Jessen, Editor-In-Chief

Articles cover case histories, clinical techniques, position papers and literature surveys.

Year Founded: 1973

4879 Journal of Speech and Hearing Research
American Speech-Language-Hearing Association
10801 Rockville Pike
Rockville, MD 20852-3226
301-897-5700
Fax: 301-571-0457; *Toll Free:* 800-638-8255
www.betterhearing.org
TTY: 301-897-5700

Nancy A. Creaghead, President
Arlene Pietranton, Executive Director
Joanne K. Jessen, Editor-In-Chief

Journal covering research in communication science.

Frequency: Bimonthly Year Founded: 1973

4880 Journal of Speech-Language-Hearing Research
American Speech-Language-Hearing Association
10801 Rockville Pike
Rockville, MD 20852-3226
301-897-5700
Fax: 301-571-0457; *Toll Free:* 800-638-8255
www.betterhearing.org
TTY: 301-897-5700

Nancy A. Creaghead, President
Arlene Pietranton, Executive Director
Joanne K. Jessen, Editor-In-Chief

Year Founded: 1973

4881 Journal of the Academy of Rehabilitation Audiology
Accident Reconstruction Associates, Inc.
4461 Hayvenhurst Ave.
Encino, CA 91436
818-783-1888
Fax: 818-783-5173
arainc@aol.com
www.ara-inc.net

Frances Laven MS, Executive Director

Professional journal providing a forum for the exchange of ideas on, knowledge of and experience with habilitative and rehabilitative aspects of audiology.

Year Founded: 1957

4882 National Association of the Deaf
National Association of the Deaf
8630 Fenton Street
Suite 820
Silver Spring, MD 20910-4504
301-587-1788
Fax: 310-587-1791
www.nad.org
TTY: 301-587-1789

Howard A. Rosenblum, CEO
Shane H. Feldman, COO
Andrew S. Phillips, Staff Attorney

Nation's largest organization safeguarding the accessibilty and civil rights of 28 million deaf and hard of hearing Americans in education, employment, health care, and tele-communications. Focuses on grassroots advocacy and empowerment, captioned media, deafness-related information and publications, legal assistance, policy development and research, public awareness, and youth leadership development.

Year Founded: 1880

4883 Perspectives in Education and Deafness
Gallaudet University
800 Florida Avenue
NE
Washington, DC 20002-3695
202-651-5000
Fax: 800-621-8476; *Toll Free:* 800-621-2736
visitors.center@gallaudet.edu
www.gallaudet.edu
TTY: 888-630-9347

Dr. T. Alan Hurwitz, President
Edward Bosso, Vice President for the Laurent C
Charity Reedy, Chief Enrollment Management Offi

A practical, reader-friendly magazine, offering help and advice in and beyond the classroom, tuned to the needs of today's students, teachers, and families.

Year Founded: 1864

4884 SHHH Journal
Self Help for Hard of Hearing People
7910 Woodmont Avenue
Suite 1200
Bethesda, MD 20814-7022
301-657-2248
Fax: 301-913-9413
national@shhh.org
www.hearingloss.org
TTY: 301-657-2249

Anna Gilmore Hall, Executive Director
Barbara Kelly, Deputy Executive Director and Ed
Lise Hamlin, Director of Public Policy

An educational journal about hearing loss for hard-of-hearing people.

Year Founded: 1979

4885 Teaching English to the Deaf as a Second Language
Gallaudet University
800 Florida Avenue
NE
Washington, DC 20002-3695
202-651-5000
Fax: 800-621-8476; *Toll Free:* 800-621-2736
visitors.center@gallaudet.edu
www.gallaudet.edu
TTY: 888-630-9347

Dr. T. Alan Hurwitz, President
Edward Bosso, Vice President for the Laurent C
Charity Reedy, Chief Enrollment Management Offi

Publishes articles of practical interest to classroom teachers of hearing impaired and second language students.

Year Founded: 1864

4886 Tinnitus Today
American Tinnitus Association
522 S.W. Fifth Ave.
Ste. 825
Portland, OR 97204
503-248-9985
Fax: 503-248-0024; *Toll Free:* 800-634-8978
tinnitus@ata.org
www.ata.org

Cara James, Executive Director
Ben Forstag, Director of Communications
Lynn Michael Allmeyer, Director of Development

Information, hearing professional referrals, support group contacts, and a bibliography service are available as well as this quarterly magazine.

28 pages Year Founded: 1971

4887 USA Deaf Sports Federation
3607 Washington Boulevard
Suite 4
Ogden, UT 84403-1761
801-393-8710
Fax: 801-393-2263
homeoffice@usadsf.org
www.usadsf.org
TTY: 801-393-7916

Dr. Joseph J Innes III, Editor

A glossy magazine called Deaf Sports Review featuring articles on all deaf sports and recreation.

4888 Volta Voices
Alexander Graham Bell Association for the Deaf
3417 Volta Place, NW
Washington, DC 20007-2753
202-337-5220
Fax: 202-337-8270
info@agbell.org
listeningandspokenlanguage.org
TTY: 202-337-5220

Alexander T. Graham, Executive Director
Judy Harrison, Director of Programs
June Martin, Development and Outreach Manager

Contains Association news and educates readers on the abilities and needs of children and adults who are deaf or hard of hearing. Includes subscription to The Valta Review, published five times a year.

Newspapers

4889 NAD Broadcaster
National Association of the Deaf
8630 Fenton Street
Suite 820
Silver Spring, MD 20910-4504
301-587-1788
Fax: 310-587-1791
www.nad.org
TTY: 301-587-1789

Howard A. Rosenblum, CEO
Shane H. Feldman, COO
Andrew S. Phillips, Staff Attorney

Newspaper for deaf and hard of hearing people, and their parents and educators.

Year Founded: 1880

4890 Tinnitus Today
American Tinnitus Association
522 S.W. Fifth Ave.
Ste. 825
Portland, OR 97204
503-248-9985
Fax: 503-248-0024; *Toll Free:* 800-634-8978
tinnitus@ata.org
www.ata.org

Cara James, Executive Director
Ben Forstag, Director of Communications
Lynn Michael Allmeyer, Director of Development

Year Founded: 1971

Newsletters, Pamphlets

4891 ADA & the Consumer Who is Deaf or Hard of Hearing
Alexander Graham Bell Association for the Deaf and
3417 Volta Place, NW
Washington, DC 20007-2753
202-337-5220
Fax: 202-337-8314
info@agbell.org
listeningandspokenlanguage.org
TTY: 202-337-5220

Donald M. Goldberg, Ph.D., President
Meredith K. Knueve Sugar, Esq., President-Elect
Alexander T. Graham, Executive Director

This brochure describes how the ADA prohibits discrimination against persons with disabilities in four main domains: employment settings, public services from state and local government agencies, public accomodations, and telecommunications.

4892 ADA and Hearing-Impaired Consumers
Alexander Graham Bell Association for the Deaf and
3417 Volta Place, NW
Washington, DC 20007-2753
202-337-5220
Fax: 202-337-8314
info@agbell.org
listeningandspokenlanguage.org
TTY: 202-337-5220

Donald M. Goldberg, Ph.D., President
Meredith K. Knueve Sugar, Esq., President-Elect
Alexander T. Graham, Executive Director

This brochure describes how the ADA prohibits discrimination against people based on impairments in their employment, state and local governments, and public accommodations.

4893 ATA Newsletter
American Tinnitus Association
522 S.W. Fifth Ave.
Ste. 825
Portland, OR 97204
503-248-9985
Fax: 503-248-0024; *Toll Free:* 800-634-8978
tinnitus@ata.org
www.ata.org

Cara James, Executive Director
Ben Forstag, Director of Communications
Lynn Michael Allmeyer, Director of Development

Information, hearing professional referrals, support group contacts, and a bibliography service are available in this quarterly magazine.

28 pages Frequency: Quarterly Year Founded: 1971

4894 Adult Bible Lessons for the Deaf
LifeWay
127 9th Avenue N
One LifeWay Plaza
Nashville, TN 37234-0162
615-251-2000
Fax: 615-251-5017; *Toll Free:* 800-458-2772
www.lifeway.com

Thom S. Rainer, President and CEO
Brad Waggoner, Executive Vice President
Tim Hill, Vice President and Chief Informa

Bible study quarterly that relates to the needs of deaf and hearing impaired persons.

Year Founded: 1891

4895 Advocacy & Access
Hearing Loss Association of America
7910 Woodmont Avenue
Suite 1200
Bethesda, MD 20814-7022
301-657-2248
Fax: 301-913-9413
national@shhh.org
www.hearingloss.org
TTY: 301-657-2249

Diana D. Bender,Ph.D., Chairperson
Margaret Wallhagen,Ph.D., Vice President
Anna Gilmore Hall, Executive Director

Year Founded: 1979

4896 Aging and Hearing Loss: Some Commonly Asked Questions
Gallaudet University
800 Florida Avenue NE
Washington, DC 20002-3695
202-651-5000
Fax: 202-651-5054
www.gallaudet.edu
TTY: 202-651-5052

Dr. T. Alan Hurwitz, President
Edward Bosso, Vice President for the Laurent C
Dr. Lynne Murray, Vice President for Development,

Discusses the hearing evaulation, tests used to determine type and extent of hearing loss and what an audiogram tells us.

Year Founded: 1864

4897 Alerting and Communication Devices for Deaf & Hard of Hearing People
Gallaudet University
800 Florida Avenue NE
Washington, DC 20002-3695
202-651-5000
Fax: 202-651-5054
www.gallaudet.edu
TTY: 202-651-5052

Dr. T. Alan Hurwitz, President
Edward Bosso, Vice President for the Laurent C
Dr. Lynne Murray, Vice President for Development,

Describes general communication in everyday life.

Year Founded: 1864

4898 All About the New Generation of Hearing Aids
Gallaudet University
800 Florida Avenue NE
Washington, DC 20002-3695
202-651-5000
Fax: 202-651-5054
www.gallaudet.edu
TTY: 202-651-5052

Dr. T. Alan Hurwitz, President
Edward Bosso, Vice President for the Laurent C
Dr. Lynne Murray, Vice President for Development,

Explains the terms digital hearing aid, and digitally controlled hearing aid.

Year Founded: 1864

4899 Americans with Disabilities Act: Selected Resources for Deaf
Gallaudet University Bookstore
800 Florida Avenue NE
Washington, DC 20002-3695
202-651-5000
Fax: 202-651-5489; *Toll Free:* 800-451-1073
www.gallaudet.edu
TDD 888-630-9347

Dr. T. Alan Hurwitz, President
Edward Bosso, Vice President for the Laurent C
Dr. Lynne Murray, Vice President for Development,

This resource identifies programs and publications specific to the ADA and deafness and also lists ADA materials and programs for people with any disability.

Year Founded: 1864

4900 Assistive Devices Demonstration Centers
Gallaudet University
800 Florida Avenue NE
Washington, DC 20002-3695
202-651-5000
Fax: 202-651-5054
www.gallaudet.edu
TTY: 202-651-5052

Dr. T. Alan Hurwitz, President
Edward Bosso, Vice President for the Laurent C
Dr. Lynne Murray, Vice President for Development,

A resource list identifying demonstration centers across the United States.

Year Founded: 1864

4901 Audio Induction Loops
Hearing Loss Association of America
7910 Woodmont Avenue
Suite 1200
Bethesda, MD 20814-7022
301-657-2248
Fax: 301-913-9413
national@shhh.org
www.hearingloss.org
TTY: 301-657-2249

Diana D. Bender,Ph.D., Chairperson
Margaret Wallhagen,Ph.D., Vice President
Anna Gilmore Hall, Executive Director

Year Founded: 1979

4902 Be in the Know: Communication Access Terms
Hearing Loss Association of America
7910 Woodmont Avenue
Suite 1200
Bethesda, MD 20814-7022
301-657-2248
Fax: 301-913-9413
national@shhh.org
www.hearingloss.org
TTY: 301-657-2249

Diana D. Bender,Ph.D., Chairperson
Margaret Wallhagen,Ph.D., Vice President
Anna Gilmore Hall, Executive Director

Year Founded: 1979

4903 Better Hearing News
Better Hearing Institute
1444 I Street, NW
Suite 700
Washington, DC 20005
202-449-1100
Fax: 202-216-9646; *Toll Free:* 800-327-
mail@betterhearing.org
www.betterhearing.org

Jerry J Rizzo, Executive Director
Ruth Bentler, Ph.D., Professor
Jennifer Bishop, J.D., Attorney

Year Founded: 1973

4904 Between Two Worlds of Hearing and Not Hearing
Hearing Loss Association of America
7910 Woodmont Avenue
Suite 1200
Bethesda, MD 20814-7022

301-657-2248
Fax: 301-913-9413
national@shhh.org
www.hearingloss.org
TTY: 301-657-2249

Diana D. Bender,Ph.D., Chairperson
Margaret Wallhagen,Ph.D., Vice President
Anna Gilmore Hall, Executive Director

Year Founded: 1979

4905 Breaking the Chain of Substance Abuse and Hearing Loss
Hearing Loss Association of America
7910 Woodmont Avenue
Suite 1200
Bethesda, MD 20814-7022
301-657-2248
Fax: 301-913-9413
national@shhh.org
www.hearingloss.org
TTY: 301-657-2249

Diana D. Bender,Ph.D., Chairperson
Margaret Wallhagen,Ph.D., Vice President
Anna Gilmore Hall, Executive Director

Year Founded: 1979

4906 CICI's Contact
Cochlear Implant Club Association
5335 Wisconsin Avenue NW
Suite 440
Washington, DC 20015-2054
202-895-2781
Fax: 202-895-2782
pwms.cici@worldnet.att.net
www.cici.org

Peg Williams, Executive Director

52 pages

4907 Canine Listener
Dogs for the Deaf
10175 Wheeler Road
Central Point, OR 97502-9360
541-826-9220
Fax: 541-826-6696; *Toll Free:* 800-990-3647
info@dogsforthedeaf.org
www.dogsforthedeaf.org

Robin Dickson, President and CEO
Janine Bol, Finance Director
John Drach, Training Director

Offers information on various dogs for the deaf that are available, hotlines, support groups and articles on the newest technology for the hard of hearing person.

Year Founded: 1977

4908 Caption Center News
Caption Center
125 Western Avenue
Boston, MA 02134-1008
617-300-3600
Fax: 617-300-1020
access@wgbh.org
www.icdri.org
TTY: 617-300-3600

Reports developments in closed captioning for persons with hearing impairments.

4909 Cellular Phones - Hearing Aid Wearers Can Use Them
Hearing Loss Association of America
7910 Woodmont Avenue
Suite 1200
Bethesda, MD 20814-7022
301-657-2248
Fax: 301-913-9413
national@shhh.org
www.hearingloss.org
TTY: 301-657-2249

Diana D. Bender,Ph.D., Chairperson
Margaret Wallhagen,Ph.D., Vice President
Anna Gilmore Hall, Executive Director

Year Founded: 1979

4910 Cochlear Impants
Alexander Graham Bell Association for the Deaf and
3417 Volta Place, NW
Washington, DC 20007-2753
202-337-5220
Fax: 202-337-8314
info@agbell.org
listeningandspokenlanguage.org
TTY: 202-337-5220

Donald M. Goldberg, Ph.D., President
Meredith K. Knueve Sugar, Esq., President-Elect
Alexander T. Graham, Executive Director

This brochure discusses how adult consumers benefit from a cochlear implant and follows the entire process of evaluation, surgery and follow-up visits.

4911 Cochlear Implants: Comprehensive Overview
Hearing Loss Association of America
7910 Woodmont Avenue
Suite 1200
Bethesda, MD 20814-7022
301-657-2248
Fax: 301-913-9413
national@shhh.org
www.hearingloss.org
TTY: 301-657-2249

Diana D. Bender,Ph.D., Chairperson
Margaret Wallhagen,Ph.D., Vice President
Anna Gilmore Hall, Executive Director

Year Founded: 1979

4912 Common Mis-Information About Hearing Loss and Hearing Aid Use
Hearing Loss Association of America
7910 Woodmont Avenue
Suite 1200
Bethesda, MD 20814-7022
301-657-2248
Fax: 301-913-9413
national@shhh.org
www.hearingloss.org
TTY: 301-657-2249

Diana D. Bender,Ph.D., Chairperson
Margaret Wallhagen,Ph.D., Vice President
Anna Gilmore Hall, Executive Director

Year Founded: 1979

4913 Communicating with People Who Have a Hearing Loss
Alexander Graham Bell Association for the Deaf and
3417 Volta Place, NW
Washington, DC 20007-2753
202-337-5220
Fax: 202-337-8314
info@agbell.org
listeningandspokenlanguage.org
TTY: 202-337-5220

Donald M. Goldberg, Ph.D., President
Meredith K. Knueve Sugar, Esq., President-Elect
Alexander T. Graham, Executive Director

This brochure describes ways to communicate more effectively with people who have hearing losses.

4914 Communication Access in Houses of Worship
Hearing Loss Association of America
7910 Woodmont Avenue
Suite 1200
Bethesda, MD 20814-7022
301-657-2248
Fax: 301-913-9413
national@shhh.org
www.hearingloss.org
TTY: 301-657-2249

Diana D. Bender,Ph.D., Chairperson
Margaret Wallhagen,Ph.D., Vice President
Anna Gilmore Hall, Executive Director

Year Founded: 1979

4915 Communication Access in Medical Facilities
Hearing Loss Association of America
7910 Woodmont Avenue
Suite 1200
Bethesda, MD 20814-7022
301-657-2248
Fax: 301-913-9413
national@shhh.org
www.hearingloss.org
TTY: 301-657-2249

Diana D. Bender,Ph.D., Chairperson
Margaret Wallhagen,Ph.D., Vice President
Anna Gilmore Hall, Executive Director

Year Founded: 1979

4916 Communication Tips to Go (Movies, Restaurants, Planes, Car...)
Hearing Loss Association of America
7910 Woodmont Avenue
Suite 1200
Bethesda, MD 20814-7022
301-657-2248
Fax: 301-913-9413
national@shhh.org
www.hearingloss.org
TTY: 301-657-2249

Diana D. Bender,Ph.D., Chairperson
Margaret Wallhagen,Ph.D., Vice President
Anna Gilmore Hall, Executive Director

Year Founded: 1979

4917 Computer-Assisted Notetaking
Hearing Loss Association of America
7910 Woodmont Avenue
Suite 1200
Bethesda, MD 20814-7022
301-657-2248
Fax: 301-913-9413
national@shhh.org
www.hearingloss.org
TTY: 301-657-2249

Diana D. Bender,Ph.D., Chairperson
Margaret Wallhagen,Ph.D., Vice President
Anna Gilmore Hall, Executive Director

How-to guide and consumer's guide to real-time notetaking.

Year Founded: 1979

4918 Consumer's Guide for Purchasing a Hearing Aid
Hearing Loss Association of America
7910 Woodmont Avenue
Suite 1200
Bethesda, MD 20814-7022
301-657-2248
Fax: 301-913-9413
national@shhh.org
www.hearingloss.org
TTY: 301-657-2249

Diana D. Bender,Ph.D., Chairperson
Margaret Wallhagen,Ph.D., Vice President
Anna Gilmore Hall, Executive Director

Year Founded: 1979

4919 Cued Speech
Hearing Loss Association of America
7910 Woodmont Avenue
Suite 1200
Bethesda, MD 20814-7022
301-657-2248
Fax: 301-913-9413
national@shhh.org
www.hearingloss.org
TTY: 301-657-2249

Diana D. Bender,Ph.D., Chairperson
Margaret Wallhagen,Ph.D., Vice President
Anna Gilmore Hall, Executive Director

Year Founded: 1979

4920 Deaf American
National Association of the Deaf
8630 Fenton Street
Suite 820
Silver Spring, MD 20910-4504
301-587-1788
Fax: 301-587-1791
www.nad.org
TTY: 301-587-1789

Christopher Wagner, President
Melissa S. Draganac-Hawk, Vice-President
Howard A. Rosenblum, Chief Executive Officer

Discusses current issues of importance to the deaf community.

Year Founded: 1880

4921 Deaf Culture Videotapes
Gallaudet University
800 Florida Avenue NE
Washington, DC 20002-3695
202-651-5000
Fax: 202-651-5054
www.gallaudet.edu
TTY: 202-651-5052

Dr. T. Alan Hurwitz, President
Edward Bosso, Vice President for the Laurent C
Dr. Lynne Murray, Vice President for Development,

This list identifies deaf culture and deaf history videotapes available from the Historic Film Collection of the National Association of the Deaf.

Year Founded: 1864

4922 Deaf Culture: Suggested Readings
Gallaudet University
800 Florida Avenue NE
Washington, DC 20002-3695
202-651-5000
Fax: 202-651-5054
www.gallaudet.edu
TTY: 202-651-5052

Dr. T. Alan Hurwitz, President
Edward Bosso, Vice President for the Laurent C
Dr. Lynne Murray, Vice President for Development,

A selected reading list providing annotations for 62 books highlighting the community, and history of deaf people.

Year Founded: 1864

4923 Deaf Episcopalian
Episcopal Conference of the Deaf
PO Box 27459
Philadelphia, PA 19118
215-247-1059
Fax: 215-247-1059
www.ecdeaf.org

Rev. Virginia Nagel, Editor
Marainne D Stephens, Religious Leader

Year Founded: 1852

4924 Deafness: A Fact Sheet
Gallaudet University
800 Florida Avenue NE
Washington, DC 20002-3695
202-651-5000
Fax: 202-651-5054
www.gallaudet.edu
TTY: 202-651-5052

Dr. T. Alan Hurwitz, President
Edward Bosso, Vice President for the Laurent C
Dr. Lynne Murray, Vice President for Development,

Year Founded: 1864

4925 Deafpride Advocate
Deafpride
1350 Potomac Avenue SE
Washington, DC 20003
202-675-6700
Fax: 202-547-0547

4926 Dealing with Anger and Echoes of a Common Fate
Hearing Loss Association of America
7910 Woodmont Avenue
Suite 1200
Bethesda, MD 20814-7022
301-657-2248
Fax: 301-913-9413
national@shhh.org
www.hearingloss.org
TTY: 301-657-2249

Diana D. Bender,Ph.D., Chairperson
Margaret Wallhagen,Ph.D., Vice President
Anna Gilmore Hall, Executive Director

Year Founded: 1979

4927 Developing an Identity for People with Hearing Loss
Hearing Loss Association of America
7910 Woodmont Avenue
Suite 1200
Bethesda, MD 20814-7022
301-657-2248
Fax: 301-913-9413
national@shhh.org
www.hearingloss.org
TTY: 301-657-2249

Diana D. Bender,Ph.D., Chairperson
Margaret Wallhagen,Ph.D., Vice President
Anna Gilmore Hall, Executive Director

Year Founded: 1979

4928 Developments in Technology
Hearing Loss Association of America
7910 Woodmont Avenue
Suite 1200
Bethesda, MD 20814-7022
301-657-2248
Fax: 301-913-9413
national@shhh.org
www.hearingloss.org
TTY: 301-657-2249

Diana D. Bender,Ph.D., Chairperson
Margaret Wallhagen,Ph.D., Vice President
Anna Gilmore Hall, Executive Director

Hearing aids and assistive devices.

Year Founded: 1979

4929 Digital Hearing Aids: An Update
Hearing Loss Association of America
7910 Woodmont Avenue
Suite 1200
Bethesda, MD 20814-7022
301-657-2248
Fax: 301-913-9413
national@shhh.org
www.hearingloss.org
TTY: 301-657-2249

Diana D. Bender,Ph.D., Chairperson
Margaret Wallhagen,Ph.D., Vice President
Anna Gilmore Hall, Executive Director

Year Founded: 1979

4930 Ear and Hearing
Gallaudet University
800 Florida Avenue NE
Washington, DC 20002-3695
202-651-5000
Fax: 202-651-5054
www.gallaudet.edu
TTY: 202-651-5052

Dr. T. Alan Hurwitz, President
Edward Bosso, Vice President for the Laurent C
Dr. Lynne Murray, Vice President for Development,

An illustrated publication of the ear and its diseases.

Year Founded: 1864

4931 Early/Mild Hearing Loss
Hearing Loss Association of America
7910 Woodmont Avenue
Suite 1200
Bethesda, MD 20814-7022
301-657-2248
Fax: 301-913-9413
national@shhh.org
www.hearingloss.org
TTY: 301-657-2249

Diana D. Bender,Ph.D., Chairperson
Margaret Wallhagen,Ph.D., Vice President
Anna Gilmore Hall, Executive Director

Year Founded: 1979

4932 Educational Perspective
Hearing Loss Association of America
7910 Woodmont Avenue
Suite 1200
Bethesda, MD 20814-7022
301-657-2248
Fax: 301-913-9413
national@shhh.org
www.hearingloss.org
TTY: 301-657-2249

Diana D. Bender,Ph.D., Chairperson
Margaret Wallhagen,Ph.D., Vice President
Anna Gilmore Hall, Executive Director

Year Founded: 1979

4933 Employers of Individuals Who are Deaf and Hard of Hearing & the ADA
Alexander Graham Bell Association for the Deaf and
3417 Volta Place, NW
Washington, DC 20007-2753
202-337-5220
Fax: 202-337-8314
info@agbell.org
listeningandspokenlanguage.org
TTY: 202-337-5220

Donald M. Goldberg, Ph.D., President
Meredith K. Knueve Sugar, Esq., President-Elect
Alexander T. Graham, Executive Director

Written for employers, this brochure discusses workplace accommodations that are required under the ADA. Most of the suggestions listed in this brochure are simple and, for the most part, relatively inexpensive to implement.

4934 Employers of Individuals with Hearing Impairments & the ADA
Alexander Graham Bell Association for the Deaf and
3417 Volta Place, NW
Washington, DC 20007-2753
202-337-5220
Fax: 202-337-8314
info@agbell.org
listeningandspokenlanguage.org
TTY: 202-337-5220

Donald M. Goldberg, Ph.D., President
Meredith K. Knueve Sugar, Esq., President-Elect
Alexander T. Graham, Executive Director

For employers, this brochure discusses workplace accommodations required by the ADA for employees with hearing impairments; communication options, procedural alterations and technologies.

4935 Endeavor
American Society for Deaf Children
800 Florida Avenue NE
Washington, DC 20002-3695
717-334-7922
Fax: 717-334-8808; *Toll Free:* 800-942-2732
asdc@deafchildren.org
www.deafchildren.org

Linda Cumbran, Operations Manager
Alicia Notarianni, Editor

Newsletter for parents of deaf children.

Year Founded: 1967

4936 Facts About Hearing Aids
Alexander Graham Bell Association for the Deaf and
3417 Volta Place, NW
Washington, DC 20007-2753
202-337-5220
Fax: 202-337-8314
info@agbell.org
listeningandspokenlanguage.org
TTY: 202-337-5220

Donald M. Goldberg, Ph.D., President
Meredith K. Knueve Sugar, Esq., President-Elect
Alexander T. Graham, Executive Director

This brochure describes defferent types of hearing aids, factors to consider when choosing a hearing aid, the best way to go about purchasing a hearing aid. It also addresses cost and provides information on hearing conservation.

4937 Facts and Fancies About Hearing Aids
American Hearing Research Foundation
310 W. Lake St.
Suite 111
Elmhurst, IL 60126
630-617-5079
Fax: 630-563-9181
american-hearing.org

Richard G. Muench, Chairman
Alan G. Micco, M.D., President
Mark R. Muench, Vice President

Offers information on types of hearing aids and hearing aid evaluations.

4938 Financial Help for Hearing Aids
Hearing Loss Association of America
7910 Woodmont Avenue
Suite 1200
Bethesda, MD 20814-7022
301-657-2248
Fax: 301-913-9413
national@shhh.org
www.hearingloss.org
TTY: 301-657-2249

Diana D. Bender,Ph.D., Chairperson
Margaret Wallhagen,Ph.D., Vice President
Anna Gilmore Hall, Executive Director

Year Founded: 1979

4939 Finding the Right Aural Rehabilitation Program
Hearing Loss Association of America
7910 Woodmont Avenue
Suite 1200
Bethesda, MD 20814-7022
301-657-2248
Fax: 301-913-9413
national@shhh.org
www.hearingloss.org
TTY: 301-657-2249

Diana D. Bender,Ph.D., Chairperson
Margaret Wallhagen,Ph.D., Vice President
Anna Gilmore Hall, Executive Director

Year Founded: 1979

4940 Forgotten Family
Hearing Loss Association of America
7910 Woodmont Avenue
Suite 1200
Bethesda, MD 20814-7022
301-657-2248
Fax: 301-913-9413
national@shhh.org
www.hearingloss.org
TTY: 301-657-2249

Diana D. Bender,Ph.D., Chairperson
Margaret Wallhagen,Ph.D., Vice President
Anna Gilmore Hall, Executive Director

Year Founded: 1979

4941 Frat
Gallaudet University
800 Florida Avenue NE
Washington, DC 20002-3695
202-651-5000
Fax: 202-651-5054
www.gallaudet.edu
TTY: 202-651-5052

Dr. T. Alan Hurwitz, President
Edward Bosso, Vice President for the Laurent C
Dr. Lynne Murray, Vice President for Development,

Offers fraternal insurance information and news about members.

Year Founded: 1864

4942 GASK Newsletter
Better Hearing Institute
1444 I Street, NW
Suite 700
Washington, DC 20005
202-449-1100
Fax: 202-216-9646
mail@betterhearing.org
www.betterhearing.org

Jerry J Rizzo, Executive Director
Ruth Bentler, Ph.D., Professor
Jennifer Bishop, J.D., Attorney

32 pages Frequency: Quarterly Year Founded: 1973

4943 Gallaudet Today
Gallaudet University
800 Florida Avenue NE
Washington, DC 20002-3695
202-651-5000
Fax: 202-651-5054
www.gallaudet.edu
TTY: 202-651-5052

Dr. T. Alan Hurwitz, President
Edward Bosso, Vice President for the Laurent C
Dr. Lynne Murray, Vice President for Development,

A university publication with both general and special issues on deafness-related topics.

Year Founded: 1864

4944 Genetics and Deafness
Gallaudet University
800 Florida Avenue NE
Washington, DC 20002-3695
202-651-5000
Fax: 202-651-5054
www.gallaudet.edu
TTY: 202-651-5052

Dr. T. Alan Hurwitz, President
Edward Bosso, Vice President for the Laurent C
Dr. Lynne Murray, Vice President for Development,

Written for deaf people and their families who wish to learn more about the relationship between heredity and deafness.

Year Founded: 1864

4945 Genetics and Hearing Loss
Hearing Loss Association of America
7910 Woodmont Avenue
Suite 1200
Bethesda, MD 20814-7022
301-657-2248
Fax: 301-913-9413
national@shhh.org
www.hearingloss.org
TTY: 301-657-2249

Diana D. Bender,Ph.D., Chairperson
Margaret Wallhagen,Ph.D., Vice President
Anna Gilmore Hall, Executive Director
Year Founded: 1979

4946 Getting Beyond Hearing Loss: A Guide for Families
Hearing Loss Association of America
7910 Woodmont Avenue
Suite 1200
Bethesda, MD 20814-7022

301-657-2248
Fax: 301-913-9413
national@shhh.org
www.hearingloss.org
TTY: 301-657-2249

Diana D. Bender,Ph.D., Chairperson
Margaret Wallhagen,Ph.D., Vice President
Anna Gilmore Hall, Executive Director
Year Founded: 1979

4947 Getting Help with a Job: Exploring Vocational Rehabilitation
Hearing Loss Association of America
7910 Woodmont Avenue
Suite 1200
Bethesda, MD 20814-7022
301-657-2248
Fax: 301-913-9413
national@shhh.org
www.hearingloss.org
TTY: 301-657-2249

Diana D. Bender,Ph.D., Chairperson
Margaret Wallhagen,Ph.D., Vice President
Anna Gilmore Hall, Executive Director
Year Founded: 1979

4948 Growing Up Hearing: A Sister's Memoir
Hearing Loss Association of America
7910 Woodmont Avenue
Suite 1200
Bethesda, MD 20814-7022
301-657-2248
Fax: 301-913-9413
national@shhh.org
www.hearingloss.org
TTY: 301-657-2249

Diana D. Bender,Ph.D., Chairperson
Margaret Wallhagen,Ph.D., Vice President
Anna Gilmore Hall, Executive Director
Year Founded: 1979

4949 Guide for Students with Hearing Loss
Hearing Loss Association of America
7910 Woodmont Avenue
Suite 1200
Bethesda, MD 20814-7022
301-657-2248
Fax: 301-913-9413
national@shhh.org
www.hearingloss.org
TTY: 301-657-2249

Diana D. Bender,Ph.D., Chairperson
Margaret Wallhagen,Ph.D., Vice President
Anna Gilmore Hall, Executive Director

Resources for college-bound students.

Year Founded: 1979

4950 Guidelines for Helping Deaf-Blind Persons
Helen Keller National Center
141 Middle Neck Road
Sands Point, NY 11050-1218
516-944-8900
Fax: 516-944-7302
hkncinfo@hknc.org

www.hknc.org
TTY: 516-944-8637

Joseph McNulty, Executive Director

Pamphlet offering information on how persons should interact with deaf-blind individuals. Includes drawings of the one hand manual alphabet.

Year Founded: 1967

4951 Hearing Aids and the Consumer: Current Wisdom
Hearing Loss Association of America
7910 Woodmont Avenue
Suite 1200
Bethesda, MD 20814-7022
301-657-2248
Fax: 301-913-9413
national@shhh.org
www.hearingloss.org
TTY: 301-657-2249

Diana D. Bender,Ph.D., Chairperson
Margaret Wallhagen,Ph.D., Vice President
Anna Gilmore Hall, Executive Director

Year Founded: 1979

4952 Hearing Alert! Informational Brochures
Alexander Graham Bell Association for the Deaf and
3417 Volta Place, NW
Washington, DC 20007-2753
202-337-5220
Fax: 202-337-8314
info@agbell.org
listeningandspokenlanguage.org
TTY: 202-337-5220

Donald M. Goldberg, Ph.D., President
Meredith K. Knueve Sugar, Esq., President-Elect
Alexander T. Graham, Executive Director

These brochures encourage early detection of hearing loss in young children. For medical facilities, speech and hearing clinics, and schools.

4953 Hearing Dogs in Public
Hearing Loss Association of America
7910 Woodmont Avenue
Suite 1200
Bethesda, MD 20814-7022
301-657-2248
Fax: 301-913-9413
national@shhh.org
www.hearingloss.org
TTY: 301-657-2249

Diana D. Bender,Ph.D., Chairperson
Margaret Wallhagen,Ph.D., Vice President
Anna Gilmore Hall, Executive Director

Year Founded: 1979

4954 Hearing Healthcare Team
Hearing Loss Association of America
7910 Woodmont Avenue
Suite 1200
Bethesda, MD 20814-7022
301-657-2248
Fax: 301-913-9413
national@shhh.org

www.hearingloss.org
TTY: 301-657-2249

Diana D. Bender,Ph.D., Chairperson
Margaret Wallhagen,Ph.D., Vice President
Anna Gilmore Hall, Executive Director

Year Founded: 1979

4955 Hearing Loss and Staying Connected: Personal Accounts
Hearing Loss Association of America
7910 Woodmont Avenue
Suite 1200
Bethesda, MD 20814-7022
301-657-2248
Fax: 301-913-9413
national@shhh.org
www.hearingloss.org
TTY: 301-657-2249

Diana D. Bender,Ph.D., Chairperson
Margaret Wallhagen,Ph.D., Vice President
Anna Gilmore Hall, Executive Director

Year Founded: 1979

4956 Hearing Loss: How to Get Help-A Guide for Consumers by Consumers
Hearing Loss Association of America
7910 Woodmont Avenue
Suite 1200
Bethesda, MD 20814-7022
301-657-2248
Fax: 301-913-9413
national@shhh.org
www.hearingloss.org
TTY: 301-657-2249

Diana D. Bender,Ph.D., Chairperson
Margaret Wallhagen,Ph.D., Vice President
Anna Gilmore Hall, Executive Director

Information on getting tested for deafness and practical advice on the next steps.

Year Founded: 1979

4957 Hearing Loss: Information for Professionals in the Aging Network
Gallaudet University
800 Florida Avenue NE
Washington, DC 20002-3695
202-651-5000
Fax: 202-651-5054
www.gallaudet.edu
TTY: 202-651-5052

Dr. T. Alan Hurwitz, President
Edward Bosso, Vice President for the Laurent C
Dr. Lynne Murray, Vice President for Development,

Introduces professionals in the aging network to the realities of hearing loss.

Year Founded: 1864

4958 Hearing Loss: Personal and Social Considerations
Hearing Loss Association of America
7910 Woodmont Avenue
Suite 1200
Bethesda, MD 20814-7022

301-657-2248
Fax: 301-913-9413
national@shhh.org
www.hearingloss.org
TTY: 301-657-2249

Diana D. Bender,Ph.D., Chairperson
Margaret Wallhagen,Ph.D., Vice President
Anna Gilmore Hall, Executive Director

Year Founded: 1979

4959 Hearing, Speech & Deafness Center(HSDC)
Newsletter
Hearing Speech and Deafness Center
1625 19th Avenue
Seattle, WA 98122-2848
206-323-5770
Fax: 206-328-6871; *Toll Free:* 888-222-5036
www.hsdc.org
TTY: 206-388-1275

Pamela Anderson, Attorney
Isavelle Banville, President
Susie Burdick, Executive Director

Bi-annual news and clinical material for members and the
community.

8 pages Year Founded: 1929

4960 How to Get the Most Out of Your Hearing Aid
Alexander Graham Bell Association for the Deaf
and
3417 Volta Place, NW
Washington, DC 20007-2753
202-337-5220
Fax: 202-337-8314
info@agbell.org
listeningandspokenlanguage.org
TTY: 202-337-5220

Donald M. Goldberg, Ph.D., President
Meredith K. Knueve Sugar, Esq., President-Elect
Alexander T. Graham, Executive Director

This informative booklet for hearing aid users tells how to
wear and adapt to your hearing aid, and provides helpful
hints on care, and troubleshooting.

4961 Inheriting Hearing Loss
Hearing Loss Association of America
7910 Woodmont Avenue
Suite 1200
Bethesda, MD 20814-7022
301-657-2248
Fax: 301-913-9413
national@shhh.org
www.hearingloss.org
TTY: 301-657-2249

Diana D. Bender,Ph.D., Chairperson
Margaret Wallhagen,Ph.D., Vice President
Anna Gilmore Hall, Executive Director

A personal narrative by SHHH Executive Director Donna
Sorkin.

Year Founded: 1979

4962 Interpreter Views
Registry of the Interpreters for the Deaf
333 Commerce Street
Suite 310
Alexandria, VA 22314

703-838-0030
Fax: 301-608-0508
www.rid.org
TTY: 703-838-0459

Shane H. Feldman, M.S., CAE, Executive Director
Matthew O'Hara, M.S., CI and, Director of Ethical
Practices Sy
Julie Schafer, Esq.,, Director of Public Policy and Ad

Information on the deaf and hard of hearing.

Frequency: Monthly

4963 Introduction to Cochlear Implants
Alexander Graham Bell Association for the Deaf
and
3417 Volta Place, NW
Washington, DC 20007-2753
202-337-5220
Fax: 202-337-8314
info@agbell.org
listeningandspokenlanguage.org
TTY: 202-337-5220

Donald M. Goldberg, Ph.D., President
Meredith K. Knueve Sugar, Esq., President-Elect
Alexander T. Graham, Executive Director

This brochure, designed for parents, explores how children
can benefit from a cochlear implant. It explains candidacy,
surgery, rehabilitation, educational emplications, and costs.

4964 It's Our Hearing Loss: What Families Need to
Know and Do
Hearing Loss Association of America
7910 Woodmont Avenue
Suite 1200
Bethesda, MD 20814-7022
301-657-2248
Fax: 301-913-9413
national@shhh.org
www.hearingloss.org
TTY: 301-657-2249

Diana D. Bender,Ph.D., Chairperson
Margaret Wallhagen,Ph.D., Vice President
Anna Gilmore Hall, Executive Director

Year Founded: 1979

4965 Large-Room Listening Systems for Hard of
Hearing People
Hearing Loss Association of America
7910 Woodmont Avenue
Suite 1200
Bethesda, MD 20814-7022
301-657-2248
Fax: 301-913-9413
national@shhh.org
www.hearingloss.org
TTY: 301-657-2249

Diana D. Bender,Ph.D., Chairperson
Margaret Wallhagen,Ph.D., Vice President
Anna Gilmore Hall, Executive Director

Year Founded: 1979

4966 Late-Deafened Adults: A Selected Annotated
Bibliography
Gallaudet University
800 Florida Avenue NE
Washington, DC 20002-3695

202-651-5000
Fax: 202-651-5054
www.gallaudet.edu
TTY: 202-651-5052

Dr. T. Alan Hurwitz, President
Edward Bosso, Vice President for the Laurent C
Dr. Lynne Murray, Vice President for Development,

A selected reading list of books and articles for late-deafened people and their families.

Year Founded: 1864

4967 Leading National Publications of and for Deaf People
Gallaudet University
800 Florida Avenue NE
Washington, DC 20002-3695
202-651-5000
Fax: 202-651-5054
www.gallaudet.edu
TTY: 202-651-5052

Dr. T. Alan Hurwitz, President
Edward Bosso, Vice President for the Laurent C
Dr. Lynne Murray, Vice President for Development,

Identifies publications with national circulations to deaf audiences.

Year Founded: 1864

4968 Listener
HEAR Center
301 E Del Mar Boulevard
Pasadena, CA 91101-2714
626-796-2016
Fax: 626-796-2320
info@hearcenter.org
www.hearcenter.org

Ellen S. Simon, Executive Director
Gayl Opatrny, Audiologist
Joanna Navarro, Audiologist

4 pages Frequency: Bimonthly Year Founded: 1954

4969 Listening
National Catholic Office for the Deaf
7202 Buchanan Street
Landover Hills, MD 20784-2236
301-577-1684
Fax: 301-577-1690
info@ncod.org
www.ncod.org

Arvilla Rank, Executive Director/Editor
Rev. Kevin C Rhoades, Episcopal Representive
Fr. Paul Zirimenya, Region I - West

Published as a pastoral service for the deaf and hard of hearing. Provides information to members and others working in ministry. Prepares an annual gathering called Pastoral Week meeting in January.

4970 Living Alone with a Hearing Loss
Hearing Loss Association of America
7910 Woodmont Avenue
Suite 1200
Bethesda, MD 20814-7022
301-657-2248
Fax: 301-913-9413
national@shhh.org

www.hearingloss.org
TTY: 301-657-2249

Diana D. Bender,Ph.D., Chairperson
Margaret Wallhagen,Ph.D., Vice President
Anna Gilmore Hall, Executive Director

Year Founded: 1979

4971 Living with Hearing Loss: Focus Group Results
Hearing Loss Association of America
7910 Woodmont Avenue
Suite 1200
Bethesda, MD 20814-7022
301-657-2248
Fax: 301-913-9413
national@shhh.org
www.hearingloss.org
TTY: 301-657-2249

Diana D. Bender,Ph.D., Chairperson
Margaret Wallhagen,Ph.D., Vice President
Anna Gilmore Hall, Executive Director

Year Founded: 1979

4972 Making New Friends
Gallaudet University
800 Florida Avenue NE
Washington, DC 20002-3695
202-651-5000
Fax: 202-651-5054
www.gallaudet.edu
TTY: 202-651-5052

Dr. T. Alan Hurwitz, President
Edward Bosso, Vice President for the Laurent C
Dr. Lynne Murray, Vice President for Development,

Identifies resources that offer opportunities for deaf people.

Year Founded: 1864

4973 Meniere's Disease
Hearing Loss Association of America
7910 Woodmont Avenue
Suite 1200
Bethesda, MD 20814-7022
301-657-2248
Fax: 301-913-9413
national@shhh.org
www.hearingloss.org
TTY: 301-657-2249

Diana D. Bender,Ph.D., Chairperson
Margaret Wallhagen,Ph.D., Vice President
Anna Gilmore Hall, Executive Director

Year Founded: 1979

4974 Meniere's Disease: Hearing Loss & Inner Ear Blood Flow
Hearing Loss Association of America
7910 Woodmont Avenue
Suite 1200
Bethesda, MD 20814-7022
301-657-2248
Fax: 301-913-9413
national@shhh.org
www.hearingloss.org
TTY: 301-657-2249

Diana D. Bender,Ph.D., Chairperson
Margaret Wallhagen,Ph.D., Vice President
Anna Gilmore Hall, Executive Director

Plus a personal narrative.

Year Founded: 1979

4975 NAD Broadcaster
National Association of the Deaf
8630 Fenton Street
Suite 820
Silver Spring, MD 20910-4504
301-587-1788
Fax: 301-587-1791
www.nad.org
TTY: 301-587-1789

Christopher Wagner, President
Melissa S. Draganac-Hawk, Vice-President
Howard A. Rosenblum, Chief Executive Officer

Association publication that provides coverage of issues, accomplishments, activities and events of importance to deaf and hard-of-hearing people, their families, and professionals.

Year Founded: 1880

4976 National Information Center on Deafness
Brochure
Gallaudet University
800 Florida Avenue NE
Washington, DC 20002-3695
202-651-5000
Fax: 202-651-5054
www.gallaudet.edu
TTY: 202-651-5052

Dr. T. Alan Hurwitz, President
Edward Bosso, Vice President for the Laurent C
Dr. Lynne Murray, Vice President for Development,

A description of services offered by NICD.

Year Founded: 1864

4977 Older Adults with Hearing Loss
Hearing Loss Association of America
7910 Woodmont Avenue
Suite 1200
Bethesda, MD 20814-7022
301-657-2248
Fax: 301-913-9413
national@shhh.org
www.hearingloss.org
TTY: 301-657-2249

Diana D. Bender,Ph.D., Chairperson
Margaret Wallhagen,Ph.D., Vice President
Anna Gilmore Hall, Executive Director

Year Founded: 1979

4978 Oral Interpreters: A Communication Option
Hearing Loss Association of America
7910 Woodmont Avenue
Suite 1200
Bethesda, MD 20814-7022
301-657-2248
Fax: 301-913-9413
national@shhh.org
www.hearingloss.org
TTY: 301-657-2249

Diana D. Bender,Ph.D., Chairperson
Margaret Wallhagen,Ph.D., Vice President
Anna Gilmore Hall, Executive Director

Year Founded: 1979

4979 Oral Interpreters: Facts for Consumers
Alexander Graham Bell Association for the Deaf and
3417 Volta Place, NW
Washington, DC 20007-2753
202-337-5220
Fax: 202-337-8314
info@agbell.org
listeningandspokenlanguage.org
TTY: 202-337-5220

Donald M. Goldberg, Ph.D., President
Meredith K. Knueve Sugar, Esq., President-Elect
Alexander T. Graham, Executive Director

This handy brochure for consumers or anyone who works with oral interpreters will answer frequently asked questions about many aspects of oral interpreting, including locating, using, and paying for an oral interpreter.

11 pages

4980 Otosclerosis
Hearing Loss Association of America
7910 Woodmont Avenue
Suite 1200
Bethesda, MD 20814-7022
301-657-2248
Fax: 301-913-9413
national@shhh.org
www.hearingloss.org
TTY: 301-657-2249

Diana D. Bender,Ph.D., Chairperson
Margaret Wallhagen,Ph.D., Vice President
Anna Gilmore Hall, Executive Director

Year Founded: 1979

4981 Ototoxic Medications: What You Should Know
Hearing Loss Association of America
7910 Woodmont Avenue
Suite 1200
Bethesda, MD 20814-7022
301-657-2248
Fax: 301-913-9413
national@shhh.org
www.hearingloss.org
TTY: 301-657-2249

Diana D. Bender,Ph.D., Chairperson
Margaret Wallhagen,Ph.D., Vice President
Anna Gilmore Hall, Executive Director

Year Founded: 1979

4982 Persuading Your Spouse/Relative/Friend to
Acknowledge a Hearing Loss and Seek Help
Hearing Loss Association of America
7910 Woodmont Avenue
Suite 1200
Bethesda, MD 20814-7022
301-657-2248
Fax: 301-913-9413
national@shhh.org
www.hearingloss.org
TTY: 301-657-2249

Diana D. Bender,Ph.D., Chairperson
Margaret Wallhagen,Ph.D., Vice President
Anna Gilmore Hall, Executive Director

Year Founded: 1979

4983 Physician Answers Your Questions About Hearing Health Care
Hearing Loss Association of America
7910 Woodmont Avenue
Suite 1200
Bethesda, MD 20814-7022
301-657-2248
Fax: 301-913-9413
national@shhh.org
www.hearingloss.org
TTY: 301-657-2249

Diana D. Bender,Ph.D., Chairperson
Margaret Wallhagen,Ph.D., Vice President
Anna Gilmore Hall, Executive Director

Year Founded: 1979

4984 Psychological Stress and Hearing Loss
Hearing Loss Association of America
7910 Woodmont Avenue
Suite 1200
Bethesda, MD 20814-7022
301-657-2248
Fax: 301-913-9413
national@shhh.org
www.hearingloss.org
TTY: 301-657-2249

Diana D. Bender,Ph.D., Chairperson
Margaret Wallhagen,Ph.D., Vice President
Anna Gilmore Hall, Executive Director

Year Founded: 1979

4985 Publications from the National Information Center on Deafness
Gallaudet University
800 Florida Avenue NE
Washington, DC 20002-3695
202-651-5000
Fax: 202-651-5054
www.gallaudet.edu
TTY: 202-651-5052

Dr. T. Alan Hurwitz, President
Edward Bosso, Vice President for the Laurent C
Dr. Lynne Murray, Vice President for Development,

Order form and explanations of NICD publications.

Year Founded: 1864

4986 Putting You in the Successful Employment Picture
Hearing Loss Association of America
7910 Woodmont Avenue
Suite 1200
Bethesda, MD 20814-7022
301-657-2248
Fax: 301-913-9413
national@shhh.org
www.hearingloss.org
TTY: 301-657-2249

Diana D. Bender,Ph.D., Chairperson
Margaret Wallhagen,Ph.D., Vice President
Anna Gilmore Hall, Executive Director

Year Founded: 1979

4987 Questions and Answers About Employment of Deaf People
Gallaudet University
800 Florida Avenue NE
Washington, DC 20002-3695
202-651-5000
Fax: 202-651-5054
www.gallaudet.edu
TTY: 202-651-5052

Dr. T. Alan Hurwitz, President
Edward Bosso, Vice President for the Laurent C
Dr. Lynne Murray, Vice President for Development,

Year Founded: 1864

4988 Questions and Answers on Hearing Loss
Hearing Loss Association of America
7910 Woodmont Avenue
Suite 1200
Bethesda, MD 20814-7022
301-657-2248
Fax: 301-913-9413
national@shhh.org
www.hearingloss.org
TTY: 301-657-2249

Diana D. Bender,Ph.D., Chairperson
Margaret Wallhagen,Ph.D., Vice President
Anna Gilmore Hall, Executive Director

Year Founded: 1979

4989 Review
House Research Institute
2100 W 3rd Street
5th Floor
Los Angeles, CA 90057-1922
213-483-4431
Fax: 213-483-8789
www.houseresearch.org

Catherine D. Meyer, Chairman
Jim Boswell, CEO
Dilys J Jones, Editor

8 pages Year Founded: 1946

4990 SHHH News
Hearing Loss Association of America
7910 Woodmont Avenue
Suite 1200
Bethesda, MD 20814-7022
301-657-2248
Fax: 301-913-9413
national@shhh.org
www.hearingloss.org
TTY: 301-657-2249

Diana D. Bender,Ph.D., Chairperson
Margaret Wallhagen,Ph.D., Vice President
Anna Gilmore Hall, Executive Director

Information about SHHH affiliates.

Year Founded: 1979

4991 Sensorineural Hearing Loss
Hearing Loss Association of America
7910 Woodmont Avenue
Suite 1200
Bethesda, MD 20814-7022
301-657-2248
Fax: 301-913-9413

national@shhh.org
www.hearingloss.org
TTY: 301-657-2249

Diana D. Bender,Ph.D., Chairperson
Margaret Wallhagen,Ph.D., Vice President
Anna Gilmore Hall, Executive Director

Year Founded: 1979

4992 Set-Ups for Speeches
Hearing Loss Association of America
7910 Woodmont Avenue
Suite 1200
Bethesda, MD 20814-7022
301-657-2248
Fax: 301-913-9413
national@shhh.org
www.hearingloss.org
TTY: 301-657-2249

Diana D. Bender,Ph.D., Chairperson
Margaret Wallhagen,Ph.D., Vice President
Anna Gilmore Hall, Executive Director

Year Founded: 1979

4993 Signaling and Assistive Listening Devices for Hearing-Impaired People
Alexander Graham Bell Association for the Deaf and
3417 Volta Place, NW
Washington, DC 20007-2753
202-337-5220
Fax: 202-337-8314
info@agbell.org
listeningandspokenlanguage.org
TTY: 202-337-5220

Donald M. Goldberg, Ph.D., President
Meredith K. Knueve Sugar, Esq., President-Elect
Alexander T. Graham, Executive Director

This illustrated pamphlet for consumers describes alarms, signalers and telephone/doorbell devices.

4994 Situation is Serious But Not Hopeless: The Psychological Benefits of Hearing Loss
Hearing Loss Association of America
7910 Woodmont Avenue
Suite 1200
Bethesda, MD 20814-7022
301-657-2248
Fax: 301-913-9413
national@shhh.org
www.hearingloss.org
TTY: 301-657-2249

Diana D. Bender,Ph.D., Chairperson
Margaret Wallhagen,Ph.D., Vice President
Anna Gilmore Hall, Executive Director

Year Founded: 1979

4995 So You Have Had an Ear Operation...What Next?
American Hearing Research Foundation
310 W. Lake St.
Suite 111
Elmhurst, IL 60126
630-617-5079
Fax: 630-563-9181
american-hearing.org

Richard G. Muench, Chairman
Alan G. Micco, M.D., President
Mark R. Muench, Vice President

Offers information on ear infections and surgery.

4996 Speech and Deafness Newsletter
Hearing Speech and Deafness Center
1625 19th Avenue
Seattle, WA 98122-2848
206-323-5770
Fax: 206-328-6871; *Toll Free:* 888-222-5036
www.hsdc.org
TTY: 206-388-1275

Pamela Anderson, Attorney
Isavelle Banville, President
Susie Burdick, Executive Director

Agency newsletter for membership and community.

8 pages Year Founded: 1929

4997 Speechreading for Better Communication
Alexander Graham Bell Association for the Deaf and
3417 Volta Place, NW
Washington, DC 20007-2753
202-337-5220
Fax: 202-337-8314
info@agbell.org
listeningandspokenlanguage.org
TTY: 202-337-5220

Donald M. Goldberg, Ph.D., President
Meredith K. Knueve Sugar, Esq., President-Elect
Alexander T. Graham, Executive Director

This brochure describes speechreading, discusses its importance to many people with hearing losses, and lists additional resources for consumers.

4998 Speechreading: Methods and Materials
Hearing Loss Association of America
7910 Woodmont Avenue
Suite 1200
Bethesda, MD 20814-7022
301-657-2248
Fax: 301-913-9413
national@shhh.org
www.hearingloss.org
TTY: 301-657-2249

Diana D. Bender,Ph.D., Chairperson
Margaret Wallhagen,Ph.D., Vice President
Anna Gilmore Hall, Executive Director

Year Founded: 1979

4999 Statewide Services for Deaf and Hard of Hearing People
Gallaudet University
800 Florida Avenue NE
Washington, DC 20002-3695
202-651-5000
Fax: 202-651-5054
www.gallaudet.edu
TTY: 202-651-5052

Dr. T. Alan Hurwitz, President
Edward Bosso, Vice President for the Laurent C
Dr. Lynne Murray, Vice President for Development,

A resource list of states that have established commissions and other offices to serve deaf people.

Year Founded: 1864

5000 Stress Management
Hearing Loss Association of America
7910 Woodmont Avenue
Suite 1200
Bethesda, MD 20814-7022
301-657-2248
Fax: 301-913-9413
national@shhh.org
www.hearingloss.org
TTY: 301-657-2249

Diana D. Bender,Ph.D., Chairperson
Margaret Wallhagen,Ph.D., Vice President
Anna Gilmore Hall, Executive Director

Year Founded: 1979

5001 Technical Assistance Resource Guide
Hearing Loss Association of America
7910 Woodmont Avenue
Suite 1200
Bethesda, MD 20814-7022
301-657-2248
Fax: 301-913-9413
national@shhh.org
www.hearingloss.org
TTY: 301-657-2249

Diana D. Bender,Ph.D., Chairperson
Margaret Wallhagen,Ph.D., Vice President
Anna Gilmore Hall, Executive Director

Includes technical assistance centers and sources of communication access products.

Year Founded: 1979

5002 Telecommunications Access Updates
Hearing Loss Association of America
7910 Woodmont Avenue
Suite 1200
Bethesda, MD 20814-7022
301-657-2248
Fax: 301-913-9413
national@shhh.org
www.hearingloss.org
TTY: 301-657-2249

Diana D. Bender,Ph.D., Chairperson
Margaret Wallhagen,Ph.D., Vice President
Anna Gilmore Hall, Executive Director

Year Founded: 1979

5003 Tinnitus
Hearing Loss Association of America
7910 Woodmont Avenue
Suite 1200
Bethesda, MD 20814-7022
301-657-2248
Fax: 301-913-9413
national@shhh.org
www.hearingloss.org
TTY: 301-657-2249

Diana D. Bender,Ph.D., Chairperson
Margaret Wallhagen,Ph.D., Vice President
Anna Gilmore Hall, Executive Director

Year Founded: 1979

5004 To Our Family Members Who Are Hard of Hearing
Hearing Loss Association of America
7910 Woodmont Avenue
Suite 1200
Bethesda, MD 20814-7022
301-657-2248
Fax: 301-913-9413
national@shhh.org
www.hearingloss.org
TTY: 301-657-2249

Diana D. Bender,Ph.D., Chairperson
Margaret Wallhagen,Ph.D., Vice President
Anna Gilmore Hall, Executive Director

Year Founded: 1979

5005 Total Access Courtroom
Hearing Loss Association of America
7910 Woodmont Avenue
Suite 1200
Bethesda, MD 20814-7022
301-657-2248
Fax: 301-913-9413
national@shhh.org
www.hearingloss.org
TTY: 301-657-2249

Diana D. Bender,Ph.D., Chairperson
Margaret Wallhagen,Ph.D., Vice President
Anna Gilmore Hall, Executive Director

Year Founded: 1979

5006 Travel Resources for Deaf and Hard of Hearing People
Gallaudet University
800 Florida Avenue NE
Washington, DC 20002-3695
202-651-5000
Fax: 202-651-5054
www.gallaudet.edu
TTY: 202-651-5052

Dr. T. Alan Hurwitz, President
Edward Bosso, Vice President for the Laurent C
Dr. Lynne Murray, Vice President for Development,

A publication list of travel industry resources for deaf and hard of hearing people.

Year Founded: 1864

5007 Troubleshooting Your Hearing Aid
Hearing Loss Association of America
7910 Woodmont Avenue
Suite 1200
Bethesda, MD 20814-7022
301-657-2248
Fax: 301-913-9413
national@shhh.org
www.hearingloss.org
TTY: 301-657-2249

Diana D. Bender,Ph.D., Chairperson
Margaret Wallhagen,Ph.D., Vice President
Anna Gilmore Hall, Executive Director

Year Founded: 1979

5008 Understanding Our Needs: Results of the SHHH Member Survey
Hearing Loss Association of America
7910 Woodmont Avenue
Suite 1200
Bethesda, MD 20814-7022
301-657-2248
Fax: 301-913-9413
national@shhh.org
www.hearingloss.org
TTY: 301-657-2249

Diana D. Bender,Ph.D., Chairperson
Margaret Wallhagen,Ph.D., Vice President
Anna Gilmore Hall, Executive Director
Year Founded: 1979

5009 Update on Captioning
Hearing Loss Association of America
7910 Woodmont Avenue
Suite 1200
Bethesda, MD 20814-7022
301-657-2248
Fax: 301-913-9413
national@shhh.org
www.hearingloss.org
TTY: 301-657-2249

Diana D. Bender,Ph.D., Chairperson
Margaret Wallhagen,Ph.D., Vice President
Anna Gilmore Hall, Executive Director
Year Founded: 1979

5010 Update: Hearing and Vision Loss
Hearing Loss Association of America
7910 Woodmont Avenue
Suite 1200
Bethesda, MD 20814-7022
301-657-2248
Fax: 301-913-9413
national@shhh.org
www.hearingloss.org
TTY: 301-657-2249

Diana D. Bender,Ph.D., Chairperson
Margaret Wallhagen,Ph.D., Vice President
Anna Gilmore Hall, Executive Director
Year Founded: 1979

5011 Using Assistive Listening Devices
Hearing Loss Association of America
7910 Woodmont Avenue
Suite 1200
Bethesda, MD 20814-7022
301-657-2248
Fax: 301-913-9413
national@shhh.org
www.hearingloss.org
TTY: 301-657-2249

Diana D. Bender,Ph.D., Chairperson
Margaret Wallhagen,Ph.D., Vice President
Anna Gilmore Hall, Executive Director
Year Founded: 1979

5012 Using Telecommunications Relay Service
Hearing Loss Association of America
7910 Woodmont Avenue
Suite 1200
Bethesda, MD 20814-7022
301-657-2248
Fax: 301-913-9413
national@shhh.org
www.hearingloss.org
TTY: 301-657-2249

Diana D. Bender,Ph.D., Chairperson
Margaret Wallhagen,Ph.D., Vice President
Anna Gilmore Hall, Executive Director
Year Founded: 1979

5013 Vestibular Disorders
Hearing Loss Association of America
7910 Woodmont Avenue
Suite 1200
Bethesda, MD 20814-7022
301-657-2248
Fax: 301-913-9413
national@shhh.org
www.hearingloss.org
TTY: 301-657-2249

Diana D. Bender,Ph.D., Chairperson
Margaret Wallhagen,Ph.D., Vice President
Anna Gilmore Hall, Executive Director
Year Founded: 1979

5014 Volta Voices
Alexander Graham Bell Association for the Deaf and
3417 Volta Place, NW
Washington, DC 20007-2753
202-337-5220
Fax: 202-337-8314
info@agbell.org
listeningandspokenlanguage.org
TTY: 202-337-5220

Donald M. Goldberg, Ph.D., President
Meredith K. Knueve Sugar, Esq., President-Elect
Alexander T. Graham, Executive Director

Contains Association news and educates readers on the abilities and needs of children and adults who are deaf or hard of hearing. Includes subscription to 'The Valta Review,' published 5 times a year.

5015 What Are TTYs? TDDs? TTs?
Gallaudet University
800 Florida Avenue NE
Washington, DC 20002-3695
202-651-5000
Fax: 202-651-5054
www.gallaudet.edu
TTY: 202-651-5052

Dr. T. Alan Hurwitz, President
Edward Bosso, Vice President for the Laurent C
Dr. Lynne Murray, Vice President for Development,

Discusses text telephones used by deaf people.

Year Founded: 1864

5016 What Do I Do with My Old Decoder?
Hearing Loss Association of America
7910 Woodmont Avenue
Suite 1200
Bethesda, MD 20814-7022
301-657-2248
Fax: 301-913-9413
national@shhh.org
www.hearingloss.org
TTY: 301-657-2249

Diana D. Bender,Ph.D., Chairperson
Margaret Wallhagen,Ph.D., Vice President
Anna Gilmore Hall, Executive Director
Year Founded: 1979

5017 What Employers Want to Know About Assistive Technology in the Workplace
Hearing Loss Association of America
7910 Woodmont Avenue
Suite 1200
Bethesda, MD 20814-7022
301-657-2248
Fax: 301-913-9413
national@shhh.org
www.hearingloss.org
TTY: 301-657-2249

Diana D. Bender,Ph.D., Chairperson
Margaret Wallhagen,Ph.D., Vice President
Anna Gilmore Hall, Executive Director
Year Founded: 1979

5018 What You Should Know About Cochlear Implants in Adults
Alexander Graham Bell Association for the Deaf and
3417 Volta Place, NW
Washington, DC 20007-2753
202-337-5220
Fax: 202-337-8314
info@agbell.org
listeningandspokenlanguage.org
TTY: 202-337-5220

Donald M. Goldberg, Ph.D., President
Meredith K. Knueve Sugar, Esq., President-Elect
Alexander T. Graham, Executive Director

This informative brochure for adults considering a cochlear implant discusses evaluation, decisionmaking, surgery, follow-up visits, and typical costs for a cochlear implant.

5019 Why People Don't Acquire and/or Wear Hearing Aids
Hearing Loss Association of America
7910 Woodmont Avenue
Suite 1200
Bethesda, MD 20814-7022
301-657-2248
Fax: 301-913-9413
national@shhh.org
www.hearingloss.org
TTY: 301-657-2249

Diana D. Bender,Ph.D., Chairperson
Margaret Wallhagen,Ph.D., Vice President
Anna Gilmore Hall, Executive Director
Year Founded: 1979

5020 Wireless Phones: Don't Mix Them Up
Hearing Loss Association of America
7910 Woodmont Avenue
Suite 1200
Bethesda, MD 20814-7022
301-657-2248
Fax: 301-913-9413
national@shhh.org
www.hearingloss.org
TTY: 301-657-2249

Diana D. Bender,Ph.D., Chairperson
Margaret Wallhagen,Ph.D., Vice President
Anna Gilmore Hall, Executive Director
Year Founded: 1979

5021 Without Sight and Sound
Helen Keller National Center
141 Middle Neck Road
Sands Point, NY 11050-1218
516-944-8900
Fax: 516-944-7302
hkncinfo@hknc.org
www.hknc.org
TTY: 516-944-8637

Joseph McNulty, Executive Director

Pamphlet offering facts, causes, types and descriptions of deaf-blindness.

Year Founded: 1967

5022 World of Sound
International Hearing Society
16880 Middlebelt Road
Suite 4
Livonia, MI 48154-3336
734-522-7200
Fax: 734-522-0200; *Toll Free:* 800-521-5247
ihsinfo.org

Thomas Higgins, President
Scott Beall, President-Elect
Kathleen Mennillo, Executive Director

The purpose of this booklet is to provide basic information for those with questions about hearing loss, hearing aids and Hearing Instrument Specialists.

Year Founded: 1951

5023 You Don't Have to Hate Meetings: Try Computer-Assisted Notetaking Instead
Hearing Loss Association of America
7910 Woodmont Avenue
Suite 1200
Bethesda, MD 20814-7022
301-657-2248
Fax: 301-913-9413
national@shhh.org
www.hearingloss.org
TTY: 301-657-2249

Diana D. Bender,Ph.D., Chairperson
Margaret Wallhagen,Ph.D., Vice President
Anna Gilmore Hall, Executive Director
Year Founded: 1979

5024 You've Done Something About It! Helpful Hints to the New Hearing Aid User
Hearing Loss Association of America
7910 Woodmont Avenue
Suite 1200
Bethesda, MD 20814-7022
301-657-2248
Fax: 301-913-9413
national@shhh.org
www.hearingloss.org
TTY: 301-657-2249

Diana D. Bender,Ph.D., Chairperson
Margaret Wallhagen,Ph.D., Vice President
Anna Gilmore Hall, Executive Director

Year Founded: 1979

5025 You, Me and Hearing Loss Makes Three
Hearing Loss Association of America
7910 Woodmont Avenue
Suite 1200
Bethesda, MD 20814-7022
301-657-2248
Fax: 301-913-9413
national@shhh.org
www.hearingloss.org
TTY: 301-657-2249

Diana D. Bender,Ph.D., Chairperson
Margaret Wallhagen,Ph.D., Vice President
Anna Gilmore Hall, Executive Director

Year Founded: 1979

Videos, Audio Tapes

5026 Assistive Devices: Doorways to Independence
Alexander Graham Bell Association for the Deaf and
3417 Volta Place, NW
Washington, DC 20007-2753
202-337-5220
Fax: 202-337-8314
info@agbell.org
listeningandspokenlanguage.org
TTY: 202-337-5220

Donald M. Goldberg, Ph.D., President
Meredith K. Knueve Sugar, Esq., President-Elect
Alexander T. Graham, Executive Director

This extensive videotape and handbook introduce auditory, visual, and vibro-tactile devices that help people with hearing losses.

67 pages

5027 Basic Course in American Sign Language Videotape Package
TJ Publishers
P.O. Box 702701
Suite 206
Dallas, TX 75370
301-585-4440
Fax: 972-416-0944; *Toll Free:* 800-999-1168
TJPubinc@aol.com
www.388.safesecureweb.com/tjpublishers/st

Angela K Thames, President
Jerald A Murphy, VP

Includes four 1-hour videotapes, plus vocabulary videotapes and two texts.

Year Founded: 1978

5028 Beginning Reading and Sign Language Video
TJ Publishers
P.O. Box 702701
Suite 206
Dallas, TX 75370
301-585-4440
Fax: 972-416-0944; *Toll Free:* 800-999-1168
www.388.safesecureweb.com/tjpublishers/st

Angela K Thames, President
Jerald A Murphy, VP

Learning Sign improves reading, motor skills and visual perception and increases language acquisition abilities. For kids from 2 to 12, this video picture book features deaf actress Susan Bressler signing over a hundred words at the zoo, at home, and around the community.

Year Founded: 1978

5029 Deaf Culture Autobiographies
Harris Communications
15155 Technology Drive
Eden Prairie, MN 55344-2273
952-388-2152
Fax: 952-906-1099; *Toll Free:* 800-825-6758
www.harriscomm.com
TTY: 800-825-9187

Robert Harris, President

Inspiring videotapes offer encouragement and enlightenment to the hearing impaired. Total of eight videotapes.

5030 Deaf Culture Series
Harris Communications
15155 Technology Drive
Eden Prairie, MN 55344-2273
952-388-2152
Fax: 952-906-1099; *Toll Free:* 800-825-6758
www.harriscomm.com
TTY: 800-825-9187

Robert Harris, President

Each video in this 5-part series features a variety of Deaf talent. It is an excellent resource for Deaf studies programs, Interpreter Preparation programs and Sign Language programs.

5031 Deaf Mosaic Series
Harris Communications
15155 Technology Drive
Eden Prairie, MN 55344-2273
952-388-2152
Fax: 952-906-1099; *Toll Free:* 800-825-6758
www.harriscomm.com
TTY: 800-825-9187

Robert Harris, President

A national magazine show produced monthly by Gallaudet University, this show has been awarded nine Emmys. As the only nation-wide program about the Deaf community, these videotapes are the best of the best from the shows programs.

5032 Diagnosis and Treatment of Unilateral Hearing Loss
American Academy of Otolaryngology
1650 Diagonal Road
Alexandria, VA 22314-2857
703-836-4444
Fax: 703-683-5100
www.entnet.org

Tom Harlow, Finance Executive

This CD-ROM focuses on evaluation and treatment of unilateral hearing loss arising from skull base lesion.

Year Founded: 1896

5033 Do You Hear That?
Alexander Graham Bell Association for the Deaf and
3417 Volta Place, NW
Washington, DC 20007-2753
202-337-5220
Fax: 202-337-8314
info@agbell.org
listeningandspokenlanguage.org
TTY: 202-337-5220

Donald M. Goldberg, Ph.D., President
Meredith K. Knueve Sugar, Esq., President-Elect
Alexander T. Graham, Executive Director

This video documents auditory-verbal therapy as it is practiced at North York General Hospital in Toronto, Canada.

5034 Getting Through Audiotape
Hearing Loss Association of America
7910 Woodmont Avenue
Suite 1200
Bethesda, MD 20814-7022
301-657-2248
Fax: 301-913-9413
national@shhh.org
www.hearingloss.org
TTY: 301-657-2249

Diana D. Bender,Ph.D., Chairperson
Margaret Wallhagen,Ph.D., Vice President
Anna Gilmore Hall, Executive Director

Simulates hearing loss for better understanding of communication dificulties. The tape features an unfair hearing test.

Year Founded: 1979

5035 Getting the Most Out of Your Hearing Aids
Hearing Loss Association of America
7910 Woodmont Avenue
Suite 1200
Bethesda, MD 20814-7022
301-657-2248
Fax: 301-913-9413
national@shhh.org
www.hearingloss.org
TTY: 301-657-2249

Diana D. Bender,Ph.D., Chairperson
Margaret Wallhagen,Ph.D., Vice President
Anna Gilmore Hall, Executive Director

Helps people new to hearing loss to accept and get the best use of their hearing aids. Open-captioned.

Year Founded: 1979

5036 Granny Good's Sign of Christmas
Gallaudet University
800 Florida Avenue NE
Washington, DC 20002-3695
202-651-5000
Fax: 202-651-5054
www.gallaudet.edu
TTY: 202-651-5052

Dr. T. Alan Hurwitz, President
Edward Bosso, Vice President for the Laurent C
Dr. Lynne Murray, Vice President for Development,

Twas The Night Before Christmas told in American Sign Language.

Year Founded: 1864

5037 HEAR's to the ADA
Hearing Loss Association of America
7910 Woodmont Avenue
Suite 1200
Bethesda, MD 20814-7022
301-657-2248
Fax: 301-913-9413
national@shhh.org
www.hearingloss.org
TTY: 301-657-2249

Diana D. Bender,Ph.D., Chairperson
Margaret Wallhagen,Ph.D., Vice President
Anna Gilmore Hall, Executive Director

A guide for consumers about communication access and the Americans with Disabilities Act. Open-captioned.

Year Founded: 1979

5038 Hearing Loss and Rehabilitation
American Academy of Otolaryngology
1650 Diagonal Road
Alexandria, VA 22314-2857
703-836-4444
Fax: 703-683-5100
www.entnet.org

Tom Harlow, Finance Executive

Slides.

Year Founded: 1896

5039 I Can Hear!
Alexander Graham Bell Association for the Deaf and
3417 Volta Place, NW
Washington, DC 20007-2753
202-337-5220
Fax: 202-337-8314
info@agbell.org
listeningandspokenlanguage.org
TTY: 202-337-5220

Donald M. Goldberg, Ph.D., President
Meredith K. Knueve Sugar, Esq., President-Elect
Alexander T. Graham, Executive Director

This inspirational video describes the auditory-verbal approach for developing speech and language for hearing impaired children and adults.

5040 I Can Hear-II
Alexander Graham Bell Association for the Deaf and
3417 Volta Place, NW
Washington, DC 20007-2753
202-337-5220
Fax: 202-337-8314
info@agbell.org
listeningandspokenlanguage.org
TTY: 202-337-5220

Donald M. Goldberg, Ph.D., President
Meredith K. Knueve Sugar, Esq., President-Elect
Alexander T. Graham, Executive Director

An exciting videotape that gives more examples of auditory-verbal therapy and a variety of kids who have been taught to speak using this method.

5041 I Only Hear You When I See Your Face
Alexander Graham Bell Association for the Deaf and
3417 Volta Place, NW
Washington, DC 20007-2753
202-337-5220
Fax: 202-337-8314
info@agbell.org
listeningandspokenlanguage.org
TTY: 202-337-5220

Donald M. Goldberg, Ph.D., President
Meredith K. Knueve Sugar, Esq., President-Elect
Alexander T. Graham, Executive Director

This video is for medical personnel providing tips on how to communicate more effectively with the hearing impaired patient.

5042 I See What You Say: Self Help Lipreading Program
Alexander Graham Bell Association for the Deaf and
3417 Volta Place, NW
Washington, DC 20007-2753
202-337-5220
Fax: 202-337-8314
info@agbell.org
listeningandspokenlanguage.org
TTY: 202-337-5220

Donald M. Goldberg, Ph.D., President
Meredith K. Knueve Sugar, Esq., President-Elect
Alexander T. Graham, Executive Director

Easy-to-follow videotape and manual for consumers teaches visual recognition of speech sounds in single words and phrases.

5043 Interview with Kirsten Gonzales
Alexander Graham Bell Association for the Deaf and
3417 Volta Place, NW
Washington, DC 20007-2753
202-337-5220
Fax: 202-337-8314
info@agbell.org
listeningandspokenlanguage.org
TTY: 202-337-5220

Donald M. Goldberg, Ph.D., President
Meredith K. Knueve Sugar, Esq., President-Elect
Alexander T. Graham, Executive Director

Interviews a longtime user and trainer of oral interpreters who offers techniques in articulation and natural gestures.

5044 Joy of Signing
Gallaudet University
800 Florida Avenue NE
Washington, DC 20002-3695
202-651-5000
Fax: 202-651-5054
www.gallaudet.edu
TTY: 202-651-5052

Dr. T. Alan Hurwitz, President
Edward Bosso, Vice President for the Laurent C
Dr. Lynne Murray, Vice President for Development,

Three tapes full of useful information to help increase skill and comfort with sign.

Year Founded: 1864

5045 Lipreading Made Easy
Alexander Graham Bell Association for the Deaf and
3417 Volta Place, NW
Washington, DC 20007-2753
202-337-5220
Fax: 202-337-8314
info@agbell.org
listeningandspokenlanguage.org
TTY: 202-337-5220

Donald M. Goldberg, Ph.D., President
Meredith K. Knueve Sugar, Esq., President-Elect
Alexander T. Graham, Executive Director

Uses actual photos of lips to teach the student to listen with their eyes.

5046 Models of Oral Interpreting
Alexander Graham Bell Association for the Deaf and
3417 Volta Place, NW
Washington, DC 20007-2753
202-337-5220
Fax: 202-337-8314
info@agbell.org
listeningandspokenlanguage.org
TTY: 202-337-5220

Donald M. Goldberg, Ph.D., President
Meredith K. Knueve Sugar, Esq., President-Elect
Alexander T. Graham, Executive Director

Modeling effective techniques, three experienced oral interpreters interpret the same lectures featuring the handling of multiple speakers, phrasing, facial expressions, and articulation.

5047 National 4th Biennial Campvention of the Deaf
National Association of the Deaf
8630 Fenton Street
Suite 820
Silver Spring, MD 20910-4504
301-587-1788
Fax: 301-587-1791
www.nad.org
TTY: 301-587-1789

Christopher Wagner, President
Melissa S. Draganac-Hawk, Vice-President
Howard A. Rosenblum, Chief Executive Officer

Depicts the big event held at the Casa De Fruta in Hollister, CA.

Year Founded: 1880

5048 People vs. Noise
Better Hearing Institute
1444 I Street, NW
Suite 700
Washington, DC 20005
202-449-1100
Fax: 202-216-9646
mail@betterhearing.org
www.betterhearing.org

Jerry J Rizzo, Executive Director
Ruth Bentler, Ph.D., Professor
Jennifer Bishop, J.D., Attorney
Year Founded: 1973

5049 Read My Lips
Alexander Graham Bell Association for the Deaf and
3417 Volta Place, NW
Washington, DC 20007-2753
202-337-5220
Fax: 202-337-8314
info@agbell.org
listeningandspokenlanguage.org
TTY: 202-337-5220

Donald M. Goldberg, Ph.D., President
Meredith K. Knueve Sugar, Esq., President-Elect
Alexander T. Graham, Executive Director

A six videotape series that takes adults from lipreading to basic words to complex phrases and sentences in a variety of real life situations.

5050 Speaking Off the Cuff
Alexander Graham Bell Association for the Deaf and
3417 Volta Place, NW
Washington, DC 20007-2753
202-337-5220
Fax: 202-337-8314
info@agbell.org
listeningandspokenlanguage.org
TTY: 202-337-5220

Donald M. Goldberg, Ph.D., President
Meredith K. Knueve Sugar, Esq., President-Elect
Alexander T. Graham, Executive Director

This videotape series features adults with hearing impairments speaking on different topics with varying degrees of speaking abilities.

5051 Teaching Strategies for the Developmentof Auditory Verbal Communication
Alexander Graham Bell Association for the Deaf and
3417 Volta Place, NW
Washington, DC 20007-2753
202-337-5220
Fax: 202-337-8314
info@agbell.org
listeningandspokenlanguage.org
TTY: 202-337-5220

Donald M. Goldberg, Ph.D., President
Meredith K. Knueve Sugar, Esq., President-Elect
Alexander T. Graham, Executive Director

This educational series of five-hour videotapes demonstrates teaching strategies for developing auditory-verbal communication in young children with severe to profound hearing loss.

5052 Telecoil: Plugging into Sound
Hearing Loss Association of America
7910 Woodmont Avenue
Suite 1200
Bethesda, MD 20814-7022
301-657-2248
Fax: 301-913-9413
national@shhh.org
www.hearingloss.org
TTY: 301-657-2249

Diana D. Bender,Ph.D., Chairperson
Margaret Wallhagen,Ph.D., Vice President
Anna Gilmore Hall, Executive Director

Guide for consumers explaining a telecoil in their hearing aid. SHHH members are featured, talking about their experiences. Includes 50 brochures. Open-captioned.

Year Founded: 1979

5053 Telecoils in Hearing Aids
Hearing Loss Association of America
7910 Woodmont Avenue
Suite 1200
Bethesda, MD 20814-7022
301-657-2248
Fax: 301-913-9413
national@shhh.org
www.hearingloss.org
TTY: 301-657-2249

Diana D. Bender,Ph.D., Chairperson
Margaret Wallhagen,Ph.D., Vice President
Anna Gilmore Hall, Executive Director
Year Founded: 1979

5054 Telling Stories
Harris Communications
15155 Technology Drive
Eden Prairie, MN 55344-2273
952-388-2152
Fax: 952-906-1099; *Toll Free:* 800-825-6758
www.harriscomm.com
TTY: 800-825-9187

Robert Harris, President

This international, award winning play, now on video, uses the symbols and myths drawn from the struggles between the world of the deaf and the world of the hearing.

5055 You Shared the World with Me Video
Alexander Graham Bell Association for the Deaf and
3417 Volta Place, NW
Washington, DC 20007-2753
202-337-5220
Fax: 202-337-8314
info@agbell.org
listeningandspokenlanguage.org
TTY: 202-337-5220

Donald M. Goldberg, Ph.D., President
Meredith K. Knueve Sugar, Esq., President-Elect
Alexander T. Graham, Executive Director

Johnny Whitaker hosts this inspiring video about having a
hearing impairment and working with the hearing impaired.

Websites

5056 ACB Government Employees
American Council of the Blind
2200 Wilson Boulevard
Suite 650
Arlington, VA 22201-3354
202-467-5081
Fax: 703-465-5085; *Toll Free:* 800-424-8666
info@acb.org
www.acb.org

Kim Charlson, President
Marlaina Lieberg, Vice President
Melanie Brunson, Executive Director

Concerns of the organization include recruitment, placement and advancement of blind and visually impaired
employees.

Year Founded: 1961

5057 ACB Radio Amateurs
American Council of the Blind
2200 Wilson Boulevard
Suite 650
Arlington, VA 22201-3354
202-467-5081
Fax: 703-465-5085; *Toll Free:* 800-424-8666
info@acb.org
www.acb.org

Kim Charlson, President
Marlaina Lieberg, Vice President
Melanie Brunson, Executive Director

A radio amateur network of blind, visually impaired and
sighted members who gather and share common problems
and solutions to help members improve radio amateurs in
getting started, provides access to educational materials in
special media and publishes a directory for the visually
impaired.

Year Founded: 1961

5058 ACB Social Service Providers
American Council of the Blind
2200 Wilson Boulevard
Suite 650
Arlington, VA 22201-3354
202-467-5081
Fax: 703-465-5085; *Toll Free:* 800-424-8666
info@acb.org
www.acb.org

Kim Charlson, President
Marlaina Lieberg, Vice President
Melanie Brunson, Executive Director

Information on blind and visually impaired social workers,
social service professionals, students pursuing careers in
social work, and other interested persons.

Year Founded: 1961

**5059 Alexander Graham Bell Association for the
Deaf and Hard of Hearing**
**Alexander Graham Bell Association for the Deaf
and**
3417 Volta Place, NW
Washington, DC 20007-2753
202-337-5220
Fax: 202-337-8314
info@agbell.org
listeningandspokenlanguage.org
TTY: 202-337-5220

Donald M. Goldberg, Ph.D., President
Meredith K. Knueve Sugar, Esq., President-Elect
Alexander T. Graham, Executive Director

Information on pediatric hearing loss, and educational issues for hearing impaired children, promotes better public
understanding of hearing loss in children and adults, provides scholarships and financial aid to families of children
with hearing loss, and promotes early detection of hearing
loss in infants.

5060 American Academy of Audiology
American Academy of Audiology
11480 Commerce Park Drive
Suite 220
Reston, VA 20191
703-790-8466
Fax: 703-790-8631; *Toll Free:* 800-222-2336
www.audiology.org

Bettie Borton, President
Erin Miller, President-Elect
M Samantha Lewis, Member-at-Large

Provides professional development, education and research
and provides increased public awareness of hearing disorders and audiologic services.

5061 American Tinnitus Association
American Tinnitus Association
522 S.W. Fifth Ave.
Ste. 825
Portland, OR 97204
503-248-9985
Fax: 503-248-0024; *Toll Free:* 800-634-8978
tinnitus@ata.org
www.ata.org

Cara James, Executive Director
Ben Forstag, Director of Communications
Lynn Michael Allmeyer, Director of Development

Provides information about tinnitus and referrals to local
contacts/support groups nationwide.

Year Founded: 1971

5062 Better Hearing Institute
Better Hearing Institute
1444 I Street, NW
Suite 700
Washington, DC 20005
202-449-1100
Fax: 202-216-9646
mail@betterhearing.org
www.betterhearing.org

Jerry J Rizzo, Executive Director
Ruth Bentler, Ph.D., Professor
Jennifer Bishop, J.D., Attorney

Information programs on hearing loss and available medical, surgical, hearing aid, and rehabilitation assistance for millions with uncorrected hearing problems.

Year Founded: 1973

5063 CAPCOM

www.capcom1.com

Presents workshops on law and the deaf and on promoting productive working relationships for the hearing impaired employees of agencies and corporations.

5064 Deafness Research Foundation
IDT
520 Broad Street
Newark, NJ 7102
973-438-1000
www.idt.net

Committed to public awareness and support for basic and clinical research into deafness and hearing disabilities.

5065 Hear Now

www.leisurelan.com/~hearnow

Committed to making technology accessible to deaf and hard of hearing individuals throughout the United States. Also raises funds to provide hearing aids, cochlear implants and related services to children and adults who have hearing losses but do not have financial resources to purchase their own devices.

5066 Hearing Education and Awareness for Elders
Hearing Education and Awareness for Rockers
443 Broadway Street

www.hearnet.com/

Kathy Peck, Co-Founder and Executive Directo
Joseph Montano, Chief of Audiology
Jerome Goldstein, Senior Executive Vice President

Educates the public about the real dangers of hearing loss resulting from repeated exposure to excessive noise levels.

Year Founded: 1988

5067 House Ear Institute
House Research Institute
2100 West Third Street
Los Angeles, CA 90057
213-483-4431
Fax: 213-483-8789
www.houseresearch.org

Catherine D. Meyer, Chairman

Year Founded: 1946

5068 National Association of the Deaf
National Association of the Deaf
8630 Fenton Street
Suite 820
Silver Spring, MD 20910-4504
301-587-1788
Fax: 301-587-1791
www.nad.org
TTY: 301-587-1789

Christopher Wagner, President
Melissa S. Draganac-Hawk, Vice-President
Howard A. Rosenblum, Chief Executive Officer

Focus on advocacy, captioned media, deafness-related information/publications, legal assistance and more.

Year Founded: 1880

5069 National Association of the Deaf Law
National Association of the Deaf
8630 Fenton Street
Suite 820
Silver Spring, MD 20910-4504
301-587-1788
Fax: 301-587-1791
www.nad.org
TTY: 301-587-1789

Christopher Wagner, President
Melissa S. Draganac-Hawk, Vice-President
Howard A. Rosenblum, Chief Executive Officer

Provides legal information about how these laws affect deaf people in jobs, education, the courts, public access and government services.

Year Founded: 1880

5070 National Information Center on Deafness
Gallaudet University
800 Florida Avenue NE
Washington, DC 20002-3695
202-651-5000
Fax: 202-651-5054
www.gallaudet.edu
TTY: 202-651-5052

Dr. T. Alan Hurwitz, President
Edward Bosso, Vice President for the Laurent C
Dr. Lynne Murray, Vice President for Development,

Provides information or referrals on questions about deafness, including general information, education, research, legislation, assistive devices and more. Offers a bibliography of readings available on 30 topics relating to deafness.

Year Founded: 1864

5071 Registry of Interpreters for the Deaf
Registry of the Interpreters for the Deaf
333 Commerce Street
Suite 310
Alexandria, VA 22314
703-838-0030
Fax: 301-608-0508
www.rid.org
TTY: 703-838-0459

Shane H. Feldman, M.S., CAE, Executive Director
Matthew O'Hara, M.S., CI and, Director of Ethical Practices Sy
Julie Schafer, Esq.,, Director of Public Policy and Ad

Professional interpreters and translators, persons with deafness or hearing impairments and professionals in related fields.

5072 Self-Help for Hard of Hearing People
Hearing Loss Association of America
www.hearingloss.org

Diana D. Bender,Ph.D., Chairperson
Margaret Wallhagen,Ph.D., Vice President
Anna Gilmore Hall, Executive Director

Promotes awareness and information about hearing loss, communication, assistive devices, and alternative communication skills through publications, exhibits and presentations.

Year Founded: 1979

5073 USA Deaf Sports Federation
www.usadsf.org

A governing body for all deaf sports and recreation in the United States.

Research Centers

5074 American Hearing Research Foundation
American Hearing Research Foundation
310 W. Lake St.
Suite 111
Elmhurst, IL 60126
630-617-5079
Fax: 630-563-9181
american-hearing.org

Richard G. Muench, Chairman
Alan G. Micco, M.D., President
Mark R. Muench, Vice President

Supports medical resarch and education into the causes, prevention, and cures of deafness, hearing losses, and balance disorders. Also keeps physicians and the public informed of the latest developments in hearing research and education.

5075 Deafness Research Foundation
Hearing Healthy Foundation
363 Seventh Avenue
10th Floor
New York, NY 10001-3904
212-257-6140
Fax: 212-599-0039; *Toll Free:* 866-454-3924
info@hearinghealthfoundation.org
hearinghealthfoundation.org

Shari Eberts, Chairman
Mark A Angelo, President
Robert Boucai, Principal

The nation's largest voluntary health organization, providing grants for fellowship, symposia, and research into causes, treatment, and prevention of all ear disorders.

Year Founded: 1958

5076 Minnesota Academy of Audiology
Minnesota Academy of Audiology
PO Box 20499
Bloomington, MN 55420
612-885-0095
Fax: 612-625-8901; *Toll Free:* 800-347-8165
www.minnesotaaudiology.org

Jennifer L. Tunnell, President
Grace L. Berry, President-Elect
John S. Tunnell, Treasurer

The Minnesota Academy of Audiology is organized for the purpose of promoting the public good by fostering the growth, development, recognition, and status of the profession of Audiology and its members. We are dedicated to providing quality hearing and balance care to our patients by enhancing our members to achieve practice objectives through education, legislation, and increased public awareness of hearing and balance disorders.

Year Founded: 2009

5077 National Center for Voice and Speech
136 South Main Street
Suite 320
Salt Lake City, UT 84101-1623
801-596-2012
Fax: 801-596-2013
www.ncvs.org

Ingo Titze, Executive Director
Lynn Maxfield, Associate Director
Darby Bailey, Program Manager

This is a consortium of institutions focusing on voice and speech disorders. The members of this consortium are the University of Iowa, the Denver Center for Performing Arts, the University of Wisconsin-Madison, and the University of Utah. NCVS trains scientists interested in careers in voice and spech research, provides continuing education for professionals, and conducts research on voice and speech production.

5078 National Institute on Deafness & Other Communication Disorders
US Department of Health & Human Services
200 Independence Avenue, S.W.
Bldg 31
Washington, DC 20201
301-496-1993
Fax: 301-402-0018; *Toll Free:* 877-696-6775
www.hhs.gov
TDD 301-402-6596

James Snow MD, Director
Martin Allen, Contact

Conducts and supports research and training with respect to disorders of hearing and other communication processes, including diseases affecting hearing, balance, voice, speech, language, touch, taste and smell through research performed in its own laboratories; a program of research grants; individual and institutional research training awards, career development awards, center grants, and contracts to public and private research institutions.

Year Founded: 1953

5079 Princeton University: Cutaneous Communication Laboratory
Psychology Department, Green Hall
5848 S. University Avenue
Chicago, IL 60637
773-702-8403
Fax: 773-702-0886
psychology.uchicago.edu

Amanda L. Woodward, Chair
Ray Weathers, Faculty Affairs
Mimi Halpern Maduff, Student Affairs

Year Founded: 1893

5080 The Graduate Center: Speech-Language-Hearing Sciences
City University of New York
365 Fifth Avenue
Room 7107
New York, NY 10016-4309
212-817-8800
Fax: 212-817-1537
www.gc.cuny.edu

Valerie Shafer, Acting Executive Officer

Programmable research of digital and auditory hearing aids and sensory aids for the speech and hearing impaired person.

Year Founded: 1957

5081 Trace Center
University of Wisconsin-Madison
1500 Highland Avenue
Room S-151
Madison, WI 53706
608-263-2400
Fax: 608-262-8848
askbucky@uwmad.wisc.edu
www.wisc.edu

Rebecca M. Blank, Chancellor
Paul M. DeLuca, Provost and Vice Chancellor for
Darrell Bazzell, Vice Chancellor for Finance and

Research and development center working with communication, control, and computer access technologies for people with disabilities.

Year Founded: 1848

5082 Yeshiva University: Institute of Communication
Disorders
Montefiore Medical Center
111 E 210th Street
Bronx, NY 10467-2401
718-920-4321
Fax: 718-405-9014; *Toll Free:* 800-636-6683
www.montefiore.org

Steven M. Safyer, President and Chief Executive Of
Phillip O. Ozuah, Executive Vice President
Joel A. Aerlman, Executive Vice President

Studies on communicative disorders including speech and hearing.

Year Founded: 1884

Heart Disease

Associations & Organizations

5083 Abrazo Arizona Heart Institute
2632 N 20th Street
Phoenix, AZ 85006
602-266-2200
Fax: 602-264-5332
azheart.com
Year Founded: 1971

5084 American Heart Association
7272 Greenville Avenue
Dallas, TX 75231
Toll Free: 800-242-8721
www.heart.org

Nancy Brown, CEO

Physicians, scientists, and laypersons. Supports research, education, and community service programs with the objective of reducing premature death and disability from cardiovascular diseases and stroke; coordinates the efforts of physicians, nurses, health professionals, and others engaged in the fight against heart and circulatory disease. Financed entirely by voluntary contributions of the public, principally during the Heart Campaign held inFebruary.

5085 Centers for Disease Control and Prevention: Heart Disease
1600 Clifton Road
Atlanta, GA 30329-4027
Toll Free: 800-232-4636
www.cdc.gov/heartdisease
TTY: 888-232-6348

Tom Frieden, Director

To create a heart-healthy and stroke-free world.
Year Founded: 1984

5086 Million Hearts
millionhearts.hhs.gov

Janet Wright, Executive Director

A national initiative of the U.S. Department of Health and Human Services to prevent heart attacks and strokes.

5087 National Heart, Lung, & Blood Institute
NHLBI Health Information Center
PO Box 30105
Bethesda, MD 20824-0105
301-592-8573
nhlbiinfo@nhlbi.nih.gov
www.nhlbi.nih.gov

Gary H. Gibbons, Director

Primary responsibility of this organization is the scientific investigation of heart, blood vessel, lung and blood disorders. Oversees research, demonstration, prevention, education, control and training activities in these fields and emphasizes the prevention and control of heart diseases.
Year Founded: 1887

5088 San Francisco Heart & Vascular Institute
Seton Medical Center
1900 Sullivan Avenue
Daly City, CA 94015

650-991-6712
Fax: 650-755-7315
seton.verity.org

5089 Texas Heart Institute
Texas Health Institute, MC 3-116
PO Box 20345
Houston, TX 77225-0345
832-355-4011
Fax: 713-791-3089
www.texasheart.org

James T. Willerson, President
David A. Ott, Surgeon-in-Chief
Year Founded: 1962

5090 The Heart Foundation
31822 Village Center Road
Suite 208
Westlake Village, CA 91361
818-865-1100
Fax: 818-530-7743
info@theheartfoundation.org
www.theheartfoundation.org

Catherine Erlinger, Executive Director

Supporting research and educating the public about heart disease and the importance of early detection.

5091 University of Tennessee Health Science Center: Division of Cardiovascular Diseases
Coleman College of Medicine Building
956 Court Avenue
Suite A312
Memphis, TN 38163
901-448-5750
Fax: 901-448-8084
www.uthsc.edu/cardiology

Karl T. Weber, Division Chief

Cardiovasular system disorders including heart disease prevention and treatment.
Year Founded: 1944

Books

5092 Adult Congenital Heart Disease: A Practical Guide
Wiley Publishing
111 River Street
Hoboken, NJ 07030-5774
201-748-6000
Fax: 201-748-6088; *Toll Free:* 877-762-2974
info@wiley.com
www.wiley.com

Stephen M. Smith, President and Chief Executive Of
Ellis E. Cousens, Executive Vice President, Chief
John Kritzmacher, Executive Vice President, Chief

This practical guide with its straighforward a,b,c approach is written for those professionals.
288 pages Year Founded: 1807

5093 Advances in Cardiac and Pulmonary Rehabilitation
Haworth Press
10 Alice Street
Binghamton, NY 13904-1503

607-722-5857
Fax: 607-722-1424; Toll Free: 800-342-9678
getinfo@haworthpress.com
www.haworthpress.com

William Cohen, Owner

Enhance your rehabilitation program with this authoritative volume.

74 pages

5094 **American Medical Association Guide to Preventing and Treating Heart Disease**
American Medical Association
515 N State Street
Chicago, IL 60610
Toll Free: 800-262-3211
www.ama-assn.org

Martin S Lipsky MD, Author
Marla Mendelson MD, Author
Stephen Havas MD, Author

Offers essential tools and timely information on the prevention and treatment of heart disease. Also features practical strategies for lifestyle changes, advice about warning signs to report to a doctor, guidance on heart-health ways to exercise, and a section on the unique risks ans symptons for women.

312 pages Year Founded: 1847

5095 **Diet & Heart Disease: It's Not What You Think**
Whitman Publications
400 Oak Hill Drive
Winona Lake, IN 46590
574-267-3941Toll free: 800-546-2995
www.whitman.com

Stephen Byrnes, Author

96 pages Year Founded: 1934

5096 **Heart Smart: A Cardiologists 5-Step Plan for Detecting, Preventing and Even Reversing Heart Disease**
Wiley Publishing
111 River Street
Hoboken, NJ 07030-5774
201-748-6000
Fax: 201-748-6088; Toll Free: 877-762-2974
info@wiley.com
www.wiley.com

Stephen M. Smith, President and Chief Executive Of
Ellis E. Cousens, Executive Vice President, Chief
John Kritzmacher, Executive Vice President, Chief

Provides the latest cutting-edge methods to treat, detect, and prevent heart disease, which is the number 1 killer in North America, Europe, and many other regions of the world. Helps readers identify their current health status through interactive quizzes and then recommends specific diagnostic procedures and lifestyle changes.

272 pages Year Founded: 1807

5097 **Heart to Heart: A Guide to the Psychological Aspects of the Disease**
Health Press
2920 Carlisle Blvd. NE
PO Box 1388
Albuquerque, NM 87110

505-888-1394
Fax: 505-983-1383; Toll Free: 877-411-0707
www.healthpress.com

Lynn Peters Adler, Author
Monica Driscoll Beatty, Author
Beverly Brown, Author

130 pages

5098 **Outliving Heart Disease**
Newmarket Press
18 East 48th Street
New York, NY 10017
212-832-3575
Fax: 212-832-3629; Toll Free: 802-388-6397
www.newmarketpress.com

Edward Coats, President & Publisher
Dr Richard A Stein, Author

Explains vascular changes that take place as you age- and how they affect your heart. The specific risk factors affecting women, African-Americans, and other group. The latest on research on statins-those miracle drugs that have revolutionized the prevention and treatment of heart disease. How to create a heart-healthy diet and cardiovascular exercise program. How depression, anxiety, and stress can impact the heart, and what you can do about it.

286 pages Year Founded: 1995

5099 **Prevent and Reverse Heart Disease: The Revolutionary, Scientifically Proven, Nutrition-Based Care**
Penguin Group USA
375 Hudson Street
New York, NY 10014-3657
212-366-2000
us.penguingroup.com

John Makinson, Chairman and Chief Executive
Coram Williams, Chief Financial Officer
David Shanks, Chief Executive Officer

320 pages Year Founded: 1838

Journals, Magazines

5100 **Heart Beat**
National Institutes of Health
31 Center Drive MSC 2486
Building 31, Room 5A52
Bethesda, MD 20892
301-592-8573
Fax: 301-592-8563
nhlbiinfo@nhlbi.nih.gov
www.nhlbi.nih.gov
TTY: 240-629-3255

Gary H. Gibbons, Director
Susan B. Shurin, Deputy Director
Nakela Cook, Chief Of Staff

Magazine for cardiology patients.

Frequency: Quarterly

Newsletters, Pamphlets

5101 American Heart Association Diet
American Heart Association
7272 Greenville Avenue
Dallas, TX 75231-4596
214-373-6300
Fax: 214-696-5211; *Toll Free:* 800-242-8721
www.heart.org

Bernie Dennis, Chairman
Mariell Jessup, President
Nancy Brown, Chief Executive Officer

An eating plan for healthy americans.

Year Founded: 1924

5102 Cholesterol and Your Heart
American Heart Association
7272 Greenville Avenue
Dallas, TX 75231
214-373-6300
Fax: 214-987-9361
www.americanheart.org

M Cass Wheeler, CEO

Offers information on lowering blood cholesterol levels.

5103 Easy Food Tips for Heart Healthy Eating
American Heart Association
7272 Greenville Avenue
Dallas, TX 75231
214-373-6300
Fax: 214-987-9361
www.americanheart.org

M Cass Wheeler, CEO

Offers food selection hints for fat-controlled meals.

5104 Exercise and Your Heart
American Heart Association
7272 Greenville Avenue
Dallas, TX 75231
214-373-6300
Fax: 214-987-9361
www.americanheart.org

M Cass Wheeler, CEO

Offers information on how to get enough exercise from daily activities, what the benefits of exercise are and what the risks of exercising are.

Research Centers

5105 American College Of Cardiology
Heart House
2400 N Street NW
Washington, DC 20037
202-375-6000
Fax: 202-375-7000; *Toll Free:* 800-253-4636
resource@acc.org
www.cardiosource.org

John Gordon Harold, MD, MAC, President
Patrick T. O'Gara, MD, FACC, Vice President
Kim Allan Williams, Sr., M, Vice President

Mission is to transform cardiovascular care and improve heart health.

Year Founded: 1949

5106 Baylor College of Medicine: DeBakey Heart Center
Texas Medical Center
2450 Holcombe Blvd.
Suite 1
Houston, TX 77021
713-791-6161
Fax: 713-793-1192
www.texasmedicalcenter.org

Robert C. Robbins, M.D., President and Chief Executive Of
William McKeon, Chief Strategy & Development Off
Denise Castillo-Rhodes, Executive Vice President and Chi

Research activities have an emphasis on therapeutic intervention and prevention of heart diseases.

Year Founded: 1905

5107 Boston University: General Clinical Research Center
Boston University Medical Campus
Boston Medical Center
Boston, MA 02118
617-638-8000
Fax: 617-414-1969
jkopp@bu.edu
www.bumc.bu.edu/

Janice Kopp, Contact
Ilga Wohlrab, Manager

Biomedical clinical research

5108 Columbia University Irving Center for Clinical Research
Presbyterian Hospital
622 W 168th Street
New York, NY 10032-3720
212-305-2071
Fax: 212-305-3213
www.novanthealth.org

Carl S. Armato, President & Chief Executive Offi
Peter S. Brunstetter, Executive Vice President & Chief
Jesse Cureton, Executive Vice President & Chief

Research center focusing on pulmonary diseases.

Year Founded: 1997

5109 General Clinical Research Center: University of California at Los Angeles
Oklahoma State University Center for Health Scien
1111 W. 17th St.
Tulsa, OK 74107
918-582-1972
Fax: 310-206-5012
info@osugiving.com
www.healthsciences.okstate.edu

Angelyn Holmes, President
Janifer Hilton, Vice President
Amanda Benn, Secretary

Cardiovascular and heart disease disorders and illness research.

5110 Harvard Thorndike Laboratory
Harvard Medical Center
25 Shattuck Street
Boston, MA 02115

617-432-1000
Fax: 617-735-4833
hms.harvard.edu

Senator William H. Frist, MD ', Chairman
John W. Rowe, MD, Vice Chairman
Neal Baer, EDM '79, AM '82,, Executive Producer
Year Founded: 1782

5111 Hope Heart Institute
The Hope Heart Institute
1380 112th Ave NE
Suite 200
Bellevue, WA 98004
425-456-8700
Fax: 425-456-8701
info@hopeheart.org
www.hopeheart.org

Craig W. Philips, Chair
Cherie Skager, MA, MNPL, Interim Executive Director
Brian Pierson, Treasurer

Heart and blood vessel research.

Year Founded: 1959

5112 Purdue University: William A Hillenbrand
Biomedical Engineering Center
AA Potter Engineering Center
701 West Stadium Ave.
Room 204
West Lafayette, IN 47907-2045
765-494-5354
Fax: 765-494-9321
dean.of.engineering@purdue.edu
engineering.purdue.edu

Leah Jamieson, Chair
William Anderson, Director of Global Engineering P
David Bahr, Head And Professor Materials Eng

Cardiology and heart disease research.

Year Founded: 1862

5113 Research and Education Institute
Harbor-UCLA Medical Center
1000 W. Carson Street
8th Floor, Room 8E8
Torrance, CA 90509
310-222-2911
Fax: 310-782-8599
www.harbor-ucla.org

Frank De Santis CAE, President
Alan Jobe, MD
Darrell W. Harrington, M.D., Director and Designated
Institut

5114 University of Alabama at Birmingham:
Congenital Heart Disease Center
Department of Surgery
600 Highland Avenue
Department of Surgery Administration MC: 7375
Madison, WI 53792
608-263-1375
Fax: 608-265-5963
kent@surgery.wisc.edu
www.surgery.wisc.edu

K. Craig Kent,MD, Chairman
Mary Marshall, Administrator
Teri J. Keeler, Chief Financial Officer

5115 University of California: Cardiovascular
Research Laboratory
Oklahoma State University Center for Health Scien
1111 W. 17th St.
Tulsa, OK 74107
918-582-1972
Fax: 310-206-5012
info@osugiving.com
www.healthsciences.okstate.edu

Angelyn Holmes, President
Janifer Hilton, Vice President
Amanda Benn, Secretary

Cellular and subcellular cardiac conditions.

5116 University of California: San Diego General
Clinical Research Center
UCSD Medical Center, 8203
200 W. Arbor Drive
San Diego, CA 92103-1910
619-543-6222
Fax: 619-543-5536
health.ucsd.edu

Paul F Viviano, Chief Executive Officer and Asso
Margarita Baggett, Chief Clinical Officer
Lori Donaldson, Chief Financial Officer

Cardiovasular and heart disease research.

Year Founded: 1962

5117 University of Iowa: Iowa Cardiovascular
Center
College of Medicine
Guys Hospital, Ground Floor
Great Maze Pond
London, SE 19RT
844-873-7388
Fax: 319-335-6969; *Toll Free:* 800-854-4461
info@collegeofmedicine.org.uk
www.collegeofmedicine.org.uk

Debbie Cragg, Chief Executive
Amanda King, Membership Secretary
Babs Guthrie, Coordinator

5118 University of Missouri: Columbia Division of
Cardiothoracic Surgery
Stanford University School of Medicine
291 Campus Drive Rm LK3C02
Li Ka Shing Building, 3rd floor
Stanford, CA 94305-5101
650-725-3900
med.stanford.edu

Phillip A. Pizzo, M.D., Dean
Dr. Jack Curtis, Contact

Cardiac surgery research.

5119 Warren Grant Magnuson Clinical Center
NIH Clinical Center
9000 Rockville Pike
Suite 3c01
Bethesda, MD 20892
301-496-2563
Fax: 301-402-2984
prpl@mail.cc.nih.gov
www.cc.nih.gov

John I. Gallin, MD, Clinical Center Director
David Henderson, MD, Deputy Director for Clinical Car
Clare Hastings, Chief Nurse Officer

Established in 1953 as the research hospital of the National Institutes of Health. Designed so that patient care facilities are close to research laboratories so new findings of basic and clinical scientists can be quickly applied to the treatment of patients. Upon referral by physicians, patients are admitted to NIH clinical studies.

Year Founded: 1944

Hypertension

Associations & Organizations

5120 American Kidney Fund
11921 Rockville Pike
Suite 300
Rockville, MD 20852
Toll Free: 800-638-8299
www.kidneyfund.org

LaVarne A. Burton, President & CEO
Donald J. Roy, EVP & COO

Fighting kidney disease through direct financial support to patients in need, health education, and prevention efforts.

5121 American Society of Hypertension
244 Madison Avenue
Suite 136
New York, NY 10016
212-696-9099
Fax: 347-916-0267
ash@ash-us.org
www.ash-us.org

Torry Mark Sansone, Executive Director

To organize and conduct educational seminars, materials, and products in all aspects of hypertension and other cardiovascular diseases.

5122 American Society of Nephrology
1510 H Street NW
Suite 800
Washington, DC 20005
202-640-4660
Fax: 202-637-9793
email@asn-online.org
www.asn-online.org

Raymond C. Harris, President
John R. Sedor, Secretary-Treasurer

Mission is to lead the fight against kidney disase and advance research.

5123 National Heart, Lung, & Blood Institute
NHLBI Health Information Center
PO Box 30105
Bethesda, MD 20824-0105
301-592-8573
nhlbiinfo@nhlbi.nih.gov
www.nhlbi.nih.gov

Gary H. Gibbons, Director

Promoting prevention and treatment of heart, lung and blood diseases.

Year Founded: 1887

5124 Pulmonary Hypertension Association
801 Roeder Road
Suite 1000
Silver Spring, MD 20910
301-565-3004
Fax: 301-565-3994; *Toll Free:* 800-748-7274
pha@phassociation.org
www.phassociation.org

Rino Aldrighetti, President & CEO

Providing hope for the pulmonary hypeertension community through support, education, and awareness.
Year Founded: 1990

5125 Wake Forest School of Medicine Hypertension and Vascular Research Center
HVRC Wake Forest School of Medicine
6 Hanes Medical Center Boulevard
Winston-Salem, NC 27157
336-716-5819
www.wakehealth.edu

This center works towards developing a comprehensive collection of basic science and clinical research in the field of hypertension.

Books

5126 Answers to 100 Questions About Hypertension
The National Organization for Rare Disorders
324 E 30th Street
New York, NY 10016-8329
212-889-3557Toll free: 800-575-9355
nathypertension@aol.com
www.nathypertension.com

Francine Rowley, Executive Director

Book describing hypertension in layman's terms.
Year Founded: 1977

5127 Conquering Hypertension: An Illustrated Guide to Understanding Treatment
Consortium Book Sales & Distribution
34 Thirteenth Avenue NE
Suite 101
Minneapolis, MN 55413
612-746-2600
Fax: 312-666-2680
hhart@cbsd.com
www.cbsd.com

Livy Traczyk, marketing
Ruth Berger, sales

168 pages

5128 Hypertension: An Integrated, Clinical Approach
Carolina Academic Division
387 Park Avenue S
Floor 5
New York, NY 10016-8810
212-779-1822
Fax: 212-779-1834
www.sc.edu

Harris Pastides, President
Michael Amiridis, Executive Vice President for Aca
Ed Walton, Chief Financial Officer

400 pages Year Founded: 1801

5129 Management of Hypertension
EMIS Medical Publishers
P.O. Box 270666
Fort Collins, CO 80527-0666
214-349-0077
Fax: 970-672-8606; *Toll Free:* 800-225-0694
www.emispub.com

Year Founded: 1977

5130 Manual of Hypertension
Wiley Publishing
111 River Street
Hoboken, NJ 07030-5774
201-748-6000
Fax: 201-748-6088; Toll Free: 877-762-2974
info@wiley.com
www.wiley.com

Stephen M. Smith, President and Chief Executive Of
Ellis E. Cousens, Executive Vice President, Chief
John Kritzmacher, Executive Vice President, Chief

Year Founded: 1807

5131 Reversing Hypertension: A Vital New Program to Prevent, Treat, and Reduce High Blood Pressure
Hachette Book Group USA
237 Park Avenue
New York, NY 10017
www.hachettebookgroupusa.com

Michael Pietsch, Chief Executive Officer
Reagan Arthur, SVP HBG & Publisher, Little, Bro
Sophie Cottrell, VP, Communications Director

Provides what causes blood pressure to rise and how to bring it down to normal levels. The natural therapy, light-on drugs, healthly lifestyle way to safely reduce blood pressure.

336 pages Year Founded: 1837

Newsletters, Pamphlets

5132 About High Blood Pressure
American Heart Association
7272 Greenville Avenue
Dallas, TX 75231
214-373-6300
Fax: 214-987-9361
www.americanheart.org

M Cass Wheeler, CEO

Offers information on what blood pressure is, risk factors and at risk persons.

5133 News Report
The National Organization for Rare Disorders
324 E 30th Street
New York, NY 10016-8329
212-889-3557Toll free: 800-575-9355
nathypertension@aol.com
www.nathypertension.com

Francine Rowley, Executive Director

Offers information and medical updates regarding hypertension.

Year Founded: 1977

Research Centers

5134 Mayo Clinic
Mayo Clinic
13400 E. Shea Blvd.
Scottsdale, AZ 85259

480-301-8000
Fax: 507-538-7802; Toll Free: 800-446-2279
mncg@mayo.edu
www.mayoclinic.org
TDD 507-284-9786

Marilyn Carlson Nelson, Chair
John H. Noseworthy, M.D., CEO and President
Shirley A. Weis, CAO and Vice President

Medical research and educaton. Includes the Mayo Nephrology Collaborative Group.

Year Founded: 1998

5135 National Insitutes of Health
National Institutes of Health
9000 Rockville Pike
Bethesda, MD 20892
301-496-4000
www.nih.gov
TTY: 301-402-9612

Francis S Collins, Director

Seeks knowledge to enhance health, lengthen life, and reduce burdens of illness and disability. Has a number of useful topics on high blood pressure.

Year Founded: 1887

5136 New York University: General Clinical Research Center
NYU Health Sciences Libraries
577 First Avenue
Room 117
New York, NY 10016-6402
212-263-5394
Fax: 212-263-8501
HSL_admin@nyumc.org
hsl.med.nyu.edu

Dr William Rom MPH, Director
Susan Firestone, Manager

Focuses in the areas of hypertension and studies into endocrinology.

5137 Wake Forest University: Arteriosclerosis Research Center
Department of Comparative Medicine
Magnuson Health Sciences Building
Room T-142, Box # 357190, Seattle
Washington, DC 98195-7190
206-543-8047
Fax: 206-685-3006
depts.washington.edu

H. Denny Liggitt, Chairman
Lillian Maggio-Price, Vice Chairman
Geogre Liu, Administrator

Hypertension research.

Impotence

Associations & Organizations

5138 American Association of Sexuality Educators, Counselors & Therapists
1444 I Street NW
Suite 700
Washington, DC 20005
202-449-1099
Fax: 202-216-9646
info@aasect.org
www.aasect.org

Konnie McCaffree, President

Promotes sexual health by advancing the fields of sexual therapy, counseling and education.

Year Founded: 1967

5139 American Urological Association
1000 Corporate Boulevard
Linthicum, MD 21090
410-689-3700
Fax: 410-689-3800; *Toll Free:* 866-746-4282
aua@auanet.org
www.auanet.org

William F. Gee, President
Manoj Monga, Secretary
Steven M. Schlossberg, Treasurer

Promotes the highest standards of urological care.

Year Founded: 1987; Number of Members: 20,000

5140 National Kidney Foundation
30 East 33rd Street
New York, NY 10016
Fax: 212-689-9261; *Toll Free:* 800-622-9010
info@kidney.org
www.kidney.org

Kevin Longino, CEO
Joseph Vassalotti, Chief Medical Officer
Petros Gregoriou, CFO

Provides information about diseases of the kidneys and urologic systems. Works on preventing kidney and urinary tract diseases.

5141 Urology Care Foundation
1000 Corporate Boulevard
Linthicum, MD 21090
410-689-3700
Fax: 410-689-3998; *Toll Free:* 800-828-7866
info@urologycarefoundation.org
www.urologyhealth.org

Richard A. Memo, Chair
Steven Schlossberg, Secretary/Treasurer

Advancing urologic research and education.

Books

5142 Overcoming Impotence: A Leading Urologist Tells You Everything You Need to Know
Prometheus Books
59 John Glenn Drive
Amherst, NY 14228-2197

716-691-0133
Fax: 716-691-0137; *Toll Free:* 800-421-0351
marketing@prometheusbooks.com
www.prometheusbooks.com

J Stephen Jones MD, Author

A user-friendly, emotionally supportive, and extremely informative that addresses the serious questions that men or their significant others may have about an increasingly common condition.

318 pages Year Founded: 1969

Journals, Magazines

5143 UrologyHealth extra
Urology Care Foundation
1000 Corporate Boulevard
Linthicum, MD 21090
Toll Free: 800-828-7866
www.urologyhealth.org/subscribe
www.urologyhealth.org/patient-magazine

John H. Lynch, Editor

A service of the Urology Care Foundation. Subscription is free.

Frequency: Quarterly

Websites

5144 Impotence Resource Center
Center for Reconstructive Urology
333 City Boulevard West
Suite 1240
Orange, CA 92868
714-456-2951
Fax: 714-456-7263
info@centerforreconstructiveurology.org
www.impotence.org

Joel Gelman, Director

5145 International Journal of Impotence Research
4 Crinan Street
The Macmillan Building
London, NI 9XM
207-833-4000
Fax: 207-843-4640
www.nature.com

Steven Inchcoombe, Managing Director
Philip Campbell, Editor-in-Chief
Christoph Hesselmann, Finance Director

Offers the latest research on men's and women's sexual function incuding important research related to cardiovascular disease, diabetes, menopause and vascular deficits.

Year Founded: 1869

5146 International Society for Sexual Medicine
International Society for Sexual Medicine
1520 AB Wormerveer
P.O. Box 94
Netherlands,
75 -47 -372
Fax: 75 -47 -371
www.issm.info

Chris McMahon, President
Wayne Hellstrom, President-Elect
David Casalod, Executive Director

Promotes research and exchange of knowledge for the clinical entity impotence throughout the internatioanl scientific community.

5147 National Institute of Diabetes & Digestive & Kidney Diseases
Bethesda, MD 20892-2560
301-496-3583
www.niddk.nih.gov

Griffin P. Rodgers, Director
Gregory Germino, Deputy Director

Provides information about diseases of the kidneys and urologic system to people with such afflictions and to their families, health care professionals, and the public. Answers inquiries; develops, reviews, and distributes publications; and works closely with professional and patient organizations and government agencies to coordinate research.

Incontinence

Associations & Organizations

5148 American Association of Clinical Urologists
1100 E Woodfield Road
Suite 350
Schaumburg, IL 60173
847-517-1050
Fax: 847-517-7229
info@aacuweb.org
www.aacuweb.org

Martin K. Dineen, President
Mark T. Edney, Secretary/Treasurer

AACU promotes and preserves professional autonomy. Provides advocacy, public policy, educational meetings and events.

Year Founded: 1968

5149 American Association of Kidney Patients
14440 Bruce B Downs Boulevard
Tampa, FL 33613
Toll Free: 800-749-2257
info@aakp.org
www.aakp.org

Diana Clynes, Interim Executive Director
Valerie Gonzalez, Director, Office Operations
Paul T Conway, President

Dedicated to improving the quality of life for kidney patients through education, advocacy, patient engagement and the fostering of patient communities.

Year Founded: 1969

5150 American Board of Urology
600 Peter Jefferson Parkway
Suite 150
Charlottesville, VA 22911
434-979-0059
Fax: 434-979-0266
info@abu.org
www.abu.org

Gerald H Jordan, Executive Secretary

The American Board of Urology (ABU) is organized to encourage study, improve standards, and promote competency in the practice of Urology.

Year Founded: 1934

5151 American Urological Association (AUA)
1000 Corporate Boulevard
Linthicum, MD 21090
410-689-3700
Fax: 410-689-3800; *Toll Free:* 866-746-4282
aua@auanet.org
www.auanet.org

William F. Gee, President
Manoj Monga, Secretary
Steven M. Schlossberg, Treasurer

Year Founded: 1987; Number of Members: 20,000

5152 International Foundation for FunctionalGastrointestinal Disorders
PO Box 170864
Milwaukee, WI 53217
414-964-1799
Fax: 414-964-7176
iffgd@iffgd.org
www.iffgd.org

Nancy J. Norton, President

Provides support and educational information for people affected by the various forms of functional bowel disorders, including irritable bowel syndrome, constipation, diarrhea, pain and incontinence.

Year Founded: 1991

5153 National Association for Continence
PO Box 1019
Charleston, SC 29402
Toll Free: 800-252-3337
www.nafc.org

Founded in 1982 as Help for Incontinent People, NAFC, with 130,000 members. Committed to alleviating the social stigma associated with bladder control problems. A leading source of education, advocacy, and support to the public and to the health professionals.

Year Founded: 1980

5154 Wound, Ostomy & Continence Nurses Society
1120 Route 73
Suite 200
Mt. Laurel, NJ 08054
Fax: 856-439-0525; *Toll Free:* 888-224-9626
wocn_info@wocn.org
www.wocn.org

Anna Shnayder, Executive Director

The WOCN Society is a professional nursing society which supports its members by promoting educational, clinical and research opportunities to advance the practice and guide the delivery of expert health care to individuals with wounds, ostomies and incontinence.

Year Founded: 1968

Books

5155 Female Urinary Incontinence
International Specialized Book Services
920 NE 58th Ave.
Suite 300
Portland, OR 97213-3640
503-287-3093
Fax: 503-280-8832; *Toll Free:* 800-944-6190
www.isbs.com

Rod Walker, Manager

156 pages Year Founded: 1974

5156 Managing Incontinence: A Guide to Living with Loss of Bladder Control
The Simon Foundation for Continence
PO Box 815
Wilmette, IL 60091
847-864-3913
Fax: 847-864-9758; *Toll Free:* 800-237-4666
cbgartley@simonfoundation.org
www.simonfoundation.org

Cheryle B Gartley, President
Daniel B. Hales, Attorney at Law
Nancy Norton, Executive Director

Seeks to bring the topic of incontinence out of the closet and remove the associated stigma; provides information to patients, their families, and the health care professionals who provide patient care.

80+ pages Year Founded: 1983

Directories

5157 The Official Patient's Sourcebook on Female Urinary Incontinence
ICON Group International
9606 Tierra Grande St.
Suite 205
San Diego, CA 92126
Fax: 858-635-9414
orders@icongroupbooks.com
www.icongrouponline.com

James N Parker MD, Editor
Philip M Parker PhD, Editor

A comprehensive manual for anyone interested in self-directed research on fully referenced with ample Internet listings and glossary. This book has ben created for patients who have decided to make education and research an integral part of the treatment process.

112 pages

Websites

5158 Simon Foundation for Continence
PO Box 815
Wilmette, IL 60091
847-864-3913
Fax: 847-864-9758; *Toll Free:* 800-237-4666
www.simonfoundation.org

Cheryl Gartley, President

Helps thousands of people to find cures and management techniques for incontinence. The mission of this Foundation is to bring the topic out of the closet, remove the stigma and educate both medical professionals and sufferers about cure, treatment and management techniques. The Foundation also operates a Helpline at the above numbers.

Year Founded: 1983

Parkinson's Disease

Associations & Organizations

5159 American Parkinson Disease Association
135 Parkinson Avenue
Staten Island, NY 10305
718-981-8001
Fax: 718-981-4399; Toll Free: 800-223-2732
apda@apdaparkinson.org
www.apdaparkinson.org

Leslie A. Chambers, President & CEO

Works to find the cure for Parkinson's disease and to alleviate the suffering of its victims by subsidizing information and referral centers and providing funds for research. Offers counseling services to patients and their families. Maintains 43 information and referral centers. Conducts symposia.

5160 American Parkinson Disease Association:Arizona
5905 E Pima Street
Tucson, AZ 85712
520-326-5400
www.apdaarizona.org

Michele Grise, Program Coordinator

5161 Baylor College of Medicine Parkinson's Disease Center & Movement Disorders Clinic
McNair Campus
7200 Cambridge Street, 9th Floor, Suite 9A
Houston, TX 77030
713-798-2273
pdcmdc@bcm.edu
www.bcm.edu/healthcare/care-centers

5162 Dallas Area Parkinsonism Society
6370 LBJ Freeway
Suite 170
Dallas, TX 75240-6400
972-620-7600
daps.us

Michael L. Miles, Executive Director

5163 Duke Neurological Disorders Clinic
Duke Health Center at Morreene Road
932 Morreene Road
Durham, NC 27705
919-668-7600
www.dukemedicine.org/treatments

A National Parkinson's Foundation Center of Excellence.

5164 Hawai'i Parkinson Association
PO Box 1312
Kailua, HI 96734
Toll Free: 808-528-0935
info@parkinsonshawaii.org
www.parkinsonshawaii.org

Kevin Lockette, President
Stephanie Cook, Secretary
Dennis Ideta, Treasurer
Year Founded: 1996

5165 Houston Area Parkinson Society
2700 Southwest Freeway
Suite 296
Houston, TX 77098
713-626-7114
Fax: 713-521-3964
www.hapsonline.org

Anne Thobae, Executive Director

5166 Johns Hopkins Parkinson's Disease & Movement Disorders Center
601 N Caroline Street
Suite 5064
Baltimore, MD 21287
410-502-0133
www.hopkinsmedicine.org

Excellence in treating, researching and teaching about movement disorders.

Year Founded: 1889

5167 Maine Parkinson Society
359 Perry Road
Bangor, ME 04401
207-992-9978
Fax: 207-262-9908; Toll Free: 800-832-4116
info@maineparkinsonsociety.org
www.maineparkinsonsociety.org

Gary Cole, President
Morgan Knox, Secretary
Eric Vogell, Treasurer

Spreading awareness and improving quality of life for people in Maine with Parkinson's.

5168 Massachusetts General Hospital MovementDisorders Unit
Massachusetts General Hospital, WACC 8-830
55 Fruit Street
Boston, MA 02114
Toll Free: 855-644-6387
www.massgeneral.org/neurology/services

Recognized as a Center of Excellence by the National Parkinson Foundation, Mass General treats patients from around the world for movement disorders.

Year Founded: 1982

5169 Michigan Parkinson Foundation
30400 Telegraph Road
Suite 150
Bingham Farms, MI 48025
248-433-1011
Fax: 248-433-1150; Toll Free: 800-852-9781
info@parkinsonsmi.org
www.parkinsonsmi.org

Deborah M. Orloff, CEO
Year Founded: 1983

5170 Mount Sinai Beth Israel Department of Neurology
Mirken Dept. of Neurology, Phillips Ambulatory Care Center
10 Union Square E, Suite 5D
New York, NY 10003
212-844-8888Toll free: 212-844-8481
www.wehealny.org/services/bi_neurology

Susan B. Bressman, Chief

5171 National Parkinson Foundation
200 SE 1st Street
Suite 800
Miami, FL 33131
Fax: 305-537-9901; *Toll Free:* 800-473-4636
contact@parkinson.org
www.parkinson.org

Paul Blom, Interim CEO

A nonprofit organization dedicated to research, diagnosis, treatment and care for men and women suffering from Parkinson's and other related neurological diseases. The Foundation also supports the Bob Hope research and rehabilitation center, which is the leading institute of its kind in the world, donating their time to Parkinson's research.

Year Founded: 1957

5172 National Parkinson Foundation: Central Savannah River Area
2406 Seminole Road
Augusta, GA 30904
706-364-1662Toll free: 800-473-4636
info@parkinsoncsra.org
www.parkinsoncsra.org

C.J. Mitchell, President

5173 National Parkinson Foundation: Greater Rochester
PO Box 23204
Rochester, NY 14692
585-234-5355Toll free: 800-473-4636
www.npfgreaterrochester.org

Dennis Whitney, President

5174 National Parkinson Foundation: Heartland
8900 State Line Road
Suite 320
Leawood, KS 66206
913-341-8828
Fax: 885-341-8885; *Toll Free:* 800-473-4636
info@parkinsonheartland.org
www.parkinsonheartland.org

Jane Ann Gorsky, Executive Director

Affiliate of the National Parkinson Foundation.

5175 National Parkinson Foundation: Minnesota
5905 Garden Valley Road
Suite 237
Minneapolis, MN 55422
763-545-1272Toll free: 800-473-4636
info@parkinsonmn.org
www.parkinsonmn.org

Julie Steen, Executive Director
Year Founded: 1995

5176 National Parkinson Foundation: Ohio
2800 Corporate Exchange Drive
Suite 265
Columbus, OH 43231
614-890-1901Toll free: 866-920-6673
comments@centralohioparkinson.org
www.centralohioparkinson.org

Bryan Alltop, Chair

5177 National Parkinson Foundation: South Florida
200 SE 1st Street
Suite 800
Miami, FL 33131
Toll Free: 800-473-4636
info@npfsouthflorida.org
www.npfsouthflorida.org

5178 National Parkinson Foundation: Western New York
300 International Drive
Suite 224
Williamsville, NY 14221
716-449-3795Toll free: 800-473-4636
cjamele@npfwny.org
www.npfwny.org

Christopher Jamele, Executive Director

5179 Northwest Parkinson's Foundation
7525 SE 24th Street
Suite 300
Mercer Island, WA 98040
206-748-9481Toll free: 877-980-7500
info@nwpf.org
nwpf.org

Steve Wright, Executive Director

Improving the quality of life for the Northwest Parkinson's disease community.

Year Founded: 1998

5180 Northwestern University Parkinson's Disease & Movement Disorders Center
710 N Lake Shore Drive
11th Floor
Chicago, IL 60611
312-503-4397
www.parkinsons.northwestern.edu

Tanya Simuni, Director

Recognized by the National Parkinson Foundation as a Center for Excellence, Northwestern University Parkinson's Disease and Movement Disorders Center conducts research to extend the knowledge and treatment of PD and other movement disorders.

5181 Parkinson Association of Northern California
1750 Prairie City Road
#130-220
Folsom, CA 95630
916-357-6641
panc@parkinsonsacramento.org
www.parkinsonsacramento.org

Nancy Kretz, President
Christine Shade, Secretary
Marianne Oliphant, Treasurer

5182 Parkinson Association of Southwest Florida
1048 Goodlette-Frank Road
Suite 201
Naples, FL 34102
239-417-3465
Fax: 239-417-3469
office@pasfi.org
www.pasfi.org

Jacqueline Urso, CEO

The Parkinson Association of Southwest Flordia is a not-for-profit organization. The mission is to promote quality of life for persons with Parkinson's Disease and their care partners. This is accomplished by providing educational, physical and social programs. The organization also provides education for the community regarding Parkinson's Disease and its effects.

5183 Parkinson Association of the Carolinas

2101 Sardis Road N
Suite 102, Box 15
Charlotte, NC 28227
704-248-3722Toll free: 866-903-7275
pac@parkinsonassociation.org
www.parkinsonassociation.org

Ann Marie Obrikat, Interim Executive Director

The Parkinson Association of the Carolinas ("PAC") was established in 2002 to serve as a resource for individuals and their families living in the Carolinas who are affected by Parkinson's disease. PAC seeks to empower these individuals and families through education, outreach and direct support.

Year Founded: 2002

5184 Parkinson Association of the Rockies

1325 South Colorado Boulevard
Suite 204B
Denver, CO 80222
303-830-1839
www.parkinsonrockies.org

Cheryl Siefert, Executive Director

5185 Parkinson Foundation of Oklahoma

720 W Wilshire Boulevard
Suite 109
Oklahoma City, OK 73116
405-810-0695
info@parkinsonoklahoma.com
parkinsonoklahoma.com

Bruce McIntyre, Executive Director
Jim Keating, Founder
Jerry Gill, President

5186 Parkinson Foundation of Western Pennsylvania

575 Lincoln Avenue
Pittsburgh, PA 15202
412-837-2542
info@pfwpa.org
pfwpa.org

Barbara Farrell, Executive Director
Year Founded: 1995

5187 Parkinson's Action Network

1025 Vermont Avenue NW
Suite 1120
Washington, DC 20005
Toll Free: 800-850-4726
parkinsonsaction.org

Ted Thompson, President & CEO

PAN works on a wide range of policy issues in order to serve the Parkinson's community.

5188 Parkinson's Association of West Michigan

260 Jefferson Avenue SE
Suite 210
Grand Rapids, MI 49503
616-954-8077
info@parkinsonswm.org
www.parkinsonswm.org

Brian Toronyi, President
Donald Michaud, Treasurer
Kim Cousineau, Secretary

The Mission of the Parkinson's Association of West Michigan (PAWM) is to provide the best information on opportunities, treatment, research, and care to people with Parkinson's and their families. PAWM is a source for Parkinson's information. Our meetings feature programs on physical and speech therapy, relaxation training, and other measures which are important in learning to live with Parkinson's. PAWM is constantly searching for and providing current information sources pertaining to research, treatment, and topics that would be of interest to people with Parkinson's, their families, and their caretakers.

Year Founded: 2009

5189 Parkinson's Association: Orange County

8555 Aero Drive
Suite 308
San Diego, CA 92123
858-273-6763
Fax: 858-273-6764; Toll Free: 877-737-7576
parkinsonsassociation.org

Lisa Fine, Executive Director

5190 Parkinson's Disease Foundation

1359 Broadway
Suite 1509
New York, NY 10018
212-923-4700
Fax: 212-923-4778; Toll Free: 800-457-6676
www.pdf.org

Robin Anthony Elliott, President
Year Founded: 1957

5191 Parkinson's Resources of Oregon

8880 SW Nimbus Avenue
Suite B
Beaverton, OR 97008
Fax: 503-594-0547; Toll Free: 800-426-6806
info@parkinsonsresources.org
www.parkinsonsresources.org

Holly Chaimov, Executive Director

Nationally recognized non-profit dedicated to improving the quality of life for people with Parkinson's in the Pacific Northwest.

Year Founded: 1980

5192 The Parkinson Alliance

PO Box 308
Kingston, NJ 08528-0308
609-688-0870
Fax: 609-688-0875; Toll Free: 800-579-8440
www.parkinsonalliance.org

Martin Tuchman, Chairman
Margaret Tuchman, President
Carol J. Walton, CEO

Raising awareness and funds for Parkinson's research.

Year Founded: 1999

5193 The Parkinson Council
111 Presidential Boulevard
Suite 141
Bala Cynwyd, PA 19004-1023
610-668-4292
Fax: 610-668-4275
info@theparkinsoncouncil.org
theparkinsoncouncil.org

Wendy R. Lewis, Executive Director

5194 The Parkinson Disease & Movement Disorders Center
Penn Medicine Neuroscience Center, Pennsylvania Hospital
330 S 9th Street, 3rd Floor
Philadelphia, PA 19107
www.pennmedicine.org/neurology

The Penn Parkinson Disease & Movement Disorders Center is recognized as a Center of Excellence by the National Parkinson Foundation.

5195 The Vanderbilt Clinic
1301 Medical Center Drive
Suite 3930
Nashville, TN 37232
615-936-0060
Fax: 615-343-2008
www.vanderbilthealth.com

P. David Charles, Director

5196 The Wisconsin Parkinson Association
2819 W Highland Avenue
Milwaukee, WI 53208
Fax: 414-312-6990; *Toll Free:* 800-972-5455
mail@wiparkinson.org
www.wiparkinson.org

Kate McDonald, President
Robert Norman, Secretary
Richard Schumann, Treasurer

The Wisconsin Parkinson Association is a regional non-profit organization assisting people who are affected by Parkinson's disease. As a Center of Excellence with the National Parkinson Foundation, the Regional Parkinson Center is a part of a nationwide effort to provide information and resources about Parkinson's Disease, to enhance public education and awareness of the disease and to support research for a cure.

Year Founded: 1984

Books

5197 100 Questions & Answers About Parkinson's Disease
Jones and Bartlett Publishers
5 Wall Street
Burlington, MA 01803
978-443-5000
Fax: 978-443-8000; *Toll Free:* 800-832-0034
info@jblearning.com
www.jbpub.com

Abraham Lieberman, Author
Marcia McCall, Author

The only text to provide the doctor and patient view, gives you authoritative, practical answers to your questions about treatment options, quality of life, sources of support, and more.

238 pages Year Founded: 1983

5198 Coping with Parkinson's Disease
American Parkinson Disease Association
135 Parkinson Avenue
Suite 4b
Staten Island, NY 10305
718-981-8001
Fax: 718-981-4399; *Toll Free:* 800-223-2732
apda@apdaparkinson.org
www.apdaparkinson.org

Fred Greene, Chairman
Patrick McDermott, Vice Chairman
Leslie A. Chambers, President & CEO

88 pages

5199 Parkinson's Disease & Movement Disorders
Lippincott Williams & Wilkins
351 W Camden Street
Baltimore, MD 21201-7912
410-949-8000
Fax: 410-528-4452; *Toll Free:* 800-638-3030
www.lww.com

640 pages Year Founded: 1998

5200 Parkinson's Disease Handbook
National Parkinson Foundation
200 SE 1st Street
Suite 800
Miami, FL 33131
305-243-6666
Fax: 305-537-9901; *Toll Free:* 800-473-4636
contact@parkinson.org
www.parkinson.org

Bernerd J. Fogel, Chairman
Joyce Oberdorf, President & CEO
Amy Gray, Vice President

A guide for patients and their families regarding the illness of Parkinson's.

Year Founded: 1957

5201 Parkinson's Disease for Dummies
For Dummies
10475 Crosspoint Boulevard
Indianapolis, IN 46256
Fax: 800-597-3299; *Toll Free:* 877-762-2974
www.dummies.com

Michele Tagliati MD, Author
Gary Guten MD, Author
Jo Horne

Discover how to keep a positive attitude and lead an active, productive life as this user-friendly, guide pilots you through the important steps toward taking charge of your condition. Provides proven coping skills, first-hand advice, and practical tools, such as worksheets to assess care options, questions to ask doctors, and current listing of care providers.

384 pages Year Founded: 1991

5202 Parkinson's Disease: 300 Tips for Making Life Easier
Demos Medical Publishing
11 West 42nd Street
15th Floor
New York, NY 10036
212-683-0072
support@demosmedical.com
www.demosmedical.com

Shelley Peterman Schwartz, Author

Helps readers lead a remarkably unlimited life. Filled with tips, techniques, and shortcuts readers will learn basic lessons for conserving time and energy, enabling them to do more of the things they want to do.

128 pages Year Founded: 1989

5203 Parkinson's Disease: A Complete Guide for Patients and Families
Johns Hopkins University Press
2715 North Charles Street
Balitmore, MD 21218-4363
410-516-6900
Fax: 410-516-6968
webmaster@jhupress.jhu.edu
www.press.jhu.edu

Kathleen Keane, Director
Erik. A. Smist, Director, Finance and Administra
Timothy D. Fuller, Chief Information Officer

Provides crucial information for managing this complex condition, including details on the use of medication, diet, exercise, complementary therapies an d surgery.

296 pages Year Founded: 1878

5204 The First Year: Parkinson's Disease: An Essential Guide for the Newly Diagnosed
Perseus Books Group
250 West 57th St.
15th Floor
New York, NY 10017
212-340-8100
special.markets@perseusbooks.com
www.perseusbooksgroup.com

David Steinberger, President & CEO
Jackie Christensen, Author

Provides guidance for the newly diagnosed step by step through their first year with Parkinson's. Also provides crucial information about the nature of the disease, treatment options, diet, exercise, charts and tables, social concerns, emotional issues, networking with others, and more.

5205 Understanding Parkinson's Disease: A Personal and Professional View
Greenwood Publishing Group
88 Post Road West
P.O. Box 5007
Westport, CT 06881-5007
203-226-3571
Fax: 203-222-1502
greenwood.enquiries@harcourt.co.uk
www.harcourt.com

Richard B Rosenbaum, Author

Topics covered include challenges of correct diagnosis, variations in prognosis, investigations of causes including exciting progress in possible toxins and genetic factors that play a role, and different treatment options including natural remedies as well as new drugs for symptom treatment.

364 pages Year Founded: 1949

Newsletters, Pamphlets

5206 American Parkinson Disease Association Newsletter
American Parkinson Disease Association
135 Parkinson Avenue
Suite 4b
Staten Island, NY 10305-1945
718-981-8001
Fax: 718-981-4399; *Toll Free:* 800-223-2732
apda@apdaparkinson.org
www.apdaparkinson.org

Fred Greene, Chairman
Patrick McDermott, Vice Chairman
Leslie A. Chambers, President & CEO

Offers information on the association activities and events, convention and legislative information, medical updates and research reports for the Parkinson's patient and their families.

5207 Basic Information About Parkinson's Disease
American Parkinson Disease Association
135 Parkinson Avenue
Suite 4b
Staten Island, NY 10305-1945
718-981-8001
Fax: 718-981-4399; *Toll Free:* 800-223-2732
apda@apdaparkinson.org
www.apdaparkinson.org

Fred Greene, Chairman
Patrick McDermott, Vice Chairman
Leslie A. Chambers, President & CEO

Offers information on the illness, incidence, treatments, education and support for both patients and professionals.

5208 Equipment and Suggestions for Persons with Parkinson's Disease
American Parkinson Disease Association
135 Parkinson Avenue
Suite 4b
Staten Island, NY 10305-1945
718-981-8001
Fax: 718-981-4399; *Toll Free:* 800-223-2732
apda@apdaparkinson.org
www.apdaparkinson.org

Fred Greene, Chairman
Patrick McDermott, Vice Chairman
Leslie A. Chambers, President & CEO

19 pages

5209 Fighting Back Against PD: One Women's Story
National Parkinson Foundation
200 SE 1st Street
Suite 800
Miami, FL 33131
305-547-6666
Fax: 305-537-9901; *Toll Free:* 800-473-4636
contact@parkinson.org
www.parkinson.org

Bernerd J. Fogel, Chairman
Joyce Oberdorf, President & CEO
Amy Gray, Vice President

One woman's battle against Parkinson's disease.

Year Founded: 1957

5210 Good Nutrition in Parkinson's Disease
American Parkinson Disease Association
135 Parkinson Avenue
Suite 4b
Staten Island, NY 10305-1945
718-981-8001
Fax: 718-981-4399; *Toll Free:* 800-223-2732
apda@apdaparkinson.org
www.apdaparkinson.org

Fred Greene, Chairman
Patrick McDermott, Vice Chairman
Leslie A. Chambers, President & CEO

Offers information on diet, nutrients, proteins and recipes for people with Parkinson's disease.

5211 How to Start a Parkinson's Disease Support Group
American Parkinson Disease Association
135 Parkinson Avenue
Suite 4b
Staten Island, NY 10305-1945
718-981-8001
Fax: 718-981-4399; *Toll Free:* 800-223-2732
apda@apdaparkinson.org
www.apdaparkinson.org

Fred Greene, Chairman
Patrick McDermott, Vice Chairman
Leslie A. Chambers, President & CEO

42 pages

5212 Parkinson Handbook: A Guide for Patients and Their Families
National Parkinson Foundation
200 SE 1st Street
Suite 800
Miami, FL 33131
305-547-6666
Fax: 305-537-9901; *Toll Free:* 800-473-4636
contact@parkinson.org
www.parkinson.org

Bernerd J. Fogel, Chairman
Joyce Oberdorf, President & CEO
Amy Gray, Vice President

Offers informative, up-to-date information on exercises, hobbies, treatments, speech impairments and psychological aspects.

Year Founded: 1957

5213 Parkinson Report
National Parkinson Foundation
200 SE 1st Street
Suite 800
Miami, FL 33131
305-547-6666
Fax: 305-537-9901; *Toll Free:* 800-473-4636
contact@parkinson.org
www.parkinson.org

Bernerd J. Fogel, Chairman
Joyce Oberdorf, President & CEO
Amy Gray, Vice President

Offers association news and events, conference and symposia news, legislative and medical updates, research reports and more for the Parkinson's patient, their families and the general public.

Year Founded: 1957

5214 Parkinson's Disease Foundation Newsletter
Parkinson's Disease Foundation
1359 Broadway
Suite 1509
New York, NY 10018
212-923-4700
Fax: 212-923-4778; *Toll Free:* 800-457-6676
info@pdf.org
www.pdf.org

Howard D. Morgan, Chairman
Constance Woodruff Atwell, Vice Chairman
Robin Anthony Elliott, President

Provides information on Parkinson's Disease Foundation events, news stories of research findings, and technical advances in the field of patient care.

Year Founded: 1957

5215 Parkinson's Disease Handbook
American Parkinson Disease Association
135 Parkinson Avenue
Suite 4b
Staten Island, NY 10305-1945
718-981-8001
Fax: 718-981-4399; *Toll Free:* 800-223-2732
apda@apdaparkinson.org
www.apdaparkinson.org

Fred Greene, Chairman
Patrick McDermott, Vice Chairman
Leslie A. Chambers, President & CEO

40 pages

5216 Parkinson's Patient: What You and Your Family Should Know
National Parkinson Foundation
200 SE 1st Street
Suite 800
Miami, FL 33131
305-547-6666
Fax: 305-537-9901; *Toll Free:* 800-473-4636
contact@parkinson.org
www.parkinson.org

Bernerd J. Fogel, Chairman
Joyce Oberdorf, President & CEO
Amy Gray, Vice President

Offers a brief overview of Parkinson's Disease causes, symptoms and treatments as well as offering an insight into statistical information on the illness.

Year Founded: 1957

5217 Parkinsons Report
National Parkinson Foundation
200 SE 1st Street
Suite 800
Miami, FL 33131
305-547-6666
Fax: 305-537-9901; *Toll Free:* 800-473-4636

contact@parkinson.org
www.parkinson.org

Bernerd J. Fogel, Chairman
Joyce Oberdorf, President & CEO
Amy Gray, Vice President

Articles, reports and news on Parkinson's disease and the activities of the National Parkinson Foundation.

32 pages Frequency: Quarterly Year Founded: 1957

5218 Patient Perspectives on Parkinson's
National Parkinson Foundation
200 SE 1st Street
Suite 800
Miami, FL 33131
305-547-6666
Fax: 305-537-9901; *Toll Free:* 800-473-4636
contact@parkinson.org
www.parkinson.org

Bernerd J. Fogel, Chairman
Joyce Oberdorf, President & CEO
Amy Gray, Vice President

Offers a brief overview of Parkinson's disease, the onset of the illness, depression, sexuality, exercise, sleep and nutrition information for daily living.

45 pages Year Founded: 1957

5219 Practical Pointers for Parkinson Patients
National Parkinson Foundation
200 SE 1st Street
Suite 800
Miami, FL 33131
305-547-6666
Fax: 305-537-9901; *Toll Free:* 800-473-4636
contact@parkinson.org
www.parkinson.org

Bernerd J. Fogel, Chairman
Joyce Oberdorf, President & CEO
Amy Gray, Vice President

Year Founded: 1957

5220 Speech & Swallowing Problems for
Parkinsonians
National Parkinson Foundation
200 SE 1st Street
Suite 800
Miami, FL 33131
305-547-6666
Fax: 305-537-9901; *Toll Free:* 800-473-4636
contact@parkinson.org
www.parkinson.org

Bernerd J. Fogel, Chairman
Joyce Oberdorf, President & CEO
Amy Gray, Vice President

Year Founded: 1957

5221 Speech Problems & Swallowing Problems In
Parkinson's Disease
American Parkinson Disease Association
135 Parkinson Avenue
Suite 4b
Staten Island, NY 10305-1945
718-981-8001
Fax: 718-981-4399; *Toll Free:* 800-223-2732
apda@apdaparkinson.org
www.apdaparkinson.org

Fred Greene, Chairman
Patrick McDermott, Vice Chairman
Leslie A. Chambers, President & CEO

Offers information on speech problems, swallowing problems, hearing impairments and facial mobility for the person with Parkinson's.

5222 Suggested Exercise Program for People with
Parkinson's Disease
American Parkinson Disease Association
135 Parkinson Avenue
Suite 4b
Staten Island, NY 10305-1945
718-981-8001
Fax: 718-981-4399; *Toll Free:* 800-223-2732
apda@apdaparkinson.org
www.apdaparkinson.org

Fred Greene, Chairman
Patrick McDermott, Vice Chairman
Leslie A. Chambers, President & CEO

Exercise program pamphlet with full illustrations explaining each exercise.

23 pages

5223 Treatment of Parkinson's Disease with
Carbidopa-Levodopa
National Parkinson Foundation
200 SE 1st Street
Suite 800
Miami, FL 33131
305-547-6666
Fax: 305-537-9901; *Toll Free:* 800-473-4636
contact@parkinson.org
www.parkinson.org

Bernerd J. Fogel, Chairman
Joyce Oberdorf, President & CEO
Amy Gray, Vice President

Offers information on treating Parkinson's Disease.

Year Founded: 1957

Research Centers

5224 California Institute for Medical Research
California Institute for Medical Research
2260 Clove Drive
San Jose, CA 95128-2637
408-998-4554
Fax: 408-998-2723
www.cimr.org

David Stevens, President
John Hotson, Vice President/Treasurer
Carol Kemper, Secretary

Medical research, including infectious diseases, stroke and cancer specializing in Parkinson's Disease related studies.

Year Founded: 1963

5225 Michael J. Fox Foundation for Parkinson's
Research
Grand Central Station
PO Box 4777
New York, NY 10163-4777
Toll Free: 800-708-7644
www.michaeljfox.org

Todd Sherer, CEO
Deborah W. Brooks, Co-Founder & Exec. Vice Chairman
Joanne Martz, Chief Financial & Admin. Officer

The largest nonprofit funder of Parkinson's research world-wide.
Year Founded: 2000

5226 Mulligan Foundation
Mulligan Foundation
10663 Nine Mile Road
Whitmore Lake, MI 48189-9130
734-449-8442
Fax: 734-449-4931
www.frostbyte.com/mulligan

5227 National Institute of Neurological Disorders & Stroke National Institute of Health / DHHS
NIH Neurological Institute
PO Box 5801
Bethesda, MD 20824-5801
301-496-5751
Fax: 301-402-2186; *Toll Free:* 800-352-9424
www.ninds.nih.gov

Story Landis, PhD, Director
Walter J. Koroshetz, Deputy Director
Caroline Lewis, Executive Officer

Mission: to reduce the burden of neurological disease.
Year Founded: 1950

5228 New York College of Osteopathic Medicine
New York Institute of Technology
1855 Broadway
61st Street
Manhattan, NY 10023-7692
212-261-1500 Toll free: 800-345-6948
asknyit@nyit.edu
www.nyit.edu

Edward Guiliano, President

Information and referral research center for Parkinson's disease patients and their families.
Year Founded: 1955

5229 Oregon Health Sciences University
Oregon Health &Science Unoversity
3181 SW Sam Jackson Park Road
Portland, OR 97239-3098
503-494-8311
www.ohsu.edu

Joe Robertson, President
James Morgan, Executive Director

Information and referral research center for Parkinson's disease patients and their families.
Year Founded: 2001

5230 Parkinson's Disease Foundation
Presbyterian Medical Center
710 W 168th Street
New York, NY 10032-3726
212-923-4700
Fax: 212-923-4778; *Toll Free:* 800-789-7366
www.pennmedicine.org

Robin Elliott, Executive Director

Raises funds for support of scientific research into causes, prevention, and cure of Parkinson's disease. Supports its

own laboratories for research in Parkinsonism. Prepares and distributes information on patient care and rehabilitation including list of clinics where treatment is available, and a list of patient selfhelp groups. Supports a brain bank to permit anatomical and chemical studies. Sponsors scientific symposia. Offers patient and family counseling and advocacy services. Maintains research advisory board. Sponsors summer fellowship program for medical students and undergraduate.
Year Founded: 1765

5231 Parkinson's Institute & Clinical Center
675 Almanor Avenue
Sunnyvale, CA 94085-2934
408-734-2800
Fax: 408-734-8455; *Toll Free:* 800-655-2273
www.thepi.org

Carrolee Barlow, Chief Executive Director

Research into new treatment options while providing comprehensive patient care.
Year Founded: 1988

5232 Presbyterian Hospital of Dallas
Texas Health Resources
8200 Walnut Hill Lane
Dallas, TX 75231-4402
214-345-6789
Fax: 214-345-2019
lindagoelzer@texashealth.org
www.texashealth.org

Britt R. Berrett, President
Cole Edmonson, Chief Nursing Officer
Aurora Estevez, Chief Medical Officer

Information and referral research center for Parkinson's disease patients and their families.
Year Founded: 1966

5233 Robert Wood Johnson University Hospital
Robert Wood Johnson University Hospital
1 Robert Wood Johnson Place
New Brunswick, NJ 08901-1966
732-828-3000
www.rwjuh.edu

Stephen K. Jones, President & CEO

Information and referral research center for Parkinson's disease patients and their families.
Year Founded: 1884

5234 San Diego Information & Referral Center
Parkinson's Association of San Diego
8555 Aero Drive
Suite 308
San Diego, CA 92123-1745
858-273-6763
Fax: 858-273-6764; *Toll Free:* 877-737-7576
contactus@parkinsonsassociation.org
www.parkinsonsassociation.org

Rick Brydges, President
David R. Higgins, Vice President
Jerry Henberger, Executive Director

Information and referral research center for Parkinson's disease patients and their families.

5235 Texas Tech University: Tarbox Parkinson's Disease Institute
Texas Tech Physicians Medical Pavilion
3601 4th Street
Lubbock, TX 79430
806-743-2669
patientservices@ttuhsc.edu
www.texastechphysicians.com

Steven L. Berk, Dean
Brent Magers, Chief Executive Officer

5236 UCSD Movement Disorder Center
UC San Diego Health
200 West Arbor Drive
San Diego, CA 92103
858-657-8540
health.ucsd.edu/specialties/neuro

Irene Litvan, Director

A National Parkinson's Foundation Center of Excellence.

5237 UCSF Parkinson's Disease Clinic & Research Center
University of California, San Francisco
505 Parnassus Avenue, Room 798-M, Box 0114
San Francisco, CA 94143-0114
415-476-9276
Fax: 415-476-3289
pdcenter.neurology.ucsf.edu

Michael J. Aminoff, Director

One of the leading neuroscience centers in the United States and a National Parkinson's Foundation Center of Excellence.

5238 University of Texas HSC at San Antonio
UT Health Center
7703 Floyd Curl Drive
San Antonio, TX 78229-3901
210-567-7000
uthscsa.edu

W A J Van Heuven, MD
Mary Etlinger DeLay, Chief of Staff, Office of the Pr
Nancy Arispe, Senior Executive Director for Co

Information and referral research center for Parkinson's disease patients and their families.

5239 Washington University Medical Center
The George Washington University
2300 Eye Street NW
Washington, DC 20037-2336
202-994-2715
Fax: 202-994-0465
smhsnews@gwu.edu
smhs.gwu.edu

Jeffrey S. Akman, M.D., Dean
Anne Banner, Executive Director
Michael Acadia, Programmer / Systems Administrat

Information and referral research center for Parkinson's disease patients and their families.

5240 William T Gossett Parkinson's Disease Center
Henry Ford Hospital Department of Neurology
2799 W Grand Boulevard
Detroit, MI 48202-2608
313-972-1693Toll free: 800-436-7936
www.henryford.com

Robert G. Riney, President and Chief Operating Of
Bill Alvin, Executive Vice President
Nancy M. Schlichting, Chief Executive Officer
Year Founded: 1997

Stroke

Associations & Organizations

5241 American Brain Foundation
201 Chicago Avenue
Minneapolis, MN 55415
americanbrainfoundation.org

The research foundation of the American Academy of Neurology.

5242 American Stroke Association
7272 Greenville Avenue
Dallas, TX 75231
Toll Free: 888-478-7653
www.strokeassociation.org

Building healthier lives free of cardiovascular diseases and stroke.

Year Founded: 1997

5243 Internet Stroke Center
UT Southwestern Medical Center
5323 Harry Hines Boulevard
Dallas, TX 75390
214-648-3111
info@strokecenter.org
www.strokecenter.org

Mark Goldberg, Director
Abner X Figueroa, Information Services
Julie Kirchem, Web Content Producer

To advance understanding of stroke research and clinical care.

5244 National Institute of Neurological Disorders & Stroke
PO Box 5801
Bethesda, MD 20824
301-496-5751 Toll free: 800-352-9424
www.ninds.nih.gov

Walter J. Koroshetz, Director

Offers advice on treatments and care of individual patients with neurological disorders and stroke.

5245 National Rehabilitation Information Center
8400 Corporate Drive
Suite 500
Landover, MD 20785
Toll Free: 800-346-2742
www.naric.com

Mark X. Odum, Project Director

Offers information about coping with stroke, rehabilitation research and disability programs.

5246 National Stroke Association
9707 E Easter Lane
Suite B
Centennial, CO 80112
Toll Free: 800-787-6537
info@stroke.org
www.stroke.org

Matt Lopez, CEO
Sharon Januchowksi, EVP

A national organization whose sole purpose is to reduce the incidence and impact of stroke by changing the way stroke is viewed and treated. NSA offers public, patient, and professional education.

Year Founded: 1984

5247 The American Stroke Foundation
5916 Dearborn Street
Mission, KS 66202
913-649-1776
americanstroke.org

Jane Savidge, Executive Director

Offering post-rehabilitation classes and wellness programs for stroke survivors.

Books

5248 Adaptive Resources Guide
National Stroke Association
9707 E Easter Lane
Suite B
Centennial, CO 80112-3754
303-649-9299
Fax: 303-649-1328; *Toll Free:* 800-787-6537
info@stroke.org
www.stroke.org

Michael D. Walker, Chairman
George Davis, Vice Chairman
James Baranski, Chief Executive Officer

A guide for stroke survivors listing adaptive resources, products, equipment, manufacturers, clothing, books and tapes.

Year Founded: 1984

5249 After a Stroke: 300 Tips to Making Life Easier
Demos Medical Publishing
11 West 42nd Street
15th Floor
New York, NY 10036
212-683-0072
support@demosmedical.com
www.demosmedical.com

Shelley Peterman Schwartz, Author

Stroke survivor and nurse Hutton gives practical tips for going through the recovery process as patient or caregiver.

Year Founded: 1989

5250 Can You Hear the Clapping of One Hand?
Learning to Live with a Stroke
Jason Aronson
PO Box 15556
NL-1001 NB
Amsterdam, NT 17405-7100
120-623-3103
Fax: 120-638-3066; *Toll Free:* 800-782-0015
mail@aronson.com
www.aronson.com

Robert D. Aronson, Director
Lisa Rooimans, Assistant
Eveline Brouwers, Project Manager

120 pages Year Founded: 1881

5251 Clinical Program for Evaluating and Managing Stroke-at-Risk Patients
National Stroke Association
9707 E Easter Lane
Suite B
Centennial, CO 80112-3754
303-649-9299
Fax: 303-649-1328; *Toll Free:* 800-787-6537
info@stroke.org
www.stroke.org

Michael D. Walker, Chairman
George Davis, Vice Chairman
James Baranski, Chief Executive Officer

Includes stroke appraisal forms and instructions for selecting patients for appraisal, evaluating stroke risk, counseling patients and motivating and reinforcing positive behavior.

Year Founded: 1984

5252 Discovery Circles
National Stroke Association
9707 E Easter Lane
Suite B
Centennial, CO 80112-3754
303-649-9299
Fax: 303-649-1328; *Toll Free:* 800-787-6537
info@stroke.org
www.stroke.org

Michael D. Walker, Chairman
George Davis, Vice Chairman
James Baranski, Chief Executive Officer

NSA's guide to organizing and facilitating stroke support groups. This detailed manual describes the support group structure and the facilitator's role.

213 pages Year Founded: 1984

5253 Helpmates
National Stroke Association
9707 E Easter Lane
Suite B
Centennial, CO 80112-3754
303-649-9299
Fax: 303-649-1328; *Toll Free:* 800-787-6537
info@stroke.org
www.stroke.org

Michael D. Walker, Chairman
George Davis, Vice Chairman
James Baranski, Chief Executive Officer

Offers advice, guidance and support for survivors and caregivers.

167 pages Year Founded: 1984

5254 Introduction to Stroke
Idyll Arbor
39129 264th Ave SE
Enumclaw, WA 98022
360-825-7797
Fax: 360-825-5670
sales@idyllarbor.com
www.idyllarbor.com

This book contains the basic information about patients with strokes that a professional needs to provide good, quality services. It is especially appropriate for someone who is just starting to work with patients who have had a stroke or for orienting interns. Three-ring binder.

945 pages Year Founded: 1967

5255 Invaluable Guide to Life After Stroke: An Owner's Manual
National Stroke Association
9707 E Easter Lane
Suite B
Centennial, CO 80112-3754
303-649-9299
Fax: 303-649-1328; *Toll Free:* 800-787-6537
info@stroke.org
www.stroke.org

Michael D. Walker, Chairman
George Davis, Vice Chairman
James Baranski, Chief Executive Officer

Practical advice and medical information to fight stroke's devastating effects.

152 pages Year Founded: 1984

5256 Life After Stroke: The Guide to Recovering
Johns Hopkins University Press
2715 North Charles Street
Baltimore, MD 21218-4363
410-516-6900
Fax: 410-516-6968
webmaster@jhupress.jhu.edu
www.press.jhu.edu

Joanne Leedom-Ackerman, Chair
Jonathan Bagger, Vice Provost Graduate Programs

Practical advice on treatment, rehabilitation, and lifestyle changes to help prevent another stroke.

Year Founded: 1878

5257 Living with Stroke: A Guide for Families
Cengage Learning
10650 Toebben Drive
Independence, KY 41051
Fax: 800-487-8488; *Toll Free:* 800-354-9706
www.cengage.com

5258 November Days
National Stroke Association
9707 E Easter Lane
Suite B
Centennial, CO 80112-3754
303-649-9299
Fax: 303-649-1328; *Toll Free:* 800-787-6537
info@stroke.org
www.stroke.org

Michael D. Walker, Chairman
George Davis, Vice Chairman
James Baranski, Chief Executive Officer

A caregiver's story of her struggle with a loved one's stroke.

225 pages Year Founded: 1984

5259 Pathways: Moving Beyond Stroke and Aphasis
National Stroke Association
9707 E Easter Lane
Suite B
Centennial, CO 80112-3754
303-649-9299
Fax: 303-649-1328; *Toll Free:* 800-787-6537
info@stroke.org
www.stroke.org

Michael D. Walker, Chairman
George Davis, Vice Chairman
James Baranski, Chief Executive Officer

A guide for those coping with issues caused by stroke and aphasia.

195 pages Year Founded: 1984

5260 Road Ahead: A Stroke Recovery Guide
National Stroke Association
9707 E Easter Lane
Suite B
Centennial, CO 80112-3754
303-649-9299
Fax: 303-649-1328; Toll Free: 800-787-6537
info@stroke.org
www.stroke.org

Michael D. Walker, Chairman
George Davis, Vice Chairman
James Baranski, Chief Executive Officer

This book offers comprehensive descriptions of stroke impairments and practical suggestions for coping, common concerns of caregivers, goal setting procedures, glossary terms and appendices.

153 pages Year Founded: 1984

5261 Stroke Book
Throndike Publishing
10 Water Street
Suite 310
Waterville, ME 04901
Fax: 800-558-4676; Toll Free: 800-223-1244
gale.printorders@cengage.com
www.thorndike.gale.com

Jamie Knobloch, Publisher
Sue Flewelling, Sales Manager
Sabine McAlpine, Key Accounts

5262 Stroke and the Family: A New Guide
Harvard University Press
79 Garden Street
Cambridge, MA 02138
617-495-2600
Fax: 617-495-5898; Toll Free: 800-405-1619
contact_hup@harvard.edu
www.hup.harvard.edu

Susan Wallace Boehmer, Editor-in-Chief
Michael Fisher, Assistant Director
Michael Aronson, Executiv Editor

To make sense of the confusing variety of diagnoses and treatment options, and goes on to explore challenges the recovering stroke patient and the recovering family will face during a long recuperation with an uncertain outcome.

Year Founded: 1913

5263 Stroke: Putting the Pieces Back Together
National Stroke Association
9707 E Easter Lane
Suite B
Centennial, CO 80112-3754
303-649-9299
Fax: 303-649-1328; Toll Free: 800-787-6537
info@stroke.org
www.stroke.org

Michael D. Walker, Chairman
George Davis, Vice Chairman
James Baranski, Chief Executive Officer

A training program designed for LTC facilities that includes audio and video tapes, student handout materials and an instructor's guide.

Year Founded: 1984

5264 Stroke: Your Complete Exercise Guide
Human Kinetics Publishers
1607 N Market Street
PO Box 5076
Champaign, IL 61820
217-351-5076
Fax: 217-351-1549; Toll Free: 800-747-4457
info@hkusa.com
www.humankinetics.com

Part of the Cooper Clinic and Research Institute Fitness Series providing exercise rehabilitation for persons suffering from strokes.

126 pages Year Founded: 1973

5265 Winning Over Stroke
National Stroke Association
9707 E Easter Lane
Suite B
Centennial, CO 80112-3754
303-649-9299
Fax: 303-649-1328; Toll Free: 800-787-6537
info@stroke.org
www.stroke.org

Michael D. Walker, Chairman
George Davis, Vice Chairman
James Baranski, Chief Executive Officer

An honest and inspiring depiction of the trials and successes of a stroke survivor. Encourages others to never give up hope on road to recovery.

110 pages Year Founded: 1984

Directories

5266 US Stroke Club Listing
National Stroke Association
9707 E Easter Lane
Suite B
Centennial, CO 80112-3754
303-649-9299
Fax: 303-649-1328; Toll Free: 800-787-6537
info@stroke.org
www.stroke.org

Michael D. Walker, Chairman
George Davis, Vice Chairman
James Baranski, Chief Executive Officer

About 1500 state stroke clubs and support groups that assist stroke survivors and their families. Entries include: Organization name, address, coordinator name, sponsor name. Lists of clubs and support groups covering a single state are available.

Year Founded: 1984

Journals, Magazines

5267 Journal of Stroke and Cerebrovascular Diseases
National Stroke Association
9707 E Easter Lane
Suite B
Centennial, CO 80112-3754
303-649-9299
Fax: 303-649-1328; *Toll Free:* 800-787-6537
info@stroke.org
www.stroke.org

Michael D. Walker, Chairman
George Davis, Vice Chairman
James Baranski, Chief Executive Officer

A multidisciplinary quarterly clinical journal devoted to all aspects of stroke.

Year Founded: 1984

Newsletters, Pamphlets

5268 African-Americans and Stroke
National Stroke Association
9707 E Easter Lane
Suite B
Centennial, CO 80112-3754
303-649-9299
Fax: 303-649-1328; *Toll Free:* 800-787-6537
info@stroke.org
www.stroke.org

Michael D. Walker, Chairman
George Davis, Vice Chairman
James Baranski, Chief Executive Officer

Year Founded: 1984

5269 Aneurysm Answers
National Stroke Association
9707 E Easter Lane
Suite B
Centennial, CO 80112-3754
303-649-9299
Fax: 303-649-1328; *Toll Free:* 800-787-6537
info@stroke.org
www.stroke.org

Michael D. Walker, Chairman
George Davis, Vice Chairman
James Baranski, Chief Executive Officer

Year Founded: 1984

5270 Atrial Fibrillation and Stroke
National Stroke Association
9707 E Easter Lane
Suite B
Centennial, CO 80112-3754
303-649-9299
Fax: 303-649-1328; *Toll Free:* 800-787-6537
info@stroke.org
www.stroke.org

Michael D. Walker, Chairman
George Davis, Vice Chairman
James Baranski, Chief Executive Officer

Year Founded: 1984

5271 Be Stroke Smart
National Stroke Association
9707 E Easter Lane
Suite B
Centennial, CO 80112-3754
303-649-9299
Fax: 303-649-1328; *Toll Free:* 800-787-6537
info@stroke.org
www.stroke.org

Michael D. Walker, Chairman
George Davis, Vice Chairman
James Baranski, Chief Executive Officer

A monthly newsletter with information on stroke, prevention, treatment, rehabilitation, resources and support for stroke survivors and caregivers.

Year Founded: 1984

5272 Be Stroke Smart - Communication
National Stroke Association
9707 E Easter Lane
Suite B
Centennial, CO 80112-3754
303-649-9299
Fax: 303-649-1328; *Toll Free:* 800-787-6537
info@stroke.org
www.stroke.org

Michael D. Walker, Chairman
George Davis, Vice Chairman
James Baranski, Chief Executive Officer

Groups of articles from the Be Stroke Smart series.

Year Founded: 1984

5273 Be Stroke Smart - Emotional Aspects
National Stroke Association
9707 E Easter Lane
Suite B
Centennial, CO 80112-3754
303-649-9299
Fax: 303-649-1328; *Toll Free:* 800-787-6537
info@stroke.org
www.stroke.org

Michael D. Walker, Chairman
George Davis, Vice Chairman
James Baranski, Chief Executive Officer

A group of 5 articles from the Be Stroke Smart series.

Year Founded: 1984

5274 Be Stroke Smart - Home and Work Adaptation
National Stroke Association
9707 E Easter Lane
Suite B
Centennial, CO 80112-3754
303-649-9299
Fax: 303-649-1328; *Toll Free:* 800-787-6537
info@stroke.org
www.stroke.org

Michael D. Walker, Chairman
George Davis, Vice Chairman
James Baranski, Chief Executive Officer

Mini-packet of articles from the Be Stroke Smart series.

Year Founded: 1984

5275 Be Stroke Smart - Prevention and Warning Signs
National Stroke Association
9707 E Easter Lane
Suite B
Centennial, CO 80112-3754
303-649-9299
Fax: 303-649-1328; *Toll Free:* 800-787-6537
info@stroke.org
www.stroke.org

Michael D. Walker, Chairman
George Davis, Vice Chairman
James Baranski, Chief Executive Officer

Mini-packet of articles from the Be Stroke Smart series.

Year Founded: 1984

5276 Be Stroke Smart - Rehabilitation Guidelines and Resources
National Stroke Association
9707 E Easter Lane
Suite B
Centennial, CO 80112-3754
303-649-9299
Fax: 303-649-1328; *Toll Free:* 800-787-6537
info@stroke.org
www.stroke.org

Michael D. Walker, Chairman
George Davis, Vice Chairman
James Baranski, Chief Executive Officer

Mini-packet of articles from the Be Stroke Smart series.

Year Founded: 1984

5277 Be Stroke Smart Series
National Stroke Association
9707 E Easter Lane
Suite B
Centennial, CO 80112-3754
303-649-9299
Fax: 303-649-1328; *Toll Free:* 800-787-6537
info@stroke.org
www.stroke.org

Michael D. Walker, Chairman
George Davis, Vice Chairman
James Baranski, Chief Executive Officer

Series of 24 articles in response to the most asked about questions about stroke.

Year Founded: 1984

5278 Brain at Risk: Understanding and Preventing Stroke
National Stroke Association
9707 E Easter Lane
Suite B
Centennial, CO 80112-3754
303-649-9299
Fax: 303-649-1328; *Toll Free:* 800-787-6537
info@stroke.org
www.stroke.org

Michael D. Walker, Chairman
George Davis, Vice Chairman
James Baranski, Chief Executive Officer

Year Founded: 1984

5279 Clinical Trials Participation
National Stroke Association
9707 E Easter Lane
Suite B
Centennial, CO 80112-3754
303-649-9299
Fax: 303-649-1328; *Toll Free:* 800-787-6537
info@stroke.org
www.stroke.org

Michael D. Walker, Chairman
George Davis, Vice Chairman
James Baranski, Chief Executive Officer

Explains what acute stroke treatment clinical trials are and how patients can participate.

Year Founded: 1984

5280 Disability Workbook for Social Security Applicants
National Stroke Association
9707 E Easter Lane
Suite B
Centennial, CO 80112-3754
303-649-9299
Fax: 303-649-1328; *Toll Free:* 800-787-6537
info@stroke.org
www.stroke.org

Michael D. Walker, Chairman
George Davis, Vice Chairman
James Baranski, Chief Executive Officer

120 pages Year Founded: 1984

5281 Guide to Understanding Stroke
National Stroke Association
9707 E Easter Lane
Suite B
Centennial, CO 80112-3754
303-649-9299
Fax: 303-649-1328; *Toll Free:* 800-787-6537
info@stroke.org
www.stroke.org

Michael D. Walker, Chairman
George Davis, Vice Chairman
James Baranski, Chief Executive Officer

Detailed color illustrations on stroke and its action for physicians to present to patients.

Year Founded: 1984

5282 Heart and Stroke Facts
American Heart Association
7272 Greenville Avenue
Dallas, TX 75231-5129
214-570-5978
Fax: 214-706-1341; *Toll Free:* 800-242-8721
www.heart.org

Bernie Dennis, Chairman
Mariell Jessup, President
Nancy Brown, CEO

Year Founded: 1924

5283 Heart and Stroke Risk Factors
American Heart Association
7272 Greenville Avenue
Dallas, TX 75231-5129

214-570-5978
Fax: 214-706-1341; *Toll Free:* 800-242-8721
www.heart.org

Bernie Dennis, Chairman
Mariell Jessup, President
Nancy Brown, CEO
Year Founded: 1924

5284 High Blood Pressure and Stroke
National Stroke Association
9707 E Easter Lane
Suite B
Centennial, CO 80112-3754
303-649-9299
Fax: 303-649-1328; *Toll Free:* 800-787-6537
info@stroke.org
www.stroke.org

Michael D. Walker, Chairman
George Davis, Vice Chairman
James Baranski, Chief Executive Officer
Year Founded: 1984

5285 Home Exercises for Stroke Survivors
National Stroke Association
9707 E Easter Lane
Suite B
Centennial, CO 80112-3754
303-649-9299
Fax: 303-649-1328; *Toll Free:* 800-787-6537
info@stroke.org
www.stroke.org

Michael D. Walker, Chairman
George Davis, Vice Chairman
James Baranski, Chief Executive Officer
Year Founded: 1984

5286 Living at Home After a Stroke
National Stroke Association
9707 E Easter Lane
Suite B
Centennial, CO 80112-3754
303-649-9299
Fax: 303-649-1328; *Toll Free:* 800-787-6537
info@stroke.org
www.stroke.org

Michael D. Walker, Chairman
George Davis, Vice Chairman
James Baranski, Chief Executive Officer
Year Founded: 1984

5287 NSA's Guide to Stroke
National Stroke Association
9707 E Easter Lane
Suite B
Centennial, CO 80112-3754
303-649-9299
Fax: 303-649-1328; *Toll Free:* 800-787-6537
info@stroke.org
www.stroke.org

Michael D. Walker, Chairman
George Davis, Vice Chairman
James Baranski, Chief Executive Officer
Year Founded: 1984

5288 Recovery After a Stroke
National Stroke Association
9707 E Easter Lane
Suite B
Centennial, CO 80112-3754
303-649-9299
Fax: 303-649-1328; *Toll Free:* 800-787-6537
info@stroke.org
www.stroke.org

Michael D. Walker, Chairman
George Davis, Vice Chairman
James Baranski, Chief Executive Officer
Year Founded: 1984

5289 Recurrent Stroke
National Stroke Association
9707 E Easter Lane
Suite B
Centennial, CO 80112-3754
303-649-9299
Fax: 303-649-1328; *Toll Free:* 800-787-6537
info@stroke.org
www.stroke.org

Michael D. Walker, Chairman
George Davis, Vice Chairman
James Baranski, Chief Executive Officer
Year Founded: 1984

5290 Reducing Risk and Recognizing Symptoms
National Stroke Association
9707 E Easter Lane
Suite B
Centennial, CO 80112-3754
303-649-9299
Fax: 303-649-1328; *Toll Free:* 800-787-6537
info@stroke.org
www.stroke.org

Michael D. Walker, Chairman
George Davis, Vice Chairman
James Baranski, Chief Executive Officer
Year Founded: 1984

5291 Stroke Connection
American Heart Association
7272 Greenville Avenue
Dallas, TX 75231-5129
214-570-5978
Fax: 214-706-1341; *Toll Free:* 800-242-8721
www.heart.org

Bernie Dennis, Chairman
Mariell Jessup, President
Nancy Brown, CEO

A forum for stroke survivors and their families to share information about coping with stroke. Provides information and referral and carriers stroke related books, videos and literature available for purchase.

Frequency: BiMonthly Year Founded: 1924

5292 Stroke Treatment and Recovery
National Stroke Association
9707 E Easter Lane
Suite B
Centennial, CO 80112-3754
303-649-9299
Fax: 303-649-1328; *Toll Free:* 800-787-6537

info@stroke.org
www.stroke.org

Michael D. Walker, Chairman
George Davis, Vice Chairman
James Baranski, Chief Executive Officer
Year Founded: 1984

5293 Stroke is a Brain Attack!
National Stroke Association
9707 E Easter Lane
Suite B
Centennial, CO 80112-3754
303-649-9299
Fax: 303-649-1328; *Toll Free:* 800-787-6537
info@stroke.org
www.stroke.org

Michael D. Walker, Chairman
George Davis, Vice Chairman
James Baranski, Chief Executive Officer
Year Founded: 1984

5294 Stroke: Clinical Updates
National Stroke Association
9707 E Easter Lane
Suite B
Centennial, CO 80112-3754
303-649-9299
Fax: 303-649-1328; *Toll Free:* 800-787-6537
info@stroke.org
www.stroke.org

Michael D. Walker, Chairman
George Davis, Vice Chairman
James Baranski, Chief Executive Officer

Offers the lates medical advances and technology news for
the health care professional.
Year Founded: 1984

5295 Stroke: Questions & Answers
National Stroke Association
9707 E Easter Lane
Suite B
Centennial, CO 80112-3754
303-649-9299
Fax: 303-649-1328; *Toll Free:* 800-787-6537
info@stroke.org
www.stroke.org

Michael D. Walker, Chairman
George Davis, Vice Chairman
James Baranski, Chief Executive Officer
Year Founded: 1984

5296 Stroke: Reducing Your Risk (Spanish)
National Stroke Association
9707 E Easter Lane
Suite B
Centennial, CO 80112-3754
303-649-9299
Fax: 303-649-1328; *Toll Free:* 800-787-6537
info@stroke.org
www.stroke.org

Michael D. Walker, Chairman
George Davis, Vice Chairman
James Baranski, Chief Executive Officer

This brochure helps persons learn what stroke is, how to
recognize warning signs, what factors affect stroke risk and
how to reduce stroke risks. Available in Spanish only.
Year Founded: 1984

5297 Understanding Speech and Language Problems
After Stroke
National Stroke Association
9707 E Easter Lane
Suite B
Centennial, CO 80112-3754
303-649-9299
Fax: 303-649-1328; *Toll Free:* 800-787-6537
info@stroke.org
www.stroke.org

Michael D. Walker, Chairman
George Davis, Vice Chairman
James Baranski, Chief Executive Officer
Year Founded: 1984

5298 What Every Family Should Know About
Stroke
National Stroke Association
9707 E Easter Lane
Suite B
Centennial, CO 80112-3754
303-649-9299
Fax: 303-649-1328; *Toll Free:* 800-787-6537
info@stroke.org
www.stroke.org

Michael D. Walker, Chairman
George Davis, Vice Chairman
James Baranski, Chief Executive Officer
Year Founded: 1984

Videos, Audio Tapes

5299 Brain at Risk: Understanding and Preventing
Stroke
National Stroke Association
9707 E Easter Lane
Suite B
Centennial, CO 80112-3754
303-649-9299
Fax: 303-649-1328; *Toll Free:* 800-787-6537
info@stroke.org
www.stroke.org

Michael D. Walker, Chairman
George Davis, Vice Chairman
James Baranski, Chief Executive Officer

Explains strokes, describes symptoms, and instructs individuals on how to reduce their risk of stroke. Available in
an opened caption version for people with hearing
impairments.
Year Founded: 1984

5300 NSA Audio Tape Series
National Stroke Association
9707 E Easter Lane
Suite B
Centennial, CO 80112-3754
303-649-9299
Fax: 303-649-1328; *Toll Free:* 800-787-6537

info@stroke.org
www.stroke.org

Michael D. Walker, Chairman
George Davis, Vice Chairman
James Baranski, Chief Executive Officer

Jackie Mayer Townsend, Miss America 1963 and a stroke survivor, shares her story and provides hope, motivation, and inspiration.

Year Founded: 1984

Research Centers

5301 American Academy of Neurology
201 Chicago Avenue
Minneapolis, MN 55415
612-928-6000
Fax: 612-454-2746; *Toll Free:* 800-879-1960
memberservices@aan.com
www.aan.com

Professional society of medical doctors specializing in brain and nervous system diseases. Maintains placement service. Sponsors research and educational programs. Compiles statistics. Publishes scientific journal.

Year Founded: 1948

5302 Cerebral Blood Flow Laboratories
Veterans Administration Medical Center
810 Vermont Avenue
NW
Washington, DC 20420
713-795-5807
Fax: 713-795-7501; *Toll Free:* 800-273-8255
www.va.gov

John S Meyer MD, Director

Offers research in cerebrovascular disorders and risk factors for stroke.

5303 Comprehensive Stroke Center of Oregon
University of Oregon Health Sciences Center
3181 SW Sam Jackson Park Road
Portland, OR 97239-3098
503-494-8311
Fax: 503-494-7556; *Toll Free:* 800-245-6478
www.ohsu.edu

Bruce Coull MD, Professor
Wayne M Clark, MD

Year Founded: 2001

5304 Cornell University Medical College: Departments of Neurology and Neuroscience
Weill Cornell Medical College
1300 York Avenue
PO Box 130
New York, NY 10065
212-746-5454
Fax: 212-746-8214
weill.cornell.edu

Sanford I. Weill, Chair
Antonio M. Gotto, Co-Chair
Robert Appel, Vice Chair

Year Founded: 1898

5305 Dana Foundation and the Dana Alliance for Brain Initiatives
The Dana Foundation and The Dana Alliance for Brai
505 Fifth Avenue
6th Floor
New York, NY 10017
212-223-4040
Fax: 212-317-8721
danainfo@dana.org
www.dana.org

Edward F Rover, Chairman & President
Barbara E Gill, Executive Vice President
Burton M Mirsky, Executive Vice President

To increase public understanding of brain-related diseases, disorders, and research.

Year Founded: 1996

5306 Duke University Medical Center
Duke University School of Medicine
DUMC 3710
PO Box 3209
Durham, NC 27710
919-684-2985
Fax: 919-684-4431
medadm@mc.duke.edu
dukemed.duke.edu

Nancy C. Andrews, Dean and Vice Chancellor for Aca
Scott Gibson, Executive Vice Dean
Edward Buckley, Vice Dean

Year Founded: 1930

5307 Hospital of the University of Pennsylvania
The Hospital of the University of Pennsylvania
3400 Spruce Street
Philadelphia, PA 19104
215-662-4000
Fax: 215-349-5165; *Toll Free:* 800-789-7366
www.uphs.upenn.edu

Francisco Gonzalez-Scarano, Professor
Ralph Muller, CEO

Year Founded: 1765

5308 Massachusetts General Departments of Neurology and Neurosurgery
Massachusetts General Hospital
55 Fruit Street
Gray 502
Boston, MA 02114
617-726-8581
Fax: 617-726-3384
www.massgeneral.org

Robert L. Martuza, Chief, Department of Neurosurger
Michael A Moskowitz MD, Professor

Year Founded: 1811

5309 Stroke Council
American Heart Association
7272 Greenville Avenue
Dallas, TX 75231
my.americanheart.org

One of 16 scientific councils of the American Heart Association, the Stroke Council supports the work of the American Stroke Association in advancing stroke research and education.

5310 University of California: Los Angeles Department of Medicine
Department of Medicine
Los Angeles, CA 90024
213-825-8858
access@mednet.ucla.edu
www.med.ucla.edu

Alan Fogelman, Executive Chair
Jan Tillisch, Executive Vice Chair
Farah Elahi, Chief Administrative Officer

5311 University of Iowa College of Medicine
University of Iowa Carver College of Medicine
451 Newton Road
200 Medicine Administration Building
Iowa City, IA 52242
319-335-9650
Fax: 319-335-7155
www.medicine.uiowa.edu

Debra A. Schwinn, Dean
Donna L. Hammond, Executive Associate Dean
Christopher Cooper, Associate Dean for Student Affai

Year Founded: 1850

5312 University of Miami School of Medicine: Department of Neurology
University of Miami
1320 S. Dixie Hwy.
Suite 701
Coral Gables, FL 33124
305-284-4443
Fax: 305-284-4985
www.miami.edu

Donna E. Shalala, President
Minor Anderson, Vice President
Thomas J. LeBlanc, Provost

Year Founded: 1925

5313 Washington University School of Medicine
Washington University of School and Medicine
660 S Euclid Avenue
Saint Louis, MO 63110-1093
314-362-8681
Fax: 314-362-4658
wumscoa@msnotes.wustl.edu
medschool.wustl.edu

Marcus Raichle MD, Contact
Janet B McGill, MD

Year Founded: 1891

Substance Abuse

Associations & Organizations

5314 ADAMHS Board of Cuyahoga County
2012 W 25th Street
6th Floor
Cleveland, OH 44113
216-241-3400
osiecki@adamhscc.org
www.adasbcc.org

Scott S Osiecki, Chief Executive Officer
Linda A Lamp, Executive Assistant
Carol A Krajewski, Executive Specialist

The Alcohol, Drug Addiction and Mental Health Services (ADAMHS) Board of Cuyahoga County is responsible for the planning, funding and monitoring of public mental health and addiction treatment and recovery services delivered to the residents of Cuyahoga County.

5315 Al-Anon Family Group Headquarters
1600 Corporate Landing Parkway
Virginia Beach, VA 23454-5617
757-563-1600
Fax: 757-563-1656; Toll Free: 888-425-2666
wso@al-anon.org
al-anon.org

A fellowship of relatives and friends of alcoholics whose lives have been affected by someone else's drinking and a self-help recovery program based on the 12 steps of Alcoholics Anonymous. The single purpose of this organization is to help families and friends of alcoholics, whether the alcoholic is still drinking or not.

5316 Alabama Division of Mental Illness and Substance Abuse Community Programs
The Alabama Department of Mental Health
100 N Union Street
P.O. Box 301410
Montgomery, AL 36130-1410
334-242-3454
Fax: 334-242-0725; Toll Free: 800-367-0955
alabama.dmh@mh.alabama.gov
www.mh.alabama.gov

Kim Boswell, Chief of Staff

Promoting the health and well-being of Alabamians with mental illnesses, developmental disabilities and substance use disorders.

5317 Alcohol Justice
24 Belvedere Street
San Rafael, CA 94901
415-456-5692
alcoholjustice.org

Karen Kuhn, Administrative Director
Bruce Lee Livingston, Executive Director

Promote evidence-based public health policies and organize campaigns with diverse communities and youth against the alcohol industry's harmful practices.

Year Founded: 1987

5318 Alcohol Research Group: Public Health Institute
Alcohol Research Group
6001 Shellmound Street
Suite 450
Emeryville, CA 94608
510-898-5800
info@arg.org
www.arg.org

Dominique Lampert, Executive Director
Thomas K Greenfield, Scientific Director
Vicky Fagan, Administrative Coordinator

ARG's mission is to improve public health through deepening our understanding of alcohol and other drug use and investigating innovative approaches to reduce its consequences for individuals, families, and communities.

Year Founded: 1959

5319 Alcohol-Drug Treatment Referral
Recovery Now
Toll Free: 800-281-4731
charliek@spencerrecovery.com
www.recoverynowtv.com

National Help and Referral Network, a nonprofit organization available 24 hours a day to assist people troubled by drug or alcohol abuse. Here to provide information on addiction treatment and support services and to help save lives and mend broken dreams.

5320 Alcoholics Anonymous
A.A. World Services, Inc.
475 Riverside Drive at W 120th Street
11th Floor
New York, NY 10115
212-870-3400
www.aa.org

Valerie O'Neill, Regional Forums Coordinator

Alcoholics Anonymous is a world-wide fellowship of men and women who have found solutions to their drinking problems. The only requirement for A.A. membership is a desire to stop drinking. There are no dues or fees; A.A. is supported by voluntary contributions of its members and groups.

Year Founded: 1935

5321 American Council on Addiction and Alcohol Problems
2376 Lakeside Drive
Birmingham, AL 35244
205-989-8177
sapacap.com

Ed Wolkin, President
William E. Day, Executive Director

Provides the forum and the mechanism through which concerned people can find common ground on alcohol and other drug problems and address these issues with a united voice. Members of the organization include 36 state temperance organizations, 22 national Christian denominations and other fraternal organizations which support the ACAP's philosophy of abstinence.

5322 American Psychological Association
750 First Street NE
Washington, DC 20002-5500

202-336-5500Toll free: 800-374-2721
www.apa.org
TDD 202-336-6123
TTY: 202-336-6123

Number of Members: 122,500+

5323 Arizona Substance Abuse Task Force
Arizona Governor's Office of Youth, Faith &
Family
1700 W Washington Street
Suite 230
Phoenix, AZ 85007
602-542-4043
azsubstanceabusepartnership@gmail.com
substanceabuse.az.gov

Debbie Moak, Director

The Arizona Substance Abuse Task Force is a coalition of
leading substance abuse experts, providers and community
members focused on addressing and reversing the growing
epidemic of drug abuse and addiction in Arizona communities by finding the best treatments and reducing barriers to
care.

5324 Arkansa Substance Abuse Prevention,
Education and Early Intervention
Arkansas Department of Human Services
305 South Palm Street
Little Rock, AR 72205
501-686-9164
Fax: 501-686-9182
jay.hill@dhs.arkansas.gov
humanservices.arkansas.gov
TDD 501-686-9176

Jay Hill, Director
Kirk Lane, State Drug Director
Pam Dobson, Assistant Clinical Director

The Division of Behavioral Health Services is responsible
for ensuring the provision of public behavioral health services, including mental health and substance abuse prevention, treatment, and recovery services throughout the State
of Arkansas. The Division supports, certifies, licenses, and
funds behavioral health providers throughout the state. In
addition, the Division of Behavioral Health Service operates two behavioral health institutions: the Arkansas State
Hospital located in Little Rock and the Arkansas Health
Center in Benton.

5325 Betty Ford Center
Eisenhower Medical Center
39000 Bob Hope Drive
PO Box 1560
Rancho Mirage, CA 92270-1375
Toll Free: 866-831-5700
www.hazeldenbettyford.org

Jim Steinhagen, Vice President Administrator
Steve Eickelberg, Medical Director

Provides effective drug and alcohol dependency treatment
services.

Year Founded: 1982

5326 California Friday Night Live Partnership
Department of Health Care Services
6200 S Mooney Boulevard
P.O. Box 5091
Visalia, CA 93278-5091

559-733-6496
Fax: 559-737-4231
www.fridaynightlive.org

Jim Kooler, Administrator
Lynne Goodwin, Program Director

These groups, located in California, are all run by students
with a faculty adviser. They arrange local alcohol and drug
free events, from dances and movies to visiting hospitalized children. Students not only have fun but they learn to
have fun sober.

Year Founded: 1984

5327 Center for Substance Abuse Prevention
1 Choke Cherry Road
Room 4-1057
Rockville, MD 20857
240-276-2420
www.samhsa.gov

Frances M. Harding, Director

This organization's goal is to connect people and resources
with innovative ideas, strategies and programs designed to
encourage creative and effective efforts aimed at reducing
and eliminating alcohol, tobacco and other drug problems
in our society.

Year Founded: 1992

5328 Center for Substance Abuse Research
4321 Hartwick Road
Suite 501
College Park, MD 20740
301-405-9770
Fax: 301-403-8342
cesar@umd.edu
www.cesar.umd.edu

Eric Wish, Director

5329 Center of Alcohol Studies
Smithers Hall
607 Allison Road
Piscataway, NJ 08854-8001
848-445-2190
Fax: 732-445-3500
alcoholstudies.rutgers.edu

Marsha Bates, Acting Director

Studies the causes and effective treatment of alcoholism.
Also operates a controlled drug-delivery research center.

5330 Cocaine Anonymous
C.A. World Services Office
21720 S Wilmington Avenue
Suite 304
Long Beach, CA 90810-1641
310-559-5833
Fax: 310-559-2554
cawso@ca.org
www.ca.org

Fellowship of men and women who share their experience,
strength and hope with each other that they may solve their
common problem and help others recover from their addiction.

Year Founded: 1982

5331 Connecticut Department of Mental Health and Addiction Services
State of Connecticut
410 Capitol Avenue
P.O. Box 341431
Hartford, CT 06134
860-418-7000 Toll free: 800-446-7348
miriam.delphin-rittmon@ct.gov
www.ct.gov/dmhas
TTY: 860-418-6707

Miriam E Delphin-Rittmon, PhD, Commissioner
Nancy Navarretta, Deputy Commissioner

The Connecticut Department of Mental Health and Addiction Services is a health care agency whose mission is to promote the overall health and wellness of persons with behavioral health needs through an integrated network of holistic, comprehensive, effective, and efficient services and supports that foster dignity, respect, and self-sufficiency.
Year Founded: 1633

5332 Cornerstone Treatment Facilities Network
159-05 Union Turnpike
116th Street
Fresh Meadows, NY 11366
Toll Free: 800-233-9999
info@cornerstoneny.com
www.cornerstoneny.com

Offers a complete integrated program for alcohol assessment, alcohol and drug rehabilitation, continuing care, community education and comprehensive family recovery.
Year Founded: 1947

5333 Delaware Division of Alcoholism, Drug Abuse & Mental Health
State of Delaware
1901 N Du Pont Highway
Main Building
New Castle, DE 19720
302-255-9399
Fax: 302-255-4428; *Toll Free:* 800-652-2929
dhss.delaware.gov

Dr. Kara Odom, Secretary

The mission is to improve the quality of life for Delaware's citizens by promoting health and well-being, fostering self-sufficiency, and protecting vilnerable populations.

5334 Dentists Concerned for Dentists
651-275-0313 Toll free: 800-632-7643
dcdmn.com

Dentists Concerned for Dentists (DCD) is a group of recovering alcoholic and chemically dependent dentists concerned about other dentists who are having problems with alcohol and/or other mood-altering drugs.
Year Founded: 1973

5335 Do It Now Foundation
Do It Now Foundation
P.O. Box 27921
Tempe, AZ 85285-7568
480-736-0599
info@doitnow.org
www.doitnow.org

James Parker, Executive Director

An information clearinghouse for service providers that publishes well-written pamphlets, booklets, and materials on chemical dependency amd recovery.
Year Founded: 1968

5336 Drug Abuse Resistance Education of America
D.A.R.E. America
P.O. Box 512090
Los Angeles, CA 90051-0090
310-215-0575
Fax: 310-215-0180; *Toll Free:* 800-223-3273
www.dare.org

Michele Leonhart, Chair
Francisco Pegueros, Secretary

D.A.R.E. is a comprehensive K-12 education program taught in thousands of schools in America and 52 other countries. D.A.R.E. curricula address drugs, violence, bullying, internet safety, and other high risk circumstances that are too often a part of students' lives.
Year Founded: 1983

5337 Drug-Free Workplace Helpline
Substance Abuse & Mental Health Services Admin.
5600 Fishers Lane
Rockville, MD 20857
Toll Free: 800-967-5752
www.samhsa.gov

A helpline for businesses to obtain information on a wide range of drug abuse related problems, issues and services.
Year Founded: 1992

5338 Families Anonymous
701 Lee Street
Suite 670
Des Plaines, IL 60016
847-294-5877
Fax: 847-294-5837; *Toll Free:* 800-736-9805
www.familiesanonymous.org

Addresses the needs of families who are concerned about a relative with a drug problem and with related behavioral problems. Offers informational packets, meetings and support networks for these families.

5339 Florida Substance Abuse and Mental Health Program (SAMH)
Florida Health
4052 Bald Cypress Way
Tallahassee, FL 32399
850-245-4444 Toll free: 800-662-4357
health@flhealth.gov
www.floridahealth.gov

Mike Carroll, Secretary
David Fairbanks, Deputy Secretary

Provides free and confidential information in English and Spanish for individuals and family members facing substance abuse and mental health issues. 24 hours a day, 7 days a week.
Year Founded: 1996

5340 Fresh Start Alcohol and Drug Recovery Group
Cambridge Health Alliance
454 Broadway
Revere, MA 02151
617-591-6051
www.challiance.org

Fresh Start is an AA-affiliated, 12-step anonymous alcohol and drug recovery peer support group. It's free and open to everyone at any stage of their recovery. Meetings every Thursday evening from 6:30 - 7:30 p.m. on the 1st floor at CHA Revere Care Center.

5341 Georgia Alcohol & Substance Abuse Prevention Project (ASAPP)
Departnment of Behavioral Health
Two Peachtree Street, NW
24th Floor
Atlanta, GA 30303
404-657-2252
dbhdd.georgia.gov

Kimberly Ryan, Chair
David Glass, Vice Chair
Ellice P Martin, Secretary

Georgia's Alcohol & Substance Abuse Prevention Project uses the Strategic Prevention Framework (SPF) and a public health approach to tackle Georgia's leading substances of abuse and misuse issues.

5342 Hawaii Alcohol and Drug Abuse Division
Department of Health
601 Kamokila Boulevard
Room 360
Kapolei, HI 96707
808-692-7506
health.hawaii.gov/substance-abuse

Virginia Pressler, MD, Director
Keith Y Yamamoto, Deputy Director

The Alcohol and Drug Abuse Division (ADAD) is the primary and often sole source of public funds for substance abuse treatment. ADAD's treatment efforts are designed to promote a statewide culturally appropriate, comprehensive system of services to meet the treatment and recovery needs of individuals and families.

5343 Hazelden Betty Ford Foundation
P.O. Box 11 CO9
15251 Pleasant Valley Road
Center City, MN 55012-0011
Toll Free: 866-286-3140
www.hazeldenbettyford.org

Dawne Calrson, VP, Human Resources
James A Blaha, VP, CFO, CAO
Jennifer Lohse, VP, General Counsel

A nonprofit organization dedicated to providing quality rehabilitation, education and professional services for chemical dependency and related addictive behaviors. Services offered include assessment and rehabilitation, family services, community prevention and professional education, counselor and clergy training and educational materials.

Year Founded: 1947

5344 Illinois Church Action on Alcohol Problems (ILCAAAP)
1132 W Jefferson Street
Springfield, IL 62702
217-546-6871Toll free: 866-940-6871
ILCAAAP@sbcglobal.net
www.ilcaaap.org

Anita Bedell, Executive Director

An interdenominational Christian agency representing church groups in Illinois. Works to prevent alcohol and

other drug-related problems through education, legislative action and public awareness.

5345 Illinois Department of Alcoholism and Substance Abuse
Illinois Department of Human Services
401 South Clinton Street
Chicago, IL 60607
Toll Free: 800-843-6154
www.dhs.state.il.us
TTY: 866-324-5553

James T Dimas, Secretary

The mission of the Division of Alcoholism and Substance Abuse is to provide a system of care along the continuum of prevention, intervention, treatment and recovery support where individuals with SUD, those in recovery and those at risk are valued and treated with dignity and where stigma, accompanying attitudes, discrimination, and other barriers to recovery are eliminated.

Year Founded: 1997

5346 Indian Health Service
5600 Fishers Lane
Rockville, MD 20857
301-443-3593
www.ihs.gov

Michael Weahkee, Acting Director
Chris Buchanan, Deputy Director
Michael Toedt, Chief Medical Director

The Indian Health Service an agency within the Department of Health Services, is responsible for providing federal health services to American indians and Alaska natives.

5347 International Lawyers in Alcoholics Anonymous
5371 Sherbrooke Street
Vancouver, BC V5W 3M6
604-644-9254
foot3@telus.net
www.ilaa.org

Barry Kerfoot, Chairman
David Crawford, Trustee
Andrea Jones, Trustee

International Lawyers in Alcoholics Anonymous is a group of recovered lawyers and judges carrying the message of recovery within our profession. Our purpose is to act as a bridge between reluctant (in denial) lawyers/judges and Alcoholics Anonymous.

Year Founded: 1975

5348 Iowa Bureau of Substance Abuse
Iowa Department of Public Health
Lucas State Office Building
321 E 12th Street
Des Moines, IA 50319
515-281-7689Toll free: 855-581-8111
idph.iowa.gov/substance-abuse

DeAnn Decker, Bureau Chief

The Bureau of Substance Abuse is part of the Division of Behavioral Health, in the Iowa Department of Public Health. The Bureau focuses on and provides oversight for all aspects related to substance abuse prevention and treatment services in Iowa, in addition to injury prevention programs. The bureau actively works to address Prevention and Treatment needs by providing focus for training efforts, identifying and securing available grant funding, monitoring grant compliance, and regulating licensure for treatment programs.

5349 Maine Association of Substance Abuse Programs
295 Water Street
Suite 200
Augusta, ME 04330
207-621-8118
Fax: 207-621-8362
mshaughnessy@masap.org
thealliancemaine.org

Malory Shaughnessy, Executive Director
Steven Cotreau, Manager
Darren Ripley, Coordinator

Statewide membership association for community behavioral health organizations that provide multi-level services, programming and coordinated leadership to ensure that Mainers have full access to the continuum of recovery-oriented systems of care for mental illness and substance use disorder - from prevention through treatment and into peer recovery support.

5350 Minnesota Recovery Connection
822 S Third Street
Suite 101
Minneapolis, MN 55415
612-584-4158
Fax: 612-886-3940
nfo@minnesotarecovery.org
minnesotarecovery.org

Julia Alexander, Co-Executive Director
Kris Kelly, Co-Executive Director
Lili Herbert, Chair

A recovery community organization serving the seven county metro area of Minnesota and supporting recovery communities in both St. Cloud and Duluth. The Minnesota Recovery Connection's mission is to strengthen the recovery community through peer-to-peer support, public education, and advocacy.

5351 Mississippi Division of Alcohol and Drug Abuse
Department of Mental Health
239 N Lamar Street
1101 Robert E. Lee Building
Jackson, MS 39201-1328
601-359-1288
Fax: 601-359-6295; *Toll Free:* 877-210-8513
www.dmh.ms.gov
TDD 601-359-6230

The Bureau of Alcohol and Drug Services has the responsibility of administering fiscal resources (state and federal) to the public system of prevention, treatment, and recovery supports for persons with substance use disorders. The overall goal of the state's substance use disorder service system is to provide quality care within a continuum of accessible community-based services including: prevention, outpatient, withdrawal management, intensive outpatient, primary and transitional residential treatment, opioid treatment services and recovery support.

Year Founded: 1974

5352 Montana Division of Addictive & Mental Disorders
Department of Public Health and Human Services
100 N Park, Suite 300
PO Box 202905
Helena, MT 59620-2905
406-444-3964
Fax: 406-444-4435
hhsamdemail@mt.gov
dphhs.mt.gov/amdd

Zoe Barnard, Administrator
Bobbi Perkins, Bureau Chief
Cindy Dallas, Office Manager

To implement and improve an appropriate statewide system of prevention, treatment, care and rehabilitation for Montanans with mental disorders or addictions to drugs or alcohol. Provides substance abuse and adult mental health services by contracting with behavioral health providers throughout Montana.

5353 Narcotics Anonymous World Services
P.O. Box 9999
Van Nuys, CA 91409
818-773-9999
Fax: 818-700-0700
fsmail@na.org
www.na.org

Narcotics Anonymous is a global, community-based organization with a multilingual and multicultural membership. NA was founded in 1953, and members hold nearly 67,000 meetings weekly in 139 countries today.

Year Founded: 1953

5354 National Association for Alcoholism andDrug Abuse Counselors
1001 N Fairfax Street
Suite 201
Alexandria, VA 22314
703-741-7686
Fax: 703-741-7698; *Toll Free:* 800-548-0497
naadac@naadac.org
www.naadac.org

Cynthia Moreno Tuohy, Executive Director
HeidiAnne Werner, Director of Operations & Finance

This organization is comprised of addiction focused professionals who enhance the health and recovery of individuals, families and communities. NAADAC's mission is to lead, unify and empower addiction focused professionals to achieve excellence through education, advocacy, knowledge, standards of practice, ethics, professional development and research.

Year Founded: 1974

5355 National Association of Addiction Treatment Providers
PO Box 6693
Denver, CO 80206
Toll Free: 888-574-1008
www.naatp.org

Marvin Ventrell, Executive Director
Katie Strand, Director of Operations

Year Founded: 1978

5356 National Association on Drug Abuse Problems
355 Lexington Avenue
2nd Floor
New York, NY 10017
212-986-1170
www.nadap.org

John A. Darin, President & CEO
Gary Stankowski, EVP
Theresa McBurnie, CFO

Provides skills evaluation, job training and job placement to recovering drug addicts in the metropolitan New York area.

Year Founded: 1971

5357 National Clearinghouse for Alcohol and Drug Information
Substance Abuse & Mental Health Administration
PO Box 2345
Rockville, MD 20847-2345
301-468-2600
Fax: 301-468-6433; Toll Free: 800-729-6686
info@health.org
www.health.org
TDD 800-487-4889

A resource for alcohol and other drug information. It carries a wide variety of publications dealing with alcohol and other drug abuse.

Year Founded: 1992

5358 National Council on Alcoholism and DrugDependence
217 Broadway
Suite 712
New York, NY 10007
212-269-7797
Fax: 212-269-7510
national@ncadd.org
www.ncadd.org

Andrew N. Pucher, President & CEO

Provides education, information, help and hope in the fight against addictions. Founded in 1944, NCADD, with its nationwide network of affiliates, advocates prevention, intervention and treatment, is committed to ridding the disease of its stigma and its sufferers of their denial and shame.

Year Founded: 1944

5359 National Crime Prevention Council
1201 Connecticut Avenue
Suite 200
Washington, DC 20036
202-466-6272
www.ncpc.org

Ann M. Harkins, President & CEO

This organization works to prevent crime and drug use in many ways, including developing materials for parents and children.

Year Founded: 1982

5360 National Families in Action
PO Box 133136
Atlanta, GA 30333-3136
404-248-9676
Fax: 404-248-1312

nfia@nationalfamilies.org
www.nationalfamilies.org

William F. Carter, Chairman
Sue Rusche, President & CEO
Carol S. Reeder, Treasurer

Offers news and information for persons interested in drug abuse prevention. Operates the Parent Corps in 9 states. Operates teh Addiction Studies Progeram for journalists and state legislatures with several University Medical Schools.

Year Founded: 1977

5361 National Institute on Drug Abuse
6001 Executive Boulevard
Rockville, MD 20852
301-443-1124
www.drugabuse.gov

Nora D. Volkow, Director

NIDA's mission is to lead the nation in bringing the power of science to bear drug abuse and addiction. The Institute operate's a toll-free hotline at the above number, with drug information and a nationwide alcohol and drug abuse treatmanet referral line.

Year Founded: 1887

5362 Nebraska Division of Alcoholism and Drug Abuse
Nebraska Department of Health & Human Services
301 Centennial Mall S
P.O. Box 94986
Lincoln, NE 68509-5026
402-471-7818
Fax: 402-471-7859
dhhs.ne.gov

Courtney N Phillips, Chief Executive Officer
Tom Williams, MD, Chief Medical Officer
Sheri Daweson, Director

Provides information on substance abuse prevention and treatment in the state of Nebraska.

5363 Nevada State Board of Examiners For Alcohol, Drug and Gambling Counselors
4600 Kietzke Lane
B-115
Reno, NV 89502
775-689-0563
Fax: 775-689-0564
agawronski@adgc.nv.gov
alcohol.nv.gov

Agata Gawronski, Executive Director
Darlene Dufault, President
Merlyn Sexton, Vice President

Mission is to reduce the impact of substance abuse in Nevada.

5364 New Jersey Division of Mental Health & Addiction Services
201 S Shore Road
Northfield, NJ 08225
609-645-5932
widitz_robert@aclink.org
www.nj.gov/health

Robert Widitz, Director

Provides information and support for prevention and treatment services for alcohol, tobacco and other drugs in New Jersey.

5365 New Mexico Behavioral Health Services
New Mexico Human Services Department
P.O. Box 2348
Santa Fe, NM 87504-2348
505-476-9266
Fax: 505-476-9277
www.hsd.state.nm.us/bhsd

Wayne Lindstrom, Director

To address need, services, planning, monitoring and continuous quality systemically across the state.

5366 New York State Office of Alcoholism and Substance Abuse Services
1450 Western Avenue
Albany, NY 12203-3526
518-473-3460
www.oasas.ny.gov

Arlene Gonzalez-Sanchez, Commissioner

To improve the lives of all New Yorkers by leading a comprehensive premier system of addiction services for prevention, treatment, and recovery.

5367 North Carolina Division of Mental Health, Developmental Disabilities and Abuse Services
Department of Human Resources
2001 Mail Service Center
Raleigh, NC 27699-2001
919-733-7011
contactdmh@dhhs.nc.gov
www.ncdhhs.gov

Providing quality support to achieve self-determination for individuals with intellectual and or developmental disabilities and quality services to promote treatment and recovery for individuals with mental illness and substance use disorders.

5368 North Dakota Mental Health & Substance Abuse
1237 W Divide Avenue
Suite 1C
Bismarck, ND 58501-1208
701-328-8920
Fax: 701-328-8969; *Toll Free:* 800-755-2719
dhsbhd@nd.gov
www.nd.gov

Provides information on substance abuse prevention and treatment in the state of North Dakota.

5369 Office of Women, Children & Families Services
Substance Abuse & Mental Health Services Admin.
5600 Fishers Lane
Rockville, MD 20857
Toll Free: 877-726-4727
www.samhsa.gov
TTY: 800-487-4889

Provides leadership and guidance in creating and maintaining an agency-wide focus for addressing the substance abuse and mental health needs of women, children, and family units.

Year Founded: 1992

5370 Office on Smoking and Health
Centers for Disease Control and Prevention
4770 Bufford Highway NE
Atlanta, GA 30341-3717
Toll Free: 800-232-4636
tobaccoinfo@cdc.gov
www.cdc.gov
TTY: 888-232-6348

Anne Schuchat, MD, Acting Director
Stephen C Redd, Deputy Director

Offers reference services to researchers through the Technical Information Center. Publishes and distributes a number of titles in the field of smoking and health.

Year Founded: 1965

5371 Oklahoma Department of Mental Health and Substance Abuse Services
2000 N Classen Boulevard
Suite E600
Oklahoma City, OK 73106
405-522-3908
Fax: 405-548-9321; *Toll Free:* 800-985-5990
boardmembers@odmhsas.org
www.odmhsas.org

Brian Bush, Chair

Provides information, assistant programs and other services to persons struggling with mental health and substance abuse in the state of Oklahoma.

5372 Oregon Alcohol and Drug Policy Commission
Department of Human Services
500 Summer Street NE
E-15
Salem, OR 97301
503-378-5796
rem.nivens@oregon.gov
www.oregon.gov/adpc
TTY: 503-945-6214

Rem Nivens, Executive Director

The Alcohol and Drug Policy Commission is an independent state government agency that was created by the Oregon Legislature to improve the effectiveness and efficiency of state and local alcohol and drug abuse prevention and treatment services.

5373 Partnership for a Drug-Free America
352 Park Avenue S
9th Floor
New York, NY 10010
212-922-1560
Fax: 212-922-1570; *Toll Free:* 855-378-4373
www.drugfree.org

Fred Muench, PhD, President & CEO
Andrea Castiello, Development Manager
Gina Samson, Chief Financial Officer

Committed to helping families whose son or daughter is struggling with substance use by empowering families with information, support and guidance to get the help their loved one needs and deserves.

5374 Pennsylvania Drug and Alcohol Programs
P.O. Box 60769
Harrisburg, PA 17106

717-526-1010
Fax: 717-526-1020
www.pacdaa.org

Cheryl Andrews, Chair
April Brown, Vice Chair
Michele Denk, Executive Director

The Pennsylvania Association of County Drug and Alcohol Administrators (PACDAA) is a professional association that represents the Single County Authorities (SCAs) across the commonwealth who receive state and federal dollars through contracts with the Department of Drug and Alcohol Programs (DDAP), to plan, coordinate, programmatically and fiscally manage and implement the delivery of drug and alcohol prevention, intervention, and treatment services at the local level.

Year Founded: 1972

5375 Phoenix House
Toll Free: 888-671-9392
www.phoenixhouse.org

Phoenix House is committed to serving those persons, families, and communities whose lives are threatened, disrupted, or otherwise burdened by addiction and related behavioral concerns.

Year Founded: 1977

5376 Pride Institute
14400 Martin Drive
Eden Prairie, MN 55344
952-353-5929
Fax: 952-934-8764; *Toll Free:* 800-547-7433
www.pride-institute.com

Rick Pliszka, Chief Executive Officer
J Heinz, Admissions Counselor
Angi Grassley, Community Relations Director

An inpatient treatment center run by and for gay men and lesbians with addiction problems. The program lasts one month and has a Twelve-Step orientation.

5377 SAMHSA Prevention of Substance Abuse and Mental Illness
Substance Abuse & Mental Health Services Admin.
5600 Fishers Lane
Rockville, MD 20857
Toll Free: 877-726-4727
www.samhsa.gov

Frances M Harding, Director
Gregory Goldstein, Deputy Director

Promotes, monitors, evaluates and coordinates programs for the prevention and treatment of alcoholism and alcohol abuse.

Year Founded: 1992

5378 SMART Recovery
Cambridge Health Alliance
195 Canal Street
1st Floor, Conference Room A/B
Malden, MA 02148
508-878-2291
www.challiance.org

Gail Cardelle, Contact

SMART Recovery is a science-based program and addresses all kinds of addictive behaviors using a four point cognitive approach: building and maintaining motivation,

coping with urges, managing thoughts, feelings and behaviors and living a balanced life. Meetings are held every Friday afternoon from noon to 1 p.m. at the CHA Malden Care Center.

5379 South Carolina Department of Alcohol & Other Drug Abuse Services
1801 Main Street
4th Floor
Columbia, SC 29201
803-896-5555
Fax: 803-896-5557
mtaylor@daodas.sc.gov
www.daodas.sc.gov

Sara Goldsby, Interim Director
Mitchell Taylor, Administrative Coordinator
Joseph Shenkar, Legal Counsel

The mission of DAODAS is to ensure the availability and quality of substance use services, improving the health status, safety, and quality of life of individuals, families, and communities across South Carolina.

5380 State University of New York at Buffalo Toxicology Research Center
3435 Main Street
Cary Room 15
Buffalo, NY 14214
716-829-2125
Fax: 716-829-2806
www.smbs.buffalo.edu/CENTERS/trc/

Paul J Kostyniak PhD, Director
James R. Olson, PhD, Associate Director

Toxicology-related research and services, including the development of tests to evaluate toxins, chemicals and drugs.

5381 Substance Abuse & Mental Health Services Administration
5600 Fishers Lane
Rockville, MD 20857
Toll Free: 877-726-4727
www.samhsa.gov

Michael E Etzinger, Executive Officer
Frances M Harding, Director
Marla Hedriksson, Director, Communications

Mission is to reduce the impact of substance abuse and mental illness on American communities.

Year Founded: 1992

5382 Susbstance Use Disorder Program, Policy and Fiscal Division
Department of Health Care Services
1501 Capitol Avenue, MS 4000
P.O. Box 997413
Sacramento, CA 95899-7413
Toll Free: 877-685-8333
www.dhcs.ca.gov

Jennifer Kent, Director

Directs prevention and treatment programs that address substance use disorders (SUD). Its core functions include developing and implementing SUD prevention strategies, reviewing and approving county SUD treatment program contracts, and granting applications submitted for state and federal funds for SUD services.

5383 Tennessee Prescription Drug Overdose Program
Tennessee Department of Health
710 James Robertson Parkway
Nashville, TN 37243
615-741-5735
Fax: 615-532-5369; *Toll Free:* 800-889-9789
tn.health@tn.gov
www.tn.gov/health

Melissa L McPheeters, PhD, Dir., Informatics & Analytics

This program is designed to combat the prescription drug overdose epidemic through education, research and communication.

5384 Texas of Mental Health & Substance Abuse Division
Texas Department of State Health Services
P.O. Box 149347
Mail Code 2053
Austin, TX 78714-9347
512-776-7111Toll free: 866-378-8440
customer.service@dshs.texas.gov
dshs.texas.gov

John William Hellerstedt, Commissioner

To improve health and well-being in Texas by providing leadership and services that promote hope, build resilience, and foster recovery.

Year Founded: 2004

5385 The Council on Alcohol and Drugs
270 Peachtree Street NW
Suite 2200
Atlanta, GA 30303-1283
404-223-2480
cwade@livedrugfree.org
www.livedrugfree.org

Chuck Wade, Executive Director & CEO
Scott E Yost, Director of Operations
Gregg G Raduka, Dir., Prevention/Intervention

The Council on Alcohol and Drugs is a substance abuse prevention and education agency that develops programs and resource material based on research on drug use and its impact on community.

Year Founded: 1969

5386 Utah Department of Human Services: Substance Abuse and Mental Health
195 North 1950 West
Salt Lake City, UT 84116
801-538-3939
Fax: 801-538-9892
dsamh@utah.gov
dsamh.utah.gov

Doug Thomas, Director
Lana Stohl, Deputy Director
Kyle Larson, Administrative Director

Oversees publicly funded prevention and treatment services through locally designed programs throughout Utah.

5387 Vermont Office of Alcohol & Drug Abuse Programs: Agency of Human Services
Vermont Department of Health
108 Cherry Street
Room 202
Burlington, VT 05402-0070
802-651-1550
AHS.VDHADAP@vermont.gov
healthvermont.gov

Mark Levine, MD, Commissioner
Tracy Dolan, Deputy Health Commissioner

Provides resources to those suffering from substance abuse across Vermont.

5388 Virginia Division of Substance Abuse Services
Department of Mental Health and Mental Retardation
1220 Bank Street
Richmond, VA 23219
804-786-3921
Fax: 804-371-6638
mellie.randall@dbhds.virginia.gov
www.dbhds.virginia.gov
TDD 804-371-8977

Mellie Randall, Administrator

In collaboration with its state and community partners, DBHDS plans, develops, directs, funds and monitors the delivery of comprehensive substance abuse services throughout the Commonwealth of Virginia.

5389 WFS' New Life Program
Women For Sobriety
P.O. Box 618
Quakertown, PA 18951
215-536-8026
Fax: 215-538-9026
contact@womenforsobriety.org
www.womenforsobriety.org

Karen Hamm, President
Rebecca Fenner, Director
Wendy Davis, Treasurer

A self-help program for women that can be used independent from AA or with AA. Groups are in many states in the United States.

Year Founded: 1975

5390 Washington Division of Alcoholism & Substance Abuse
Washington Department of Social & Mental Health
Toll Free: 877-501-2233
www.dshs.wa.gov

Robin Arnold-Williams, Secretary
Tracy Guerin, Chief Of Staff

Provide a basic overview of alcohol/substance abuse system and guidelines to assist in determining if a client is in need of alcohol or substance abuse treatment.

5391 West Virginia Division of Alcohol and Drug Abuse
WV Bureau for Behavioral Health
350 Capitol Street
Room 350
Charleston, WV 25301

304-356-4811
Fax: 304-558-1008
www.dhhr.wv.gov/bhhf

Nancy Sullivan, Commissioner

Responsible for prevention, control, treatment, rehabilitation, educational research and planning for substance abuse related services.

5392 Wisconsin Bureau of Substance Abuse Services
Wisconsin Department of Health Services
1 West Wilson Street
Madison, WI 53703
608-266-9485
scott.stokes@wi.gov
www.dhs.wisconsin.gov/substabuse
TTY: 800-947-3529

Scott Stokes, Contact

Privodes resources and treatment services for persons suffering of substance abuse problems.

5393 Women for Sobriety
P.O. Box 618
Quakertown, PA 18951
215-536-8026
Fax: 215-538-9026
contact@womenforsobriety.org
www.womenforsobriety.org

Karen Hamm, President
Rebecca Fenner, Director
Wendy Davis, Treasurer

A national organization with local units that address the specific needs of women with alcohol-related problems.

Year Founded: 1975

5394 Workplace Program
Substance Abuse & Mental Health Services Admin.
5600 Fishers Lane
Rockville, MD 20857
Toll Free: 877-726-4727
www.samhsa.gov

Ron Flegel, Director

This program sets standards for drug testing in workplace settings.

Year Founded: 1992

5395 Wyoming Behavioral Health Division
Wyoming Department of Health
6101 Yellowstone Road
Suite 220
Cheyenne, WY 82002
307-777-6494
Fax: 307-777-5849; *Toll Free:* 800-535-4006
health.wyo.gov/behavioralhealth

Chris Newman, Administrator

Oversees programs and grants for communities to provide outpatient and regional mental health and substance use treatment services and supports, including Court Supervised Treatment programs, that are accessible, affordable and provided in the least restrictive and most appropriate environment.

Books

5396 A Resource Guide for Drug Management Programs for Older Persons
Administration on Aging

Marjorie Bogaert-Tullis, Author

5397 Addiction and Responsibility
Crossroad Publishing Company
370 Lexington Avenue
New York, NY 10017-6503
212-532-3650
Fax: 212-532-4922; *Toll Free:* 800-395-

Anyone who has wrestled with such basic questions about addiction such as: Is drug addiction a behavior disorder or a character flaw? Is it genetic or learned? What is it like to be addicted? will find welcome answers in this groundbreaking philosophical inquiry into the addictive mind. The author helps readers understand addiction.

192 pages

5398 Addictions Counseling
Crossroad Publishing Company
370 Lexington Avenue
New York, NY 10017-6503
212-532-3650
Fax: 212-532-4922; *Toll Free:* 800-395-

A practical guide to counseling people with chemical and other addictions.

144 pages

5399 Addictive Personality
Hazelden
15251 Pleasant Valley Road
PO Box 11
Center City, MN 55012-0011
651-213-4200
Fax: 651-213-4793; *Toll Free:* 800-257-7810
info@hazelden.org
www.hazelden.org

Mark Mishek, President & CEO
James A. Blaha, Vice President
Sharon Birnbaum, Corporate Director

Understanding how an individual becomes an addict through examination of addiction's causes, stages of development, and consequences. Second edition further refines these ideas and includes the most recent information on the addictive process, cultural influences on addictive behaviors, recovery, genetic factors in addiction, mental health issues, and new research findings.

130 pages Year Founded: 1947

5400 Addictive Thinking Understanding Self-Deception
Hazelden
15251 Pleasant Valley Road
PO Box 11
Center City, MN 55012-0011
651-213-4200
Fax: 651-213-4793; *Toll Free:* 800-257-7810
info@hazelden.org
www.hazelden.org

Mark Mishek, President & CEO
James A. Blaha, Vice President
Sharon Birnbaum, Corporate Director

Illustrates the irrational perspective and complicated, contradictory thinking patterns of addictive thinking, and demonstrates how they lead to low self-esteen, addiction, and relapse. Revised edition includes expanded information on depression and affective disorders, the relationship between addictive thinking and relapse, and the new research related to the origins of addictive thinking.

140 pages Year Founded: 1947

5401 Al-Anon Family Groups - Classic Edition
Al-Anon Family Group Headquarters
1600 Corporate Landing Parkway
Virginia Beach, VA 23454-5617
757-563-1600
Fax: 757-563-1655; *Toll Free:* 800-356-9996
wso@al-anon.org
www.al-anon.alateen.org

Basic book that explains the purpose of fellowship, how it works and how it is held in unity. Includes real life stories by husbands, wives, parents and children of those who suffer from alcoholism.

177 pages

5402 Alcoholics Anonymous, The Big Book
Hazelden
15251 Pleasant Valley Road
PO Box 11
Center City, MN 55012-0011
651-213-4200
Fax: 651-213-4793; *Toll Free:* 800-257-7810
info@hazelden.org
www.hazelden.org

Mark Mishek, President & CEO
James A. Blaha, Vice President
Sharon Birnbaum, Corporate Director

Classic text that guides Alcoholics Anonymous programs and describes how millions of men and women have recovered from alcoholism.

575 pages Year Founded: 1947

5403 Blueprint for Progress: Al-Anon's Fourth Step Inventory
Al-Anon Family Group Headquarters
1600 Corporate Landing Parkway
Virginia Beach, VA 23454-5617
757-563-1600
Fax: 757-563-1655; *Toll Free:* 800-356-9996
wso@al-anon.org
www.al-anon.alateen.org

A practical guide in taking the Fourth Step. Shows the way toward becoming self-nurturing while making a fearless moral search of ourselves.

64 pages

5404 Body, Mind and Spirit
Hazelden
15251 Pleasant Valley Road
PO Box 11
Center City, MN 55012-0011
651-213-4200
Fax: 651-213-4793; *Toll Free:* 800-257-7810

info@hazelden.org
www.hazelden.org

Mark Mishek, President & CEO
James A. Blaha, Vice President
Sharon Birnbaum, Corporate Director

Addressing such issues as self-esteem, fear, anger, and spirituality, these 366 daily meditations and affirmations integrate the physical, mental, and spiritual aspects of healing from addiction.

410 pages Year Founded: 1947

5405 Came to Believe
Alcoholics Anonymous
PO Box 459
Grand Central Station
New York, NY 10163
212-870-3400
Fax: 212-870-3137
www.aa.org

Greg Muth, Manager

A collection of stories by AA members who write about what the phrase spiritual awakening means to them.

120 pages Year Founded: 1950

5406 Concepts of Chemical Dependency, Third Edition
Brooks/Cole Publishing Company
511 Forest Lodge Road
Pacific Grove, CA 93950-5040
408-373-0728
Fax: 408-375-6414
bc-info@brookscole.com
www.cengage.co.in

A useful introduction to the basics of chemical dependency focusing on one substance at a time as it presents the facts about the most common chemicals of abuse and their effects.

473 pages

5407 Day at a Time Daily Reflections for Recovering People
Hazelden
15251 Pleasant Valley Road
PO Box 11
Center City, MN 55012-0011
651-213-4200
Fax: 651-213-4793; *Toll Free:* 800-257-7810
info@hazelden.org
www.hazelden.org

Mark Mishek, President & CEO
James A. Blaha, Vice President
Sharon Birnbaum, Corporate Director

Offers inspiration and hope for people recovering from chemical dependency or other addictions. Each daily passage reinforces the message of Twelve Step recovery.

384 pages Year Founded: 1947

5408 Day by Day
Hazelden
15251 Pleasant Valley Road
PO Box 11
Center City, MN 55012-0011
651-213-4200
Fax: 651-213-4793; *Toll Free:* 800-257-7810

info@hazelden.org
www.hazelden.org

Mark Mishek, President & CEO
James A. Blaha, Vice President
Sharon Birnbaum, Corporate Director

A book of daily meditations for recovering addicts that reinforce Narcotics Anonymous principles and objectives.

400 pages Year Founded: 1947

5409 Dual Disorders Recovery Book
Hazelden
15251 Pleasant Valley Road
PO Box 11
Center City, MN 55012-0011
651-213-4200
Fax: 651-213-4793; *Toll Free:* 800-257-7810
info@hazelden.org
www.hazelden.org

Mark Mishek, President & CEO
James A. Blaha, Vice President
Sharon Birnbaum, Corporate Director

Helps individuals with dual disorders develop a plan for daily living through a specially designed Twelve-Step program.

242- pages Year Founded: 1947

5410 Each Day a New Beginning
Hazelden
15251 Pleasant Valley Road
PO Box 11
Center City, MN 55012-0011
651-213-4200
Fax: 651-213-4793; *Toll Free:* 800-257-7810
info@hazelden.org
www.hazelden.org

Mark Mishek, President & CEO
James A. Blaha, Vice President
Sharon Birnbaum, Corporate Director

Promotes the development of a significant spiritual core for recovery that can be enhanced throughout the rest of the victims lives.

400 pages Year Founded: 1947

5411 Eye Opener
Hazelden
15251 Pleasant Valley Road
PO Box 11
Center City, MN 55012-0011
651-213-4200
Fax: 651-213-4793; *Toll Free:* 800-257-7810
info@hazelden.org
www.hazelden.org

Mark Mishek, President & CEO
James A. Blaha, Vice President
Sharon Birnbaum, Corporate Director

Daily meditations about understanding the Alcoholics Anonymous program, writen by a favorite early AA member and author.

380 pages Year Founded: 1947

5412 Gentle Path Through the Twelve Steps
Hazelden
15251 Pleasant Valley Road
PO Box 11
Center City, MN 55012-0011
651-213-4200
Fax: 651-213-4793; *Toll Free:* 800-257-7810
info@hazelden.org
www.hazelden.org

Mark Mishek, President & CEO
James A. Blaha, Vice President
Sharon Birnbaum, Corporate Director

This workbook provides a unique set of structured forms and exercises to help recovering people integrate the Twelve Steps into all aspects of their lives.

224- pages Year Founded: 1947

5413 Getting Started in AA
Hazelden
15251 Pleasant Valley Road
PO Box 11
Center City, MN 55012-0011
651-213-4200
Fax: 651-213-4793; *Toll Free:* 800-257-7810
info@hazelden.org
www.hazelden.org

Mark Mishek, President & CEO
James A. Blaha, Vice President
Sharon Birnbaum, Corporate Director

Practical suggestions for staying sober, summaries of AA principles, concepts and slogans, and a historical overview to help the reader understand the spirit of the program.

211- pages Year Founded: 1947

5414 God Grant Me the Laughter: A Treasury of Twelve Step Humor
Hazelden
15251 Pleasant Valley Road
PO Box 11
Center City, MN 55012-0011
651-213-4200
Fax: 651-213-4793; *Toll Free:* 800-257-7810
info@hazelden.org
www.hazelden.org

Mark Mishek, President & CEO
James A. Blaha, Vice President
Sharon Birnbaum, Corporate Director

Hearty cartoons and humorous anecdotes clearly demonstrate how readers' lives today contrast with their drinking and drug using in the past.

200- pages Year Founded: 1947

5415 Good First Step
Hazelden
15251 Pleasant Valley Road
PO Box 11
Center City, MN 55012-0011
651-213-4200
Fax: 651-213-4793; *Toll Free:* 800-257-7810
info@hazelden.org
www.hazelden.org

Mark Mishek, President & CEO
James A. Blaha, Vice President
Sharon Birnbaum, Corporate Director

Features a structured format and emphasis on the meaning of the First Step to help build a solid foundation for recovery.

60 - pages Year Founded: 1947

5416 Grateful to Have Been There
Hazelden
15251 Pleasant Valley Road
PO Box 11
Center City, MN 55012-0011
651-213-4200
Fax: 651-213-4793; *Toll Free:* 800-257-7810
info@hazelden.org
www.hazelden.org

Mark Mishek, President & CEO
James A. Blaha, Vice President
Sharon Birnbaum, Corporate Director

Aide and executive secretary to AA's co-founder, Bill W. for 20 years, Wing shares her memories and impressions of 42 years of involvement with the Fellowship.

150 pages Year Founded: 1947

5417 How Al-Anon Works for Families & Friends of Alcoholics
Al-Anon Family Group Headquarters
1600 Corporate Landing Parkway
Virginia Beach, VA 23454-5617
757-563-1600
Fax: 757-563-1655; *Toll Free:* 800-356-9996
wso@al-anon.org
www.al-anon.alateen.org

Everything you wanted to know about Al-Anon and more. This is the one book that has it all.

400 pages

5418 I'm Black and I'm Sober
Hazelden
15251 Pleasant Valley Road
PO Box 11
Center City, MN 55012-0011
651-213-4200
Fax: 651-213-4793; *Toll Free:* 800-257-7810
info@hazelden.org
www.hazelden.org

Mark Mishek, President & CEO
James A. Blaha, Vice President
Sharon Birnbaum, Corporate Director

An autobiography written by a recovering African American woman who discusses the impact of discrimination and the obstacles faced through the journey back to sobriety.

279 pages Year Founded: 1947

5419 In God's Care
Hazelden
15251 Pleasant Valley Road
PO Box 11
Center City, MN 55012-0011
651-213-4200
Fax: 651-213-4793; *Toll Free:* 800-257-7810
info@hazelden.org
www.hazelden.org

Mark Mishek, President & CEO
James A. Blaha, Vice President
Sharon Birnbaum, Corporate Director

Excellent relaxation and education tool for clients working on their Second and Third Steps.

400- pages Year Founded: 1947

5420 Keep It Simple
Hazelden
15251 Pleasant Valley Road
PO Box 11
Center City, MN 55012-0011
651-213-4200
Fax: 651-213-4793; *Toll Free:* 800-257-7810
info@hazelden.org
www.hazelden.org

Mark Mishek, President & CEO
James A. Blaha, Vice President
Sharon Birnbaum, Corporate Director

Daily prayers that help clients learn to ask for help and to turn their self-will over to a Higher Power.

400- pages Year Founded: 1947

5421 Keep Quit
Hazelden
15251 Pleasant Valley Road
PO Box 11
Center City, MN 55012-0011
651-213-4200
Fax: 651-213-4793; *Toll Free:* 800-257-7810
info@hazelden.org
www.hazelden.org

Mark Mishek, President & CEO
James A. Blaha, Vice President
Sharon Birnbaum, Corporate Director

Daily motivational guide to help the new nonsmoker understand the craving for nicotine and learn how to break the rituals and patterns associated with relapse.

300 pages Year Founded: 1947

5422 Life of My Own: Daily Meditations on Hope and Acceptance
Hazelden
15251 Pleasant Valley Road
PO Box 11
Center City, MN 55012-0011
651-213-4200
Fax: 651-213-4793; *Toll Free:* 800-257-7810
info@hazelden.org
www.hazelden.org

Mark Mishek, President & CEO
James A. Blaha, Vice President
Sharon Birnbaum, Corporate Director

Offers daily access to strength, serenity and insight in our relationships with chemically dependent people.

400- pages Year Founded: 1947

5423 Little Red Book
Hazelden
15251 Pleasant Valley Road
PO Box 11
Center City, MN 55012-0011
651-213-4200
Fax: 651-213-4793; *Toll Free:* 800-257-7810
info@hazelden.org
www.hazelden.org

Mark Mishek, President & CEO
James A. Blaha, Vice President
Sharon Birnbaum, Corporate Director

A primer for members of Alcoholics Anonymous. Each page acts as a study guide to the Big Book and its teachings.

164 pages Year Founded: 1947

5424 Living Sober
Hazelden
15251 Pleasant Valley Road
PO Box 11
Center City, MN 55012-0011
651-213-4200
Fax: 651-213-4793; Toll Free: 800-257-7810
info@hazelden.org
www.hazelden.org

Mark Mishek, President & CEO
James A. Blaha, Vice President
Sharon Birnbaum, Corporate Director

Offers clients sound advice about how to stay sober.

88 pages Year Founded: 1947

5425 Lois Remembers
Al-Anon Family Group Headquarters
1600 Corporate Landing Parkway
Virginia Beach, VA 23454-5617
757-563-1600
Fax: 757-563-1655; Toll Free: 800-356-9996
wso@al-anon.org
www.al-anon.alateen.org

The memoirs of a co-founder of Al-Anon. Lois tells her personal story and recalls the eventful years before and after the funding of AA and Al-Anon.

204 pages

5426 My Mind is Out to Get Me: Humor and Wisdom in Recovery
Hazelden
15251 Pleasant Valley Road
PO Box 11
Center City, MN 55012-0011
651-213-4200
Fax: 651-213-4793; Toll Free: 800-257-7810
info@hazelden.org
www.hazelden.org

Mark Mishek, President & CEO
James A. Blaha, Vice President
Sharon Birnbaum, Corporate Director

500 inspirational sayings and slogans that reflect both the lighter side of living a sober life and the profound wisdom offered in recovery. Each quote has been drawn from the wisdom of Alcoholics Anonymous.

180 pages Year Founded: 1947

5427 Narcotics Anonymous
Hazelden
15251 Pleasant Valley Road
PO Box 11
Center City, MN 55012-0011
651-213-4200
Fax: 651-213-4793; Toll Free: 800-257-7810
info@hazelden.org
www.hazelden.org

Mark Mishek, President & CEO
James A. Blaha, Vice President
Sharon Birnbaum, Corporate Director

Men and women describe the N.A. program and how it works.

289 pages Year Founded: 1947

5428 One Day at a Time in Al-Anon
Al-Anon Family Group Headquarters
1600 Corporate Landing Parkway
Virginia Beach, VA 23454-5617
757-563-1600
Fax: 757-563-1655; Toll Free: 800-356-9996
wso@al-anon.org
www.al-anon.alateen.org

Inspirational daily readings cover various aspects of the Al-Anon philosophy and relate it to everyday situations. Large print.

376 pages

5429 Passages Through Recovery
Hazelden
15251 Pleasant Valley Road
PO Box 11
Center City, MN 55012-0011
651-213-4200
Fax: 651-213-4793; Toll Free: 800-257-7810
info@hazelden.org
www.hazelden.org

Mark Mishek, President & CEO
James A. Blaha, Vice President
Sharon Birnbaum, Corporate Director

Guides clients through the six stages of recovery.

130- pages Year Founded: 1947

5430 Program for You
Hazelden
15251 Pleasant Valley Road
PO Box 11
Center City, MN 55012-0011
651-213-4200
Fax: 651-213-4793; Toll Free: 800-257-7810
info@hazelden.org
www.hazelden.org

Mark Mishek, President & CEO
James A. Blaha, Vice President
Sharon Birnbaum, Corporate Director

Study guide interpreting the original AA program as described in Alcoholics Anonymous and helps apply the wisdom to everyday life.

183 pages Year Founded: 1947

5431 Quit & Stay Quit: A Personal Program to Stop Smoking
Hazelden
15251 Pleasant Valley Road
PO Box 11
Center City, MN 55012-0011
651-213-4200
Fax: 651-213-4793; Toll Free: 800-257-7810
info@hazelden.org
www.hazelden.org

Mark Mishek, President & CEO
James A. Blaha, Vice President
Sharon Birnbaum, Corporate Director

Guide to nicotine recovery offerring an effective long-term program to quit by showing readers how smoking has subtly shaped their values, attitudes, and lives.

196 pages Year Founded: 1947

5432 Quit Smoking Manual
American Lung Association
55 W. Wacker Drive
Suite 1150
Chicago, IL 60601
212-315-8700
Fax: 202-452-1805
www.lung.org

Ross P. Lanzafame, Chair
Kathryn A. Forbes, Vice Chair
Harold Wimmer, President and CEO

Original self-help smoking cessation manual showing the public how to quit smoking in 20 days.

64 pages

5433 Recovery Journal for Exploring Who I Am
Hazelden
15251 Pleasant Valley Road
PO Box 11
Center City, MN 55012-0011
651-213-4200
Fax: 651-213-4793; Toll Free: 800-257-7810
info@hazelden.org
www.hazelden.org

Mark Mishek, President & CEO
James A. Blaha, Vice President
Sharon Birnbaum, Corporate Director

Introduces clients to journal writing as an effective therapeutic adjunct for addiction recovery.

48 pages Year Founded: 1947

5434 Shame Faced
Hazelden
15251 Pleasant Valley Road
PO Box 11
Center City, MN 55012-0011
651-213-4200
Fax: 651-213-4793; Toll Free: 800-257-7810
info@hazelden.org
www.hazelden.org

Mark Mishek, President & CEO
James A. Blaha, Vice President
Sharon Birnbaum, Corporate Director

Discusses the relationship between shame and chemical dependency.

28 - pages Year Founded: 1947

5435 Skeptic's Guide to the Twelve Steps
Hazelden
15251 Pleasant Valley Road
PO Box 11
Center City, MN 55012-0011
651-213-4200
Fax: 651-213-4793; Toll Free: 800-257-7810
info@hazelden.org
www.hazelden.org

Mark Mishek, President & CEO
James A. Blaha, Vice President
Sharon Birnbaum, Corporate Director

Investigates each of the Twelve Steps to gain a deeper understanding of a Higher Power.

241- pages Year Founded: 1947

5436 Sober But Stuck
Hazelden
15251 Pleasant Valley Road
PO Box 11
Center City, MN 55012-0011
651-213-4200
Fax: 651-213-4793; Toll Free: 800-257-7810
info@hazelden.org
www.hazelden.org

Mark Mishek, President & CEO
James A. Blaha, Vice President
Sharon Birnbaum, Corporate Director

Collection of personal stories by men and women who are long-time members of Alcoholics Anonymous. Each story shows the antidotes and resources which helped members break through the barriers that limited their enjoyment of a sober life.

215 pages Year Founded: 1947

5437 Social Policy Prevention Handbook
African American Family Services
2616 Nicollet Avenue
Minneapolis, MN 55408-1628
612-871-7878
Fax: 612-871-2567
www.aafs.net

Thomas Adams, Chief Executive Officer
Bernice Mack, Contact
Julie Jones, Manager

A manual that details IBCA's community based approach to the development of alcohol and drug abuse prevention strategies.

24 pages Year Founded: 1975

5438 Substance Abuse Intervention, Prevention, Rehabilitation and Systems Change
Columbia University Press
61 West 62nd Street
New York, NY 10023
212-459-0600
Fax: 800-351-5073; Toll Free: 800-343-4499
customer@wiley.com
www.cup.columbia.edu

Approach of social work practice with substance-abusing clients, bridging clinical, community, and social policy approaches in order to place individual addiction in its sociopolitical context.

Year Founded: 1893

5439 Turnabout
Women For Sobriety
PO Box 618
Quakertown, PA 18951
215-536-8026
Fax: 215-536-9026; Toll Free: 800-333-1606
WFSobriety@aol.com
www.womenforsobriety.org

This is the story of the founder of Women for Sobriety and her struggle to quit drinking.

183 pages

Directories

5440 National Conference on Drug Abuse Research & Practice
Substance Abuse & Mental Health Services Administr
1 Choke Cherry Road
Room 13C-05
Rockville, MD 20857
301-443-8956
Fax: 301-443-9050; *Toll Free:* 877-726-4727
dgoodman@samhsa.hhs.gov
www.samhsa.gov
TDD 800-487-4889

Pamela S. Hyde, Administrator
Kana Enomoto, Principal Deputy Administrator
Marla Hedriksson, Director

Offers summaries of workshops, forums, dinner speeches and sessions presented at the National Conference on Drug Abuse Research and Practice.

275 pages Year Founded: 1992

5441 National Directory of Drug and Alcohol Abuse Treatment and Programs
Office of Applied Studies
5600 Fishers Lane
Room 16-105
Rockville, MD 20857
301-443-0525
Fax: 301-443-9847; *Toll Free:* 800-662-4357
www.findtreatment.samhsa.gov
TDD 800-487-2889

Deborah Trunzo, DASIS Team Leader
Gerri Scott-Pinkney, DASIS Team

11,000 listings of substance abuse treatment facilities across the nation.

550 pages Frequency: Annual

Journals, Magazines

5442 ACAP Recap
American Council on Alcohol Problems
2376 Lakeside Drive
Birmingham, AL 35244
205-989-8177
Fax: 314-739-0848
sapacap.com

Mark Creech, President
Ed Wolkin, President-Elect
William E. Day, Executive Director

Offers information on organization activities and events, updates on resources and publications and legislative information for affiliate executives.

Year Founded: 1895

5443 American Issue
American Council on Alcohol Problems
2376 Lakeside Drive
Birmingham, AL 35244
205-989-8177
Fax: 314-739-0848
sapacap.com

Mark Creech, President
Ed Wolkin, President-Elect
William E. Day, Executive Director

Offered to contributors of the organization.

Year Founded: 1895

Newsletters, Pamphlets

5444 AA Member - Medications and Other Drugs
Alcoholics Anonymous
PO Box 459
Grand Central Station
New York, NY 10163
212-870-3400
Fax: 212-870-3137
www.aa.org

Greg Muth, Manager

Report from a group of doctors in Alcoholics Anonymous.

Year Founded: 1950

5445 AA Service Manual/Twelve Concepts for World Service
Alcoholics Anonymous
PO Box 459
Grand Central Station
New York, NY 10163
212-870-3400
Fax: 212-870-3137
www.aa.org

Gret Muth, Manager

This manual opens with a history of AA services.

Year Founded: 1950

5446 AA and the Armed Services
Alcoholics Anonymous
PO Box 459
Grand Central Station
New York, NY 10163
212-870-3400
Fax: 212-870-3137
www.aa.org

Greg Muth, Manager

Personal stories tell how men and women in the military can beat a drinking problem.

Year Founded: 1950

5447 AA and the Gay/Lesbian Alcoholic
Alcoholics Anonymous
PO Box 459
Grand Central Station
New York, NY 10163
212-870-3400
Fax: 212-870-3137
www.aa.org

Greg Muth, Manager

Excerpts from experience, strength and hope of sober gay and lesbian alcoholics.

Year Founded: 1950

5448 AA as a Resource for Health Care Professionals
Alcoholics Anonymous
PO Box 459
Grand Central Station
New York, NY 10163
212-870-3400
Fax: 212-870-3137
www.aa.org

Greg Muth, Manager

Information about the Fellowship and describes some approaches that health care professionals use in referring problem drinkers to AA.

Year Founded: 1950

5449 AA for the Native North American
Alcoholics Anonymous
PO Box 459
Grand Central Station
New York, NY 10163
212-870-3400
Fax: 212-870-3137
www.aa.org

Greg Muth, Manager

Addressed to and contains stories by Native American AA members.

Year Founded: 1950

5450 AA for the Woman
Alcoholics Anonymous
PO Box 459
Grand Central Station
New York, NY 10163
212-870-3400
Fax: 212-870-3137
www.aa.org

Greg Muth, Manager

Relates the experiences of alcoholic women, all ages and from all walks of life.

Year Founded: 1950

5451 AA in Correctional Facilities
Alcoholics Anonymous
PO Box 459
Grand Central Station
New York, NY 10163
212-870-3400
Fax: 212-870-3137
www.aa.org

Greg Muth, Manager

Experience based on the functioning of AA groups in prisons, with institutional opinions recommending AA as a helpful ally.

Year Founded: 1950

5452 AA in Treatment Facilities
Alcoholics Anonymous
PO Box 459
Grand Central Station
New York, NY 10163

212-870-3400
Fax: 212-870-3137
www.aa,org

Greg Muth, Manager

Shares experiences of treatment facility administrators and of AA's who have carried the message into these facilities.

Year Founded: 1950

5453 Al-Anon Fact File
Al-Anon Family Group Headquarters
1600 Corporate Landing Parkway
Virginia Beach, VA 23454-5617
757-563-1600
Fax: 757-563-1655; *Toll Free:* 800-356-9996
wso@al-anon.org
www.al-anon.alateen.org

Factual information for the general public, media, professional community and those working in the field of alcohol treatment.

16 pages

5454 Al-Anon Focus
Al-Anon Family Group Headquarters
1600 Corporate Landing Parkway
Virginia Beach, VA 23454-5617
757-427-0680
Fax: 757-563-1655; *Toll Free:* 800-356-9996
wso@al-anon.org
www.al-anon.alateen.org

Recovering alcoholics find help in Al-Anon.

6 pages

5455 Al-Anon Is for Men
Al-Anon Family Group Headquarters
1600 Corporate Landing Parkway
Virginia Beach, VA 23454-5617
757-563-1600
Fax: 757-563-1655; *Toll Free:* 800-356-9996
wso@al-anon.org
www.al-anon.alateen.org

Straightforward questions to help men identify their reactions to alcoholism in another person.

6 pages

5456 Al-Anon Newcomer Packet
Al-Anon Family Group Headquarters
1600 Corporate Landing Parkway
Virginia Beach, VA 23454-5617
757-563-1600
Fax: 757-563-1655; *Toll Free:* 800-356-9996
wso@al-anon.org
www.al-anon.alateen.org

Material specifically for the newcomer to Al-Anon packed in a handsome sleeve. Members can add local meeting information and literature of special interest.

8 pages

5457 Al-Anon Spoken Here
Al-Anon Family Group Headquarters
1600 Corporate Landing Parkway
Virginia Beach, VA 23454-5617
757-563-1600
Fax: 757-563-1655; *Toll Free:* 800-356-9996

wso@al-anon.org
www.al-anon.alateen.org

Why are Al-Anon meetings the way they are? Questions and answers that lead to a better understanding of the importance of keeping Al-Anon.

8 pages

5458 Al-Anon and Professionals
Al-Anon Family Group Headquarters
1600 Corporate Landing Parkway
Virginia Beach, VA 23454-5617
757-563-1600
Fax: 757-563-1655; *Toll Free:* 800-356-9996
wso@al-anon.org
www.al-anon.alateen.org

Questions and answers to help members and professionals learn how Al-Anon cooperates with the professional community.

5459 Al-Anon, Newcomer's Packet
Al-Anon Family Group Headquarters
1600 Corporate Landing Parkway
Virginia Beach, VA 23454-5617
757-563-1600
Fax: 757-563-1655; *Toll Free:* 800-356-9996
wso@al-anon.org
www.al-anon.alateen.org

Material specifically for the newcomer to Al-Anon packed in a handsome sleeve.

5460 Al-Anon, You, and the Alcoholic
Al-Anon Family Group Headquarters
1600 Corporate Landing Parkway
Virginia Beach, VA 23454-5617
757-563-1600
Fax: 757-563-1655; *Toll Free:* 800-356-9996
wso@al-anon.org
www.al-anon.alateen.org

Answers the most frequently asked questions about Al-Anon and how it helps families deal with problems brought about by alcoholism.

12 pages

5461 Alateen Talks Back on Higher Power
Al-Anon Family Group Headquarters
1600 Corporate Landing Parkway
Virginia Beach, VA 23454-5617
757-563-1600
Fax: 757-563-1655; *Toll Free:* 800-356-9996
wso@al-anon.org
www.al-anon.alateen.org

Members express views on the God of their understanding.

32 pages

5462 Alcohol Alert #11: Estimating the Cost of Alcohol Abuse
National Clearinghouse for Alcohol and Drug Info.
1 Choke Cherry Road
PO Box 2345
Rockville, MD 20857
301-468-2600
Fax: 301-468-2600; *Toll Free:* 877-726-4727
webmaster@samhsa.hhs.gov
beta.samhsa.gov

TDD 800-487-4889
TTY: 800-487-4889

Daryl W. Kade, Chief Financial Officer and Dire
Kana Enomoto, Principal Deputy Administrator
Pamela S. Hyde, Administrator

Discusses the various problems of estimating the cost of alcohol abuse.

Year Founded: 1992

5463 Alcohol Alert #15: Alcohol and AIDS
National Clearinghouse for Alcohol and Drug Info.
1 Choke Cherry Road
PO Box 2345
Rockville, MD 20857
301-468-2600
Fax: 301-468-2600; *Toll Free:* 877-726-4727
webmaster@samhsa.hhs.gov
beta.samhsa.gov
TDD 800-487-4889
TTY: 800-487-4889

Daryl W. Kade, Chief Financial Officer and Dire
Kana Enomoto, Principal Deputy Administrator
Pamela S. Hyde, Administrator

Discusses the relationship between alcohol consumption and HIV infection and AIDS.

Year Founded: 1992

5464 Alcohol Alert #16: Moderate Drinking
National Clearinghouse for Alcohol and Drug Info.
1 Choke Cherry Road
PO Box 2345
Rockville, MD 20857
301-468-2600
Fax: 301-468-2600; *Toll Free:* 877-726-4727
webmaster@samhsa.hhs.gov
beta.samhsa.gov
TDD 800-487-4889
TTY: 800-487-4889

Daryl W. Kade, Chief Financial Officer and Dire
Kana Enomoto, Principal Deputy Administrator
Pamela S. Hyde, Administrator

Defines moderate drinking and explores the benefits and risks associated with moderate drinking.

Year Founded: 1992

5465 Alcohol Alert #17: Treatment Outcome Research
National Clearinghouse for Alcohol and Drug Info.
1 Choke Cherry Road
PO Box 2345
Rockville, MD 20857
301-468-2600
Fax: 301-468-2600; *Toll Free:* 877-726-4727
webmaster@samhsa.hhs.gov
beta.samhsa.gov
TDD 800-487-4889
TTY: 800-487-4889

Daryl W. Kade, Chief Financial Officer and Dire
Kana Enomoto, Principal Deputy Administrator
Pamela S. Hyde, Administrator

Discusses purpose, methodology, randomization, blinding, followup and what treatment outcome research reveals.

Year Founded: 1992

5466 Alcohol Alert #18: The Genetics of Alcoholism
National Clearinghouse for Alcohol and Drug Info.
1 Choke Cherry Road
PO Box 2345
Rockville, MD 20857
301-468-2600
Fax: 301-468-2600; *Toll Free:* 877-726-4727
webmaster@samhsa.hhs.gov
beta.samhsa.gov
TDD 800-487-4889
TTY: 800-487-4889

Daryl W. Kade, Chief Financial Officer and Dire
Kana Enomoto, Principal Deputy Administrator
Pamela S. Hyde, Administrator

Presents the results of studies that investigate the role of genes and the environment in the development of alcoholism.

Year Founded: 1992

5467 Alcohol Alert #21: Alcohol and Cancer
National Clearinghouse for Alcohol and Drug Info.
1 Choke Cherry Road
PO Box 2345
Rockville, MD 20857
301-468-2600
Fax: 301-468-2600; *Toll Free:* 877-726-4727
webmaster@samhsa.hhs.gov
beta.samhsa.gov
TDD 800-487-4889
TTY: 800-487-4889

Daryl W. Kade, Chief Financial Officer and Dire
Kana Enomoto, Principal Deputy Administrator
Pamela S. Hyde, Administrator

Year Founded: 1992

5468 Alcohol Alert #23: Alcohol and Minorities
National Clearinghouse for Alcohol and Drug Info.
1 Choke Cherry Road
PO Box 2345
Rockville, MD 20857
301-468-2600
Fax: 301-468-2600; *Toll Free:* 877-726-4727
webmaster@samhsa.hhs.gov
beta.samhsa.gov
TDD 800-487-4889
TTY: 800-487-4889

Daryl W. Kade, Chief Financial Officer and Dire
Kana Enomoto, Principal Deputy Administrator
Pamela S. Hyde, Administrator

Year Founded: 1992

5469 Alcohol Alert #24: Animal Models in Alcohol
Research
National Clearinghouse for Alcohol and Drug Info.
1 Choke Cherry Road
PO Box 2345
Rockville, MD 20857
301-468-2600
Fax: 301-468-2600; *Toll Free:* 877-726-4727
webmaster@samhsa.hhs.gov
beta.samhsa.gov
TDD 800-487-4889
TTY: 800-487-4889

Daryl W. Kade, Chief Financial Officer and Dire
Kana Enomoto, Principal Deputy Administrator
Pamela S. Hyde, Administrator
Year Founded: 1992

5470 Alcohol Alert #25: Alcohol-Related Impairment
National Clearinghouse for Alcohol and Drug Info.
1 Choke Cherry Road
PO Box 2345
Rockville, MD 20857
301-468-2600
Fax: 301-468-2600; *Toll Free:* 877-726-4727
webmaster@samhsa.hhs.gov
beta.samhsa.gov
TDD 800-487-4889
TTY: 800-487-4889

Daryl W. Kade, Chief Financial Officer and Dire
Kana Enomoto, Principal Deputy Administrator
Pamela S. Hyde, Administrator

Year Founded: 1992

5471 Alcohol Alert #26: Alcohol and Hormones
National Clearinghouse for Alcohol and Drug Info.
1 Choke Cherry Road
PO Box 2345
Rockville, MD 20857
301-468-2600
Fax: 301-468-2600; *Toll Free:* 877-726-4727
webmaster@samhsa.hhs.gov
beta.samhsa.gov
TDD 800-487-4889
TTY: 800-487-4889

Daryl W. Kade, Chief Financial Officer and Dire
Kana Enomoto, Principal Deputy Administrator
Pamela S. Hyde, Administrator

Year Founded: 1992

5472 Alcohol Alert #27: Alcohol Medication
Interactions
National Clearinghouse for Alcohol and Drug Info.
1 Choke Cherry Road
PO Box 2345
Rockville, MD 20857
301-468-2600
Fax: 301-468-2600; *Toll Free:* 877-726-4727
webmaster@samhsa.hhs.gov
beta.samhsa.gov
TDD 800-487-4889
TTY: 800-487-4889

Daryl W. Kade, Chief Financial Officer and Dire
Kana Enomoto, Principal Deputy Administrator
Pamela S. Hyde, Administrator

Year Founded: 1992

5473 Alcohol and Drug Abuse in Black America: A
Guide for Community Action
African American Family Services
310 Groveland Avenue South
Suites 1 & 7
Minneapolis, MN 55403
612-813-5034
Fax: 651-925-0044
www.aafs.net

Thomas Adams, Chief Executive Officer
Bernice Mack, Contact
Julie Jones, Manager

A booklet giving a description of the history and the current manifestations of alcohol and drug problems in Black America with a discussion of strategies for fundamental change.

24 pages Year Founded: 1975

5474 Alcoholics Anonymous and Employee Assistance Program
Alcoholics Anonymous
Grand Central Station
PO Box 459
New York, NY 10163
212-870-3400
Fax: 212-870-3137
www.aa.org

Greg Muth, Manager

Of interest to management and union officials, this pamphlet gives concise descriptions of the help AA can offer to the alcoholic employee.

Year Founded: 1950

5475 Alcoholism Tends to Run in Families
National Clearinghouse for Alcohol and Drug Info.
1 Choke Cherry Road
PO Box 2345
Rockville, MD 20857
301-468-2600
Fax: 301-468-2600; Toll Free: 877-726-4727
webmaster@samhsa.hhs.gov
beta.samhsa.gov
TDD 800-487-4889
TTY: 800-487-4889

Pamela S. Hyde, Administrator
Kana Enomoto, Principal Deputy Administrator
Daryl W. Kade, Chief Financial Officer and Dire

Provides answers and questions about how to help children of alcoholics and where to find resources for additional information.

Year Founded: 1992

5476 Alcoholism, a Merry-Go-Round Named Denial
Al-Anon Family Group Headquarters
1600 Corporate Landing Parkway
Virginia Beach, VA 23454-5617
757-563-1600
Fax: 757-563-1655; Toll Free: 800-356-9996
wso@al-anon.org
www.al-anon.alateen.org

Dramatic explanations that help family members and friends see the roles they play in the problems of alcoholism.

18 pages

5477 Alcoholism: The Family Disease
Al-Anon Family Group Headquarters
1600 Corporate Landing Parkway
Virginia Beach, VA 23454-5617
757-563-1600
Fax: 757-563-1655; Toll Free: 800-356-9996
wso@al-anon.org
www.al-anon.alateen.org

A treasury of information and inspiration, purpose of the Al-Anon program, actual stories for people who found serenity in Al-Anon.

5478 Anonymity
Al-Anon Family Group Headquarters
1600 Corporate Landing Parkway
Virginia Beach, VA 23454-5617
757-563-1600
Fax: 757-563-1655; Toll Free: 800-356-9996
wso@al-anon.org
www.al-anon.alateen.org

Offers information on Al-Anon and Alateen traditions and what a big factor anonymity plays for members.

6 pages

5479 Basic Al-Anon Program Card
Al-Anon Family Group Headquarters
1600 Corporate Landing Parkway
Virginia Beach, VA 23454-5617
757-563-1600
Fax: 757-563-1655; Toll Free: 800-356-9996
wso@al-anon.org
www.al-anon.alateen.org

Wallet card with the Preamble, Twelve Steps, Twelve Traditions and Serenity Prayer.

5480 Breaking the Chain of Substance Abuse and Hearing Loss
Hearing Loss Association of America
7910 Woodmont Avenue
Suite 1200
Bethesda, MD 20814-7022
301-657-2248
Fax: 301-913-9413
national@shhh.org
www.hearingloss.org
TTY: 301-657-2249

Anna Gilmore Hall, Executive Director
Barbara Kelley, Deputy Executive Director and Ed
Lise Hamlin, Director of Public Policy
Year Founded: 1979

5481 Chemical Dependency Pamphlets
Greenhaven Press
P.O. Box 9187
Farmington Hills, MI 48333-9187
858-485-7424
Fax: 800-414-5043; Toll Free: 800-877-4253
www.gale.cengage.com/greenhaven/

Bruce Glassman, Owner

Pamphlet titles included in this set are: What are the causes of chemical dependency?; Is smoking harmful?; How harmful is alcohol?; Should drug laws be reformed?; Should pregnant women be prosecuted for drug abuse?; and How can chemical dependency be reduced?.

Year Founded: 1974

5482 Chemical Dependency and the African American
Hazelden
15251 Pleasant Valley Road
PO Box 11
Center City, MN 55012-0011

651-213-4200
Fax: 651-213-4793; *Toll Free:* 800-257-7810
info@hazelden.org
www.hazelden.org

Mark Mishek, President & CEO
James A. Blaha, Vice President
Sharon Birnbaum, Corporate Director

Reviews the impact alcohol and other drug abuse has on African American communities.

66 pages Year Founded: 1947

5483 Chemical Dependency: An Acceptable Disease
Hazelden
15251 Pleasant Valley Road
PO Box 11
Center City, MN 55012-0011
651-213-4200
Fax: 651-213-4793; *Toll Free:* 800-257-7810
info@hazelden.org
www.hazelden.org

Mark Mishek, President & CEO
James A. Blaha, Vice President
Sharon Birnbaum, Corporate Director

Help persons identify and acknowledge their chemical dependency.

14 pages Year Founded: 1947

5484 Concepts: Al-Anon's Best Kept Secret?
Al-Anon Family Group Headquarters
1600 Corporate Landing Parkway
Virginia Beach, VA 23454-5617
757-563-1600
Fax: 757-563-1655; *Toll Free:* 800-356-9996
wso@al-anon.org
www.al-anon.alateen.org

An illustrated introduction to Al-Anon's third legacy - service. The Concepts are the Twelve Steps and Traditions expanded to the business level.

16 pages

5485 Cooperating with the Professional
Al-Anon Family Group Headquarters
1600 Corporate Landing Parkway
Virginia Beach, VA 23454-5617
757-563-1600
Fax: 757-563-1655; *Toll Free:* 800-356-9996
wso@al-anon.org
www.al-anon.alateen.org

All the information you need to get started in Al-Anon CPC service.

5486 Crack Cocaine - The Big Lie
National Clearinghouse for Alcohol and Drug Info.
1 Choke Cherry Road
PO Box 2345
Rockville, MD 20857
301-468-2600
Fax: 301-468-2600; *Toll Free:* 877-726-4727
webmaster@samhsa.hhs.gov
beta.samhsa.gov
TDD 800-487-4889
TTY: 800-487-4889

Pamela S. Hyde, Administrator
Kana Enomoto, Principal Deputy Administrator
Daryl W. Kade, Chief Financial Officer and Dire

Offers information on what crack and cocaine are, how strong the addictions are from these drugs, how they affect the body and other risks in taking cocaine and crack.

Year Founded: 1992

5487 Crossing the Line Between Social Drinking and Alcoholism
Hazelden
15251 Pleasant Valley Road
PO Box 11
Center City, MN 55012-0011
651-213-4200
Fax: 651-213-4793; *Toll Free:* 800-257-7810
info@hazelden.org
www.hazelden.org

Mark Mishek, President & CEO
James A. Blaha, Vice President
Sharon Birnbaum, Corporate Director

20 pages Year Founded: 1947

5488 Denial
Hazelden
15251 Pleasant Valley Road
PO Box 11
Center City, MN 55012-0011
651-213-4200
Fax: 651-213-4793; *Toll Free:* 800-257-7810
info@hazelden.org
www.hazelden.org

Mark Mishek, President & CEO
James A. Blaha, Vice President
Sharon Birnbaum, Corporate Director

Describes denial and its role in the five-stage acceptance process.

Year Founded: 1947

5489 Depression and Recovery From Chemical Dependency
Hazelden
15251 Pleasant Valley Road
PO Box 11
Center City, MN 55012-0011
651-213-4200
Fax: 651-213-4793; *Toll Free:* 800-257-7810
info@hazelden.org
www.hazelden.org

Mark Mishek, President & CEO
James A. Blaha, Vice President
Sharon Birnbaum, Corporate Director

Outlines depression's warning signs.

Year Founded: 1947

5490 Detaching with Love
Hazelden
15251 Pleasant Valley Road
PO Box 11
Center City, MN 55012-0011
651-213-4200
Fax: 651-213-4793; *Toll Free:* 800-257-7810
info@hazelden.org
www.hazelden.org

Mark Mishek, President & CEO
James A. Blaha, Vice President
Sharon Birnbaum, Corporate Director

Addresses the essential recovery tools clients need to cope with addiction and detach from the problem.

Year Founded: 1947

5491 Detachment
Al-Anon Family Group Headquarters
1600 Corporate Landing Parkway
Virginia Beach, VA 23454-5617
757-563-1600
Fax: 757-563-1655; *Toll Free:* 800-356-9996
wso@al-anon.org
www.al-anon.alateen.org

Everything you always wanted to know about detachment in an easy-to-use leaflet.

5492 Did You Grow Up with a Problem Drinker?
Al-Anon Family Group Headquarters
1600 Corporate Landing Parkway
Virginia Beach, VA 23454-5617
757-563-1600
Fax: 757-563-1655; *Toll Free:* 800-356-9996
wso@al-anon.org
www.al-anon.alateen.org

20 personal questions help individuals decide if they can benefit from Al-Anon.

5493 Do You Think You're Different?
Alcoholics Anonymous
Grand Central Station
PO Box 459
New York, NY 10163
212-870-3400
Fax: 212-870-3137
www.aa.org

Greg Muth, Manager

Speaks to newcomers who may wonder how AA can work for someone different.

Year Founded: 1950

5494 Does She Drink Too Much?
Al-Anon Family Group Headquarters
1600 Corporate Landing Parkway
Virginia Beach, VA 23454-5617
757-563-1600
Fax: 757-563-1655; *Toll Free:* 800-356-9996
wso@al-anon.org
www.al-anon.alateen.org

Does a woman in your life drink too much? Men who found answers in Al-Anon share what has helped them.

12 pages

5495 Don't Lose a Friend to Drugs
National Crime Prevention Council
2001 Jefferson Davis Highway
Suite 901
Arlington, VA 22202-4801
202-466-6272
Fax: 202-296-1356
www.ncpc.org

David A. Dean, Chairman
Robert F. Diegelman, Vice Chairman
Ann M. Harkins, President & CEO

Offers practical advice to teenagers on how to say no to drugs, how to help a friend who uses drugs and how to initiate community efforts to prevent drug use.

Year Founded: 1979

5496 Drug Abuse Health Pamphlets
Greenhaven Press
P.O. Box 9187
Farmington Hills, MI 48333-9187
858-485-7424
Fax: 800-414-5043; *Toll Free:* 800-877-4253
www.gale.cengage.com/greenhaven/

Bruce Glassman, Owner

Offers informational pamphlets such as: How should the war on drugs be waged?; Are international drug campaigns effective?; Should drug testing be used?; What should be done about the drug problem in sports? and How should drugs be legally prescribed?.

Year Founded: 1974

5497 Drug Free Zones: A Manual
African American Family Services
310 Groveland Avenue South
Suites 1 & 7
Minneapolis, MN 55403
612-813-5034
Fax: 651-925-0044
www.aafs.net

Thomas Adams, Chief Executive Officer
Bernice Mack, Contact
Julie Jones, Manager

This booklet describes a variety of strategies concerned citizens are using to reclaim their neighborhoods from rampant drug abuse and dealing.

24 pages Year Founded: 1975

5498 Employer's Guide to Dealing with Substance Abuse
National Clearinghouse for Alcohol and Drug Info.
1 Choke Cherry Road
PO Box 2345
Rockville, MD 20857
301-468-2600
Fax: 301-468-2600; *Toll Free:* 877-726-4727
webmaster@samhsa.hhs.gov
beta.samhsa.gov
TDD 800-487-4889
TTY: 800-487-4889

Pamela S. Hyde, Administrator
Kana Enomoto, Principal Deputy Administrator
Daryl W. Kade, Chief Financial Officer and Dire

Instructs employers in setting up comprehensive alcohol and other drug programs in the workplace.

18 pages Year Founded: 1992

5499 Enabling
Hazelden
15251 Pleasant Valley Road
PO Box 11
Center City, MN 55012-0011
651-213-4200
Fax: 651-213-4793; *Toll Free:* 800-257-7810
info@hazelden.org
www.hazelden.org

Mark Mishek, President & CEO
James A. Blaha, Vice President
Sharon Birnbaum, Corporate Director

Describes problems families encounter when they focus their lives on their chemically dependent family member.

Year Founded: 1947

5500 Facts About Alcohol Abuse
Medical Arts Center Hospital
159-05 UNION TURNPIKE
Fresh Meadows, NY 11366
718-906-6700
Fax: 718-906-6840
www.cornerstoneny.com

Michael Richards, Data Processing Executive

A question and answer pamphlet that offers information on alcohol abuse and the effects the abuse has on the family unit.

Year Founded: 1974

5501 Family Denial
Hazelden
15251 Pleasant Valley Road
PO Box 11
Center City, MN 55012-0011
651-213-4200
Fax: 651-213-4793; *Toll Free:* 800-257-7810
info@hazelden.org
www.hazelden.org

Mark Mishek, President & CEO
James A. Blaha, Vice President
Sharon Birnbaum, Corporate Director

Describes ways for families to recognize denial, examine common fears that cause denial and develop methods for overcoming it.

Year Founded: 1947

5502 Free to Care
Hazelden
15251 Pleasant Valley Road
PO Box 11
Center City, MN 55012-0011
651-213-4200
Fax: 651-213-4793; *Toll Free:* 800-257-7810
info@hazelden.org
www.hazelden.org

Mark Mishek, President & CEO
James A. Blaha, Vice President
Sharon Birnbaum, Corporate Director

Explores today's definition of family and new attitudes about gender, technology, single-parents, relatives and friends.

Year Founded: 1947

5503 Freedom From Despair
Al-Anon Family Group Headquarters
1600 Corporate Landing Parkway
Virginia Beach, VA 23454-5617
757-563-1600
Fax: 757-563-1655; *Toll Free:* 800-356-9996
wso@al-anon.org
www.al-anon.alateen.org

A message of hope for those faced with a problem they can't solve alone.

4 pages

5504 Grieving
Hazelden
15251 Pleasant Valley Road
PO Box 11
Center City, MN 55012-0011
651-213-4200
Fax: 651-213-4793; *Toll Free:* 800-257-7810
info@hazelden.org
www.hazelden.org

Mark Mishek, President & CEO
James A. Blaha, Vice President
Sharon Birnbaum, Corporate Director

Outlines the five-phase grieving process for clients and the significance of each.

Year Founded: 1947

5505 Guidance on Our Journeys
Hazelden
15251 Pleasant Valley Road
PO Box 11
Center City, MN 55012-0011
651-213-4200
Fax: 651-213-4793; *Toll Free:* 800-257-7810
info@hazelden.org
www.hazelden.org

Mark Mishek, President & CEO
James A. Blaha, Vice President
Sharon Birnbaum, Corporate Director

Examines the relationship between the recovering person and his or her sponsor.

Year Founded: 1947

5506 Guide for the Family of the Alcoholic
Al-Anon Family Group Headquarters
1600 Corporate Landing Parkway
Virginia Beach, VA 23454-5617
757-563-1600
Fax: 757-563-1655; *Toll Free:* 800-356-9996
wso@al-anon.org
www.al-anon.alateen.org

A clear and realistic look at alcoholism, problems encountered by those close to the alcoholic and choices available to the family.

16 pages

5507 Homeward Bound
Al-Anon Family Group Headquarters
1600 Corporate Landing Parkway
Virginia Beach, VA 23454-5617
757-563-1600
Fax: 757-563-1655; *Toll Free:* 800-356-9996
wso@al-anon.org
www.al-anon.alateen.org

A booklet designed to help beginners make the transition from the family treatment setting to Al-Anon. Contains forty members' personal sharings, a basic glossary of Al-Anon terms, brief explanations of Al-Anon slogans and helpful suggestions for newcomers.

48 pages

5508 How Drug Abuse Takes Profit Out of Buisness
National Clearinghouse for Alcohol and Drug Info.
1 Choke Cherry Road
PO Box 2345
Rockville, MD 20857

301-468-2600
Fax: 301-468-2600; *Toll Free:* 877-726-4727
webmaster@samhsa.hhs.gov
beta.samhsa.gov
TDD 800-487-4889
TTY: 800-487-4889

Pamela S. Hyde, Administrator
Kana Enomoto, Principal Deputy Administrator
Daryl W. Kade, Chief Financial Officer and Dire

Answers employers questions about substance abuse in the workplace.

Year Founded: 1992

5509 How to Get the Most Out of Group Therapy
Hazelden
15251 Pleasant Valley Road
PO Box 11
Center City, MN 55012-0011
651-213-4200
Fax: 651-213-4793; *Toll Free:* 800-257-7810
info@hazelden.org
www.hazelden.org

Mark Mishek, President & CEO
James A. Blaha, Vice President
Sharon Birnbaum, Corporate Director

Answers clients' questions about going to and getting help from group therapy.

Year Founded: 1947

5510 I Can't Be Addicted Because...
Hazelden
15251 Pleasant Valley Road
PO Box 11
Center City, MN 55012-0011
651-213-4200
Fax: 651-213-4793; *Toll Free:* 800-257-7810
info@hazelden.org
www.hazelden.org

Mark Mishek, President & CEO
James A. Blaha, Vice President
Sharon Birnbaum, Corporate Director

Focuses on denial and elaborates on its most common forms.

Year Founded: 1947

5511 Ice Storm
Hazelden
15251 Pleasant Valley Road
PO Box 11
Center City, MN 55012-0011
651-213-4200
Fax: 651-213-4793; *Toll Free:* 800-257-7810
info@hazelden.org
www.hazelden.org

Mark Mishek, President & CEO
James A. Blaha, Vice President
Sharon Birnbaum, Corporate Director

Prepares treatment professionals for the complications of one of the most recently synthesized drugs - ice.

Year Founded: 1947

5512 If Someone Close to You Has a Problem with Alcohol or Other Drugs
National Clearinghouse for Alcohol and Drug Info.
1 Choke Cherry Road
PO Box 2345
Rockville, MD 20857
301-468-2600
Fax: 301-468-2600; *Toll Free:* 877-726-4727
webmaster@samhsa.hhs.gov
beta.samhsa.gov
TDD 800-487-4889
TTY: 800-487-4889

Pamela S. Hyde, Administrator
Kana Enomoto, Principal Deputy Administrator
Daryl W. Kade, Chief Financial Officer and Dire

This booklet is aimed at the general public and gives support and suggestions on coping with someone close who has an alcohol or drug problem.

Year Founded: 1992

5513 If You Are a Professional, AA Wants to Work with You
Alcoholics Anonymous
Grand Central Station
PO Box 459
New York, NY 10163
212-870-3400
Fax: 212-870-3137
www.aa.org

Greg Muth, Manager

Directed at professionals of all types who deal with alcoholics.

Year Founded: 1950

5514 If Your Parents Drink Too Much
Al-Anon Family Group Headquarters
1600 Corporate Landing Parkway
Virginia Beach, VA 23454-5617
757-563-1600
Fax: 757-563-1655; *Toll Free:* 800-356-9996
wso@al-anon.org
www.al-anon.alateen.org

Alateen's cartoon booklet.

24 pages

5515 Index to Alcoholics Anonymous
Hazelden
15251 Pleasant Valley Road
PO Box 11
Center City, MN 55012-0011
651-213-4200
Fax: 651-213-4793; *Toll Free:* 800-257-7810
info@hazelden.org
www.hazelden.org

Mark Mishek, President & CEO
James A. Blaha, Vice President
Sharon Birnbaum, Corporate Director

Features page and line references to the topics discussed in Alcoholics Anonymous, the Big Book.

Year Founded: 1947

5516 Institutions Discount Package
Al-Anon Family Group Headquarters
1600 Corporate Landing Parkway
Virginia Beach, VA 23454-5617
757-563-1600
Fax: 757-563-1655; *Toll Free:* 800-356-9996
wso@al-anon.org
www.al-anon.alateen.org

A sampling of literature for Institutions groups and service projects.

5517 Institutions Service Kit
Al-Anon Family Group Headquarters
1600 Corporate Landing Parkway
Virginia Beach, VA 23454-5617
757-563-1600
Fax: 757-563-1655; *Toll Free:* 800-356-9996
wso@al-anon.org
www.al-anon.alateen.org

All the information needed to get started in Al-Anon Institutions service.

5518 Is AA for Me?
Alcoholics Anonymous
Grand Central Station
PO Box 459
New York, NY 10163
212-870-3400
Fax: 212-870-3137
www.aa.org

Greg Muth, Manager

An illustrated easy to read version of the 12 questions in Is AA for You? pamphlet.

32 pages Year Founded: 1950

5519 Is AA for You?
Alcoholics Anonymous
Grand Central Station
PO Box 459
New York, NY 10163
212-870-3400
Fax: 212-870-3137
www.aa.org

Greg Muth, Manager

Symptoms of alcoholism are summed up in 12 questions most AA's had answered to identify themselves as alcoholics.

Year Founded: 1950

5520 Is There an Alcoholic in Your Life?
Alcoholics Anonymous
Grand Central Station
PO Box 459
New York, NY 10163
212-870-3400
Fax: 212-870-3137
www.aa.org

Greg Muth, Manager

Explains the AA program as it affects anyone close to an alcoholic.

Year Founded: 1950

5521 It Happened to Alice
Alcoholics Anonymous
Grand Central Station
PO Box 459
New York, NY 10163
212-870-3400
Fax: 212-870-3137
www.aa.org

Greg Muth, Manager

Easy to read comic-book style format for women alcoholics.

Year Founded: 1950

5522 It Sure Beats Sitting in a Cell
Alcoholics Anonymous
Grand Central Station
PO Box 459
New York, NY 10163
212-870-3400
Fax: 212-870-3137
www.aa.org

Greg Muth, Manager

An illustrated pamphlet which presents the experience of seven inmates who found AA while in prison. It also offers suggested dos and don'ts for staying sober after release.

Year Founded: 1950

5523 Let's Talk
Hazelden
15251 Pleasant Valley Road
PO Box 11
Center City, MN 55012-0011
651-213-4200
Fax: 651-213-4793; *Toll Free:* 800-257-7810
info@hazelden.org
www.hazelden.org

Mark Mishek, President & CEO
James A. Blaha, Vice President
Sharon Birnbaum, Corporate Director

Offers 12 guidelines to promote effective communication between parent and child.

Year Founded: 1947

5524 Letter to a Woman Alcoholic
Alcoholics Anonymous
Grand Central Station
PO Box 459
New York, NY 10163
212-870-3400
Fax: 212-870-3137
www.aa.org

Greg Muth, Manager

Describes with sensitive understanding the problem of the alcoholic woman.

Year Founded: 1950

5525 Letting Go of the Need to Control
Hazelden
15251 Pleasant Valley Road
PO Box 11
Center City, MN 55012-0011
651-213-4200
Fax: 651-213-4793; *Toll Free:* 800-257-7810

info@hazelden.org
www.hazelden.org

Mark Mishek, President & CEO
James A. Blaha, Vice President
Sharon Birnbaum, Corporate Director

Discusses how control issues are common among chemically dependent people.

Year Founded: 1947

5526 Little More About Alcohol
Alcohol Research Information Service
1120 E Oakland Avenue
Lansing, MI 48906-5513
517-485-9900Toll free: 888-696-4222
niaaaweb-r@exchange.nih.gov
www.niaaa.nih.gov

Robert Hammond, Manager

A cartoon character explains the facts about alcohol and its effects on the body.

5527 Living Sober
Alcoholics Anonymous
Grand Central Station
PO Box 459
New York, NY 10163
212-870-3400
Fax: 212-870-3137
www.aa.org

Greg Muth, Manager

Practical book demonstrating through simple examples, how AA members throughout the world live and stay sober one day at a time.

88 pages Year Founded: 1950

5528 Living in a Shelter
Al-Anon Family Group Headquarters
1600 Corporate Landing Parkway
Virginia Beach, VA 23454-5617
757-563-1600
Fax: 757-563-1655; *Toll Free:* 800-356-9996
wso@al-anon.org
www.al-anon.alateen.org

5529 Living with Sobriety: Another Beginning
Al-Anon Family Group Headquarters
1600 Corporate Landing Parkway
Virginia Beach, VA 23454-5617
757-563-1600
Fax: 757-563-1655; *Toll Free:* 800-356-9996
wso@al-anon.org
www.al-anon.alateen.org

This book is for everyone who is trying to accept change, let go of guilt and resentment, deal with disappointments, improve communication and learn to be happy.

48 pages

5530 Look at Cross-Addiction
Hazelden
15251 Pleasant Valley Road
PO Box 11
Center City, MN 55012-0011
651-213-4200
Fax: 651-213-4793; *Toll Free:* 800-257-7810
info@hazelden.org
www.hazelden.org

Mark Mishek, President & CEO
James A. Blaha, Vice President
Sharon Birnbaum, Corporate Director

Discusses cross-addiction, denial, coping skills and avoidance.

Year Founded: 1947

5531 Look at Relapse
Hazelden
15251 Pleasant Valley Road
PO Box 11
Center City, MN 55012-0011
651-213-4200
Fax: 651-213-4793; *Toll Free:* 800-257-7810
info@hazelden.org
www.hazelden.org

Mark Mishek, President & CEO
James A. Blaha, Vice President
Sharon Birnbaum, Corporate Director

Addresses emotional consequences of relapse, such as decreased feelings of self-esteem and self-confidence.

Year Founded: 1947

5532 Managing Cocaine Cravings
Hazelden
15251 Pleasant Valley Road
PO Box 11
Center City, MN 55012-0011
651-213-4200
Fax: 651-213-4793; *Toll Free:* 800-257-7810
info@hazelden.org
www.hazelden.org

Mark Mishek, President & CEO
James A. Blaha, Vice President
Sharon Birnbaum, Corporate Director

Offers clients hands-on plan to help them stay away from cocaine.

Year Founded: 1947

5533 Marijuana
Hazelden
15251 Pleasant Valley Road
PO Box 11
Center City, MN 55012-0011
651-213-4200
Fax: 651-213-4793; *Toll Free:* 800-257-7810
info@hazelden.org
www.hazelden.org

Mark Mishek, President & CEO
James A. Blaha, Vice President
Sharon Birnbaum, Corporate Director

Outlines the physical and psychological effects of marijuana unique to episodic and chronic use.

65 pages Year Founded: 1947

5534 Media Kit
Al-Anon Family Group Headquarters
1600 Corporate Landing Parkway
Virginia Beach, VA 23454-5617
757-563-1600
Fax: 757-563-1655; *Toll Free:* 800-356-9996
wso@al-anon.org
www.al-anon.alateen.org

An attractive silver folder containing information necessary to work with radio and TV stations.

5535 Member's Eye View of Alcoholics Anonymous
Alcoholics Anonymous
Grand Central Station
PO Box 459
New York, NY 10163
212-870-3400
Fax: 212-870-3137
www.aa.org
Greg Muth, Manager

Designed to explain to people in the helping professionals how AA works.

30 pages Year Founded: 1950

5536 Members of the Clergy Ask About Alcoholics Anonymous
Alcoholics Anonymous
Grand Central Station
PO Box 459
New York, NY 10163
212-870-3400
Fax: 212-870-3137
www.aa.org
Greg Muth, Manager

Introduction to AA for members of the clergy unfamiliar with the Fellowship.

Year Founded: 1950

5537 Memo to an Inmate Who May Be an Alcoholic
Alcoholics Anonymous
Grand Central Station
PO Box 459
New York, NY 10163
212-870-3400
Fax: 212-870-3137
www.aa.org
Greg Muth, Manager

A message from AA's who have themselves been inmates. Their personal stories offer a new outlook to inmate alcholics who want to know who AA can help.

Year Founded: 1950

5538 Men: Newcomer's Packet
Al-Anon Family Group Headquarters
1600 Corporate Landing Parkway
Virginia Beach, VA 23454-5617
757-563-1600
Fax: 757-563-1655; *Toll Free:* 800-356-9996
wso@al-anon.org
www.al-anon.alateen.org

For men who are not sure Al-Anon is for them, this collection offers a realistic look at alcoholism and straightforward answers to frequently asked questions.

5539 Message to Correctional Facilities Administrators
Alcoholics Anonymous
Grand Central Station
PO Box 459
New York, NY 10163

212-870-3400
Fax: 212-870-3137
www.aa.org
Greg Muth, Manager

Information about what AA is and can do, and how groups function in correctional facilities.

Year Founded: 1950

5540 Military Packet
Al-Anon Family Group Headquarters
1600 Corporate Landing Parkway
Virginia Beach, VA 23454-5617
757-563-1600
Fax: 757-563-1655; *Toll Free:* 800-356-9996
wso@al-anon.org
www.al-anon.alateen.org

For those in the armed services with loved ones or colleagues who are alcoholic, here's a collection that says, Al-Anon can help.

5541 Moment to Reflect on Codependency
Hazelden
15251 Pleasant Valley Road
PO Box 11
Center City, MN 55012-0011
651-213-4200
Fax: 651-213-4793; *Toll Free:* 800-257-7810
info@hazelden.org
www.hazelden.org
Mark Mishek, President & CEO
James A. Blaha, Vice President
Sharon Birnbaum, Corporate Director

A collection of four booklets offering meditations that emphasize and reinforce self-esteem for young people recovering from addiction.

Year Founded: 1947

5542 Moment to Reflect on Self-Esteem
Hazelden
15251 Pleasant Valley Road
PO Box 11
Center City, MN 55012-0011
651-213-4200
Fax: 651-213-4793; *Toll Free:* 800-257-7810
info@hazelden.org
www.hazelden.org
Mark Mishek, President & CEO
James A. Blaha, Vice President
Sharon Birnbaum, Corporate Director

Focuses on the fundamental recovery issue of self-esteem.

Year Founded: 1947

5543 NIDA Capsules
National Clearinghouse for Alcohol and Drug Info.
1 Choke Cherry Road
PO Box 2345
Rockville, MD 20857
301-468-2600
Fax: 301-468-2600; *Toll Free:* 877-726-4727
webmaster@samhsa.hhs.gov
beta.samhsa.gov
TDD 800-487-4889
TTY: 800-487-4889

Pamela S. Hyde, Administrator
Kana Enomoto, Principal Deputy Administrator
Daryl W. Kade, Chief Financial Officer and Dire

Year Founded: 1992

5544 Newcomer Asks
Alcoholics Anonymous
Grand Central Station
PO Box 459
New York, NY 10163
212-870-3400
Fax: 212-870-3137
www.aa.org

Greg Muth, Manager

Gives straightforward answers on 15 points that once puzzled many of us.

Year Founded: 1950

5545 Now What Do I Do for Fun?
Hazelden
15251 Pleasant Valley Road
PO Box 11
Center City, MN 55012-0011
651-213-4200
Fax: 651-213-4793; *Toll Free:* 800-257-7810
info@hazelden.org
www.hazelden.org

Mark Mishek, President & CEO
James A. Blaha, Vice President
Sharon Birnbaum, Corporate Director

Explores the dilemma of finding new interests in recovery after completing treatment.

Year Founded: 1947

5546 Older Adults After Treatment
Hazelden
15251 Pleasant Valley Road
PO Box 11
Center City, MN 55012-0011
651-213-4200
Fax: 651-213-4793; *Toll Free:* 800-257-7810
info@hazelden.org
www.hazelden.org

Mark Mishek, President & CEO
James A. Blaha, Vice President
Sharon Birnbaum, Corporate Director

Discusses aftercare issues, such as family relations, health, medication and relapse.

Year Founded: 1947

5547 Older Adults in Treatment
Hazelden
15251 Pleasant Valley Road
PO Box 11
Center City, MN 55012-0011
651-213-4200
Fax: 651-213-4793; *Toll Free:* 800-257-7810
info@hazelden.org
www.hazelden.org

Mark Mishek, President & CEO
James A. Blaha, Vice President
Sharon Birnbaum, Corporate Director

Examines past beliefs about addiction and defines chemical dependency as a disease.

Year Founded: 1947

5548 Our World Service Office
Al-Anon Family Group Headquarters
1600 Corporate Landing Parkway
Virginia Beach, VA 23454-5617
757-563-1600
Fax: 757-563-1655; *Toll Free:* 800-356-9996
wso@al-anon.org
www.al-anon.alateen.org

Briefly describes the function and services of Al-Anon's international clearinghouse, the World Service Office.

8 pages

5549 Preventing Relapse
Hazelden
15251 Pleasant Valley Road
PO Box 11
Center City, MN 55012-0011
651-213-4200
Fax: 651-213-4793; *Toll Free:* 800-257-7810
info@hazelden.org
www.hazelden.org

Mark Mishek, President & CEO
James A. Blaha, Vice President
Sharon Birnbaum, Corporate Director

Offers practical information and personal stories to help clients better understand the relapse process.

28 pages Year Founded: 1947

5550 Purpose and Suggestions
Al-Anon Family Group Headquarters
1600 Corporate Landing Parkway
Virginia Beach, VA 23454-5617
757-563-1600
Fax: 757-563-1655; *Toll Free:* 800-356-9996
wso@al-anon.org
www.al-anon.alateen.org

A brief introduction to Al-Anon with down-to-earth suggestions for making improvements.

6 pages

5551 Put on the Brakes Bulletin: Take a Look at College Drinking
National Clearinghouse for Alcohol and Drug Info.
1 Choke Cherry Road
PO Box 2345
Rockville, MD 20857
301-468-2600
Fax: 301-468-2600; *Toll Free:* 877-726-4727
webmaster@samhsa.hhs.gov
beta.samhsa.gov
TDD 800-487-4889
TTY: 800-487-4889

Pamela S. Hyde, Administrator
Kana Enomoto, Principal Deputy Administrator
Daryl W. Kade, Chief Financial Officer and Dire

This second edition continues CSAP's campaign to raise awareness about the problems of college drinking.

Year Founded: 1992

5552 Quick List to Build Pride in Your Communities
National Clearinghouse for Alcohol and Drug Info.
1 Choke Cherry Road
PO Box 2345
Rockville, MD 20857
301-468-2600
Fax: 301-468-2600; *Toll Free:* 877-726-4727
webmaster@samhsa.hhs.gov
beta.samhsa.gov
TDD 800-487-4889
TTY: 800-487-4889

Pamela S. Hyde, Administrator
Kana Enomoto, Principal Deputy Administrator
Daryl W. Kade, Chief Financial Officer and Dire

This parent guide is an adaptation of CSAP's Be Smart!
Quick List: 10 Steps to Help Your Child Say No.
Year Founded: 1992

5553 Relapse and the Addict
Hazelden
15251 Pleasant Valley Road
PO Box 11
Center City, MN 55012-0011
651-213-4200
Fax: 651-213-4793; *Toll Free:* 800-257-7810
info@hazelden.org
www.hazelden.org

Mark Mishek, President & CEO
James A. Blaha, Vice President
Sharon Birnbaum, Corporate Director

Identifies specific stages and triggers of relapse.
Year Founded: 1947

5554 Releasing Anger
Hazelden
15251 Pleasant Valley Road
PO Box 11
Center City, MN 55012-0011
651-213-4200
Fax: 651-213-4793; *Toll Free:* 800-257-7810
info@hazelden.org
www.hazelden.org

Mark Mishek, President & CEO
James A. Blaha, Vice President
Sharon Birnbaum, Corporate Director

Discusses anger as a normal feeling and how anger can endanger recovery.
Year Founded: 1947

5555 Research on Drugs and the Workplace
National Clearinghouse for Alcohol and Drug Info.
1 Choke Cherry Road
PO Box 2345
Rockville, MD 20857
301-468-2600
Fax: 301-468-2600; *Toll Free:* 877-726-4727
webmaster@samhsa.hhs.gov
beta.samhsa.gov
TDD 800-487-4889
TTY: 800-487-4889

Pamela S. Hyde, Administrator
Kana Enomoto, Principal Deputy Administrator
Daryl W. Kade, Chief Financial Officer and Dire

Discusses prevalence and costs to society of drug use in the
workplace, along with information on employee assistance
programs, drug testing, grants and additional resources.
Year Founded: 1992

5556 Sexual Intimacy and the Alcoholic Relationship
Al-Anon Family Group Headquarters
1600 Corporate Landing Parkway
Virginia Beach, VA 23454-5617
757-563-1600
Fax: 757-563-1655; *Toll Free:* 800-356-9996
wso@al-anon.org
www.al-anon.alateen.org

Sex and alcohol? Al-Anon members face this personal
problem when they apply to the Al-Anon program indexed.
48 pages

5557 So You Love an Alcoholic
Al-Anon Family Group Headquarters
1600 Corporate Landing Parkway
Virginia Beach, VA 23454-5617
757-563-1600
Fax: 757-563-1655; *Toll Free:* 800-356-9996
wso@al-anon.org
www.al-anon.alateen.org

First steps to a changed attitude toward the alcoholic.
6 pages

5558 Sponsorship: What It's All About
Al-Anon Family Group Headquarters
1600 Corporate Landing Parkway
Virginia Beach, VA 23454-5617
757-563-1600
Fax: 757-563-1655; *Toll Free:* 800-356-9996
wso@al-anon.org
www.al-anon.alateen.org

An important part of getting the program and then giving it
away is sponsorship.
12 pages

5559 Stress in Recovery
Hazelden
15251 Pleasant Valley Road
PO Box 11
Center City, MN 55012-0011
651-213-4200
Fax: 651-213-4793; *Toll Free:* 800-257-7810
info@hazelden.org
www.hazelden.org

Mark Mishek, President & CEO
James A. Blaha, Vice President
Sharon Birnbaum, Corporate Director

Outlines methods for clients to overcome stress in their
daily lives.
Year Founded: 1947

5560 Substance Abuse Funding News
CD Publications
2222 Sedwick Drive
Durham, NC 27713
301-588-6380
Fax: 301-588-6385; *Toll Free:* 855-237-1396
info@cdpublications.com
www.cdpublications.com

Michael Gerecht, President
Mike Gerecht, Publisher

Detailed coverage of private and federal funding opportunities for alcohol, tobacco and drug abuse programs. Plus advice on successful grantseeking strategies and news affecting your programs.

Year Founded: 1961

5561 This Is AA
Alcoholics Anonymous
Grand Central Station
PO Box 459
New York, NY 10163
212-870-3400
Fax: 212-870-3137
www.aa.org

Greg Muth, Manager

A pamphlet offering an introduction to the AA recovery program.

Year Founded: 1950

5562 This Is Al-Anon
Al-Anon Family Group Headquarters
1600 Corporate Landing Parkway
Virginia Beach, VA 23454-5617
757-563-1600
Fax: 757-563-1655; *Toll Free:* 800-356-9996
wso@al-anon.org
www.al-anon.alateen.org

Explains Al-Anon through the Opening/Welcome, Preamble, Serenity Prayer, Twelve Steps and Traditions.

16 pages

5563 Three Talks to Medical Societies
Alcoholics Anonymous
Grand Central Station
PO Box 459
New York, NY 10163
212-870-3400
Fax: 212-870-3137
www.aa.org

Greg Muth, Manager

Contains Bill Wilson's, the co-founder of AA, principles borrowed from medicine and religion and a summary of AA's first 23 years.

Year Founded: 1950

5564 Three Views of Al-Anon
Al-Anon Family Group Headquarters
1600 Corporate Landing Parkway
Virginia Beach, VA 23454
757-563-1600
Fax: 757-563-1655; *Toll Free:* 800-356-9996
wso@al-anon.org
www.al-anon.alateen.org

AA members tell how Al-Anon and AA cooperate to help alcoholics and their families.

8 pages

5565 Time to Start Living
Alcoholics Anonymous
Grand Central Station
PO Box 459
New York, NY 10163

212-870-3400
Fax: 212-870-3137
www.aa.org

Greg Muth, Manager

Addresses the older alcoholic, with nine stories of men and women who came to AA after the age of 60 (large print edition is also available).

Year Founded: 1950

5566 Twelve Steps Illustrated
Alcoholics Anonymous
Grand Central Station
PO Box 459
New York, NY 10163
212-870-3400
Fax: 212-870-3137
www.aa.org

Greg Muth, Manager

An easy-to-read version of AA's twelve steps.

Year Founded: 1950

5567 Twelve Steps and Traditions
Al-Anon Family Group Headquarters
1600 Corporate Landing Parkway
Virginia Beach, VA 23454-5617
757-563-1600
Fax: 757-563-1655; *Toll Free:* 800-356-9996
wso@al-anon.org
www.al-anon.alateen.org

Handy guide to understanding and using Al-Anon's Steps and Traditions in our daily lives.

32 pages

5568 Twelve Steps for Tobacco Users
Hazelden
15251 Pleasant Valley Road
PO Box 11
Center City, MN 55012-0011
651-213-4200
Fax: 651-213-4793; *Toll Free:* 800-257-7810
info@hazelden.org
www.hazelden.org

Mark Mishek, President & CEO
James A. Blaha, Vice President
Sharon Birnbaum, Corporate Director

Presents the Surgeon General's findings that classify nicotine as an addictive substance.

25 pages Year Founded: 1947

5569 Understanding Depression and Addiction
Hazelden
15251 Pleasant Valley Road
PO Box 11
Center City, MN 55012-0011
651-213-4200
Fax: 651-213-4793; *Toll Free:* 800-257-7810
info@hazelden.org
www.hazelden.org

Mark Mishek, President & CEO
James A. Blaha, Vice President
Sharon Birnbaum, Corporate Director

29 pages Year Founded: 1947

5570 Understanding Major Anxiety Disorders and and Addiction
Hazelden
15251 Pleasant Valley Road
PO Box 11
Center City, MN 55012-0011
651-213-4200
Fax: 651-213-4793; *Toll Free:* 800-257-7810
info@hazelden.org
www.hazelden.org

Mark Mishek, President & CEO
James A. Blaha, Vice President
Sharon Birnbaum, Corporate Director

36 pages Year Founded: 1947

5571 Understanding Ourselves and Alcoholism
Al-Anon Family Group Headquarters
1600 Corporate Landing Parkway
Virginia Beach, VA 23454-5617
757-563-1600
Fax: 757-563-1655; *Toll Free:* 800-356-9996
wso@al-anon.org
www.al-anon.alateen.org

Explains how compulsion, obsession and denial affect those close to an alcoholic as well as the alcoholic.

6 pages

5572 Understanding Personality Problems and Addiction
Hazelden
15251 Pleasant Valley Road
PO Box 11
Center City, MN 55012-0011
651-213-4200
Fax: 651-213-4793; *Toll Free:* 800-257-7810
info@hazelden.org
www.hazelden.org

Mark Mishek, President & CEO
James A. Blaha, Vice President
Sharon Birnbaum, Corporate Director

Describes common features of personality problems, such as self-centeredness and setting boundaries.

28 pages Year Founded: 1947

5573 Understanding Post-Traumatic Stress Disorder and Addiction
Hazelden
15251 Pleasant Valley Road
PO Box 11
Center City, MN 55012-0011
651-213-4200
Fax: 651-213-4793; *Toll Free:* 800-257-7810
info@hazelden.org
www.hazelden.org

Mark Mishek, President & CEO
James A. Blaha, Vice President
Sharon Birnbaum, Corporate Director

17 pages Year Founded: 1947

5574 Up Front Drug Information
Adfam
25 Corsham Street
Apt 602
London, FL 33137-2696

207-553-7640
Fax: 207-253-7991
admin@adfam.org.uk
www.adfam.org.uk

Joss Gaynor, Director of Policy and Regional
Omar Amin, Director of Finance and Administ
Oliver French, Policy and Communications Coordi

Provides information on drugs and drug referrals.

Year Founded: 1984

5575 What Are the Signs of Alcoholism?
Hazelden
15251 Pleasant Valley Road
PO Box 11
Center City, MN 55012-0011
651-213-4200
Fax: 651-213-4793; *Toll Free:* 800-257-7810
info@hazelden.org
www.hazelden.org

Mark Mishek, President & CEO
James A. Blaha, Vice President
Sharon Birnbaum, Corporate Director

Self-test for clients to review the role of alcohol in their lives.

Year Founded: 1947

5576 What Do You Do About the Alcoholics' Drinking?
Al-Anon Family Group Headquarters
1600 Corporate Landing Parkway
Virginia Beach, VA 23454-5617
757-563-1600
Fax: 757-563-1655; *Toll Free:* 800-356-9996
wso@al-anon.org
www.al-anon.alateen.org

Shows errors most people make in trying to cope with the problem of alcoholism before Al-Anon.

8 pages

5577 What Happened to Joe?
Alcoholics Anonymous
Grand Central Station
PO Box 459
New York, NY 10163
212-870-3400
Fax: 212-870-3137
www.aa.org

Greg Muth, Manager

Dramatic story of a young construction worker and his drinking problem, told in brightly colored comic book style.

Year Founded: 1950

5578 What Is AA ?
Hazelden
15251 Pleasant Valley Road
PO Box 11
Center City, MN 55012-0011
651-213-4200
Fax: 651-213-4793; *Toll Free:* 800-257-7810
info@hazelden.org
www.hazelden.org

Mark Mishek, President & CEO
James A. Blaha, Vice President
Sharon Birnbaum, Corporate Director

Answers the basic questions about Alcoholics Anonymous.

Year Founded: 1947

5579 What Is NA ?
Hazelden
15251 Pleasant Valley Road
PO Box 11
Center City, MN 55012-0011
651-213-4200
Fax: 651-213-4793; *Toll Free:* 800-257-7810
info@hazelden.org
www.hazelden.org

Mark Mishek, President & CEO
James A. Blaha, Vice President
Sharon Birnbaum, Corporate Director

Helps clients evaluate their addiction to narcotics and answers their questions about N.A.

Year Founded: 1947

5580 When I Got Busy, I Got Better
Al-Anon Family Group Headquarters
1600 Corporate Landing Parkway
Virginia Beach, VA 23454-5617
757-563-1600
Fax: 757-563-1655; *Toll Free:* 800-356-9996
wso@al-anon.org
www.al-anon.alateen.org

Tried and true methods of building self-esteem and confidence while getting rid of anxiety and guilt.

64 pages

5581 When You Go Back to Work
Hazelden
15251 Pleasant Valley Road
PO Box 11
Center City, MN 55012-0011
651-213-4200
Fax: 651-213-4793; *Toll Free:* 800-257-7810
info@hazelden.org
www.hazelden.org

Mark Mishek, President & CEO
James A. Blaha, Vice President
Sharon Birnbaum, Corporate Director

Stories demonstrating co-workers' attitudes clients may face upon their return to work.

Year Founded: 1947

5582 Where Do I Go From Here?
Alcoholics Anonymous
Grand Central Station
PO Box 459
New York, NY 10163
212-870-3400
Fax: 212-870-3137
www.aa.org

Greg Muth, Manager

For people leaving treatment facilities, single-sheet flyer tells of continuing help offered by outside AAs.

Year Founded: 1950

5583 Why Is Al-Anon Anonymous?
Al-Anon Family Group Headquarters
1600 Corporate Landing Parkway
Virginia Beach, VA 23454-5617
757-563-1600
Fax: 757-563-1655; *Toll Free:* 800-356-9996
wso@al-anon.org
www.al-anon.alateen.org

Stresses the importance of preserving anonymity of Al-Anon and AA members.

8 pages

5584 Workers at Risk: Drugs and Alcohol onthe Job
National Clearinghouse for Alcohol and Drug Info.
1 Choke Cherry Road
PO Box 2345
Rockville, MD 20857
301-468-2600
Fax: 301-468-2600; *Toll Free:* 877-726-4727
webmaster@samhsa.hhs.gov
beta.samhsa.gov
TDD 800-487-4889
TTY: 800-487-4889

Pamela S. Hyde, Administrator
Kana Enomoto, Principal Deputy Administrator
Daryl W. Kade, Chief Financial Officer and Dire

Gives facts about drugs in the workplace and suggests appropriate behavior for employees who are confronted with a coworker's use of alcohol or other drugs.

Year Founded: 1992

5585 You Can Help Your Community Get Rid of Drugs
National Clearinghouse for Alcohol and Drug Info.
1 Choke Cherry Road
PO Box 2345
Rockville, MD 20857
301-468-2600
Fax: 301-468-2600; *Toll Free:* 877-726-4727
webmaster@samhsa.hhs.gov
beta.samhsa.gov
TDD 800-487-4889
TTY: 800-487-4889

Pamela S. Hyde, Administrator
Kana Enomoto, Principal Deputy Administrator
Daryl W. Kade, Chief Financial Officer and Dire

Supports drug abuse treatment and explains how drug use can create problems for your community.

Year Founded: 1992

5586 Your Job and HIV: Are There Risks?
American Red Cross
2025 E Street, NW
17th Floor
Washington, DC 22209-3110
703-312-8724
Fax: 703-312-8738; *Toll Free:* 800-733-2767
www.redcross.org

Bonnie McElveen-Hunter, Chairman
Gail J. McGovern, President & CEO
Dale P. Bateman, Chief Audit Executive

Year Founded: 1881

Videos, Audio Tapes

5587 Alcoholics Anonymous: An Inside View
Alcoholics Anonymous
Grand Central Station
PO Box 459
New York, NY 10163
212-870-3400
Fax: 212-870-3137
www.aa.org

Greg Muth, Manager

Depicts alcoholics, recovering in A.A., going about their daily lives, attending A.A. meetings, and other gatherings.

Year Founded: 1950

5588 Art of Living with Change: Turning Your Good Intentions Into Progress...
Hazelden
15251 Pleasant Valley Road
PO Box 11
Center City, MN 55012-0011
651-213-4200
Fax: 651-213-4793; *Toll Free:* 800-257-7810
info@hazelden.org
www.hazelden.org

Mark Mishek, President & CEO
James A. Blaha, Vice President
Sharon Birnbaum, Corporate Director

Video. 45 minutes
Year Founded: 1947

5589 Bill Discusses the Twelve Traditions
Alcoholics Anonymous
Grand Central Station
PO Box 459
New York, NY 10163
212-870-3400
Fax: 212-870-3137
www.aa.org

Greg Muth, Manager

Bill W. tells how the principles safe-guarding A.A. unity developed.

Year Founded: 1950

5590 Bill's Own Story
Alcoholics Anonymous
Grand Central Station
PO Box 459
New York, NY 10163
212-870-3400
Fax: 212-870-3137
www.aa.org

Greg Muth, Manager

Co-founder Bill W. tells of his drinking and recovery.
Year Founded: 1950

5591 Caring for Ourselves: Hope for Healthy Relationships
Hazelden
15251 Pleasant Valley Road
PO Box 11
Center City, MN 55012-0011
651-213-4200
Fax: 651-213-4793; *Toll Free:* 800-257-7810

info@hazelden.org
www.hazelden.org

Mark Mishek, President & CEO
James A. Blaha, Vice President
Sharon Birnbaum, Corporate Director

Video. 50 minutes
Year Founded: 1947

5592 Hope: Alcoholics Anonymous
Alcoholics Anonymous
Grand Central Station
PO Box 459
New York, NY 10163
212-870-3400
Fax: 212-870-3137
www.aa.org

Greg Muth, Manager

Explains the principles of AA: what it is, steps, traditions, sponsorship, and basic recovery tools.

Year Founded: 1950

5593 Markings on the Journey
Alcoholics Anonymous
Grand Central Station
PO Box 459
New York, NY 10163
212-870-3400
Fax: 212-870-3137
www.aa.org

Greg Muth, Manager

Videocassette depicts 45 years of AA history, using rare materials from our archives.

Year Founded: 1950

Websites

5594 Al-Anon
Al-Anon Family Group Headquarters
1600 Corporate Landing Parkway
Virginia Beach, VA 23454-5617
757-563-1600
Fax: 757-563-1655; *Toll Free:* 800-356-9996
wso@al-anon.org
www.al-anon.alateen.org

The single purpose of this organization is to help families and friends of alcoholics, whether the alcoholic is still drinking or not.

5595 American Council for Drug Education
Phoenix House
New York, NY
www.phoenixhouse.org

Howard Meitiner, President and Chief Executive Of
Mitchell S. Rosenthal, Founder, Executive Director
Andrew Kolodny, Chief Medical Officer

This organization provides information on drug use, develops media campaigns, reviews scientific findings, publishes books and offers films and curriculum materials for prevention.

Year Founded: 1967

5596 CSAP State Liason Program
National Clearinghouse for Alcohol and Drug Info.
1 Choke Cherry Road
PO Box 2345
Rockville, MD 20857
301-468-2600
Fax: 301-468-2600; *Toll Free:* 877-726-4727
webmaster@samhsa.hhs.gov
beta.samhsa.gov
TDD 800-487-4889
TTY: 800-487-4889

Pamela S. Hyde, Administrator
Kana Enomoto, Principal Deputy Administrator
Daryl W. Kade, Chief Financial Officer and Dire

This program is designed to support alcohol and other drug abuse prevention efforts in the States.
Year Founded: 1992

5597 Center for Substance Abuse Prevention
National Clearinghouse for Alcohol and Drug Info.
1 Choke Cherry Road
PO Box 2345
Rockville, MD 20857
301-468-2600
Fax: 301-468-2600; *Toll Free:* 877-726-4727
webmaster@samhsa.hhs.gov
beta.samhsa.gov
TDD 800-487-4889
TTY: 800-487-4889

Pamela S. Hyde, Administrator
Kana Enomoto, Principal Deputy Administrator
Daryl W. Kade, Chief Financial Officer and Dire

This organization's goal is to connect people and resources with innovative ideas, strategies and programs designed to encourage creative and effective efforts aimed at reducing and eliminating alcohol, tobacco and other drug problems in our society.
Year Founded: 1992

5598 Cocaine Anonymous
CAWSO
21720 S. Wilmington Ave.
Ste. 304
Long Beach, CA 90810-1641
310-559-5833
Fax: 310-559-2554
www.ca.org

A support group based on the twelve steps of Alcoholics Anonymous that focuses specifically on problems of cocaine addiction.

5599 DrugAbuse.com
Toll Free: 888-744-0069
drugabuse.com

5600 Food and Drug Administration
U.S. Food and Drug Administration
10903 New Hampshire Avenue
Silver Spring, MD 20993-0002
301-575-0156Toll free: 888-463-6332
www.fda.gov

Margaret A. Hamburg, Commissioner of Food and Drugs
Walter S. Harris, Deputy Commissioner for Operatio
Sally Howard, Deputy Commissioner for Policy,

The FDS is responsible for protecting the public health by assuring the safety, efficacy, and security of human and veterinary drugs, biological products, medical devices, our nation's food supply, cosmetics, and products that emit emit radiation.
Year Founded: 1848

5601 Health Answers
HealthAnswers Education
410 Horsham Road
Horsham, PA 19044
215-442-9010
Michael.tague@healthanswers.com
www.healthanswers.com

Michael Tague, Managing Director

Information on substance abuse, including articles and resources.

5602 Healthlink USA
HealthLink USA
e-mail: contact@healthlinkusa.com
www.healthlinkusa.com

Excellent health information concerning treatment, cures, prevention, diagnosis, risk factors, research, support groups, email lists, personal stories and much more. Updated regularly.

5603 National Clearinghouse for Alcohol and Drug Information
National Clearinghouse for Alcohol and Drug Info.
1 Choke Cherry Road
PO Box 2345
Rockville, MD 20857
301-468-2600
Fax: 301-468-2600; *Toll Free:* 877-726-4727
webmaster@samhsa.hhs.gov
beta.samhsa.gov
TDD 800-487-4889
TTY: 800-487-4889

Pamela S. Hyde, Administrator
Kana Enomoto, Principal Deputy Administrator
Daryl W. Kade, Chief Financial Officer and Dire
Year Founded: 1992

5604 National Council on Alcoholism and Drug Dependence
National Council on Alcoholism and Drug Dependence
217 Broadway
Suite 712
New York, NY 10007
212-269-7797
Fax: 212-269-7510
national@ncadd.org
www.ncadd.org

William H. Foster, President and CEO
Jayne Restivo, Director of Development
Leah Brock, Director of Affiliate Relations

Provides education, information, help and hope in the fight against addictions. Nationwide network of affiliates, advocates prevention, intervention and treatment, and is committed to ridding the disease of its stigma and its sufferers of their denial and shame.
Year Founded: 1935

5605 Peter Lamy Center for Drug Therapy and Aging
University of Maryland School of Pharmacy
20 North Pine Street Baltimore
Maryland, MD 21201
410-706-7650
Fax: 410-706-4012
www.pharmacy.umaryland.edu

Natalie D. Eddington, Dean and Professor
William J. Cooper, Senior Associate Dean for Admini
Richard Dalby, Associate Dean for Academic Affa

The Lamy Center is dedicated to improving drug therapy for aging adults through innovative research, education and clinical initiatives.

Year Founded: 1841

5606 Substance Abuse and Mental Health Services Administration
National Clearinghouse for Alcohol and Drug Info.
1 Choke Cherry Road
PO Box 2345
Rockville, MD 20857
301-468-2600
Fax: 301-468-2600; *Toll Free:* 877-726-4727
webmaster@samhsa.hhs.gov
beta.samhsa.gov
TDD 800-487-4889
TTY: 800-487-4889

Pamela S. Hyde, Administrator
Kana Enomoto, Principal Deputy Administrator
Daryl W. Kade, Chief Financial Officer and Dire

The goal of this organization is to reduce incidence and prevalence of mental disorders and substance abuse and improve treatment outcomes for persons suffering from addictive and mental health problems and disorders.

Year Founded: 1992

Research Centers

5607 American Academy of Addiction Psychiatry
American Academy of Addiction
400 Massasoit Ave
Suite 307 - 2nd Floor
East Providence, RI 02914
401-524-3076
Fax: 401-272-0922
info@aaap.org
www.aaap.org

Kathryn Cates-Wessel, Executive Director
Isabel Vieira, Director of Education and Progra
Miriam Giles, Director of Professional Develop

Psychiatrists and other health care and mental health professionals treating people with addictions. Promotes excellence in the treatment of addictions; seeks to insure availability of addiction treatment programs; encourages improvement in the training of health and mental health care providers treating people with addictions.nsulting services to public policy makers. Serves as a clearinghouse on addictions and their treatment; provides support and assistance to addictions research.

5608 Center for Alcohol & Addiction Studies
Brown University
PO Box G-B
Providence, RI 02912
401-863-1000
Fax: 401-444-1850
denise_bayles@brown.edu
brown.edu

Christina Paxson, President
Mark S. Schlissel, Provost
Elizabeth Huidekoper, Executive Vice President

The Center for Alcohol and Addiction Studies, through its affiliation with the Brown Medical School, occupies a unique position within the University. The Center brings together more that 90 faculty and professional staff members, from 11 University departments and eight affiliated hospitals, to promote the identification, prevention, and effective treatment of alcohol and other substance abuse.

Year Founded: 1764

5609 Center for Applied Prevention Research
Community Prevention Initiative
708 College Ave.
Suite 106
Santa Rosa, CA 95404
877-568-4227
Fax: 707-568-3810
www.ca-cpi.org

Jo%ol L. Phillips, Executive Director
Kerrilyn Scott-Nakai, CPI and SIG Project Director
Joanne Oshel, Technical Assistance and Data Co

Prevention of alcohol and drug abuse is the main focus of the research studies.

5610 Ernest Gallo Clinic and Research Center
San Francisco General Hospital
5858 Horton Street
Suite 200
Emeryville, CA 94608-2007
510-985-3100
Fax: 510-985-3101
ngreen@gallo.ucsf.edu
www.galloresearch.org

John A. De Luca, Chairman of the Board and Presid
William R. Sawyers, Chief Administrative Officer, Ex
Howard L. Fields, MD, PhD, Chief Scientific Officer

Alcoholism studies with a special emphasis on genetics.

Year Founded: 1980

5611 Hamot Medical Center: Research Department
UPMC Hamot
200 Lothrop St.
Pittsburgh, PA 15213-2582
412-647-8762
Fax: 814-877-7590; *Toll Free:* 800-533-8762
www.upmc.com

Desmond J. McDonald, Chairman
V. James Fiorenzo, President
Christopher Larson, DMD, MD, President of the Medical Staff,

Drug evaluations and medical products.

Year Founded: 1881

5612 Hazeldon Foundation: Library and Information Resources
Hazelden
15251 Pleasant Valley Road
PO Box 11
Center City, MN 55012-0011
651-213-4200
Fax: 651-213-4793; *Toll Free:* 800-257-7810
info@hazelden.org
www.hazelden.org

Mark Mishek, President & CEO
James A. Blaha, Vice President
Sharon Birnbaum, Corporate Director

Since its 1949 founding in a rural Minnesota lakeside farmhouse, Hazelden has grown into one of the world's largest, most respected, and best-known private alcohol and drug rehabilitation centers in the world. Thousands of people from all 50 states and 42 foreign countries have turned to Hazelden to find expertise, quality care, and leading authorities on addiction and recovery issues. Our mission today remains the same as our early founders had dreamed - to help alcoholics and addicts who need help.

Year Founded: 1947

5613 Interdisciplinary Program in Cell and Molecular Pharmacology
Medical University of South Carolina
171 Ashley Avenue
Charleston, SC 29425
843-792-1414
Fax: 843-792-2475
academicdepartments.musc.edu

Dr. Harry Margolis, Chariman
Mark S. Southmann, Interim President and Vice Presi
Lisa Montgomery, Executive Vice President

Research into pharmacology and toxicology.

Year Founded: 1824

5614 Johns Hopkins Behavioral Pharmacology Research Unit
School of Medicine
4940 Eastern Avenue
Baltimore, MD 21224-2735
410-550-0616
Fax: 410-550-0030
www.hopkinsmedicine.org

Paul B. Rothman, Chief Executive Officer
Ronald R. Peterson, Executive Vice President
William A. Baumqartner, Senior Vice President

Year Founded: 1889

5615 Maine State Office of Substance Abuse: Information and Resource Center
Substance Abuse
41 Anthony Ave.
#11 State House Station
Augusta, ME 04333-0011
207-287-2595
Fax: 207-287-4334
osa.ircosa@maine.gov
www.maine.gov
TTY: 800-606-0215

Guy Cousins, Director
Geoff Miller, Associate Director
Christine Theriault, Prevention Team Manager

The Maine Office of Substance Abuse is the single state administrative authority responsible for the planning, development, implementation, regulation, and evaluation of substance abuse services. The Office provides leadership in substance abuse prevention, intervention, and treatment. Its goal is to enhance the health and safety of Maine citizens through the reduction of the overall impact of substance use, abuse, and dependency.

Year Founded: 1979

5616 Narcotic and Drug Research
Informa Healthcare
11 Beach Street
New York, NY 10013-2429
212-966-8700
Fax: 212-334-8058
informahealthcare.com

Douglas S Lipton PhD, Director
Arthur Liu, CEO

Nonprofit organization that is devoted to drug abuse education, treatment and prevention.

5617 National Clearinghouse for Alcohol and Drug Information Library (NCADI)
Substance Abuse & Mental Health Services Offices
1 Choke Cherry Road
PO Box 2345
Rockville, MD 20857
301-468-2600
Fax: 301-468-2600; *Toll Free:* 877-726-4727
webmaster@samhsa.hhs.gov
beta.samhsa.gov
TDD 800-487-4889
TTY: 800-487-4889

Pamela S. Hyde, Administrator
Kana Enomoto, Principal Deputy Administrator
Daryl W. Kade, Chief Financial Officer and Dire

National Clearinghouse for Alcohol and Drug Information (NCADI) is the Nation's one-stop resource for information about substance abuse prevention and addiction treatment. We staff both English- and Spanish-speaking information specialists who are skilled at recommending appropriate publications, posters, and videocassettes; conducting customized searches; providing grant and funding information; and referring people to appropriate organizations. The NCADI library has hundreds of journals, newspapers, magazines, and reference books, plus equipment for reviewing audiotapes and videotapes.

Year Founded: 1992

5618 National Development and Research Institutes: Library/Resource Center
National Development and Research Institute
71 West 23rd Street
8th Floor
New York, NY 10010
212-845-4400
Fax: 212-438-0894
www.ndri.org

Natalie Becker, PhD, President
Erik M. Bagin, Vice President
JoAnn Y. Sacks, PhD, Executive Director

Year Founded: 1967

5619 National Institute on Drug Abuse Addiction Research Center Library (NIDA)
National Institute on Drug Abuse
6001 Executive Boulevard
Room 5213, MSC 9561
Bethesda, MD 20892-9561
301-443-1124
Fax: 410-550-1438
mpfeiffe@intra.nida.nih.gov
www.drugabuse.gov

Nora Volkow, Director
Wilson Compton, Deputy Director
Glenda Conroy, Associate Director

NIDA's mission is to lead the Nation in bringing the power of science to bear on drug abuse and addiction. Recent scientific advances have revolutionized our understanding of drug abuse and addiction. The majority of these advances, which have dramatic implications for how to best prevent and treat addiction, have been supported by the National Institute on Drug Abuse (NIDA). NIDA supports over 85 percent of the world's research on the health aspects of drug abuse and addiction. NIDA supported science addresses the most fundamental and essential questions about drug abuse, ranging from the molecule to managed care, and from DNA to community outreach research.

5620 Office of Applied Studies
Substance Abuse & Mental Health Services Offices
1 Choke Cherry Road
PO Box 2345
Rockville, MD 20857
301-468-2600
Fax: 301-468-2600; *Toll Free:* 877-726-4727
webmaster@samhsa.hhs.gov
beta.samhsa.gov
TDD 800-487-4889
TTY: 800-487-4889

Pamela S. Hyde, Administrator
Kana Enomoto, Principal Deputy Administrator
Daryl W. Kade, Chief Financial Officer and Dire

Provides the leadership needed for collecting data on mental illness and substance abuse, including incidence and prevalence studies.

Year Founded: 1992

5621 Ohio State University: Division of Clinical Trials
The Ohio State University
281 W. Lane Ave.
Columbus, OH 43210-1239
614-292-8600
Fax: 614-292-7232; *Toll Free:* 800-854-4461
www.ohio-state.edu

Wolfgang Sadee, Professor/Chairman
Melinda Church, Vice President
Glen Apseloff MD, Clinical Trials

Clinical studies and clinical pharmacology research.

5622 Research Institute on Alcoholism
1021 Main Street
Buffalo, NY 14203-1016
716-887-2566
Fax: 716-887-2252
webmaster@ria.buffalo.edu
www.ria.buffalo.edu

Kenneth E. Leonard, Director
Kimberly S. Walitzer, Deputy Director
Laurie L. Wikander, Grants and Contracts Officer

Research center within the University at Buffalo. The State University of New York.

Year Founded: 1970

5623 Ruth E Golding Clinical Pharmacokinetics Laboratory
College of Pharmacy
1295 N. Martin
PO Box 210207
Tucson, AZ 85721
520-626-1427
Fax: 520-626-2466
gandolfi@pharmacy.arizona.edu
www.pharmacy.arizona.edu

Michael Mayersohn, Head Master
Ivo Abraham, PhD, RN, Professor, Director
Monica Adams, PharmD, Medication Management Specialist

Conducts studies of drugs in humans and animals.

5624 Southern California Research Institute
Journal Studies on Alcohol and Drugs
11912 W Washington Boulevard
Los Angeles, CA 90066-5816
213-427-3200
Fax: 310-398-6651
www.jsad.com

Dr. M Burns, Director
Dirk Stoehr, Manager

Effects of alcohol and drugs on behavior studies.

Year Founded: 1940

5625 Stanford Center for Research in Disease Prevention
Stanford University School of Medicine
211 Quarry Road
Suite 302
Palo Alto, CA 94304-1426
650-723-6028
Fax: 650-725-6906
stanfordmedicine.org

Philip A. Pizzo, Former Dean
John W Farquhar MD, Director
Jackie Keeling, Manager

Prevention and control of alcohol and drug abuse related disorders.

5626 Substance Abuse and Mental Health Services Administration
Substance Abuse & Mental Health Services Offices
1 Choke Cherry Road
PO Box 2345
Rockville, MD 20857
301-468-2600
Fax: 301-468-2600; *Toll Free:* 877-726-4727
webmaster@samhsa.hhs.gov
beta.samhsa.gov
TDD 800-487-4889
TTY: 800-487-4889

Pamela S. Hyde, Administrator
Kana Enomoto, Principal Deputy Administrator
Daryl W. Kade, Chief Financial Officer and Dire

The goal of this organization is to reduce incidence and prevalence of mental disorders and substance abuse and improve treatment outcomes for persons suffering from addictive and mental health problems and disorders.

Year Founded: 1992

5627 University of Alabama: Center for Alcohol and Addiction Studies

3211 Providence Drive
Anchorage, AK 99508-4614
907-786-1805
Fax: 907-786-4866

Dennis Fisher, Director

Basic, applied and evaluative research into alcohol and substance abuse.

5628 University of Delaware: Center for Drug and Alcohol Studies
University of Delaware

77 E Main Street
Newark, DE 19716
302-831-2792
Fax: 302-831-3307
butzin@udel.edu
www.udel.edu/butzin/cdas.html

Patrick T. Harker, President
Domenico Grasso, Provost
Alan Brangman, Vice President

Substance abuse research

Year Founded: 1991

5629 University of Michigan Alcohol Research Center
University of Michigan Health System

1500 E. Medical Center Drive
Suite 2a
Ann Arbor, MI 48109
734-615-0863
Fax: 734-615-6085; *Toll Free:* 855-855-0863
zuckerra@umich.edu
www.med.umich.edu

Ora Hirsch Pescovitz, Executive Vice President
Douglas L. Strong, Chief Executive Officer
James O. Woolliscroft, Dean

Alcohol abuse among the elderly, including the relationship of alcohol and aging on the central nervous system. Also does general research pertaining to the effects of alcholoism and drug abuse.

5630 University of Missouri: Kansas City Drug Information Service
University of Missouri

2411 Holmes Street
Suite Mg-2000
Kansas City, MO 64110
816-235-1000
webmaster@umkc.edu
www.umkc.edu

Patrick J Bryant PharmD, Director
Antoine D Richardson PharmD, Assistant Director
Cydney E McQueen PharmD, Assistant Director

Literature research and evaluation of clinical drug problems and questions.

5631 University of Tennessee Drug Information Center
UT Health Science Center

920 Madison Ave.
Suite 210
Memphis, TN 38163
901-448-8423
Fax: 901-524-4545
www.uthsc.edu
TDD 901-448-7382

Dr. Peter A Chyka, Director
Cheryl R. Scheid, Vice Chancellor
Sonya G. Smith, Associate Vice Chancellor

Year Founded: 1911

5632 University of Utah: Center for Human Toxicology
Center for Human Toxicology

417 Wakara Way
Suite 2111
Salt Lake City, UT 84112
801-581-5117
Fax: 801-581-5034
pharmacy.utah.edu

Dennis Crouch, Director
Diana Wilkins, Director
Douglas Rollins MD, Associate Director

Clinical, forensic and toxicology research.

Year Founded: 1973

5633 University of Washington: Alcohol & Drug Abuse Institute Library
University of Washington

1107 Northeast 45th Street, Suite 120
Box 354805
Seattle, WA 98105-4631
206-543-0937
Fax: 206-543-5473
library@adai.uw.edu
lib.adai.washington.edu/

Nancy Sutherland, Director
Meg Brunner, Librarian
Jennifer Velotta, Clearinghouse Manager

The ADAI Library collection represents the spectrum of research and scientific literature on alcohol and other drug use from all relevant disciplines, including medicine, nursing, social work, criminal justice, sociology and psychology.

Year Founded: 1975

5634 University of Wisconsin: Milwaukee Medicinal Chemistry Group
Medical College of Wisconsin

8701 Watertown Plank Road
PO Box 413
Milwaukee, WI 53226
414-955-8296
www.mcw.edu

John R. Raymond, President and CEO
Dr. Kerschne , Dean and Executive Vice Presiden
G. Allen Bolton, Senior Vice President and COO

Research on drugs, including studies of valium receptors.
Year Founded: 1893

5635 Veterans Administration Medical Center: Research Service
U.S. Department of Veterans Affairs
810 Vermont Avenue, NW
Washington, DC 20420
217-442-8000
Fax: 217-431-6523
www.va.gov

Eric K. Shinseki, Secretary of Veterans Affairs
Jose D. Riojas, Chief of Staff
Stephen W. Warren, Executive in charge for Informat

Alcoholism and rehabilitation research.

Year Founded: 1636

Visually Impaired

Associations & Organizations

5636 1-800-BRAILLE
Braille Institute
741 North Vermont Avenue
Los Angeles, CA 90029
323-663-1111
Fax: 323-663-0867; *Toll Free:* 800-272-4553
la@brailleinstitute.org
www.brailleinstitute.org

Peter A. Mindnich, President

A toll free information and referral service that provides
callers with information on the Braille Institute's programs
and resources, as well as referrals to other local agencies
and organizations for the visually impaired.

Year Founded: 1927

5637 ACB Government Employees
American Council of the Blind
1703 North Beauregard Street
Suite 420
Alexandria, VA 22201
202-467-5081
Fax: 202-465-5085; *Toll Free:* 800-424-8666
info@acb.org
www.acb.org

Renee M. Zelickson, President

Promotes the recruitment, placement and advancement of
blind and visually impaired employees in federal, state, local and county government agencies.

5638 ACB Radio Amateurs
American Council of the Blind
1703 North Beauregard Street
Suite 420
Alexandria, VA 22201
202-467-5081
Fax: 703-465-5085; *Toll Free:* 800-424-8666
acbra@acb.org
www.acbhams.org

John Glass, President
Steve Dresser, Vice President
Mike Duke, Treasurer

An organization consisting of blind, visually impaired and
sighted members who gather to participate in amateur radio
operations.

5639 Achromatopsia Network
PO Box 214
Berkeley, CA 94701-0214
510-540-4700
Fax: 510-540-4767
www.achromat.org

The Achromatopsia Network is an information network for
individuals, families and professionals concerned with
achromatopsia. It is committed to providing information
about achromatopsia, producing resources designed to meet
the needs of affected individuals, and promoting awareness
of the eye condition.

5640 Alliance on Aging and Vision Loss
American Council of the Blind
1703 North Beauregard Street
Suite 420
Alexandria, VA 22201
202-467-5081
Fax: 202-465-5085; *Toll Free:* 800-424-8666
info@acb.org
www.acb.org

John Huffman, President

Advocates, educates, and welcomes anyone who has experienced aging and the loss of sight, and visually impaired
people who are compelled to help others with blindness.

5641 American Academy of Ophthalmology
American Academy of Ophthalmology
PO Box 7424
San Francisco, CA 94120-7424
415-561-8500
Fax: 415-561-8533
aaoe@aao.org
www.aao.org

William L. Rich III, President
David W. Parke II, Chief Executive Officer

Serves to advance the ophthalmology profession and promote education resources on ophthalmology.

Year Founded: 1896

5642 American Action Fund for Blind Children and
Adults
American Action Fund for Blind Children and
Adults
1800 Johnson Street
Baltimore, MD 21230
410-659-9315
actionfund@actionfund.org
www.actionfund.org

Barbara Loos, President
Romana Walhof, First Vice President
Sandra Halverson, Second Vice President

Serves to provide consultation services, braille assistance,
specialized aids, and education resources for blind and
deaf-blind children and adults.

Year Founded: 1919

5643 American Association of Blind Teachers
865-692-4888
www.blindteachers.net

Membership organization of blind teachers, professors and
instructors in all levels of education. Provides support and
information regarding professional responsibilities, classroom techniques, national testing methods and career obstacles. Publishes The Blind Educator, national magazine
specifically for blind educators.

Year Founded: 1940

5644 American Association of Visually Impaired
Attorneys
American Council of the Blind
1703 North Beauregard Street
Suite 420
Alexandria, VA 22311
202-467-5081
Fax: 703-465-5085; *Toll Free:* 800-424-8666

info@acb.org
www.acb.org

Charles Nabarrete, President

Membership includes licensed attorneys, judges, law professors, students and other interested people concerned with law school admission tests and bar exams, private sector and government employment relations and specialized work techniques for the blind and visually impaired.

Year Founded: 1969

5645 American Association of the Deaf-Blind
American Association of the Deaf-Blind
PO Box 24493
Federal Way, WA 98093
301-495-4403
Fax: 301-495-4404
aadb-info@aadb.org
www.aadb.org

Mark Gasaway, President
Adam Drake, Treasurer

A national consumer organization dedicated to helping deaf-blind persons become productive and independent members of the community.

5646 American Board of Ophthalmology
The American Board of Ophthalmology
111 Presidential Boulevard
Suite 241
Bala Cynwyd, PA 19004-1075
610-664-1175
Fax: 610-664-6503
info@abop.org
www.abop.org

Nancy A. Hamming, Chair
Paul P. Lee, Vice Chair
John G. Clarkson, Executive Director

Implements certification programs that serve to enhance the quality of ophthalmic practice.

Year Founded: 1916

5647 American Council of Blind Lions
American Council of the Blind
148 Vernon Avenue
Louisville, KY 40206
502-897-1472
info@acb.org
www.acb.org

June Lenk, President

Educates Lions Club members about the needs and capabilities of blind people, promotes the exchange of information concerning opportunities for the blind and visually impaired among ACB Lions, and encourages blind people to become involved in local clubs and other civic activities.

Year Founded: 1971

5648 American Council of the Blind
1703 N Beauregard Street
Suite 420
Alexandria, VA 22201
202-467-5081
Fax: 703-465-5085; *Toll Free:* 800-424-8666
info@acb.org
www.acb.org

Kim Charlson, President
Ray Campbell, Secretary
Carla Ruschival, Treasurer

Advocates for the acceptance of blind and visually impaired people and strives to achieve equality of opportunity and improved quality of life for members of the blind community.

Year Founded: 1961

5649 American Foundation for the Blind
2 Penn Plaza
Suite 1102
New York, NY 10121
212-502-7600
Fax: 888-545-8331
www.afb.org

Carl R. Augusto, President and CEO
Rick Bozeman, Chief Financial Officer
Kelly Bleach, Chief Administrative Officer

The American Foundation for the Blind, the organization for which Helen Keller worked for over 40 years of her life, is a national, nonprofit organization whose mission is to eliminate barriers and ensure equality of opportunity for blind and visually impaired people. AFB is headquartered in New York City and maintains offices in Atlanta, Dallas, Huntington, San Francisco and Washington, DC.

Year Founded: 1921

5650 American Foundation for the Blind: Atlanta
American Foundation for the Blind
739 West Peachtree Street Northwest
Suite 250
Atlanta, GA 30308
404-525-2303
Fax: 646-478-9260
literacy@afb.net
www.afb.org

Carl R. Augusto, President and CEO
Rick Bozeman, Chief Financial Officer
Kelly Bleach, Chief Administrative Officer

Provides information, referral, and assistive technology services for adults and children, as well as education and training services for professionals.

Year Founded: 1921

5651 American Foundation for the Blind: Center on Vision Loss
American Foundation for the Blind
11030 Ables Lane
Dallas, TX 75229
214-352-7222
Fax: 646-478-9260
dallas@afb.net
www.afb.org

Cynthia Watson, Director

Seeks to help people with vision loss to live independently by offering resource information, professional services and related products and devices.

Year Founded: 1921

5652 American Foundation for the Blind: Huntington
American Foundation for the Blind
1000 Fifth Avenue
Suite 350
Huntington, WV 25701
304-523-8651
Fax: 646-478-9260
www.afb.org

Carl R. Augusto, President and CEO
Rick Bozeman, Chief Financial Officer
Kelly Bleach, Chief Administrative Officer

Includes AFB Tech, the technology arm of the American Foundation for the Blind focused on giving people with vision loss access to critical technology products, and AFB CareerConnect, a web-based program designed to help blind and visually impaired people with employment.

Year Founded: 1921

5653 American Foundation for the Blind: Public Policy Center
American Foundation for the Blind
1660 L Street Northwest
Suite 513
Washington, DC 20036
202-469-6831
Fax: 646-478-9260
afbgov@afb.net
www.afb.org

Mark Richert, Director
Rebecca Sheffield, Senior Policy Researcher

Partners with policymakers in Congress and the Executive Branch as well as organizations and advocates to work towards achieving equal rights for Americans with vision loss. Offers information resources and advocacy services to blind and visually impaired persons.

Year Founded: 1921

5654 American Macular Degeneration Foundation
American Macular Degeneration Foundation
PO Box 515
Northampton, MA 01061-0515
413-268-7660Toll free: 888-622-8527
www.macular.org

Chip Goehring, President
Mark Torrey, Vice President
Sidney S. Schreiber, Scientific Advisor

A non-profit organization dedicated to treating and curing macular degeneration through education, funds, and scientific research.

Year Founded: 1998

5655 American Optometric Association
American Optometric Association
243 North Lindbergh Boulevard
Floor 1
St. Louis, MO 63141-7881
800-365-2219
www.aoa.org

Steven A. Loomis, President
Christopher Quinn, Vice President
Samuel D. Pierce, Secretary-Treasurer

Seeks to provide strong eye and vision care to the public.

Year Founded: 1898

5656 American Printing House for the Blind
The American Printing House for the Blind, Inc.
1839 Frankfort Avenue
PO Box 6085
Louisville, KY 40206-0085
502-895-2405
Fax: 502-899-2284; *Toll Free:* 800-223-1839
info@aph.org
www.aph.org

Craig Meador, President
W. Barrett Nichols, Chairman

Offers products and services to visually impaired people, including educational and independent living products, product training programs, and accessible publications in braille, recorded, large print and computer file formats. APH's Research Department is dedicated to the ongoing development of products designed to advance the independence of people who are blind and visually impaired.

Year Founded: 1858

5657 American Society of Contemporary Medicine, Surgery & Ophthalmology
7250 N Cicero Avenue
Lincolnwood, IL 60712-1643
847-677-9093
iaos@aol.com
ascmso.accountsupport.com

Randall Bellows, Director

Ophthalmologists interested in promoting clinical investigative advances in ophthalmology. Offers continuing medical education courses approved by the American Council for Continuing Medical Education (ACCME) on new opthalmic developments in medical, therapeutic, diagnostic, and surgical procedures.

5658 American Society of Ophthalmic Registered Nurses
American Academy of Ophthalmology
655 Beach Street
San Francisco, CA 94109
415-561-8513
Fax: 415-561-8531
asorn@aao.org
www.asorn.org

Barbara Ann Harmer, President
Nancy Haskell, Secretary-Treasurer

Organization dedicated to uniting nurses specializing in the field of ophthalmology and providing quality patient care. ASORN conducts educational programs focused on ophthalmology, including courses, webinars and annual meetings; produces ophthalmic nursing publications; offers continuing education resources for ophthalmic nurses; and represents members' interests before government agencies and professional associations.

Year Founded: 1976

5659 Arizona Center for the Blind and Visually Impaired
Arizona Center for the Blind and Visually Impaired
3100 East Roosevelt Street
Phoenix, AZ 85008
602-273-7411
www.acbvi.org

Paul K. Batt, Chair
Alexia Matek, Vice Chair
Steve Welker, Secretary

Promotes the independence of the blind and visually impaired and works towards the acceptance and integration of blind and visually impaired people within the community. Provides services for legally blind and visually impaired individuals as well as those with degenerative eye conditions.

Year Founded: 1947

5660 **Arizona Industries for the Blind**
Arizona Industries for the Blind
515 North 51st Avenue
Suite 130
Phoenix, AZ 85043
602-771-9100
Fax: 602-353-5701
www.azdes.gov/aib/

Richard Monaco, General Manager
Lorraine Hudspeth, Controller
Larry Mann, Information Technology Manager

Provides blind people in Arizona with employment opportunities and offers programs and services to help blind individuals develop their employability skills.

Year Founded: 1952

5661 **Arizona Rehabilitation Services Administration, Services for the Blind/Visually Impaired & Deaf**
Arizona Rehabilitation Services Administration
1789 West Jefferson Street
Phoenix, AZ 85007
602-542-3332
Fax: 602-542-3778
des.az.gov
TDD 520-628-6864

Letitia Labrecque, Administrator
Karin Grandon, Program Manager
Paul Howell, Statewide Supervisor

Seeks to help visually impaired individuals coming to terms with the emotional and social effects of blindness. Assists clients with developing the skills necessary to live independently through the provision of rehabilitation counseling, services and resources.

5662 **Arkansas Lighthouse for the Blind**
6818 Murray Street
Little Rock, AR 72209
501-562-2222
Fax: 501-246-8079
info@arkansaslighthouse.org
www.arkansaslighthouse.org

Lighthouse for the Blind employs workers who are blind and visually impaired, along with sighted workers as needed, to manufacture diverse products and provide business services through the Contact Center. Rehabilitation professionals and other Lighthouse supporters throughout the state refer potential employees.

Year Founded: 1940

5663 **Associated Services for the Blind and Visually Impaired**
919 Walnut Street
Philadelphia, PA 19107

215-627-0600
Fax: 215-922-0692
asbinfo@asb.org
www.asb.org

Patricia C. Johnson, President & CEO
Richard Forsythe, Director, Braille Division
David Goldfield, Computer Technology Instructor

Provides rehabilitation and education services designed to help clients to adapt to visual impairment; computer training programs at the Computer Technology Department that assist clients with computer use; and books and magazines in braille, large print and audio formats at the Free Library of Philadelphia's Library for the Blind and Physically Handicapped.

Year Founded: 1874

5664 **Association for Education & Rehabilitation of the Blind & Visually Impaired**
Association for Education & Rehabilitation
1703 North Beauregard Street
Suite 440
Alexandria, VA 22311
703-671-4500
Fax: 703-671-6391; Toll Free: 877-492-2708
aer@aerbvi.org
www.aerbvi.org

Christy Shepard, President
Lou Tutt, Executive Director
Ginger Croce, Deputy Executive Director

Provides tools and services to educators and rehabilitation professionals with the objective of promoting services for visually impaired individuals.

Year Founded: 1984

5665 **Association for Macular Diseases**
The Association for Macular Diseases, Inc.
210 East 64th Street
New York, NY 10065
212-605-3719
Fax: 212-606-3795
www.macula.org

Bernard Landou, President
Mary Fern Breheney, Director
Patricia Dahl, Director

A nonprofit organization serving as a resource for patients with degernative eye conditions. Conducts research and offers educational resources on macular disease, including updates on medical advances and developments. Seeks to provide support to individuals with macular disease as well as the professional community.

Year Founded: 1978

5666 **Association for Research in Vision and Ophthalmology**
1801 Rockville Pike
Suite 400
Rockville, MD 20852
240-221-2900
Fax: 241-221-0370
arvo@arvo.org
www.arvo.org

Iris M. Rush, Executive Director
Joanne Olson, Deputy Executive Director

Research organization dedicated to conducting eye and vision research and advancing the treatment of eye disorders.

Year Founded: 1928; Number of Members: 12,000

5667 Association for Vision Rehabilitation and Employment

174 Court Street
Binghamton, NY 13901-3514
607-724-2428
Fax: 607-771-8045
avreinfo@avreus.org
www.avreus.org

Jenn Small, Chief Operating Officer
Anthony Saccento, Chief Financial Officer
Ken Fernland, President & CEO

To assist people who are blind or visually impaired attain or maintain economic and personal independence.

5668 Association for the Blind & Visually Impaired of Greater Rochester

422 South Clinton Avenue
Rochester, NY 14620
585-232-1111Toll free: 800-646-8166
www.seegreatthings.com

Mike Norris, Chair
A. Gidget Hopf, President & CEO
George Klemann, Chief Financial Officer

Social enterprise focused on empowering blind and visually impaired people to be independent, productive and self-sufficient individuals.

Year Founded: 1911

5669 Association for the Blind Charleston
Association for the Blind and Visually Impaired

One Carriage Lane
Building A
Charleston, SC 29407
843-723-6915
info@abvisc.org
abvisc.org

Julius J Anderson, Jr, President
Clay W Hershey, Vice President
Fleetword S Hassell, Secretary

Mission is to empower individuals with blindness and visual impairment to lead safe, dignified, independent and rewarding lives and to prevent vision loss for adults in South Carolina.

Year Founded: 1936

5670 Association for the Blind and Visually Impaired
Association for the Blind and Visually Impaired

456 Cherry Street Southeast
Grand Rapids, MI 49503
616-458-1187
Fax: 616-458-7113; *Toll Free:* 800-466-8084
abvi@abvimichigan.org
www.abvimichigan.org

Eric Smith, Chair
Kathleen VanderVeen, Vice Chair
Richard A. Stevens, Executive Director

Offers rehabilitation services to advance the independence of visually impaired people. Advocates for an inclusive community consisting of educational resources on blind-

ness and accommodations that directly acknowledge the needs of those who are blind and visually impaired.

Year Founded: 1913

5671 Aurora of Central New York

518 James Street
Suite 100
Syracuse, NY 13203-2282
315-422-7263
Fax: 315-422-4792
auroracny@auroraofcny.org
www.auroraofcny.org
TDD 315-422-9746
TTY: 315-422-9746

Jeanne Matthews-Fox, Chair
John McCormick, Vice Chair
Deb Chaiken, President

To promote independence, opportunity and full-access for individuals of all ages with vision or hearing loss, while both organizations will realize expanded capacity.

Year Founded: 1917

5672 Beaver County Association for the Blind

616 Fourth Street
Beaver Falls, PA 15010-4704
724-843-1111
bcab@bcblind.org
www.bcblind.org

Allen Connely, Executive Director

To provide services to blind and visually impaired persons to promote independence, provide services to prevent blindness and provide employment opportunities to persons who are blind or disabled.

Year Founded: 1947

5673 Bestwork Industries for the Blind

1940 Olney Avenue
Suite 200
Cherry Hill, NJ 08003
856-424-2510
info@bestworkindustries.org
www.bestworkindustries.org

Belinda S Moore, President
Steven McLaughlin, VP, Finance & Operations
Jacqueline Luke-Herman, Operations Manager

To improve the quality of life for individuals who are blind or visually impaired by providing employment opportunities in a supportive work setting.

Year Founded: 1981

5674 Blair/Clearfield Association for the Blind
Visually Impaired

300 5th Avenue
Altoona, PA 16602-2730
814-944-3197
Fax: 814-944-2021
gpattie@bcabvi.org
bcabvi.org

Gloria Pattie, Chief Executive Officer
Dr. Greg Caldwell, President
Allen Stevens, Vice President

Individuals interested in helping to meet the needs of the visually impaired. Promotes blindness prevention. Sponsors errand, life skills training, radio reading, and transportation services. Provides public education information.

5675 Blind & Vision Rehabilitation Services of Pittsburgh
1816 Locust Street
Pittsburgh, PA 15219
412-368-4400
epetach@pghvis.org
www.bvrspittsburgh.org

Louis A Lobes, Jr., MD, Chairman
Joe Gordon, Vice Chairman
Erika M Petach, President

For more than 100 years, Blind and Vision Rehabilitation Services of Pittsburgh has empowered people who are blind, deaf blind or vision impaired to become independent. Their mission is to change the lives of persons with vision loss and other disabilities by fostering independence and individual choice.

Year Founded: 1910

5676 Blind Association of Western New York
Olmsted Center For Sight
1170 Main Street
Buffalo, NY 14209
716-882-1025
www.olmstedcenter.org

Phillip Catanese, Chair
Kevin J Cross, Vice Chair
George Wands, Treasurer

Sponsors rehabilitation, education, vocation, employment services, housing, adult day health care, and programs for the blind and visually impaired.

Year Founded: 1907

5677 Blind Enterprises of Oregon
6540 SE Foster Road
Portland, OR 97206-4662
503-774-6387
Fax: 503-774-0585
nametapes@blindenterprises.org
www.blindenterprises.com

Tami Foss, Executive Director
Year Founded: 1988

5678 Blind Industries and Services of Maryland
3345 Washington Boulevard
Baltimore, MD 21227
410-737-2600
Fax: 410-737-2665; *Toll Free:* 888-322-4567
info@bism.org
www.bism.org

Frederick J Puente, President
Dr. Michael Gosse, Chairman

A not-for-profit organization dedicated to providing career and training resources to blind residents of Maryland.

Year Founded: 1908

5679 Blind Rehabilitation Services
U.S. Department of Veterans Affairs
www.rehab.va.gov

To provide personal and social adjustment programs and medical or health-related services for eligible blind veter-

ans at selected VA Medical Centers maintaining blind rehabilitation centers.

5680 Blind Service Association
17 North State Street
Suite 1050
Chicago, IL 60602
312-236-0808
dgrossman@blindserviceassociation.org
www.blindserviceassociation.org

Linda Schwartz, President
Carol Menner, MD, Executive Vice President
Debbie Grossman, Executive Director

Individuals who promote the welfare of blind and partially blind persons through voluntary service or financial support. Through its service program, the association maintains reading rooms for daily oral readings of textbooks and work-related material primarily to blind students, senior citizens, and business and professional people; records textbooks on cassette tapes for blind people's home, study, work and leisure needs; supplies visual aids, field trips, and other assistance to blind and visually handicapped children in Chicago, IL schools; helps maintain eye clinics in hospitals; helps support recreational programs for visually impaired minors and workshop program for the blind retarded; sponsors cultural activities for blind adults and provides tickets for some events; provides emergency relief for blind in need of assistance and cooperates with other charitable agencies in referral cases.

Year Founded: 1924

5681 Blinded Veterans Association
125 N West Street
3rd Floor
Alexandria, VA 22314
Fax: 202-371-8258; *Toll Free:* 800-669-7079
bva@bva.org
www.bva.org

Joe Parker, National President
Paul Mimms, National Vice President
Brigitte Jones, Administrative Director

Offers service programs without cost to blinded veterans. The Field Service program provides counseling to veterans and their families. The organization also offers a peer support program, volunteer service program, advocacy for blind veterans and their families, as well as a Blind Hockey team.

Year Founded: 1945

5682 Bosma Industries for the Blind
BOSMA Enterprises
6270 Corporate Drive
Indianapolis, IN 46278
317-684-0600Toll free: 866-602-6762
info@bosma.org
www.bosma.org

Lou Moneymaker, President & CEO
Doug Pingel, Vice President of Operations
Teresa Watson, Chief Financial Officer

Dedicated to providing assistance to persons with vision loss achieve professional and personal independence.

Year Founded: 1915

5683 Braille Institute
741 N Vermont Avenue
Los Angeles, CA 90029
323-663-1111
Fax: 323-663-0867
la@brailleinstitute.org
brailleinstitute.org

Peter A. Mindnich, President

Dedicated to providing blind and visually impaired men, women and children with the training, programs and services they need to enjoy productive lives. Services offered include child development, youth programs, library services and adult education.

Year Founded: 1927

5684 Braille Institute Library
Braille Institute
741 N Vermont Avenue
Los Angeles, CA 90029
323-663-1111
Fax: 323-663-0867
la@brailleinstitute.org
www.brailleinstitute.org

Peter A. Mindnich, President

Discs, cassettes, braille, Optacon, home visits, braille writer, reference materials on blindness and other handicaps. Closed-circuit TV, Optacon, braille writer, and large print copier also available. Home visits and cassette books are part of special services offered.

Year Founded: 1927

5685 Braille Revival League
American Council of the Blind
1703 N Beauregard Street
Suite 420
Alexandria, VA 22311
202-467-5081
Fax: 703-465-5085; *Toll Free:* 800-424-8666
info@acb.org
braillerevivalleague.org

Paul Edwards, President
Denise Colley, First Vice President
May Davis, Second Vice President

Encourages blind people to read and write in braille, advocates for mandatory braille instruction in educational facilities for the blind, strives to make available a supply of braille materials from libraries and printing houses and more.

5686 Brevard Association for the Advancement of the Blind
674 S Patrick Drive
Satellite Beach, FL 32937-3873
321-773-7222
baabhelpfortheblind.org

Volunteers providing educational services to the blind and visually impaired. Transfers books and magazines to audio tapes. Offers independent living programs.

Year Founded: 1966

5687 Bureau of Education and Services for the Blind (DESB)
Department of Rehabilitation Services
184 Windsor Avenue
Windsor, CT 06095

860-602-4000
Fax: 860-602-4020; *Toll Free:* 800-842-4510
brian.sigman@CT.GOV
www.ct.gov/besb
TDD 860-602-4221

Brian S. Sigman, Executive Director

Provides resources, comprehensive low vision services, specialized education services, life skills training, case management, and vocational services to individuals of all ages who are legally blind and to children who are visually impaired.

5688 Canine Companions for Independence
PO Box 446
Santa Rosa, CA 95402-0446
Toll Free: 800-572-2275
www.cci.org

Paul Mundell, CEO
Alan Feinne, CFO

5689 Carroll Center for the Blind
770 Centre Street
Newton, MA 02458
617-969-6200
Fax: 617-969-6204; *Toll Free:* 800-852-3131
carroll.org

Joseph F. Abely, President
Katherine L. Leahy, CFO

Assists blind and visually impaired adults and adolescents to adjust to loss of vision. The goal of this dynamic program is to help the person become more independent, to restore self-confidence, prepare for employment and improve the quality of life. Programs of individual counseling are offered as part of the program.

Year Founded: 1936

5690 Carroll Job Management Preparation Program
Carroll Center for the Blind
770 Centre Street
Newton, MA 02458-2597
617-969-6200Toll free: 800-852-3131
marianne.gilmore@carroll.org
carroll.org

Marianne Gilmore, Director

Provides training for persons who are blind and visually impaired to develop work skills, including technology training, vocational transition, job coaching, orientation and mobility instruction, and business development.

5691 Catholic Guild for the Blind
Catholic Charities of the Archdiocese of New York
1011 1st Avenue
6thFloor
New York, NY 10022
Toll Free: 888-744-7900
www.catholiccharitiesny.org

Kevin Sullivan, Executive Director

A nonprofit organization under the sponsorship of the Catholic Charities of the Archdiocese of New York. Daily living skills, orientation and mobility training, communication skills and bilingual preparation for high school equivalency diplomas are among the programs designed to help visually impaired people maintain their independence.

Year Founded: 1812

5692 Center for Vision Loss
845 W Wyoming Street
Allentown, PA 18103
610-433-6018
Fax: 610-433-4856
doug.yingling@centerforvisionloss.org
centerforvisionloss.org

Doug Yingling, Executive Director
Ruth Weber, Business Administrator
Dennis Zehner, Development Director

Provides a comprehensive set of preventative, rehabilitative, support and social services enabling blind and visually impaired customer to achieve their personal goals and restore quality of life consistent with those goals.

5693 Center for the Blind and Visually Impaired
100 W 15th Street
Chester, PA 19013
610-874-1476
Fax: 610-874-6454
cbvi@cbvi.net
cbvi.net

Multiservice agency with specialized services for people who have lost or are losing vision.

Year Founded: 1941

5694 Central Association for the Blind and Visually Impaired
507 Kent Street
Utica, NY 13501
315-797-2233
Fax: 315-797-2244; *Toll Free:* 877-719-9996
www.cabvi.org

Edward P Welsh, Chair
James B Turnbull, Vice Chair
Rudy D'Amico, President and CEO

A not-for-profit agency that serves people who are blind or visually impaired, from newborns to the elderly. CABVI offers vision rehabilitation, employment and technology services personally tailored to meet each individual's needs.

Year Founded: 1929

5695 Chester County Branch Pennsylvania Association for Blind
71 S First Avenue
Coatesville, PA 19320-3461
610-384-2767
Fax: 610-384-8005
info@chescoblind.org
www.chescoblind.org
TTY: 610-384-7224

Charles S Frank Jr, President
Mark Z McGill, First Vice President
Robert L Milliken, Executive Director

Sponsors employment workshops and counseling programs to support the blind and visually impaired to promote self-reliance and independence.

Year Founded: 1948

5696 Chicago Lighthouse for People who areBlind or Visually Impaired
1850 W Roosevelt Road
Chicago, IL 60608-1298

312-666-1331
Fax: 312-243-8539
chicagolighthouse.org
TDD 312-957-4865

Janet P Szlyk, PhD, President & CEO
Pamela Tully, EVP, Chief Operating Officer
Mary Lynne Januszewski, EVP, Chief Financial Officer

An organization offering progressive programs for the blind, visually impaired, deaf-blind and multi-disabled children and adults, including vocational programs, computer and office skills training, job placement, independent living skills, orientation and mobility training, counseling, and low vision adaptation.

Year Founded: 1906

5697 Christian Record Services for the Blind
5900 S 58th Street
Suite M
Lincoln, NE 68516
402-488-0981
Fax: 402-488-7582
info@christianrecord.org
www.christianrecord.org

Diane Thurber, President
Lonnie Kreiter, Vice President of Finance
Daniel R Jackson, Chair

Organization that provides interdenominational services to the visually impaired. Produces materials in large print, braille and on cassette. Membership includes access to lending library and information about summer camps for the blind upon request.

Year Founded: 1899; Number of Members: 20,000

5698 Cincinnati Association for the Blind and Visually Impaired
2045 Gilbert Avenue
Cincinnati, OH 45202
513-221-8558Toll free: 888-687-3935
info@cincyblind.org
www.cincyblind.org

John Mitchell, President & CEO
Ginny Backscheider, Director Of Program Services
Jennifer Dubois, VP, Administration & CFO

A not-for-profit organization offering comprehensive vision rehabilitation services for people of all ages who are blind or visually impaired.

Year Founded: 1911

5699 Clearinghouse for Specialized Media and Technology
California Department of Education
1430 N Street
Sacramento, CA 95814-5901
916-319-0881
csmt@cde.ca.gov
www.cde.ca.gov

Assists schools and students in the identification and acquisition of textbooks, reference books and study materials in aural media, braille, large print and electronic media access technology.

5700 Cleveland Sight Center
1909 E 101st Street
Cleveland, OH 44106

216-791-8118
info@clevelandsightcenter.org
www.clevelandsightcenter.org
TTY: 216-791-8119

Larry Benders, President & CEO

Mission is to empower people who are blind or have low vision to realize their full potential and to shape the community's vision of that potential.

Year Founded: 1906

5701 Clovernook Center for the Blind and Visually Impaired

7000 Hamilton Avenue
Cincinnati, OH 45231
513-522-3860
Fax: 513-728-6229
www.clovernook.org

Christopher Faust, President & CEO

Offers various library services, information and resources for the blind and visually impaired.

Year Founded: 1903

5702 Columbia Lighthouse for the Blind

8757 Georgia Avenue
Suite 805
Silver Spring, MD 20910
301-589-0894
Fax: 877-595-9228
info@clb.org
www.clb.org

Anthony J Cancelosi, President & CEO

Offers persons who are blind and visually impaired in the areas of DC, Maryland and Virginia, training in assistive technology, career development and rehabilitation and offers services such as braille production, speakers bureau, visionaries store, volunteer assistance, low-vision clinics and Columbia Extension recreational activities.

Year Founded: 1900

5703 Connecticut Braille Association

44 Imperial Avenue
Westport, CT 06880
203-227-5243
micki1@juno.com
www.afb.org

Micki McCabe, Computer Coordinator

Serves the visually impaired, with special emphasis on aid for children and young adults in school.

Year Founded: 1921

5704 Dallas Lighthouse for the Blind

4306 Capitol Avenue
Dallas, TX 75204
214-821-2375
info@dallaslighthouse.org
www.dallaslighthouse.org

Hugh McElroy, Chief Executive Officer
Greg Bogard, Chief Financial Officer
Maria MacMullin, Vice President, Development

Serves adults and senior citizens with vision disabilities. Programs include vocational rehabilitation, independent living rehabilitation and employment. Services include orientation and mobility skills training, information and referral, case work services, personal and social adjustment

counseling, employment readiness training, on-the-job training, job placement assistance, technology training, adult basic education, Braille instruction.

Year Founded: 1931

5705 Delaware Association for the Blind

2915 Newport Gap Pike
Wilmington, DE 19808
302-998-5913
Fax: 302-691-5810; *Toll Free:* 888-777-3925
blindsightdelaware.org

Lewis K Rolph, Jr, President
William E Bartlett, Vice President
James Law, Secretary

Provides recreational and counseling services not provided by the government to the blind and visually impaired.

Year Founded: 1909

5706 Delaware Division for the Visually Impaired
University of Delaware

461 Wyoming Road
Newark, DE 19716
302-831-0354
Fax: 302-831-4690
www.dati.org
TTY: 800-870-3284

State agency serving the visually impaired persons from birth, with or without other handicaps. Services offered include educational, computer training, employment and pre-vocational training.

Year Founded: 1991

5707 Diabetes Action Network
National Federation of the Blind

3101 NE 87th Avenue
Vancouver, WA 98662-6832
360-576-5965
nfb.org/diabetics

Michael Freeman, President

The NFB Diabetes Action Network educates, empowers, and inspires people living with diabetes and its complications.

5708 Ed Lindsey Industries of the Blind

4110 Charlotte Avenue
Nashville, TN 37209-3706
615-627-4012
Fax: 615-627-4015
abroughton@elifortheblind.org

W Allen Broughton, Executive Vice President

Offers daily independent living skills training, as well as workforce training, for blind and visually impaired persons.

Year Founded: 1982

5709 Evansville Association for the Blind

500 N Second Avenue
Evansville, IN 47710
812-422-1181
karlahorrell@evansvilleblind.org
www.evansvilleblind.org

Karla Horrell, Exectuvie Director

The low vision support group is open to all ages with a wide range of vision problems. Members recieve a monthly calendar and newsletter to inform participants on the social, entertainment, and informational events at the Association. Low vision aids are available at the Low Vision Center

Year Founded: 1923

5710 Eye Bank Association of America

1015 18th Street NW
Suite 1010
Washington, DC 20036
202-775-4999
Fax: 202-429-6036
info@restoresight.org
restoresight.org

Kevin P. Corcoran, President & CEO
Bernie Dellario, Director of Finance

Not-for-profit organization dedicate to the restoration of sight through the promortion and advancement of eye banking. Promotes research and professional education with a newsletter, brochures and pamphlets.

5711 EyeCare America
American Academy of Opthalmology

PO Box 7424
San Francisco, CA 94120-7424
415-561-8500
Fax: 415-561-8533
www.aao.org/eyecare-america

Ophthalmologists dedicated to ensuring eye care for the elderly, particularly those who are economically disadvantaged. Provides medical and surgical eye care to individuals 65 and over who normally would not have access or the means to consult an ophthalmologist. Disseminates information on participating physicians and eye diseases of the aging. Offers referral services. A project of the Foundation of the American Academy of Ophthalmology.

Year Founded: 1985

5712 Fidelco Guide Dog Foundation

103 Vision Way
Bloomfield, CT 06002
860-243-5200
Fax: 860-769-0567
info@fidelco.org
www.fidelco.org

Eliot D Russman, President & CEO
Julie M Unwin, Chief Operating Officer
Gregg Barratt, Chief of Staff

Purpose is to breed, train and place Fidelco German shepherd guide dogs with blind persons throughout the Northeast. Provides training services to blind persons, reviews performance of the guide dog teams to see that satisfactory level of achievement is maintained, utilizes genetic processes and clinical methods to improve and refine the breed and maintains an ongoing program for development and improvement of training methods.

Year Founded: 1960

5713 Foundation Fighting Blindness

7168 Columbia Gateway Drive
Suite 100
Columbia, MD 21046
410-423-0600Toll free: 800-683-5555
info@FightBlindness.org
www.blindness.org
TDD 800-683-5551

Benjamin R Yerxa, PhD, Chief Executive Officer
Stephen M Rose, PhD, Chief Research Officer
Brian Mansfield, Deputy Chief Research Officer

Provides information and referral services and support networks for individuals with retinitis pigmentosa and their families. The main focus of the Foundation is to fund research on the causes, cures, and prevention of retinites pigmentosa, Usher syndrome, and related reetinal degenerations.

Year Founded: 1971

5714 Friends for Sight

6715 S 1300 E
Suite 250
Salt Lake City, UT 84121
801-524-2020Toll free: 800-675-LOOK
2020@friendsforsight.org
www.friendsforsight.org

Frances Larsen, Chair
Greg Reid, Chair Elect
Kate C. Edwards, Executive Director

Individuals wishing to prevent loss of eyesight. Works to preserve sight and prevent blindness through comprehensive eye screening programs. Offers educational programs and self-help support groups. Makes available free glaucoma and ambloyopia, visual acuity, screening; operates speakers' bureau.

Year Founded: 1955

5715 Friends of Tennessee School of the Blind

P.O. Box 140057
Nashville, TN 37214-0057
615-231-7307
info@friendsoftsb.org
www.friendsoftsb.org

Jim Oldham, President
DeeGee Lester, Vice President
Sue Glore, Treasurer

A non-profit organization assisting Tennessee School for the Blind with the purchase of equipment, materials and enrichment activities. The mission of Friends of Tennessee School for the Blind is to supplement state appropriations by enhancing and enriching the educational, vocational, special skills and social development of students enrolled at the Tennessee School for the Blind.

Year Founded: 1997

5716 Friends-In-Art
American Council of the Blind

521 Oxford Circle
Birmingham, AL 35209
205-942-1987
lynnsbrc@gmail.com
www.friendsinart.com/drupal

Lynn Hedi, President

Aims to enlarge the art experience of blind people, encourages blind people to visit museums, galleries, concerts, the theater, etc., offers consultation to program planners in establishing accessible art and museum exhibits and presents Performing Arts Showcases.

5717 Georgia Industries for the Blind

700 Faceville Highway
Bainbridge, GA 39819

Toll Free: 800-605-7260
GIB_customer_Service@gvs.ga.gov
gvs.georgia.gov/georgia-industries-blind

Sean T Casey, Executive Director
Kevin Harris, Deputy Executive Director

Employs people who are blind in two locations across the
state: Bainbridge and Griffin.

Year Founded: 1937

5718 Glaucoma Support Groups
Glaucoma Research Foundation
251 Post Street
Suite 600
San Francisco, CA 94108
415-986-3162Toll free: 800-826-6693
grf@glaucoma.org
www.glaucoma.org

Andrew Iwach, Chair
Thomas M Brunner, President & CEO
Ruth D Williams, MD, Vice Chair

A peer support service for glaucoma patients and their families. The Network provides meaningful, helpful answers to
questions from individuals concerned about vision and
glaucoma.

Year Founded: 1978

5719 Greater Detroit Agency for the Blind and
Visually Impaired
16625 Grand River Avenue
Detroit, MI 48227
313-272-3900
Fax: 313-272-6893
information@gdabvi.org
gdabvi.org

William Van Winkle, Chairman
Frederick J Simpson, Vice Chairman
Leonard W Robinson, Secretary

Provides rehabilitation and daily living skills training to
blind and visually impaired senior citizens.

Year Founded: 1961

5720 Guide Dog Foundation for the Blind
371 E Jericho Turnpike
Smithtown, NY 11787-2976
631-930-9000
Fax: 631-930-9009; *Toll Free:* 800-548-4337
info@guidedog.org
www.guidedog.org

Don Dea, Chair
Gretchen G Evans, Vice Chair
Wells B. Jones, Chief Executive Officer

Provides guide dogs for the blind. All programs, including
training with instructor and guide dog, transportation to and
from the foundation, and aftercare are free.

Year Founded: 1946

5721 Guide Dog Users, Inc. (GDUI)
3603 Morgan Way
Imperial, MO 63052
Toll Free: 866-799-8436
guidedogusersinc.org

Penny Reeder, President

Promotes the acceptance of blind people and their dogs,
works for enforcement and expansion of laws admitting

guide dogs into public places, advocates for quality training
and follow-up services.

5722 Guide Dogs for the Blind
350 Los Ranchitos Road
San Rafael, CA 94903
415-499-4000
Fax: 415-499-4035; *Toll Free:* 800-295-4050
www.guidedogs.com

Christine Benninger, Chief Executive Officer
Cathy Martin, Treasurer & CFO
Susan Armstrong, VP, Training Operations, Oregon

Offers educational materials, transportation, seminars and
newsletters for the blind.

Year Founded: 1942

5723 Guiding Eyes for the Blind
611 Granite Springs Road
Yorktown Heights, NY 10598
914-245-4024
Fax: 914-245-1609; *Toll Free:* 800-942-0149
www.guidingeyes.org

Thomas Panek, Chief Executive Officer

Provides the means for blind and visually impaired individuals to achieve mobility, independence and companionship
through the use of professionally bred and trained guide
dogs. Each month Guiding Eyes graduates approximately
12 guide dog/student teams. The guide dogs, 26 day residential training program, special needs program and home
training programs are free of charge.

5724 Helen Keller National Center for Deaf-Blind
Youths & Adults
141 Middle Neck Road
Sands Point, NY 11050
516-944-8900
hkncinfo@hknc.org
www.helenkeller.org

Joseph F. Bruno, President & CEO
Marc Feldman, CFO

Provides diagnostic, evaluation, short term comprehensive
rehabilitation and personal adjustment training. A technical
assistance center is offered providing assistance to public
and private agencies and to parent groups who work towards community integration and the enhancement of the
quality of life. A national parent network is also provided
that develops and shares information about advocacy,
legislation, new services and achievements.

Year Founded: 1967

5725 Helen Keller National Center: East Central
14440 Cherry Lane Court
Suite 214
Laurel, MD 20707
240-786-6534
www.helenkeller.org
TTY: 240-786-6847

Cynthia Ingraham, Regional Representative

Regional representatives help deaf-blind individuals access
programs and services in DE, DC, MD, PA, VA, and WV.

5726 Helen Keller National Center: Great Plains
450 E Park Street
Olathe, KS 66061

913-677-4562
www.helenkeller.org

Beth Jordan, Regional Representative

Regional representatives help deaf-blind individuals access programs and services in IA, KS, MO, and NE.

5727 Helen Keller National Center: Mid-Atlantic
144 Middle Neck Road
Sand Point, NY 11050
516-944-8900
www.helenkeller.org

Ryan Odland, Regional Representative

Regional representatives help deaf-blind individuals access programs and services in NJ, NY, PR, and VI.

5728 Helen Keller National Center: New England
175 North Beacon Road
Watertown, MA 02472
617-923-1600
www.helenkeller.org

Steve Perreault, Regional Representative

Regional representatives help deaf-blind individuals access programs and services in CT, ME, MA, NH, RI, and VT.

5729 Helen Keller National Center: North Central
485 Avenue of the Cities
Suite 5
East Moline, IL 61244
419-951-6020
www.helenkeller.org

Judy Knisely, Regional Representative

Regional representatives help deaf-blind individuals access programs and services in IL, IN, MI, MN, OH, and WI.

5730 Helen Keller National Center: Northwest
1620 18th Avenue
Suite 201
Seattle, WA 98122
206-324-9120
www.helenkeller.org
TTY: 206-324-1133

Dorothy Walt, Regional Representative

Regional representatives help deaf-blind individuals access programs and services in AK, ID, OR, and WA.

5731 Helen Keller National Center: Rocky Mountain
190 E 9th Avenue
Suite 150
Denver, CO 80203
303-934-9037
www.helenkeller.org
TTY: 303-934-9037

Ryan Odland, Regional Representative

Regional representatives help deaf-blind individuals access programs and services in CO, MT, ND, SD, UT, and WY.

5732 Helen Keller National Center: South Central
PO Box 152080
Austin, TX 78715
516-393-7997
www.helenkeller.org

Molly Sinanan, Regional Representative

Regional representatives help deaf-blind individuals access programs and services in AR, LA, NM, OK, and TX.

5733 Helen Keller National Center: Southeast
PO Box 380
Concord, GA 30206
516-393-7733
www.helenkeller.org

Barbara Posner, Regional Representative
Marilyn Trader, Regional Representative

Regional representatives help deaf-blind individuals access programs and services in AL, FL, GA, KY, MS, NC, SC, and TN.

5734 Helen Keller National Center: Southwest
9939 Hibert Street
Suite 108
San Diego, CA 92131
858-578-1600
www.helenkeller.org
TTY: 858-578-1600

Cathy Kirscher, Regional Representative

Regional representatives help deaf-blind individuals access programs and services in AZ, CA, HI, NV, Guam, and Samoa.

5735 Ho'opono Services for the Blind
600 Kapi'olani Boulevard
Suite 305
Honolulu, HI 96813
808-586-9745 Toll free: 808-586-5269
smitchell@dhs.hawaii.gov
humanservices.hawaii.gov
TTY: 808-586-5269

Albert Perez, Administrator

Provides services to blind and visually impaired persons in Adjustment to Blindness, Vocational Rehabilitation, Low Vision evaluation and assistance. Offers work assesment and vending training.

Year Founded: 1994

5736 Ho'opono Workshop for the Blind
600 Kapi'olani Boulevard
Suite 305
Honolulu, HI 96813
808-586-9745 Toll free: 808-586-5269
smitchell@dhs.hawaii.gov
humanservices.hawaii.gov
TTY: 808-586-5269

Albert Perez, Administrator

Offers workshops for job placement and maintenance support, Older Blind training services, help with applying for Library for the Blind services, Home Care Referral, Tax Filing Assistance, free presentations on blindess education and the prevention of blindess, and youth activities.

Year Founded: 1994

5737 Horizons for the Blind
125 Erick Street
A103
Crystal Lake, IL 60014-4401
815-444-8800
Fax: 815-444-8830
mail@horizons-blind.org
www.horizons-blind.org

Camille Caffarelli, Executive Director
Jeff T. Thorsen, First Vice President/Treasurer
Keith Myers, Second Vice President

Braille and large print books on recipes, crafts, healthy living and poetry; monthly magazine and tactile pictures.

Year Founded: 1977

5738 IFB Solutions

7730 North Point Drive
Winston Salem, NC 27106-3310
336-759-0551
Fax: 336-759-0990; *Toll Free:* 800-242-7726
ifbsolutions.org

Ann Johnston, Chairman
Tim Nerhood, Vice Chairman
David Horton, President & CEO

Formerly known as the Winston-Salem Industries for the Blind, IFB Solutions provides employment opportunities for the blind and visually impaired persons.

Year Founded: 1936

5739 Idaho Commission for the Blind and Visually Impaired

341 W Washington Street
P.O. Box 83720
Boise, ID 83702-0012
208-334-3220
Fax: 208-334-2963; *Toll Free:* 800-542-8688
bcunningham@icbvi.idaho.gov
www.icbvi.state.id.us

Britt Raubenheimer, Chair
Mike Gibson, Vice Chair
Beth Cunningham, Administrator

Independent living services for individual over 55 years of age. Orientation and mobility, adaptive technology, cooking, braills, money management, advocacy, and related services. Peer support group services available.

Year Founded: 1967

5740 Illinois Society for the Prevention of Blindness

211 West Wacker Drive
Suite 1700
Chicago, IL 60606
312-363-6029
www.eyehealthillinois.org

Mary Elizabeth White, President
Charles S Bouchard, MD, Vice President
Elyse Fineman, Executive Director

To prevent the tragedy of needless blindness. Dedicated to the care, protection, and preservation of sight, ISPB programs stress education, eye safety, information and research.

Year Founded: 1916

5741 Independent Living Services for Older Individuals who are Blind
US Department of Education OSERS

400 Maryland Avenue SW
PCP, Room 5155
Washington, DC 20202
202-245-7454
suzanne.mitchell@ed.gov
www.ed.gov

Suzanne Mitchell, Administrator

To provide independent living services to older blind individuals, i.e., individuals aged 55 or older, whose severe visual impairments make gainful employment extremely

difficult to attain but for whom independent living in their own homes and communities is feasible.

Year Founded: 1980

5742 Indiana County Association for the Blind
Pennsylvania Association for the Blind

555 Gettysburg Pike
Suite A300
Mechanicsburg, PA 17055
717-766-2020
Fax: 717-766-2099
info@pablind.org
www.pablind.org

To provide support to its statewide network of member agencies, empowering them to help Pennsylvanians prevent, prepare for and manage vision loss. Services include daily living workshops, orientation and mobility instructions, counseling and case management, low vision examinations, in-home supportive services, and more.

Year Founded: 1910; Number of Members: 25

5743 Insight

43 Jefferson Boulevard
Warwick, RI 02888
401-941-3322
Fax: 401-941-3356
insightri@gmail.com
www.in-sight.org

Robert Tyler, Jr, Chairman
Melissa Burnett-Testa, Vice Chairman
Christopher Butler, Executive Director

Sponsors rehabilitation and vocational programs for blind and visually impaired individuals in Rhode Island and southeastern Massachusetts. Seeks to enable blind and visually impaired persons to become more active, independent, and productive.

Year Founded: 1905

5744 International Braille and Technology Center for the Blind
National Federation of the Blind

200 East Wells Street
at Jernigan Place
Baltimore, MD 21230
410-659-9314
Fax: 410-685-5653
access@nfb.org
nfb.org

Clara Van Gerven, Contact

World's largest and most complete evaluation and demonstration center of all assistive technology used by the blind from around the world. Includes all Braille, synthetic speech, print-to-speech scanning, internet and portable devices and programs. Available for tours by appointment to blind persons, employers, technology manufacturers, teachers, parents and those working in the assistive technology field.

Year Founded: 1940

5745 Iowa Regional Library for the Blind & Physically Handicapped
Iowa Department for the Blind

524 4th Street
Des Moines, IA 50309-2364

515-281-1333
Fax: 515-281-1263; *Toll Free:* 800-362-2587
library@blind.state.ia.us
idblibrary.blind.state.ia.us
TDD 515-281-1355

Sarah Wilford, Director
Gail Stricker, Instructional Material Center

Offers services to blind and visually-impaired individuals; provides counseling, educational, recreational, rehabilitation, home visits, computer training, and professional training services. Access to Braillewriters, magnifiers, closed-circuit TV, large print photocopiers, cassette, Braille, large print books, cassette magazines, descriptive videos, and other reference materials on blindness and handicaps.

Year Founded: 1958

5746 Jewish Braille Institute International
110 E 30th Street
New York, NY 10016
212-889-2525
Fax: 212-689-3692; *Toll Free:* 800-433-1531
admin@jbilibrary.org
www.jbilibrary.org

Ellen Isler, President & CEO
Israel A. Taub, VP & CFO

Supplies books and reading material of Jewish interest in braille, on audio cassette and in large print. Provides various services free of charge to those in more than 50 countries.

Year Founded: 1931

5747 Kansas Association for the Blind andVisually Impaired
712 S Kansas Avenue
Suite 410
Topeka, KS 66603
785-235-8990Toll free: 800-799-1499
kabvi@att.net
www.kabvi.com

Ann Byington, President
Phyllis Schmidt, Membership Secretary
Bob Chaffin, Treasurer

KABVI strives to increase the independence, opportunity, and quality of life for all the blind and visually impaired Kansans, and to assist them in taking their rightful place as equals among their sighted peers.

Year Founded: 1920

5748 Kansas City Association for the Blind
Alphapointe
7501 Prospect Avenue
Kansas City, MO 64132-2103
816-421-5848
Fax: 816-237-2019
info@alphapointe.org
www.alphapointe.org

David Westbrook, Chairman
Jill Forrest, Vice Chair
Reinhard Mabry, President & CEO

The Alphapointe Foundation strives to meet the needs of the vision loss community by building awareness, funding, and expanding resources, including rehabilitation and education.

Year Founded: 1911

5749 Kansas Division of Services for the Blind
Kansas Department for Children & Families
555 S Kansas
3rd Floor
Topeka, KS 66603
785-368-7471
Fax: 785-368-7467; *Toll Free:* 866-213-9079
www.dcf.ks.gov
TTY: 785-368-7478

Gina Meier-Hummel, Secretary

Offers services for the totally blind, legally blind, visually impaired, mentally retarded blind and more with health, counseling, educational, recreational, rehabilitation, computer training and professional training services.

5750 Kentucky Division: Prevent Blindness America
Prevent Blindness America
211 West Wacker Drive
Suite 1700
Chicago, IL 60606
312-363-6040Toll free: 800-331-2020
info@preventblindness.org
www.preventblindness.org

Richard Sanchez, Chairman
Hugh Parry, President & CEO
Jeff Todd, Chief Operating Officer

Prevent Blindness America is the nation's volunteer eye health and safety organization dedicated to fighting blindness and saving sight. Focused on promoting a continuum of vision care.

Year Founded: 1908

5751 Kentucky Office for the Blind
Kentucky Career Center
275 East Main Street
Mail Stop 2 E-J
Frankfort, KY 40621
502-564-4754
Fax: 502-564-2951; *Toll Free:* 800-321-6668
cora.mcnabb@ky.gov
workforce.ky.gov

Cora McNabb, Executive Director

Provides career services and assistance to adults with severe visual handicaps who want to become productive in the home or work force. Also provides the Client Assistance Program established to provide advice, assistance and information available from rehabilitation programs to persons with handicaps.

5752 Learning Ally
20 Roszel Road
Princeton, NJ 08540
Toll Free: 800-221-4792
www.learningally.org

Andrew Friedman, President & CEO
Harold J Logan, Chair
Therese Llorente, Vice Chair

Provides recorded and computerized textbooks, library services and other educational resources to people who cannot effectively read standard print because of a visual impairment, learning disability or other physical disability. RFB&D also provides bibliographic reference services and acts as a recording service for additional titles.

5753 Lighthouse Center for Vision Loss
4505 W Superior Street
Duluth, MN 55807
218-624-4828
Fax: 218-624-4479; *Toll Free:* 800-422-0833
info@lcfvl.org
www.lcfvl.org
TTY: 218-624-8822

Linda Goese, President
James Kelm, Vice President
Mary Junnila, Executive Director

The Lighthouse Center for Vision Loss offers training and a variety of services to 1,500 individuals with vision loss each year. Services include: vision rehabilitation, low vision optometric exams, occupational therapy, home and workplace adaptations, community and business education, etc.

Year Founded: 1919

5754 Lighthouse Guild
250 West 64th Street
New York, NY 10023
212-769-6200 Toll free: 800-284-4422
info@lighthouseguild.org
www.lighthouseguild.org

Alan R Morse, President & CEO
Mark G Ackermann, EVP & COO
Christina Wonge, CFO & GuildNet COO

The Lighthouse Guild is a leading not-for-profit vision & healthcare organization.

Year Founded: 1905

5755 Lighthouse for the Blind of Fort Worth
912 West Broadway
Fort Worth, TX 76104
817-332-3341
Fax: 817-332-3456
rmaloney@lighthousefw.org
lighthousefw.org

Platt Allen, III, President & CEO
Rheana Maloney, Executive Assistant
Lisa Fellers, Head of Development

For over 80 years Lighthouse Fort Worth has provided services to assist legally and totally blind individuals to achieve their highest level of personal and economic self-sufficiency consistent with their specific skills, general abilities and interests.

Year Founded: 1935

5756 Lighthouse of Oakland County
46156 Woodward Avenue
P.O. Box 430508
Pontiac, MI 48342
248-920-6000
info@lighthouseoakland.org
www.lighthouseoakland.org

Rick David, Chief Executive Officer
Wilma Abney, Chief Programs Officer
Liz McLachlan, Chief Development Officer

Lighthouse of Oakland County serves residents of southeastern Michigan who are facing economic hardship by providing the support and resources they need to move from crisis towards self-sufficiency.

Year Founded: 1972

5757 Louisiana Association for the Blind
1750 Claiborne Avenue
Shreveport, LA 71103
318-635-6471
Fax: 318-635-8901; *Toll Free:* 877-913-6471
www.lablind.com

Libby Murphy, President & CEO
Doug Young, SVP, Operations
Tom Tyler, VP, Sales & Business Development

Dedicated to improving the quality of life for the blind through training, services and employment. As a part of National Industries for the Blind (NIB), LAB participates in the nation's AbilityOne program, providing quality products to the government made by Americans with visual and other severe disabilities.

Year Founded: 1927

5758 Louisiana Center for the Blind
101 South Trenton Street
Ruston, LA 71270
318-251-2891
Fax: 318-251-0109; *Toll Free:* 800-234-4166
info@louisianacenter.org
www.louisianacenter.org

Pam Allen, Executive Director

Provides adult rehabilitation training for the blind. Conducts summer children's programs. Sponsors seminars.

5759 Maine Division for the Blind & Visually Impaired Services
Bureau of Rehabilitation Services
150 State House Station
Augusta, ME 04333-0150
207-623-6799
Fax: 207-287-5292
www.maine.gov
TTY: 207-623-6799

John Butera, Commissioner

Comprehensive services for visually impaired and blind individuals of all ages.

5760 Maryland Society for Sight
1313 W Old Cold Spring Lane
Baltimore, MD 21209-4989
410-243-2020
Fax: 410-889-2505
info@mdsocietyforsight.org
www.mdsocietyforsight.org

Audrey E Novak, Executive Director

To preserve sight by providing early detection of conditions that can lead to blindness and through public education on the causes of blindness.

Year Founded: 1909

5761 Massachusetts Association for the Blind
200 Ivy Street
Brookline, MA 02446
617-738-5110
Fax: 617-738-1247
bsalisbury@mabcommunity.org
www.mabcommunity.org

Michael O'Friel, President
Karen Quigley, Vice President
Barbara Salisbury, Chief Executive Officer

Provides services to the blind, visually impaired, multihandicapped, or individuals with traumatic brain injury. Promotes self-reliance, equal opportunities, and community participation. Specializes in: recruiting and matching volunteers with consumers; braille, recording, and assistance supplies for the visually impaired; education for multi-handicapped children (visual impairment not required or adolescents with traumatic brain injury); information and referrals; residential and work services for adults with mental retardation.

Year Founded: 1903

5762 Media Access Group
WBGH
1 Guest Street
Boston, MA 02135
617-300-2000
access@wgbh.org
www.wgbh.org

Jonathan C. Abbott, President & CEO
Benjamin Godley, Chief Operating Officer
David Bernstein, Vice President/General Manager

Media Access Group at WGBH has been pioneering and delivering accessible media to disabled adults, students, and their families, teachers, and friends for over 30 years and is made up of the Caption Center, Descriptive Video Service, and National Center for Accessible Media. Founded in 1993, NCAM is a research, development, and advocacy entity that works to make existing and emerging technologies more accessible to all audiences.

5763 Miami Lighthouse for the Blind and Visually Impaired
601 SW 8th Avenue
Miami, FL 33130
305-856-2288
Fax: 305-285-6967
info@miamilighthouse.org
www.miamilighthouse.org

Virginia A Jacko, President & CEO
Richard Fernandez, Chief Financial Officer
Lynda Medina, Executive Assistant

Miami Lighthouse for the Blind and Visually Impaired is the oldest and largest private agency in Florida to serve people of all ages who are blind or visually impaired. Services include rehabilitation, eye health care, and education that promote independence.

5764 Minnesota State Services for the Blind
Employment and Economic Development Department
2200 University Avenue W
Suite 240
Saint Paul, MN 55114
651-539-2300
mn.gov/deed

Kathy McGillivray, Chair, Community Center
Robert Hobson, Chair, Employment
Kotumu Kamara, Chair, Minority Outreach

State agency serving blind and visually impaired persons with rehabilitation, information access, assistive technology, training, and job placement services, with an extensive Older Blind Program.

5765 Mississippi Industries for the Blind
2501 N West Street
Jackson, MS 39216
601-984-3200
sales@msblind.org
www.msblind.org

Sandra Hall, Chair
Pshon Barrett, Vice Chair
Michael Chew, Executive Director

The missions is to provide viable work opputunities for Mississippians who are blind or visually impaired.

5766 Missouri Rehabilitation Services for the Blind
P.O. Box 2320
615 Howerton Court
Jefferson City, MO 65102-2320
573-751-4249
Fax: 573-751-4984
askrsb@dss.mo.gov
www.dss.mo.gov
TDD 800-735-2966
TTY: 800-735-2966

Eric Greitens, Governor

Offers services for the totally blind, legally blind, visually impaired, mentally retarded blind and more with health, counseling, educational, recreational, rehabilitation, computer training and professional training services.

5767 Mobile Association for the Blind
2440 Gordon Smith Drive
Mobile, AL 36617
www.mobileblind.org/aboutus

Offers work adjustment training, job placement, activities of daily living, mobility, communication skills and sheltered employment for adults who are visually impaired and for persons with other disabilities.

Year Founded: 1926

5768 National Association of Blind Lawyers
National Federation of the Blind
1660 South Albion Street
Suite 918
Denver, CO 80222-4046
303-504-5979
Fax: 303-757-3640
www.blindlawyer.org

Scott C. LaBarre, President

Provides support and information regarding employment, techniques used by the blind, advocacy, laws affecting the blind, current information about the American Bar Association and other issues for blind lawyers.

5769 National Association of Blind Merchants
National Federation of the Blind
16 Linsley Place
Metuchen, NJ 08840-2532
Toll Free: 877-521-8363
www.blindmerchants.org

Nicky Gacos, President

Provides information regarding rehabilitation, social security, tax and other issues which directly affect blind merchants. Serves as advocacy and support group.

5770 National Association of Blind Office Professionals
National Federation of the Blind
7001 Hamilton Avenue
Unit 2
Cincinnati, OH 45231
513-931-7070
lhall007@cinci.rr.com

Lisa Hall, President

5771 National Association of Blind Rehabilitation Professionals
National Federation of the Blind
3230 Grove Avenue
Richmond, VA 23221
804-371-3323
melody.lindsey@dbvi.virginia.gov

Melody Roane, President

5772 National Association of Blind Students
nabslink.org

Sean Whalen, President

Works to facilitate progress toward full accessibility of college programs and facilities, provides opportunities for discussion of issues important to students and assists with National Student Seminars.

Year Founded: 1967

5773 National Association of Blind Veterans
National Federation of the Blind
PO Box 784957
Winter Garden, FL 34778
321-948-1466
president@nabv.org
nabv.org

Dwight Sayer, President

5774 National Association of Guide Dog Users
National Federation of the Blind
1003 Papaya Drive
Tampa, FL 33619
813-626-2789 Toll free: 888-624-3841
info@nagdu.org
www.nagdu.org

Marion Gwizdala, President

Provides information and support for guide dog users and works to secure high standards in guide dog training. Addresses issues of discrimination of guide dog users and offers public education about guide dog use.

5775 National Association of Parents of Children with Visual Impairments (NAPVI)
Lighthouse Guild
15 W 65th Street
New York, NY 10023
Toll Free: 800-562-6265
napvi@lighthouseguild.org
www.lighthouseguild.org

Susan LaVenture, Executive Director

A partnership organization with the National Eye Health Education Program and the National Agenda for the Education of Children and Youths with Visual Impairments including those with multiple disabilities.

5776 National Association to Promote the Use of Braille
National Federation of the Blind
200 East Wells Street
at Jernigan Place
Baltimore, MD 21230
410-659-9314
Fax: 410-685-5653
www.nfbcal.org

Nadine Jacobson, President
Jennifer Dunnam, Secretary
Warren Figueiredo, Treasurer

Dedicated to securing improved Braille instruction, increasing the number of Braille materials available to the blind and providing information about the importance of Braille in securing independence, education and employment for the blind.

5777 National Braille Association
95 Allens Creek Road
Bldg. 1, Suite 202
Rochester, NY 14618
585-427-8260
Fax: 585-427-0263
www.nationalbraille.org

Whitney Gregory, President
David Shaffer, Executive Director

The National Braille Association provides continuing education to those who prepare braille by sponsoring workshops and publishing manuals for the production of technical and nontechnical materials. Direct services to the blind include a print-to-braille transcription service and duplication of braille materials from our collection of textbooks, music, technical tables, and general interest materials.

Year Founded: 1945

5778 National Captioning Institute
3725 Concorde Pkwy
Suite 100
Chantilly, VA 20151
703-917-7600
Fax: 703-917-9853
mail@ncicap.org
www.ncicap.org

Gene Chao, Chairman & CEO
Jill Toschi, President & COO
Meredith Patterson, Director of Production

NCI provides closed-captioning technology and related services to the broadcast, cable and home video industries for the benefit of people who are deaf and hard of hearing and others who can benefit from the service. In addition, NCI provides access to televised and recorded video programming for people who are blind or have low vision.

Year Founded: 1979

5779 National Eye Health Education Program
National Eye Institute
31 Center Drive
MSC 2510
Bethesda, MD 20892-2510
301-496-3583
nei.nih.gov/nehep

Offers information and support for persons with vision disorders, including Retinitis Pigmentosa.

5780 National Federation of the Blind
200 East Wells Street
at Jernigan Place
Baltimore, MD 21230
410-659-9314
Fax: 410-685-5653
nfb@nfb.org
nfb.org

Mark Riccobono, President
James Gashel, Secretary
Jeannie Massay, Treasurer

The largest membership organization of blind people in the nation, with chapters in every state and approximately 50,000 individual members. It seeks to integrate the blind into society on the basis of equality with the sighted so that the blind are seen as normal, participating citizens. 50,000 members and 700 local chapters.

Year Founded: 1940; Number of Members: 50,000+

5781 National Federation of the Blind Amateur Radio Division
National Federation of the Blind
15 Charles Plaza
Apartment 803
Baltimore, MD 21201
765-977-1683
rachel@olivero.us

Rachel Olivero, President

5782 National Federation of the Blind SeniorsDivision
National Federation of the Blind
7634 Carla Road
Pikesville, MD 21208-4409
410-602-9030
nfb.org/seniors

Ruth Sager, President

Membership organization of elderly blind persons providing support and information to other blind seniors. Issues include concerns such as remaining active in community and social life, maintaining private homes or living in retirement communities or nursing homes, learning the techniques used by the blind, independently caring for oneself and maintaining a positive approach to vision loss.

5783 National Federation of the Blind in Communities of Faith
National Federation of the Blind
8023 Grandview Lane
Overland Park, KS 66204
303-842-9661
tanderson81452@gmail.com

Tom Anderson, President

5784 National Federation of the Blind in Computer Science
National Federation of the Blind
400 Central Avenue SE
Unit 201
Albuquerque, NM 87102
505-508-1978
curtischong@earthlink.net

Curtis Chong, President

New technologies, to secure access to current technology and to develop new ways of using current or new technologies by the blind.

5785 National Federation of the Blind of Alabama
5209 Sterling Glen Drive
Pinson, AL 35126-7612
e-mail: joy.harris@dwx.com
www.nfbal.org

Joy Harris, Contact

5786 National Federation of the Blind of Alaska
2225 Arctic Boulevard
Apartment 215
Anchorage, AK 99503
e-mail: packeet1@gmail.com
www.alaskanfb.org

Tracy Packee, President

5787 National Federation of the Blind of Arizona
9014 East Bellevue Street
Tucson, AZ 85715-5652
520-733-5894
krezguy@cox.net
www.az.nfb.org

Bob Kresmer, President

5788 National Federation of the Blind of Arkansas
2360 Wedington Drive
Fayetteville, AR 72701
e-mail: tosheeler@cox.net

Terry Sheeler, President

5789 National Federation of the Blind of California
3934 Kern Court
Pleasanton, CA 94588
e-mail: mwillows@sbcglobal.net
www.nfbcal.org

Mary Willows, President

5790 National Federation of the Blind of Colorado
1660 South Albion Street
Suite 918
Denver, CO 80222
e-mail: slabarre@labarrelaw.com
www.nfbco.org

Scott C. LaBarre, President

5791 National Federation of the Blind of Connecticut
477 Connecticut Boulevard
Suite 217
East Hartford, CT 06108
860-289-1971
personal.edward@gmail.com
www.nfbct.org

Edward Shaham, President

5792 National Federation of the Blind of Delaware
24 Monterry Drive
Newark, DE 19713
302-368-2963
kat.bottner@gmail.com
www.nfbdelaware.org

Kathryn Bottner, President

5793 National Federation of the Blind of Florida
14919 SW 90th Terrace
Miami, FL 33196-1463
e-mail: valkemadenise@aol.com
www.nfbflorida.org

Denise Valkema, President

5794 National Federation of the Blind of Georgia
1901 Montreal Road
Suite 102
Tucker, GA 30084
404-371-1000
Fax: 404-371-1002
gscott@nfbga.org
www.nfbga.org

Garrick Scott, President

5795 National Federation of the Blind of Hawaii
PO Box 4372
Honolulu, HI 96812-4372
808-595-6123
nanifife@aol.com
hawaii.nfb.org

Nani Fife, President

5796 National Federation of the Blind of Idaho
1320 E Washington Street
Boise, ID 83712
208-345-3906
danalynard@q.com
www.nfbidaho.org

Dana Ard, President

5797 National Federation of the Blind of Illinois
3410 North Lake Shore Drive
Apartment 4-L
Chicago, IL 60657
e-mail: davant1958@gmail.com
www.nfbofillinois.org

Denise Avant, President

5798 National Federation of the Blind of Indiana
6010 Winnpenny Lane
Indianapolis, IN 46220-5253
317-205-9226
rb15@iquest.net
www.nfb-in.org

Ron Brown, President

5799 National Federation of the Blind of Iowa
1486 S 1st Avenue
Unit 5
Iowa City, IA 52240
319-321-8769
dprime27@gmail.com
www.nfbi.org

Donna Prime, President

5800 National Federation of the Blind of Kansas
120 E 1st Street
Apartment 3-C
Wichita, KS 67202
e-mail: topage@swbell.net
www.nfbks.org

Tom Page, President

5801 National Federation of the Blind of Kentucky
210 Cambridge Drive
Louisville, KY 40214-2809
e-mail: cathyj1949@gmail.com
www.nfbofky.org

Cathy Jackson, President

5802 National Federation of the Blind of Louisiana
605 University Boulevard
Ruston, LA 71270-4862
318-251-1511
pallen@louisianacenter.org
www.nfbla.org

Pam Allen, President

5803 National Federation of the Blind of Maine
33 Morse Avenue
Lewiston, ME 04240
207-212-1455
leonproctorjr@yahoo.com
www.nfb-me.org

Leon Proctor Jr., President

5804 National Federation of the Blind of Maryland
9013 Nelson Way
Columbia, MD 21045-5148
410-645-0632
nfbmd@earthlink.net
www.nfbmd.org

Sharon Maneki, President

5805 National Federation of the Blind of Massachusetts
9 Quail Run
Hingham, MA 02043
617-752-1116
aruell@comcast.net
www.nfbma.org

Amy Ruell, President

5806 National Federation of the Blind of Michigan
7189 Connors Road
Munising, MI 49862
e-mail: president.nfb.mi@gmail.com
www.nfbmi.org

Larry Posont, President

5807 National Federation of the Blind of Minnesota
100 E 22nd Street
Minneapolis, MN 55404
612-872-9363
jennifer.dunnam1829@gmail.com
www.nfbmn.org

Jennifer Dunnam, President

5808 National Federation of the Blind of Mississippi
268 Lexington Avenue
Jackson, MS 39209-5431
sgleese@city.jackson.ms.us

Sam Gleese, President

5809 National Federation of the Blind of Montana
3105 4th Avenue S
Great Falls, MT 59405-3331

406-454-3096
breslauerj@gmail.com
www.nfbofmt.org

Joy Breslauer, President

5810   National Federation of the Blind of Nebraska
411 North 75th
Lincoln, NE 68505
e-mail: amy.buresh74@gmail.com
www.ne.nfb.org

Amy Buresh, President

5811   National Federation of the Blind of Nevada
6955 N Durango Drive
Suite 1115-356
Las Vegas, NV 89149
e-mail: kimie.beverly@gmail.com
www.nfbnevada.org

Kimie Beverly, President

**5812   National Federation of the Blind of North
Carolina**
137 Kristens Court Drive
Mooresville, NC 28115
e-mail: weddington.sharon@gmail.com
www.nfbofnc.org

Sharon Weddington, President

5813   National Federation of the Blind of Ohio
PO Box 82055
Columbus, OH 43202
614-935-6965
peduffy63@gmail.com
www.nfbohio.org

Eric Duffy, President

5814   National Federation of the Blind of Oklahoma
505 Baker Street
Norman, OK 73072
405-600-0695
jeannie.massay@nfbok.org
www.nfbok.org

Jeannie Massay, President

5815   National Federation of the Blind of Oregon
5005 Main Street
Springfield, OR 97478
541-653-9153
president@nfb-oregon.org
www.nfb-oregon.org

Carla McQuillan, President

**5816   National Federation of the Blind of
Pennsylvania**
1500 Walnut Street
Suite 200
Philadelphia, PA 19102
215-988-0888
president@nfbp.org
www.nfbp.org

James Antonacci, President

5817   National Federation of the Blind of Puerto Rico
PO Box 9023531
Old San Juan Station
San Juan, PR 00902-3531
e-mail: arguza@attglobal.net
www.nfbpr.org

Alpidio Rolon, President

**5818   National Federation of the Blind of Rhode
Island**
69 Fourth Street
East Providence, RI 02914
401-433-2606
silvara@cox.net
www.nfbri.org

Grace Pires, President

**5819   National Federation of the Blind of South
Carolina**
847 Jefferson Street
West Columbia, SC 29169
803-254-3777
frankcoppel@att.net
www.nfbofsc.org

Frank Coppel, President

5820   National Federation of the Blind of Tennessee
4113 Tea Garden Way
Antioch, TN 37013-5440
615-412-9632
nfb.tennessee@gmail.com
www.nfb-tn.org

James Brown, President

5821   National Federation of the Blind of Texas
1600 E Highway 6
Suite 215
Alvin, TX 77511
281-968-7733
ncrosby@nfbtx.org
www.nfbtx.org

Norma Crosby, President

5822   National Federation of the Blind of Utah
1751 Park Street
Salt Lake City, UT 84105
e-mail: baconev@yahoo.com
www.nfbutah.org

Everette Bacon, President

5823   National Federation of the Blind of Vermont
PO Box 1043
Milton, VT 05468
802-730-6537
ibretthess@aol.com
www.nfbvt.org

Brett Hess, President

5824   National Federation of the Blind of Virginia
1305 Prince Edward Street
Fredericksburg, VA 22401
e-mail: michaelgkasey@verizon.net
www.nfbv.org

Michael Kasey, President

5825 National Federation of the Blind of Washington
3200 California Avenue SW
Apartment 35
Seattle, WA 98116-3361
e-mail: mjc59@comcast.net
www.nfbw.org

Marci Carpenter, President

5826 National Federation of the Blind of West Virginia
401 E Olive Street
Apartment 1-A
Bridgeport, WV 26330
e-mail: cs.nfbwv@frontier.com
www.nfbwv.org

Charlene Smyth, President

5827 National Federation of the Blind of Wisconsin
27824 Nuthatch Road
Kendall, WI 54638
608-758-4800
johnfritz66@gmail.com
www.nfbwis.org

John Fritz, President

5828 National Federation of the Blind of Wyoming
6611 King Salmon Drive
Casper, WY 82604
e-mail: rreed@wyoassist.com
www.nfbwyoming.org

Richard Reed, President

5829 National Federation of the Blind of theDistrict of Columbia
PO Box 29141
c/o Robert Ash
Washington, DC 20017
e-mail: callaway.shawn@gmail.com
www.nfbdc.org

Shawn M. Callaway, President

5830 National Federation of the Blind: Agriculture & Equestrian Division
National Federation of the Blind
3510 Bedford Circle
Carlsbad, CA 92008
760-505-8500
regenerative@earthlink.net

Fred Chambers, President

5831 National Federation of the Blind: Assistive Technology Trainers Division
National Federation of the Blind
880 S 39th Street
Lincoln, NE 68510-3522
402-488-8610
nancy.l.coffman@gmail.com

Nancy Coffman, President

5832 National Federation of the Blind: Community Service Division
National Federation of the Blind
1440 Palou Avenue
San Francisco, CA 94124

415-215-9809
president@nfbcommunityservice.org

Darian Smith, President

5833 National Federation of the Blind: Deaf-Blind Division
National Federation of the Blind
216 W McNeal Street
Millville, NJ 08332
856-765-0601
cheiro_alice@aol.com

Alice Eaddy, President

5834 National Federation of the Blind: HumanServices Division
National Federation of the Blind
1003 Papaya Street
Tampa, FL 33619
813-625-1850
merrys@verizon.net

Merry C. Schoch, President

Organization of blind persons working in counseling, personnel, psychology, social work, psychiatry, rehabilitation and other social science and human resource fields. Provides resources regarding blindness-related techniques and methods used in these fields.

5835 National Federation of the Blind: Krafters Division
National Federation of the Blind
465 Highland Avenue
Stratford, CT 06614-3222
e-mail: blindhands@aol.com
www.krafterskorner.org

Joyce Kane, President

5836 National Federation of the Blind: Missouri
3910 Tropical Lane
Columbia, MO 65202-6205
e-mail: gwunder@earthlink.net
www.nfbmo.org

Gary Wunder, President

5837 National Federation of the Blind: New Hampshire
12 Summer Street
Apartment A
Keene, NH 03431
603-357-4080
cemcnabb21@yahoo.com
www.nfbnh.org

Cassandra McKinney, President

5838 National Federation of the Blind: New Jersey
254 Spruce Street
Bloomfield, NJ 07003-3644
973-743-0075
nfbnj1@verizon.net
www.nfbnj.org

Joe Ruffalo, President

5839 National Federation of the Blind: New Mexico
700 New York Avenue
Alamogordo, NM 88310

e-mail: avigil74@gmail.com
www.nfbnm.org

Adelmo Vigil, President

5840 National Federation of the Blind: New York
PO Box 205666
Sunset Station
Brooklyn, NY 11220
718-567-7821
office@nfbny.org
www.nfbny.org

Carl Jacobsen, President

5841 National Federation of the Blind: NorthDakota
909 8th Street S
Fargo, ND 58103
e-mail: mota1252@gmail.com
www.nfbnd.org

Milton Ota, President

5842 National Federation of the Blind: Performing Arts Division
National Federation of the Blind
1626 University Avenue
Apartment B-1
Columbia, MO 65201
314-610-7740
www.nfbpad.org

Julie McGinnity, President

Offers support and information regarding copyright, publishing, promotion and other career details.

5843 National Federation of the Blind: Public Employees Division
National Federation of the Blind
4301 Clogston Avenue NE
Bremerton, WA 98310
e-mail: ieweich@budworks.net

Ivan Weich, President

Focuses on issues such as changes in governmental hiring and retention practices, new job skills needed for the future, government employment downsizing, new electronic means of finding public sector jobs, self-advocacy and career planning strategies.

5844 National Federation of the Blind: Science and Engineering Division
National Federation of the Blind
10955 Deering Street
San Diego, CA 92126
e-mail: johnmillerphd@hotmail.com

John Miller, President

This is a strong support group to encourage blind persons in pursuit of these careers, many of which have been considered not possible for the blind in the past.

5845 National Federation of the Blind: SouthDakota
903 Fulton Street
Rapid City, SD 57701
605-721-3311
gatorbumps@rushmore.com
www.nfbofsd.org

Kenneth Rollman, President

Blind persons and interested sighted people. Promotes continuing public education on visual impairments and the circumstances of the visually impaired. Works towards the attainment of equality, security, and opportunity for all blind persons. Provides speakers.

5846 National Federation of the Blind: Writers' Division
National Federation of the Blind
208-339-2430
www.writers.nfb.org

Eve Sanchez, President

Covers various aspects of this business, including selling your work, publishing, technology, motivation and discovering writing and publishing resources.

5847 National Industries for the Blind
1310 Braddock Place
Alexandria, VA 22314-1691
703-310-0500
www.nib.org

Kevin A. Lynch, President & CEO
Angela Hartley, EVP & Chief Program Officer
Steven T. Brice, VP & CFO

A nonprofit organization that represents over 100 associated industries serving people who are blind in thirty-six states. These agencies serve prople who are blind or visually impaired and help them to reach their full potential. Services include job and family counseling, job skills training, instruction in Braille and other communication skills, children's programs and more.

5848 National Library Service for the Blind and Physically Handicapped
Library of Congress
1291 Taylor Street NW
Washington, DC 20542
202-707-5100
Fax: 202-707-0712; *Toll Free:* 800-424-8567
nls@loc.gov
www.loc.gov/nls
TDD 202-707-0744

Administers a national library service that provides braille and recorded books and magazines on free loan to anyone who cannot read standard print because of visual or physical disabilities.

5849 National Organization of Blind Educators
National Federation of the Blind
200 East Wells Street
at Jernigan Place
Baltimore, MD 21230
410-659-9314
Fax: 410-685-5653
blindeducators.org

Cayte Mendez, President
Arthur Jacobs, Treasurer

Provides support and information regarding professional responsibilities, classroom techniques, national testing methods and career obstacles. Publishes The Blind Educator, national magazine specifically for blind educators.

5850 Nebraska Commission for the Blind & Visually Impaired
4600 Valley Road
Suite 100
Lincoln, NE 68510-4844
402-471-2891
Fax: 402-471-3009; *Toll Free:* 877-809-2419
kathy.stephens@nebraska.gov
ncbvi.nebraska.gov

Carlos Servan, Executive Director
Kathy Stephens, Administrative Assistant
Carrie DeFreece, Business Manager

The NCBVI works to help blind and visually impaired Nebraskans achieve full and rewarding lives through independent living skills and assisting with finding employment in Nebraska and across the country.

5851 Nevada's Bureau of Services to the Blind and Visually Impaired
NV Dept of Employment, Training & Rehabilitation
500 East Third Street
Carson City, NV 89713
775-687-6860
www.detr.state.nv.us
TTY: 775-684-8400

Offers services for the totally blind, legally blind, visually impaired, mentally retarded blind and more with health, counseling, educational, recreational, rehabilitation, computer training and professional training services.

5852 New Eyes for the Needy
New Eyes
549 Millburn Avenue
Short Hills, NJ 07078
973-376-4903
info@new-eyes.org
www.new-eyes.org

Susan Dyckman, President
Marianne Muench Busby, Vice President
Sondra Kasdon, Treasurer

Provides new glasses for those with low vision who may not be able to afford them.
Year Founded: 1932

5853 New Hampshire Association for the Blind
25 Walker Street
Concord, NH 03301
603-224-4039
services@futureinsight.org
futureinsight.org

Nate Abbott, Chair
Timothy Murray, Vice Chair
David Morgan, President & CEO

Provides rehabilitation services to blind and visually impaired New Hampshire residents in their homes, workplaces, and communities. Maintains Access Center, which produces large print, braille and audio tape materials for corporations and individuals.
Year Founded: 1912

5854 New Jersey Blind Citizens Association
18 Burlington Avenue
Leonardo, NJ 07737

732-291-0878
adminassist@njbca.org
www.njbca.org

Stacey Stefanski, Director
Robyne Hastick, Administrative Assistant

Organization dedicated to improving the lives of the blind. Services available to blind men, women, and couples age 18 and over who are legally blind and residents of New Jersey. Summer vacation program and day camp program. Both programs inlcude: mobility training, Braille lessons, social and recreational activities.
Year Founded: 1910

5855 New Mexico Commission for the Blind
Commission for the Blind
2200 Yale Boulevard SE
Albuquerque, NM 87106
505-841-8844Toll free: 888-513-7968
www.cfb.state.nm.us

Arthur Schreiber, Chairman
Greg Trapp, Executive Director

Offers services for the totally blind, legally blind, visually impaired, mentally retarded blind and more with health, counseling, educational, recreational, rehabilitation, computer training and professional training services.

5856 NewView Oklahoma
501 N Douglas Avenue
Oklahoma City, OK 73106
855-811-9699Toll free: 888-522-4644
info@newviewoklahoma.org
nvoklahoma.org

Lauren Branch, President & CEO
John Wilson, Chief Financial Officer
Dennis Loney, VP, Operations/Bsn. Developement

NewView Oklahoma focuses on Providing jobs in manufacturing, management, administrative and rehabilitation for people who are blind and vision-impaired.
Year Founded: 1949

5857 North Central Sight Services
2121 Reach Road
P.O. Box 3292
Williamsport, PA 17701
570-323-9401
Fax: 570-323-8194; *Toll Free:* 866-320-2580
ncss@ncsight.org
www.ncsight.org

Gregory Stapp, Chair
Debra Bowes, Vice Chair
Robert B. Garrett, President

To provide blindness prevention education, vision screenings, services and employment to individuals who are blind or visually impaired in the communities of Bradford, Centre, Clinton, Lycoming, Sullivan, and Tioga Counties.

5858 North Country Association for the Visually Impaired (NCAVI)
22 US Oval
Suite B-15
Plattsburgh, NY 12903
518-562-2330
Fax: 518-562-2331
ncavi2001@yahoo.com
www.ncavi.org

Amy L Kretser, Executive Director
Colleen Sheehan, President
Robert Poulin, Vice President

A private not-for-profit organization dedicated to assisting people who are blind, legally blind, or visually impaired with attaining or maintaining personal independence.

Year Founded: 1988

5859 Northeastern Association of the Blind at Albany

301 Washington Avenue
Albany, NY 12206
518-463-1211
www.naba-vision.org

Richard A Frankle, Chair
Robin M Pellegrino, Vice Chair
Takla Awad, Treasurer

Commited to helping blind or visually impaired individuals remain independent by providing individualized rehabilitation, low vision equipment, adaptive technology, vocational assessment, and job placement services.

Year Founded: 1908

5860 Oklahoma Department of Rehabilitation Services: Visually Impaired

3535 NW 58th Street
Suite 500
Oklahoma City, OK 73112
405-951-3400 Toll free: 800-845-8476
www.okdrs.org

Noel Tyler, Director

Expands opportunities for employment, independent life and economic self-sufficiency by helping Oklahomans with disabilities bridge barriers to success in the workplace, school and at home.

5861 Olmsted Center for Sight

1170 Main Street
Buffalo, NY 14209
716-882-1025
Fax: 716-882-5577
olmstedcenter.org

Tammy Owen, President & CEO
Franca Trincia, CFO

Sponsors rehabilitation, education, vocation, employment services, housing, adult day health care, and programs for the blind and visually impaired.

Year Founded: 1907

5862 Oregon State Commission for the Blind

535 SE 12th Avenue
Portland, OR 97214-2408
971-673-1588
Fax: 503-234-7468; *Toll Free:* 888-202-5463
ocb.mail@state.or.us
www.oregon.gov/blind

Dacia Johnson, Executive Director
Gail Stevens, Chief Financial Officer
Angel Hale, Dir., Rehabilitation Services

To provide services to Oregon's citizens who experience vision loss and need specialized training and support to live full and productive lives. The agency receives policy direction and oversight from a seven member Commission representing consumer organizations, education, ophthalmology/optometry, business and individual citizens.

5863 Pasadena Braille Club

386 S Los Robles Avenue
Pasadena, CA 91101-3216
626-793-7636

Blind and visually impaired persons in the Pasadena, CA area. Provides assistance to blind persons by offering educational, rehabilitation, and social activities. Teaches braille, mobility, and independent living skills.

5864 Pennsylvania Bureau of Blindness and Visual Services

PA Department of Labor & Industry
www.pa.gov

W Gerard Oleksiak, Secretary
Tom Wolf, Governor

Provides services to Pennsylvanians who are blind and visually impaired to promote economic and social independence in their daily life activities. Services include vocational rehabilitation to help working age Pennsylvanians gain employment; older blind independent living services (age 55 and up); children's services (birth to age 17); services to adults with multiple disabilities.

Year Founded: 1913

5865 Pioneers: A Volunteer Network

1801 California Street
Suite 225
Denver, CO 80202
303-571-1200
Fax: 888-477-3351; *Toll Free:* 800-872-5995
info@pioneersvolunteer.org
www.pioneersvolunteer.org

Charlene Hill, Executive Director

Pioneers is a network of volunteers in Canada and the United States who effect tangible change in our communities by answering the call of those in need.

Year Founded: 1911

5866 Pony Express Association of the Blind

Missouri Council of the Blind
5453 Chippewa
St. Louis, MO 63109
314-832-7172 Toll free: 800-342-5632
phylaron@bbwi.net
www.missouricounciloftheblind.org

Phyllis Zirkle, President

Visually impaired persons; interested others. Promotes the interests of the visually impaired; monitors legal activity effecting the blind; conducts social activities.

Year Founded: 1956

5867 Prevent Blindness America

211 W Wacker Drive
Suite 1700
Chicago, IL 60606
312-363-6001
Fax: 312-363-6052; *Toll Free:* 800-331-2020
info@preventblindness.org
www.preventblindness.org

Hugh Parry, President & CEO
Jerome Desserich, VP & CFO
Jeff Todd, COO

Dedicated to fighting blindness, saving sight and promoting a continuum of vision care.

Year Founded: 1908

5868 Prevent Blindness Connecticut
Prevent Blindness America
211 W Wacker Drive
Suite 1700
Chicago, IL 60606
312-363-6040Toll free: 800-331-2020
info@preventblindness.org
www.preventblindness.org

Richard Sanchez, Chairman
Hugh Parry, President & CEO
Jeff Todd, Chief Operating Officer

Preserves and enhances visual health through eye screenings, education, safety activities and support of research. Places special emphasis on preschool children, the elderly, and individuals at risk for eye injuries throughout Connecticut.

Year Founded: 1908

5869 Prevent Blindness Iowa
Prevent Blindness America
1111 9th Street
Suite 250
Des Moines, IA 50314-2585
515-244-4341
Fax: 515-244-4718; *Toll Free:* 800-329-8782
mail@preventblindnessiowa.org
iowa.preventblindness.org

Jeanne Burmeister, Executive Director

To prevent blindness, preserve sight and enhance and extend the quality of vision for all Iowans.

Year Founded: 1958

5870 Prevent Blindness Nebraska
Prevent Blindness America
211 W Wacker Drive
Suite 1700
Chicago, IL 60606
312-363-6040Toll free: 800-331-2020
info@preventblindness.org
www.preventblindness.org

Richard Sanchez, Chairman
Hugh Parry, President & CEO
Jeff Todd, Chief Operating Officer

Volunteers and service organizations. Seeks to improve eye health awareness and prevent unnecessary blindness through education, health training, and mass screenings. Provides information and referral services. Conducts public awareness campaign on eye health and safety topics; operates speakers' bureau; audio-visual lending library.

Year Founded: 1908

5871 Prevent Blindness North Carolina
Prevent Blindness America
4011 WestChase Boulevard
Suite 225
Raleigh, NC 27607-3978
919-755-5044
Fax: 919-755-5013
info@pbnc.org
www.preventblindness.org

Richard Sanchez, Chairman
Hugh Parry, President & CEO
Jeff Todd, Chief Operating Officer

Volunteers working to prevent blindness and preserve maximum vision. Conducts glaucoma and preschool vision screenings and eye safety campaigns. Issues publications and certifications for vision screeners.

Year Founded: 1908

5872 Prevent Blindness Northern California
550 Kearny Street
Suite 1000
San Francisco, CA 94108
415-567-7500
Fax: 415-567-7600; *Toll Free:* 800-338-3041
q@eyeinfo.org
northerncalifornia.preventblindness.org

Richard Sanchez, Chair
Hugh Parry, President & CEO
Jeff Todd, Chief Operating Officer

Individuals interested in preventing blindness and preserving sight through research and education programs. Provides preschool vision and adult vision screening services and eye safety programs.

Year Founded: 1966

5873 Prevent Blindness Ohio
1500 W 3rd Avenue
Suite 200
Columbus, OH 43212
614-464-2020
Fax: 614-481-9670; *Toll Free:* 800-301-2020
info@pbohio.org
ohio.preventblindness.org

Richard Sanchez, Chair
Hugh Parry, President & CEO
Jeff Todd, Chief Operating Officer

Volunteers. Works to preserve sight and prevent blindness. Conducts charitable activities.

5874 Prevent Blindness Tennessee
Prevent Blindness America
211 W Wacker Road
Suite 1700
Chicago, IL 60606
312-363-6040Toll free: 800-331-2020
info@preventblindness.org
www.preventblindness.org

Richard Sanchez, Chair
Hugh Parry, President & CEO
Jeff Todd, Chief Operating Officer

Individuals interested in preventing blindness and preserving sight through research, education programs, and community service. Conducts charitable activities.

Year Founded: 1908

5875 Prevent Blindness Texas
Prevent Blindness America
2202 Waugh Drive
Houston, TX 77006
713-526-2559
Fax: 713-529-8310; *Toll Free:* 888-98S-IGHT
info@preventblindnesstexas.org
texas.preventblindness.org

Heather Shirk Patrick, President & CEO
Craig Windon, Director of Finance
Monica Seanz, VP, Programs

The mission of Prevent Blindness Texas is to prevent blindness and preserve sight.

Year Founded: 1965

5876 Prevention of Blindness Society of Metropolitan Washington

233 Massachusetts Avenue NE
Washington, DC 20002
202-234-1010
Fax: 202-234-1020
www.youreyes.org

Caren Forsten, Co-Executive Director
Michele D Hartlove, Co-Executive Director
Donald A Gagliano, MD, President

Organization provides comprehensive information on vision problems, macular degeneration, glaucoma, diabetic retinopathy, eyeglasses, other vision correction, and a directory of professional members. Provides services in the entire Metropolitan Area, including Northern Virginia, surburan Maryland, and Washington, DC.

Year Founded: 1936

5877 Research to Prevent Blindness

360 Lexington Avenue
Floor 22
New York, NY 10017-6528
212-752-4333Toll free: 800-621-0026
inforequest@rpbusa.org
www.rpbusa.org/rpb

Diane S Swift, Chairman
Brain F Hofland, PhD, President
David H Brenner, Vice President and Secretary

National voluntary health foundation supported by foundations, corporations, and voluntary gifts and bequests from individuals. Established to stimulate basic and applied research into the causes, prevention and treatment of blinding eye diseases.

Year Founded: 1960

5878 Sight into Sound

3935 Essex Lane
Houston, TX 77027
713-622-2767
info@sightintosound.org
sightintosound.org

Mary Farish Johnston, President

Formerly known as Taping for the Blind, Sight into Sound records reading material on audiotape, copied onto cassettes, for use by blind and physically handicapped persons. Promotes increased interest in and use of, free audio materials. Books, textbooks and technical manuals are recorded and sent to the Library of Congress for duplication and distribution on cassette tapes to 50 regional libraries.

Year Founded: 1967

5879 Sight-Loss Support Group of Central Pennsylvania

P.O. Box 782
Lemont, PA 16851
814-238-0132
office@slsg.org
www.slsg.org

William Muzzy, President
Jesse Smith, Treasurer
Rana Arnold, Co-Founder

The Sight-Loss Support Group of Central PA is a non-profit, self-help organization comprised of people personally coping with sight loss and those with a desire to assist those with sight loss. The Group offers peer counseling, including vision rehabilitation referral services, community outreach educational events as well as direct accessibility support in the form of guides and audio describers for local cultural events.

Year Founded: 1982

5880 South Texas Lighthouse for the Blind

4421 Agnes Street
Corpus Christi, TX 78405
361-883-6553
info@stlb.net
www.stlb.net

Nicky Ooi, Chief Executive Officer

The mission of South Texas Lighthouse for the Blind is to employ blind or visually impaired persons, provide training and resources to help build communities towards a more blind-friendly environment, and to empower persons who are blind or visually impaired.

Year Founded: 1964

5881 Southern Tier Association for the Visually Impaired

719 Lake Street
Elmira, NY 14901-2538
607-734-1554
Fax: 607-734-9467
info@st-avi.org
st-avi.org

Brian Bleiler, President
Cherie Losey, Vice President
Timothy Hertlein, President & CEO

The Southern Tier Association for the Visually Impaired (STAVI) has been serving the local blind and visually impaired community for over 90 years. Providing support, employment and rehabilitation services to Chemung, Schuyler and Steuben Counties.

Year Founded: 1921

5882 St. Louis Society for the Blind

8770 Manchester Road
St. Louis, MO 63144
314-968-9000
www.slsbvi.org

Greg Levine, Chair
Michael McKinnis, Vice Chair
David Ekin, President

Offers rehabilitation and education services to blind and visually impaired adults.

Year Founded: 1911

5883 Tampa Lighthouse for the Blind

1106 W Platt Street
Tampa, FL 33606-2142
813-251-2407
Fax: 813-254-4305
www.tampalighthouse.org

Jennifer Brooks, Rehabilitation Service Manager
Kathy Laubenthal, Executive Secretary
Sheryl Brown, Executive Director

Provides employment opportunites and maximize independence for persons who are blind or visually impaired.

Year Founded: 1940

5884 Tennessee Council of the Blind
American Council of the Blind
1703 N Beauregard Street
Suite 420
Alexandria, VA 22311
844-304-2006Toll free: 800-424-8666
president@tennesseecounciloftheblind.org
tennesseecounciloftheblind.org

Carol Francisco, President

The Tennessee Council of the Blind is a not-for-profit membership organization whose members are concerned about the dignity and well-being of blind people. An affiliate of the American Council of the Blind, the TCB works to expand the social, economic, and cultural opportunities for blind persons in Tennessee.

Year Founded: 1961

5885 The Iris Network
189 Park Avenue
Portland, ME 04102
207-774-6273
Fax: 207-774-0679
ashah@theiris.org
www.theiris.org

James E. Phipps, Executive Director
Year Founded: 1905

5886 The Lighthouse for the Blind
2501 S Plum Street
Seattle, WA 98144
Fax: 206-329-3397; *Toll Free:* 800-914-7307
thelighthousefortheblindinc.org

Bennett Prows, Chair
George Abbott, Vice Chair
Barbara Ross, President

The Lighthouse for the Blind, Inc. is a manufacturing organization with over 50 years of experience in precision machining. The Lighthouse's mission is to create and enhance opportunities for independence and self-sufficiency of people who are blind, DeafBlind, and blind with other disabilities.

Year Founded: 1914

5887 The Lighthouse of Houston
3602 West Dallas
Houston, TX 77019
713-527-9561
Fax: 713-284-8451
custserv@houstonlighthouse.org
www.houstonlighthouse.org

Gibson DuTerroil, President

The Lighthouse of Houston is a private, nonprofit education and service center dedicated to assisting blind and visually impaired people to live independently. The Lighthouse offers a wide variety of educational programs, community services and outpatient rehabilitation for the blind and visually impaired.

Year Founded: 1939

5888 The Metropolitan Washington Ear
12061 Tech Road
Silver Spring, MD 20904
301-681-6636
Fax: 301-625-1986
information@washear.org
www.washear.org

Paul W Schroeder, Chairman
Freddie L Peaco, President
Neely Oplinger, Executive Director

A nonprofit organization providing reading and information services for the blind, visually impaired and physically disabled persons who cannot effectively read print, see plays, watch television programs or view museum exhibits. This organization provides radio reading services, dial-in telephone newspaper service, National Symphony Orchestra program notes on audio cassette and raised line and large print atlases and books.

Year Founded: 1974

5889 The Metropolitan Washington Ear, Inc.
12061 Tech Road
Silver Spring, MD 20904
301-681-6636
Fax: 301-625-1986
information@washear.org
www.washear.org

Neely Oplinger, Executive Director
Nora Hart, Development Officer
Rene Schecker, Dial In Program Manager

A nonprofit organization providing reading and information services for the blind, visually impaired and physically disabled persons who cannot effectively read print, see plays, watch television programs or view museum exhibits. This organization provides radio reading services, dial-in telephone newspaper service, National Symphony Orchestra program notes on audio cassette and raised line and large print atlases and books.

Year Founded: 1974

5890 The Seeing Eye
P.O. Box 375
Morristown, NJ 07963-0375
973-539-4425
info@seeingeye.org
www.seeingeye.org

Thomas Duffy, Chairman
James A Kutsch, PhD, President & CEO
Julie H Carroll, Secretary

Breeds, raises, and trains puppies to become Seeing Eye dogs. Instructs blind people in the proper use, handling, and care of the dogs.

Year Founded: 1929

5891 Travis Association for the Blind
Austin Lighthouse
2307 Business Center Drive
P.O. Box 3297
Austin, TX 78764-3297
512-442-2329
Fax: 512-442-5498
info@austinlighthouse.org
www.austinlighthouse.org

Jerry A Mayfield, Executive Director
Donald Harcum, Chief Financial Officer
Tim Brevard, Controller

Assists blind and visually impaired men and women to gain work skills and prepare them for job experience.

Year Founded: 1934

5892 Tri-State Independent Blind Society

1068 Cedar Cross Road
Dubuque, IA 52003
563-556-8746
Fax: 563-556-3592
emailus@tristateblind@gmail.com
www.tristateblind.org

Debra Gagne, President
Linda Manders, Vice President
Pam Gagne, Treasurer/Secretary

Blind and visually impaired persons in Iowa, Wisconsin, and Illinois. Provides education, training, referral, and low vision services to visually impaired citizens and their families. Services include braille and cooking classes, cane travel, emergency transportation to and from activities, and training classes.

Year Founded: 1973

5893 United Blind Industrial Workers of America
National Federation of the Blind

810 22nd Street S
Arlington, VA 222025
703-379-1141

Sandy Halverson, Chair

Membership organization of blind persons employed in industrial and manufacturing work or in government job programs for the blind. Dedicated to protecting the rights of blind workers in salary, job stability, advancement and labor issues.

5894 United States Association for Blind Athletes

1 Olympic Plaza
Colorado Springs, CO 80909
719-866-3224
Fax: 719-866-3400
www.usaba.org

Michael Bina, PhD, President
Larry Dickerson, Vice President
Mark A Lucas, Executive Director

Supports and empowers Americans who are blind and visually impaired to experience life-changing opportunities in sports, recreation and physical activities, thereby educating and inspiring the nation.

Year Founded: 1976

5895 VOICEcorps Reading Service Inc.
Ohio Radio Reading Services

2955 W Broad Street
Columbus, OH 43204
614-274-7650Toll free: 614-274-9430
voicecorps@voicecorps.org
voicecorps.org

Voicecorps is a 24/7 radio station for the Columbus, central and southern Ohio region that provides access to print for people who cannot read the printed word. The radio schedule features newspapers, magazines, assorted periodicals/journals and books.

Year Founded: 1975

5896 Vermont Division for the Blind and Visually Impaired

HC 2 South
280 State Drive
Waterbury, VT 05671-2050
802-241-0328
Fax: 802-241-0341; *Toll Free:* 888-405-5005
dbvi.vermont.gov

Fred Jones, Director

DBVI is the designated state unit to provide vocational rehabilitation and independent living services to eligible Vermonters who are blind and visually impaired.

5897 Virginia Association for Education & Rehabilitation of the Blind & Visually Impaired

1703 N Beauregard Street
Suite 440
Alexandria, VA 22311
703-671-4500
Fax: 703-671-6391
aer@aerbvi.org
aerbvi.org

Joe Catavero, President
Laura Bozeman, Secretary
Jennifer Wheeler, Treasurer

The only professional membership organization dedicated to the advancement of education and rehabilitation of blind and visually impaired children and adults in Virginia.

Year Founded: 1984

5898 Virginia Department for the Blind & Vision Impaired

397 Azalea Avenue
Richmond, VA 23227
804-371-3140
Fax: 804-371-3157; *Toll Free:* 800-622-2155
ray.hopkins@dbvi.virginia.gov
www.vdbvi.org

Raymod E Hopkins, Commissioner

Offers services for the totally blind, legally blind, visually impaired, mentally retarded blind and more with health, counseling, educational, recreational, rehabilitation, computer training and professional training services.

5899 Virginia Industries for the Blind

397 Azalea Avenue
Richmond, VA 23227
Toll Free: 855-842-7867
matt.koch@dbvi.virginia.gov
www.vibonline.org

Matt Koch, General Manager

To employ and develop Virginians who are blind, visually impaired or deaf/blind to achieve their desired level of employment through the manufacture and delivery of quality products and services.

Year Founded: 1922

5900 Vision Rehabilitation Service Providers
American Council of the Blind

1703 N Beauregard Street
Suite 420
Alexandira, VA 22311

202-467-5081
Fax: 703-465-5085; Toll Free: 800-424-8666
info@acb.org
www.acb.org

Kim Charlson, President
Dan Spoone, First Vice President
Eric Bridges, Executive Director

Blind and visually impaired social workers, social service professionals, students pursuing careers in social work, and other interested persons are members of this organization. Works to promote full participation by visually impaired social services professionals in the field of social welfare.

5901 VisionCorps

244 N Queen Street
Lancaster, PA 17603
717-291-5951
info@visioncorps.net
www.visioncorps.net

Zach Klipa, Chair
Steve Klipa, Vice Chair
Dennis Steiner, President and CEO

A nonprofit organization dedicated to the empowerment of people who are blind or visually impaired and help them attain independence.

Year Founded: 1926

5902 Visually Impaired Veterans of America

American Council of the Blind
1703 N Beauregard Street
Suite 420
Alexandria, VA 22311
918-346-0274Toll free: 800-424-8666
d.l.dowland@sbcglobal.net
www.acb.org

David Dowland, Acting Vice President

Directs members to resources, promotes the rights of visually impaired veterans to receive all benefits, encourages research and development of new products for blind people.

Year Founded: 1961

5903 Vizavance

50 Penn Place
1900 NW Expressway, Suite R110
Oklahoma City, OK 73118
405-848-7123
Fax: 405-848-6935
info@vizavance.org
www.vizavance.org

Dainna Bonfiglio, President & CEO
Brandon Miller, Director of Development (Tulsa)
Melanie Gamble, Director of Programs

Vizavance, formerly Prevent Blindness Oklahoma, is a nonprofit organization dedicated to advancing children's education through vision.

Year Founded: 1965

5904 WEYE Seeing Eye Radio

Goodwill
570 E Waterloo Road
Akron, OH 44319
330-724-6995Toll free: 800-989-8428
dbinkley@goodwillakron.org
www.goodwillakron.org

Dave Binkley, Manager

WEYE offers a means for delivery of vital information to individuals with visual and other physical impairments. The service has been broadcasting topical and local information to print-impaired individuals over a secondary channel of WZIP-FM in North Central Ohio and Clear Channel in the Mansfield area. Programming includes in-depth coverage of local newspapers along with readings from magazines, and best-selling books presented in series.

Year Founded: 1983

5905 Washington Department of Services for the Blind

4565 7th Avenue SE
Lacey, WA 98503
360-725-3830
Fax: 360-407-0679
info@dsb.wa.gov
www.dsb.wa.gov

Lou Oma Durand, Executive Director

Provides training, counseling, and support to help Washington residents of all ages, who are blind or visually impaired, pursue employment, education, and independent living.

5906 Washington-Greene County Branch of the Pennsylvania Association for Blind

Pennsylvania Association for the Blind
555 Gettysburg Pike
Suite A300
Mechanicsburg, PA 17055
717-766-2020
Fax: 717-766-2099
info@pablind.org
www.pablind.org

To provide support to its statewide network of member agencies, empowering them to help Pennsylvanians prevent, prepare for and manage vision loss. Services include daily living workshops, orientation and mobility instructions, counseling and case management, low vision examinations, in-home supportive services, and more.

Year Founded: 1910

5907 West Tennessee Lions Volunteer Blind Industries

758 W Morris Boulevard
Morristown, TN 38101
423-714-1673
lvbi.org

Factory director mattress outlets providing blind people with employment opportunities.

Year Founded: 1951

5908 West Texas Lighthouse for the Blind

2001 Austin Street
San Angelo, TX 76903
325-653-4231
Fax: 325-657-9367
customerservice@lighthousefortheblind.org
www.lighthousefortheblind.org

Steve Cecil, Chairman
Barbara Rogers, Secretary
David Wells, Executive Director

West Texas Lighthouse for the Blind provides employment for the blind and visually impaired.

5909 Wisconsin Enterprises for the Blind
Industries for the Blind
445 S Curtis Road
West Allis, WI 53214
Toll Free: 800-642-8778
info@ibmilw.com
www.ibmilwaukee.com

CJ Lange, President & CEO
Cindy Pinkley, Controller
Patrick Crain, Chief Manufacturing Officer

Provide and grow employment opportunities for people who are blind in both the manufacturing of products and fulfillment of services that meet customer needs.

Year Founded: 1948

5910 Michigan Bureau of Services for Blind Persons
Department of Licensing & Regulatory Affairs
201 N Washington Square
2nd Floor, P.O. Box 30652
Lansing, MI 48909
517-373-2062
Fax: 517-335-5140; *Toll Free:* 800-292-4200
martinr15@michigan.gov
www.michigan.gov/BSBP
TTY: 517-373-4025

Shelly Edgerton, Director
Allan Pohl, Deputy Director & CFO
Kim Gaedeke, Acting Deputy Director

The Michigan Bureau of Services for Blind Persons (BSBP) believes in the capacity of people who are blind or visually impaired to achieve employment and independence. BSBP provides training and other services that empower people to achieve their individual goals.

Year Founded: 2012

Books

5911 A Picture is Worth a Thousand Words for
Blind and Visually Impaired Persons Too!
American Foundation for the Blind/AFB Press
2 Penn Plaza
Suite 1102
New York, NY 10121
212-502-7600
Fax: 888-545-8331; *Toll Free:* 232-304-
literacy@afb.net
www.afb.org

Carl R. Augusto, President & CEO
Kelly Bleach, Chief Administrative Officer
Rick Bozeman, Finance Director, Chief Financia

Audiodescription - the art of describing in words for visually impaired viewers the visual aspects seen in television, film, etc. - is highlighted in this book for the blind and visually impaired person.

32 pages Year Founded: 1921

5912 A Step-By-Step Guide to Personal Management
for Blind Persons
American Foundation for the Blind/AFB Press
2 Penn Plaza
Suite 1102
New York, NY 10121
212-502-7600
Fax: 888-545-8331; *Toll Free:* 232-304-

literacy@afb.net
www.afb.org

Carl R. Augusto, President & CEO
Kelly Bleach, Chief Administrative Officer
Rick Bozeman, Finance Director, Chief Financia

A manual of techniques in the areas of hygiene, grooming, clothing, shopping and child care.

136 pages Year Founded: 1921

5913 AFB Directory of Services for Blind and
Visually Impaired Persons in the US
American Foundation for the Blind
2 Penn Plaza
Suite 1102
New York, NY 10121
212-502-7600
Fax: 888-545-8331; *Toll Free:* 800-232-5463
literacy@afb.net
www.afb.org

Carl Augusto, President & CEO
Kelly Bleach, Chief Administrative Officer
Rick Bozeman, Finance Director, Chief Financia

Information concentrates on over 1,500 government and national voluntary agencies, as well as other organizations which serve blind and visually impaired persons.

664 pages Year Founded: 1921

5914 APH Catalog of Accessible Books for People
who are Visually Impaired
American Printing House for the Blind
1839 Frankfort Avenue
P.O. Box 6085
Louisville, KY 40206-0085
502-895-2405
Fax: 502-899-2284; *Toll Free:* 800-223-1839
info@aph.org
www.aph.org

Tuck Tinsley, President

Offers thousands of selections and publishers of large type and braille books for persons with visual impairments.

Year Founded: 1858

5915 Access to Art: A Museum Directory for the
Blind and Visually Impaired People
American Foundation for the Blind
2 Penn Plaza
Suite 1102
New York, NY 10121
212-502-7600
Fax: 888-545-8331; *Toll Free:* 800-232-5463
literacy@afb.net
www.afb.org

Carl Augusto, President & CEO
Kelly Bleach, Chief Administrative Officer
Rick Bozeman, Finance Director, Chief Financia

Details the access facilities of over 300 museums, galleries and exhibits in the United States. Also included are organizations offering art-related resources such as, art classes, competitions and traveling exhibits.

144 pages Year Founded: 1921

5916 Age-Related Macular Degeneration
National Association for Visually Handicapped
22 W 21st Street
Floor 6
New York, NY 10010-6943
212-889-3141
Fax: 212-727-2931
kcampbell@lighthouse.org
lighthouse.org/navh

Ann Illuzzi, Manager

A large booklet offering information, with illustrations and up-to-date research, on macular degeneration. Also available in Russian. Revised in 1999.

Year Founded: 1905

5917 Aging Eye and Low Vision
Lighthouse International
111 E 59th Street
The Sol and Lillian Goldman Building
New York, NY 10022-1202
212-821-9200
Fax: 212-821-9707; *Toll Free:* 800-829-0500
info@lighthouse.org
www.lighthouse.org
TTY: 212-821-9713

A free study guide for physicians on common age-related vision disorders.

Year Founded: 1905

5918 Art and Science of Teaching Orientation and Mobility to Persons with Visual Impairments
American Foundation for the Blind/AFB Press
2 Penn Plaza
Suite 1102
New York, NY 10121
212-502-7600
Fax: 888-545-8331; *Toll Free:* 232-304-
literacy@afb.net
www.afb.org

Carl R. Augusto, President & CEO
Kelly Bleach, Chief Administrative Officer
Rick Bozeman, Finance Director, Chief Financia

Comprehensive decription of the techniques of teaching orientation and mobility, presented along with considerations and strategies for sensitive and effective teaching. Hardcover. Paperback also available.

200 pages Year Founded: 1921

5919 Being in Touch
Gallaudet Univ. Press c/o Chicago Distrib. Center
800 Florida Avenue, NE
Washington, DC 20002-3695
202-651-5000
Fax: 800-621-8476; *Toll Free:* 800-621-2736
president@gallaudet.edu
www.gallaudet.edu
TTY: 888-630-9347

Dr. T. Alan Hurwitz, President
Stephen Weiner, Provost
Edward Bosso, Vice President for the Laurent C

Provides information on hearing and vision loss.

80 pages

5920 Berthold Lowenfeld on Blindness and Blind People
American Foundation for the Blind/AFB Press
2 Penn Plaza
Suite 1102
New York, NY 10121
212-502-7600
Fax: 888-545-8331; *Toll Free:* 232-304-
literacy@afb.net
www.afb.org

Carl R. Augusto, President & CEO
Kelly Bleach, Chief Administrative Officer
Rick Bozeman, Finance Director, Chief Financia

These writings of the pioneering educator, author and advocate range over a forty-year period include various ground-breaking papers for the blind educator, a rememberance of Helen Keller and other essays on education, sociology and history.

254 pages Year Founded: 1921

5921 Blindness: What it is, What it Does and How to Live with it
American Foundation for the Blind/AFB Press
2 Penn Plaza
Suite 1102
New York, NY 10121
212-502-7600
Fax: 888-545-8331; *Toll Free:* 232-304-
literacy@afb.net
www.afb.org

Carl R. Augusto, President & CEO
Kelly Bleach, Chief Administrative Officer
Rick Bozeman, Finance Director, Chief Financia

A classic work on how blindness affects self-perception and social interaction and what can be done to restore basic skills, mobility, daily living and an appreciation of life's pleasures.

396 pages Year Founded: 1921

5922 Burns Braille Transcription Dictionary
American Foundation for the Blind/AFB Press
2 Penn Plaza
Suite 1102
New York, NY 10121
212-502-7600
Fax: 888-545-8331; *Toll Free:* 232-304-
literacy@afb.net
www.afb.org

Carl R. Augusto, President & CEO
Kelly Bleach, Chief Administrative Officer
Rick Bozeman, Finance Director, Chief Financia

A handy, portable guide that is a quick reference for anyone who needs to check print-to-braille and braille-to-print meanings and symbols. Paperback.

96 pages Year Founded: 1921

5923 Career Perspectives: Interviews with Blind and Visually Impaired Professionals
American Foundation for the Blind/AFB Press
2 Penn Plaza
Suite 1102
New York, NY 10121
212-502-7600
Fax: 888-545-8331; *Toll Free:* 232-304-

literacy@afb.net
www.afb.org

Carl R. Augusto, President & CEO
Kelly Bleach, Chief Administrative Officer
Rick Bozeman, Finance Director, Chief Financia

Profiles of 20 successful archivers who describe in their own words what it takes to pursue and attain professional success in a sighted world. Available in large print, cassette and braille.

96 pages Year Founded: 1921

5924 Cataracts
National Association for Visually Handicapped
22 W 21st Street
Floor 6
New York, NY 10010-6943
212-889-3141
Fax: 212-727-2931
kcampbell@lighthouse.org
lighthouse.org/navh

Ann Illuzzi, Manager

A booklet offering information about Cataracts, diagnosis and treatment of this common condition.

Year Founded: 1905

5925 Comprehensive Examination of Barriers to Employment Among Persons who are Blind or Impaired
Mississippi State University
108 Herbert - South, Room 150 Industrial Education Department Building
PO Box 6189
Mississippi State, MS 39762-6189
662-325-2001
Fax: 662-325-8989; *Toll Free:* 800-675-7782
nrtc@colled.msstate.edu
www.blind.msstate.edu
TDD 662-325-2694

Douglas Bedsaul, Research and Training Coordinato
Jacqui Bybee, Research Associate II
Anne Carter, Research and Training Coordinato

A multi-phase research project designed to: identify barriers to employment; identify and develop innovative successful strategies to overcome these barriers; develop methods for others to utilize these strategies; disseminate this information to rehabilitation providers; replicate the use of selected strategies in other settings.

90 pages

5926 Contrasting Characteristics of Blind and Visually Impaired Clients
Rehab/Training Center on Blindness and Low-Vision
108 Herbert - South, Room 150 Industrial Education Department Building
PO Box 6189
Mississippi State, MS 39762-6189
601-325-2001
Fax: 662-325-8989; *Toll Free:* 675-778-
nrtc@colled.msstate.edu
www.blind.msstate.edu
TDD 662-325-2694

Douglas Bedsaul, Research and Training Coordinato
Jacqui Bybee, Research Associate II
Anne Carter, Research and Training Coordinato

This report examines cases in the National Blindness and Low Vision Employment Database to identify and profile environmental and personal characteristics of clients who are blind or visually impaired and who were achieving successful and unsuccessful retention of competitive jobs. A total of 787 cases were analyzed.

44 pages

5927 Coping with Vision Loss: Maximizing What You See & Do
Hunter House Publishers
PO Box 2914
Alameda, CA 94501
510-865-5282
Fax: 510-865-4295; *Toll Free:* 800-266-5592
ordering@hunterhouse.com
www.hunterhouse.com

Christina Sverdrup, Customer Service Manager
Bill Chapman EdD, Author

Helps readers with severe vision loss maximize the use of their remaning visual perception.

304 pages Year Founded: 1999

5928 Data on Blindness and Visual Impairment in the US: A Resource Manual
American Foundation for the Blind
2 Penn Plaza
Suite 1102
New York, NY 10121
212-502-7600
Fax: 888-545-8331; *Toll Free:* 800-232-5463
literacy@afb.net
www.afb.org

Carl Augusto, President & CEO
Kelly Bleach, Chief Administrative Officer
Rick Bozeman, Finance Director, Chief Financia

Provides facts and figures for long-range planning, preparing grant proposals and legislative services.

412 pages Year Founded: 1921

5929 Eye and Your Vision
National Association for Visually Handicapped
22 W 21st Street
Floor 6
New York, NY 10010-6943
212-889-3141
Fax: 212-727-2931
kcampbell@lighthouse.org
lighthouse.org/navh

Ann Illuzzi, Manager

A large booklet offering information, with illustrations, on the eye. Includes information on protection of eyesight, how the eye works and vision disorders. Available in Russian and Spanish also.

Year Founded: 1905

5930 Finding Wheels: A Curriculum for Nondrivers with Visual Impairments for Gaining Control
AFB Press
2 Penn Plaza
Suite 1102
New York, NY 10121
212-502-7600
Fax: 888-545-8331; *Toll Free:* 232-304-
literacy@afb.net
www.afb.org

Carl R. Augusto, President & CEO
Kelly Bleach, Chief Administrative Officer
Rick Bozeman, Finance Director, Chief Financia

It is designed to be used by teachers, child-care workers, houseparents or others who are responsible for helping students to develop daily living skills. It is a set of suggested goals and objectives.

Year Founded: 1921

5931 Foundations of Rehabilitation Counseling with Persons who are Blind
American Foundation for the Blind/AFB Press
2 Penn Plaza
Suite 1102
New York, NY 10121
212-502-7600
Fax: 888-545-8331; *Toll Free:* 232-304-
literacy@afb.net
www.afb.org

Carl R. Augusto, President & CEO
Kelly Bleach, Chief Administrative Officer
Rick Bozeman, Finance Director, Chief Financia

Rehabilitation professionals have long recognized that the needs of people who are blind or visually impaired are unique and require a special knowledge and expertise to provide and coordinate rehabilitation services.

477 pages Year Founded: 1921

5932 If Blindness Comes
National Federation of the Blind
200 East Wells Street
at Jernigan Place
Baltimore, MD 21230
410-659-9314
Fax: 410-685-5653
nfb.org

Mark Riccobono, President

An introduction to issues relating to vision loss and provides a positive, supportive philosophy about blindness. It is a general information book which includes answers to many common questions about blindness, information about services and programs for the blind and resource listings. Contact the Materials Center.

Year Founded: 1940

5933 If Blindness Strikes; Don't Strike Out
Charles C Thomas Publisher
2600 S 1st Street
Springfield, IL 62704-4730
217-789-8980
Fax: 217-789-9130; *Toll Free:* 800-258-8980
books@ccthomas.com
www.ccthomas.com

Michael P Thomas, President

This book is a storehouse of information on daily life for the visually impaired and those around them. From opticons and laser canes to housekeeping to travel, the author describes how to successfully cope with the problems posed by visual impairment and blindness.

316 pages

5934 Intervention Practices in the Retention of Competitive Employment Among Individuals who are Blind
Mississippi State University
108 Herbert - South, Room 150 Industrial Education
Department Building
PO Box 6189
Mississippi State, MS 39762-6189
601-325-2001
Fax: 662-325-8989; *Toll Free:* 675-778-
nrtc@colled.msstate.edu
www.blind.msstate.edu
TDD 662-325-2694

Douglas Bedsaul, Research and Training Coordinato
Jacqui Bybee, Research Associate II
Anne Carter, Research and Training Coordinato

This study investigated the methods by which an individual can retain competitive employment after the onset of a significant vision loss. Interviews were conducted with 89 rehabilitation counselors across the US. Strategies that contribute to successful job retention were identified as well as best rehabilitation practices in job retention.

60 pages

5935 Issues in Aging and Vision: A Curriculum for University Programs and In-Service Training
American Foundation for the Blind
2 Penn Plaza
Suite 1102
New York, NY 10121
212-502-7600
Fax: 888-545-8331
literacy@afb.net
www.afb.org

Carl R. Augusto, President & CEO
Kelly Bleach, Chief Administrative Officer
Rick Bozeman, Finance Director, Chief Financia

Provides information involving university programs in gerontology, training programs and related areas.

224 pages Year Founded: 1921

5936 Large Print Loan Library
National Association for Visually Handicapped
22 W 21st Street
Floor 6
New York, NY 10010-6943
212-889-3141
Fax: 212-727-2931
kcampbell@lighthouse.org
lighthouse.org/navh

Ann Illuzzi, Manager

A huge large print catalog of all the publications, fiction and non-fiction, cassette tapes, books-on-tape and videos available for the visually impaired from the loan library of the National Association for the Visually Handicapped.

100 pages Year Founded: 1905

5937 Library Resources for the Blind and Physically Handicapped
National Library Service for the Blind
1291 Taylor Street NW
Washington, DC 20011
202-707-5100
Fax: 202-707-0712; Toll Free: 800-424-8567
nls@loc.gov
www.loc.gov/nls
TDD 202-707-0744

Frank Cylke, Executive Director

5938 Life of My Own Daily Meditations on Hope and Acceptance
Hazelden
15251 Pleasant Valley Road
PO Box 11
Center City, MN 55012-0011
651-213-4200
Fax: 651-213-4793; Toll Free: 800-257-7810
info@hazelden.org
www.hazelden.org

Mark Mishek, President & CEO
James A. Blaha, Vice President
Sharon Birnbaum, Corporate Director

Offers daily access to strength, serenity, and insight in our relationships with chemically dependent people.

400 pages Year Founded: 1947

5939 Lifestyles of Employed Legally Blind People
Rehab Research & Training Center on Blindness
108 Herbert - South, Room 150 Industrial Education Department Building
PO Box 6189
Mississippi State, MS 39762-6189
601-325-2001
Fax: 662-325-8989; Toll Free: 675-778-
nrtc@colled.msstate.edu
www.blind.msstate.edu
TDD 662-325-2694

Douglas Bedsaul, Research and Training Coordinato
Jacqui Bybee, Research Associate II
Anne Carter, Research and Training Coordinato

Results from a telephone survey show that visually impaired respondents are involved in a wide variety of activities with little restrictions on their range of activities. Sighted respondents tended to spend more time in child care, obtaining goods and services, attending to self-care activities, and engaging in social activities, while visually impaired respondents spent more time in education and passive activities. This report is a study of ex

193 pages

5940 Living with Low Vision: A Resource Guide for People with Sight Loss
Resources for Rehabilitation
22 Bonad Road
Winchester, MA 01890-1302
781-368-9094
Fax: 781-368-9096
info@rfr.org
www.rfr.org

Susan L. Greenblatt, Editor

A large print resource directory that helps people with sight loss locate the services and products that they need to keep reading, working and enjoying life.

272 pages

5941 Low Vision: Reflections of the Past, Issues for the Future
American Foundation for the Blind/AFB Press
2 Penn Plaza
Suite 1102
New York, NY 10121
212-502-7600
Fax: 888-545-8331; Toll Free: 232-304-
literacy@afb.net
www.afb.org

Carl R. Augusto, President & CEO
Kelly Bleach, Chief Administrative Officer
Rick Bozeman, Finance Director, Chief Financia

Background papers and a strategies section are used to identify the shifting needs of visually impaired persons and the resources that may be needed to address them. Paperback.

Year Founded: 1921

5942 Making Life More Livable
American Foundation for the Blind/AFB Press
2 Penn Plaza
Suite 1102
New York, NY 10121
212-502-7600
Fax: 888-545-8331
literacy@afb.net
www.afb.org

Carl R. Augusto, President & CEO
Kelly Bleach, Chief Administrative Officer
Rick Bozeman, Finance Director, Chief Financia

Shows how simple adaptations in the home and environment can make a big difference in the lives of blind and visually impaired older persons. The suggestions offered are numerous and specific, ranging from how to mark food cans for greater visibility to how to get out of the shower safley. Large print.

132 pages Year Founded: 1921

5943 National Braille Press
88 Saint Stephen Street
Boston, MA 02115-4312
617-266-6160
Fax: 617-437-0456; Toll Free: 888-965-8965
contact@nbp.org
www.nbp.org

Brian A. MacDonald, President
Diane L. Croft, Publisher

Promoting the literacy of blind children through braille and providing access to information that empowers blind people to actively engage in work, family, and community affairs.

5944 Perigee Visual Dictionary of Signing
Harris Communications
15155 Technology Drive
Eden Prairie, MN 55344-2273
952-906-1180
Fax: 952-906-1099; Toll Free: 800-825-6758

www.harriscomm.com
TTY: 800-825-9187

Robert Harris, President
Bill Williams, National Sales Manager

An A-to-Z guide to American Sign Language vocabulary.

450 pages Year Founded: 1982

5945 Picture is Worth a Thousand Words for Blind and Visually Impaired Persons
American Foundation for the Blind
2 Penn Plaza
Suite 1102
New York, NY 10121
212-502-7600
Fax: 888-545-8331; *Toll Free:* 800-232-5463
literacy@afb.net
www.afb.org

Carl R. Augusto, President & CEO
Kelly Bleach, Chief Administrative Officer
Rick Bozeman, Finance Director, Chief Financia

Audiodescription - the art of describing in words for visually impaired viewers the visual aspects seen in television, film, etc. - is highlighted in this book for the blind and visually impaired person.

32 pages Year Founded: 1921

5946 Prescriptions for Independence
American Foundation for the Blind/AFB Press
2 Penn Plaza
Suite 1102
New York, NY 10121
212-502-7600
Fax: 888-545-8331; *Toll Free:* 232-304-
literacy@afb.net
www.afb.org

Carl R. Augusto, President & CEO
Kelly Bleach, Chief Administrative Officer
Rick Bozeman, Finance Director, Chief Financia

Easy-to-read manual on how older visually impaired persons can pursue their interests and activities in community residences, senior centers, long-term care facilities and other community settings. Paperback.

Year Founded: 1921

5947 Providing Services for People with Vision Loss: Multidisciplinary Perspective
Resources For Rehabilitation
22 Bonad Road
Winchester, MA 01890-1302
781-368-9094
Fax: 781-368-9096
info@rfr.org
www.rfr.org

Susan L. Greenblatt, Editor

A collection of articles by ophthalmologists and rehabilitation professionals, including chapters on operating a low vision service, starting self-help programs, mental health services, aids and techniques that help people with vision loss.

136 pages

5948 Referring Blind and Low Vision Patients for Rehabilitation Services
American Foundation for the Blind
2 Penn Plaza
Suite 1102
New York, NY 10121
212-502-7600
Fax: 888-545-8331; *Toll Free:* 800-232-5463
literacy@afb.net
www.afb.org

Carl R. Augusto, President & CEO
Kelly Bleach, Chief Administrative Officer
Rick Bozeman, Finance Director, Chief Financia

Clear information on such basic topics as the objectives of low vision services, what's covered in the examinations, what rehabilitation services do and how to locate these services.

Year Founded: 1921

5949 Rehabilitation Resource Manual: Vision
Resources for Rehabilitation
22 Bonad Road
Winchester, MA 01890-1302
781-368-9094
Fax: 781-368-9096
info@rfr.org
www.rfr.org

Susan L. Greenblatt, Editor

Publication includes: Descriptions of information sources, products, and publications in North America for people who are visually impaired or blind. Entries include: Company or organization name, address, phone, fax, description, prices of product or publication.

Frequency: Biennial

5950 Smith Kettlewell Rehabilitation Engineering Research Center
Smith-Kettlewell Eye Research Institute
2318 Fillmore Street
San Francisco, CA 94115-1813
415-345-2000
Fax: 415-345-8455
rerc@ski.org
www.ski.org
TTY: 415-345-2290

Arthur Jampolsky, President
John Brabyn, Executice Director/CEO
Ruth S. Poole, Chief Operating Officer

Reports on technology and devices for persons with visual impairments.

5951 Unseen Minority: A Social History of Blindness in the United States
American Foundation for the Blind/AFB Press
2 Penn Plaza
Suite 1102
New York, NY 10121
212-502-7600
Fax: 888-545-8331; *Toll Free:* 232-304-
literacy@afb.net
www.afb.org

Carl R. Augusto, President & CEO
Kelly Bleach, Chief Administrative Officer
Rick Bozeman, Finance Director, Chief Financia

A lively narrative, peppered with anecdotes, recounts how the blind overcame discrimination to gain full participation in the social, educational, economic and legislative spheres. Hardcover.

573 pages Year Founded: 1921

5952 Vision and Aging: Crossroads for Service Delivery
American Foundation for the Blind
2 Penn Plaza
Suite 1102
New York, NY 10121
212-502-7600
Fax: 888-545-8331; Toll Free: 800-232-5463
literacy@afb.net
www.afb.org

Carl R. Augusto, President & CEO
Kelly Bleach, Chief Administrative Officer
Rick Bozeman, Finance Director, Chief Financia

An overview of the service delivery systems in the aging and blindness fields that covers the essential issues concerning vision loss among older persons in this country, the growth of visual impairments in the elderly, and the policy and service questions.

392 pages Year Founded: 1921

5953 Vision and Aging: Issues in Social Work Practice
Haworth Press
10 Alice Street
Binghamton, NY 13904-1503
607-722-5857
Fax: 607-771-0012; Toll Free: 800-429-6784
www.impresaitalia.info

Jackie Blakeslee, Advertising
William Cohen, Owner

Responds to the needs of the growing population of blind or severely disabled elderly.

196 pages

5954 Visual Impairment: An Overview
American Foundation for the Blind/AFB Press
2 Penn Plaza
Suite 1102
New York, NY 10121
212-502-7600
Fax: 888-545-8331; Toll Free: 232-304-
literacy@afb.net
www.afb.org

Carl R. Augusto, President & CEO
Kelly Bleach, Chief Administrative Officer
Rick Bozeman, Finance Director, Chief Financia

An overall look at the most common forms of vision loss and their impact on the individual. Includes drawings as well as photographs that stimulate how people with vision loss see. Paperback.

56 pages Year Founded: 1921

5955 Visually Impaired Seniors as Senior Companions: A Reference Guide
American Foundation for the Blind/AFB Press
2 Penn Plaza
Suite 1102
New York, NY 10121

212-502-7600
Fax: 888-545-8331; Toll Free: 232-304-
literacy@afb.net
www.afb.org

Carl R. Augusto, President & CEO
Kelly Bleach, Chief Administrative Officer
Rick Bozeman, Finance Director, Chief Financia

This useful guide describes the Senior Companion Program that is intended to broaden opportunities for older persons with disabilities. Appendix includes training materials, evaluation forms, recruitment and public relations information.

108 pages Year Founded: 1921

Directories

5956 AFB Directory of Services for Blind and Visually Impaired Persons in the US
American Foundation for the Blind
2 Penn Plaza
Suite 1102
New York, NY 10121
212-502-7600
Fax: 888-545-8331; Toll Free: 800-232-5463
literacy@afb.net
www.afb.org

Carl R. Augusto, President & CEO
Kelly Bleach, Chief Administrative Officer
Rick Bozeman, Finance Director, Chief Financia

Information concentrates on over 1,500 government and national voluntary agencies, as well as other organizations which serve blind and visually impaired persons.

664 pages Year Founded: 1921

5957 APH Catalog of Accessible Books for People Who Are Visually Impaired
American Printing House for the Blind
1839 Frankfort Avenue
P.O. Box 6085
Louisville, KY 40206-0085
502-895-2405
Fax: 502-899-2284; Toll Free: 800-223-1839
info@aph.org
www.aph.org

Tuck Tinsley, President

Offers thousands of selections and publishers of large type and braille books for persons with visual impairments.

Year Founded: 1858

5958 Access Travel: Airports
Airport Council International - North America
1615 L Street NW
Suite 300
Washington, DC 20036
202-293-8500
Fax: 202-331-1362; Toll Free: 888-424-7767
nzimini@aci-na.org
www.aci-na.org

Kevin M. Burke, President & CEO
Deborah McElroy, Executive Vice President
Nancy Zimini, Senior Vice President

About 553 airports worldwide; dot matrix tabulation. Entries include: Airport name, location, TDD and toll free numbers of hotels and rental cars, indication of presence or absence of about 60 facilities and services of special importance to persons in wheelchairs and to blind, deaf, and elderly persons.

50 pages Year Founded: 1948

5959 Access to Art: A Museum Directory for Blind & Visually Impaired People
American Foundation for the Blind
2 Penn Plaza
Suite 1102
New York, NY 10121
212-502-7600
Fax: 888-545-8331; *Toll Free:* 800-232-5463
literacy@afb.net
www.afb.org

Carl R. Augusto, President & CEO
Kelly Bleach, Chief Administrative Officer
Rick Bozeman, Finance Director, Chief Financia

Details the access facilities of over 300 museums, galleries and exhibits in the United States. Also included are organizations offering art-related resources such as, art classes, competitions and traveling exhibits.

144 pages Year Founded: 1921

5960 Address List: Regional and Subregional Libraries for the Blind and Physically Handicapped
Nat Lib Serv for the Blind/Physically Handicapped
101 Independence Ave, SE
Washington, DC 20540
202-707-5000
Fax: 202-707-0712; *Toll Free:* 800-424-8567
nls@loc.gov
www.loc.gov

Frank Cylke, Executive Director
James H. Billington, Librarian

143 state and local libraries that serve blind and physically handicapped persons as part of the Library of Congress co-operating network. Entries include: Name, address, contact name, phone.

25 pages Frequency: Semiannual Year Founded: 1814

5961 Blindness and Visual Impairments: National Organizations
Nat Lib Svc for the Blind & Physically Handicapped
101 Independence Ave, SE
Washington, DC 20540
202-707-5000
Fax: 202-707-0712; *Toll Free:* 800-424-8567
nls@loc.gov
www.loc.gov

Frank Cylke, Executive Director
James H. Billington, Librarian

Organizations providing services and publications listing sources of products and information for blind and visually-impaired individuals; state-level agencies that administer public programs providing special education and rehabilitation services. Entries include: Organization or agency name, address, phone, descriptions of services and publications.

33 pages Year Founded: 1814

5962 Braille Catalog of General Interest Items
National Braille Association
95 Allens Creek Road
Bldg. 1, Suite 202
Rochester, NY 14618
585-427-8260
Fax: 585-427-0263
www.nationalbraille.org

Jan Carroll, President
Whitney Williams, President-Elect
Cindi Laurent, Vice President

Lists hundreds of titles of fiction and non-fiction books offered in large print, braille or on cassette to visually impaired readers.

Year Founded: 1945

5963 Carolyn's Low Vision Solutions
1415 57th Avenue W
Bradenton, FL 34207-3646
941-739-5555
Fax: 941-739-5503; *Toll Free:* 800-648-2266
info@carolynscatalog.com
www.carolynscatalog.com

Carolyn Tojek, President
John Colton, Owner

Free mail-order catalog of items for visually impaired people.

5964 Directory of Resources for the Blind & Visually Impaired
John Milton Society for the Blind
475 Riverside Drive
Suite 455
New York, NY 10115
212-870-3335
Fax: 212-870-3229
www.jmsblind.org

Darcy Quigley, Mailing Contact/Editor

Over 100 church and secular publications available in Braille, large type, and on cassette for the visually impaired; transcription services, organizations who provide camps and other associations assisting the visually impaired. Entries include: Organization name, address, phone, financial data, description of product/service.

125 pages

5965 Library Resources for the Blind and Physically Handicapped
National Library Service for the Blind
1291 Taylor Street NW
Washington, DC 20011
202-707-5100
Fax: 202-707-0712; *Toll Free:* 800-424-8567
nls@loc.gov
www.loc.gov/nls
TDD 202-707-0744

Frank Cylke, Executive Director

57 regional and 85 subregional libraries, and 4 machine-lending agencies in the United States, Puerto Rico, the US Virgin Islands, and Guam that provide a free library service of Braille and recorded books and magazines to visually and physically handicapped persons; other agencies distributing Braille materials and talking book machines are also indicated. Entries include: Name of library, address, phone, fax, in-WATS number, e-mail address, TDD

number (for the deaf), name of librarian, name of contact for machines (if any), hours of operation, list of book collections (includes disc, cassette, Braille, large type), list of special collections (films, foreign language cassettes), list of special services.

91 pages Frequency: Annual

5966 Living with Low Vision: A Resource Guide for People with Sight Loss
Resources for Rehabilitation
22 Bonad Road
Winchester, MA 01890-1302
781-368-9094
Fax: 781-368-9096
info@rfr.org
www.rfr.org

Susan L. Greenblatt, Editor

Resources and services for people with vision loss, including national organizations, publications, distributors of large print publications, reading services, technological aids, and organizations and publications for groups such as the elderly, adolescents, veterans, and those with hearing loss as well. Entries include: Company or organization name, address, phone, fax, e-mail address and web sites, description, price of product or publication. Printed in large print.

288 pages Frequency: Biennial

5967 New Vision Store
919 Walnut Street
Philadelphia, PA 19107-5237
215-629-2990
webmaster@thenewvisionstore.com
www.thenewvisionstore.com

Store and catalog for individuals with visual impairments, listing visual aids, magnifiers, large print books and more.

30 pages

5968 Visual Aids and Informational Material
National Association for Visually Handicapped
22 W 21st Street
Floor 6
New York, NY 10010-6943
212-889-3141
Fax: 212-727-2931
kcampbell@lighthouse.org
lighthouse.org/navh

Ann Illuzzi, Manager

A complete listing of the visual aids NAVH carries such as magnifiers, talking clocks, large print playing cards, etc.

65 pages Year Founded: 1905

Journals, Magazines

5969 Aging & Vision News
Lighthouse International
111 E 59th Street
The Sol and Lillian Goldman Building
New York, NY 10022-1202
212-821-9200
Fax: 212-821-9707; *Toll Free:* 800-829-0500
info@lighthouse.org
www.lighthouse.org
TTY: 212-821-9713

Intended for professionals engaged in research, education or service delivery in the field of vision and aging.

Year Founded: 1905

5970 Aging and Vision: Declarations of Independence
American Foundation for the Blind/AFB Press
2 Penn Plaza
Suite 1102
New York, NY 10121
212-502-7600
Fax: 888-545-8331; *Toll Free:* 232-304-
literacy@afb.net
www.afb.org

Carl R. Augusto, President & CEO
Kelly Bleach, Chief Administrative Officer
Rick Bozeman, Finance Director, Chief Financia

A very personal look at five older people who have successfully coped with visual impairmant and continue to lead active, satisfying lives. Their stories are not only inspirational, but also provide practical, down-to-earth suggestions for adapting to vision loss later in life. 18 minute video tape. Also available in PAL, $52.95, 0-89128-276-9.

Year Founded: 1921

5971 American Printing House for the Blind
American Printing House for the Blind
1839 Frankfort Avenue
P.O. Box 6085
Louisville, KY 40206-0085
502-895-2405
Fax: 502-899-2284; *Toll Free:* 800-223-1839
info@aph.org
www.aph.org

Tuck Tinsley, President
Fred Gissoni, Customer Support

The world's largest company devoted solely to producing products for people who are visually impaired. We manufacture books and magazines in braille, large type and recorded form from over 200 vendors across the US. We also make a wide range of educational and daily living aids, such as braille paper and styluses, talking book equipment, and synthetic speech computer products. APH also offers LOUIS, an electronic database that lists accessible b

Year Founded: 1858

5972 Blindness, A Family Matter
American Foundation for the Blind/AFB Press
2 Penn Plaza
Suite 1102
New York, NY 10121
212-502-7600
Fax: 888-545-8331; *Toll Free:* 232-304-
literacy@afb.net
www.afb.org

Carl R. Augusto, President & CEO
Kelly Bleach, Chief Administrative Officer
Rick Bozeman, Finance Director, Chief Financia

A frank exploration of the effects of an individual's visual impairment on other members of the family and how those family members can play a positive role in the rehabilitation process. Features interviews with three families whose 'success stories' provide advice and encouragement, as well as interviews with newly blinded adults currently involved in a rehabilitation program. 23 minute video tape. Also available in PAL, $49.95, 0-89128-271-8.

Year Founded: 1921

5973 Braille Book Review
National Library Service for the Blind
1291 Taylor Street NW
Washington, DC 20011
202-707-5100
Fax: 202-707-0712; *Toll Free:* 800-424-8567
nls@loc.gov
www.loc.gov/nls
TDD 202-707-0744

Frank Cylke, Executive Director

New braille books and product news.

5974 Braille Forum
American Council of the Blind
2200 Wilson Boulevard
Suite 650
Arlington, VA 22201-3354
202-467-5081
Fax: 703-465-5085; *Toll Free:* 800-424-8666
info@acb.org
www.acb.org

Kim Charlson, President
Jeff Thom, Vice President
Melanie Brunson, Executive Director

Offered in print, braille, cassette, IBM computer disk, and e-mail. $25 per format per year for companes and non-US residents.

48 pages Year Founded: 1961

5975 Braille Mirror
Braille Institute Press
741 N Vermont Avenue
Los Angeles, CA 90029-3514
323-660-3880
Fax: 323-663-0867; *Toll Free:* 800-272-4533
www.brailleinstitute.org

Lester M. Sussman, Chairman
Leslie M. Stocker, President
Peter A. Mindnich, Executive Vice President

General interest magazine (Braille).

Year Founded: 1919

5976 Braille Monitor
National Federation of the Blind
200 East Wells Street
at Jernigan Place
Baltimore, MD 21230
410-659-9314
Fax: 410-685-5653
gwunder@nfb.org
nfb.org

Gary Wunder, Editor

Covering events and activities of the National Federation of the Blind as well as issues and concerns of the blind.

5977 Bulletin
National Association for Visually Handicapped
22 W 21st Street
Floor 6
New York, NY 10010-6943

212-889-3141
Fax: 212-727-2931
kcampbell@lighthouse.org
lighthouse.org/navh

Ann Illuzzi, Manager

Annual report offering information on Association activities and events, conferences, vision aids and resources for the visually impaired.

Year Founded: 1905

5978 Choice Magazine Listening
Choice Magazine Listening
85 Channel Drive
Port Washington, NY 11050-2278
516-883-8280
Fax: 516-944-6849; *Toll Free:* 888-724-6423
choicemag@aol.com
www.choicemagazinelisting.org

Pamela Loeser, Editor-in-Chief
Ann Schlegel-Kyrkostas, Associate Editor
David Graham Page, Associate Editor

A free audio anthology available to visually impaired/physically disabled or dyslexic persons nationwide. Playable on the special free 4-track cassette playback equipment which is provided by the Library of Congress through the National Library Service. Each issue free to keep; bimonthly — six times yearly.

Year Founded: 1962

5979 Dialogue
Blindskills
PO Box 5181
Salem, OR 97304-0181
503-581-4224
Fax: 503-581-0178; *Toll Free:* 800-860-4224
info@blindskills.com
www.blindskills.com

Carol M McCarl, Founder and Publisher Emeritus
B. T. Kimbrough, Editor/Executive Director
Phyllis Schmidt, Office Assistant

Bimonthly magazine written by and for visually impaired people, available in large print, audio cassette, Braille, disk and via e-mail. It features articles on adapting to life with low vision, techniques of daily living, careers, education, sports and recreation, technology tips and reviews, and descriptions of new products and services designed for visually impaired people.

Frequency: Bimonthly Year Founded: 1983

5980 Gleams Newsletter
Glaucoma Research Foundation
251 Post Street
Suite 600
San Francisco, CA 94108
415-986-3162
Fax: 415-986-3763; *Toll Free:* 800-826-6693
question@glaucoma.org
www.glaucoma.org

Andrew Iwach,MD, Chairman
Robert L. Stamper,MD, Vice Chair
Thomas M. Brunner, President & CEO

Offers updated and medical information on vision loss and glaucoma. Included are legislative information, professional articles and book reviews.

Year Founded: 1978

5981 Guideway
Guide Dog Foundation for the Blind
371 E Jericho Turnpike
Smithtown, NY 11787-2976
631-930-9000
Fax: 631-930-9009; Toll Free: 800-548-4337
info@guidedog.org
www.guidedog.org

James C. Bingham, Chairman
Alphonce J. Brown, Jr., ACFRE, Vice Chair
Wells B. Jones, Chief Executive Officer

Offers updates and information on the foundation's activities and guide dog programs. In print form but is also available on cassette.

Frequency: Quarterly

5982 Hub
SPOKES Unlimited
1006 Main Street
PO Box 7896
Klamath Falls, OR 97601
541-883-7547
Fax: 541-885-2469
www.spokesunlimited.org

Meg Graf, Resource Librarian
Wendy Howard, Executive Director

Newsletter on rehabilitation, peer counseling, blindness, visual impairments, information and referral.

5983 Illinois Braille Messenger
Illinois Council For The Blind
217 Monroe, Suite 95
PO Box 1336
Springfield, IL 62705-1336
217-512-4967
icb@icbonline.org
www.icbonline.org

Rachel Schroeder, President
Marla Chorney, 1st Vice President
Tom Jones, 2nd Vice President

5984 Insight
US Association of Blind Athletes
33 N Institute Street
Colorado Springs, CO 80903-3508
719-630-0422
Fax: 719-630-0616
www.usaba.org

Dave Bushland, President
Tracie Foster, Vice President
Mark A. Lucas, MS, Executive Director

Magazine reporting on news and activities of the US Association of Blind Athletes.

Frequency: Quarterly

5985 Jewish Braille Review
Jewish Braille Institute Of America
110 E 30th Street
New York, NY 10016-7375
212-889-2525
Fax: 212-689-3692; Toll Free: 800-433-1531
admin@jbilibrary.org
www.jbilibrary.org

Judy E. Tenney, Chairman
Ellen Isler, President & CEO
Israel A. Taun, Vice President & CFO

Magazine for the blind. Printed in braille.

Year Founded: 1931

5986 Journal of Visual Impairment and Blindness
American Foundation for the Blind
2 Penn Plaza
Suite 1102
New York, NY 10121
212-502-7600
Fax: 888-545-8331; Toll Free: 800-232-5463
literacy@afb.net
www.afb.org

Carl R. Augusto, President & CEO
Kelly Bleach, Chief Administrative Officer
Rick Bozeman, Finance Director, Chief Financia

The peer reviewed, interdisciplinary, scholarly journal for special educators, rehabilitators, mobility instructors, low vision specialists, technologists and others who care about new possibilities who are blind and visually impaired; the impact of public policy on services and people; new approaches to working with students and clients; new directions in service delivery world-wide and the latest news on products and programs, technology and activities around the world.

Frequency: Monthly Year Founded: 1921

5987 Journal of Visual Impairments and Blindness
Sheridan Press
PO Box 465
Hanover, PA 17331
717-632-3535
Fax: 717-633-8929
www.sheridan.com

Joan Davidson, President
Jane Erin, Editor-in-Chief
Sharon Shively, Managing Editor

Published in braille, regular print and on ASC II disk and cassette, this journal contains a wide variety of subjects including rehabilitation, psychology, education, legislation, medicine, technology, employment, sensory aids and childhood development as they relate to visual impairments. $90 Annual individual subscription, $125 Annual institutional subscription.

64 pages

5988 Lifeglow
Christian Record Service
4444 South 52nd Street
PO Box 6097
Lincoln, NE 68506-0097
402-488-0981
Fax: 402-488-7582
info@christianrecord.org
www.christianrecord.org

Dan Jackson, Chairman
Tom Lemon, Vice Chairman
Lawrence Pitcher, President

Magazine for the blind. Printed in braille and large print.

Frequency: Bimonthly Year Founded: 1899

5989 Lion's Club Headquarters
Lions Clubs International
300 W 22nd Street
Oak Brook, IL 60523-8842
630-571-5466
Fax: 630-571-8890
www.lionsclubs.org

Barry J. Palmer, International President
Joseph Preston, First Vice President
Dr. Jitsuhir Yamada, Second Vice President

Publications for the blind from this large international organization dedicated to the largest blindness prevention program ('SightFirst').
Year Founded: 1917

5990 Long Cane News
American Foundation for the Blind/AFB Press
2 Penn Plaza
Suite 1102
New York, NY 10121
212-502-7600
Fax: 888-545-8331; *Toll Free:* 232-304-
literacy@afb.net
www.afb.org

Carl R. Augusto, President & CEO
Kelly Bleach, Chief Administrative Officer
Rick Bozeman, Finance Director, Chief Financia
Year Founded: 1921

5991 Low Vision Questions and Answers:
Definitions, Devices, Services
American Foundation for the Blind/AFB Press
2 Penn Plaza
Suite 1102
New York, NY 10121
212-502-7600
Fax: 888-545-8331; *Toll Free:* 232-304-
literacy@afb.net
www.afb.org

Carl R. Augusto, President & CEO
Kelly Bleach, Chief Administrative Officer
Rick Bozeman, Finance Director, Chief Financia

What does low vision mean? What do low vision services cost? What diseases cause low vision? Answers to these and other questions are presented in a comprehensive format with accompanying photographs. $50.00/pack of 25.
21 pages Year Founded: 1921

5992 Magazines in Special Media
National Library Service for the Blind
1291 Taylor Street NW
Washington, DC 20011
202-707-5100
Fax: 202-707-0712; *Toll Free:* 800-424-8567
nls@loc.gov
www.loc.gov/nls
TDD 202-707-0744

Frank Cylke, Executive Director
Frequency: Biennial

5993 Matilda Ziegler Magazine for the Blind
Matilda Ziegler Magazine for the Blind
80 8th Avenue
Suite 1304
New York, NY 10011-7161

212-242-0263
Fax: 212-633-1601
www.matildaziegler.com

Gregory Evanina, Owner
Michael Mellor, Editor

Publication presenting general interest articles, humor, fiction, and poetry from newspapers, magazines, and books. Also includes news and information of special interest to people with vision problems.
Frequency: Monthly

5994 Musical Mainstream
National Library Service for the Blind
1291 Taylor Street NW
Washington, DC 20011
202-707-5100
Fax: 202-707-0712; *Toll Free:* 800-424-8567
nls@loc.gov
www.loc.gov/nls
TDD 202-707-0744

Frank Cylke, Executive Director

Articles selected from print music magazines.

5995 NLS News
National Library Service for the Blind
1291 Taylor Street NW
Washington, DC 20011
202-707-5100
Fax: 202-707-0712; *Toll Free:* 800-424-8567
nls@loc.gov
www.loc.gov/nls
TDD 202-707-0744

Frank Cylke, Executive Director

Newsletter on current program developments.

5996 NLS Update
National Library Service for the Blind
1291 Taylor Street NW
Washington, DC 20011
202-707-5100
Fax: 202-707-0712; *Toll Free:* 800-424-8567
nls@loc.gov
www.loc.gov/nls
TDD 202-707-0744

Frank Cylke, Executive Director

Newsletter on the services volunteer activities.

5997 Not Without Sight
American Foundation for the Blind/AFB Press
2 Penn Plaza
Suite 1102
New York, NY 10121
212-502-7600
Fax: 888-545-8331; *Toll Free:* 232-304-
literacy@afb.net
www.afb.org

Carl R. Augusto, President & CEO
Kelly Bleach, Chief Administrative Officer
Rick Bozeman, Finance Director, Chief Financia

This video describes the major types of visual impairment and their causes and effects on vision, while camera simulations approximate what people with each impairmant actually see. Also demonstrates how people with low vision make the best use of the vision they have. 20 minute video tape. Also available in PAL, $52.95, 0-89128-272-6.

Year Founded: 1921

5998 Opportunity
National Industries For The Blind
1310 Braddock Place?
PO Box 969
Alexandria, VA 22314-1691
703-310-0500
Fax: 973-595-9122
www.nib.org

George J Mertz, President/CEO

Offers information and articles on the newest technology, equipment, services and programs for blind and visually impaired persons.

5999 Our Special
National Braille Press
88 Saint Stephen Street
Boston, MA 02115-4302
888-965-8965
Fax: 617-437-0456; *Toll Free:* 800-548-7323
orders@nbp.org
www.nbp.org

Paul Parravano, Chairman
David S. Kennedy, Vice Chair
Brian A. Mac Donald, President

General interest Braille magazine for blind women.

6000 Out of Left Field
American Foundation for the Blind/AFB Press
2 Penn Plaza
Suite 1102
New York, NY 10121
212-502-7600
Fax: 888-545-8331; *Toll Free:* 232-304-
literacy@afb.net
www.afb.org

Carl R. Augusto, President & CEO
Kelly Bleach, Chief Administrative Officer
Rick Bozeman, Finance Director, Chief Financia

Illustrates how youngsters who are blind or visually impaired integrated with their sighted peers in a variety of recreational and athletic activities. 17 minute video tape. Also available in PAL, $33.95, 0-89128-270-X.

Year Founded: 1921

6001 Quarterly Update
National Association for Visually Handicapped
22 W 21st Street
Floor 6
New York, NY 10010-6943
212-889-3141
Fax: 212-727-2931
kcampbell@lighthouse.org
lighthouse.org/navh

Ann Illuzzi, Manager

Quarterly newsletter offering information on new products for the visually impaired, advances in medical treatments, new books available in the NAVH large print loan library and any new/updated booklets. Free.

Year Founded: 1905

6002 Recorded Periodicals
Associated Services for the Blind and Visually Imp
919 Walnut Street
Philadelphia, PA 19107-5237
215-627-0600
Fax: 215-922-0692
asbinfo@asb.org
www.asb.org

Patricia C. Johnson, President & Chief Executive Offi
Ron Conklin, Agency IT Manager and Site Evalu
Tim McGovern, Human Relations

A subscription service of Associated Services for the Blind, these periodicals provide 21 magazines through this subscription service. A magazine list can be sent, in both large print and on audio cassette.

Year Founded: 1874

6003 Recording for the Blind News
Learning Ally
20 Roszel Road
Princeton, NJ 8540
609-452-0606
Fax: 609-987-8116
info@rfbd.org
www.learningally.org

Andrew Friedman, President & CEO
Jim Halliday, Executive Vice President
Connie Murphy, Chief Development and Community

6004 Seeing Clearly
National Association for Visually Handicapped
22 W 21st Street
Floor 6
New York, NY 10010-6943
212-889-3141
Fax: 212-727-2931
kcampbell@lighthouse.org
lighthouse.org/navh

Ann Illuzzi, Manager

This newsletter offers short stories, news, medical updates, assistive device information, poems, resources, crossword puzzles and more for the visually impaired.

Year Founded: 1905

6005 Seeing Eye Guide
Seeing Eye
10 Washington Valley Rd.
PO Box 375
Morristown, NJ 07963
973-539-4425
Fax: 973-539-0922
info@seeingeye.org
www.seeingeye.org

Lewis M. Chakrin, Chairman
Peter N. Crnkovich, Vice Chairman
James A. Kutsch, Jr., Ph.D, President and Chief Executive Of

Newsletter.

8 pages Frequency: 4 Year Founded: 1929

6006 Smith-Kettlewell Technical File
Smith-Kettlewell Eye Research Institute
2318 Fillmore Street
San Francisco, CA 94115-1813

415-345-2000
Fax: 415-345-8455
rerc@ski.org
www.ski.org
TTY: 415-345-2290

Arthur Jampolsky, President
John Brabyn, Executice Director/CEO
Ruth S. Poole, Chief Operating Officer

Magazine reporting on technology and devices for visually impaired persons.

6007 Tactic
Clovernook Home And School For The Blind
7000 Hamilton Avenue
Cincinnati, OH 45231-5240
513-522-3860
www.clovernook.org

Year Founded: 1903

6008 Talking Book Topics
National Library Service for the Blind
1291 Taylor Street NW
Washington, DC 20011
202-707-5100
Fax: 202-707-0712; *Toll Free:* 800-424-8567
nls@loc.gov
www.loc.gov/nls
TDD 202-707-0744

Frank Cylke, Executive Director

Offers hundreds of listings of books, fiction and nonfiction, for adults and children on cassette. Also offers listings on foreign language books on cassette, talking magazines and reviews.

6009 Tract Messenger
Lutheran Braille Evangelism Association
1740 Eugene Street
White Bear Lake, MN 55110-3312
651-426-0469
mail@lbea.org
www.lbea.org

Dennis Hawkinson, Contact

Religious magazine in Braille.

Frequency: Monthly Year Founded: 1952

6010 USABA Newsletter
US Association of Blind Athletes
33 N Institute Street
Colorado Springs, CO 80903-3508
719-630-0422
Fax: 719-630-0616
www.usaba.org

Dave Bushland, President
Tracie Foster, Vice President
Mark A. Lucas, MS, Executive Director

Covers news, announcements and activities of the Association.

6011 Update (Library of Congress)
National Library Services Blind & Physically Hand.
1291 Taylor Street NW
Washington, DC 20011
202-707-5100
Fax: 202-707-0712; *Toll Free:* 800-424-8567

nls@loc.gov
www.loc.gov/nls
TDD 202-707-0744

Frank Cylke, Executive Director

Magazine reporting on current information on library services for disabled individuals.

Frequency: Quarterly

6012 Vision
National Catholic Office for the Deaf
7202 Buchanan Street
Landover Hills, MD 20784-2236
301-577-1684
Fax: 301-577-1690
info@ncod.org
www.ncod.org

Rev. Kevin C Rhoades, Episcopal Representative
Fr. Paul Zirimenya, Region I - West
Arvilla Rank, Executive Director/Editor

Published as a pastoral service for the deaf and hard of hearing.

16 pages

6013 Vision Enhancement, Journal
Vision World Wide
5707 Brockton Drive
Apt 302
Indianapolis, IN 46220-5481
317-254-1332
Fax: 317-251-6588; *Toll Free:* 800-431-1739
www.visionww.org

Patricia Price, President/Managing Editor

Provides information through helplines, a website, internet lists, information packets, and comprehensive quarterly journal, Vision Enhancement (available in large print, audiocassette, and computer disk) - all designed to inform, encourage, and support individuals with vision loss, family members, and professionals who serve them. Aim is to enhance everyday living so as to make it possible to maintain an independent lifestyle.

68-75 pages Frequency: 4

6014 Visions
Easter Seals Inc.
233 South Wacker Drive
Suite 2400
Chicago, IL 60606-4703
312-726-6200
Fax: 312-726-1494; *Toll Free:* 800-221-6827
www.easterseals.com

Richard W. Davidson, Chairman
Sandra L. Bouwman, 1st Vice Chairman
Joseph G. Kern, 2nd Vice Chairman

Magazine concerning the National Easter Seal Society's activities.

Frequency: Quarterly Year Founded: 1907

6015 Voice of Vision
GW Micro
725 Airport North Office Park
Fort Wayne, IN 46825-6707
260-489-3671
Fax: 260-489-2608

sales@gwmicro.com
www.gwmicro.com

Doug Geoffray, Vice President Development
Dan Weirich, VP Sales And Marketing
Lois Baich, Orders And Production

Offers product reviews, product announcements, tips for making systems or applications more accessible, or explanations of concepts of interest to any computer user or would-be computer user. This association newsletter is available in braille, in large print, on audio cassette and on 3.5 or 5.25 IBM format diskette.

Year Founded: 1990

6016 We Can Do It Together!
American Foundation for the Blind/AFB Press
2 Penn Plaza
Suite 1102
New York, NY 10121
212-502-7600
Fax: 888-545-8331; *Toll Free:* 232-304-
literacy@afb.net
www.afb.org

Carl R. Augusto, President & CEO
Kelly Bleach, Chief Administrative Officer
Rick Bozeman, Finance Director, Chief Financia

This video illustrates a transdisciplinaty team orientation and mobility program for students with severe visual and multiple impairments, covering both adapted communication systems used to teach mobility skills and basic indoor mobility in the school. For mobility instructors, administrators, teachers of the visually and severely handicapped, occupational, physical and speech therapists and parents. Discussion guide included. 10 minute video t

Year Founded: 1921

Newspapers

6017 NFB-Newsline
National Federation of the Blind
200 East Wells Street
at Jernigan Place
Baltimore, MD 21230-4914
Toll Free: 866-504-7300
nfb.org

Mark Riccobono, President

Nation's only digital talking newspaper service for the blind. Allows the blind to read the full text of leading national and local newspapers by using a touch-tone telephone. Service is free of charge and available 24 hours a day, 7 days per week.

Newsletters, Pamphlets

6018 A Patient's Guide to Visual Aids and Illumination
National Association for Visually Handicapped
22 W 21st Street
Floor 6
New York, NY 10010-6943
212-889-3141
Fax: 212-727-2931

kcampbell@lighthouse.org
lighthouse.org/navh

Ann Illuzzi, Manager

A reference booklet offering information on aids for the visually impaired.

Year Founded: 1905

6019 ACB Reports
American Council of the Blind
2200 Wilson Boulevard
Suite 650
Arlington, VA 22201-3354
202-467-5081
Fax: 202-467-5085; *Toll Free:* 800-424-8666
info@acb.org
www.acb.org

Kim Charlson, President
Jeff Thom, First Vice President
Melanie Brunson, Executive Director

Radio news feature program for radio information services.

Year Founded: 1961

6020 AFB News
American Foundation for the Blind
2 Penn Plaza
Suite 1102
New York, NY 10121
212-502-7600
Fax: 888-545-8331; *Toll Free:* 800-232-5463
literacy@afb.net
www.afb.org

Carl R. Augusto, President & CEO
Kelly Bleach, Chief Administrative Officer
Rick Bozeman, Finance Director, Chief Financia

National newsletter for general readership about blindness and visual impairments featuring people, programs, services and activities.

12 pages Year Founded: 1921

6021 ALDA News
Association of Late-Deafened Adults
8038 Macintosh Lane
Suite 2
Rockford, IL 61107
815-332-1515
info@alda.org
www.alda.org
TTY: 815-332-1515

Steve Larew, President

6022 Age-Related Macular Degeneration
National Eye Institute, Information Office
31 Center Drive
MSC 2510
Bethesda, MD 20892-2510
301-496-5248
Fax: 301-402-1065
2020@nei.nih.gov
www.nei.nih.gov

Dr. Paul A. Sieving, Director
Dr. Deborah Carper, Deputy Director
Dr. Richard Fisher, Associate Director for Science P

6023 Aging and Vision
American Foundation for the Blind
2 Penn Plaza
Suite 1102
New York, NY 10121
212-502-7600
Fax: 888-545-8331; *Toll Free:* 800-232-5463
literacy@afb.net
www.afb.org

Carl R. Augusto, President & CEO
Kelly Bleach, Chief Administrative Officer
Rick Bozeman, Finance Director, Chief Financia

Booklet offering information on the causes of vision loss
with aging, cataracts, macular degeneration, lighting, vision
aids and more for the elderly persons.

Year Founded: 1921

6024 Aging and Vision News
National Center for Vision and Aging
800 2nd Avenue
New York, NY 10017-4709
212-808-0077Toll free: 800-334-5497
www.palmcoasteyecenter.com

Sang Park, Owner

6025 BVA Bulletin
Blinded Veterans Association
477 H Street NW
Washington, DC 20001-2694
202-371-8880
Fax: 202-371-8258; *Toll Free:* 800-669-7079
BVA@BVA.ORG
www.bva.org

Mark Cornell, National President
Reverend Rob Dale Stamper, National President
Thomas H Miller, Executive Director

Year Founded: 1945

6026 Books are Fun for Everyone
National Library Service for the Blind
1291 Taylor Street NW
Washington, DC 20011
202-707-5100
Fax: 202-707-0712; *Toll Free:* 800-424-8567
nls@loc.gov
www.loc.gov/nls

Frank Cylke, Executive Director

6027 Braille Book Review
National Library Service for the Blind
1291 Taylor Street NW
Washington, DC 20011
202-707-5100
Fax: 202-707-0712; *Toll Free:* 800-424-8567
nls@loc.gov
www.loc.gov/nls

Frank Cylke, Executive Director

New braille books and product news.

6028 Braille: An Extraordinary Volunteer
Opportunity
National Library Service for the Blind
1291 Taylor Street NW
Washington, DC 20011

202-707-5100
Fax: 202-707-0712; *Toll Free:* 800-424-8567
nls@loc.gov
www.loc.gov/nls

Frank Cylke, Executive Director

6029 Bulletin
National Association for Visually Handicapped
22 W 21st Street
Floor 6
New York, NY 10010-6943
212-889-3141
Fax: 212-727-2931
kcampbell@lighthouse.org
lighthouse.org/navh

Ann Illuzzi, Manager

Annual report offering information on Association activities and events, conferences, vision aids and resources for
the visually impaired.

Year Founded: 1905

6030 Cataracts
National Eye Institute, Information Office
31 Center Drive
MSC 2510
Bethesda, MD 20892-2510
301-496-5248
Fax: 301-402-1065
2020@nei.nih.gov
www.nei.nih.gov

Dr. Paul A. Sieving, Director
Dr. Deborah Carper, Deputy Director
Dr. Richard Fisher, Associate Director for Science P

Provides information about this common condition and its
treatment.

6031 Classification of Impaired Vision
National Association for Visually Handicapped
22 W 21st Street
Floor 6
New York, NY 10010-6943
212-889-3141
Fax: 212-727-2931
kcampbell@lighthouse.org
lighthouse.org/navh

Ann Illuzzi, Manager

Describes various degrees of impaired vision.

Year Founded: 1905

6032 Communicating with People Who Have
Trouble Hearing & Seeing: A Primer
National Association for Visually Handicapped
22 W 21st Street
Floor 6
New York, NY 10010-6943
212-889-3141
Fax: 212-727-2931
kcampbell@lighthouse.org
lighthouse.org/navh

Ann Illuzzi, Manager

Line drawings that depict problems for those with both deficiencies.

Year Founded: 1905

6033 D.V.H. Quarterly
University of Arkansas At Little Rock
2801 S University Avenue
Little Rock, AR 72204-1099
501-683-7397
Fax: 501-683-7679
ualr.edu

Joel E. Anderson, Chancellor
Zulma Toro, Executive Vice Chancellor and Pr
Robert H. Adams, Vice Chancellor for Finance and

Offers information on upcoming events, conferences and
workshops on and for visual disabilities. Book reviews, information on the newest resources and technology, educational programs, want ads and more.

6034 Department for the Blind & Physically
Handicapped
South Carolina Library
1430 Senate Street
Columbia, SC 29201-3710
803-734-4611
Fax: 803-734-4610; *Toll Free:* 800-922-7818
TDD 813-734-7298

James B Johnson Jr, Executive Director

4 pages Frequency: Quarterly

6035 Diabetes, Vision Impairment and Blindness
American Foundation for the Blind
2 Penn Plaza
Suite 1102
New York, NY 10121
212-502-7600
Fax: 888-545-8331; *Toll Free:* 800-232-5463
literacy@afb.net
www.afb.org

Carl R. Augusto, President & CEO
Kelly Bleach, Chief Administrative Officer
Rick Bozeman, Finance Director, Chief Financia

A presentation of how chronic diabetes affects vision and
how diabetes can be managed at home by blind and visually impaired individuals.

32 pages Year Founded: 1921

6036 Diabetic Retinopathy
National Association for Visually Handicapped
22 W 21st Street
Floor 6
New York, NY 10010-6943
212-889-3141
Fax: 212-727-2931
kcampbell@lighthouse.org
lighthouse.org/navh

Ann Illuzzi, Manager

Describes types of this disease and methods of treatment.
Year Founded: 1905

6037 Directory of Services for Blind and Visually
Impaired Persons in the United States and
Canada
American Foundation for the Blind
2 Penn Plaza
Suite 1102
New York, NY 10121

212-502-7600
Fax: 888-545-8331; *Toll Free:* 800-232-5463
literacy@afb.net
www.afb.org

Carl R. Augusto, President & CEO
Kelly Bleach, Chief Administrative Officer
Rick Bozeman, Finance Director, Chief Financia

624 pages Year Founded: 1921

6038 Diseases of the Macula
National Association for Visually Handicapped
22 W 21st Street
Floor 6
New York, NY 10010-6943
212-889-3141
Fax: 212-727-2931
kcampbell@lighthouse.org
lighthouse.org/navh

Ann Illuzzi, Manager

Describes various conditions which affect the macular area
and hot to best maximize the use of residual peripheral
vision.

Year Founded: 1905

6039 Dog Sponsorship Program
Guide Dog Foundation for the Blind
371 E Jericho Turnpike
Smithtown, NY 11787-2976
631-930-9000
Fax: 631-930-9009; *Toll Free:* 800-548-4337
info@guidedog.org
www.guidedog.org

James C. Bingham, Chairman
Alphonce J. Brown, Jr., ACFRE, Vice Chair
Wells B. Jones, Chief Executive Officer

Offers information to an individual or an organization that
wishes to sponsor a guide dog.

6040 Don't Lose Sight of Age-Related Macular
Degeneration
National Eye Institute, Information Office
31 Center Drive
MSC 2510
Bethesda, MD 20892-2510
301-496-5248
Fax: 301-402-1065
2020@nei.nih.gov
www.nei.nih.gov

Dr. Paul A. Sieving, Director
Dr. Deborah Carper, Deputy Director
Dr. Richard Fisher, Associate Director for Science P

6041 Don't Lose Sight of Cataracts
National Eye Institute, Information Office
31 Center Drive
MSC 2510
Bethesda, MD 20892-2510
301-496-5248
Fax: 301-402-1065
2020@nei.nih.gov
www.nei.nih.gov

Dr. Paul A. Sieving, Director
Dr. Deborah Carper, Deputy Director
Dr. Richard Fisher, Associate Director for Science P

6042 Don't Lose Sight of Glaucoma
National Eye Institute, Information Office
31 Center Drive
MSC 2510
Bethesda, MD 20892-2510
301-496-5248
Fax: 301-402-1065
2020@nei.nih.gov
www.nei.nih.gov

Dr. Paul A. Sieving, Director
Dr. Deborah Carper, Deputy Director
Dr. Richard Fisher, Associate Director for Science P

6043 Eye-Q Test
National Association for Visually Handicapped
22 W 21st Street
Floor 6
New York, NY 10010-6943
212-889-3141
Fax: 212-727-2931
kcampbell@lighthouse.org
lighthouse.org/navh

Ann Illuzzi, Manager

Five questions and answers to assist in knowing more about vision.

Year Founded: 1905

6044 Facts: Books for Blind and Physically Handicapped Individuals
National Library Service for the Blind
1291 Taylor Street NW
Washington, DC 20011
202-707-5100
Fax: 202-707-0712; *Toll Free:* 800-424-8567
nls@loc.gov
www.loc.gov/nls

Frank Cylke, Executive Director

6045 Facts: Music for Blind and Physically Handicapped Individuals
National Library Service for the Blind
1291 Taylor Street NW
Washington, DC 20011
202-707-5100
Fax: 202-707-0712; *Toll Free:* 800-424-8567
nls@loc.gov
www.loc.gov/nls

Frank Cylke, Executive Director

6046 Facts: Playback Machines and Accessories Provided On Free Loan
National Library Service for the Blind
1291 Taylor Street NW
Washington, DC 20011
202-707-5100
Fax: 202-707-0712; *Toll Free:* 800-424-8567
nls@loc.gov
www.loc.gov/nls

Frank Cylke, Executive Director

6047 Facts: Sources for Purchase of Cassette& Disc Players From NLS
National Library Service for the Blind
1291 Taylor Street NW
Washington, DC 20011

202-707-5100
Fax: 202-707-0712; *Toll Free:* 800-424-8567
nls@loc.gov
www.loc.gov/nls

Frank Cylke, Executive Director

6048 Family Guide - Growth & Development of the Partially Seeing Child
National Association for Visually Handicapped
22 W 21st Street
Floor 6
New York, NY 10010-6943
212-889-3141
Fax: 212-727-2931
kcampbell@lighthouse.org
lighthouse.org/navh

Ann Illuzzi, Manager

Offers information for parents and guidelines in raising a partially seeing child.

Year Founded: 1905

6049 Fighting Blindness News
RP Foundation Fighting Blindness
7168 Columbia Gateway Drive
Suite 100
Columbia, MD 21046
410-423-0600
Fax: 410-771-9470; *Toll Free:* 800-683-5551
www.blindness.org
TDD 410-363-7139

William T. Schmidt, Chief Executive Officer
James W. Minow, Chief Development Officer
Stephen M. Rose, Ph.D., Chief Research Officer

Offers information on medical updates, donor programs, assistive devices, resources and clinical trial information for persons with visual impairments, blindness and retinal degenerative diseases.

6050 General Facts and Figures on Blindness
Prevent Blindness America
211 West Wacker Drive
Suite 1700
Chicago, IL 60173-5624
847-843-2020
Fax: 847-843-8458
info@preventblindness.org
www.preventblindness.org

6051 Gift of Sight
RP Foundation Fighting Blindness
1401 W Mount Royal Avenue
Baltimore, MD 21217-4245
410-225-9409
Fax: 410-771-9470; *Toll Free:* 800-683-

A pamphlet offering information on the Retina Donor Program, which studies diseased, human retinal tissue in their search for a cure of retinal degenerative diseases.

6052 Glaucoma
Foundation for Glaucoma Research
200 Pine Street
Suite 200
San Francisco, CA 94104-2704
415-986-3162
Fax: 415-986-3763

Offers information on what glaucoma is, the causes, treatments, types of glaucoma, eye exams and prevention.

6053 Glaucoma - the Sneak Thief of Sight
National Association for Visually Handicapped
22 W 21st Street
Floor 6
New York, NY 10010-6943
212-889-3141
Fax: 212-727-2931
kcampbell@lighthouse.org
lighthouse.org/navh

Ann Illuzzi, Manager

A pamphlet describing the disease, treatment and medications.

Year Founded: 1905

6054 Guide Dog Foundation Flyer
Guide Dog Foundation for the Blind
371 E Jericho Turnpike
Smithtown, NY 11787-2976
631-930-9000
Fax: 631-930-9009; *Toll Free:* 800-548-4337
info@guidedog.org
www.guidedog.org

James C. Bingham, Chairman
Alphonce J. Brown, Jr., ACFRE, Vice Chair
Wells B. Jones, Chief Executive Officer

Offers information on the programs and services provided by the Foundation.

6055 Guidelines for Comprehensive Low Vision Care
National Association for Visually Handicapped
22 W 21st Street
Floor 6
New York, NY 10010-6943
212-889-3141
Fax: 212-727-2931
kcampbell@lighthouse.org
lighthouse.org/navh

Ann Illuzzi, Manager

A description of the proper method to conduct a low vision evaluation.

Year Founded: 1905

6056 Guild Briefs
Guild for the Blind
180 N Michigan Avenue
Suite 1700
Chicago, IL 60601-7479
312-236-8569
Fax: 312-236-8128

David Tabak, Executive Director

8-16 pages Frequency: Monthly

6057 Heartbreak of Being A Little Bit Blind
National Association for Visually Handicapped
22 W 21st Street
Floor 6
New York, NY 10010-6943
212-889-3141
Fax: 212-727-2931
kcampbell@lighthouse.org
lighthouse.org/navh

Ann Illuzzi, Manager

Summary of what it means to have impaired vision with illustrations. Free for members; 50 cents for non-members.

Year Founded: 1905

6058 History and Use of Braille
American Council of the Blind
2200 Wilson Boulevard
Suite 650
Arlington, VA 22201-3354
202-467-5081
Fax: 202-467-5085; *Toll Free:* 800-424-8666
info@acb.org
www.acb.org

Kim Charlson, President
Jeff Thom, First Vice President
Melanie Brunson, Executive Director

Year Founded: 1961

6059 How Does a Blind Person Get Around?
American Foundation for the Blind
2 Penn Plaza
Suite 1102
New York, NY 10121
212-502-7600
Fax: 888-545-8331; *Toll Free:* 800-232-5463
literacy@afb.net
www.afb.org

Carl R. Augusto, President & CEO
Kelly Bleach, Chief Administrative Officer
Rick Bozeman, Finance Director, Chief Financia

Offers information on daily living as a blind person.

Year Founded: 1921

6060 How to Develop a Self-Help Group for Elders Losing Eyesight
National Association for Visually Handicapped
22 W 21st Street
Floor 6
New York, NY 10010-6943
212-889-3141
Fax: 212-727-2931
kcampbell@lighthouse.org
lighthouse.org/navh

Ann Illuzzi, Manager

The pioneer for development of self-help groups, using the NAVH model, this publication is designed to help start and facilitate self-help groups.

Year Founded: 1905

6061 How to Use Your Low Vision Glasses
National Association for Visually Handicapped
22 W 21st Street
Floor 6
New York, NY 10010-6943
212-889-3141
Fax: 212-727-2931
kcampbell@lighthouse.org
lighthouse.org/navh

Ann Illuzzi, Manager

A line drawing showing the correct way to benefit from low vision glasses.

Year Founded: 1905

6062 In Focus
National Association for Visually Handicapped
22 W 21st Street
Floor 6
New York, NY 10010-6943
212-889-3141
Fax: 212-727-2931
kcampbell@lighthouse.org
lighthouse.org/navh

Ann Illuzzi, Manager

Offers information on new items for the partially seeing, advances made in treatments and medical science, stories and poems from readers, humor and crossword puzzles for young adults.

Year Founded: 1905

6063 InSight
Prevent Blindness America
211 West Wacker Drive
Suite 1700
Chicago, IL 60606
847-843-2020
Fax: 847-843-8458; *Toll Free:* 800-331-2020
info@preventblindness.org
www.preventblindness.org

Paul G. Howes, Chairman
Hugh Parry, President & CEO
Sally Atherton, Ph.D, Executive Director

Year Founded: 1908

6064 Information on Glaucoma
Glaucoma Research Foundation
251 Post Street
Suite 600
San Francisco, CA 94108
415-986-3162
Fax: 415-986-3763; *Toll Free:* 800-826-6693
question@glaucoma.org
www.glaucoma.org

Andrew Iwach,MD, Chairman
Robert L. Stamper,MD, Vice Chair
Thomas M. Brunner, President & CEO

Year Founded: 1978

6065 Information on Macular Degeneration
American Council of the Blind
2200 Wilson Boulevard
Suite 650
Arlington, VA 22201-3354
202-467-5081
Fax: 202-467-5085; *Toll Free:* 800-424-8666
info@acb.org
www.acb.org

Kim Charlson, President
Jeff Thom, First Vice President
Melanie Brunson, Executive Director

Year Founded: 1961

6066 It's All Right to Be Angry
National Association for Visually Handicapped
22 W 21st Street
Floor 6
New York, NY 10010-6943
212-889-3141
Fax: 212-727-2931

kcampbell@lighthouse.org
lighthouse.org/navh

Ann Illuzzi, Manager

A helpful pamphlet describing reactions to learning to live with vision impairment.

Year Founded: 1905

6067 JBI Points
Jewish Braille Institute of America
110 E 30th Street
New York, NY 10016-7393
212-889-2525
Fax: 212-689-3692; *Toll Free:* 800-433-1531
www.jewishvirtuallibrary.org

Ellen Isler, President

8 pages Year Founded: 1993

6068 Jewish Guild for the Blind Newsletter
Jewish Guild for the Blind
15 W 65th Street
New York, NY 10023-6601
212-769-6200
Fax: 212-769-6266; *Toll Free:* 800-284-4422
info@jewishguild.com
www.guildhealth.org

Pete Williamson, Editor
Alan Morse, Manager

8-12 pages Frequency: Quarterly Year Founded: 1914

6069 Know Your Eye
American Council of the Blind
2200 Wilson Boulevard
Suite 650
Arlington, VA 22201-3354
202-467-5081
Fax: 202-467-5085; *Toll Free:* 800-424-8666
info@acb.org
www.acb.org

Kim Charlson, President
Jeff Thom, First Vice President
Melanie Brunson, Executive Director

Year Founded: 1961

6070 Large Print Loan Library Catalog
National Association for Visually Handicapped
22 W 21st Street
Floor 6
New York, NY 10010-6943
212-889-3141
Fax: 212-727-2931
kcampbell@lighthouse.org
lighthouse.org/navh

Ann Illuzzi, Manager

Listing of over 7,000 commercially published and NAVH large print books available through NAVH on a loan basis. Includes a limited selection of titles available for purchase.

Year Founded: 1905

6071 Long Cane News
American Foundation for the Blind
2 Penn Plaza
Suite 1102
New York, NY 10121

212-502-7600
Fax: 888-545-8331; *Toll Free:* 800-232-5463
literacy@afb.net
www.afb.org

Carl R. Augusto, President & CEO
Kelly Bleach, Chief Administrative Officer
Rick Bozeman, Finance Director, Chief Financia

Year Founded: 1921

6072 Low Vision Questions and Answers
American Foundation for the Blind
2 Penn Plaza
Suite 1102
New York, NY 10121
212-502-7600
Fax: 888-545-8331; *Toll Free:* 800-232-5463
literacy@afb.net
www.afb.org

Carl R. Augusto, President & CEO
Kelly Bleach, Chief Administrative Officer
Rick Bozeman, Finance Director, Chief Financia

What does low vision mean? What do low vision services cost? What diseases cause low vision? Answers to these and other questions are presented in a comprehensive format with accompanying photographs.

21 pages Year Founded: 1921

6073 Lutheran Braille Evangelism Association
Lutheran Braille Evangelism Association
1740 Eugene Street
White Bear Lake, MN 55110-3312
651-426-0469
mail@lbea.org
www.lbea.org

Dennis Hawkinson, Executive Director

2 pages Frequency: Quarterly Year Founded: 1952

6074 Magnifier Highlights
Independent Living Aids
137 Rano Rd
Buffalo, NY 14207
516-937-1848
Fax: 516-937-3906; *Toll Free:* 800-537-2118
techsupport@independentliving.com
www.independentliving.com

Marvin Sandler, President

Full line of maginifiers, ranging from high-powered vision aids to hoppy instruments and accessories

6075 Music Is for Everyone
National Library Service for the Blind
1291 Taylor Street NW
Washington, DC 20011
202-707-5100
Fax: 202-707-0712; *Toll Free:* 800-424-8567
nls@loc.gov
www.loc.gov/nls

Frank Cylke, Executive Director

6076 Musical Mainstream
National Library Service for the Blind
1291 Taylor Street NW
Washington, DC 20011
202-707-5100
Fax: 202-707-0712; *Toll Free:* 800-424-8567

nls@loc.gov
www.loc.gov/nls

Frank Cylke, Executive Director

Articles selected from print music magazines.

6077 NLS News
National Library Service for the Blind
1291 Taylor Street NW
Washington, DC 20011
202-707-5100
Fax: 202-707-0712; *Toll Free:* 800-424-8567
nls@loc.gov
www.loc.gov/nls

Frank Cylke, Executive Director

Newsletter on current program developments.

6078 NLS Update
National Library Service for the Blind
1291 Taylor Street NW
Washington, DC 20011
202-707-5100
Fax: 202-707-0712; *Toll Free:* 800-424-8567
nls@loc.gov
www.loc.gov/nls

Frank Cylke, Executive Director

Newsletter on the services volunteer activities.

Frequency: Quarterly

6079 Opportunity
National Industries For The Blind
1310 Braddock Place?
PO Box 969
Alexandria, VA 22314-1691
703-310-0500
Fax: 973-595-9122
www.nib.org

George J Mertz, President/CEO

Offers information and articles on the newest technology, equipment, services and programs for blind and visually impaired persons.

Frequency: Quarterly

6080 Patient's Guide to Visual Aids and Illumination
National Association for Visually Handicapped
22 W 21st Street
Floor 6
New York, NY 10010-6943
212-889-3141
Fax: 212-727-2931
kcampbell@lighthouse.org
lighthouse.org/navh

Ann Illuzzi, Manager

A reference booklet offering information on aids for the visually impaired.

Year Founded: 1905

6081 Prevent Blindness News
Prevent Blindness America
211 West Wacker Drive
Suite 1700
Chicago, IL 60606
847-843-2020
Fax: 847-843-8458; *Toll Free:* 800-331-2020

info@preventblindness.org
www.preventblindness.org

Paul G. Howes, Chairman
Hugh Parry, President & CEO
Sally Atherton, Ph.D, Executive Director

Offers information and articles on eye safety, programs and services of the Society, conferences and seminars on safety in the workplace, sports eye safety information and more.

12-14 pages Frequency: Three Year Founded: 1908

6082 Puppy Walker Brochure
Guide Dog Foundation for the Blind
371 E Jericho Turnpike
Smithtown, NY 11787-2976
631-930-9000
Fax: 631-930-9009; Toll Free: 800-548-4337
info@guidedog.org
www.guidedog.org

James C. Bingham, Chairman
Alphonce J. Brown, Jr., ACFRE, Vice Chair
Wells B. Jones, Chief Executive Officer

Offers information on being a volunteer Puppy Walker family.

6083 Reading Is for Everyone
National Library Service for the Blind
1291 Taylor Street NW
Washington, DC 20011
202-707-5100
Fax: 202-707-0712; Toll Free: 800-424-8567
nls@loc.gov
www.loc.gov/nls

Frank Cylke, Executive Director

6084 Reading with Low Vision
National Library Service for the Blind
1291 Taylor Street NW
Washington, DC 20011
202-707-5100
Fax: 202-707-0712; Toll Free: 800-424-8567
nls@loc.gov
www.loc.gov/nls

Frank Cylke, Executive Director

6085 Recording for the Blind News
Learning Ally
20 Roszel Road
Princeton, NJ 8540
609-452-0606
Fax: 609-987-8116
info@rfbd.org
www.learningally.org

Andrew Friedman, President & CEO
Jim Halliday, Executive Vice President
Connie Murphy, Chief Development and Community

6086 Reference and Information Services from NLS
National Library Service for the Blind
1291 Taylor Street NW
Washington, DC 20011
202-707-5100
Fax: 202-707-0712; Toll Free: 800-424-8567
nls@loc.gov
www.loc.gov/nls

Frank Cylke, Executive Director

6087 Referring Blind and Low Vision Patients for Rehabilitation Services
American Foundation for the Blind
2 Penn Plaza
Suite 1102
New York, NY 10121
212-502-7600
Fax: 888-545-8331; Toll Free: 800-232-5463
literacy@afb.net
www.afb.org

Carl R. Augusto, President & CEO
Kelly Bleach, Chief Administrative Officer
Rick Bozeman, Finance Director, Chief Financia

Clear information on such basic topics as the objectives of low vision services, what's covered in the examinations, what rehabilitation services do and how to locate these services.

Year Founded: 1921

6088 Resource List for Persons with Low Vision
American Council of the Blind
2200 Wilson Boulevard
Suite 650
Arlington, VA 22201-3354
202-467-5081
Fax: 202-467-5085; Toll Free: 800-424-8666
info@acb.org
www.acb.org

Kim Charlson, President
Jeff Thom, First Vice President
Melanie Brunson, Executive Director

Year Founded: 1961

6089 Seeing
National Association for Visually Handicapped
22 W 21st Street
Floor 6
New York, NY 10010-6943
212-889-3141
Fax: 212-727-2931
kcampbell@lighthouse.org
lighthouse.org/navh

Ann Illuzzi, Manager

This newsletter offers short stories, news, medical updates, assistive device information, poems, resources, crossword puzzles and more for the visually impaired.

Frequency: Biannually Year Founded: 1905

6090 Seeing Clearly
National Association for Visually Handicapped
22 W 21st Street
Floor 6
New York, NY 10010-6943
212-889-3141
Fax: 212-727-2931
kcampbell@lighthouse.org
lighthouse.org/navh

Ann Illuzzi, Manager

This newsletter for adults offers information on new items, advances in medical treatments and science, stories, crosswords, poems, humor and more.

Year Founded: 1905

6091 Sharing Solutions: A Newsletter for Support Groups
Lighthouse International
111 E 59th Street
The Sol and Lillian Goldman Building
New York, NY 10022-1202
212-821-9200
Fax: 212-821-9707; *Toll Free:* 800-829-0500
info@lighthouse.org
www.lighthouse.org
TTY: 212-821-9713

A newsletter for members and leaders of support groups for older adults with impaired vision. The letter provides a forum for support groups members to network and share information, printed in a very large type format.

Year Founded: 1905

6092 Smith-Kettlewell Technical File
Smith-Kettlewell Eye Research Institute
2318 Fillmore Street
San Francisco, CA 94115-1813
415-345-2000
Fax: 415-345-8455
rerc@ski.org
www.ski.org
TTY: 415-345-2290

Arthur Jampolsky, President
John Brabyn, Executice Director/CEO
Ruth S. Poole, Chief Operating Officer

6093 Talking Book Topics
National Library Service for the Blind
1291 Taylor Street NW
Washington, DC 20011
202-707-5100
Fax: 202-707-0712; *Toll Free:* 800-424-8567
nls@loc.gov
www.loc.gov/nls

Frank Cylke, Executive Director

Offers hundreds of listings of books, fiction and nonfiction, for adults and children on cassette. Also offers listings on foreign language books on cassette, talking magazines and reviews.

6094 Talking Books for Senior Adults
National Library Service for the Blind
1291 Taylor Street NW
Washington, DC 20011
202-707-5100
Fax: 202-707-0712; *Toll Free:* 800-424-8567
nls@loc.gov
www.loc.gov/nls

Frank Cylke, Executive Director

6095 The Blind Educator
National Organization of Blind Educators
2214 Emerson Avenue S
Apartment 4
Minneapolis, MN 21230
410-659-9314
Fax: 410-685-5653
shekoenig@msn.com
nfb.org/blind-educator

Sheila Koenig, President

Newsletter of the National Organization of Blind Educators, a division of the National Federation of the Blind.

6096 Vision Over 50
American Optometric Association
243 N Lindbergh Boulevard
Floor 1
Saint Louis, MO 63141-7881
314-991-4100
Fax: 314-991-4101; *Toll Free:* 800-365-2219
slthomas@aoa.org
www.aoa.org

Mitchell T. Munson, O.D, President
David A. Cockrell, O.D., President-Elect
Steven A. Loomis, O.D., Vice President

Offers information among adults over 50, medicare coverage, eye examinations, and tips for better seeing.

6097 Visions World Wide
Vision World Wide
5707 Brockton Drive
Apt 302
Indianapolis, IN 46220-5481
317-254-1332
Fax: 317-251-6588; *Toll Free:* 800-431-1739
www.visionww.org

62-78 pages Frequency: Quarterly

6098 Voice of Vision
GW Micro
725 Airport North Office Park
Fort Wayne, IN 46825-6707
260-489-3671
Fax: 260-489-2608
sales@gwmicro.com
www.gwmicro.com

Doug Geoffray, Vice President Development
Dan Weirich, VP Sales And Marketing
Lois Baich, Orders And Production

Offers product reviews, product announcements, tips for making systems or applications more accessible, or explanations of concepts of interest to any computer user or would-be computer user. This association newsletter is available in braille, in large print, on audio cassette and on 3.5 or 5.25 IBM format diskette.

Year Founded: 1990

6099 Volunteer at Your Braille and Talking Book Library
National Library Service for the Blind
1291 Taylor Street NW
Washington, DC 20011
202-707-5100
Fax: 202-707-0712; *Toll Free:* 800-424-8567
nls@loc.gov
www.loc.gov/nls

Frank Cylke, Executive Director

6100 Wings for the Future
American Printing House for the Blind
1839 Frankfort Avenue
P.O. Box 6085
Louisville, KY 40206-0085
502-895-2405
Fax: 502-899-2284; *Toll Free:* 800-223-1839

info@aph.org
www.aph.org

Tuck Tinsley, President

This booklet offers an introduction to the American Printing House For The Blind's programs, services, tools, aids and more.

13 pages Year Founded: 1858

6101 Without Sight and Sound
Helen Keller National Center for Deaf-Blind Youths
141 Middle Neck Road
Suite 3214
Sands Point, NY 11050
240-786-6534
Fax: 516-944-7302
hkncinfo@hknc.org
www.hknc.org
TDD 240-786-6847
TTY: 516-944-8637

Joseph McNulty, Executive Director

Pamphlet offering facts, causes, types and descriptions of deaf-blindness.

Year Founded: 1967

Videos, Audio Tapes

6102 Making Life More Livable
American Foundation for the Blind/AFB Press
2 Penn Plaza
Suite 1102
New York, NY 10121
212-502-7600
Fax: 888-545-8331; *Toll Free:* 800-232-5463
literacy@afb.net
www.afb.org

Carl R. Augusto, President & CEO
Kelly Bleach, Chief Administrative Officer
Rick Bozeman, Finance Director, Chief Financia

Shows how simple adaptations in the home and environment can make a big difference in the lives of blind and visually impaired older persons. The suggestions offered are numerous and specific, ranging from how to mark food cans for greater visibility to how to get out of the shower safley. Large print.

132 pages Year Founded: 1921

6103 Visions
Visions/Services for the Blind & Visually Impaired
500 Greenwich Street
Floor 3
New York, NY 10013-1354
212-625-1616
Fax: 212-219-4078; *Toll Free:* 888-245-8333
info@visionsvcb.org
www.visionsvcb.org

Nancy T. Jones, President
Richard P. Simon, Vice President
Burton M. Strauss, Jr., Treasurer

Offers rehabilitation services for older blind persons in New York City; self study kits on audio cassette for blind and visually impaired persons in the areas of personal management, mobility training, and sensory development.

Year Founded: 1923

Websites

6104 ACB Government Employees
American Council of the Blind
2200 Wilson Boulevard
Suite 650
Arlington, VA 22201-3354
202-467-5081
Fax: 202-467-5085; *Toll Free:* 800-424-8666
info@acb.org
www.acb.org

Kim Charlson, President
Jeff Thom, First Vice President
Melanie Brunson, Executive Director

Concerns of the organization include recruitment, placement and advancement of blind and visually impaired employees.

Year Founded: 1961

6105 ACB Radio Amateurs
American Council of the Blind
2200 Wilson Boulevard
Suite 650
Arlington, VA 22201-3354
202-467-5081
Fax: 202-467-5085; *Toll Free:* 800-424-8666
info@acb.org
www.acb.org

Kim Charlson, President
Jeff Thom, First Vice President
Melanie Brunson, Executive Director

A radio amateur network of blind, visually impaired and sighted members who gather and share common problems and solutions to help members improve radio amateurs in getting started, provides access to educational materials in special media and publishes a directory for the visually impaired.

Year Founded: 1961

6106 ACB Social Service Providers
American Council of the Blind
2200 Wilson Boulevard
Suite 650
Arlington, VA 22201-3354
202-467-5081
Fax: 202-467-5085; *Toll Free:* 800-424-8666
info@acb.org
www.acb.org

Kim Charlson, President
Jeff Thom, First Vice President
Melanie Brunson, Executive Director

Information on blind and visually impaired social workers, social service professionals, students pursuing careers in social work, and other interested persons.

Year Founded: 1961

6107 American Blind Lawyers Association
American Council of the Blind
2200 Wilson Boulevard
Suite 650
Arlington, VA 22201-3354
202-467-5081
Fax: 202-467-5085; *Toll Free:* 800-424-8666
info@acb.org
www.acb.org

Kim Charlson, President
Jeff Thom, First Vice President
Melanie Brunson, Executive Director

Information on law school admission tests and bar exams, private sector and government employment relations and specialized work techniques for the blind and visually impaired.

Year Founded: 1961

6108 American Council of Blind Lions
American Council of the Blind
2200 Wilson Boulevard
Suite 650
Arlington, VA 22201-3354
202-467-5081
Fax: 202-467-5085; Toll Free: 800-424-8666
info@acb.org
www.acb.org

Kim Charlson, President
Jeff Thom, First Vice President
Melanie Brunson, Executive Director

Information concerning Club activities in the field of work for the blind and encourages blind people to join Lions Clubs and other civic activities.

Year Founded: 1961

6109 American Printing House for the Blind
American Printing House for the Blind
1839 Frankfort Avenue
P.O. Box 6085
Louisville, KY 40206-0085
502-895-2405
Fax: 502-899-2284; Toll Free: 800-223-1839
info@aph.org
www.aph.org

Tuck Tinsley, President

This organization promotes the independence of blind persons by providing special media, tools and materials needed for education and life.

Year Founded: 1858

6110 Blinded Veterans Association
Blinded Veterans Association
477 H Street NW
Washington, DC 20001-2694
202-371-8880
Fax: 202-371-8258; Toll Free: 800-669-7079
BVA@BVA.ORG
www.bva.org

Mark Cornell, National President
Reverend Rob Dale Stamper, National President
Thomas H Miller, Executive Director

Offers two main service programs without cost to blinded veterans. Field service program provides counseling to veterans and families, and information on benefits and rehabilitation.

Year Founded: 1945

6111 Braille Revival League
American Council of the Blind
2200 Wilson Boulevard
Suite 650
Arlington, VA 22201-3354

202-467-5081
Fax: 202-467-5085; Toll Free: 800-424-8666
info@acb.org
www.acb.org

Kim Charlson, President
Jeff Thom, First Vice President
Melanie Brunson, Executive Director

Information for people to read and write in braille, advocates for mandatory braille instruction in educational facilities for the blind, strives to make available a supply of braille materials from libraries and printing houses and more.

Year Founded: 1961

6112 Guide Dog Foundation for the Blind
Guide Dog Foundation for the Blind
371 E Jericho Turnpike
Smithtown, NY 11787-2976
631-930-9000
Fax: 631-930-9009; Toll Free: 800-548-4337
info@guidedog.org
www.guidedog.org

James C. Bingham, Chairman
Alphonce J. Brown, Jr., ACFRE, Vice Chair
Wells B. Jones, Chief Executive Officer

Furnishes guide dogs, free of charge, to qualified people who seek independence, mobility and companionship.

6113 Guide Dog Users
American Council of the Blind
2200 Wilson Boulevard
Suite 650
Arlington, VA 22201-3354
202-467-5081
Fax: 202-467-5085; Toll Free: 800-424-8666
info@acb.org
www.acb.org

Kim Charlson, President
Jeff Thom, First Vice President
Melanie Brunson, Executive Director

Promotes the acceptance of blind people and their dogs, works for enforcement and expansion of laws admitting guide dogs into public places, advocates for quality training and follow-up services.

Year Founded: 1961

6114 Independent Visually Impaired Enterprisers
American Council of the Blind
2200 Wilson Boulevard
Suite 650
Arlington, VA 22201-3354
202-467-5081
Fax: 202-467-5085; Toll Free: 800-424-8666
info@acb.org
www.acb.org

Kim Charlson, President
Jeff Thom, First Vice President
Melanie Brunson, Executive Director

Information on rehabilitation facilities for all types of business enterprises and publicizes the capabilities of blind and visually impaired business persons.

Year Founded: 1961

6115 Lighthouse International
Lighthouse International
111 E 59th Street
The Sol and Lillian Goldman Building
New York, NY 10022-1202
212-821-9200
Fax: 212-821-9707; *Toll Free:* 800-829-0500
info@lighthouse.org
www.lighthouse.org
TTY: 212-821-9713

Offers information about vision impairment and vision rehabilitation, and provides referrals to services and support groups nationwide.

Year Founded: 1905

6116 National Association for Visually Handicapped
National Association for Visually Handicapped
22 W 21st Street
Floor 6
New York, NY 10010-6943
212-889-3141
Fax: 212-727-2931
kcampbell@lighthouse.org
lighthouse.org/navh

Ann Illuzzi, Manager

Serves the partially seeing (not totally blind) with informational literature, newsletters for adults and children, educational outreach, referrals, counsel and guidance.

Year Founded: 1905

6117 National Captioning Institute
www.ncicap.org

Advocates captioned television for people who want to see, as well as hear, the dialogue of a television program. It not only enables deaf and hard-of-hearing people to understand all of a program's content, but it is also beneficial for new Americans learning English as a second language, as well as children learning to read.

6118 National Library Service for the Blind and Physically Handicapped
National Library Service for the Blind
1291 Taylor Street NW
Washington, DC 20011
202-707-5100
Fax: 202-707-0712; *Toll Free:* 800-424-8567
nls@loc.gov
www.loc.gov/nls

Frank Cylke, Executive Director

Administers a national library service that provides braille and recorded books and magazines on free loan to anyone who cannot read standard print because of visual or physical disabilities who are eligible residents of the United States or American citizens living abroad.

6119 Vision World Wide
www.visionww.org

Aims is to enhance everyday living so as to maintain an independent lifestyle. It also serves as a consumer protection against misrepresentation and fraud.

6120 Visually Impaired Data Processors International
American Council of the Blind
2200 Wilson Boulevard
Suite 650
Arlington, VA 22201-3354
202-467-5081
Fax: 202-467-5085; *Toll Free:* 800-424-8666
info@acb.org
www.acb.org

Kim Charlson, President
Jeff Thom, First Vice President
Melanie Brunson, Executive Director

Provides for the exchange of work technique ideas and works with agencies to increase the availability of braille and recorded materials.

Year Founded: 1961

6121 Visually Impaired Veterans of America
American Council of the Blind
2200 Wilson Boulevard
Suite 650
Arlington, VA 22201-3354
202-467-5081
Fax: 202-467-5085; *Toll Free:* 800-424-8666
info@acb.org
www.acb.org

Kim Charlson, President
Jeff Thom, First Vice President
Melanie Brunson, Executive Director

Promotes the rights of visually impaired veterans to receive all benefits, encourages research and development of new products for blind people.

Year Founded: 1961

Research Centers

6122 Baylor College of Medicine: Cullen Eye Institute
The Cullen Eye Institute
6565 Fannin Street
NC-205
Houston, TX 77030-2703
713-798-4951
Fax: 713-798-4364
pa-webteam@bcm.edu
www.bcm.edu

Dan B Jones MD, Chairperson

Research activities focus on restoring vision and preventing blindness through a better understanding of the disease.

Year Founded: 1936

6123 Berman-Gund Laboratory for the Study of Retinal Degenerations
Massachusetts Eye and Ear
243 Charles Street
Boston, MA 02114-3002
617-523-7900
Fax: 617-573-3444
www.masseyeandear.org

Wycliffe Grousbeck, Chairman
John Fernandez, President & CEO
Sunil Eappen, M.D., Chief Medical Officer

Year Founded: 1824

6124 Dean A McGee Eye Institute
Oklahoma Health Center Location
608 Stanton L Young Boulevard
Oklahoma City, OK 73104-5065
405-271-6060
Fax: 405-271-4442; *Toll Free:* 800-787-9012
www.mei.org

Mr. David E. Rainbolt, Chairman
Gregory L. Skuta, MD, President and Chief Executive Of
Matthew D. Bown, Executive Vice President

Basic and clinical investigations in visual sciences.

Year Founded: 1965

6125 Glaucoma Foundation
The Glaucoma Foundation
80 Maiden Lane
Suite 700
New York, NY 10038
212-285-0080
Fax: 212-260-1002; *Toll Free:* 800-832-3926
info@glaucomafoundation.org
www.glaucomafoundation.org

Scott R. Christensen, President & Chief Executive Offi
Marianne Howard, Director of Outreach Programs
Angela Cooley, Director of Fundraising

Hotline provides answers to questions and makes referrals.
The Foundation supports research into the causes and treatment of glaucoma. Publishes free copies of About Glaucoma and Glaucoma Medications-Purpose and Side Effects.

6126 Glaucoma Research Foundation
Glaucoma Research Foundation
251 Post Street
Suite 600
San Francisco, CA 94108
415-986-3162
Fax: 415-986-3763; *Toll Free:* 800-826-6693
question@glaucoma.org
www.glaucoma.org

Andrew Iwach,MD, Chairman
Robert L. Stamper,MD, Vice Chair
Thomas M. Brunner, President & CEO

A national organization dedicated to protecting the sight of people with glaucoma through research and education. The Foundation conducts and supports research that contributes to improved patient care and a better understanding of the disease process. Provides education, advocacy and emotional support to patients and their families.

Year Founded: 1978

6127 Johns Hopkins University: Dana Center for Preventive Ophthalmology
Dana Center for Preventive Ophthalmology
600 North Wolfe Street
Wilmer Suite 122
Baltimore, MD 21287-9019
410-955-6100
Fax: 410-955-9777
www.hopkinsmedicine.org

Harry A Quigley, Director
Cindy Difernando, Manager

Year Founded: 1979

6128 National Eye Institute
National Institutes of Health
9000 Rockville Pike
Bldg 31
Bethesda, MD 20892
301-496-0417
www.nih.gov

Dr. Francis Collins, Director
Lawrence A. Tabak, D.D.S.; Ph.D., Principal Deputy Director
Kathy Hudson, Ph.D, Deputy Director for Science, Out

Mission is to discover safe and effective methods to prevent, diagnose and treat diseases and disorders of the visual system. In this way the Institute helps to prevent, reduce and possibly eliminate blindness and visual impairment.

Year Founded: 1887

6129 National Glaucoma Research
BrightFocus Foundation
22512 Gateway Center Drive
Clarksburg, MD 20871-2005
301-948-3244
Fax: 301-258-9454; *Toll Free:* 800-437-2423
jphilabaum@brightfocus.org
www.brightfocus.org

Dave Marks, Vice President of Finance and Ad
Jill Philabaum, Information and Donor Services C
Donna Callison, Vice President of Development

Offers up to date information on research, treatments, and publications. Also provides a free newsletter, National Glaucoma Research Report.

6130 Schepens Eye Research Institute
Schepens Eye Research Institute, Massachusetts Eye
20 Staniford Street
Boston, MA 02114-2508
617-912-0100
Fax: 617-523-3463
www.schepens.harvard.edu

Michael Gilmore, President
Mary E. Leach, Director of Public Affairs
Frances Ng, Director of Human Resources

Prominent center for research on eye, vision, and blinding diseases; dedicated to reserach that improves the understanding, management, and prevention of eye diseases and visual deficiencies; fosters collaboration among its faculty members; trains young scientists and clinicians from around the world; promotes communication with scientists in allied fields; leader in the worldwide dispersion of basic scientific knowledge of vision.

6131 Smith-Ketterwell Eye Research Institute
Smith-Kettlewell Eye Research Institute
2318 Fillmore Street
San Francisco, CA 94115-1813
415-345-2000
Fax: 415-345-8455
rerc@ski.org
www.ski.org
TTY: 415-345-2290

Arthur Jampolsky, President
John Brabyn, Executice Director/CEO
Ruth S. Poole, Chief Operating Officer

Dedicated to research on human vision. The Institute was founded to encourage a productive collaboration between the medical clinic and scientific laboratory. Research is conducted with clinical studies which relate directly to the diagnosis and treatment of eye diseases, the development of devices and vocational programs to aid the partially sighted and basic research to understand how the eye and brain work for both the clinical and rehabilittation programs.

6132 University of Illinois at Chicago: Lions of Illinios Eye Research Institute

UIC Eye Center
1855 West Taylor Street, m/c 648
Room 3.138
Chicago, IL 60612-3731
312-996-6591
Fax: 312-996-7770
eyeweb@uic.edu
chicago.medicine.uic.edu

Dimitri T. Azar, Dean
Todd Van Neck, Associate Dean for Administratio
Larry Tobacman, Senior Associate Dean for Resear

Visual impairments and blindness research, including glaucoma studies.

288 pages

6133 University of Miami: Bascom Palmer Eye Institute

Department of Ophthalmalogy
900 N.W. 17th Street
Miami, FL 33136-1015
305-326-6000
Fax: 305-326-6306; Toll Free: 800-329-7000
bascompalmer.org

John G Clarkson MD, Chairman

Clinical and basic research into blindness and visual impairments.

6134 Warren Grant Magnuson Clinical Center

10 Center Drive
Bldg 61
Bethesda, MD 20892
301-496-2563
Fax: 301-402-2984
prpl@mail.cc.nih.gov
www.cc.nih.gov

John I. Gallin,MD, Clinical Center Director
David Henderson, MD, Deputy Director for Clinical Car
Clare Hastings,Ph.D,RN,FAAN, Chief Nurse Officer

Established in 1953 as the research hospital of the National Institutes of Health. Designed so that patient care facilities are close to research laboratories so new findings of basic and clinical scientists can be quickly applied to the treatment of patients. Upon referral by physicians, patients are admitted to NIH clinical studies.

Year Founded: 1944

6135 Yale University: Vision Research Center

Yale School of Medicine
333 Cedar Street
New Haven, CT 06510-3218
203-785-2020
Fax: 203-785-7090; Toll Free: 800-395-7949
medicine.yale.edu

James C. Tsai, Chairman
Pam Burkheiser, Manager

Vision including studies on growth and development.

Assisted Living Facilities

Alabama

6136 Azalea Manor
Azalea Manor
557 E Waterman Street
Marietta, GA 30060
770-428-0331
Fax: 205-485-9652
azaleamanor1@bellsouth.net
www.azalea-manor.com

Mark Watkins, Admnistrator

Specializes in caring for residents who have special care needs.

Year Founded: 1983

6137 Fair Haven Retirement Community
Methodist Homes of Alabama & Northwest Florida
1424 Montclair Road
Birmingham, AL 35210-2208
205-956-4150
Fax: 205-951-7681
methodisthomes.org

Christopher Tomlin, President, CEO & CFO
Michael D. Giles, Senior Vice President, COO & Gen
Regina T. Lawler, Vice President, Dir. of Informat

Offers quality assisted living services. We provide 70 assisted living units.

Year Founded: 1961

6138 Gardens of Clanton
The Gardens of Clanton
850 Scott Drive
Clanton, AL 35045-8725
205-280-0084
Fax: 205-280-0449
www.seniorlivingguide.com

Robert O'Malley, President & CEO
John Brennan, IT Development Director
Vicki Moseley, Administrator

Offers quality assisted living services.

6139 Gordon Oaks Convalescent Center
3151 Knollwood Drive
Mobile, AL 36693-2753
251-661-7608
Fax: 334-602-9146
www.thirdage.com

Sondra Forsyth, Co-Editor-in-Chief
Jane Farrell, Co-Editor-in-Chief
Lois Joy Johnson, Beauty and Fashion Director??

Gordon Oaks provides for the residents' wide variety of daily needs from within the community.

Year Founded: 1997

6140 Homestead Village of Fairhope
Homestead Village
924 Plantation Boulevard
Fairhope, AL 36532-2952
251-929-0250
Fax: 251-929-0259; *Toll Free:* 800-395-3864

info@hvfairhope.com
www.hvfairhope.com

Malissa Hubert, Marketing Director

Located on a 17-acre campus community providing a variety of residential options for seniors. An array of services and amenities are offered to promote each resident's sence of security while promoting healthy and fulfilling lifestyles. Residents can easily maintain their individual lifestyles while enjoying the comfort of knowing assistance is close at hand.

6141 Kirkwood by the River
Kirkwood by the River
3605 Ratliff Road
Birmingham, AL 35210-4512
205-956-2184
Fax: 205-956-0990
lellison@kirkwoodbytheriver.com
www.kirkwoodbytheriver.com

Sandi Hall, Marketing Director

Kirkwood by the River is a non profit continuing care retirement community located on 120 beautiful wooded acres in the foothills of the Appalachians. Incorporated as a Presbyterian Homes of Birmingham and sponsored by Independent Presbyterian Church, it is open to all people regardless of church affiliation. An applicant or spouce must be at least sixty-two to move into kirkwood.

Year Founded: 1980

6142 Knowlwood Assisted Living
Knowlwood Assisted Living
4804 Highway 25
Montevallo, AL 35115
205-665-5955
Fax: 205-665-2855
Kathykno@knowlwood.com
www.knowlwood.com

Kathy Turner, Owner

We are a state licensed facility, providing 24 hour care to senior citizens needing assistance.

6143 Liveoak Village
Livesoak Village
300 Village Square
Foley, AL 36535
251-971-1940
Fax: 251-971-1944; *Toll Free:* 877-231-6981
info@liveoakvillage.com
www.liveoakvillage.com

Doug Warren, President & CEO
Richard Denham, Manager
Kim Willingham, Broker

Our goal is to create a community that ofers our families fredom to live the retirement lifestyle they have always wanted.

Year Founded: 2007

6144 Morningside of Decatur
Five Star Quality Care
2115 Point Mallard Drive SE
Decatur, AL 35601-6765
256-350-0089
Fax: 256-350-1530
www.morningsideofdecatur.com

Lanette Arnold, Executive Director

We are uniquely designed to provide different levels of assisted living.

6145 Mount Royal Towers
Rolling Hills Ranch - Chula Vista
850 Duncan Ranch Road
Chula Vista, CA 91914
619-482-8000
Fax: 205-871-3111
www.healthcaregrp.com/mountroyal/index

W. Major Chance, Founder/Chief Executive Officer
B. Renee Barnard, President/Chief Financial Office
Todd A. Shetter, Chief Operating Officer

Mount Royal Towers Retirement Community has a full continuum of health care on site including Independent Living, Independent Plus, Skilled Nursing and ActivCare Residential Alzheimer's Care. Whether you require personal assistance or full fursing care, you'll find courteous and caring staff and a safe, secure enviroment.

Year Founded: 1981

6146 Murray House
Murray House
1257 Government Street
Mobile, AL 36604-2410
251-432-2272
Fax: 251-432-1935
pauldeanna@bellsouth.net
www.murray-house.org

Rev. Thomas Heard, President
Stacy Reckeweg, Vice President
Joe Basenberg, Vice President

Offers quality assisted living services.

Year Founded: 1829

6147 North Mobile Retirement Center
North Mobile Retirement Ctr
300 Baker Road
Satsuma, AL 36572-2446
334-679-9192
Fax: 334-679-9868
www.seniorhousingnet.com

Elizabeth Frye, Administrator

Assisted living facility with a 40 bed capacity.

6148 Saint Martins in the Pines
St. Martin's
4941 Montevallo Road
Birmingham, AL 35210
205-956-9440
Fax: 205-956-9124
www.stmartins.ws

Terry Rogers, President and Chief Executive Of
Mike Faulkner, Chief Financial Officer
Chris Barnett, Director of The Pines Rehab Cent

To serve God through a ministry that provides a continuum of care and quality of life to aging individuals and their families.

Year Founded: 1957

6149 Somerby at Jones Farm
AssistedLivingWay.com
2815 Carl T Jones Drive SE
Huntsville, AL 35802-1258
256-881-6111
Fax: 256-881-8748
www.thirdage.com

Sondra Forsyth, Co-Editor-in-Chief
Jane Farrell, Co-Editor-in-Chief
Lois Joy Johnson, Beauty and Fashion Director??

The Apartment Homes are designed for those who still enjoy an independent lifestyle and want to be an integral part of a state of the art, service-oriented community. The homes offer comfort and convenience in an ideal setting with a variety of plans to accommodate different needs and desires.

Year Founded: 1997

6150 Somerset Assited Living Facility
Assisted Living Facility
815 John D Odom Road
Dothan, AL 36303-9347
334-671-1176
Fax: 334-793-9104; *Toll Free:* 866-333-6002
www.assistedlivingfacilities.org

Sheila Cobb, Manager

Provides assisted living residential services. This includes assistance with medication, bathing, dressing, meal preparation, laundry, recreational activities and supervision. 16 bed capacity.

6151 Village at Cook Springs
Village at Cook Springs
415 Cooks Spring Road
Pell City, AL 35125-4312
205-338-2221
Fax: 205-814-3189
VillageInfo@nolandhealth.com
www.villageatcooksprings.com

Assisted Living residents enjoy the independence of their own suite, while knowing they have special assistance from a caring staff when needed.

6152 Westminster Village
Westminster Village
500 Spanish Fort Boulevard
Spanish Fort, AL 36527-5018
251-626-2900
Fax: 334-626-8529; *Toll Free:* 800-843-3740
melanie.thornton@wvsf.us
www.westminstervillageal.com

Ben McKibbens, Chairman
James Bledsoe, Vice Chairman
Robert S. Edington, Corporate Counsel

The only community on the Alabama Gulf Coast to offer the full continuum of Life Care services on one campus.

Alaska

6153 Anchorage Pioneers' Home
923 W 11th Avenue
Anchorage, AK 99501-4306
907-276-3414
Fax: 907-343-7291

david_frain@health.state.ak.us
www.alaska.gov

David Frain, Administrator

Assisted living home for Alaskans age 65 and over including Alzheimer's and related dementia care.

6154 Chugiak-Eagle River Senior Center

22424 North Birchwood Loop
Chugiak, AK 99567-6476
907-688-2677
Fax: 907-688-1319
csc@mtaonline.net
www.chugiak-seniors.org

Linda Hendrickson, Executive Director
Monika Dahlberg, Development Director
Patti Riggs, Program Director

Providing senior independent housing (43 units), low income senior housing (20 units), assisted living (20 units), congregate community meals, meals on wheels, transportation, adult day care, senior activities and wellness clinics.

6155 Juneau Pioneers Home

4675 Glacier Highway
Juneau, AK 99801-9518
907-586-3740
Fax: 907-780-4765
rosemary_gute-gruening@admin.state.ak.us
juneauempire.com

Jill Sandelben, Administrator
Ruston Burton, Publisher
Kathryn Nickerson, Advertising Manager

Offers quality assisted living services.

6156 Marlow Manor/Manor Management

Marlow Manor Assisted Living
2030 Muldoon Road
Anchorage, AK 99504-3611
907-338-8708
Fax: 907-338-8627
Theresa@marlowmanor.com
www.marlowmanor.com

Theresa A Brisky, RN, BSN, Executive Administrator
Lisa Gilligan, RN, Director Resident Services
Norma Reece, Facility Manager

Forty eight assisted living community for seniors. Four of the apartments are designated for dementia care on a secured floor.

6157 Tranquility Manor

Tranquility Manor Estates
1950 Hemmer Road
Palmer, AK 99645-8624
907-746-4220
Fax: 907-746-4207
www.tranquilitymanorllc.com

Catherine Korman, Administrator
Bruce Korman, Manager

Offers quality assisted living services.
Year Founded: 2003

6158 Outlook Pointe at Mountain Home

Elmcroft Senior Living
9510 Ormsby Station Road
Louisville, KY 40223
502-753-6000
Fax: 502-753-6100
outlook@mtnhome.com
www.elmcroftal

Diane West, Contact
Erica Warmoth, Contact

An assisted living community dedicated to the independence, dignity and purpose of every residence. Outlook Pointe offers truly worry-free assisted living.

6159 West Shores Retirement Community

West Shores
2607 Albert Pike Road
Hot Springs, AR 71913-4501
501-767-1200
Fax: 501-767-2083; Toll Free: 800-818-1201
www.capitalsenior.com/westshores

Nina Alter, Executive Director

Offers a lifestyle that is genuinely inviting with a combination of comfort and freedom. In addition to luxurious surrounding and friendly people, we offer the special accomodations and considerations that allow your retirement to be worry free.

6160 ALC Copper Hills House

12234 E North Frontage Road
Yuma, AZ 85367
928-305-0892
Fax: 520-342-1768
www.alcoo.com

Mary Ward, Executive Director

Offers quality assisted living services.

6161 Bethesda Gardens

Bethesda Senior Living
15475 Gleneagle Dr
Colorado Springs, CO 80921
719-481-5481
Fax: 719-488-6080
phinfo@ba.org
www.bethesdaseniorliving.com

Dennis Smith, Administrator

Offers quality assisted living services.

6162 Broadway Proper

Leisure Care, LLC
1601 Fifth Avenue
Suite 1900
Seattle, WA 98101
206-436-7827
Fax: 206-436-7705
mhiatt@leisurecare.com
www.leisurecare.com

Dan Madsen, Chief Executive Officer

Features apartment homes in a fun and active retirement community.

Year Founded: 1976

6163 Care with Love
Care With Love
813 E Belmont Avenue
Phoenix, AZ 85020-4102
602-618-6445
Fax: 602-216-0291
lgorodishter@cox.net
www.carewithlove.net

Lana Akhenblit, Contact

An alternative, state licensed, care facility capable of handling residents at a skilled care level.

6164 Desert Point-La Reserve
Leisure Care, LLC
1601 Fifth Avenue
Suite 1900
Seattle, WA 98101
206-436-7827
Fax: 206-436-7705; *Toll Free:* 800-327-3490
www.leisurecare.com

Dan Madsen, Chief Executive Officer

Located in the foothills of the Santa Catalina Mountain Range in Oro Valley, and offers luxurious apartment homes.

Year Founded: 1976

6165 Emerald Springs Retirement & Assisted Living Community
1475 S 46th Avenue
Yuma, AZ 85364-4010
928-257-1689
Fax: 928-329-7717
www.seniorlifestyle.com

Bill Kalpan, Chairman
Joni DeLuca, President and Chief Executive Of
Keven J. Bennema, Executive Vice President, Chief

Our appartments are fully carpeted with individual climate control and emergency call systems. At Emerald Springs, you will enjoy the privacy of your own individual apartment within a community of care and support.

6166 Emeritus at Catalina Foothills
Senior Lifestyle
3701 N Swan Road
Tucson, AZ 85718-6968
520-299-7755
Fax: 520-229-7827
www.emeritus.com

Teresa Warren, Executive Director

Offers quality assisted living services.

Year Founded: 1985

6167 Forum at Tucson
The Forum at Tucson
2500 N Rosemont Boulevard
Tucson, AZ 85712-2167
520-320-6532
Fax: 520-319-4076
www.theforumattucson.com

Kay Warren, Administrator

Offers quality assisted living services.

6168 La Posada
La Posada
350 E Morningside Road
Green Valley, AZ 85614
520-648-8131
Fax: 520-648-8397
www.laposadagv.com

Lisa Israel, President/CEO
Joni Condit, Vice President & COO
Paul Ide, Vice President & CFO

Maximizes the well being and care of seniors.

Year Founded: 1987

6169 La Siena
La Siena
909 East Northern Avenue
Phoenix, AZ 85020
602-870-5500
Fax: 602-870-5501
info@srg-llc.com
www.srgseniorliving.com

Michael S. Grust, President and Chief Executive Of

Retirement living center.

6170 McDowell Village
McDowell Village
8300 East McDowell Road
Scottsdale, AZ 85257
480-559-8137
www.mcdowellvillage.com

Debbie Whipple, General Manager
Michael Bergmans, Guest Services Manager
Thomas Miranda, Chef

Designed to offer a full complement of services for independent seniors who want to spend their time having fun.

6171 SunQuest Village of Yuma
SunQuest Village of Yuma
265 E 24th Street
Yuma, AZ 85364
928-344-8680
Fax: 928-344-4985
www.sunquestvillage.com

Linda Gwinn, Administrator

Offers quality assisted living services.

6172 Villa Hermosa
La Siena
6300 East Speedway Blvd
Tucson, AZ 85710
520-329-4038
info@srg-llc.com
www.srgseniorliving.com

Michael S. Grust, President and Chief Executive Of

Retirement living center.

California

6173 Aegis Escondido
Ageis Living
17602 NE Union Hill Road
Redmond, WA 92025

760-735-8084
Fax: 760-735-8182; *Toll Free:* 866-688-5829
www.aegisliving.com

Dwayne Clark, Chairman and CEO
David Ford, Vice Chairman
Jerry Meyer, President and Chief Operating Of

Offers a range of lifestyle options including retirement living and assisted living.

6174 Aegis Gardens
Ageis Living
36281 Fremont Boulevard
Fremont, CA 94536
510-739-0909
Fax: 510-739-0946; *Toll Free:* 866-688-5829
www.aegisliving.com

Dwayne Clark, Chairman and CEO
David Ford, Vice Chairman
Jerry Meyer, President and Chief Operating Of

A unique retirement community offering assisted living and Alzheimer's care and is dedicated to the Asian culture. Located close to shopping, medical centers and our sister community, Aegis of Fermont. Those who call Aegis Gardens Home will feel enveloped in the Asian culture through the interiors, landscaping and authentic Asian cusine.

6175 Aegis at Shadowridge
Ageis Living
1440 S. Melrose Drive
Oceanside, CA 92056
760-444-0758
Fax: 760-806-9508; *Toll Free:* 866-688-5829
www.aegisliving.com

Dwayne Clark, Chairman and CEO
David Ford, Vice Chairman
Jerry Meyer, President and Chief Operating Of

Located centrally to Carlsbad, Oceanside and Vista and is the beneficiary of the warm California Climate. Aegis at Shadowridge is committed to being an active part of the North Country community by providing education and leadership on senior issues, and helping wherever we can promote quality of life for the elderly and their families.

6176 Aegis of Aptos
Ageis Living
125 Heather Terrace
Aptos, CA 95003
831-706-2977
Fax: 831-684-2719; *Toll Free:* 866-688-5829
www.aegisliving.com

Dwayne Clark, Chairman and CEO
David Ford, Vice Chairman
Jerry Meyer, President and Chief Operating Of

Assisted living with separate wings for Alzheimer's and dementia care.

6177 Aegis of Carmichael
Ageis Living
4050 Walnut Avenue
Carmichael, CA 95608
916-231-9427
Fax: 916-972-1060; *Toll Free:* 866-688-5829
www.aegisliving.com

Dwayne Clark, Chairman and CEO
David Ford, Vice Chairman
Jerry Meyer, President and Chief Operating Of

Situation in a quite residential neighborhood where there are 48 assisted living apartments which are a mix of one bedrooms and spacious studios, plus 27 apartments for residents with alzheimer's disease or other dementia.

6178 Aegis of Chino Hills
Ageis Living
14837 Peyton Drive
Chino Hills, CA 91709
909-614-4050
Fax: 909-597-3383; *Toll Free:* 866-688-5829
www.aegisliving.com

Dwayne Clark, Chairman and CEO
David Ford, Vice Chairman
Jerry Meyer, President and Chief Operating Of

Choose from different apartments. Some offering spacious kitchens and fireplaces, garages and carports.

6179 Aegis of Concord
Ageis Living
4756 Clayton Road
Concord, CA 94521
925-692-5838
Fax: 925-692-0071; *Toll Free:* 866-688-5829
www.aegisliving.com

Dwayne Clark, Chairman and CEO
David Ford, Vice Chairman
Jerry Meyer, President and Chief Operating Of

Offers seven different floor plans all featuring nine foot ceilings with crown molding and private balconies.

6180 Aegis of Corte Madera
Ageis Living
5555 Paradise Drive
Corte Madera, CA 94925
415-927-4200
Fax: 415-927-4244; *Toll Free:* 866-688-5829
www.aegisliving.com

Dwayne Clark, Chairman and CEO
David Ford, Vice Chairman
Jerry Meyer, President and Chief Operating Of

Located in a quiet residential neighborhood convenient to great shopping, bay trails and beautiful view of Mt. Tamalpais. Here we feature services for independent living and Alzheimer's care.

6181 Aegis of Dana Point
Ageis Living of Dana Point
26922 Camino De Estrella
Dana Point, CA 92624-1603
949-340-8558
Fax: 949-488-2669
www.aegisofdanapoint.com

Sondra Brakeville, Executive Director

Knows the importance of recognizing, celebrating, and honoring people's lives.

6182 Aegis of Fremont
Ageis Living
3850 Walnut Avenue
Fremont, CA 94538

510-584-9526
Fax: 510-739-1559; *Toll Free:* 866-688-5829
www.aegisliving.com

Dwayne Clark, Chairman and CEO
David Ford, Vice Chairman
Jerry Meyer, President and Chief Operating Of

Assisted living services and dedicated care for individuals living with Alzheimer's or dementia.

6183 Aegis of Granada Hills
Ageis Living
10801 Lindley Avenue
Granada Hills, CA 91344
818-275-4700
Fax: 818-363-1933; *Toll Free:* 866-688-5829
www.aegisliving.com

Dwayne Clark, Chairman and CEO
David Ford, Vice Chairman
Jerry Meyer, President and Chief Operating Of

Provides assisted living services and dedicated care especially designed for residents with Alzheimer's or other dementia.

6184 Aegis of Laguna Niguel
Ageis Living
32170 Niguel Road
Laguna Niguel, CA 92677
949-340-9152
Fax: 949-496-8181; *Toll Free:* 866-688-5829
www.aegisliving.com

Dwayne Clark, Chairman and CEO
David Ford, Vice Chairman
Jerry Meyer, President and Chief Operating Of

Aegis of Laguna Niguel is nestled in the beautiful and residential Beacon Hill area. Located in a special place and surrounded by some of the finest senior housing anywhere, it has become the preferred choice for those who seek the best in assisted living services and also for those residents with Alzheimer's disease or other dementia. The quality of care there is rated with the very best.

6185 Aegis of Moraga
Ageis Living
950 Country Club Drive
Moraga, CA 94556
925-478-7327
Fax: 925-377-7929; *Toll Free:* 866-688-5829
www.aegisliving.com

Dwayne Clark, Chairman and CEO
David Ford, Vice Chairman
Jerry Meyer, President and Chief Operating Of

Located close to shopping, banking, and walking trails. Temperatures are typically warm and moderate in this part of California so it allows residents to enjoy an exceptional climate in a lovely part of the country.

6186 Aegis of Napa
Ageis Living
2100 Redwood Road
Napa, CA 94558
707-780-3206
Fax: 707-251-1410; *Toll Free:* 866-688-5829
www.aegisliving.com

Dwayne Clark, Chairman and CEO
David Ford, Vice Chairman
Jerry Meyer, President and Chief Operating Of

Enhance resident care, promote independence, and celebrate residents' lives.

6187 Aegis of Pleasant Hill
Ageis Living
1660 Oak Park Boulevard
Pleasant Hill, CA 94523
925-588-7030
Fax: 925-939-2785; *Toll Free:* 866-688-5829
www.aegisliving.com

Dwayne Clark, Chairman and CEO
David Ford, Vice Chairman
Jerry Meyer, President and Chief Operating Of

Situated in a quite residential neighborhood, there are 50 assisted living apartments, a mix of one bedrooms and spacious studios, plus 29 apartments for residents with Alzheimer's or dementia.

6188 Aegis of San Francisco
Ageis Living
2280 Gellert Boulevard South
San Francisco, CA 94080
650-242-4154
Fax: 650-952-5186; *Toll Free:* 866-688-5829
www.aegisliving.com

Dwayne Clark, Chairman and CEO
David Ford, Vice Chairman
Jerry Meyer, President and Chief Operating Of

Provides different levels of assisted living services.

6189 Aegis of San Rafael
Ageis Living
111 Merrydale Road
San Rafael, CA 94903
415-233-6693
Fax: 415-472-3969; *Toll Free:* 866-688-5829
www.aegisliving.com

Dwayne Clark, Chairman and CEO
David Ford, Vice Chairman
Jerry Meyer, President and Chief Operating Of

Assisted living services specifically designed to meet your individual needs.

6190 Aegis of Ventura
Ageis Living
4964 Telegraph Road
Ventura, CA 93003-8181
805-290-1953
Fax: 805-650-6283; *Toll Free:* 866-688-5829
www.aegisliving.com

Dwayne Clark, Chairman and CEO
David Ford, Vice Chairman
Jerry Meyer, President and Chief Operating Of

Offers assisted living services and specially designed care for those living with Alzheimer's or other dementia.

6191 Alpine View Lodge
The Alpine View Lodge
973 Arnold Way
Alpine, CA 91901

619-445-5291
Fax: 619-659-0617
www.alpineviewlodge.com

Linda Cioffi, Administrator

Offers residential living, specializing in dementia and Alzheimer's care.

6192 Atherton Baptist Homes
Atherton Baptist Homes
214 South Atlantic Boulevard
Alhambra, CA 91801
626-863-1224
Fax: 626-576-0857; *Toll Free:* 800-340-4178
www.abh.org

Dennis McFadden, President/CEO
Jackie Pascual, CFO

Offers residents freedom from the day-to-day chores necessary to run a home but still offers the benefits of an fulfilling lifestyle.

Year Founded: 1914

6193 Belmont Village Cardiff by the Sea
Belmont Village
3535 Manchester Avenue
Cardiff By The Sea, CA 92007
760-436-8900
www.belmontvillage.com

Patricia G. Will, Co-Founder and President

Location is convenient to worship and is less than two miles south of the El Camino Real retail corridor.

6194 Belmont Village Crown Cove
Belmont Village
3901 E Coast Highway
Corona del Mar, CA 92625
949-760-2800
www.belmontvillage.com

Patricia G. Will, Co-Founder and President

Located in the seaside village of Corona del Mar, overlooking the Pacific Ocean.

6195 Belmont Village Westwood
Belmont Village
10475 Wilshire Blvd
Los Angeles, CA 90024
310-475-7501
www.belmontvillage.com

Patricia G. Will, Co-Founder and President

Located along Wilshire Boulevard's Golden Mile, and adjacent to the Westwood United Methodist Church.

6196 Belmont Village at Sabre Springs
Belmont Village
13075 Evening Creek Drive South
San Diego, CA 92128
858-486-5020
Fax: 858-486-3540
www.belmontvillage.com

Patricia G. Will, Co-Founder and President
Inan Linton, Community Manager

Offers residents a more dignified, independent life in a comfortable residential neighborhood setting.

6197 Belmont Village of Burbank
Belmont Village
455 E Angeleno Avenue
Burbank, CA 91501
818-972-2405
Fax: 323-874-4123
www.belmontvillage.com

Patricia G. Will, Co-Founder and President
Jane Hirsch, Manager

Offers residents a more dignified, independent life in a comfortable residential neighborhood setting.

6198 Belmont Village of Encino
Belmont Village
15451 Ventura Blvd
Sherman Oaks, CA 91403
818-788-8870
Fax: 818-380-0205
kgarnett@belmontvillage.com
www.belmontvillage.com

Patricia G. Will, Co-Founder and President
Ken Garnett, Executive Director
Venca Avivi, Director

Located on the prime residential areas of Encino and Sherman Oaks in the San Fernando Valley.

6199 Belmont Village of Hollywood Hills
Belmont Village
2051 N Highland Avenue
Los Angeles, CA 90068
323-874-7711
Fax: 323-874-4123
www.belmontvillage.com

Patricia G. Will, Co-Founder and President
Tom Park, Executive Director
Stephanie Sanchez, Director

Offers residents a more dignified, independent life in a comfortable residential neighborhood setting.

6200 Belmont Village of Rancho Palos Verdes
Belmont Village
5701 Crestridge Road
Rancho Palos Verdes, CA 90275
310-377-9977
Fax: 310-377-4499; *Toll Free:* 866-965-2891
www.belmontvillage.com

Patricia G. Will, Co-Founder and President
Judith Uy-Villaruz, Executive Director
Rene Navarrette, Coordinator

Located in a beautiful Palos Verdes peninsula residential neighborhood, overlooking the ocean and Greater Los Angeles basin.

6201 Belmont Village of San Jose
Belmont Village
500 S Winchester Boulevard
San Jose, CA 95128
408-984-4767
sambrose@belmontvillage.com
www.belmontvillage.com

Patricia G. Will, Co-Founder and President
Scott Ambrose, Executive Director
Eloisa Abayan, Director

Offers residents a more dignified, independent life in a comfortable residential neighborhood setting.

6202 Belmont Village of Sunnyvale
Belmont Village
1039 E. El Camino Real
Sunnyvale, CA 94087
408-720-8498
Fax: 408-720-8499
rlieberman@belmontvillage.com
www.belmontvillage.com

Patricia G. Will, Co-Founder and President
Rich Lieberman, Executive Director
Zenaida Jarin, Director

Offers residents a more dignified, independent life in a comfortable residential neighborhood setting.

6203 British Home in California
The British Home in California, Ltd.
647 Manzanita Avenue
Sierra Madre, CA 91024
626-355-7240
Fax: 626-355-7267
info@britishhome-ca.us
www.britishhome-ca.us

We are uniquely designed to provide different levels of assisted living services from minimum daily supervision to 24 hour care.

Year Founded: 1931

6204 Broadview Residential Care Center
535 W Broadway
Glendale, CA 91204
818-246-4951
Fax: 818-243-0437
www.thebroadview.net

Marcia Spears Cihon, Administrator

Specialize in caring for elderly with mild dementia who need a helping hand with their daily routine. Also able to help seniors recovering from sugery.

6205 Californian Retirement Residence
The Californian Assisted Living and Dementia Care
1224 Cottonwood Street
Woodland, CA 95695
530-666-2433
Fax: 530-666-2458
www.thecalifornian.net

Offers expanded assisted living area; nonambulatory residents; secured Alzhimer's special care,

6206 Campbell Adult Center
The City of Campbell
70 N. First St.
C-33
Campbell, CA 95008
408-866-2100
Fax: 408-374-6965
hr@cityofcampbell.com
www.cityofcampbell.com

JoElle Hernandez, Chairman
Susan E. Blake, Vice Chair
Michael Kotowski, Mayor

For individuals over 50 years of age. Provides programs and services to assist older adults in remaining independent and improve their quality of life.

6207 Chancellor Health Care
An Assisted Living Community
990 East Del Mar Boulevard
Pasadena, CA 91106
707-687-1919
Fax: 707-687-1912
amy.c@chancellorhealthcare.com
www.chancellorhealthcare.com

Michael Augsburger, Administration
Jeanne Murdoch, Quality Operations

The goal is to provide exceptional care for residents and to be recognized as the premier provider in the senior housing and care industry.

Year Founded: 1992

6208 Chancellor Place of Chino Hills
An Assisted Living Community
6500 Butterfield Ranch Road
Chino Hills, CA 91709-6379
909-606-2553
Fax: 707-573-1929
amy.c@chancellorhealthcare.com
www.chancellorhealthcare.com

Allan Slight, Administrator

We provide different levels of assisted living services. Our goal is to provide exceptional care for residents, and to be recognized as the provider in the long term care industry.

Year Founded: 1992

6209 Chancellor Place of Lodi
An Assisted Living Community
990 East Del Mar Boulevard
Pasadena, CA 91106
707-687-1919
Fax: 707-687-1912
amy.c@chancellorhealthcare.com
www.chancellorhealthcare.com

We provide different levels of assisted living services.

Year Founded: 1992

6210 Chancellor Place of Murrieta
An Assisted Living Community
990 East Del Mar Boulevard
Pasadena, CA 91106
707-687-1919
Fax: 707-687-1912
amy.c@chancellorhealthcare.com
www.chancellorhealthcare.com

We provide different levels of assisted living services.

Year Founded: 1992

6211 Chancellor Place of Pasadena
An Assisted Living Community
990 East Del Mar Blvd
Pasadena, CA 91106
626-577-0215
amy.c@chancellorhealthcare.com
www.chancellorhealthcare.com

We provide different levels of assisted living services.

Year Founded: 1992

6212 Chancellor Place of Windsor
An Assisted Living Community
990 East Del Mar Boulevard
Pasadena, CA 91106
707-687-1919
Fax: 707-687-1912
amy.c@chancellorhealthcare.com
www.chancellorhealthcare.com

We provide different levels of assisted living services.

Year Founded: 1992

6213 CiminoCare
CiminoCare
7501 Sunrise Blvd
Citrus Heights, CA 95610
916-486-9639
Fax: 916-486-9675; *Toll Free:* 855-224-6466
mark@CiminoCare.com
www.ciminocare.com

Mark Cimino, CEO & Director
Wilma Cimino, Co-Founder & Director
John Cimino, Co-Founder & Director

An array of programs designed with the individual's capabilities in mind. Dignified living blended with old world hospitality.

Year Founded: 1973

6214 Cordia Senior Living
Cordia Corporate
197 Eighth Street
Suite 900
Charlestown, MA 02129
617-886-0200
Fax: 916-780-3331
www.cordiaseniorliving.com

Karen Anderson, President/CEO
Eustace Theodore, PhD, Vice President, Organizational a
Anne Tobin, Vice President, Human Resources

Comitted to creating opportunities for seniors to continue to lead meaningful lives.

6215 Country Village Senior Services
Country Village Apartments
10250 Country Club Drive
Suite H
Mira Loma, CA 91752-1329
951-681-5718
Fax: 951-681-5773; *Toll Free:* 877-700-4556
www.countryvillageseniorliving.com

Pat Shivers, Manager

Afternoons by appointment and scheduled meetings, information and assistance for residents of this retirement community, linkage with Social Security, DPSS, Public Health, Mental Health, Legal Services, Office on Aging, Nutrition Counseling, planning with Doctors Discharge Planners for homecare, extensive use of volunteers for meal delivery, telephone reassurance, transportation, roster of available homemakers, support group for caregivers, educational lectures and videos. Must be 55+ and resident.

6216 Courtyards at Pine Creek
Courtyards at Pine Creek
1081 Mohr Lane
Concord, CA 94518

925-798-3900
Fax: 925-798-0773
susan@courtyardsatpinecreek.com
www.courtyardsatpinecreek.com

Steve Millard, Executive Director
Alicia Holman, Health Service Director
Susan R McLaughlin, Community Relations Director

An assisted living community committed to assisting our residents through the natural aging process with grace, a little humor, and the utmost dignity. The delicate balance of enriching their independence while maintaining their safety is our ongoing challenge.

6217 Crown Cove
Crown Cove Cottages
4752 Highway #1
Granville Ferry, RR2
Nova Scotia, CA 92625
902-532-7976
Fax: 949-760-2888; *Toll Free:* 888-627-5653
vacation@crowncove.ca
www.crowncove.ca

Vicki Kaiser, Manager

Assisted living program is designed for residents who need help with the activities of daily living, but do not require intensive nursing intervention.

6218 Cypress Court Escondido
Cypress Court
1255 N Broadway
Escondido, CA 92026-2863
760-747-1940
Fax: 760-747-3723
cypresscourt@kiscosl.com
www.kiscoseniorliving.com

Stuart Ostseld, Manager

Cypress Court caters to residents who value their freedom and independence, yet need an occasional helping hand. Here you'll find all the comforts of home designed expressly to meet the needs and interests of independent seniors.

6219 Emeritus at Alhambra
Emeritus Senior Living
3131 Elliott Avenue
Suite 500
Seattle, WA 98121
206-298-2909
Fax: 626-570-5254; *Toll Free:* 800-429-4828
www.emeritus.com

Residents receive assistance as needed with medication management and the activities of daily living.

6220 Emeritus at Garden Manor
Emeritus Senior Living
3131 Elliott Avenue
Suite 500
Seattle, WA 98121
206-298-2909
Fax: 714-636-0978; *Toll Free:* 800-429-4828
www.emeritus.com

Monica Negrete, Manager

We are passionately commited to providing care and services of the highest quality and value in a safe, supportive, residential environment, promoting the health, independence and social interaction of seniors.

6221 Emeritus at Orange
Emeritus Senior Living
3131 Elliott Avenue
Suite 500
Seattle, WA 98121
206-298-2909
Fax: 714-639-0833; *Toll Free:* 800-429-4828
www.emeritus.com
Berneice Holmes, Administrator

Private and semi-private apartments complement the homey atmosphere of the beautifully decorated common areas. Residents of Summerville at Orange enjoy three delicious meals a day, snacks, social activities and easy access to medical care. For those needing an extra hand, Summerville's assisted living program offers help with bathing, dressing, grooming and other activities of daily living.

6222 Emeritus at Valley View
Emeritus Senior Living
3131 Elliott Avenue
Suite 500
Seattle, WA 98121
206-298-2909
Fax: 714-891-3052; *Toll Free:* 800-429-4828
www.emeritus.com
Lori Loucks, Executive Director

We are committed to providing care and services of the highest quality and value in a safe supportive, residential enviroment, promoting the health, independence and social interaction of seniors.

6223 Emeritus at Victorian Court
Emeritus Senior Living
3131 Elliott Avenue
Suite 500
Seattle, WA 98121
206-298-2909
Fax: 909-391-8587; *Toll Free:* 800-429-4828
www.emeritus.com
Kim Weidman, Executive Director

Should you ever need extra support, we're a fully licensed assisted living community, so we can give you personalized services.

6224 Emeritus at Villa De Anza
Emeritus Senior Living
3131 Elliott Avenue
Suite 500
Seattle, WA 98121
206-298-2909
Fax: 909-685-8453; *Toll Free:* 800-429-4828
www.emeritus.com
Lori McCracken, Executive Director

In addition to numerous social activities, residents of Emeritus at Villa de Anza benefit from easy access to shopping, movie theatres and golf courses. Each private apartment features high ceilings and air conditioning. For those needing extra care, Summerville's assisted living program offers help with bathing, dressing, grooming and other activities of daily living.

6225 Eskaton Cameron Park Lodge
Eskaton Administrative Center
5105 Manznita Avenue
Carmichael, CA 95608
916-334-0810
Fax: 530-672-0390
Info@eskaton.org
www.eskaton.org
Todd Murch, President & Chief Executive Offi
Bill Pace, Chief Financial Officer
Besty Donovan, Chief Operating Officer

Our philosophy is to blend up-to-the-minute health technology with a home-like environment to enhance the independence and quality of life for each resident in the comfort of his or her own home.

Year Founded: 1968

6226 Eskaton Gold River Lodge
Eskaton Administrative Center
5105 Manznita Avenue
Carmichael, CA 95608
916-334-0810
Info@eskaton.org
www.eskaton.org
Todd Murch, President & Chief Executive Offi
Bill Pace, Chief Financial Officer
Besty Donovan, Chief Operating Officer

We blend up-to-the-minute health technology with a home-like environment to enhance the independence and quality of life of each resident in the comfort of his or her own home. Our community includes cozy touches like fireplaces and warm-water spas. Each resident room is personally identified with a customized shadow box just outside his or her door. Our grounds are carefully manicured and feature walkways and courtyards.

Year Founded: 1968

6227 Fairwinds-Ivey Ranch
Leisure Care, LLC
1601 Fifth Avenue
Suite 1900
Seattle, WA 98101
206-436-7827
Fax: 206-436-7705; *Toll Free:* 800-327-3490
www.leisurecare.com
Dan Madsen, Chief Executive Officer

Our community's inviting atmosphere is complemented by regularly scheduled social and recreational activities designed to fit a variety of lifestyles. Residents are free to enjoy life at their pace, participating in activities, or spending time with a friend. Peace of mind can also be enjoyed knowing that our staff is available 24 hours a day to answer questions and that every apartment is equipped with an emergency communication system.

Year Founded: 1976

6228 Fairwinds-West Hills
Leisure Care, LLC
1601 Fifth Avenue
Suite 1900
Seattle, WA 98101
206-436-7827
Fax: 206-436-7705; *Toll Free:* 800-327-3490
www.leisurecare.com

Dan Madsen, Chief Executive Officer
Patricia Luc, General Manager
Rick Waugh, Contact

Offers luxurious studio, one-and two-bedroom apartment homes in a fun and active retirement community.

Year Founded: 1976

6229 Fairwinds-Woodward Park
Leisure Care, LLC
1601 Fifth Avenue
Suite 1900
Seattle, WA 98101
206-436-7827
Fax: 206-436-7705; *Toll Free:* 800-327-3490
www.leisurecare.com

Dan Madsen, Chief Executive Officer

Offers luxurious studio, one-and two-bedroom apartment homes in a fun and active retirement community.

Year Founded: 1976

6230 Fountaingrove Lodge
Ageis Living
4210 Thomas Lake Harris Drive
Santa Rosa, CA 95403
707-584-6595
Fax: 707-756-1121; *Toll Free:* 866-688-5829
www.aegisliving.com

Dwayne Clark, Chairman and CEO
David Ford, Vice Chairman
Jerry Meyer, President and Chief Operating Of

The Lodge is the nation's first lesbian, gay, bisexual and transgendered independent senior community with the option of continuing care services.

6231 Fountains at Sea Bluffs
Watermark Retirement Communities
25411 Sea Bluffs Drive
Dana Point, CA 92629
949-443-9543
Fax: 949-443-0290; *Toll Free:* 800-846-4440
www.watermarkcommunities.com

David Freshwater, Chairman
David Barnes, President
Rick Kamminga, Chief Operating Officer

Emphasize proactive wellness through prevention, education and socialization.

6232 Garden of Palms
Garden of Palms
1025 N Fairfax Avenue
Los Angeles, CA 90046
323-656-7900
Fax: 323-656-9321
info@gardenofpams.com
www.gardenofpalms.com

Murielle Chocron, Executive Director
Susan Glaser, Regional Director

Every aspect of living at Garden of Palms has been planned to ensure maximum enjoyment and comfort - nurturing the spirit, emotional and physical well being of our residents while providing support to their families. Our residents with Alzheimer's live in The Gardens where they benefit from a specially designed program for individuals with memory loss.

6233 Gardens at Hillsborough Village
Brookdale-Senior Living Solutions
11918 Central Avenue
Chino, CA 91710-1914
866-785-9025Toll free: 855-444-7658
info@brookdaleliving.com
www.brookdaleliving.com

Mark Ohlendorf, Co-President
John P. Rijos, Co-President
W.E. Sheriff, Chief Executive Officer

Daily activities which encourage and promote socialization, independence and dignity.

6234 Gardens at Park Balboa
The Garden at Park Balboa
7046 Kester Avenue
Van Nuys, CA 91405
818-787-0462
Fax: 818-787-7472
info@parkbalboa.com
www.parkbalboa.com

Garrett Loube, President
Maru Cohen, Executive Director
W.E. Sheriff, Chief Executive Officer

In addition to independent living, we offer our residents assisted living services and Safe Haven, a secure environment for those facing Alzheimer's Disease and dementia.

6235 Gardens of Santa Monica
Brookdale-Senior Living Solutions
851 Second Street
Santa Monica, CA 90403
866-785-9025
Fax: 310-394-5002; *Toll Free:* 855-444-7658
info@brookdaleliving.com
www.brookdaleliving.com

Gary Lachs, Director of Marketing

The Gardens of Santa Monica (formerly Pacific Gardens) is the perfect place to enjoy the best in retirement living, offering Independent and Assisted Living tailored to suit your unique needs. Located a few blocks from beaches, restaurants, the Santa Monica Pier and the Promenade. The Gardens provides an exceptional retirement lifestyle.

6236 Gardens of Tarzana
Brookdale-Senior Living Solutions
18700 Burbank Boulevard
Tarzana, CA 91356-3367
866-785-9025
Fax: 818-342-0298; *Toll Free:* 855-444-7658
info@brookdaleliving.com
www.brookdaleliving

Sarah S Laloyan, Executive Director

California senior living in a beautiful setting with lush grounds.

6237 Grossmont Gardens
ActivCare Living
9619 Chesapeake Drive
Suite 103
San Diego, CA 92123
858-565-4424
Fax: 619-461-7736
activcareliving.com

W. MAJOR CHANCE, Founder/Chief Executive Officer
B. RENEE BARNARD, President/Chief Financial Office
D. KEVIN MORIARTY, Vice President of Development

Grossmont Gardens offers a retirement lifestyle on a nine-acre garden community that will inspire you to enjoy the various daily activities. You will also feel assured knowing that there is qualified, professional staff on campus to provide multilevel health care services.

Year Founded: 1988

6238 Heritage Estates
Heritage Estates
900 E Stanley Blvd
Livermore, CA 94550
925-373-3636
www.HeritageEstatesRetirement.com

Offers luxurious apartment homes in a fun and active retirement community.

6239 Heritage Estates Senior Apartments
Leisure Care, LLC
1601 Fifth Avenue
Suite 1900
Seattle, WA 98101
206-436-7827
Fax: 206-436-7705; Toll Free: 800-327-3490
www.leisurecare.com

Dan Madsen, Chief Executive Officer

Offers luxurious apartment homes in a fun and active retirement community.

Year Founded: 1976

6240 Heritage Pointe
Heritage Pointe Drive
27356 Bellogente
RR1 DeWinton
Alberta, CA 92691-6341
403-256-9192
Fax: 403-256-4494
inform@heritagepointe.com
www.heritagepointe.com

Carol Oxtoby, President &CEO
Alexis Johnston, Director of Finance and Administ
E. H. (Ted) Stack, Vice President Land Development

A non-profit, 200-resident community providing independent, assisted and memory care services for the elderly, while incorporating Jewish traditions and lifestyles.

6241 Hollenbeck Palms
Hollenbeck Palms
573 S Boyle Avenue
Los Angeles, CA 90033-3897
323-263-6195
Fax: 323-264-6955
holpalms@aol.com
www.hollenbeckpalms.com

William G Heideman, President & CEO
Morris Shockley, Vice President & Treasurer
Camile Goldsmith, RN, MN, Director of Nursing

To accommodate our members' changing needs, three levels of continuing care are available: Independent Residential Living, Assisted Residential Living and Skilled Nursing Care. Transition from one level of care to another may be temporary or longer term. The goal of our entire staff is to

ensure that our members lives as independently and comfortably as possibly.

6242 Integrated Care Communities
Integrated Care Communities
14315 Nason Street
Moreno Valley, CA 92555
951-247-6115
Fax: 951- 24- 561; Toll Free: 866-391-8742
lrodriguez@icare.bz
www.icarecommunities.com

Carl Rowe, Executive Director
Phillip Saucedo, President & CFO
Meghan O'Connor, Administrator

Guests include high care, frail-elderly and those suffering from memory impairment, Alzheimer's and related dementias.

6243 Las Villas De Carlsbad
ELMCROFT Senior Living Communities
9510 Ormsby Station Road
Louisville, KY 40223
502-753-6000
Fax: 502-753-6100
www.elmcroft.com

Rudy Littlefield, Administrator

Las Villas de Carlsbad is a multi-level retirement community that offers independent residential living apartments catering to active seniors who desire the comfort of home. Residential assisted living is available for those who may require additional services in the privacy of their own apartment. The Health Center is available for those who require more care featuring 24-hour nursing care.

6244 Las Villas Del Norte
ActivCare Living
9619 Chesapeake Drive
Suite 103
San Diego, CA 92123
858-565-4424
Fax: 760-741-0221
www.activcareliving.com

W. MAJOR CHANCE, Founder/Chief Executive Officer
B. RENEE BARNARD, President/Chief Financial Office
D. KEVIN MORIARTY, Vice President of Development

As a resident of Las Villas del Norte, you'll enjoy an active lifestyle, comfortable apartment living and the shared pride of living in a community of caring neighbors and staff members. You'll also feel secure knowing that optional health care services are available, should the need arise.

Year Founded: 1988

6245 Linda Valley Care Center
An Assisted Living Community
990 East Del Mar Boulevard
Pasadena, CA 91106
707-687-1919
Fax: 707-687-1912
amy.c@chancellorhealthcare.com
www.chancellorhealthcare.com

We develop and manage long term care communities which include high-quality housing, support services, and skilled nursing care.

Year Founded: 1992

6246 Linda Valley Villa
An Assisted Living Community
990 East Del Mar Boulevard
Pasadena, CA 91106
707-687-1919
Fax: 707-687-1912
amy.c@chancellorhealthcare.com
www.chancellorhealthcare.com

An independent living community in Loma Linda.

Year Founded: 1992

6247 Newport Beach Plaza
Leisure Care, LLC
1601 Fifth Avenue
Suite 1900
Seattle, WA 98101
206-436-7827
Fax: 206-436-7705; *Toll Free:* 800-327-3490
www.leisurecare.com

Dan Madsen, Chief Executive Officer

Offers luxurious apartment homes in a fun and active retirement community.

Year Founded: 1976

6248 O'Connor Woods
O'Connor Woods
3400 Wagner Heights Road
Stockton, CA 95209-4843
209-956-3400
Fax: 209-952-6201; *Toll Free:* 800-249-6637
info@oconnorwoods.org
www.oconnorwoods.org

Scot Sinclair, Executive Director
Eric Sholty, Associate Executive Director
Marcia Fitzgerald, Senior Administrator

0'Connor Woods is a multi-level retirement community designed for active seniors. O'Connor Woods offers residents the services and amenities to match their personal interests.

6249 Palo Alto Commons
Palo Alto Commons
4075 El Camino Way
Palo Alto, CA 94306-4005
650-494-0760
Fax: 650-494-0942
marketing@paloaltocommons.com
www.paloaltocommons.com

Mary Lou Marshall, Marketing Director
Joyce Chang

A unique concept in senior living offering personalized care in a gracious residential setting, located in Northern California. It's where our lovely home-like environment, cozy private apartments and supportive personal care services provide a positive and affordable alternative.

6250 Rehman Retirement Resorts-Poway
Gate Manor Poway
13110 Gate Drive
Poway, CA 92064-5126
619-928-4026
Fax: 858-780-0222
StephanieStephens619@gmail.com
www.gatemanorpoway.com

Jamal Khalid, CEO

Offers seniors quality residential health care facilities.

6251 Renaissance at the Gables
RENAISSANCE AT THE GABLES
2340 SW 32nd Avenue
Miami, FL 33145
305-445-1313
Fax: 626-303-8655
info@renaissancemiami.com
renaissancemiami.com

C.C. Da Silva, Executive Director

In addition to independent living, we are proud to offer residents our Heritage Personal Care Program. Heritage is designed for those who require additional care to meet their daily living needs.

6252 Rio Las Palmas
Rio Las Palmas
877 E March Lane
Stockton, CA 95207-5800
209-957-4711
Fax: 209-957-1407
www.riolaspalmasretirement.com

Sam Ogden, Manager

With a three story lobby waterfall, independent senior living and assisted living apartments offer an exciting array of social activities for active seniors.

6253 San Clemente Villas by the Sea
San Clemente Villas
660 Camino De Los Mares
San Clemente, CA 92673-1800
949-489-3400
Fax: 949-234-0081
www.sanclementevillas.com

Aileen Brazeau, Owner

Free to spend quality time with family and friends. Providing a full social calendar of culturally enriching social activities, special events, physical fitness in our Fitness room and swimming in our beautifully designed pool and Jacuzzi, arts and crafts and socializing with friendly neighbors and caring staff.

6254 Springfield Place
Leisure Care, LLC
1601 Fifth Avenue
Suite 1900
Seattle, WA 98101
206-436-7827
Fax: 206-436-7705; *Toll Free:* 800-327-3490
www.leisurecare.com

Dan Madsen, Chief Executive Officer

Our Assisted Living staff provides personalized services to those who may need special care and support with their daily activities of living.

Year Founded: 1976

6255 St. Paul's Senior Homes & Services
ST. Paul's Senior Homes & Services
328 Maple Street
San Diego, CA 92103
619-232-2996
Fax: 619-239-1256
www.stpaulseniors.org

Justin Weber, Director of Marketing & PR

St. Paul's Senior Homes & Services is a full-service, non-profit retirement community with independent assisted living and skilled nursing communities as well as an intergenerational day care program ans Program of All-Inclusive Care for the Elderly (PACE). St. Paul's provides affordable and comprehensive programs in a non-denominational environment with great value placed on optimal independence at all stages of life.

6256 St. Regis
St. Regis
23950 Mission Boulevard
Hayward, CA 94544-1052
510-881-7888
Fax: 510-582-0812
stregiscenter@aol.com
www.starwoodhotels.com

Shabbir Chinikamwala, Administrator

Full service assisted living residence, centrally located in Hayward on 5 acres with a park like setting. Independent living for dementia care.

6257 Sunny View Manor
Sunny View Retirement Community
22445 Cupertino Road
Cupertino, CA 95014-1097
408-454-5600
Fax: 408-255-6015
tbowman@frontporch.net
www.sunny-view.org

Tim Bowman, Contact

Our special care unit is designed exclusively for individuals with Alzhimer's disease or with related memory impairment disorders.

Year Founded: 1964

6258 Sunrise at Yorba Linda
Sunrise Senior Living, LLC
7900 Westpark Drive
Suite T-900
McLean, VA 22102
703-273-7500
Fax: 703-744-1601
www.sunriseseniorliving.com

Penny McIntyre, Chief Executive Officer
Marc Richards, Chief Financial Officer
Chris Winkle, Chief Operating Officer

To champion quality of life for all seniors.

Year Founded: 1981

6259 Sunshine Care Mountain Vistas
Sunshine Care
12695 Monte Vista Road
Poway, CA 92064-2524
858-674-1255
Fax: 858-674-1282; *Toll Free:* 800-811-9595
info@sunshinecare.com
www.suneshincare.com

Adrienne Lake French, Director Community Relations

Offers one-on-one individual care. Bright, airy rooms and individualized care programs by our specially trained staff, cater to our residents.

Year Founded: 1990

6260 Trinity House
Retirement Housing Foundation
2701 Capitol Avenue
Sacramento, CA 95816
916-446-4806
Fax: 916-446-9947
www.rhf.org

Rev. Dr. Joh Trnka, Chairman
Christina E. Potter, Vice Chairman
Rev. Dr. Lav Joseph, President & CEO

Provides housing and services for older adults including persons with various disabilities and low-income families.

6261 Villa Capri at Varenna
Oakmont Senior Living
220 Concourse Blvd
Santa Rosa, CA 95403
707-535-3200
Fax: 707-526-9099
Chris.Kasulka@oakmontmg.com
www.oakmontseniorliving.com

William P. Gallaher, Founder
Sam Faye, Executive Director

Provides care, but more importantly they provide respect and friendship.

Year Founded: 1997

6262 Villa Santa Barbara
Capital Senior Living
14160 Dallas Pkwy
Suite 300
Dallas, TX 75254
972-770-5600
Fax: 972-770-5666; *Toll Free:* 800-635-1232
www.capitalsenior.com

Larry Cohen, Chief Executive Officer
Keith Johannessen, President and Chief Operating Of
Ralph Beattie, Executive Vice President and Chi

Provides quality housing and services to enrich the daily lives of our senior residents by providing an environment that stimulates them physically, mentally, and emotionally.

Year Founded: 1990

Colorado

6263 Anam Chara Homes
Anam Chara
1795 Quince Avenue
Boulder, CO 80304
303-442-4484
home@anamchara.org
www.anamchara.org

Anam Chara operates two homes for elders who are unable to live alone. The homes are in residential neighborhoods, and the focus is on family and community. The approach to care is holistic, with self-reliance being held as long as possible.

6264 Argyle Square
The Argyle-Affordable Assisted Living in Denver
4115 West 38th Street
Denver, CO 80212

303-455-9513
Fax: 303-433-7127
www.TheArgyle.org

Janis Mueller, Executive Director
Heather Adair, Assistant Executive Director
Tracy Stutsman, Director of Activities

The Argyle Square provides delightful apartment-style living for the individual who needs some assistance, but does not require ongoing medical care. Our facility has 109 studio apartments.

Year Founded: 1874

6265 Atria Inn at Lakewood
ATRIA SENIOR LIVING, INC.
555 South Pierce Street
Lakewood, CO 80226-3470
303-742-4800
www.atriaassistedliving.com

We are dedicated to being the senior living community of choice where residents have all the conveniences and comforts of home, and the right amount of assistance with activities of daily living.

6266 Beatrice Hover Assisted Living
Hover Community Inc
1401 Elmhurst Drive
Longmont, CO 80503
303-772-9292
Fax: 303-772-4016
hover@hovercommunity.org
www.hovercommunity.org

Bob Roggow, Chairman
Larry Schluntz, Vice Chairman
Liza Czolowski, Executive Director

Dedicated to providing retirement living with dignity in every aspect of life. The private suites in the Beatrice Hover Assisted Living Residence vary in size, floor plan and monthly rates. All are combination living room/bedroom suites with full private baths.

6267 Broadmoor Court
Bethesda Adult Community
2045 Roanoke Street
Colorado Springs, CO 80906
719-471-2285
www.bethesdaadultcommunities.com

Cindy Batey, Executive Director

Broadmoor Court is an assisted-living community with a wide variety of services, which makes this community an easy choice for those who need the added advantages of assisted living.

6268 Collinwood
Bethesda Adult Community
5055 South Lemay Avenue
Fort Collins, CO
970-223-3552
www.bethesdaadultcommunities.com

Kristen Jacoby, Executive Director

Provides both independent and assisted living services. Collinwood offers six apartment styles to choose from for a total of 87 units.

6269 Emeritus at Highline
Emeritus Senior Living
3131 Elliott Avenue
Suite 500
Seattle, WA 98121
206-298-2909
Fax: 714-636-0978; *Toll Free:* 800-429-4828
www.emeritus.com

Promises to become an extended family to the seniors entrusted in our care and to our residents who have chosen independent retirement living.

6270 Golden Pond
Golden Pond Retirement Community
1270 North Ford Street
Golden, CO 80403
303-271-0430
Fax: 303-278-0623
info@goldenpondliving.com
www.goldenpondliving.com

Karen Jenkins, Executive Director
Dan Whittle, Assistant Executive Director
Nancy Wyatt, Health Services Director, LPN

The goal is to ensure and preserve each resident's privacy, dignity, independence and well-being.

6271 Grand Villa
Bethesda Adult Community
2680 North 15th Street
Grand Junction, CO 81506
970-241-9706
gvinfo@ba.org
www.bethesdaadultcommunities.com

Judith Shue, Executive Director

An assisted living community of 45 apartment units in two styles. The assisted living community is dedicated to promoting independence and nuturing each resident by offering many features and services.

6272 Granville Assisted Living Center
The Granville Assisted Living Center
1325 Vance Street
Lakewood, CO 80214
303-274-4400
Fax: 303-274-4100
info@thegranvilleassisted.com
www.thegranvilleassisted.com

Sara Tatlor, Executive Director
Joe Whitney, Director of Resident Services
Lesley Brown, Medication Coordinator

The Granville Assisted Living Center provides a residential setting for elderly individuals and couples who need supportive services to maintain their independence.

6273 Harvard Square
Leisure Care, LLC
1601 Fifth Avenue
Suite 1900
Seattle, WA 98101
206-436-7827
Fax: 206-436-7705; *Toll Free:* 800-327-3490
www.leisurecare.com

Dan Madsen, Chief Executive Officer

Offers apartment homes in a fun and active retirement community.

Year Founded: 1976

6274 MacKenzie Place: Colorado Springs
Leisure Care, LLC
1601 Fifth Avenue
Suite 1900
Seattle, WA 98101
206-436-7827
Fax: 206-436-7705; *Toll Free:* 800-327-3490
www.leisurecare.com

Dan Madsen, Chief Executive Officer

Retirement living community.

Year Founded: 1976

6275 MacKenzie Place: Fort Collins
Leisure Care, LLC
1601 Fifth Avenue
Suite 1900
Seattle, WA 98101
206-436-7827
Fax: 206-436-7705; *Toll Free:* 800-327-3490
www.leisurecare.com

Dan Madsen, Chief Executive Officer

Retirement living community.

Year Founded: 1976

6276 Nightingale Suites at Springwood
SpringWood Retirement
6550 Yank Way
Arvada, CO 80004-2298
303-424-6550
Fax: 303-778-0299
www.SpringwoodRetirement.com

Pat Gallinger, Executive Director
Susan Walker, Marketing Director
Gene Guerink, Campus Social Director

The Suites are comfortable, with many built-in features.
Each opens onto a cheerful common area where residents
may gather to work on projects, talk and develop friendships. Residents can also take advantage of the award-winning food services along with an excellent activity
program.

Year Founded: 1986

6277 Sterling House of Arvada
Brookdale-Senior Living Solutions
851 Second Street
Santa Monica, CA 90403
866-785-9025
Fax: 310-394-5002; *Toll Free:* 855-444-7658
info@brookdaleliving.com
www.brookdaleliving.com

Mark Schulte, Co-CEO
Mark W Ohlendorf, Co-President
John P Rijos, Co-President

Our assisted living programs and communities provide
housing, care and services to older adults who want to retain their independence while receiving daily support, but
don't require the skilled care provided in nursing homes.

6278 Sunrise of Boulder
Sunrise Senior Living, LLC
7900 Westpark Drive
Suite T-900
McLean, VA 22102
703-273-7500
Fax: 703-744-1601
www.sunriseseniorliving.com

Penny McIntyre, Chief Executive Officer
Marc Richards, Chief Financial Officer
Chris Winkle, Chief Operating Officer

Sunrise's assisted living options offer personalized assistance, supportive services and compassionate care in a professionally managed, carefully designed, community
setting. It's the perfect alternative for seniors who can no
longer live on their own at home, yet don't need 24-hour,
complex medical supervision.

Year Founded: 1981

6279 View Pointe
Bethesda Adult Community
555 South Rockrimmon Boulevard
Colorado Springs, CO 80919
719-528-8000
www.bethesdaadultcommunities.com

Leslie Eldridge, Executive Director
Judith Teel, Health Services Director

Provides both independent and assisted living services.
View Pointe offers 21 assisted living apartments.

6280 Winslow Court
Leisure Care, LLC
1601 Fifth Avenue
Suite 1900
Seattle, WA 98101
206-436-7827
Fax: 206-436-7705; *Toll Free:* 800-327-3490
disner@stellarliving.com
www.leisurecare.com

Dan Madsen, Chief Executive Officer

Offers comfortable studio, and one-and tow-bedroom apartment homes in a fun and active retirement community.

Year Founded: 1976

Connecticut

6281 Academy Point at Mystic
Academy Point at Mystic
20 Academy Lane
Mystic, CT 06355-2557
860-245-8915
Fax: 860-536-2245
www.academypointatmystic.com

Bollie Pollard Johnson, Executive Director

Academy Point at Mystic offers senior families the rental
of an apartment, personal care services, 3 meals served
daily in an elegant dining room, housekeeping and linen
service and security in a homelike environment.

6282 Arbors at Hop Brook
Arbors of Hop Brook Retirement Community
403 W Center Street
Manchester, CT 06040-4700

860-647-9343
www.arborsct.com

Chante Drasdis, Director
Paul T Lisstro, Manager
Suzanne Sorensen, Retirement Counselor

Arbors offers a stress free lifestyle with security, companionship, services and access to long term and rehabilitative health care.

Year Founded: 1988

6283 Arden Courts Alzheimer's Assisted Living
Arden Courts
45 South Road
Farmington, CT 06032-2022
860-677-4060
Fax: 860-677-2795; *Toll Free:* 888-478-2410
www.arden-courts.com/

Ron Bowen, Executive Director

Provides a safe and pleasing home for individuals with memory loss including individuals diagnosed with Alzheimer's disease.

6284 Atria Crossroads Place
ATRIA SENIOR LIVING, INC.
1 Beechwood Drive
Waterford, CT 06385-2831
860-444-6700
Fax: 860-443-6880
www.atriaseniorliving.com

Kathy Ryan, Executive Director

Offers elegant rental apartments, personal care assistance, and a full continuum of care should health needs change, including a special, secure memory impaired neighborhood.

6285 Atria at Stratford
ATRIA SENIOR LIVING, INC.
6911 Main Street
Stratford, CT 06614-1360
203-380-0006
Fax: 203-380-0007
www.atriaseniorliving.com

David Vail, Executive Director

At Atria Stratford we encourage each and every resident to take the time to do the things they enjoy. And if that requires a little extra assistance at times, then we're always there to help. Because the safety of our residents and the peace of mind of their family members come first and foremost at Atria.

6286 Crescent Point at Niantic
Crescent Point
417 Main Street
Niantic, CT 06357
860-451-9094
www.crescentpointatniantic.com

Offers exceptional assisted living services in a residential living environment. Crescent Point captures the spirit of village convenience and accessibility.

6287 Curtis Home
The Curtis Home
380 Crown Street
Meriden, CT 06450-6497

203-237-4338
Fax: 203-630-1127
info@thecurtishome.org
www.thecurtishome.org

Paul Sprague, Executive Director

Provides specialized care for the elderly of Greater Meriden, Wallingford, Cheshire, and all of Connecticut.

Year Founded: 1884

6288 Edgehill Health Center
Edgehill
122 Palmers Hill Road
Stamford, CT 06902-2134
203-323-2323
Fax: 203-323-6437; *Toll Free:* 800-721-8068
www.edgehillcommunity.com/

Robert Newcomer, Administrator

6289 Elim Park Baptist Home
Elim Park
140 Cook Hill Road
Cheshire, CT 06410
203-272-3547
Fax: 203-271-7753
elimpark.org/

Pauline Pavasaris Parrish, Director of Marketing
Sarah Ranchinsky, Marketing & Admissions Coordinat
Nicole Caccomo, Marketing & Admissions Coordinat

6290 Emeritus at Litchfield Hills
Emeritus Senior Living
3131 Elliott Avenue
Suite 500
Seattle, WA 98121
206-298-2909
Fax: 714-636-0978; *Toll Free:* 800-429-4828
litchfieldhills-crd@emeritus.com
www.emeritus.com

Beth Prevo, Community Relations Director

Assisted living and memory care community.

6291 Emeritus at Rocky Hill
Emeritus Senior Living
3131 Elliott Avenue
Suite 500
Seattle, WA 98121
206-298-2909
Fax: 714-636-0978; *Toll Free:* 800-429-4828
www.emeritus.com

Promises to become extended family to the seniors entrusted in their care. Offers retirement living, assisted living, Alzheimer's and memory care, short stay/respite care, and on-site rehabilitation.

6292 Essex Meadows
Essex Meadows
30 Bokum Road
Essex, CT 06426-1509
860-767-7201
Fax: 860-767-0014; *Toll Free:* 888-377-3972
hinesk@essexmeadows.com
www.essexmeadows.com

Jennifer Rannestad, Administrator

Our large selection of 188 apartment homes gives you choices about the way you will reflect your individuality and sense of style. The services and amenities have been chosen to serve your needs and desires: first-class dining, numerous and varied activities, meticulous housekeeping, 24-hour security, health care, and maintenance of grounds and buildings.

Year Founded: 1971

6293 Evergreen Woods
Evergreen Woods
88 Notch Hill Road
N Branford, CT 06471-1846
203-488-8000
Fax: 203-488-9429
info@evergreenwoods.com
www.evergreenwoods.com

Jeannie Kinnard, Administrator

Our finely crafted lifestyle is a perfect balance of privacy and hospitality, freedom and security. It expertly comple-ments who you are and the way you live. More importantly, our lifestyle inspires you to be yourself.

6294 Gables at Farmington
Brookdale-Senior Living Solutions
851 Second Street
Santa Monica, CA 90403
866-785-9025
Fax: 310-394-5002; *Toll Free:* 855-444-7658
info@brookdaleliving.com
www.brookdaleliving.com

Mark Schulte, Co-CEO
Mark W Ohlendorf, Co-President
John P Rijos, Co-President

Whether you're ready to simplify your life, eliminate the daily demands of home ownership or simply need a little assistance with day-to-day activities, The Gables at Farmington is the perfect solution.

6295 Greens at the Greenwich
The Greens at Greenwich
1155 King Street
Greenwich, CT 06831-3246
203-531-5500
Fax: 203-531-1224
info@thegreensatgreenwich.com
www.thegreensatgreenwich.com

Sherry Dey, Executive Director

6296 Heights at Avery Heights
Avery Heights
705 New Britain Avenue
Hartford, CT 06106-4039
860-527-9126
Fax: 860-525-2090; *Toll Free:* 860-953-1201
mmiller@churchhomes.org
www.AveryHeights.org

Mary C Miller, Director Admissions/Marketing
Patrick Gilland, CEO

Offering a full continuum of care, seniors at lifestyle options for older adults including Independent and assisted living; subacute care, comprehensive medical care and rehabilita-tion for seniors.

6297 Laurel Gardens at Milford
Laurel Gardens
334 Kennett Pike
Chadds Ford, PY 19317
610-388-4100
Fax: 610-388-4103; *Toll Free:* 800-758-7685
info@jacksbistrode.com
www.laurel-gardens.com

Bonnie Pollard, Executive Director

Offer elegant rental apartments, personal care assistance, and a full continuum of care should health needs change over time.

Year Founded: 1966

6298 Laurel Gardens of Avon
Laurel Gardens
334 Kennett Pike
Chadds Ford, PY 19317
610-388-4100
Fax: 610-388-4103; *Toll Free:* 800-758-7685
info@jacksbistrode.com
www.laurel-gardens.com

Jennie Eisenhaure, Executive Director

Elegant rental apartments, personal care assistance, and a full continuum of care should health needs change, includ-ing a special, secure memory impaired neighborhood.

Year Founded: 1966

6299 Maple Woods at Hamden Benchmark Assisted Living
Benchmark Senior Living
40 William Street
Suite #350
Wellesley, MA 02481
781-489-7100
Fax: 781-489-7200
www.benchmarkseniorliving.com

Greg Jimmie, Executive Director
Tawana Joyner, Community Relations Director

Offer elegant rental apartments, personal care assistance, and a full continuum of care shoudl health needs change over time.

6300 Miller Memorial Community
360 Broad Street
Meriden, CT 06450
203-237-8815
Fax: 203-630-3714
www.millercommunity.org

Cindy Hamel, Director Marketing
Nancy Luddy, Director Admissions
Brandon Munson, Administrator

Year Founded: 1976

6301 Mulberry Gardens of Southington
Mulberry Gardens of Southington
58 Mulberry Street
Plantsville, CT 06479-1704
860-276-1020
Fax: 860-378-1024
terzakm@mulberrygardens.org
www.mulberrygardens.org

Perry Phillips, Executive Director
Marie Terzak, Retirement Counselor

Offers supportive living environments as well as specialized care for those with early memory loss.

6302 Orchards at Southington
The Orchards at Southington
34 Hobart Street
Southington, CT 06489-3322
860-628-5656
Fax: 860-628-5311; *Toll Free:* 888-340-2775
www.southingtonorchards.org/

Audrey Vinci, Executive Director

The Orchards at Southington offers a service-rich environment which allows seniors the freedom to do the things they enjoy most without all the worry of upkeep, security, or unexpected financial burdens of owning their own home. In addition, The Orchards offers residents and their families peace of mind in knowing that assisted living is available within the community should the need arise.

6303 Pomperaug Woods
Pomperaug Woods
80 Heritage Road
Southbury, CT 06488-3851
203-267-2835
Fax: 203-264-2155
www.pomperaugwoods.com

Nancy Hughan, Marketing Director
Kevin Moshier, Administrator

Continuing care retirement community.

6304 Shady Oaks Assisted Living
Shady Oaks Assisted Living
344 Stevens Street
Bristol, CT 06010-2769
860-583-1526
Fax: 860-583-1297
info@shadyoaksassistedliving.com
www.shadyoaksassistedliving.com/

Kay Belanger, Owner

6305 Spring Meadows at Trumbull
Capital Senior Living Corporation
6949 Main Street
Trumbull, CT 06611-6304
203-261-0006
Fax: 203-452-0549; *Toll Free:* 877-648-1989
www.capitalsenior.com/

Mindy Stollman, Manager

Today's seniors are bringing a new attitude to retirement living — they want to live where they can enjoy not just services and security but also independence, wellness, and lifelong opportunities for growth and learning. We are dedicated to helping our residents make the most out of retirement.

6306 Suffield by the River
Suffield by the River
7 Canal Road
Suffield, CT 06078-1970
860-668-6672
Fax: 860-668-4770
suffieldbytheriver.com/

Celia Moffie, Owner

6307 Sunrise Assisted Living of Stamford
Sunrise of Stamford
251 Turn of River Road
Stamford, CT 06905-1320
203-968-8393
Fax: 203-968-8348
www.sunriseseniorliving.com/

Jenifer Salamino, Executive Director

Sunrise is built on a commitment to our residents and their families. We believe no two people are alike, so the services and attention we provide should never be exactly the same. That's also why we offer a variety of lifestyle, service and care options. By providing these choices, we not only offer solutions for today, but we provide the security of knowing that there are options for tomorrow.

6308 Tower One/Tower East
Tower One/Tower East
18 Tower Lane
New Haven, CT 06519-1764
203-772-1816
Fax: 203-785-8280
info@towerone.org
www.towerone.org

Alan Siegal, Chairman
Bruce Spiewak, Vice Chairman
Mark Garilli, President/CEO

The mission of the Towers organization is to provide older persons of varying means with high quality living arrangements and services based upon Jewish values and traditions.

6309 Village at Brookfield Common
The Village at Brookfield Common
246a Federal Road
Brookfield, CT 06804-2652
203-885-7460
Fax: 203-775-1786
www.villageatbrookfieldcommon.com/

Diane Vaseturo, Executive Director

6310 Village at Buckland Court
The Village at Buckland Court
432 Buckland Road
South Windsor, CT 06074-3741
860-281-2498
Fax: 860-644-7360
www.villageatbucklandcourt.com/

Tom Sebula, Administrator

Our unique, maintenance-free catered living options allow you to pursue your interests, form lasting friendships and experience the retirement lifestyle of your dreams. Enjoy the peace of mind that comes from our full range of services supporting the health and wellness of all our residents.

6311 Village at East Farms
The Village at East Farms
180 Scott Road
Waterbury, CT 06705-3284
203-721-7998
Fax: 203-754-4331
www.villageateastfarms.com/

Perry Phillips, Manager

Our unique, maintenance-free catered living options allow you to pursue your interests, form lasting friendships and experience the retirement lifestyle of your dreams. Enjoy the peace of mind that comes from our full range of services supporting the health and wellness of all our residents.

6312 Village at South Farms
The Village at South Farms
645 Saybrook Road
Middletown, CT 06457-4746
860-342-8033
Fax: 860-346-6225
www.villageatsouthfarms.com/

Richard Damarjian, Administrator

Our unique, maintenance-free catered living options allow you to pursue your interests, form lasting friendships and experience the retirement lifestyle of your dreams. Enjoy the peace of mind that comes from our full range of services supporting the health and wellness of all our residents.

Delaware

6313 Elder Wood Village of Dover
Elderwood
21 N State Street
Dover, DE 19901-3802
302-674-2144
www.elderwood.com

Marijane Copes, Administrator

6314 Forwood Manor Assisted Living
Forwood Manor
1912 Marsh Road
Wilmington, DE 19810-3954
302-529-1600
Fax: 302-529-1250
www.forwoodmanorde.com/

Gail Deerdorff, Contact

6315 Foulk Manor North
Foulk Manor North
1212 Foulk Road
Wilmington, DE 19803-2797
302-478-4296
Fax: 302-478-2956
www.foulkmanornorth.com/

Virginia Grey, Executive Director

We pride ourselves in our ability to offer freedom of choice to our residents. Beginning with various apartment selections, and including fine dining and activities, all areas of our service and hospitality are delivered according to our residents' unique needs and preferences.

6316 Foulk Manor South
Foulk Manor South
407 Foulk Road
Wilmington, DE 19803-3899
302-655-6249
Fax: 302-655-5451
www.foulkmanorsouth.com/

Gregory Artis, Executive Director

We pride ourselves in our long-standing reputation for excellent care, as one of the friendliest retirement communities in North Wilmington. Our residents and their families especially appreciate our delicious meals, the cleanliness of our community and the creativity of our activity programming.

6317 Gardens at White Chapel
Emeritus at White Chapel
200 E Village Road
Newark, DE 19713-3845
302-352-2942
Fax: 302-368-5660
www.emeritus.com

Phillip Santoro, Executive Director

6318 Green Meadows at Dover
Emeritus at Dover
150 Saulsbury Road
Dover, DE 19904-2776
302-352-2943
Fax: 302-674-3341
www.emeritus.com

Marijames Copes, Contact
Donna Winegar, Executive Director

6319 Heritage at Milford
Genesis HealthCare
500 S Dupont Highway
Milford, DE 19963-1758
302-422-8700
Fax: 302-422-8744
www.genesishcc.com/

Doris Schonbrunner, MSM, NHA, Executive Director
Cathy Wetherill, Resident Care Director
Melissa Heverin, Guest Services Director

6320 Methodist Country House
ACTS Retirement-Life Communities
4830 Kennett Pike
Wilmington, DE 19807-1899
302-654-5101
Fax: 302-426-8108
www.actsretirement.org/

Donald L. Davis, CPA, Chairman
Thomas A. Dunn, III, Vice Chairman
H. Bruce Detweiler, CPA, Managing Director & President

Senior citizen retirement and long term care facility offering: food, medical care, skilled nursing, activities, & housekeeping.

Year Founded: 1972

6321 Millcroft Assisted Living
Millcroft
255 Possum Park Road
Newark, DE 19711-3877
302-366-0160
Fax: 302-366-7634
www.millcroftseniorliving.com/

Steve Rovner, Contact
Annie Cantylmagli, Executive Director

6322 Seaford Center Assisted Living
Genesis HealthCare
1100 Norman Eskridge Highway
Seaford, DE 19973-1724

302-629-3575
Fax: 302-629-0561
www.genesishcc.com/

Doris Schonbrunner, MSM, NHA, Executive Director
Cathy Wetherill, Resident Care Director
Melissa Heverin, Guest Services Director

6323 Shipley Manor Assisted Living
Shipley Manor
2723 Shipley Road
Wilmington, DE 19810-3251
302-479-0111
Fax: 302-479-5880
www.shipleymanorseniorliving.com/

Kathy Scott, Contact
Roger Connell, Executive Director

6324 Somerford House
Somerford House & Place Newark
501 S Harmony Road
Newark, DE 19713-3338
302-266-9255
Fax: 302-266-9250
www.somerfordplacenewark.com/

Joyce Medkeff, Executive Director

6325 Somerford Place
Somerford House & Place Newark
4175 Ogletown Road
Newark, DE 19713
302-283-0540
Fax: 302-283-0543
www.somerfordplacenewark.com/

6326 Westminster Village
Westminster Village in Dover
1175 McKee Road
Dover, DE 19904-2268
302-744-3600
Fax: 302-774-3540; *Toll Free:* 866-710-3101
kkerstetter@presbyterianseniorliving.org
www.wmvdover.org/

Robert Kratz, Executive Director

Florida

6327 Abbey Delray Health Center
Abbey Delray
2000 Lowson Boulevard
Delray Beach, FL 33445-6095
561-454-2000Toll free: 800-936-7397
info@AbbeyDelray.com
www.abbeydelray.com

Tim Smith, Owner

We've gone to great lengths to create a community that lets you take a permanent vacation from everyday worries. Living at Abbey Delray means giving up the worrisome responsibilities of maintaining a house. Instead you can spend more of your time the way you want. Socializing and pursuing the activities you enjoy. From housekeeping and maintenance services to scheduled transportation and delicious dining.

6328 Alderman Oaks Retirement Center
Alderman Oaks Retirement Residence, Inc.
727 Hudson Avenue
Sarasota, FL 34236-7785
941-955-9099
Fax: 941-316-7878
info@aldermanoaks.com
www.aldermanoaks.com

Rusty Blix, Administrator
Don Fitts, Director Of Marketing

Both residents and their family find it comforting to know that help, if needed, is only seconds away. Most of the time residents feel better because they eat regular, healthy, and delicious meals. Transportation often helps residents to be more active than they have been for years, and it's nice to have energy to do things you enjoy.

Year Founded: 1997

6329 Alterra Sterling House of Tavares
Pennsylvania - Alterra Sterling House of Tavares
2232 Dora Avenue
Tavares, FL 32778-5708
352-343-2500
Fax: 352-343-2971
shtavares@assisted.com
www.assisted.com/

Debbie Flaherty, Executive Director

6330 Aviva - A Campus for Senior Life
1951 N Honore Avenue
Sarasota, FL 34235-9117
941-225-9369
Fax: 941-377-1893
marketing@avivaseniorlife.org
www.avivaseniorlife.org

Jay Solomon, Chief Executive Officer
Jean Kramer, Chief Operating Officer
David Larson, Chief Financial Officer

Welcome to Aviva - A Campus for Senior Life, Sarasota's only rental senior community offering all levels of living. Live life to the fullest in our warm, intellectually stimulating environment which attracts educated and curious individuals. Aviva is the perfect blend of resort-style living, lifelong learning, and innovative health and wellness programs to engage the mind, body and spirit.

Year Founded: 1993

6331 Bahia Oaks Lodge
Brookdale-Senior Living Solutions
851 Second Street
Santa Monica, CA 90403
866-785-9025
Fax: 310-394-5002; *Toll Free:* 855-444-7658
info@brookdaleliving.com
www.brookdaleliving.com

Mark Schulte, Co-CEO
Mark W Ohlendorf, Co-President
John P Rijos, Co-President

6332 Bay Breeze Nursing & Retirement Center
Bay Breeze Nursing and Retirement Center
3387 Gulf Breeze Parkway
Gulf Breeze, FL 32563-3360

850-932-9257
Fax: 850-932-5989; *Toll Free:* 800-881-9905
www.gchc.com

Jamie Richardson, Administrator

6333 Bay Village of Sarasota
Bay Village of Sarasota
8400 Vamo Road
Sarasota, FL 34231-7807
941-966-5611
Fax: 941-966-4040
info@bayvillage.org
www.bayvillage.org

Jack McClelland, Administrator
Susan Richardson, Contact

Bay Village of Sarasota, Inc., is a not-for-profit, accredited continuing care retirement community, which offers its residents a gracious home and a full array of services for senior living. It combines elegance and security with continuing healthcare provided by its Health Care Clinic, Home Health Services, Assisted Living Facility, and Licensed Skilled Nursing Center.

6334 Bristol Park of Coral Springs
2975 NW 99th Way
Coral Springs, FL 33065-5084
954-255-5557
Fax: 954-255-6821
www.bristol-park.com

Sheryl James, Administrator
Terri D'Alessandro, Assistant Administrator
Carolynn Alongi, Marketing

Assisted Living.

6335 Clare Bridge of Bradenton: A Brookdale Senior Living Community
6101 Pointe West Boulevard
Bradenton, FL 34209-5534
866-276-2858
Fax: 941-795-8317; *Toll Free:* 877-400-5296
info@brookdaleliving.com
www.brookdaleliving.com

T. Andrew Smith, Chief Executive Officer
Mark W. Ohlendorf, Co-President and CFO
Gregory B. Richard, Chief Operating Officer

Memory care residence for those with cognitive loss or memory impairment.

6336 Clare Bridge of Leesburg
710 S Lake Street
Leesburg, FL 34748-7316
866-382-0867Toll free: 877-400-5296
info@brookdaleliving.com
www.brookdaleliving.com

T. Andrew Smith, Chief Executive Officer
Mark W. Ohlendorf, Co-President and CFO
Gregory B. Richard, Chief Operating Officer

6337 Clare Bridge of Tequesta
211 Village Boulevard
Tequesta, FL 33469-9321
866-832-5214Toll free: 877-400-5296
info@brookdaleliving.com
www.brookdaleliving.com

T. Andrew Smith, Chief Executive Officer
Mark W. Ohlendorf, Co-President and CFO
Gregory B. Richard, Chief Operating Officer

6338 Coral Landing Assisted Living Residences
2820 Old Moultrie Road
Saint Augustine, FL 32086-5454
904-794-2273
Fax: 904-794-2465
corallanding@seniorcaregroup.com
www.corallanding.com

Janet Pierce, Administrator

Located in a natural setting that feels like home where you get assistance with dignity and compassion. All the services and amenities you expect and deserve such as transportation to events and outings as well as indoor activities and intresting events.

6339 Coral Plaza Retirement Residence
5850 Margate Boulevard
Margate, FL 33063-7861
954-970-0053
Fax: 954-971-7961
www.mylivewell.org

Campbell Epes, Owner

6340 Court at Plam Aire
2701 N Course Drive
Pompano Beach, FL 33069-3089
954-975-8900
Fax: 954-975-8933
www.thecourtatpalmaire.com

Debbie Ormos, Administrator

6341 Crown Pointe of Sebring
5005 Sun N Lake Boulevard
Sebring, FL 33872-2175
863-386-1060
Fax: 863-386-4925
www.crownpointecommunities.com

Renee Marley, LPN, Executive Director

6342 Cypress Village
4600 Middleton Park Circle E
Jacksonville, FL 32224-6624
866-360-3923Toll free: 800-228-6163
info@brookdaleliving.com
www.brookdaleliving.com

T. Andrew Smith, Chief Executive Officer
Mark W. Ohlendorf, Co-President and CFO
Gregory B. Richard, Chief Operating Officer

The campus has a wide variety of living accommodations, ranging from single family homes or apartments to a health center with skilled nursing care and assisted living. Most importantly, however, it is a community that encourages residents to pursue all kinds of activities, so the lifestyle is anything but retiring. This is a retirement community designed for people 55 years of age or older.

6343 Donnelly Place-A Classic Residence by Hyatt
2792 Donnelly Drive
Lantana, FL 33462-6431
561-966-4600
Fax: 407-330-3941; *Toll Free:* 866-961-5314
www.viliving.com

Penny Smith, Executive Director
Craig Koff, Care Center Administrator
Barbara Kelley, Sales Director

Donnelly Place offers assisted living, memory support/Alzheimer's care and skilled nursing care with the Hyatt Touchr on the campus of the award-winning Lakeside Village life care community.

6344 East Ridge Retirement Village

19301 SW 87th Avenue
Cutler Bay
Miami, FL 33157-8984
305-256-3564
Fax: 305-256-3516; Toll Free: 800-605-7778
info@eastridgerc.com
www.eastridgeatcutlerbay.com

Ken Kremer, Executive Director

Our amenities and calendar of activities offer a wide variety of recreational, entertaining and educational opportunities. Conveniences such as a branch bank, sundries shop, beauty salon and barber shop, make it easier to accomplish the tasks and errands of everyday living.

6345 Emeritus @ Altamonte Springs

433 Orange Drive
Altamonte Springs, FL 32701-5377
407-287-6328
Fax: 407-260-0392
www.altamontespringsseniorliving.com

Vernon Campbell, Executive Director

6346 Epworth Village Retirement Community

5300 W 16th Avenue
Hialeah, FL 33012-2104
305-556-3500
Fax: 305-556-0887
israelmimi@epworthrc.com
www.epworthvillagerc.com

K C Cross, CEO

6347 Florida Living Center

3355 E Semoran Blvd
Apopka, FL 32703-6062
407-862-6263
Fax: 407-862-4188
www.floridalivingnursing.com

Jeannie De Prada, Administrator

6348 Forest Trace at Inverrary

5500 NW 69th Avenue
Lauderhill, FL 33319-7266
954-572-1800
Fax: 954-572-4752; Toll Free: 800-648-8060
www.foresttrace.com

Stanley R. Rosenthal, Owner's Representative
Elaine Grossinger Etess, Director of Hospitality

Forest Trace is a luxury, resort-style retirement community in Fort Lauderdale, Florida, providing full-service housing, assisted living, nursing home and lifestyle services to senior adults.

Year Founded: 1920

6349 Fountainview by Marriott

111 Executive Center Drive
West Palm Beach, FL 33401-4801

561-697-5500
Fax: 561-697-5897
www.fountainviewretirement.com

Carole Williams, Human Resources Executive

6350 Freedom Inn at Tarpon Springs

1651 S Pinellas Avenue
Tarpon Springs, FL 34689-1946
866-557-6378
Fax: 727-945-9219; Toll Free: 888-891-7207
rsmith@brookdaleliving.com
www.brookdaleliving.com

T. Andrew Smith, Chief Executive Officer
Mark W. Ohlendorf, Co-President and CFO
Gregory B. Richard, Chief Operating Officer

6351 Golden Cove Assisted Living Facility

918 Egan Drive
Orlando, FL 32822-6018
407-281-1886
Fax: 407-281-7176
goldencovealf.com

Yolette Precil, Owner

6352 Gulf Coast Village Assisted Living

1333 Santa Barbara Boulevard
Cape Coral, FL 33991-2803
239-772-1333
www.gulfcoastvillage.com

Richard Heath, Contact

Year Founded: 1999

6353 Gulf Coast Village Retirement Community

1333 Santa Barbara Boulevard
Cape Coral, FL 33991-2803
239-772-1333
www.gulfcoastvillage.com

Richard Heath, Executive VP

Gulf Coast Village is a retirement community built around the idea of living life to the fullest. We want you to spend your time enjoying life instead of worrying about all the little details. Here you'll have plenty of time to enjoy yourself, and you'll be able to keep your mind on what's important, because we take care of everything else.

Year Founded: 1999

6354 Hampton Manor Belleview

10590 SE 62nd Avenue Road
Belleview, FL 34420-3004
352-245-6201
Fax: 352-245-9188
www.hamptonmanor.net

Sandy Glidden, Executive Director
Monica Blood, Nurse Care Manager
Linda McSorley, Activities Coordinator

6355 Harbor Place at Port St Lucie

3700 SE Jennings Road
Port St Lucie, FL 34952-7778
888-649-3685
Fax: 772-398-8689
madeline_sottile@lcca.com
retirementresort.com

Sharon Wilford, Manager

6356 Henderson Village
125 S. Langston Circle Perry
Georgia, FL 31069
478-988-8696
Fax: 478-988-9009; *Toll Free:* 888-615-9722
www.hendersonvillage.com

Jose Gonzalez, General Manager
Alex Gonzalez, Executive Chef
Linda Keen, Executive Housekeeper

6357 Heritage Oaks Senior Housing
Tallahassee, FL 32309-2221
850-668-4004
Fax: 850-668-4426
info@heritageoaks.com
www.theallegro.com

Karen Pinney, Manager

Inspired senior living.

6358 Heron House
512 Simonton Street
Key West, FL 33040
305-294-9227
Fax: 941-955-7576; *Toll Free:* 800-294-1644
www.heronhouse.com

Robin Jones, Executive Director

Heron House is an assisted living community you will be proud to call home. Our unique approach to assisted living is simply better by design. Heron House was built to provide affordable luxury and quality care in an environment that was created specifically with you in mind. From your residence to the countless in-house amenities, you'll find that Heron House has included the details that make the difference.

6359 Homewood Residence at Boca Raton
9591 Yamato Road
Boca Raton, FL 33434-5549
866-439-6115
Fax: 561-477-1665; *Toll Free:* 877-259-6225
www.brookdaleliving.com

Paul Markowitz, Manager

Here, in a community of friendly neighbors and supportive staff, you'll discover for yourself just how much the ARC commitment will mean to you.

6360 Homewood Residence at Boynton Beach
2400 S Congress Avenue
Boynton Beach, FL 33426-7461
866-568-2678
Fax: 561-733-0229; *Toll Free:* 877-259-6226
www.brookdaleliving.com

Chris Spencer, Administrator

6361 Homewood Residence at Delray Beach
8020 W Atlantic Avenue
Delray Beach, FL 33446-9713
866-686-6547
Fax: 561-498-3161; *Toll Free:* 877-259-8068
www.brookdaleliving.com

Kim Welsch, Executive Director

As an American Retirement Corporation community, we are committed to offering you a living environment that maintains the highest standards while providing a personal touch.

6362 Homewood Residence at Freedom Plaza
3910 Galen Court
Sun City Center, FL 33573-6817
877-767-0039
Fax: 813-634-1548
www.brookdaleliving.com

Sally Nichols, Contact
Trenna Russ, Manager

6363 Inn at University Village
2650 Ohio State Drive Massillon
Ohio, FL 44646
330-837-3000
Fax: 813-975-5141
www.innatuniversityvillage.com

Denise Beck, Executive Director
Tonya Fusko, Director of Marketing and Admiss
Bonita Yeager, Director of Nursing

6364 John Knox Village of Central Florida
698 Monastery Road
Orange City, FL 32763-6220
386-775-0788
Fax: 386-775-4604; *Toll Free:* 800-344-4504
info@johnknox.com
www.johnknox.com

Lester Barker, Contact

Our residents enjoy a wide selection of social, recreational and cultural activities, the security of life-care and the fellowship of good friends.

Year Founded: 1972

6365 John Knox Village of Florida
651 SW 6th Street
Pompano Beach, FL 33060-3700
954-783-4000
Fax: 954-783-4011; *Toll Free:* 800-998-5669
www.johnknoxvillage.com

William G Knibloe, Chair
Dirk DeJong, Vice Chair
WD Lepin, Secretary

6366 John Knox Village of Tampa Bay
4100 E Fletcher Avenue
Tampa, FL 33613-4864
813-632-2306
Fax: 813-632-2446
www.johnknoxvillage.com

Joyce E Knowles, CEO
Suresh Pai, Executive Director

6367 Kiva of Mount Dora
505 E 9th Avenue
Mount Dora, FL 32757-4937
352-383-5005
Fax: 352-735-1350
kivaofmtdora@gmail.com
www.kivaofmountdora.com

Julie Young, Administrator

6368 Mangrove Bay
110 E Mangrove Bay Way
Jupiter, FL 33477-6401
888-325-1869
Fax: 561-575-4341
www.seniorlifestyle.com

Kathy Wise, Executive Director

6369 Marriott's Brighton Garden of Port St Lu cie
1699 SE Lyngate Drive
Port St Lucie, FL 34952-5016
772-335-9990
Fax: 772-335-9993
www.gardensofportstlucie.com

Lona Aiken, Administrator

6370 Marriott's Brighton Gardens of WPB
2090 N Congress Avenue
West Palm Beach, FL 33401-8210
561-686-5100
Fax: 561-686-9530

Cathy Davis, President

6371 Masonic Home of Florida
3201 1st Street NE
St Petersburg, FL 33704-2299
727-822-3499
Fax: 727-821-6775; *Toll Free:* 866-868-6749
masonichm@aol.com
www.masonichomeofflorida.org

James W Ford, Chairman

The Masonic Home of Florida offers care on two levels: skilled nursing for residents who require round-the-clock care and assisted living for residents who need little or no supervision. More than 140 staff members, under the direction of career professionals in geriatric disciplines, join together to create a lifestyle through which residents can reach their full potential.

Year Founded: 1990

6372 Mayflower Assisted Living Facility
1620 Mayflower Court
Winter Park, FL 32792-2500
407-672-1620
Fax: 407-671-6336; *Toll Free:* 800-228-6518
info@themayflower.com
www.TheMayflower.com

David McGuffin, CEO

The Mayflower is structured to permit residents to enjoy their retirement years with grace, dignity, independence and security; to ensure that all residents are treated equally; to provide services which meet the physical, spiritual, social and psychological needs of the residents; to create an environment which will enrich the lives of people who live and work at the Mayflower.

6373 Mease Manor
700 Mease Plaza
Dunedin, FL 34698-6680
727-738-3240
www.measemanor.com

Jack Norton, Contact

6374 Merrill Gardens at Lutz
414 Chapman Road E
Lutz, FL 33549-5779
813-909-9679
Fax: 813-948-2878
www.merrillgardens.com

Cathy Bennick, Community Relations Director
Michael Cavallo, Manager

Merrill Gardens community living for seniors is a place where you're absolutely free to be yourself. You can enjoy the quiet comforts of independent living, participate in our active retirement community, or both. The choice is yours, and it's just one of the many choices you'll find all around you.

6375 Moorings Park
120 Moorings Park Drive
Naples, FL 34105-2188
239-643-9111Toll free: 866-802-4302
www.mooringspark.org

Guenther Gosch, Executive Director

6376 Northpark-A Classic Residence by Hyatt
2480 N Park Road
Hollywood, FL 33021-3744
954-963-0200
Fax: 954-961-1266; *Toll Free:* 800-989-9159
www.viliving.com

Nancy Bubick, Executive Director

In addition to apartments for independent living, NorthPark features an assisted living center, where trained professionals provide a helping hand with bathing, dressing, grooming and supervising medications. For residents with memory impairments such as Alzheimer's disease, NorthPark offers a memory support center.

6377 Orlando Lutheran Towers
300 E Church Street
Orlando, FL 32801-3551
407-422-4103Toll free: 800-859-1033
marketing@orlandolt.com
www.orlandolt.com

Alicia Labrecque, Executive Director
Kerry Gerrity, Executive Director

6378 Spring Hills Lake Mary Assisted Living and Memory Care
3655 W Lake Mary Boulevard
Lake Mary, FL 32746-3497
321-710-8513
Fax: 407-688-2550
dfowler@spring-hills.net
www.spring-hills.com

Alex C Markowits, CEO

6379 Sterling Aventura
2777 NE 183rd Street
Aventura, FL 33160-2165
888-337-7480
Fax: 305-918-0099
www.seniorlifestyle.com

Mary Buchanan, Executive Director

The Sterling Aventura offers the very finest available in independent and assisted living housing. Every aspect of our community has been meticulously planned to provide discriminating seniors the luxury and gracious lifestyle they expect and deserve.

6380 Sunrise Atrium of Boca Raton
1080 NW 15th Street
Boca Raton, FL 33486-1311
888-337-1033
Fax: 561-750-6746
www.seniorlifestyle.com

Christopher Kochan, Administrator

6381 Victoria Villa Assisted Living
5151 SW 61st Avenue
Davie, FL 33314-5303
954-791-8881
Fax: 954-791-1157
victoriavilla@live.com
www.victoriavilla.com

Lucie Eichler, President
Hungria Medina , Staff Superviso

6382 Westminster Towers
1330 India Hook Rd
Rock Hill, SC 29732
800-345-6026
Fax: 407-849-0900; *Toll Free:* 803-328-5000
www.westminstertowers.org

Tony Fountain, CEO
Mandy Stamper, Campus Administrato

Georgia

6383 Belmont Village at Buckhead
5455 Glendridge Drive NE
Atlanta, GA 30342
404-252-6271
www.belmontvillage.com

Offers convenient access to healthcare, places of worship, shopping and restaurants.

6384 Belmont Village at Johns Creek
4315 Johns Creek Parkway
Suwanee, GA 30024
770-813-9505
www.belmontvillage.com

Offers easy access to shopping, dining, healthcare and places of worship.

6385 Mount Carmel Personal Care
3084 Mount Carmel Road
Hampton, GA 30228-2881
770-946-3376
Fax: 770-946-8214
www.mountcarmelassistedliving.com

Mouhad Khouri, Administrator

Provide a caring home where residents can live in a low stress and secured environment with dignity, comfort and the assurance that help is always available.

6386 Plantation South at Duluth
3450 Duluth Park Lane
Duluth, GA 30096-3257
678-534-5075
Fax: 770-497-8278
www.plantationsouth-duluth.com

Margaret Lynn, Contact
Jan Boatright, Executive Director

Personalized care and supportive surroundings help create the ideal environment for meeting professional care needs. Friendly, caring, and specially trained staff members are here round the clock to provide the assistance necessary to deal with minor health matters, medications and more. Residents enjoy a home environment that nourishes their interests, satisfies their needs and maintains their independence.

6387 Plantation South at Dunwoody
4594 Barclay Drive
Dunwoody, GA 30338-5883
678-534-5072
Fax: 770-936-9614
www.plantationsouth-dunwoody.com

Kristi Foster, Contact

Personalized care and supportive surroundings help create the ideal environment for meeting personal care needs.

6388 Remington House
1504 Renaissance Drive NE
Conyers, GA 30012-3895
888-327-0405
Fax: 770-761-4509
www.seniorlifestyle.com

Patricia White, Executive Director

6389 Savannah Court
395 Alafaya Woods
Blvd Oviedo, Fl 32765
407-278-7237
Fax: 770-977-2240
www.savannahcourtoviedo.com

Kathryn Chandler, Executive Director

Compassionate and highly trained staff provides assistance with the activities of daily living to ensure the highest quality of life. Residents enjoy safety, security and socialization with a quality-dining program, creative activities and personalized care program.

6390 Southern Plantation
580 Tommy Lee Fuller Drive
Loganville, GA 30052-3928
888-336-5033
Fax: 770-466-2220
www.seniorlifestyle.com

Anita Khan, Executive Director

This family owned and operated retirement community offers independent living in the cottages and villas, as well as assisted living in the manor house and alzheimer's care in the carriage house.

6391 Tapestry House
2725 Holcomb Bridge Road
Alpharetta, GA 30022-6812
770-649-0808
Fax: 770-649-0807
www.tapestryhouseassistedliving.com

Katherine Liabastre, Contact
Thomas Comte, President

Mission is to love, respect, and be caring.

6392 Yellow Brick House
52 W Beaver Creek Rd #4
Richmond Hill, CA 30058-4441
800-263-3247
Fax: 770-482-4981; *Toll Free:* 905-474-0124
www.yellowbrickhouse.org

Lorris Herenda, Executive Director

Offers a friendly helping hand to seniors in need of security, social opportunities and services. Family owned and operated with the help of a dependable and caring staff.

Idaho

6393 Aarenbrooke Place: Ashley Manor
North Cloverdale
Boise, ID 83713
208-376-1300
Fax: 208-376-3242; *Toll Free:* 888-376-7298
contactAM@ashleycares.com
www.caravita.com

Vickie McCuistion, Administrator
Gary May, Manager

We provide clean, homelike living environments with loving ,caring staff we truly strive to be a part of your family. Our dream has always been to provide the kind of care to our residents that will make a positive difference to them and their families.

6394 Alterra Wynwood at Twin Falls
1367 Locust Street N
Twin Falls, ID 83301-3451
877-776-6691
Fax: 208-735-0900
www.brookdaleliving.com

Anita Burdick, Administrator

6395 Annabelle House
917 E Ustick Road
Caldwell, ID 83605-6357
208-455-2324
Fax: 208-442-3371
www.alcco.com

Shirley Farley, Administrator

6396 Apple Valley Residential Care
18524 Corwin Rd
Apple Valley, CA 92307
760-242-3188
Fax: 208-365-2854
www.valleycrestseniorliving.com

Viki McCuistion, Manager

6397 Ashley Manor Care Centers-Harmony
2703 Harmony Avenue
Boise, ID 83706-5025
208-331-9228
Fax: 208-331-9145
skolnes@ashleycares.com
www.ashleycares.com

Priscilla Landeros, Manager
Sara Kolnes, Director of Admissions

6398 Ashley Manor Care Centers-Highmont
11099 W Highmont Drive
Boise, ID 83709-7702
208-377-4107
Fax: 208-377-3413
dbender@ashleycares.com
www.ashleycares.com

Diane Bender, Director of Admissions

6399 Ashley Manor Care Centers-Nampa
69 S Midland Boulevard
Nampa, ID 83651-2422
208-461-1452
Fax: 208-422-4307

sbell@ashleycares.com
www.ashleycares.com

Summer Bell, Director of Admissions

6400 Ashley Manor-Beverly Hills
861 Beverly Hills Drive
Payette, ID 83661-3065
208-642-1711
Fax: 208-642-0127
www.ashleycares.com

Holly Krasowski, Director of Admissions

6401 Aspen Grove Assisted Living-Lava Hot Sprrings
580 W Elm Street
Lava Hot Springs, ID 83246
208-776-5899
Fax: 208-776-5899
www.agingcare.com

Sally Nichols, Administrator

6402 Beehive Homes of Grangeville
709 W North 2nd Street
Grangeville, ID 83530-1174
208-983-3793
Fax: 208-983-3762
beehivehomes.com

Gary Ghramm, Owner
Linda Ghramm, Owner
Diane Walker, President

The mission of Bee Hive Homes is to provide assistance with the activities of daily living in a respectful, dignified manner in a home like setting to the frail elderly who choose to retain their independence and dignity to the fullest measure possible.

6403 Beehive Homes of Idaho I
1081 Fairwood Court
Meridian, ID 83646-1443
208-936-4525
Fax: 208-888-4791
ccastagneto@beehivehomes.com
beehivehomes.com

Cory Castagneto, Owner
Linda Palmer, Owner
Dawn Lindsay, Owner

The mission of Bee Hive Homes is to provide assistance with the activities of daily living in a respectful, dignified manner in a home like setting to the frail elderly who choose to retain their independence and dignity to the fullest measure possible.

6404 Beehive Homes of Idaho II
2321 Kenmere Drive
Meridian, ID 83646-1675
208-888-3699
Fax: 208-888-3699
ccastagneto@beehivehomes.com
beehivehomes.com

Cory Castagneto, Owner
Linda Palmer, Owner
Tanya Ripley, Manager

The mission of Bee Hive Homes is to provide assistance with the activities of daily living in a respectful, dignified manner in a home like setting to the frail elderly who choose to retain their independence and dignity to the fullest measure possible.

6405 Beehive Homes of Idaho VI
652 S Main Street
Star, ID 83669-5253
208-286-7783
Fax: 208-286-7783
ccastagneto@beehivehomes.com
beehivehomes.com

Cory Castagneto, Owner
Linda Palmer, Owner
Diana Rushin, Manager

The mission of Bee Hive Homes is to provide assistance with the activities of daily living in a respectful, dignified manner in a home like setting to the frail elderly who choose to retain their independence and dignity to the fullest measure possible.

6406 Beehive Homes of North Idaho
2100 E Sherman Avenue
Coeur D Alene, ID 83814-5335
208-763-3622
Fax: 208-765-3396
beehivehomes.com

Gary Ghramm, Owner

6407 Beehive Homes-Mountain Home
940 W 8th S
Mountain Home, ID 83647-3681
208-587-1308
Fax: 208-587-1316
beehivehomes.com

6408 Bridgeview Estates
1828 Bridgeview Boulevard
Twin Falls, ID 83301-3051
208-736-3933
Fax: 208-736-3941
www.bridgeviewretirement.com

Lori Bentzler, Executive Director

6409 Brookside Landing
431 Johnson Avenue
Orofino, ID 83544-9516
208-476-2000
Fax: 208-476-7748
www.brooksidelanding.com

Jill Tyler, Administrator

6410 Burley Care Assisted Living
1729 Miller Avenue
Burley, ID 83318-2338
208-678-9474
Fax: 208-678-3727
www.safehavenhealthcare.org

Renee Mai, Contact
Carol Gonzales, Administrator

6411 Capital City Assisted Living-Spaulding
PO Box 5394
Boise, ID 83705
208-384-1393
Fax: 208-333-0636
www.capitalsenior.com

6412 Cenoma House
1930 Heyburn Avenue E
Twin Falls, ID 83301-4921
208-735-9796
Fax: 208-736-7471; *Toll Free:* 208-420-8384
www.cenomahouse.com

Linda Biain, Owner
Linda Biain, Administrator

6413 Clearwater House Assisted Living Concept
715 W Comstock Avenue
Nampa, ID 83651-8406
208-463-1732
Fax: 208-463-9381
clearwatermail@alcco.com
www.alcco.com

Stacey Stallings, Executive Director

6414 Coeur D'Alene Home
624 W. Harrison Avenue
Coeur d'Alene, ID 83814-2361
208-664-8119
Fax: 208-666-0749
rdearing@cdaseniorliving.org
www.cdahomes.org

Mike Grabenstein, Administrator

Our ecumenical mission is to provide a not-for-profit housing campus, offering Christian care without discrimination, for our elderly and disadvantaged residents.

6415 Cotttages of Emmett
411 E 12th Street
Emmett, ID 83617-3628
208-365-9490
Fax: 208-323-5593
www.assistedlivingidaho.com

Garold Maxwell, Owner
Mark Maxwell, President

6416 Creekside Care Center
9107 N. Davis Rd
Stockton, CA 95209-1807
209-478-6488
Fax: 208-324-8536
www.genesishcc.com

Judy Treloar, Administrator
Stephen Lofy, Program Director

6417 Desano Place Residential Care
218 West B Street
Shoshone, ID 83352
888-848-5698
Fax: 208-886-2737
terri@pendleton.myrf.net
www.agingcare.com

Terri Pendleton RN, Owner/Administrator

9-bed residential care.

6418 Edgewood Spring Creek Senior Living American Falls
653 N Eagle Road
Eagle, ID 83616-5007
208-938-5578
Fax: 208-938-1589

joyce.foster@scmanor.com
www.edgewoodseniorliving.com

Joyce Foster, Executive Director

6419 Fairwinds-Coeur d'Alene
2340 West Seltice Way
Coeur d'Alene, ID 83814
208-765-5505
www.leisurecare.com

Offers luxurious apartment homes in a fun and active retirement community.

6420 Fairwinds-Sand Creek
3310 Valencia Drive
Idaho Falls, ID 83404
208-542-6200
www.leisurecare.com

Offers luxurious apartment homes in a fun and active retirement community.

6421 Heritage Retirement Center-Boise
1777 S Curtis Road
Boise, ID 83705-2708
208-376-4191
Fax: 208-376-9512
www.heritagewoodstone.com

Cathy Lynch, Administrator

6422 Heritage Retirement Center-Twin Falls
622 Filer Avenue W
Twin Falls, ID 83301-4533
208-733-9064
Fax: 208-733-0343
www.heritagewoodstone.com

Dorkis Knowles, Contact

Recognize the uniqueness of each perso, the mission is to maximize independence in aging by assisting residents to live with dignity in a secure, home-like environment.

6423 Highland Estates
2050 Hiland Avenue
Burley, ID 83318-2761
208-678-4411
Fax: 208-678-4470
www.highlandretirement.com

Lisa Oaks, Executive Director

6424 Highland Hills
1501 Baldy Avenue
Pocatello, ID 83201-7117
208-366-0076
Fax: 208-237-3889
www.emeritus.com

Robyn Smith, Administrator

6425 Hillcrest
1093 S Hilton Street
Boise, ID 83705-1971
208-901-8875
Fax: 208-345-0178
www.boiseassistedlivingservice.com

Eric Bultez, Manager

6426 Indianhead Estates
590 W Indianhead Road
Weiser, ID 83672-1512
208-549-3455
Fax: 208-549-3483
www.indianheadestates.net

Patricia Caroll, Contact
Renee Edwards, Owner

6427 Joyce's Orchard Residential Care Home
615 Cedar Avenue
Lewiston, ID 83501-5121
208-746-5695
Fax: 208-798-4667
www.seniorhomeblog.com

Joy Dunlap, Manager

6428 Karcher Estates
1127 Caldwell Boulevard
Nampa, ID 83651-1719
208-465-4935
Fax: 208-465-4953
www.karcherestates.com

Donna Lant, Administrator

Experience is a fundamental benefit when choosing a Frontier Management, LLC community. Our team has the expertise in retirement living and assisted living to meet your needs. Our entire company is dedicated to those who have selected one of our communities as home for themselves or their loved ones.

Year Founded: 1990

6429 Legends Park Assisted Living Community
1820 W Golf Course Road
Coeur D Alene, ID 83815-1627
866-939-1721
Fax: 208-765-6587
www.seniorhomes.com

Trudie Chamberlain, Manager

6430 Lincoln Court
850 Lincoln Drive
Idaho Falls, ID 83401
208-419-0281
www.stellarliving.com

Offers a luxurious studio, and one-and two-bedroom apartment homes in a fun and active retirement community.

6431 Living Springs
1605 N Catherine Street
Post Falls, ID 83854-7237
208-773-6145
Fax: 208-773-1138
lsjag.alice@yahoo.com
www.livingspringshome.com

Alice Thibault, Administrator/Owner
Jennifer Trefz, Administrator/Owner
Gary Trefz, Owner

Assisted Living.

6432 Loyaton of Coeur d'Alene
205 E Anton Avenue
Coeur D Alene, ID 83815-3721

208-366-0078
Fax: 208-765-4352
www.emeritus.com

Tambra Maple, Contact
Jodie Lynch, Administrator

ttractive apartment homes. Delicious, restaurant-style dining. Housekeeping and laundry services. Personal care and assistance, if needed, from skilled caregivers and licensed specialists. A daily offering of fun and enlightening activities. You'll find all these things, and more, in Emeritus communities.

6433 Odd Fellows Home of Idaho
206 E Walulla St
Idaho City, ID 83631
208-459-7601
Fax: 208-459-0139
www.idahoheritage.org
Year Founded: 1875

6434 Paramount Parks at Boise
10250 W Smoke Ranch Drive
Boise, ID 83709-1467
208-350-6347
Fax: 208-322-2345
overlanded@islllc.com
overlandcourtseniorliving.com

Tamara McCann, Manager

6435 Parkwood Meadows Assisted Living Community
1885 Parkwood Street
Idaho Falls, ID 83401-6135
208-523-7800
Fax: 208-523-2240
www.prestigecare.com

Kaddy Fyfe, Executive Director

6436 Pine Brook Assisted Living
636 E. 1st South Rigby
Idaho Falls, ID 83442
208-745-0100
Fax: 208-542-6028
pinebrookif@msn.com
pinebrookassistedliving.com

Ron Hedelius, Owner
Michelle Allen, Administrative Assistant

Providing care in a home like environment for Alzheimer/Dementia and elderly.

6437 Pine Brook Assisted Living Center
636 E 1st Street
Rigby, ID 83442-5502
208-745-0100
Fax: 208-745-8364
www.pinebrookassistedliving.com

Fawn Hedelius, Manager/Owner
Ron Hedelius, Owner/Administrator

Care for elderly, dementia and alzheimers.

6438 Plantation Place Retirement & Assisted Living
3921 N Kessinger Lane
Garden City, ID 83703-3003

208-853-7300
Fax: 208-853-9328
www.edgewoodseniorliving.com

Phil Gisi, Owner/Chief Executive Officer
Russell G Kubik, Vice President

6439 Prestige Assisted Living at Autumn Wind
200 W Beech Street
Caldwell, ID 83605-5692
208-459-3335
Fax: 208-459-3300
www.prestigecare.com

Kerri Wells, Executive Director

6440 Quail Ridge Assisted Living
12401 Trail Oak Dr
Oklahoma City, OK 73120
405-755-5775
Fax: 208-233-8797
www.quailridgeassistedliving.com

Jonathan Levey, Co-Owner
Skye Melvin, Executive Director

6441 Ridge Wind Assisted Living
4080 Hawthorne Road
Chubbuck, ID 83202-2746
208-366-0000
Fax: 208-237-6024
www.emeritus.com

Sandy Guidinger, Administrator

6442 Spring Creek Manor Assisted Living
653 N Eagle Road
Eagle, ID 83616-5007
208-938-5578
Fax: 208-938-1589
eagle@scmanor.com
www.scmanor.com

Laura Lee Mathias, Administrator
Jessica Tatum, Clinical Services Manager

6443 Spring Creek Manor-American Falls
605 Hillcrest Avenue
American Falls, ID 83211-1365
208-226-1856
Fax: 208-226-1842
www.edgewoodseniorliving.com

Joyce Foster, Executive Director

6444 Spring Creek Manor-Soda Springs
425 S Spring Creek Drive
Soda Springs, ID 83276-1628
208-547-0257
Fax: 208-547-4027
www.edgewoodseniorliving.com

Randy Hill, Executive Director

6445 Stoney Creek Living Center
3808 N 2538 E
Twin Falls, ID 83301
208-736-5705
Fax: 208-736-3848
stoneycreeklivingcenter@gmail.com
www.stoneycreeklivingcenter.com

Daivd Weight, Administrator

6446 Sunbridge Living Center-Meridian Careand Rehabilitation
1351 West Pine
Meridian, ID 83642-2062
208-888-7049
Fax: 208-888-7246
www.genesishcc.com

Joe Rudd, Administrator

6447 SunnyRidge Rehabilitation & Retirement Center
2609 Sunnybrook Drive
Nampa, ID 83686-6399
208-467-7298
Fax: 208-463-0901
www.genesishcc.com

David Chinchurreta, Executive Director
Roxie Tracy, Admissions Director

Caring is the key in life.

6448 Sylvan House
660 W Honeysuckle Avenue
Hayden, ID 83835-9759
208-762-4097
Fax: 208-772-9335
www.alcco.com

Tanya Wilson, Manager

6449 Turtle & Crane Assisted Living
1950 1st Street
Idaho Falls, ID 83401-4342
208-557-0186
Fax: 208-529-4063
www.turtleandcraneonfirst.com

Sumiko Mitchell, Manager

6450 Warren House
1301 Bennett Avenue
Burley, ID 83318-2675
208-677-8212
Fax: 208-677-9022
www.alcco.com

Jim Serve, Administrator

6451 Willow Park Assisted Living
2600 N Milwaukee Street
Boise, ID 83704-5784
208-373-1234
Fax: 208-375-1316
willowpark2@rgnt.com
www.willowparkseniorliving.com

Bryan Elliott, Manager

Personal care assistance around the clock, medication assistance, weekly housekeeping, and apartment maintenance are only some of the amenities and services included in your basic monthly rent at Willow Park. From Tai Chi to painting, residents are having fun while improving their flexibility, mobility and emotional well-being.

6452 Willowbrook Assisted Living
1871 Julie Lane
Twin Falls, ID 83301-3525
208-736-3727
Fax: 208-732-6047

willowbrook@cableone.net
www.willowbrookassistedliving.com

Kevin Haight, Owner/Administrator

6453 Willows
898 S Meridian Street
Blackfoot, ID 83221-2660
208-782-1478
Fax: 208-785-0090
willows5@TrueYellow.net
www.willowsliving.net

Bill Hines, CEO

Illinois

6454 Addolorata Villa
555 McHenry Road
Wheeling, IL 60090-3899
847-537-2900
Fax: 847-215-5805
fcinfo@franciscanservices.com
www.addoloratavilla.com

Maggie Turk, Contact
Larry Carlson, Executive Officer

Offers elegant living accommodations, amenities and a positive environment to enjoy life to the fullest.

6455 Belmont Village at Geneva Road
545 Belmont Lane
Carol Stream, IL 60188
630-510-1515
Fax: 630-510-0633
www.belmontvillage.com

Offers residents a more dignified, independent life in a comfortable residential neighborhood setting.

6456 Belmont Village of Buffalo Grove
500 McHenry Road
Buffalo Grove, IL 60089
847-537-5000
Fax: 847-537-7260
www.belmontvillage.com

Seniors community that sets a new standard in Assisted Living. Offers residents a more dignified, independent life in a comfortable residential neighborhood setting.

6457 Belmont Village of Glenview
2200 Golf Road
Glenview, IL 60025
847-657-7100
Fax: 847-657-7171
www.belmontvillage.com

Offers residents a more dignified, independent life in a comfortable residential neighborhood setting.

6458 Belmont Village of Oak Park
1035 Madison Street
Oak Park, IL 60302
708-848-7200
www.belmontvillage.com

Convenient to shops, galleries and museums.

6459 Bethesda Home and Retirement Center
2833 N Nordica Avenue
Chicago, IL 60634-4794

773-622-6144
Fax: 773-622-8261
www.bethesdahome.com

Julie Boggess, Administrator
Paul Roberts, Financial Officer

Offering continuum of care, this facility is located in an attractive and quiet residential neighborhood with access to shopping, local churches and civic activites.

6460 Bethlehem Woods Retirement Community
1571 W Ogden Avenue
La Grange Park, IL 60526-1723
708-579-3663
Fax: 708-579-7159
www.presencehealth.org

Sandra Bruce, CEO

Located on 42 wooded acres we offer elegant independent living residentces, while enhanced supportive living services are also provided. We are dedicated to assuring you wellness, independence, security and spiritual comfort.

6461 Concord Place Retirement & Assisted Living Community
401 W Lake Street
Northlake, IL 60164-2436
708-562-9000
Fax: 708-409-2750
www.concordplace.com

Cheryl Cohen, Manager

Assisted living at the most affordable rental prices combined with quality support services.

6462 Cordia Senior Residence
865 N Cass Avenue
Westmont, IL 60559
630-887-7000
Fax: 630-887-7577; *Toll Free:* 866-430-2890
www.cordia.biz

Teresa Rogala, Acting Executive Director

Through our staff, programming and residential environment, we encourage residents to live their lives to their fullest potential.

6463 Devonshire of Hoffman Estates
1515 Barrington Road
Hoffman Estates, IL 60169-5021
847-490-5800
Fax: 847-490-5830
www.brookdaleliving.com

Jennifer Gamache, Manager

Our approach to senior living, which combines a variety of services ranging from independent living to personal assistance, enables us to accommodate the changing needs of our residents. In the event that needs change, we can arrange services to accommodate every situation.

6464 Fountains at Crystal Lake-The Inn
965 N Brighton Circle
Crystal Lake, IL 60012-2036
815-893-7216
Fax: 815-477-6502; *Toll Free:* 800-382-1308
www.watermarkcommunities.com

Michael Ross, Executive Director

The Inn offers a lovely, amenity-rich environment in which residents can enjoy privacy, independence and freedom of choice while receiving all the care and support they need.

6465 Hearthstone of Arlington Heights
800 W Oakton Street
Arlington Heights, IL 60004-4602
888-958-2690
Fax: 847-368-3702
www.seniorcareauthority.com

Vicki Schlomann, Executive Director

Offers the independent senior peace of mind. Apartments in a wide choice of floor plans are accented with beautiful sitting areas, porches and a fine dining room.

6466 Holland Home Assisted Living
16300 Louis Avenue
South Holland, IL 60473-2281
708-596-3050
Fax: 708-596-3067
www.providencelifeservices.com

Wayne Rost, Administrator

Program serves those people needing help with daily tasks such as dressing, bathing, and medication supervision.

6467 Kenwood of Lake View
3121 N Sheridan Road
Chicago, IL 60657-4945
773-404-9800
Fax: 773-404-7898
www.brookdaleliving.com

Anna Anderson, Owner

Our approach to senior living, which combines a variety of services ranging from independent living to personal assistance, enables us to accommodate the changing needs of our residents. In the event that needs change, we can arrange services to accommodate every situation.

6468 Lake Barrington Woods
22320 Classic Court
Lake Barrington, IL 60010-5903
847-842-8900
Fax: 847-381-7253; *Toll Free:* 888-223-9663
lbw@parkside-sr.com
www.parksidesenior.com

Cheryl Black, Executive Director

Offers independent living and assisted living. Whatever your interests, you'll find endless opportunities for exceptional retirement living at Lake Barrington Woods.

6469 Marian Village
15624 Marian Dr
Homer Glen, IL 60491
708-226-3780
Fax: 847-215-5805
fcinfo@franciscanservices.com
www.marianvillage.com

Larry Carlson, Executive Director

At Marian Village, whether you are an active senior looking for just the right place to enjoy your retirement or a person needing a little assistance, our comprehensive range of supportive services are designed to fit your individual needs.

6470 Moorings of Arlington Heights
811 E Central Road
Arlington Heights, IL 60005-3244
847-956-4304
Fax: 847-956-4451; *Toll Free:* 800-445-8431
www.presbyterianhomes.org

Pat Walsh, Executive Director

Residents are able to receive light assistance in a residential setting. Private rooms as well as two room suites are available.

6471 North Shore Retirement Hotel
1611 Chicago Avenue
Evanston, IL 60201-6019
847-864-6400
Fax: 847-864-0947
www.retirementhotel.com

Margaret Gergen, Manager

Each resident has a lovely, fully-furnished private apartment with daily maid service and three delicious meals a day.

6472 Norwood Park Home
6016 N Nina Avenue
20
Chicago, IL 60631-2498
773-631-4856
Fax: 773-631-4850
www.norwoodcrossing.org

Marcia R Hagopian, Executive Director

Not-for-profit residence for seniors, offering private suites in assisted living with emergency call system in a clean, family atmosphere. Provides continuum of care, including skilled nursing in addition to hospice and respite services.

6473 Provena Fox Knoll Retirement
421 N Lake Street
Aurora, IL 60506-4180
630-844-0380
Fax: 630-844-0702
www.provenia.org/foxknoll

Sue Hanegraaf, Marketing Coordinator
Michele Hilger, Marketing Coordinator
Carol Ricken, Executive Director

A friendly, faith based senior community offering Independent Living, Assisted Living, Residential Memory care, and Respite (short term) Care. spacious 1 and 2 bedroom assisted living suites, all with private bathrooms and in their own unique environments. Array of social, spiritual and physical activities to choose from, plus private transportation, to meet the needs, interests, hobbies and talents of today's vibrant seniors.

6474 Saint Andrew Life Center
7000 N Newark Avenue
Niles, IL 60714-4577
847-647-8332
Fax: 708-647-7073
www.provenia.org

Jean Kennedy, Contact
Nikki Curth, Administrator

Provides independent living, assisted living, or 24-hour nursing care with an intermediate care facility and a wellness center.

6475 Spring Meadows Libertyville
901 Florsheim Drive
Libertyville, IL 60048-5200
847-816-6644
Fax: 847-816-6633
www.capitalsenior.com/springmeadowsatlib

Mary Jester, Executive Director

6476 St. James Villas
1251 E Richton Road
Crete, IL 60417-1623
708-672-6700
Fax: 708-672-4939; *Toll Free:* 800-524-6126
www.trilogyhs.com

Tina Strimbu, Executive Director

Offer 60 one-story apartment-like units for residents needing a certain level of personal care and supervision.

6477 Sunrise Assisted Living of Naperville
960 E Chicago Avenue
Naperville, IL 60540
630-579-5937
Fax: 630-579-1772
naperville.dcr@sunriseseniorliving.com
www.sunriseseniorliving.com

Mark Blau, Executive Director
Laura Wolst, Director Community Relations
Julie Gimpel, Director Community Relations

6478 Sunrise Senior Living of Naperville
960 E Chicago Avenue
Naperville, IL 60540
630-579-1400
Fax: 630-579-1772
naperville.dos@sunriseseniorliving.com
www.sunrisenaperville.com

Jennifer Marlette, Executive Director
Laura Wolst, Director of Sales

Sunrise is built on a commitment to our residents and their families. We believe no two people are alike, so the services and attention we provide should never be exactly the same. That's also why we offer a variety of lifestyle, service and care options. By providing these choices, we not only offer solutions for today, but we provide the security of tomorrow.

Year Founded: 1999

6479 Sunrise of Bloomingdale
129 E Lake Street
Bloomingdale, IL 60108-1104
630-295-8600
Fax: 639-295-8498
www.sunriseseniorliving.com

Penny McIntyre, Chief Executive Officer
Marc Richards, Chief Financial Officer
Chris Winkle, Chief Operating Officer

For residents with memory impairment, Sunrise offers an innovative program called Reminiscence.

6480 Sunrise of Buffalo Grove
180 W Half Day Road
Buffalo Grove, IL 60089-6552
847-478-8484
Fax: 847-478-2039
www.sunriseseniorliving.com

Joann Guarneri, Executive Director
Penny McIntyre, Chief Executive Officer
Marc Richards, Chief Financial Officer

Sunrise is built on a commitment to our residents and their families. We believe no two people are alike, so the services and attention we provide should never be exactly the same. That's also why we offer a variety of lifestyle, service and care options. By providing these choices, we not only offer solutions for today, but we provide the security of knowing that there are options for tomorrow.

6481 Sunrise of Crystal Lake

751 E Terra Cotta Avenue
Crystal Lake, IL 60014-3604
815-444-6600
Fax: 815-444-6600
www.sunriseseniorliving.com

Beth Johnston, Executive Director
Penny McIntyre, Chief Executive Officer
Marc Richards, Chief Financial Officer

Sunrise is built on a commitment to our residents and their families. We believe no two people are alike, so the services and attention we provide should never be exactly the same. That's also why we offer a variety of lifestyle, service and care options. By providing these choices, we not only offer solutions for today, but we provide the security of knowing that there are options for tomorrow.

6482 Sunrise of Flossmoor

19715 Governors Highway
Flossmoor, IL 60422-1794
708-798-1600
Fax: 708-798-3406
www.sunriseseniorliving.com

John Brimm, Executive Director
Penny McIntyre, Chief Executive Officer
Marc Richards, Chief Financial Officer

6483 Sunrise of Glen Ellyn

95 Carleton Avenue
Glen Ellyn, IL 60137-5500
630-469-5555
Fax: 630-469-0922
www.sunriseseniorliving.com

Christine Umbdenstock, Executive Director
Penny McIntyre, Chief Executive Officer
Marc Richards, Chief Financial Officer

Sunrise is built on a commitment to our residents and their families. We believe no two people are alike, so the services and attention we provide should never be exactly the same. That's also why we offer a variety of lifestyle, service and care options. By providing these choices, we not only offer solutions for today, but we provide the security of knowing that there are options for tomorrow.

6484 Sunrise of Gurnee

500 N Hunt Club Road
Gurnee, IL 60031-2416
847-856-8100
Fax: 847-856-8188
www.sunriseseniorliving.com

Rita Jedkins, Executive Director
Penny McIntyre, Chief Executive Officer
Marc Richards, Chief Financial Officer

Sunrise is built on a commitment to our residents and their families. We believe no two people are alike, so the ser-

vices and attention we provide should never be exactly the same. That's also why we offer a variety of lifestyle, service and care options. By providing these choices, we not only offer solutions for today, but we provide the security of knowing that there are options for tomorrow.

6485 Sunrise of Naperville-North

535 W Ogden Avenue
Naperville, IL 60563-3286
630-305-9400
Fax: 630-305-9444
www.sunriseseniorliving.com

Georgean Sweiss, Executive Director
Penny McIntyre, Chief Executive Officer
Marc Richards, Chief Financial Officer

Sunrise is built on a commitment to our residents and their families. We believe no two people are alike, so the services and attention we provide should never be exactly the same. That's also why we offer a variety of lifestyle, service and care options. By providing these choices, we not only offer solutions for today, but we provide the security of knowing that there are options for tomorrow.

6486 Sunrise of Palos Park

12828 S La Grange Road
Palos Park, IL 60464-2247
708-361-3577
Fax: 708-361-3889
www.sunriseseniorliving.com

Kathleen Roloff, Executive Director
Penny McIntyre, Chief Executive Officer
Marc Richards, Chief Financial Officer

6487 Sunrise of Park Ridge

1725 Ballard Road
Park Ridge, IL 60068-1005
847-824-1724
Fax: 847-824-9864
www.sunriseseniorliving.com

Denny Zook, Executive Director
Penny McIntyre, Chief Executive Officer
Marc Richards, Chief Financial Officer

Sunrise is built on a commitment to our residents and their families. We believe no two people are alike, so the services and attention we provide should never be exactly the same. That's also why we offer a variety of lifestyle, service and care options. By providing these choices, we not only offer solutions for today, but we provide the security of knowing that there are options for tomorrow.

6488 Sunrise of Schaumburg

790 N Plum Grove Road
Schaumburg, IL 60173-4764
847-517-9700
Fax: 847-517-8701
www.sunriseseniorliving.com

Desma Thrist, Executive Director
Penny McIntyre, Chief Executive Officer
Marc Richards, Chief Financial Officer

Sunrise is built on a commitment to our residents and their families. We believe no two people are alike, so the services and attention we provide should never be exactly the same. That's also why we offer a variety of lifestyle, service and care options. By providing these choices, we not only offer solutions for today, but we provide the security of knowing that there are options for tomorrow.

6489 Sunrise of Willowbrook
6300 Clarendon Hills Road
Willowbrook, IL 60527-2133
630-734-9954
Fax: 630-734-9956
www.sunriseseniorliving.com

Penny McIntyre, Chief Executive Officer
Marc Richards, Chief Financial Officer
Chris Winkle, Chief Operating Officer

Sunrise is built on a commitment to our residents and their families. We believe no two people are alike, so the services and attention we provide should never be exactly the same. That's also why we offer a variety of lifestyle, service and care options. By providing these choices, we not only offer solutions for today, but we provide the security of knowing that there are options for tomorrow.

6490 The Park at Vernon Hills
145 N Milwaukee Avenue
Vernon Hills, IL 60061-4170
855-350-3800
Fax: 847-793-2471
www.brookdaleliving.com

6491 Victorian Inn at Victorian Village
12600 Renaissance Circle
Lockport, IL 60491-5891
708-301-0800
Fax: 708-301-2493
www.providencelifeservices.com

Mike Venzon, Administrator

Provides convenient and comfortable living arrangements with choice of studio, one bedroom or shared suite settings.

6492 Village Woods
2681 Route 394
Crete, IL 60417-4353
708-672-6111
Fax: 708-672-8914
vw@provlife.com
www.providencelifeservices.com

Tom Travato, Manager

6493 Westbridge Assisted Living
500 Wyndemere Circle
Wheaton, IL 60187-2451
630-923-8016
Fax: 630-690-2362; *Toll Free:* 866-933-4797
www.wyndemereseniorliving.com

Shirley Pollard, Executive Director

Residents at this premier assisted living facility receive a helping hand with daily tasks and enjoy a variety of activities, amenities and services.

Indiana

6494 Atria Eastlake Terrace
3109 E Bristol Street
Elkhart, IN 46514-4372
574-266-4508
www.atriaassistedliving.com

Come to Atria Eastlake Terrace's traditionally designed, one-story building offering an active, carefree lifestyle for today's seniors. Assisted living care plans are designed to promote independence and enhance the quality of life of our residents.

6495 Bethesda Gardens at the Crossings
Bethesda Adult Community
1450 E Crossing Boulevard
Terre Haute, IN 47802-5316
812-298-8209
Fax: 812-298-9190
www.bethesdaadultcommunities.com

Gaynell McKenzie, Executive Director

This 70-unit apartment complex has five assisted living apartment styles.

6496 Meridan Oaks
1251 West 96th Street
Indianapolis, IN 46260
317-575-9200
Fax: 317-575-8209; *Toll Free:* 877-771-8285
www.emeritus.com

Daniel R Baty, Chairman/CEO
Raymond B Brandstrom, Vice Chairman/VP Finance
Gary Becker, SVP Operations

Meridan Oaks' commitment to our residents is to provide a nuturing environment that preserves dignity, fosters independence, encourages freedom of choice, promotes emotional well being and includes family and friends.

6497 Shamrock Gardens
17650 Generations Drive
South Bend, IN 46635
574-271-1151
www.shamrockgardens.net

Richard Herath, Administrator
Joan Ross, LPN, Director Nursing
Kelly Buwa, Activities Director

A licensed residential care (Assisted Living) facility offering a supportive environment while maximizing independence.

6498 Sunrise of Carmel
301 Executive Drive
Carmel, IN 46032
317-580-0389
Fax: 317-843-9790
www.sunriseseniorliving.com

Paul J Klaassen, Founder/Chairman/CEO
Teresa M Klaassen, Founder/Chief Cultural Officer
Thomas B Newell, President

Our care is designed to meet the individualized needs of each of our residents.

6499 Towne Centre
7250 Arthur Boulevard
Merrillville, IN 46410-3766
219-736-2900
Fax: 219-736-2209
www.capitalsenior.com

Michael D Moore, Executive Vice President
Nitsa Foundos, Contact

6500 3801 Grand
3801 Grand Avenue
Des Moines, IA 50312-2800
515-255-3499
Fax: 515-255-9344
www.3801grand.com

Mary Ann Larsen, Manager

You want to remain in charge of your life, and needing help with activities of daily living should not change that. Our certified facility offers a supportive environment that empowers tenants to remain as independent and autonomous as possible. You and your family can relax, knowing that professional staff is available to meet scheduled and unscheduled needs.

6501 AASE Hougen Assisted Living
4 Ohio Street
Decorah, IA 52101-1516
563-382-3603
Fax: 563-382-3606
www.aasehaugen.com

Sue Bjelland, Administrator

6502 Allen House
1406 E 19th Street
Atlantic, IA 50022-2897
712-243-3820
Fax: 712-243-6707
www.alcco.com/location/allen-house

6503 Arbor Heights at University
233 University Avenue
Des Moines, IA 50314-3124
515-284-1280
Fax: 515-284-0127
www.universityparkdsm.com

Ron Osby, Administrator

6504 Arlin Flack Assisted Living
911 Ridgewood Drive
Decorah, IA 52101-2354
563-382-8787
Fax: 563-382-8788
barthelloeshome@yahoo.com
www.barthelloeshome.com

Karl Jacobsen, Administrator

6505 Arlington Place of Grundy Center
95 D Avenue
Grundy Center, IA 50638-1950
319-824-5674
Fax: 319-824-5676
www.arlingtonplaceretirement.com

Teri Hook, Administrator

6506 Arlington Place of Red Oak
800 E Ratliff Road
Red Oak, IA 51566-5102
712-623-1999
Fax: 712-623-2007
www.arlingtonplaceretirement.com

Di Smith, Manager

6507 Bickford Assisted Living of Fort Dodge
1536 20th Avenue N
Fort Dodge, IA 50501-7134
515-573-3300
Fax: 515-576-1593
www.enrichinghappiness.com

Cheryl Cherry, CRD
Candy Egdorf, Director

6508 Bickford Cottage-Ames
2418 Kent Avenue
Ames, IA 50010-7119
515-233-6000
Fax: 515-268-9817
www.enrichinghappiness.com

Susan Doran, Contact
Kelley Loenser, Manager

6509 Bickford Cottage-Davenport
4040 E 55th Street
Davenport, IA 52807-2905
563-322-0000
Fax: 319-441-0758
www.enrichinghappiness.com

Laura Brock, Executive Director

6510 Bickford Cottage-Marshalltown
101 New Castle Road
Marshalltown, IA 50158-5241
641-753-5700
Fax: 641-753-0829
www.enrichinghappiness.com

Patricia Hayes, Manager

6511 Bickford Cottage-Muscatine
2807 Cedar Street
Muscatine, IA 52761-2276
563-263-6600
Fax: 563-263-3508
www.enrichinghappiness.com

Bobbe Kreiger, Executive Director

6512 Brickford Cottage
5101 University Avenue
Cedar Falls, IA 50613-6246
319-266-6800
Fax: 319-277-1294
www.enrichinghappiness.com

Jill Knipp, Executive Director

6513 Brickford Cottage-Burlington
3301 Sterling Driveive
Burlington, IA 52601-8660
319-754-7500
Fax: 319-754-0447
www.enrichinghappiness.com/branch/bickfo

Christa Poggemiller, Director

6514 Brickford Cottage-Clinton
1150 13th Avenue N
Clinton, IA 52732-3490
563-242-2400
Fax: 319-242-7620
www.enrichinghappiness.com

Kim Schaffer, Director

6515 Brickford Cottage-Iowa City
3500 Lower West Branch Road
Iowa City, IA 52245-4106
319-351-3200
Fax: 319-351-6861
www.enrichinghappiness.com/branch/bickfo

Barbara Faust, Executive Director

6516 Brickford Cottage-West Des Moines
5050 Hawthorne Drive
W Des Moines, IA 50265-5353
515-657-6401
Fax: 515-223-0151
www.enrichinghappiness.com

Jenny Knust, Contact
Kris Lange, Manager

6517 Calvin Community Assisted Living Service
4210 Hickman Road
Des Moines, IA 50310-3333
515-277-6141
Fax: 515-271-0933
info@calvincommunity.org
www.calvincommunity.org

Debra Peterson, Administrator

Our mission is to provide, on a nonprofit basis, services to older adults in a caring, Christian community designed to meet their physical, social, spiritual and psychological needs and contribute to their health, security and happiness. We offer a full range of living options to give you just the right amout of assistance when you need it.

6518 Cardinal Grove
1355 Division Street
Garner, IA 50438-1968
641-923-2114
Fax: 641-923-0074
www.abcmcorp.com

6519 Char-Mac Assisted Living
200 E Char Mac Drive
Lawton, IA 51030-8171
712-944-4893
Fax: 712-944-4853
www.lawtonia.com
www.char-mac.com

Jeanine Chartier, Owner

6520 Clover Ridge
205 Ehlers Lane
Maquoketa, IA 52060-9615
563-652-2125
Fax: 563-625-0147
www.cloverridgeplace.com

Nancy Miller, Contact
Lynne Popp, Manager

6521 Cornerstone Assisted Living
Good Shepherd Inc
302 2nd Street NE
PO Box 1707
Mason City, IA 50402-1707
641-424-1740
Fax: 641-424-4260
info@goodshepherd-inc.com
www.goodshepherd-inc.com

Diane Horning, CEO
Michael Svejda, Administration

A not-for-profit corporation consisting of 200 dually certified long term care beds, 93 assisted living apartments and 230 independent senior apartments.

6522 Cottage Grove Place
2115 1st Avenue SE
Cedar Rapids, IA 52402-6358
319-363-2420
Fax: 319-297-5555
www.cottagegroveplace.com

Abby Bruce, Executive Director
Michelle Milcoff, Marketing Director

6523 Country Manor Memory Care
900 W 46th Street
Davenport, IA 52806-4362
563-284-2789
Fax: 319-391-6267
www.countrymanormemorycare.com

Tammy Humphreys, Contact

6524 Courtyard
401 W 10th Avenue N
Clear Lake, IA 50428-4202
641-357-1648
Fax: 641-357-7154
www.abcmcorp.com

6525 Davenport Lutheran Assisted Living
1130 W 53rd Street
Davenport, IA 52806-2401
563-391-5342
Fax: 563-386-1056
s.hopp@lhaa-e.org
www.lhaa-e.org

Shelley Hopp, Administrator

6526 Eiler House
920 W Garfield Street
Clarinda, IA 51632-2072
712-542-5508
Fax: 712-542-2587
www.alcco.com

Joy Cox, Manager

6527 Elm Crest Retirement Community
2104 12th Street
Harlan, IA 51537-2025
712-755-5174
Fax: 712-755-5654
www.abhomes.net

Tron Dandy, Administrator

6528 Elm Heights Assisted Living
56 Elm St
Topsham, ME 4086
207-725-1134
Fax: 866-531-8540
jill@elmstassistedliving.com
www.elmstassistedliving.com

Jill Wallace, Owner

6529 Fleur Heights Care Center
4911 SW 19th Street
Des Moines, IA 50315-4484
515-285-2559
Fax: 515-285-6487
jstoker@pacificahealth.com
www.pacificahealth.com

John Beaudette, Administrator

6530 Floyd House
403 C Street
Sergeant Bluff, IA 51054
712-943-7025
Fax: 712-943-7172
www.alcco.com/location/floyd-house

Geane Figg, Administrator

6531 Forest Plaza Assisted Living
635 Highway 9 E
Forest City, IA 50436
641-585-1555
Fax: 641-585-2522
lonny@forestplaza.biz
www.forestplaza.biz

Lonny Smith, Owner

6532 Garnett Place
202 35th Street Drive SE
Cedar Rapids, IA 52403-1353
319-362-3630
Fax: 319-365-7936
www.garnettplace.net

Justine Omar, Contact
Melissa Reed, Manager

6533 Glenwood Place
2907 S 6th Street
Marshalltown, IA 50158-4687
641-752-8410
Fax: 641-752-8515
www.glenwoodplaceal.net

Patt Holder, Contact
Amy Edmonson, Manager

6534 Greenfield Manor Assisted Living
615 SE Kent Street
Greenfield, IA 50849-9499
641-743-6131
Fax: 641-343-7090
www.greenfieldiowa.com

Suzie Morgan, Administrator

6535 Hawthorne Inn at Windmill
1500 1st Avenue
Coralville, IA 52241-1192
319-337-6320
Fax: 319-337-3099
www.windmillpointe.net

Anne Stramel, Manager

6536 Heartland Care Center Assisted Living
604 E Fenton Street
Marcus, IA 51035-7170
712-376-2500
Fax: 712-376-2512
www.heartlandcarecenter.com

Luanne Rogge, Administrator

6537 Heritage House
1200 Brookridge Circle
Atlantic, IA 50022-2346
712-243-1850
Fax: 712-243-3418
www.wesleylife.org

Damon Buskohl, Administrator
Bob Johannsen, Executive Director

6538 Holy Spirit
1701 W 25th Street
Sioux City, IA 51103-1705
712-252-2726
Fax: 712-252-2728
www.holyspiritretirementhome.com

Patrick Tomscha, Administrator

6539 Homestead Acres
2306 State Street
Guthrie Center, IA 50115-8896
641-332-2204
Fax: 515-747-8717
www.thenewhomestead.org

Nancy Wells, Social Worker
Barbara Howell, Administrator
Maradith Janssen, Manager

The assisted living offered by Homesteaad Acres provides a community for older adults who want to live an independent lifestyle but need some assistance with life's daily tasks. You will have the security of knowing that certified staff is available 24 hours a day to meet your needs.

We ar pages

6540 Jersey Ridge
5605 Jersey Ridge Road
Davenport, IA 52807-3132
563-355-2027
Fax: 563-441-9227
jrplacemarketing@yahoo.com
www.jerseyridgeplace.com

Karen McCoy, Contact

6541 Jewish Senior Life Center
900 Polk Boulevard
Des Moines, IA 50312-2225
515-255-5433
Fax: 515-255-1920
www.seniorlifecenter.org

Stephen Blend, Executive Director

6542 Kensington
2210 Avenue H
Fort Madison, IA 52627-4000
319-372-4233
Fax: 319-372-7940
rbenda@kensington-evergreen.com
www.kensington-evergreen.com

Rachel Benda, Director

Treating people like family.

6543 Keystone Senior Suites
250 5th Street
Keystone, IA 52249-9521

319-442-3234
Fax: 319-442-3236
www.keystonecarecenter.co

Sue Meyer, Administrator

6544 Lakeview Lodge
312 Southbrooke Drive
Waterloo, IA 50702-5804
319-291-1300
Fax: 319-291-1360
www.friendshipvillageiowa.com

Kathy Martin, Executive Director

6545 Lakeview Village
9100 Park Street
Lenexa, KS 66215
913-888-1900
Fax: 319-622-6458
www.lakeviewvillage.org

Rod Buch, CEO

6546 Lutheran Home Apartments
2421 Lutheran Drive
Muscatine, IA 52761
563-263-1241
Fax: 319-472-3070
www.lutheran-homes.org

Kim Emerick, Administrator

6547 Madison Square Assisted Living
209 W Jefferson Street
Winterset, IA 50273-1676
515-462-5087
Fax: 515-462-5151
www.madisonsquare.iowacare.com

Elecia Henke, Manager

6548 Maple Manor Village
345 Parrott Street
Aplington, IA 50604-1014
319-347-1502
Fax: 319-347-6347
www.abcmcorp.com

Sharon Quail, Administrator

6549 Martina Place
5815 Winwood Drive
Johnston, IA 50131-1666
515-251-7999
Fax: 515-331-8860
glarew@mercydesmoines.org
www.mercydesmoines.org

Sharon Brown, Executive Director

6550 Meadows
200 McCarren Drive
Manchester, IA 52057-1874
563-927-6467
Fax: 563-927-8437
www.goodneighborsociety.org

Elaine Seaman, Operator
Leslie Nussle, Manager

6551 Meadows Assisted Living
528 N Kelly Street
Shell Rock, IA 50670-1006

319-885-4141
Fax: 319-885-6596
Betty.Oren@tealwoodcc.com
www.twdcc.com

Betty Oren, Administrator

6552 Meth-Wick Community
1224 13th Street NW
Cedar Rapids, IA 52405-2499
319-365-9171
Fax: 319-363-5312
www.methwick.org

Robin Mixdorf, President
Ron Jaeger, CFO
Teresa Dusil, Director of Operations

6553 Mill Pond Assisted Living
1201 SE Mill Pond Court
Ankeny, IA 50021-6534
515-964-2273
Fax: 515-965-3100
www.mill-pond.org

Daniel A Lindh, CEO
Mark T Meyer, CFO
Janna R Severance, Secretary

6554 Monticello Nursing and Rehab Center
500 Pinehaven Drive
Monticello, IA 52310-2049
319-465-5415
Fax: 319-524-3001
www.monticellocampus.com

Dave Chensvold, Administrator

6555 Mulberry Place
11 Deborah Drive
Bloomfield, IA 52537-1174
641-664-2523
Fax: 515-664-2929
www.abcmcorp.com

Beth Owens, Administrator

6556 Northern Hills
4002 Teton Trce
Sioux City, IA 51104-4387
712-239-9402
Fax: 712-255-9799
www.northernhills.biz

Gary Troth, Executive Director

6557 Oaknoll Assisted Living
701 Oaknoll Drive
Iowa City, IA 52246-5168
319-351-1720
Fax: 319-351-6772
www.oaknoll.com

Patricia Heiden-Ringham, Executive Director

Our Assisted Living area provides services and programs
that support residents who may need additional assistance
in their daily lives. With the option of assisted living, our
residents will maintain their independence and dignity
while living in their own apartment.

6558 Oakwood Place Assisted Living at Ridgecrest Village
4130 Northwest Boulevard
Davenport, IA 52806-4243
563-391-3430
Fax: 563-388-3287
BMorrison@ridgecrestvillage.org
www.ridgecrestvillage.org

Shelley H Wicks, Administrator
Bert Vigen, Executive Director

Life Care is a unique concept that truly benefits Ridgecrest residents. There is a wonderful peace of mind knowing that although you may not ever need nursing care services, you have immediate access to excellent care...just in case. And you are insulated from escalating private pay charges in a nursing home.

6559 Park Place Estates
900 Lincoln Street NE
Le Mars, IA 51031-3345
712-546-6793
Fax: 712-578-5214
ppe@floydvalleyhospital.org
www.parkplaceestates.org

Judith Roddy, Executive Director

We offer affordable assisted living options for adult seniors who do not require skilled nursing care. Our residents appreciate a secure, comfortable environment with maintenance-free living and the camaraderie of a friendly community.

6560 Perry Lutheran Home Assisted Living
2323 Willis Avenue
Perry, IA 50220-2148
515-465-5342
Fax: 515-465-5344
deb.steadman@perrylutheranhome.org
www.perrylutheranhome.org

Doug Wood, Contact

6561 Premier Estates
1510 S Carroll Street
Rock Rapids, IA 51246-2099
712-472-4100
Fax: 712-472-4231
someone@premierestates.com
www.premierestatesrockrapids.com

Gary Durbin, Administrator

6562 Ramsey Home
1611 27th Street
Des Moines, IA 50310-5499
515-274-3612
Fax: 515-274-8004
www.crmscommunities.com/ramseyvillage

Karen Broman, Administrator

6563 Ridgeway Place
155 E Ridgeway Avenue
Waterloo, IA 50702-5000
319-272-2622
Fax: 319-272-2633
RidgewayPlace@fm-inc.org
www.fm-inc.org/ridgewayplace.html

Colleen O'Connell, Manager

6564 River Hills Village
20 Village Circle
Keokuk, IA 52632-2059
319-524-5772
Fax: 319-524-3001
www.riverhillsvillage.com

Cindy Shriver, Administrator

6565 Riverview Terrace
1301 Saint Luke Drive
Spencer, IA 51301-6043
712-262-5931
Fax: 712-262-4743
www.stlukelh.com

Nancy Ketcham, Executive Director

6566 Senior Suites
4700 84th Street
Urbandale, IA 50322-7352
515-270-9700
Fax: 515-270-9582
www.seniorsuitesofurbandale.com

Demaris Luttengger, Administrator

6567 Silvercrest Ames Assisted Living
1325 Coconino Road
Suite 300
Ames, IA 50014-7842
515-292-2858
Fax: 515-296-2134
www.retirementcommunity.com

Karen Eubank, Executive Director

Independent Living with Assistance:24 Hour Certified Staffing, Restaurant Style Dining, Schedule Transportation, Weekly Housekeeping, Planned Activities and Outings, Secure Enclosed Courtyard, Beauty and Barber Shop, RN Monitoring and Assessment

6568 Silvercrest Assisted Living: Garner Farms
1575 W 53rd Street
Davenport, IA 52806-2448
563-386-9196
Fax: 563-445-7397
www.garnerfarms.com

Pat Day, Owner

We tailor our residents' care plans to provide just the right amount of assistance for a comfortable lifestyle. Services are based on assessment at admission and varying intervals. Type of services include assistance with bathing, dressing, medication, orientation, continence managment and reassurance.

6569 Silvercrest Legacy Pointe
1020 S Scott Boulevard
Iowa City, IA 52240-2944
319-341-0911
Fax: 402-493-8069
www.legacypointeiowa.com

David Burkhart, Manager

Silvercrest Legacy Pointe Assisted Living is thoughtfully designed with an environment of ease with high-standard services and beautiful furnishings. An array of carefully chosen amenities are available to enhance day-to-day living along with social activity and convenient personal services. Our residents can expect to enjoy a quality home-like lifestyle, which recognizes individuality, privacy, choice, and dignity.

6570 Skiff Medical Center Assisted Living
204 N 4th Avenue E
Newton, IA 50208-3135
641-792-1273
Fax: 641-792-4603; *Toll Free:* 888-792-1273
www.skiffmed.com

Patti Hayes, Director
Eric Lothe, CEO

6571 Sunnybrook Assisted Living
3000 W. Madison Ave
Fairfield, IA 52556-4736
641-469-5778
Fax: 641-469-5578
fairfield@sunnybrookseniorliving.com
www.sunnybrookseniorliving.com

Betty D Howell, Administrator

6572 Sunset Park Place
3730 Pennsylvania Avenue
Dubuque, IA 52002-3701
563-583-7939
Fax: 563-365-2982
www.sunsetparkplace.net

Janet Marxen, Contact
Jerry Bell, Manager

6573 Swan House
1024 E 12th Street
Carroll, IA 51401-3913
712-792-6974
Fax: 712-792-9811
swanhouse@alcco.com
www.alcco.com/location/swan-house

Nancy Snyder, Administrator

6574 The Villages at Marion
365 Marion Boulevard
Marion, IA 52302-3139
319-377-9808
Fax: 319-377-9821
info@marionvillages.com
www.marionvillages.com

Sharlynn Page, Marketing Coordinator
Cindy Dason, Executive Director

The Villages at Marion provides senior independent housing (Village Place) and assisted living including Memory Care and Respite care (Village Ridge).

6575 Valley Lodge Assisted Living
12415 N 103rd Ave.
Sun city, AZ 85351
623-933-0137
Fax: 623-933-0130
info@sunvalleylodge.org
www.sunvalleylodge.org

Loretta Frahm, Manager
Year Founded: 1965

6576 Valley View Manor Assisted Living
2421 Lutheran Drive
Muscatine, IA 52761-9382

563-263-1241
Fax: 563-263-5180
www.lutheran-homes.org

Sheryl Wieskamp, Contact
Eric Thomas, Administrator

6577 Waukon Living Center
209 2nd Avenue SW
Waukon, IA 52172-1900
563-568-2915
Fax: 319-245-1684
www.waukonlivingcenter.com

Diane Erickson, Owner

6578 Wel-Life at Alta
705 W 7th Street
Alta, IA 51002-1525
712-200-2620
Fax: 712-286-2620
www.welcov.com

Sheila Thomson, Manager

We are a family-oriented health care provider, dedicated to excellence, whose mission is to enhance the lives of those we serve by providing quality care with respect, dignity and kindness.

6579 Wel-Life at Spirit Lake
1819 23rd Street
Spirit Lake, IA 51360-7096
712-336-3553
Fax: 712-336-4478
www.welcov.com

Kim Ingwersen, Manager

6580 Wesley Acres Memorial Loss Center
3520 Grand Avenue
Des Moines, IA 50312-4359
515-271-6500
Fax: 515-271-6898
www.wesleylife.org

Rob Kretzinger, CEO
Janet Simpson, Administrator

6581 Western Home Communities
420 E 11th Street
5500 S Main Street
Cedar Falls, IA 50613-3364
319-277-2141
Fax: 319-277-5158
www.westernhomecommunities.org

Kris Hansen, CEO
Jerry Harris, COO

A charitable, Christian service organization which assertively seeks to develop fulfilling lifestyles for seniors, their families and the employees. Now serves nearly 800 residdents in villas, town homes, apartments, assisted living and nursing care.

Year Founded: 1912

6582 Willow Pointe
17396 Kingbird Avenue
Mason City, IA 50401-9251
641-423-7722
Fax: 641-421-8078

nursing@willowpointeseniorliving.com
www.willowpointeseniorliving.com

Rick Burke, Contact

Kansas

6583 Alterra Sterling House of Abilene II
1102 N Vine Street
Abilene, KS 67410-4015
877-712-9913
Fax: 785-263-2455; *Toll Free:* 785-263-7800
www.brookdaleliving.com

Alterra Sterling House is an assisted living residence that provides housing and assistance to older adults who want to retain their independence while receiving the daily support they need. The intimate setting for those with limited mobility, as well as specialized programming, help residents maximize independence and quality of life.

6584 Alterra Sterling House of Arkansas
402 E Windsor Road
Arkansas City, KS 67005-3894
877-712-9918
Fax: 620-442-1230
www.brookdaleliving.com

Janice Thomas, Exeuctive Director

Alterra Sterling House is an assisted living residence that provides housing and assistance to older adults who want to retain their independence while receiving the daily support they need. The intimate setting for those with limited mobility, as well as specialized programming, help residents maximize independence and quality of life.

6585 Alterra Sterling House of Derby
1709 East Walnut Grove Rd
Derby, KS 67037-3555
877-713-0924
Fax: 316-788-1239
www.brookdaleliving.com

Bruce Monrue, Executive Director

Alterra Sterling House is an assisted living residence that provides housing and assistance to older adults who want to retain their independence while receiving the daily support they need. The intimate setting for those with limited mobility, as well as specialized programming, help residents maximize independence and quality of life.

6586 Alterra Sterling House of Emporia
1200 W 12th Avenue
Emporia, KS 66801-2557
877-713-0926
Fax: 620-342-2762
www.brookdaleliving.com

Lori Wisdom, Executive Director

Alterra Sterling House is an assisted living residence that provides housing and assistance to older adults who want to retain their independence while receiving the daily support they need. The intimate setting for those with limited mobility, as well as specialized programming, help residents maximize independence and quality of life.

6587 Alterra Sterling House of Fairdale
2251 E Crawford Street
Salina, KS 67401-1317

877-713-0931
Fax: 785-825-8284
www.brookdaleliving.com

Ben Schmitz, Executive Director

6588 Alterra Sterling House of Great Bend
1206 Patton Road
Great Bend, KS 67530-3190
877-713-0957
Fax: 620-792-5955
www.brookdaleliving.com

Jim Herman, Executive Director

Alterra Sterling House is an assisted living residence that provides housing and assistance to older adults who want to retain their independence while receiving the daily support they need. The intimate setting for those with limited mobility, as well as specialized programming, help residents maximize independence and quality of life.

6589 Alterra Sterling House of Hays
1801 E 27th Street
Hays, KS 67601-2136
877-713-0963
Fax: 785-628-0830
www.brookdaleliving.com

Lisa Leiker, Executive Director

Alterra Sterling House is an assisted living residence that provides housing and assistance to older adults who want to retain their independence while receiving the daily support they need. The intimate setting for those with limited mobility, as well as specialized programming, help residents maximize independence and quality of life.

6590 Alterra Sterling House of Junction
1022 Caroline Avenue
Junction City, KS 66441-5230
855-350-3800
Fax: 785-762-6222
www.brookdaleliving.com

Joye Gfeller, Manager

6591 Alterra Sterling House of Lenexa II
8740 Caenen Lake Road
Lenexa, KS 66215-2069
913-894-0014
Fax: 913-894-9147

Deb Hatlestad, Executive Director

6592 Alterra Sterling House of McPherson
1460 N Main Street
McPherson, KS 67460-1917
877-713-1016
Fax: 620-241-7406
www.brookdaleliving.com

Joan Diehl, Executive Diretor

Alterra Sterling House is an assisted living residence that provides housing and assistance to older adults who want to retain their independence while receiving the daily support they need. The intimate setting for those with limited mobility, as well as specialized programming, help residents maximize independence and quality of life.

6593 Alterra Sterling House of Salina
1200 E Kirwin Avenue
Salina, KS 67401-6333

877-713-1869
Fax: 785-825-8284
www.brookdaleliving.com

Christen Robinson, Manager

Alterra Sterling House is an assisted living residence that provides housing and assistance to older adults who want to retain their independence while receiving the daily support they need. The intimate setting for those with limited mobility, as well as specialized programming, help residents maximize independence and quality of life.

6594 Alterra Sterling House of Wichita

918 Midwestern Parkway
Wichita Falls, TX 76302-2110
866-658-2216
Fax: 316-684-6612
www.brookdaleliving.com

Michael Agpoon, Executive Director

Alterra Sterling House is an assisted living residence that provides housing and assistance to older adults who want to retain their independence while receiving the daily support they need. The intimate setting for those with limited mobility, as well as specialized programming, help residents maximize independence and quality of life.

6595 Andover Court Assisted Living

721 W 21st Street
Andover, KS 67002-8491
316-733-2662
Fax: 316-733-6754
www.andovercourtretirement.com

Janet Garretson, General Manager

From around-the-clock nursing services to retirement living, Life Care Centers of America offers a full continuum of care for today's seniors. We also ease the challenges of the caregiver with specialty services such as home care, rehabilitation services and respite care.

6596 Assisted Lifestyles Of KS Inc.

625 N Lincoln Street
Olathe, KS 66061-2501
913-829-6920
Fax: 913-829-6993
www.assistedlifestyles.com

Diane Klemm, Contact/Executive Director
Gary Aull, Owner

43 bed assisted living.

6597 Atria Assisted & Retirement Living

3515 SW 6th Avenue
Topeka, KS 66606-1900
785-783-5894
Fax: 785-234-4002
www.atriaseniorliving.com

Jared Holroyd, Executive Director

6598 Brookside Assisted Living

702 W 7th Street
Overbrook, KS 66524-9496
785-665-3246
Fax: 785-665-3247
www.alfa.org

Scott Averill, Executive Director

6599 Carriage House of Greensburg

723 S Elm Street
Greensburg, KS 67054-1910
620-723-3400
Fax: 620-723-3436
www.lakepointnc.com

Steve Dawson, Administrator

6600 Cedar Lake Village

15325 S Lone Elm Road
Olathe, KS 66061-5416
913-780-9916
Fax: 913-768-8903
info@cedarlakevillagekc.org
www.cedarlakevillagekc.org

Joanna Randall, Executive Director

6601 Cedarview Assisted Living

2929 Sternberg Drive
Hays, KS 67601-2055
785-628-3200
Fax: 316-628-4833
www.cedarviewassistedliving.com

Treva Benoit, Executive Director

6602 Chaucer Estates-Retirement

10550 E 21st St N Unit 404
Wichita, KS 67206-3511
316-630-8111
Fax: 316-630-6193
www.meridiansenior.com

Don Schmidt, Owner

6603 Cornerstone Assisted Living

3750 Lawndale Lane N
Plymouth, MN 55446-0333
763-550-0333
Fax: 316-636-2576
www.elimcare.org

Ellie Garrett, Executive Director

6604 Cornerstone Ridge Plaza

3636 N Ridge Road
Apt 400
Wichita, KS 67205-1221
316-462-3636
Fax: 316-462-3676
Dane.Stember@viachristi.org
www.via-christi.org

Monty Warren, Manager

6605 Elm Grove Estates

2416 Brentwood Street
Hutchinson, KS 67502-5000
913-904-0484
Fax: 620-663-6602
www.emeritus.com

For seniors who want the convenience of retirement community living, for families caring for an aging adult, or for people with Alzheimer's, Elm Grove Estates offers a world of options - all designed to help residents maintain as much independence as possible. There are no hidden costs, buy-in fees or pre-paid leases; everything is included for one monthly fee.

6606 Fort Scott Presbyterian Village
2401 Horton Street
Fort Scott, KS 66701-3178
620-223-5550
Fax: 620-223-7800
www.fortscottpresbyterianvillage.org

Ginger Dierksen, Administrator

6607 Gran Villas-Atchison
1635 Riley Street
Atchison, KS 66002-1518
913-367-2077
Fax: 913-367-1755
www.granvillasatchison.com

Garen Cox, CEO

Offers personal and health care services to a residential environment, assisted living centers enable frail individuals to remain independent and to avoid institutionalization for as long as possible. Offering community living and minimal supervision, assisted living provides the solution for the active senior who should not be living alone.

6608 Gran Villas-Hiawatha
400 Kansas Avenue
Hiawatha, KS 66434-1954
785-742-4566
Fax: 913-742-4573
www.seniorhousingnet.com

Michelle Catrell, Manager

Offers personal and health care services to a residential environment, assisted living centers enable frail individuals to remain independent and to avoid institutionalization for as long as possible. Offering community living and minimal supervision, assisted living provides the solution for the active senior who should not be living alone.

6609 Gran Villas-Neodesha
400 Fir Street
Neodesha, KS 66757-1298
620-325-2244
Fax: 620-325-2762
www.ks-neodesha.doctors.at/dr/gran-villa

Terri Greaves, Manager

Offers personal and health care services to a residential environment, assisted living centers enable frail individuals to remain independent and to avoid institutionalization for as long as possible. Offering community living and minimal supervision, assisted living provides the solution for the active senior who should not be living alone.

6610 Homestead of Auburn Assisted Living
280 Valley Springs Drive
Auburn, KS 66402-9464
785-256-7100
Fax: 785-256-7902
www.midwesthealth.ppi.net

Kate Clemmons, Director

6611 Linwood Place I & II
1509 Linn Street
Valley Falls, KS 66088-1185
888-563-0251
Fax: 785-945-3684
www.assistedlivinginfo.com

Marilyn Zieg, Owner

6612 Meadows
1201 Martindale Street
Burlington, KS 66839-2400
620-364-8861
Fax: 620-364-5504
www.coffeyhealth.org

Elaine Seamen, Manager

6613 Overland Park Place
6555 W 75th Street
Overland Park, KS 66204-3019
913-383-9876
Fax: 913-383-9875
www.overlandparkplace.com

Jennifer Evers, Administrator

6614 Park View Assisted Living
750 N Missouri Street
Ulysses, KS 67880-1868
620-424-2000
Fax: 620-424-3699
www.legacypv.com

Billie Upshaw, Administrator

6615 Redbud Plaza
205 W 9th Street
Onaga, KS 66521-9625
785-889-4142
Fax: 785-889-4172
info@chcsks.org
www.chcs-ks.org

Linda Werren, Executive Director

Redbud Plaza Assisted Living Center is a unique home away from home. It's a warm friendly place with all the comforts of home without worries. Our personal caregivers believe in providing our residents with the very best services. We take pride in giving you the assistance you need and the companionship you desire.

6616 Rolling Hills Assisted Living Apartments
2410 SW Urish Road
Topeka, KS 66614-4347
855-886-4874
Fax: 785-271-2496
www.seniorliving.net

Brian Falk, Administrator

Rolling Hills Assisted Living is home for a group of friendly, retired people who share a desire for independent living with the comfort of 24-hour health care. Residents have independence in their own apartments while enjoying the benefits of many support services.

6617 Shawnee Heartland Assisted Living
16207 Midland Drive
Shawnee, KS 66217-9499
913-248-6600
Fax: 913-789-8989
www.shawneeheartlandal.com

Phyllis Hornbaker, Owner

6618 Twin Oaks Assisted Living
657 W Eisenhower Road
Lansing, KS 66043-2204
877-559-5291
Fax: 913-727-1722
www.seniorliving.net

Debbie Eyerly, Executive Director

Superior care is continued at Twin Oaks Retirement Community with our exceptional Assisted Living facility. Medication assistance, nursing and social services are only some of the needs we assist our residents with every day. Our professional staff includes 24-hour nursing and home health care specialists ready to help each resident.

6619 Vintage Park at Lenexa
8710 Caenen Lake Road
Lenexa, KS 66215-2069
913-894-6979
Fax: 913-894-0901
www.vintageparklenexa.com

Jayne Heilman, Executive Director

6620 Vintage Park of Atchison
1301 N 4th Street
Atchison, KS 66002-1207
913-367-2655
Fax: 913-367-0642
www.vintageparkassistedliving.com

Cindy Weigman, Administrator

Vintage Park Assisted Living offers security, independence, comfort, beautiful surroundings and local worry-free living. Filled with your own furnishings, our home provides a family-oriented atmosphere and peace of mind to those who need some assistance with their activities of daily living.

6621 Vintage Park of Baldwin City
321 Crimson Avenue
Baldwin City, KS 66006-4157
785-594-4255
Fax: 785-594-2280
www.vintageparkassistedliving.com

Sue Brown, Administrator

Vintage Park Assisted Living offers security, independence, comfort, beautiful surroundings and local worry-free living. Filled with your own furnishings, our home provides a family-oriented atmosphere and peace of mind to those who need some assistance with their activities of daily living.

6622 Vintage Park of Gardner
869 S Juniper Ter
Gardner, KS 66030-1468
913-856-7643
Fax: 913-884-4582
www.vintageparkassistedliving.com

Mitzie Terrell, Administrator
Marilyn McDonald, Manager

Vintage Park Assisted Living offers security, independence, comfort, beautiful surroundings and local worry-free living. Filled with your own furnishings, our home provides a family-oriented atmosphere and peace of mind to those who need some assistance with their activities of daily living.

6623 Vintage Park of Louisburg
202 S Rogers Road
Louisburg, KS 66053-4064
913-837-5133
Fax: 913-837-5169
www.vintageparkassistedliving.com

Ava Purvis, Administrator

Vintage Park Assisted Living offers security, independence, comfort, beautiful surroundings and local worry-free living. Filled with your own furnishings, our home provides a family-oriented atmosphere and peace of mind to those who need some assistance with their activities of daily living.

6624 Vintage Park of Paola
601 N East Street
Paola, KS 66071-1183
913-557-0202
Fax: 913-294-5187
www.vintageparkassistedliving.com

Tina Rhoades, Administrator

Vintage Park Assisted Living offers security, independence, comfort, beautiful surroundings and local worry-free living. Filled with your own furnishings, our home provides a family-oriented atmosphere and peace of mind to those who need some assistance with their activities of daily living.

6625 Vintage Place of Derby
1701 Walnut Grove Road
Derby, KS 67037-3528
316-788-9600
Fax: 316-788-9775
www.foundationproperties.net

Lori Mouak, Executive Director

6626 Vyne at Meadows Park
1221 W Maple Street
Wichita, KS 67213-3915
316-729-2400
Fax: 316-729-2403

Shiela Landis, Executive Director

6627 Waterfront Inn Assisted Living
900 N Bayshore Drive
Wichita, KS 67212-4807
316-945-3344
Fax: 316-945-3344
www.vintageparkwaterfront.com

Karen Loy, Manager

6628 Wheat Ridge Acres
707 Wheat Ridge Circle
Goodland, KS 67735-2256
785-899-0100
Fax: 785-899-0277

Donna Swagger, Exective Director

6629 Woodridge Estates
329 Kay Lane
Parsons, KS 67357-3501
620-421-4700
Fax: 620-421-2666

Don Woodworth, Owner

Kentucky

6630 Baptist Homes
489 Castle Shannon Boulevard
Pittsburgh, PA 15234

412-563-6550
Fax: 270-726-4188
www.baptisthomes.org

James B Lewis, President
Amy Arnold, Manager

Our goal is to provide a continuum of quality care to all of our residents through caring, qualified professionals, state-of-the-art facilities and support services

6631 Belmont Village at St Matthews
4600 Bowling Boulevard
Louisville, KY 40207-5155
502-721-7500
Fax: 502-896-8224
www.belmontvillage.com

Sheila Carter, Manager

Located in St. Matthews residential neighborhood of Louisville.

6632 Four Courts Senior Center
2100 Millvale Road
Louisville, KY 40202
502-451-0990
Fax: 502-459-1018
www.shcofcherokeepark.com

Deborah May, Executive Director

Provides the community's seniors with a continuum of care - from personal and intermediate to skilled nursing home care - along with a complete program of activities.

6633 Frontier Nursing Service
132 FNS Drive
Wendover, KY 41775-8921
606-672-2317
Fax: 606-672-3022
fnstours@yahoo.com
www.frontiernursing.org

Barb Gibson, Director

Provides health care to persons in approximately 1000 square miles of eastern Kentucky using a 40-bed hospital, two primary care centers, three rural health clinics, and a home health agency.

6634 Liberty Ridge
701 Liberty Ridge Lane
Lexington, KY 40509-4461
859-543-9449
Fax: 859-543-0059; *Toll Free:* 800-264-0840
www.libertyridge.com

Dan Wilkerson, Executive Director

6635 McCready Manor
300 Stocker Drive
Richmond, KY 40475-4304
859-625-1400
Fax: 606-625-1623
ckelly@standrewsplace.org
www.standrewsplace.org

Gil Shew, Administrator

6636 McDowell Place of Danville
1181 Ben Ali Drive
Danville, KY 40422-8939

859-239-4663
Fax: 859-238-0171
www.emhealth.org

Susan Matherly, Administrator

Our community offers assistance with some daily activities as well as security for your peace of mind and that of your family. McDowell Place of Danville is spacious, comfortable, and finely appointed to make your stay, or that of a loved one, as pleasant as possible.

6637 Morningside Paducah
1700 Elmdale Road
Paducah, KY 42003-5517
270-534-9173
Fax: 270-554-7126
jacksong@lifetrust.com
www.morningsideofpaducah.com

Gerry Jackson, Contact

6638 Morningside of Bowling Green
981 Campbell Lane
Bowling Green, KY 42104-4136
270-746-9600
Fax: 270-842-4104
www.morningsideofbowlinggreen.com

Melissa Kincaid, Executive Director

6639 River's Bend Retirement Community
300 Beech Street
Kuttawa, KY 42055-6214
270-388-2868
Fax: 270-684-6283
www.riversbendrc.org

Tammy Workman, Administrator

6640 Weley Manor
5012 E Manslick Road
Louisville, KY 40219-5100
502-969-3277
Fax: 502-966-0819
www.wesman.org

Jerry L Hoganson,, President

Louisiana

6641 Arbor of Natchitoches
1907 Highway 1 S
Natchitoches, LA 71457
318-356-0016
Fax: 318-323-0016

Angie Ingram, Manager

6642 Arbor of Ruston
4518 Highway 80
Ruston, LA 71270-8952
318-251-3116
Fax: 318-251-3152
information@arborandterraceofruston.com
www.arborandterraceofruston.com

6643 Assisted Living Center at St James Place
333 Lee Drive
Baton Rouge, LA 70808-4980

225-215-4500
Fax: 225-215-4515; *Toll Free:* 800-460-7007
www.stjamesplace.org

Enjoy the freedom to travel, to discover new friendships, to pursue outside interests and personal growth. St. James Place provides a variety of services and amenities that encourage residents to maintain their zest for living active and interesting lives.

6644 Azalea Estates of Gonzales
2305 S Purpera Avenue
Gonzales, LA 70737-5416
225-644-1028
Fax: 225-647-9520; *Toll Free:* 800-567-0650
www.azaleaestates.com

Lorraine Lavigne, Manager

6645 Azalea Estates of Monroe
4380 Old Sterlington Road
Monroe, LA 71203-2359
318-343-1626
Fax: 318-345-4825
www.azaleaestates.com

Bonnie Westmoreland, Executive Director

6646 Azalea Estates of New Iberia
1318 Andre Street
New Iberia, LA 70563-2148
337-364-1695
Fax: 337-367-8280; *Toll Free:* 888-364-1695
www.azaleaestates.com

Christine Thibodeaux, Executive Director

6647 Azalea Estates of Shreveport
516 E Flournoy Lucas Road
Shreveport, LA 71115-3856
318-797-2408
Fax: 317-797-8540
www.azaleaestates.com

Cheryl Foster, Manager

6648 Cornerstone Village
103 W Martial Avenue
Lafayette, LA 70508-6719
337-981-5335
Fax: 337-269-1255

Lance Linscombe, Administrator

6649 Cornerstone Village South
103 W Martial Avenue
Lafayette, LA 70508-6719
337-981-5335
Fax: 337-981-0775

Lance Linscombe, Administrator

6650 Grand Cove
1525 W McNeese Street
Lake Charles, LA 70605-4293
337-474-6000
Fax: 337-478-7522
www.grandcovecenter.com

Randy Stelly, Administrator

6651 Haven at Windermere
8225 Ymca Plaza Drive
Baton Rouge, LA 70810

225-769-9996
Fax: 225-819-1334
lisa.kirby@thehavenbr.com
www.thehavenbr.com

Annette Willis, Contact
Thomas Elkins, Owner

6652 Kingsley Place at Alexandria
351 Windermere Boulevard
Alexandria, LA 71303-2600
225-036- 349
Fax: 318-443-2366
www.emeritus.com

Judy White, Executive Director

6653 Kingsley Place at Lafayette
215 W Farrel Road
Lafayette, LA 70508-7019
504-335-2796
Fax: 337-993-0071
www.emeritus.com

Madeline Husband-Ardoin, Executive Director

6654 Kingsley Place at Shreveport
7110 University Drive
Shreveport, LA 71105-5034
504-335-2794
Fax: 318-524-2300
www.emeritus.com

Bridget Lyman, Executive Director

If your loved one has difficulties with bathing, dressing, remembering medications or has memory impairment, a retirement community may not offer enough support, a nursing home may be too much care and home health may lack a sense of community or social interaction. Assisted Living often offers just the right amount of care in the right type of setting.

6655 Lakewood Quarters Retirement Community
8585 Summa Avenue
Baton Rouge, LA 70809
225-767-7877
Fax: 225-767-7807
www.azaleaestates.com

Regina McMakin, Admissions
Terri Achette, Executive Director

Lakewood Quarters is a retirement living community, especially designed to combine independence with individualized assistance. When residents begin relying on family or friends for added support for everyday activities, the home-like setting of Lakewood Quarters can provide a welcome alternative. Lakewood also offers a secure Alzheimer's wing to the retirement community.

6656 Live Oak Village of Slidell
2200 Gause Boulevard E
Slidell, LA 70461-4223
985-781-4545
Fax: 985-781-8786
LiveOakSlidell.DCR@SlidellSeniorLiving.com
www.slidellseniorliving.com

Tara Picou, Administrator

Our Principles of Service are encouraging independence, enabling freedom of choice, preserving dignity, celebrating individuality, nurturing the spirit and involving family and friends. All Sunrise team members are trained to provide services and care in a manner that supports these principles and furthers Sunrise's mission.

6657 Maison Oaks Assisted Living
504 W 5th Street
La Place, LA 70068-3940
985-653-8858
Fax: 225-652-9583
www.twinoaksnursing.com

Guy Birch, Administrator

6658 Montclair Park Assisted Living
9100 E Kings Highway
Shreveport, LA 71115-2766
318-797-1114
Fax: 318-797-1158
www.montclair-park.com

David Abdehou, Contact
Melanie Bond, Executive Director

6659 Oakmont Estate
204 Cocoville Road
Mansura, LA 71350-4266
318-240-7424
Fax: 877-280-0573
oestates@bellsouth.net
www.oakmontassistedliving.com

Joseph Loughman, Contact

6660 Oakwood Village
4400 McHugh Road
Zachary, LA 70791-5324
225-658-8888
Fax: 225-658-8211
www.oakwood-living.com

Milton Ourso, Owner

Our mission is to serve older or infirm persons through loving, caring Christian communities, respinding to thier physical, social, emotional, intellectual and spiritual needs, and to encourage a sense of independence, individuality, dignity and worth throughout life.

6661 Pratt-Stanton Manor
1224 Saint Charles Avenue
New Orleans, LA 70130-4396
504-525-0895
Fax: 504-525-0895

Michael Calhoun, Executive Director

6662 Regency Place
14333 Old Hammond Highway
Baton Rouge, LA 70816-1146
225-272-1401
Fax: 225-527-2933
gsider@cypresshealthgroup.com
www.cypresshealthcare.net

Heather Marsh, Marketing Executive

6663 Rosewood Retirement & Assisted Living Community
203 Rue Fountaine
Lafayette, LA 70508-5775
337-981-0333
Fax: 337-988-1706
www.rosewoodretirement.com

Nicol Hannie, Owner

6664 Russ House
165 Jefferson Avenue
Ruston, LA 71270-7067
318-251-9068
Fax: 318-251-9060
www.alcco.com

Claire Givens, Executive Director

6665 Southside Gardens Assisted Living Center
4536 Perkins Road
Baton Rouge, LA 70808-3057
225-928-1600
Fax: 225-922-9945
www.southsidegardens.com

Becky Gammon, Executive Director

6666 St Francis Villa Assisted Living
10411 Jefferson Highway
New Orleans, LA 70123-1865
504-738-1060
Fax: 504-738-9870
rhyman@stfrancisvilla.com
www.stfrancisvilla.com

Greg Deris, Owner

6667 St Joesph Manor
1201 Cardinal Drive
Thibodaux, LA 70301-4880
985-446-9050
Fax: 985-449-0047
www.stjosephmanor.org

Rev. Msgr. F Amedee, Executive Director
Jerald P Block, President

6668 Summerville at Kenner
1600 Joe Yenni Boulevard
Kenner, LA 70065-1380
504-704-5136
Fax: 504-467-1017
www.emeritus.com

Deeni Shannon, CEO

6669 Sunrise Assisted Living of Baton Rouge
8502 Jefferson Highway
Baton Rouge, LA 70809-2230
225-932-9400
Fax: 255-932-9409
www.sunriseseniorliving.com

Sally King, Executive Director

6670 Terrace of Shreveport
8950 E Kings Highway
Shreveport, LA 71115-2704
318-323-2115
Fax: 318-323-6281

6671 Terreboone House
1163 Museum Drive
Houma, LA 70360-5910
985-580-0620
Fax: 985-223-4502
www.alcco.com

Jessica Ledt, Executive Director

6672 Village in the Oaks
75520 Highway 1081
Covington, LA 70435-2604
985-871-0111
Fax: 985-875-0009
www.villageintheoaks.com

Myriam Ruppel, Director
Donna Baldus, Manager

Independent and assisted living retirement community.

6673 Ville Ste Marie Senior Living Community
4112 Jefferson Highway
Jefferson, LA 70121-1500
504-834-3164
Fax: 504-849-0608
vsmseniors@aol.com
www.VilleSteMarie.com

Aurora Alleman, Marketing/Community Relations
Barbara Eschete, General Manager

87 unit independent and assisted living complex.

6674 Willamsburg Senior Living Community
5445 Government Street
Baton Rouge, LA 70806-6000
225-929-8917
Fax: 225-928-3284
www.williamsburgseniorlivingcommunity.co

Dwyane Disotell, Manager

6675 Windsor Senior Living Community
1770 N Causeway Boulevard
Mandeville, LA 70471-3168
985-624-8040
Fax: 985-624-8822
www.windsorseniorliving.com

Sondra Bellott, Administrator

Maryland

6676 Asbury Methodist Village
201 Russell Avenue
Gaithersburg, MD 20877-2801
301-216-4103
Fax: 301-216-4392
www.asburymethodistvillage.org

Edwin D Thomas III, CEO

6677 Blossom Place at Edenton
5901 Genesis Lane
Frederick, MD 21703-5104
301-694-7813
Fax: 301-694-0745

Rayann Butler, Administrator

6678 Brighton Gardens at Friendship Heights
5555 Friendship Boulevard
Chevy Chase, MD 20815-7243
301-656-1900
Fax: 301-656-5840
www.sunriseseniorliving.com

Jim Hackett, Executive Director

6679 Brighton Gardens of Columbia
7110 Minstrel Way
Columbia, MD 21045-5426
410-884-0773
Fax: 410-884-0776
www.sunriseseniorliving.com

Steve Gaylor, Manager

6680 Buckinghams Choice
3200 Baker Circle
Adamstown, MD 21710-9653
301-874-5630
Fax: 301-631-5491; *Toll Free:* 800-409-6111
Fullerd@emaseniorcare.org
www.emaseniorcare.org

Donna M Fuller, Director Marketing
Collier Baird, Executive Director

Continuing care retirement community.

6681 Byron House
9210 Kentsdale Drive
Potomac, MD 20854-4529
301-469-9400
Fax: 301-765-8112
www.victoryhousing.org

Sharon Borowiec, Manager

6682 Copper Ridge
710 Obrecht Road
Sykesville, MD 21784-7650
410-795-8808
Fax: 410-795-8893; *Toll Free:* 800-531-6539
www.copperidge.org

Cheryl Fisher, Director Addmissions
Marcie Koenig, Executive Director

Dedicated exclusively to care for persons with Alzheimer's disease and dementia.

6683 Edenwald Retirement Community
800 Southerly Road
Towson, MD 21286-8403
410-339-6000
Fax: 410-823-1845
marketing@edenwald.org
www.edenwald.org

Diana Fusting, Marketing Director
Sal Molite Jr, President
Anne Almirovdis

Continuing care retirement community.

6684 General German Aged Peoples Home
800 Southerly Road
Towson, MD 21286-8403
410-823-1341
Fax: 410-583-8786
www.edenwald.org

Sal Molite Jr, President

6685 Heartfields Hall at Heartlands
3004 N Ridge Road
Ellicott City, MD 21043-3381
Fax: 410-461-8233; *Toll Free:* 888-461-9494
www.heartlandsseniorlivingvillage.com

Joyce Marier, Marketing Director
Nanci Target, Executive Director
Debbie Davis

Heartlands Senior Living Village is a rental retirement community that offers full continuum of care, including independent living apartments, cottages and assisted living suites. Heartlands' features and amenities are bound to keep you vigorous with a great activities program, indoor swimming pool, onsite Wellness Center and the taste of delightful restaurant style dishes prepared by our experienced chefs.

6686 Heartfields at Frederick
1820 Latham Drive
Frederick, MD 21701-9395
301-663-8800
Fax: 301-663-8801
www.heartlandsseniorlivingvillage.com

Heather Junta, Executive Director

6687 Hearthhomes Resedence Bay Ridge I
3023a Arundel on the Bay Road
Annapolis, MD 21403-4301
410-974-8208
Fax: 410-974-8210
lkat@hearthomesassistedliving.com.
www.hearthomesassistedliving.com

Lakeshia Hooper, Administrator

6688 Hearthhomes Residence Piney Orchard
8735 Piney Orchard Parkway
Odenton, MD 21113-2245
410-695-0366
Fax: 410-695-0286
www.hearthomesassistedliving.com

Jaime Weyaled, Owner

6689 Hillhaven Assisted Living
3210 Powder Mill Road
Adelphi, MD 20783-1029
301-937-3939
Fax: 301-937-8798
www.hillhaven.com

Joyce Milin, President

6690 Homewood at Crumland Farms
7407 Willow Road
Frederick, MD 21702-2500
301-694-7292
Fax: 301-293-6331
www.homewood.com

Eric Nichols, Manager

6691 Homewood of Williamsport
16505 Virginia Avenue
Williamsport, MD 21795-1321
301-582-1472
Fax: 301-582-1805
www.homewood.com

Richard Lenehan, Executive Director
Anne Whitman, Director Marketing

Continuing care retirement community offering independent cottages and apartments, assisted living and nursing care.

6692 Independence Court of Hyattsville
5821 Queens Chapel Road
Hyattsville, MD 20782-3867
301-699-7900
Fax: 301-864-9514
www.independencecourt.com

Yveonne Coram, Administrator

6693 Kensington Park Woodlands-Groves
3620 Littledale Road
Kensington, MD 20895-3434
301-946-7700
Fax: 301-929-4030
marketing@kensingtonretirement.com
www.kensingtonretirement.com

George Oxx, Executive Director

6694 Lifesprings Eldercare I
4107 Buck Creek Road
Temple Hills, MD 20748-4930
301-449-0322
Fax: 301-449-0046
info@lifespringelderacre.com
www.lifespringseldercare.com

Faye Hutchinson, Owner

6695 Oakcrest Village
8800 Walther Boulevard
Parkville, MD 21234-9001
800-918-7135
Fax: 410-665-7481
www.ericksonliving.com

Gary Hibbs, Executive Director

6696 Renaissance Gardens at Charlestown
709 Maiden Choice Lane
Catonsville, MD 21228-3632
410-737-8922
Fax: 410-737-8817
www.thecareexperts.com

Taryn Toman, Health Care Counselor
Michael Conord, Manager

Features all private Assisted Living apartments and private and semi-private Long-Term Care rooms; full-time, on-site staff doctors with nurses on duty 24-hours a day. Short-Term Rehab (physical, speech and occupational therapy); dementia and Alzheimer's care also available. Renaissance Gardens, the choice you can feel good about.

6697 Renaissance Gardens at Oak Crest
8832 Walther Boulevard
Parkville, MD 21234-9020
410-882-3295
Fax: 410-657-3545
www.thecareexperts.com

Randi Bershak, Health Care Counselor
Mark Erickson, Executive Director

Features all private Assisted Living apartments and all private Long-Term Care rooms; full-time, on-site staff doctors with nurses on duty 24-hours a day. Short-Term Rehab (physical, speech and occupational therapy); dementia and Alzheimer's care also available. Renaissance Gardens, the choice you can feel good about.

6698 Renaissance Gardens at Riderwood
3160 Gracefield Road
Silver Spring, MD 20904-1986
301-572-8420
Fax: 301-572-8416
www.thecareexperts.com

Elena Price, Health Care Counselor
Timothy Sanna, Manager

Features all private Assisted Living apartments and all private Long-Term Care rooms; full-time, on-site staff doctors with nurses on duty 24-hours a day. Short-Time Rehab (physical, speech and occupational therapy); dementia and Alzheimer's care also available. Renaissance Gardens, the choice you can feel good about.

6699 Ronald Park Place
830 W 40th Street
Baltimore, MD 21211-2116
410-243-5800
Fax: 401-243-4929
www.rolandparkplace.org

John R Collins, Financial Officer
Daniel S Hudson, Managing Principal

Massachusetts

6700 Alden Place
391 Alden Road
Fairhaven, MA 02719-4405
508-994-9238
Fax: 508-994-9239

Susan Mosher, Executive Director

6701 Allerton House at Central Park
43 School House Road
Weymouth, MA 02188-4142
781-335-8666
Fax: 781-335-7666
aewing@welchhrg.com
www.welchhrg.com

Albert C Ewing Jr, Marketing Director

6702 Allerton House at Hancock Park
164 Parkingway Street
Quincy, MA 02169-5020
617-471-2600
Fax: 617-773-1115
krichards@welchhrg.com
www.welchhrg.com

Kelly Richards, Marketing Director

6703 Allerton House at Harbor Park
15 Condito Road
Hingham, MA 02043-1753
781-749-3322
Fax: 781-749-3330
ctaylor@welchhrg.com
www.welchhrg.com

Carol Taylor, Marketing Director

6704 Allerton House at the Village at Duxbury
290 Kingstown Way
Duxbury, MA 02332-4635
781-585-7136
Fax: 781-582-2274

IOsadcia@villageatduxbury.com
www.welchhrg.com

Irene O Sadcia, Marketing Director

6705 Arbors at Amherst
130 University Drive
Amherst, MA 01002-2296
413-548-6800
Fax: 413-548-6888
amherst@arborsassistedliving.com
www.arborsassistedliving.com

Carol Gianthetti, Executive Director

6706 Artia in Falmouth
339 Gifford Street
Falmouth, MA 02540-2913
508-444-0340
Fax: 508-548-2996
www.atriaseniorliving.com

Joan Houlihan, Manager

6707 Atrium at Cardinal Drive
153 Cardinal Drive
Agawam, MA 01001-2182
413-342-1329
Fax: 413-821-9912
www.atriumatcardinaldrive.com

6708 Atrium at Drum Hill Alzheimer's Dementia Assisted Living
2 Technology Drive
N Chelmsford, MA 01863-2400
978-674-5295
Fax: 978-934-0022
www.atriumatcardinaldrive.com

Susan Antkowiak, Admissions Director
Avril Taylor, Admissions Coordinator
Joanne Thomas

The Atrium is a specifically designed assisted living facility exclusively for those with Alzheimer's Disease, dementia and related memory impairments. Within our safe and secure environment, Alzheimer specific activity programs promote resident's functional abilities, well-being and happiness. Our trained staff provide each resident with 24-hour assistance and supervision with daily living needs.

6709 Atrium at Faxon Woods
2003 Falls Boulevard
Quincy, MA 02169-8202
617-237-6370
Fax: 671-471-6335
www.atriumatcardinaldrive.com

Susan Loiurio, Manager

6710 Atrium at Veronica Drive
1 Veronica Drive
Danvers, MA 01923-5213
978-705-1322
Fax: 978-646-9393
www.atriumatcardinaldrive.com

Jan Chiampa, Executive Director

6711 Avery Crossing
110 West Street
Needham, MA 02494-1399

781-444-6655
Fax: 781-444-2794
www.averycrossings.com

Elayne Labrecque, Executive Director

6712 Bertram House of Swampscott
565 Humphrey Street
Swampscott, MA 01907-2600
781-595-1991
Fax: 781-595-1999
www.sunriseseniorliving.com

Walter Berdachowski, Executive Director

6713 Billerica Crossings
20 Charnstaff Lane
Billerica, MA 01821-6702
978-600-8503
Fax: 978-667-0890
www.billericacrossings.com

Sarah Barber, Executive Direcctor

6714 Briarwood Continuing Care Retirement Community
65 Briarwood Circle
Worcester, MA 01606-1249
508-852-2670
Fax: 508-856-0309
caking@briarwoodsl.com
www.briarwoodretirement.com

Paul Bowler, CEO

6715 Cadbury Commons at Cambridge
66 Sherman Street
Cambridge, MA 02140-3527
617-868-0575
Fax: 617-868-0023
www.cadburycommons.com

Steve Elswig, Executive Director

6716 Cambridge Homes
360 Mount Auburn Street
Cambridge, MA 02138-5599
617-876-0369
Fax: 617-876-6432
info@thecambridgehomes.org
www.seniorlivingresidences.com

Helene Quinn, Executive Direcctor

6717 Cameron House
109 Housatonic Street
Lenox, MA 01240-2633
413-637-3100
Fax: 413-525-8153

Barbara Comalli, Executive Director

6718 Carmel Terrace
933 Central Street
Framingham, MA 01701-4813
508-788-8000
Fax: 508-626-1603
www.carmelterrace.org

Sister Gustin, Executive Director

6719 Chelmsford Crossings
199 Chelmsford Street
Chelmsford, MA 01824-2306
978-250-8855
Fax: 978-250-2750
www.chelmsfordcrossings.com

Margaret Palm, Executive Director

6720 Christopher Heights Assisted Living
20 Mary Scano Drive
Worcester, MA 01605-2892
508-792-1456
Fax: 508-792-3156
www.christopherheights.com

Wendi B Willette, Executive Director

6721 Christopher Heights of Webster
Thompson Road
Webster, MA 01570
508-949-0400
Fax: 508-792-3156
www.christopherheights.com

Thomas McMullen, Executive Director

6722 Cohen Florence Levine Estates
201 Captains Row
Chelsea, MA 02150-4068
617-887-0826
Fax: 617-884-8661
info@chelseajewish.org
www.florencechafetzhome.org

Betsy Mullen, Executive Director

6723 Concord Park Assisted Living
68 Commonwealth Avenue
Concord, MA 01742-2967
978-369-4728
Fax: 978-369-5381
info@concordpark.net
www.seniorlivingresidences.com

Nancy Crowley, Manager

6724 Country Club Heights
3 Rehabilitation Way
Woburn, MA 01801-6050
781-935-4094
Fax: 781-938-5571; *Toll Free:* 800-533-0861
galles@bvsl.net
www.woburnma.brightviewseniorliving.com

Daniella Guarracino, Manager

6725 Davis Manor
200 Harvard Road
Lancaster, MA 01523-2505
978-368-6590
Fax: 781-368-6590
www.davismanor.org

Sharon Brennan, Director

6726 Decatur House
176 Main Street
Sandwich, MA 02563-2269
508-888-6404
Fax: 508-833-2781
decatur@decaturhouse.com
www.decaturhouse.com

Linda Austin, Executive Director

6727 Draper Place at Hopedale
25 Hopedale Street
Hopedale, MA 01747-1734
508-876-2833
Fax: 508-482-0600; *Toll Free:* 800-854-0576
www.atriaseniorliving.com

Brian Pillo, Manager

6728 Emmanuel House Residence
25 E Nilsson Street
Brockton, MA 02301-6604
508-588-5334
Fax: 508-588-8775
www.emmanuelhs.org

Sara Goverman, Executive Director

6729 Falls at Cordingly Dam
2300 Washington Street
Newton, MA 02462-1472
617-454-4808
Fax: 617-928-0697
www.fallsatcordinglydam.com

Susan Cwieka, Executive Director

6730 Forge Hill Senior Living Community
4 Forge Hill Road
Franklin, MA 02038-3162
508-570-2192
Fax: 508-541-6591
www.forgehill.com

Carol O'Connor, Marketing Director
Arlene Lowney, Executive Director

Independent assisted living mamory impaired program.

6731 Gabriel House of Fall River
261 Oliver Street
Fall River, MA 02724-2917
888-563-0251
Fax: 508-677-2973
www.assistedlivinginfo.com

Dennis Etzkorn, Manager

6732 Goddard House in Brookline
165 Chestnut Street
Brookline, MA 02445-7573
617-731-8500
Fax: 617-731-5188
info@goddardhouse.org
www.goddardhouse.org

Nancy Shapiro, Executive Director

6733 Grace Morgan House
489 Prospect Street
Methuen, MA 01844-7511
978-682-4324
Fax: 978-682-4802
www.gracemorganhouse.com

Scott Erickson, Owner

6734 Grey & Emil Eisenber Assisted Living Residence
631 Salisbury Street
Worcester, MA 01609-1120

508-757-0981
Fax: 508-757-7080
www.eisenbergal.com

Steve Willens, Chief Executive Officer

6735 Grove Manor Estates Assisted Living
160 Grove Street
Braintree, MA 02184-7216
781-843-3700
Fax: 781-843-3744
info@assistedlivingfacilitybraintree.com
www.assistedlivingfacilitybraintree.com

Anthony Franchi Jr, Owner

6736 Harbor Point at Centerville
22 Richardson Road
Centerville, MA 02632-2453
508-827-2422
Fax: 508-862-9887
www.harborpointatcenterville.com

Jamie Matthews, Executive Director

6737 Haverhill Crossings
254 Amesbury Road
Haverhill, MA 01830-2348
978-228-5039
Fax: 978-556-1601
www.haverhillcrossings.com

Shelli Hermance, Executive Director

6738 Hearthstone at New Horizons
400 Hemenway Street
Marlborough, MA 01752-6771
508-460-5000
Fax: 580-460-0270
www.countrycommunities.com

Maureen Diana, Executive Director

6739 Heatherwood Assisted Living
100 Heatherwood
Yarmouth Port, MA 02675-1444
508-362-4400
Fax: 508-375-0479; *Toll Free:* 800-852-0365
info@heatherwoodsenior.com
www.heatherwoodsenior.com

Bob La Crosse, Manager

6740 Henrietta Brewer House
11 Macs Lane
Vineyard Haven, MA 02568-5573
508-693-4500
Fax: 508-693-5754
hbhi@comcast.net
www.henriettabrewerhouse.com

Ellen Gerstmar, Owner

6741 Heritage Woods Assisted Living
462 Main Street
Agawam, MA 01001-1869
413-786-9704
Fax: 413-789-8366
genesishcc.com

Theresa Bollea, Executive Director

Offers a dynamic lifestyle that promotes mind, body and spirit wellness to maximize independence. Has been registered with The Eden Alternative longer than any other assisted living community in the country.

6742 Heritage at Cleveland Circle
50 Sutherland Road
Brighton, MA 02135-7132
617-396-4031
Fax: 617-566-1752
www.chestnutparkatclevelandcircle.com

Neil Tockman, President

6743 Heritage at Danvers
9 Summer Street
Danvers, MA 01923-1558
978-705-1330
Fax: 978-774-5454
www.putnamfarm-danvers.com

Chris Sintros, Manager

6744 Heritage at Falmouth
140 Ter Heun Drive
Falmouth, MA 02540-2531
508-457-6400
Fax: 508-457-6437
www.capecodhealth.org

Margret Corrideau, Manager

6745 Heritage at Framingham
747 Water Street
Framingham, MA 01701-3208
508-788-6050
Fax: 508-788-6601
www.heritageassistedliving.com

Ellen Adam, Executive Director

6746 Heritage at North Andover
700 Chickering Road
North Andover, MA 1845
978-291-5071
Fax: 978-683-0330
www.ashlandfarmatnorthandover.com

Steve Ostrander, Executive Director

6747 Herrick House
89 Herrick Street
Beverly, MA 01915-2767
978-922-1999
Fax: 978-922-3402
www.theherrickhouse.org

Sandra Earl, Executive Director

6748 Landmark at Fall River
400 Columbia Street
Fall River, MA 02721-1500
508-324-7960
Fax: 508-324-7961
www.landmarkseniorliving.com

Kathleen Cardenas, Executive Director

6749 Landmark at Ocean View
3 Essex Street
Beverly, MA 01915-4527
978-927-4227
Fax: 978-921-4885
www.landmarkseniorliving.com

Gayel Cote, Marketing Director
Steve Galante, Executive Director

6750 Leominster Crossings
1160 Main Street
Leominster, MA 01453-8709
978-751-3230
Fax: 978-537-2421
www.leominstercrossings.com

Thomas Burns, Executive Director

6751 Longmeadow Place at Burlington
42 Mall Road
Burlington, MA 01803-4568
781-995-2842
Fax: 781-270-9009; Toll Free: 800-854-0576
www.atriasseniorliving.com

Kellie McHugh, Executive Director

6752 Longwood Place at Reading
75 Pearl Street
Reading, MA 01867-2689
781-944-9200
Fax: 781-942-3833
info@longwoodplaceatreading.com
www.longwoodplaceatreading.com

Frank Petras, Executive Director

6753 Manor on the Hill
450 N Main Street
Leominster, MA 01453-5499
978-537-1661
Fax: 978-840-3341
manoronthehill1@aol.com
www.manoronthehill.com

Bharti Bhakta, Administrator
Pauls Doucet, Director

Provides residents with a level of service that continually exceeds their expectations. Believes in offering a variety of tools and supportive services designed to meet each individual's needs so that the residents can maintain maximum independence and personal dignity.

6754 Maplewood Place at Malden
295 Broadway
Malden, MA 02148-4535
781-218-3308
Fax: 781-324-5335; Toll Free: 800-854-0576
www.atriasseniorliving.com

Sara Rizzari, Executive Director

6755 Marina Place at Quincy
4 Seaport Drive
North Quincy, MA 02171-1591
617-830-7921
Fax: 617-770-3682; Toll Free: 800-854-0576
www.atriasseniorliving.com

Maria Lastoria, Executive Director

6756 Marland Place at Andover
15 Stevens Street
Andover, MA 01810-3599
978-357-8628
Fax: 978-475-5818; Toll Free: 800-854-0576
www.atriasseniorliving.com

Marilyn Stasonis, Executive Director

6757 Marriott Mapleridge of Plymouth
97 Warren Avenue
Plymouth, MA 02360-2425
508-746-9733
Fax: 508-746-9683
www.caremavens.com

Karen Foley, Executive Director

6758 Mason Wright Retirement Community
74 Walnut Street
Springfield, MA 01105-2179
413-733-1517
Fax: 413-747-8357
www.masonwright.org

Lisa Walters Vucco, Manager

6759 Mayflower Place
579 Buck Island Road
W Yarmouth, MA 02673-3200
508-790-0200
Fax: 508-790-0004
www.mayflowerplace.com

Peg Holmes, Executive Director

6760 Meadow Lodge at Drum Hill
4 Technology Drive
N Chelmsford, MA 01863-2438
985-377-1621
Fax: 978-453-9143
www.emeritus.com

Evelyn Whiteway, Executive Director

6761 Merrimack Place
85 Storey Avenue
Newburyport, MA 01950-3571
978-378-3276
Fax: 978-462-7325; *Toll Free:* 800-854-0576
www.atriaseniorliving.com

Donna Byrnes, Executive Director

6762 New Horizons at Choate
21 Warren Avenue
Woburn, MA 01801-4981
781-932-8000
Fax: 781-938-8355
nhc@cummings.com
www.newhorizonsatchoate.org

Christine Coakley, Executive Dirctor

6763 New Horizons at Marlboro
400 Hemenway Street
Marlborough, MA 01752-6771
508-460-5000
Fax: 508-460-7682
www.countrycommunities.com

Robert O'Connor, Manager

6764 New Pond Village
180 Main Street
Walpole, MA 02081-4020
508-660-1555
Fax: 508-668-8893
pwelsh@bvsl.net
www.norwoodma.brightviewseniorliving.com

Peter Welsh, President

6765 Norumbega Point at Weston
99 Norumbega Road
Weston, MA 02493-2482
781-899-5505
Fax: 781-899-3673
info@norumbegapoint.com
www.norumbegapoint.com

Betsy O'Brien, Executive Director

6766 Orchard Hill At Sudbury
761 Boston Post Road
Sudbury, MA 01776-3384
978-443-0080
Fax: 978-443-7277
www.orchard-hill.com

Clifford T Hughes, Owner

Orchard Hill of Sudbury is a small, unique privately owned home-like setting on a ten acre site near the historic Wayside Inn. The award winning, elegant, farmhouse style mansion house has spacious studio and 1 bedroom apartments in the midst of beautifully landscaped grounds and an orchard bordered by a stream and surrounded by neighborhoods. A full range of personal care services for the health and wellness needs of individuals is included in the base monthly fee. Orchard HIll is the first assisted living in MA to offer a telehealth kiosk that monitors health parameters and transmits the health data directly to the residents' physicians, helping to reduce the number of hospitalizations.

6767 Orchard Valley at Wilbraham
2387 Boston Road
Wilbraham, MA 01095-1246
413-366-1794
Fax: 413-596-4181
www.orchardvalleyatwilbraham.com

Nancy Harper, Manager

6768 Pinehill at Kimball Farms
235 Walker Street
Lenox, MA 01240-2762
413-637-7000
Fax: 413-637-7277
www.kimballfarms.org

Albert Ingegni, Executive Director

6769 Pines of Tewksbury
2580 Main Street
Tewksbury, MA 01876-3155
978-657-0800
Fax: 978-657-8087
www.tewksbury.patch.com

Jennifer King, Executive Director

6770 Plymouth Crossings
157 South Street
Plymouth, MA 02360-7605
508-503-1457
Fax: 508-830-4748
www.plymouthcrossings.com

Susan Lubke, Executive Director

6771 Renaissance Gardens at Brooksby Village
400 Brooksby Village Drive
Peabody, MA 01960-1447

978-536-7920
Fax: 978-536-7922
www.thecareexperts.com

Deb Laflamme, Health Care Counselor

Features all private Assisted Living apartments and all private Long-Term Care rooms; full-time, on-site staff doctors with nurses on duty 24-hours a day. Short-Time Rehab (physical, speech and occupational therapy); dementia and Alzheimer's care also available. Renaissance Gardens, the choice you can feel good about.

6772 Ruth's House

780 Converse Street
Longmeadow, MA 01106-1719
413-567-6212
Fax: 413-567-4380
info@jewishgeriatric.org
www.jewishgeriatric.org

Linda Donoghue, Manager

6773 Salisbury Assisted Living Center

19 Beach Road
Salisbury, MA 01952-2014
978-463-9809
Fax: 978-463-3009
www.assistedlivingcenter.org

Arthur Signorelli, President

6774 Sarawood Retirement Home

1 Loomis Avenue
Holyoke, MA 01040-2000
413-532-7879
Fax: 413-535-2015
www.sarawood.net

William G Lyons, Owner

6775 Scandinavian Living Center

206 Waltham Street
Newton, MA 02465-1733
617-527-6566
Fax: 617-527-2078
www.slcenter.org

Joseph Carella, Executive Director

6776 Shrewsbury Crossing

311 Main Street
Shrewsbury, MA 01545-2298
508-925-7791
Fax: 508-845-2101
www.shrewsburycrossings.com

Robert Moran, Executive Director

6777 Southgate at Shrewsbury

30 Julio Drive
Shrewsbury, MA 01545-3054
508-842-8331
Fax: 508-842-8331
www.southgateatshrewsbury.com

Donald Flanagan, President

6778 Springhouse Retirement Community

46 Allandale Street
Boston, MA 02130-3466
617-522-0043
Fax: 617-522-0893

cgulman@springhouseboston.org
www.springhouseinfo.org

Catherine Gulman, Marketing Director
Kathy Foley, Executive Director

6779 Standish Village at Lower Mills

1190 Adams Street
Dorchester Center, MA 02124-5772
617-298-5656
Fax: 617-298-2508
www.seniorlivingresidences.com

Kim Diaz, Executive Director

6780 Sunrise Assisted Living at Gardner Park

73 Margin Street
Peabody, MA 01960-1877
978-532-3200
Fax: 978-532-3211
www.sunriseseniorliving.com

Carol Styczo, Executive Director

6781 Sunrise Assisted Living of Cohasset

125 King Street
Cohasset, MA 02025-1364
781-383-6300
Fax: 781-383-2830
www.sunriseseniorliving.com

Denise Baxter, Executive Director

6782 Sunrise Assisted Living of Norwood

86 Saunders Road
Norwood, MA 02062-3249
781-762-1333
Fax: 781-255-7493
www.sunriseseniorliving.com

Patricia Blackburn, Executive Director

6783 Sunrise Assisted Living of Wayland

285 Commonwealth Road
Wayland, MA 01778-5042
508-652-6300
Fax: 508-655-6608
www.sunriseseniorliving.com

Eileen Mahoney, Executive Director

6784 Tatnuck Park at Worcester

340 May Street
Worcester, MA 01602-1800
774-312-6020
Fax: 508-755-6333
www.tatnuckparkworcester.com

Lonna Greco, Executive Director

6785 Traditions of Wayland

10 Green Way
Wayland, MA 01778-2616
508-358-0700
Fax: 508-358-4726
www.traditionsofwayland.com

Judy Huber, Executive Director

6786 Victorian of Chatham

389 Orleans Road
Chatham, MA 02633

508-945-1211
Fax: 508-945-2245
www.aurumnetwork.com

Ann Lavalle, Executive Director

6787 Village at Farm Pond
300 West Farm Pond Road
Framingham, MA 01702-6286
508-409-4673
Fax: 508-620-6580
www.emeritus.com

Roald Rolfson, Executive Director

6788 Village at Willow Crossings
25 Cobb Street
Mansfield, MA 02048-2541
508-964-0382
Fax: 508-261-8844
www.villageatwillowcrossings.com

Don Walsh, Executive Director

6789 Westfield Meadows
74 Old Holyoke Road
Westfield, MA 01085-1487
413-562-6940
Fax: 413-564-0175

Mary Ellen Morissette, Resident Manager
John Shannon, Owner

Westfield Meadows is an Assisted Living Residence, licensed by the Commonwealth of Massachsetts providing 24 hour service, three meals per day, laundry service and other needs to all Tenants which include Medicaid eligible individuals.

6790 Whitcomb House
245 West Street
Milford, MA 01757-2201
508-634-2440
Fax: 508-473-6366
www.capitalsenior.com

Chris Dulaney, Owner

6791 Whitney Place at Natick
3 Vision Drive
Natick, MA 01760-2078
508-655-9767
Fax: 508-655-1661; *Toll Free:* 800-372-3800
www.salmonhealthandretirement.com

Donna Deleo, Manager

6792 Woodbridge Assisted Living
240 Lynnfield Street
Peabody, MA 01960-5052
978-532-4411
Fax: 978-532-2407
www.avivliving.org

Harriet Flashenberg, Executive Director

6793 Woods at Eddy Pond
667 Washington Street
Auburn, MA 01501-2722
508-409-4674
Fax: 508-832-8488
www.emeritus.com

Steven Sacco, Executive Director

6794 Youville House Assisted Living Residence
1573 Cambridge Street
Cambridge, MA 02138-4377
617-491-1234
Fax: 617-491-8838
www.youvilleassistedliving.org

Joanne Parsons, Executive Director

6795 Youville Place
10 Pelham Road
Lexington, MA 02421-8400
781-861-3535
Fax: 781-862-4289
www.youvilleassistedliving.org

Joanne Scianna, Manager

Michigan

6796 Ann Arbor Center for Independent Living
2568 Packard Street
Ann Arbor, MI 48104-6852
734-971-0277
Fax: 734-971-0826
www.aacil.org

James K Magyar, President/CEO
Tom Hoatlin, Director Development

The Ann Arbor Center for Independent Living assists people with disabilities and their families in living full and productive lives. Our mission is to assure the equality of opportunity, full participation, independent living and economic self-sufficiency of people with disabilities in our community.

6797 Argentine Care Center
9051 Silver Lake Road
Linden, MI 48451-9730
810-735-9487
Fax: 810-735-9035
www.argentinecarecenter.com

Emil Kovacs, Owner

6798 Burcham Hills Retirement Center
2700 Burcham Drive
East Lansing, MI 48823-3898
517-351-8377
Fax: 517-351-1738
www.brookdaleliving.com

Pam Ditri, Executive Director

6799 CQC Stephenson Home
120 N Locust Street
Adrian, MI 49221-2855
517-265-8185
Fax: 517-265-8186

Theresa Chang, Administrator

6800 Cherrywood Nursing & Living Center
2372 Fiften Mile Road
Sterling Heights, MI 48310
586-978-2280
Fax: 810-978-8407
www.cherrywoodnursing.com

Greg Trombley, Administrator

6801 Clark Retirement Community
1551 Franklin Street SE
Grand Rapids, MI 49506-8203
616-452-1568
Fax: 616-452-0428
www.clarkretirement.org

Robert Perl, Executive Director

A not-for-profit, continuing care retirement community, offering a full complement of services and residential options from independent and assisted living to skilled nursing and short term rehabilitation.

6802 Covenant Village of the Great Lakes
2520 Lake Michigan Drive NW
Grand Rapids, MI 49504-4696
616-735-4541
Fax: 616-735-4546
www.covenantretirement.com

Steven Karnes, Campus Administrator
Deborah May, Marketing Director

6803 Fairview Living Centre
441 E Main Street
Centreville, MI 49032-9626
269-467-9575
Fax: 616-467-7077
www.atriumlivingcenters.com

Vickie Cox, Executive Director

6804 Fountains at Franklin
28301 Franklin Road
Southfield, MI 48034-1672
248-809-1076
Fax: 248-368-1874
www.watermarkcommunities.com

Cathy Lubanski, Executive Director

Offers different and better choices for extraordinary assisted living.

6805 Fraser Villa: A Mercy Living Center
33300 Utica Road
Fraser, MI 48026-2017
586-293-3300
Fax: 582-293-6949
www.trinityseniorsanctuary.org

Gail Fliwinski, Administrator

6806 Gilbert Residence
203 S Huron Street
Ypsilanti, MI 48197-5422
734-482-9498
Fax: 734-482-1848
www.gilbertresidence.com

Maryjo Gibbons, Administrator

6807 Glacier Hills Retirement Center
1200 Earhart Road
Ann Arbor, MI 48105-2768
734-663-5202
Fax: 734-769-0058
info@glacierhills.org.
www.glacierhills.org

Ray Rabidoux, CEO

6808 Hazel I Findlay Country Manor
1101 S Scott Road
Saint Johns, MI 48879-9039
989-224-8936
Fax: 989-224-9423
www.hazelfindlay.com

Mary Ann Bond, Administrator

6809 Heartland HCC-Crestview
625 36th Street SW
Wyoming, MI 49509-4004
616-531-0200
Fax: 616-531-0407
www.heartland-manorcare.com

Deborah Gross, Administrator

6810 Hume Home of Muskegon
1244 W Southern Avenue
Muskegon, MI 49441-2271
231-755-1715
Fax: 231-755-3155
www.humehomeassistedliving.org

Barbara Betts, Administrator

6811 Ingham Regional Assisted Living
6429 Earlington Lane
Lansing, MI 48917-8279
517-321-3391
Fax: 517-321-3646
www.inghamal.com

Lolaurie Shepard, Executive Director

A warm, award winning home with whole life assisted living and memory care suites available.

6812 Jackson Friendly Home
435 W North Street
Jackson, MI 49202-3390
517-784-1377
Fax: 517-784-1235
info@jacksonfriendlyhome.org
www.jacksonfriendlyhome.org

Donna Luckadoo, Administrator

6813 John George Home
1501 E Ganson Street
Jackson, MI 49202-3593
517-783-4134
Fax: 517-783-0872
www.johngeorgehomeinc.wildapricot.org

Karrie Good, Administrator

6814 McLaren Homewood Village
4444 W Court Street
Flint, MI 48532-4329
810-720-5184
Fax: 810-720-5187
www.arclp.com

Deanna Colby, Executive Director
Teresa McCulloch Stilson, Community Relations
Coordinator
Tina Olshove

Assisted Living and Alzheimer's/Dementia community.

6815 Meadows at Silver Maples
100 Silver Maples Drive
Chelsea, MI 48118-1192
734-475-4111
Fax: 734-475-4112; *Toll Free:* 800-213-0442
www.silvermaples.org

Jerry Wilcznski, CEO

6816 Northpointe Woods Assisted Living
700 N Avenue G
Battle Creek, MI 49017
269-964-7625
Fax: 616-964-4973
www.northpointewoods.org

Nancy Kruse, Executive Director

6817 Park Village Pines
2920 Crystal Lane
Kalamazoo, MI 49009-2195
269-372-1928
Fax: 616-372-0638
www.parkvillagepines.org

Wilson Haarsma, Executive Director

6818 Pilgram Manor
2000 Leonard Street NE
Grand Rapids, MI 49505-5894
616-458-1133
Fax: 616-458-8900
www.pilgrimmanor.org

Karen Messick, Administrator

6819 Plymouth Inn
205 N Haggerty Road
Plymouth, MI 48170-6131
734-451-0700
Fax: 734-451-0727
www.plymouthinn.net

William Gala, Manager

6820 Porter Hills Presbyterian Village
3600 E Fulton Street
Grand Rapids, MI 49546-1322
616-949-4975
Fax: 616-954-1795
www.porterhills.org

Bette Morris, Executive Director

6821 Renaissance Gardens at Henry Ford Village
15101 Ford Road
Dearborn, MI 48126-4611
313-584-1700
Fax: 313-846-7731
www.thecareexperts.com

Kristine Anderson, Health Care Counselor
Larry Vidovish, President

Features all private Assisted Living apartments and all private Long-Term Care rooms; full-time, on-site staff doctors with nurses on duty 24-hours a day. Short-Time Rehab (physical, speech and occupational therapy); dementia and Alzheimer's care also available. Renaissance Gardens, the choice you can feel good about.

6822 Rest Haven Home
1424 Union Avenue NE
Grand Rapids, MI 49505-5152

616-363-6819
Fax: 616-363-1658
www.resthavenhomes.com

Greg Tracy, Administrator

6823 Riverview Manor
55378 Wilbur Road
Three Rivers, MI 49093-8815
269-279-7441
Fax: 269-279-7244
rvadmi@gracehc.com
www.riverviewmanor.com

Jennifer Beam, Administrator

6824 Rose Garden Home
3391 Prairie Street SW
Grandville, MI 49418-1992
616-538-1914
Fax: 616-831-2444

Sue Wedekind, Executive Director

6825 Saginaw Geriatrics Home
1413 Gratiot Avenue
Saginaw, MI 48602-2699
989-793-3471
Fax: 989-793-7090
SaginawGeriatrics@yahoo.com
www.saginawgeriatrics.com

George Pike, Administrator

6826 St Ann's Home
2161 Leonard Street NW
Grand Rapids, MI 49504-3891
616-453-7715
Fax: 616-453-7359
www.stannshome.com

Steve Rolston, Administrator

6827 St Anne's Mead Retirement Home
16106 W 12 Mile Road
Southfield, MI 48076-2974
248-557-1221
Fax: 248-557-3142
www.stannesmead.org

Rick Mehrer, Administrator

6828 St Joesph's Home for the Aged
4800 Cadieux Road
Detroit, MI 48224-2293
313-882-3800
Fax: 313-882-5940
info@stjosephmanor.com
www.stjosephmanor.com

Carolyn Ford, Administrator

6829 Sunrise Assisted Living at Farmington Hills
29681 Middlebelt Road
Farmington Hills, MI 48334-2313
248-538-9200
Fax: 248-538-0411
www.sunriseseniorliving.com

Patricia Henning, Executive Director

6830 Sunrise Assisted Living at Northville
16100 N Haggerty Road
Plymouth, MI 48170-4857

734-420-4000
Fax: 734-420-5468
www.sunriseseniorliving.com

Tricia McTaggart, Manager

6831 Sunrise Assisted Living of Ann Arbor
2190 Ann Arbor Saline Road
Ann Arbor, MI 48103-9710
734-327-1350
Fax: 734-327-1351
www.sunriseseniorliving.com

6832 Sunrise Assisted Living of Rochester
500 E University Drive
Rochester, MI 48307-2110
248-601-9000
Fax: 248-601-9001
www.sunriseseniorliving.com

Karen Parrott, Executive Director

6833 Sunrise Assisted Living of Troy
6870 Crooks Road
Troy, MI 48098-1704
248-293-1200
Fax: 248-293-1201
www.sunriseseniorliving.com

Kathy Szajna, Executive Director

6834 Sunrise Assisted Living of West Bloomfield
7005 Pontiac Trl
W Bloomfield, MI 48323-2181
248-738-8101
Fax: 248-738-8177
www.sunriseseniorliving.com

Suzanne Withorn, Executive Director

Assisted living and memory care.

6835 Thurston Woods Village: The Villa
307 N Franks Avenue
Sturgis, MI 49091-1298
269-651-7841
Fax: 616-651-2050
www.thurstonwoods.org

Theo Omo, CEO

6836 Waltonwood of Royal Oak
2450 W 13 Mile Road
Royal Oak, MI 48073-3004
800-239-1396
Fax: 248-549-6426
www.waltonwood.com

Jean Brace, Administrator

6837 Woodhaven Retirement Community
29667 Wentworth Street
Livonia, MI 48154-6231
734-261-9000
Fax: 734-261-9003
www.woodhaven-retirement.com

Randy Gasser, Executive Director

6838 Woodside at Friendship Village
1390 N Drake Road
Kalamazoo, MI 49006-3940
269-381-8837
Fax: 616-381-7129

info@woodsidefvk.com
www.woodsidefvk.com

Stan Clouse, CEO

Assisted living is an ideal solution for people who wish to maintain their privacy and independence yet receive the help they need with daily life.

Minnesota

6839 Almond House
802 28th Street SE
Brainerd, MN 56401-6308
218-825-9255
Fax: 218-822-3068
www.dibbern.com

Sue Johnson, Owner

6840 Alterra Clare Bridge Cottage of West St Paul
315 Thompson Avenue E
West Saint Paul, MN 55118-3239
877-712-9819
Fax: 651-453-1806
www.brookdaleliving.com

Gayle Sajewicz, Executive Director

Alterra Sterling House is an assisted living residence that provides housing and assistance to older adults who want to retain their independence while receiving the daily support they need. The intimate setting for those with limited mobility, as well as specialized programming, help residents maximize independence and quality of life.

6841 Alterra Clare Bridge Cottage-Owatonna
364 Cedardale Drive SE
Owatonna, MN 55060-4467
855-308-0670
Fax: 507-446-8601
www.brookdaleliving.com

Emily Shelstad, Executive Director

Alterra Sterling House is an assisted living residence that provides housing and assistance to older adults who want to retain their independence while receiving the daily support they need. The intimate setting for those with limited mobility, as well as specialized programming, help residents maximize independence and quality of life.

6842 Alterra Clare Bridge of Eagan
1365 Crestridge Lane
Eagan, MN 55123-1042
877-712-9776
Fax: 651-686-7778
www.brookdaleliving.com

Andrea Schroetke, Executive Director

Alterra Sterling House is an assisted living residence that provides housing and assistance to older adults who want to retain their independence while receiving the daily support they need. The intimate setting for those with limited mobility, as well as specialized programming, help residents maximize independence and quality of life.

6843 Alterra Clare Bridge of North Oaks
300 Village Center Drive
North Oaks, MN 55127-3021

877-712-9792
Fax: 651-482-8333
www.brookdaleliving.com

Alterra Sterling House is an assisted living residence that provides housing and assistance to older adults who want to retain their independence while receiving the daily support they need. The intimate setting for those with limited mobility, as well as specialized programming, help residents maximize independence and quality of life.

6844 Alterra Clare Bridge of Plymouth
15855 22nd Avenue N
Plymouth, MN 55447-6452
877-712-9795
Fax: 763-476-5900
www.brookdaleliving.com

Heather Roduenz, Executive Director

Alterra Sterling House is an assisted living residence that provides housing and assistance to older adults who want to retain their independence while receiving the daily support they need. The intimate setting for those with limited mobility, as well as specialized programming, help residents maximize independence and quality of life.

6845 Alterra Sterling House of Apple Valley
14625 Pennock Avenue
Apple Valley, MN 55124-3502
952-891-2711
Fax: 952-953-3132
www.centennial-house.org

Janis Rivers, Administrator

6846 Alterra Sterling House of Blaine
1005 Paul Parkway NE
Blaine, MN 55434-3926
877-713-0049
Fax: 763-755-6400
www.brookdaleliving.com

Joy Williams, Executive Director

Alterra Sterling House is an assisted living residence that provides housing and assistance to older adults who want to retain their independence while receiving the daily support they need. The intimate setting for those with limited mobility, as well as specialized programming, help residents maximize independence and quality of life.

6847 Alterra Sterling House of Faribault
935 Spring Road
Faribault, MN 55021-6975
877-713-0934
Fax: 507-333-2557
www.brookdaleliving.com

Jeff Treml, Manager

Alterra Sterling House is an assisted living residence that provides housing and assistance to older adults who want to retain their independence while receiving the daily support they need. The intimate setting for those with limited mobility, as well as specialized programming, help residents maximize independence and quality of life.

6848 Alterra Sterling House of Inver Grove Heights
5891 Carmen Avenue
Inver Grove Heights, MN 55076-4414
877-713-0967
Fax: 651-306-1020
www.brookdaleliving.com

Jeannie Gatlin, Manager

Alterra Sterling House is an assisted living residence that provides housing and assistance to older adults who want to retain their independence while receiving the daily support they need. The intimate setting for those with limited mobility, as well as specialized programming, help residents maximize independence and quality of life.

6849 Alterra Sterling House of West St Paul
305 Thompson Avenue E
West Saint Paul, MN 55118-3239
877-713-2740
Fax: 651-453-1804
www.brookdaleliving.com

Mary Bryan-Day, Manager

Alterra Sterling House is an assisted living residence that provides housing and assistance to older adults who want to retain their independence while receiving the daily support they need. The intimate setting for those with limited mobility, as well as specialized programming, help residents maximize independence and quality of life.

6850 Alterra Sterling House-Brooklyn Center
6001 Earle Brown Drive
Brooklyn Center, MN 55430-2522
763-566-1495
Fax: 763-566-1625

Anne Nowatzki, Administrator

6851 Alterra Sterling House-Mankato
100 Teton Lane
Mankato, MN 56001-4827
877-713-0990
Fax: 507-386-1174
www.brookdaleliving.com

Shawn Soucek, Executive Director

Alterra Sterling House is an assisted living residence that provides housing and assistance to older adults who want to retain their independence while receiving the daily support they need. The intimate setting for those with limited mobility, as well as specialized programming, help residents maximize independence and quality of life.

6852 Alterra Sterling House-Sauk Rapids
1325 Summit Avenue N
Sauk Rapids, MN 56379-2545
877-713-1870
Fax: 320-203-8207
www.brookdaleliving.com

Amanda Chirsten, Manager

Alterra Sterling House is an assisted living residence that provides housing and assistance to older adults who want to retain their independence while receiving the daily support they need. The intimate setting for those with limited mobility, as well as specialized programming, help residents maximize independence and quality of life.

6853 Alterra Sterling House-Winona
835 E Belleview Street
Winona, MN 55987-4502
877-713-2748
Fax: 507-454-5466
www.brookdaleliving.com

Bernadette Merchlewitz, Manager

Alterra Sterling House is an assisted living residence that provides housing and assistance to older adults who want to retain their independence while receiving the daily support they need. The intimate setting for those with limited mobility, as well as specialized programming, help residents maximize independence and quality of life.

6854 Alterra Sterling-Owatonna
334 Cedardale Drive SE
Owatonna, MN 55060-4467
877-713-1037
Fax: 507-451-7083
www.brookdaleliving.com

Deidra Burke, Executive Director

Alterra Sterling House is an assisted living residence that provides housing and assistance to older adults who want to retain their independence while receiving the daily support they need. The intimate setting for those with limited mobility, as well as specialized programming, help residents maximize independence and quality of life.

6855 Alterra Wynwood of Rochester
3035 Salem Meadows Dr SW
Rochester, MN 55902-2847
507-252-5400
Fax: 507-252-5500
www.assistedlivingathome.com

Cheryl Saballa, Executive Director

6856 Arlington Place
21 16th Avenue SE
Saint Joseph, MN 56374-9789
320-363-1313
Fax: 320-363-1021
www.arlingtonplacemn.com

Mary Hawkins, Executive Director

6857 Arrowhead Senior Living Community
601 Grant Avenue
Eveleth, MN 55734-1314
218-741-9800
Fax: 218-749-8929
mariacarehome@aol.com
www.arrowheadseniorliving.com

Maria Istrate, Owner

6858 Assisted Living in Heritage Hall
11501 Masonic Home Drive
Minneapolis, MN 55437-3661
952-948-7000
Fax: 952-948-6210; *Toll Free:* 800-869-8665
www.mnmasonichomes.org

6859 Assumption Court
615 N 1st Street
Shakopee, MN 55379
320-348-2358
Fax: 952-496-2013
www.assumptionhome.org

Jan Luthens, Administrator

6860 Auburn Courts
501 Oak Street N
Chaska, MN 55318-2646

952-448-9303
Fax: 952-892-0305
www.auburnhomes.org

Wayne Ward, Administrator

6861 Barrett Assisted Living Community
310 2nd Street
Barrett, MN 56311-4505
320-528-2371
Fax: 320-528-2642
barrett@runestone.net
www.barrettmn.com

Vern Junker, Owner

6862 Brickford Cottage
4020 Indian Hills Drive
Saint Paul, MN 55108
712-239-2065
Fax: 712-239-3417
www.enrichinghappiness.com

6863 Brooks of St Paul
2480 Saint Paul Road
Owatonna, MN 55060-2455
507-446-0611
Fax: 507-446-5858
JamesGross@ecumen.org
www.brooksowatonna.org

Sue Doty, Manager

6864 Bryant House
1520 Wyman Avenue
Maple Plain, MN 55359-9446
763-479-1993
Fax: 763-479-3656
www.elimcare.org

Kay Olson, Manager

6865 Callista Court
1455 W Broadway Street
Winona, MN 55987-2392
507-457-0280
Fax: 507-494-5117
www.saintanneofwinona.org

Sue Wilber, Manager

6866 Care-Age Country Home
18846 Eagle Bend Road
Park Rapids, MN 56470-2073
218-732-3721
Fax: 218-732-1208
www.careagecountryhome.com

Chris Niemeyer, Owner

6867 Carefree Living America-Brainerd
2723 Oak Street
Brainerd, MN 56401-3818
218-829-8622
Fax: 218-829-4463
www.carefreeliving.com

Angela Sandelin, Manager

6868 Carefree Living America-Burnsville
600 E Nicollet Boulevard
Burnsville, MN 55337-6739

952-892-5559
Fax: 952-892-1585
www.carefreeliving.com

Tim McLain, Manager

6869 Carefree Living of America-St Cloud
1225 E Division Street
Saint Cloud, MN 56304
320-251-6483
Fax: 320-251-2714
www.carefreeliving.com

Linda Corrigan, Manager

6870 Catholic Eldercare at Home
817 Main Street NE
Minneapolis, MN 55413-1900
612-379-1370
Fax: 612-362-2449
www.catholiceldercare.org

Paula Finn, Executive Director

6871 Cedar Crest Estate
225 Shady Ridge Road NW
Hutchinson, MN 55350-1407
320-587-7077
Fax: 320-587-4299
www.cedarcrestmn.com

Roz Ewald, Owner
Dede Fischer, Assitant Manager

To offer a clean, homelike atmosphere for the people in the estate's care. Dedicated to helping residents maintain their independence. Provides friendly, honest, respectful care ensuring residents a sense of security and peace of mind.

6872 Cedars of Austin
700 1st Drive NW
Austin, MN 55912-3095
507-437-3246
Fax: 507-437-3248
info@cedarsofaustin.com???
www.cedarsofaustin.com

Lisa Nelson, Director

6873 Centennial Villa Assisted Living
660 Park Street E
Annandale, MN 55302-3057
320-274-5031
Fax: 320-274-3631
www.ahcsmn.org

Mark D. Miller, Chairman
Roger Miller, Vice Chairman

6874 Central Todd County Care Center
406 Highway 71 E
Clarissa, MN 56440-2000
218-756-3636
Fax: 218-756-3639
www.ctcccinc.com

Margaret Taggart, Administrator

6875 Chandler Place
3701 Chandler Drive NE
Minneapolis, MN 55421-4413
612-788-7321
Fax: 612-913-5370
www.chandlerplacesenior.com

Whiteny Stickland, Director

6876 Clearwater Suites Assisted Living
1902 7th Avenue E
Alexandria, MN 56308-2364
320-759-2121
Fax: 320-759-2120
www.edgewoodseniorliving.com

Doris Denal, Director Operations

6877 Commons on Marice
1380 Marice Drive
Eagan, MN 55121-9748
651-688-9999
Fax: 651-688-7888
www.commonsonmarice.com

Kezia Wicklander, Manager

6878 Copperfield Hill Phase II
4020 Lakeland Avenue N
Robbinsdale, MN 55422-5800
763-277-1001
Fax: 763-533-6146
www.copperfieldhill.com

Shae Rodger, Executive Director

6879 Country Neighbors
206 3rd Avenue SE
Mapleton, MN 56065-9746
507-524-4990
Fax: 507-524-3239
Amanda.Beavens@ecumen.org
www.countryneighbors.org

Traci A Birr, Manager

6880 Country Neighbors-Le Center
175 E Derrynane Street
Le Center, MN 56057-1603
507-357-4104
Fax: 651-766-4310
ChristiCarter@ecumen.org
www.countryneighbors.org

Anne Casper, Manager

6881 Country Villa
7475 Country Club Drive
Minneapolis, MN 55427-4622
763-512-1579
Fax: 763-540-6899
asamrock@extendicare.com
www.countryv.com

Arlene Samrock, Marketing Director
Ned Ammons, Manager

Assisted living community.

6882 Edgewood Vista
4195 Westberg Road
Hermantown, MN 55811-3916
218-723-8905
Fax: 218-723-4051
www.edgewoodseniorliving.com

Carolyn Fisher, Administrator

6883 Edgewood Vista-Virginia
705 17th Street N
Virginia, MN 55792-2176

218-741-7106
Fax: 218-741-7229
www.edgewoodseniorliving.com

Julie Winans, Administrator

6884 English Rose Suites

7409 Gleason Road
Minneapolis, MN 55439-2557
952-983-0412
Fax: 952-938-2548
www.englishrosesuites.com

Jon D. Rappaport, CEO

6885 Evergreen Knoll

1309 14th Street
Cloquet, MN 55720-2562
218-878-3302
Fax: 218-878-3340
www.evergreenknoll.org

Terri Langevin, Manager

6886 Evergreens of Moorhead

502 3rd Avenue South
Moorhead, MN 56560-2703
218-233-1535
Fax: 218-291-1162
www.evergreensofmoorhead.org

Michelle Seibel, Manager

6887 Galeon Assisted Living

410 W Main Street
Osakis, MN 56360-8243
320-859-2142
Fax: 320-859-6293
www.galeonmn.com

Angie Reinke, Social Services Director
Sheila Roering RN, Housing Services Director

Apt style assisted living with 24hr staff and residential style memory care assisted living.

6888 Gianna Homes-Sursum Corda

4605 Fairhills Road E
Minnetonka, MN 55345-3502
952-988-0953
Fax: 952-988-6935
anne@giannahomes.org
www.giannahomes.org

Anne Marie Hansen, Owner

6889 Granite Falls Senior Services

345 10th Avenue
Granite Falls, MN 56241-1719
320-564-3308
Fax: 320-564-3111
www.granitefallshealthcare.com

Tammy Tammen, Manager

6890 Guardian Angels Elem HomeCare

400 Evans Avenue NW
Elk River, MN 55330-2699
763-241-0654
Fax: 763-241-0274
lbrabec@gaehc.org
www.guardianangelsmn.org

Linda Olson, President

6891 Guardian Angels Elim HomeCare & Hospice

403 Main Street
Elk River, MN 55330
763-241-0654
Fax: 763-241-0274

Linda Olson, Director of Homecare/Hospice
Gary Hjelmsted, Administrator
Andrea Jung, Director of Business Development

Establishe in 1991, Guardian Angels + Elim Home Care and Hospice is part of a full continuum of care. We are a small home town agency with local employees serving local residents. Our Home Care has experts in chronic disease management, and our hospice has an Honor Our Veterans Program. We have numerous employees that habe been with the company for more than a decade. We are living our mission with a family of services that support 6 counties inthe north west metro. We are growing strong by sharing our faith based mission with our clients, their families, and the communities we serve. Our mission is to share Christ's love by providing holistic and compassionate care to adults with chronic illness, recent acute illness, and to those facing end of life.

Year Founded: 1991

6892 Healtheast Residence on Humboldt

514 Humboldt Avenue
Saint Paul, MN 55107-4013
651-220-1700
Fax: 651-220-1724
www.cerenityseniorcare.org

Peter Schuna, Administrator

6893 Healtheast Residence-White Bear Lake

4615 2nd Avenue
White Bear Lake, MN 55110-3375
651-232-1867
Fax: 651-232-1878
www.cerenityseniorcare.org

Trudy Fuller, Manager

6894 Heritage House Assisted Living Facility

5825 Saint Croix Avenue N
Golden Valley, MN 55422-4419
763-544-1555
Fax: 763-544-8032

Lynette Clausen, Manager

6895 Hillcrest Rehabilitation & Healthcare Center

15409 Wayzata Boulevard
Wayzata, MN 55391-1402
952-473-5466
Fax: 952-473-6842
GLC02232@goldenliving.com
www.local.goldenlivingcenters.com

Lisa Harrell, Executive Director

6896 Hub City Developmental

Linden & Front Street
Slayton, MN 56172
507-836-1055
Fax: 507-836-1075

Cathy Kor, Manager

6897 Interim Assisted Care
2200 University Avenue W
Suite 160
Saint Paul, MN 55114-8769
651-917-3634
Fax: 651-917-3620
www.interimhealthcare.com

Grace Boatman, Manager

6898 Interlachen Senior Suites
5240 Interlachen Boulevard
Edina, MN 55436-1427
952-848-8765
Fax: 952-848-8765
www.start.cortera.com

6899 Johnson Park Place
1011 E Elm Street
Redwood Falls, MN 56283-1300
507-627-8121
Fax: 507-637-4446
www.good-sam.com

Sandi Reck, Manager

6900 Jones Harrison Residence Assisted Living
3700 Cedar Lake Avenue
Minneapolis, MN 55416-4240
612-920-2030
Fax: 612-225-1190
info@jonesharrison.org
www.jones-harrison.org

Joanne Buytendorp, Administrator
Year Founded: 1888

6901 Just Like Home
PO Box 770
Albert Lea, MN 56007
507-383-2697
Fax: 507-373-1961
jlhpassistedliving@gmail.com
www.justlikehomeplace.com

Rollie Keyeski, Manager
Year Founded: 1952

6902 Kenwood Heritage Living
400 15th Avenue SW
Austin, MN 55912-3232
507-434-7255
Fax: 507-434-7201
www.ecumen.org

James Ingersoll, Administrator

6903 Kenwood Retirement Community
825 Summit Avenue
Minneapolis, MN 55403-4141
612-374-8100
Fax: 612-377-3600
jvolkenant@thekenwood.org
www.thekenwood.net

Jennifer S Volkenant, Executive Director
Karen Edberg, Marketing Director

6904 Keystone Bluffs
2528 Trinity Road
Duluth, MN 55811-3315

218-727-2800
Fax: 218-727-2850
www.keystonebluffs.com

6905 Kingsway Assisted Living
357 Kings Road
Schenectady, NY 12304
518-393-4304
Fax: 518-393-4315
manor@kingswaycommunity.com
www.kingswaycommunity.com

6906 Knutson Place Apartments
901 Luther Place
Albert Lea, MN 56007-1500
507-373-8226
Fax: 507-373-8226
www.stjohnsofalbertlea.org

Scot Spates, Administrator
Sandy Nelson, Director of Nursing

6907 La Bonnie Vie
6443 Westchester Circle
Minneapolis, MN 55427-4966
612-735-8480
Fax: 763-544-0202
www.labonneviemn.com

Tammy Tuntilla, Owner

6908 Lakeside Manor
4831 London Road
Duluth, MN 55804-2499
218-525-2784
Fax: 218-525-3411
www.lakesidemanormn.com

Tom Kolar, Owner

6909 Lakewood Pine Senior Housing
1702 Airport Road
Staples, MN 56479-3345
218-894-4460
Fax: 218-894-4453
www.lakewoodhealthsystem.com

6910 Laurels Edge
77 Stadium Road
Mankato, MN 56001-6099
507-387-2133
Fax: 507-387-1135
dfontaine@throcompany.com
www.throcompany.com

Christopher Thro, President
Susan Kratzke, Vice President

6911 Loving Residence
1760 Perlich Avenue
Red Wing, MN 55066-2978
651-388-1650
Fax: 651-388-1684
www.lovingresidence.com

Sandy McDonald, Manager

6912 Lutheran Home: Cedar Haven
630 and 640 Reed Street
Mankato, MN 56001

507-625-1512
Fax: 507-388-6428
msnyder@tlha.org
www.tlha.org

Mariann Snyder, Administrator
Wendy Allen, RN/DON

Provides for the spiritual, physical, mental and emotional needs of people entrusted to our care.

6913 Lutheran Memorial Retirement Center
PO Box 480
Twin Valley, MN 56584
218-584-5181
Fax: 218-584-5304
www.lutheranlivingcenter.com

Dwight Fulie, Executive Director

6914 Maranatha Place
5401 69th Avenue North
Brooklyn Center, MN 55429-4508
763-549-9600
www.maranathaphs.com

6915 Margaret Place
1555 118th Lane NW
Coon Rapids, MN 55448-7579
763-754-2505
Fax: 763-754-0332
www.marytinc.com

Mary Tjosvole, Owner

6916 Martin Luther Care Center
1401 E 100th Street
Bloomington, MN 55425-2614
952-888-7751
Fax: 952-888-5465
www.martinluthercampus.com

Jody Barney, Administrator

6917 May Creek Lodge Assisted Living
303 10th Street S
Walker, MN 56484
218-547-4515
Fax: 218-547-4713
www.maycreekcampus.com

Ann Noland, Owner

6918 McCarthy Manor
2221 N Arlington Avenue
Duluth, MN 55811-2029
218-722-1501
Fax: 218-722-1501
www.mccarthymanor.com

John Hansen, Administrator

6919 Meadow Woods
1301 E 100th Street
Bloomington, MN 55425-2625
952-888-1010
Fax: 952-888-4323
www.martinluthercampus.com

Bev Heise, Executive Director

6920 Meadows of Worthington
1801 Collegeway
Worthington, MN 56187-3075

507-372-7838
Fax: 507-372-7804
www.ecumenmeadows.org

Patricia Hendersciedt, Executive Director

6921 Meadows on Main
611 S Main Street
Renville, MN 56284-1816
320-329-3788
Fax: 320-329-3678
www.sfhs.org

Jane Dikken, Manager

6922 Mother of Mercy Nursing & Retirement Center
230 Church Avenue
Albany, MN 56307
320-845-2195
Fax: 320-845-7092
www.motherofmercymn.org

Bob Wikan, Administrator

6923 North Oaks on Emerson
2912 Fremont Avenue North
Minneapolis, MN 55411-1300
612-521-2929
Fax: 612-287-3505
www.stolafcommunitycampus.org

Deanna Winge, Manager

6924 Northfield Parkview
900 Cannon Valley Drive
Northfield, MN 55057-3300
507-645-9511
Fax: 507-645-0117
info@northfieldretirement.org
www.northfieldretirement.org

Kyle Nordine, Executive Director

6925 Northside Retirement Home
102 E Line Ave, Sapulpa
Sapulpa, OK 74066
918-224-0833
Fax: 918-227-2405
www.northsidenursinghome.com

Ernie Jonson III, Administrator

6926 Oak Hill Living Center Assisted Living
1314 8th North Street
New Ulm, MN 56073-1554
507-233-0800
Fax: 507-354-2751
info@oakhillsnewulm.com
www.oakhillsnewulm.com

6927 Oak Park Place-Albert Lea
1615 Bridge Avenue
Albert Lea, MN 56007-2111
507-373-5600
Fax: 507-373-1121
www.oakparkplace.com

Jessica Richards, Director Housing
Stephanie Erdman RN, Director Resident Care Services
Joyce Nixon, Exeuctive Director

Assisted living community with memory are providing independence when you want it and assistance when you need it.

6928 Oak Ridge Assisted Living-Hastings
1128 Bahls Drive
Hastings, MN 55033-4500
651-438-0418
Fax: 651-438-0419
www.oakridgeassistedliving.org

Diane Fiala, Administrator

6929 Oak Ridge Place
6060 Oxboro Avenue N
Stillwater, MN 55082-6123
651-439-8034
Fax: 651-439-8305
www.oakridgeplace.net

David Smith, Manager

6930 Oakenwald Terrace
218 Winona Streeet SE
Chatfield, MN 55923-1238
507-867-3806
Fax: 507-867-3806
info@oakenwaldterrace.com
www.oakenwaldterrace.com

Marion Lund, Owner

6931 Oaks
945 Century Avenue SW
Hutchinson, MN 55350-3788
320-234-9791
Fax: 320-234-6008
www.ecumenoaksandpines.org

Joyce Aakre, Executive Director

6932 Osseo Gardens
525 2nd Street SE
Osseo, MN 55369-1658
763-315-4869
Fax: 763-315-0050
sarah.lien@vqpm.com
www.osseogardensassistedliving.com

Sarah Lien, Director

6933 Our House
204 14th Street NW
Austin, MN 55912-4645
507-437-2179
Fax: 507-437-2310
mdunlop@ourhousesl.com
www.ourhousesl.com

Shannon Pacholl, Manager

6934 Parker Oaks Assisted Living
211 6th Street NW
Winnebago, MN 56098-1067
507-893-3171
Fax: 507-893-3174
agronewold@parkeroaks.com
www.parkeroaks.com

Anna Gronewold, Manager

6935 Parkwood Apartments
505 S 2nd Street
Belview, MN 56214-1003
507-938-3020
Fax: 507-938-3019
www.parkviewseniorlivingbelview.com

Paula Pohlen, Manager

6936 Pines
1508 North Highway
Jackson, MN 56143-1095
507-847-5762
Fax: 507-847-5763
www.good-sam.com

Mary Lou Drahota, Manager

6937 Pioneer Estates of Minnesota
8751 Preserve Boulevard
Eden Prairie, MN 55344-5301
952-914-0934
Fax: 952-943-2563
christine@pioneerestatesofmn.com
www.pioneerestatesofmn.com

Christine Rowland, Owner

10 bed residential care home.

6938 Pioneer Senior Cottages
1131 Mabelle Avenue South
Fergus Falls, MN 56537-3758
218-998-1500
Fax: 218-998-9972
www.pioneercare.org

6939 Prairie Senior Cottages-Alexandria
814 McKay Avenue
Alexandria, MN 56308-2362
320-763-8244
Fax: 320-763-8255
kayla@prairieseniorcottages.com
www.prairieseniorcottages.com

Jenny Jones, Executive Director

6940 Prairie Senior Cottages-Hutchinson
1310 Bradford Street SE
Hutchinson, MN 55350-3302
320-587-5508
Fax: 320-587-7419
john@prairieseniorcottages.com
www.prairieseniorcottages.com

6941 Prairie Senior Cottages-Willmar
1701 19th Avenue SW
Willmar, MN 56201-4944
320-235-6022
Fax: 320-235-6029
becky@prairieseniorcottages.com
www.prairieseniorcottages.com

Becky Holmgrem, Executive Director

6942 Presbyterian Assisted Living Homecare
1910 County Road D W
Saint Paul, MN 55112-3503
651-631-6200
Fax: 651-631-6094
www.phsroseville.com

Scott Welter, Administrator

6943 Primrose
1360 Adams Street
Mankato, MN 56001-4298

507-388-9292
Fax: 507-388-9292
www.primroseretirement.com

Brooke Britton, Manager

6944 Rakhma Peace Home
4953 Aldrich Avenue S
Minneapolis, MN 55419-5352
612-824-2345
Fax: 612-824-3165
www.rakhma.org

Bryan Shirley, Co-Chair

6945 Regina Retirement Center
1175 Nininger Road
Hastings, MN 55033-1056
651-480-4100
Fax: 651-480-4212
www.reginamedical.org

Mark Wilson, CEO

6946 Reminiscence Home
34388 County Road 233
Grand Rapids, MN 55744-5324
218-327-4954
Fax: 218-327-4954
www.seniorlifestyle.com

Linda Carraevu, Owner

6947 Ridgeway on German
715 S German Street
New Ulm, MN 56073-4403
507-354-7400
Fax: 507-359-5711
Ridgeway@newulmtel.net
www.ridgewaynewulm.org

Kyla Franta, Manager

6948 Roseview Court Care Agency
425 N Badger Street
Caledonia, MN 55921-1567
507-725-3351
Fax: 507-724-5142
www.caledoniacareandrehab.com

Marian Rauk, Administrator

6949 Rosewood Estate-Highland
750 Mississippi River Boulevard S
Saint Paul, MN 55116-1006
651-698-1111
Fax: 651-698-8688
www.sunriseseniorliving.com

Scott Mixer, Manager

6950 Ruth Homes
1306 Lincoln Lane
Hastings, MN 55033-1068
651-437-8446
Fax: 651-437-0265
www.ruthhomes.com

Jane Hausman, Owner

6951 Samaritan Bethany Terrace
101 NW 7th St Suite 20
Rochester, MN 55901-6817

507-289-5042
Fax: 507-289-6001
www.samaritanbethany.com

Sue Knutson, Administrator

6952 Senior Suites of New Brighton
805 6th Avenue NW
Saint Paul, MN 55112-2717
651-633-7200
Fax: 651-697-7377
www.newbrightoncarecenter.com

Michael Chies, Administrator

6953 Skylight Gardens
501 1st Street N
Saint Cloud, MN 56303-4705
320-259-4584
Fax: 320-259-6159
michelle.mace@vqpm.com
www.stcloudseniorliving.com

Michael Pattee, Manager

6954 Solbakken
7733 W 99th Street Circle
Minneapolis, MN 55438-2079
952-943-8485
Fax: 952-943-2941
adams@solbakkeninc.com
www.solbakkeninc.com

6955 St Anns Residence
330 E 3rd Street
Duluth, MN 55805-1846
218-727-8831
Fax: 218-727-8833
www.stanns.com

Traci Jaszczak, CEO
Stephane Maki, Administrator

Independent and assisted living for senior citizens.

6956 St Benedicts Senior Community
1810 Minnesota Boulevard
Saint Cloud, MN 56304-2436
320-252-0010
Fax: 320-654-2351
www.centracare.com

Linda Doerr, Executive Director

6957 Sterling Park Commons
142 North First Street
Waite Park, MN 56387-1225
320-252-9595
Fax: 320-252-5629
www.twdcc.com

Carla Brunn, Manager

6958 Stevens Residence
3704 Cardinal Road
Minnetonka, MN 55345-2204
952-930-9144
Fax: 952-930-9184
www.stevensresidence.com

6959 Sunrise Assisted Living of Buffalo
201 1st Street NE
Buffalo, MN 55313-1550

763-682-5489
Fax: 763-682-6511
www.sunriseseniorliving.com

Cheryl Klinkhammer, Executive Director

6960 Sunrise Assisted Living of Edina
7128 France Avenue S
Edina, MN 55435-4301
952-927-8000
Fax: 952-927-6400
www.sunriseseniorliving.com

Renae Witschen, Executive Director

6961 Sunrise Assisted Living-Roseville
255 Snelling Avenue N
Saint Paul, MN 55104-5327
651-636-4800
Fax: 651-636-4809
www.sunriseseniorliving.com

Anneliese Soldner, Executive Director

6962 Sunrise Cottage of Mankato
300 Bunting Lane
Mankato, MN 56001-7020
507-345-8787
Fax: 507-345-8870
www.sunriseseniorliving.com

Kim Alinder, Executive Director

6963 Sunrise Cottages of Rochester
4220 55th Street NW
Rochester, MN 55901-8900
507-286-8528
Fax: 507-286-8527
www.sunriseseniorliving.com

Alicia Adams, Executive Director

6964 Sunrise Village
1125 9th Street SE
Willmar, MN 56201-4683
320-235-1602
Fax: 320-235-4517
www.sunriseseniorliving.com

Angie Gerhardson, Manager

6965 The Country Place
23110 347th Street SE
Erskine, MN 56535-9491
218-687-2288
Fax: 218-687-3278
countryplace@gvtel.com
pioneercountryplace.com

Karen ne Friedley RN, Housing Manager
Assisted living.

6966 The Lodge of Winthrop
Good Samaritan Society
204 S County Road 33
Winthrop, MN 55396
507-647-3980
Fax: 507-647-3982
pmorson@good-sam.com
www.good-sam.com

Pam Morson, Senior Living Manager

A senior living resource that offers valuable choices to the community. Bridges the gap between full independence and traditional skilled nursing care. Offers independence of 24 hour staffing and Good Samaritan caring.

6967 Thorne Crest Retirement Center
1201 Garfield Avenue
Albert Lea, MN 56007-3637
507-373-2311
Fax: 207-377-1216
www.thornecrest.net

Karolee Coppoc, Administrator

6968 Valley View Estates
1104 4th Avenue NE
Long Prairie, MN 56347
320-732-3516
Fax: 320-732-7018
sheilatowle@hotmail.com
www.valleyviewassistedliving.com

Chuck Lane, Owner

6969 Valleyview Board and Lodge
4061 W 173rd Street
Jordan, MN 55352-8318
952-492-6160
Fax: 952-492-6446
www.valleyviewofjordan.biz

Grace Guemple, Administrator

6970 Villa St Vincent
516 Walsh Street
Crookston, MN 56716-2757
218-281-3424
Fax: 218-281-4755
www.pws.bhshealth.com

Michael Siekas, Administrator

6971 Volunteers of America of Minnesota
5905 Golden Valley Road
Suite 110
Minneapolis, MN 55422-4490
763-546-3242
Fax: 612-546-2774
www.voamn.org

Mike Weber, CEO

6972 Wellington
2235 Rockwood Avenue
Saint Paul, MN 55116-3175
651-699-2664
Fax: 651-699-9726
www.wellingtonresidence.com

Kim Webster, Manager

6973 Wellstead of Rogers
20600 S Diamond Lake Road
Rogers, MN 55374-4515
763-428-1981
Fax: 763-428-3792
www.wellsteadofrogers.com

Tom Wiskow, Owner

6974 Wesley Residence
5601 Grand Avenue
Duluth, MN 55807-2545

218-628-2307
Fax: 218-628-9623
www.athomeliving.org

6975 Westwood Place
209 Jefferson Avenue SW
Watertown, MN 55388-8100
952-955-1399
Fax: 952-955-1399
www.westwoodplaceliving.com

Deanne Beito, Manager

6976 Wilder Assisted Living Programs
451 Lexington Pkwy
Saint Paul, MN 55104
651-280-2000
Fax: 651-772-5227
www.wilder.org

Jane Vohs, Manager

6977 Wilds of Sand Prairie
700 Knight Street
Saint Peter, MN 56082-1739
507-931-4375
Fax: 651-766-4477
www.ecumensandprairie.org

Kristi Keller-Smith, Manager

6978 Wildwood Grove
412 E Main Street
Le Roy, MN 55951-6740
507-324-9515
Fax: 507-324-5355
wildwoodgrove@frontiernet.net
www.wildwoodgrovemn.com

Laurie Schwarck, Executive Director

6979 Woodland Good Samaritan Village Apartments
200 Buffalo Hills Lane
Brainerd, MN 56401-4555
218-829-1429
Fax: 218-829-4815
www.good-sam.com

Michael Deuth, Religious Leader

6980 Woodland Manor
610 Summit Drive
Fairmont, MN 56031-2247
507-235-6606
Fax: 507-235-3995
www.lumhsi.org

Sue Owens RN, Director
Robert Lake, Administrator

Missouri

6981 Autumn Ridge
300 Autumn Ridge Drive
Herculaneum, MO 63048
636-931-8400
Fax: 636-933-3975; *Toll Free:* 877-231-1243
www.emeritus.com

Daniel R Baty, Chairman/CEO
Raymond R Brandstrom, Vice Chairman/VP Finance
Gary Becker, SVP Operations

Assisted living services are designed with a focus on wellness to help residents maintain or improve their health.

6982 Autumn View Gardens
Bethesda Adult Community
16219 Autumn View Terrace
Ellisville, MO 63011
636-458-5225
www.bethesdaadultcommunities.com

Cathy Krege, Executive Director

Provides assisted living in a secure environment for individuals with Alzheimer's disease or related dementia.

6983 Fairwinds-River's Edge
600 River's Edge Drive
St. Charles, MO 63303
636-754-0100
www.leisurecare.com

Offers luxurious apartment homes in a fun and active retirement community.

6984 Gardens Assisted Living
Bethesda Adult Community
1302 West Sunset
Springfield, MO 65807
417-889-7600
Fax: 417-889-7681; *Toll Free:* 800-274-7132
www.bethesdaadultcommunities.com

Brian Miller, Executive Director

Provides assisted living in a secure environment for individuals with Alzheimer's disease or related dementia.

6985 McKnight Place Assisted Living
Three McKnight Place
Saint Louis, MO 63124
314-997-5333
www.mpassistedliving.com

Christie Wolff, LNHA, Administrator
Patti Romeo, Admissions Coordinator/SS
Patrick Majors, MD, Medical Director

We provide complete assisted living services for seniors who want to remain independent, but need extra attention and care.

6986 Saint Louis Altenheim
5408 South Broadway
Saint Louis, MO 63111
314-353-7225
Fax: 314-353-7389
knewell@stlouisaltenheim.com
www.altenheim-stlouis.com

Kathy Clark, Administrator
Kay Newell, Director Marketing
Margie Batha, Director Nursing

St. Louis Altenheim is a continuing care residence with style. We offer services to meet each resident's needs, while maintaining the highest level of privacy, respect and individuality. Our goal is to enhance the quality of life for each resident at every level of care.

6987 Sunrise Senior Living
2100 Swope Drive
Independence, MO 64057-2808
816-257-5100
Fax: 816-257-2442
www.sunriseseniorliving.com

Paul J Klaassen, Founder/Chairman/CEO
Teresa M Klaassen, Founder/Chief Cultural Officer
Thomas B Newell, President

The Fountains at Greenbriar offers extraordinary rental retirement living in a quaint, suburban setting that is ideally located to all the area has to offer. The Fountains at Greenbriar can be tailored to meet your needs and desires.

Montana

6988 Aspen Meadows Retirement Community
3155 Avenue C
Billings, MT 59102-8109
406-656-8818
Fax: 406-656-9552; Toll Free: 800-325-1774
www.billingsclinic.com

Anne Gonzalez, Administrator

6989 Bee Hive Homes of Flathead County
660 13th St W
Columbia Falls, MT 59912
406-892-4100
Fax: 405-755-4483
www.beehivehomes.com

Ron Cattron, Owner
Claudia Cattron, Owner
Kathleen Jacobs, Administrator

The mission of Bee Hive Homes is to provide assistance with the activities of daily living in a respectful, dignified manner in a home like setting to the frail elderly who choose to retain their independence and dignity to the fullest measure possible.

6990 Buffalo Hill Terrace
40 Claremont Street
Kalispell, MT 59901-3527
406-752-9624
Fax: 406-752-9609
www.ilcorp.org

Carol Cockrell, Manager

6991 Edgewood Vista
1011 Cardinal Drive
Belgrade, MT 59714-8373
406-388-9439
Fax: 406-388-7722
www.edgewoodseniorliving.com

Glenda Elkins, Manager

6992 Grand Park Assisted Living Community
1221 28th Street W
Billings, MT 59102-3790
406-652-6989
Fax: 406-652-4879
www.marquiscompanies.com

Judy Annin, Manager

6993 Hamilton House
9430 Haggerty Lane
Bozeman, MT 59715-9263
406-586-9459
Fax: 406-586-9459
www.hamiltonhouseassistedliving.com

Don Hamilton, Owner

6994 Heritage Acres Assisted Living
200 N Mitchell Avenue
Hardin, MT 59034-1696
406-665-2802
Fax: 406-665-3809
www.bighornhospital.org

Paula Small-Plenty, Administrator

6995 Hillside Place
4720 23rd Avenue
Missoula, MT 59803-1163
406-251-5100
Fax: 406-251-4278
www.hillsidesenior.com

6996 Hunters Glen at Grizzly Peak
3620 American Way
Missoula, MT 59808-1379
406-542-7009
Fax: 406-542-7094
www.emeritus.com

Janice Barber, Executive Director

6997 Lodge at Lone Tree Creek
1015 7th Avenue SW
Sidney, MT 59270-4900
406-488-4682
Fax: 406-488-2260
www.lodgeatlonetree.org

Tawnya Gurney, Executive VP

6998 Montana Masonic Home
2010 Masonic Home Road
Helena, MT 59602-9514
406-458-5431
Fax: 406-458-9322
masonichome@mhmt.org
www.mhmt.org

Gale Evans, Administrator

6999 Prestige Assisted Living at Kalispell
125 Glenwood Drive
Kalispell, MT 59901-6075
406-756-1818
Fax: 406-756-0583
www.prestigecare.com

Patty Cordell, Executive Director

7000 River Ridge
1415 Yellowstone River Road
Billings, MT 59105-1834
406-245-9330
Fax: 406-245-4219
www.welcov.com

Loree Aman, Manager

7001 Springmeadows
3175 Graf Street
Bozeman, MT 59715-7160
406-586-2423
Fax: 406-582-0032
www.emeritus.com

Penelope Watkins, Executive Director

7002 Waterford on Saddle Drive
915 Saddle Drive
Helena, MT 59601-5754
406-449-4900
Fax: 406-449-4999; *Toll Free:* 800-336-0716
www.touchmarkhelena.com

Steve Nistler, Executive Director

North Carolina

7003 Abbotswood at Irving Park Assisted Living
3504 Flint Street
Greensboro, NC 27405-3488
336-282-8870
Fax: 336-282-9148
irvingpark@kiscosl.com
www.kiscosl.com

Julie Butel Grimmett LPC, Marketing Director
Grege Woodward, Executive Director

Our vision is to grow as a unique and enduring company dedicated to meeting the changing needs of our residents and their families. To create a collaborative environment where associates are appreciated and inspired to develop as individuals where strengths and abilities are nurtures and rewarded. A company of high quality retirement communities and services delivered with a warm and friendly feeling.

7004 Abington Place of Gastonia
1680 S New Hope Road
Gastonia, NC 28054-5854
855-350-3800
Fax: 704-886-4848
www.brookdaleliving.com

Patti Lineberger, Executive Director

7005 Ahoskie House
407 Loftin Lane S
Ahoskie, NC 27910-3447
252-862-4700
Fax: 252-862-4800
www.meridiansenior.com

7006 Alterra Clare Bridge of Asheville
4 Walden Ridge Drive
Asheville, NC 28803-8583
877-938-8655
Fax: 828-687-0511
www.brookdaleliving.com

Kevin Parries, Administrator
Susan Woofter, Executive Director

7007 Alterra Clare Bridge of Cary
7870 Chapel Hill Road
Cary, NC 27513-5428

919-852-1355
Fax: 919-852-0899
brookdaleliving.com

Heidi Keys, Marketing Manager

7008 Alterra Clare Bridge of Charlotte
5326 Park Road
Charlotte, NC 28209-3648
704-544-7255
Fax: 704-544-6965
www.brookdaleliving.com

7009 Alterra Clare Bridge of Greensboro
3896 N Elm Street
Greensboro, NC 27455-2596
336-286-1235
Fax: 336-286-1252
www.brookdaleliving.com

7010 Alterra Clare Bridge of Wilmington
3501 Converse Drive
Wilmington, NC 28403-6179
877-938-8659
Fax: 910-790-5662
www.brookdaleliving.com

Esther Hynes, Manager

7011 Alterra Clare Bridge of Winston Salem
275 S Peace Haven Road
Winston Salem, NC 27104-4419
877-938-7119
Fax: 336-659-6474
www.brookdaleliving.com

Scott Steckey, Manager

7012 Alterra Sterling House of Goldsboro
1800 N Berkeley Boulevard
Goldsboro, NC 27534-3368
877-713-0955
Fax: 919-759-1927
www.brookdaleliving.com

Troy Smothers, Executive Director

7013 Alterra Sterling House of Greenville
2105 W Arlington Boulevard
Greenville, NC 27834-5744
877-713-0959
Fax: 252-758-3738
www.brookdaleliving.com

Troy Smothers, Executive Director

7014 Alterra Sterling House of Hickory
910 29th Avenue NE
Hickory, NC 28601-1135
877-713-0966
Fax: 828-328-6090
www.brookdaleliving.com

Sheila Madigan, Executive Director

7015 Alterra Sterling House of New Bern
1336 S Glenburnie Road
New Bern, NC 28562-2624
877-713-1029
Fax: 252-638-2063
www.brookdaleliving.com

Donna Le Blanc, Executive Director

7016 Alterra Sterling House of Shelby
1425 E Marion Street
Shelby, NC 28150-4979
877-713-1871
Fax: 704-471-9935
www.brookdaleliving.com

Elsie Carter, Executive Director

7017 Alterra Wynwood of Chapel Hill
2220 Farmington Drive
Chapel Hill, NC 27517-7843
877-713-2893
Fax: 919-933-1543
www.brookdaleliving.com

Agnes Mauro, Finance Executive

7018 Alterra Wynwood of Greensboro
3896 N Elm Street
Greensboro, NC 27455-2596
336-286-1235
Fax: 336-286-1252
www.nursinghomeoptions.org

7019 Arbor Terrace of Asheville
3199 Sweeten Creek Road
Asheville, NC 28803-2136
828-681-5533
Fax: 828-681-5554; *Toll Free:* 888-214-6884
spegg@arborcompany.com
www.arborterrace-asheville.com

Nancy Miller, Executive Director

Provides a warm, nurturing environment in gracious sur-roundings, encouraging individual responsibility and free-dom of choice, and creates a home atmosphere where residents make decisions regarding their daily lives.

7020 Arbors at Carriage Club of Charlotte
5800 Old Providence Road
Charlotte, NC 28226-6872
704-365-8551
Fax: 704-366-4914
www.brookdaleliving.com

Jackie Pittman, Executive Director

7021 Ardenwoods
2400 Appalachian Boulevard
Arden, NC 28704-8327
828-684-0040
Fax: 828-684-7800
www.ardenwoodsatsaveryscreek.com

The warmth of our intimate community is enhanced by our gracious, professional staff. Not only do they know you by name and take care of daily chores such as housekeeping, home maintenance and lawn care, but they also remember your special preferences. It's these thougtfull touches that make living at Ardenwoods so wonderful.

7022 Asheville Manor
308 Overlook Road
Arden, NC 28704
877-938-7079
Fax: 828-684-1917
www.brookdaleliving.com

Chris Szalony, Executive Director

7023 Ashland Healthcare
215 Badger Street
West Jefferson, NC 28694
573-657-2877
Fax: 336-246-2169
www.brookdaleliving.com

7024 Atria Assisted Retirement Living Merrywood
3600 Park Road
Charlotte, NC 28209-4102
704-523-4949
Fax: 704-527-8866
atriaassistedliving.com

Connie Brown, Executive Director

Retirement living at Atria MerryWood means enjoying a wonderful sence of independence, along with an active community life with social, recreational and cultural events available both within our community and in town. We also offer assisted living services.

7025 Bell House
2400 Summit Avenue
Greensboro, NC 27405-5014
336-621-0938
Fax: 336-621-0947
www.bellhouseinc.org

Linda Gordon, Executive Director

7026 Blakey Hall Assisted Living
501 Manning Avenue
Elon College, NC 27244-9136
336-506-2300
Fax: 336-506-2455
www.bhhamlet.com

John Ketcham, Owner

Our purpose is to care for residents in an environment that encourages them to make the most of their abilities. We want them to feel they are engaged in meaningful activities and not merely passing time.

7027 Bradford Village East
413 N Main Street
Kernersville, NC 27284-2643
336-993-4696
Fax: 336-993-8957
gloria@bradfordvillage.org
www.bradfordvillage.org

Mark Mitchel, Administrator

7028 Bradford Village West
602 Piney Grove Road
Kernersville, NC 27284-2333
336-993-8711
Fax: 336-993-8499
gloria@bradfordvillage.org
www.bradfordvillage.org

Mark Mitchell, Administrator

7029 Bridging the Gap of Care
56 W Vineyard Lane
Hayesville, NC 28904-5603
828-389-8350
Fax: 828-389-9064
ipenland@frontier.com
www.btgcares.com

Irene Penland, Owner

7030 Brighton Gardens by Marriott-Greensboro
1208 New Garden Road
Greensboro, NC 27410-2679
336-297-4700
Fax: 336-297-1244
www.sunriseseniorliving.com

Debbie Ankrom, Manager

7031 Brighton Gardens by Marriott-Raleigh
3101 Duraleigh Road
Raleigh, NC 27612-4189
919-571-1123
Fax: 919-571-9091
www.sunriseseniorliving.com

Greg Fox, Manager

7032 Brighton Gardens of Winston Salem
2601 Reynolda Road
Winston Salem, NC 27106-3863
336-722-2224
Fax: 336-722-7212
www.sunriseseniorliving.com

Mary Locicero, Executive Director

At Sunrise Senior Living we take living personally. That's why we offer our seniros a variety of living arrangements, amenities, services, meal plans, social activities and care. It's a broad range of options that help seniors enjoy a full life - all on their own terms.

7033 Brookstone Haven Residential Care
501 Pointe South Drive
Randleman, NC 27317-9503
336-495-2800
Fax: 336-495-4865
www.mytahome.com

David Dean Wilson, Owner

7034 Burlington Manor
3615 S Mebane Street
Burlington, NC 27215-5221
855-350-3800
Fax: 336-584-9026
www.brookdaleliving.com

Tammy Conklin, Executive Director

7035 Cardinal Care Center-Hendersonville
1000 W Allen Street
Hendersonville, NC 28739-4881
828-693-3388
Fax: 828-697-5461
www.cardinalcarecenter.com

Sandee Barnwell, Administrator

7036 Carillon Assisted Living of Asheboro
2925 Zoo Parkway
Asheboro, NC 27205-1410
336-633-7600
Fax: 336-633-7621
www.cardinalcarecenter.com

7037 Carillon Assisted Living of Cramer Mountain
500 Cramer Mountain Road
Cramerton, NC 28032-1663
704-823-0500
Fax: 704-823-0504
www.carillonassistedliving.com

Charlene Swilling, Marketing
Zerina Francum, Executive Director

Carillon facilities provide assistance with activities of daily living and a secure dementia care unit.

7038 Carillon Assisted Living of Newton
1088 Radio Station Road
Newton, NC 28658-9478
828-466-7474
Fax: 828-466-7477
www.carillonassistedliving.com

7039 Carillon Assisted Living of Shelby
1550 Charles Road
Shelby, NC 28152-7036
704-471-2828
Fax: 704-471-2829
www.carillonassistedliving.com

7040 Carillon of Salisbury
1915 Mooresville Road
Salisbury, NC 28147-8813
704-633-4666
Fax: 704-633-6400
www.carillonassistedliving.com

Wendy Hooper, Executive Director

7041 Carmel Hills
2801 Carmel Road
Charlotte, NC 28226-6393
704-364-8302
Fax: 704-364-8819
info@carmelhills.org
www.carmelhills.org

Richard Todd, Administrator

7042 Carolina House of Asheboro
514 Vision Drive
Asheboro, NC 27203-3895
855-350-3800
Fax: 336-683-0073
www.brookdaleliving.com

Ellen Hill, Sales Director

7043 Carolina House of Cary
111 Macarthur Drive
Cary, NC 27513-8900
877-712-9732
Fax: 919-460-4505
www.brookdaleliving.com

Rhonda Quattlebaum, Sales Director
Matt Cross, Executive Director

7044 Carolina House of Durham
4434 Ben Franklin Blvd
Durham, NC 27704
877-712-9734
Fax: 919-479-9977
www.brookdaleliving.com

Allison Lee, Sales Director
Angela Wright, Manager

7045 Carolina House of Elizabeth City
401 Hastings Lane
Elizabeth City, NC 27909-3327

877-938-7006
Fax: 252-331-0334
www.brookdaleliving.com

Sharee Wilder, Executive Director

7046 Carolina House of Forest City
493 Piney Ridge Road
Forest City, NC 28043-9017
877-938-7008
Fax: 828-288-1178
www.brookdaleliving.com

Tina Rippy, Executive Director

7047 Carolina House of Greenville
2715 Dickinson Avenue
Greenville, NC 27834-5099
877-938-7010
Fax: 252-353-6577
www.brookdaleliving.com

Randy Jackson, Executive Director

7048 Carolina House of Lexington
161 Young Drive
Lexington, NC 27292-4435
877-938-6801
Fax: 336-224-1448
www.brookdaleliving.com

Cindy Smith, Executive Director

7049 Carolina House of Pinehurst
17 Regional Drive
Pinehurst, NC 28374-8650
877-938-7113
Fax: 910-235-0650
www.brookdaleliving.com

James Floyd, Executive Director

7050 Carolina House of Reidsville
2931 Vance Street Extension
Reidsville, NC 27320-9409
877-938-6803
Fax: 336-349-2240
www.brookdaleliving.com

Becky Vance, Executive Director

7051 Carolina House of Smithfield
830 Berkshire Road
Smithfield, NC 27577-4729
877-938-7012
Fax: 919-989-3032
www.brookdaleliving.com

Kathy Vidal, Executive Director

7052 Carolina House of Wake Forest
611 Brooks Street
Wake Forest, NC 27587-2978
877-712-9735
Fax: 919-562-4687
www.brookdaleliving.com

Greg Fox, Executive Director

7053 Carolina Inn at Village Green
405 Forsythe Street
Fayetteville, NC 28303-5488

910-829-0100
Fax: 910-829-7100
www.carolinainnnc.com

Franklin Clark, Owner

7054 Carolina Village
600 Carolina Village Road
Hendersonville, NC 28792-2845
828-692-6275
Fax: 828-692-7876
www.carolinavillage.com

Doley Bell, Administrator

A non profit, continuing care for the retired.

7055 Carriage Club of Charlotte
5800 Old Providence Road
Charlotte, NC 28226-6872
704-365-8551
Fax: 704-366-4270
www.brookdaleliving.com

Jackie Pittman, Executive Director

7056 Cedar Rock Assisted Living
PO Box 1237
Mocksville, NC 27028-1237
336-751-1515
Fax: 336-751-1621

Sheila Simons, Owner

7057 Champions at Porters Neck
1007 Porters Neck Road
Wilmington, NC 28411-7383
910-686-6462
Fax: 918-686-8320
www.thedaviscommunity.org

Charles Long, Chief Executive
Diane Blake, Administrator

7058 Chancellor Gardens of Charlotte
9120 Willow Ridge Road
Charlotte, NC 28210-8313
704-540-0098
Fax: 704-540-9020
www.southernassisted.com

7059 Charlotte Square
5820 Carmel Road
Charlotte, NC 28226-8106
704-544-4979
Fax: 704-540-7883
www.capitalsenior.com

Alverita Peeples, Manager

7060 Chatham Creek Rest Home
809 W Chatham Street
Cary, NC 27511-3136
919-469-9309
Fax: 919-469-4565
www.Depaul.org

Terri Zimmerman, Administrator

7061 Cherry Springs Village
2222 N Main Street
Hendersonville, NC 28792-2438

828-698-6501
Fax: 828-698-6504
www.cherryspringsvillage.com

Angela White, Owner

Cherry Springs offers a wide range of social activites and special events designed to promot active involvement. Transportation is provided for medical appointments outside the facility.

7062 Churchhill Assisted Living Residences
140 Carriage Club Drive
Mooresville, NC 28117-9002
704-658-1200
Fax: 704-814-0350
www.emeritus.com

7063 Clare Bridge of Chapel Hill
2230 Farmington Drive
Chapel Hill, NC 27517-7843
877-712-9775
Fax: 919-493-7123
www.brookdaleliving.com

Mary Casey, Executive Director

7064 Clemmons Village
6401 Holder Road
Clemmons, NC 27012-9207
336-766-2990
Fax: 336-766-2138
www.clemmonsvillage1.com

Kathy Edens, Owner

7065 Colonial Manor Rest Home
160 Health Care Drive
Rutherfordton, NC 28139-8058
828-287-7353
Fax: 828-286-4890

James E Yelton, Owner

7066 Community Care of Haywood
67 Loving Way
Clyde, NC 28721-9471
828-452-3822
Fax: 828-452-3820
www.comcarenc.com

Mary Allen, Manager

Our facilities are licensed and monitored monhly by the state.

7067 Concord Place
2452 Rock Hill Church Road
Concord, NC 28027-8048
855-350-3800
Fax: 704-786-3173
www.brookdaleliving.com

Kellee Armsworthy, Executive Director
Beverly Register, Administrator

7068 Country Sunshine Rest Home
148 Cox Avenue
Richlands, NC 28574-6163
910-324-1121
Fax: 910-324-5371

Debbie Moscow, Manager

7069 Countryside Living
5383 Us Highway 117 N
Pikeville, NC 27863-9443
919-242-6369
Fax: 919-242-9884
www.countyside-living.com

Marsha Sauls, Administrator

7070 Countrytime Inn
602 Brevard Street
Kings Mountain, NC 28086-8692
704-739-2760
Fax: 704-789-4775
www.meridiansenior.com

Tahir Majeed, Executive Director

7071 Crescent View Retirement Community
2533 Hendersonville Road
Arden, NC 28704-8583
828-687-0068
Fax: 828-684-8929
www.lsanc.net

Jerry Bramley, Chair

7072 Croasdaile Village
2600 Croasdaile Farm Parkway
Durham, NC 27705-1397
919-384-2475
Fax: 919-384-2513
www.croasdailevillage.com

Carol Roycroft, Marketing Director

7073 Cross Road Retirement Community
1302 Old Cox Road
Asheboro, NC 27205-9466
336-629-7811
Fax: 336-629-6264
crrc@triad.rr.com
www.cross-road.org

Janet Harllee, Admissions/Marketing
Steve Rumbley, Administrator

Provides a safe and comfortable environment for seniors.

7074 Discovery Program at Burlington Manor
3619 S Mebane Street
Burlington, NC 27215-5221
336-538-0367
Fax: 336-538-1724
www.southernassisted.com

Tammy Conklin, Office Manager
Marilyn Williams, Executive Director

7075 Eden Estates
314 W Kings Highway
Eden, NC 27288-5012
855-350-3800
Fax: 336-623-5144
www.brookdaleliving.com

Tammy Martin, Executive Director

7076 Eden Gardens of Statesville
2147 Davie Avenue
Statesville, NC 28625-9200
704-878-0123
Fax: 704-878-8689

Danny Boone, Manager

7077 Edengardens of Concord
15801 Zion Chuch Road E
Concord, NC 28085
704-782-1100
Fax: 704-721-3144

Chuck Pierce, Executive Director

7078 Elms at Tanglewood
3750 Harper Road
Clemmons, NC 27012-8682
336-766-2131
Fax: 336-766-2160
www.elmsattanglewood.com

Charlotte Tullock, Administrator

Our mission is to provide quality, professional assisted care in a comfortable, nurturing, homelike environment, an atmosphere of respect and warmth and dignity, where our residents can feel a sense of purpose and community.

7079 Fountains at the Albemarle Inn
200 Trade Street
Tarboro, NC 27886-5055
252-377-4396
Fax: 252-823-6555
www.watermarkcommunities.com

Christopher Casteel, Executive Director

We offer a lovely, amenity-rich environment in which residents can enjoy privacy, independence and freedom of choice while receiving all the care and support they need.

7080 Gaston Manor
1717 Union Road
Gastonia, NC 28054-5583
855-350-3800
Fax: 704-865-1548
www.brookdaleliving.com

Diane Payne, Executive Director

7081 Gaston Place
1750 Robinwood Road
Gastonia, NC 28054-1664
855-350-3800
Fax: 704-864-4448
www.brookdaleliving.com

Hal Shoup, Executive Director

7082 Greenbrier
703 S Walnut Street
Fairmont, NC 28340-1837
910-628-9021
Fax: 910-628-7441
www.depaul.org

Laura Hardison, Administrator

7083 Greensboro Manor
5809 Old Oak Ridge Road
Greensboro, NC 27410-9265
877-938-7071
Fax: 336-856-1060
www.brookdaleliving.com

Carol Royals, Executive Director

7084 Greensboro Place on Lawndale
4400 Lawndale Drive
Greensboro, NC 27455-1819
877-938-7073
Fax: 336-286-3005
www.brookdaleliving.com

Jo Frazier, Sales Director
Patricia McCulloh, Executive Director

7085 Haven in the Village at Carolina Place
13150 Dorman Road
Pineville, NC 28134-9327
704-540-0155
Fax: 704-540-7769
www.havencarolinaplace.com

Nancy Nye, Manager

7086 Haywood Lodge & Retirement Center
251 Shelton Street
Waynesville, NC 28786-3362
828-456-8365
Fax: 828-456-6792; *Toll Free:* 888-238-0103
www.haywoodlodge.com

Aaron Crawford, Owner

Our mission is to provide the highest standard of care possible for our residents while maintaining a high quality of life, independence and self-esteem. Our dedicated staff works closely with outside health professionals to meet the specific needs of each resident.

7087 HeartFields Assisted Living at Cary
1050 Cresent Drive
Cary, NC 27511
919-852-5757
Fax: 919-852-2628
www.heartforseniors.com

Denise Alala, Executive Director

HeartFields provides seniors the perfect blend of comfort, care and choice. The heart of our program rests on providing just the right level of personalized services, while allowing residents to be as independent as possible.

7088 Heritage Place
325 N Cool Spring Street
Fayetteville, NC 28301-5197
910-323-4925
Fax: 910-678-8673
www.heritage-place.com

Shelia Sorkin, Executive Director

7089 Heritage Woods
3812 Forrestgate Drive
Winston Salem, NC 27103-3036
336-768-2011
Fax: 336-760-4258
www.kiscoseniorliving.com

7090 Hickory Manor
2530 16th Street NE
Hickory, NC 28601-7603
828-324-5400
Fax: 828-326-9770
www.brookdaleliving.com

BJ Fore, Sales Director
Jeff Dula, Executive Director

7091 High Point Manor
201 W Hartley Drive
High Point, NC 27265-2843
877-938-6827
Fax: 336-885-5817
www.brookdaleliving.com

Kimberly Hemric, Executive Director

7092 High Point Place
1568 Skeet Club Road
High Point, NC 27265-9530
855-350-3800
Fax: 336-869-0062
www.brookdaleliving.com

Gina Floyd, Executive Director
Trudy Snuggs, Manager

7093 Homeplace of Burlington
118 Alamance Road
Burlington, NC 27215
336-227-2328
Fax: 336-227-2329
www.homeplaceofburlington.com

7094 Homeplace of New Bern
1309 McCarthy Boulevard
New Bern, NC 28562
252-637-7133
Fax: 336-378-9705
www.homeplaceofnewbern.com

Steven D Bell, Owner

7095 Homestead Hills Assisted Living
3250 Homestead Club Drive
Winston Salem, NC 27103-6445
336-659-0708
Fax: 336-659-8506
Info@Homestead-Hills.com
www.homestead-hills.com

Phyllis Shore, Executive Director

7096 Inn at Quail Haven
155 Blake Boulevard
Pinehurst, NC 28374-8497
910-295-2294
Fax: 910-295-2379
www.umrh.org

Myron Dice, Administrator

The Inn provides respite care, skilled nursing, rehabilitative and restorative servivces. Residents recieve truly individualized service from a staff of caring, competent professionals in an atmosphere of genuine warmth and compassion.

7097 Kerner Ridge Assisted Living
250 Hopkins Road
Kernersville, NC 27284-9314
336-993-1881
Fax: 336-993-2592
www.ridgecare.com

Mary Spainhour, Administrator

7098 Laurels in Highland Creek
6101 Clarke Creek Parkway
Charlotte, NC 28269-6936
704-947-8050
Fax: 704-947-2363
www.highlandcreekseniorliving.com

Jennifer Davidson, Executive Director

7099 Laurels in the Village at Carolina Place
13180 Dorman Road
Pineville, NC 28134-9327
704-540-8007
Fax: 704-540-8088
www.laurelscarolinaplace.com

Stacy Gatto, Executive Director

We offer licensed nursing professionals on-site 24 hours a day/7 days a week, alcove, companion, one and two bedroom apartments with kitchenettes, a personal emergency call system, individually controlled thermostats for comfort as well as home cooked meals, scheduled transportation, activities and housekeeping services.

7100 Lawyers Glen Retirement Living Center
10830 Lawyers Road
Charlotte, NC 28227
704-545-9555
Fax: 704-545-2075
johnelliotte@lawyersglen.com
www.lawyersglen.com

The campus is dedicated to our philosophy: to enhance independence, productivity, security, and dignity while providing affordable healthcare to promote comfort, conveniences, companionship and place of mind and to provide for social, emotional, physical and spiritual well-being of our residents. To fulfill this mission, Lawyers Glen will cater to the desired lifestyle of its residents by proviging the highest quality and best services available.

7101 Little Flower Assisted Living Residence
8700 Lawyers Road
Charlotte, NC 28227-8740
704-545-7005
Fax: 704-545-7016
www.premierseniorliving.com

Doloris Brown, Administrator

7102 Marriotts Brighton Gardens of Charlotte
6000 Park South Drive
Charlotte, NC 28210-3298
704-643-1400
Fax: 704-643-9400
www.sunriseseniorliving.com

Lynne Napoli, Manager

7103 Mars Hill Retirement Community
170 S Main Street
Mars Hill, NC 28754-6622
828-689-7970
Fax: 828-689-7972; *Toll Free:* 888-420-6983
tammie.chandler@marshillretire.com
www.marshillretire.com

Tammie S Chandler, Marketing Director
Richard Pridgen, Administrator
Gail Blankenship, Office Manager

Mars Hill offers a cost-effective quality care that is personalized for the individuals needs, fosters independence for each resident, treats each resident with dignity and respect, promotes individuality of each resident, allows each resident choice of care and lifestyle, protects each resident's right to privacy, provides a safe residential environment, and makes the assisted living residence a valuable community asset.

7104 Maryfield
109 Penny Road
High Point, NC 27260-2611
336-821-4000
Fax: 336-886-4036
www.pennybyrnatmaryfield.org

Sylvia Wunch, Staff Development
Lucy Hennessy, Manager

Provides assisted living accommodations to residents who need a little help to remain independent. Our assisted living wing provides residents with a higher level of independence and activity range. Residents enjoy privacy, independence and have many choices in their desired activites.

7105 North Carolina Assisted Living Association
1306 Annapolis Drive
Suite 120
Raleigh, NC 27608-2136
919-467-2486
Fax: 919-467-5132
info@ncassistedliving.org
www.ncassistedliving.org

Jerry Cooper, Executive Director
Kathy Rodgers, Meeting/Membership Coordinator

7106 Oak Hill Living Center
PO Box 759
Angier, NC 27501
919-639-9000
Fax: 919-639-9435
www.oakhillliving.com

Christopher Strickland, Administrator

7107 Piedmont Christian Home
1510 Deep River Road
High Point, NC 27265-3400
336-883-6023
Fax: 336-883-6024
www.piedmonthome.com

Bonnie Smith, Owner

7108 Ridge Crest Retirement
100 Ridgecrest Drive
Mount Airy, NC 27030-9196
336-786-9100
Fax: 336-786-2899
www.ridge-crest.com

Laney Johnson, Executive Director

7109 Salisbury Gardens
2201 Salisbury Boulevard
Salisbury, NC 28147
855-350-3800
Fax: 704-639-1146
www.brookdaleliving.com

Lou Cranford, Executive Director

7110 Samaritan Place Assisted Living
52 Lower Grassy Branch Road
Asheville, NC 28805-1639

828-298-7592
Fax: 828-298-2637
www.good-sam.com

Tammy Wise, Manager

Our mission statement is to provide caring assistance in daily living with dignity and respect while promoting individual independence.

7111 Shallotte Assisted Living
520 Mulberry Street
Shallotte, NC 28470-4586
910-754-6621
Fax: 910-754-6621
www.shallotteassisted.com

Denise Kirby, Manager

7112 Spring Arbor of Apex
901 Spring Arbor Court
Apex, NC 27502-4951
919-805-3861
Fax: 919-303-0659
apexinfo@hhhunt.com
www.springarborliving.com

Sandy Gegax, Executive Director

7113 Spring Arbor of Herdersonville
1820 Pisgah Drive
Hendersonville, NC 28791-3759
828-633-4050
Fax: 828-692-8922
hendersonvilleinfo@hhhunt.com
www.springarborliving.com

Jeffrey Marhafer, Executive Director

7114 Spring Arbor of Kinston
3207 Carey Road
Kinston, NC 28504-1205
252-558-1194
Fax: 252-523-8074
kinstoninfo@hhhunt.com
www.springarborliving.com

Cynthia Sparks, Administrator

7115 Spring Arbor of Raleigh
1810 N New Hope Road
Raleigh, NC 27604-8305
919-805-3858
Fax: 919-250-0247
raleighinfo@hhhunt.com
www.springarborliving.com

Pam Mayo, Executive Director

7116 Spring Arbor of Rocky Mount
1251 S Winstead Avenue
Rocky Mount, NC 27803-1557
252-969-0990
Fax: 252-443-3113
rockymountinfo@hhhunt.com
www.springarborliving.com

Rebecca Holoman, Administrator

7117 Spring Arbor of Wilmington
809 John D Barry Drive
Wilmington, NC 28412
910-249-4823
Fax: 910-799-8210

wilmingtoninfo@hhhunt.com
www.springarborliving.com
Loretta Evans, Administrator

7118 Spring Arbor of Wilson
2045 Ward Boulevard
Wilson, NC 27893-2873
252-289-1970
Fax: 252-234-0001
wilsoninfo@hhhunt.com
www.springarborliving.com

Eve Artis, Executive Director

Pur dedicated team nurtures our residents independence by promoting dignity and choice within a setting of professional, compassionate care. Assistance is always offered, never imposed and our full-service lifestyle offers our residents and their families the time to focus on opportunities, not challenges.

7119 Statesville Place
2806 Peachtree Road
Statesville, NC 28625-8204
855-350-3800
Fax: 704-872-1992
www.brookdaleliving.com

Karen Cline, Executive Director

7120 Sterling House of Rocky Mount, Brookdale Senior Living
650 Goldrock Road
Rocky Mount, NC 27804-8804
252-446-6005
Fax: 252-446-0974
www.brookdaleliving.org

Crystal Boettcher, Executive Director

Enriching the lives of those that aer seved with compassion, respect, excellence and integrity.

7121 Sunrise Assisted Living at Eastover
3610 Randolph Road
Charlotte, NC 28211-1318
704-366-2550
Fax: 704-366-4041
www.sunriseseniorliving.com

Carrie Dellinger, Executive Director

At Sunrise Senior Living we take living personally. Thats why we offer our seniors a variety of living arrangements, amenities, services, meal plans, social activities and care. It's a broad range of options that help seniors a full life, all on their own terms.

7122 Sunrise Assisted Living of Raleigh
4801 Edwards Mill Road
Raleigh, NC 27612-4417
919-787-0777
Fax: 919-787-6105
www.sunriseseniorliving.com

Karen Sherman, Executive Director

7123 Sunrise Assisted Living of South Charlotte
5515 Rea Road
Charlotte, NC 28226-3446
704-544-2094
Fax: 704-544-6530
www.sunriseseniorliving.com

Rita Shew, Executive Director

At Sunrise Senior Living we take living personally. That's why we offer our seniors a variety of living arrangements, amenities, services, meal plans, social activities and care. It's a broad range of options that help seniors enjoy a full life, all on their own terms.

7124 Sunrise of Providence
5114 Providence Road
Charlotte, NC 28226-5852
704-365-5252
Fax: 704-365-4306
www.sunriseniorliving.com

Nancy Myer, Manager

At Sunrise Senior Living we take living personally. That's why we offer our seniors a variety of living arrangements, amenities, services, meal plans, social activities and care. It's a broad range of options that help seniors enjoy a full life, all on their own terms.

7125 Trinity Oaks Retirement Community
728 Klumac Road
Salisbury, NC 28144-5720
704-633-1002
Fax: 704-636-5038
apressly@trinityoaks.net
www.trinityoaks.net

Mike Walsh, Executive Director

North Dakota

7126 Baptist Home of Kenmare
PO Box 787
Kenmare, ND 58746
701-385-4941
Fax: 701-385-4215
www.abhomes.net

Karen Schwartz, Asministrator

Attention to physical well-being is an important aspect of life at the Baptist Home with weekly exercise opportunities. Delicious, balanced meals are enjouyed daily by residents of the Baptist Home of Kenmare.

7127 Bethany Homes
201 University Drive S
Fargo, ND 58103-8299
701-239-3000
Fax: 701-239-3237
www.bethanyhomes.org

Ray Weisgarber, Executive Director

We dedicate outselves to making Bethany a place where residents can live in comfort and dignity in a communiyt that is shaped by Christian concern.

7128 Bethel Lutheran Home
1515 Second Avenue
Williston, ND 58801
701-572-6766
Fax: 701-572-7579
home.att.net/~bethel/

Kurt Stoner, Administrator

Our Mission at Bethel Lutheran is dedicated to serving the physical, emotional and spiritual needs of each aging person regardless of race, color, sex, religion, age, national origin or handicap by striving to provide the highest quality facilities, personal care and programs out of obedience to and love for christ in order to enhance the dignity, self worth and purpose of life for each individual who enters the sphere of Bethel's influence.

7129 Devils Lake Good Samaritan

302 7th Avenue NE
Devils Lake, ND 58301-2516
701-662-6580
Fax: 701-662-6580
www.good-sam.com

Karen Boulden, Administrator

7130 Edgewood Vista - Minot

800 16th Ave SE
Minot, ND 58701-5933
701-852-1399
Fax: 701-383-0613
www.edgewoodseniorliving.com

Becky Rotvedt, Administrator

Edgewood Vista exists to provide personalized care in settings designed specifically for Elderly, including those with Alzheimer's Disease or other forms of fementia. Our individualizes approach provides a high quality, safe, home-like setting to Seniors who choose to no longer reside alone, but who can live better in social settings. Through empathetic hearts we eill serve the needs of our residents 24 hours a day.

7131 Edgewood Vista of Bismark

3406 Dominion Street
Bismarck, ND 58503-5577
701-258-7489
Fax: 701-258-7491
www.edgewoodvista.com

Dale Klein, President

Edgewood Vista exists to provide personalized care in settings designed specifically for Seniors, including those with Alzheimer's Disease or other forms of dementia. Our individualized approach provides a high quality, safe, home-like setting to Seniros who choose to no longer redside alone, but who can live better in social residential settings. Through empathetic hearts we will serve the needs of our residents 24 hours a day.

7132 Ellendale Evergreen Place

241 Main Street
Ellendale, ND 58436-7103
701-349-3611
Fax: 701-349-4656
nd.gov/dhs/services/disabilities

Tony Hanson, Manager

To provide room and board, and health, social, and personal care to assist the residents to attain or maintain their highest level of functioning, consistent with the resident assessment and care plan, to five or more residents not related by blood or marraige to the owner or manager. The services are provided on a 24-hour bases within the facility, either directly or through contract, and include assistance with activities of daily living andprovision of leisure, recreational and therapeutic activities, as well as of nutritional needs and medication administration.

7133 Golden Acres Manor

PO Box 261
Carrington, ND 58421
701-652-3117
Fax: 701-652-3118
www.goldenacresmanor.com

Allan Metzger, Administrator

This organization was formed to enhance the lives of residents of Golden Acres Manor by making possible the purchase of special needs equipment, furnishings, etc. which the nursing home would not otherwise be able to fund.

7134 Good Shepherd Home

709m 4th Avenue NE
Watford City, ND 58854-7628
701-444-2331
Fax: 701-842-4629

Kris Pacheco, Administrator

7135 Harolds Haaland Home

1025 3rd Ave S
Rugby, ND 58368-2118
701-776-5203
Fax: 701-776-6688
www.nd.gov/dhs/services/disabilities

Mark Weber, Manager

Our mission is to provide quality medical care, as reflected by the needs and demographics of north central North Dakota. Although we are determined to be self-supporting, our Christian dedication is primarliy to provide an array of quality services for patients and residents regardless of race, color, creed, or disability.

7136 Luther Memorial Home

750 Main Street E
Mayville, ND 58257-1698
701-786-3401
Fax: 701-786-9022
activities@luthermemorialhome.com,
www.luthermemorialhome.com

Brett Ulrich, Administrator

7137 Maddock Memorial Home

301 Roosevelt Avenue
Maddock, ND 58348-7138
701-438-2641
Fax: 701-438-2641

Beth Olsen

7138 Manor St Joesph

404 4th Avenue
Edgeley, ND 58433-7417
701-493-2477
Fax: 701-493-2477
www.edgeley.com

Tammy Jangula, Administrator

7139 Marian Manor

604 E Ash Avenue
Glen Ullin, ND 58631-7138
701-348-3107
Fax: 701-348-3080
www.marianmanorhc.com

Rod Auer, Administrator

7140 Marillac Manor
1016 N 28th Street
Bismarck, ND 58504
701-258-8702
Fax: 701-223-3127
www.bismarck.sanfordhealth.org

Pheobe Schwartze, Admissions
Grant Wilz, Administrator

7141 Noonan Good Samaritan Center
PO Box 69
Noonan, ND 58765
701-925-5670
Fax: 701-925-5718
www.good-sam.com

Elaine Heide, Administrator

The mission of the Society is to share God's love in word and deed by providing shelter and supportive services to older persons and others in need.

7142 Old Fellows Home
1107 Walnut Street E
Devils Lake, ND 58301-3240
701-662-3330
Fax: 701-662-6672
ndioof@gondtc.com

Mark Ulrich, Administrator

7143 Park River Good Samaritan
301 S Highway 12b
Park River, ND 58270-4134
701-284-7115
Fax: 701-284-7117
gss6300@good-sam.com

David Carda, Administrator

Our center provides physical, occupational and speech therapy services; a full range of activities; delicious meals; an on-site chaplain; and the living care of a dedicated and comapssionate staff.

7144 Primrose Retirement Center
1144 College Drive
Bismarck, ND 58501-1212
701-222-8183
Fax: 701-250-9719
bismarck@primroseretirement.com
www.primroseretirement.com

Chuck Wolfgram, Manager

7145 Redwood Village
PO Box 339
Wilton, ND 58579
701-734-6409
Fax: 701-523-4139
www.prideinc.org

Judy Pepple, Administrator

7146 Riverview Place
5300 12th Street S
Fargo, ND 58104-6427
701-237-4700
Fax: 701-235-5738
www.riverviewplace.org

Jeff Pederson, President
Kristine Christensen, Controller

7147 Sheridan Memorial Home
610 S Main
McClusky, ND 58463
701-363-2203
Fax: 701-363-2703

Theresa Jorgenson, Administrator

7148 St Catherine's Living Center
1307 7th Street N
Wahpeton, ND 58075-3624
701-642-6667
Fax: 701-642-2485
pws.bhshealth.com

Steve Williams, Manager

7149 Tufte Manor
3300 Cherry Street
Grand Forks, ND 58201-7699
701-775-2581
Fax: 701-775-2259
www.valleymemorial.org

Garth Rydland, CEO
Nancy Andrews, Director

7150 Valley View Heights
2500 Valleyview Avenue
Bismarck, ND 58501-3090
701-221-3018
Fax: 701-221-3023
www.valleyviewheights.com

Robert R Thompson, CEO

7151 Waterford at Hardwoodgroves
1200 Harwood Drive S
Fargo, ND 58104-6298
701-476-1200
Fax: 701-476-1201
www.touchmarkfargo.com

Kari Dick, Executive Director

7152 Waterford on West Century
1000 W Century Avenue
Bismarck, ND 58503
701-323-7000
Fax: 701-221-2525
www.touchmarkfargo.com

Arlene Farnsworth, Executive Director

7153 Wheatland Terrace
4006 24th Avenue S
Grand Forks, ND 58201-8871
701-787-7621
Fax: 701-787-7564
nanadrews@valleymemorial.org
www.valleymemorial.org

Greg Hanson, CEO
Nancy Andrews, Administrator
Nancy Hartvikson, Director Personal Services

We are committed to providing quality care and servicves from a Christian perspective in an environment designed to enhance the dignity and independence of those we serve.

Nebraska

7154 Ambassabor Nebraska City Assisted Living
1800 14th Avenue
Nebraska City, NE 68410-1159
402-873-6650
Fax: 402-873-6621
www.ambhealthsys.com

Mike Brogman, Executive Director

7155 An Angels Touch
1113m N 85th Street
Omaha, NE 68114-2916
402-672-9580
Fax: 402-697-1311
nangelstouchinc@hotmail.com
www.anangelstouchinc.com

Judy Allington, Owner

7156 Bell View Rehabilitation Center
1702 Hillcrest Drive
Bellevue, NE 68005-3652
402-291-8500
Fax: 402-291-8500
www.bellevueclinic.com

Jolene Robert, Owner

7157 Bethany Home
515 W 1st Street
Minden, NE 68959-1401
308-832-1595
Fax: 308-832-0662
www.kearneyhub.com

James Dyck, Administrator

7158 Beverly Square Scottsbluff
111 W 36th Street
Scottsbluff, NE 69361-4623
308-635-2019
Fax: 308-635-2458

Jay Cooburn, Administrator

7159 Blue Valley Riverside Apartments
715 S 1st Street
Hebron, NE 68370-2006
402-768-6073
Fax: 402-768-6014

Michelle Plock, Manager

7160 Brighton Gardens of Omaha
9220 Western Avenue
Omaha, NE 68114-2297
402-393-7313
Fax: 402-393-7340
www.sunriseseniorliving.com

Diane Ross, Executive Director

7161 Carter House
1028 Joann Drive
Blair, NE 68008-2725
402-426-1977
Fax: 402-426-0322
www.alcco.com

Susan McDunn, Manager

7162 Centennial Park Retirement Village
510 Centennial Circle
North Platte, NE 69101-6520
308-534-7000
Fax: 308-534-8216
www.centennialparkretirement.com

Bob Tank, Administrator

7163 Chapion Home - Mental Health Assisted Living
602 S Wabash Avenue
PO Box 1197
Hastings, NE 68962
402-463-6021
Fax: 402-463-7011

Vivian Sullivan, Administrator
Gary Barrera, Owner

Assisted living for adults with mental disabilities.
Year Founded: 1999

7164 Chapion Home of Hastings
602 S Wabash Avenue 1Po Box 1197
Hastings, NE 68901-6152
402-463-6021
Fax: 402-463-7011
www.championhomesmentalhealthalf.net

Vivian Sullivan, Administrator
Gary Barrera, Owner

7165 Chrisoma West Assisted Living
1923 W 4th Avenue
Holdrege, NE 68949-3113
308-995-4493
Fax: 308-995-8702
www.chrisoma.com

Don Bakke, Administrator

7166 Christian Homes Assisted Living Center
1927 W 4th Avenue
Holdrege, NE 68949-3114
308-995-4493
Fax: 308-995-8702
www.chrisoma.com

Don Bakke, Administrator

7167 Clark Jeary Home
1313 Eldon Drive
Lincoln, NE 68510-5024
402-489-0331
Fax: 402-489-0462
www.clarkjeary.com

Kathleen Pearson, Administrator

7168 Comfortcare Homes of Nebraska
2315 South 168th Street
Omaha, NE 68130
402-445-4474
Fax: 402-397-1114
tomr@cchne.com
www.cchne.com

Tom Ruffino, Executive Director

7169 Community Pride Care Center
901 S 4th Street
Battle Creek, NE 68715-3035

402-675-2955
Fax: 402-675-2965

Steve Freese, Administrator

7170 Cottonwood House

3271 29th Avenue
Columbus, NE 68601-3811
402-562-9136
Fax: 402-563-2097
www.alcco.com

Patti Stuthman, Administrator

7171 Cottonwood Villa

450 S Main Street
Ainsworth, NE 69210-1701
402-387-1000
Fax: 402-238-1015
info@cottonwoodvilla.com
www.cottonwoodvilla.com

Ann Fiala, Administrator
Heidi O'Dea, Coordinator

7172 Countryside Home

703 N Main Street
Madison, NE 68748-6061
402-454-3373
Fax: 402-454-9021
www.lifeatcountryside.com

Dolores Woodruff, Manager

7173 Crossroads Assisted Living

150 W 24th Street
Alliance, NE 69301-2156
308-762-1615
Fax: 308-762-1621

Felisha Hoagland, Administrator

7174 Crowell Home Health Services

245 S 22nd Street
Blair, NE 68008-1811
402-426-2177
Fax: 402-426-2577
billwill@crowellhome.com
wwwcrowellhome.com

Terry Wulf, Asst Administrator

The home provides a compassionate care for seniros. We offer a full time physical, occupational, and speech therapies, that are available on site to help residents maintain the highest level of independence possible.

7175 Custer Care Center

346 N 16th Avenue
Broken Bow, NE 68822-1422
308-872-6303
Fax: 308-872-5236
www.custercare.com

Jeanette Denson, Executive Director

Our mission is to provide high quality and reliable services and to maintain the clients independence in their home or at the Center.

7176 East Park Villa

1704 L Street
Aurora, NE 68818-2100

402-694-2300
Fax: 402-694-2305
www.memorialcommunityhealth.org

7177 Eastmont Towers

6315 O Street
Lincoln, NE 68510-2237
402-489-6591
Fax: 402-486-2331
www.eastmonttowers.com

7178 Edgewood Vista Columbus

3386 53rd Avenue
Columbus, NE 68601-1512
402-564-3785
Fax: 402-564-4157
www.edgewoodvista.com

Patty Voichoskie, Manager

We provide personalized care in settings designed sepcifically for the Elderly, including those with Alzheimer's Disease or other forms of dementia. Our individualized approach provides a high quality, safe, home-like setting to Seniors who choose to no longer reside alone, but who can live better in social residential settings.

7179 Edgewood Vista Grand Island

214 Piper Street
Grand Island, NE 68803-4027
308-384-0717
Fax: 308-384-0728
www.edgewoodvista.com

Faye Roebuck, Manager

We provide personalized care in settings designed specifically for the Elderly, including those with Alzheimer's Disease or other forms of dementia. Our individualized approach provides a high quality, safe, home like setting to Seniors who choose to on longer reside alone, but who can live better in social residential settings.

7180 Edgewood Vista Norfolk

1109 Oasewalk Avenue
Norfolk, NE 68701
402-371-0052
Fax: 402-371-0053
www.edgewoodvista.com

Ann Saegebarth, Manager

We provide personalized care in settings designed specigically for the Elderly, including those with Alzheimer's Disease or other forms of dementia. Our individualized approach provides a high quality, safe, home-like setting to Seniors who choose to no longer reside alone, but who can live better in social residential settings.

7181 Edgewood Vista of Fremont

2910 N Clarkson Street
Fremont, NE 68025-2399
402-753-8800
Fax: 402-753-8801
www.edgewoodvista.com

7182 Edgewood Vista of Hastings

2400 W 12th Street
Hastings, NE 68901-3501
402-462-4633
Fax: 402-462-6828
www.edgewoodvista.com

Tami Newbery, Manager

We provide personalized care in settings designed specifically for the Elderly, inculding those with Alzheimer's Disease or other forms of dementia. Our individualized approach provides a high quality, safe, home like setting to Seniors who choose to no longer reside alone, but who can live better in social residential settings.

7183 Edgewood Vista of Omaha
17620 Poppleton Avenue
Omaha, NE 68130-4614
402-333-5749
www.edgewoodvista.com

Marysue Pook, Manager

We provide personalized care in settings designed specifically for the Elderly, including those with Alzheimer's Disease or other forms of dementia. Our individualized approach provides a high quality, safe, home like setting to Seniors who choose to no longer reside alone, but who can live better in social residential settings.

7184 El Dorado Manor Nursing Home
Junction Highway 25 & 34
Trenton, NE 69044
308-334-5241
www.eldoradomanor.com

Sandra Brunkhorst, Administrator

7185 Emerald Court
315 W 33rd Street
Scottsbluff, NE 69361-4359
308-220-4007

Arlene Miller, Manager

7186 Florence Home Assisted Living
7915 N 30th Street
Omaha, NE 68112-2418
402-827-6000
Fax: 402-827-6005
www.omahaseniorcare.org

Dr Greg Witte, Administrator
Timothy Malloy, Medical Director
Steve Hess, CEO

7187 Garden Square of Crete
1405 Hickory Avenue
Crete, NE 68333-1955
402-826-2241
Fax: 402-826-2775

Jane Boden, Administrator

7188 Gateway Manor
225 N 56th Street
Lincoln, NE 68504-3577
402-464-6371
Fax: 402-467-0299
www.gatewayseniorliving.com

Linda Tisdel, Executive Director

7189 Gold Crest Retirement Center
200 Levi Lane
Adams, NE 68301-8830
402-988-7115
Fax: 402-988-2111
www.goldcrest.net

Heath Boddy, Executive Director

7190 Golden Manor Assisted Living
3853 Decatur Street
Omaha, NE 68111-4015
402-551-2484
Fax: 402-551-1114
www.goldenmanoromaha.com

Rachel Pinkerton, Executive Director

7191 Good Samaritan Society-Prairie View Gardens
1705 Prairie View Place
Kearney, NE 68845-8300
308-865-2650
Fax: 308-865-2657; *Toll Free:* 866-337-6408
www.good-sam.com

Rita Weber, Executive Director

We encorauge residents to live life to the fullest as independently as possible while offering personalized assistance, with daily living needs. We also offer an innovative program of care called Reminiscence in separate, secure area for residents with Alzheimer's disease or other types of memory impairments.

7192 Good Samaritan Towers
423 Boyd Avenue
Alliance, NE 69301-3668
308-762-8970
Fax: 308-762-7740
www.good-sam.com

Wayne McLaughlin, Manager

The mission of the Society is to share God's love in a word and deed by providing shelter and supportive services to older persons and others in need.

7193 Good Shepherd Lutheran Home
2242 Wright St
Blair, NE 68008-1192
402-426-4663
Fax: 402-426-1988
www.goodshepherdblair.com

Lois Pfeiffer, Administrator

7194 Gordon Countryside Care
500 E 10th Street
Gordon, NE 69343-1160
308-282-0806
Fax: 308-282-0251
www.gordonmemorial.org

Krissa Rucker, Administrator

7195 Gramercy Hill
600 a Street
Lincoln, NE 68502-1119
402-483-1010
Fax: 402-483-2197
www.gramercyhill.com

Carol Rafat, Manager

We are a community that offers you the opportunity to live to life you've always wanted.

7196 Grand Island Veterand Home
2300 W Capital Avenue
Grand Island, NE 68803-2097

308-385-6252
Fax: 308-385-6257
joanne.badura@nebraska.gov
dhhs.ne.gov

Allen M Thompkins, MD

7197 Greene House
600 Church Street
Seward, NE 68434-1099
402-643-9111
Fax: 402-643-9128
www.alcco.com

Terry Schoen, Manager

7198 Hastings Homestead
1116 Sycamore Avenue
Hastings, NE 68901-3380
402-461-3841
Fax: 402-461-4398
www.midwesthealth.ppi.net

Tammy Price, Executive Director

7199 Haven Manor Assisted Living
730 Larkspur Drive
Hickman, NE 68372
402-792-3088
Fax: 402-434-2683
www.havenmanor.com

Gus Peach, Administrator

7200 Hester Memorial Home
407 Dakota Street
Benkelman, NE 69021
308-423-2179
Fax: 308-423-2177
admin@bwtelcom.net
www.rhdconsult.com

Janice Edwards, Administrator

7201 Hickory Villa
7315 Hickory Street
Omaha, NE 68124-1678
402-392-0767
www.bethesdaseniorliving.com

Monte McVey, Administrator

Hickory Villa has been providing assisted living services to the Omaha community since 1988. This community is also one of the most affordable homes, with rates tailored to a wide range of income.

7202 Hidden Pines Assisted Living Community
309 W 7th Street
McCook, NE 69001-3507
308-345-4600
www.hillcrestnh.org

Peggy Rogers, Administrator

7203 Highland House
PO Box 241
Spencer, NE 68777
402-589-0025

Pam Vanderwerf, Manager

7204 Homestead
4205 6th Avenue
Kearney, NE 68845-3470
308-234-5600
Fax: 308-236-6663

Tanya Stephens, Executive Director

7205 Hospice House
7415 Cedar Street
Omaha, NE 68124-2367
402-343-8600
www.hospicehouseomaha.org

Cindy Alloway, VP
Rosemary Lebeda, Director

The in patient hospice facility is primarily designed to care for those who do not have a caregiver at home. We are also able to provide respite care for caregivers, five days at a time. For patients already in out home program who develop symptoms that cannot be managed adequatley at home, or for those caregivers who are unable to provide care anylonger at home, then Hospice is the place to be.

7206 Immanuel Trinity Village
522 W Lincoln Street
Papillion, NE 68046-3121
402-614-5500
www.immanuelcommunities.com

Cheri Mundt, Executive Director

7207 Imperial Manor Nursing Home
PO Box 757
Imperial, NE 69033
308-882-5333

Diane Cooper, Administrator

7208 Improved Living
114 S 9th Street
Norfolk, NE 68701-5165
402-371-3712

Donna Finkral, Manager

7209 Kimball County Manor Nusing Home
810 E 7th Street
Kimball, NE 69145-1699
308-235-4693
www.kcmanor.com

Bev Schnell, Administrator

7210 Kirkwood House
514 E 6th Street
Wayne, NE 68787-2211
402-375-2515
www.r-way.org

Jeannia Bressler, Manager

7211 Legacy
5600 Pioneers Boulevard
Lincoln, NE 68506-5172
402-436-3000
Fax: 402-436-3013
www.legacyretirement.com

Jay Bohlken, Executive Director

7212 Legacy Terrace
5700 Fremont Street
Lincoln, NE 68507-1674
402-464-5700
Fax: 402-464-5825
www.legacyretirement.com

John Kopetzky, Administrator

7213 Madison House
1120 N 1st Street
Norfolk, NE 68701-2926
402-644-4567
Fax: 402-644-8111
www.alcco.com

Stephanie Hoff, Executive Director

7214 Madonna Assisted Living
5401 South St
Lincoln, NE 68506-2028
402-413-3000
Fax: 402-486-8464; *Toll Free:* 800-676-5448
www.madonna.org

7215 Mahoney House
1810 E 12th Street
York, NE 68467-2241
402-362-5538
Fax: 402-362-5690
www.alcco.com

Kristi Roberts, Manager

7216 Meadows
500 S 18th Street
Norfolk, NE 68701-4543
402-371-1730
Fax: 402-644-4702
meadows@cableone.net

Jan Nixon, Executive Director

7217 Merrick Manor Assisted Living
1415 16th Street
Central City, NE 68826-1836
308-946-2624
Fax: 308-946-5700

Gene Church, Manager

7218 Methodist Memorial Homes
1320 11th Avenue
Holdrege, NE 68949-1999
308-995-8631
Fax: 308-995-8636
www.holdregehomes.org

Kevin Moriarty, Administrator

7219 Morton House
1500 14th Avenue
Nebraska City, NE 68410-1150
402-873-5551
Fax: 402-873-5994
www.alcco.com

Candy Herzog, Executive Director

7220 New Cassel Retirement Center
900 N 90th Street
Omaha, NE 68114-2704
402-393-2277
Fax: 402-393-3784
www.newcassel.org

Joe Schulte, Religious Leader

7221 Norfolk Homestead
3614 Koenigstein Avenue
Norfolk, NE 68701-8010
402-379-9622
Fax: 402-379-4794
info@norfolkhomestead.com
www.norfolkhomestead.com

Gayle Wright, Executive Director
Kim Summers, Assistant Executive Director
Char Brewer, Resident Care Coordinator

Our mission is to create an environment in which residents can continue to enjoy thier individuality, their independence, and their dignity in a secure, supportive environment. The Homestead represents our proud achievement of this mission.

7222 Northridge Retirement Community
5410 17th Avenue
Kearney, NE 68845-8305
308-698-5410
Fax: 308-698-5157
www.norhtridgeretirement.com

Deb Prange, Administrator

Our modern, well-appointed facility, beautiful spacious grounds and friendly capable staff provide our independent and assisted living residents freedom and piece of mind. From out comfortable apartments and suites to out very own Main Street, you will find that Northridge feels just like home.

7223 Nye Square Retirement Community
2230 N. Somers Ave
Fremont, NE 68025-2589
402-753-1400
Fax: 402-721-1447
info@nyeseniorservices.com
www.nyeseniorservices.com

Russ Peterson, Manager

7224 Oakland Heights
207 S Engdahl Avenue
Oakland, NE 68045-1419
402-685-5683
Fax: 402-685-5684

Dee Bailey, Administrator

7225 Oaks Retirement Center
1500 Vintage Hill Drive
Wayne, NE 68787-1227
303-552-5963
Fax: 402-375-3579
www.emeritus.com

Susan Wells, Administrator

7226 Our Homes
2445 R Street
Lincoln, NE 68503-3000
402-474-4922
Fax: 402-474-4923

Mary O'Shea, Owner

7227 Paddock Kensington
105 N 6th Street
Beatrice, NE 68310-3994
402-228-2000
Fax: 402-228-3287
tkeslar@kensington-evergreen.com
www.kensington-evergreen.com

Diana Meyer, Executive Director
Laurie Leners, Resident Services

The Paddock-Kinsington strives to provide each of its residents with a healthy, safe, enjoyable place to live. Meeting your expectations and daily needs is out highest priority. The Paddock-Kensington strives to make the most of living each day, by encouraging as well as supporting — the way families do.

7228 Park Avenue Estates
1811 Ridgeway Drive
Lexington, NE 68850-1188
303-552-5960
Fax: 308-324-5181
www.emeritus.com

Arletta Childress, Administrator

7229 Parkview Lodge Asssited Living
307 Conrad Street
Rushville, NE 69360
308-327-2248
Fax: 308-327-2066

Karen Edwards, Administrator

7230 Parsons House on Eagle Run
14325 Eagle Run Drive
Omaha, NE 68164-5435
402-498-9554
Fax: 402-498-0047
info@parsonshouseoneaglerun.com
www.parsonshouseoneaglerun.com

Penny Coatman, Executive Director

At Parsons House, service is not simply limited to a laundry list of offerings. Its a philosophy that's put into action in all we do to make livinghere at first choice, not a last resort. That's why you will find that we not only provide these types of assistance, we also tailor how they are delievered to demonstrate that the resident is always at the center of our focus.

7231 Pathfinder House
3010 N Clarkson Street
Fremont, NE 68025-7709
402-721-7714
Fax: 402-727-4225
www.alcco.com

Linda Parker, Administrator

7232 Pender Care Center
200 Valley View Drive
Pender, NE 68047-4443
402-385-3072
Fax: 402-385-2603
www.pendercommunityhospital.com

Pat Licthy, Administrator

7233 Plum Creek Care Center
1505 N Adams Street
Lexington, NE 68850-1255

308-324-5531
Fax: 308-324-5630
www.welcov.com

Keith Sladky, Manager

Plum Creek Care Center is a cozy skilled nursing facility with a caring home environment. Rehabilitation services at plum creek focus on assisting patients in becoming as independent and safe as they can be in their everyday funcional activities. Plum Creek offers Physical Therapy, Occupational Therapy, and Speech-Language Pathology to Care Center Patients as well as outpatients.

7234 Prairie Pines Lodge
900 W 7th Street
Chadron, NE 69337-2500
308-432-4305
Fax: 308-432-2737
www.chadronhospital.com

Tom Serres, Manager

Prairie Pines is devoted to improving the choices for better housing alternatives for the retired citizens of the Chadron area. Prairie Pines offers both housing and services tailored to each individual's needs, with the best of retiement living: security, peach of mind, and the absence of worry and responsibility in a comforatble setting.

7235 Prairie Village Retirement
3000 39th Avenue
Columbus, NE 68601-2250
402-563-4213
Fax: 402-563-9314
www.pvrc.net

Rich Widga, Executive Director

7236 Prairie Winds
603 W 6th Street
Doniphan, NE 68832-9677
402-845-4500
Fax: 402-845-4501
pwadministrator@hamilton.net
www.prairiewindsalc.com

Tammy Price, Manager

7237 Precious Time
2124 N. Broadwell
109
Grand Island, NE 68803
308-384-4590
Fax: 308-389-9015
judy@precioustimesgi.com
www.precioustimesgi.com

Jeanie Cooper, Owner

7238 Premier Estates
2895 We Street
North Platte, NE 69101
308-534-2200
Fax: 308-537-6477
www.premierestatesnorthplatte.com

Ruth Sands Jerke, Administrator

7239 Quality Living
6404 N 70th Plz
Omaha, NE 68104-1075

402-573-3700
Fax: 402-573-3792
www.qliomaha.com

Kim Hoogeveen, CEO

7240 Regency Square Care Center
3501 Dakota Avenue
South Sioux City, NE 68776-3699
402-494-4273
Fax: 402-494-7267
info@regencysquarecare.com
www.regencysquarecare.com

Greg Gregerson, Administrator

7241 Remington Heights Retirement Center
12606 W Dodge Road
Omaha, NE 68154-2349
402-493-5807
Fax: 402-493-3967
www.remingtonheightsretirement.com

Amy Birkel, Executive Director

7242 Riverside Lodge Retirement Community
404 Woodland Drive
Grand Island, NE 68801-8813
308-382-1657
Fax: 308-381-1863
www.riversidelodge.ne

Jan Thayer, Owner

7243 Royale Oaks
4801 N 52nd Street
Omaha, NE 68104-2229
402-557-6860
Fax: 402-827-6065
www.omahaseniorcare.org

Lois Siestima, Administrator

7244 Saunders House
1313 N Hackberry Street
Wahoo, NE 68066-1148
402-443-3333
Fax: 402-443-5578
www.alcco.com

Angi Streek, Administrator

7245 Seneca Sunrise
710 Grand Avenue
Ravenna, NE 68869-1100
308-452-4444
Fax: 308-452-4452
www.senecasunrise.com

Linda Zinnell, Owner

7246 Senior Living Choices at Curtis
217 Crook Avenue
Curtis, NE 69025-9531
308-367-4259
Fax: 308-367-4387
www.curtisseniorliving.com

Steve Krull, Owner

Senior Living Choices offers Assisted Living and Independent Cottages. Small facility with that homey atmosphere. Qualified staff 24-7, LPN part time. Medicaid waiver, Helping hands caring heart.

7247 Silvercrest at Fountain View
5710 S. 108th St
Omaha, NE 68137-3547
402-596-9033
Fax: 402-593-8010
www.fountainviewseniorliving.com

Shelly Watson, Executive Director

7248 Silvercrest at Miracle Hills Assisted Living
11909 Miracle Hills Drive
Omaha, NE 68154-4408
402-431-0011
Fax: 402-431-9257
www.waterfordatmiraclehills.com

Pearl Guy, Executive Director

7249 Skyline Retirement Community
7300 Graceland Drive
Omaha, NE 68134-4358
402-572-5750
Fax: 402-572-5777
www.skylinerc.com

Tim Smith, Executive Director

Our warm and inviting community encourages active independent seniros to flourish. We offer convenient services and amenities to make life a little easier and more enjoyable. We also offer day trips, group dinners at local restaurants and outings to the symphony, theaters and museums, all with the convenience of regularly scheduled transportation.

7250 Southview Heights Nursing Home
5110 S 49th Street
Omaha, NE 68117-2159
402-731-2118
Fax: 402-233-0782
www.southviewheightsomaha.com

Paul Randazzo, Administrator

7251 St Joseph Tower Assisted Living
2205 S 10th Street
Omaha, NE 68108-1155
402-952-5000
Fax: 402-952-5117
www.stjosephtower.com

Tracy Lichti, Executive Director

7252 St Joseph's Retirment Community
430 N Monitor
West Point, NE 68788-1593
402-372-2404
Fax: 402-372-2360
www.fcswp.org/sjrc/

Emy Beth Furrer, Administrator

7253 St Joseph's Villa
927 7th Street
David City, NE 68632-1398
402-367-3045
Fax: 402-367-3730
www.adorers.org/stjosephsvilla/page1

Joyce Stewart, Administrator

We are in existance to imitate the compassionate Jesus by creating a home for aging men and women where they feel secure, loved and respected. We enable residents to live thier lives to the fullest while preparing themselves for a new dimenstion-life after death. We also maintain a warm, friendly, clean, orderly, safe, and comfotable environment.

7254 St Josephs Nursing Home
401 N 18th Street
Norfolk, NE 68701-3686
402-644-7375
Fax: 402-379-4867
frhs.org/about-us

Bill Disch, Administrator

7255 St Luke's Countryside Villa
2300 E 32nd Street
Kearney, NE 68847-1910
308-236-9395
Fax: 308-237-3799
www.good-sam.com

Racy Bauer, Manager

Offers independent as assisted living for seniors on a budget.

Nevada

7256 Aegis of Las Vegas
9100 West Desert Inn Road
Las Vegas, NV 89117
702-472-8505
Fax: 702-240-3072
www.aegisliving.com

Debra Moore, Executive Director

Offers dedicated care to help make life more comfortable and secure. Our community has outdoor grounds with plenty of walking paths and sitting areas to enjoy the warm, sunny weather.

7257 Plaza at Sun Mountain
6031 W Cheyenne Avenue
Las Vegas, NV 89108-4200
www.adultcareconsultants.org/plaza

The Plaza at Sun Mountain Independent and Assistd Living offers affordable elegance and gracious living to fit your lifestyle. You will enjoy the riches of retirement with continuing privacy and independence with as much or as litle assistance as you choose.

7258 Prestige Assisted Living
1050 E Lake Mead Parkway
Henderson, NV 89015-3200
702-564-1771
Fax: 702-567-1985
www.prestigecare.com

Sarah Delamarter, President

We are uniquely designed to provide different levels of assisted living, from minimum daily supervision to personal 24-hour care.

7259 Silver Rose Manor
1490 Grimes Street
Fallon, NV 89406-3103
775-423-4137
www.silverrosemanor.com

Dell Williams, Owner

Silver Rose Manor provides a home-like, family oriented atmosphere for adults in need of assistance. Visitors are always welcome and residents are free to come and go at will. Residents are provided with three healty, home-cookes meals a day. Everyone is encourages to participate in the exercise classes which meet three days a week. Additionally, transportation is provided for local doctor visites and all medication is supervised.

New Jersey

7260 Acorn Glen
775 Mount Lucas Road
Princeton, NJ 08540-1954
609-430-4000
Fax: 609-430-4001
www.assisted.com

Jack Occonor, Owner

We are one of the nation's leading providers of assisted living residences for the physically frail elderly and the nation's largest iperator of freestanding residences for individuals with Alzheimer's disease or other forms of memory loss. The companies mission has remained steadfast: to maximize the quality of life and dignity of older adults.

7261 Allendale Community for Mature Living
85 Harreton Road
Allendale, NJ 07401-1317
201-825-0660
www.allendalecommunity.com

Michael Giancarlo, Administrator

7262 Alterra Clare Bridge Cottage of Monroe
1648 S Black Horse Pike
Williamstown, NJ 08094-9247
856-740-9400
www.upspring.com

Alane Melendez, Executive Director

7263 Alterra Clare Bridge of Hamilton
1645 Whitehorse
Trenton, NJ 08619
609-586-4000
www.assisted.com

Nicole Salvi, Executive Director

We are one of the nation's leading providers of assisted living residences for the physically frail elderly and the nation's largest operator of freestanding residences for individuals with Alzheimer's disease or other forms of memory loss. The company's mission has remained steadfast: to maximize the quality of life and dignity of older adults.

7264 Alterra Clare Bridge of Westhampton
480 Woodlane Road
Mount Holly, NJ 08060-3828
609-877-0555
www.assisted.com

Ted Hamilton, Manager

We are one of the nation's leading providers of assisted living residences for the physically frail elderly and the nation's largest operator of freestanding residences for individuals with Alzheimer's disease or other forms of memory loss. The company's mission has remained steadfast: to maximize the quality of life and dignity of older adults.

7265 Alterra Sterling House of Florence
901 Broad Street
Florence, NJ 08518-2813
609-499-6662
www.assisted.com

Joel Davey, Manager

We are one of the nation's leading providers of assisted living residences for the physically frail elderly and the nation's largest operator of freestanding residences for individuals with Alzheimer's disease or other forms of memory loss. The company's mission has remained steadfast: to maximize the quality of life and dignity of older adults.

7266 Alterra Wynwood of Emerson
590 Old Hook Road
Emerson, NJ 07630-1378
201-986-9009
www.assisted.com

Dana Smiles, Manager

We are one of the nation's leadng providers of assited living residences for the physically frail elderly and the nation's largest operator of freestanding residences for individuals with Alzheimer's disease or other forms of memory loss. The company's mission has remaines steadfast: to maximize the quality of life and dignity of older adults.

7267 Alterra Wynwood of Galloway
820 Hamburg Tpke
Wayne, NJ 07470-2019
973-942-4800
www.assisted.com

Gilbert Santa, Executive Director

We are one of the nation's leading providers of assisted living residences for the physically frail elderly and the nation's largest operator of freestanding residences for individuals with Alzheimer's disease or other forms of memory loss. The company's mission has remained steadfast: to maximise the quality of life and dignity of older adults.

7268 Arbor Glen
100 Monroe Street
Bridgewater, NJ 08807-5002
908-595-6500
Fax: 908-595-6515
marketing@arborglen.org
www.arborglen.org

Thomas Mondloch, CEO

7269 Arden Courts of Whippany
18 Eden Lane
Whippany, NJ 07981-1402
973-581-1800
Fax: 973-581-1979
www.arden-courts.com/whippany

Kathy Harrison, Executive Director

7270 Assisted Living at Spring Oak
1611 S Main Road
Vineland, NJ 08360-6513

856-507-1505
Fax: 856-507-1528
alvineland@earthlink.net
www.springoak.net

Dawn Lavoir, Resident Relations Specialist
Dawn Watkins, Administrator
Trish Benfor, Administrative Assistant

Assisted Living

7271 Atria Tinton Falls
44 Pine Street
Tinton Falls, NJ 7753
732-361-2820
Fax: 732-918-1952
www.atriaseniorliving.com

Carolann Koerner, Executive Director

7272 Avalon at Bridgewater
565 Route 28
Bridgewater, NJ 08807
908-707-8800
Fax: 908-707-9805
www.bridgewayseniorcare.com

Julia Paima, Executive Director

7273 Bayside Manor
7 Laurel Avenue
Keansburg, NJ 07734-1122
732-471-1600
Fax: 732-471-1077
care@baysidemanor.com
www.baysidemanor.com

Joseph A Cappadona, Owner

7274 Bey Lea Village Nursing & Rehabilitation Center
Revera Health Systems
1351 Old Freehold Road
Toms River, NJ 08753-2795
732-240-0090
Fax: 732-244-8551
www.reverabeylea.com

Michael Norbury, Administrator
Melissa Johnson, Admissions Director

Bey Lea Village is a skilled nursing center that offers quality long-term and subacute care and specializes in Alzheimer's and related dementia care throughout all states of the disease. Using the collaborative efforts of our interdisciplinary team, we provide a wide range of comprehensive care and services to meet the specific needs of each resident.

7275 Brandall Estates
432 Central Avenue
Linwood, NJ 08221-1372
609-926-4663
Fax: 609-926-5354
www.brandycare.com/communities/Brandall

Peter Burke, Executive Director
Sherry Sullivan, Associate Executive Director

7276 Brandywine Assisted Living at Middlebrook Cross
2005 Route 22 W
Bridgewater, NJ 08807

732-868-8181
Fax: 732-868-8178
www.brandycare.com/communities/Middlebro

Richard Heaney, Executive Director

7277 Brandywine Assisted Living at Moorestown

1205 N Church Street
Moorestown, NJ 08057-1198
856-778-0600
Fax: 856-778-4544
www.brandycare.com/communities/Moorestow

Chris Gillies, Executive Director
Holly BakemanTkac, Director of Community Relations

7278 Brandywine Assisted Living at the Gables

515 Jack Martin Boulevard
Brick, NJ 08724-7744
732-836-1400
Fax: 732-836-9600
www.brandycare.com/communities/Gables

Marilyn Goldstein, Executive Director
Linda Melendez Keating, Director of Community Relations

7279 Brighton Gardens of Edison

1801 Oak Tree Road
Edison, NJ 08820-2772
732-767-1031
Fax: 732-767-0835
www.sunriseseniorliving.com

Sanford Mann, Executive Director

7280 Brighton Gardens of Florham Park

21 Ridgedale Avenue
Florham Park, NJ 07932-2336
973-966-8999
Fax: 973-966-8998
www.sunriseseniorliving.com

George Edson, Executive Director

7281 Brighton Gardens of Middletown

620 Highway 35
Middletown, NJ 07748-4224
732-275-0790
Fax: 732-275-0797
middletown.dcr2@sunriseseniorliving.com
www.sunriseseniorliving.com

Patsy Distler, Director of Community Relations
Tom Kessler, Manager

Assisted Living and Alzheimer's Care.

7282 Brighton Gardens of Paramus

186 Paramus Road
Paramus, NJ 07652-1309
201-251-9600
Fax: 201-251-0776
www.sunriseseniorliving.com

Wilson Anhar, Executive Director

7283 Brighton Gardens of Saddle River

5 Boroline Road
Upper Saddle River, NJ 07458-2343
201-818-8680
Fax: 201-818-7875
sunriseseniorliving.com

Samantha Lawrence, Executive Director

7284 Brighton Gardens of West Orange

220 Pleasant Valley Way
West Orange, NJ 07052-2997
973-731-9840
Fax: 973-731-9170
www.sunriseseniorliving.com

Merri Buckstone, Executive Director

7285 Bristol Glen

200 Bristol Glen Drive
Newton, NJ 07860-2329
973-300-5788
Fax: 973-579-2351
snorton@bristolglen.org
www.umh-nj.org/bristolglen

G Scott Norton, Executive Director
James W McCracken, Administrator
Jeffrey J Quinn, Marketing Director

7286 Cardinal Retirement Village

455 Hurffville Crosskeys Road
Sewell, NJ 08080-2328
856-582-5292
Fax: 856-582-5026
www.cardinalvillage.com

Skip Broomall, Owner

7287 Chelsea at East Brunswick

606 Cranbury Road
E Brunswick, NJ 08816-5422
732-651-6100
Fax: 732-651-6446
www.chelseaseniorliving.com

Gloria Petro, Executive Director

7288 Chelsea at Fanwood

295 South Avenue
Fanwood, NJ 07023-1357
908-654-5200
Fax: 908-789-0451
www.chelseaal.com

Jennifer Ricci, Manager

We the staff, will provide a comfortable, safe and secure home to our residents in a caring atmosphere of respect and dignity. Through individualized support and health care services, encouragement of maximum independence, emphasis on freedom of choice and protection of privacy, our residents will enjoy the greatest quality life possibel.

7289 Chelsea at Montville

165 Changebridge Road
Montville, NJ 07045-9563
973-882-0800
Fax: 973-402-4132
www.chelseaal.com

Chris Nichols, Manager

We, the staff, will provide a comfortable, safe, and secure home to our residents in a caring atmosphere of respect and dignity. Through individualized support and health care services, encouragement of maximum independence, emphasis on freedom of choice and protection of privacy, our residents will enjoy thr greatest quality of life.

7290 Chelsea at Tinton Falls

1 Hartford Drive
Tinton Falls, NJ 07701

732-933-4700
Fax: 732-933-0999
www.chelseaseniorliving.com

Eileen Weller, Community Relations Director

Assisted Living, Respite, Separate Memory Impaired Unit, near Jersey shore.

7291 Chestnut Hill Residence
338 Chestnut Street
Passaic, NJ 07055-3158
973-777-7800
Fax: 937-778-9013
salc@chestnuthillcc.net
www.chestnuthillcc.net

Michael Mazzola, Administrator

7292 Collinswood Manor
460 Haddon Avenue
Collingswood, NJ 08108-1336
856-854-4331
Fax: 856-854-0879
www.umh-nj.org

Barbara Wrzeszcz, Marketing Director

7293 Elms of Cranbury
61 Maplewood Avenue
Cranbury, NJ 08512-3237
609-395-0641
Fax: 609-395-8200
www.elmsofcranbury.com

Anita M Dietrick, Owner

We provide the highest levels of care in a warm, comfortable and personal environment.

7294 Father Hudson House
111 Dehart Place
Elizabeth, NJ 07202-1224
908-353-6060
Fax: 908-353-4504
www.centerforhope.com

Sally Sinclair, Manager

7295 Fountains at Cedar Parke
114 Hayes Mill Road
Atco, NJ 08004-2457
856-753-2000
Fax: 856-753-2333
www.centerforhope.com

Jennifer Kelley, Executive Director

7296 Francis Asbury Manor
70 Stockton Avenue
Ocean Grove, NJ 07756-1150
732-774-1316
Fax: 732-776-6313
www.umh-nj.org

Diane Scott, Executive Director

7297 Green Acres Manor
1931 Lakewood Road
Toms River, NJ 08755-1211
732-286-2323
Fax: 732-914-9095
www.greenacresmanor.net

Tejas Patel, Administrator

7298 Haven at Holiday Manor
1700 Route 37 W
Toms River, NJ 08757-2347
732-341-0880
Fax: 732-341-3506
www.hovnanianseniorhousing.com

Barbara Estabrook, Administrator

7299 Heritage Assisted Living at Hammonton
45 Route 206
Hammonton, NJ 08037-2722
609-561-8977
Fax: 609-564-1158
www.heritagealf.com

Diane Welke, Administrator

7300 House of the Good Shepherd
798 Willow Grove Street
Hackettstown, NJ 07840-1721
908-684-5900
Fax: 908-979-7030
www.hotgs.org

Fred Heleine, Executive Director

7301 Independence Manor at Hunterdon
188 State Route 31
Flemington, NJ 08822-5764
908-788-4893
Fax: 908-788-3783
www.independencemanor.com

Gary Nagle, Owner

7302 Job Haines Home
250 Bloomfield Avenue
Bloomfield, NJ 07003-5689
973-743-0792
Fax: 973-743-1135
dplotnick@earthlink.net
www.job-haines.org

Donna Plotnick, Marketing Director
Noreen Haveron, Executive Director

Emphasizes three ideals; dignity, independence and individuality. Residents are encouraged to make the Home their home.

7303 Liberty Manor Assisted Living Residence
49 Lasatta Avenue
Englishtown, NJ 07726-1656
732-786-1000
Fax: 732-786-0689
www.libertymanor.com

Noreen Heller, Administration

We are dedicated to making your family member feel every bit a part of ours. Those who join our family recieve individualized attention, patient support, and warm companionship. And while we are there whenever we're needed, we are always carful to respect privacy and protect independence.

7304 Mill Gardens at Midland Park
36 Faner Road
Midland Park, NJ 07432-1719
201-493-7400
Fax: 201-493-7374
info@millgardens.net
www.millgardens.net

Nicholas Drivanos, Executive Director

7305 Newseasons of Cherry Hill
490 Cooper Landing Road
Cherry Hill, NJ 08002-2560
856-482-9300
Fax: 856-482-9330
www.cherryhillseniorliving.com

Peggy O'Neill, Manager

7306 Newseasons of Voorhees
501 Laurel Oak Road
Voorhees, NJ 08043-4418
856-566-2340
Fax: 856-566-2341
www.fivestarseniorliving.com

Allyson Buscher, Administrator

Assisted living offers all the attention you'd expect from traditional nursing home care, but in a beautiful, home-like setting. Assisted living communities emphasize a warm and comfortable physical environment through the style of dining areas and services, social and recreational activities, common areas for group or private socializing and ongoing accessibility to community resources and health professionals.

7307 Orchards at Bartley Assisted Living
100 N County Line Road
Jackson, NJ 08527-1264
732-370-4700
Fax: 732-370-8872
info@bartleyhealthcare.com
www.bartleyhealthcare.com

Phil Scalo, CEO

7308 Renaissance Gardens at Seabrook
3002 Essex Road
Tinton Falls, NJ 07753-7758
732-643-2060
Fax: 732-643-2081
www.thecareexperts.com

Steve Olsen, Health Care Counselor
Ben Unkle, Executive Director

Features all private Assisted Living apartments and all private Long-Term Care rooms; full-time, on-site staff doctors with nurses on duty 24-hours a day. Short-Time Rehab (physical, speech and occupational therapy); dementia and Alzheimer's care also available. Renaissance Gardens, the choice you can feel good about.

7309 Rose Hill Assisted Living
1150 Washington Boulevard
Trenton, NJ 08691-3154
609-371-7007
Fax: 609-371-7027
www.rosehillassistedliving.com

Georgeann Polito, Administrator

7310 Shores at Wesley Manor
22nd Bay Aveunenue
Ocean City, NJ 08226
609-399-8505
Fax: 609-391-8411
www.umh-nj.org

Sue Handron, Executive Director

7311 Spring Hills at Morristown
17 Spring Place
Morristown, NJ 07960-3947
973-539-3370
Fax: 973-539-9210
www.spring-hills.com

Tanya Massicot, Sales Executive

7312 Spring Meadows at Summit
41 Springfield Avenue
Summit, NJ 07901-4038
908-522-8852
Fax: 908-522-8862
www.capitalsenior.com

Mary Majors, Executive Director

7313 Summerville at Hillsborough
600 Auten Road
Somerville, NJ 08876
908-431-1403
Fax: 908-431-1304
www.sslusa.com

We provide care for residence with Alzheimer's disease and other forms of memory impairments. All Summerville communities are designed to provide a comfortable residential envioronment for seniors, with a distinct hospitality feel. Summerville residents from independent to frail, enjoy services tailored to meet their individual needs and preferences.

7314 Summerville at Stafford
1275 Route 72 W
Manahawkin, NJ 08050-2473
609-741-3059
Fax: 609-597-9898
www.emeritus.com

Shaun Lynch, Executive Director

7315 Summerville at Voorhees
1301 Laurel Oak Road
Voorhees, NJ 08043-4339
856-679-0964
Fax: 856-783-8484
www.emeritus.com

Kevin Summerville, Vice President

7316 Sunnyside Manor
2501 Ramshorn Drive
Manasquan, NJ 08736-2133
732-528-9311
Fax: 732-528-9026
sunnyside_manor@aol.com.
www.sunnysidemanornj.com

John Keane, Owner

7317 Sunrise Assisted Living East Brunswick
190 Summerhill Road
East Brunswick, NJ 08816-4908
732-613-1355
Fax: 732-613-1365
www.sunriseseniorliving.com

Sundeep Jeste, Executive Director

7318 Sunrise Assisted Living of Edgewater
351 River Road
Edgewater, NJ 07020-1028

201-941-6111
Fax: 201-941-6638
www.sunriseseniorliving.com
Edward Midgley, Executive Director

7319 Sunrise Assisted Living of Morris Plains
209 Littleton Road
Morris Plains, NJ 07950-2934
973-538-7878
Fax: 973-359-0994
www.sunriseseniorliving.com

7320 Sunrise Assisted Living of Mt Laurel
400 Fern Brook Lane
Mount Laurel, NJ 08054-9542
856-222-1213
Fax: 856-802-9749
www.sunriseseniorliving.com
Bruce Bosco, Executive Director

7321 Sunrise Assisted Living of Paramus
567 Paramus Road
Paramus, NJ 07652-1708
201-493-9889
Fax: 201-493-0888
www.sunriseseniorliving.com
Donna Zayat, Executive Director

7322 Sunrise Assisted Living of Wall
2600 Allaire Road
Wall Township, NJ 07719-9568
732-282-1700
Fax: 732-282-1720
www.sunriseseniorliving.com
David Woodward, Executive Director

7323 Sunrise Assisted Living of West Essex
47 Greenbrook Road
Fairfield, NJ 07004-3890
973-228-7890
Fax: 973-228-7918
www.sunriseseniorliving.com
Richard Caminiti, Executive Director

7324 Sunrise Assisted Living of Westfield
240 Springfield Avenue
Westfield, NJ 07090-1023
908-317-3030
Fax: 908-789-5778
www.sunriseseniorliving.com
Andrew Harris, Executive Director

7325 Sunrise of Old Tappan
195 Old Tappan Road
Old Tappan, NJ 07675-7042
201-750-1110
Fax: 201-750-1191
www.sunriseseniorliving.com
Richard Lombardo, Executive Director

7326 Sunrise of Wayne
184 Berdan Avenue
Wayne, NJ 07470-3232
973-628-4900
Fax: 973-633-0680
www.sunriseseniorliving.com

Anna Marie Novak, Executive Director

7327 Sunrise of Woodbury Lake
752 Cooper Street
Deptford, NJ 08096-2521
856-848-8777
Fax: 856-848-3171
www.sunriseseniorliving.com
Anda Constina, Executive Director

7328 Surnise of Woodcliff Lake
430 Chestnut Ridge Road
Woodcliff Lake, NJ 07677-7604
201-782-1888
Fax: 201-782-1899
www.sunriseseniorliving.com
Gina Bizzarro, Executive Director

7329 Twin Cedars
1456 Glassboro Road
Wenonah, NJ 08090-1606
856-468-6824
Fax: 856-468-6318
Adeline Murphy, Owner

7330 Victoria Mews Assisted Living
51 N Main Street
Boonton, NJ 07005-8740
973-263-3000
Fax: 973-263-3107
vdalia@victoriamews.net
www.victoriamews.net
Anthony Bastardi, Owner

7331 Whispering Knoll Assisted Living
62 James Street
Edison, NJ 08820-3938
732-744-5541
Fax: 732-906-4908
www.whisperingknoll.org

Rose Chavez, Executive Director

We offer an alternative for people who are looking for that special place to call home. With a dedicated staff of professionals, assistance is always available, 24 hours a day, seven days a week. Our housekeeping staff can assist you with any or all of your needs, and out health care staff provides nursing assistance around the clock. There is also an emergency call and repsonse system installed in every suite.

7332 Willows at Holmdel Assisted Living Community
713 N Beers Street
Holmdel, NJ 07733-1503
732-335-4405
Fax: 732-962-7441
pbrown@bchs.com
www.bchs.com

Patricia Brown LSW, CALA, Director Marketing
Cathy Movny, Administrator

Assisted living and a secure community for Alzheimer's care.

New Mexico

7333 Acantilado Vista
920 Riverview Drive SE
Rio Rancho, NM 87124
505-896-3000
www.leisurecare.com

Offers resort style living in an active retirement community.

New York

7334 Atria Forest Hills
10825 Horace Harding Expy
Corona, NY 11368-4532
718-760-4600
Fax: 804-550-9314
www.chelseaseniorliving.com

Susan Koster, Executive Director

Offers a unique supportive living environment with all the comforts of home.

7335 Bellevue Manor Assisted Living Community
4330 Onondaga Boulevard
Syracuse, NY 13219-3030
315-277-8019
Fax: 315-468-5108
www.emeritus.com

David Quirello, Administrator

7336 Birchwood Assisted Living and Physical Rehabilitation
423 Clay Pitts Road
East Northport, NY 11731-3801
631-368-5252
Fax: 631-368-3128
www.birchwoodsuites.com

James Steffens, Owner

7337 Briarwood Manor
1001 Lincoln Avenue
Lockport, NY 4094-6142
716-433-1513
Fax: 716-433-8142
www.assistedlivinglockportny.com

Charly Wiech, Activities Director
Mark Ferreri, Assistant Administrator

7338 Bronxwood Home for the Aged
799 E Gun Hill Road
Bronx, NY 10467-6192
718-881-9100
Fax: 718-515-0150

Betty Bonta, Administrator

Socially active adults will find a myriad of supervised activities and services.

7339 Clark Meadows
Ferris Hills at West Lake, One Ferris Hills, Canandaigua
Canandaigua, NY 14424-1754
585-393-4330
Fax: 585-393-0567
www.clarkmeadows.com

Dan Goldstein, Executive Director

7340 Country House in Westchester
2000 Baldwin Road
Yorktown Heights, NY 10598-4010
914-962-3625
Fax: 914-962-4130; *Toll Free:* 800-362-1957
astone@countryhouseretirement.com
www.countryhouseretirement.com

Anita R Stone, Administrator
Sherry Weber, Admissions Associate
Maureen Hildebrand, Case Manager

At the Country House, you can enjoy retiremet living in th comfort and privacy of your own charming studio or suite - with added security of knowing that our Health Services Department and other staff are available around the clock to serve you, should you need assistance.

7341 Dosberg Manor Adult Home
2700 North Forest Road
Getzville, NY 14068-1556
716-639-3311
Fax: 716-639-3309
www.weinbergcampus.org

David Dunkelman, President

7342 Elm York Home for Adults
10030 Ditmars Boulevard
East Elmhurst, NY 11369-1395
718-446-7900
Fax: 718-446-7938
www.elmyork.com

Tibor Klein, Owner

7343 Empire State Association of Assisted Living
646 Plank Road
Suite 207
Clifton Park, NY 12065
518-371-2573
Fax: 518-371-3774
nyasstliv@aol.com
www.ny-assisted-living.org

Jim Kane Jr, President
Jim Vitale, Executive Vice President
Lisa Newcomb, Executive Director

Dedicated to strengthening New York State's assisted living industry and promoting the best interests of providers and residents.

Number of Members: 20,000

7344 Fountains at Millbrook
Watermark Retirement Communities
79 Flint Road
Millbrook, NY 12545-6410
845-677-8550
Fax: 845-677-8630
dslocum@watermarkcommunities.com
www.watermarkcommunities.com

Deborah Slocum, Administrator

Our continuum of care gives residents the ability to choose the service program that best suits their current lifestyle and to add more services as their needs change.

7345 Hillcrest Spring
5052 Upper Market Street
Amsterdam, NY 12010

518-843-3770
Fax: 518-843-3878
www.hillcrestspringresidential.com

Catherin Sha, Administrator

7346 Long Island Living Program Assisted Living
431 Beach 20th Street
Far Rockaway, NY 11691
718-327-2700
Fax: 718-327-2223
ahe1836@aol.com
www.livingcenteralp.com

Amram Shetrit, Administrator

The Long Island Living Center Adult Home has extended our services to include an Assisted Living Program. We offer personalized attentive care to the frail and elderly i n a homelike atmosphere. Our retirement home is non-sectarian and is designed to help meet the physical, emotional and social needs of the elderly. For those eligible, wh have a Medicard funded program. All rates include 3 delicious Kosher meals, recreation, synagogue on premises. Housekeeping, laundry, physical therapy and beauty salon services as well as 24 hour secured environment.

7347 Maplewood Residence
225 Bennett Road
Buffalo, NY 14227-1528
716-681-9480
Fax: 716-681-8762
www.elderwood.com

Patrice Evans, Administrator

7348 New Central Manor Assisted Living Progra
1509 Central Avenue
Far Rockaway, NY 11691-4001
718-471-7700
Fax: 718-471-7732

Alex Klein, Manager

7349 Palm Beach Home for Adults
2900 Bragg Street
Brooklyn, NY 11235-1199
718-891-8400
Fax: 718-769-1006

Shimon Lefkowitz, Executive Director

Offers you a luxurious lifestyle in a secure and caring environment.

7350 Regency at Glen Cove
94 School Street
Glen Cove, NY 11542-2513
516-674-3007
Fax: 516-674-4144
Beth@theregencyatglencove.com
www.theregencyatglencove.com

Beth Dressler, Administrator

At the Regency, you can relax, while our exclusive MediComfort program, customized to provide for each resident's individual needs, ensures that you retain the level of independence that you are use to, all while preserving your dignity and privacy. From personal care assistance to health care monitoring and management, everything is taken care of. The Regency's devoted and caring staff go out of their way to enhance residents day to day living.

7351 Savoy at Little Neck Assusted Living Community
5515 Little Neck Parkway
Little Neck, NY 11362-2244
718-423-7900
Fax: 718-423-5050
www.brandycare.com

Joanna Laba, Executive Director

7352 Scharome Manor Home for Adults
631 Foster Avenue
Brooklyn, NY 11230-1398
718-859-2400
Fax: 718-859-4412
www.scharomemanor.com

Leo Rosenson, Owner

7353 Seneca Lake Terrace Adult Residential Community
3670 Pre Emption Road
Geneva, NY 14456-9138
315-789-4162
Fax: 315-781-1494
cjv2552@dreamscape.com
www.senecalaketerrace.com

Chris Vitale, Administrator

Our home provides quality care in a home-like supportive environment to ensure independence, dignity, privacy, and individuality.

7354 Shire at Culverton Adult Home
2515 Culver Road
Rochester, NY 14609-1751
585-467-4544
Fax: 585-698-2975
info@ShireatCulverton.com
www.shireatculverton.com

Tracy Vogl, Administrator

7355 Tanglewood Manor
560 Fairmount Avenue
Jamestown, NY 14701-2797
716-483-2876
Fax: 716-483-2832
www.tanglewoodmanor.com

Terri Ingersoll, Administrator

Tanglewood Manor was created to be a community that feels functious like family. Care programs offered include Assisted Living, Adult Day Care, Respite Care and Private Care.

7356 Tappan Zee Manor
51 Mountainview Avenue
Nyack, NY 10960-1709
845-353-6100
Fax: 845-353-1660
info@tzmanor.com
www.tzmanor.com

Michele Rothbuan, Manager

7357 Vassar-Warner Home
52 S Hamilton Street
Poughkeepsie, NY 12601-4198

845-454-3754
Fax: 845-454-6967
www.vassarwarner.org

Karen Harvatin, Executive Director

Ohio

7358 Alterra Sterling House of Alliance
1277 S Sawburg Road
Alliance, OH 44601-5750
877-712-9917
Fax: 330-821-5587
www.brookdaleliving.com

Andrea Williams, Executive Director

7359 Alterra Sterling House of Springfield
3270 Middle Urbana Road
Springfield, OH 45502-9285
855-350-3800
Fax: 937-390-7805
www.brookdaleliving.com

Michael Campbell, Executive Director

7360 Anchor Lodge Retirement Village
3756 W Erie Avenue
Lorain, OH 44053-1298
440-244-2019
Fax: 440-244-5612

Staci Lehmkuhl, Administrator

7361 Anna Maria of Aurora
889 N Aurora Road
Aurora, OH 44202-9503
330-562-6171
Fax: 330-562-3572
www.annamariaofaurora.com

George Norton, Owner

7362 Apostolic Christian Home
10680 Steiner Road
Rittman, OH 44270-9714
330-927-1010
Fax: 330-937-1020
www.apostolichome.com

David Maletich, Administrator

7363 Arbors at Clyde Assisted Living Center
700 Helen Street
Clyde, OH 43410-2051
419-547-9595
Fax: 419-547-1605
www.extendicare.com

Bonnie Stephanian, Administrator

7364 Arbors at Dayton Residential Care
320 Albany Street
Dayton, OH 45408-1402
937-496-6200
Fax: 937-496-1990
www.extendicareus.com

Ed Roberts, Administrator

7365 Arbors at Fairlawn Residential Care
575 Scleveland Massillon Road
Fairlawn, OH 44333

330-666-5866
Fax: 330-666-3215
www.extendicareus.com

Monica Herberth, Administrator

7366 Arbors at Marietta Residential Care
400 17th Street
Marietta, OH 45750
740-373-3597
Fax: 740-373-3597
www.extendicareus.com

7367 Arden Courts of Parma
9205 W Sprague Road
N Royalton, OH 44133-1208
440-886-5858
Fax: 440-886-5880
www.arden-courts.com/parma

Meredith Pasco, Executive Director

7368 Aspen Woodside Village
19455 Rockside Road
Bedford, OH 44146-2000
440-439-8666
Fax: 440-439-7352
www.aspenretirement.com

Jill Risner, Administrator

7369 Bayley Place
990 Bayley Place Drive
Cincinnati, OH 45233-1655
513-347-5500
Fax: 513-347-5553
www.bayleyplace.org

Adrain Walsh, Administrator

Bayley PLace is a non profit ministry of the Sisters of Charity, that is a continuing care retirmenet community that offers a full spectrum of health and wellness lifestyle options. Bayley Place meets the changing needs of today's mature adults. Our beautiful campus includes maintenance free cottages, assisted living apartments, Alzheimer's and Dementia care, nursing care, Eldermont Adult Day Program, Community Outreach Services and more.

7370 Berea Lake Towers Retirement Community
4 Berea Commons
Berea, OH 44017-2524
440-243-9050
Fax: 440-243-3049
www.berealaketowers.com

Tammy Cummins, Administrator

Berea Lake Towers is committed to providing the highest quality and most cost effective services possible to its clients and residents community. Through our commitment, Berea Lake Towers will strive to enhance its position as a predominant provider of health care and management services.

7371 Berkley Square Retirement Community
100 Berkley Drive
Hamilton, OH 45013-1787
513-856-8600
Fax: 513-856-8324
information@colonialseniors.org
www.berkeleysquareretirement.com

James Mayer, Administrator

7372 Blossom Hill Care Center
12496 Princeton Road
Huntsburg, OH 44046-9792
440-635-5567
Fax: 440-338-7833
www.blossomhillhealthcare.com

Donald Gray, Owner

7373 Breckenridge Village
36855 Ridge Road
Willoughby, OH 44094-4198
440-942-0093
www.breckenridgeohio.org

David Schell, Executive Director

7374 Briarfield Manor Residential Care
461 S Canfield Niles Road
Youngstown, OH 44515-4089
330-270-3468
Fax: 330-270-3479
www.briarfield.net

Diane Reese, Administrator

Briarfield Health Care Centers are dedicated to offering a variety of health services that meet the rehabilitation, nursing, psychological, social and spiritual needs of the community we serve. We recognize the importance of meeting individual needs by offering our experience and knowledge in cooperation with clients and residents in setting realistic expecations for their outcomes and quality of life in an environment of comapssion and dignity.

7375 Briarwood
3700 Englewood Drive
Stow, OH 44224-3223
330-688-1828
Fax: 330-688-2071
www.thebriarwood.com

Jonathan Trimble, President

7376 Brookhaven the Lifecare Community
804 Vinnie Connecticut
Brookville, OH 45309
937-833-2133
Fax: 937-297-6904
www.brookhavenoh.org

Mike McKinniss, Administrator

7377 Brookside Estates
15435 Bagley Road
Middleburg Heights, OH 44130-4827
440-299-2061
Fax: 440-887-1126; *Toll Free:* 877-839-0591
www.emeritus.com

Mary Kelly, Executive Director

We offer the perfect complement of housing, health care, support services, meals, activities and many extra amenities for seniors who can no longer live on their own, but want to maintain their independence. These are all provided in one customized Service Care Plan, all for one affordable monthly fee. Our community also has a licensed nurse on staff.

7378 Canton Christian Home
2550 Cleveland Ave NW
Canton, OH 44709-3371

330-456-0004
Fax: 330-452-9951
info@cantonchristianhome.org
www.cantonchristianhome.org

Tom Strobl, Administrator

The mission of Canton Christian Home is to provide the highest level of quality care and services to older adults, compassionately meeting their needs in a Christian home-like environment, and promoting their health, security, happiness, and usefulness in longer living.

7379 Canton Regency Retirement Community
4515 22nd Street NW
Canton, OH 44708-1573
330-477-7664
Fax: 330-477-9634
www.capitalsenior.com/cantonregency/

Alan Gruber, Administrator

7380 Capital Senior Living Corp. Woodlands of Shaker Heights
16333 Chagrin Boulevard
Shaker Heights, OH 44120
216-751-0930
Fax: 216-751-0980; *Toll Free:* 800-635-1232
www.capitalsenior.com

An assisted living and memory care community that offers a bed-and-breakfast-style environment. Staff are on call 24 hours a day to provide care plans tailored for each individual resident.

7381 Commons of Providence
5000 Providence Drive
Sandusky, OH 44870-1410
419-624-1171
Fax: 419-624-0302
www.commonsatsandusky.org

Jane E Windisch, Marketing Director
Rick Didomienico, Executive Director

7382 Community's Hearth & Home
550 W Harding Road
Springfield, OH 45504-1709
937-399-8622
Fax: 937-399-8863
www.chancellorhealth.com/nursing_home/

Kim Henry, Executive Director

7383 Cottingham Retirement Community
3995 Cottingham Drive
Cincinnati, OH 45241-1686
513-563-3600
Fax: 513-563-3601
cotadmin@deaconessltc.org
www.cottinghamrc.org

Margie Berryman, Executive Director

We are committed to providing the highest quality of care to our residents and thier families. This care is to be provided with dediction to spiritual values, compassion, customer service and continuous improvement, public accountability, respect, teamwork and finanial strength. We are also dedicated to maximizing the abilities of our valued employees and to being a productive, responsible member of each community we serve.

7384 Delaware Court
4 New Market Drive
Delaware, OH 43015-4282
740-369-6400
Fax: 740-369-6401
courts.delaware.gov

Ken Levering, Administrator

7385 East Park Retirement Community
6360 Elmdale Road
Brook Park, OH 44142-4075
216-267-7067
Fax: 216-267-0603
www.sovereignhealthcare.com/EastPkRETIRE

Pat Zingale, Executive Director

East Park Care Center is designed with the resident in mind. Accommodations include private and semi-private suites. A family/resident lounge encourages families and friends to enjoy private visits.

7386 Elms Retirement Village
136 S Main Street
Wellington, OH 44090-1344
440-647-2414
Fax: 440-647-9004
sales@thejohnkinchgroup.co.uk
www.elmsretirementpark.co.uk

Stuart Kinch, Managing Director
Tracey Coulson, Director
Ann Kinch, Sales and Advertising Manager

7387 Emeritus at Mentor Assisted Living
5700 Emerald Court
Mentor, OH 44060-1870
440-354-5499
Fax: 440-354-5422; *Toll Free:* 800-429-4828
www.emeritus.com

Stephanie Siegel, Director of Community Relations
Terry Sombat, Executive Director
Nancy Brothers RN, Director of Resident Care

The community is known for its warmth and hospitality, with beautiful common areas including a parlor, library, and two courtyards. In addition, the community is complemented with both private and semi-private suites for residents to comfortably enjoy. Summerville provides an on-site healthcare professional 24 hours a day to assist those residents who may needs extra care with their activities of daily living.

7388 Genoa Retirement Village Assisted Living
300 Cherry Street
Genoa, OH 43430-1823
419-855-7755
Fax: 419-855-4047
www.genoahs.com

Julie McKitrick, Administrator

7389 Good Shepherd Home
PO Box 163
Ashford, KT 44830-3255
419-435-1801
Fax: 419-435-1594; *Toll Free:* 800-298-8090
goodshepherdhomes.org.uk

Chris Widman, Administrator

7390 Inn at Belden Village
3927 38th Street NW
Canton, OH 44718-2900
330-493-0096
Fax: 330-493-9600
www.innatbeldenvillage.com

Nan Gammill, Executive Director
Deborah Sims, Business Director
Melissa Surratt, Marketing Director

The Village was designed to give as mich assistance as one watns, while carefully preserving dignity. We believe every life deserves to be cherished, needs to be cared for, and longs to be needed. We know every person desires independence, the freedom to choose, a sense of dignity and self-esteem.

7391 Kendal at Oberlin
600 Kendal Drive
Oberlin, OH 44074-1900
440-775-0094
Fax: 440-775-9820
admissions@kao.kendal.org
www.kao.kendal.org
TDD 440-775-9817

Barbara Thomas, Executive Director

Kendal at Oberlin offers independent living in spacious cottages and apartments.

7392 Kingston Residence of Perrysburg
333 E Boundary Street
Perrysburg, OH 43551-2861
419-872-6200
Fax: 419-872-6209
krp@kingstonhealthcare.com
www.kingstonhealthcare.com

It has been our goal to create an environment that went well beyond making our residents feel welcome or comfortable. Our caring and attentive staff and you will realize this is a place that successfully balances the delacate requirements of independence and assistance.

7393 Landing of Canton
4550 Hills and Dales Road NW
Canton, OH 44708-1508
330-409-4187
Fax: 330-477-5327
www.thelandingofcanton.com

Chanin McElroy, Executive Director
Darlene Fleming, Marketing Director
Colleen Gulling, Office Manager

Emertius Assisted Living operates the Landing of Canton. They provide cost-effective quality care that is personalized for individual needs, fosters independence for each resident, treats each resident with dignity and respect, promotes the individuality of each resident, allows each resident choice of care and lifstyle, protects each residents right to privacy, nurtures the spirit of each resident, and provides a safe, residential environment.

7394 Laurel Lake Retirement Community
200 Laurel Lake Drive
Hudson, OH 44236-2156
330-650-2100
Fax: 330-655-1738
info@laurellake.org
www.laurellake.com

David Oster, President

Our community offers you a gracious and comfortable home, first class support services, and an active community life to fulfill your social recreational and spiritual needs. The following services and amenities will make your life at Laurel Lake more carefree and convenient.

7395 Life Center at Wesley Ridge
2225 State Route 256
Reynoldsburg, OH 43068-9538
614-759-0023
Fax: 614-501-1413; *Toll Free:* 855-636-2225
www.wesleyridge.com

Elizabeth Vogt, President

At Life Center clients recieve and individualized plan of day time care in a well supervides environment. Clients are able to socialize in a comfrotable yet, stimulating atmosphere which offers social and therapeutic activities based on individual interests and needs. Clients are helped to maintain maximun functioning, health and wellness through nursing care and rehabilitative services.

7396 Light of Hearts Villa
283 Union Street
Bedford, OH 44146-4578
440-232-1991
Fax: 440-232-1782
information@lightofheartsvilla.org
www.lightofheartsvilla.org

Helen T Scasny, Administrator

We provide three meals per day, daily housekeeping, daily personal care, weekly laundry as needed, and medication monitoring.

7397 Lincoln Park Manor
694 Isaac Prugh Way
Kettering, OH 45429-3481
937-298-0594
Fax: 937-297-4199
info@lincolnparkseniors.com
www.lincolnparkseniors.com

Anita Theis, Manager

We offer the best in resident care that is provided by our professional staff. Individual needs, raging from advances in medical attention to a friendly helping hand are provided in warm, homelike surroundings.

7398 Lochaven Apartments
99 Lochview Drive
Newport News, VA 23602
757-595-2190
Fax: 419-224-2761
www.lochavenapartments.com

Jean Shellenbarger, Executive Director

7399 Lodge of Montgomery
12050 Montgomery Road
Cincinnati, OH 45249-2003
513-683-9966
Fax: 513-683-3709

Tawnya Hensely, Executive Director

7400 Lutheran Home at Toledo Assisted Living
2021 N. McCord Road
Toledo, OH 43615

419-861-4991
Fax: 419-693-1026
www.lutheranhomessociety.org

Robin Burkett, Director

7401 Mallard Crove Seniors Community
1410 Mallard Cove Drive
Cincinnati, OH 45246-3943
513-772-6655
Fax: 513-772-7908

Barb Lingby, Administrator

7402 Manor at the Meadows
301 W Western Reserve Road
Youngstown, OH 44514-3527
330-726-7110
Fax: 330-726-2517

7403 Maple Knoll Village-Beecher Place
11100 Springfield Pike
Cincinnati, OH 45246-4112
513-782-2400
Fax: 513-782-2717
www.mapleknoll.org

7404 Marymount Place
5200 Marymount Village Drive
Garfield Heights, OH 44125-2952
216-332-1100
Fax: 216-587-8212
info@marymountplace.org
www.marymountplace.com

Peggy Mathews, Administrator

Our mission is to offer older adults housing and supportive services enhancing the physical, social and spiritual needs of each individual while recognizing one's privacy, dignity, and personal choice.

7405 Mayfair Village Retirement Community
3011 Hayden Road
Columbus, OH 43235-7250
614-889-6202
Fax: 614-889-7532

Jamie Foley, Manager

7406 Meadows at Friendship Village
6000 Riverside Drive
Dublin, OH 43017-1492
614-717-0000
Fax: 614-764-7466

Alyson Hoover, Executive Director

7407 Mennonite Memorial Home
410 W Elm Street
Bluffton, OH 45817-1199
419-358-1015
Fax: 419-358-1919
www.mhcoliving.org

Lynn Thompson, Administrator

7408 Mount Royal Villa
13900 Bennett Road
N Royalton, OH 44133-3897
440-237-7966
Fax: 440-237-2558

Matt Haynes, Administrator

7409 National Church Residences Mill Run
3550 Fishinger Boulevard
Hilliard, OH 43026
614-771-0100
Fax: 614-529-2584
screamer.nationalchurchresidences.org
www.nationalchurchresidences.org

Linda Rochrenbeck, Administrator

7410 Oakwood Village
1500 Villa Road
Springfield, OH 45503-1656
937-390-9000
Fax: 937-390-9333
www.oakwoodvillage.net

7411 Ohio Assisted Living Association
1335 Dublin Road
Suite 221b
Columbus, OH 43215-7013
614-481-1950
Fax: 614-481-1954
oala@ohioassistedliving.org
www.ohioassistedliving.org

Jean Thompson, Executive Director

7412 Ohio Masonic Home
2655 W National Road
Springfield, OH 45504-3617
937-325-1531
Fax: 937-325-5238; *Toll Free:* 877-679-4869
www.ohiomasonichome.org

David Bannerman, CEO

7413 Omni West
3259 Vestal Road
Youngstown, OH 44509-1000
330-793-4404
Fax: 330-793-6004

Melanie Thirion, Executive Director

7414 Otterbein Portage Valley
20311 Pemberville Road
Pemberville, OH 43450-9413
419-833-7000
Fax: 419-833-5763
www.otterbein.org

Tom Keith, Executive Director

7415 Paisley House for Aged Women
1408 Mahoning Avenue
Youngstown, OH 44509-2595
330-799-9431
Fax: 330-799-8810

Audean Patterson, Executive Director

7416 Patriot Ridge Community
789 Stoneybrook Trail
Fairborn, OH 45324-6099
937-878-0262
Fax: 937-878-8407
www.patriotridgecommunity.org

Greg Nijak, Administrator

7417 Pebble Creek Senior Care Residence
670 Jarvis Road
Akron, OH 44319-2538
330-645-0200
Fax: 330-645-2010

Jim Egli, Manager

7418 Rittenhouse Senior Living of Middletown
880 East Swedesford Road
Suite 210
Wayne, PA 45044-4991
484-831-5310
Fax: 484-831-5398
koneeal@rittenhousesl.com
www.rittenhousesl.com

Arlene Edwards, Executive Director
Kristen O'Neal, Marketing Director

To maximize the quality of life and dignity of older adults
in the area. Provides residents with a secure, enriched environment, delivering assistance based on the principles of
care, respect, understanding and compassion while encouraging and promoting independence.

7419 Rockmill Springs Assisted Living
3682 Dolson Court
Carroll, OH 43112-9721
740-654-4529

Danielle Ashbaugh, Manager

7420 Rutherford House
805 S Buchanan Street
Fremont, OH 43420-4992
419-334-6962
Fax: 419-332-7346

Judy Rendon, Executive Director

7421 Sara Moore Home
26 N Union Street
Delaware, OH 43015-1922
740-362-9641
Fax: 740-369-2834

Lisa Graham, Manager

7422 Shepherd of the Valley Howland
4100 N River Road NE
Warren, OH 44484-1041
330-856-9232
Fax: 330-856-2571
www.shepherdofthevalley.com

Lisa Graham, Manager

7423 Shepherd of the Valley Lutheran Retirmen
1500 McKinley Avenue
Niles, OH 44446-3718
330-544-0771
Fax: 330-544-6840
www.shepherdofthevalley.com

Lisa Graham, Manager

7424 St Augustine Health Campus
7801 Detroit Avenue
Cleveland, OH 44102-2813
216-939-7600
Fax: 216-634-2717
www.staugministries.org

Karen McCarthy, Chairperson
Edward Hack, Vice Chairman
Linda Sheehan, Secretary

7425 Summit Villa Assisted Living
330 Southwest Avenue
Tallmadge, OH 44278-2235
330-633-4723
Fax: 330-633-5012
mkt@tandemhealthcare.com
www.tandemhealthcare.com

Doug Pearson, Executive Director

7426 Sunrise Assisted Living
216000 Detroit Road
Rocky River, OH 44116
440-356-9797
Fax: 440-356-9997
www.sunriseseniorliving.com

Penny Mcintyre, CEO
Chris Winkle, COO

Our residents maintain their independence in a secure home like setting, with individualized service plans dedicated to their specific needs.

7427 Sunrise Assisted Living at Bexley
2600 E Main Street
Bexley, OH 43209-2446
614-235-3900
Fax: 614-235-1919
bexley.ed@sunriseseniorliving.com
www.sunriseseniorliving.com

Penny Mcintyre, CEO
Chris Winkle, COO

At sunrise we take living personally. That's why we offer our seniors a variety of living arrangements, amentities, services, meal plans, social activities, and care. It's a broad range of options that help seniors enjoy a full life - all on their own terms.

7428 Sunrise Assisted Living at Finneytown
9101 Winton Road
Cincinnati, OH 45231-3829
513-729-5233
Fax: 513-729-5234
www.sunriseseniorliving.com

Penny Mcintyre, CEO
Chris Winkle, COO

7429 Sunrise Assisted Living of Bath
101 N Cleveland Massillon Road
Akron, OH 44333-2422
330-666-7011
Fax: 330-665-1493
www.sunriseseniorliving.com

Penny Mcintyre, CEO
Chris Winkle, COO

Our assisted living provides the ideal solution for seniors who need some help with daily activities.

7430 Sunrise Assisted Living of Cuyahoga Falls
1500 State Road
Cuyahoga Fls, OH 44223-1302
330-929-8500
Fax: 330-929-2090
www.sunriseseniorliving.com

Penny Mcintyre, CEO
Chris Winkle, COO

We pride ourselves in being an alternative to nursing home care by providing care and services with a personalized touch in an environment that looks and feels like home.

7431 Sunrise Assisted Living of Englewood
95 W Wenger Road
Englewood, OH 45322-2723
937-836-9617
Fax: 937-836-9616
www.sunriseseniorliving.com

Penny Mcintyre, CEO
Chris Winkle, COO

7432 Sunrise Assisted Living of Hamilton
896 NW Washington Boulevard
Hamilton, OH 45013-1281
513-893-9000
Fax: 513-893-9001
www.sunriseseniorliving.com

Penny Mcintyre, CEO
Chris Winkle, COO

7433 Sunrise Assisted Living of Kenwood
9090 Montgomery Road
Cincinnati, OH 45242-7712
513-745-9292
Fax: 513-745-9666
www.sunriseseniorliving.com

Penny Mcintyre, CEO
Chris Winkle, COO

We pride ourselves in our customer service and the outstanding quality of life we provide for our residents.

7434 Sunrise Assisted Living of Oakwood
1701 Far Hills Avenue
Dayton, OH 45419-2532
937-294-1772
Fax: 937-294-1134
www.sunriseseniorliving.com

Penny Mcintyre, CEO
Chris Winkle, COO

7435 Sunrise Assisted Living of Parma
7766 Broadview Road
Parma, OH 44134-6743
216-447-8909
Fax: 216-328-9272
www.sunriseseniorliving.com

Penny Mcintyre, CEO
Chris Winkle, COO

7436 Sunrise Assisted Living of Wooster
1615 Cleveland Road
Wooster, OH 44691-2335
330-262-1615
Fax: 330-264-1666
www.sunriseseniorliving.com

Penny Mcintyre, CEO
Chris Winkle, COO

We pride ourselves in our great reputation in the community for being the place to live if you need assistance.

7437 Sunrise at Tucker Creek
6525 N High Street
Worthington, OH 43085-4045
614-846-6500
Fax: 614-845-6654
www.sunriseseniorliving.com

Penny Mcintyre, CEO
Chris Winkle, COO

7438 Sunrise of Gahanna
775 E Johnstown Road
Gahanna, OH 43230-2115
614-418-9775
Fax: 614-418-9799
www.sunriseseniorliving.com

Penny Mcintyre, CEO
Chris Winkle, COO

7439 Sunrise of Poland
335 W McKinley Way
Youngstown, OH 44514-1681
330-707-1313
Fax: 330-707-1411
www.sunriseseniorliving.com

Penny Mcintyre, CEO
Chris Winkle, COO

7440 Sunrise on the Scioto
3500 Riverside Drive
Upper Arlington, OH 43221-1753
614-457-3500
Fax: 614-457-4300
www.sunriseseniorliving.com

Penny Mcintyre, CEO
Chris Winkle, COO

7441 Vancrest Assisted Living
10357 Van Wert Decatur Road
Van Wert, OH 45891-9209
419-238-4646
Fax: 419-238-5727
www.vancrest.com

Mick Murphy, Administrator

7442 Villas at St Therese Assisted Living
25 Noe Bixby Road
Columbus, OH 43213-1411
614-864-3576
Fax: 614-864-3577
srfcasey@inbox.com
villasatsttthereseassistedliving.com

Sister Michaels, Administrator

7443 Washington County Home
Rr 10
Box 124
Marietta, OH 45750-9156
740-373-2028
Fax: 740-373-2094

7444 Wedgewood Estates of Mansfield
600 Timble Road
Mansfield, OH 44906
419-756-7400
Fax: 418-756-5891

William Casto, Owner

7445 Westlake Village
28550 Westlake Village Drive
Westlake, OH 44145-3880
440-892-4200
Fax: 440-892-4756

Sharon Essi, Administrator

7446 Willow Knoll Retirement Community
4400 Vannest Avenue
Middletown, OH 45042-2770
513-422-5600
Fax: 513-422-6532

7447 Worthington Christian Village
165 Highbluffs Boulevard
Columbus, OH 43235-1400
614-846-6076
Fax: 614-842-9541

Brian Cooper, Administrator

Oklahoma

7448 Alterra Clare Bridge Oklahoma City
12401 Dorset Drive
Oklahoma City, OK 73120-9190
405-752-4220
Fax: 405-752-2771

Anita Burkhaulter, Executive Director

7449 Alterra Sterling House of Bartlesville
3737 Camelot Drive
Bartlesville, OK 74006-7589
918-333-9400
Fax: 918-330-9503

Carrie Kruouac, Manager

7450 Alterra Sterling House of Bethany
4101 N Council Road
Bethany, OK 73008-3108
405-787-9200
Fax: 405-787-9208

Carrie Elmore, Executive Director

7451 Alterra Sterling House of Claremore
1605 Oklahoma 88
Claremore, OK 74017-4843
918-343-3300
Fax: 918-343-9840; *Toll Free:* 866-485-4911

Norma Muller, Manager

7452 Alterra Sterling House of Durant
1500 N 19th Avenue
Durant, OK 74701-2152
580-931-0600
Fax: 580-931-8030
www.assisted.com

Willie Ferguson, Residence Director

Assisted living at its finest. We take care of memory care
residents, incontinence, dementia, etc.

7453 Alterra Sterling House of Edmond
116 West Danforth Rd.
Edmond, OK 73003-5280
405-330-9100
Fax: 405-330-9102; *Toll Free:* 866-485-4911

Lynnette Streobele, Administrator

7454 Alterra Sterling House of Enid
4613 W Willow Road
Enid, OK 73703-2757
580-237-0700
Fax: 580-237-0767

Glenda Kouba, Executive Director

7455 Alterra Sterling House of Lawton
6302 SW Lee Boulevard
Lawton, OK 73505-9103
580-536-6800
Fax: 580-536-6924

Lynette Carter, Executive Director

Provides housing and assistance to older adults who want to reatin their independence while recieving the daily support they need.

7456 Alterra Sterling House of Midwest City
615 W Blueridge Drive
Midwest City, OK 73110-1241
405-741-2000
Fax: 405-741-2926; Toll Free: 866-821-5543

Kara Bolino, Executive Director

7457 Alterra Sterling House of Muskogee
3211 Chandler Road
Stillwater, OK 74075
405-624-1616
Fax: 405-624-1619

Misty Keeble, Executive Director

7458 Alterra Sterling House of Norman
1701 Alameda Street
Norman, OK 73071-3078
405-573-9200
www.assisted.com

Mary Stacey, Executive Director

7459 Alterra Sterling House of Oklahoma City
7535 W Hefner Road
Oklahoma City, OK 73162-4462
405-773-8300
Fax: 405-755-5631

Anita Burkhalter, Executive Director

7460 Alterra Sterling House of Ponca City
1500 Bradley Avenue
Ponca City, OK 74604-2524
580-765-9900
Fax: 580-762-1915

Tammie McWilliams, Executive Director

7461 Alterra Sterling House of Shawnee
3947 N Kickapoo Avenue
M
Shawnee, OK 74804-1708
405-275-7747
Fax: 405-275-7973

Bryan Hiel, Executive Director

7462 Alterra Sterling House of Weatherford
800 Gartrell Place
Weatherford, OK 73096-2074
580-772-6600
Fax: 580-772-0484; Toll Free: 866-928-5630

Charlene Jantz, Manager

7463 Alterra Sterling of ADA
801 Stadium Driveive
Shawnee, OK 74801
405-275-7747
Fax: 405-275-7971

Bryan Hiel, Executive Director

7464 Ambassadors Courtyards
1380 E 61st Street
Tulsa, OK 74136-693
918-743-7887
Fax: 918-293-3050
www.ambassadorscourtyardstulsa.com

Phoebe Blackwell, Administrator

7465 Angel House Residential Assisted Living
10018 E 29th Street
Tulsa, OK 74129-4409
918-664-1215
Fax: 918-664-2575

Rita Cook, Owner

7466 Arbor House Assisted Living Center
4501 W Main Street
Norman, OK 73072-4459
405-292-9200
Fax: 405-292-5672

Angie Nance, Administrator

7467 Brighton Gardens of Oklahoma City
12928 N May Avenue
Oklahoma City, OK 73120
405-748-6464
Fax: 405-748-6551

Luella Nabors, Executive Director

7468 Brighton Gardens of Tulsa
5211 S Lewis Avenue
Tulsa, OK 74105-6556
918-743-2700
Fax: 918-743-1343

Matt Hoskin, Manager

7469 Brookridge Retirement Community
7802 Quanah Parker Trailway
Lawton, OK 73505
580-536-9700
Fax: 580-536-7954

Ronnie Stringer, Administrator

7470 Country Wood Manor Living Center
1604 S 13th Street
Kingfisher, OK 73750-4619
405-375-5232
Fax: 405-375-5830

Vickie Trent, Manager

7471 Crystal Place Assisted Living Center
400 SW 79th Street
Oklahoma City, OK 73139-8120
405-616-1980
Fax: 405-616-2985

Natalie Jewel, Administrator

7472 Crystalwood Assisted Living Center
2610 Reardon Road
Woodward, OK 73801-5846
580-256-4001
Fax: 580-256-7289

Ginger Canico, Manager

7473 Davis Home
1900 Margaret St
PO Box 205
Steubenville, OH 43952
740-283-3131
Fax: 740-283-3944
www.davishomes-inc.com

7474 Dogwood Creek Retirement Center
3230 E Shawnee Road
Muskogee, OK 74403-1813
918-683-5100
Fax: 918-683-5113

Kim McConnell, Administrator

7475 Emerald Square Assisted Living Center
701 N Council Road
Oklahoma City, OK 73127-4980
405-787-4466
Fax: 405-789-8101
info@emerald-square.com
www.emerald-square.com

Mary Harris, Administrator

Emerald Square provides assistance with bathing and dressing, medication administration, housekeeping, laundry and physician appointment transportation.

7476 Forest Glade Retirement Center II
2500 N Glade Avenue
Bethany, OK 73008-7905
405-495-7100
Fax: 405-495-7458
www.forestgladeok.com

Charlotte Fulbright, Administrator

7477 Forest Hills Health Care Center
4300 W Houston Street
Broken Arrow, OK 74012-4519
918-254-5000
Fax: 918-250-2538

Carla Jackson, Administrator

7478 Frances Strietel Villa
2300 W Broadway Street
Collinsville, OK 74021-1625
918-371-2545
Fax: 918-371-0564

Ron Hoffman, Administrator

7479 Gardens Assisted Living
1302 W Sunset
Springfield, MO 65807

417-889-7600
Fax: 918-224-6287
www.bethesdaseniorliving.com

Jeanne Taylor, Administrator

7480 Golden Oaks Village
5801 N Oakwood Road
Enid, OK 73703-9344
580-234-2817
Fax: 580-233-3426

Wesley Kroeker, Owner

7481 Green County Village Assisted Living
1027 Swan Drive
Bartlesville, OK 74006-5048
918-335-2086
Fax: 918-335-3254

Wes Ramsey, Administrator

7482 Hearthstone at Quail Springs
14300 N Portland Avenue
Oklahoma City, OK 73134-4030
405-755-6469
Fax: 405-755-6474
www.hearthstoneassisted.com

Karen Lorimor, Manager

To provide quality and affordable assisted iving care and services that offer value and exceed the expectations of our residents and their families.

7483 Heartsworth House
821 N Foreman Street
Vinita, OK 74301-1434
918-256-7856
Fax: 918-256-3703

Pam Wolfe, Administrator

7484 Heritage Assisted Living Center
9025 NW Expressway Street
Yukon, OK 73099-8374
405-722-5552
Fax: 250-798-8842

Curtis Aduddell, Owner

7485 Jefferson's Garden
15401 N Pennsylvania Avenue
Edmond, OK 73013-1514
405-715-1717
Fax: 405-715-9017

Carl Balaban, Director
Judith Wartman, Manager
Kay Coldiron, Social Services

Independent homes assisted living mamory care and fitness center for seniors.

7486 Manchester House
2333 Manchester Drive
Oklahoma City, OK 73120-3791
405-775-9009
Fax: 405-775-9292
www.manchesterhouse.uk.com

Shelee Stewart, Manager

7487 Mansion at Waterford
6110 N Pennsylvania Avenue
Oklahoma City, OK 73112-7361
405-848-1817
Fax: 405-607-0006

7488 Mustang Manor Assisted Living
1017 W State Highway 152
Mustang, OK 73064-2310
405-376-5600
Fax: 405-376-3867

Sandra Killian, Administrator

7489 Oklahoma Methodist Manor
4134 E 31st Street
Tulsa, OK 74135-1599
918-743-2565
Fax: 918-743-1782

Steve Dickey, Administrator

7490 Parke Senior Living
7821 E 76th Street
Tulsa, OK 74133-3680
918-249-1262
Fax: 918-250-9666
www.theparkeassistedliving.com

7491 Plantation House-Okmulgee
1001 S Belmont Avenue
Okmulgee, OK 74447-6300
918-756-1253
Fax: 918-756-2764

Sherri Powell, Administrator

7492 Rambling Oaks Assisted Living Center
1060 Rambling Oaks Drive
Norman, OK 73072-4187
405-360-4755
Fax: 405-292-5191

Dirk O'Hara, Owner

7493 Renaissance of Ponca City
2616 Turner Street
Ponca City, OK 74604-2203
580-765-5900
Fax: 580-765-5916
www.renaissanceok.com

George Rahme, Owner

7494 Schallmo Assisted Living Center
101 Naylor Street
Okeene, OK 73763-9107
580-822-4437
Fax: 580-822-3010; *Toll Free:* 580-822-4661
www.okeenhospital/assistedliving.com

Mattie Tucker, Administrator

We provide meals, houskeeping, laundry and medication over site, and other amenities. Your loved one will feel secure with our state of the art security system. We encourage them to be involved in the social activities, their care and peronal needs.

7495 Smith Manor
1103 Birch Street
Perry, OK 73077-6269

580-336-1119
Fax: 580-336-2285

7496 Sommerset Assisted Living Residences
1601 SW 119th Street
Oklahoma City, OK 73170-4902
405-691-9221
Fax: 405-691-9253
www.sommersetassistedliving.com

Diana Hendrix, Administrator

7497 Sycamore Square Assisted Living
850 N Clear Springs Road
Mustang, OK 73064-1513
405-376-2872
Fax: 405-376-5868

Kathy Hankey, Executive Director

7498 Tamarack Retirement Center
1224 E Tamarack Road
Altus, OK 73521-1234
580-379-6990
Fax: 580-481-2345
www.retireattamarack.com

Kay Stewart, Manager

We are dedicated to making your life easy and comforatble.

7499 Ten Oaks at Merrill Gardens Community
3610 SE Huntington Circle
Lawton, OK 73501-8444
580-353-1190
Fax: 580-353-1006

Tracy Cantwell, Executive Director

7500 The Gardens Healthcare
1165 South Brenner Road
Sapulpa, OK 74066
918-224-0600
Fax: 918-224-6287
valerie@gardenstulsa.com
www.gardentulsa.com

Valerie Donaldson, Administrator
Sheri Lambky, Director of Nursing
Judy Edwards, Admission Coordinator

Long term care and skilled nursing and rehab facility featuring newly remodeled therapy gym and private suites for skilled patients.

7501 Unlimited Care-Richmond Hills
7002 S Richmond Avenue
Tulsa, OK 74136-4603
918-499-1988
Fax: 918-499-1992

Tammry R Skalenda, Owner

7502 Village of Lee Retirement Center
6920 SW Lee Boulevard
Lawton, OK 73505-9104
580-536-4848
Fax: 580-536-0304

Connie Greb, Administrator

7503 Vyne at Cedar Ridge
14701 E 86th Street N
Owasso, OK 74055-8474

918-461-1955
Fax: 918-249-8829

Jackie Bell, Executive Director

7504 Welch Assisted Living Center
320 NE Saint Louis Avenue
Welch, OK 74369-9301
918-788-3377
Fax: 918-788-3379

Jayne McCarty, Administrator

7505 Windsor Manor Assisted Living
608 S 15th Street
Indianola, IW 50125
515-961-8900
Fax: 515-333-1942
gayla.gilliland@windsor-manor.com
www.windsor-manor.com

Judith Wartman, Administrator

7506 the Retirement Village at Copper Lake
1600 Lakeshore Drive
Edmond, OK 73013-3006
405-340-5121
Fax: 405-359-0202

Chris Kincaid, Executive Director

Oregon

7507 Adams House
121 Cordelia Drive
Myrtle Creek, OR 97457-7411
541-863-4444
Fax: 541-863-7978
www.adamshousealf.org

Susan Lebengood, Executive Director

7508 Alderwood Assisted Living
131 Alder Street
Central Point, OR 97502-2225
541-664-3757
Fax: 541-664-8527

Dee Lopez, Administrator

Now you can live in lovely surroundings while recieveing the extra help you might need to keep your independence without leaving your community.

7509 Alpine House Assisted Living
2901 Tremainsville Rd.
Toledo, OH 43613
541-432-7402
Fax: 419-724-3672
info@alpinehouse.net
www.alpinehouse.net

Margo Peppers, Executive Director

7510 Alpine Springs Assisted Living and Cottages
3760 N Clarey Street
Eugene, OR 97402-8744
541-607-9525
Fax: 541-607-5838

Jill Krupoff, Administrator

7511 Aspen Court
470 NE Oak Street
Madras, OR 97741-2201
541-475-6425
Fax: 541-475-6001

7512 Astor House
999 Klaskanine Avenue
Astoria, OR 97103-5131
503-325-6970
Fax: 503-325-9555

Debra Hart, Executive Director

7513 Avamere at Hillsboro
2000 SE 30th Avenue
Hillsboro, OR 97123-4120
503-693-9944
Fax: 503-640-6654
www.avamereathillsboro.com

Sarah Silva, Executive Director

7514 Avamere at Newberg
730 Foothills Drive
Newberg, OR 97132-6004
503-554-0767
Fax: 503-554-0436
www.avamereatnewberg.com

Virginia Gaines, Administrator

7515 Avamere at Sandy
17727 SE Langensand Road
Sandy, OR 97055-6487
503-668-4199
Fax: 503-668-7758

Connie Easter, Manager

7516 Avamere at Sherwood
16500 SW Century Drive
Sherwood, OR 97140-6100
503-625-7333
Fax: 503-625-6565
www.avamereatsherwood.com

Lissa Watts, Executive Director

7517 Awbrey House
2825 Neff Road
Bend, OR 97701-7914
541-317-8464
Fax: 541-317-4147

Suzanne Travis, Executive Director

7518 Bridgewood Rivers
1901 NW Hughwood Avenue
Roseburg, OR 97470-9970
541-440-1914
Fax: 541-440-9009

Teresa Courtney, Manager

7519 Brookside House
3550 SW Canal Boulevard
Redmond, OR 97756-8947
541-923-2068
Fax: 541-923-7335
Rooms@Brooksidehouselodging.com
www.brooksidehouselodging.com

Barb Thompson, Administrator

7520 Cambridge Terrace Assisted Living
2800 14th Avenue SE
Albany, OR 97322-7079
541-928-9494
Fax: 541-812-9198
administratorct@mtwestret.com

Kay Hayez-Rodiguez, Administrator

Provides the services you need, delicious meals, and a host of amenities in a gracious setting that has been designed with your comfort and security in mind.

7521 Canfield Place Retirement
14570 SW Hart Road
Beaverton, OR 97007-7000
503-626-5100
Fax: 503-526-3803
www.leisurecare.com

Offers a luxurious studio and one-and two bedroom apartment homes in a fun and active retirement community.

7522 Carriage House
150 SE Williamson Drive
Prineville, OR 97754-9115
541-416-0500
Fax: 541-416-1445

Kristy Spindler, Manager

7523 Cedar Village Assisted Living Community
4452 Lancaster Drive NE
Salem, OR 97305-1551
971-239-5538
Fax: 503-390-9152
www.cedarvillageseniorliving.com

Ryan Bethke, Administrator

7524 Cherry Wood Village
10610 SE Clay Street
Portland, OR 97216-3187
503-946-0225
Fax: 503-946-0207
www.gebnerationcilc.com

Jim Norris, Marketing Director
Tory Thompson, Marketing Associate
Traci Manley, President

Cherry Wood Village is convenienty locates in southeast Portland near the Adventist Medical Center and professional buildings. The nearby Gateway business district offers a wide variety of shopping opportunities. Cherry Wood Village is serves by Tri-Met buses and is locates near light rail trains, which literally put the city of Portland at your door step.

7525 Churchill Clubhouse Estates
1919 Bailey Hill Road
Eugene, OR 97405-1139
541-485-8320
Fax: 541-484-8405

Larry Boman, Administrator

7526 Clackamas Woods Assisted Living
14314 SE Webster Road
Milwaukie, OR 97267-1910
503-654-3413
Fax: 503-353-0225

Lisa Maynard, Manager

7527 Cornell Estates Living Center
1005 NE 17th Avenue
Hillsboro, OR 97124-2701
503-640-2884
Fax: 503-693-1037
marketing@cornell-estates.com
www.cornell-estates.com

Debbie Van Dynn, Administrator

7528 Courtyard Senior Living
6323 SE Division Street
Portland, OR 97206-1385
503-772-9795
Fax: 503-788-8711

Pam Urico, Administrator

7529 Dallas Retirement Assisted Living Facility
340 NW Brentwood Avenue
Dallas, OR 97338-1066
503-831-0214
Fax: 503-831-0278

David Parrett, Executive Director

7530 Davenport House
930 Oak Street
Silverton, OR 97381-1813
503-873-7162
Fax: 503-873-6672

Jama Plummer, Administrator

7531 Deerfield Village
5770 SE Kellogg Creek Drive
Milwaukie, OR 97222-2128
503-653-4064
Fax: 503-659-4525

Denise Cockreham, Manager

7532 Dorian Place
375 N Dorian Drive
Ontario, OR 97914-1805
541-889-8545
Fax: 541-889-7340

Ashley Holiday, Administrator

7533 Douglas House
419 Amelia Street,
Key West, FL 33060
305-294-5269
Fax: 305-292-7665; *Toll Free:* 800-833-0372
www.douglashouse.com

Judy Cain, Manager

7534 Emerald Valley
4450 W Amazon Drive
Eugene, OR 97405-4558
541-345-9668
Fax: 541-345-1190

Elizabeth Moss, Manager

7535 Forest Grove Beehive
2122 Hawthorne Street
Forest Grove, OR 97116-1778
503-357-6409
Fax: 503-357-9046

Kathleen Leatham, Administrator

7536 Fountains at Town Center Village

8607 SE Causey Avenue
Happy Valley, OR 97086-7579
503-654-4500
Fax: 503-786-1232

Town Center Village offers a full range of housing and services designed for comfort, enjoyment and a sense of community. The complex contains a variety of housing units, fitness and health care facilities - to serve a wide range of interests and needs of retired adults. A highly trained staff is available to provide the level of services that best suit your lifestyle, from housekeeping and meal preparation to personal fitness training.

7537 Gibson Creek Retirement and Assisted Living

1615 Brush College Road NW
Salem, OR 97304-1400
503-361-8599
Fax: 503-371-1160

Laura Miller, Administrator

7538 Gilman Park

2205 Gilman Drive
Oregon City, OR 97045-1563
503-563-4764
Fax: 503-667-1183
www.gilmanpark.com

Elaine Rust, Administrator

7539 Grace House

380 NW 6th Avenue
Estacada, OR 97023-7713
503-630-5341
Fax: 503-630-5348

Catherine Hammell, Administrator

7540 Grande Ronde Retirement Residence

1809 Gekeler Lane
La Grande, OR 97850-3375
541-963-4700
Fax: 541-963-6519
www.frontiermgmt.com

John Lamoreau, Administrator

Grande Ronde is more than a place to live - it's a community. You can enjoy our salon, our library, our gardens, and our recreational rooms and lounges. Grande Ronde is filled with live, family, friends, and a sense of pride.

7541 Greenridge Estate at Mountain Park, UC

4 Greenridge Drive
Lake Oswego, OR 97035-1400
503-635-8818
Fax: 503-635-6857
www.greenridgeestates.net

Rebecca Rhineheimer, Administrator
Megann Nudo, Community Relations Director
Sharon Tonack, Office Manager

7542 Grove Assisted Living Community

2112 Oak Street
Forest Grove, OR 97116-2044
503-359-1002
Fax: 503-359-0615; *Toll Free:* 800-652-0750

Sherry Ward, Manager

The Grove is a unique assisted living opportunity for those who value their independence, yet may need additional support with the details of daily living. We provide services designed to help people remain independent while living in their own apartments as long as possible.

7543 Harvest Homes

1331 Cole Road
Delanson, NY 12053
518-895-2341
Fax: 503-289-6473
info@harvesthomes.com
www.harvesthomes.com

Lynda Moyer, Owner

7544 Hearthstone of Beaverton

12520 SW Hart Road
Beaverton, OR 97008-5783
503-641-0911
Fax: 503-641-1118
www.hearthstonealc.com

Mike Magill, Business Manager
Suzie Reeb, Activities Director
Susan Magnuson, Administrator

Hearthstone of Beaverton is a privately owned non smoking assisted living community where seniors are served with love, respect and integrity. We endeavor to serve the whole person promoting physical mental, spiritual and emotional wellness.

7545 Heights Assisted Living

3000 SW 32nd Street
Redmond, OR 97756-8321
541-923-5452
Fax: 541-923-0280

Joyce Werner, Administrator

7546 Heritage Place Assisted Living

100 6th Avenue W
Bandon, OR 97411
541-347-7502
Fax: 541-347-1412; *Toll Free:* 800-819-1001

Betty Peper, Administrator

We have a professional staff that is knowledgeable, skilled, and compassionate to the needs of our residents. We combine the dignity and independence of a homelike environment with the quality and care that allows our residents to enjoy to richness of like and wonders of the surrounding area.

7547 Hermiston Terrace Assisted Living Facility

980 W Highland Avenue
Hermiston, OR 97838-2146
541-567-3141
Fax: 541-567-2282

Charotte King, Administrator

7548 Heron Pointe Retirement & Assisted Living

504 Gwinn Street E
Monmouth, OR 97361-1571
503-838-6850
Fax: 503-838-6443

John Kaiser, Administrator

7549 Hillside Communities
1020 Raleigh Drive,
Carrollton, TX 75007
503-472-9534
Fax: 972-492-3131; *Toll Free:* 800-275-2384
www.hillsidecarrollton.com

Jacklyn Friedman, Manager

7550 Hillside House Assisted Living Center
1400 SE 19th Street
Lincoln City, OR 97367-2333
541-994-8028
Fax: 541-994-8331

Sandra Taylor, Manager

7551 Homewood Heights Assisted Living Facility
17999 SE River Road
Milwaukie, OR 97267-5885
503-659-6600
Fax: 503-659-8193

Eric Murk, Executive Director

7552 Huffman House
1307 N College Street
Newberg, OR 97132-7395
503-537-0422
Fax: 503-538-1584

Terry Hacker, Administrator

7553 Inland Point Assisted Living
2290 Inland Drive
North Bend, OR 97459-1240
541-756-0176
Fax: 541-756-8405
www.sunholdingscorp.com

Chris Cooney, Manager

We assist you with activities of daily living, such as dressing, grooming, and bathing, but will encourage you to do as much as you can for yourself. We will help you to remain as independent as possible.

7554 Jackson House
300 Suncrest Road
Talent, OR 97540-7601
541-512-9474
Fax: 541-512-9340

Ivy Olvera, Administrator

7555 Jennings McCall Center II
2221 Oak Street
Forest Grove, OR 97116-2048
503-357-4499
Fax: 503-359-4468
rean@jenningsmccall.com

Doris Kinzle, Manager

7556 Johnson Assisted Living
10801 NE Weidler Street
Portland, OR 97220-3066
503-255-0685
Fax: 503-256-1140

Steve Williams, Administrator

7557 Johnson Assisted Living Center
10801 NE Weidler Street
Portland, OR 97220-3066
503-255-0685
Fax: 503-256-1140

Steve Williams, Administrator

7558 Junction City Retirement & Assisted Living Facility
500 E 6th Avenue
Junction City, OR 97448-1557
541-995-0278
Fax: 541-998-3747

Gary Heagy, Administrator

7559 Juniper House
301 SW 28th Drive
Pendleton, OR 97801-1871
541-278-0666
Fax: 541-278-1578

Toni Sims, Manager

7560 Kilchis House
4212 Marolf Place
Tillamook, OR 97141-3257
503-842-2204
Fax: 503-815-1694

Carol Helser, Manager

7561 Lakeside Assisted Living Community
1109 S. Schumaker Dr.
Salisbury,, MD 21804
410-749-4480
Fax: 410-546-9710

John Buckley, Administrator

7562 Lakewood Pointe Assisted Living
524 N G Street
Lakeview, OR 97630-1400
541-947-2060
Fax: 541-947-4902

Lisa Powell, Manager

7563 Lancaster Assisted Living
4138 Market Street NE
Salem, OR 97301-2065
503-364-3383
Fax: 503-371-0498

Judy Belt, Manager

7564 Lancaster Village
4138 Market Street NE
Salem, OR 97301-2065
503-364-3383
Fax: 503-364-6433

Judy Belt, Manager

7565 Lancaster Woods
4398 Glencoe Street NE
Salem, OR 97301-2172
503-581-4239
Fax: 503-581-5052

Linda Fortune, Administrator

7566 Lone Oak Assisted Living
2615 Lone Oak Way
Eugene, OR 97404-2554
541-321-0983
Fax: 541-461-0539
www.loneoakassistedliving.com

Amanda Boehlke, Executive Director

7567 MacDonald Residence
605 NW Couch Street
Portland, OR 97209-3646
503-241-7374
Fax: 503-241-7375

David Berger, Manager

We provide in a caring environment which promotes good
health, tolerance, and respect for the value of every individual. The Residence offers assisted livng for older adults
with disabilities who want to retain their independence
while receiving services they need.

7568 Macklyn House
755 Elk Drive
Brookings, OR 97415-9066
541-469-7182
Fax: 541-469-5672

Kathy McCourt, Executive Director

7569 Magnolia Gardens Assisted Living Facilities
3800 62nd Avenue N.
Pinellas Park,, FL 33781
727-489-6440
Fax: 727-489-6452
www.magnoliagardensassistedliving.com

Carmen Dake, Owner

7570 Markham House
1601 Fifth Avenue,
Suite 1900
Seattle, WA 98101
206-436-7827
Fax: 206-436-7705
www.leisurecare.com

Offers luxurious apartment homes in a fun and active retirement community.

7571 Marquis Vintage Suites at Forest Grove
3336 19th Avenue
Forest Grove, OR 97116-1913
503-359-1129
Fax: 503-357-4449

Lynn Cole, Executive Director

7572 Mary's Woods at Marylhurst
17400 Holy Names Drive
Lake Oswego, OR 97034-5187
503-635-7381
Fax: 503-675-2015; *Toll Free:* 800-968-8678
www.maryswoods.com

Marvin Kaiser, CEO
Diane Hood, COO
Roswitha Frawley, Mission Director

This facility has been developed to help residents preserve
their active lifestyles by offering assistance with activities
of daily living.

7573 McKillop Residence Assisted Living Facility
500 SE Conifer Circle
Sublimity, OR 97385-9523
503-769-0900
Fax: 503-769-0950

Maurice Reece, Owner

7574 Meadow Creek Village Assisted Living Residence
3988 12th Street SE
Salem, OR 97302
503-375-9732
Fax: 503-375-2144
www.reveraliving.com/meadowcreek

Deborah Goodard, Manager

7575 Meadowbrook Place
4000 Cedar Street
Baker City, OR 97814-1649
541-523-6333
Fax: 541-523-9166

Gayle Gazley, Administrator

7576 Northridge Center
3737 S Pacific Highway
Medford, OR 97501-8958
541-535-5497
Fax: 541-535-1221
www.northridgecenter.net

Les Connell, Owner

7577 Oaks at Lebanon
621 W Oak Street
Lebanon, OR 97355-1725
541-258-7777
Fax: 541-258-7255
www.oaksatlebanon.com

Angie Kutsch, Executive Director

The Oaks was created to help you maintain your independence. We offer assisted living services which may include
friendly reminders, assistance with bathing, dressing or
personal hygiene, medication monitoring, personal laundry,
plus much more.

7578 Ocean Crest Retirement & Assisted Living Facility
192 Norman Avenue
Coos Bay, OR 97420-4732
541-888-2255
Fax: 541-888-3598

Karla Dieterich, Administrator

7579 Parkhurst House
2450 May Street
Hood River, OR 97031-7747
541-387-4600
Fax: 541-387-4472

Tim Dufour, Executive Director

7580 Pheasant Pointe Assisted Living
835 E Main Street
Molalla, OR 97038-9164
971-216-4220
Fax: 503-829-7392
www.pheasantpointeseniorliving.com

Patricia Clark, Executive Director

7581 Powell Valley ASL & ALZ Care Community
4001 SE 182nd Avenue
Gresham, OR 97030-5063
503-665-2496
Fax: 503-661-9872

Karla Cheney, Administrator

7582 Prairie House Retirement & Assisted Community
51485 Morson Street
La Pine, OR 97739-9481
541-536-8559
Fax: 541-536-1373
www.prairiehousealf.com

Betty Musselman, Administrator

7583 Princeton Village
14370 SE Oregon Trail Drive
Clackamas, OR 97015-6290
503-558-1215
Fax: 503-558-8425

Cara Koenig, Administrator

7584 Providence Benedictine Orchard House
550 S Main Street
Mount Angel, OR 97362-9540
503-845-2544
Fax: 503-845-2560
www.providence.org

Deana Wentworth, Manager

Providence Benedictine Orchard House is state licensed as assisted living and offers different levels of personal care services. Residents have private apartments with full bathrooms (roll in showers), three daily meals, snacks, routine personal care services, weekly housekeeping and linen services, social activities and unlimited use of many of Orchard House's other amenities.

7585 Providence Brookside Manor
1550 Brookside Drive
Hood River, OR 97031-8553
541-387-6370
Fax: 541-387-2728
www.providence.org

Mary Delarue, Administrator

Providence Brookside Manor is an Assisted Living and Alzheimer's Dementia Residential Care Facility, located in senic Hood River, Oregon - the heart of the Columbia River Gorge. Our facility is conveniently locates next to Down Manor Retirement Community and more.

7586 Quail Run Assisted Living at Mennonite Village
2525 47th Avenue SE
Albany, OR 97322-8842
541-928-1122
Fax: 541-917-1393
www.mennonitevillage.org

Mary Ellen Lind, Administrator

We offer a community for seniros that is alive with activity, light, energy, and nature. We respect our seniors for their lifetime of accomplishments, their past and present talents, and the life lessions that have to share. We honor and nourish each individual's spiritual life.

7587 Rackleff House
655 SW 13th Avenue
Canby, OR 97013-4052
503-263-6123
Fax: 503-263-6502
www.rackleffplace.net

Kim Lewis, Administrator

7588 Regent at Regency Park Assisted Living
8300 SW Barnes Road
Portland, OR 97225-6300
503-292-8444
Fax: 503-292-8409

Susan Magnuson, Marketing Executive

Independent living, assisted care, memory care, adult day stay memory care.

7589 Ridgeview Assisted Living
872 Golf View Drive
Medford, OR 97504-9651
541-779-2208
Fax: 541-779-2384

Dan Gregory, President

7590 Rose Arbor Assisted Living
6033 E Arbor Avenue
Meza, AZ 85206
480-630-3647
Fax: 541-564-8178
www.arborroseseniorcare.com

Paula Oltman, President

Home-like apartment living for 32 seniors/disabled adults. personal services available according to level of need. Managed & operated by owners.

7591 Rose Valley Assisted Living Facility
33800 SE Frederick Street
Scappoose, OR 97056-3831
503-543-4646
Fax: 503-543-4648

Jamie Harwood, Administrator

7592 Sawyer House
160 Lombard Loop Rd
Zillah, WA 98953
509-853-5095
Fax: 514-338-0387
info@sawyerhouseofyakima.com
www.sawyerhouseofyakima.com

Tris Legacy, Administrator

7593 Settler's Park Assisted Living & Memory Care
2895 17th Street
Baker City, OR 97814-1245
541-523-0200
Fax: 541-523-0268

Michael Shoemaker, Administrator

7594 Shore Pines Assisted Living
93975 Ocean Way
Gold Beach, OR 97444-8521
541-247-0333
Fax: 541-247-9213

Nancy Tiovannetti, Administrator

7595 Silver Creek Assisted Living
6630 Crumpler Blvd.
Woodburn, MS 38654
662-895-8952
Fax: 662-895-8966; *Toll Free:* 662-895-8952
www.silvercreekseniorliving.com
Wayne Buckles, Administrator

7596 Skylark Assisted Living
900 Skylark Place
Ashland, OR 97520-9640
541-552-1713
Fax: 541-552-1058
Bob Bolling, Administrator

7597 Spencer House
411 SE 35th Street
Newport, OR 97366-9700
541-867-7400
Fax: 541-867-7401
Susan Cain, Administrator

7598 Spring Village
1420 Redwood Circle
Grants Pass, OR 97527-5536
541-474-0200
Fax: 541-956-0190
Christina Liddycoat, Administrator

7599 Spruce Point
375 9th Street
Florence, OR 97439-9470
541-997-6111
Fax: 541-997-5747
info@sprucepoint.com
www.sprucepointinn.com
Toni Underwood, Marketing Director
BJ Rollins, General Manger
Shirley Moore, Resident Care Coordiantor

Spruce Point offers a new resident-focused alternative - independent living supported by a wide range of personal services.

7600 St Anthony Village
3560 SE 79th Avenue
Portland, OR 97206-2372
503-775-4414
Fax: 503-771-9689
Melodi Kellenbeck, Administrator

7601 Summit Assisted Living
127 SE Wilson Avenue
Bend, OR 97702-1788
541-317-3544
Fax: 541-330-0121
www.summitalf.com
Flora Meisner, Administrator

7602 Summit Springs Assisted Living Facility
133 S Church Street
Condon, OR 97823
541-384-2101
Fax: 541-384-2102
Persis Dyer, Administrator

7603 Sun Terrace Hermiston
1550 NW 11th Street
Hermiston, OR 97838-6692
541-564-2595
Fax: 541-564-3087
www.regencysunterracehermiston.com
Laura Young, Administrator

7604 Suzanne Elise Assisted Living
101 Forest Drive
Seaside, OR 97138-7867
503-738-0307
Fax: 503-717-8102
Mike Maltman, Owner

7605 Tanner Spring
23000 Horizon Drive
West Linn, OR 97068-8247
503-655-4373
Fax: 503-655-4175
www.tannerspringalf.com/
Wendell White, CEO

7606 Terwilliger Plaza
2425 SW Terwilliger Boulevard
Portland, OR 97201
503-226-4911
Fax: 503-299-4803
Dee Sellner, Executive Director

7607 Timberhill Place
989 NW Spruce Avenue
Corvallis, OR 97330-2182
541-753-1767
Fax: 541-757-3528
www.timberhillplace.com/

7608 Valley View Assisted Living
112 NW Valley View Drive
John Day, OR 97845-1286
541-575-3533
Fax: 541-575-2366
Barbara Weeks, Administrator

7609 Well Springs Assisted Living Facility
2104 W Idaho Avenue
Ontario, OR 97914-1991
541-889-3020
Fax: 541-889-3020
Larry Chandler, Administrator

7610 Wiley Creek Community
4901 Highway 20
Sweet Home, OR 97386-3240
541-367-1800
Fax: 541-367-1700
Margaret Champion, Manager

Residents enjoy Wiley Creek's special services, including daytime excursions, delicious food, a respect for an individual's privacy, and friendly, professional staff. And your small pet is welcome at Wiley Creek.

7611 Willamette Manor
176 W C Street
Lebanon, OR 97355-3193

541-258-8178
Fax: 541-258-8197
www.willamettemanor.org

Jacine Vanatte, Administrator

7612 Willamette View
12705 SE River Road
Portland, OR 97222-8096
503-654-6581
Fax: 503-652-6801; *Toll Free:* 800-446-0670
info@willametteview.org
www.willametteview.org

James Mertz, CEO

A multi-licensed assisted living facility that offers skilled care.

7613 Willamette View Health Center
13145 SE River Road
Portland, OR 97222-8030
503-353-7000
Fax: 503-652-6255

Karen Stahlecker, Administrator

7614 Wilsonville
7600 SW Vlahos Drive
Wilsonville, OR 97070-5480
503-582-9414
Fax: 503-582-9236

Linda Swanson, Administrator

7615 Woodland Heights
9355 SW McDonald Street
Tigard, OR 97224-5906
503-684-9696
Fax: 503-684-9892

Jerry Crowe, Owner

7616 Woodside Assisted Living Community
4851 Main Street
Springfield, OR 97478-6057
541-747-1887
Fax: 541-747-0181
www.woodsideseniorcommunities.org

Grace Geil, Administrator

Pennsylvania

7617 Alterra Wynnwood of Northampton Manor
65 Newtown Richboro Road
Richboro, PA 18954-1726
215-357-6565
Fax: 215-953-6700

7618 Artman Lutheran Home
250 N Bethlehem Pike
Ambler, PA 19002-3597
215-643-6333
Fax: 215-643-6249
www.artmanhome.com

Luanne Fisher, CEO

Our care is designed to meet a wide variety of individual needs while providing peace of mind for our residents and their family members.

7619 D'Youville Manor
1750 Quarry Road
Yardley, PA 19067-3910
215-579-1750
Fax: 215-579-3054
www.dyouville.org

Cecile Shocket, Administrator

Offers assisted living with personalized, loving care.

7620 Deer Meadows
8301 Roosevelt Boulevard
Philadelphia, PA 19152-2006
215-624-7575
Fax: 215-624-7020

Offer a supportive environment with a staff that is dedicated and responsive to each resident's needs.

7621 Grand Residence at Upper St. Clair
45 McMurray Road
Upper St Clair, PA 15241-1649
412-833-2500
Fax: 412-833-8826

Bill Polachek, Owner

Variety of programs and services aimed at fostering the strong sense of independence that has been developed over a lifetime.

7622 Masonic Retirement Community of Lafayette Hill
801 Ridge Pike
Lafayette Hill, PA 19444-1723
610-828-5760
Fax: 619-828-2803

Adrienne Staudenmayer, Administrator

7623 Residence
4004 Linglestown Road
Harrisburg, PA 17112-1017
717-549-9400
Fax: 717-441-8583

Residential independent and assisted living and respite care will be provided.

7624 Residence at Glen Riddle
263 Glen Riddle Road
Media, PA 19063-5810
610-358-9933
Fax: 619-358-5815
www.glenriddleseniorliving.com/

Lisa Grech, Executive Director

The Residence offers several types of accommodations within each of our retirement communities. We also provide the kind of exceptional amenities you would expect from the assisted living industry.

7625 Willow Lake
1120 York Road
Willow Grove, PA 19090-1334
215-830-0433
Fax: 215-830-0693

Renee Ackerman, President

Offers quality care with supportive service's designed to maintain a resident's independence.

7626 Bay Spring Village
147 Bay Spring Avenue
Barrington, RI 02806-1370
401-246-2500
Fax: 401-246-2145

Gerald Paulhus, Executive Director

7627 Better Days Residential
240 Central Avenue
Pawtucket, RI 02860-2319
401-728-2671
Fax: 401-726-0848

Sandra Greco, Owner

7628 Blackstone Valley Assisted Living
649 Broad Street
Central Falls, RI 02863-2803
401-725-7045
Fax: 401-725-0004

Concetta DiCenzo

7629 Blenheim Newport Residential Retirement Community
303 Valley Road
Middletown, RI 02842-5272
401-849-0031
Fax: 401-849-0199
www.blenheimnewport.com

Warren Strong, Executive Director

7630 Brick Manor Residential Care
29 9th Street
Providence, RI 02906-2926
401-331-6288
Fax: 401-861-3499

Agnes Wrzesien, Administrator

7631 Cortland Place
20 Austin Avenue
Greenville, RI 02828-1449
401-949-3880
Fax: 401-949-4170
www.cortlandplace.com/

Norman Audino, Owner

7632 Darlington Assisted Living Centers
123 Armistice Boulevard
Pawtucket, RI 02860-3207
401-725-2400
Fax: 401-722-3677

Margret Bubis, Administrator

Darlington is a small assisted living residence where residents enjoy a home-like environment and atmosphere with very personalized attention. Our primary goal is to create a carefree lifestyle for older individuals where all their daily needs are met.

7633 Elms Retirement Home
22 Elm Street
Westerly, RI 02891-2159
401-596-4630
Fax: 401-348-0113

Robert Elmer, Admiistrator

7634 Emerald Bay Manor
10 Old Diamond Hill Road
Cumberland, RI 02864-4611
401-333-3393
Fax: 401-333-6021

Richard Fishpaw, Executive Director

From independent living to assistedliving to the availability of skilled nursing care, Emerlad Bay Manor has it all. You have the option of selecting your private apartment from a variety of spacious and distinctive studios and one bedroom floor plans. Each feature has a full private bath, individual climate controls, spacious closets, emergency call systems and room for your furnishings.

7635 Ethan Place
85 Ethan Street
Warwick, RI 02888-3905
401-781-0172
Fax: 401-781-0479

Peggy Richard, Executive Director

7636 Evergreen Assisted Living Home
116 Greene Street
Woonsocket, RI 02895-4508
401-769-6869
Fax: 401-765-5906

Susan Cornell, Manager

7637 Forest Farm Assisted Living
191 Forest Avenue
Middletown, RI 02842-7415
401-849-9929
Fax: 401-849-9345

Nancy Nelson Caswell

7638 Manchester Manor
12 Manchester Street
Pawtucket, RI 02860-2016
401-725-8390
Fax: 401-755-1559

Frances Goulet, Owner

7639 Pocasset Lodge Assisted Living
14 Old Pocasset Lane
Johnston, RI 02919-3143
401-272-0690
Fax: 401-272-2659

7640 Scandinavian Home
1811 Broad Street
Cranston, RI 02905-3533
401-461-1433
Fax: 401-461-4005
www.scandinavianhome.com

J Chris Woulfe, Executive Director
Linda Tucker, Administrator

Our mission is to provides a continuum of excellent health care to individuals through their stages of life in a warm homelike atmosphere. Resident dignity and quality of life are emphasized. Although Scandinavian traditions are recognized, admissions to our facility is open to all persons. A cooperative approach with resdients and their families is utilized to maximize the strengths of each resident.

7641 The Elms Retirement Campus
22 Elm Street
Westerly, RI 02891
401-596-4630
Fax: 401-348-0113
mtaylor.elmal@verizon.net
www.elmsassistedliving.com

Mark Taylor, Administrator

Independent, assisted living, and memory care for seniors.

7642 Tockwotten Home
75 E Street
Providence, RI 02903-4499
401-272-5280
Fax: 401-421-0550
www.tockwotton.org

Kevin McKay, Administrator
Robert Martin, Assisted Living Administrator

Founded in 1856, Tockwotton Home provides skilled nursing and assisted living. Tockwotton Home is a 501 (c)(3) Non-Profit.

7643 United Methodist Retirement Center
40 Irving Avenue
E Providence, RI 02914-2301
401-438-4456
Fax: 401-431-9166

Karen Smith, Executive Director

7644 Victoria Court
55 Oaklawn Avenue
Cranston, RI 02920-9334
401-946-5522
Fax: 401-942-5582
www.victoriacourt.biz/

Carolyn Delfino, Administrator

7645 Villa at St Antoine
400 Mendon Road
N Smithfield, RI 02896-6945
401-767-2574
Fax: 401-767-2581
www.hotel-villa-saint-antoine.com

Mary Ann Altruie, Executive Director

7646 Village at Elmhurst
700 Smith Street
Providence, RI 02908-3500
401-521-0090
Fax: 401-453-2514
www.villageretirement.com

Chris Stack, Executive Director

We provide residents exceptional access to medical resources. Our unique, maintenance-free catered living options allow you to pursue your interests, from lasting friends and experience the retirement lifestyle of your dreams. Our residents enjoy the peace of mind that comes from our full range of services supporting the health and wellness.

7647 Village at Hillsgrove
75 Minnesota Avenue
Warwick, RI 02888-6023

401-737-7222
Fax: 401-737-9702
www.villagereitrement.com

Teri Le, Executive Director

The Village at Hillsgrove is a lively suburban hideaway, convenient to shop, amenities and the airport. Our unique, maintenance free catered living options allow you to pursue your interests, form lasting friendships and experience the retirement lifestyle of your dreams. Our residents enjoy the peace of mind that comes from our full range of services supporting the health and wellness.

7648 Warren Manor I
682 Pleasant Dr
Warren, PA 16365
814-723-7060
Fax: 401-232-9240

Ann Marie Coleman, Administrator

7649 West Bay Manor
2783 W Shore Road
Warwick, RI 02889-8659
401-739-7300
Fax: 401-738-3488

Cheryl Kingma, Administrator

7650 Willows Assisted Living
898 S. Meridian
Blackfoot, I 83221
208-782-1478
Fax: 401-247-9030
www.willowsliving.net

Marey Beth Lefchuet, Owner

7651 Wyndemere Woods
1044 Mendon Road
Woonsocket, RI 02895-3997
401-762-4226
Fax: 401-766-5548

Jeffrey Roy, Owner

South Dakota

7652 Avera Bormann Manor
501 N 4th Street
Parkston, SD 57366-2008
605-928-3384
Fax: 605-928-7368

Gail Walker, Administrator

7653 Avera Brady Assisted Living
1414 W Cedar Avenue
Mitchell, SD 57301-3868
605-996-7702
Fax: 605-996-0039
www.avera.org

Veronica Smith, Administrator

7654 Avera Gettysburg Hospital
606 E Garfield Avenue
Gettysburg, SD 57442-1325
605-765-2461
Fax: 605-765-2704
www.avera.org/st-marys-pierre/gettysburg

Mark Schmidt, Executive Director

7655 Avera Mother Joseph Manor Retirement Community
1002 N Jay Street
Aberdeen, SD 57401-2439
605-622-5850
Fax: 605-622-5851
www.avera.org

Tom Snyder, Administrator

7656 Avera Prince of Peace Retirement Community
4504 S Prince of Peace Place
Sioux Falls, SD 57103-5865
605-322-5600
Fax: 605-332-5622
www.avera.org

Lavonne Gaspar, Administrator

7657 Avera St Benedict Assisted Living
401 W Glynn Drive
Parkston, SD 57366-9605
605-928-3718
Fax: 605-928-7368
www.avera.org

Gale Walker, CEO

7658 B and C Resthome
341 9th Street
Sturgis, SD 57785-1117
605-720-3659
Fax: 605-720-4384

7659 Bennett County Healthcare Center
102 Major Allen
PO Box 70D
Martin, SD 57551
605-685-6622
Fax: 605-685-1166
www.bennettcountyhospital.com

Ethel Frein, CEO
Judy Soderlin, CFO
Denise Juhnke, Revenue Manager

7660 Bethel Suites
911 S Egan Avenue
Madison, SD 57042-3315
605-256-4539
Fax: 605-256-4007

Jim Iverson, Administrator

7661 Bethesda Towne Square
1425 15th Avenue SE
Aberdeen, SD 57401-7726
605-225-7600
Fax: 605-225-7585
info@bha.cc
www.bha.cc

Gina Sommers, Manager

7662 Carousel Living Center
PO Box 100
Faulkton, SD 57438
605-598-6262
Fax: 605-598-6260

Ken Barotholmew, Manager

7663 Cedar View Assisted Living
225 14th Avenue NE
Watertown, SD 57201-1207
605-882-8419
Fax: 605-882-4961

Nancy Wittmeier, Manager

7664 Cottages at Fairmont Grand
417 E Fairlane Drive
Rapid City, SD 57701-7207
605-348-1040
Fax: 605-399-1471

The Cottages at Fairmont Grand Manor are a unique part of Regional Senior Care Living Facilities. The Cottages specialize in the care of residential with Alzheimer's and other Dementia-realted disorders. We call this focused level of care Enhanced Care.

7665 Edgewood Vista of Sioux Falls
3409 E. 5th Street
Sioux Falls, SD 57103
605-275-0074
Fax: 605-275-0076
edgewoodseniorliving.com

Alyce Dobson, Manager

Edgewood Vista exists to provide personalized care in setting designed specifically for Elderly, including those with Alzheimer's Disease of other forms of dementia. Our individualized apporoach provides a high quality, safe, homelike setting to Seniors who choose to no longer reside alone, but who can live better in social residential settings.

7666 Estelline Nursing and Care Center
PO Box 130
Estelline, SD 57234
605-873-2278
Fax: 605-873-2989

Michael Ward

7667 Evergreen Assisted Living
801 Gregory Street
Normal, IL 61701
309-451-9355
Fax: 605-882-8556
www.evergreenplaceassistedliving.com/

Terri Lynn M Becker, Administrator

7668 Fairmont Grand Manor
417 E Fairlane Drive
Rapid City, SD 57701-7207
605-399-1551
Fax: 605-399-1471

Fay Kuhn, Manager

7669 Fay Wookey Memorial Assisted Living Center
700 N Smith Street
Clark, SD 57225-1120
605-532-5799
Fax: 605-532-1320; *Toll Free:* 605-881-1663

Gail Wookey, Owner

7670 Foothills Assisted Living
999 West Union Rd
West Union, SC 29696

864-638-4370
Fax: 605-347-2333
www.foothillsassistedlivingsc.com/

7671 Fox Run Residences
301 Fox Run Drive
Rapid City, SD 57701-2313
605-342-4552
Fax: 605-343-3816

7672 Golden Prairie Manor
1145 Prairie Drive
Winner, SD 57580
605-842-0508
Fax: 605-842-0508

Shawna Kaiser, Manager

7673 Greater Fall River Health Care Services
209 N 16th Street
Hot Springs, SD 57747-1374
605-745-3159
Fax: 605-745-3957

7674 Heritage Senior Living
211 NW 1st Street
Madison, SD 57042-2884
605-256-1525
Fax: 605-256-1535
www.heritagesenior.com

Jo Ann Cassanova, Manager

7675 Herreid Good Samaritan Center
PO Box 8
Herreid, SD 57632
605-437-2425
Fax: 605-437-2950

Mary Mitzel, Administrator

7676 Hilda's Heritage Home
220 S Lincoln Street
Lennox, SD 57039-2306
605-647-5515
Fax: 605-647-5502

Edith Buseman, Owner

7677 Homestead Assisted Living
300 W Hazel Avenue
Howard, SD 57349-8700
605-785-3310
Fax: 605-785-3310

7678 Inn on Westport
4000 S Westport Avenue
Sioux Falls, SD 57106-2300
605-362-1210
Fax: 605-361-8866
www.innonwestport.com

Michele Rassamussen, Sales and Marketing Director

7679 Kirkwood Manor
2590 Loop 337 N
Box 208
New Braunfels, TX 57732
830-620-0509
Fax: 605-578-7789
www.kirkwoodmanor.net

7680 Lakeside Assisted Living Residence
1010 W 5th Street
Redfield, SD 57469-2026
605-472-2191
Fax: 605-472-2194

7681 Marion Assisted Living Center
200 Eisenhower Dr
Marion, KS 66861
620-382-3000
Fax: 888-382-3001
www.seniorsinmarion.com

Paul I Engbrecht, Administrator

7682 Marshall County Healthcare Center
413 9th Street
Britton, SD 57430-2274
605-448-2253
Fax: 605-448-2304

Stephanie Reasy, Administrator

7683 Morningside Manor Assisted Living
700 Babcock Road
San Antonio, TX 78201
605-934-2011
Fax: 605-934-9923; *Toll Free:* 888-505-4085
Info@MMLiving.org
www.mmliving.org

Todd Willson, Administrator

7684 Morningside Manor Assisted Living II
700 Babcock Road
San Antonio, TX 78201
605-934-2011
Fax: 605-934-9923; *Toll Free:* 888-505-4085
Info@MMLiving.org
www.mmliving.org

Desile Carlis, Administrator

7685 Morningstar Assisted Living
700 Babcock Road
San Antonio, TX 78201
605-934-2011
Fax: 605-341-5736; *Toll Free:* 888-505-4085
Info@MMLiving.org
www.mmliving.org

Linda Slezak, Administrator

7686 Orchard Hills
200 W 10th Street
Dell Rapids, SD 57022-1264
605-428-6200
Fax: 605-428-6201

Carmen Stoebner, Administrator

7687 Park Place Assisted Living
6900 37TH Floor S
Seattle, WA 98118
206-722-7275
Fax: 605-692-5982
parkplace@rhf.org
www.parkplaceassistedliving.org/

Diane Stroschein, Manager

7688 Parkview Apartments Assisted Living
PO Box 327
Wakonda, SD 57073
605-267-2081
Fax: 605-267-2690

Becky McManus, Administrator

7689 Prairie Crossings
901 14th Avenue NE
Suite A
Watertown, SD 57201-6820
605-882-2045
Fax: 605-229-6673
leasing@terrafirma-co.com
www.prairiecrossing.com

Glenda Soine, Manager

7690 Prairie Crossings-Huron
901 14th Avenue NE
Suite A
Watertown, SD 57201-6820
605-882-2045
Fax: 605-352-4873
www.prairiecrossing.com

Glenda Soine, Manager

7691 Prairie Crossings-Mitchell
2211 N Wisconsin Street
Mitchell, SD 57301-1074
605-996-2048
Fax: 605-996-2074
www.prairiecrossing.com

Donna Weiland, Manager

7692 Prairie Crossings-Sioux Falls
1806 S Dorothy Avenue
Sioux Falls, SD 57106-3826
605-361-0056
Fax: 605-361-0158
www.prairiecrossing.com

Mary Besson, Manager

7693 Prairie Crossings-Watertown
424 9th Street SE
Watertown, SD 57201-4554
605-882-9003
Fax: 605-882-9433
www.prairiecrossing.com

7694 Prairie Good Samaritan Center Assisted Living
421 E 4th Street
Miller, SD 57362-1599
605-853-2701
Fax: 605-583-5370
www.prairiecrossing.com

James Gisi, Administrator

7695 Prairie Homes Assisted Living
1463 Kenwood Dr
Menasha, WI 57078-4000
920-969-0526
Fax: 605-260-6133
www.prairiehomeassistedliving.com

John H. McCarthy, Executive Director

7696 Prairie Sunset Village
PO Box 580
Mobridge, SD 57601
605-845-3692
Fax: 605-845-7905

Angie Svihovec, CEO

The facility is equipped with emergency responce buttons
in each apartment and secured access after hours with
24-hour staff available to respond to the tenants needs.

7697 Prairie View Assisted Living Center
500 East McNair St
Winnebago, IL 61088
81- 33- 180
Fax: 605-778-6718
www.prairieviewwinnebago.com

Virginia Banek, Owner

7698 Primrose Assisted Living
224 E Minnesota Street
Rapid City, SD 57701-7734
605-342-6699
Fax: 605-342-1092
www.primroseretirement.com

Lynn Ivey, Manager

7699 Primrose Place
1801 3rd Avenue SE
Aberdeen, SD 57401-5049
605-226-1515
Fax: 605-226-1515
www.primroseplace.net/

Deb Rice, Manager

7700 Riverview Health Services
611 E 2nd Avenue
Flandreau, SD 57028-1399
605-997-2481
Fax: 605-997-2488
www.riverviewhealth.com

Jo Ann Lind, Administrator

We provide skilled nursing home care, home health, independent living apartments, and an extensive rehabilitative
therapy program (in and out patient).

7701 Riverview Retirement Home
1801 E. Upriver Dr,
Spokane, WA 99207
605-734-5447
Fax: 605-734-5852
www.riverviewretirement.org

Dwain Blackwell, Owner

7702 Rosholt Care Center Assisted Living Center
85 1st Avenue East
PO Box 108
Rosholt, SD 57260
605-537-4272
Fax: 605-537-4335
contact@rosholtcarecenter.com
www.rosholtcarecenter.com

Tina Muller, Administrator

7703 Salem Mennonite Home
106 W 7th Street
Freeman, SD 57029-2319
605-925-4994
Fax: 605-925-4764
www.salemmenno.mennonite.net

Stewart Hofer, Administrator

7704 Sandstone Manor
16677 NE Russell
Portland, OR 97230
50- 2-3 07
Fax: 605-642-4819
www.sandstonemanornow.com

Nancy Barron, Owner

7705 Scotland Good Samaritan Center Assisted Living Center
130 6th Street
Scotland, SD 57059
605-583-2216
Fax: 605-583-2256
good-sam.com/index.php/locations/scotlan

7706 Shelby Good Samaritan Center Assisted Living
4861 Lincoln Ave.
Selby, SD 57472
605-649-7663
good-sam.com/index.php/locations/selby

Jill Hoogeveen, Administrator

7707 Springfield Assisted Living Center
701 Pine Street
Springfield, SD 57062
605-369-5445
Fax: 605-369-2868
www.springfieldsd.com

Charlene Tjeerdsma, Manager

7708 Stoneybrook Suites of Watertown
500 16th Avenue
Watertown, NE 57201
605-882-0013
Fax: 605-884-1930
www.stoneybrooksuites.com

Beth Reynolds, Manager
Deb Whitlock, Administration

7709 Sun Dial Manor
410 Second Street
PO Box 337
Bristol, SD 57219
605-492-3615
Fax: 605-492-3616
sundial@nvc.net
www.sundialmanor.com

Peggy Pearson, Administrator
Year Founded: 1965

7710 Trail Ridge Retirement Community Assisted Living Center
3408 W Ralph Rogers Road
Suite 100
Sioux Falls, SD 57108

605-339-4847
Fax: 605-373-0088
www.trailridgeretirement.net

Al Svennes, Administrator
Bonnie Berghorst, Director of Marketing
Jason Honey, Senior Living Counselor
Year Founded: 1930

7711 Victorian
1321 Columbus Street
Rapid City, SD 57701
605-342-1913
Fax: 605-348-2078
hunekel@midconetwork.com
www.victorianassistedliving.net

Lavon Huneke, Manager
Year Founded: 1997

7712 Waterford at All Saints
111 W 17th Street
Sioux Falls, SD 57104-4972
605-335-1117
Fax: 605-335-1100; *Toll Free:* 800-713-1117
www.touchmarksiouxfalls.com

Werner G. Nistler Jr., Founder and CEO
Bernie L. Neil, Executive Vice President
Thomas L. Biel, Executive Vice President

Tennessee

7713 Adamsplace Assisted Living
1927 Memorial Boulevard
Murfreesboro, TN 37129-1545
615-904-2449
Fax: 615-867-5223
www.adamsplace.org

Buckley Winfree, Administrator

7714 Allen Morgan Health Center at Trezevant Manor
177 North Highland Street
Memphis, TN 38111-4747
901-325-4000
Fax: 901-325-4023
dcongleton@trezevantmanor.org
www.trezevantmanor.org

Charley Tirrell, Administrator
Year Founded: 1977

7715 Asbury Acres
2648 Sevierville Road
Maryville, TN 37804-3643
865-984-1660
Fax: 865-982-1617
www.asburyplace.org/

Bernie Bowman, CEO

7716 Atria Weston Place
2900 Lake Brook Boulevard
Knoxville, TN 37909-1140
865-584-9857
Fax: 865-588-6223
www.atriaseniorliving.com/atria-weston-p

Leigh Ann Garrett, Executive Director

7717 Baptist Assisted Living Center
PO BOX 728
Brentwood, TN 37024-0728
615-371-2050
Fax: 615-371-2042
tbah@tnbaptist.org
www.tnbaptisthomes.org

Dr. C. Kenny Cooper, President - Treasurer

7718 Belmont Village of Green Hills
8554 Katy Freeway
Suite 200
Houston, TX 77024
713-463-1700
Fax: 713-647-9601
www.belmontvillage.com

7719 Belmont Village of Memphis
8554 Katy Freeway
Suite 200
Houston, TX 77024
713-463-1700
Fax: 713-647-9601
www.belmontvillage.com

7720 Hearthside at Castle Heights
215 Castle Heights Avenue
Lebanon, TN 37087-3418
615-443-1994
Fax: 614-443-7548
info@HearthsideLiving.com

Sarah C Johnston, Administrator
Brian McDonald, Executive Director
Betty Kelley, Activity Director

Dedicated to providing care and compassion to those who
choose to make this place their home.

7721 Homewood Residence at Deane Hill
401 Catherine McAuley Way
Knoxville, TN 37919
865-690-4070
Fax: 865-690-4076
www.brookdaleliving.com/homewood-residen

Monica Casey, Manager

7722 Knollwood Manor
405 Times Avenue
Lafayette, TN 37083-1247
615-666-3170
Fax: 615-666-9146
www.knollwoodtn.com

Linda Austin, Administrator
Beverly Walker

7723 Life Care Center of Sparta
3570 Keith Street
PO Box 3480
Cleveland, TN 37320-3480
423-472-9585
Fax: 931-738-9455
www.lcca.com/140/

Sabra York, Executive Director
Cathy Howe, Director

7724 Manorhouse Assisted Living
8501 S Northshore Drive
Knoxville, TN 37922-6006
865-670-0504
Fax: 864-670-2745
knoxville.executive.director@manorhouseretire
www.manorhouseretirement.com

Bridgete Duver, Manager

7725 Martin Boyd Christian Home
6845 Standifer Gap Road
Chattanooga, TN 37421-1476
423-892-1020
Fax: 423-499-8734
snjohnston@epbfi.com
www.martinboydhome.com

Sandra Johnston, Director
Allen Womack, President
Ken Wilson, Vice President

7726 Morningside of Gallatin
1085 Hartsville Pike
Gallatin, TN 37066-2501
615-230-5600
Fax: 615-230-4499
www.morningsideofgallatin.com

Sharon Spears, Executive Director

7727 NHC Place Farragut
120 Cavette Hill Lane
Knoxville, TN 37934-6674
865-777-4000
Fax: 865-777-4994
klane@nhcfarragut.com
www.nhcfarragut.com

Karla Lane, Administrator
Vivian Akins, Admissions Director
Karen Jackson, Director of Nursing
Year Founded: 1998

7728 Oak Ridge Retirement Community
12925 Yonge Street
Ontario, L4E3G4
905-773-4220
Fax: 865-483-3118
www.oakridgesretirement.com

Toni Ladd, Administrator

7729 Outlook Pointe at Oak Ridge
124 Randolph Road
Oak Ridge, TN 37830
865-482-9251
Fax: 865-481-3988
orfrontn@aol.com
www.oakridgefloralcompany.com

Christina Trenthran, Administrator
Year Founded: 1986

7730 Park Place Retirement Community
31 Executive Park Drive
Hendersonville, TN 37075-3463
615-822-6002
Fax: 615-822-3765
www.parkplaceret.com

Nancy Jenkins, Manager

7731 Regency House Assisted Living
2062 Hamill Road
Hixson, TN 37343
423-870-0050
Fax: 423-490-2161
ldiener@veritasincare.com
www.regencyhouse-hixson.com

Rhonda Donald, Manager

7732 Shelbyville Residential Care
895 Union Street
Shelbyville, TN 37160-2607
931-536-1577
Fax: 931-685-6950
www.americareusa.net

Mary Ann Steelman, Administrator

7733 Southern Living Center of Lebanon
900 Coles Ferry Pike
Lebanon, TN 37087-5677
615-210-2991
Fax: 615-443-7502
www.southernmlc.com

Cheryl Pendergrass, Executive Director
Jennifer Bradshaw, Executive Director
Kim Gulley, Director of Windchester

7734 Uplands Retirement Village
PO Box 168
Pleasant Hill, TN 38578
931-277-3518
Fax: 931-277-5396
www.uplandsvillage.com

Rev. Lyle Weible, Chairman
Richard Woodard, Executive Director
Tracey Barnes, Director of Sales and Marketing
Year Founded: 1884

7735 Waverly Gardens
6312 seven Corners Centre
161
Falls Church, VA 22044-2409
703-237-5606
Fax: 901-360-9044
www.greenfieldseniorliving.com

Patricia Bray, Administrator

Offers affordable rental apartments, restaurat style dining, housekeeping, planned social activities, and resident services.

Texas

7736 Arden Courts Alzheimer's Assisted Living
11630 Four Iron Drive
Austin, TX 78750-3100
512-918-2800
Fax: 512-835-8814; *Toll Free:* 888-478-2410
www.arden-courts.com

7737 Arkansas House
350 State Capitol
500 Woodlane Avenue
Little Rock, AR 72201-1037

501-682-6211
Fax: 817-861-4645
www.arkansashouse.org

Lynne Walraven, Executive Director
Number of Members: 100

7738 Ashwood Retirement & Assisted Living
12151 Hunters Chase Drive
Austin, TX 78729-7960
512-336-4100
Fax: 512-336-4155
kedwards@ashwoodassitedliving.com
www.ashwoodliving.com

Tommy Wood, Administrator

7739 Atria in Kingwood
2401 Green Oak Drive
Kingwood, TX 77339-2075
281-359-8959
Fax: 281-359-1237
www.atriaseniorliving.com

Paula Brown, Executive Director

7740 Atria in West Chase
11424 Richmond Avenue
Houston, TX 77082-2507
281-617-2196
Fax: 281-370-4846
www.atriaseniorliving.com

Kim Parnel, Executive Director

7741 Barton Hills Assisted Living
1606 Nash Avenue
Austin, TX 78704-3332
512-441-6000
Fax: 512-441-2205
www.bartonhillsal.com/assisted-living-se

Belinda Huerta, Administrator

7742 Barton House
7000 East Mountain View Road
Scottsdale, AZ 85253
480-607-2898
Fax: 512-833-0060
www.thebartonhouse.com

Kim Greenwood, Administrator
Jennifer Scott, Manager
Joycelen Lankford, Activity Director

We tailor the care of each of our residents to his or her needs. This highly personlized program is made possible by our small size and unusually high staff ratio. Our philosophy of care is really quite simple. Focus on strengths, rather than weaknesses. Never stop communitcating, and be kind always.

7743 Barton House at First Colony
7000 East Mountain View Road
Scottsdale, AZ 85253
480-607-2898
Fax: 281-313-2505
www.thebartonhouse.com

Jane Relton, Administrator

7744 Bellaire Lodge
6125 Edloe
Houston, TX 77005
713-665-4100
Fax: 713-776-1816
www.bellairelodge.org

Jeffrey Thomson, WM
Gary Krzywicki, Secretary
Graham Cull, SW

Year Founded: 1953

7745 Belmont Village at West University
8554 Katy Freeway
Suite 200
Houston, TX 77024
713-463-1700
Fax: 713-647-9601
www.belmontvillage.com

At Bellmont Village, we take great care to balance the independence our seniors desire with the support they need. Belmont Village programs and services have been designed to provide a sense of well-being for all residents, with a common support system that is thoughtful and sensitive to seniors at every turn.

7746 Braeswood Personal Care Homes
3519 South Braeswood
Houston, TX 77025
713-666-6545
Fax: 713-838-2220
bpchi@aol.com
www.braeswoodhomes.com

Susan S Di Filippo, Administrator

The Braeswood Home is an assisted living facility that provides residential and personalized support services to older adults, the frail elderly, and those who need assistance with activities of daily living, but do not need skilled medical care.

7747 Brookwood Community
1752 Fm 1489 Road
Brookshire, TX 77423-8809
281-375-2100
Fax: 281-375-2160
www.brookwoodcommunity.org

Stephen C Beasley, Chairman
David R Streit, Vice Chairman
Dea L. Larson, Treasurer

Year Founded: 1985

7748 Buckner Retirement Services
600 N Pearl Street
Suite 2000
Dallas, TX 75201-2874
214-758-8031
Fax: 972-519-9765; *Toll Free:* 855-264-8783
foundation@buckner.org
www.buckner.org

Albert L Reyes, President & CEO

We care for senior adlults, and care about them too. Rich in heritage and tradition, Buckner has provided care for senior adults for 100 years. That long history of caring for and about people has helped us create an atmosphere of warmth and friendship.

7749 Buckner Villas
1110 Tom Adams Drive
Austin, TX 78753
512-836-1515
Fax: 512-834-9763; *Toll Free:* 800-381-4551
www.bucknervillas.org

Doyle Antle, Administrator

Year Founded: 1879

7750 Cambridge Square Retirement Center
2700 Avenue N
Rosenberg, TX 77471-4507
281-344-8444
Fax: 281-344-8444
cambridgesquareliving.com

Maxine Hunter, Administrator
Maria Elena Edwards, Activity Director
Jessica Morales, Resident Care Supervisor

7751 Caruth Haven Court
5585 Caruth Haven Lane
Dallas, TX 75225-8157
972-587-7544
Fax: 214-368-8998
www.caruthhavencourt.com

Christy Connor, Executive Director
Eilleen Aldridge, Director of Marketing
Dick Blaylock, Owner

7752 Chandler Assisted Living
1510 Howard Street
San Antonio, TX 78212-3444
210-737-5200
Fax: 210-737-5221
www.mmliving.org/communities/chandler-es

7753 Colonial Oaks at First Colony
13825 Lexington Boulevard
Sugar Land, TX 77478-5364
281-277-0900
Fax: 281-277-3674
kimberly@colonialoaks.org
www.colonialoaks.org

Clarissa Woods, Executive Director

Year Founded: 1977

7754 Eastman Estates
2920 N Eastman Road
Longview, TX 75605-5099
903-416-8376
Fax: 903-757-2491
www.emeritus.com/retirement-communities-

Andy Bynum, Executive Director

7755 Eden Home
118 Avenue Aristide Briand
Montrouge, TX 92120
830-625-6291
Fax: 830-620-7786
www.edenhome.com

Laurence Dahl, Executive Director

7756 Five Star Personal Care Homes
12610 Silver Spur
Austin, TX 78727-4345

512-388-5943
Fax: 512-454-5502

Terry Yates, Owner

7757 Gardens of Richardson
1111 W Shore Drive
Richardson, TX 75080-4917
972-783-8000
Fax: 972-783-4267
www.gardensofrichardson.com

Colleen Holliday, Director of Nursing
Sylvia Rocker, Assisted Living Director
Wanda Ledford, Administrator

7758 Good Place Assisted Living
7801 N. Richland Boulevard
North Richland Hills, TX 76180-6415
817-581-6310
Fax: 817-581-0608
www.capitalsenior.com

Gilbert Gutierrez, Executive Director

7759 Grace House of Lake Travis
11825 Bee Caves Road
Bee Cave, TX 78738-5302
512-402-0968
Fax: 512-402-0950
info@gracehouse.com
www.gracehouse.com

Jud Wyatt, President

7760 Harbourview Assisted Living of League City
300 Enterprise Avenue
League City, TX 77573-2936
281-334-4243
Fax: 281-334-8016
mminer@regentcare.biz
harbourviewcarecentre.com

Leslie Burns, Administrator

7761 Heights Assisted Living
3000 SW 32nd Street
Redmond, OR 97756
541-923-5452
Fax: 210-822-3698
www.heightsal.com

Beverly Moore, Manager

7762 Heritage at Gaines Ranch
4409 Gaines Ranch Loop
Austin, TX 78735-6555
512-721-3100
Fax: 512-899-1711; *Toll Free:* 866-404-0741
www.brookdaleliving.com

Linda Blyson, Administrator

7763 Heritage at Tomball
1221 Graham Drive
Tomball, TX 77375-6407
281-401-5400
Fax: 281-357-2280
www.sagora.com

7764 Incarnate Word Personal Care Facility
4707 Broadway Street
San Antonio, TX 78209-6215

210-829-7561
Fax: 210-828-0020
info@iwretire.org
www.iwretire.org

Alma Cosme, Community Relations Director
Jeanette Eisenmenger, Resident Services Director
Ronald Mazuca, Development Director
Number of Members: 1988

7765 Independence Hill Assisted Living
20450 Huebner Road
San Antonio, TX 78258-3942
210-615-4000
Fax: 210-615-4289; *Toll Free:* 888-810-5768
indpendencehill.com

Michelle Houriet, Manager

7766 Individual Care of Texas
1655 Private Road 2530
Quinlan, TX 75474-5459
903-356-4526
Fax: 903-356-4544
info@individualcareoftx.com
www.individualcareoftx.com

Velma Boyd, Executive Director

7767 Inn at Los Patios
8700 Post Oak Lane
San Antonio, TX 78217-5134
210-829-7357
Fax: 210-829-8238
www.theinatlospatios.com

Sandra Dietz, Manager
Number of Members: 1990

7768 Jefferson Place Assisted Living
911 S Jefferson Street
La Grange, TX 78945-3105
979-968-9161
Fax: 979-968-6962
jefforsonplace@cmaaccess.com
www.srnctx.com

Virginia Munoz, Administrator

7769 Kensington Cottages at Quail Creek
6811 Plum Creek Drive
Amarillo, TX 79124-1602
806-553-6642
Fax: 806-351-1310
www.cottageholdingsltd.com

Penny Glaesman, Executive Director

7770 Kings Manor Personal Care Home
400 Ranger Drive
Hereford, TX 79045-2812
806-364-0661
Fax: 806-364-0675
www.kmmrs.com

Shelly Moss, Executive Director
Jim Layman, Chief Financial Officer
Larry Carlson, Director of Maintenance
Number of Members: 1962

7771 Lexington Place
1737 North Loop West
Houston, TX 77008
713-869-5551
Fax: 713-869-3230
lexingtonplacehouston.com

Jesse Sias, Administrator
Dr. Carlos Herrera, Medical Director
Kellie Hawkins, Finance Director

7772 Lodge at Leon Springs
24137 Boerne Stage Road
San Antonio, TX 78255-9517
210-698-9365
Fax: 210-698-0353
mary@thelodgeatleonsprings.com
www.boerneassistedliving.com

Dana Tucker, Manager

7773 Marbridge Ranch
2310 Bliss Spillar Road
Manchaca, TX 78652-4400
512-282-1144
Fax: 512-282-3723
info@marbridge.com
www.marbridge.com

C David Perry, Chairman
Thomas H Leyden, Secretary
James Stacey, President
Number of Members: 1953

7774 Merrill Gardens at Denton, an Assisted Living Community
1938 Fairview Avenue E
Suite 300
Seattle, WA 98102
206-676-5300
Fax: 206-676-5353; *Toll Free:* 800-379-8831
www.merrillgardens.com

Tiffany White, Executive Director

We are a lovely, active retirement community that mirrors the warmth and friendship of the city of Denton. We offer our residents enticing activities and meals. For independent seniors or those who need a little assistance, we offer an environment that's one of a kind.

7775 Merrill Gardens at North Richland Hills
1938 Fairview Avenue E
Suite 300
Seattle, WA 98102
206-676-5300
Fax: 206-676-5353; *Toll Free:* 800-379-8831
www.merrillgardens.com

Martha Mattison, Manager

Conveniently located in the heart of the Dallas/Fort Worth Metroplex, Merrill Gardens at North Richland Hills is near shopping, entertainment, churches and fantasitc medical services.

7776 Merrill Gardens at Round
1938 Fairview Avenue E
Suite 300
Seattle, WA 98102

206-676-5300
Fax: 206-676-5353; *Toll Free:* 800-379-8831
www.merrillgardens.com

Sarah Boone, Manager

Our residents enjoy a wide variety of activities to accomodate an independent lifestyle. Our staff and friendly neighboring community make Round ROck an ideal place to retire.

7777 Merrill Gardens at San Antonio
1938 Fairview Avenue E
Suite 300
Seattle, WA 98102
206-676-5300
Fax: 206-676-5353; *Toll Free:* 800-379-8831
www.merrillgardens.com

Natalie Wright, Administrator

Our atmosphere encouraged independence, however Assisted living services are also available.

7778 Merrill Gardens at San Marcos
1938 Fairview Avenue E
Suite 300
Seattle, WA 98102
206-676-5300
Fax: 206-676-5353; *Toll Free:* 800-379-8831
www.merrillgardens.com

Angie Smerz, Manager

Offers independenct and assisted living services to meet your changing needs. Enjoy convenient month to month rental anytime dining, weekly housekeeping, schedules transportation and a variety of activities.

7779 Morningside Manor
13251 W 64th Ave
Arvada, CO 80004
303-425-5616
Fax: 210-731-1060
www.themorningsidemanor.com

Bob Hultgren, Administrator

7780 Oak Park Retirement Center
408 South Oak Park Avenue
Oakpark, IL 60302
708-386-4040
Fax: 817-763-3841
www.oakparkarms.com

Moses Williams Jr, Executive Director
Bonnie Benson, Assisstant Director
Heather Lindstorm, Director of Storm

7781 Oak Shadows Allendale
4801 Allendale Road
Houston, TX 77017-5421
713-941-7700
Fax: 713-941-0173
info@oakshadows.com
www.oakshadows.com

Penny Clark, Administrator
Rick Wolf, Maintenance Supervisor
Wanda Saucier, Assistant Supervisor
Number of Members: 1987

7782 Oak Wood Acres
7123 Crossroads Boulevard
Brentwood, TN 37027
615-771-9949
Fax: 830-980-4985
info@celebration tn.com
celebrationhomes.com

Randal B Smith, President
Corey W Craig, Vice President
Lloyd H Craig, Secretary

7783 Oak Wood Place
603 Wood Street
Athens, TX 75751
903-675-2002
Fax: 903-677-0659
www.oakwoodplace.com

David Daniels, Owner

7784 Pafford Place
615 County Road, 340A
Burnet, TX 78611
512-756-7854
Fax: 512-759-8088
www.paffordplace.com

Janie Pafford, Owner

7785 Park Place Retirement
31 Executive Park Drive
Hendersonville, TN 37075
615-822-6002
Fax: 281-970-6455
www.parkplaceret.com

Sue Winder, Marketing Director
Ken Quiring, Administrator

7786 Park Place Retirement Residence of Friendswood
1310 S Friendswood Drive
Friendswood, TX 77546-4968
281-648-5454
Fax: 281-648-5455
www.parkplaceseniorliving.com

Betty Martin, Administrator

7787 Park Place Retirement Residence of Stafford
11919 W Airport Boulevard
Stafford, TX 77477-2415
281-240-1707
Fax: 281-240-0140
www.simranhomes.com

Jim Hussey, Manager

7788 Parkwood Place
300 N Bynum Street
Lufkin, TX 75904-2722
336-526-6000
Fax: 936-637-2368
www.parkwoodliving.org

Terri Hutcherson, Administrator

7789 Quality Personal Care Home
139 Dean Drive Suite 4
Clarksville, TS 37040
931-906-0085
Fax: 931-906-0095

spears@qpcare.com
www.qpcare.com

Bertriche Ahamba, Manager

7790 Regency of El Paso
1600 Utica Avenue South
9th floor
St Louis Park, MN 55416
763-533-3179
Fax: 915-584-5115; *Toll Free:* 800-787-6456
regency@regencybeauty.com
www.regency.edu

Joy Gaylord, President & CEO
Mark Carani, Campus Operations
Andrea Fike, General Counsel
Year Founded: 2002

7791 Remington Park
1 Remington Pl
Oklahoma City, OK 73111
405-424-1000
Fax: 281-420-9465
mailto:contact@remingtonpark.com
www.remingtonpark.com

Ran lLeonard, Chairman
Bradon Burton, Vice Chairman
Mel Bollenbach, Secretary
Year Founded: 1988

7792 Sabine House
58 Rue du Garde Chasse
93260 Les Lilas
France, TX 77632-1200
141-832-200
Fax: 409-883-8302
www.sabinehouse.net

Thelma Swearingen, Administrator

7793 San Antonio Jewish Senior Services
13409 NW Millitary Hwy
Suite 210
San Antonio, TX 78231
210-616-4811
letyv@sajss.com
www.sajss.com

Stacey Kline Schwartz, Executive Director
Lety P Vargas, Executive Assistant
Lauren Sandoval, Special Projects

San Antonio Jewish Senior Services is a nonprofit organization that addresses the needs and enriches the lives of San Antonio Jewish seniors by creating and fostering connections between Jewish seniors and both the Jewish and broader community. SAJSS does this both directly and indirectly by offering programs, resources and assistance to the Jewish senior community, and education to those in the non-Jewish community that deal with seniors. SAJSS also serves as an educational resource for caregivers.

7794 Serenity Gardens Personal Care
600 Leslie Drive
Kerrville, TX 78028
570-373-3000
Fax: 570-373-3784
tshingara@serenitygardensal.com
www.serenitygardensal.com

Linda Stewart, Administrator

7795 Silverado Senior Living-Cypresswood
10225 Cypresswood Drive
Houston, TX 77070
281-955-0880
Fax: 981-955-1270; *Toll Free:* 832-604-4499
www.silveradosenior.com

Chris Holland, Administrator
Dr. Janette Nguyen, Medical Director
Leslie Love, Director of Health Services

At Silverado, we are committed to helping your loved one maintain the best health possible with no physical restraints and minimal use of medications. At Silverado Senior Living, we feel that no one should face this disease alone. That's why we take special care to offer support to the families of our assisted living residents. At Silverado, we do more than jyst welcome their residents, we welcome their families as well.

7796 Silverado Senior Living-Sugarland
1221 Seventhth Street
Sugar Land, TX 77478
281-201-1510
Fax: 281-277-1020
www.silveradosenior.com

Tana McMillon, Administrator
Suleman Lalani, Medical Director
Dr. Stanley Fisher, Medical Director

At silverado we are committed to helping your loved one maintain the best health possible with no physical restraints and minimal use of medications. At Silverado Senior Living we feel that no one should face this disease alone. We at Silverado do more than just welcome its residents, we welcome their families as well.

7797 Southern Knights Assisted Living Center
27919 Johnson Road
Tomball, TX 77375
281-351-8575
Fax: 281-351-1129
www.southernknightsalc.com

Elizabeth Howe, Owner

7798 Summer Glen Senior Living
2920 Forest Lane
Dallas, TX 75234
972-241-4100
Fax: 972-241-4464
summerglenseniorliving.com

Maggie Dunegan, Administrator

7799 Summer Ridge Assisted Living & Retirement Community
3020 Ridge Road
Rockwall, TX 75032
972-771-2800
Fax: 972-771-0340
webmaster@scc-texas.com
www.scc-texas.com

Marcela Wenzel, Executive Director
Year Founded: 1978

7800 Summit at Lakeway
1915 Lohmans Crossing Road
Lakeway, TX 78734
512-261-7146
Fax: 512-261-7149; *Toll Free:* 866-659-5537
info@brookdaleliving.com
www.brookdaleliving.com

Rose Vera, Manager
T Andrew Smith, Chief Executive Officer
Mark W Ohlendorf, Chief Financial Officer

The Summit Assisted Living Residences provides extra help you may need with you daily activities, while you maintain the privacy, dignity and independence that means so much to you.

7801 Summit at Northwest Hills
5715 Mesa Drive
Austin, TX 78731
512-454-5900
Fax: 512-419-1484; *Toll Free:* 866-659-6483
info@brookdaleliving.com
www.brookdaleliving.com

Annette McDonald, Manager
T Andrew Smith, Chief Executive Officer
Mark W Ohlendorf, Chief Financial Officer

7802 Touch of Home
4301 Crestridge Drive
Round Rock, TX 78681
512-773-5820
Fax: 512-218-0039
sharon@touchofhome.net
www.touchofhome.net

Sharon Scott, Owner and Administrator
Theresa Scott, Co Owner

7803 Twelve Oaks Irving Assisted Living Center
820 N Britain Road
Irving, TX 75061-7675
972-721-1500
Fax: 972-438-4074; *Toll Free:* 877-978-3338
www.seniorcarecompass.com

7804 Valley Ranch Retirement Center
38 Mockingbird Land Highway
Camp Wood, TX 78833
830-597-4123
Fax: 830-597-6337
www.wysk.com

David L Wright, Managing Member
Peggy L Wright, Managing Member

7805 Waterford Assisted Living
301 S.Sixth Street
Waterford, WI 53185
262-534-4800
Fax: 817-303-9478
info@waterfordseniorliving.com
www.waterfordseniorliving.com

7806 Waterford at Plano
3401 Premier Drive
Plano, TX 75023
972-423-7400
Fax: 972-423-8898
www.capitalsenior.com

Larry Cohen, Chief Executive Officer
Keith Johannesen, President
Ralph Beattie, Executive Vice President

Retirement/Assisted Living Community

7807 Weelington at Arapaho
600 W Arapaho Road
Richardson, TX 75080
469-330-2800
Fax: 469-330-2299; Toll Free: 800-635-1232
www.capitalsenior.com

Susan Sergent, Executive Director

7808 Wesley Village
2800 Loy Lake Road
Denison, TX 75020
903-465-6463
Fax: 903-465-6498
www.wesleyvillage.org

Kathy Busbey, Executive Director
Lori Cannon, President
Preston Parrish, Vice President

Year Founded: 1987

7809 Whitley Place
Whitley Pl Dr.
Prosper, TX 75078
817-379-0795
Fax: 817-337-1032
www.whitleyplace.com

Dara Chapman, Administrator

7810 Wildflower House
706 Red Coat Drive
Temple, TX 76504-2200
254-742-1581
Fax: 254-742-0425; Toll Free: 888-252-5001
www.alcco.com

Melissa Collins, Administrator

Year Founded: 2006

Virginia

7811 Green Hill Home for Adults
2904 Double Cabin Road
Hillsville, VA 24343-4768
276-728-7094
Fax: 276-728-9997
info@greenhillhfa.com
www.greenhillhfa.com

7812 Mayflower
One Mayflower Dr.
St. Louis, Mo 63026-2934
540-463-3161
Fax: 540-464-3214
www.mayflower.com

H. Daniel McCollister, Chairman & CEO
Kim Hurt, Manager

Year Founded: 1927

7813 Orange County Home for Adults
120 Dogwood Lane
Orange, VA 22960-1096

540-672-2611
Fax: 540-672-3187
www.dogwoodvillageocva.org

Tom Czelusta, Chairman
Lee Frame, Vice Chairman
Vernon M. Baker, Administrator

Year Founded: 1970

7814 Pulaski Retirement Community
2847 Penn Forest Blvd.
Suite 201
Roanoke, VA 24018
540-980-8535
Fax: 540-980-1876
www.rui.net

Janet Beahm, Executive Director
Kim Greene, Director Of Nursing

Independant and assisted living community

7815 Rappahannock Westminster-Canterbury
132 Lancaster Drive
Irvington, VI 22480
804-438-4000
Fax: 804-438-4027; Toll Free: 800-792-1444
marketing@rw-c.org
www.embracelifeatrwc.org

Stuart Bunting, President

7816 Renaissance Gardens at Greenspring
7410 Spring Village Drive
Springfield, VA 22150-4487
703-436-4515
Fax: 703-923-4651; Toll Free: 800-917-3049
www.thecareexperts.com

Jim Davis, Chairman
R. Alan Butler, Chief Executive Officer
Gerald F Doherty, General Councel

Features all private Assisted Living apartments and all private Long-Term Care rooms; full-time, on-site staff doctors with nurses on duty 24-hours a day. Short-Time Rehab (physical, speech and occupational therapy); dementia and Alzheimer's care also available. Renaissance Gardens, the choice you can feel good about.

Year Founded: 1983

7817 Shelby Manor Group Home
14184-22 Mile Road
Shelby, MI 48315
586-532-9461
Fax: 586-532-0987
dannywheatley@sbcglobal.net
www.shelbymanor.net

7818 Shenandoah Valley Village
9137 N Congress Street
New Market, VA 22844-9543
540-740-8100
Fax: 540-740-9380
brpress@ntelos.net
www.shenandoahvalleyweb.com

Tom Rice, Administrator

7819 St. Luke's Assisted Living
2359 Jefferson Hwy
Waynesboro, VA 22980-6540

540-943-9049
Fax: 540-943-9405
stlukesinc.com

Victor Shifflet, Owner
Pat Shifflet, Owner

7820 Westwood Center
Westwood Medical Park
Bluefield, VA 24605
276-322-5439
Fax: 540-322-5442; *Toll Free:* 866-745-
www.genesishcc.com/Westwood

Susan Williams, Administrator
Kathleen Keene, Director of Nursing
Tracy Freund, Admissions Director

7821 Whatland Hills Retirement Center
7486 Lee Highway
Radford, VA 24141-8579
540-639-2411
Fax: 540-639-9128
Stay in Touch @Commonwealth
www.commonwealthal.com

Richard J Brewer, President & CEO
Victoria L Morris, Chief Financial Officer
Earl Parker, Chief Operating Officer

7822 Willows at Meadow Branch
1881 Harvest Drive
Winchester, VA 22601-6350
540-667-3000
Fax: 540-667-2174
dma@thewillows-mb.com
www.thewillowsatmeadowbranch.com

Linda M Duvall, Administrator
Tammi Collins, Director of Marketing & Nursing
Charity Balentine, Director of Nursing

Senior assisted living facility.

Washington

7823 Aegis Lodge
12629 116th Avenue NE
Kirkland, WA 98034
425-947-0105
Fax: 425-823-2881
www.aegisliving.com

Dwayne Clark, Founder & CEO
Kathy Stewart, R. N. & General Manager
Rob Johnston, Executive Director

Year Founded: 1997

7824 Aegis Senior Living of Shoreline
14900 First Avenue NE
Shoreline, WA 98155
206-279-3448
Fax: 206-306-1064
www.aegisliving.com

Dwayne Clark, Founder & CEO
Terri Schmidgall, Resident Services Director
Susan Roberts, Marketing Director

Offers assisted living services within a comfortable community and dedicated care for those living with Alzheimer's or dementia.

Year Founded: 1997

7825 Aegis at Northgate
11039 17th Avenue NE
Seattle, WA 98125
206-452-0291
Fax: 206-440-1613
www.aegisliving.com

Dwayne Clark, Founder & CEO
Debra Moore, Executive Director
Judy Adams, Executive Director

Offers assisted living services tailored to meet each individual's needs.

Year Founded: 1997

7826 Aegis of Bothell
10605 NE 185th Street
Bothell, WA 98011
425-298-3977
Fax: 425-481-9782
www.aegisliving.com

Dwayne Clark, Founder & CEO
Roxanna Lee O'Neal, Activities Director
Karl Miller, Executive Director

Aegis of Bothell also provides dedicated care for individuals living with Alzheimer's or other dementia.

Year Founded: 1997

7827 Aegis of Edmonds
21500 72nd Avenue W
Edmonds, WA 98026
425-329-7292
Fax: 425-776-3622
www.aegisliving.com

Dwayne Clark, Founder & CEO
Wendy Mcilnay, Executive Director

Year Founded: 1997

7828 Aegis of Issaquah
780 NW Juniper Street
Issaquah, WA 98027
425-298-3969
Fax: 425-391-8804
www.aegisliving.com

Dwayne Clark, Founder & CEO
Melisa Mather, Marketing Director
Jim Cox, Executive Director

Offers assisted living services and dedicated care for those with Alzheimer's or other dementia.

Year Founded: 1997

7829 Aegis of Kent
10421 SE 248th Street
Kent, WA 98030
253-243-0054
Fax: 253-520-0360
www.aegisliving.com

Dwayne Clark, Founder & CEO
Emma Cronin, Executive Director

Offers assisted living services and dedicated care for those with Alzheimer's or other dementia.

Year Founded: 1997

7830 Aegis of Kirkland
13000 Totem Lake Boulevard NE
Kirkland, WA 98034-2982
425-903-3092
Fax: 425-823-8227
www.aegisliving.com

Dwayne Clark, Founder & CEO
Saroeun Khan, Activities Director
Kathy Stewart, Executive Director

Aegis living is a national leader in independent and assisted living with a premier Alzheimer's and dementia care program. Assisted Living communities are newly constructed and specially designed for seniors who need a little help with assisted-living services or for those who need dementia care.

Year Founded: 1997

7831 Aegis of Lynnwood
18700 44th Avenue West
Lynnwood, WA 98037
425-329-7289
Fax: 425-744-1506
www.aegisliving.com

Dwayne Clark, Founder & CEO
Elizabeth Hudson, Activities Director
Larry Smith, Executive Director

Year Founded: 1997

7832 Aegis of Redmond
7480 West Lake Sammamish
Parkway NE
Redmond, WA 98052
425-786-2040
Fax: 425-882-1823
www.aegisliving.com

Dwayne Clark, Founder & CEO
Glen Lewis, General Manager
Jason Porter, Executive Director

Offers programs for residents with Alxheimer's disease or other dementia.

Year Founded: 1997

7833 Aegis of Shoreline (Callahan House)
15100 First Avenue NE
Shoreline, WA 98155
206-452-0285
Fax: 206-417-9711
www.aegisliving.com

Dwayne Clark, Founder & CEO
Peter Koshi, Activities Director
Jarrett Houser, Executive Director

Offers assisted living services within a comfortable community and dedicated care for those living with Alzheimer's or dementia.

Year Founded: 1997

7834 Brighton Court
6520-196th Street SW
Lynnwood, WA 98036
425-775-4440
information@leisurecare.com
www.leisurecare.com

Dan Madsen, CEO

Offers luxurious apartment homes in a fun and active retirement community.

7835 Brittany Park
17143 133rd Avenue NE
Woodinville, WA 98072
425-402-7100
information@leisurecare.com
www.leisurecare.com

Dan Madsen, CEO

Offers luxurious apartment homes in a fun and active retirement community.

7836 Eagle Meadows Assisted Living Community
550 East Whitman
College Place, WA 99324
509-302-2208
www.eaglemeadowsalf.com
TDD 199- -

Dan Baty, Chairman
Granger Cobb, President & CEO
Robert C Bateman, Executive VP & CFO

Our goal at Eagle Meadows is to meet each resident's individuals needs while maintaining the highest level of choice, dignity, privacy and respect - all in a homelike atmosphere. Assisted Living at Eagle Meadows is designed for senior adults who wish to maintain their independent lifestyle but may need some additional assistance to do so.

7837 Fairwinds-Redmond
9988 Avondale Rd NE
Redmond, WA 98052
425-558-4700
information@leisurecare.com
www.leisurecare.com

Dan Madsen, CEO

Offers luxurious apartment homes in a fun and active retirement community.

7838 Fairwinds-Spokane
520 East Holland Avenue
Spokane, WA 99218
509-468-1000
information@leisurecare.com
www.leisurecare.com

Dan Madsen, CEO

Offers spacious apartment homes in a fun and active retirement community.

7839 Farrington Court
516 Kenosia Avenue
Kent, WA 98030
253-852-2737
information@leisurecare.com
www.leisurecare.com

Dan Madsen, CEO

Offers luxurious apartment homes in a fun and active retirement community.

7840 Hawthorne Court
524 North Ely
Kennewick, WA 99336
509-783-8313
information@leisurecare.com
www.leisurecare.com

Dan Madsen, CEO

Offers luxurious apartment homes in a fun and active retirement community.

7841 Living Court Assisted Living Community
7700 NE Parkway Dr
Suite 300
Vancouver, WA 98662-6654
800-476-9108
Fax: 360-825-6272
www.prestigecare.com

Sarah Delamarter, President

We are uniquely designed to provide different levels of assisted living, from minimum daily supervision to 24-hour care.

7842 Olympics West Retirement Inn
JEA Senior Living
12115 NE 99th Street
Suite 1800
Vancouver, WA 98682
360-943-9900
Fax: 360-956-0699; *Toll Free:* 800-254-9442
info@jeacorp.com
www.jeaseniorliving.com

Jerry Erwin, President & CEO
Cody Erwin, Chief Operating Officer
John McNeil, VP of Operations

JEA Senior Living offers personalized services that allow our residents to benefit from individualized care. Personalized assistance is provided in activities of daily living. We offer 89 beds for Assisted Living.

7843 Queen Anne Manor
100 Crockett Street
Seattle, WA 98109-2514
206-282-5001
Fax: 206-282-9064
www.qamanor.com

Carole Kelley, Executive Director
Sonja Bring, Resident Services Director
Patricia Del Von Nadon, Marketing Director

Offers a safe and comfortable assisted living community centrally located on Queen Anne hill in a beautiful turn of the century historic building.

7844 Regency Samaritan House
704 North 16th Avenue
Yakima, WA 98902
509-453-6357
Fax: 509-457-4438
www.regencysamaritanhouse.com

Samaritan House is an assisted living community that prides itself on personal care with a personal touch. Our community is small, allowing our staff to spend time with every resident.

7845 Regency on Whidbey
3326 160th Ave SE
Suite 120
Bellevue, WA 98008
425-392-4066
www.regencywhidbey.com/assisted

Ann Votava, Administrator
Leta Benfield, RN, Residents Services Coordiantor
Heidi Kuzina, Activities Director

The individual and specific needs of each resident, determined by their personal assessment, are the foundation of our resident care plans, designed to meet these needs. We offer five levels of care to better serve a resident's special needs.

7846 Tapestry at Village Gate West
5129 Dundas Street West
Toronto ON, ZZ M9A 0B3
416-777-2911
information@leisurecare.com
www.leisurecare.com

Dan Madsen, CEO

Retirement living community.

7847 The Bellettini
1115 108th Avenue NE
Bellevue, WA 98004
425-450-0800
information@leisurecare.com
www.leisurecare.com

Dan Madsen, CEO

Retirement living community.

7848 Three Links Center
Washington Odd Fellows Home
815 Forest Avenue
Northfield, MN 55057-1643
507-664-8800
Fax: 507-645-0942; *Toll Free:* 877-311-2786
threelinks.org

Patricia Vincent, CEO
John Brigham, Administrator
Joani Wicklund, Director Admissions

A non-proft retirement facility offering three levels of care: independent apartments, assisted living, and skilled nursing.

7849 Van Mall
7808 NE 51st Street
Vancouver, WA 98662
360-896-9140
information@leisurecare.com
www.leisurecare.com

Dan Madsen, CEO

Offers luxurious apartment homes in a fun and active retirement community.

7850 Washington Oakes
1717 Rockefeller Avenue
Everett, WA 98201
425-339-3300
information@leisurecare.com
www.leisurecare.com

Dan Madsen, CEO

Retirement living community.

Wyoming

7851 Aspen Wind Assisted Living
4010 N College Drive
Cheyenne, WY 82001-1960
307-778-9511
Fax: 307-772-0977
edgewoodseniorliving.com

Brandy Roland, Business Officer Director
Tony Sanchez, Dining Service Director
Donald Swenson, Environmental Service Director

7852 Garden Square of Casper
1950 South Beverly Street
Casper, WY 82601
307-215-5024
Fax: 307-472-1152
www.gardensquarecasper.com

Liz Krise Thompson, Administrator
Tammy Krauter, Dietary Manager
Chuck Sweatland, Maintenance Director

7853 Meadow Wind Assisted Living
3955 E 12th Street
Casper, WY 82609-3114
307-577-3045
Fax: 307-266-3370
www.edgewood-emg.com

Josaphine Ingram, Administrator

7854 Point Frontier Retirement Community
1406 Prairie Avenue
Cheyenne, WY 82009-4855
307-635-6953
Fax: 307-635-3566
www.pointefrontierretirement.com

Rich Pfeiffer, Manager

7855 Sierra Hills
4606 N College Drive
Cheyenne, WY 82009-5456
307-638-7798
Fax: 307-638-7919
edgewoodseniorliving.com

Elizabeth Marzluf, Clinical Service Director
Jody Bowen, Business Office Director
Tony Conley, Dining Services Director

7856 Spring Wind Assisted Living
1072 N 22nd Street
Laramie, WY 82072-5303
307-755-5811
Fax: 307-755-0478
edgewoodseniorliving.com

Karol Hodges, Clinical Service Director
Denise Deem, Marketing Director
Ron Schriner, Business Office Director

Independent Living Centers

Alabama

7857 Independent Living Center
5301 Moffett Road
Suite 110
Mobile, AL 36618-2926
251-460-0301
Fax: 251-341-1267
www.ilcmobile.org
TDD 251-460-0301
TTY: 251-460-2872

Michael Davis, Executive Director
Barbara Hattier, Assistant Director/Interpreter
Brandy Goodson, Program Manager YAAP

The Independent Living Center of Mobile/ILC, and its partner, the Birmingham Independent Living Center (BILC), offer choices of living options for people with disabilities and an array of services to help nursing home residents move to the community. Choosing where to live is a basic right of all Americans. But for people with disabilities who live in nursing homes, the opportunity to weigh community options is often limited. ILC strives to foster and promote programs which empower persons with disabilities to attain their maximum degree of independence. Services include independent living skills, peer support and advocacy, in addition to providing information and referral services.

7858 Independent Living Center-Jasper
300 Birmingham Ave.
Po Box 434
Jasper, AL 35502
205-387-0159
Fax: 205-387-1594
ilcwalker@bellsouth.net
www.birminghamilc.org
TDD 205-387-0162

Grahm Sisson, President
Phil Klebine, Vice President
Milton Moats, Treasurer

The Birmingham Independent Living Center in Jasper encourages people with disabilities to support one another in reaching their own independent living goals. The Center also promotes equal access and disability rights through advocacy and public awareness activities. A majority of staff, decision-making staff, and board members are people with disabilities. Consumers, not professionals, set their own independent living goals. Consumers are offered the option of developing an independent living plan; however, consumers may elect to waive such a plan and receive services. Independent living is based upon peer relationships, and principles of integration, consumer control, cross-disability, and equal access. All services are community-based and non-residential in nature. At the core of independent living is advocacy. Equal access is promoted within the Center and in the community. Mission is to empower people with disabilities to fully participate in the community.

7859 Montgomery Independent Living Center
600 South Court Street
Montgomery, AL 36104
334-240-2520
Fax: 334-240-6869

mcil@bellsouth.net
www.birminghamilc.org

Grahm Sisson, President
Phil Klebine, Vice President
Milton Moats, Treasurer

The Montgomery Independent Living center, a branch of the Birmingham Independent Living Center, encourages people with disabilities to support one another in reaching their own independent living goals. The Center also promotes equal access and disability rights through advocacy and public awareness activities. A majority of staff, decision-making staff, and board members are people with disabilities. Consumers, not professionals, set their own independent living goals. Consumers are offered the option of developing an independent living plan; however, consumers may elect to waive such a plan and receive services. Independent living is based upon peer relationships, and principles of integration, consumer control, cross-disability, and equal access. All services are community-based and non-residential in nature. At the core of independent living is advocacy. Equal access is promoted within the Center and in the community. Mission is to empower people with disabilities to fully participate in the community.

Alaska

7860 Access Alaska-Anchorage
1217 East 10th Avenue
Anchorage, AK 99501
907-248-4777
Fax: 907-263-1942; *Toll Free:* 800-770-4488
info@accessalaska.org
www.accessalaska.org
TTY: 907-248-8799

Lorali Simon, President
Mike Mclane, Vice President
Jim Babb, Secretary

Access Alaska is a private, non-profit, consumer-controlled organization that provides independent living services to people who experience a disability. As an Independent Living Center, our mission is to encourage & promote the total integration of people who experience a disability to live independently in the community of their choice. Through our assistance and support individuals with disabilities can identify and obtain needed services inan effort to maintain their independence as opposed to living in an institution. Access Alaska was formed in 1983 to serve the Anchorage area. Services were later expanded in 1984 and 1998 when offices were opened in Fairbanx and Matanuska-Susitna Valley.

Year Founded: 1983

7861 Access Alaska-Fairbanks
526 Gaffney Road
Suite 100
Fairbanks, AK 99701
907-479-7940
Fax: 907-474-4052; *Toll Free:* 800-770-7940
info@accessalaska.org
www.accessalaska.org

Lorali Simon, President
Mike Mclane, Vice President
Jim Babb, Secretary

Access Alaska is a private, non-profit, consumer-controlled organization that provides independent living services to people who experience a disability. As an Independent Living Center, our mission is to encourage and promote the total integration of people who experience a disability to live independently in the community of their choice. Through our assistance and support individuals with disabilities can identify and obtain needed services inan effort to maintain their independence as opposed to living in an institution. Access Alaska was formed in 1983 to serve the Anchorage area. Services were later expanded in 1984 and 1998 when offices were opened in Fairbanks and the Matanuska-Susitna Valley.

Year Founded: 1983

7862 Kenai Peninsula Independent Living Center-Homer

3953 Bartlett Street
PO Box 2474
Homer, AK 99603-2474
907-235-7911
Fax: 907-235-6236; Toll Free: 800-770-7911
ilc@xyz.net
www.peninsulailc.org
TTY: 206-455-8955

Joyanna Geisler, Executive Director

The Kenai Peninsula Independent Living Center is a non-profit organization run by the persons with disabilities for persons with disabilities. Our primary goal is to assist persons with impairments to live as independently as possible in their own homes and in the communities of their choice. Independent Living Center offices are located in Homer, Soldotna, and Seward Alaska. We provide direct service to the entire Kenai Peninsula and outreach service to Kodiak Island and the Valdez-Cordova region. Contact any office for more information.

7863 Kenai Peninsula Independent Living-Central Peninsula

47255 Princeton Avenue,
Suite 8
Soldotna, AK 99669-1907
907-262-6333
Fax: 907-260-4495
ilc@xyz.net
www.peninsulailc.org
TTY: 206-452-0143

Joyanna Geisler, Executive Director

The Keni Peninsula Independent Living Center is a non-profit organization run by persons with disabilities for persons with disaibilites. Our primary goal is to assist persons with impairments to live as independently as possible in their own homes and in the communities of their choice. Independent Living Center offices are located in Homer, Soldotna, and Seward Alaska. We provide direct service to the entire Keni Peninsula and outreach serviceto Kodiak Island and the Valdez-Cordova region. Contact any office for more information.

7864 Seward Independent Living Center

201 Third Avenue, Suite 101B
PO Box 3523
Seward, AK 99664-3523
907-224-8711
Fax: 907-224-7793
www.peninsulailc.org
TTY: 907-224-8711

Joyanna Geisler, Executive Director

The Kenai Peninsula Independent Living Center is a non-profit organization run by persons with disabilities for persons with disabilities. Our primary goal is to assist persons with impairments to live as independently as possible in their own homes and in the communities of their choice. Independent Living Center offices are located in Homer, Soldotna, and Seward Alaska. We provide direct service to the entire Kenai Peninsula and outreach service to Kodiak Island and the Valdez-Cordova region. Contact any office for more information.

7865 Southeast Alaska Independent Living (SAIL)

602 Dock Street
Suite 107
Ketchikan, AK 99901-6072
907-225-4735
Fax: 907-247-4753; Toll Free: 888-452-7245
ketchikan@sailinc.org
www.sailinc.org
TTY: 907-225-4735

Robert Purvis, President
Jeff Irwin, Vice President
Mary Gregg, Treasurer

Incorporated in 1992, SAIL is a private nonprofit organization that provides consumer-directed independent living services to people with disabilities throughout Southeast Alaska. SAIL offers an array of disability related services including loans of hearing, vision, and assistive devices, accessable home modifications and advocacy.

7866 Southeast Alaska Independent Living Center (SAIL)

3225 Hospital Drive
Suite 300
Juneau, AK 99801-8080
907-586-4920
Fax: 907-586-4980; Toll Free: 800-478-7245
info@sailinc.org
www.sailinc.org
TTY: 907-523-5285

Robert Purvis, President
Jeff Irwin, Vice President
Mary Gregg, Treasurer

Incorporated in 1992, SAIL is a private nonprofit organization that provides consumer-directed independent living services to people with disabilities throughout Southeast Alaska. SAIL offers an array of nonresidential disability related services and maintains three offices for your convenience, in the communities of Juneau, Sitka, and Ketchikan. The primary purpose of SAIL is to empower consumers with disabilities by providing services and information to support them in making choices that will positively affect their independence and productivity in society. SAIL serves all people with physical and mental disabilities regardless of race, ancestry, color, religion, age, marital status, sexual preference, gender and/or income.

7867 Southeast Alaska Living Center (SAIL)

514 Lake St.
Suite C
Sitka, AK 99835-7701
907-747-6859
Fax: 907-747-6783; Toll Free: 888-500-7245
sitka@sailinc.org
www.sailinc.org
TTY: 907-747-6859

Robert Purvis, President
Jeff Irwin, Vice President
Mary Gregg, Treasurer

Incorporated in 1992, SAIL is a private nonprofit organization that provides consumer-directed independent living services to people with disabilities throughout Southeast Alaska. SAIL offers an array of nonresidential disability related services and maintains three offices for your convenience, in the communities of Juneau, Sitka, and Ketchikan. The primary purpose of SAIL is to empower consumers with disabilities by providing services and information to support them in making choices that will positively affect their independence and productivity in society. SAIL serves all people with physical and mental disabilities regardless of race, ancestry, color, religion, age, marital status, sexual preference, gender and/or income.

Arizona

7868 Arizona Bridge to Independent Living

1229 East Washington Street
Phoenix, AZ 85034-1101
602-296-0551
Fax: 602-256-0184; *Toll Free:* 800-280-2245
azbridge@abil.org
www.abil.org

Lynn Larson, Chairman
Mary Slaughter, Vice Charman
Steven Tait, Treasurer

Arizona Bridge to Independent Living (ABIL), offers and promotes programs designed to empower people with disabilities to take personal responsibility so they may achieve or continue independent lifestyles within the community. ABIL offers services to facilitate implementation of the Americans with Disabilities Act (ADA) throughout the state including ADA training, technical assistance and materials to businesses and persons with disabilities onthe requirements and options of the ADA. We offer advocacy services with the intent of facilitating cooperative compliance. ABIL provides ADA counseling on larger projects such as facilities surveys and job accommodations. In addition, ABIL offers a variety of opportunities for consumers to have input into the laws, policies and procedures that affect their lives. Through the use of self, one on one, systems, legislative and community Advocacy, cooking skills, self-advocacy, household management, communication skills and stress management. ABIL assists motivated consumers in developing self-determined goals to gain greater independence.ABIL's consumers participate in shaping the future of our community. ndependent Living is the freedom to direct one's own life. Each individual has the right to optimize their personal ability and fully integrate into the community. ABILis independent living skills instruction includes: use of community resources, budgeting, transportation skills,

Year Founded: 1981

7869 DIRECT Independent Living Center

1023 North Tyndall Avenue
Tucson, AZ 85719-4446
520-624-6452
Fax: 520-792-1438; *Toll Free:* 800-342-1853
direct@directilc.org
www.directilc.org

Wendy Dewey, Executive Director
Eugene Y. Mar, President
Tony Langan, Vice President

DIRECT Center for Independence, Inc. is a consumer-directed, community-based advocacy organization, that promotes independent living and offers a variety of programs for all people with disabilities which encourages them to achieve their full potential and to participate in the community. Direct Center for Independence, Inc., came into existence as Metro Independent Living Center in 1980. It was the first agency of its kind in Arizona serving asa non-residential Independent Living Center operated by and for persons with disabilities. The Center became incorporated and got its 501(c)(3) status as an independent, non-profit agency in 1994. The Center has a variety of programs including independent living skills, information and referral, peer counseling services, mentoring services, personal care assistance, and the transit solutions program.

7870 New Horizons Disability Empowerment Center - Prescott Valley

8085 East Manley Dr.
Prescott Valley, AZ 86314
928-772-1266
Fax: 928-772-3808; *Toll Free:* 800-406-2377
nhilc@cableone.net
www.newhorizonsilc.org
TTY: 928-772-1266

Vicky McLane, Board President
Nick Perry, VP
Liz Toone, Executive Director

New Horizons provides services and advocacy to empower and enable people with disabilities to self-determine the goals and activities of their lives in family, home, community and workplace. New Horizons provides the following services free to anyone with a disability: independent living skills; training-home management, cooking, cleaning, budgeting, etc.; Social Security benefits planning and work incentives assistance; information and referral; peer support and guidance in addition to community education public seminars and employment evaluation and training programs.

7871 New Horizons Independent Living Center - Prescott Valley

8085 East Manley Dr.
Prescott Valley, AZ 86314
928-772-1266
Fax: 928-772-3808; *Toll Free:* 800-406-2377
nhilc@cableone.net
www.newhorizonsilc.org
TTY: 927-772-8870

Liz Toone, Executive Director
Vicky McLane, President
Nick Perry, Vice President

Year Founded: 1992

7872 Services Maximizing Independent Living and Empowerment (SMILE)

1929 South Arizona Avenue
Suite 12
Yuma, AZ 85364-4603
928-329-6681
Fax: 520-329-6715; *Toll Free:* 855-209-8363
SMILE1929@adelphia.net

www.smile-az.org
TDD 928-782-7458

Kathryn Robins, Executive Director
Laura Duval, Assistive Technology Specialist

SMILE's mission is to provide the catalyst for community change and life altering experiences and thereby empower individuals with significant disabilities, throughout Yuma and La Paz Counties: to function independently; to live safely, with dignity; and, to enjoy full access to one's communities. Services include independent living skills training; information and referral; peer support groups, and benefits planning, assistance and outreach.

7873 Statewide Independent Living Council (SILC)
5025 E Washington Street
Suite 214
Phoenix, AZ 85034
602-262-2900
Fax: 602-271-4100
silc@azsilc.org
www.azsilc.org
TDD 602-542-6049
TTY: 602-262-2900

Tony DiRienzi, Executive Director
Linda Jane Austen, Executive Assistant
Dan Bercovich, Program Co-ordinator

A non profit organization consisting of a council of advocates appointed by the governor of the state of Arizona. Their role is to advocate for the development of networks of programs, services, and options designed to empower Arizonans with disabilities to live independently in their community. The vision of the council is that all Arizonans with disabilities are treated equally and included fully in a society that embraces freedom of choice and integration so that people with disabilities can be responsible for the achievement of their potential. The goal of the independent living movement is integration and full inclusion of individuals with disabilities into the mainstream of society.

Arkansas

7874 Division of Aging and Adult Services - Elder Choices
Arkansas Department of Human Services
PO Box 1437
Slot S-530
Little Rock, AR 72203-1437
501-682-2441
Fax: 501-682-8155
aging.services@arkansas.gov
www.arkansas.gov

Krista Hudges, Director
Connie Parker, Assisstant Director
Herb Sanderson, Executive Director

ElderChoices is Arkansas' Medicaid home and community-based waiver designed for its elderly population. ElderChoices, implemented July 1, 1991, is designed for persons who due to physical, cognitive or medical reasons, require a level of assistance that would have to be provided in a nursing facility, if it were not for the services offered through this program. The program is designed to assist elderly persons reside in their own homes, or livewith relatives or caregivers for as long as possible, if that is their choice. ElderChoices has provided services to more than 13,000 elderly Arkansans since 1991. There are currently

6,368 recipients participating in the program with a statewide total of 276 providers of service. In addition to ElderChoices services, waiver recipients may receive other Medicaid covered services such as physician visits, some prescription drugs, personal care and others.

Year Founded: 1966

7875 Mainstream Living
300 South Rodney Parham Road
Suite 5
Little Rock, AR 72205-4774
501-280-0012
Fax: 501-280-9267; *Toll Free:* 800-371-9026
mainstreamlr@sbcglobal.net
www.mainstreamilrc.com
TDD 501-280-9262

Rita Byers, Executive Director

Mainstream is dedicated to the concept of consumer directed service delivery in that each consumer has control of his or her life, the services, support, and advocacy that they receive. The type of services a consumer receives are conducted within the framework of a written individual Independent Living Plan (ILP). These plans are developed by the consumer him/herself with the assistance of a qualified Mainstream staff member. The mission of Mainstream is to provide advocacy, peer support, and services which will enable people with severe disabilities to live independently in the community. The organization will work to achieve the integration of people with disabilities into the mainstream of society.

7876 Sources for Community Independent Living Services (SOURCES)
1918 North Birch Avenue
Fayetteville, AR 72703-3911
479-442-5600
Fax: 479-442-5192; *Toll Free:* 888-284-7521
jmather@arsources.org
www.arsources.org
TDD 479-251-1378
TTY: 479-439-8314

Brent Williams, President
Burke Fanari, Secretary
Elise Burt, Treasurer

It is the mission of SOURCES to promote the independence of persons with disabilities by facilitating and supporting their full integration and participation in all aspects of community life. SOURCES will provide services, support, and advocacy for persons with disabilities, their families, and the community at large. SOURCES is dedicated to the Independent Living Philosophy and the concept of consumer-directed service delivery: each consumer has control of his or her own life. All services and activities reflect this concept. Services include information and referral; peer support; independent living skills training, and advocacy.

California

7877 (RICV) Resources for Independence Central Valley
710 West 18th Street
Suite #5
Merced, CA 95340
209-383-1683
Fax: 209-725-9153; *Toll Free:* 800-244-2274

info@ricv.org
www.ricv.org

Bob Hand, Executive Director
Anuradha Gajaraj-Lopez, Executive Assistant
Joseph Cody, Dir. Technology & Resources

Encouraging people with disabilities to be in control of their lives and to live more independently through a diverse range of choices and opportunities.

7878 CCCIL-Central Coast Center for Independenet Living - Capitola
1395 41st Avenue
Suite 101
Capitola, CA 95010-3930
831-462-8720
Fax: 831-462-8727
cccil@cccil.org
www.cccil.org
TDD 831-462-8729

Jennifer Williams, President
Brenda Cardoza, Information and Referral
Elsa Quezada, Executive Director

Services include advocacy, housing assistance, personal assistance, peer support, living skills, skills training, and community advocacy. Serves Santa Cruz, Monterey and San Benito counties.

Year Founded: 1984

7879 California Foundation for Independent Living Centers (CFILC)
1234 H Street
Suite 100
Sacramento, CA 95814-2494
916-325-1690
Fax: 916-325-1699
CFILC@cfilc.org
www.cfilc.org
TTY: 916-325-1695

Robert Hand, Chairperson
Ana Acton, Vice Chairperson
Susan Rotchy, Treasurer

The California Foundation for Independent Living Centers, based in Sacramento, Calif., is a statewide, non-profit trade organization made up of 25 Independent Living Centers. Through unified action, CFILC envisions civil rights for all people with disabilities. CFILC'S mission is to support independent living centers in their local communities through advocating for systems change & promoting access & integration for people with disabilities.

Year Founded: 1976

7880 California State Independent Living Council (SILC)
1600 K Street
Suite 100
Sacramento, CA 95814-4020
916-445-0142
Fax: 916-445-5973; *Toll Free:* 866-866-7452
www.calsilc.org
TTY: 866-745-2889

David Wilder, Chairman
Liz Pazdral, Executive Director
Kathleen Derby, Legislative Analyst

In cooperation with the state Department of Rehabilitation, the SILC prepares a State Plan for Independent Living

which sets the policy and funding levels for the state's network of Independent Living Centers (ILCs) and services. To help guide this policy, the SILC solicits continual public feedback on the effectiveness of independent living services and the changing needs of the community. In addition to preparing and updating the State Plan for Independent Living, the SILC monitors the implementation of it. The SILC also coordinates with similar agencies and councils at the state and federal levels to increase communication and help assure that services to people with disabilities are delivered effectively. SILC strongly supports a society where persons with disabilities have the choice to live without barriers and to fully participate in all aspects of the community that includes equal opportunity; equal access; self determination; self sufficiency and independence.

7881 Center for Independent Living (CIL)
2539 Telegraph Avenue
Berkeley, CA 94704-2997
510-649-1100
Fax: 510-649-1717
theshop@cilberkeley.org
www.cilberkeley.org
TTY: 510-848-3101

Henry Leng, President
Hank Stratford, Treasurer
Jan Garrett, Executive Director

The Center for Independent Living (CIL) is a national leader in supporting disabled people in their efforts to lead independent lives. As an organization founded by people with disabilities, CIL understands the challenges faced by their consumers. CIL strives toward the achievement of immediate and long-term solutions - be it assistance with finding housing or a job, equipping a home with assistive technologies, or enhancing independent living skills. CIL's consumer services give people with disabilities the tools and resources they need to achieve independence. All of these services are free and feature advocacy, counseling, education and referrals. Additionally, these services are offered in multiple languages.

7882 Center for Independent Living - Central Coast/Hollister (CCCIL)
318 Cayuga St
Suite 208
Salinas, CA 93901
831-757-2968
Fax: 831-757-5549
cccil@cccil.org
www.cccil.org
TDD 831-757-3949

Jennifer Williams, President
Brenda Cardoza, Information and Referral
Elsa Quezada, Executive Director

Services include advocacy, education and support to all people with disabilities, their families and their community, such as independent living information, housing assistance, living and life skills training and technology support. Serves Santa Cruz, Monterey and San Benito counties.

Year Founded: 1984

7883 Center for Independent Living-Oakland
1904 Franklin Street
Suite 320
Oakland, CA 94612

510-763-9999
Fax: 510-763-4910
info@cilberkeley.org
www.cilberkeley.org
TTY: 510-444-1837

Henry Leng, President
Hank Stratford, Treasurer
Jan Garrett, Executive Direrctor

The Center for Independent Living (CIL) is a national leader in supporting disabled people in their efforts to lead independent lives. As an organization founded by people with disabilities, CIL understands the challenges faced by their consumers. This motivates CIL to achieve immediate and long-term solutions - be it assistance with finding housing or a job, equipping a home with assistive technologies, or enhancing independent living skills. CIL's consumer services give people with disabilities the tools and resources they need to achieve independence. All of these services are free and feature advocacy, counseling, education and referrals. Additionally, these services are offered in multiple languages.

7884 Community Access Center

6848 Magnolia Avenue
Suite 150
Riverside, CA 92506-2858
951-274-0358
Fax: 951-274-0833
execdir@ilcac.org
www.ilcac.org
TTY: 951-274-0834

Mark Dyer, President
Janet Newcomer, Vice President
Perry Halterman, Secretary

The primary purpose of Community Access Center is to empower consumers with disabilities by providing services and information to support them in making choices that will positively affect their independence and productivity in society and in advocating to achieve complete social, economic, and political integration. The Community Access Center implements this vision by providing information, supportive services and independent living skills training.

7885 Community Resources for Independent Living

439 A Street
Hayward, CA 94541-5013
510-881-5743
Fax: 510-881-1593
info@cril-online.org
crilhayward.org
TTY: 510-881-0218

Sheri Burns, Executive Director
P. Michael Galvan, Program Director
April Monroe, Finance Director

Community Resources for Independent Living is founded on the principles of independent living philosophy. Independent living philosophy concentrates on inclusive communities, choice, equality, diversity, empowerment and independence. CRIL offers independent living services at no charge to persons with disabilities living in southern and eastern Alameda County. In order to become a CRIL consumer, an individual must have a disability and be pairedwith an Independent Living (IL) Coordinator.

7886 Dayle McIntosh Center for the Disabled

150 West Cerritos Avenue
Bldg 4
Anaheim, CA 92805-6546
714-772-8285
Fax: 714-772-8292
www.daylemc.org
TTY: 714-772-8366

Bill Chrisner, Executive Director

The mission of the Dayle McIntosh Center (DMC) is to advance empowerment and inclusion of all persons with disabilities. Dayle McIntosh Center (DMC) was named in memory of a young woman with a severe physical disability who worked to found the Center in 1977. DMC is the largest Independent Living Center in California. Independent Living is a philosophy and a movement of people with disabilities who work for self-determination, equal opportunity,and self respect. A non-residential facility, DMC exists to succeed in every arena they desire.

7887 Dayle McIntosh-South County

24031 El Toro Road
Suite 300
Laguna Hills, CA 92653
949-460-7784
Fax: 949-855-8742
www.daylemc.org
TDD 714-663-2087
TTY: 949-855-6749

Bill Chrisner, Executive Director

The mission of the Dayle McIntosh Center is to advance empowerment and inclusion of all persons with disabilities. Dayle McIntosh Center (DMC) was named in memory of a young woman with a severe physical disability who worked to found the Center in 1977. DMC is the largest Independent Living Center in California. Independent Living is a philosophy and a movement of people with disabilities who work for self-determination, equal opportunity, and self respect. A non-residential facility, DMC exists to succeed in every arena they desire.

7888 IL Resources of Contra Costa County-Fairfield

1545 Webster Street
Suite C
Fairfield, CA 94533-4917
707-435-8174
Fax: 707-435-8177
info@ilrcoco-sol.org
ilrcoco.sol.org
TTY: 510-794-5562

Eli Gelardin, Interim Executive Director
Claude Battaglia, Program Director
Susan Rotchy, Program Manager

Services include education, peer support and advocacy for social and politiacl integration.

7889 Independent Living Center of Kern County

5251 Office Park Drive
Suite 200
Bakersfield, CA 93309
661-325-1063
Fax: 661-325-6702; *Toll Free:* 800-529-9541
info@ilcofkerncounty.org
www.ilcofkerncounty.org
TTY: 661-399-8966

Jimmie Soto, Executive Director
Tammy Hartsch, Finance Manager
Laura Rodriguez, Program Manager

The Independent Living Center of Kern County empowers people with disabilities to grow creatively, professionally, and personally; and educates the community about disability-related issues.

Year Founded: 1981

7890 Independent Living Center of Southern California (ILCSC)
14407 Gilmore Street
Suite 101
Van Nuys, CA 91401-1481
818-785-6934
Fax: 818-785-0330; *Toll Free:* 800-524-5272
ilcsc@ilcsc.org
www.ilcsc.org
TTY: 818-785-7097

Norma Vescovo, CEO
Humberto Quintanar, Board-Directors President
Michael A Hansel, Board-Directors Vice President

A non-profit consumer-based, non-residential agency providing a wide range of services to a growing population of people with disabilities. ILCSC is dedicated to empowerin persons with disabilities to excercise independence, professionally, personally and creatively, while striving to educate the community on their needs.

Year Founded: 1976

7891 Independent Living Center-Lancaster
1505 West Avenue J
Suite 102
Lancaster, CA 93534
661-942-9726
Fax: 661-945-5690
ilcsclanc@ilcsc.org
www.ilcsc.org
TTY: 661-723-2509

Norma Vescovo, CEO
Humberto Quintanar, Board-Directors President
Michael A Hansel, Board-Directors Vice President

A non-profit consumer-based, non-residential agency providing a wide range of services to a growing population of people with disabilities. ILCSC is dedicated to empowering persons with disabilities to excercise independence, professionally, personally, and creatively, while striving to educate the community on their needs.

Year Founded: 1976

7892 Independent Living Center-Santa Clarita
23560 Lyons Avenue
Suite 201
Santa Clarita, CA 91321-2521
661-290-2569
Fax: 661-290-2556
ilcscsc@ilcsc.org
www.ilcsc.org
TTY: 661-290-2420

Norma Vescovo, CEO
Humberto Quintanar, Board-Directors President
Michael A Hansel, Board-Directors Vice President

A non-profit, consumer-based, non-residential agency providing a wide range of services to a growing population of people with disabilities. ILCSC is dedicated to empowering

persons with disabilities to excercise independence, professionally, personally, and creatively, while striving to educate the community on their needs.

Year Founded: 1976

7893 Independent Living Resource Center (ILRCSF)
649 Mission Street
3rd Floor
San Francisco, CA 94105-4128
415-543-6222
Fax: 415-543-6318
info@ilrcsf.org
www.ilrcsf.org
TTY: 415-543-6698

Katherine Martinez, President
Sandy O'Neill, Vice President
Sam Ruben, Secretary

Independent Living Resource Center San Francisco (ILRCSF) is a disability rights advocacy and support organization. Our mission is to ensure that people with disabilities are full social and economic partners, within their families and within a fully accessible community. ILRCSF's mission is achieved by: systems change; community education; partnerships with business, community organizations and government; and consumer directed services. We work to empower individuals and community, so that all people with disabilities have as full, productive and independent lives as they so chose. ILRCSF programs and services include information and referrals, assistive technology education and support, peer counseling, system change advocacy, housing counseling, benefits and employment planning, and individual advocacy benefits eligibility.

Year Founded: 1976

7894 Independent Living Resource of Contra Costa County
1850 Gateway Blvd
Suite 120
Concord, CA 94520
925-363-7293
Fax: 925-363-7296
www.ilrscc.org
TDD 925-363-7293
TTY: 925-363-7293

Susan Rotchy, Executive Director

Services include advocacy and support for complete social and political integration, assistive technology training, information and referrals and peer support.

Year Founded: 1976

7895 Independent Living Resources Center-Santa Maria
327 East Plaza Drive
Suite 3A
Santa Maria, CA 93454-6930
805-925-0015
Fax: 805-349-2416
jblack@ilrc-trico.org
www.ilrc-trico.org
TTY: 805-354-5948

Jo Black, Executive Director
Elizabeth Houston, Comm. Living Advocate-Deaf
Jennie Morales, Interpreter Advocate

The Independent Living Resource Center, Inc., is an organization of, by and for persons with disabilities who reside or work in our service area. Our purpose is to assist and encourage individuals to achieve their optimal level of self-sufficiency while eliminating the architectural, communication and attitudinal barriers which prevent them from full participation in the community. Services include that of independent living skills training, advocacy, assistive technology, information and referral, peer and benefits counseling, American Sign Language interpreter, and communications access assistance.

7896 Independent Living Resources Center-Santa Barbara

423 West Victoria Street
Santa Barbara, CA 93101-3619
805-963-0595
Fax: 805-963-1350
info@ilrc-trico.org
www.ilrc-trico.org
TTY: 805-284-9051

Josephine Black, Executive Director
Jennifer Griffin, Business Manager
Kathleen Riel, Program Manager

The Independent Living Resource Center, Inc., is an organization of, by and for persons with disabilities who reside or work in our service area. Our purpose is to assist and encourage individuals to achieve their optimal level of self-sufficiency while eliminating the architectural, communication and attitudinal barriers which prevent them from full participation in the community. Services include that of independent living skills training, advocacy, assistive technology, benefits and peer counseling, American Sign Language interpreting, information and referral, and, communications access.

7897 Independent Living Resources Center-Ventura

1802 Eastman Avenue
Suite 112
Ventura, CA 93003-5759
805-650-5993
Fax: 805-650-9278
jblack@ilrc-trico.org
www.ilrc-trico.org
TTY: 805-256-1036

Jo Black, Executive Director
Carol Baizer, Comm. Living Advocate-Benefits
Jennifer Martinez, Information & Referral Specialis

The Independent Living Resource Center, Inc., is an organization of, by and for persons with disabilities who reside or work in our service area. Our purpose is to assist and encourage individuals to achieve their optimal level of self-sufficiency while eliminating the architectural, communication and attitudinal barriers which prevent them from full participation in the community. Services include that of independent living skills training, advocacy, assistive technology, communications access assistance, American Sign Language interpreting, information and referrals, and peer and benefits counseling.

7898 Independent Living Services of Northern California

1161 East Avenue
Chico, CA 95926-1018
530-893-8527
Fax: 530-893-8574; Toll Free: 800-464-8527
info@ilsnc.org

www.ilsnc.org
TTY: 830-593-8527

Sarah Bates, President
Brandi Zellers, Vice President
Eddie Evans, Secretary

Services include living skills training, peer counseling, housing assistance and a newsletter.

Year Founded: 1976

7899 Placer Independent Resource Services/PIRS

11768 Atwood Road
Suite 29
Auburn, CA 95603-9074
530-885-6100
Fax: 530-885-3032; Toll Free: 800-833-3453
lbrewer@pirs.org
www.pirs.org
TTY: 530-885-0326

Dawn Davidson, President
Jerry Henry, Vice President
Paula Mosqueda, Secretary

Placer Independent Resource Services (PIRS) advocates for the rights of people with disabilities, educates the community about disability issues, and provides services to persons with disabilities to live independent, productive lives. Any person with a disiability is eligible for our services. Services are free of charge.

7900 Resources for Independent Living

420 I Street Level B
Suite 3
Sacramento, CA 95814-2319
916-446-3074
Fax: 916-446-2443
francesg@ril-sacramento.org
www.ril-sacramento.org
TTY: 916-446-3074

Ramona Garcia, Chairperson
Joanne Bodine, Treasurer
Larry Stenzel, Secretary

Resources for Independent Living/ RIL supports and promotes the socio-economic independence of persons with disabilities by providing peer-supported, consumer-directed independent living services and advocacy. The majority of the policy-making board is comprised of individuals with disabilities thereby making the decision-making process both innovative and highly effective. RIL provides numerous services including that of information and referral, advocacy and legislative monitoring, peer counseling and assistive technology in addition to independent living skills training.

7901 Rolling Start

570 West 4th Street
Suite 107
San Bernardino, CA 92401-1438
909-884-2129
Fax: 909-386-7446
support@rollingstart.com
www.rollingstart.org
TDD 909-884-7396

John Anaya, Chairperson
Theresa Ramirez, Vice Chairman
Virginia R Macy, Secretary/Treasurer

Rolling Start Center for Independent Living was incorporated in October of 1977. The center was established as a grassroots organization manned mostly by volunteers who were also persons with disabilities. The philosophy of the center has always been to empower individuals with all types of disabilities to be the best they can be. The driving force of the center is teaching people with disabilities to advocate for what they need to be productive members within the communities in which they live. The core services which Rolling Start currently provides are: independent living skills training; assistive technology; information and referral; systems and individual advocacy; peer counseling; personal assistant referral, and, housing information.

7902 Salinas-Central Coast Center for Independent Living

234 Capitol Street
Suites A&B
Salinas, CA 93901-2600
831-757-2968
Fax: 831-757-5549
cccil@cccil.org
www.cccil.org
TDD 831-757-3949

Jennifer Williams, President
Brenda Cardoza, Information and Referral
Elsa Quezada, Executive Director

A non-profit organization founded in Santa Cruz County in 1984 as a grassroots organization dedicated to serving the unmet needs of people with disabilities. CCCIL moved its main office to Salinas in 1994.

7903 Westside Center for Independent Living

12901 Venice Boulevard
Los Angeles, CA 90066-3509
310-390-3611
Fax: 310-390-4906; *Toll Free:* 888-851-9245
development@wcil.org
www.wcil.org
TTY: 310-398-9204

Mary Ann Jones, Executive Director
Robin Hargrove, Development Director
Aliza Barzilay, Associate Director

The Westside Center for Independent Living was founded in 1976 as a non-residential, public-benefit corporation to enable people with disabilities and seniors in the Los Angeles community to live more independent, self supporting and satisfying lives. The mission of the Westside Center for Independent Living is to empower people with disabilities to reach their independent living goals through a variety of non-residential programs and services. WCIL advocates, educates and provides primarily peer-conducted services to its consumers and the community. WCIL is staffed primarily by people with disabilities. Through their guidance and support, consumers gain the confidence to take the first steps toward their own independence. WCIL has helped over 30,000 people achieve this goal by providing a wide range of services, including benefits and housing advocacy, peer counseling, personal assistance services, independent living skills training, job training and placement and information and referral.

Colorado

7904 Atlantis Community, Inc.

201 S Cherokee Street
Denver, CO 80223
303-733-9324 Toll free: 877-262-6525
atlantiscommunity.org

Candie Dalton, Executive Director
Cherish Marquez, Operations Coordinator
Paige Gallaher, Independent Living Manager

Atlantis Community supports the right of people with disabilities to take control over their own lives with full and informed consent, primarily by providing a variety of consumer-directed services-from advocacy to education to transitioning people out of nursing homes and into their very own apartments.

Year Founded: 1974

7905 Center For People With Disabilities

615 North Main Street
Longmont, CO 80501
303-772-3250
Fax: 303-772-5125
info@cpwd.org
www.cpwd-ilc.org
TTY: 719-546-1867

Larry Williams, Executive Director

Private, non-profit corporation that provides services to maximize the independence of individuals with disabilities and the accessibility of the communities they live in.

7906 Center for Independence

740 Gunderson Avenue
Grand Junction, CO 81501-4647
970-241-0315
Fax: 970-245-3341; *Toll Free:* 800-613-2271
info@cfigj.org
www.cfigj.org/temp
TTY: 970-245-3341

Bill Queen, President
Tom Kenyon, Vice President
Linda Taylor, Executive Director

A non-profit, non-residential, grassroots, State-of-Colorado certified independent living center, assisting people with disabilities since 1982. CFI is governed by people with disabilities and upholds the independent living philosophy that people with disabilities have the right to self-determination, and the right to live their lives independently and with dignity to their fullest potential.

Connecticut

7907 Center for Disability Rights
Connecticut Tech Act Project

23 West Market Street
Suite 103
Corning, NY 14830
607-654-0030
Fax: 607-936-1258
cdr7077@aol.com
www.cdrnys.org
TTY: 203-934-7079

Robert Defelice, Board Chairman
Carmen Hernandaz, Board Vice Chair
Murray Stahl, Treasurer

The Center for Disability Rights, in conjunction with the Connecticut Tech Art Project, provides information and guidance on the Americans with Disabilities Act, Section 508, and accessible information technology to individuals living in New England. In addition, the Center also provides information on the Assistive Technology Loan Program which is sponsored by the Connecticut Department of Social Services, Bureau of Rehabilitation Services in partnership with People's Bank. Assistive technology is any tool, device or equipment designed to help you develop, maintain or improve your ability to function daily. It could range from small, inexpensive kitchen gadgets that help you cook to a van adapted with special controls to help you drive independently. Hearing aids, motorized wheelchairs, computers controlled by voice or other special switch and augmentative alternative communication tools are included in a long list of assistive technology devices. The Peer Technology Counselors at the Center for Disability Rights can provide individuals with information about vendors who sell assistive technology and other funding sources.

7908 Center for Independent Living of Northwestern Connecticut
1183 New Haven Road
Suite 200
Naugatuck, CT 06770
203-729-3299
Fax: 203-729-2839
www.members.aol.com/indnw
TDD 203-729-1281

Eileen Healey, Executive Director
Scott M Robbins, Program Director
Luann Scarola, Administrative Assistant

Independence Northwest, is part of the nationwide network of Centers for Independent Living that grew out of the disability rights movement of the early 1970's. Centers for Independent Living are directed, managed and staffed to a substantial degree by qualified persons with severe disabilities. A majority of the staff and board of directors at Independence Northwest are persons with disabilities. Independence Northwest provides services in suchareas as peer counseling, advocacy, independent living skills training and information and referral. In addition, we also provide services to the community in the form of disability awareness programs and technical assistance in such areas as architectural barrier removal and community organizing.

7909 Disability Resource Center of Fairfield County (DRCFC)
Connecticut Tech Art Project
80 Ferry Boulevard
Suite 210
Stratford, CT 06615
203-378-6977
Fax: 203-375-2748
info@drcfc.org
www.drcfc.org
TDD 203-378-3248

Thomas D, President
Margaret A, Vice President
William A, Treasurer

Disability Resource Center of Fairfield County (DRCFC) provides the means to put the values of Independent Living into action by providing individuals with empowerment and working for change in the attitudinal and physical barriers that face people with disabilities in the community. Services provided by DRCFC include that of information and referral, technical assistance and training, independent living skills training, disability awareness, peer support, systems advocacy and resource assistance.

7910 Independence Unlimited Inc.
151 New Park Avenue
Suite D
Hartford, CT 06106-2170
860-523-5021
Fax: 860-523-5603
clow@independenceunlimited.org
independenceunlimited.org
TTY: 860-523-2021

Kay Carver, Chairperson
Diana LaRocco, Vice Chairperson
Robin Trowbridge, Treasurer/Secretary

Independent Living is a philosophy that challenges the social attitudes and physical barriers that stigmatize and exclude people with disabilities from the community. Independence Unlimited is commited to increasing the independence of people with disabilities by assisting individuals in identifying and accessing services and supports, benefits, assistive technology, housing, personal assistance services, and other resources.

Delaware

7911 Carelink Community Support Services
1510 Chester Pike Ste 600
Eddystone, PA 19022
610-874-1119
Fax: 302-429-8031
admin@carelinkservices.org
www.carelink-svs.org
TDD 302-429-8034

James McDonald, Chair
Ted Pendergrass, Vice Chair
Scot Stetka, Treasurer

CareLink provides a growing array of vocational, care management, residential, and day rehabilitation programs. Services are flexible and individually tailored to the interests, needs and goals of each person served. At CareLink, we encourage people to be active participants in their own recovery. By building upon strengths, residents can become more independent and effective in managing their own lives. A comprehensive assessment is completedwith the consumer. This leads to the development of an individualized personal plan that can include services such as monitoring living and vocational arrangements, skill training, financial stewardship, and providing crisis management services. Our rehabilitation services and professional staff provide the supports that people with serious mental illness, physical disabilities and other developmental challenges need to be active, productive members of their communities. Our mission is to serve individuals who need specialized supports to achieve recovery, wellness and self-determination.

Florida

7912 Caring and Sharing Center for Independent Living
12552 Belcher Road South
Largo, FL 33773
727-539-7550
Fax: 727-539-7588; *Toll Free:* 866-539-7550
cascil@cascil.org
www.cascil.org
TDD 727-577-0065

Jack Humburg, Chairman
Barbara Page, Vice Chairman
Barbara Dandro, Treasurer

Caring & Sharing Center for Independent Living, Inc. (CASCIL) is a consumer controlled, community based, 501(c)(3), cross-disability organization that promotes the empowerment and self-determination of persons with disabilities through its services and advocacy. A majority of the staff and board of directors are persons with significant disabilities. The independent philosophy espouses the position that persons with disabilities, as well as society, benefit from living and functioning within the community as opposed to being maintained in an institutional setting. The mission of the Caring & Sharing Center for Independent Living, Inc. (CASCIL) is to assist persons with all types of disabilities and their families, to achieve the greatest degree of self-determination in accessibility, advocacy, education, employment, and place of residence in keeping with the consumer's freedom of choice.

7913 Center for Independent Living of North Central Florida-Ocala
3445 Northeast 24th Street
Ocala, FL 34470-3921
352-368-3788
Fax: 352-629-0098
carol@cilncf.org
www.cilncf.org
TDD 352-368-2969
TTY: 352-368-2969

Ken Osfield, President
Claudia Munnis, Vice President
Alan West, Treasurer

A consumer driven, community based, non-residential private not-for-profit organization. The CILNCF serves 16 counties in the North Central Florida region from 4 locations. We are a consumer controlled organization and have at least 51 % people with disabilities comprising our governing board of directors as well as staff. Our center delivers the 4 core services of Advocacy, Information and Referral, Peer Support, and Independent Living Skills Education.

7914 Center for Independent Living of Broward
4800 N State Road 7
Suite 102
Ft. Lauderdale, FL 33319
954-722-6400
Fax: 954-735-1958; *Toll Free:* 888-722-6400
www.cilbroward.org
TTY: 954-735-1958

Karen Dickerhoof, Executive Director
William Knight, Deputy Director
Terry Keter, Program Director

Services include advocacy, information and referrals, independent living skills and peer counseling.

7915 Center for Independent Living of Jacksonville
2709 Art Museum Drive
Jacksonville, FL 32207-5036
904-399-8484
Fax: 904-396-0859; *Toll Free:* 888-427-4313
info@cilj.com
www.cilj.com
TTY: 904-398-6322

Michael Whitchurch, President
Jim Murphy, Treasurer
Mary Randall, Secretary

A consumer driven, community based, non-residential, private not-for-profit organization. We serve as a resource agency serving people with disabilities in 5 counties throughout Northeast Florida. ILRC is guided by its mission statement: To empower all people with a disability (as defined in the American's With Disabilities act (ADA) or Rehab act of 1973), to live independent and self-empower lives.

Year Founded: 1991

7916 Center for Independent Living of Northern Florida / Ability 1st
1823 Buford Court
Tallahassee, FL 32308-1544
850-575-9621
Fax: 850-576-5740
judithbarrett@ability1st.info
www.ability1st.info
TDD 850-575-5245

Judith Barrett, Executive Director
Steve Amnott, Director Of Finance & Admin.
Anne Leigh Keller, Office Manager

Offers advocacy, information and referrals, independent living skills and peer counseling. Mission is to empower persons with disabilities to live independently and participate actively in their community.

7917 Center for Independent Living of South Florida
6660 Biscayne Boulevard
Miami, FL 33138-6285
305-751-8025
Fax: 305-751-8944
Info@soflacil.org
www.soflacil.org
TDD 305-751-8891
TTY: 305-751-8025

Kelly Greene, Executive Director
Alvin W Roberts, President
Gregg Goldfarb, Vice President

Empowers people with disabilities of all ages to reach their highest level of achievement and to advocate for systemic change that results in access, equality, inclusion, integration, independence, and choice for all peope with disabilities.

7918 Center for Independent Living-Central Florida
720 North Denning Drive
Winter Park, FL 32789-3095
407-623-1070
Fax: 407-623-1390
info@cilorlando.org

www.cilorlando.org
TTY: 407-623-1185

Elizabeth Howe, Executive Director
Jason Venning, Development Director
Dan Ryan, Operations Director

The Center for Independent Living in Central Florida Inc. (CIL) is a private non-profit organization that was founded in 1976 by Central Floridians dedicated to helping people with disabilities achieve their self-determined goals for independent living. CIL is a consumer-driven organization whose philosophy is based on peer role models: people with disabilities empowering people with disabilities and their families on the road to independence.

7919 Center for Independent Living-Northwest Florida

3600 North Pace Boulevard
Pensacola, FL 32505-6625
850-595-5566
Fax: 850-595-5560; Toll Free: 877-245-2457
www.cilnwf.org
TDD 850-595-5566

Susan Patterson, President
Nancy Wise, Secretary
John Bouchard, Treasurer

The Center for Independent Living is a consumer-controlled, community-based cross-disibility, nonresidentail private non-profit agency that is designed and operated within a local community by individuals with disabilities and provides an array of independent living services. Our goal is to secure for all people with disabilities the opportunity to choose and realize their goals of where and how they live, learn, work and play. Also to assure that the consumer has optimal controll over all their services and options. You are not charged for our four core services.

7920 Coalition for Independent Living Options

6800 Forest Hill Boulevard
West Palm Beach, FL 33413
561-966-4288
Fax: 561-641-6619; Toll Free: 800-683-7337
cilo2000@bellsouth.net
www.cilo.org
TTY: 561-641-6538

Genevieve Cousminer, Executive Director
Scott M Shoemaker, President
Sharon D Eusanio, Vice President

The objectives of the Coalition for Independent Living Options (CILO) are: to increase advocacy efforts with public & private entities to promote independence for people with disabilities; to increase visibility & viability of CILO; to expand services in all geographic areas; to increase collaboration with other agencies; to diversify funding through resource development, and, to increase diversity in board, staff & consumers. Services provided by CILO include that of independent living skills training, information and referral, advocacy, and peer support.

7921 Florida Independent Living Council

1018 Thomasville Road
Suite 100A
Tallahassee, FL 32303
850-488-5624
Fax: 850-488-5881; Toll Free: 877-822-1993
www.flailc.org
TTY: 850-488-5624

Molly Gosline, Executive Director
Donald Dawkins, Advocacy Coordinator
Kristi Chapman, Consumer Advocacte

The Florida Independent Living Council is a statewide council established by federal mandate and Florida Statute. FILC's purpose is to promote independent living opportunities for persons with disabilities throughout the state of Florida. This includes the promotion of a direct service philosophy that is consumer controlled and directed. The Council also works to insure: that persons with disabilities have an opportunity for input into the development of a state plan for Independent Living Services; that the independent living needs of people with disabilities are identified and met; and that advocacy on behalf of independent living programs and consumers is initiated and carried out.

7922 Self-Reliance

8901 North Armenia Avenue
Tampa, FL 33604-1041
813-375-3965
Fax: 813-975-3970
sriadmin@self-reliance.org
www.self-reliance.org
TTY: 813-375-3972

Joseph DiDomenico, Executive Director

Self Reliance, Inc. Center for Independent Living is a non-profit 501C3 organization established in 1978. Our mission is to promote independence through empowering persons with disabilities and improving the communities in which they live. We are a cross disability agency providing services to both children and adults with disabilities (regardless of age and type of disability) to identify and overcome barriers to independence in their lives. Services are provided free of charge. Self Reliance is one of 17 Centers for Independent Living statewide. Mandated by the Federal Government, Centers For Independent Living provide four core services to individuals with disabilities. The core services are Advocacy - giving aid to a cause; active verbal support for a cause or position. Peer Support & Mentoring - talking to a person with a disability who can understand and encourage you in your decicommunity independence.sion-making and quest for independence. Independent Living Skills Training - individual and group training in areas such as job readiness, home management, parenting, transportation, healthcare and other areas as needed. Information & Referral - learn about community resources and how to connect with valuable services to achieve your goals towards

7923 Space Coast Center for Independent Living

2700 Judge Fran Jamieson Way
Viera, FL 32940
321-633-1000
Fax: 321-633-6472
llfowler@bellsouth.net
ese.brevard.k12.fl.us/icb/scc
TTY: 321-784-9008

Larry Fowler, Executive Director
Pamela Treadwell, Director
Sherri Hayes, Administrative Secretary

Information & referral, independent living skills training, advocacy, peer support, social/recreational opportunities, low-cost wheelchair accessible transportation, sign language interpreter referral services, specialized telephones &Æequipment for people who are deaf, hard of hearing, deaf/blind or speech impaired, high school transitioning services, accessibility services, volunteer program, notary services.

7924 Suncoast Center for Independent Living

3281 17th Street
P O Box 52649
Sarasota, FL 34235
941-351-9545
Fax: 941-316-9320
info@scil4u.org
www.scil4u.org
TTY: 941-351-9943

Candy Partee, Chairman
Fredd Atkins, Vice Chairperson
Vicke Mack, Treasurer

Offers advocacy for the elimination of social and physical barriers for people with disabilities. Provides peer counseling, equipement and building of access ramps.

Georgia

7925 Access Center for Independent Living

901 S Ludlow ST
Dayton, OH 45402-2614
937-341-5202
Fax: 937-341-5217; *Toll Free:* 937-341-5218
info@acils.com
www.acils.com
TTY: 770-534-6656

Alan R Cochrun, Executive Director
Greg Davis, Accountin/Human Resources
Greg Karmer, Assistant Director

Offers advocacy, information and referrals, independent living skills and peer support.

7926 Georgia Statewide Independent Living Council

755 Commerce Drive
Suite 415
Decatur, GA 30030-1852
770-270-6860
Fax: 770-270-5957; *Toll Free:* 888-288-9780
ppuckett@silcga.org
www.silcga.org
TTY: 770-270-5671

Patricia Puckett, Executive Director
Colleen Caffrey, Business Manager
Sherita Robinson, Administrative Assistant

The SILC of Georgia is a nonprofit, non-governmental, consumer-controlled organization that plays the vital role of providing disability information, financial support, and technical assistance to a network of seven Centers for Independent Living (CILs) located throughout the state. Centers for Independent Living are non-residential, community-based organizations, governed and staffed by people with disabilities, that offer a wide variety of services to consumers with disabilities and their families. The foundation of these services is the peer-to-peer relationship, where people with disabilities act as mentors for other people with disabilities, showing them by example how to help themselves and to live independently. The core services that CILs provide are: Individual Advocacy and Systems Advocacy; Peer Counseling; Information and Referral; and Independent Living Skills Training. Whileo educate the public about our services and the unique needs of people with disabilities. We do this by conducting and publishing the re-

sults of public opinion polls, disseminating information on a variety of issues and advocating for social change. the SILC of Georgia is a private, non-profit organization, it is also a Governor-appointed body. Board members are composed of members from across the state who represent a broad range of disabilities and backgrounds, and who are knowledgeable about centers for independent living and independent living services. SILC of Georgia's purpose is also t

7927 Living Independence for Everyone (LIFE) Center for Independent Living

5105 Paulsen Street
Suite 143-B
Savannah, GA 31405
912-920-2414
Fax: 912-920-0007; *Toll Free:* 800-948-4824
www.lifecil.com
TTY: 912-920-2419

Fran Todd, Executive Director
Susan Dawson, Assisstant Director
John-Paul Berlon, President

Living Independence for Everyone (L.I.F.E) is a small non-profit advocacy organization dedicated to empowering people with disabilities to achieve equal rights, equal opportunities and integration into the community. L.I.F.E. Inc. is operated by and for people with disabilities. Our organization embraces the independent living philosophy. This philosophy is based on the core of independent living concepts of consumer controll, self advocacy, community change, and cross-disability participation. One of the bases of the IL philosophy is that everyone, no matter what his or her disability, has the right to maker his or hew own informed decisions.

7928 Walton Options for Independent Living

948 Walton Way
Augusta, GA 30901
706-724-6262
Fax: 706-724-6729
tjohnston@waltonoptions.org
www.waltonoptions.org
TTY: 706-261-0206

Tiffany Johnston, Administration
Deversly Holloway, Assistive Technology Specialist
Judy Bartee, Administration

Walton Options for Independent Living was established September of 1994 in Augusta, Georgia to serve 30 counties in north eastern Georgia and 10 counties in western South Carolina as a private, nonprofit, consumer-controlled (meaning that the organization is governed by a majority of people who have disabilities), nonresidential Center for Independent Living, as defined by the Rehabilitation Act of 1973, as amended. The mission of Walton Optionsis to empower persons of all ages with all types of disabilities to reach their highest level of independence, including community inclusion and employment. Over 70% of the Board and Staff at Walton Options are people with disabilities. The name of the organization came from George Walton, a native Augustan who was the youngest signer of the Declaration of Independence.

Hawaii

7929 Regency at Hualalai
75-181 Hualalai Road
Kailua Kona, HI 96740-1787
808-329-7878
Fax: 808-329-7838
marketing@retirementhawaii.com
www.regencyhualalai.com

Lisa Fujikawa, Genral Manager

Regency at Hualalai's assisted living options offer personalized assistance, supportive services and compassionate care in a professionally managed, carefully designed, community setting. It's the perfect alternative for seniors who can no longer live on their own at home, yet don't need 24-hour, complex medical supervision. The Regency is a place where seniors can enjoy catered independent living, or various levels of assisted living, based ontheir individual needs. The setting of the Regency at Hualalai is within the comfortable atmosphere of a retirement community that is complemented by personal senior care services provided by a kind and helpful staff.

7930 Statewide Independent Living Council-Hawaii
Davies Pacific Center
841 Bishop Street, Suite 201
Honolulu, HI 96813
808-585-7452
Fax: 808-585-7453
www.hisilc.org

Sheryl Nelson, Executive Director
Jennifer Hausler, Chaiman
Beverly Wong, Secretary

The Statewide Independent Living Council of Hawaii is made up of representatives from around the State, appointed by the Governor. The majority of our Council is represented by persons with disabilities. It is a not for profit, non-Governmental, consumer controlled organization, which develops, monitors and evaluates the federally-funded State Plan for Independent Living in the State of Hawaili. It promotes the independent living philosophy statewide and provides support and technical assistance to the Independent Living Center in Hawaii, which consists currently of five community based organizations run by and for people with disabilities. The mission of SILC-Hawaii is to promote independent living and the integration of persons with disabilities into the community and to aid individuals in achieving their goals and basic human rights.

Idaho

7931 Disability Action Center Northwest
505 N Main St
Moscow, ID 83843-2906
208-883-0523
Fax: 208-883-0524; *Toll Free:* 800-475-0070
moscow@dacnw.org
www.dacnw.org
TTY: 208-883-0523

Mark Leeper, CEO
Steven Cor, PAS Program Manager
Krista Kramer, IL Planning Coordinator

Disability Action Center NW Inc. is a non-profit community partnership working to promote the independence and equality of all individuals with disabilities in all aspects of society. Utilizing our collective power, we provide information and referral services while fostering attitudes, policies, and environments of equality and freedom. DAC strives to create a compassionate and accessible place for people with disabilities. We encourage people with disabilities to take controll of their lives and to live life to the fullest.

7932 IMPACT
2735 East Broadway
Alton, IL 62002-1859
618-462-1411
Fax: 618-474-5309
www.incil.org

Cathy Contarino, Executive Director

The Illinois Network of Centers for Independent Living (INCIL) is a statewide organization made up of 24 Centers for Independent Living (CILs) in Illinois. INCIL coordinates the activities and efforts of all CILs, resulting in a stronger, more unified voice to promote the needs and priorities of the CILs and the people they serve. Operated by the executive directors of these CILs, this aggressive core of leadership advocates for and works to ensure that all people are treated with respect and given the same opportunities in life, regardless of their abilities.

7933 Living Independence Network (LINC)
1878 West Overland Road
Boise, ID 83705-2408
208-336-3335
Fax: 208-384-5037
info@lincidaho.org
www.lincidaho.org
TTY: 208-336-3335

Roger Howard, Executive Director

Living Independence Network Corporation (LINC) is a non-profit organization empowering people with disabilities to achieve their desired level of independence. LINC promotes personal growth and freedom of choice through advocacy, netoworking, public awareness and modification of environments.

7934 Statewide Independent Living Council-Idaho
816 West Bannock Street
P.O.Box 83720
Boise, ID 83720-9601
208-334-3800
Fax: 208-334-3803; *Toll Free:* 800-487-4866
silc@silc.idaho.gov
www.silc.idaho.gov
TDD 208-334-3800

Robbi Barrutia, Executive Director
Shirley Wentland, Financial Specialist
Jami Davis, Manageent Assistant

The Idaho State Independent Living Council (SILC) whose service is provided to acquaint the disability community and service providers to our organization, which advocates for equal opportunity, equal access, self-determination, independence and choice for people with disabilities. The focus of the SILC is to maximize opportunity and to incorporate people with disabilities into all walks of life by empowering them. The Idaho SILC provides leadership development opportunities to empower grassroots advocates, who, in turn, will develop systemic changes in public policy to positively impact people with disabilities.

Illinois

7935 Access Living of Chicago

115 West Chicago Avenue
Chicago, IL 60654
312-640-2100
Fax: 312-640-2101; *Toll Free:* 800-613-8549
generalinfo@accessliving.org
www.accessliving.org
TTY: 312-640-2102

Benjamin Lumicao, Board Chairman
Michael K. Santay, Treasurer
Brad Markham, Secretary

Established in 1980, Access Living is a non-residential Center for Independent Living for people with all types of disabilities, providing services that promote the independence and the inclusion of people with disabilities in every aspect of community life. Access Living follows the independent living philosophy that calls for community-based, consumer-controlled service and advocacy programs that emphasize a cross-disability and self-help approach. All services are provided at no charge to our Consumers. Access Living is a cross-disability organization governed and staffed by a majority of people with disabilities. Access Living fosters the dignity, pride, and self-esteem of people with disabilities and enhances the options available to them so they may choose and maintain individualized and satisfying lifestyles. Access Living recognizes the innate rights, abilities, needs and diversity of people with disabilities, works toward their integration into community life and serves as an agent of social change.

7936 Center For Independent Living-Jacksonville

15 Permac Road
Jacksonville, IL 62650-2071
217-245-8371
Fax: 217-245-1872; *Toll Free:* 888-317-3287
info@jacil.org
www.jacil.org
TTY: 217-245-8371

Vicki Mullis, President
Phil Foxworth, Vice President
Ruth Linear, Secretary

The Jacksonville Area Center for Independent Living (JACIL) is organized to serve people with disabilities in Morgan, Scott, Cass and Mason counties. JACIL is committed to enabling persons with disabilities to gain effective control and direction of their lives in the home, in the workplace and in the community. The JACIL goal is to stimulate and promote a growing sense of personal dignity through individualized programs designed to provide the the tools necessary for maximum independence and community participation. Services provided by JACIL include that of information and referral, independent living skills training, individual and systems advocacy, and, peer counseling.

7937 Illinois-Iowa Center for Independent Living (IICIL)

3708 11th Street
Po Box 6156
Rock Island, IL 61231

309-793-0090
Fax: 309-793-5198; *Toll Free:* 877-541-2505
iicil@iicil.com
www.iicil.com
TTY: 309-793-0090

Liz Sherman, Executive Director
Shirley Holgorsen, Staff Assistant
Tammy Duet, Staff Associate

The mission of the IICIL is to create and maintain independence options for people with disabilities by advocating for civil rights, providing services, and promoting full participation of disabled individuals in all aspects of the community. IICIL provides a number of consumer directed services, including information and referral, advocacy, independent living skills training, and peer support, which are mandated by the Rehabilitation Act of 1973. In addition to these services, we also have a fully accessible computer lab, state of the art information and referral library, TTY/Amplified Phone acquisition, Low tech devices for people who have low vision or blind, Braille and transcription, Sign language and Spanish interpreters, Technical assistance on disability laws and policy, Disability Awareness Training, Accessibility audits, and a host of volunteer opportunities for consumers and other interested persons.

7938 LIFE Center for Independent Living

2201 Eastland Drive
Suite 1
Bloomington, IL 61704-7923
309-663-5433
Fax: 309-663-7024; *Toll Free:* 888-543-3245
lifecil@lifecil.org
www.lifecil.org
TTY: 309-663-5433

Gail Kear, Executive Director
Jill Doran, Associate Director
Brianne Anderson, Office Manager

LIFE Center for Independent Living advances equality and integration of all persons with disabilities. To achieve this mission, we: promote local, state and national advocacy; educate persons with disabilities about their rights and responsibilities; provide support services, and Raise community awareness about disability issues. LIFE Center for Independent Living serves persons of all ages with all kinds of disabilities in DeWitt, Ford, Livingston and McLean Counties in Illinois. We also provide community services that promote accessibility and break down attitudinal barriers. Services include that of information and referral, independent living skills training, advocacy, community reintegration, peer mentoring support, communication services and benefits counseling.

7939 Lake County Center for Independent Living (LCCIL)

377 North Seymour Avenue
Mundelein, IL 60060-2322
847-949-4440
Fax: 847-949-4445
info@lccil.org
www.lccil.org/
TDD 847-388-0776
TTY: 847-949-4440

Anita Gorski, Executive Director
Donna Shalala, Community Integration Director

Lake County Center for Independent Living (LCCIL) is a disability rights organization governed and staffed by a majority of people with disabilities. Lake County Center for Independent Living offers services and advocacy that promote a fully accessible society, which expects participation by persons with disabilities. LCCIL's vision is that people with disabilities are involved in every aspect of society and have the freedom and opportunity to control their own lives. It is the belief of LCCIL that the quality of life is important for all people including people with disabilities. Services include that of information and referral, independent living skills training, advocacy, community reintegration, deaf services and peer counseling.

7940 Opportunities for Access
4206 Williamson Place
Suite 3
Mount Vernon, IL 62864-2352
618-244-9212
Fax: 618-244-9310
spud@ofacil.org
www.ofacil.org/
TDD 618-244-7400
TTY: 618-244-9575

Michael Egbert, Executive Director

Opportunities for Access strives to empower persons with disabilities to increase their opportunities to access all aspects of community life, serving the counties of: Clinton, Edwards, Hamilton, Jefferson, Marion, Wabash, Washington; Wayne, and White. Services include that of peer advisory, system advocacy, information and referral, independent living skills training, interpreter referral, housing referral, community integration, and adaptive equipment selection.

7941 Options Center for Independent Living
22 Heritage Drive
Suite 107
Bourbonnais, IL 60914-2510
815-936-0100
Fax: 815-936-0117
optionscil@optionscil.org
www.optionscil.org
TTY: 815-936-0132

Options Center for Independent Living (CIL) is a non-residential, not-for-profit organization that promotes independent living for persons of all ages who have disabilities. Community-based, our service area encompasses Kankakee and Iroquois Counties. Options CIL is a consumer-based organization that is managed and controlled by persons who have disabilities. In fact, over 50 percent of our volunteer board of directors and staff are individuals with disabilities. Options Center for Independent Living (CIL) believes that persons with disabilities have the right to make choices about their own lives and to experience life as active participants in society. Services include that of independent living skills training, community integration, referrals for sign language interpreters, a TTY distribution and training center, peer support and advocacy, in addition to having an assistive technologcenter.

7942 Persons Assuming Control of their Environment (PACE)
1317 East Florida
Urbana, IL 61801-6043
217-344-5433
Fax: 217-344-2414
info@pacecil.org
www.pacecil.org

TDD 217-244-5024
TTY: 217-344-5024

Evelyn Brown, President
Fred Neuburt, Vice President
Becca Hardy, Secretary

PACE provides services which assist people with disabilities in achieving or maintaining independence. People with disabilities direct our services in that our board and staff are mandated to be at least 51% people with disabilities. Services include that of access and advocacy, independent living counseling, information and referral, skills training, specialty services, interpreter referral, housing referral, and community intergration.

7943 Progress Center for Independent Living
7521 Madison Street
Forest Park, IL 60130-1407
708-209-1500
Fax: 708-209-1735
info@progresscil.org
www.progresscil.org/
TDD 708-209-1826
TTY: 708-209-1826

Horacio Esparza, Executive Director
Rebecca Thompson, Program Director
Lucille Burns, Office Manager

Progress Center directly assists persons with disabilities to establish lives in the community, providng serves and support to people with disabilities of all ages to increase and maintain their independence, in addition to assisting families and communities. The Progress Center provides the services of independent living skills training, advocacy, information and referral, and peer counseling, in addition to community integration and housing referral.

7944 RAMP
202 Market Street
Rockford, IL 61107-3954
815-968-7467
Fax: 815-968-7612
www.rampcil.org
TTY: 815-968-2401

Julie Bosma, Executive Director
Amy Morris, Development Director
Jackie Sundquist, Services Director

Established in 1980, RAMP Inc, is a non-profit, non-residential Center for Independent Living (CIL). RAMP advocates for and serves people with disabilities and their communities in Boone, DeKalb, Stephenson and Winnebago Counties from offices in Belvidire, DeKalb, Freeport and Rockford. At no cost to the individual, we serve with the purpose of increasing the ability of people with disabilities to become productive, contributing and self-directing members of society. We also educate businesses, service providers and public entities on disability issues and help them to comply with the technical requirements of the Americans with Disabilities Act and other disability related laws and standards.

7945 Regional Access & Mobilization Project (RAMP)
115 N First Street
Dekalb, IL 60115-9637
815-756-3202
Fax: 815-758-3556

www.rampcil.org
TTY: 815-756-4263

Julie Bosma, Executive Director
Amy Morris, Development Director
Jackie Sundquist, Services Director

Established in 1980, RAMP, Inc. is a non-profit, non-residential Cener for Independent Living (CIL). RAMP advocates for and serves people with disabilities and their communities in Boone, DeKalb, Stephenson and Winnebago Counties from offices in Belvidere, DeKalb, Freeport and Rockford. At no cost to the individual, we serve with the purpose of increasing the ability of people with disabilities to become productive, contributing and self-directing members of society. We also educate businesses, service providers and public entities on disability issues and help them to comply with the technical requirements of the Americans with Disabilities Act and other disability related laws and standards.

7946 Soyland Access to Independent Living
2449 Federal Drive
Decatur, IL 62526-5924
217-876-8888
Fax: 217-876-7245; Toll Free: 800-358-8080
jwooters@decatursail.com
www.decatursail.com
TDD 217-876-8888
TTY: 217-876-8888

Jeri J. Wooters, Executive Director
Rich Adams, Visual Servives Director
Laverla Carrington, Interpreter/Advocate for Blind

As an advocacy agency, Soylant Acess to Independent Living (SAIL) is a community-based, non-residential Center for Independent Living (CIL). Its purpose is to promote and practice independent living for all people with disabilities. The organization strives to encourage and assist people with disabilities to gain effective controll of their lives by participation in all aspects of society to their fullest extent possible, especially in performingroutine daily activities. The organization promotes personal dignity of people with disabilities and develops community awareness by providing training, direct services and information.

7947 Springfield Center for Independent Living (CIL)
330 S Grand Avenue W
Springfield, IL 62704-1318
217-523-2587
Fax: 217-523-0427; Toll Free: 800-841-6167
www.sil.org
TTY: 217-523-6304

Fedrick A Boswell, Executive Director
Kenneth Schmitt, Associate Executive Director
Eleanor L Berry, CFO

The Statewide Independent Living Council of Illinois (SILC), formed in 1993, is a not-for-profit statewide planning organization. The Federal Rehabilitation Act requires each state to create an autonomous Statewide Independent Living Council to develop a state plan for independent living services and Centers for Independent Living. The Statewide Independent Living Council of Illinois (SILC), formed in 1993, is a not-for-profit statewide planningorganization. The Federal Rehabilitation Act requires each state to create an autonomous Statewide Independent Living Council to develop a state plan for independent living services and Centers for Independent

Living. Through the state plan, SILC works to expand existing Centers for Independent Living (CILs) and independent living services. SILC also supports the development of new programs where services are not currently available. The Councilworks to ensure that independent living services and CILs are accessible by all persons with disabilities.

7948 Will-Grundy Center for Independent Living
2415-a West Jefferson Street
Joliet, IL 60435-6464
815-729-0162
Fax: 815-729-3697
pamwgcil@smcglobal.net
www.will-grundycil.org
TTY: 815-729-2085

Pam Heavens, Executive Director
Missy Martin, Program Manager
Robert Smith, President

As people with disabilities and their advocates, the Will-Grundy Center for Independent Living strives for equality and empowerment of persons with disabilities in the Will and Grundy County areas. As people with disabilities and their advocates, the Will-Grundy Center for Independent Living strives for equality and empowerment of persons with disabilities in the Will and Grundy County areas, inform persons with disabilities of their rights, educate them about their responsibilities, provide support services, promote advocacy, and raise community awareness about disability issues. Services include that of individual advocacy and systems advocacy, information referral, independent living skills training, peer support, deaf services and interpreter services.

Indiana

7949 Cameron Woods
416 E Maumee Street
Angola, IN 46703-8808
260-665-2141
Fax: 260-665-2879
www.cameronmch.com

Gregory T Burns, President/CEO

Cameron Woods is a spacious residential community, conveniently located in a natural setting just north of Angola, offering assisted living alternatives. Designed to provide a sense of security while helping residents maintain their independence, Cameron Woods offers a choice of apartment styles, care levels and financial options to suit the individual needs of each resident. A wide range of additional services is also available.

7950 Crown Point Senior Living-Anderson
1836 S.Patriot Drive
Yorktown, IN 47396
765-641-9995
Fax: 765-622-0340
www.crownpointecommunities.com/

Emily Carroll, Executive Director

Crownpointe can provide custom services individually designed for each person's lifestyle. Independent living services include a choice of apartments in studio, 1 bedroom or 2 bedroom styles, with all utilities included, three restaurant meals per day served to your table, cable tv, life enrichment activities, on site postal and copy services, 24 hour staff and security, weekly wellness clinic by staff registered nurse, emergency response pendant, apartment maintenance, trash removal and grounds keeping, housekeeping and linen service, in addition to the availibility of local transportation.

7951 Heritage Park Independent Living Apartments
2001 Hobson Road
Fort Wayne, IN 46805
260-484-9557Toll free: 888-788-2501
info@americansrcommunities.com
americansrcommunities.com

Kim Hues, Manager

Senior Independent and Assisted Living Apartments are available in studio as well as one or two bedroom floor plans, furnished and decorated as you so desire, making a familiar and comfortable atmosphere where family members and friends can visit. Our residents enjoy the company of their neighbors while enjoying three meals a day offered in our unique, restaurant-style dining rooms. There are many opportunities to participate in a wide range of planned social activities, scheduled transportation to shopping, restaurants and appointments. We continue to add services designed to keep our residents as active as they desire while having the comfort and security of living in a senior community.

7952 Indianapolis Resource Center for Independent Living (IRCIL)
5302 East Washington Street
Indianapolis, IN 46219
317-926-1660
Fax: 317-926-1687; *Toll Free:* 866-794-7245
info@abilityindiana.com
ablityindiana.com
TTY: 317-926-1660

Melissa Madill, Executive Director
Trish Langford, Office Manager
Quiana Anderson, Office Assistant

Since 1987, IRCIL has provided services, support and information to people with disabilities to help insure equal access to all aspects of community life. Additionally, IRCIL provides education and advocacy to all members of the community to help increase awareness and break down barriers that impede inclusion. IRCIL is a consumer-controlled organization. No less than 51% of our staff and governing board are persons with a disability to insure that the will and needs of people with disabilities are reflected in all we do. IRCIL was established to assist people with disabilities in developing the supports they need to assure full inclusion in community life. Services include that of information and referral, peer counseling, independent living skills training, individual and systems advocacy, services for people who are blind or visually impaired, braille reproduction, and benefits planning.

7953 Park Square Manor
6990 East County Road 100 North
Avon, IN 46123
317-272-7300
Fax: 317-272-7400
nsigler@5sqc.com
www.parksquareseniorliving.com

Nancy Sigler, Executive Director

Park Square Manor is an independent and asssited living community that provides numerous services including that

of advocacy for support, information and referral, independent living skills training, peer support, orientation and mobility, and public education and development.

7954 Southern Indiana Center For Independent Living
1494 W.Main Street
P O Box 308
Mitchell, IN 47446
812-277-9626
Fax: 812-277-9628; *Toll Free:* 800-845-6914
www.sicilindiana.org
TTY: 812-277-9627

Albert Tolbert, Executive Director

SICIL is a consumer controlled, community based, cross-disability, non-residential and not-for-profit organization that promotes and practices the philosophy of independent living: consumer control, peer support, self-help, self-determination, equal access, and individual and community advocacy.

7955 St Paul Hermitage
501 N 17th Avenue
Beech Grove, IN 46107
317-786-2261
Fax: 317-782-1411
www.stpaulhermitage.org

Sr. Sharon Bierman, Administrator

From the beginning, St. Paul Hermitage has been recognized as a leader in the area of healthcare for the aged and infirm. The Hermitage offers a truly Christian atmosphere.

Iowa

7956 Central Iowa Center for Independent Living
655 Walnut Street
Suite 131
Des Moines, IA 50309
515-243-1742
Fax: 515-243-5385; *Toll Free:* 888-503-2287
www.centraliowacil.com
TTY: 515-243-2177

Robert Jepson, Manager

The Central Iowa Center for Independent Living is a community based, non-residential program serving persons with disabilities. Our board of directors is composed of a majority of persons who have disabilities. CICIL is dedicated to assisting all persons, regardless of disability in making choices about their own lives and in experiencing success as active participants in society. CICIL serves people of all ages and disabilities. We also work with public officials, service providers and businesses that require technical assistance in responding to the needs of persons with disabilities. Services to individuals and families are provided free of charge or at a reduced rate.

7957 SILC-Iowa Department for the Blind
524 4th Street
Des Moines, IA 50309-2364
515-281-1333
Fax: 515-281-1263; *Toll Free:* 800-362-2587
information@blind.state.ia.us
www.idbonline.org
TTY: 515-281-1355

Richard Sorey, Director
Bruce Snethen, Deputy Director

The Iowa Department for the Blind provides programs that offer the specialized, integrated services that blind and severely visually impaired Iowans need to live independently and work competitively. It is the Department's belief that with the right training and opportunity, people who are blind can become full, contributing members of their communities. Services include a vocational rehabilitation program, an independent living program, assistive devices and technology services, in addition to a library for the blind and physically handicapped.

7958 Southwest Iowa Center for Independent Living
League of Human Dignity
1520 Avenue M
Council Bluffs, IA 51501
712-323-6863
Fax: 712-323-6811
Cinfo@leagueofhumandignity.com
leagueofhumandignity.com/text/index.html

Mike Schafer, Executive Director

The League of Human Dignity is an organization of people concerned about the rights and quality of life for people with disabilities. League members collaborate to ensure social, economic, and political equality for persons with disabilities. We believe in emphasizing likeness not difference, ability not disability, normality not abnormality, and integration not segregation. We work toward independent living for people who have disabilities. League members are people from the citizenry, government, and the business community who recognize that human dignity comes only through equal opportunity for all citizens. We recognize that society as a whole benefits when all its members are enabled to contribute freely in accordance with their potential and without regard to their disabilities. The mission of the League of Human Dignity is to actively promote the full integration of individuals with disabilities into society. To this end, we will advocate their needs and rights, and provide quality services to involve these persons in becoming and remaining independent citizens. Services include that of information and referral, systems advocacy, individual advocacy, peer suport, and independent living skills training.

7959 Three Rivers Center for Independent Living
Gordon Recovery Center
800 5th Street
Stuie 131
Sioux City, IA 51101-1315
712-255-1065
Fax: 866-616-2526
www.members.aol.com/trilc/

Becky Cadwell, President
Eleanor Luse, Vice President
Amanda Beller, Secretary/Treasurer

A non-profit, non residential, consumer driven organization committed to providing and increasing consumer designed services and community awareness regarding disabilities through the development of collaborations and partnerships.

Kansas

7960 Independent Living Resource Center
3033 West 2nd Street North
Wichita, KS 67203-5357
316-942-6300
Fax: 316-942-2078; *Toll Free:* 800-479-6861
www.ilrcks.org
TTY: 316-942-6300

James Thayer, President
John Brennan, Vice President
Jane Mobley, Secretary/Treasurer

The mission of Independent Living Resource Center, Inc. (ILRC) is to empower people with disabilities to lead independent lives by providing advocacy, community education and direct services. ILRC is a consumer-focused, consumer-directed organization. Over half of the ILRC Board of Directors and staff have disabilities and they are committed to assisting others in choosing and achieving a desired level of independence in their daily lives. Consumers, board members and all ILRC employees work to improve the availability of affordable, accessible housing and transportation for people with disabilities, increase the accessibility of the community, and advocate for supports that assist people with disabilities to remain in the home setting of their choice. Services include that of information and referral, advocacy, independent living skills training, and peer support.

7961 Independent Living of Northeast Kansas
521 Commercial
Suite C
Atchison, KS 66002
913-367-1830
Fax: 913-367-1430; *Toll Free:* 888-845-2879
ilcnek@sbcglobal.net
www.ableks.org
TTY: 913-367-1830

Ken Gifford, President & CEO

The Independent Living Center of Northeast Kansas is not-for-profit agency providing services within the State of Kansas. Funding for programs and services comes through grants from the Kansas Department of Social and Rehabilitation Services Division of Community Supports and Services, and also the Kansas Department of Rehabilitation Services. The mission of the Indepedent Living Center of Northeast Kansas is to assist people with disabilitiesto live an integrated, quality life with dignity, respect, and independence. Services include that of information and referral, peer support, independent living skills training, home and community based services, and vocational training.

7962 Living Independently in Northwest Kansas (LINK)
2401 East 13th Street
Hays, KS 67601
785-625-6942
Fax: 785-346-5260; *Toll Free:* 800-569-5926
brianatwell@linkinc.org
www.linkinc.org
TTY: 785-346-5865

Brian Atwell, Executive Director
Judy Droppleman, Manager

LINK promotes and supports the civil rights of people with disabilities and empowers them to achieve a life of indepedence and equality. Services include that of information and referral, independent living skills training, peer support, advocacy in addition to community based services and a newsletter.

Year Founded: 1979

7963 Resource Center for Independent Living
1137 Laing Street
PO Box 257
Osage City, KS 66523-1013
785-528-3105
Fax: 785-528-3665; *Toll Free:* 800-580-7245
info@rcilinc.org
www.rcilinc.org
TDD 785-528-3106

Chad Wilkins, Executive Director
Becky Brewer, Director Of Operations
Mike Pitts, Director Of Finance

RCIL, Inc. is committed to working with individuals, families, and communities to promote independent living and individual choice to persons with disabilities. Services include that of information and referral, advocacy, independent living skills training, peer counseling, deinstitutionalization, build a ramp program, RC@Home, financial management services, blind and low vision, durable medical equipment loan program, Kansas equipment exchange,assistive Technology for Kansas, braille translation services.

7964 Southeast Kansas Independent Living (SKIL)
1801 Main
PO Box 957
Parsons, KS 67357-1034
620-421-5502
Fax: 620-421-3705; *Toll Free:* 800-688-5616
skil@skilonline.com
www.skilonline.com
TDD 620-421-0983

Sheri Coatney, CEO

Southeast Kansas Independent Living, Inc. (SKIL) is a private, not-for-profit corporation devoted to meeting the needs of individuals with disabilities and to serving them, their families and communities. Services include that of independent livings skills, advocacy, peer counseling, assistive technology, in addition to home and community based services.

7965 Statewide Independent Living Council of Kansas
420 S.E.6th Avenue
Suite 2000
Topeka, KS 66607
785-234-6990
Fax: 785-215-6631
shannon.jones@silck.org
www.silck.org
TDD 785-234-6990

Shannon Jones, Executive Director
Chris Owens, Board-Directors Chairman
Robert C Harder, Board-Directors Treasurer

The vision of the State Plan for Independent Living in Kansas (SILCK) s an inclusive community which would enable Kansans to live in the environment of their choice. Independent living demands consumer empowerment, control, equal access, and integration. The plan shall insure that there are civil rights in place for total integration. The mission of the SILCK is to: develop a state plan through exter-

nal input, which ensures independent living for Kansans; advocate for the accomplishment of the state plan objectives; monitor, review, and evaluate the implementation of the plan; and to be a statewide catalyst for independent living.

7966 Three Rivers
504 Miller Drive
PO Box 408
Wamego, KS 66547-0408
785-456-9915
Fax: 785-456-9923; *Toll Free:* 800-555-3994
reception@threeriversinc.org
www.threeriversinc.org
TTY: 785-456-9915

Audrey Schremmer Phillips, Executive Director
Erica Christie, Director of Support & Services
Kristi Harmer, Senior Accountant

The Center manages programs in independent living which offer an array of services for individuals requiring assistance with personal, nursing/medical, and social needs. These services allow individuals to remain in their own home as an alternative to costly institutional care and include independent living skills training, information and referral, advocacy and peer support.

Year Founded: 1986

7967 Three Rivers-Manhattan
200 Southwind Pl.
Suite 103
Manhattan, KS 66502-5058
785-537-8985
Fax: 785-537-3435; *Toll Free:* 877-714-7272
reception@threeriversinc.org
www.threeriversinc.org
TDD 785-537-8985

Audrey Schremmer Phillips, Executive Director
Erica Christie, Director of Support & Services
Kristi Harmer, Senior Accountant

The Center manages programs in independent living which offer an array of services for individuals requiring assistance with personal, nursing/medical, and social needs. These services allow individuals to remain in their own home as an alternative to costly institutional care. Services include that of information and referral, advocacy, independent living skills training, and peer counseling.

Year Founded: 1986

7968 Topeka Independent Living Resource Center
501 Southwest Jackson Street
Suite 100
Topeka, KS 66603-3300
785-233-4572
Fax: 785-233-1561
tilrc@tilrc.org
www.tilrc.org
TDD 785-233-4572
TTY: 785-233-1815

Michael Oxford, Executive Director
Ami Hyten, Assistant Executive Director
Evan Korynta, Operations Manager

The Topeka Independent Living Resource Center is a civil and human rights organization. Our mission is to advocate for justice, equality and essential services for a fully integrated and accessible society for all people with disabilities. Services include that of information and referral, peer counseling, legal advocacy, independent living skills training and communications services.

Year Founded: 1980

Kentucky

7969 Center for Accessible Living

1051 North 16th Street
Suite C
Murray, KY 42071-1698
270-753-7676
Fax: 270-753-7729; *Toll Free:* 888-261-6194
calmur@calky.org
www.calky.org
TDD 270-767-0549

Jeanne M Gallimore, Branch Director
Carissa Johnson, Employment Specialist
John Canter, Benefits Specialist

The Center for Accessible Living (CAL) is a disability resource center for people with disabilities, governed by people with disabilities. It operates on a cross disability basis, which means that individuals will be served regardless of type of disability. Experienced staff provides information, advocacy and services that create opportunities for people with disabilities to live as independently as possible. Independent living for people with disabilities means having the opportunity and responsibility to make decisions as well as to exercise their right to control their own lives. The Center for Accessible Living promotes equal access and the ultimate goal of equal and independent status for all people with disabilities by encouraging awareness, involvement, and support for the rights of all people with disabilities by the entire community. Services include that of independent living skills training, advocacy, information and referral, and peer counseling.

7970 Center for Accessible Living-Louisville

305 West Broadway
Suite 200
Louisville, KY 40202
502-589-6620
Fax: 502-589-3980; *Toll Free:* 888-813-8497
webinfo@calky.org
www.calky.org
TTY: 502-589-6690

Jan Day, CEO
David Allgood, Community Advocate
Kelly Peace, Interpreter Coordinator

The Center for Accessible Living (CAL) is a disability resource center for people with disabilities, governed by people with disabilities. It operates on a cross disability basis, which means that individuals will be served regardless of type of disability. Experienced staff provides information, advocacy and services that create opportunities for people with disabilities to live as independently as possible. Independent living for people with disabilities means having the opportunity and responsibility to make decisions as well as to exercise their right to control their own lives. The Center for Accessible Living promotes equal access and the ultimate goal of equal and independent status for all people with disabilities by encouraging awareness, involvement, and support for the rights of all people with disabilities by the entire community. Services include that of independent living skills training, advocacy, information and referral, and peer counseling.

7971 Independence Place

1093 S. Broadway
Suite 1218
Lexington, KY 40504
859-266-2807
Fax: 859-335-0627; *Toll Free:* 877-266-2807
info@independenceplaceky.org
www.independenceplaceky.org
TTY: 877-266-2807

Michael Fein, Chairman
Carla Webster, Vice Chairman
Cindy Paulding, Treasurer

The philosophy of the Independent Living Center stresses the importance of all persons to be as responsible as possible for their own needs despite personal and external barriers. Also, to be free from over-dependence on others and on society as a whole. Independence Place aids individuals in attaining these goals by helping them make the necessary changes in themselves and their environment, thereby enhancing their integrity and maintaining controll of their own life.

Year Founded: 1995

7972 Pathfinders for Independent Living

105 East Mound Street
Harlan, KY 40831
606-573-5777
Fax: 606-573-5739; *Toll Free:* 877-240-PATH
pathfinders@harlanonline.net
www.pathfindersilc.org
TTY: 606-573-5777

Rosezella B Qualls, Chairperson
Patrick Perry, Vice-Chairperson

Works toward achieving equal participation in all communities for people with disabilities.

Louisiana

7973 New Horizons

8508 Line Avenue
Suite D
Shreveport, LA 71116
318-671-8131
Fax: 318-688-7823; *Toll Free:* 877-219-7327
nhilc@nhilc.org
www.nhilc.org
TTY: 318-671-8131

Gale Dean, Executive Director
Joy Lennon, Office Manager
Kimberly Sisco, Administrative Assistant

New Horizons was established as an independent living center in 1984 and is an association of adults with disabilities working to improve the quality of life for all who have disabilities. New Horizons believes that the quality of life for persons with disabilities improves directly as they exert control over their lives through independent living. New Horizons is a non-residential independent living center that offers a variety of programs and services for persons with disabilities including that of information and referral, independent living skills training, advocacy and peer counseling. New Horizons is a consumer-driven organization, which means the consumer is in the driver's seat. The majority of both New Horizons staff and Board of Directors for New Horizons are people with disabilities themselves.

7974 Resources for Independent Living - Baton Rouge

3233 S. Sherwood Forest Blvd
Suite 101 A
Baton Rouge, LA 70816
225-753-4772
Fax: 225-753-4831; *Toll Free:* 877-505-2260
contact@noril.org
www.noril.org
TTY: 225-753-4831

Yavorika Archaga, Executive Director

Consumers have access to a variety of services provided by Resources for Independent Living/RIL within the southeast region of Louisiana. RIL provides quality services to individuals with disabilities to assist with living independently, including that of information and referral, advocacy, peer support and independent living skills training.

Maine

7975 ALPHA One

127 Main Street
South Portland, ME 04106-2639
207-767-2189
Fax: 207-799-8346; *Toll Free:* 800-640-7200
webmaster@alphaonenow.org
www.alphaonenow.com
TTY: 207-767-5387

Dennis Fitzgibbons, Executive Director

Alpha One annually assists more than 4,000 people of all ages, including children and the elderly, with a range of disabilities: mobility impairments, traumatic brain injury, deafness, blindness, other vision and hearing impairments, developmental disabilities, mental illness, mental retardation, and AIDS. For more than two decades, Alpha One has been responsive to the needs of individuals with disabilities, initiating, advocating for, and implementing systems change to overcome the barriers that prevent people with disabilities from living independently. Alpha One offers a variety and depth of independent living services: information and referral, outreach, advocacy, one-to-one and group peer support, consumer-directed personal assistance services, assistive technology financing, access design, resume workshops, and independent living skills instruction. Alpha One's adapted driver assessment and education service enables people to learn to drive using adaptive equipment. Alpha One Medical, Alpha One's wholly-owned subsidiary, is a durable medical equipment sales and service company with locations in South Portland, and Lewiston, Maine.

Year Founded: 1978

7976 Maine Department of Labor: BRS: Division of Vocational Rehabilitation Independent Living Services Program

150 State House Station
Augusta, ME 04330-0150
207-623-6799Toll free: 800-698-4440
mdol@maine.gov
www.maine.gov/rehab/
TTY: 207-287-5292

The Independent Living Services (ILS) Program assists people who have significant disabilities to live more independently in their homes and communities. The program provides and arranges needed IL services subject to the availability of funds. The program is also an advocacy program for people with disabilities and their families. All ILS Program services are carried out through an Independent Living Plan that is mutually agreed upon by theconsumer and the IL counselor. The four core services that every Independent Living Center provides are: information and referral; individual independent living skills training; peer counseling; and individual and systems advocacy.

7977 Shalom House

106 Gilman Street
Po Box 560
Portland, ME 04102
207-874-1080
Fax: 207-874-1077
generalmail@shalomhouseinc.org
www.shalomhouseinc.org
TDD 207-842-6888

Susan Litchman, President
Jay Waterman, Vice-President
Kieith O'Blenis, Secretary

Shalom House offers hope for adults living with severe mental illness by providing a choice of quality housing and support services that help people lead stable and fulfilling lives in the community. Shalom House helps hundreds of people with serious mental illness each year by providing affordable housing where people can escape the stress of homelessness, hunger, and isolation. Once basic housing needs have been met, peoples' lives can become more stable. Shalom House's mission is to help people address personal goals, receive services, take medication, and once again become a vital part of the community.

Year Founded: 1972

Maryland

7978 Deaf Independent Living Association

806 Snow Hill Road
Salisbury, MD 21804
410-742-5052
Fax: 410-543-4874
dila@dila.org
www.dila.org

Lance MacAllister, Chairman
Max Verbits, President
Sherry Perkins, Secretary

Deaf Independent Living Association, Inc. (DILA) was established in 1982. DILA offers a variety of services, including employment support, residential support, information and referral and communication resources, for Eastern Shore residents with hearing loss. Above all DILA strives to promote active, independent living among the people we serve. The mission is to promote access to the services and resources for the Eastern Shore residents who are deaf or hard of hearing and provide opportunities for full participation in all aspects of community life.

Year Founded: 1982

7979 Independence Now

12301 Old Columbia Pike
Suite 101
Silver Spring, MD 20904
301-277-2839
Fax: 301-625-9777

INfo@innow.org
www.innow.org

Robert Watson, President
Cindy Buddington, Vice-President
Regina Lee-Byrd, Secretary

Established 1995, Independence Now (IN) is a nonprofit organization created by people with disabilities. Independence Now is a non-residential Center for Independent Living (CIL), one of more than 400 in the United States that provides an array of services to people with all types of disabilities who live in Montgomery and Prince George's Counties. The majority of our staff and Board of Directors have disabilities. Independence Now promotes the independent living philosophy and equal access for all people with disabilities. The mission of Independence Now (IN) is to facilitate independent thought and action by people with disabilities promoting the principle that each person has value. To this end, we provide the tools for individuals to develop and discover their power to control their interactions with the environment, their families and their communities.

7980 Oasis Senior Advisors

Toll Free: 888-455-5838
info@oasisssenioradvisors.com
www.oadsissenioradvisors.com

Shawn Charles, Owner

Oasis Senior Advisors help seniors find housing. They are a local, community based organization with locations across the country, dedicated to simplifying the process of selecting a senior housing facility for individuals and their family members.

7981 Resources for Independence

30. N. Mechanic Street
Unit B
Cumberland, MD 21502
301-784-1774
Fax: 301-784-1776; *Toll Free:* 800-371-1986
www.rficil.org

Lori Magruder, Executive Director
John Michaels, Assisstant Director
Robert Cannon, Resource Developer

Offers a strong consumer voice on a wide range of national, state and local issues for people with disabilities.

Massachusetts

7982 AD LIB Incorporated

215 North Street
Pittsfield, MA 01201-4629
413-442-7047
Fax: 413-443-4338; *Toll Free:* 800-232-7047
adlib@adlibcil.org
www.adlibcil.org
TTY: 413-442-7158

Linda Febles, President
Michael Hinkley, Vice-President
Shannon Miller, Secretary/Clerk

Offers information and referrals, independent living skills training, advocacy and peer counseling for the residents of Berkshire County. A private non-profit, community based, consumer controlled, Independent Living Center. The Center provides independent living and specialized services for people with disabilities in Berkshire County. Adlib empow-

ers people with disabilities to live more independently and have controll of their own lives.

7983 Boston Center for Independent Living

60 Temple Place
Fifth Floor
Boston, MA 02111-1324
617-338-6665
Fax: 617-338-6661; *Toll Free:* 866-338-8085
info@bostoncil.org
www.bostoncil.org
TTY: 617-338-6662

Sergio Goncalves, Chairman
Linda Landry, Vice Chairman
Stacey Zelbow, Treasurer

The Boston Center for Independent Living is a frontline civil rights organization led by people with disabilities that advocates to eliminate discrimination, isolation and segregation by providing advocacy, information and referral, peer support, skills training, and PCA services in order to enhance the independence of people with disabilities.

7984 Center for Living and Working

484 Main Street
Suite 345
Worcester, MA 01608-1824
508-798-0350
Fax: 508-797-4015; *Toll Free:* 800-570-4020
opsearch@centerlw.org
www.centerlw.org
TDD 508-762-1164
TTY: 508-755-1003

Cindy Purcell, President
Marry Ann Donovan, Treasurer
Ed Roth, Secretary/Clerk

Center for Independent Living and Working is a non-profit Independent Living Center, incorporated in 1975, which takes its direction from persons with disabilities. We advocate to empower persons with disabilities to take active roles in their lives and in the community in which they live. We provide comprehensive and innovative programs and services in order to maximize individual independence and opportunities. We are driven by the belief thatpeople with disabilities must always be equal members of society with equal access.

7985 DEAF Inc.

215 Brighton Avenue
Allston, MA 02134-2000
617-254-4041
Fax: 617-254-7091; *Toll Free:* 800-866-5195
info@deafinconline.org
www.deafinconline.org
TTY: 617-254-4041

Sharon L Applegate, Executive Director
Thomas Keydel, President
Kendra Timko-Hochkeppel, Treasurer

D.E.A.F., Inc. encourages and empowers Deaf, Hard of Hearing, Deaf/Blind and Late-Deafened individuals to lead independent and productive lives. We offer a comprehensive package of programs and services in a supportive community environment that is linguistically and culturally accessible for Deaf, Hard of Hearing, Deaf/Blind and Late-Deafened individuals from diverse ethnic and cultural populations.

Year Founded: 1977

7986 Independent Living Center of the North Shore & Cape Ann
27 Congress Street
Suite 107
Salem, MA 01970-5577
978-741-0077
Fax: 978-741-1133; *Toll Free:* 888-751-0077
information@ilcnsca.org
www.ilcnsca.org
TTY: 978-741-1735

Lisa Orgettas, Executive Director

The Independent Living Center of the North Shore and Cape Ann Inc. is a service and advocacy center run by and for people with disabilities. ILCNSCA supports the struggle of people who have all types of disabilities to live independently and participate fully in community life. ILCNSCA pursues this mission through a combination of self-advocacy services and community action. Self-advocacy services are designed to enable participants to develop the skills and knowledge necessary to achieve personal independence. ILCNSCA also organizes and supports collective action by people with disabilities aimed at positive social change, the elimination of discriminatory barriers, and the creation of a supportive and fully accessible community environment.

Year Founded: 1987

7987 Massachusetts Statewide Independent Living Council (MASILC)
280 Irving Street
Framingham, MA 01702
508-620-7452
Fax: 508-620-7450; *Toll Free:* 866-662-7452
info@masilc.org
www.masilc.org
TTY: 508-620-7452

Pam Burkley, SILC Chair
James R Clark, MASILC Coordinator

The Massachusetts Statewide Independent Living Council (MASILC) is a Governor appointed Council. Members include persons who are knowledgeable about centers for independent living and the services they provide. The Council was established by Executive Order No.373 of William F. Weld, Governor of the Commonwealth of Massachusetts on September 26, 1994. The Council includes representation of individuals with a range of physical and mental disabilities from the various geographic areas within the Commonwealth of Massachusetts. The Council along with the Designated State Units (Massachusetts Rehabilitation Commission and Massachusetts Commission for the Blind) Jointly develops and submits the State Plans required in section 704 of the Rehab Act. It is also charged with monitoring, reviewing, and evaluating the implementation of the State Plan for Independent Living as well as coordinatingactivities with the State Rehabilitation Advisory Council established under section 105 and other State Councils that address the needs of specific disability populations and issues under other federal laws.

7988 MetroWest Center for Independent Living
280 Irving Street
Framingham, MA 01702-7306
508-875-7853
Fax: 508-875-8359
info@mwcil.org

www.mwcil.org
TTY: 508-875-7853

Paul Spooner, Executive Director
Youcef J Bellil, President
Michael Kennedy, Vice President

Independent Living Philosophy maintains that individuals with disabilities have the right to choose services that they want to receive and to make decisions about how they live their lives. Consistent with this philosophy, Metro West Center for Independent Living / MWCIL assists consumers in achieving the goals that they have set for themselves by providing training, information, and support. MWCIL's mission is twofold: to help individuals with disabilities become productive and contributing members of the community and to eliminate barriers within the community that impede this process.

7989 Northeast Independent Living Program
20 Ballard Road
Lawrence, MA 01843-1018
978-687-4288
Fax: 978-689-4488
help@nilp.org
www.nilp.org
TTY: 978-687-4288

June Cowen, Executive Director
Kevin Hatch, Vice Chairman
Fran Kuchar, President

The Northeast Independent Living Program, Inc. is a consumer controlled Independent Living Center providing Advocacy and Services to people with all disabilities in the greater Merrimack Valley who wish to live as independently as possible in the community. Services include that of information and referral, independent living skills training, advocacy, and peer counseling.

7990 Southeast Center for Independent Living
66 Troy Street Merrill Building
Suite 3
Fall River, MA 02720-3015
508-679-9210
Fax: 508-677-2377
scil@secil.org
www.secil.org
TTY: 508-679-9210

Lisa M. Pitta, Executive Director
Damase Cote, President
Paul Remy, Vice President

The Philosophy of Independent Living, maintains that individuals with disabilities have the right to choose services and make decisions for themselves. This belief is the foundation and guiding principle of all of SCIL's policies and operations. SCIL provides training, information and support to help consumers achieve individual goals, experience personal growth and participate fully in community life. Services include that of information referral, independent living skills training, advocacy, and peer counseling.

Year Founded: 1986

7991 Stavros Center for Independent Living
210 Old Farm Road
Amherst, MA 01002-3045
413-256-0473
Fax: 413-256-0190; *Toll Free:* 800-804-1899
info@stavros.org

www.stavros.org
TTY: 413-256-0473

Glenn Hartmann, President
Nancy Bazanchuk, Vice President
Donna M Bliznak, Treasurer

Stavros Center for Independent Living was established in 1974 as a 501 c 3 not-for-profit organization. We are a grass-roots advocacy organization that works for justice and access for people with disabilities in western Massachusetts. It is our goal at Stavros to give people with disabilities the tools to take charge of their life choices, act on their own behalf, and overcome situations that reduce their potential for independence. Independent Living Services enable people with disabilities to live in an environment that encourages and supports the rights of people with disabilities to achieve and maintain a sense of autonomy in their lives. Our advocates accomplish this by providing counseling, skills training, general encouragement and support to people with disabilities in need of such assistance.

Year Founded: 1974

Michigan

7992 Ann Arbor Center for Independent Living
3941 Research Park Drive
Ann Arbor, MI 48108
734-971-0277
Fax: 734-971-0826
cilstaff@aacil.org
www.aacil.org
TTY: 734-971-0310

James Magyar, President/CEO
Tom Tomsik, Chairperson
Michael Harris, Treasurer

The Ann Arbor Center for Independent Living assists people with disabilities and their families in living full and productive lives. Our mission is to assure the equality of opportunity, full participation, independent living and economic self-sufficiency of people with disabilities in our community. The Ann Arbor Center for Independent Living utilizes the independent living model, a well-demonstrated and effective four-pronged advocacy and service delivery strategy. Fueled by a consumer-driven philosophy, we provide four core services required of all Centers for Independent Living along with several other services. The four core services are: information and referral, peer support, advocacy, and independent living skill development. The cornerstone of our approach requires that services are provided by people with disabilities for people with a full range of physical, cognitive, sensory (hearing and vision), and/or mental and emotional disabilities.

Year Founded: 1976

7993 Blue Water Center for Independent Living Center
310 Water Street
Port Huron, MI 48060-5431
810-987-9337
Fax: 810-987-9548; *Toll Free:* 800-527-2167
www.bwcil.org
TTY: 800-527-2167

Angela Hoff, Executive Director
Karen Massaro Mundt, Board-Directors President
Edward N. McGraw, Treasurer

The Blue Water Center for Independent Living is a consumer-based organization designed to serve persons with disabilities who have physical, psychiatric, sensory, cognitive, and multiple disabilities through the provision of advocacy, information and referral, service provision, and the promotion of needed services so to maximize the individual's optimal level of independence. The philosophy of the Blue Water Center for Independent Living is that every person has the right to control and self-direct his or her own life. Through the provision of advocacy, information and promotion of needed resources, people with disabilities can maximize their optimal level of ability.

7994 Capital Area Center for Independent Living
2812 N Martin Luther King
Jr Blvd
Lansing, MI 48906
517-999-2760
Fax: 517-999-2767; *Toll Free:* 800-649-3777
info@cacil.org
www.cacil.org
TDD 800-649-3777

Ellen Weaver, Executive Director
Al Swain, Associate Director
Marsha Moers, Community Advocacy

The Capital Area Center for Independent Living (CACIL) was established in 1976 to empower people with disabilities to take control of their lives. Independent Living is the principle that individuals with any disability, to the fullest extent possible, shall work, live in their own homes, raise families, and participate in the everyday activities of life. CACIL is one of nearly four hundred Independent Living Centers (CILs) around the country that were created under the Rehabilitation Act of 1973 and funded by the taxpayers of America. These centers can be easily distinguished from other service agencies by the extent of involvement of people with disabilities. CILs have a majority of people with disabilities on their governing boards, and they hire qualified people with disabilities to fill management and service delivery positions. Core services include information and referral, community awareness and advocacy, individual skills development, and peer support.

Year Founded: 1976

7995 Disability Advocates of Kent County
3600 Camelot Drive Southeast
Grand Rapids, MI 49546-8103
616-949-1100
Fax: 616-949-7865
contact@dakc.us
www.dakc.us
TTY: 616-949-1100

David Bulkowski, Executive Director
Debra Hines, President
Cameron Young, Vice President

Disability Advocates of Kent County empowers independence for persons with disabilities and leads the community towards equal opportunity for all.

Year Founded: 1981

7996 Disability Network Oakland & Macomb
16645 15 Mile Road
Clinton Township, MI 48035
586-268-4160
Fax: 586-285-9942; *Toll Free:* 800-284-2457

info@dnom.org
www.dnom.org

Andrew Maurer, Chairperson
Randy Charon, Vice Chairperson
Mark Cronmiller, Secretary

The Oakland and Macomb Center for Independent Living is committed to assisting people with disabilities to achieve independence through participation, choice and self-determination working to establish a supportive and unified community inclusive of people with disabilities. The Oakland & Macomb Center for Independent Living (OMCIL) is a consumer driven, non-residential, community based organization helping people with disabilities live independently and become participating members of society. The Staff and Board, most of whom are people with disabilities, are strongly committed to supporting others in their efforts toward independence. Since its founding in 1987, OMCIL has been advocating for changes to make the community accessible to people with disabilities, and offering a core of services which include: peer support, independent living skills training, individual and systems advocacy, information and referral. This comprehensive package of services to people with all disabilities is offered in the belief that it is the most effective way to serve consumers who have complex needs.

7997 Disability Network of Mid-Michigan

1705 South Saginaw Road
Suite C
Midland, MI 48640
989-835-4041
Fax: 989-835-8121; *Toll Free:* 800-782-4160
info@dnmm.org
www.dnmm.org
TTY: 989-835-4043

David Emmel, Executive Director
Steven Locke, Associate Director
Terri Cady, Program Leader

The Disability Network of Mid-Michigan promotes and encourages independence for all peoples with disabilities.

7998 Disability Network-Lakeshore Center for Independent Living

426 Century Lane
Holland, MI 49423-3079
616-396-5326
Fax: 616-396-3220; *Toll Free:* 800-656-5245
info@dnlakeshore.org
www.dnlakeshore.org/dnn
TTY: 616-396-5326

Michelle Chaney, President/Treasurer
Fred L Johnson, Vice President
Rev Terry De Young, Secretary

Disability Network/Lakeshore opened in Holland in 1992 under the name Lakeshore Center for Independent Living, as part of a state and national network serving people with disabilities. Our passionate and committed staff offer expertise on wide-ranging disability issues. Serving Allegan and Ottawa counties, Disability Network concentrates its efforts on building communities that work. Disability Network assists over 2,500 individuals with disabilities and their families on an annual basis, connecting them with supports and services as well as providing training and mentoring. Staff members are specialists in the areas of housing, employment, transportation, accessibility, educa-

tion, transition, and long-term supports. We also provide general information and referral services.

Minnesota

7999 Freedom Resource Center for Independent Living

2701 9th Avenue S
Suite H
Fargo, ND 58103
701-478-0459
Fax: 701-478-0510; *Toll Free:* 800-450-0459
freedom@freedomrc.org
www.freedomrc.org
TTY: 701-478-0459

Joyce Wolter, Executive Director

Provides a number of services for people with disabilities, their families and friends, service providers and interested community members. These services include information and referral, independent living skills, peer support, advocacy and support services, and personal care attendant programs. Each Center is an individual nonprofit agency and provides additional services.

Year Founded: 1981

8000 Metropolitan Center for Independent Living (MCIL)

530 Robert Sreet North
Saint Paul, MN 55104-3834
651-646-8342
Fax: 651-603-2006
mcil@mcil-mn.org
www.mcil-mn.org
TTY: 651-603-2001

David Hancox, Executive Director

MCIL is a Twin Cities metro-based, non-profit consumer-directed organization founded in 1981. MCIL is dedicated to the full promotion of the independent living (IL) philosophy by supporting individuals with disabilities in their personal efforts to pursue self-directed lives.

8001 Options Interstate Resource Center for Independent Living

318 Third Street NW
East Grand Forks, MN 56721-1887
218-773-6100
Fax: 218-773-7119; *Toll Free:* 800-726-3692
options@myoptions.info
www.macil.org/options.html
TTY: 218-773-6100

Randy Sorensen, Executive Director

Options provides people with disabilities advocacy, information, skills training and peer mentoring relationships to help them achieve their personal goals of how and where they live their lives. Options serves the eleven county region of Northwestern Minnesota and the eight county region of Northeastern North Dakota.

8002 Southeastern Minnesota Center for Independent Living

2720 North Broadway
Rochester, MN 55906
507-285-1815
Fax: 507-288-8070; *Toll Free:* 888-460-1815
semcil.uhhc@semcil.org

www.semcil.org
TTY: 507-285-0616

Vicki Dalle Molle, Executive Director

The Southeastern Minnesota Center for Independent Living, Inc. which was founded in 1981, is a non profit organization that assists people with disabilities to become independent and productive community members. Our Independent Living and Personal Care Assistant Programs promote self-sufficiency and help assure that persons with a disability have the same opportunities as members of the general public. SEMCIL is located in Rochester, MN and hasoffices in Goodhue and Winona Counties. In 1980, a small group of community members - with the mission of creating or sustaining independence for all persons with disabilities-wrote a grant that got us started and formed our first Board of Directors. Their vision led to the establishment of the Rochester Center for Independent Living (RCIL) in 1981. SEMCIL offers numerous programs focused on living independently and becoming an active community member through various independent living programs. Services include that of information and referral, advocacy, peer counseling, assistive technology, and independent living skills training.

8003 Southern Minnesota IL Enterprises and Services (SMILES)

709 South Front Street
Suite 7
Mankato, MN 56001-3804
507-345-7139
Fax: 507-345-8429; *Toll Free:* 888-676-6498
smiles@smilescil.org
www.smilescil.org
TTY: 507-345-7139

Brian Koch, President
Nate Clark, Vice President
Dan Robinson, Treasurer

SMILES Center for Independent Living was established in 1988 to provide services for people with disabilities in the nine county region of South Central Minnesota. SMILESÆis a non-profit, non-residential center funded through private and public foundation grants, government and community grants, the United Way, fees for service, and public contributions. Since January 1990 hundreds have found asistance in their efforts to make positive life choices. Because consumers, parents, professionals, and community advocates saw a need for a support system that would empower people with disabilities to build independent, fulfilling lives, resulting in the birth of the center 15 years ago.

8004 Southwest Center for Independent Living

109 South Fifth Street
Suite 700
Marshall, MN 56258-1298
507-532-2221
Fax: 507-532-2222; *Toll Free:* 800-422-1485
swcil@swcil.com
www.swcil.com/
TTY: 507-532-2221

Steve Thovson, Executive Director

Since independent living is a dynamic process, SWCIL is dedicated to working with and responding to the ever changing needs of persons with disabilities in southwestern Minnesota. We strive to provide services, supports, and resources, as defined necessary by consumers, that will lead

to the creation or enhancement of independent living options. We are committed to providing education and awareness to promote society acceptance, inclusion, andequal access for all persons with disabilities. Independent living programs offer a wide range of supportive services that are provided as a means to assist people with disabilities in obtaining and maintaining the greatest control over their lives. Independent living philosophy is based on the concept that persons with disabilities have the right to choose and live a lifestyle free from discrimination and segregation. Our services are designedsumer in establishing and achieving their independent living goals. Core services include that of information and referral, advocacy, independent living skills training, and peer support.to meet the specific needs of persons with all types of disabilities. Consumers are responsible to develop and control their own goal-oriented service plans. In addition, consumers are able to choose where their services are provided be it within the home, school or community Staff members provide assistance, support and encouragement to the con

Mississippi

8005 LIFE of South Mississippi

1304 Vine Street
Jackson, MS 39202
601-969-4009
Fax: 601-969-1662; *Toll Free:* 800-748-9398
lifeofms@aol.com
www.lifeofms.com
TDD 800-748-9398
TTY: 800-748-9398

Christi Dunaway, Executive Director
Augusta Smith, Assistant Director
Cindy Haslob, LIFE Regional Coordinator

The purpose of Living Independence For Everyone is to empower people with significant disabilities to be as independent and as fully involved in their communities as they can and want to be. The primary goal of LIFE is to assist in the independent living empowerment of people with significant disabilities by: Providing or coordinating the provision of devices, equipment, aids, modifications, or other services or forms of support that improve their capacity to live independently; Supplying information and referral services to allow sufficient access and utilization of available assistance; Furnishing peer counseling and guidance, encourage, establish, and maintain independent living attitudes and philosophies; Rendering advocacy support on and individual or systems-wide basis; Providing skills training instruction to improve specific independent living abilities and competencies; and, Contributing any other help that aids people with significant disabilities in acquiring, retaining, or enhancing their capacity to live independently.

Missouri

8006 Access II Independent Living Center

101 Industrial Parkway
Gallatin, MO 64640-1489
660-663-2423
Fax: 660-663-2517; *Toll Free:* 888-663-2423
access@accessii.org
www.accessii.org
TDD 660-663-2663

Heather Swymeler, Executive Director
Vickie Tolen, Independent Living Specialist
Georgia Jackson, Independent Living Specialist

The Mission of Access II is to remove architectural and attitudinal barriers that limit the independence of persons with disabilities, promote a positive change in attitudes about disability and persons with disabilities, and encourage greater independence for persons with disabilities within our communities. As a Center for Independent Living, Access II is committed to the provision of a full range of independent living services. Core services include that of information and referral, independent living skills training, peer counseling, in addition to consumer and community advocacy.

8007 Bootheel Area Independent Living Services (BAILS)

719 Teaco Road
Box 326
Kennett, MO 63857-0326
573-888-0002
Fax: 573-888-0708; *Toll Free:* 888-449-0949
tshaw@bails.org
www.bails.org
TTY: 573-888-0002

Tim Shaw, Executive Director
Tommie Brown, Access/Assistive Technology
Sherry Dollins, Intake Specialist

Offers information and referrals, advocacy, independent living skills and peer counseling. BAILS goal is to foster an open, barrier free society for all people regardless of their disability. All persons regardless of disability, are entitles to and should have equal access to the rights and responsibilities that other citizens are provided; to be an active and productive member of society as they choose.

8008 Delta Center for Independent Living

PO Box 550
St. Peters, MO 63376
636-926-8761
Fax: 636-447-0341; *Toll Free:* 866-727-3245
info@dcil.org
www.dcil.org
TTY: 636-926-8761

Mike Bender, President
Bob Zeffert, Treasurer
Catherine Davis, Secretary

Delta Center for Independent Living partners with people with disabilities and their communities to remove barriers and promote positive changes leading to greater independence for all. Delta Center is a consumer-controlled, not-for-profit agency that provides non-residential, community-based services for persons with all types of disabilities residing in the Missouri counties of St. Charles, Lincoln and Warren. Delta Center was formed in 1997 by a group of local citizens with disabilities and other persons concerned about disability issues. Helping those with physical and mental impairment, the Delta Center for Independent Living Services in St. Louis County, St. Charles County, Franklin County, Warren County, and Lincoln County can assist in maintaining and improve the ability to live independently. Core services include that of information and referral, peer support, advocacy, skillstraining for independent living, in addition to assistive technology.

8009 Disability Resource Association

420B South Truman Boulevard
Crystal City, MO 63019-1726
636-931-7696
Fax: 636-931-9400
dra@disabilityresourceassociation.org
www.disabilityresourceassociation.org
TTY: 636-937-9019

Craig Henning, Executive Director
Nancy Pope, Assistant Director
Suzan Weller, Director Of Programing

The independent living concept is based on the philosophy that people with all types of disabilities should have the same civil rights as those without disabilities. They have a right to control their lives based on options that minimize their reliance on others. Core services provided by Disability Resource Association (DRA) include that of information and referral, independent living skills, advocacy, and peer support. DRA is a member of the Missouri Statewide Independent Living Council, the purpose of which is to gather and disseminate information, conduct studies and analyses, develop model policies, conduct training on independent living issues, provide outreach to unserved and underserved populations, and work to expand and improve independent living services.

8010 Disabled Citizens Alliance for Independence-DCAI

8 Missouri Avenue
PO Box 675
Viburnum, MO 65566-0675
573-244-3315
Fax: 573-244-5609; *Toll Free:* 800-844-3316
dcitizen@misn.com
dcai.us/web/
TTY: 573-244-3315

Richard Blakely, Executive Director
Norma Moore, President
Elizabeth Broughton, Vice President

Disabled Citizens Alliance for Independence (DCIA) supports the vision that the independent living concept is based on the philosophy in which people with all types of disabilities should have the same civil rights as those without disabilities. They have a right to control their lives based on options that minimize their reliance on others. Core services provided by DCIA include that of information and referral, advocacy, independent living skills training, and peer support. DCAI is a member of the Missouri Statewide Independent Living Council, the mission of which is to gather and disseminate information, conduct studies and analyses, develop model policies, conduct training on independent living issues, provide outreach to unserved and underserved populations, and work to expand and improve independent living services.

8011 Independent Living Center

2639 East 34th Street
Joplin, MO 64804-4313
417-659-8086
Fax: 417-659-8087; *Toll Free:* 800-346-8951
jflowers@ilcenter.org
www.ilcenter.org
TTY: 417-659-8702

Jeff Flowers, Executive Director
Stephanie Brady, Director of Programs
Stormi Nordstrom, Office Manager

Offers information and referrals, advocacy, independent living skills training and peer support for individuals with disabilities. The mission of the Independent Living Center is to remove all barriers that limit the independence of persons with disabilities.

8012 Independent Living Resource Center

1760 Southridge Dr.
Jefferson City, MO 65109
573-556-0400
Fax: 573-556-0402; *Toll Free:* 877-627-0400
admin@ilrcjcmo.org
www.ilrcjcmo.org/
TTY: 573-634-3876

Stephanie Cooper, Executive Director
B.J Davis, President
Donna Borgmeyer, Vice President

Independent Living Resource Center, Inc. (ILRC) is a consumer controlled, not-for-profit agency that provides community-based services for persons with all types of disabilities. ILRC was incorporated June 28, 1996 by a group of citizens with disabilities and others concerned about disability issues. All ILRC programs are consumer-controlled. Consumers make all decisions in individual and group activities and staff assists and/or advocates as requested. In minimizing reliance on others, consumers learn to manage their own lives and make key decisions, which increases their independence and move toward self-determination. People with disabilities know their needs best and have the right to make decisions regarding their daily lives. Independent Living Resource Center, Inc. promotes a barrier-free environment, free of both architectural and attitudinal barriers that place limits on the independence of persons with disabilities. ILRC encourages greater independence for persons with disabilities within our community. Core services include that of information and referral, advocacy, peer counseling, and independent living skills training, in addition to assistive technology.

Year Founded: 1972

8013 Living Independently for Everyone (LIFE)

725 E Karsch Blvd.
Po Box 967
Farmington, MO 63640-1125
573-756-4314
Fax: 573-756-3507; *Toll Free:* 800-596-7273
tima@lifecilmo.org
www.lifecilmo.org
TTY: 573-760-1402

Robert Mooney, Chair
Roy Henson, Vice Chair
Jill Wolk, Secretary/Treasurer

Independent Living is based on the concept that a person with a disability can lead a constructive life as a functioning member of his/her community. It affirms that ones worth as a vital human being is not diminished because of a disability. Building skills and confidence to live an independent lifestyle requires special programs - programs that provide peer support, assistance in purchasing needed equipment, hiring and managing a personal careattendant and a whole spectrum of services provided by professional persons. These programs and services are offered through Centers for Independent Living. L.I.F.E is the Independent Living Center serving St. Francois, Madison and St. Genevieve counties in southeast Missouri. Core services provided by L.I.F.E. include that of information and

referral, advocacy, peer support, and independent living skills training.

Year Founded: 1997

8014 Midland Empire Resources for Independent Living (MERIL)

4420 South 40th Street
Saint Joseph, MO 64503
816-279-8558
Fax: 816-279-1550; *Toll Free:* 800-242-9326
meril@meril.org
www.meril.org
TTY: 816-579-4943

Tom Sinclair, Chairman
Dr. Bob Bush, Vice-Chairman
Jaren Pippit, Secretary

MERIL is a community-based, non-residential program, designed to promote independent living and to enhance the quality of life for persons with disabilities by empowering them to control and direct their lives and thus participate actively and independently in society. Our area is predominately rural and includes the nine-county area of Andrew, Atchison, Buchanan, Clinton, Holt, Nodaway, DeKalb, Gentry and Worth counties. Northwest Missouri has a high population of people with disabilities because of the extensive mental health services that exist here. MERIL also serves a large population of Deaf and hard of hearing persons and traumatic brain injury survivors. MERIL provides core services which include that of information and referral, advocacy, peer counseling and independent living skills training.

8015 NorthEast Independent Living Services (NEILS)

909 Broadway
Suite 350
Hannibal, MO 63401
573-221-8282
Fax: 573-221-9445; *Toll Free:* 877-713-7900
neils@neilscenter.org
www.neilscenter.org/
TTY: 573-221-8282

Brooke Kendrick, Executive Director
Rose McNally, President
Dawn Davis, Vice President

NorthEast Independent Living Services (N.E.I.L.S) was incorporated on May 2, 1994. N.E.I.L.S. began as a group of people with diverse physical disabilities who started a grassroots effort to educate the community about disability related issues in the Northeast Missouri areas. In February, 1996, N.E.I.L.S. received funding and opened for services. N.E.I.L.S. offers a full range of programs for individuals with a disability and any family members, employers, and/or co-workers with disability concerns. Four core services provided by NorthEast Independent Living Services (N.E.I.L.S) include that of information and referral, advocacy, independent living skills training and peer counseling, in addition to assistive technology support.

Year Founded: 1994

8016 On My Own

111 North Elm Street
Nevada, MO 64772-2609
417-667-7007
Fax: 417-667-6262; *Toll Free:* 800-362-8852
www.onmyowninc.com

Jennifer Gundy, Executive Director

A non-residential, Independent Living Center providing programs to persons with disabilities, core services of which include that of information and referral, advocacy, peer counseling, and independent living skills training. Advocacy works in partnership with consumers to resolve incidents of discrimination and denial of services through mediation with governments, business, and service providers. In addition, a clearing house of information concerning disabilities is available for access. Support in the form of one-on-one counseling and group counseling is available to assist individuals, families and groups with disability related problems and personal issues.

8017 Ozark Independent Living

109 Aid Avenue
West Plains, MO 65775
417-257-0038
Fax: 417-257-2380; *Toll Free:* 888-440-7500
info@ozarkcil.com
ozarkcil.com/index.php
TDD 417-256-8714

Clifford Steelman, Chair
Jeanne McLaughlin, President
Scott Schneider, Director of Business

Independent Living supports people with disabilities in having the opportunity to make their own decisions about things that affect their lives. Independent Living also supports self determination, the right and opportunity to try a course of action, and the freedom to fail and learn from your mistakes. The Independent Living philosophy believes in consumer power, self reliance, political and economic rights. Services are provided by people withdisabilities. Ozark Independent Living (OIL) was created to provide independent living services to persons with disabilities who reside in the following counties in Missouri: Oregon, Ozark, Shannon, Wright, Howell, Texas, and Douglas. OIL is non-profit, non-residential supported by grants, donations, and volunteers in addition to being funded by a grant from the Dept. of Elementary and Secondary Education and Vocational Rehabilitation of Missouri. OIL provides the core services of information and referral, peer support, independent living skills, and advocacy.

Year Founded: 1996

8018 Paraquad

5240 Oakland Avenue
Saint Louis, MO 63110
314-289-4200
Fax: 314-289-4201
contactus@paraquad.org
www.paraquad.org
TTY: 314-289-4252

John Sondag, Chairman
J. Gibson Henderson, Vice Chairman
Nancy Klepper, Secretary

Paraquad, Inc. is a private, not-for-profit community-based Center for Independent Living. Paraquad was founded in 1970 and is a St. Louis organization where professional independent living services are provided by staff members with disabilities. The fact that directors as well as staff members have disabilities enables us to establish keen insight into the ever-changing needs of individuals with all types of disabilities and to develop programs that respond to those needs. Paraquad's programs are created by staff, based on input from participants and have evolved and expanded along with the needs of the disability community. Paraquad exists for the sole purpose of offering services that assist people with disabilities to live independently in society. Our mission is fulfilled through direct and in-direct services as well as advocacy initiatives which shape our public policy agenda. Core services provided by Paraquad include that of information and referral, advocacy, peer counseling and independent living skills training.

8019 Rural Advocates for Independent Living (RAIL)

P.O.Box 98
Green City, MO 63545
660-874-4111
Fax: 660-665-9849
admin@nemr.net
www.nemr.net
TTY: 660-627-0614

Theresa Myers, Executive Director
Jean Robbins, Assistant to Executive Director
Carolyn Chambers, Legislative Specialist

RAIL's Mission is to assist persons with disabilities to live as independently as they choose within the communities of their choice. RAIL supports people in accomplishing this through: Peer Support - The RAIL staff helps organize formal support groups throughout our service area; Advocacy - RAIL helps those with disablilites learn their rights and how to exercise them for themselves; Information and Referral - RAIL provides persons with disablitities with information on programs, services and products that can help them live more independently; Independent Living Skills Training - Independent Living Specialists (ILS) help persons with disabilities learn specific skills they need to live as independently as they wish. These could include: Rearranging their living environment, using assistive devices, and learning activities to increase their independence.

8020 SEMO Alliance for Disability Independence (SADI)

1913 Rusmar Avenue
Cape Girardeau, MO 63703
573-651-6464
Fax: 573-651-6565; *Toll Free:* 800-898-7234
www.sadi.org
TTY: 573-651-6464

Steve Hodges, President
Jeff Harms, Vice President
Miriam Ganiel, Secretary

A community based, non-profit, nonresidential center for independent living. SADI is committed to providing services to persons with disabilities to enable them to remain in their own home and community, and not in an institution. Oue service area is predominantly rural. Information and referral services are offered to anyone living in the Southeast Missouri counties of Bollinger, Cape Girardeau, Mississippi, Perry, Scott, and city of Sikeston

Year Founded: 1949

8021 Services for Independent Living

1401 Hathman Place
Columbia, MO 65201
573-874-1646
Fax: 573-874-3564
www.silcolumbia.org
TTY: 573-874-4121

Tec Chapman, Executive Director
Cheryl Price, President
Dan Dunham, Vice President

Services for Independent Living (SIL) is a not-for-profit center for independent living (CIL). As a CIL, 51 percent or more of the agency's Board of Directors and staff are persons with disabilities who have personally experienced the attitudinal and physical barriers associated with having a disability. SIL educates people with disabilities about the many opportunities available in their community, enabling them to make more informed choices. People with disabilities have control over their lives through informed choices. SIL empowers people with disabilities, encouraging them to become informed and thereby control their lives. Change occurs on an individual and systems level through information, education, and advocacy. The core services provided by SIL are that of information and referral, advocacy, peer counseling, and independent living skills training.

8022 Southwest Center for Independent Living (SCIL)
2864 South Nettleton Avenue
Springfield, MO 65807
417-886-1188
Fax: 417-886-3619; *Toll Free:* 800-676-7245
scil@swcil.org
www.swcil.org
TTY: 417-886-1188

Dr. Amy C Lewis, President
Mark Grantham, Vice President
Pat Killingsworth, Secretary

The Southwest Center for Independent Living (SCIL) is a private, not-for-profit agency which was established in 1985 in Springfield, MO to provide services, advocacy, and resources for people with any disability in Southwest Missouri. SCIL is one of over 300 independent living centers around the country. People with disabilities serve on our board of directors and make up much of our staff. SCIL serves the counties of Christian, Dallas, Greene, Lawrence, Polk, Stone, Taney, and Webster. The mission of SCIL is to promote a barrier-free environment for all disabilities through public education and advocacy for social change, and to provide a full range of independent living services which will assist each in meeting his or her goals for independence. The basic consumer core services provided by SCIL include that of information and referral, advocacy, independent living skills training, and that of peer counseling, in addition to assistive technology support.

8023 Tri-County Center for Independent Living
1420 Hwy 72 East
Rolla, MO 65401-3638
573-368-5933
Fax: 573-368-5991
Douglas@fidmail.com
www.tricountycenter.com
TTY: 573-368-5933

Victoria Evans, Executive Director

Independent Living is having the opportunity to make decisions that affect your life - limited only in the same manner as a person without a disability. Tri-County Center for Independent Living is a not-for-profit organization designed to assist persons with disabilities to achieve and maintain as much independence as they wish and in the setting of their choice. The Center provides services to people with disabilities to enable them to live independently in their own homes. Core services provided by the Center include that of information and referral, advocacy, peer support and independent living skills training.

8024 West Central Independent Living Solutions (WCILS)
710 N College Street
Suite D
Warrensburg, MO 64093
660-422-7883
Fax: 660-422-7895; *Toll Free:* 800-236-5175
wils@iland.net
www.w-ils.org/
TTY: 660-422-7894

Kathy Kay, Executive Director
Cindy Price, Director of Programs
Julie Steele, Human Resources

Independent Living Centers (ILCs) help people with disabilities achieve or maintain more self-sufficient and productive lives in their communities. people with disabilities are assisted in exploring alternatives to institutionalization and are encouraged to make their own decisions about how they will live. ILCs directly provide or coordinate through referral those services, which assist people in increasing their abilities to exercise controlover their lives. Control over one's life means having a choice of acceptable options that minimize reliance on others in making decisions and performing every day activities. This includes managing one's own affairs, participating in day-to-day community life and fulfilling a range of social roles. West-Central Independent Living Solutions works to empower people with disabilities to become more independent by providing independent living skil ls training, peer support, information and referral and advocacy.

Montana

8025 Living Independently for Today & Tomorrow (LIFTT)
1201 Grand Avenue
Suite 1
Billings, MT 59102
406-259-5181
Fax: 406-259-5259; *Toll Free:* 800-669-6319
www.liftt.org
TTY: 406-245-1225

Dan MacDonald, President
Lavonne Kautzman, Vice President
Mary Westwood, Secretary

LIFTT's Independent living program works with people with disabilities so they can live independently and have access to the community. LIFTT staff, most of whom have disabilities, serve as mentors to people as they work to achieve the goals they have set for themselves. Core services provided by LIFTT include that of information and referral, advocacy, peer support and independent living skills training, in addition to guidance on accessibility and benefits counseling.

8026 Montana Independent Living Project
825 Great Northern Blvd
Helena, MT 59601-4768
406-442-5755
Fax: 406-442-1612; *Toll Free:* 800-735-6457
bmaffit@milp.us

www.milp.us
TTY: 406-442-5756

Bob Maffit, Executive Director
Betty Bergstrom, Chief Financial Officer
Les Clark, Independent Living Specialist

The philosophy of independent living promotes consumer control, peer support, self-help, self-determination, equal access, and individual and systems advocacy in order to maximize the leadership, empowerment, independence, and productivity of individuals with disabilities. Full inclusion and integration of individuals with disabilities into the mainstream of American society is primary. This philosophy is implemented through the Montana Independent Living Council and the network of Montana centers for independent living. The four centers and their satellites provide statewide coverage with centers situated in Great Falls, Helena, Missoula, Billings, Glasgow, Miles City, Glendive, Kalispell, Ronan, and Hamilton. Services include information and referral, individual and systems advocacy, peer support and independent living skills training in addition to assistive technology support.

8027 North Central Independent Living Services

1120 25th Avenue Northeast
Black Eagle, MT 59414
406-452-9834
Fax: 406-453-3940; Toll Free: 800-823-6245
ropper@mt.gov
www.dphhs.mt.gov
TTY: 406-452-9834

Richard Opper, Director
Sheila Lopach, Executive Assisstant
Deb Sloat, Human Resourcr Manager

The philosophy of independent living promotes consumer control, peer support, self-help, self-determination, equal access, and individual and systems advocacy in order to maximize the leadership, empowerment, independence, and productivity of individuals with disabilities. Full inclusion and integration of individuals with disabilities into the mainstream of American society is primary. This philosophy is implemented through the Montana Independent Living Council and the network of Montana centers for independent living. The four centers and their satellites provide statewide coverage with centers situated in Great Falls, Helena, Missoula, Billings, Glasgow, Miles City, Glendive, Kalispell, Ronan, and Hamilton. Services include that of information referral, advocacy, peer support and independent living skills training in addition to assistive technology support.

8028 Summit Independent Living Center-Kalispell

1203 Highway 2 W.
Suite 901
Kalispell, MT 59901-6020
406-257-0048
Fax: 406-257-0634; Toll Free: 800-995-0029
kalispell@summitilc.org
www.summitilc.org
TTY: 406-257-0048

Flo Kiewel, Country Co-ordinator
Gab Skibsrub, Board-Directors Kalispell Branch

Summit Independent Living Center Inc. is a non-profit non-residential program serving people with mobility impairments, neurological disorders, hearing impairments, learning disabilities, visual impairments and other disabling conditions. Summit's mission is to promote community

awareness, equal access, and the independence of people with disabilities through advocacy, education and the advancement of civil rights.

8029 Summit Independent Living Center-Missoula

700 Southwest Higgins Avenue
Suite 101
Missoula, MT 59803
406-728-1630
Fax: 406-829-3309; Toll Free: 800-398-9002
missoula@summitilc.org
www.summitilc.org
TTY: 406-728-1630

Mike Mayer, Executive Director
Kathy Boyer, Secretary

Summit Independent Living Cener, Inc. is a non-profit, non-residential program serving people with mobility impairments, neurological disorders, hearing impairments, learning disabilities, visual impairments, and other disabling conditions. Summit's mission is to promote community awareness, equal access, and the independence of people with disabilities through advocacy, education and the advancement of civil rights.

8030 Summit Independent Living Center-Ronan

111 Second Avenue Southwest
Ronan, MT 59864-2707
406-676-0190
Fax: 406-676-0190; Toll Free: 866-230-6936
ronan@summitilc.org
www.summitilc.org/
TTY: 406-676-0190

Gary Stevens, Director
Scott Williamson, Country Co-ordinator
Scott Williamson, Country Co-ordinator

Summit Independent Living Cener, Inc. is a non-profit, non-residential program serving people with mobility impairments, neurological disorders, hearing impairments, learning disabilities, visual impairments and other disabling conditions. Summit's mission is to promote community awareness, equal access, and the independence of people with disabilities through advocacy, education and the advancement of civil rights.

North Carolina

8031 Disability Rights And Resources

5801 Executive Center Drive
Suite 101'
Charlotte, NC 28212-8870
704-537-0550
Fax: 704-566-0507; Toll Free: 800-755-5749
mailto@disability-rights.org
www.disability-rights.org
TTY: 704-537-0550

Julia Sain, Executive Director
Maura Chavez, President
James Davis, Vice President

PAL's mission and purpose is to guard the civil rights of people with disabilities as we empower ourselves and others to live as we choose. At least 51% of PAL's staff is living with a disability and serve a four-county service area including Mecklenburg, Cabarrus, Gaston and Union counties. Core services include that of information and referral, advocacy, peer support and independent living skills training.

Year Founded: 1980

North Dakota

8032 Dakota Center for Independent Living

3111 East Broadway Avenue
Bismarck, ND 58501
701-222-3636
Fax: 701-222-0511; *Toll Free:* 800-489-5013
www.dakotacil.org/
TDD 701-222-3636

Robin Werre, President
Diane Tomlin, Vice President
Carol Mihulka, Secratary/Treasurer

The Dakota Center for Independent Living advocates for community based services and training opportunities that assist people with disabilities to live more independently. Outreach services are provided in eighteen south west and south central N.D. counties, and on the Standing Rock and the southern part of the Fort Berthold Native American reservations. The Dakota Center for Independent Living believes in self-determination for people with disabilities and creates the environment in which it is achieved. Services include that of information and referral, advocacy, independent living skills training, and peer support.

Year Founded: 1980

8033 Freedom Resource Center for Independent Living

2701 9th Avenue S
Suite H
Fargo, ND 58103
701-478-0459
Fax: 701-478-0510; *Toll Free:* 800-450-0459
freedom@freedomrc.org
www.freedomrc.org
TTY: 800-450-0459

Nate Aalgaard, Executive Director
Mikara Kverno, Information Specialist
Joyce Wolter, Independent Living Advocate

Freedom resource center is an independent non-profit organization, serving people of all ages and all disabilities. The mission of the Freedom Resource Center is to work toward equality and inclusion for people with disabilities through programs of empowerment, community education, and systems change.

8034 Independence

300 3rd Avenue Southwest
Suite F
Minot, ND 58701-4308
701-839-4724
Fax: 701-838-1677; *Toll Free:* 800-377-5114
independencecil@independencecil.org
www.independencecil.org/
TDD 701-839-4724

Susan Ogurek, Chairman
Heather Wittliff, Vice Chairman
Scott Burlingame, Executive Director

Independence, Inc, is a private non-profit corporation devoted to meeting the needs of individuals with disabilities and serving them, their families and communities. The mission is to advocate for the freedom of choice for individuals

with disabilities to live independently through the removal of barriers.

Year Founded: 1995

Nebraska

8035 Center for Independent Living of Central Nebraska

3204 College Street
Grand Island, NE 68803
308-382-9255
Fax: 308-384-7832; *Toll Free:* 877-400-1004
www.cilne.org
TTY: 308-382-9255

Joni Thomas, Executive Director
Irene Britt, Western Program Manager
Wendy Space, Independent Living Specialist

The Center for Independent Living of Central Nebraska provides a comprehensive set of services designed to enable persons with disabilities to exercise control over their lives based on their choices of acceptable options that minimize their reliance on other people in making decisions and in performing everyday activities. This includes their managing their affairs, fulfilling the range of social roles, making decisions that lead to self-determination and minimizing their physical and psychological dependence on others. Our center will always strews that independence is not a matter of ability or limitation, but is instead a matter of making educated choices. Services include that of information and referral, advocacy, independent living skills training, and peer support.

8036 League of Human Dignity Independent Living Center

1701 P Street
Lincoln, NE 68508-1799
402-441-7871
Fax: 402-441-7650
info@leagueofhumandignity.com
www.leagueofhumandignity.com
TTY: 402-441-7871

Mike Schafer, CEO

The League of Human Dignity is an organization of people concerned about the rights and quality of life for people with disabilities. League members collaborate to ensure social, economic, and political equality for persons with disabilities. We believe in emphasizing likeness not difference, ability not disability, normality not abnormality, and integration not segregation. We work toward independent living for people who have disabilities. Themission of the League of Human Dignity is to actively promote the full integration of individuals with disabilities into society. To this end, we will advocate their needs and rights, and provide quality services to involve these persons in becoming and remaining independent citizens. Services include that of information and referral, systems advocacy, individual advocacy, independent living skills training, and peer support.

Nevada

8037 Northern Nevada Center for Independent Living
999 Pyramid Way
Sparks, NV 89431-4471
775-353-3599
Fax: 702-353-3588
info@nncil.org
www.nncil.org/
TTY: 775-353-3599

Lisa Bonie, Executive Director
Hilda Velasco, Operations Manager
Joni Inglis, Independent Living Advocate

The Northern Nevada Center for Independent Living is a consumer-controlled, community-based, cross-disability, nonresidential, private, nonprofit agency that is designed and operated within the local community by individuals with disabilities. The Center provides an array of independent living services including the core services of information and referral, independent living skills training, peer counseling, and individual and systems advocacy. The purpose of the independent living program is to maximize the leadership, empowerment, independence, and productivity of individuals with disabilities and to integrate these individuals into the mainstream of American society.

Year Founded: 1982

8038 Southern Nevada Center for Independent Living
2950 S Rainbow Boulevard
Suite 220
Las Vegas, NV 89146
702-889-4216
Fax: 702-889-4574; *Toll Free:* 800-870-7003
sncil.sncil.org
www.sncil.org
TTY: 702-889-4216

Elliott Yug, President
William Sheehan, Vice President
Gary Cottino, Treasurer

SNCIL is founded on the belief that independent living is about consumer control. Guided by the Independent Living and People First Philosophy, the majority of board, staff and volunteers are individuals with disabilities. SNCIL provides services designed to empower people with disabilities to: make individual choices, assume responsibility to direct their lives, manager their own affairs, fulfill social roles, and achieve independent lifestyles in the community.

Year Founded: 1984

New Hampshire

8039 Granite State Independent Living Center
21 Chenell Drive
Concord, NH 03301
603-228-9680
Fax: 603-225-3304; *Toll Free:* 800-826-3700
info@gsil.org
www.gsil.org
TTY: 888-396-3459

Ron Page, Chair
Ken Traum, Vice Chair
Dan Hebert, 2nd Vice Chair

AÆstatewide non-profit, service and advocacy organization that provides tools for living life on your own terms-so you can navigate your own live and participate as fully as you choose in your community, just like everyone else.

New Jersey

8040 Alliance for Disabled in Action
629 Amboy Avenue
Lower Level
Edison, NJ 08837
732-738-4388
Fax: 732-738-4416
adacil@adacil.org
www.adacil.org
TTY: 732-738-9644

Colleen Roche, Chair
Bernard Zuckerman, Treasurer
Natalia Lapidus, Secretary

The Alliance for Disabled in Action, Inc. (ADA) is a private, not-for-profit center for independent living serving people in Middlesex, Somerset and Union Counties of New Jersey. Initially created in 1986 as an Independent Living Resource Center (as part of JFK Johnson Rehabilitation), the Alliance was incorporated as a separate, private non-profit organization in 1991. The Alliance provides information & referral, peer support, advocacy and Independent Living Skill training to people with all disabilities of all ages to increase their independence in all aspects of integrated community life. We respond to their families, businesses, and governments to enable them to better meet the needs of people with disabilities. We educate and influence our community in pursuit of full inclusion. People with disabilities should be empowered to control the direction of their own lives. This means corts and promote self-reliance. CILs advocate for the inclusion and integration of people with disabilities in all aspects of community living.hoosing their goals, plotting their course and taking responsibility for their actions and results. People with disabilities have the right to make their own choices and decisions and the right to make mistakes and learn/benefit from those mistakes. Centers for Independent Living foster independence facilitate the development of networks and supp

8041 Heightened Independence & Progress (HIP)
131 Main Street
Suite 120
Hackensack, NJ 07601-7182
201-996-9100
Fax: 201-996-9422
ber@hipcil.org
www.hipcil.org
TDD 201-996-9424

Jean Csaposs, Chair
Lottie Esteban, First Vice Chair
Betty A Fetzer, Second Vice Chairman

Centers for independent living (CILs) are private, nonprofit corporations that provide services to maximize the independence of individuals with disabilities and the accessibility of the communities they live in. Heightened Independence and Progress (HIP) is designed and operated within a local community by individuals with disabilities, providing an array of independent living services, including the core services of information and referral, independent living skills training, peer counseling, and individual and systems advocacy. The purpose of the independent living programs is to maximize the leadership, empowerment, independence, and productivity of individuals with disabilities and to integrate these individuals into the mainstream of American society.

8042 Heightened Independence & Progress-Hudson (HIP Hudson)

35 Journal Square
Suite 703
Jersey City, NJ 07306
201-533-4407
Fax: 201-533-4421
hud@hipcil.org
www.hipcil.org
TDD 201-533-4409
TTY: 201-533-4409

Jean Csaposs, Chair
Lottie Esteban, First Vice Chair
Betty A Fetzer, Second Vice Chairman

Centers for independent living (CILs) are private, nonprofit corporations that provide services to maximize the independence of individuals with disabilities and the accessibility of the communities they live in. Heightened Independence and Progress (HIP Hudson) is designed and operated within a local community by individuals with disabilities, providing an array of independent living services, including the core services of information and referral, independent living skills training, peer counseling, and individual and systems advocacy. The purpose of the independent living programs is to maximize the leadership, empowerment, independence, and productivity of individuals with disabilities and to integrate these individuals into the mainstream of American society.

8043 Moceans Center for Independent Living

279 Broadway 2nd Floor
Suite 201
Long Branch, NJ 07740-6941
732-571-4884
Fax: 732-571-4003
moceans@moceanscil.org
www.moceanscil.org
TDD 732-571-4878
TTY: 732-571-4878

Darryl Banks, Chair
Patricia McShane, Executive Director
Maureen Poling, Secretary

Centers for independent living (CILs) are private, nonprofit corporations that provide services to maximize the independence of individuals with disabilities and the accessibility of the communities they live in. MOCEANS Center for Independent Living is designed and operated within a local community by individuals with disabilities, providing an array of independent living services, including the core services of information and referral, independent living skills training, peer counseling, and individual and systems advocacy. The purpose of the independent living programs is to maximize the leadership, empowerment, independence, and productivity of individuals with disabilities and to integrate these individuals into the mainstream of American society.

8044 Progressive Center for Independent Living (PCIL)

1262 Whitehorse Hamilton Road
Suite 102, Bldg A
Hamilton, NJ 08690

609-581-4500
Fax: 609-581-4555; *Toll Free:* 877-917-4500
info@pcil.org
www.pcil.org
TTY: 609-581-4550

Scott Elliott, Executive Director
Eric Laufenberg, President
Norman Smith, Vice President

Centers for independent living (CILs) are private, nonprofit corporations that provide services to maximize the independence of individuals with disabilities and the accessibility of the communities they live in. Progressive Center for Independent Living (PCIL) is designed and operated within a local community by individuals with disabilities, providing an array of independent living services, including the core services of information and referral, independent living skills training, peer counseling, and individual and systems advocacy. The purpose of the independent living programs is to maximize the leadership, empowerment, independence, and productivity of individuals with disabilities and to integrate these individuals into the mainstream of American society.

Year Founded: 1996

New Mexico

8045 Ability Center for Independent Living

715 East Idaho Avenue
Bldg 3E
Las Cruces, NM 88001
575-526-5016
Fax: 575-526-1202; *Toll Free:* 800-376-4372
freedom@theabilitycenter.org
www.theabilitycenter.org
TTY: 505-526-5016

Ruth D Rodriguez, President
Cesasr Rodriguez, Vice-President
Rev. C. Neil Gibbs, Treasurer

The Ability Center for Independent Living (TACIL) is a center for independent living (CIL), and is a private, nonresidential, nonprofit New Mexico corporation. The purpose of a CIL is to provide a variety of services to promote independence, self-reliance, and community integration. The Ability Center strives to enable persons with disabilities to gain effective control and direction of their own lives. The Ability Center attempts to stimulate and promote a growing sense of personal dignity and responsible community participation of persons with disabilities through training, community development, and direct services. The Ability Center seeks to meet the unserved needs of persons with disabilities living in the counties of Catron, Doña Ana, Grant, Hidalgo, Luna, Otero, and Sierra, New Mexico. Our Advocacy, Informational & Referral program provides the four core services of the Rehabilitation Act of 1992 to individuals of all ages and disabilities. These services are advocacy, information and referral, peer counseling, and life skills training.

Year Founded: 1989

8046 New Vistas Independent Living Center

1205 Parkway Drive
Suite A
Santa Fe, NM 87507
505-471-1001
Fax: 505-471-4427; *Toll Free:* 800-737-0330

info@newvistas.org
www.newvistas.org
TTY: 505-471-1001

William A Moffett, President
Victor Ortega, Vice President
Gay Romero, Secretary/Treasurer

Centers for independent living (CILs) are private, nonprofit corporations that provide services to maximize the independence of individuals with disabilities and the accessibility of the communities they live in. New Vistas Independent Living Center offers services for people with all types of disabilities. Independence and community integration are promoted by providing options in the following areas: information and referral, advocacy, independent livings skills training, and peer support services.

Year Founded: 1971

New York

8047 Access to Independence and Mobility (AIM
271 East 1st Street
Corning, NY 14830-2924
607-962-8225
Fax: 607-937-5125
www.aimcil.com
TTY: 607-962-8225

Rene Snyder, Executive Director
Sabrina Mineo-O'Connell, President
George Spisack, Vice President

It is AIM's goal to enable the consumer to live an independent and comfortable lifestyle in the security of their home environment so they may feel dignity and pride in their achievements while controlling their own care. AIM is a human service agency with offices in Bath, Corning, Elmira and Hornell serving people whose lives have been affected by disability. AIM is a part of a national network of organizations called Independent Living Centers(ILC). An ILC is a nonresidential resource center run by and for people with a personal knowledge of disabilities. Our emphasis is on acknowledging consumers as unique individuals. Therefore, we often offer services and programs to meet specific requests. Our emphasis is on acknowledging consumers as unique individuals. Therefore, we often offer services and programs to meet specific requests. For instance, depending on a consumer's situation, wedent living skills such as money management, attendant care supervision and employment skills.may actively assist him or her in securing legal, civil, social or economic rights. Perhaps an individual's needs are more tangible - we can provide information on topics such as availability of accessing housing, sign language interpreters or TDDs. We can also help individual consumers access learning experiences and/or training to develop indepen

8048 Access to Independence and Mobility-Bath (AIM)
117 East Steuben Street
Bath, NY 14810
607-776-3838
Fax: 607-776-3838
www.aimcil.com
TDD 607-776-3838

Rene Snyder, Executive Director
Sabrina Mineo-O'Connell, President
George Spisack, Vice President

It is AIM's goal to enable the consumer to live an independent and comfortable lifestyle in the security of their home environment so they may feel dignity and pride in their achievements while controlling their own care. AIM is a human service agency with offices in Bath, Corning, Elmira and Hornell serving people whose lives have been affected by disability. AIM is a part of a national network of organizations called Independent Living Centers(ILC). An ILC is a nonresidential resource center run by and for people with a personal knowledge of disabilities. Our emphasis is on acknowledging consumers as unique individuals. Therefore, we often offer services and programs to meet specific requests. For instance, depending on a consumer's situation, we may actively assist him or her in securing legal, civil, social or economic rights. Perhaps an individual's needs are more tangible - we can provide information on topics such as availability of accessing housing, sign language interpreters or TDDs. We can also help individual consumers access learning experiences and/or training to develop independent living skills such as money management, attendant care supervision and employment skills.

8049 Auburn Options for Independence
75 Genesee Street
Auburn, NY 13021-3667
315-255-3447
Fax: 315-255-0836; *Toll Free:* 800-496-9148
gguy@optionsforindependence.org
www.optionsforindependence.org/
TTY: 315-255-3447

Greg Guy, Executive Director
Nancy Wise, Chairperson
Judy Dove, First Vice-Chairperson

Options For Independence is an Independent Living Center which assists people with disabilities to gain opportunities, make their own decisions, pursue activities and become part of community life. We provide a variety of services to all people with disabilities, their family and friends in Cayuga and Seneca Counties. Services include that of information and referral, advocacy, independent living skills training, and peer support. Additionally, the Center also has a Resource Library in which we continually develop and collect information and subscribe to a variety of journals and disability related periodicals, including a magazine written in Braille for use. Options also has a selection of books on tape and the necessary equipment to use them from the Library of Congress Talking Book Program that may be borrowed by customers.

8050 Bronx Independent Living Services
4419 Third Avenue
Suite 2C
Bronx, NY 10457
718-515-2800
Fax: 718-515-2803
www.bils.org
TTY: 718-515-2803

Brett L Eisenberg, Executive Director
Barbara Linn, President
Anita Richichi, Vice President

Bronx Independent Living Services, Inc. (BILS) is a not-for-profit community agency serving people with all kinds of disabilities. Our mission is to empower people with disabilities toward living independent lives. We assist individuals by providing advocacy, peer counseling, housing information, and independent living training/counseling. We also work to educate and advocate for legislative and social change so that people who have disablties can live more independently. We educate people about their civil and human rights, and work on providing access to the tools and means necessary to insure those rights. A part of the international Independent Living movement, we are oriented towards self-help and control by those who are actually concerned.

8051 Brooklyn Center for Independence of the Disabled

27 Smith Street
Suite 200
Brooklyn, NY 11201
718-998-3000
Fax: 718-998-3743
advocate@bcid.org
www.bcid.org
TTY: 718-998-7406

Zainab Jama, Executive Director

The Brooklyn Center for Independence of the Disabled, Inc. (BCID) is a non-profit, grass roots organization operated by a majority of people with disabilities since 1956. We are dedicated to guaranteeing the civil rights of people with disabilities. We exist to improve the quality of life of Brooklyn residents with disabilities through programs that empower them to gain greater control of their lives and achieve full and equal integration into society. We accomplish this through our services, our advocacy for systems change to remove physical, attitudinal and communication barriers to people with disabilities, and through our education and awareness programs.

Year Founded: 1956

8052 Capital District Center for Independent Living

875 Central Avenue
South 3
Albany, NY 12206
518-459-6422
Fax: 518-459-7847
info@cdciweb.com
www.cdciweb.com/index.html
TDD 518-459-6422

Laurel Lei Kelley, Executive Director
Dawn Werner, Deputy Director
Judy Zuchero, Program Director

Established in 1979, Capital District Center for Independence, Inc., one of 37 Independent Living Centers (ILC) in New York State, was initially known as Wheels to Independence. Upon incorporation in 1980, the name was officially changed to better reflect the wide range of services provided by the ILC. The Center is a non-residential, community based organization, which primarily serves Albany and Schenectady Counties; however some programs extend beyond these regions. By assisting people with disabilities to acquire self-advocacy skills and by teaching through example (peer advocacy), consumers achieve greater control over the direction of their lives. Staff and volunteers strive to educate community leaders and the general public in the areas of inclusion and universal access to enlist their support in the removal of attitudinal, economic and structural

barriers, which prevent equalparticipation of people with disabilities in all aspects of community life.

8053 Catskill Center for Independence

6104 State Highway 23
Oneonta, NY 13820-5247
607-432-8000
Fax: 607-432-6907
ccfi@ccfi.us
www.ccfi.us
TTY: 607-432-8000

Chris Zachmeyer, Executive Director
Edward Lynch, Operations Manager
Charles Reichardt, Systems Advocate

Independent living centers are consumer driven What this means is that at least 50% of our governing board must be a person with a disability. Many of us who work at the Center are also people with disabilities. So independent living centers are run by people with disabilities for people with disabilities. We assist people with disabilities to achieve independence in everyday life. The Catskill Center for Independence is one of thirty-seven independent centers located throughout the state of New York. The Center provides a variety of services to individuals with disabilities who reside in Delaware, Otsego, or Schoharie County. The Center also provides information, training and other disability related assistance to family members and friends of people with disabilities, employers, landlords, government and other agencies and members of both the private and business sectors of our community.

8054 Center for Independence of Disabled in New York (CIDNY)

841 Broadway
Suite 301
New York, NY 10003
212-674-2300
Fax: 212-254-5953
info@cidny.org
www.cidny.org
TTY: 212-674-5619

Martin Eichel, President
Anne M Davis, Vice President
John O Neill, Vice President

The Center for Independence of the Disabled, New York's (CIDNY) goal is to ensure full integration, independence and equal opportunities for all people with disabilities by removing barriers to the social, economic, cultural and civic life of the community. CIDNY is a non-profit organization founded in 1979. We are part of the Independent Living Cenres movement- a national network of grassroots and community-based organizations that enhance opportunities for all people with disabilities to direct their own lives.

Year Founded: 1978

8055 Finger Lakes Independence Center

215 5th Street
Ithaca, NY 14850-3403
607-272-2433
Fax: 607-272-0902
flic@clarityconnect.com
www.fliconline.org

Lenore Schwager, Executive Director

The Finger Lakes Independence Center assists all people with disabilities, their families and friends to promote independence and make informed decisions in pursuit of their goals. Our services are free of charge. We primarily serve residents of Tompkins, Cortland and Schuyler counties. We believe that a society which is inclusive of people with disabilities is beneficial to all of its members. Furthermore, we believe that individual and group attitudes toward people with disabilities often create closed social structures and architectural barriers which are detrimental to all members of society. The mission of the Finger Lakes Independence Center is to work toward the elimination of these obstacles, to empower people with disabilites, and thereby create an inclusive society.

8056 Harlem Independent Living Center

289 Saint Nicholas Avenue
Suite 21 Lower Level Between 124 & 125 Street
New York, NY 10027
212-222-7122
Fax: 212-222-7199; *Toll Free:* 800-673-2371
www.hilc.org
TTY: 212-222-7198

Christina Curry, Executive Director

The mission of the Harlem Independent Living Center is to create an accessible society where persons with disabilities realize their full potential throughout their lives. Services include information and referral, advocacy, independent living skills training, and peer support.

8057 Independent Center-Southern Tier

135 East Frederick
St. Binghamton, NY 13904
607-724-2111
Fax: 607-722-3600; *Toll Free:* 877-722-9150
stic@stic-cil.org
www.stic-cil.org
TTY: 677-242-2111

Maria Dibble, Executive Director

In addition to providing services, the Southern Tier Independence Center is a gathering place for people and information. Our joint efforts in understanding the issues and concerns of people with disabilities can pave the way to this more accessible world. Services include that of information and referral, advocacy, independent living skills training, and peer support.

8058 Independent Living Center of Hudson Valley

802 Columbia Street
Hudson, NY 12534
518-828-4886
Fax: 518-828-2592
jbachman@ilchv.org
www.ilchv.org
TTY: 518-828-6293

Denise A Figueroa, Executive Director
Vincent Reiter, Personal Assistance Services
Arlene Burt, Peer Advocate

The Independent Living Center of the Hudson Valley is rooted in a philosophy of self reliance and self determination. We offer the following services to individuals with disabilities and their families: advocacy; peer counseling; benefits advisement; information and referral; housing information; consultation on architectural barriers; transportation; independent livings skills training; employment services; and personal assistance services.

Year Founded: 1987

8059 Independent Living of the Hudson Valley

15-17 Third Street
Troy, NY 12180
518-274-0701
Fax: 518-274-7944
admin@ilchv.org
www.ilchv.org
TTY: 518-274-0701

Denise A Figueroa, Executive Director
Vincent Reiter, Personal Assistance Services
Arlene Burt, Peer Advocate

The Independent Living Center of the Hudson Valley is rooted in a philosophy of self reliance and self determination. We offer the following services to individuals with disabilities and their families: advocacy; peer counseling; benefits advisement; information and referral; housing information; consultation on architectural barriers; transportation; living skills training; employment services, and personal assistance services.

Year Founded: 1987

8060 Long Island Center for Independent Living

3601 Hempstead Turnpike
Suite 208 & 500
Levittown, NY 11756-1331
516-796-0144
Fax: 516-520-1247
licil@aol.com
www.licil.net
TTY: 516-796-0135

Patricia Moore, Executive Director
Joan Lynch, Deputy Director

The Long Island Center for Independent Living, is committed to the empowerment of consumers with disabilities. LICIL staff functions as ambassadors to the belief that individuals with disabilities have a responsibility to take an active role in their own lives and a self-determined view of their futures. Services include that of information and referral, advocacy, independent living skills training, and peer support.

8061 Massena Independent Living Center

43 Broadway
Suite 1
Saranac Lake, NY 12983
518-891-5295
Fax: 518-891-5293
info@tlcil.org
www.tlcil.org
TTY: 518-891-5293

Michael Northrop, President
Carol Techman, Vice President
Beatrice Beguin, Secretary

AÆprivate non-for-profit Organization that remains true to our mandate to be Consumer controlled and operated (by and for the people with disabilities). Incorporated in 1987, MILC has assisted thousands of North Country residents to increase their independence and access to community life. The MILC hs the important but unfulfilled Mission of working to ensure that we and our nation's more than 45 million fellow people experiencing disabilities are one day able to participate in, and be considered as equals in, all areas and aspects of the American way of life.

8062 New York State Independent Living Council
111 Washington Avenue
Suite 101
Albany, NY 12210-2280
518-427-1060
Fax: 518-427-1139; *Toll Free:* 888-469-7452
nysilc@nysilc.org
www.nysilc.org
TTY: 518-427-1060

Denise A Figueroa, Chair
Susan Gray, Vice Chair
Brad Williams, Executive Director

The New York State Independent Living Council, Inc. is made up of representatives, a majority of whom have disabilities, from around the State, who are appointed by the Board of Regents. It is a not-for-profit, non-Governmental, consumer controlled organization which monitors the federally funded Independent Living Centers in New York State, promotes the independent living philosophy statewide, and provides support and technical assistance to the entire network of Independent Living Centers (ILC) in New York State.

8063 North Country Center for Independence
80 Sharron Avenue
Plattsburgh, NY 12901-3827
518-563-9058
Fax: 518-563-0292
andrew@ncci-online.com
www.ncci-online.com
TTY: 518-563-9058

Robert Poulin, Executive Director
Ted Graser, President
Kathy Latinville, Vice President

The Mission of the North Country Center for Independence is to empower people with disabilities to live more independent and productive lives, and to promote beneficial policies and community understanding of disability issues. All people have value, should be treated with respect, and have the right to make choices about their own lives. People with disabilities are limited mainly by the barriers they encounter in society. If they have the knowledge, tools and freedom they need, all pepople with disabilities can live independently, carry out the responsibilities of citizenship and reach their full potential.

8064 Northern Regional Center for Independent Living
210 Court Street
Suite 107
Watertown, NY 13601-4546
315-785-8703
Fax: 315-785-8612; *Toll Free:* 800-583-8703
nrcil@nrcil.net
www.nrcil.net
TDD 315-785-8703
TTY: 315-785-8703

Brenda Campany, Executive Director
Ronald Griffin, President
Michael Simmons, Vice President

Northern Regional Center for Independent Living is a disability rights and resource center that promotes community efforts to end discrimination, segregation, and prejudice against people with disabilities. NRCIL serves people with disabilities and their families in Jefferson and Lewis counties. Services include that of information and referral, advocacy, independent living skills training, and peer counseling.

8065 Olean Center
512 West State Street
Olean, NY 14760-2544
716-373-4602
Fax: 716-373-4604
info@oleanilc.org
www.oleanilc.org/
TTY: 716-373-4602

Leonard Liguori, Executive Director
Marcella M Richmond, President
Christina Veno, Vice President

Directions in Independent Living can help people with disabilities learn to have more control over their own lives and to live more independently in their communities. Basic core services include that of information and referral, advocacy, independent living skills training, and peer support.

Year Founded: 1988

8066 Regional Center for Independent Living
497 State Street
Rochester, NY 14608
585-442-6470
Fax: 585-271-8558
rcil@rcil.org
www.rcil.org
TTY: 585-442-6470

Bruce Darling, Executive Director
Shelly Perrin, Chairperson
Bobbi Wallach, Vice Chairperson

The mission of the Regional Center for Independent Living is to empower people with disabilities to self-advocate, to live independently and to enhance the quality of community life. Our services and programs are primarily of an advocacy nature (both individual and systems). We seek to overcome the barriers faced by people with disabilities who choose to live independently. The independent living philosophy supports persons with disabilities having opportunities to make decisions that affect their lives just as their nondisabled counterparts do.

8067 Resource Center for Accessible Living
727 Ulster Avenue
Kingston, NY 12401
845-331-0541
Fax: 845-331-2076
office@rcal.org
www.rcal.org/
TTY: 845-331-8680

Paula Kindos, President
Bernadette Mueller, Vice President
Darlene Donofrio, Vice President

RCAL is a non-profit, community based service and advocacy organization run by and for people with any type of disability. Since 1983, RCAL has been dedicated to assisting and empowering individuals, of all ages, to live independently and participate in all aspects of community life. RCAL, as an Independent Living Center, has a long tradition of consumer controlled and directed service delivery. This approach, combined with OMRDD's newer PersonalCentered Planning ensures that participants will get the assistance in areas of their choice. It is the RCAL's philosophy that people with disabilities can and should make their own choices and decisions, and take control of all issues that affect their daily lives-education, employment, housing, healthcare, recreation, etc.

8068 Resource Center for Independent Living
497 State Street
Rochester, NY 14608
585-442-6470
Fax: 585-271-8558
rcil@rcil.com
www.rcil.com
TDD 315-797-5837
TTY: 585-442-6470

Bruce Darling, Executive Director
Shelly Perrin, Chairperson
Bobbi Wallach, Vice Chairperson

RCIL is a civil rights organization offering a wide range of independent living and advocacy services for and — most importantly — with people with disabilities. To support these goals, RCIL helps individuals of all ages and types of disability obtain the community supports and services they need to live independently including that of information and referral, advocacy, independent living skills training, and peer support.

8069 Resource Center for Independent Living (RCIL)
497 State Street
Rochester, NY 14608
585-442-6470
Fax: 585-271-8558
www.rcil.com/
TTY: 585-442-6470

Bruce Darling, Executive Director
Shelly Perrin, Chairperson
Bobbi Wallach, Vice Chairperson

Resource Center for Independent Living (RCIL) is a civil rights organization offering a wide range of independent living and advocacy services for and — most importantly — with people with disabilities. To support these goals, RCIL helps individuals of all ages and types of disability obtain the community supports and services they need to live independently. Services include that of information and referral, advocacy, independent living skills training and peer support.

8070 Rockland Independent Living Center
873 Route 45
Suite 108
New City, NY 10956
845-624-1366
Fax: 845-624-1369
info@rilc.org
www.rilc.org
TTY: 845-426-3053

George Hoehmann, Executive Director / CEO
David Goldwasser, President
Patricia Ranieri, First Vice President

The Rockland Independent Living Center (RILC) is a not-for profit agency serving all individuals with disabilities. RILC is one of 37 Independent Living Centers in NY State helping to promote the philosophy of consumer empowerment and control. This includes all areas of life education, recreation, employment, housing, and community involvement. RILC opened its doors in October 1986 as a result of the hard work and perseverance of several individ-

uals who were committed to removing architectural, attitudinal and legislative barriers to accessibility.

8071 Westchester Disabled on the Move
984 North Broadway
Suite LL10
Yonkers, NY 10701
914-968-4717
Fax: 914-968-6137
info@wdom.org
www.wdom.org
TDD 914-968-4717
TTY: 914-968-4717

Melvin R Tanzman, Executive Director
Gail Caetenuto Cohn, President
Mattie Trupia, Vice President

Westchester Disabled on the Move is a notfor-profit community based organization. It is a non-residentail center for people with disabilities. WDOMI is part of a network of Independent Living Centers dedicated to independence and equal rights for individuals with disabilities. Westchester Disabled On the Move, Inc. is staffed and governed primarily by people with disabilities. The programs and services of WDOMI are free to consumers with disabilities and their families. WDOMI does not discriminate based on age, sex, disability, race or ethnicity, sexual orientation or religion.

8072 Westchester Independent Living Center
200 Hamilton Avenue
White Plains, NY 10601-1812
914-682-3926
Fax: 914-682-8518
www.wilc.org
TDD 914-682-0926

Joe Bravo, Executive Director
Mildred Caballero Ho, Deputy Executive Director
Gerard Fleming, President

The Westchester Independent Living Center, Inc. (WILC) is a not-for-profit, community-based advocacy and resource center that serves people with all types of disabilities. It is part of a national network of centers that provide a wide spectrum of non-residential and non-medical services including that of information and referral, advocacy, independent living skills training, and peer support.

Year Founded: 1981

Ohio

8073 Ability Center of Greater Toledo
5605 Monroe Street
Sylvania, OH 43560-2793
419-885-5733
Fax: 419-882-4813; *Toll Free:* 866-885-5733
tharrington@abilitycenter.org
www.abilitycenter.org
TTY: 419-885-5733

Tim Harrington, Executive Director
Lisa Justice, Executive Assisstant
Dale Abell, Director Of Program Development

The Ability Center is a non-profit independent living center in Northwest Ohio. The Center serves seven Ohio counties: Defiance, Fulton, Henry, Lucas, Ottawa, Williams and Wood; with satellite offices in Defiance and Ottawa counties. Our mission is to assist people with disabilities to live their lives as independently as possible. We do this by providing several core services including that of information and referral, advocacy, independent living skills training, and peer support.

8074 Access Center for Independent Living

901 S Ludlow St
Dayton, OH 45402-2614
937-341-5202
Fax: 937-341-5217
info@acils.com
www.acils.com
TTY: 937-341-5218

Alan R Cochrun, Executive Director
Greg Kramer, Senior IL Specialist/Assist. Dir
Maria Matzik, Events Coordinator

The mission of the Access Center for Independent Living (ACIL) is to ensure that people with disabilities have full and complete access to the community in which they reside. The four core programs provided by the Center are that of advocacy, information and referral, independent living skills training, and peer support.

Year Founded: 1984

8075 Center for Independent Living Options (CILO)

2031 Auburn Avenue
Cincinnati, OH 45219
513-241-2600
Fax: 513-241-1707
cilo@cilo.net
www.cilo.net
TTY: 513-241-7170

Lin Laing, Executive Director
Justin Bifro, President
Brian Frazier, Vice President

The Center for Independent Living Options (CILO) is dedicated to helping individuals who have physical, sensory, cognitive, and/or phychological disabilities to maintain active, productive lives of their choosing. In fact, we are who we serve. We are governed, managed, and staffed by a majority of professionals with disabilities. This gives us personal insight into the issues that people with disabilities face. Our mission is to break down architectural and attitudinal barriers, build bridges to understanding, and create options and choices in the continuous process of empowerment of persons with disabilities.

8076 Society for Equal Access Independent Living Center

1458 5th St. NW
New Philadelphia, OH 44663-1224
330-343-3668
Fax: 330-343-3721; *Toll Free:* 888-213-4452
drenicker@seailc.org
seailc.org/
TDD 330-602-2557

Dianne Renicker, Executive Director
Scott Huston, President
Edna Fillinger, Vice President

The Society for Equal Access works with individuals with disabilities to help them become more independent. Our agency assists with Peer Support, Advocacy, Information and Referral and Independent Living Skills. Our goal is to move individuals with disabilties in the direction of independence and help them become active members within the community.

8077 Tri-County Independent Living Center

680 East Market Street
Suite 205
Akron, OH 44304-1640
330-762-0007
Fax: 330-762-7416
rose@tcilc.org
www.tcilc.org
TTY: 800-750-0750

Rose Juriga, Executive Director

Founded in 1985, Tri-County Independent Living Center, Inc. is a non-residential, non-profit 501(c)(3) organization whose Board of Directors and staff is comprised of a majority of persons with various disabilities. Tri-County's mission is to empower citizens with disabilities to be in charge of their lives and participate as members of their communities. Through our collective strength, we advocate for the elimination of societal barriers and strive to achieve community accessibility and acceptance. Services include that of information and referral, advocacy, independent living skills training, community education and technical assistance, and peer support.

Oklahoma

8078 Ability Resources

823 South Detroit Avenue
Suite 110
Tulsa, OK 74120-4223
918-592-1235
Fax: 918-592-5651; *Toll Free:* 800-722-0886
clawson@ability-resources.org
www.ability-resources.org

Carla Lawson, Executive Director
Debby Newman, Office Manager
Tita Talbot, Finance Manager

Ability Resources' mission is to assist people with disabilities in attaining and maintaining their personal independence. One way this can be achieved is in the creation of an environment in which people with disabilities can exercise their rights to control and direct their own lives. Services include that of information and referral, advocacy, independent living skills training, and peer support.

8079 Progressive Independence

121 North Porter Avenue
Norman, OK 73071-5834
405-321-3203
Fax: 405-321-7601
www.progind.org
TDD 800-801-3203
TTY: 405-321-2942

Scott Spray, Chairperson
Teresa Tisdell, Vice-Chairman
Mark Newman, Treasurer

Offers information and referrals, advocacy, peer counseling and independent living skills training.

Oregon

8080 Eastern Oregon Center for Independent Living

1021 SW 5th Avenue
Ontario, OR 97914

541-889-3119
Fax: 541-889-4647; *Toll Free:* 866-248-8369
eocil@eocil.org
www.eocil.org
TTY: 541-889-3119

Drea Williams, President
Carolyn Haney, Vice President
Kirt Toombs, CEO

Eastern Oregon Center for Independent Living (EOCIL) is a nonprofit community-based resource and advocacy center that promotes independent living and equal access for all persons with disabilities. Based in Ontario, Oregon, with a second office in Pendleton, it serves consumers in 10 eastern Oregon counties. EOCIL operates from a philosophy of consumer control, peer models and self-advocacy. The desired outcome of all EOCIL independent living services is to improve the individual's ability to function, continue functioning, or move toward functioning independently in his or her family or community.

8081 Holiday Retirement Communities
5885 Meadows Road
Suite 500
Lake Oswego, OR 97035
Toll Free: 800-322-0999
info@holidaytouch.com
www.holidaytouch.com

Jack R Callison, Chief Executive Officer
Kai Hsiao, President
Scott Shanaberger, Chief Financial Officer

Holiday Retirement sets out to create an independent living lifestyle unlike anything seniors have ever experienced before: cheerful communities filled with friendly, accepting neighbors, dedicated satff, and opportunities for personal growth. They have 300 Holiday Retirement communities across the United States and Canada.

Year Founded: 1971

8082 Independent Living Resources, Inc. (ILR)
1839 NE Couch Street
Portland, OR 97232
503-232-7411
Fax: 503-232-7480
info@ilr.org
www.ilr.org
TDD 503-232-8408
TTY: 503-232-8408

Barry Fox Quamee, Executive Director
Barbara Norris, Office Manager
May Altman, Associate Director

Independent Living Resources (ILR) is a non-profit organization dedicated to helping people with disabilities. The agency provides services using both staff and volunteers. By offering the core services of Advocacy, Information and Referral, Peer Counseling, and Skills Training, ILR continues to help over 3000 people annually. Its mission is to promote the philosophy of Independent Living by creating opportunities, encouraging choices, advancingequal access, and furthering the level of independence for all people with disabilities.

Year Founded: 1957

8083 SPOKES Unlimited
1006 Main Street
Klamath Falls, OR 97601-6003

541-883-7547
Fax: 541-885-2469
www.spokesunlimited.org
TTY: 541-883-7547

Wendy Howard, Executive Director

Offers information and referrals, advocacy, peer counseling and independent living skills training.

Pennsylvania

8084 Anthracite Region Center for Independent Living
8 West Broad Street
Suite 228
Hazleton, PA 18201-7801
570-455-9800
Fax: 570-455-1731; *Toll Free:* 800-777-9906
www.anthracitecil.org
TDD 800-777-9906
TTY: 570-455-9800

Irene Mordosky, President
Margo Madden, Vice President
Rand Martin, Treasurer

The mission of the Anthracite Region Center for Independent Living is to enable individuals with disabilities to attain their highest possible level of independence.

8085 Center for Independent Living of Central Pennsylvania
207 House Avenue
Suite 107
Camp Hill, PA 17011-4908
717-731-1900
Fax: 717-731-8150; *Toll Free:* 800-323-6060
office@cilcp.org
www.cilcp.org
TTY: 717-737-1335

Theotis Braddy, Executive Director

The Center For Independent Living of Central Pennsylvania (CILCP)is a non-profit, nonresidential organization established for and by people with disabilities. To empower people with disabilities to fully participate in all aspects of society is the guiding principal of the CILCP. The mission of the Center is to advance the rights of persons with disabilities through the elimination and prevention of barriers that people with disabilities experience. Community participation is an integral part of the Center's activities.

8086 Citizens for Independence and Access
150 Roosevelt Avenue
Suite 300
York, PA 17401-9311
717-849-0991
Fax: 717-849-0996; *Toll Free:* 800-956-0099
hhillary@verizon.net
www.livingwellwithadisability.org
TDD 717-840-9753
TTY: 717-757-4556

Hillary Hasson, Executive Director

8087 Community Resources for Independence
3410 West
12th Street
Erie, PA 16505

814-838-7222
Fax: 814-835-5104; *Toll Free:* 800-530-5541
www.crinet.org
TTY: 814-838-8115

Timothy J Finegan, Executive Director
William Essigman, Administrative Program Manager
Carl Berry, Human Resources Director

Mission statement of the Community Resources for Independence, Inc. is that the we will strive, in partnership with others, to empower people with disabilities to become fully integrated into society.

8088 Freedom Valley Disability Enablement
3607 Chapel Road
Newtown Square, PA 19073-3602
610-353-6640
Fax: 610-353-6753; *Toll Free:* 800-427-4754
facopefvdc@msn.com
www.livingwellwithadisability.org
TDD 610-353-6753
TTY: 610-353-8900

Ann Cope, Executive Director

Offers information and referrals, advocacy, peer counseling, and independent living skills training.

8089 Lehigh Valley Center for Independent Living
435 Allentown Drive
Allentown, PA 18109
610-770-9781
Fax: 610-770-9801; *Toll Free:* 800-495-8245
info@lvcil.org
www.lvcil.org
TTY: 610-770-9789

Rev. Joy Lynn Wyler, President
Ham Malek, Vice President
Dr. Lisa Marie McCauley, Treasurer

The Lehigh Valley Center for Independent Living, Inc. (LVCIL) is proud to be one of Pennsylvania's 18 centers for Independent Living. LVCIL is a private non-profit organization. We are both staffed and governed, at all times, by a majority of persons with disabilities. All Centers for Independent Living place the greatest emphasis on consumer self-determination, we are not here to make decisions for our consumers, but to provide information and resources to allow consumers to make independent decisions. We also work to increase inclusion in our community whether it is in housing, transportation, voting rights, employment, or many other ideas.

Year Founded: 1990

8090 Liberty Resources
714 Market Street
Suite 100
Philadelphia, PA 19106
215-634-2000
Fax: 215-634-6628; *Toll Free:* 888-634-2155
LRinc@libertyresources.org
www.libertyresources.org
TDD 215-634-6630

Mary Ellen Caffrey, Co-chairman
James K Goodwin, Co-chairman
Melissa Monser, Vice Chairperson

Liberty Resources, Inc. is a non-profit, Consumer driven organization that advocates and promotes Independent Living for persons with disabilities. More than 50 percent of

our Board as well as 50 percent of our employees are persons with disabilities. Liberty Resources, Inc. is the Center for Independent Living for the Philadelphia area, which advocates for and works with persons with disabilities to ensure their civil rights and equal access to all aspects of live in our community. It is our hope that the Center will be seen as the major point of entry into the community for people with disabilities, in Philadelphia and the surrounding area, a place where an individual can make contact and receive the services they need, or are referred to appropriate organizations in the community.

Year Founded: 1980

8091 Life and Independence for Today
503 East Arch Street
Saint Marys, PA 15857-1779
814-781-3050
Fax: 814-781-1917; *Toll Free:* 800-341-5438
lift@liftcil.org
www.liftcil.org

Robert Mecca, Executive Director
Stephen DePrater, President
Linda McKinstry, Vice President

Life and Independence for Today (LIFT) is a non-profit organization developed by people with disabilities for people with disabilities. As a Center for Independent Living (CIL) LIFT offers services to enable people with disabilities to achieve new goals and broaded their horizons. It enables them to achieve and maintain self-sufficient and productive lives. Most services are provided free of charge and availiable to all age groups.

8092 Northeast Pennsylvania Center for Independent Living
1142 Sanderson Avenue
Scranton, PA 18509
570-344-7211
Fax: 570-344-7218; *Toll Free:* 800-344-7211
nepacilinfo@nepacil.org
www.mycil.org
TTY: 570-344-5275

Daniel Loftus, Executive Director

The Northeast Pennsylvania Center for Independent Living was established to assist in removing barriers and expanding independent living options availiable to people with disabilities in the counties of Bradford, Columbia, Lackawanna, Luzerne, Monroe, Pike, Sullivan, Susquehanna, Wayne and Wyoming. The individual controls and directs the services he or she receives to establish a more independent lifestyle.

8093 Three Rivers Center for Independent Living
900 Rebecca Avenue
Pittsburgh, PA 15221
412-371-7700
Fax: 412-371-9430; *Toll Free:* 800-633-4588
sholbrook@trcil.org
trcil.myfastsite.net/
TTY: 412-371-6230

Stan Holbrook, Executive Director

The mission of the Three Rivers Center for Independent Living is to empower people with disabilities to enjoy self-directed, personally meaningful lives by providing outstanding consumer controlled services and by advocating for effective community change.

Year Founded: 1983

8094 Tri-County Partnership for Independent Living
69 East Beau Street
Washington, PA 15301-4711
724-223-5115
Fax: 724-223-5119; *Toll Free:* 877-889-0965
www.tripil.com
TDD 724-228-4028
TTY: 724-228-4028

Gerald Longsretch, Chairperson
Larry Smith, Vice Chairperson
Kathleen Kleinmann, CEO/Executive Director

The mission/purpose of TRPIL is to teach ourselves about the past, present, and future prospects of the Independent living movement as part of the disability and equal rights movement; to share ideas towards the building of a common vision for Independent Living in Pennsylvania; and to strengthen our sense of community and common purpose as part of the local, state, national, and international independent living movement.

Rhode Island

8095 Ocean State Center for Independent Living
1944 Warwick Avenue
Warwick, RI 02289
401-738-1013
Fax: 401-738-1083; *Toll Free:* 866-857-1161
info@oscil.org
www.oscil.org
TTY: 401-738-1015

Lorna Ricci, Executive Director

Ocean State Center for Independent Living (OSCIL) is a consumer controlled, community based, nonprofit organization established to provide a range of independent living services to enhance, through self direction, the quality of life of Rhode Islanders with significant disability and to promote integration into the community.

Year Founded: 1988

8096 PARI Independent Living Center
500 Prospect Street
Pawtucket, RI 02860-6259
401-725-1966
Fax: 401-725-2104
info@pari-ilc.org
www.pari-ilc.org
TDD 401-725-1966

Leo Canuel, Executive Director

PARI was incorporated in 1980 as a consumer-directed Independent Living Center. Our staff works with people with any kind of disability to identify goals and provide training, equipment, advocacy, and counseling to help them to achieve their goals. Whether the consumer is seeking medical resources, new ways of performing activities of daily life, transportation, housing, or ways of becoming involved in the community, the PARI Independent LivingCenter is the individual's professional resource for reaching independence. The Independent Living Center is a unique concept in non-residential resources for the person with a disability. PARI is a private, not for profit, community based agency whose programs and policies are determined by people with disabilities.

Year Founded: 1980

Tennessee

8097 Jackson Center for Independent Living
1981 Hollywood Drive
Jackson, TN 38305-2743
731-668-2211
Fax: 731-668-0406
information@jcil.tn.org
www.j-cil.com
TTY: 731-668-2211

Glen Barr, Executive Director

The Jackson Center for Independent Living (JCIL) is a nonprofit, tax deductible United Way agency. We work with people with significant disabilities and the Deaf Community in achieving their Independent Living goals while assisting the community in eliminating barriers to Independent Living.

8098 Memphis Center for Independent Living
1633 Madison Avenue
Memphis, TN 38104-2506
901-726-6404
Fax: 901-726-6521; *Toll Free:* 800-848-0298
mcil@mcil.org
www.mcil.org

Kevin Lofton, Chair
Marvin Glenn Bailey, Vice Chair
Deborah Cunningham, Executive Director

The Memphis Center for Independent Living works so that people with disabilities in the Memphis area may live independently. We believe that there is nothing more disabling then pity. People with disabilities are a powerful and significant part of the community, yet; as a group our social roles have been marginalized by bigotry, discrimination, poverty, isolation, dependency and pity. Americans with disabilities have not had access to transportation, housing and employment that other citizens have enjoyed; MCIL will change that.

Texas

8099 ABLE
1931 E 37th Street
Suite 1
Odessa, TX 79762
432-580-3439
Fax: 432-580-0208
info@ablecenterpb.org
ablecenterpb.org

Marylin Hancock M.Ed, Executive Director
Daniel Panter B.S., Transition/Relocation Specialist
Kathleen Story M.A., Independent Living Specialist

ABLE is dedicated to the idea that everyone should be living life to its fullest potential. We provide activities, education, and peer counseling for undividual desiring to soar above all expectations. ABLE is about focusing on abilities. ABLE teaches people to live independently, assists in providing support to promote independence.

8100 Coalition for Barrier Free Living: Houston Center for Independent Living
6201 Bonhomme Road
Suite 150
South Houston, TX 77036

713-974-4621
Fax: 713-974-6927
hcil@neosoft.com
www.coalitionforbarrierfreeliving.com
TTY: 713-974-2703

Sandra Bookman, Executive Director
Tony Koosis, Director Programs/Services

Advocacy organization for people with disabilities. Mission is to promote the full inclusion, equal opportunity and participation of persons with disabilities in every aspect of community life. We believe that people with disabilities have the right to make choices affecting their lives, a right to take risks, a right to fail, and a right to succeed

8101 REACH of Plano Resource Center on Independent Living
720 E Park Blvd
Suite 104
Plano, TX 75074-8844
972-398-1111
Fax: 972-398-9649
reachplano@reachcils.org
www.reachcils.org

Charlotte A Stewart, Executive Director
Susan Reukema, Assisstant Director
Cynthia Rogers, Office Manager

REACH is a nonprofit organization with the goal of advocating for and empowering people with disabilities to take charge of their lives and participate actively in community life. The centers are non-residential resource agencies which provide services for people with disabilities and education to the community on disability related topics. The Centers are governed and staffed by a majority of people with disabilities who bring a wide range of knowledge and experience to their work in assisting other people with disabilities.

8102 Reach Resource Center on Independent Living
1000 Macon Street
Suite 200
Fort Worth, TX 76102-4501
817-870-9082
Fax: 817-877-1622
reachftw@reachcils.org
www.reachcils.org
TTY: 817-870-9086

Charlotte A Stewart, Executive Director
Robin Lassiter, Assistant Director
Karen Williams, Community Living Specialist

REACH is a nonprofit organization with the goal of advocating for and empowering people with disabilities to take charge of their lives and participate actively in community life. REACH centers are non-residential resource agencies which provide services for people with disabilities and education to the community on disability related topics. The Centers are governed and staffed by a majority of people with disabilities who bring a wide range ofknowledge and experience to their work in assisting other people with disabilities.

8103 Reach of Denton Resource Center on Independent Living
405 S Elm Street
Suite 202
Denton, TX 76201-6068

940-383-1062
Fax: 940-383-2742
reachden@reachcils.org
www.reachcils.org
TDD 817-383-1062

Charlotte A Stewart, Executive Director
Missy Dickenson, Assistant Director
Becky Teal, Office Manager

REACH Inc. is a nonprofit organization with the goal of advocating for and empowering people with disabilities to take charge of their lives and participate actively in community life. REACH Centers are non-residential resource agencies which provide services for people with disabilities and education to the community on disability related topics. The Centers are governed and staffed by a majority of people with disabilities who bring a wide range of knowledge and experience to their work in assisting other people with disabilities.

8104 SAILS
1028 S Alamo Street
San Antonio, TX 78210-1170
210-281-1878
Fax: 210-281-1759; *Toll Free:* 800-474-0295
www.sailstx.org
TDD 210-281-1878

Patricia Byrd, Chair
Dennis Wolf, Vice Chair
Kitty L Brietzke, Executive Director

San Antonio Independent Living Center (SAILS) is a non-profit and federally designated Center for Independent Living aimed at those who reside in the Bexar county and 27 additional counties area. SAILS helps individuals with any disability: mental, physical, cognitive, or sensory, We can assist you or your family member by teaching independent living skills, providing up-to-date information and referrals, and training individuals on how to advocate for themselves.

Year Founded: 1981

Utah

8105 OPTIONS for Independence-Northern Utah Center For Independent Living
1095 N Main Street
Logan, UT 84341-2215
435-753-5353
Fax: 435-753-5390
jbiggs@optionsind.org
www.optionsind.org
TTY: 435-753-5353

Cheryl Atwood, Executive Director

OPTIONS for Independence (OPTIONS) is a nonresidential Independent Living Center where people with disabilities can learn skills to gain more control and independence over their lives. The mission of OPTIONS for Independence is to raise the vision and capability of the community at large to the point where people of all abilities will have equal access.

Year Founded: 1982

8106 Tri-County Independent Living Center
2726 Washington Blvd. (Rear)
Ogden, UT 84401

801-612-3215
Fax: 801-612-3732; *Toll Free:* 866-734-5678
www.tri-county-ilc.com
TTY: 801-612-3215

Andy Curry, Executive Director

The mission of the Tri-County Independent Living Council is to enhance independent living for all persons with disabilities.

8107 Utah Independent Living Center

3445 S Main Street
Salt Lake City, UT 84115-4418
801-466-5565
Fax: 801-466-2363; *Toll Free:* 800-355-2195
uilc@uilc.org
www.uilc.org
TDD 801-466-5565

Mark Christiansen, Chairperson
Richard Fox, Vice Chaiperson
Debra Mair, Executive Director

The Utah Independent Living Center (UILC) is a private, non-profit, non-residential facility that teaches independent living skills to people with disabilities. The UILC was the first center in Utah and has been serving the community since 1982. The UILC is committed to providing services needed by people with disabilities to function more independently in their families and communities. In order to be eligible to receive UILC services, a personmust have a physical of mental disability which impairs activities of daily living and a reasonable expectation exists that UILC services will increase independence.

8108 Utah Statewide Independent Living Council

150 South 600 East
Suite 5C
Salt Lake City, UT 84102
801-463-1592
Fax: 801-463-1683
byoung@usilc.org
www.usilc.org
TDD 801-463-1592

Lester Ruesch, Chair
Donna McCormick, Vice Chair
William Young, Executive Director

The Utah Statewide Independent Living Council is a private, nonprofit organization. The USILC mission is to promote full inclusion, independence and empowerment of people with disabilities through advocacy/system change, planning/organization, education, networking, resource development and independent living service enhancement.

Virginia

8109 Appalachian Independence Center

230 Charwood Drive
Abingdon, VA 24210-2566
276-628-2979
Fax: 276-628-4931
aicadmin@ntelos.net
www.aicadvocates.org
TTY: 276-676-0920

Greg Morrell, Executive Director
Scarlett Cox, Operations Director
Donna Buckland, Development Director

Appalachian Independence Center, Inc. (AIC) was founded in 1988 by a group of local citizens who had a desire to make sure services were availiable to people with disabilities and to help them learn about community services specific to their needs. AIC s a non-profit, non residential center for independent living which receives some of its funding from the State of Virginia and United Way. However, it is an independent organization governed by aboard of directors made up of local citizens, a majority of whom have disabilities themselves. This assures that AIC is in touch with the needs of people with disabilities in our community.

8110 Blue Ridge Independent Living Center

1502B Williamson Road NE
Roanoke, VA 24012-5100
540-342-1231
Fax: 540-342-9505; *Toll Free:* 866-244-0740
brilc@brilc.org
www.brilc.org
TTY: 540-342-1231

Karen Michalski Karney, Executive Director
Sallee Ebbett, Finance & Operations Manager
Katherine Wells, Program Services Manager

The Blue Ridge Independent Living Center assists people with disabilities to live independently. The Center also serves the community at large by helping to create an environment that is accessible to all. The Center, established in 1989, is a private, non-profit community agency with non-residential programs. Support for service is received from state and federal sources and donations from regional business and individuals. The Center is governed by a Board of Directors with a majority of members having disabilities.

Year Founded: 1989

8111 Endependence Center

6300 E Virginia Beach Boulevard
Norfolk, VA 23502-2827
757-461-8007
Fax: 757-455-8223
ecinorf@endependence.org
www.endependence.org
TDD 757-461-7527
TTY: 757-461-7527

Stephen Johnson, Executive Director
Michael Wang, President
Chris Dailey, Vice President

The Endependence Center, Incorporated (ECI) is a consumer controlled, community-based, cross-disability, non-residential, private, non-profit Center for Independent Living (CIL) operated by and for individuals with disabilities in South Hampton Roads, including the cities of Chesapeake, Norfolk, Portsmouth, Franklin, Suffolk, Virginia Beach and Isle of Wight County. ECI provides an array of independent living services to individuals with disabilities and to the community. The purposes of the ECI are 2 fold; to prepare individuals and to prepare the community for full integration of persons with disabilities into society.

8112 Endependence Center of Northern Virginia

2300 Clarendon Blvd
Suite 305
Arlington, VA 22201-3001
703-525-3268
Fax: 703-525-3585

info@ecnv.org
www.ecnv.org
TTY: 703-525-3553

David Burds, Executive Director
Marcie Goldstein, President
Lee Page, Vice President

ENDependence Center of Northern Virginia (ECNV) is a community-based resource and advocacy center which is managed by and for people with disabilities.ECNV promotes independent living (IL) philosophy and equal access for all persons with disabilities and, like the nearly 400 centers for independent living across the country, ECNV grew from local disability rights and self help movements. We operate from a philosophy of consumer controll and peer-to-peer relationships to empower people with physical, mental, cognitive and sensory disabilities to direct their own lives.

8113 Junction Center for Independent Living
PO Box 1210
Norton, VA 24273
276-679-5988
Fax: 276-679-6569
www.junctioncenter.org
TDD 540-523-1798

Dennis Horton, Executive Director

JCIL's mission is to assist people who have significant disabilities to live independently in the least restrictive and most integrated environment possible. The Junction Center for Independent Living is a non-profit, non-residential program which provides services to persons with disabilities, their families, and their community.

8114 Resources For Independent Living
4009 Fitzhugh Avenue
Suite 100
Richmond, VA 23230-3953
804-353-6503
Fax: 804-358-5606
info@ril-va.org
www.ril-va.org
TDD 804-353-6583

Marianne Miller, Chair
Tom Allen, Secretary/Treasurer
Sandra Wagener, Executive Director

The Central Virginia Independent Living Center, Inc. (CVILC) was established in February, 1983. It is a community based, non-profit, non-residential program which provides services to persons with a disability, their family, and the community. In 2003, we changed our name to Resources for Independent Living to better reflect our mission. Our mission is assisting persons who are severely disabled to live independently in the community and to encourage necessary change within the community so independent living is a possiblity.

Vermont

8115 Vermont Center for Independent Living
11 E State Street
Montpelier, VT 05602-3008
802-229-0501Toll free: 800-639-1522
info@vcil.org
www.vcil.org
TTY: 802-229-0501

Sarah Launderville, Executive Director
Marty Roberts, President
Sam Liss, Vice President

The Vermont Center for Independent Living (VCIL) works to promote the dignity, independence, and civil rights of Vermonters with disabilities. VCIL is committed to cross-disability services, the promotion of active citizenship, and working with others to create services that support self-determination and full participation in community life. Founded in 1979, VCIL is a statewide, nonprofit organization directed and staffed by individuals with disabilities. VCIL believes that individuals with disabilities have the right to live with dignity and with appropriate support in their own homes, fully participate in their communities, and to controll and make decisions about their lives.

West Virginia

8116 North Central West Virginia Center for Independent Living
601-603 E Brockway Avenue
Suite A26
Morgantown, WV 26505
304-296-6091Toll free: 800-834-6408
cchantler@nwvcil.org
www.nwvcil.org

Jan Derry, Executive Director
William Lindley, President
Mary Slanbinski, Vice President

Northern West Virginia Center for Independent Living is an advocacy resource center for persons with disabilities and the communities in which they live, not a social service agency. We want our consumer to be independent, not dependent on us for their independence. We do all that is possible to ensure that consumers have the skills and information they need to make informed choices and assist communities to better meet the needs of their citizens with disabilities.

Wisconsin

8117 Access to Independence
3810 Milwaukee St
Madison, WI 53714
608-242-8484
Fax: 608-242-0383; *Toll Free:* 800-362-9877
info@accesstoind.org
www.accesstoind.org
TTY: 608-242-8485

Jason B, Assisstant Director
Geri , Finance/HR

Access to independence promotes the integration of people with disabilities into communities, which have a wealth of opportunities. The mission of Access to Independence is to join with people with disabilities to create access to the community through education, action, and choice.

8118 Appalachian Center for Independent Living
4710 Chimney Drive
Suite C
Charleston, WV 25302-4804
304-965-0376
Fax: 304-965-0377; *Toll Free:* 800-642-3003
acil@yahoo.com
www.mtstcil.org/contact_wvcils.html

TDD 800-642-3003
TTY: 304-965-0377

Larry E Paxton, Executive Director

To promote the interdependence, productivity and quality of life of individuals with disabilities through empowerment, integration and inclusion.

8119 Center for Independent Living for Western Wisconsin
2920 Schneider Avenue East
Menomonie, WI 54751
715-233-1070
Fax: 715-233-1083; *Toll Free:* 800-228-3287
cilww@cilww.com
www.cilww.com
TDD 715-233-1070
TTY: 715-233-1070

Tim Sheehan, Executive Director
Kay Sommerfeld, Assistant Director
Tammy Grage, Fiscal & Human Resources Manager

The Center for Independent Living for Western Wisconsin (CILWW) advocates for the full participation in society of all persons with disabilities. Our goal is empowering individuals to exercise choices to maintain or increase their independence. Our strategy is providing consumer-driven services at no cost to persons with disabilities in Western Wisconsin.

8120 Independence First
540 South 1st Street
Milwaukee, WI 53204-1516
414-291-7520
Fax: 414-291-7525
www.independencefirst.org
TTY: 414-291-7520

Lee Schulz, Executive Director
John Schmid, Chair
Judy Murphy, Vice Chair

Independence First is a non-profit agency directed by, and for the benefit of, persons with disabilities, primarily serving the 4 country metropolitan Milwaukee area. Our agency mission is to effctively facilitate empowerment of individuals with disabilities through education, advocacy, independent living services, and coalition building. We promote diversity and multicultural participation in our operation and services.

8121 Independent Living Resources
4439 Mormon Coulee Road
La Crosse, WI 54650
608-787-1111
Fax: 608-787-1114; *Toll Free:* 888-474-5745
advocacy@ilresources.org
www.ilresources.org
TTY: 608-787-1148

Kathy Knoble-Iverson, Executive Director
Alicia Oliver, Assistant Dir. of IL Programs
Lori Dubczak, Marketing & Fundraising Coord.

ILR provides information about disability-related issues, resources and service to people with disabilities, families, professionals and the general public. ILR provides services to individuals of all ages, all disabilities and often with no cost to the individual or their family. ILR also provides personal care, supportive home care and companion care.

8122 Independent Living Resources-La Crosse
4439 Mormon Coulee Road
La Crosse, WI 54601-8220
608-787-1111
Fax: 608-787-1114; *Toll Free:* 888-474-5745
advocacy@ilresources.org
www.ilresources.org
TTY: 608-787-1148

Kathy Knoble-Iverson, Executive Director
Patrick Dienger, President
Mike Bowers, Vice President

8123 Independent Living Resources-Richland
149 E Mill Street
Suite A
Richland Center, WI 53581-2261
608-647-8053
Fax: 608-647-7783; *Toll Free:* 877-471-2095
advocacy@ilresources.org
www.ilresources.org
TTY: 608-647-8053

Kathie Knoble-Iverson, Executive Director
Patrick Dienger, President
Mike Bowers, Vice President

Independent Living Resources is committed to community diversity through advocacy, choice and education resulting in empowerment for individuals with disabilities.

8124 Midstate Independent Living Consultants-Stevens Point
3262 Church Street
Suite 1
Stevens Point, WI 54481-5321
715-344-4210
Fax: 715-344-4414; *Toll Free:* 800-382-8484
milc@milc-inc.org
www.milc-inc.org
TDD 715-344-4210
TTY: 715-344-4210

Jenny Fasula, Executive Director
Evelyn Buckles, Assistant Director
Laurie Lane, Program Manager

MILC is a private non-profit agency serving persons with disabilities of all ages. MILC is operated by staff and board composed primarily of people with disabilities. MILC services are consumer directed working together with staff to meet goals. You are eligible for services if you are a person with a disability and you reside in Adams, Florence, Forest, Langdale, Lincoln, Marathon, Oneida, Portage, Taylor, Vilas or Wood counties.

8125 Midstate Independent Living-Rhinelander
PO Box 369
Rhinelander, WI 54501
715-369-5040
Fax: 715-369-5043; *Toll Free:* 800-311-5044
milc@milc-inc.org
www.milc-inc.org
TDD 715-369-5040

Jenny Fasula, Executive Director
Evelyn Buckles, Assistant Director
Laurie Lane, Program Manager

MILC is a private non-profit agency serving persons with disabilities of all ages. MILC is operated by staff and board composed primarily of people with disabilities. MILC services are consumer directed working together with staff to meet goals. You are eligible for services if you are a person with a disability and you reside in Adams, Florence, Forest, Langdale, Lincoln, Marathon, Oneida, Portage, Taylor, Vilas, or Wood counties.

8126 North County Independent Living-Ashland
422 3rd Street W
Suite 114
Ashland, WI 54806-1573
715-682-5676
Fax: 715-682-3144; *Toll Free:* 800-499-5676
www.northcountryil.com
TTY: 715-682-5676

John Nedden-Durst, Disability Navigator
Stewart Holman, Independent Living Specialist

North Country Independent Living empowers people with disabilities. The mission is broad based, allowing North Country Independent Living to respond to a variety of needs. The philosophy promotes people with disabilities being active participants in daily living and being given the same opportunities and choices as others. This philosophy is promoted through consumer choice and controll. People with disabilities are active participants within theagency. The majority of the Board of Directors and staff are people with disabilities.

8127 North County Independent Living-Superior
69 N 28th Street
Suite 28
Superior, WI 54880
715-392-9118
Fax: 715-392-4636; *Toll Free:* 800-924-1220
ncil@superior-nfp.org
www.northcountryil.com
TTY: 715-392-9118

John Nousaine, Director
Gloria Johnson, Assistant Director
Nickoel Anderson, Accountant

North Country Independent Living empowers people with disabilities. The mission is broad based, allowing North Country Independent Living to respond to a variety of needs. The philosophy promotes people with disabilities being active participants in daily living and being given the same opportunities and choices as others. This philosophy is promoted through consumer choice and control. People with disabilities are active participants within theagency. The majority of the Board of Directors and staff are people with disabilities.

8128 Options for Independent Living-Appleton
820 W College Avenue
Suite 5
Appleton, WI 54914-5275
920-997-9999
Fax: 920-997-9381
info@optionsil.com
www.optionsil.com
TDD 920-997-9999

Thomas J Diedrick, Director
Mary Ann Toma, President
Keith Pamperin, Vice President

Options for Independent Living, Inc. is a non-profit organization committed to empowering people with disabilities to lead independent and productive lives in their community through advocacy, the provision of information, education, technology and related services. As part of the independent

living philosophy of consumer directed services, Options staff will provide information so consumers can make informed choices and achieve their objectives.The direction and development of Options is determined by a Board of Directors comprised primarily of individuals with disabilities. Options is committed to hiring staff with disabilities.

8129 Options for Independent Living-Green Bay
555 Country Club Road
Po Box 11967
Green Bay, WI 54307-1967
920-490-0500
Fax: 920-490-0700; *Toll Free:* 888-465-1515
info@optionsil.com
www.optionsil.com
TTY: 920-490-0600

Thomas J Diedrick, Director
Mary Ann Toma, President
Keith Pamperin, Vice President

Options for Independent Living, Inc. is a non-profit organization committed to empowering people with disabilities to lead independent and productive lives in their community through advocacy, the provision of information, education, technology and related services. As part of the independent living philosophy of consumer directed services, Options staff will provide information so consumers can make informed choices and achieve their objectives.The direction and development of Options is determined by a Board of Directors comprised primarily of individuals with disabilities. Options is committed to hiring staff with disabilities.

Legal Aid Resources

Alabama

8130 Alabama Department of Senior Services
600 Dexter Avenue
Montgomery, AL 36130-1851
334-242-7100
Fax: 334-353-0004; *Toll Free:* 877-425-2243
www.alabama.gov

Linda Adams, Scheduling Director
David Perry, Chief to staff
Wanda Kelly, Executive Assisstant to Governor

The Alabama Department of Senior Services receives its primary funding under Title III of the Older Americans Act of 1965, as amended. Under the terms of that Legislation, the Alabama Department of Senior Services supports a network of agencies and programs throughout the State of Alabama for the following purposes: secure and maintain independence and dignity of older persons; remove social and individual barriers; assure the provision of a continuum of care for the vulnerable elderly; and develop comprehensive, coordinated systems for older persons.

8131 Alabama Disabilities Advocacy Program (ADAP)
Alabama Protection and Advocacy Agency
P O Box 870395
Tuscalossa, AL 35487-0395
205-348-4928
Fax: 205-348-3909; *Toll Free:* 800-826-1675
adap@adap.ua.edu
www.adap.net
TDD 205-348-9484

Ellen Gillespie, Executive Director
James Tucker, Associate Director
Patrick Hackney, Sr. Staff Attorney

The Alabama Disabilities Advocacy Program (ADAP) is part of the nationwide federally mandated protection and advocacy (P&A) system. ADAP's mission is to provide quality, legally-based advocacy services to Alabamians with disabilities in order to protect, promote and expand their rights. ADAP's vision is one of a society where persons with disabilities are valued and exercise self-determination through meaningful choices, and have equality of opportunity.

8132 Alabama State Bar: Elder Law
415 Dexter Avenue
PO Box 671
Montgomery, AL 36014
334-269-1515
Fax: 334-261-6310; *Toll Free:* 800-354-6154
ed.patterson@alabar.org
www.alabar.org

Keith B Norman, Executive Director
Dorothy Johnson, Director of Admissions
Laura Calloway, Director of Service Programs

Formed in the early part of 1997 and the newest section of the Alabama State Bar, the Elder Law's mission is to develop, promote and enhance the quality of legal services for the elderly in Alabama.

8133 Legal Services for the Elderly: Area Agency on Aging
1075 S. Brannon STAND Road
Dothan, AL 36305
334-793-6843
robert.crowder@adss.alabama.gov
www.sarcoa.org/area_agencies.html

Robert Crowder, Executive Director
Dana Eidson, Director of Finance and Administ
Melinda Glover, Director of Resources & Activiti

The Area Agency on Aging seeks to keep area seniors independent, active and healthy through the many available services including legal assistance, meals and transportation.

8134 West Alabama Regional Commission's Senior Programs: Legal Counsel for the Elderly (WARC)
4200 Highway 69 North
Suite 1, P.O. Box 509
Northport, AL 35476-0509
205-333-2990
warc@westel.org
www.warc.info/index.php

Craig Patterson, Chairperson
Keith Mahaffey, Vice Chairman
Robert Lake, Secretary

West Alabama Regional Commission's programs for senior citizens are broad and inclusive. Depending upon individual circumstances, a senior citizen in West Alabama can get advice on health insurance, legal counseling, a home-delivered meal, help with household chores, discounted prescription medicines, placement in a part-time job, and many other services. Legal Counsel for the Elderly provides assistance with a wide variety of issues including health care, public benefits, and protective services. The program is funded through West Alabama Regional Commission by Older Americans Act funds. No legal fees are charged, but contributions are welcomed.

Alaska

8135 Alaska Commission on Aging: Alaska Department of Health & Social Services
150 Third Street
PO Box 110693
Juneau, AK 99811-0693
907-465-3250
Fax: 907-465-1398
hss.acoa@alaska.gov
www.alaskaaging.org/

William J Streur, Commissioner
Sana Efird, Assisstant Commissioner
Ree Sailors, Deputy Commisioner

The Alaska Commission on Aging (ACoA) advocates for state policy, public and private partnerships, state/federal projects and citizen involvement that assists each of us to age successfully in our homes, in our communities or as near as possible to our communities and families. Our work involves planning, advocacy, and interagency collaboration on issues and state and federal services affecting older Alaskans.

8136 Alaska Legal Services Corporation: Elder Law Project
1016 West 6th Avenue
Suite 200
Anchorage, AK 99501
907-272-9431
Fax: 907-279-7417; *Toll Free:* 888-478-2572
anchorage@alsc-law.org
www.alsc-law.org

Nikole Nelson, Executive Director

Legal services are provided to residents 60 years old and over. Issues include income maintenance, health care, housing, consumer wills, family caregiver matters, and information and referral on other legal issues.

Year Founded: 1967

8137 Alaska Legal Services Corporation: Senior Legal Services Project
1016 West 6th Avenue
Suite 200
Anchorage, AK 99501-1963
907-272-9431
Fax: 907-279-7417; *Toll Free:* 888-478-2572
anchorage@alsc-law.org
www.alsc-law.org

Nikole Nelson, Executive Director
Greg Razo, President
Janell Hafner, Vice President

Year Founded: 1967

8138 Disability Law Center Of Alaska
3330 Arctic Boulevard
Suite 103
Anchorage, AK 99503
907-565-1002
Fax: 907-565-1000; *Toll Free:* 800-478-1234
akpa@dlcak.org
www.dlcak.org

Tracy Barbeent, President
Kim Rion, Vice President
Sarah Randolph-Andrew, Secretary

Part of a nationwide system that provides protection and advocacy for the legal, civil and human rights of persons with disabilities.

8139 Elderlaw Project
1016 West 6th Avenue
Suite 200
Anchorage, AK 99501
907-272-9431
Fax: 907-279-7417; *Toll Free:* 888-478-2572
anchorage@alsc-law.org
www.alsc-law.org

Nikole Nelson, Executive Director
Greg Razo, President
Janell Hafner, Vice President

This program has 9 offices located throughout Alaska - Anchorage, Bethel, Dillingham, Fairbanks, Juneau, Ketchikan, Kotzebue, and Nome. The program provides services to low income persons of all ages, with special attention given to seniorsan their family caregivers. Areas of interest include public benefits, wills, consumer issues, landlord/tenant, and caregiver issues.

Year Founded: 1967

8140 Advocates for the Disabled
2200 N Central Ave
Suite 211
Phoenix, AZ 85004-1431
602-212-2600
Fax: 602-263-8845
www.cirs.org/homepage/advocates/

Adrienne Howell, President
Bonnie Temme, Vice President
Dennis A Bourgeois, Treasurer

Advocates services are establish the eligibility of individuals seeking benefits, manage benefits, educate the public how to obtain and use benefits, and to advoctae for the right to receive benefits. Providing social services. Provides a finding service.

Year Founded: 1964

8141 Arizona Center for Disability Law
3839 N 3rd Street
Suite 209
Phoenix, AZ 85012-2069
602-274-6287
Fax: 602-274-6779; *Toll Free:* 800-927-2260
www.acdl.com

Henry G Hawkins, Executive Director
Peri Jude Radecic, Public Advocacy Director
Kris Stocking, Finance & Admin. Director

A non profit law firm dedicated to protecting the rights of individuals with a wide range of disabilities.

8142 Arizona Department of Economic Security: Division of Aging and Community Services
Aging and Adult Administration
5025 E Washington Street
Suite 202
Phoenix, AZ 85034
602-274-6287
Fax: 602-274-6779; *Toll Free:* 800-927-2260
https://www.azdes.gov/

Rex Critchfield, Acting Assistant Director

The Aging and Adult Administration provides information and services to seniors within Arizona through Adult Protective Services, Benefits Counseling, Long Term Care Ombudsman Program, Legal Services Assistance, and the Home and Community Living Supports / Mature Workers Programs. Each of these services assists in accomplishing the administration's number one goal to provide opportunities for keeping vulnerable adults and older persons in their homes and communities.

Year Founded: 1974

8143 Arizona Elder Abuse and Fraud Taskforce Committee
Office of the Attorney General
Consumer Protection & Advocacy Section
1275 West Washington
Phoenix, AZ 85007-2926
602-542-5025
Fax: 602-542-4085; *Toll Free:* 800-352-8431
aginfo@azag.gov
www.azag.gov/
TDD 877-815-8390

Janice K Brewer, Governor
Clarence H Carter, Director
Sharon E Sergent, Deputy Director of Programs

8144 Arizona Protection and Advocacy Agency: Arizona Center for Disability Law
5025 E Washington Street
Suite 202
Phoenix, AZ 85034
602-274-6287
Fax: 602-274-6779; *Toll Free:* 800-927-2260
www.azdisabilitylaw.org

Henry G Hawkins, Executive Director
Peri Jude Radecic, Public Advocacy Director
Kris Stocking, Finance & Admin. Director

The Arizona Center for Disability Law advocates for the legal rights of persons with disabilities to be free from abuse, neglect and discrimination and to have access to education, health care, housing and jobs, and other services in order to maximize independence and achieve equality. The Arizona Center for Disability Law (the Center) is a federally-designated Protection and Advocacy System for the State of Arizona. Protection and Advocacy Systems (P&As) throughout the United States assure that the human and civil rights of persons with disabilities are protected. In creating Protection and Advocacy Systems, Congress gave them unique authorities and responsibilities, including the power to investigate reports of abuse and neglect and violations of the rights of persons with disabilities. P&As are also authorized to pursue appropriate legal and administrative remedies on behalf of persons with disabilities to insure the enforcement of their constitutional and statutory rights.

Year Founded: 1974

8145 DNA People's Legal Services
PO Box 306
Window Rock, AZ 86515-0306
928-871-4151
Fax: 928-871-5036; *Toll Free:* 800-789-7287
lhenry@dnalegalservices.org
www.dnalegalservices.org/

Chee Smith, President
Bill Cooke, Vicepresident
Amanda Lomayesva, Secretary

Offers legal assistance to Native Americans.

Year Founded: 1967

8146 Legal Advocate Program: Pinal-Gila Council for Senior Citizens
Area Agency on Aging
8969 W. McCartney Road
Casa Grande, AZ 85194-7432
520-836-2758
Fax: 520-421-2033; *Toll Free:* 800-293-9393
info@pgcsc.org
www.pgcsc.org

Olivia Guerrero, President/CEO

Year Founded: 1974

8147 National Academy of Elder Law Attorneys
1577 Spring Hill Road
Suite 220
Vienna, VA 22182

703-942-5711
Fax: 703-563-9504
naela@naela.org
www.naela.com/

Peter G. Wacht, CAE, Executive Director
Ann Watkins, Operations Manager
Amelia Seaton, Administrative Specialist

Provides legal advocacy, guidance and services to enhance the lives of older people with special needs.

8148 Southern Arizona Legal Aid (SALA)
2343 East Broadway Bvld
Suite 200
Tucson, AZ 85719-6007
520-623-9465
Fax: 520-620-0443; *Toll Free:* 800-640-9465
www.sazlegalaid.org/

Anthony L. Young, Esq., Executive Director
Doris Lee Butler, Chief Operations Officer
Rose Marie Castro, Chief Financial Officer

Offers workshops and representation for people with disabilities.

Year Founded: 1951

8149 T.A.S.A. Taskforce Against Senior Abuse
Office of the Attorney General
Consumer Protection & Advocacy Section
1275 West Washington
Phoenix, AZ 85007-2926
602-542-2124
Fax: 602-542-4579; *Toll Free:* 800-352-8431
seniorabuse@azag.gov
www.azag.gov/
TDD 877-815-8390

Tom Horne, Chief Legal Officer/Attorney Gen
Tom Chenal, Director of T.A.S.A.

Addresses the problems of elder abuse and exploitation. The direct services component uses in-house attorneys in areas such as licensing, nursing home regulation, adult protective services, civil rights, and criminal fraud.

8150 William E Morris Institute for Justice
202 East McDowell Road
Suite 257
Phoenix, AZ 85004
602-252-3432
Fax: 602-257-8138
ajinstitu@qwestoffice.net
www.MorrisInstituteforJustice.org/

Ellen Sue Katz, Litigation Director/ Administrat

Offers legal services for seniors in need.

Arkansas

8151 Arkansas Department of Health & Human Services: Division of Aging and Adult Services
700 main Street
P O Box 1437, Slot S-530
Little Rock, AR 72203-1437
501-682-2441
Fax: 501-682-8155
aging.services@arkansas.gov
www.das.ar.gov

Krista Hughes, Executive Director
Connie Parker, Assistant Director
Stephenie Blocker, Assistant Director

Year Founded: 1965

8152 Arkansas Protection and Advocacy Agency: Disability Rights Center

1100 North University
Suite 201
Little Rock, AR 72207
501-296-1775
Fax: 501-296-1779; *Toll Free:* 800-482-1174
panda@arkdisabilityrights.org
www.arkdisabilityrights.org/
TDD 800-482-1174

Nan Ellen, Executive Director
Joyce Soularie, Chairperson
Kim Weser, Secretary

8153 Arkansas Volunteer Lawyers for the Elderly (AVLE)

1300 W. 6th St.
Little Rock, AR 72201
501-376-3423
Fax: 501-376-3664; *Toll Free:* 800-952-9243
www.arlegalservices.org/Home/

Lee Richardson, Executive Director
Sarah Sparkman, Staff Attorney

Serves elderly in 67 Arkansas counties. Legal services and area agency on aging staff conduct initial intake and send cases to AVLE, where coordinator refers them to panel of 600 volunteer attorneys.

8154 Center for Arkansas Legal Services

1300 W. 6th St.
Little Rock, AR 72201
501-376-3423
Fax: 501-376-3664; *Toll Free:* 800-952-9243
www.arlegalservices.org/Home/

Lee Richardson, Executive Director
Sarah Sparkman, Staff Attorney

8155 Legal Aid of Arkansas

714 South Main Street
Jonesboro, AR 72401
870-972-9224
Fax: 870-910-5562; *Toll Free:* 800-952-9243
www.arlegalservices.org/Home/

Lee Richardson, Executive Director
Sarah Sparkman, Staff Attorney

Legal Aid of Arkansas 501(c)3 is a nonprofit organization that provides free legal services to low-income Arkansans in non-criminal cases, ranging from family to consumer and housing to individual rights cases. LAA serves 31 counties within Arkansas. Their vision is to improve the lives of low-income Arkansans by championing equal access to justice for all regardless of economic or social circumstances.

California

8156 Bet Tzedek Legal Services

3250 Wilshire Blvd
3rd Floor
Los Angeles, CA 90010

323-939-0506
Fax: 213-471-4568
www.bettzedek.org/

Sandore E Samuels, President & CEO
Elissa D. Barrett, Vice President and General Couns
Ileana Prado, Vice President of Operations

Bet Tzedek is one of the nation's premier legal services organizations, providing free assistance to more than 10,000 people of every racial and religious background at its headquarters in the Fairfax area and its office in North Hollywood and at more than 30 senior centers throughout Los Angeles County. With a dedicated staff of over 55 and more than 400 active volunteers, Bet Tzedek makes a crucial difference in the lives of the most vulnerable members of the community.

8157 California Department of Aging

1300 National Drive
Suite 200
Sacramento, CA 95834-1992
916-419-7500
Fax: 916-928-2267
lconnoll@aging.ca.gov
www.aging.ca.gov/
TDD 800-735-2929

Lora Connolly, Director
Diane Paulsen, Acting Chief Deputy Director

The California Department of Aging serves as both a unifying force for services to seniors and adults with disabilities and as a focal point for federal, state and local agencies which serve the elderly and adults with disabilities in California. It fulfills the goals outlined in the Older Americans Act and also acts as an advocate for seniors and adults with disabilities by striving to develop an environment which respects and values the state's older residents and adults with disabilities. As the designated State Unit on Aging, the California Department of Aging is part of the California Health and Human Services Agency. The Department administers Older Americans Act programs for supportive services, in-home services, congregate and home-delivered meals and a system of multipurpose senior centers. It also administers the program for community service employment; programs for advocaivities, the Department works closely with private and public sector aging advocates.cy and protection; and programs which provide health insurance counseling, case management, Alzheimer's Day Care Resource Center and Adult Day Health Care services. Further, it performs a wide range of functions related to advocacy, planning, coordination, interagency linkages, information sharing, brokering, monitoring and evaluation. In its act

8158 California State Bar Committee on Legal Problems of Aging

180 Howard Street
San Francisco, CA 94105
415-538-2000Toll free: 800-843-9053
feedback@calbar.ca.gov
www.calbar.ca.gov/calbar

Thomas G Stolpman, Executive Director

The Commission on Legal Problems of the Elderly (Commission) is an entity of the American Bar Association (ABA). Its goal is to examine and respond to law-related needs of older persons in the United States through policy development, education, and the provision of technical assistance. The Commission does not provide direct legal services or make referrals to private lawyers. The Commission can, however, help connect individuals with the freelegal services/legal aid programs serving older persons in the area in which they live.

Year Founded: 1927

8159 Central California Legal Services

2115 Kern Street
Suite 1
Fresno, CA 93721
559-570-1200
Fax: 559-570-1254; *Toll Free:* 800-675-8001
cclsinfo@centralcallegal.org
www.centralcallegal.org
TTY: 559-570-1256

William Eric McComas, President
David Rodriguez, Vicepresident
Chris A Schneider, Executive Director

8160 Council on Aging of Sonoma County

30 Kawana Springs Rd
Santa Rosa, CA 95404
707-525-0143
Fax: 707-525-0454; *Toll Free:* 800-675-0143
www.councilonaging.com

Corrine Lorenzen, Chair
Deborah Roberts, Vice Chair
Bonnie Burrell, Secretary

The Council on Aging offers our senior clients timely legal services and advice to contribute to their sense of well being and support their independence and security. Those in social or financial need receive priority. To be eligible for our legal services you must be a Sonoma County resident 60 years of age or older. Our part-time Senior Legal Services staff includes an attorney, three paralegals, and an office manager.

8161 Disability Rights Education and Defense Fund

3075 Adeline Street
Suite 210
Berkeley, CA 94703
510-644-2555
Fax: 510-841-8645; *Toll Free:* 800-348-4232
info@dredf.org
www.dredf.org
TTY: 510-841-8645

Susan Henderson, Executive Director
Arlene B. Mayerson, Directing Attorney
Linda D. Kilb, Director, Legal Services Trust F

A national law and policy center dedicated to protecting and advancing civil rights of people with disabilities through legislation, litigation, formal and informal advocacy and education and training of people with disabilities, parents of children with disabilities, advocates and attorneys.

8162 Hawkins Center of Law and Services for the Disabled

101 Broadway Avenue
Suite 1
Richmond, CA 94804-1911
510-232-6611
info@hawkinscenter.org
www.hawkinscenter.org/

Linda Mills, Contact

The Hawkins Center works to improve the health and financial stability of people with disabilities. In partnership with service organizations, The Hawkins Center provides high quality legal, social, and educational services, and advocates for changes in policy. In all its programs, the agency promotes dignity, respect, and fairness for people with disabilities.

8163 Inland Counties Legal Services for Seniors

715 North Arrowhead Avenue
Suite 113
San Bernardino, CA 92401
909-884-8615 Toll free: 800-677-4257
www.inlandlegal.org/

George S Theios, President
Barbara A Purvis, Vice President
Forest E Wright, Treasurer

Inland Counties Legal Services provides free civil legal assistance to seniors who are 60 years or older who reside in Riverside and San Bernardino Counties. Elder law advocates travel to senior and community centers throughout both counties to give legal counsel and assistance. Priority is given to elder abuse cases, including matters involving financial, emotional and mental abuse as well as physical abuse, and help seniors with government andpublic benefits.

8164 Legal Assistance to the Elderly

100 McAllister Street
San Francisco, CA 94102
415-861-4444
Fax: 415-861-6458
info@laesf.org
www.laesf.org

Roger Levin, President
Tom Weathered, Vice Presiident
Mary Foran, Secretary

Provides advice and representation to San Francisco residents age sixty and over experiencing problems with their housing, public benefits, health care or who are experiencing physical or financial abuse.

8165 Legal Services for Seniors

21 West Laurel Avenue
Suite 83
Salinas, CA 93906
831-442-7700
www.legalservicesforseniors.org/

Don Leach, President
John Kesecker, Co-Vice President
Michael Leavy, Co-Vice President

8166 Los Angeles County Bar Association: Elderline Public Council

321 North Clark Street
Chicago, IL 60654
312-988-5000 Toll free: 312-988-5000
abaelderly@abanet.org
www.abanet.org/aging/states/california06

Charles P Sabatino, Director ABA Law/Aging Cmmsn
Erica F Wood, Asst. Director ABA Law/Ag Csm
Holly Robinson, Associate Staff Director

Elderline is a Legal Referral for the Elderly Program. A phone counselor recieves calls and makes referrals for cases involving property, consumer problems, landlord-tenant problems, uninsured torts, uncontested probate, uncontested guardianship and conservatorship, grandparents rights, and tax.

Year Founded: 1878

8167 Senior Adults Legal Assistance (SALA)
160 East Virginia Street
Suite 260
San Jose, CA 95112
408-295-5991
Fax: 408-295-7401; *Toll Free:* 650-969-8656
www.sala.org/

Dan Hoffman, Board President
Naomi Comfort, Board Vice President
Kevin Comstock, Board Secretary

Year Founded: 1973

8168 Senior Citizens Legal Services
5151 Murphy Canyon Road
Suite 110
San Diego, CA 92123
858-565-1392
Fax: 858-565-1394
www.seniorlaw-sd.org/metro.html

Carolyn L Reilly, Program Director
Jaime Levine, Staff Attorney

Senior Citizens Legal Services provides free legal services to San Diego County senior citizens age 60 or older.

8169 Senior Law Project
255 North Forbes Street
Second Floor
Lakeport, CA 95453
707-263-2580
Fax: 707-263-0348; *Toll Free:* 800-260-4703
Alicia.Flores@lakecountyca.gov
www.co.lake.ca.us/

Jeff Rein, Deputy Admin Officer

Lake County Community Action Agency through the Senior Law Project, provides seniors with assistance regarding Social Security, SSI, Medi-Cal, Medicare, Landlord/Tenant problems, Elder Abuse, Consumer Protection and planning for incapacity and long-term care.

8170 Senior Legal Center of Northern California
1370 West Street
Redding, CA 96001
530-241-3565
Fax: 530-241-3982; *Toll Free:* 800-822-9687
www.lsnc.net

Thomas M Welsh, Contact

In Lassen, Modoc, Shasta, Siskiyou, and Trinity counties, the Senior Legal Hotline is available for legal advice or brief assistance by phone.

8171 Volunteer Lawyers Project for the Elderly
321 North Clark Street
Suite 200
Chicago, IL 60654
312-988-5000
Fax: 209-441-7215; *Toll Free:* 312-988-5000
www.abanet.org/aging/states/

Chris A Schnieder, Directing Attorney

Provides counseling on issues such as housing, consumer, domestic relations, simple wills, and tort defense litigation.

Services are free to residents of Fresno County whose incomes are within Legal Services Croporation guidelines.

8172 Western Law Center for Disability Rights
800 South Figueroa St
Suite 200
Los Angeles, CA 90017
213-736-1031
Fax: 213-736-1428
DRLC@lls.edu
www.disabilityrightslegalcenter.org/
TTY: 213-736-8310

Paula D Pearlman, Executive Director
Michael McDonough, President of the Board
Harvey Saferstein, Vice President

The Western Law Center for Disability Rights provides legal representation in accordance with the Americans With Disabilities Act of 1990 to people with a wide range of disabilities; provides information to people with cancer or with disabilities; advocates on behalf of disabled people through class-action lawsuits; and mediates disputes disabled people have with employers and others.

Year Founded: 1975

Colorado

8173 Boulder County Aging Services Division: Elder Rights Program
3482 North Broadway
PO Box 471
Boulder, CO 80306-0471
303-441-3570
Fax: 303-441-4550
bcaaa@co.boulder.co.us
www.co.boulder.co.us/cs/ag/

Rosemary Williams MSW, Division Manager

The mission of Boulder County Aging Services Division is to promote the health and well-being of older adults by building on individual, family, and community strengths. Free and confidential services advocating for the rights of older adults in Boulder County are available.

8174 Colorado Department of Human Services: Division of Aging and Adult Services
1575 Sherman Street
10th Floor
Denver, CO 80203
303-866-5700
Fax: 303-866-2696; *Toll Free:* 888-866-4243
cdhs_communications@state.co.us
www.cdhs.state.co.us/aas/
TTY: 303-866-2850

Scott Thoemke, Executive Director

The Division of Aging and Adult Services (AAS) will efficiently and effectively provide human services in support of independent living, self-sufficiency, safety and dignity goals. These goals are on behalf of adults who have disabilities or functional impairments or are otherwise at risk. The Division of Aging and Adult Services provides oversight for and coordination of programs that allow the elderly and adults with disabilities to live independently. These programs are administered through the County Departments of Social (Human) Services or through regional Area Agencies on Aging.

8175 Colorado Protection and Advocacy Agency: The Legal Center at Grand Junction
455 Sherman Street
Suite 130
Denver, CO 80203-4403
303-722-0300
Fax: 303-722-0720; *Toll Free:* 800-288-1376
tlcmail@thelegalcenter.org
www.thelegalcenter.org

Mary Anne Harvey, Executive Director
Randy Chapman, Director of Legal Services

Works for systematic change that will improve the quality of life for seniors and those with disabilities.

Year Founded: 1976

8176 Larimer County Office on Aging (LCOA)
200 W Oak Street
Fort Collins, CO 80521
970-498-7000
Fax: 970-498-6455
www.larimer.org/humanservices/seniors/

Karen A Wagner, Commissioner
Margaret Long, Executive Director

The Larimer County Office on Aging (LCOA), in the Larimer County Department of Human Services, is a comprehensive planning unit that advocates for the concerns of older adults and caregivers. LCOA will assist older adults, age 60 and over, in maintaining health, dignity, independence, and quality of life, by advocating, planning, coordinating, and delivering services and programs, with emphasis on meeting the needs of those who are socially and/or economically disadvantaged.

Year Founded: 1861

8177 Legal Center for People with Disabilities and Older People
455 Sherman Street
Suite 130
Denver, CO 80203-4403
303-722-0300
Fax: 303-722-0720; *Toll Free:* 800-288-1376
tlcmail@thelegalcenter.org
www.thelegalcenter.org/contact.html
TTY: 303-722-3619

Mary Anne Harvey, Executive Director
Randy Chapman, Director of Legal Services
Mark Ivandick, Office Managing Attorney

Provides legal representation to persons with disabilities, their advocates, including parents, guardians and family members concerned with the rights and responsibilities of persons with disabilities, when the disability is central to rather than incidental to the legal dispute; special knowledge of the disabling condition is required; and special knowledge of the applicable law is required.

Year Founded: 1976

Connecticut

8178 Center for Medicare Advocacy
PO Box 350
Willimantic, CT 06226-0350
860-456-7790
Fax: 860-456-2614; *Toll Free:* 800-262-4414

mshepard@medicareadvocacy.org
www.medicareadvocacy.org

Judith Stein, Executive Director/Attorney
Brad Plebani, Deputy Director
Margaret M Murphy, Associate Director

8179 Connecticut Department of Social Services: Elderly Services Division
25 Sigourney Street
Hartford, CT 06106
860-424-5274
Fax: 860-424-5301; *Toll Free:* 866-218-6631
ctelderlyserv.dss@po.state.ct.us
www.ctelderlyservices.state.ct.us/

Stephanie Marino, Program Manager

Connecticut's Aging Services Division is committed to serving seniors by supporting and promoting programs that serve the growing needs of the aging community in all five regions of Connecticut. The Aging Services Division is the component within DSS which ensures that Connecticut's elders have access to the supportive services necessary to live with dignity, security and independence. The Division is responsible for planning, developing, and administering a comprehensive and integrated service delivery system for elderly persons in Connecticut. To accomplish this, the Division conducts needs assessments, surveys methods of service administration, evaluates and monitors such services, maintains information and referral services, and develops, coordinates, and/or collaborates with other appropriate agencies to provide outreach, social, housing, transportation, health, educational, cultural and nutritional programs that help Connecticut's elderly residents.

8180 Connecticut Lawyers' Legal Aid to the Elderly Program (CLLAEP)
Law and Regulatory Affairs
321 North Clark Street
Suite 200
Chicago, IL 60654
312-988-5000Toll free: 312-988-5000
www.abanet.org/aging/states/

Charles P Sabatino, ABA Law/Aging Director
Erica F Wood, Assistant Director ABA Law/Aging
Holly Robinson, Staff Director ABA Law/Aging

Staffed by Hartford-area lawyers from corporate law departments and private law firms, the program offers free legal assistance to low-income elderly in the Greater-Hartford/Middletown areas.

8181 Connecticut Protection and Advocacy Agency: Office of Protection and Advocacy for Persons with Disabilities
60-B Weston Street
Hartford, CT 06120-1551
860-297-4300
Fax: 860-566-8714; *Toll Free:* 800-842-7303
james.mcgaughey@po.state.ct.us
www.state.ct.us/opapd/
TTY: 860-842-7303

James D McGaughey, Executive Director

The Office of Protection and Advocacy for Persons with Disabilities is an independent State agency created to safeguard and advance the civil and human rights of people with disabilities in Connecticut. Part of a nationwide network of protection and advocacy systems, we operate under both State and federal legislative mandates to provide information, referral, and advocacy services; pursue legal and administrative remedies on behalf of people with disabilities who experience disability-related discrimination; selectively investigate complaints from people with disabilities and into allegations of abuse and neglect with respect to adults who have mental retardation, and for people in psychiatric facilities; and, provide public education and training on disability issues and to inform policy makers about issues affecting people with disabilities.

8182 Legal Assistance for Elders in Connecticut
Connecticut Elder Law Program

62 Washington Street
Middletown, CT 06457
860-344-0447Toll free: 800-453-3320
www.ctelderlaw.org/

Marvin Farbman, Executive Director

Provides comprehensive, current information on elder law, government programs and legal assistance for residents of Connecticut age 60 and older. Services include free counseling and representation on many Elder Law issues such as Medicaid and other government programs, patients' rights, nursing home issues.

8183 Legal Services Programs for Elders: Bridgeport

211 State Street
Bridgeport, CT 06604
203-336-3861Toll free: 800-453-3320
www.ctelderlaw.org/

Marvin Farbman, Executive Director

Provides comprehensive, current information on elder law, government programs and legal assistance for residents of Connecticut age 60 and older. Services include free counseling and representation on many Elder Law issues such as Medicaid and other government programs, patients' rights, nursing home issues.

8184 Legal Services Programs for Elders: Hartford

80 Jefferson Street
Hartford, CT 06106
860-541-5000Toll free: 800-453-3320
www.ctelderlaw.org/

Marvin Farbman, Executive Director

Provides comprehensive, current information on elder law, government programs and legal assistance for residents of Connecticut age 60 and older. Services include free counseling and representation on many Elder Law issues such as Medicaid and other government programs, patients' rights, nursing home issues.

8185 Legal Services Programs for Elders: Waterbury

85 Central Avenue
Waterbury, CT 06702
203-756-8074Toll free: 800-453-3320
www.ctelderlaw.org/

Marvin Farbman, Executive Director

Provides comprehensive, current information on elder law, government programs and legal assistance for residents of Connecticut age 60 and older. Services include free counseling and representation on many Elder Law issues such as Medicaid and other government programs, patients' rights, nursing home issues.

8186 Legal Services Programs for Elders: Willimantic

872 Main Street
Willimantic, CT 06226
860-456-1761Toll free: 800-453-3320
www.ctelderlaw.org/

Marvin Farbman, Executive Director

Provides comprehensive, current information on elder law, government programs and legal assistance for residents of Connecticut age 60 and older. Services include free counseling and representation on many Elder Law issues such as Medicaid and other government programs, patients' rights, nursing home issues.

8187 New Haven Legal Assistance Association (LAA)

426 State Street
New Haven, CT 06112
203-946-4811Toll free: 800-453-3320
www.ctelderlaw.org/

Marvin Farbman, Executive Director

Provides comprehensive, current information on elder law, government programs and legal assistance for residents of Connecticut age 60 and older. Legal Services include free counseling and representation on many Elder Law issues such as Medicaid and other government programs, patients' rights, nursing home issues.

8188 No Longer Disabled: The Federal Courts
Greenwood Publishing Group

130 Cremona Drive
Santa Barbara, CA 93117
805-968-1911
Fax: 866-270-3856; *Toll Free:* 800-368-6868
CustomerService@abc-clio.com
www.greenwood.com/

Susan Gluck Mezey, Author
Ron Maas, VP Planning Greenwood Publishing

This book is a case study of judicial policy making. It focuses on the role of adjudication in the making and refining of federal policy.

208 pages

Delaware

8189 Community Legal Aid Society: Dover

100 West 10th Street
Suite 801
Wilmington, DE 19801
302-575-0660
Fax: 302-575-0840
clasinc@declasi.org
www.declasi.org
TDD 302-575-0696
TTY: 302-575-0696

James G. McGiffin, Jr., Esq., Senior Staff Attorney

Services provides by the Elder Law Program include that of powers of attorney and advance health care directives (formerly known as Living Wills); consumer problems such as debt collection and home repair cases; housing problems such as evictions, and, benefits issues such as Medicaid and Social Security. The Elder Law Program also conducts community legal education workshops for older people about legal problems that occur with advancing age.

8190 Community Legal Aid Society: Georgetown
100 West 10th Street
Suite 801
Wilmington, DE 19801
302-575-0660
Fax: 302-575-0840
clasincc@declasi.org
www.declasi.org
TDD 302-575-0696
TTY: 302-575-0696

Eleanor M. Kiesel, Esq., Managing Attorney

Services provides by the Elder Law Program include that of powers of attorney and advance health care directives (formerly known as Living Wills); consumer problems such as debt collection and home repair cases; housing problems such as evictions, and, benefits issues such as Medicaid and Social Security. The Elder Law Program also conducts community legal education workshops for older people about legal problems that occur with advancing age.

8191 Community Legal Aid Society: Wilmington
100 West 10th Street
Suite 801
Wilmington, DE 19801
302-575-0660
Fax: 302-575-0840
clasincc@declasi.org
www.declasi.org
TDD 302-575-0696
TTY: 302-575-0696

Pattrick Gallagher, President
Judith Scarborough, Vice President
Rodger D Smith, Immediate Past President

Services provides by the Elder Law Program include that of powers of attorney and advance health care directives (formerly known as Living Wills); consumer problems such as debt collection and home repair cases; housing problems such as evictions, and, benefits issues such as Medicaid and Social Security. The Elder Law Program also conducts community legal education workshops for older people about legal problems that occur with advancing age.

8192 Delaware Bar Association Committee on Law and the Elderly
405 N King Street
Suit 100
Wilmington, DE 19801
302-658-5279
Fax: 302-658-5212; *Toll Free:* 800-292-7869
www.dsba.org/SecComm/sections.htm

Gregory B Williams, President
Yvonne Saville, President Elect
Richard A Forsten, Vice President-At-Large

The Committee produces a handbook for senior citizens, coordinates the publication of a bar journal on legal problems of the elderly, advises the bar on legislation affecting the elderly, sponsors two continuing legal education seminars, and sponsors three call-in nights for senior citizens.

8193 Delaware Division of Services for Aging and Adults with Physical Disabilities
1901 North DuPont Highway
New Castle, DE 19720
302-255-9040
Fax: 302-255-4429; *Toll Free:* 800-223-9074

DSAAPDinfo@state.de.us
www.dhss.delaware.gov/dhss/dsaapd/

Rita M Landgraf, Secretary
Charles E Hayward, Director
Jane J Gallivan, Director

The Delaware Division of Services for Aging and Adults with Physical Disabilities (DSAAPD) carries out a broad range of activities to assist older persons and adults with physical disabilities. The Division operates a number of programs, including the Adult Protective Services Program, the Long Term Care Ombudsman Program, the Community Services Program, the Delaware Medicare Fraud Alert Program, the Delaware Money Management Program, and Joining Generations. In addition, the Division provides services such as information and assistance, caregiver support, and health promotion. The Division also contracts with agencies around the State to provide many home and community-based services. Finally, the Division advocates on behalf of older persons and adults with physical disabilities to create a broader awareness of the needs of these populations within Delaware.

District of Columbia

8194 AARP Legal Advocacy Group
601 E Street NW
Washington, DC 20049
202-434-2120
Fax: 202-434-6424; *Toll Free:* 888-687-2277
tosborne@aarp.org
www.aarp.org/states/dc/dc-lce/

Wayne Moore, Director
Thomas Osborne, Senior Attorney
William Novelli, CEO

Operates a public interest litigation unit, provides technical assistance on legal hotlines, supports a discount legal services program for AARP membersand operates a national legal training program.

8195 Administrative Advocacy Clinic/Advocates for Older People
2121 Eye Street
Washington, DC 20052
202-994-1000
Fax: 202-676-5269
susanjones@law.gwu.edu
www.gwu.edu/~ccommit/law.htm

Susan R Jones, Clinic Director
Steven Knap, President

George Washington University Law students provide services for indigent and elderly Washington residents who are pursuing their entitlements to various government rights and benefits before local and federal agencies and courts. Services include free legal assistance, public benefits, wills, income tax return preparation and other legal problems for D.C. residents ages 55 and older.

8196 District of Columbia Bar: Individual Rights Section
321 North Clark Street
Chicago, IL 60654
312-988-5000
Fax: 202-626-3471; *Toll Free:* 312-988-5000
kmazzaferri@dcbar.org
www.abanet.org/irr/html or www.dcbar.org

Katherine A Mazzaferri, Executive Director
Al Wilcox, Director of Operations
Cynthia G Kuhn, Communications Director

Created in 1966, the Section of Individual Rights and Responsibilities provides leadership within the ABA and the legal profession in protecting and advancing human rights, civil liberties, and social justice. The Section fulfills this role by raising and addressing often complex and difficult civil rights and civil liberties issues in a changing and diverse society, and ensuring that protection of individual rights remains a focus of legal and policy decisions.

8197 District of Columbia Office on Aging

500 K Street
Washington, DC 20002
202-724-5622
Fax: 202-724-4979
dcoa@dc.gov
dcoa.dc.gov/dcoa/site/default.asp
TTY: 202-724-8925

E. Veronica Pace, Executive Director

The mission of the District of Columbia Office on Aging is to advocate, plan, implement, and monitor programs in health, education, employment, and social services which promote longevity, independence, dignity, and choice for our senior citizens. The Office on Aging also funds a Senior Service Network comprising 20 community-based, nonprofit organizations that provide direct services to the District's elderly citizens. The 30 community-based, education, government, and private organizations that make up the Senior Service Network operate more than 40 programs for older persons. Crucial to the Network are five Lead Agencies that offer a broad range of legal, nutrition, social, and health services. The goal of these six agencies is to enhance the quality of life for older adults and their families throughout all eight wards of the District of Columbia. The agencies accomplish this goal through widespread distribution of information about the variety of services and programs offered seniors throughout the city and ways to access them.

8198 Equal Employment Advisory Council

1501 M Street, NW
Suite 400
Washington, DC 20005
202-629-5650
Fax: 202-629-5651
info@eeac.org
www.eeac.org/

Joseph S Lakis, President
Cory Siansky, Vice President
Judy C Jackson, Vice President

A nonprofit association for the purpose of monitoring federal equal employment litigation and filing amicus curiae briefs in precedent-setting cases. Also file comments on equal opportunity employment and affirmative action regulatory proposals and monitors judicial developments.

Year Founded: 1976

8199 Federal Bar Association

1220 North Fillmore St.
Ste. 444
Arlington, VA 22201
571-481-9100
Fax: 571-481-9090

fba@fedbar.org
www.fedbar.org/

Karen Silberman, Executive Director
Stacy King, Deputy Executive Director
April Davis, Staff Accountant

Attorneys employed by the federal government as legislators, judges, lawyers, or members of quasi-judicial boards and commissions; those with previous government legal experience; and those with a substantive interest in federal law and who practice before a federal court or agency. Over 100 specialized committees, operating through 24 Sections and Divisions, provide various programs such as continuing legal education and professional and community service.

8200 Legal Counsel for the Elderly

601 East Street NW
Washington, DC 20049
202-434-2120
Fax: 202-434-6424; Toll Free: 888-687-2277
tosborne@aarp.org
www.aarp.org/states/dc/dc-lce/

Thomas Osborne, Directing Attorney
William Novelli, CEO
Erik Olsen, President Board of Directors

Provides free legal services to Washington, DC residents aged 60 and older, with priority given to low income persons. Serves as the Long-Term Care Ombudsman for DC by advocating for residents of nursing homes and board and care homes.

8201 Paralyzed Veterans of America (PVA)

801 18th Street NW
Washington, DC 20006-3517
202-872-1300
Fax: 202-785-4452; Toll Free: 800-424-8200
info@pva.org
www.pva.org/
TDD 800-795-4327

Bill Lawson, President
Homer S. Townsend, Jr., Executive Director

The Paralyzed Veterans of America, a congressionally chartered veterans service organization founded in 1946, has developed a unique expertise on a wide variety of issues involving the special needs of our members- veterans of the armed forces who have experienced spinal cord injury or dysfunction.

8202 US Department of Labor

200 Constitution Avenue NW
Frances Perkins Building
Washington, DC 20210
202-693-6000
Fax: 202-219-7312
www.dol.gov/
TTY: 877-889-5627

Elaine L Chao, Secretary of Labor
Paul T Conway, Chief of Staff
Ruth D Knouse, Executive Secretariat Director

The Department of Labor (DOL) fosters and promotes the welfare of the job seekers, wage earners, and retirees of the United States by improving their working conditions, advancing their opportunities for profitable employment, protecting their retirement and health care benefits, helping employers find workers, strengthening free collective bargaining, and tracking changes in employment, prices, and other national economic measurements. In carrying out this mission, the Department administers a variety of Federal labor laws including those that guarantee workers' rights to safe and healthful working conditions; a minimum hourly wage and overtime pay; freedom from employment discrimination; unemployment insurance; and other income support.

8203 Veterans' Advocate
2001 S Street NW
PO Box 65762
Washington, DC 20009-1157
202-265-8305
Fax: 202-328-0063
info@nvlsp.org
www.nvlsp.org/

Ronald S Flagg, Chairman
Rafael B Acosta, Member
Ronald B Abrams, Co-Director

Non-profit veterans law firm. Recruits volunteer lawyers to handle cases before the US Court of Veterans Claims. Engages in many activities around Agent Orange and VA reform. Publishes the only treatise on veteran's law.

8204 Washington D.C. Protection and Advocacy Agency
University Legal Services
220 I Street Northeast
Suite 130
Washington, DC 20002
202-547-0198
Fax: 202-547-2662
jbrown@uls-dc.org
www.uls-dc.org

Jane M Brown Esq., Executive Director
Andrew Martin, TP Program Manager
Alicia C. Johns, AT Program Director

Provides litigation services and technical assistance for seniors and those with disabilities.

8205 Washington Watch
United Cerebral Palsy Association
1825 K Street NW
Suite 600
Washington, DC 20006
202-776-0406
Fax: 202-776-0414; *Toll Free:* 800-872-5827
info@ucp.org
www.ucp.org/
TDD 202-973-7197

Woody Connette, Chair
Ian Ridion, Vice Chair
Mark Boles, Treasurer

Provides information on national legislation and regulatory affairs, updates on disability and social service fields.

24-36 pages

Florida

8206 Bay Area Legal Services
1302 N 19th Street
Suite 400
Tampa, FL 33605-5230
813-232-1343
Fax: 813-229-1403; *Toll Free:* 800-625-2257

jreed@bals.org
www.bals.org/About%20Us

Richard C Woltmann, Executive Director
Judy Reed, Development Director Assistant

People served through this program receive legal advice over the phone and forms and informational materials by mail when needed. They are also referred for necessary social services and extended legal representation, when appropriate.

8207 Florida Legal Services: Tallahassee Office
2425 Torreya Drive
Tallahassee, FL 32303
850-385-7900
Fax: 850-385-9998
kent@floridalegal.org
www.floridalegal.org/tallahas.htm

Kent Spuhler, Executive Director
Anne Swerlick, Deputy Director of Advocacy, Sta
Barbara O Stean, Deputy Direco of Finance

The Tallahassee office is the main office of Florida Legal Services (FLS) of which the staff advocates have expertise in all the major legal areas impacting the elderly and low income community in Florida. Policy advocacy, legislation and administration are major responsibilities for all of the advocates in the Tallahassee office. The staff is available for consultation with all those providing civil legal assistance to elderly, low income and disadvantaged persons in Florida. Statewide training and technical assistance is coordinated from the Tallahassee office.

8208 Senior Citizen Law Project
Coast to Coast Legal Aid of South Florida
491 North State Road 7
Plantation, FL 33317
954-765-8955
www.coasttocoastlegalaid.org

Steven Jaffe, Chair
Jeffrey M Wank, Vice Chair
Sherylle Francis, Secretary

The Senior Citizen Law Project provides legal advice and representation to Broward County residents who are 60 years of age or older. The Project offers services in the following areas: public/subsidized housing, eviction defence, landlord/tenant, food stamps, social security, medicaid and medicare, long term medical care, foreclosure defence, bankruptcy, debt collection defence, abuse and exploitation, and assistance to individuals seeking citizenship to qualify for pubic benefits.

Year Founded: 2003

8209 University of South Florida Library: Special Collections Department
4202 East Fowler Avenue
Tampa, FL 33620-9951
813-974-2729
Fax: 813-396-9006
www.lib.usf.edu/spccoll/edu/spccoll

Thomas Jay Kemp, University Librarian
Paul Eugen Camp, University Librarian
Merell Dickey, Development Director

The mission of the University of South Florida (USF) Library is to provide public services that focus on relevant collections and in addition facilitate the optimal use of resources, services, and facilities which support the university community's teaching, research and service initiatives. The Special Collections Department of the USF Libraries Digital Collections contain a wide range of digital content, including images, audio, video, full text, E-Journals, E-Books, articles, indexes, and collection guides. Many of the Tampa Library Special Collections Department collections may also contain a limited number of representative digital samples from the individual collections.

Year Founded: 1962

Georgia

8210 Atlanta Legal Aid Society: Atlanta

151 Spring Street Northwest
Atlanta, GA 30303
404-524-5811
pmckay_alas@yahoo.com
www.atlantalegalaid.org/

Rita A Sheffey, President Executive Committee
Stephen Krumm, Managing Attorney Law Project
Cheri Tipton, Managing Attorney Senior Hotline

Atlanta Legal Aid Society's primary function is to provide referrals and legal representation to people who otherwise cannot obtain access to the court system - the poor, minorities, the elderly, those disabled by mental illness or long term diseases, and recent immigrants. They come to us for help in meeting their basic needs, protecting their homes and safeguarding their families. In addition to the issues covered through special projects, we offer assistance with simple legal matters, such as drafting wills and seeking redress for substandard consumer goods. Staff attorneys are also available to speak publicly about legal issues.

8211 Atlanta Legal Aid Society: Decatur

246 Sycamore Street
Decatur, GA 30030-3434
404-377-0701
pmckay_alas@yahoo.com
www.atlantalegalaid.org/

Rita A Sheffey, President Executive Committee
Stephen Krumm, Managing Attorney Law Project
Cheri Tipton, Managing Attorney Senior Hotline

Atlanta Legal Aid Society's primary function is to provide referrals and legal representation to people who otherwise cannot obtain access to the court system - the poor, minorities, the elderly, those disabled by mental illness or long term diseases, and recent immigrants. They come to us for help in meeting their basic needs, protecting their homes and safeguarding their families. In addition to the issues covered through special projects, we offer assistance with simple legal matters, such as drafting wills and seeking redress for substandard consumer goods. Staff attorneys are also available to speak publicly about legal issues.

8212 Atlanta Legal Aid Society: East Point

1514 East Cleveland Avenue
Suite 100
East Point, GA 30344
404-669-0233
pmckay_alas@yahoo.com
www.atlantalegalaid.org/

Rita A Sheffey, President Executive Committee
Stephen Krumm, Managing Attorney Law Project
Cheri Tipton, Managing Attorney Senior Hotline

Atlanta Legal Aid Society's primary function is to provide referrals and legal representation to people who otherwise cannot obtain access to the court system - the poor, minorities, the elderly, those disabled by mental illness or long term diseases, and recent immigrants. They come to us for help in meeting their basic needs, protecting their homes and safeguarding their families. In addition to the issues covered through special projects, we offer assistance with simple legal matters, such as drafting wills and seeking redress for substandard consumer goods. Staff attorneys are also available to speak publicly about legal issues.

8213 Atlanta Legal Aid Society: Lawrenceville

185 Central Avenue
Suite T-704
Atlanta, GA 30303
404-335-2789
pmckay_alas@yahoo.com
www.atlantalegalaid.org/

Rita A Sheffey, President Executive Committee
Stephen Krumm, Managing Attorney Law Project
Cheri Tipton, Managing Attorney Senior Hotline

Atlanta Legal Aid Society's primary function is to provide referrals and legal representation to people who otherwise cannot obtain access to the court system - the poor, minorities, the elderly, those disabled by mental illness or long term diseases, and recent immigrants. They come to us for help in meeting their basic needs, protecting their homes and safeguarding their families. In addition to the issues covered through special projects, we offer assistance with simple legal matters, such as drafting wills and seeking redress for substandard consumer goods. Staff attorneys are also available to speak publicly about legal issues.

8214 Atlanta Legal Aid Society: Marietta

30 South Park Square
Marietta, GA 30090
770-528-2565
pmckay_alas@yahoo.com
www.atlantalegalaid.org/

Rita A Sheffey, President Executive Committee
Stephen Krumm, Managing Attorney Law Project
Cheri Tipton, Managing Attorney

Atlanta Legal Aid Society's primary function is to provide referrals and legal representation to people who otherwise cannot obtain access to the court system - the poor, minorities, the elderly, those disabled by mental illness or long term diseases, and recent immigrants. They come to us for help in meeting their basic needs, protecting their homes and safeguarding their families. In addition to the issues covered through special projects, we offer assistance with simple legal matters, such as drafting wills and seeking redress for substandard consumer goods. Staff attorneys are also available to speak publicly about legal issues.

8215 Georgia Division for Aging Services

Two Peachtree Street Northwest
33rd Floor
Atlanta, GA 30303-3142
404-657-5258
Fax: 404-657-5285; *Toll Free:* 866-552-4464
magreene@dhr.state.ga.us
aging.dhr.georgia.gov/portal/site

Maria Greene, Executive Director

The Georgia Department of Human Resources, Division of Aging Services (DAS) administers a statewide system of services for senior citizens, their families and caregivers, working with other aging agencies and organizations to effectively and efficiently respond to the needs of elderly Georgians. DAS meets the challenge of Georgia's growing older population through continued service improvement and innovation.

8216 Georgia Protection and Advocacy Agency
150 East Ponce de Leon Avenue
Suite 430
Decatur, GA 30030
404-885-1234
Fax: 404-378-0031; *Toll Free:* 800-537-2329
info@thegao.org
www.thegao.org/
TDD 404-885-1234

Ruby Moore, Executive Director
Denise Quigley, Director of Resource Advocacy
Naomi Walker, Program Director

Hawaii

8217 Hawaii Disability Rights Center: Honolulu
Hawaii Protection and Advocacy Agency
1132 Bishop Street
Suite 2102
Honolulu, HI 96813
808-949-2922
Fax: 808-949-2928; *Toll Free:* 800-882-1057
info@hawaiidisabilityrights.org
www.HawaiiDisabilityRights.org
TDD 808-949-2922

Bowles Bud, Executive Director
Kirby Shaw, Vice President
pauline Arellano, Director Client Services

Hawaii Disability Rights Center (HDRC is the designated Client Assistance Program (CAP) and Protection and Advocacy (P&A) System for Hawaii's estimated 180,000 residents with disabilities. We strive to serve as many individuals with disabilities with as many different legal rights issues as our resources will allow; and to achieve the following outcomes to advance the human, civil and legal rights of people with disabilities: freedom from abuse and neglect; accessible communities; independence, productivity, integration and inclusion, and, self determination.

8218 Legal Aid Society of Hawaii
305 Wailuku Drive
Hilo, HI 96720-2488
808-961-2851
Fax: 808-969-3983; *Toll Free:* 808-934-0678
www.legalaidhawaii.org/

Susan Ichinose, President
Jodi Shin Yamamoto, Esq., Vice President/ Treasurer
Joseph boivin, Esq., Vice President/ Treasurer

Serves older persons in Hawaii. Developed a long-term care planning presentation that discusses options for financing long-term care, living wills, powers of attorney, joint accounts, representative payees, due process in public benefits, and estate planning.

Year Founded: 1950

8219 Legal Aid Society of Hawaii: Hilo
305 Wailuku Drive
Hilo, HI 96720-2448

808-961-2851
Fax: 808-969-3983; *Toll Free:* 808-934-0678
www.legalaidhawaii.org/

Susan Ichinose, President
Jodi Shin Yamamoto, Esq., Vice President/ Treasurer
Joseph boivin, Esq., Vice President/ Treasurer

Serves older persons in Maui County. Provides ongoing outreach and community education programs regarding Medicaid, living wills, powers of attorney.

Year Founded: 1950

8220 Legal Aid Society of Hawaii: Honolulu
924 Bethel Street
Honolulu, HI 96813
Fax: 808-527-8088; *Toll Free:* 808-536-4302
www.legalaidhawaii.org/

Susan Ichinose, President
Jodi Shin Yamamoto, Esq., Vice President/ Treasurer
Joseph boivin, Esq., Vice President/ Treasurer

Serves older persons in Maui County. Provides ongoing outreach and community education programs regarding Medicaid, living wills, powers of attorney.

Year Founded: 1950

8221 Legal Aid Society of Hawaii: Kaunakakai
19-23 Ala Malama Street
Kaunakakai, HI 96748-0427
Fax: 808-553-5809; *Toll Free:* 808-553-3251
www.legalaidhawaii.org/

Susan Ichinose, President
Jodi Shin Yamamoto, Esq., Vice President/ Treasurer
Joseph boivin, Esq., Vice President/ Treasurer

Serves older persons in Maui County. Provides ongoing outreach and community education programs regarding Medicaid, living wills, powers of attorney.

Year Founded: 1950

8222 Legal Aid Society of Hawaii: Lanai City
730 Lanai Avenue
Suite 129
Lanai City, HI 96763-0315
Fax: 808-565-6089; *Toll Free:* 808-565-6089
www.legalaidhawaii.org/

Susan Ichinose, President
Jodi Shin Yamamoto, Esq., Vice President/ Treasurer
Joseph boivin, Esq., Vice President/ Treasurer

Serves older persons in Maui County. Provides ongoing outreach and community education programs regarding Medicaid, living wills, powers of attorney.

Year Founded: 1950

8223 Legal Aid Society of Hawaii: Lihu'e
3016 Umi Street
Suite 220
Lihu'e, HI 96766
808-245-4728
Fax: 808-246-8824; *Toll Free:* 808-245-7580
www.legalaidhawaii.org/

Susan Ichinose, President
Jodi Shin Yamamoto, Esq., Vice President/ Treasurer
Joseph boivin, Esq., Vice President/ Treasurer

Serves older persons in Maui County. Provides ongoing outreach and community education programs regarding Medicaid, living wills, powers of attorney.

Year Founded: 1950

8224 Legal Aid Society of Hawaii: Maui
2287 Main Street
Wailuku, HI 96793-1655
808-242-0724
Fax: 808-244-5856
www.legalaidhawaii.org/

Susan Ichinose, President
Jodi Shin Yamamoto, Esq., Vice President
Joseph boivin, Esq., Secretary/Treasurer

Serves older persons in Maui County. Provides ongoing outreach and community education programs regarding Medicaid, living wills, powers of attorney.

8225 Legal Aid Society of Hawaii: Maui County
2062 W. Vineyard Street
Suite 200
Wailuku, HI 96793
808-244-3731
Fax: 808-244-5856; *Toll Free:* 808-242-0724
www.legalaidhawaii.org/

Susan Ichinose, President
Jodi Shin Yamamoto, Esq., Vice President/ Treasurer
Joseph boivin, Esq., Vice President/ Treasurer

Year Founded: 1950

8226 University of Hawaii at Manoa: William S Richardson School of Law
2515 Dole Street
Honolulu, HI 96822-2328
808-956-6544
Fax: 808-956-9439
uhelp@hawaii.edu
www.hawaii.edu/uhelp/UHELP_whatis.html

James H Pietsch, Executive Director
John W. Gilm Saedene Ota, Vice Chai, James H. Q. Lee, Vice Chair

Operates an elder law clinic and an elder law unit that provide legal services to older persons. The Elder Law Clinic is a law school educational program with the primary responsibility of training law students in the Elder Law area.

Idaho

8227 Idaho Commission on Aging
341 W. Washington
3rd Floor
Boise, ID 83702
208-334-3833
Fax: 208-334-3033; *Toll Free:* 800-926-2588
ICOA@aging.idaho.gov
www.idahoaging.com/

Sam Haws, Administrator
Jeff Weller, Deputy Administrator
Kevin Bittner, Administrative Services

The Idaho Commission on Aging (ICOA) is the sole state agency designated under the Older Americans Act to administer programs and services for Idahoans 60 years of age and older. Located under the oversight of the Executive Office of the Governor, the ICOA plans and coordinates, funds, and monitors a statewide program of services to meet present and future needs of older Idahoans. Its second responsibility is to advocate for Idaho's elderly to secure existing rights, benefits and services under Federal, State and local law and to gain crucial new programs.

8228 Idaho Senior Legal Hotline
Idaho Legal Aid Services, Inc.
1447 S Tyrell Lane
Boise, ID 83706
208-345-0106 Toll free: 866-345-0116
www.idaholegalaid.org

Jim Cook, Executive Director
Howard Belodoff, Associate Director
Bev Allen, Executive Assistant

A hotline available to provide legal advice to individuals aged 60 and up. Idaho Legal Aid Services, Inc. is a non-profit law firm and community education organization providing access to justice for low income Idahoans.

Illinois

8229 AIDS Legal Council of Chicago
180 North Michigan Avenue
Suite 2110
Chicago, IL 60601
312-427-8990
Fax: 312-427-8419; *Toll Free:* 866-506-3038
info@aidslegal.com
www.aidslegal.com

Ann Hilton Fisher, Esq., Executive Director
Todd A Solomon, President
D Matthew Feldhaus, Vice President

Legal advice and services for persons who are HIV positive or have AIDS, and their companions, families, etc., regarding HIV-related legal matters.

Year Founded: 1987

8230 Center for Medicare and Medicaid Services (CMS)
Chicago Region 5 Office
233 North Michigan Avenue
Suite 600
Chicago, IL 60601-5519
312-886-6432
Fax: 312-353-0252; *Toll Free:* 800-465-3203
www.CMS.gov

Jackie Garner, Regional Administrator
Gwen Sampson, Deputy Regional Administrator

The Chicago Regional Office (Region 5) should be your initial point of contact on any Medicare, Medicaid, or State Child Health Insurance Program (SCHIP), issue in the following states: Illinois, Indiana, Michigan, Minnesota, Ohio and Wisconsin.

Year Founded: 1965

8231 Chicago Kent Law School Information Center
Illinois Institute of Technology
565 West Adams Street
Chicago, IL 60661
312-906-5000
Fax: 312-906-5280
kstivers@kentlaw.edu
library.kentlaw.edu/

Keith Stiverson, Library Director
JoAnn Hounshell, Associate Director
Deborah Ginsberg, Head of Research, Faculty Servic

Information on federal and Illinois law, law and aging, international relations law, financial services law, business and management, environmental law.

8232 Chicago Lawyers' Committee For Civil Rights Under Law

100 North LaSalle Street
Suite 600
Chicago, IL 60602-2403
312-630-9744
Fax: 312-630-1127
clccrul@aol.com
www.clccrul.org/index.html

Max A Stein, President
Nancy L Maldonado, Vice President
Eric J Gorman, Treasurer

Legal aid, including class action suits and impact cases concerning the rights of persons with disabilities and their families.

Year Founded: 1969

8233 Council for Disability Rights

30 East Adams
Suite 1130
Chicago, IL 60603
312-444-1967
Fax: 312-444-1977
www.disabilityrights.org

Josephine E Holzer, Executive Director/Editor
Dorie Stewart, Information Specialist
Mary Beth Gahan, Disability Consultant

Promotes human rights of persons with disabilities and their families. Offers a job placement service, legal referrals, information services, a website and monthly newsletter (CDR Reports).

Year Founded: 1981

8234 Disabled Americans Rally for Equality

4752 South Kilpatrick Avenue
Chicago, IL 60632-4833
773-873-8703
Fax: 773-873-7818

Dennis Schreiber, Coordinator

Promotes awareness and lobbies for disabled persons rights.

8235 Equip for Equality: Chicago Advancing the Human & Civil Rights of People with Disabilities in IL

20 North Michigan Avenue
Suite 300
Chicago, IL 60602
312-341-0022
Fax: 312-541-7544; *Toll Free:* 800-537-2632
contactus@equipforequality.org
www.equipforequality.org
TTY: 800-610-2779

Zena Naiditch, President/CEO

The mission of Equip for Equality is to advance the human and civil rights of children and adults with physical and mental disabilities in Illinois. It is the only statewide, cross-disability, comprehensive advocacy organization providing self-advocacy assistance, legal services, and disability rights education while also engaging in public policy

and legislative advocacy and conducting abuse investigations and other oversight activities.

8236 Equip for Equality: Rock Island Advancing the Human & Civil Rights of People with Disabilities in IL

20 North Michigan Avenue
Suite 300
Chicago, IL 60602
312-341-0022
Fax: 312-541-7544; *Toll Free:* 800-537-2632
contactus@equipforequality.org
www.equipforequality.org
TTY: 800-610-2779

Zena Naiditch, President/CEO

The mission of Equip for Equality is to advance the human and civil rights of children and adults with physical and mental disabilities in Illinois. It is the only statewide, cross-disability, providing self-advocacy assistance, legal services, and disability rights education while also engaging in public policy and legislative advocacy and conducting abuse investigations and other oversight activities.

8237 Equip for Equality: Springfield Advancing the Human & Civil Rights of People with Disabilities in IL

20 North Michigan Avenue
Suite 300
Chicago, IL 60602
312-341-0022
Fax: 312-541-7544; *Toll Free:* 800-537-2632
contactus@equipforequality.org
www.equipforequality.org
TTY: 800-610-2779

Zena Naiditch, President/CEO

The mission of Equip for Equality is to advance the human and civil rights of children and adults with physical and mental disabilities in Illinois. It is the only statewide, cross-disability, comprehensive advocacy organization providing self-advocacy assistance, legal services, and disability rights education while also engaging in public policy and legislative advocacy and conducting abuse investigations and other oversight activities.

8238 Guardianship Services Associates

41 South Boulevard
Oak Park, IL 60302
708-386-5398
Fax: 708-386-5970
GSAoakpark@aol.com

Robert R Wohlgemuth, Director

Information and counseling on guardianship issues. Can provide direct assistance in obtaining guardianship for disabled adults.

8239 Illinois Department on Aging

One Natural Resources Way
Suite 100
Springfield, IL 62702-1271
217-785-3356
Fax: 217-785-4477; *Toll Free:* 800-252-8966
aging.ilsenior@illinois.gov
www.state.il.us/aging/
TTY: 888-206-1327

John K. Holton, Director

The mission of the Illinois Department on Aging is to serve and advocate for older Illinoisans and their caregivers by administering programs and promoting partnerships that encourage independence, dignity, and quality of life.

8240 Pro Bono Center for Disability and Elder Law (CDEL): Lifelong Lawyers Project
Chicago Bar Association Senior Lawyers Committee
321 South Plymouth Court
Chicago, IL 60604
312-554-2000
Fax: 312-554-1203
proos@chicagobar.org
www.chicagobar.org/

J Timothy Eaton, President
Daniel Cotter, First Vice President
Patricia Brown, Second Vice President

The Pro Bono Center for Disability and Elder Law (CDEL) identifies, protects and advances the legal rights of persons with disabilities and the elderly by providing free, high quality legal services. CDEL bills itself as a pro bono law firm, and the spectrum of pro bono opportunities available is extensive and varied. Whether you choose direct legal services or community outreach activities, the staff will provide everything needed to accommodateindividual schedule and service requirements.

8241 Senior Citizens' Wills Program: Chicago Bar Association
321 South Plymouth Court
Chicago, IL 60604
312-554-2000
tmurphy@chicagobar.org
www.chicagobar.org/

J Timothy Eaton, President
Daniel Cotter, First Vice President
Patricia Brown, Second Vice President

Provides senior citizens with access to low-cost wills and other important legal services.

8242 US Department of Health and Human Services: Office for Civil Rights
100 South Grand Avenue East
Springfield, IL 62762
312-353-5160
Fax: 312-886-1718; *Toll Free:* 800-843-6154
www.state.il.us/agency/dhs/592ycrnp.html

Donna Morros Weinstein, Regional Chief Counsel

Enforces the Rehabilitation Act of 1973, prohibiting discrimination against handicapped persons by recipients of federal funding.

Indiana

8243 Aging and In Home Services of Northeast Indiana
Indiana Area Agency on Aging
2927 Lake Avenue
Fort Wayne, IN 46805
260-745-1200
Fax: 260-422-4916; *Toll Free:* 800-552-3662
info@agingihs.org
www.agingihs.org/

Connie Wolfe, President

The Indiana Association of Area Agencies on Aging (IAAAA) advocates for quality programs and services for older adults and persons with disabilities. IAAAA believes in the individual's right to: choose among health care alternatives to maintain independence and dignity; practice healthy lifestyles to have a happier, healthier, and longer life; and, be educated about services and alternatives available.

8244 Indiana Division of Aging
Indiana Family & Social Services Administration
33 North Central Avenue
Suite 317
Medford, IN 97501
800-362-8837
Fax: 317-232-7867
info@ltcoptions.com
www.ltcoptions.com

Faith Laird, Director
Karen Filler, Deputy
Nick Petrone, Deputy

The Indiana Division of Aging (IDA) provides a broad range of in-home and community based services to older adults and persons of all ages with disabilities. Services provided focus on prevention, early intervention, protection and advocacy. The Division collaborates with communities, local organizations, and other units of government to provide services to individuals and their families.

8245 Indiana Protection and Advocacy Agency
4701 North Keystone Avenue
Suite 222
Indianapolis, IN 46205
317-722-5555
Fax: 317-722-5564; *Toll Free:* 800-622-4845
kpedevilla@ipas.IN.gov
www.IN.gov/ipas
TDD 317-722-5555

Tom Gallagher, Executive Director

IPAS was created in 1977 by state law (IC. 12-28-1-6 as amended) to protect and advocate the rights of people with disabilities and is Indiana's federally designated Protection and Advocacy (P&A) system and client assistance program.

Year Founded: 1977

8246 Northwest Indiana Community Action Corp
Indiana Area Agency on Aging
5240 Fountain Drive
Crown Point, IN 46307
219-794-1829
Fax: 219-932-0566; *Toll Free:* 800-826-7871
director@nwi-ca.org
www.nwi-ca.com
TTY: 888-814-7597

Karen Evans, Board President
Jennifer Malone, Director Elderly Services
Ida Parker, Board Vice President

The Indiana Association of Area Agencies on Aging (IAAAA) advocates for quality programs and services for older adults and persons with disabilities. IAAAA believes in the individual's right to: choose among health care alternatives to maintain independence and dignity; practice healthy lifestyles to have a happier, healthier, and longer life; and, be educated about services and alternatives available.

8247 Resources For Enriching Adult Learning(REAL)
Indiana Area Agency on Aging
1151 South Michigan Street
PO Box 1835
South Bend, IN 46634-1835
574-284-7928
Fax: 574-284-2642; *Toll Free:* 800-552-7928
www.realservicesinc.com

Steven Watts, Chairperson
Mary Downes, Treasurer
Rebecca Zaseck, Secretary

The Indiana Association of Area Agencies on Aging (IAAAA) advocates for quality programs and services for older adults and persons with disabilities. IAAAA believes in the individual's right to: choose among health care alternatives to maintain independence and dignity; practice healthy lifestyles to have a happier, healthier, and longer life; and, be educated about services and alternatives available.

Year Founded: 1966

8248 Senior Law Project
Indiana Legal Services, Inc.
151 N Delaware
Suite 1800
Indianapolis, IN 46204
317-631-9410
Fax: 317-631-9775; *Toll Free:* 800-869-0212
www.indianalegalservices.org

Jon Laramore, Executive Director

Offers legal representation, consultation, and advice to individuals aged 60 and over in areas such as estate planning, public benefits, housing, consumer, and family.

Year Founded: 1966

8249 Southwestern Indiana Mental Health Center
415 Mulberry Street
Evansville, IN 47713-1298
812-423-7791
Fax: 812-422-7558
www.southwestern.org/

Tonee Brinkman, Contact

The mission of Southwestern shall be to provide quality mental health services to the citizens of Gibson, Posey, Vanderburgh and Warrick counties. The services provided shall be consistent with demonstrated community needs and prudent utilization of Southwestern's resources. The services shall be reasonably available and accessible to all citizens and shall be provided in an environment in which the rights of individual patients are recognized aNd respected.

Year Founded: 1978

Iowa

8250 Elderbridge-Area Agency on Aging: Legal Referral Panel
22 North Georgia Avenue
Suite 216
Mason City, IA 50401
641-424-0678
Fax: 641-424-2927; *Toll Free:* 800-243-0678
rthompson@elderbridge.org
www.elderbridge.org

Mick Tagesen, Executive Director

The Panel accepts cases in which the clients are not eligible for free legal services, yet cannot afford to retain a private attorney.

Year Founded: 1973

8251 Help Legal Assistance: Senior Citizens Law Project
Jesse M. Parker Building
510 East 12th Street
Suite 2
Des Moines, IA 50319-9025
515-725-3333
Fax: 515-725-3300; *Toll Free:* 800-532-3213
www.iowalegalaid.org/hotline/

Dennis Groenenboom, Executive Director

The Legal Hotline is the first place to go to get information and advice about elder law issues. The Legal Hotline is a special project of Iowa Legal Aid that provides legal advice and other services to Iowans who are 60 or older. The Hotline's services are free and confidential. By getting legal advice when you need it, you can prevent and resolve legal problems, avoid being victimized, remain independent and make better life planning decisions.

8252 Iowa Department on Aging: Legal Assistance
Jesse M. Parker Building
510 East 12th Street
Suite 2
Des Moines, IA 50319-9025
515-725-3333
Fax: 515-725-3300; *Toll Free:* 800-532-3213
Deanna.Clingan@iowa.gov
www.aging.iowa.gov
TTY: 515-725-3302

John McCalley, Executive Director
Deanna Clingan-Fischer, Legal Assistance Developer

Provides advocacy, educational, prevention and health promotion services for older Iowans, their families and caregivers through partnerships with Area Agencies on Aging and other stakeholders.

8253 Iowa State Bar: Young Lawyer Section Committee on Delivery of Legal Services to the Elderly
625 East Court Avenue
Suite 3700
Des Moines, IA 50309-8004
515-243-3179
Fax: 515-243-2511; *Toll Free:* 800-457-3729
isba@iowabar.org
www.iowabar.org

Wiliam J Miller, Committee Chair
Dwight Dinkla, Executive Director
Harry Shipley, Assisstant Executive Director

The services to the elderly committee is a volunteer organization of lawyers who are interested in ensuring that the legal needs and rights of older iowans are met.

8254 Seneca Area Agency on Aging
Iowa Department of Elder Affairs
117 North Cooper Street
Ottumwa, IA 52501
641-681-2270
Fax: 641-682-2445; *Toll Free:* 800-642-6522
seneca@seneca-aaa.org
www.seneca-aaa.org

Connie Holland, Chief Executive Director
Christta Meritt, Chief Operating Officer
Lisa Crews, Financial Officer

Seneca Area Agency on Aging advocates for and provides assistance to older persons in a non-discriminatory manner, working toward fostering and maintaining independence while preserving the dignity of each individual and focusing on their quality of life.

8255 Siouxland Aging Services
2301 Pierce Street
Sioux City, IA 51104
712-279-6900
Fax: 712-233-3415; *Toll Free:* 800-432-9209
siouxlandaging@siouxlandaging.org
www.SiouxlandAging.org

Terry Amburn, Chairperson
John Twombly, Vice Chair
Lorraine Davis, Secretary

The mission of Siouxland Aging Services is to: secure and maintain maximum independence and dignity in a home environment for older individuals capable of self care with appropriate supportive services; remove individual and social barriers to economic and personal independence for older individuals; and, provide a continuum of care for the vulnerable elderly.

8256 Winifred Law Opportunity Center
1553 Broadwaay
Pella, IA 50219
641-628-1162
Fax: 641-628-8682
www.christianopportunity.org/

Ron Groenenboom, President
Bob Kroese, Vice President
Mike Maakestad, Secretary

The Christian Opportunity Center sTrives to provide quality support to people with disabilities and is also committed to the Christian values of the founding fathers.

Year Founded: 1969

Kansas

8257 Elder Law Hotline
Kansas Legal Services
712 S Kansas Avenue
Suite 200
Topeka, KS 66603
Toll Free: 888-353-5337
www.kansaslegalservices.org

Marilyn Harp, Executive Director

Elder Law Hotline is funded by the Kansas Bar Foundation. Hotline attorneys answer questions in civil cases for Kansans age 60 or older. Cases may be referred to a local Senior Citizens Law Project attorney or a private attorney through the Elder Law Panel, arranged together with the Kansas Bar Association.

8258 Kansas Department of Aging: Legal Assistance Services for Older Adults (KDOA)
Kansas Department on Aging
503 South Kansas Avenue
Topeka, KS 66603-3404
785-296-4986
Fax: 785-296-0256
www.agingkansas.org/

Kathleen Sebelius, KDOA Governor
Kathy Greenlee, KDOA Acting Secretary

Legal assistance services provide access to the system of justice by offering advice and representation by a legal provider. This provider acts as an advocate for the social and economically needy older individual to ensure gaining access to essential services or financial resources, and protecting their rights to be autonomous and to retain their dignity.

8259 Kansas Protection and Advocacy Agency & Disability Rights Center of Kansas
635 SW harrison St
Suite 100
Topeka, KS 66603
785-273-9661
Fax: 785-273-9414; *Toll Free:* 877-776-1541
rocky@drckansas.org
www.drckansas.org
TDD 877-335-3725

Rocky Nichols, Executive Director
Debbie White, Deputy Director
Lane Williams, Deputy Director, legal Division

The Disability Rights Center of Kansas (DRC), is a public interest legal advocacy agency empowered by federal law to advocate for the civil and legal rights of Kansans with disabilities. DRC is the Official Protection and Advocacy System for Kansas and is a part of the national network of federally mandated and funded protection and advocacy systems. As such, DRC advocates for the rights of Kansans with disabilities under state or federal laws (ADA, the Rehabilitation Act, Federal Medicaid Act, Kansas Act Against Discrimination, etc.).

8260 Senior Citizen Law Project Kansas
Kansas Legal Services
712 S Kansas Avenue
Suite 200
Topeka, KS 66603
785-233-2068Toll free: 785-354-8311
www.kansaslegalservices.org

Marilyn Harp, Executive Director

Provides services in a wide range of civil legal issues to persons age 60 and older. Its goal is to target the more at risk elderly residents who are in the greatest social and economic need. Priorities include assuring that seniors obtain the cash and medical assistance needed for their wellbeing. Another focus is on stopping financial, physical or psychological abuse of elders. SCLP also has a broad public teaching program. The program helps elders and workers serving the elderly by teaching about elders' rights and protections under the law.

Kentucky

8261 Kentucky Bar Association: Committee on Legal Concerns of Elderly Clients
514 West Main Street
Frankfort, KY 40601-1883
502-564-3795
Fax: 502-564-3225
webmaster@kybar.org
www.kybar.org/

J Frank Burnette, Director
Charlene S Jones, Information Systems Manager
Peggy Morris, Administrator

Produces a handbook on eight broad law-related areas for the elderly, including information and referral sections, a reading list, and a resource guide.

8262 Kentucky Bar Association: Senior Lawyers Section
514 West Main Street
Frankfort, KY 40601-1883
502-564-3795
Fax: 502-564-3225
webmaster@kybar.org
www.kybar.org/

George Rabe, Executive Director

The Senior Lawyers Section of the Kentucky Bar Association is comprised of lawyers 55 years old and older that includes senior practicing attorneys as well as retired and semi-retired lawyers. The section provides a common forum for exchanging ideas and promotes and provides continuing education for retired or semi-retired lawyers and fosters excellence and professionalism.

8263 Kentucky Legal Aid
1122 Jefferson Street
Paducah, KY 42001
270-442-5518Toll free: 866-452-9243
www.klaid.org/

Jeffrey A Been, Executive Director/Attorney
Ronald E Marstin, Managing Attorney
S. Stewart Pope, Advocacy Director/Attorney

The mission of Kentucky Legal Aid (KLA) is to assist and to enable low-income families, as well as the elderly, disabled and other vulnerable individuals in South Central and Western Kentucky, to resolve legal problems that are barriers to self-sufficiency, and to provide these individuals an opportunity for an improved quality of life. KLA utilizes attorneys and other staff to provide direct legal assistance; coordinates referrals to volunteer (pro bono) attorneys; and also addresses these client needs through programs for Benefits Counseling and Domestic Violence Assistance.

Year Founded: 1977

8264 Kentucky Protection and Advocacy Agency
100 Fair Oaks Lane
3rd Floor
Frankfort, KY 40601
502-564-2967
Fax: 502-564-0848; *Toll Free:* 800-372-2988
www.kypa.net
TDD 800-372-2988

Marsha Hochensmith, Executive Director

Protection and Advocacy (P&A) is an independent state agency that was designated by the Governor as the protec-

tion and advocacy agency for Kentucky. P&A's staff includes professional advocates and attorneys. Advocates work together with people who have disabilities to promote and protect their legal rights in addition to providing information and referral services regarding an individual's rights under disability laws.

Louisiana

8265 AIDSLAW of Louisiana
2601 Tulane Ave
Suite 500
New Orleans, LA 70119-6439
501-821-2601
Fax: 504-821-2040
info@noaidstf.org
www.aidslaw.org/

Sergio Farfan, Co Chair
Helen Seigal, Co Chair
Troy Scroggins, Vice Chair

Second year of funding for new legal agency serving persons affected by HIV/AIDS.

8266 Acadiana Legal Service Corporation
1020 Surrey Street
Lafayette, LA 70502
337-237-4320
Fax: 337-237-8839; *Toll Free:* 800-256-1175
alsclaf@la-law.org
www.la-law.org/locations.html

Joseph R Oelkers, III, Executive Director
Sharon Jones, Administrative Director
Cathy Davis, Secretary

Provides support and services to those with disabilities and the senior population.

Year Founded: 1974

8267 Baton Rouge Advocacy Center
8325 Oak Street
Augusta, LA 70118
318-227-6186
Fax: 318-227-1841; *Toll Free:* 800-960-7705
advocacycenter@advocacyla.org
www.advocacyla.org
TTY: 855-861-3577

Glyn Butler, Client Advocate

The Advocacy Center believes in the dignity of every life, and in the freedom of all people to experience the highest degree of self-determination. Embracing this philosophy, the Advocacy Center protects and advocates for the human and legal rights of persons living in Louisiana who are elderly or disabled.

Year Founded: 1977

8268 Lafayette Advocacy Center
8325 Oak Street
Augusta, LA 70118
318-227-6186
Fax: 318-227-1841; *Toll Free:* 800-960-7705
advocacycenter@advocacyla.org
www.advocacyla.org
TTY: 855-861-3577

Suzanne Chevallier, Program Director

The Advocacy Center believes in the dignity of every life, and in the freedom of all people to experiencethe highest degree of self-determination. Embracing this philosophy, the Advocacy Center protects and advocates fo the human and legal rights of persons living in Louisianna who are elderly or disabled.

Year Founded: 1977

8269 New Orleans Advocacy Center
8325 Oak Street
New Orleans, LA 70118
504-522-2337
Fax: 318-227-1841; *Toll Free:* 800-960-7705
advocacycenter@advocacyla.org
www.advocacyla.org/
TTY: 855-861-3577

Lois Simpson, Executive Director
Charles Tubre, Program Director

The Advocacy Center serves individuals with disabilities and senior citizens as New Orleans and Louisiana struggle to rebuild.

Year Founded: 1977

8270 Shreveport Advocacy Center
8325 Oak Street
New Orleans, LA 70118
318-227-6186
Fax: 318-227-1841; *Toll Free:* 800-960-7705
advocacycenter@advocacyla.org
www.advocacyla.org
TTY: 855-861-3577

Lois Simpson, Executive Director
Freddie Pincus, President
Denver D Nobles Jr, Advisory Council Co-Chair

The Advocacy Center believes in the dignity of every life, and in the freedom of all people to experience the highest degree of self-determination. Embracing this philosophy, the Advocacy Center protects and advocates for the human and legal rights of persons living in Louisiana who are elderly or disabled.

Year Founded: 1977

Maine

8271 Legal Services for the Elderly: Augusta
5 Wabon Street
Augusta, ME 04330
207-621-0087
Fax: 207-621-0742; *Toll Free:* 800-750-5353
www.mainelse.org/

Jaye Martin, Executive Director
Stanley N Marshall Jr, Chairman
Donald Dufour, Finance Manager

Legal Services for the Elderly provides persons age 60 and over with free legal advice regarding health care, health insurance, medicare (including part d), MaineCare (medicaid), social security and other public benefits.

8272 Maine Protection and Advocacy Agency Disability Rights Center: Augusta Office
24 Stone Street
Suite 204
Augusta, ME 04330

207-626-2774
Fax: 207-621-1419; *Toll Free:* 800-452-1948
advocate@drcme.org
www.drcme.org
TDD 800-452-1948

Richard O Meara, President
Penny Plourde, ice resident
Corin Swift, Secretary

The mission of the Disability Rights Center is to advance and enforce the rights of individuals with disabilities. In working with and on behalf of people with disabilities, we are committed to the principles that people with disabilities can make choices and that they are entitled to enjoy life's benefits as full and equal members of Maine's communities.

8273 Maine State Bar Association: Section on Elder Law
PO Box 788
Augusta, ME 04332
207-622-7523
Fax: 207-623-0083
info@mainebar.org
www.mainebar.org/sections

Julie G Rowe, Executive Director
Diana Dusini, President
David Levesque, President Elect

Projects include community education events for seniors, continuing legal education on elder law, legislation, formulation of ethical guidelines in representing older people, and a series of elder law techniques and management.

Maryland

8274 Maryland Disability Law Center
1500 Union Avenue
Suite 2000
Baltimore, MD 21211
410-727-6352
Fax: 410-727-6389; *Toll Free:* 800-233-7201
www.mdlcbalto.org/
TDD 410-235-5387

Laurence Eisenstein, Esq., Chairman
Virginia Knowlton, Executive Director
Lorraine Cheehan, Deputy Director Public Policy

8275 Maryland Legal Aid Bureau: Annapolis
229 Hanover Street
Annapolis, MD 21401
410-972-2700
Fax: 410-951-7818; *Toll Free:* 800-666-8330
www.mdlab.org

Wilhelm H Joseph, Jr., Esq., Executive Director
Cheryl Hystad, Esq., Advocacy Director
Gustava Taler, Esq, COO

The Legal Aid Bureau has been providing free civil legal services in Maryland for low-income people, children and the elderly since 1911. Legal Aid handles civil, not criminal, cases. Priorities for general civil legal services are family/domestic, housing, income maintenance (public benefits), and consumer/finance.

8276 Maryland Legal Aid Bureau: Baltimore
500 East Lexington Street
Baltimore, MD 21202

410-951-7777
Fax: 410-951-7818; *Toll Free:* 800-999-8904
www.mdlab.org

Wilhelm H Joseph Jr., Esq., Executive Director
Cheryl Hystad, Esq., Advocacy Director
Gustava Taler, Esq, COO

The Legal Aid Bureau has been providing free civil legal services in Maryland for low-income people, children and the elderly since 1911. Legal Aid determines financial eligibility for general legal services based on income and assets available to the household, using the Federal Poverty Income Guidelines (except for specialized services where eligibility conditions, such as age, are set by the terms of the grants). Legal Aid handles civil, not criminal, cases. Priorities for general civil legal services are family/domestic, housing, income maintenance (public benefits), and consumer/finance.

8277 Maryland State Bar Association of Legal Services
520 West Fayette Street
Baltimore, MD 21201
410-685-7878
Fax: 410-685-1016; *Toll Free:* 800-492-1964
president@msba.org
www.msba.org/about/service.htm

Paul V Carlin, Executive Director
Michael J Baxter, President
Pamila J Brown, Secretary

The Sixty Plus Program provides reduced fee wills, health care and financial powers of attorney, living wills, intra-family deeds, and small estate administration for financially eligible elderly persons.

Massachusetts

8278 Bristol Elder Services
1 Father Devalles Blvd.
Suite 101
Fall River, MA 02723
508-675-2101
Fax: 208-324-4619; *Toll Free:* 800-462-4632
info@bristolelder.org
www.bristolelder.org
TTY: 508-646-9704

Melanie Minutelli-Ramos, Grants Manager/Planner
Margaret Pilkington, Program Director

Founded in 1973, Bristol Elder Services, Inc. (Bristol) is a not-for-profit corporation, designated as an Aging Services Access Point and Area Agency on Aging. Bristol recieves state and federal monies to assist elders in maintaining their independence in the community. Bristol serves as the entry point for elder services in southeastern Massachusetts. Additionally, through the federal Older Americans Act, Bristol coordinates and funds an array of community programs designed to bridge the gaps in services and promote independence for elders. Bristol offers many services for elders and their caregivers.

Number of Members: 1973

8279 Commonwealth of Massachusetts Executive Office of Elder Affairs
One Ashburton Place
Fifth Floor
Boston, MA 02108

617-727-7750
Fax: 617-727-9368; *Toll Free:* 800-243-4636
elder.affairs@state.ma.us
www.mass.gov/
TTY: 800-872-0166

Elana Margolis, Chief of Staff
Je'Lesia M. Jones, Communication Director
Jennifer Davis Carey, Secretary

The vision of the Executive Office of Elder Affairs is to ensure that elders in Massachusetts have the supports necessary to maintain their well being and dignity. In addition, the Office of Elder Affairs promotes the independence and well-being of elders and people needing medical and social supportive services by providing advocacy, leadership, and management expertise to maintain a continuum of services responsive to the needs of our constituents, their families, and caregivers.

8280 Disability Law Center (DLC)
11 Beacon Street
Suite 925
Boston, MA 02108
617-723-8455
Fax: 617-723-9125; *Toll Free:* 800-872-9992
mail@dlc-ma.org
www.dlc-ma.org
TDD 617-227-9464

Alan Kerzin, Executive Director

Provides support that allows those with disabilities to participate fully and equally in the social and economic life of Massachusett.

8281 Greater Boston Legal Services: Elderly Unit
197 Friend Street
Boston, MA 02114
617-371-1234
Fax: 617-371-1222; *Toll Free:* 800-323-3205
www.gbls.org
TDD 617-371-1228

Robert Sable, Executive Director
Daniel Manning, Associate Director
Sonia Marcquez, Director of Human Resources

GBLS represents individuals and families, assisting with individual client needs as well as systemic problems. We also represent community groups and provide community legal education. We give advice and represent people in court, before agencies, and before city councils and the state legislature.

Number of Members: 1976

8282 Legal Assistance Corporation of Central Massachusetts: Senior Citizens Community Legal Aid (CLA)
P O Box 34441
LA, CA 90034
310-474-3600
Fax: 508-752-5918; *Toll Free:* 855-252-5342
klee@cla-ma.org
www.communitylegal.org
TTY: 508-755-3260

Jonathan Mannina, Executive Director

Provides free legal assistance to elders on many issues including benefits, housing, civil matters, Medicaid/Medicare eligibility, and elder abuse and nursing home issues. Also conducts education programs and distributes literature on critical topics.

8283 Massachusetts Mutual Life Insurance Company Law Library

1295 State Street
Springfield, MA 01111-0001
413-788-8411
Fax: 413-744-6114
www.massmutual.com

Roger W Crandall, Chairman
Robert J Casale, Executive Vice President
Susan m Cicco, Vice President

Law - insurance, taxation, securities, real estate, pensions; litigation.

8284 Mount Ida College: National Center for Death Education

777 Dedham Street
Newton Centre, MA 02459-3310
617-928-4500
Fax: 617-928-4713
jharding@mountida.edu
www.mountida.edu/ncde

Judith Harding, Coordinator Resources/Director
Barry Brown, President

The National Center for Death Education (NCDE) is an educational center dedicated to promoting knowledge and understanding in the field of Thanatology. NCDE aims to help people enhance their own awareness of death as well as provide them with the resources to support the dying and grieving of all ages. We provide ongoing learning opportunities for professional caregivers and others designed for acquiring and maintaining a current knowledge base, as well as developing creative and useful skills for providing care associated with end of life, bereavement and loss.

Year Founded: 1984

8285 Sturgis Library

3090 Main Street
P O Box 606
Barnstable, MA 02630
508-362-6636
Fax: 508-362-5467
sturgislibrary@comcast.net
www.sturgislibrary.org/

Ted Lowrie, Library Director
Sue Angus, Vice president
John Ehret, Treasurer

Sturgis Library, a historic public library in the village of Barnstable, Massachusetts is dedicated to promoting the study of Cape Cod history and genealogy while serving the needs of a contemporary community.

Year Founded: 1963

8286 Volunteer Lawyers Project of the Boston Bar Association

29 Temple Place
Boston, MA 02111-1340
617-423-0648
Fax: 617-423-0061

Mary M Connolly, Executive Director
Legal services for elgible clients.

8287 Berrien County Legal Services: Senior Law Center

89 Ionia Avenue
Suite 400
Grand Rapids, MI 49503
616-774-0672
Fax: 616-983-1045; *Toll Free:* 888-418-1311
amin@legalaidwestmich.net
www.legalaidwestmich.org/

Paul T Vlachos, President
Preston Hopson Jr, Treasurer
Brian P McMahon, Vice President

For more than 30 years, Legal Services Corporation funded agencies in Western Michigan have provided free legal assistance to low income persons and Seniors in non-criminal, non-fee generating matters. Legal Aid of Western Michigan currently serves people in 17 counties in the lower Western part of Michigan.

8288 Center for Elder Rights + Advocacy, aproject at Elder Law of Michigan (CERA)

3815 West St. Joseph Street
Suice C-200
Lansing, MI 48917
Toll Free: 866-949-2372
info@ceraresource.com
www.legalhotlines.org

Kath L. Morris, Director

The Center for Elder Rights Advocacy (CERA) is supported by a grant from the United States Administration on aging. CERA provides technical assistance to managers of non profit legal hotlines, legal programs planning to develop a legal hotline, and others interested in integrating a legal hotline into their legal services delivery system,

8289 Elder Law of Michigan: Legal Hotline for Michigan Seniors

3815 West Street
Suite C200
Lansing, MI 48917
517-485-9164
Fax: 517-372-0792; *Toll Free:* 866-400-9164
info@elderslaw.org
www.elderslaw.org/

Keith Moris, President
Talbott C Smith, Director
Forest Harper, Vice President

8290 Michigan Protection & Advocacy Service: Livonia

4095 Legacy Parkway
Suite 500
Lansing, MI 48911
517-487-1755
Fax: 517-487-0827; *Toll Free:* 800-288-5923
ecerano@mpas.org
www.mpas.org/

Elmer L Cerano, Executive Director
Kate Pew Walters, President
Thomas Landry, 1st Vice President

Michigan Protection and Advocacy Service strives to advance the dignity, equality, self-determination, and expressed choices of individuals. Michigan Protection and

Advocacy Service, Inc. (MPAS) promotes, expands and protects the human and legal rights of people by providing them with information and advocacy.

8291 Michigan Protection and Advocacy Service: Lansing
4095 Legacy Parkway
Suite 500
Lansing, MI 48911
517-487-1755
Fax: 517-487-0827; *Toll Free:* 800-288-5923
ecerano@mpas.org
www.mpas.org/
TDD 517-487-1755

Elmer L Cerano, Executive Director
Kate Pew Walters, President
Thomas Landry, 1st Vice President

Michigan Protection and Advocacy Service strives to advance the dignity, equality, self-determination, and expressed choices of individuals. Michigan Protection and Advocacy Service, Inc. (MPAS) promotes, expands and protects the human and legal rights of people by providing them with information and advocacy.

8292 State Bar of Michigan: Senior Justice Committee
Michael Franck Building
306 Townsend Street
Lansing, MI 48933-2012
517-346-6300
Fax: 517-482-6248; *Toll Free:* 800-968-1442
www.michbar.org/programs/

Brian D Einhorn, Chairman
Thomas C Rombach, President Elect
Lori A Buiteweg, Vice President

Committee deals in pro bono, education of public and legal community, legislative activities, and long-range planning.

Minnesota

8293 Minneapolis Age & Opportunity Center
1807 Nicollet Avenue South
Minneapolis, MN 55403
612-863-1000
Fax: 612-863-1451
www.abanet.org/aging/

Jack L Rives, Exective Director

The Minneapolis Age and Opportunity Center offers and coordinates an impressive array of services for its home-bound and disabled clients ranging from legal assistance to home-delivered meals, from skilled nursing to home maintenance.

Number of Members: 1878

8294 Minnesota Board on Aging
Elmer L Andersen Human Services Building
540 Cedar Street
St. Paul, MN 55155
651-431-2500
Fax: 651-431-7543; *Toll Free:* 800-882-6262
mba@state.mn.us
www.mnaging.org/
TTY: 800-627-3529

Jean Wood, Executive Director
Don Samuelson, Chair

The Minnesota Board on Aging (MBA) is the gateway to services for seniors and their families. MBA listens to senior concerns, researches for solutions, and proposes policy to address senior needs. In addition, MBA administer funds from the Older Americans Act that provide a spectrum of services to seniors, including Senior LinkAge LineT, Insurance Counseling and more. First established in 1956, the MBA is one of the pioneers in the field of agingworks closely with its Area Agencies on Aging, which are located throughout the state, to provide services that seniors need.

Number of Members: 1956

Mississippi

8295 Mississippi Council on Aging
750 North State Street
Jackson, MS 39202
601-359-4925
Fax: 601-359-4370; *Toll Free:* 800-345-6347
Mdunn-tutor@mdhs.state.ms.us
www.mdhs.state.ms.us/aas.html

Marion Dunn Totor, Ph.D, Executive Director

The mission of the Division of Aging and Adult Services is to protect the right of older citizens while expanding their opportunities and access to quality services. Our vision is for each older citizen to live the best life possible. The Division of Aging and Adult Services plans, coordinates and advocates for, and ensures the provision of services to all older Mississippians.

8296 NMRLS - Northern Mississippi Rural Legal Services: Clarksdale Office
5 County Road 1014
P O Box 76
Oxford, MS 38655
662-234-8731
Fax: 662-236-3263; *Toll Free:* 800-898-8731
www.nmrls.com/Elder.htm

Willie James Perkins, Chairperson
Katherine Weathersby, Vice Chairperson
Barbara Brooks, Advisory Committee

In 1985 NMRLS initiated its Elder Law Project, which has been ongoing for fifteen years. The project was developed to enhance the delivery of high quality legal services to the elderly population in the NMRLS service area. Through the project, NMRLS makes special efforts to overcome the access barriers which increase the difficulty older persons have in obtaining legal representation. Also, outreach is accomplished through community education activities and training on legal rights of older persons, which is provided each year to groups of older persons, advocates for older persons, and/or providers of social services for older persons.

Number of Members: 1966

8297 Northern Mississippi Rural Legal Services (NMRLS): Elder Law Project - Oxford (Administrative) Office
5 County Road 1014
PO Box 76
Oxford, MS 38655

933

662-234-8731
Fax: 662-236-3263; *Toll Free:* 800-898-8731
www.nmrls.com/Elder.htm

Willie James Perkins, Chairperson
Katherine Weathersby, Vice Chairperson
Barbara Brooks, Advisory Committee

In 1985 NMRLS initiated its Elder Law Project, which has been ongoing for fifteen years. The project was developed to enhance the delivery of high quality legal services to the elderly population in the NMRLS service area. Through the project, NMRLS makes special efforts to overcome the access barriers which increase the difficulty older persons have in obtaining legal representation. Also, outreach is accomplished through community education action activities and training on legal rights of older persons, which is provided each year to groups of older persons, advocates for older persons, and/or providers of social services for older persons.

Number of Members: 1966

Missouri

8298 Gateway Older Adult Legal Services

200 North Broadway
Suite 950
Saint Louis, MO 63102
314-534-0404
Fax: 314-652-8308; *Toll Free:* 888-782-8380
www.gatewaylegal.org

Michael Ferry, Executive Director
Philip Senturia, Managing Attorney

Screens cases and makes referrals to a small number of volunteer attorneys in St. Louis.

8299 Legal Aid of Western Missouri: Kansas City

1125 Grand Boulevard
Suite 1900
Kansas City, MO 64106
816-474-9868
www.lawmo.org/

Jerome T Wolf, Co-Chair
Jack Bangert, Co-Chair

Legal Aid of Western Missouri (LAWMo) has been providing essential legal services to low-income and elderly citizens since 1964. LAWMo staff attorneys, paralegals and volunteers assist over 20,000 people each year with problems that seriously affect their ability to provide for themselves and their families.

8300 Missouri Division of Senior & Disability Services

912 Wildwood
PO Box 570
Jefferson City, MO 65102-0570
573-751-6400
Fax: 573-751-6010; *Toll Free:* 800-235-5503
info@health.mo.gov
www.healh.mo.gov

Gail Vasterling, Director
Nikki Loethen, Chief
Ellie Glenn, Legislative Liaison

The Missouri Department of Health and Senior Services (DHSS) provides Adult Protective Services (APS) to eligible adults living in the community with consideration to the following rights: self-determination; protection; confidentiality; obtaining assistance and participating in care planning; and refusal of services and/or medical treatment.

8301 Missouri Protection and Advocacy

925 South Country Club Drive
Jefferson City, MO 65109
573-893-3333
Fax: 573-893-4231; *Toll Free:* 866-777-7199
mopasjc@embarqmail.com
www.moadvocacy.org
TDD 800-735-2966

Joe Wrinkle, Chairman
Barbara H French, Vice Chair
Susan Pritchard-Green, Secretary/Treasurer

Missouri Protection and Advocacy Agency (MO P&A) is a Federally mandated system in the state of Missouri which provides protection of the rights of persons with disabilities through legally based advocacy. MO P&A was established in 1977 to address public outcry in response to the abuse, neglect and lack of programming in institutions for persons with disabilities.

Montana

8302 Montana Advocacy Program

1022 Chestnut Street
Helena, MT 59601
406-449-2344
Fax: 406-449-2418; *Toll Free:* 800-245-4743
advocate@disabilityrightsmt.org
www.mtadv.org/
TDD 406-449-2344

Diana Tavary, Board of Director
Susie Mcintyre, Board of Directors
Will Warberg, Board of Directors

8303 Montana Legal Services Association: Helena

616 Helena Avenue
Suite 100
Helena, MT 59601
406-442-9830
www.mtlsa.org/

Dan McLean, President
Stacey Gordon, Vice President
James A Patten, Secretary

The Montana Legal Services Association (MLSA) is a federally and privately funded program that provides free legal assistance in civil cases to low-income people and the elderly.

8304 Montana Legal Services Developer Program & Office on Aging

111 North Sanders
PO Box 4210
Helena, MT 59604
406-444-5622
Fax: 406-444-1910; *Toll Free:* 800-332-2272
www.dphhs.mt.gov
TTY: 406-444-2590

Richard Opper, Director
Sheila Lopach, Executive Assisstant
Jon Ebelt, Public Information Officer

The Montana Legal Services Developer in the Office on Aging, provides elder law training and resources for seniors, family members and social outreach workers. The program also develops pro bono and local legal services referrals, training materials and telephone assistance to seniors on related matters.

Nebraska

8305 Division of Aging and Disability Services: Legal Services for Older Adults
Nebraska Department of Health & Human Services
301 Centennial Mall South, 5t Floor
Nebraska
Lincoln, NE 68509
402-471-3121
Fax: 402-471-4619; *Toll Free:* 800-942-7830
dhhs.ne.gov/Pages/contact.aspx#mainConte

Joann Weis, Executive Director
Bob Leopold, Interim Deputy Director
Joann Schaefer, M.D., Chief Medical Officer

Legal assistance is a service provided through Nebraska's eight Area Agencies on Aging. It is authorized by the federal Older Americans Act and helps older Nebraskans increase their financial and legal security. Legal assistance providers regularly visit senior centers around the state to share information. As needed, providers will visit with people in their home or in a nursing home, assisted living facility, or hospital. Common areas of assistance include wills, health care powers of attorney, durable powers of attorney, and other substitute decision-making forms. Each person's situation is unique and important to these providers.

8306 Nebraska Advocacy Services Center for Disability Rights, Law and Advocacy
134 South 13th Street
Suite 600
Lincoln, NE 68508
402-474-3183
Fax: 402-474-3274; *Toll Free:* 800-422-6691
info@disabilityrightsnebraska.org
www.nebraskaadvocacyservices.org
TDD 402-474-3183

Jill Flagel, Chairperson
Mary Angus, Vice Chairperson
Graciela Sharif, Secretary

Nebraska Advocacy Services. Inc. (NAS), The Center for Disability Rights, Law and Advocacy, is a private non-profit organization designated by the Governor to protect and advocate for the rights of Nebraskans with significant physical or mental disabilities. Established in 1977, NAS is the protections and advocacy system in the State of Nebraska. We work with people who have disabilities to secure their rights and to achieve a vision which is supportive of the ideals of interdependence, productivity, human dignity, personal inttegrity and full participation for individuals with disabilities in thier community.

Year Founded: 1977

8307 Nebraska Bar Association: Elderlaw Committee
635 S 14th Street Suite 200
PO Box 81809
Lincoln, NE 68508

402-475-7091
Fax: 402-457-7098; *Toll Free:* 800-927-0117
jschoenike@nebar.com
www.nebar.com/

Liz Neeley, Executive Director
G. Michael Fenner, President
Amie C Martinez, Presedent Elect

Sponsors annual legal fairs around the state and continuing legal education sessions for Nebraska attorneys.

Nevada

8308 Nevada Department of Health & Human Services: Division for Aging Services
3416 Goni Road
Building D, Suite 132
Carson City, NV 89706
775-687-4210
Fax: 775-687-0574
dascc@aging.nv.gov
aging.state.nv.us/index.htm

Mike Willden, Director
Ellen Crecelius, Deputy Director
Carol Sala, Administrator

The mission of the Aging and Disability Services Division is to develop, coordinate and deliver a comprehensive support service system in order for Nevada's senior citizens to lead independent, meaningful and dignified lives. The Division for Aging Services in the State of Nevada, Department of Health and Human Services, represents Nevadans aged 60 years and older. We assist our seniors in every step of the service continuum from safeguarding thefostering their self-sufficiency, providing counseling to advocating on their behalf.

8309 Nevada Disability Advocacy & Law Center Sparks Office/Northern Nevada
1865 Plumas Street
Suite 2
Reno, NV 89509
775-333-7878
Fax: 775-786-2520; *Toll Free:* 800-992-5715
reno@ndalc.org
www.ndalc.org

Jack Mayes, Executive Director
Charles Wilber, Fiscal Director

The Nevada Disability Advocacy & Law Center (NDALC) is a private, nonprofit organization and serves as Nevada's federally-mandated protection and advocacy system for the human, legal, and service rights of individuals with disabilities. NDALC was designated as Nevada's protection and advocacy system by the Governor in March 1995 and is funded by Federal grants and charitable, tax deductible contributions of private citizens. Services provided byNDALC include information and referral; education and training; negotiation or mediation; investigation of reported or suspected abuse or neglect; legal counsel, technical assistance, and litigation services; and technical assistance about policy, administration, and legislative developments.

8310 Nevada Disability Advocacy and Law Center (NDLAC)
6039 Eldora Avenue
Suite C, Box 3
Las Vegas, NV 89146

702-257-8150
Fax: 702-257-8170; *Toll Free:* 888-349-3843
lasvegas@ndalc.org
www.ndalc.org

Jack Mayes, Executive Director
Charles Wilber, Fiscal Director

The Nevada Disability Advocacy & Law Center (NDALC) is a private, nonprofit organization and serves as Nevada's federally-mandated protection and advocacy system for the human, legal, and service rights of individuals with disabilities. NDALC was designated as Nevada's protection and advocacy system by the Governor in March 1995 and is funded by Federal grants and charitable, tax deductible contributions of private citizens. Services provided by NDALC include information and referral; education and training; negotiation or mediation; investigation of reported or suspected abuse or neglect; legal counsel, technical assistance, and litigation services; and technical assistance about policy, administration, and legislative developments.

8311 Senior Citizens Law Project
495 S Main Street
Las Vegas, NV 89101-2927
702-229-6596
www.lasvegasnevada.gov/

Sheri Cane Vogel, Senior Citizen Project Director

The Senior Citizens Law Project provides free legal counsel and assistance to Clark County residents age 60 and older. Donations are accepted. Clients are responsible for applicable filing fees and other court costs. Services include legal advocacy/assistance in civil areas of law including simple wills, long-term health care planning issues, consumer disputes and small claims instructions, intervention in elder abuse, landlord/tenant and mobile home problems, homesteads, social security problems and other government benefits problems. Also helps with preparation of documents for handling medical/legal issues in the event that the client is unable to do so.

New Hampshire

8312 Bureau of Elderly & Adult Services
New Hampshire Division of Health & Human Services
129 Pleasant Street
Concord, NH 03301-3852
603-271-8140
Fax: 603-271-4643
www.dhhs.state.nh.us/DHHS/BEAS/

Kathleen F Otte, Bureau Director
Susan Lombard, Operations Director

The Bureau of Elderly and Adult Services provides a variety of social and long-term supports to adults age 60 and older and to adults between the ages of 18 and 60 who have a chronic illness or disability. These services range from home care, meals on wheels, care management, transportation assistance and assisted living to nursing home care. Legal support services, advocacy for disabled adults, information and assistance regarding Medicare, and information about volunteer opportunities are also important support services provided in the community by BEAS. All services and supports are intended to assist people to live as independently as possible in safety and with dignity.

8313 New Hampshire Legal Assistance
1361 Elm Street
Suite 307
Manchester, NH 03101-1333
603-668-2900
Fax: 603-625-1840; *Toll Free:* 800-562-3174
officemanager@nhla.org
www.nhla.org/

Mark C Rouvalis, Chairperson
James D Kerouac, President
Elizabeth M Leonard, Vice President

New Hampshire Legal Assistance provides free legal help to low-income and elderly persons who cannot afford a private attorney. NH Legal Assistance handles legal matters involving health care, domestic violence, public and private housing issues, food stamps, welfare, unemployment compensation, utility shut-off and nursing home problems.Operates a senior citizens law project including a senior legal hotline.

8314 New Hampshire Protection and Advocacy
Agency: Disabilities Rights Center
18 Low Avenue
Concord, NH 03301-4971
603-228-0432
Fax: 603-225-2077; *Toll Free:* 800-834-1721
advocacy@drcnh.org
www.drcnh.org
TDD 603-228-0432

Richard Cohen, Executive Director
Paul Levy, President
Joanne Malloy, Vice President

The Disabilities Rights Center (DRC) is New Hampshire's designated Protection and Advocacy agency and authorized by federal statute to pursue legal, administrative and other appropriate remedies on behalf of individuals with disabilities. The DRC is a statewide organization that is independent from state government or service providers. The Disabilities Rights Center is dedicated to eliminating barriers existing in New Hampshire to the full and equal enjoyment of civil and other legal rights by people with disabilities.ASL Version for Deaf/HH Community. The DRC provides information, referral, advice, and legal representation and advocacy to individuals with disabilities on a wide range of disability-related problems.

New Jersey

8315 Essex County Bar: Elder Law Committee
354 Eisenhower Parkway
Plaza II
Livingston, NJ 07039
973-622-6207
Fax: 973-533-6720
info@essexbar.com
www.essexbar.com/

Stacie L Powers, Chairperson
Thomas F Quinn, President
Judith A Hartz, Vice President

Committee sponsors annual seminars on legal issues. Issues include rights of the elderly, living wills, and home equity and income.

8316 Legal Services of New Jersey: Atlantic City

PO Box 1357
Edison, NJ 08818-1357
609-348-4200Toll free: 888-576-5529
www.lsnj.org/

Douglas E Gershuny, Deputy Director
Trinna Rodgers, Managing Attorney

8317 Legal Services of New Jersey: Edison

PO Box 1357
Edison, NJ 08818-1357
732-572-9100Toll free: 888-576-5529
legalhelp@lsnj.org
www.lsnj.org/

Melville D Miller Jr, President/General Counsel

8318 New Jersey Protection and Advocacy Agency

210 South Broad Street
3rd Floor
Trenton, NJ 08608
609-292-9742
Fax: 609-777-0187; *Toll Free:* 800-922-7233
advocate@drnj.org
www.drnj.org/
TTY: 609-633-7106

Joseph B Young, Executive Director
Walter Anthony Woodberry, Chair
Kathleen F Wood, Vice Chair

Provides legal advocacy and representation for those with disabilities.

Year Founded: 1994

8319 New Jersey State Bar Association: Committee on the Elderly

One Constitution Square
New Brunswick, NJ 08901-1520
732-249-9500
Fax: 732-249-2815
jbluriesq@aol.com
njsba.com/committees_sections/index.cfm

Ralph J Lamparello, President
Miles S Winder, 1st Vice President
Thomas H Prol, 2nd Vice President

The Committee operates a Senior Citizens Referral Panel in conjunction with the Office on Aging. Reviews and comments on issues of special concern to the elderly, their families and caregivers. Disseminates timely information on legal topics vitally important to the elderly.

Year Founded: 1899

8320 Office on Aging: Senior Citizens Referral Panel
Burlington County Bar Association

1050 Connecticut Avenue
Suite 400
Washington, DC 20036
202-662-8690
Fax: 202-662-8698
aging@americanbar.org
www.americanbar.org/content/aba/groups/l

Joyce Miller, Contact

Approximately 50 attorneys work at a reduced fee for seniors. The committee operates a Senior Citizens Referral Panel in conjunction with the New Jersey Office on Aging. The committee has a public guardianship project, funded

by the Office on Aging, to assist the New Jersey Mental Health Agency in adult guardianship proceedings.

Year Founded: 1878

New Mexico

8321 Native American Disability Law Center

3535 East 30th Street
Suite 201
Farmington, NM 87402
505-566-5880
Fax: 505-566-5889; *Toll Free:* 800-862-7271
info@nativedisabilitylaw.org
www.nativedisabilitylaw.org

Therese Yanan, Executive Director/Attorney
Alexis DeLaCruz, Staff Attorney
Steve Tarnowski, Staff Attorney

Advocates so that the rights of Native Americans with disabilities are enforced, strengthened and brought in harmony with their community. Service area: within the Navajo Nation and Hopi tribe. Service type: The Native American Disability Law Center (The Law Center) provides legal representation for individuals with disabilities in various areas, such as abuse, neglect, special education, civil rights and discrimination, vocational rehabilitation, and employment.

Number of Members: 11

8322 New Mexico Aging & Long-Term Services Department: Elderly and Disability Services Division

Toney Anaya Building
2550 Cerrillos Road
Santa Fe, NM 87505
505-476-4799Toll free: 866-451-2901
marise.mcfadden@state.nm.us
www.nmaging.state.nm.us/

Marise McFadden, Director
Doyle Smith, Deputy Director
Gino Rinaldi, Cabinet Secretary

The Elderly and Disability Services Division has programs that provide support to enable older adults and individuals with disabilities to remain in their own homes and communities or to return to their homes from a nursing facility or institution. The Division also advocates for each consumer to live in the least restrictive environment, and provides education and training for consumers, case managers, and direct service providers.

Year Founded: 2004

8323 State Bar of New Mexico: Elder Law Section

5121 Masthead Northeast
PO Box 92860
Albuquerque, NM 87109
505-797-6000
Fax: 505-828-3765; *Toll Free:* 800-876-6227
sbnm@nmbar.org
www.nmbar.org

Mary H Smith, Chair
Mary Ann Green, Finance Officer
Joe Conte, Executive Director

Advisory committee to the Lawyer Referral Project for the Elderly, their mission is to facilitate and improve the law and practice of law in areas of particular concern to the el-

derly, including preserving and enhancing the rights of
physically and mentally challenged individuals with respect
to care, housing and asset management and to lead, coordinate and serve as a coordinating agent and clearinghouse
for the efforts of the various agencies involved in service to
the elderly.

8324 State Bar of New Mexico: Lawyer Referral for the Elderly Program

5121 Masthead Northeast
PO Box 92860
Albuquerque, NM 87109
505-797-6000
Fax: 505-828-3765; *Toll Free:* 800-876-6227
sbnm@nmbar.org
www.nmbar.org

Mary H Smith, Chair
Mary Ann Green, Finance Officer
M Dwight Hurst, Executive Director

Statewide referral project serving elderly in all 33 counties
in New Mexico. Project is based in State Bar Complex in
Albuquerque, with regional offices in Northern and Southern New Mexico.

New York

8325 Association of the Bar of the City of New York: Committee for Senior Volunteer Lawyers

42 West 44th Street
New York, NY 10036-6604
212-382-6600
Fax: 212-398-6634
bopotowsky@nycbar.org
www.nycbar.org

Bret Parker, Executive Director
Carey R Dunne, President
Mark C Morrill, Vice President

Provide services for senior lawyers; conduct programs for
assistance to and of interest to senior lawyers; consider and
promote programs for the benefit of the bar, law schools,
law students, and the community, utilizing the services and
experience of senior lawyers, both on a volunteer or com-
pensated basis; and to act as the voice of senior lawyers
within the Association of the Bar.

8326 Legal Services for the Elderly

40 Worth Street
Suite 606
New York, NY 10013
646-442-3600
Fax: 212-719-1939
info@LegalServicesNYC.org
www.legalservicesnyc.org

Raun J Rasmussen, Executive Director
Joseph S Genova, Chair
Michael D Young, Vice Chair

Lawyers who advise on and litigate cases concerning problems of the elderly. Funded through the Legal Services Corporation in New York City, attorney fees, grants, and the
state of New York. Conducts research, litigation, and educational programs.

8327 Legal Services for the Elderly, Disabled or Disadvantaged of Western New York

40 Worth Street
Suite 606
New York, NY 10013
646-442-3600
Fax: 212-719-1939
info@LegalServicesNYC.org
www.legalservicesnyc.org

Raun J Rasmussen, Executive Director
Joseph S Genova, Chair
Michael D Young, Vice Chair

It is the mission of Legal Services for the Elderly, Disabled
or Disadvantaged of Western New York, Inc. (LSED) to
improve the quality of life, primarily for elderly persons,
but also disabled persons, in Western New York by providing free legal services in those areas which generally have
a significant impact on their lives. These areas include
health care, housing, income maintenance, family law and
protective services. LSED's primary goal is to use the legal
system to assure that older people in our community may
live with dignity.

8328 National Organization of Social Security Claimants' Representatives

560 Sylvan Avenue
Suite 2200
Englewood Cliffs, NY 07632
201-567-4228
Fax: 845-735-8812; *Toll Free:* 201-567-1542
nosscr@nosscr.org
www.nosscr.org/

Barbara Silverstone, Executive Director
Cynthia Berger, President
Timothy Cuddigan, Vice President

Professional organization of attorneys who represent claimants before the Social Security Administration. The National Organization of Social Security Claimants'
Representatives (NOSSCR) is committed to providing the
highest quality representation and advocacy on behalf of
persons who are seeking Social Security and Supplemental
Security Income.

Year Founded: 1979

8329 New York Legal Aid Society

199 Water Street
New York, NY 10038
212-577-3300
Fax: 212-509-8761; *Toll Free:* 888-218-6974
www.legal-aid.org/

Richard J Davis, Chair
Douglas F Curtis, Vice Chair
Blaine V Frogg, President

The Legal Aid Society is the nation's oldest and largest
provider of legal services to the indigent. Founded in 1876,
the Society provides a full range of civil legal services, as
well as criminal defense work, and juvenile representation
in Family Court, ensuring that poverty is not a barrier to
accessing the justice system. Our core service is to provide
free legal assistance to New Yorkers who live at or below
the poverty level and cannot afford to hire a lawyer when
confronted with a legal problem. Through neighborhood
and court-based offices in 18 facilities in the five boroughs
of New York City, more than 800 lawyers working with approximately 600 paraprofessionals and other supporting
staff, handle 300,000 cases annually. Legal Aid's fiscal

budget is $140 million; 90% from public funding, principally for criminal defense work and representation of juveniles in child protective and delinquency matters. The remaining funding comes from the fund-raising activities of the organization, which include private donations from law firms, associates, corporations, foundations, individuals and special events. The largest source of current support is the New York legal community.

Year Founded: 1876

8330 New York State Bar Association: Elder Law Section

1 Elk Street
Albany, NY 12207
518-463-3200
Fax: 518-463-5993
sbsc@nysba.org
www.nysba.org/

Patricia K Bucklin, Esq., Executive Director
John A Williams Jr., Esq., Associate Executive Director
David M Schraver, President

The Elder Law Section provides services and opportunities for involvement on issues relating to Elder Law, for members of the New York State Bar Association. Among activities, the Section presents educational programs and publishes materials on practice, procedure and developments to enhance the competence and skill of lawyers who practice in this field and improve their ability to deliver the most efficient and highest quality services to theirclients; prepare studies, analyses and recommendations to seek improvement in the law and procedure relating to elder law; and undertake projects to increase the understanding of senior citizens, their families and the general pubic concerning legal issues affecting the elderly.

8331 New York State Commission On Quality of Care and Advocacy for Persons with Disabilities

161 Delaware Avenue
Delmar, NY 12054
518-549-0200
Fax: 518-388-2890; *Toll Free:* 800-522-4369
www.justicecenter.ny.gov/
TDD 800-624-4143
TTY: 800-522-4369

Jeff Wise, Executive Director

The New York State Commission on Quality of Care and Advocacy for Persons with Disabilities (CQCAPD) is an independent, New York State government agency charged with improving the quality of life for New Yorkers with disabilities and protecting their rights.

8332 New York State Office for the Aging

2 Empire State Plaze
Albany, NY 12223-1251
518-474-7012
Fax: 518-474-1398; *Toll Free:* 800-342-9871
mike.burgess@ofa.state.ny.us
www.aging.ny.gov/NYSOFA/ContactNYSOFA.cf

Mike Burgess, Director

The New York State Office for the Aging is part of the Executive Department and is the designated State Unit on Aging under the Older Americans Act of 1965, as amended. It is the mission of the New York State Office for the Aging to help older New Yorkers to be as independent as possible for as long as possible through advocacy, development and

delivery of cost-effective policies, programs and services which support and empower the elderly and their families, in partnership with the network of public and private organizations which serve them. The New York State Office for the Aging was created by Executive Order of the Governor in 1961 and was one of the first State Units on Aging in the Nation. In 1965 the Office was made an independent agency in the Executive Department and became the central State agency to plan and coordinate programs and services for the aging at all levels in both the public and private sectors.

8333 Samuel Sadin Institute on Law & Rights of Older Adults

2180 Third Avenue
8th Floor
New York, NY 10035
212-396-7835
Fax: 212-396-7852
www.brookdale.org/iol/index.html

Jean Callahan, Director
Debra Studer Sacks, LPN/J.D., Senior Staff Attorney
Sara Meyers, J.D., Staff Attorney

The Sadin Institute on Law, Public Policy & Aging (The Law Institute) is a division of the Brookdale Center on Aging of Hunter College. We are a leader in providing services for professionals who assist older persons in securing their rights and public benefits. Since it's inception in 1977, the Law Institute's goal has been to ensure that impoverished older persons receive access to public benefits and entitlements. To this end, the Institute acts as a legal support program for social workers, paralegals, attorneys and other professionals engaged in providing advocacy assistance to the elderly poor.

North Carolina

8334 Cumberland County Coordinating Council for Older Adults: Elderly Law Unit

339 Devers Street
Fayetteville, NC 28303-4750
910-484-0111
Fax: 910-484-0627
www.ccccooa.org/

Dennis R Bowen, Executive Director

Refers cases to a panel of participating attorneys, on both a pro bono and reimbursement basis.

8335 Legal Aid of North Carolina

224 South Dawson Street
PO Drawer 1731
Raleigh, NC 27602
919-828-4647
Fax: 919-839-8370
www.legalaidnc.org/

Charles R Holton, Chair
Georgiana L Yonuschot, Vice Chair
Ellen Sheppard, Secretary

Legal Aid of North Carolina (LANC) is a statewide, non-profit, 501(c)3 law firm that provides free legal services in civil matters to low-income people in order to ensure equal access to justice and to remove legal barriers to economic opportunity. Legal Aid of NC is committed to equal justice for all people. We help children, families, individuals and migrant workers solve problems that affect their basic needs, such as housing, safety from domesstic violence or abuse, health care (Medicare or Medicaid), subsistence income (SSI or SSDI), environmental safety and consumer loan problems.

8336 Legal Services for the Elderly
1431 Elizabeth Avenue
Charlotte, NC 28204-2506
704-971-2621
Fax: 704-971-0180; *Toll Free:* 800-738-3868
lseval@earthlink.net
www.legalaidnc.org

Valerie Egzibher, Director

Provides legal assitance to those with disabilities.

8337 Mecklenburg County Bar: Volunteer Lawyers Program and Services for the Elderly
1123 South Church Street
Suite 103
Charlotte, NC 28203
704-375-8624
Fax: 704-333-6209
www.meckbar.org

Nancy Roberson, Executive Director
Jennifer Howle, Volunteer Lawyers Coordinator
Sally Larsen, Lawyer Referral Coordinator

Coordinator screens and refers clients to panel of over 80 volunteer attorneys throughout Mecklenberg County who provide pro bono representation to elderly citizens over 60 years of age, and children through three programs. They are the Volunteer Lawyers Program (VLP), Legal Services for the Elderly (LSE), and The Children's Law Center (CLC). Opportunities available through pro bono service in Mecklenburg County encompass numerous areas of civillaw, including domestic or family law, real estate, bankruptcy, wills and estates, landlord-tenant, consumer, and social security disability law.

8338 North Carolina Division of Aging and Adult Services
2101 Mail Service Center
Raleigh, NC 27699-2101
919-855-3400
Fax: 919-733-0443
melvinna.adams@dhhs.nc.gov
www.ncdhhs.gov/aging/

Dennis Streets, Division Director
Debbie Brantley, Elder Rights Section Chief
Steve Freedman, Service Operations Chief

The mission of the North Carolina Division of Aging and Adult Services is to promote independence and enhance the dignity of North Carolina's older and disabled persons and their families through a community-based system of opportunities, services, benefits, and protections; to ready younger generations to enjoy their later years; and to help society and government plan and prepare for the changing demographics.

8339 Onslow Coordinating Council on Aging
4024 Richlands Highway
PO Box 982
Jacksonville, NC 28540
910-455-2747
Fax: 910-455-0781
www.onslowcountync.gov/Seniors/

Chrishtine Kinnett, Director

The Onslow County Senior Services provides for the needs of the elderly population of Onslow County, keeping them active and involved in the community and preventing pre-mature institutionalization. The objective is to meet the needs of the older adult population of Onslow County through direct programs and services, advocacy, community involvement or referral to additional resources.

North Dakota

8340 Legal Services of North Dakota
PO Box 1893
Bismarck, ND 58502-1893
701-222-2110
Fax: 701-222-2110; *Toll Free:* 800-634-5263
lluchsinger@legalassist.org
www.legalassist.org/

Jim Fitzsimmons, Executive Director
Ricahrd R Lemay, Litigation Director
Lois Luchsinger, Intake Coordinator

Legal Services of North Dakota provides civil legal services for disadvantaged elderly or low-income North Dakotans who cannot afford an attorney.

8341 North Dakota Aging Services Division
600 East Boulevard Avenue,
Dept. 325
Bismarck, ND 58505-0250
701-328-2310
Fax: 701-328-2359; *Toll Free:* 800-472-2622
dhseo@nd.gov
www.nd.gov/dhs
TTY: 701-328-3480

Maggie Anderson, Executive Director
Debra McDermott, Chief Financial Officer
Marcie Wuitschick, Director

The Department of Human Services' Aging Services Division administers programs and services that help older adults and people with physical disabilities to live safely and productively in the least restrictive, appropriate setting. In addition, the Department of Human Services operates a Senior Information and Assistance Service funded under the Older Americans Act, called Senior Info-line that can link seniors, adult children, caregivers, professionals, and others up with information about important services that can help older adults and people with disabilities to live independently or meet their changing needs. This database of information is free and confidential.

8342 North Dakota Lawyer Referral and Information Service: Elder Law Panel
504 North Washington Street
PO Box 2136
Bismarck, ND 58501
701-255-1404
Fax: 701-224-1621; *Toll Free:* 800-472-2685
bill@sband.org
www.sband.org

Tony J Weiler, Executive Director
Nancy Morris, President
Jack McDonald, President - Elect

The State Bar Association of North Dakota offers a statewide pro bono and reduced fee panel for seniors emphasizing service to rural and low-income individuals. Legal Assistance refers clients to statewide panel of attorneys.

8343 North Dakota Protection and Advocacy Agency
400 East Broadway
Suite 409
Bismarck, ND 58501
701-328-2950
Fax: 701-328-3934; *Toll Free:* 800-472-2670
info@sband.org
www.ndpanda.org
TDD 800-366-6888

Teresa Larsen, Executive Director

The North Dakota Protection & Advocacy Project (P&A) is a state agency whose purpose is to advocate for, and protect the legal rights of, people with disabilities. The Protection & Advocacy Project is concerned with asserting the human, civil and legal rights of people with disabilities, especially those who are not able to protest deprivations on their own behalf. The Project operates in a manner which is consistent with the belief that people with disabilities have the same legal and constitutional rights and guarantees as every other American citizen. The Project believes that people with disabilities should be empowered to advocate on their own behalf to the extent possible. Services provided by the Project shall promote consumer control in decision-making and focus on the empowerment of people with disabilities in order to foster independence, productivity and integration into the community.

Ohio

8344 Ohio Department of Aging
50 West Broad Street
9th Floor
Columbus, OH 43215-3363
614-466-5500
Fax: 614-466-5741; *Toll Free:* 800-266-4346
jsmith@age.state.oh.us
aging.ohio.gov/home
TTY: 614-466-5500

Merle Grace Kearns, Director
Jason Smith, Chief of Staff
Roland Hornbostel, Deputy Director of Policy

The Ohio Department of Aging strives to help our citizens live active, healthy and independent lives. We accomplish this by providing services, information and supports to help older Ohioans remain engaged in their communities as long as possible. The Ohio Department of Aging works closely with statewide agencies, advocates and service providers to advocate for and serve older Ohioans.

8345 Ohio Protection and Advocacy Agency: Ohio Legal Rights Service (OLRS)
8 East Long Street
Suite 500
Columbus, OH 43215
614-466-7264
Fax: 614-644-1888; *Toll Free:* 800-282-9181
CKnight@olrs.state.oh.us
ohio.gov
TDD 614-466-7264

Carolyn S Knight, Executive Director
William Crum, Commission Chairman

The Ohio Legal Rights Service (OLRS) is an independent state agency and the federally and state designated Protection and Advocacy System for people with disabilities in the State of Ohio. The mission of the OLRS is to protect and guarantee the human, civil, and legal rights of Ohioans with disabilities.

8346 Pro Seniors
7162 Reading Road
Suite 1150
Cincinnati, OH 45237
513-345-4160
Fax: 513-621-5613; *Toll Free:* 800-488-6070
www.proseniors.org/

Rhonda Y Moore, Executive Director
Laurie Crothers, Controller
Diane C Kleinfelter, Resource Development Manager
Year Founded: 1975

Oklahoma

8347 Legal Aid Services of Oklahoma
Oklahoma City Law Center
151 West 30th Street
10th Floor
New York, NY 10001
405-521-1302
Fax: 405-557-0023; *Toll Free:* 800-421-1641
www.lawhelp.org/

Jack L Brown, President
Richard Mitchell, Vice President
Lucille Logan, Secretary/Treasurer

Provides legal assistance to seniors regardless of income.

8348 Oklahoma Aging Services Division
Oklahoma Department of Human Services
2401 Northwest 23rd Street
Suite 40
Oklahoma City, OK 73107
405-522-3069
Fax: 405-521-2086; *Toll Free:* 800-211-2116
www.okdhs.org

Carey D Garland, Director
Robert E Adams, Support Services Unit Director
Stacy Gholson, Finance Director

The Oklahoma Aging Services Division provides leadership in issues of concern to older Oklahomans, helps to develop community-based systems which support independence and protect the quality of life of older persons and helps to promote citizen involvement in planning and delivering those services.

8349 Oklahoma Department of Mental Health and Substance Abuse Services (ODMHSAs)
1200 Northeast 13th Street
PO Box 53277
Oklahoma City, OK 73117
405-522-3908
Fax: 405-552-3650; *Toll Free:* 800-522-9054
ok.gov/odmhsas/
TDD 405-522-3851

J Andy Sullivan, Chairperson
Gail Wood, Vice Chairperson

The ODMHSAS was established through the Mental Health Law of 1953, although publicly supported services to Oklahomans with mental illness date back to early statehood. Today, ODMHSAS delivers services in the areas of mental health, substance abuse, and domestic violence and sexual assault. A governing board provides oversight regarding Department functions and activity related to the care, treatment, and recovery of persons suffering from mentalillness and substance abuse. The Board is responsible for appointing the Commissioner of Mental Health and Substance Abuse Services.

Year Founded: 1950

8350 Oklahoma Disability Law Center: Oklahoma City
Oklahoma Protection and Advocacy Agency
2915 Classen Boulevard
300 Cameron Building
Oklahoma City, OK 73106
405-525-7755
Fax: 405-525-7759; *Toll Free:* 800-880-7755
Kayla@okdlc.org
www.oklahomadisabilitylaw.org
TDD 800-880-7755

Kayla Bower, Program Director

The Mission of the Oklahoma Disability Law Center, Inc. is to protect, promote and expand the rights of people with disabilities. The ODLC mission reflects a belief that people with disabilities are entitled to be treated with dignity and respect; to be free from abuse, neglect, exploitation and discrimination. The ODLC mission also reflects the belief that people with disabilities are entitled to equal rights and to equally effective access to the same opportunities as are afforded to other members of society. Since 1977, ODLC has helped people with disabilities achieve equality, inclusion in society and personal independence without regard to disabling conditions. We are a system of protection and advocacy for people with disabilities in the State of Oklahoma. We are federally funded through the Administration for Children and Families, the Center for Mental Health Services of the Department of Health and Human Services, and the Department of Education. ODLC is a member of the National Disability Rights Network.

Year Founded: 1977

8351 Oklahoma Disability Law Center: Tulsa
Oklahoma Protection and Advocacy Agency
2915 Classen Boulevard
300 Cameron Building
Oklahoma City, OK 73106
405-522-3908
Fax: 405-552-3650; *Toll Free:* 800-522-9054
Kayla@okdlc.org
www.oklahomadisabilitylaw.org
TDD 405-522-3851

Kayla Bower, Program Director

The Mission of the Oklahoma Disability Law Center, Inc. is to protect, promote and expand the rights of people with disabilities. The ODLC mission reflects a belief that people with disabilities are entitled to be treated with dignity and respect; to be free from abuse, neglect, exploitation and discrimination. The ODLC mission also reflects the belief that people with disabilities are entitled to equal rights and to equally effective access to the same opportunities as are afforded to other members of society. Since 1977, ODLC has helped people with disabilities achieve equality, inclusion in society and personal independence without regard to disabling conditions. We are a system of protection and advocacy for people with disabilities in the State of Oklahoma. We are federally funded through the Administration for Children and Families, the Center for Mental Health Ser-

vices of the Department of Health and Human Services, and the Department of Education. ODLC is a member of the National Disability Rights Network.

Oregon

8352 Lane County Law and Advocacy Center: Senior Law Service
376 East 11th Avenue
Eugene, OR 97401
541-485-1017
Fax: 541-342-5091; *Toll Free:* 800-575-9283
www.lclac.org/

Laurence Hamblen, Regional Director
Ralph Saltus, Program Director
Jean Beachdel, Senior Law Service Director

Provides legal assistance for senior citizens.

8353 Legal Aid Services of Oregon: Senior Law Project
Multnomah County Office
921 Southwest Washington
Suite 500
Portland, OR 97205
503-224-4086
Fax: 503-220-2480
www.oregonlawhelp.org/OR/index.cfm

Lynn Spruill, CEO

The Senior Law Project (SLP) is a volunteer lawyer program that is operated by Legal Aid Services of Oregon. The SLP has provided legal assistance to seniors since 1978. Lawyers initially meet with clients for 30-minute appointments at nine senior centers in Multnomah County.

8354 Oregon State Bar: Rights of Persons with Disabilities Section
16037 SW Upper Boones Ferry Road
PO Box 231935
Tigard, OR 97224
503-620-0222
Fax: 503-684-1366; *Toll Free:* 800-452-8260
info@osbar.org
www.osbar.org/index.html

Sylvia Stevens, Executive Director
Tom Kranovich, President
Patrick Ehlers, Vice President

Plays an active role in the passage of guardianship legislation.

Pennsylvania

8355 Allegheny County Area Agency on Aging
441 Smithfield Street
Pittsburgh, PA 15222-2219
412-350-5460
Fax: 412-350-3091
SeniorLine@dhs.county.allegheny.pa.us
www.alleghenycounty.us
TDD 412-350-2727
TTY: 412-350-2727

Pat Sullivan, Chair

Our mission is to enhance the quality of life of all older Pennsylvanians by empowering diverse communities, the family and the individual. The Area Agency on Aging is an office of the Allegheny County Department of Human Services. Its purpose is to provide programs and services that enable the older adults of Allegheny County to maintain their independence, and to have safe, healthy lifestyles with the type of care that is needed.

8356 Bucks County Legal Aid Society: Social Security Referral Panel
625 Swede Strret
Norristown, PA 19401
610-275-5400
Fax: 610-275-5406; *Toll Free:* 877-429-5994
www.lasp.org/

Elizabeth Fritsch, Executive Director
Ronald R Bolig, President
Nancy R Paul, Vice President

Provides legal assistance to those with disabilities and senior citizens.

8357 Chester County Services for Senior Citizens
15 West Gay Street
West Chester, PA 19380-2616
610-692-1889
Fax: 610-692-9546; *Toll Free:* 610-692-1889
whoffman@chescobar.org
www.chescobar.org/public/probono/

Wendy C Hoffman, Executive Director
Lisa Comber Hall, President
Craig A Styer, President Elect

Reduced fee panel sponsored by the Chester County Bar Association and Services for Senior Citizens.

8358 Disabilities Rights Network of Pennsylvania
1315 Walnut Street
Suite 500
Philadelphia, PA 19107-4798
215-238-8070
Fax: 215-772-3126
drnpa-phila@drnpa.org
www.drnpa.org

Judy Banks, CEO
Ken Oakes, Chair
Nicole Turman, Vice Chair

The Disabilities Rights Network of Pennsylvania (DRN) is a non profit statewide public interest law firm that provides legal assistance and other services to individuals with disabilities, their organizations, their families, and their advocates. DRN's main purpose is to advocate for the civil rights of persons with mental and physical disabilities, especially their right to live as integral parts of their communities. DRN works to ensure that people with disabilities have equal and unhindered access to employment, transportation, public accommodations, and government services; to enforce their rights to vocational, habilitative, post-secondary educational, health, and other services; and to protect them from abuse and neglect.

8359 Disability Rights Network of PA
1414 North Cameron Street
2nd Floor
Harrisburg, PA 17103
717-236-8110
Fax: 717-236-0192; *Toll Free:* 800-692-7443
drnpa-hbg@drnpa.org

www.drnpa.org
TDD 877-375-7139

Judy Banks, CEO
Ken Oakes, Chair
Nicole Turman, Vice Chair

DRN works directly and through its legal subcontractors to make systemic changes that will remove barriers to people with disabilities and their ability to live and thrive in their communities.

8360 Pennsylvania Bar Association: Elder Law Section
100 South Street
PO Box 186
Harrisburg, PA 17101
717-238-6715
Fax: 717-238-1204; *Toll Free:* 800-932-0311
info@pabar.org
www.pabar.org/

C Dale McClain, Chairman
Richard Thomas Murphy, Secretary
Katherine C Pearson, Treasurer

The Elder Law Section shall assist members of the legal community, the elderly population and those associated with the elderly community by developing educational programs focusing on advancements in elder law. The committee shall study, review and make recommendations concerning legislation affecting the elder community.

8361 Pennsylvania Department of Aging: Legal Services and Assistance
Commonwealth of Pennsylvania
555 Walnut Street
5th Floor
Harrisburg, PA 17101-1919
717-783-1550
Fax: 717-783-6842
aging@pa.gov
www.aging.state.pa.us/aging/cwp/

Nora Dowd-Eisenhower, Secretary of Aging
Gary Miller, Communications/Press Director
William Johnston-Walsh, Deputy Secretary

The mission of the Department of Aging/Legal Services and Assistance, is to enhance the quality of life of all older Pennsylvanians by empowering diverse communities, the family and the individual. Legal Assistance includes legal advice and representation by an attorney (and, to the extent feasible, counseling or other appropriate assistance by a paralegal or law student under the supervision of an attorney), as well as benefits and rights counseling or representation by a non-lawyer to older people with social or economic needs. These cases are only on non-fee generating (unless adequate representation is unavailable from private attorneys) and civil legal problems.

8362 Senior Citizens Judicare Project
1101 Market Street
11th Floor
Philadelphia, PA 19107-2934
215-238-8943
Fax: 215-238-1159
www.scjudicare.org

Mary A Scherf, Executive Director
Angel Recchia, Manager
Karen Buck, Senior Law Center Director

Provides pro bono and reduced fee representation. For the past 20 years, the Senior Citizen Judicare Project has been dedicated to meeting the legal needs of the elderly living on limited incomes in Philadelphia. Judicare provides legal representation and counsel, community education, outreach and advocacy for Philadelphia's senior citizens, through the energies of its legal staff and panel of approximately100 practitioners. Since its founding in1978, Judicare has provided free legal services to more than 26,000 needy seniors, educated more than 65,000 seniors through community-based education, and assisted over 100,000 seniors by providing advice, information and referral services.

Rhode Island

8363 Rhode Island Protection and Advocacy Agency: Rhode Island Disability Law Center

275 Westminister Street
Suite 401
Providence, RI 02903-3434
401-831-3150
Fax: 401-274-5568; *Toll Free:* 800-733-5332
info@ridlc.org
www.ridlc.org
TDD 401-831-5335

Ray Bandusky, Executive Director

The mission of the Rhode Island Disability Law Center is to assist people with differing abilities in their efforts to achieve full inclusion in society and to exercise their civil and human rights through the provision of legal advocacy. Services include individual representation to protect rights or to secure benefits and services; self-help information; educational programs; and administrative and legislative advocacy.

South Carolina

8364 South Carolina Bar Association: Elder Law Committee

950 Taylor Street
Columbia, SC 29201
803-799-6653
Fax: 803-799-4118
scbar-info@scbar.org
www.scbar.org

Alice F Paylor, President
Anne S Ellefson, Treasurer
Leah B Moody, Secretary

The Elder Law Committee provides education to members of the Bar and the public on issues affecting the elderly, monitors legislation and proposes statutory changes and publishes the South Carolina Senior Citizens Handbook.

8365 South Carolina Centers for Equal Justice (SCCEJ)

2109 Bull Street
PO Box 1445
Columbia, SC 29201
803-799-9668
Fax: 803-799-1781; *Toll Free:* 888-799-9668
andrealoney@sccej.org
www.sccej.org/locations.htm

Jim O Stuckey, President
Velma McDonald, First Vice President
Maridolores Valentin, Vice President

8366 South Carolina Lieutenant Governor's Office on Aging

1301 Gervais Street
Suite 350
Columbia, SC 29201
803-734-9900
Fax: 803-734-9887; *Toll Free:* 800-868-9095
askus@aging.sc.gov
www.aging.sc.gov

Glenn McConnell, Lieutenant Governor
William Gambrel, Medicaid Control Unit
Denny W Neilson, Legislative Committee Aging

The Lieutenant Governor's Office on Aging is the statewide leader for advocating, planning and developing resources in partnership with individuals and communities to meet the present and future needs of 660,000 older South Carolinians and their caregivers; to develop and coordinate a comprehensive continuum of care system; and to promote education, research and training in the field of gerontology. The Lieutenant Governor's Office on Aging works with a network of regional and local organizations to develop and manage programs and services to improve the quality of life of South Carolina's older citizens, and to help them remain independent in their homes and communities. The Lieutenant Governor's Office on Aging, through its administration of the Older Americans Act programs, aids 34,000 older adults who have the greatest social, economic, and health needs, and rural and low-income minority elders. Additionally, the Lieutenant Governor's Office on Aging works with many other state agencies, as well as with the private sector, to coordinate the needs and interests of older adults and to develop new resources.

South Dakota

8367 South Dakota Department of Social Services: Legal Services for the Elderly

700 Governors Drive
Pierre, SD 57501
605-773-3165
Fax: 605-773-6834; *Toll Free:* 866-854-5465
ASA@state.sd.us
dss.sd.gov/contactus/

Kim Malsam, Secretary
Lynne Valenti, Deputy Secretary
Amy Iversen, Deputy Secretary

Adult Services and Aging (ASA) provides opportunities that enable disabled adults and older South Dakotans to live independent, meaningful and dignified lives while maintaining close family and community ties. Through various programs, ASA provides or purchases services for disabled adults and older persons who are determined eligible for the programs. ASA field staff directly provide assessment and case management services to evaluate the needsof the individual. Based on the assessment, appropriate services are authorized and an Individual Care Plan is developed with the needs of the individual specifically identified. Social workers may also work with community groups and organizations to identify needs of older citizens.

8368 South Dakota Protection and Advocacy Services
221 South Central Avenue
Suite 38
Pierre, SD 57501
605-224-8294
Fax: 605-224-5125; *Toll Free:* 800-658-4782
keanr@sdadvocacy.com
www.sdadvocacy.com
TDD 605-224-8294

Robert J Kean, Executive Director

South Dakota Advocacy Services is South Dakota's designated protection and advocacy (P&A) system. P&A systems are mandated under various federal statues to provide legal representation and other advocacy services to all eligible persons with disabilities. These services are provided through a variety of vehicles: individual representation, educating policy makers, advocacy for groups, information and referral services, rights education and self advocacy training. The fundamental mission of the P&A system is to respond to allegations of abuse, neglect and violations of the rights of persons with disabilities, including discrimination based on disability. P&As devote considerable resources to develop capacities of persons with disabilities, ensuring full access to inclusive educational programs, financial entitlement programs (e.g., Medicaid and Social Security), health care, accessible housing, and productive employment opportunities.

Year Founded: 1977

Tennessee

8369 Disability Law & Advocacy Center of Tennessee (DLAC)
2416 21st Avenue South
Suite 100
Nashville, TN 37212-1257
615-298-1080
Fax: 615-298-2046; *Toll Free:* 800-342-1660
GetHelp@DLACTN.org
www.dlactn.org
TTY: 888-852-2852

Shalini Rose, Chair
Ebony Gilbert, Vice Chair
Mary Collins, Treasurer

Disability Law & Advocacy Center of Tennessee (DLAC) advocates for the rights of Tennesseans with disabilities to ensure they have an equal opportunity to be productive and respected members of our society.

Year Founded: 1978

8370 Legal Aid of East Tennessee (LAET)
502 South Gay Street
Suite 404
Knoxville, TN 37902
865-637-0484
Fax: 865-525-1162
dyoder@laet.org
www.laet.org

Marilyn L Hudson, President
Donald F Mason, President Elect
Marshall H Peterson, Secretary

The mission of Legal Aid of tennessee is to ensure justice for elderly, abused and low-income people by providing broad scope of civil legal assistance and advocacy. LAET has been part of the community fabric of east Tennessee for nearly 50 years, serving 26 counties from Chattanooga to Bristol.

8371 Nashville Bar Association (NBA): Young Lawyers Division (YLD)
150 4th Avenue North
Suite 1050
Nashville, TN 37219
615-242-9272
Fax: 615-255-3026
www.nashvillebar.org

Gigi Woodruff, Executive Director
Charles Grant, President
Edward D Lanquist, President - Elect

The Young Lawyers Division (YLD) of the NBA takes an active role in Bar programs and in other community activities. Some of their projects include programs for the elderly, the homeless, youth, and other groups with special needs. Honored in 1999, by Lexis for their outstanding work with the Tornado Hotline.

8372 Northwest Assistance for the Elderly Project
Northwest Tennessee Area Agency on Aging
124 Weldon Drive
PO Box 963
Martin, TN 38237-0963
731-587-4213
Fax: 731-588-5833
laverdia.mccullough@tn.gov
www.state.tn.us/comaging/localarea.html

Ken Kisiel, Chair
Patricia Miller, Vice Chair
Susan Hill, Director

The Northwest Assistance for the Elderly Project offers legal advice and education in these matters: food stamps, Social Security, SSI, Medicaid, TennCare, Medicare, nursing home care and access, boarding home care, federally subsidized housing, utilities, age discrimination, cases involving the immediate risk of loss of housing; adult abuse, neglect and exploitation; and medical collection actions threatening access to health care. Additionally, it offers advice, education and preparation of health care power of attorney and living will documents for elderly who are homebound, institutionalized or terminally ill. Representation is available in some cases that involve these areas of the law and to assist persons who wish to contest or defend against conservatorship actions. Also, project staff may serve as guardians-ad-litem in conservatorship actions. Legal representation in other matters is restricted due to limited staff availability.

Year Founded: 1963

8373 Tennessee Commission on Aging and Disability
9th Floor
Nashville, TN 37243-0860
615-741-2056
laverdia.mccullough@tn.gov
www.state.tn.us/comaging/

Ken Kisiel, Chair
Patricia Miller, Vice Chair
Susan Hill, Director

The Tennessee Commission on Aging and Disability is working for adults with disabilities and older Tennesseans by providing leadership and guidance for a system that promotes health, dignity, independence and security through an array of community and in-home services, the protection of rights and the implementation of best practices.

8374 Tennessee Justice Center
301 Charlotte Avenue
Nashville, TN 37201
615-255-0331
Fax: 615-255-0354; *Toll Free:* 877-608-1009
info@tnjustice.org
www.tnjustice.org/

Gordon Bonnyman, Executive Director

Year Founded: 1995

8375 West Tennessee Legal Services (WTLS)
210 West Main Street
PO Box 2066
Jackson, TN 38301
731-423-0616
Fax: 731-423-2600; *Toll Free:* 800-372-8346
wtls@wtls.org
www.wtls.org

Catherine B Clayton, Executive Director

Helping people access legal rights.

Year Founded: 1978

Texas

8376 Dallas Young Lawyers Association: Committee on Legal Aid to the Elderly
2101 Ross Avenue
Dallas, TX 75201
214-220-7420
Fax: 214-220-7422
chad@appeal.pro
www.dayl.com

Sarah Rogers, President
Meyling Ly, President Elect
Jonathan Childers, Vice President

The Committee sponsors a speakers bureau in which attorneys talk with seniors in nursing homes, churches, nutrition sites, and senior centers concerning advance directives, guardianship, etc.

Year Founded: 1920

8377 Houston Bar Association: Judicare Program for the Elderly
1001 Fannin
Suite 1300
Houston, TX 77002
713-759-1133
Fax: 713-759-1710
www.hba.org

Kay Sim, Executive Director
David Chaumette, President
M. Carter Crow, President Elect

Senior citizens have unique legal needs. Through this program, volunteer attorneys help income-eligible seniors with legal problems, including wills and medical directives. A free Elder Law Handbook is available in English, Spanish, Korean, and Mandarin Chinese to answer many legal questions facing the seniors and their caregivers.

Year Founded: 1870

8378 State Bar of Texas: Texas Young Lawyers Association
1414 Colorado
4th Floor
Austin, TX 78701
512-427-1529
Fax: 512-427-4117; *Toll Free:* 800-204-2222
www.tyla.org

Karen Crump, President
Krishty Blachard, President
Cameron J Cox, Chair

Produces the booklet Rights and Needs of Senior Citizens in Texas.

Year Founded: 1930

8379 Texas Legal Services Center: Legal Hotline for Older Texans
815 Brazos Street
Suite 1100
Austin, TX 78701-2509
512-477-3950
Fax: 512-477-6576; *Toll Free:* 800-622-2520
www.tlsc.org/hotline.html

Randall Chapman, Executive Director
Krishty Blachard, President
Cameron J Cox, Chair

The Legal Hotline is a project of Texas Legal Services Center. The Hotline receives funding from the Texas Department on Aging, through the HICAP Program, coordinating services with the Texas Department on Aging and the Texas Department of Insurance for elderly clients needing benefits analysis and legal advice. We provide legal information and advice in obtaining benefits such as Medicaid for Qualified Medicare Beneficiaries, food stamps, elderly housing assistance, and SSI; we are also able to answer other legal questions. Common concerns include debt collection, advance planning and estate planning issues, powers of attorney, and housing and consumer problems. In addition, we are able to send informational publications to Texans age sixty (60) and older on a variety of topics such as alternatives to guardianship, wills and probate, public benefits, consumer and debtor rights, health care rights, and nursing homes.

Year Founded: 1977

8380 Texas Protection and Advocacy Agency North Texas Regional Office: Dallas
1420 West Mockingbird Lane
Suite 450
Dallas, TX 75247-4932
214-630-0916
Fax: 214-630-3472; *Toll Free:* 800-880-2884
infoai@advocacyinc.org
www.disabilityrightstx.org/

Betty Black, Executive Director

Advocacy, Inc. is a nonprofit corporation funded by the United States Congress to protect and advocate for the legal rights of people with disabilities in Texas. Program services include that of education, Medicaid issues, housing discrimination, community services, transportation, and accessible public accommodations.

Utah

8381 Utah Department of Human Services Division of Aging and Adult Services
Legal Services for Older Adults in Utah
195 North 1950 West
Salt Lake City, UT 84116
801-538-3991
Fax: 801-538-4395; *Toll Free:* 801-520-2777
esollis@utah.gov
www.hs.utah.gov

Ann Silverberg, Executive Director

The Division administers the Adult Protective Services program to protect seniors and disabled adults from abuse, neglect, or exploitation. Trained staff within a statewide system of offices, working in cooperation with local law enforcement, investigate cases involving seniors and disabled adults. Adult Protective Services workers provide services designed to assist victims and prevent further abuse, neglect, and exploitation.

8382 Utah State Bar: Senior Legal Clinic Program Salt Lake County
645 South 200 East
Salt Lake City, UT 84111
801-531-9077
Fax: 801-531-0660; *Toll Free:* 801-532-1234
info@utahbar.org
www.utahbar.org

Stephen M Jennings, Chairman

The Needs of the Elderly Committee of the Utah State Bar runs this program. Volunteer attorneys meet with senior citizens at senior citizen centers within Salt Lake County. Volunteers meet one-on-one with six clients for 20 minute consultations, over a two hour period. The goal is not to provide in-depth legal advice, but to determine whether the individual has a legal problem and then to identify potential legal services to address the problem. The volunteers do not need to have specialized knowledge of the legal issues affecting elderly persons.

8383 Utah State Bar: Young Lawyers Section
645 South 200 East
Salt Lake City, UT 84111
801-537-9077
Fax: 801-531-0660; *Toll Free:* 801-532-1234
info@utahbar.org
www.utahbar.org

David R Hall, President
Stephanie Wilkins-Pugsley, President Elect
H Craig Hall Jr, Secretary

Produces the Utah Senior Citizens' Handbook: A Guide to Laws and Programs Affecting Senior Citizens. Includes sections on health care, financial assistance, estate planning, protective arragements and services, housing and landlord-tenant relations, rights and protection, and a resource directory. Also has a series of lectures at senior centers throughout the state focused on consumer fraud.

Vermont

8384 Disability Rights Vermont
141 Main Street
Suite 7
Montpelier, VT 05602

802-229-1355
Fax: 802-229-1359; *Toll Free:* 800-834-7890
www.disabilityrightsvt.org

Ed Paquin, Executive Director
Sarah Wendell - Launderville, President
David Gallagher, Vice President

Disability Rights Vermont is a statewide agency dedicated to advancing the rights of people with mental health and disabilities issues. The organization works towards a system that honors the dignity and needs of all people with disabilities.

8385 Funeral Consumers Alliance
PO Box 144
Plainfield, VT 05667-0144
802-482-3437
Fax: 802-482-5246; *Toll Free:* 855-698-8322
VT-FCA@myfairpoint.net
vermontfca.org

Dave Grundy, President

Mediates funeral complaints, monitors funeral industry practices and works to protect consumer rights. Local affiliates in most states.

8386 Senior Citizens Law Project of Vermont Legal Aid
264 North Winooski Avenue
PO Box 1367
Burlington, VT 05401
Fax: 802-651-4130; *Toll Free:* 800-639-8857
www.vtlawhelp.org

Michael Benvenuto, Executive Director

Senior Citizens Law Project of Vermont, working in conjunction with the Administration on Aging, supports efforts to provide seniors with legal advice on topics such as wills, power of attorney and health care paperwork.

Virginia

8387 AACD Legal Series
5999 Stevenson Avenue
Alexandria, VA 22304-3300
703-823-9800
Fax: 800-472-2329; *Toll Free:* 800-347-6647
webmaster@counseling.org
www.counseling.org
TDD 703-823-6862

Richard Yep, Executive Director
Cirecie A West, President
Robert L Smith, President Elect

Offering three volumes: Preparing for Court Appearances; Documentation in Counseling Records; and The Counselor and The Law.

Year Founded: 1952

8388 Arlington County Bar Association: Legal Services of Northern Virginia
1425 North Courthouse Road
Suite 1800
Arlington, VA 22201
703-228-3390
Fax: 703-228-7360
arlingtonbar.org/Services.html

Matthew Foley, President
Jason Rucker, President Elect
Susan Earman, Secretary

Helps to plan the annual Arlington Law Day for the Elderly and co-sponsors education sessions for professionals and service providers on advance directives and the Patient Self Determination Act.

Year Founded: 1926

8389 National Center for State Courts

300 Newport Avenue
Williamsburg, VA 23185-4147
Fax: 757-220-0449; *Toll Free:* 800-616-6164
www.ncsc.org/

Micahel G Heavican, Chair
Zygmont A Pines, Vice Chair
Mary McQueen, President

Develops a national clearinghouse and resource center for local and state courts to focus on requirements and methods of compliances with ADA.

8390 National Right to Work Legal Defense and Education Foundation

8001 Braddock Road
Springfield, VA 22160
703-321-8510
Fax: 703-321-9319; *Toll Free:* 800-336-3600
info@nrtw.org
www.nrtw.org

Raymond J Lajeunesse Jr, VP / Legal Director
Richard J Clair, Corporate Counsel/Staff Attorney

Seeks to assist employees whose human civil rights are being violated.

8391 Virginia Department for the Aging

1610 Forest Avenue
Suite 100
Henrico, VA 23229
804-662-9333
Fax: 804-662-9354; *Toll Free:* 800-552-3402
aging@vda.virginia.gov
www.vda.virginia.gov/

Rothrock James A, Commissioner

The Virginia Department for the Aging (VDA) works with 25 local Area Agencies on Aging (AAAs) as well as various other public and private organizations to help older Virginians, their families and loved ones find the services and information they need to lead healthy and independent lives as they grow older. VDA's mission is to foster the dignity, independence, and security of older Virginians by promoting partnerships with families and communities. The Department for the Aging is designated by the federal government as the agency to oversee all state programs using funds provided by the federal Older Americans Act and the Virginia General Assembly. Area Agencies on Aging contract with the Department to provide services for older Virginians and their families in communities throughout Virginia.

8392 Virginia Protection and Advocacy Agency

1910 Byrd Avenue
Suite 5
Richmond, VA 23230
804-225-2042
Fax: 804-662-7057; *Toll Free:* 800-552-3962

info@dLCV.org
www.vopa.state.va.us
TDD 804-225-2042

Miller Colleen, Executive Director
Darrel T Masan, Chairperson
Angela Thanyachareon, Vice Chairperson

The Virginia Office for Protection and Advocacy (VOPA) helps with disability-related problems like abuse, neglect, and discrimination in addition to assisting people with disabilities to obtain services and treatment. Through zealous and effective advocacy and legal representation, VOPA strives to protect and advance legal, human, and civil rights of persons with disabilities; combat and prevent abuse, neglect, and discrimination; and promote independence, choice, and self-determination for persons with disabilities.

8393 Virginia Protection and Advocacy Agency: Virginia Beach

1910 Byrd Avenue
Suite 5
Richmond, VA 23230
804-225-2042
Fax: 804-662-7057; *Toll Free:* 800-552-3962
info@dLCV.org
www.vopa.state.va.us
TDD 804-225-2042

Miller Colleen, Executive Director
Darrel T Masan, Chairperson
Angela Thanyachareon, Vice Chairperson

The Virginia Office for Protection and Advocacy (VOPA) helps with disability-related problems like abuse, neglect, and discrimination in addition to assisting people with disabilities to obtain services and treatment. Through zealous and effective advocacy and legal representation, VOPA strives to protect and advance legal, human, and civil rights of persons with disabilities; combat and prevent abuse, neglect and discrimination; and promote independence, choice, and self-determination by persons with disabilities.

Washington

8394 Disabilities Law Project: Washington
Alliance of People With Disabilities

1120 E Terrace Street
Suite 100
Seattle, WA 98005
206-545-7055
Fax: 206-545-7059; *Toll Free:* 866-545-7055
info@disabilitypride.org
www.disabilitypride.org/
TDD 206-633-6637
TTY: 206-632-3456

Jeanne Sloannecker, President
Steve Lewis, Vice President
Toby Wills, Treasurer

The Disabilities Law Project offers legal advice and representation in situations where an individual has been discriminated against because of his or her disability.

Year Founded: 1977

8395 Northwest Justice Project: Olympia

711 Capitol Way South
Suite 704
Olympia, WA 98501

360-753-3610
Fax: 360-753-0174; *Toll Free:* 888-212-0380
www.nwjustice.org/

Cesar E. Torres, Executive Director
Christina Gerrish, President
John S Tracy, Vice President

The Northwest Justice Project (NJP) is a not-for-profit statewide organization that provides free civil legal services to low-income people from ten offices and two satellite locations throughout the state of Washington. Each year, NJP assists more than 18,000 people in need of critical legal assistance. Clients in need of interpreter services in order to access legal services through NJP are entitled to those services. NJP strives to secure justice in a democratic society by working for equal access to the legal system by empowering low-income persons and communities through education about their legal rights and obligations, and by promoting respect for human dignity through legal advocacy.

8396 Northwest Justice Project: Seattle
401 Second Avenue S
Suite 407
Seattle, WA 98104
206-464-1519
Fax: 206-624-7501; *Toll Free:* 888-201-1012
www.nwjustice.org/

Cesar E. Torres, Executive Director
Christina Gerrish, President
John S Tracy, Vice President

The Northwest Justice Project (NJP) is a not-for-profit statewide organization that provides free civil legal services to low-income people from ten offices and two satellite locations throughout the state of Washington. Each year, NJP assists more than 18,000 people in need of critical legal assistance. Clients in need of interpreter services in order to access legal services through NJP are entitled to those services. NJP strives to secure justice in a democratic society by working for equal access to the legal system by empowering low-income persons and communities through education about their legal rights and obligations, and by promoting respect for human dignity through legal advocacy.

8397 Northwest Justice Project: Vancouver
500 West 8th Avenue
Suite 275
Vancouver, WA 98660
360-693-6130
Fax: 360-693-6352; *Toll Free:* 888-201-1020
www.nwjustice.org/

Cesar E. Torres, Executive Director
Christina Gerrish, President
John S Tracy, Vice President

The Northwest Justice Project (NJP) is a not-for-profit statewide organization that provides free civil legal services to low-income people from ten offices and two satellite locations throughout the state of Washington. Each year, NJP assists more than 18,000 people in need of critical legal assistance. Clients in need of interpreter services in order to access legal services through NJP are entitled to those services. NJP strives to secure justice in a democratic society by working for equal access to the legal system by empowering low-income persons and communities through education about their legal rights and obligations, and by

promoting respect for human dignity through legal advocacy.

West Virginia

8398 West Virginia Protection and Advocacy Agency
1207 Quarrier Street
Ste 400
Charleston, WV 25301-1842
304-346-0847
Fax: 304-346-0867; *Toll Free:* 800-950-5250
wvainfo@wvadvocates.org
www.wvadvocates.org

Clarice Hausch, Executive Director
Terry Dilcher, President
Cathy Reed, President Elect

West Virginia Advocates (WVA) protects and advocates for the human and legal rights of persons with disabilities. Services are based on the principles of equality, equity and fairness; meaningful choice and empowerment; individuality and independence; cultural competency; and, access and privacy.

8399 West Virginia Senior Legal Aid
235 High Street
Suite 519
Morgantown, WV 26505-5454
304-296-0082
Fax: 304-296-2746; *Toll Free:* 800-229-5068
seniorlegalaid@yahoo.com
www.seniorlegalaid.org/

Cathy McConnell, Esq, Executive Director
Robert M Bastress, President
Beverly D Kerr, Secretary
Year Founded: 1967

Wisconsin

8400 Elder Law Center: Coalition of Wisconsin Aging Groups
2850 Dairy Drive
Suite 100
Madison, WI 53718
608-224-0606 Toll free: 800-366-2990
cwag@cwag.org
www.cwag.org

Arlene Meyer, Chair
Leigh Roberts, Vice Chair
A.J.Nino Amato, Prseident/Executive Director

Benefit specialists provide information, counseling, and representation to county citizens age 60 and older with problems of public benefits and health care financing. Trains AARP volunteers to provide information and counseling on Medicare and Medicaid. Also collaborates on publications with the Center for Public Representation.

8401 Milwaukee Young Lawyers Association: Committee on Legal Services to the Elderly
424 East Wells Street
Milwaukee, WI 53202
414-274-6760
Fax: 414-274-6765
info@milwbar.org
www.milwbar.org

Beth E Hanan, President
David G Peterson, President Elect
Marcia F Drame, Vice President

Operates a lawyer referral service in which seniors recieve half-hour consultations. Also provides a speakers bureau, on ongoing Senior Center Counseling Program at three senior centers, and a question and answer booklet on wills and probates.

Year Founded: 1858

8402 State Bar of Wisonsin

5302 Eastpark Boulevard
Madison, WI 53718-2101
608-257-3838
Fax: 608-257-5502; *Toll Free:* 800-728-7788
service@wisbar.org
www.wisbar.org/

Patrick J. Fiedler, President
George C. Brown, Executive Director

The Elder Law Section works to develop and improve the laws that affect the elderly, and promotes high standards of ethical performance and technical expertise for those who practice in the area. The section sponsors CLE programs at State Bar conventions, monitors proposed state legislation and publishes a newsletter.

8403 Wisconsin Bar Association: Elder Law

5302 Eastpark Boulevard
Madison, WI 53718-2101
608-257-3838
Fax: 608-257-5502; *Toll Free:* 800-728-7788
service@wisbar.org
www.wisbar.org

Green Bay, Chair
Robert R Gagan, President Elect

Year Founded: 1803

8404 Wisconsin Department of Health and Human Services: The State Bureau on Aging

1 West Wilson Street
Madison, WI 53703
608-266-1865
DHSDLTCAging@wisconsin.gov
dhfs.wisconsin.gov/aging/
TTY: 888-701-1251

Dennis Smith, Secretary

County and tribal benefit specialists assist older persons who are having a problem with their private or government benefits. The benefits specialists are often called red tape cutters because they are experts at helping older persons with the extensive and complicated paperwork that is often required in benefit programs. They help older persons figure out what benefits they are entitled to and tell them what they must do to receive them. Benefit specialists receive ongoing training and are monitored by attorneys knowledgeable in elder law. The attorneys are also available to assist older persons in need of legal representation on benefit matters.

Wyoming

8405 State of Wyoming Aging Division

6101 Yellowstone Road
Room 259B
Cheyenne, WY 82002

307-777-7986
Fax: 307-777-5340; *Toll Free:* 900-442-2766
wyaging@wyo.gov
www.wyomingcompany.com

Bob Peck, CFO
Lee Clabots, Deputy Director

Allotments for vulnerable elder rights protection activities has several components: the Long Term Care Ombudsman advocates on behalf of older persons in institutions or receiving long term care in -home services and their families; the Legal Assistant Developer program provides, on a statewide basis, the protection of rights of vulnerable older persons; and,the Legal Services program provides legal assistance services to older Americans. To be eligible for these services a client must be over 60 years of age, a spouse of an individual over 60 years of age, or a disabled person living in senior housing attached to a congregate meals site.

8406 West Virginia Bureau of Senior Services

1900 Kanawha Boulevard East
Holly Grove, Building #10
Charleston, WV 25305-0160
304-558-3317
Fax: 304-558-5609; *Toll Free:* 877-987-3646
www.wvseniorservices.gov

Sandra Vanin, Commissioner
Janet H Frazier, Chairperson

The West Virginia Bureau of Senior Services is a cabinet-level agency within State Government and acts as the lead entity for programs serving older West Virginians. A Commissioner appointed by the Governor is the chief administrative officer and oversees all program and fiscal operations. In addition to agency staff members, the Bureau consists of a 15-member Advisory Council on Aging. The Bureau of Senior Services administers a wide range of programs available through the area agencies on aging and the providers operating on the local level.

Libraries & Information Centers

Alabama

8407 Alabama Institute for Deaf and Blind
PO Box 698
205 South Street
Talladega, AL 35160
256-761-3551
Fax: 256-761-3337
tlacy@aidb.state.al.us
www.aidb.org

Teresa Lacy, Librarian
John Mascia, President

Book collection includes discs, cassettes, braille and large print. Also closed-circuit TV and magnifiers.

Year Founded: 1858

8408 Alabama Regional Library for the Blind and Physically Handicapped
Alabama Public Library Service
6030 Monticello Drive
Montgomery, AL 36130-6000
334-213-3900
Fax: 334-213-3993; *Toll Free:* 800-723-8459
fzaleski@apls.state.al.us
www.apls.state.al.us

Mitchell Rebecca, Director
Ralya Kelyn, Assisstant Director

Special format material for US citizens unable to use standard print due to visual or physical impairment.

8409 Auburn University: Special Collections& Archives
231 Mell Street
Auburn University
Auburn, AL 36849-5606
334-884-4500
Fax: 334-844-4424; *Toll Free:* 800-446-0387
libwebm@auburn.edu
www.lib.auburn.edu

Dwayne Cox, Department Head
Lynn Williams, Librarian

Houses published and unpublished materials which, because of their uniqueness or condition, require special care and handling.

8410 Houston-Love Memorial Library
445 North Oates Street
Dothan, AL 36303
334-793-9767
Fax: 334-793-6645
dhcls@dhcls.org
dhcolibrary.org

Steve Roy, Chairman
Myrtis Merrow, Librarian
Bettye Forbus, Executive Director

Offers an extensive selection of reading material via cassette recordings and brochures for various activities; braille is also available if requested. The cassette recordings are provided along with cassette players if the patron qualifies for the services.

Year Founded: 1903

8411 Samford University Library Special Collections
800 Lakeshore Drive
Birmingham, AL 35229
205-726-2748
Fax: 205-870-2642
library.samford.edu

Kim Herndon, Dean of University Library
Lori Northup, Associate Dean
Eric Allen, Secretary

The mission of the Special Collection is: to collect and preserve special materials through providing a secure and protected environment for the conservation and use of the sources; to provide access and organization for manuscripts and other archival materials; to promote and support the research, teaching programs and scholarship of the University; to project the image of Samford University as an institution of higher learning; and to serve asas the repository for the Samford University archives and for the Alabama Baptist Historical Collection.

Year Founded: 1957

8412 US Deptartment of Veterans Affairs: Central Alabama Veterans Health Care System
215 Perry Hill Road
Montgomery, AL 36109-3725
334-272-4670
Fax: 334-260-4125; *Toll Free:* 800-214-8387
www.centralalabama.va.gov

Eric K Shinseki, Secretary
Sloan D Gibson, Deputy Secretary
James R Talton, Director

Medicine, allied health sciences.

Year Founded: 1997

8413 US Deptartment of Veterans Affairs: Medical Center Library
700 19th Street S
Birmingham, AL 35233-1927
205-933-8101
Fax: 205-933-4484
www.birmingham.va.gov

Eric K Shinseki, Secretary
Sloan D Gibson, Deputy Secretary
Thomas C Smith, Director

Medicine, nursing, hospital administration.

8414 US Deptartment of Veterans Affairs:Alabama Veterns Health Care System
2400 Hospital Road
Tuskegee, AL 36083-5001
334-727-0550
Fax: 334-724-2793; *Toll Free:* 800-214-8387
www.centeralalabama.va.gov

Eric K Shinseki, Secretary
Sloan D Gibson, Deputy Secretary
James R Talton, Director

Medicine, patient education, psychiatry, geriarics.

Alaska

8415 Alaska State Library Talking Book Center
344 W 3rd Avenue
Suite 125
Anchorage, AK 99501-2338

907-269-6575
Fax: 907-269-6580
aslanc@alaska.gov
library.alaska.gov

Patience Frederiksen, Regional Librarian
Beverly Griffin, Manager

The Talking Book Center provides library service and special materials to Alaskans whose visual or physical handicaps prevent them from reading standard print materials. The center provides books and magazines on audio and Braille, as well as necessary playback equipment, to eligible patrons.

Arizona

8416 Arizona State Braille and Talking Book Library
1030 N 32nd Street
Phoenix, AZ 85008-5108
602-255-5578
Fax: 602-286-0444; *Toll Free:* 800-255-5578
btbl@lib.az.us
www.azlibrary.gov/braille/

Linda A Montgomery, Library Director
Linda Montgomery, Executive Director

Cassette and braillle books, for blind, visually impaired and physically disabled who are unable to use standard print books.

8417 Flagstaff City-Coconino County Library for the Visually & Physically Impaired
300 W Aspen Avenue
Flagstaff, AZ 86001-5304
928-779-7670
Fax: 928-774-9573
www.flagstaffpubliclibrary.org
TDD 928-213-2417

Kay Whitaker, Executive Director

Reference materials on blindness and other handicaps, braille writer, magnifiers and kurzweil reading machine.

8418 Mesa Arizona Regional Family History Center
41 South Hobson
Mesa, AZ 85204
480-964-1200
Fax: 480-964-7137
admin@mesarfhc.org
www.mesarfhc.org/

Glenn E Scott, Director

The Mesa Arizona Regional Family History Center is a branch of the Family History Library in Salt Lake City, Utah that offers patrons a variety of resources including free Internet access, workshops and classes in addition to having commercial CD's with genealogical research data.

Year Founded: 1923

8419 Phoenix Public Library: Special Needs Center
1221 N Central Avenue
Phoenix, AZ 85004-1867
602-261-8690
Fax: 602-261-8836
www.phoenixpubliclibrary.org

Mimi McCain, Supervisor

Offers services and resources of the Phoenix Public Library accessible to people with disabilities. Books and periodicals

in large print, sign language, braille, resource directories and disability information. Information also available on video and DVS.

8420 Pima Council on Aging
8467 E Broadway Boulevard
Tucson, AZ 85710-4009
520-790-7262
Fax: 520-790-7577
help@pcoa.org
www.pcoa.org

Dr. Palmer Evans, Chairman
Terrence H Allen, First Vice Chairman
Frank Watts, Second Vice Chairman

Serves as an advocate, planner, developer and provider of services and programs for Pima County's older citizens and their families. Since 1967, individuals, regardless of background or income, have turned to the council for relevant information about how to prepare for events and chantes that accompany their maturity.

8421 Prescott Talking Book Library
215 E Goodwin Street
Prescott, AZ 86303-3911
928-777-1500
ask.librarian@prescott-az.gov.
www.prescottlibrary.info

Toni Kaus, Library Director
Roger Saft, Director

Home visits, book discussion groups, magnifiers, braille writers and reference materials on blindness and other handicaps.

8422 Travis L Williams Family Services Center
200 W. Washington Street
Phoenix, AZ 85003
602-262-6011
Fax: 602-534-2785
contactus@phoenix.gov
phoenix.gov/CITZASST/famtlw.html
TTY: 602-534-5500

Joseph Kress, Executive Director

Travis L. Williams Family Services Center operates in partnership with public and private agencies to provide a comprehensive array of onsite services to meet the emergency needs of low-income Phoenix residents. Examples of assistance provided include: budgeting, education and job training referrals, social and life-skills development, client advocacy, technical assistance, resource development, counseling and direct services to become self-sufficient/self-supporting. Services may include information and referral, emergency financial assistance for eligible clients experiencing a crisis with utilities and rent. Emergency food boxes and bus tickets are available for qualifying individuals.

8423 US Department of Veterans Affairs: Northern Arizona VA Health Care System
500 Highway 89 N
Prescott, AZ 86313
928-445-4860
Fax: 928-776-6094; *Toll Free:* 800-273-8255
www.prescott.va.gov

Thomas Hogan, Deputy Assistant Secretary
R Allen Pittman, Administration Assist Secretary
Donna K Jacobs, Director

Medicine, nursing, surgery, dentistry, allied health sciences, administration.

8424 US Department of Veterans Affairs: Phoenix Medical Center Library
650 E Indian School Road
Phoenix, AZ 85012-1839
602-277-5551
Fax: 602-222-6472; *Toll Free:* 800-554-7174
www.phoenix.va.gov

Eric K Shinseki, Secretary
Sloan D Gibson, Deputy Secretary
Lance E Robinson, Associate Director

Medicine, nursing, allied health sciences.

8425 US Department of Veterans Affairs: Tucson Medical Center Library
3601 S 6th Avenue
Tucson, AZ 85723
520-792-1450
Fax: 520-629-4638; *Toll Free:* 800-470-8262
www.tucson.va.gov

Eric K Shinseki, Secretary
Sloan D Gibson, Deputy Secretary
Joanthan H Gardner, Director

Medicine, nursing, surgery, neurology, psychiatry, radiology, management, patient health education.

Arkansas

8426 Educational Services for the Visually Impaired
2042 Wildwood Avenue
Sute 112
Sherwood, AR 72120
501-835-5448
Fax: 501-835-6840
esvi.org

Jame Caton, Director

Offers textbooks, braille books and more to the visually impaired grades K-12 in the Arizona area.

8427 Northwest Ozarks Regional Library for the Blind and Handicapped
2423 E Robinson Ave
Springdate, AR 72764
479-756-5901
Fax: 501-442-6254; *Toll Free:* 800-865-5901
www.ozark.org

Jerre VanHoose, Chairperson
Lorl Ericson, Vice Chair
Mike Lanier, Secretary

Offers a summer reading program, closed-circuit TV, magnifiers, braille writers and large print books.

8428 US Department of Veterans Affairs Hospital Libraries
4300 W 7th Street
Little Rock, AR 72205-5446
501-324-5234
Fax: 501-671-2528
www.va.gov

Eric K Shinseki, Secretary
Sloan D Gibson, Deputy Secretary
Jose D Riojas, Chief to Staff

Medicine, surgery, nursing, psychiatry, psychology, social work, dietetics.
Year Founded: 1811

8429 US Department of Veterans Affairs Medical Center Library Service
1100 N College Avenue
Fayetteville, AR 72703-1944
479-443-4301
www.va.gov

Eric K Shinseki, Secretary
Sloan D Gibson, Deputy Secretary
Jose D Riojas, Chief to Staff

Medicine, nursing, allied health sciences, and psychology.
Year Founded: 1811

California

8430 Books Aloud Library
PO Box 5731
San Jose, CA 95150-5731
408-808-2613
Fax: 408-808-2625
info@booksaloud.org
www.booksaloud.org

Joyce Meurer, Executive Director
John A Leventon, Production Manager
Nancy R Consentino, Office Manager

Blind, braille, talking books.

8431 California State Library: Braille & Talking Book Library
PO Box 942837
Sacramento, CA 94237-0001
916-654-7843
www.library.ca.gov

Christopher Berger, Senior Librarian
Olena Bilyk, Web Developer
Emily Blodget

Blind; braille; talking books.

8432 Eureka Ward Family History Center
Church of Jesus Christ of Latter Day Saints
3441 Edgewood Road
Eureka, CA 95501-2756
707-443-7411
Fax: 707-443-7411
www.lds.org/

Thomas S Monson, President

Family search computer programs, all Microfilms and Microfiche available for a small rental fee. Assists patrons with their family histories through a collection of films, microfiche, books and periodicals of family history subjects.

8433 Fresno County Free Library: Talking Book Library for the Blind
770 N San Pablo Avenue
Fresno, CA 93728-3640
559-488-3217
Fax: 559-488-1971
www.fresnolibrary.org

Laurel Prysiazny, Librarian

Blind; braille; talking books.

8434 Oakland Public Library
125 14th Street
Oakland, CA 94612-4397
510-238-3134
Fax: 510-238-2125
lcutler@oaklandlibrary.org
www.oaklandlibrary.org

Gerry Garzon, Director of Library Services
Jamie Turbak, Associate Director
Gene Tom, Chief Financial Officer

Services and materials for people that are deaf, hard of
hearing or have speech disorders.

Year Founded: 1878

8435 Salk Institute for Biological Studies Library
10010 N Torrey Pines Road
La Jola, CA 92037
858-453-4100
Fax: 858-452-7472
webmaster@salk.edu
www.salk.edu

William R Brody, President
Marsha A Chandler, Executive Vice President
Jennefer Collins, Vice President

Molecular biology, genetics, neuroscience, AIDS, Alzheimer's disease, biochemistry, cancer, neurobiology, plant biology, structural biology, virology.

**8436 San Francisco Public Library for the Blind and
Print Handicapped**
100 Larkin Street
San Francisco, CA 94102-4733
415-557-4400
sfpl.org
TTY: 415-557-4433

Luis Herrera, Librarian
Toni Bernardi, Special Projects Manager
Karen Strauss, Chief of Man

Foreign-language books on cassette, children's books on
cassettes and more.

**8437 San Francisco Public Library: Talking Books
Program & Blind Services Center**
100 Larkin Street
San Francisco, CA 94102-4733
415-557-4400
sfpl.org
TTY: 415-557-4433

Luis Herrera, Librarian
Toni Bernardi, Special Projects Manager
Karen Strauss, Chief of Man

Blind; braille; talking books.

8438 San Jose State University Library
150 E Fernando st
San Jose, CA 95112
408-808-2100
www.sjlibrary.org

Donna Pontau, Reference Librarian
Don Kassing, President

Information on physical disabilities, accessibility and learning disabilities.

Year Founded: 1977

**8439 US Department of Veteran Affairs: Palo Alto
Health Care and Medical Information Service**
3801 Miranda Avenue
Palo Alto, CA 94304-1207
650-493-5000
Fax: 650-852-3228; *Toll Free:* 800-455-0057
www.paloalto.va.gov

Eric K Shinseki, Secretary
Sloan D Gibson, Deputy Secretary
Jose D Riojas, Chief to Staff

Medicine, behavioral sciences.

Year Founded: 1776

**8440 US Department of Veterans Affairs: H Earl
Gordon Medical Library**
810 Vermont Avenue
Washington, DC 20420
310-235-7421
Fax: 310-268-4919; *Toll Free:* 800-827-1000
www.vacareers.va.gov

Eric K Shinseki, Secretary
Sloan D Gibson, Deputy Secretary
Jose D Riojas, Chief to Staff

Clinical medicine, surgery, dentistry, nursing, epilepsy, geriatrics, nutrition, social work.

Year Founded: 1776

**8441 US Department of Veterans Affairs: Loma
Linda Medical Center Library Service**
810 Vermont Avenue
Washington, DC 20420
479-443-4301
Fax: 909-422-3106; *Toll Free:* 800-827-1000
www.va.gov

Eric K Shinseki, Secretary
Sloan D Gibson, Deputy Secretary
Jose D Riojas, Chief to Staff

Medicine.

Year Founded: 1811

**8442 US Department of Veterans Affairs: Long
Beach Medical Center Library Service**
810 Vermont Avenue
Washington, DC 20420
562-826-8000
Fax: 310-494-5447; *Toll Free:* 800-827-1000
www.va.gov

Eric K Shinseki, Secretary
Sloan D Gibson, Deputy Secretary
Jose D Riojas, Chief to Staff

Medicine and allied health sciences, patient education.

Year Founded: 1811

**8443 US Department of Veterans Affairs: San Diego
Medical Center Library Service**
810 Vermont Avenue
Washington, DC 20420
479-443-4301
Fax: 858-552-7452; *Toll Free:* 800-827-1000
www.va.gov

Eric K Shinseki, Secretary
Sloan D Gibson, Deputy Secretary
Jose D Riojas, Chief to Staff

Medicine, patient education, management, self development, EEO, ethics.

Year Founded: 1811

8444 US Department of Veterans Affairs: San Francisco Medical Center Library Service
810 Vermont Avenue
Washington, DC 20420
479-443-4301
Fax: 415-750-6919; *Toll Free:* 800-827-1000
www.va.gov

Eric K Shinseki, Secretary
Sloan D Gibson, Deputy Secretary
Jose D Riojas, Chief to Staff

Health sciences.

Year Founded: 1811

8445 University of California: Mount Zion Medical Center
Harris M Fishbon Memorial Library
1600 Divisadero Street
San Francisco, CA 94115-3010
415-567-6600
Fax: 415-776-0689
mountzion.ucsfmedicalcenter.org

Gail Sorrough, Director

Medicine, geriatrics, cardiology, pediatrics, and psychiatry.

Year Founded: 1864

8446 VA Central California Health Care System
Heartland Regional Network Library
2615 E Clinton Avenue
Fresno, CA 93703-2223
559-228-5341
Fax: 559-228-6924
assist@heartlandlibraries.org
www.heartlandlibraries.org/

Jo Ellen Misakian, Executive Director
Cynthia Meyer

Medicine, nursing, allied health sciences.

8447 Vacaville Public Library: Town Square
1 Town Square Place
Vacaville, CA 95688
707-469-4590Toll free: 866-572-7587
www.solanolibrary.com

Jim Dunbar, President
Constance Boulware, Vice President
Cherelyn Ellington, Secretary

Provides senior programs and services to Californians.

Year Founded: 1914

Colorado

8448 AMC Cancer Research Center Medical Library
Medical Library
250 Williams Street
Atlanta, GE 30303
303-239-3422
Fax: 303-233-9562; *Toll Free:* 800-525-3777
www.cancer.org

Doris Borchert, Librarian
David Silberberg, President

Cancer - research, prevention, control.

8449 Colorado Department of Social Service Library
1575 Sherman Street
Denver, CO 80203-1702
303-866-5700
Fax: 303-866-4047
cdhs_communications@state.co.us
www.cdhs.state.co.us

Mary V McGhee, Division Directr
Tammy Humphrey, Program assistant
Jean Mc Allister, Special Projects Coordinater

Social work, public and social welfare, psychology, sociology, child welfare, adoption, foster care, aged, child development, handicapped, crime and juvenile delinquency, group work and community organizations.

8450 Colorado School for the Deaf and Blind Media Center
33 N Institute Street
Colorado Springs, CO 80903-3599
719-578-2100
Fax: 719-578-2239
csdbsupt@csdb.org
www.csdb.org

Mr David Ek, Chairperson

Books of interest to deaf and blind children; professional books on deafness and blindness for staff and parents.

8451 Penrose Hospital: Webb Memorial Library
Margery Reed Professional Building
2222 N Nevada Avenue
Colorado Springs, CO 80907-6736
719-776-5288
Fax: 719-776-5028
webblibrary@centura.org
www.penrosestfrancis.orgwww.penrosestfra

Rick O'Connell, President/CEO

Consumer health collection with materials for health related issues.

8452 US Department of Veterans Affairs: Denver Medical Center Library
1055 Clermont Street
Denver, CO 80220-3808
303-399-8020
Fax: 303-393-4647; *Toll Free:* 888-336-8262
www.denver.va.gov

Eric K Shinseki, Secretary
Sloan D Gibson, Deputy Secretary
Jose D Riojas, Chief to Staff

Medicine and allied clinical sciences.

Year Founded: 1811

8453 US Department of Veterans Affairs: Grand Junction Medical Center Library Service
2121 North Avenue
Grand Junction, CO 81501-6428
970-242-0731
Fax: 970-244-1303; *Toll Free:* 866-206-6415
www.grandjunction.va.gov

Eric K Shinseki, Secretary
Sloan D Gibson, Deputy Secretary
Jose D Riojas, Chief to Staff

Medicine, surgery.

Year Founded: 1811

8454 US Department of Veterans Affairs: Southern Colorado Healthcare System
810 Vermont Avenue
Washington, DC 20420
303-761-0117
Fax: 303-781-9378; *Toll Free:* 800-827-1000
www.va.gov

Eric K Shinseki, Secretary
Sloan D Gibson, Deputy Secretary
Jose D Riojas, Chief to Staff

Psychiatry, nursing, geriatrics, psychology.

Year Founded: 1811

8455 University of Colorado: Science Libaray
12950 E Mountview Blvd
Aurora, CO 80045
303-724-2152
Fax: 303-724-2166
david.fagerstrom@spot.colorado.edu
hslibrary.ucdenver.edu

David M Fagerstrom, Contact
Shaun Baber, Library Technician
Jo Hall, Catloger

General science; botany; chemistry; biochemistry; biology - molecular, cellular, developmental, environmental, organismic, population; psychology; pharmacy; speech pathology; audiology; artificial intelligence; exercise physiology; nutrition; zoology.

Year Founded: 1924

8456 Weld Library District: Lincoln Park Branch Library
919 7th Street
Greeley, CO 80631-3967
970-506-8460
Fax: 970-506-8461
www.mylibrary.us/

Charlene Parker, Library Branch Manager
Janine Reid, Executive Director

Located in historic downtown Greeley, the Lincoln Park Branch Library serves as a neighborhood library with an emphasis on popular materials. The Lincoln Park Branch features the largest collection of large print books in the District plus the largest collection of books and media in Spanish. The 14,000 square foot facility maintains an up-to-date selection of popular, high-demand fiction known as Express Books, that are available for immediate checkout. In addition, the Branch also has strong collections of books and media for children and teens. The Lincoln Park Branch offers a wide variety of quality programs for children, adults, and teens that encourage reading, literacy, education, and cultural diversity.

Connecticut

8457 Connecticut Society to Prevent Blindness
231 Capitol Avenue
Hartford, CT 06106
860-757-6500Toll free: 860-266-6733
webmaster@ct.gov
www.ctstatelibrary.org

Gordon Reddick, Director
Kris Abery, Deputy Director
Kathy Hotchkiss, Readers Advisor

Offers braille and large print books, large-print photocopiers, cassettes, talking books, home services and more for the visually impaired.

8458 Connecticut State Library for the Blindand Physically Handicapped
198 West Street
Rocky Hill, CT 06067-3598
860-721-2020
Fax: 860-721-2056; *Toll Free:* 800-842-4516
www.cslib.org/lbph.htm

Gordon Reddick, Director/Librarian
Kathy Hotchkiss, Deputy Director/Librarian
Nilda Martinez, Reader Advisor

This service lends books and magazines in braille or recorded formats along with the necessary playback equipment, FREE, for any Connecticut adult or child who is unable to read regular print due to a visual or physical disability. All materials are mailed to and from library patrons by postage-free mail.

8459 Hartford Hospital Health Science Libraries
80 Seymour Street
Hartford, CT 06102-5037
860-545-5000
Fax: 860-545-5066
library@harthosp.org
www.harthosp.org

Stuart Markowitz, President
Jeffry A Flaks, EVP & COO
Gerald J Boisvert, VP & CFO

Clinical medicine, nursing, education, administration, gerontology, allied health specialties.

Year Founded: 1854

8460 Hartford Hospital: Gerontology Resource Center
Hartford Hospital, Jefferson House
80 Seymour Street
Hartford, CT 06102-5037
860-545-5000
Fax: 860-545-5066
www.harthosp.org

Stuart Markowitz, President
Jeffry A Flaks, EVP & COO
Gerald J Boisvert, VP & CFO

Geriatrics, gerontology.

Year Founded: 1854

8461 US Department of Veterans Affairs, Health & Science Library
555 Willard Avenue
Newington, CT 06111-2631
860-667-6702
Fax: 860-667-6767; *Toll Free:* 800-827-1000
www.vba.va.gov/ro/hartford/index.htm

Erik K Shinseki, Secretary
Sloan D Globson, Deputy Secretary
Jose D Riojas, Chief to Staff

8462 University of Connecticut Health Center: Center on Aging
263 Farmington Avenue
Farmington, CT 06030-5215
860-679-3956
Fax: 860-679-1867
www.uconn-aging.uchc.edu/

George A Kuchel MD, Director
Cherell A Curtis, Admininstrative Manager

Committed to providing high quality comprehensive care for older adults. Consultative, specialty services are available along with educational activities.

8463 University of Connecticut in Storrs: Homer Babbidge Library
369 Fairfield Way
Storrs, CT 06269-9016
860-486-2518
Fax: 860-486-0584
www.lib.uconn.edu

Paul Kobulnicky, Director

Resource section for the aging on health information, nutrition and drug information.

Delaware

8464 Delaware Division of Libraries for the Blind and Physically Handicapped
121 Martin Luther King
North Dover, DE 19901-7430
302-736-4748
Fax: 302-736-6787
debph@lib.de.us
libraries.delawaregov

Lee Steele, Librarian

Provides books in Braille and audio books on record and cassette for the blind and physically handicapped residents of Delaware.

8465 US Department of Veterans Affairs: Health Administration Medical Center
1601 Kirkwood Highway
Wilmington, DE 19805-4917
302-994-2511
Fax: 302-633-5516
www.hud.gov/offices/

Shaun Donovan, Secretary
Jennifer Ho, Senior Advisor to the Secretary
Ted Tozer, President

General medicine, surgery, dentistry, nursing, allied health sciences.

Year Founded: 1965

District of Columbia

8466 American Association of Retired Persons: Research Information Center
601 E Street NW
B-3
Washington, DC 20049
202-434-3525Toll free: 888-687-2277
member@aarp.org

www.aarp.org
TTY: 877-434-7598

Robert G Romasco, President
Jeannine English, President Elect
Gail E Aldrich, Board Chair

Social gerontology, retirement, pre-retirement planning, voluntarism, and association management.

8467 American Health Care Association: Information Resource Center
1201 L Street NW
Washington, DC 20005-4046
202-842-4444
Fax: 202-842-3860

Dave Kyllo, Vice President

Geriatrics and gerontology, health and health care, Medicaid, Medicare, nursing, nursing homes, assisted living.

8468 Association for Gerontology in Higher Education
1220 L St. NW
Washington, DC 20005-4018
202-289-9806
Fax: 202-289-9824
www.aghe.org

M Angela Baker, Director
Janet C Frank, President
Donna L Wagner, President

Aging - education, training programs, courses.

8469 District of Columbia Public Library: Blind and Physically Handicapped
901 G Street NW
Room 215
Washington, DC 20001-4531
202-727-2142
Fax: 202-727-1129
lbph.dcpl@dc.gov
www.disability.gov
TDD 202-727-2145
TTY: 202-727-2255

Grace J Lyons, Contact
Phillip Long-Cross, Manager

Senior Mobile Service Bookmobile serves 18 senior residential complexes with programs, large and regular print book collection. Washington Lifelong Learning Center serves as educational clearinghouse for low or no cost programs for seniors

8470 District of Columbia Public Library: Librarian for the Deaf Community
901 G Street NW
Room 410
Washington, DC 20001-4531
202-727-2142
Fax: 202-727-1129
www.dclibrary.org

Janice Rosen, Librarian Service to the Deaf
Phillip Long-Cross, Manager

Offers reference services through TDD, portable TDD for public use at pay phone, signers for library programs, sign language classes, information about deafness, print and non-print materials for persons who are deaf.

8471 Employee Benefit Research Institute Library
1100 13th St,NW
Suite 878
Washington, DC 20005
202-659-0670
Fax: 202-775-6312
info@ebri.org
www.ebri.org

Jeanette B Hull, Head Librarian
Dallas Salisbury, President

Pension plans, health care benefits, employee benefits, retirement income.

8472 Gallaudet University Library Deaf Collection
800 Florida Avenue NE
Washington, DC 20002-3600
202-651-5220
Fax: 202-651-5213
www.gallaudet.edu

John M Day, University Librarian
Dr. Robert R Davila, President

Deaf culture and history, deaf community, sign language and audiology.

8473 Howard University Social Work Library
500 Howard Place NW
Washington, DC 20059
202-806-7250
Fax: 202-806-7234
www.howard.edu/library

Howard Dodson, Director
Arthuree R. Wright, Assistant Director
Ciarra Hearn, Administrative Assistant

Social work theory and practice; social policy, planning, administration; social welfare problems of black community; urban-oriented problems; human development; women's issues; gerontology.

8474 Ivins, Phillips, Barker Library
1700 Pennsylvania Avenue NW
Washington, DC 20006-4704
202-393-7600
Fax: 202-393-7601
www.ipbtax.com/cm/custom

Eric Fox, Manager
Pensions, taxation.

8475 Judge David L Bazelon Center for Mental Health Law
1101 15th Street NW
Suite 1212
Washington, DC 20005
202-467-5730
Fax: 202-223-0409
pubs@bazelon.org
www.bazelon.org
TDD 202-467-4232

Ira Burnim,, Executive Director
Jennifer Mathis, Deputy Legal Director
Karen Smith,, Executive Assistant

National litigation and support center for people with mental disabilities. Offers a variety of publications, handbooks, issue papers and manuals to help advocate for, implement, enforce and comply with federal laws and court orders on

early intervention, discrimination based on a label of mental illness, fair housing, cultural competence of service systems, SSI for children, children's mental health care, rights of elders, and other legal issues.

8476 Laurent Clerc National Deaf Education Center
800 Florida Avenue NE
Washington, DC 20002
202-651-5031
Fax: 202-651-5101
clerccenter.gallaudet.edu
TTY: 202-651-5636

Margaret Halau, PhD, Director Outreach & Research
Janne M Harrelson, Drctr National Mission Planning
Nicole Sutliffe, Manager Reporting and Projects

Provides information and assistance on hearing disability related problems. Operates a legal clinic for deaf and hard of hearing persons.

8477 National Academy of Social Insurance
1776 Massachusetts Avenue NW
Suite 615
Washington, DC 20036-1912
202-452-8097
Fax: 202-452-8111
nasi@nasi.org
www.nasi.org

Nonprofit, nonpartisan organization made up of the nation's leading experts on social insurance. Its mission is to promote understanding and informed policymaking on social insurance and related programs through research, public education, training, and the open exchange of ideas.

8478 National Association of the Deaf: Legal Defense Fund
800 Florida Avenue NE
PO Box 2304
Washington, DC 20002
202-651-5343
www.nad.org

Nancy J Bloch, CEO

Represents deaf and hearing-impaired persons with discrimination complaints in the areas of employment, education, housing, health, welfare, and social services.

8479 National Civil Rights Clearinghouse Library
US Commission on Civil Rights
624 9th Street NW
Room 600
Washington, DC 20425
202-376-7700
Fax: 202-376-7597
www.usccr.gov

Barbara J Fontana, Librarian
Kenneth L Marcus, Executive Director

Civil rights, economics, education, sex discrimination, law, equal employment, fair housing.

8480 National Information Center on Deafness
31 Center Drive,
MSC 2320
Bethesda, MD 20892-2320
202-651-5000
Fax: 202-651-5054
nidcdinfo@nidcd.nih.gov
www.nidcd.nih.gov

Loraine DiPietro, Director
Susan Ripley, Manager

Deafness, hearing loss.

8481 National Library Service for the Blind and Physically Handicapped
US Library of Congress
1291 Taylor Street NW
Washington, DC 20542
202-707-5100
Fax: 202-707-0712; *Toll Free:* 888-657-7323
nls@loc.gov
www.loc.gov/nls

Frank Cylke, Executive Director

To provide library service (books and magazines on cassette and in braille) to the blind and physically handicapped residents of the United States and its territories, and to American citizens living abroad. An applicant must provide a certificate, from a competent authority, of his inability to read or manipulate convential printed material. Program is free. See Libraries chapter for state listings.

8482 Pension Benefit Guaranty Corporation, Office of the General Counsel Library
1200 K Street NW
Suite 340
Washington, DC 20005-4026
202-326-4020
Fax: 202-326-4111
www.pbgc.gov

Lynn Artabane, Documents Librarian
Vince Snowbarger, Deputy Executive Director
Richard Macy, Chief Operating Officer

Pension law, pensions.

8483 US Department of Veterans Affairs, Medical Center Library Section
50 Irving Street NW
Washington, DC 20422
202-745-8000
Fax: 202-745-8530; *Toll Free:* 877-328-2621
www.washingtondc.va.gov

Iris Renner, Administrative Librarian

General medicine, surgery.

8484 US Equal Employment Opportunity Commission
Library
1801 L Street NW
Room 6502
Washington, DC 20507
202-366-4070
Fax: 202-663-4629
www.eeoc.gov

Susan D Taylor, Library Director

Employment discrimination, minorities, women, aged, persons with disabilities, labor law, civil rights.

8485 US Social Security Administration: Washington
Library
500 E Street SW
9th Floor
Washington, DC 20254

202-358-6276
Fax: 202-358-6193
www.ssa.gov

US and international Social Security programs, retirement, economics, disability insurance, income maintenance, pension benefits, health insurance, medical care.

Florida

8486 Broward County Talking Book Library
115 S Andrews Avenue
Fort Lauderdale, FL 33301-1830
954-831-4000
www.broward.org

Barbara Kelly, Librarian
Marianne Caldron, Executive Director

Reference materials on blindness and other handicaps, films, closed-circuit TV, discs, cassettes and a book discussion group is offered.

8487 Florida Department of Labor and Employment Security
Bureau of Braille & Talking Book Library Services
421 Platt Street
Daytona Beach, FL 32114-2803
386-239-6000
Fax: 386-239-6069; *Toll Free:* 800-226-6075
opac_librarian@dbs.fldoe.org
dbs.myflorida.com/library

Jane Karp, Library Program Administrator

Recreational reading material for people with print disabilities, blindness, physical disabilities, rehabilitation.

8488 Florida Division of Blind Services
Regional Library
421 Platt Street
Daytona Beach, FL 32114-2803
386-239-6000
Fax: 850-239-6069
TDD 800-226-6079

Mike Gunde, Librarian
Jane Karp, Administrator

Discs, cassettes, closed-circuit TV, large-print photocopier, films, children's books on cassettes and more.

8489 Florida Instructional Materials Center for the Visually Impaired
4210 West Bay Villa Avenue
Tampa, FL 33611-1206
813-837-7826
Fax: 813-837-7979
www.fimcvi.org

Suzanne Dalton, Supervisor

Operates a clearinghouse depository and production center for braille, large print and recorded texts. Provides assistance in assessment of materials and specialized apparatus, organizes volunteers for material production and more for the visually handicapped.

8490 Florida School for the Deaf and Blind
Library for the Deaf
207 San Marco Avenue
St Augustine, FL 32084-2799

904-827-2200
Fax: 386-865-4203
www.fsdb.k12.fl.us

Linda L Zimmerman, Head Librarian
E Dillingham, Administrator

Education of the deaf (pre-kindergarten through high school), sign language and the deaf, fiction and nonfiction (low level, high interest).

8491 Hillsborough County Talking Book Library
Tampa-Hillsborough County Public Library
900 N Ashley Drive
Tampa, FL 33602-3704
813-273-3652
Fax: 813-272-5728
www.hcplc.org/hcplc/liblocales
TDD 813-273-3610

Kurt Jasielonis, Contact
Joe Stines, Executive Director

Books on cassette tape free on loan to people with print disablities. A branch of the National Library Service for the Blind and Handicapped.

8492 Jacksonville Public Library
2809 Commonwealth Avenue
Jacksonville, FL 32254-2599
904-384-7424
jpl.coj.net

Gloria Zittrauer, Librarian
Anthony Jackson, Manager

Discs, cassettes, reference materials on blindness and other handicaps and children's books on cassettes.

8493 Miami-Dade Public Library: Genealogy
Collection
101 West Flagler Street
Miami, FL 33130-1504
305-375-2665
Fax: 305-375-3048
florida@mdpls.org
www.mdpls.org

Sam Boldrick, Librarian IV

A complete collection of the U.S. Census for all states and for all available years is housed in this extensive reference department. Other important microfilm holdings include the U.S. City Directories covering major cities from 1860 through 1935, and immigration lists. The Family Search Database worldwide is also available. The book collection, with publications on nearly every state in the Union, emphasizes the Eastern Atlantic States.

1913

8494 Orange County Library System Audio-Visual
Department
101 E Central Boulevard
Orlando, FL 32801-2429
407-835-7323
www.ocls.info
TDD 407-425-5668

Sally Fry, Contact
Maryann Hodel, Manager

8495 Orange County Library System: Genealogy
Department
101 East Central Boulevard
Orlando, FL 32801-2429
407-835-7323
Fax: 407-425-6779
www.ocls.lib.fl.us

Mary Anne Hodel, Library Director/CEO
Gregg Gronlund, Genealogy Director

The core of the Genealogy Collection, located on the fourth floor of the Orlando Public Library, was a 1923 gift of Captain Charles Albertson, an avid genealogist. In 1929, the Library became the official repository of the Florida State Society of the Daughters of the American Revolution. The collection now contains more than 25,000 books and bound periodicals, 10,000 microfiche and over 15,000 reels of microfilm.

1923

8496 Sylvester Comprehensive Cancer Center,
Cancer Information Service
1550 NW 10th Avenue
Suite 200a
Miami, FL 33136-1013
305-243-4821
Fax: 305-243-6678
www.cancer.gov

Jo Beth Speyer, Director
Julie Kornfeld, Executive Director

Information on treatment prevention screening and clinical trials.

8497 Talking Book Library, Miami and Dade Public
Library System
2455 NW 183rd Street
Miami Gardens, FL 33056-3641
305-751-8687
Fax: 305-757-8401; *Toll Free:* 800-451-9544
talkingbooks@mdpls.org
www.mdpls.org

Barbara Moyer, Librarian

Library services for people with visual or physical disabilities.

8498 Talking Books Library for the Blind and
Physically Handicapped
Palm Beach County Library Annex
7950 Central Industrial Drive
Suite 104
Riviera Beach, FL 33404-3439
561-996-9644
Fax: 561-845-4640

Pat Mistretta, Librarian

Library services for people with disabilities.

8499 US Department of Veterans Affairs Medical
Library
1201 NW 16th Street
Miami, FL 33125-1624
305-575-3150
Fax: 305-324-3118
www.va.gov

Susan Harker, Chief Librarian
Stephen Lucas, CEO

Medicine, nursing, psychology, allied health sciences.

8500 US Department of Veterans Affairs and Center Learning Resources Service Library
801 S Marion Street
Lake City, FL 32025
386-755-3016
Fax: 386-758-3218
www.va.gov

Susan Lescenski, Chief LRS

Medicine, surgery, nursing, and allied health sciences; hospital administration; patient education; ambulatory care.

8501 US Department of Veterans Affairs, Hospital Library
1601 SW Archer Road
Gainesville, FL 32608-1135
352-376-1611
Fax: 352-374-6148
www.va.gov

Marylyn E Gresser, Chief Library Service
Frederick L Malphurs, CEO

Health education, neurology, surgery, internal medicine, nursing, pathology, pharmacology, ophthalmology, psychiatry, radiology.

8502 US Department of Veterans Affairs: Medical Library
PO Box 5005
Bay Pines, FL 33744-5005
727-398-9366
Fax: 727-398-9366
www.va.gov

Diana F Akins, Chief Library Service

Medicine, surgery, psychiatry, nursing, radiology, consumer health.

8503 US Department of Veterans Affairs: Medical Library
James a Haley Veterans Hospit
Tampa, FL 33612
813-972-7531
Fax: 813-978-5917
www.va.gov

Nancy Bernal, Chief Librarian

Internal medicine, psychiatry, nursing, surgery, geriatrics, allied health.

8504 University of Florida: Center for Governmental Responsibility
PO Box 117621
Gainesville, FL 32611-7621
352-273-0835
Fax: 352-392-1457
www.law.ufl.edu

Jon Mills, Director
JoAnn Klein, Development Director
Timothy McLendon, Staff Attorney

Florida's oldest legal and public policy research institute. Provides students with the opportunity to conduct research with staff attorneys on issues of state, national, and international importance.

8505 West Florida Regional Library
222 West Main Street
Pensacola, FL 32502-4822
850-435-1603
Fax: 850-435-1603; *Toll Free:* 850-435-1611
www.cityofpensacola.com

Martha Lazor, Librarian
Eugene Fischer, Manager

Offers children's print/braille books.

Georgia

8506 Bainbridge Subregional Library for the Blind
SW Georgia Regional Library
301 S Monroe Street
Bainbridge, GA 39819-4029
229-248-2680
Fax: 229-248-2670
www.swgrl.org

Susan Whittle, Subregional Librarian/Director

8507 Cave Spring Library
17 Cedartown Street
Cave Spring, GA 30124-2702
706-777-3346
Fax: 706-777-0947
www.cavespringlibrary.org

Katie Faught, Branch Manager
Steve Head, Manager

Summer reading programs, braille writer, magnifiers, closed-circuit TV, large-print photocopier, cassette books and magazines, children's books on cassette, home visits and other reference materials on blindness and other handicaps.

8508 Cedartown Library
245 East Avenue
Cedartown, GA 30125-3001
770-748-5644
Fax: 770-748-4399
www.cedartownlibrary.org

Sharon Cleveland, Branch Manager

Summer reading programs, braille writer, magnifiers, closed-circuit TV, large-print photocopier, cassette books and magazines, children's books on cassette, home visits and other reference materials on blindness and other handicaps.

8509 Hall County Library System
127 N Main Street
Gainesville, GA 30501
770-532-3311
Fax: 770-532-4305
www.hallcountylibrary.org/

Adrian Mixson, Director

Summer reading programs, braille writer, magnifiers, closed-circuit TV, large-print photocopier, cassette books and magazines, children's books on cassette, home visits and other reference materials on blindness and other handicaps.

8510 Oconee Regional Library
801 Bellevue Avenue
Dublin, GA 31021

478-272-5710
Fax: 478-275-5381
www.laurens.public.lib.ga.us

Susan Williams, Librarian

Summer reading programs, braille writer, magnifiers, closed-circuit TV, large-print photocopier, cassette books and magazines, children's books on cassette, home visits and other reference materials on blindness and other handicaps.

8511 Rockmart Library

316 North Piedmont Avenue
Building 201
Rockmart, GA 30153-2938
770-684-3022
Fax: 770-684-7876
www.rockmartlibrary.org

Ann Wheeler, Branch Manager

Summer reading programs, braille writer, magnifiers, closed-circuit TV, large-print photocopier, cassette books and magazines, children's books on cassette, home visits and other reference materials on blindness and other handicaps.

8512 Rome Subregional Library Service for People with Disabilities

205 Riverside Parkway
2nd Floor
Rome, GA 30161-2922
706-236-4618
Fax: 706-236-4631; *Toll Free:* 800-201-5757
www.rome-lpd.org

Deana Wallace, Coordinator
Susan Sexton Cooley, Executive Director

Patrons may borrow all types of popular interest books. Readers may also receive over 40 popular magazines and local newspapers recorded on cassette. Special equipment needed to play casettes is loaned indefinitely to readers as long as they continue to be active readers. Equipment is repaired at no charge to the patron.

8513 SWGA Library for Accessible Services

SW Georgia Regional Library
301 S Monroe Street
Bainbridge, GA 39819
229-248-2680
Fax: 229-248-2670
www.swgrl.org

Susan Whittle, Subregional Librarian/Director

Discs, cassettes, summer reading programs, closed-circuit TV, magnifiers and more.

8514 US Department of Veterans Affairs Medical Center Library

1 Freedom Way
Augusta, GA 30904-6285
706-823-2238
Fax: 706-823-3920
www.va.gov

Elizabeth Northington, Chief Library Section
Earl Payne, Manager

Medicine, nursing, psychiatry, allied health sciences.

8515 US Department of Veterans Affairs: Carl Vinson Medical Center Library

1826 Veterans Boulevard
Dublin, GA 31021-3620
478-272-1210
Fax: 478-277-2717; *Toll Free:* 800-595-5229
www.dublin.va.gov

Steve Toepper, Chief Library Service
Benjamin Harrell, Manager

Medicine, nursing and allied health sciences.

8516 US Department of Veterans Affairs: Medical Center Medical Library

1670 Clairmont Road
Decatur, GA 30033-4004
404-321-6111
Fax: 404-728-7781
www1.va.gov/atlanta/

Rita L Clifton, Manager Medical Library
Thomas Cappello, CEO

Medicine, health and social sciences.

Idaho

8517 US Department of Veterans Affairs: Medical Center Library

500 W Fort Street
Boise, ID 83702-4501
208-334-1707
Fax: 208-422-1390
gordon.carlson@med.va.gov
www.va.gov

Gordon Carlson, Chief Librarian

Clinical medicine.

Illinois

8518 Adler School of Professional Psychology

Sol and Elaine Mosak Library
17 North Dearborn Street
Chicago, IL 60602
312-662-4000
Fax: 312-662-4099
www.adler.edu

Karen Drescher, Director
Raymond Crossman, President

Psychology, psychotherapy, substance abuse, gerontology, marriage and family, gender and culture, psychiatry, education.

8519 Alzheimer's Association: Green-Field Library

252 N Michigan Avenue
Floor 17
Chicago, IL 60601-7633
312-335-9602
Fax: 866-699-1238; *Toll Free:* 800-272-3900
greenfield@alz.org
www.alz.org

Mary Ann Urbashich, Manager

Alzheimer's disease, gerontology, aging.

8520 Catholic Guild for the Blind
1011 First Avenue
11th Floor
New York, NY 10022
312-236-8569
Fax: 312-236-8128; *Toll Free:* 888-744-900
www.catholiccharitiesny.org

David Tabak, Executive Director

Offers books in braille and large print, cassettes and a lending library.

8521 Du Page Library
System Center
127 S 1st Street
Geneva, IL 60134-2771
630-232-8457
Fax: 603-232-0699
www.dupagels.lib.il.us

Pamela Feather, Executive Director
Shirley May Byrnes, Executive Director

Library science.

8522 Hopedale Medical Complex: Medical Library
107 Tremont Avenue
Hopedale, IL 61747
309-449-3321
Fax: 309-449-5441
www.hopedalmedicalcomplex.com

Karen J Nordstrom, DDS

Geriatrics, substance abuse, rehabilitation.

8523 Illinois Institute of Technology: Chicago Kent Law School Information Center
565 W Adams Street
Chicago, IL 60661-3652
312-906-5600
Fax: 312-906-5685
www.kentlaw.edu

Prof. Mickie Voges Piatt, Director
Keith Ann Stiverson, Executive Director

Federal and Illinois law, law and aging, international relations law, financial services law, business and management, environmental law.

8524 McDermott, Will & Emery Library
227 W Monroe Street
46th Floor
Chicago, IL 60606-5096
312-984-3289
Fax: 312-984-2094
www.mwe.com

Louis J Covotsos, Director Legal Information
Harvey W Freishtat, CEO

Federal, state, foreign taxation; American and English probate law; litigation; pension; real estate.

8525 Mid-Illinois Talking Book Center
600 High Point Lane
Suite 2
East Peoria, IL 61611-9397
309-353-5444
Fax: 309-353-8281; *Toll Free:* 800-426-0709
info@illinoistalkingbooks.org
www.illinoistalkingbooks.org

Lori Bell, Librarian

Summer reading programs, cassette books and magazines, children's books on cassette, reference materials on blindness and other handicaps.

8526 Provena-Mercy Center Medical Library
19065 Hickory Creek Drive
Suite 300,
Mokena, IL 60448
708-478-6300
Fax: 630-801-2687
www.provena.org

Janet Leach, Library Manager

Medicine, psychiatry, nursing, hospital administration.

8527 Shawnee Library System
607 S Greenbriar Road
Carterville, IL 62918-1600
618-985-3711
Fax: 618-985-4211
www.shawls.lib.il.us

Kristi Gorden, Librarian
Thomas Joe Harris, Executive Director

Summer reading programs, braille writer, magnifiers, closed-circuit TV, large-print photocopier, cassette books and magazines, children's books on cassette, home visits and other reference materials on blindness and other handicaps.

8528 Skokie Accessible Library Services
Skokie Public Library
5215 Oakton Street
Skokie, IL 60077-3680
847-673-7774
Fax: 847-673-7797
www.skokielibrary.info

Carolyn Anthony, Executive Director
Gary Gustin, Librarian

Library services for people with disabilities, including electronic aids, materials in special formats, programs and special services, and access to the North Suburban Library System.

8529 US Department of Veterans Affairs: Chicago Health Care System-West Side Division
820 S Damen Avenue
Chicago, IL 60612-3728
312-886-6503
Fax: 312-633-2110
www.va.org

Susan L Thompson, Deputy Chief Library Service
Christopher Fox, Manager

Medicine and allied health sciences.

8530 US Department of Veterans Affairs: Hospital Library
W Main Street, 142-D
Marion, IL 62959
618-993-4114
Fax: 618-993-4176
www.va.org

Arlene M Dueker, Chief Library Service

Medicine, surgery.

8531 US Department of Veterans Affairs: Library Services
Edward Hines Jr Medical Cente
5000 South 5th Avenue
Hines, IL 60141
708-202-8387
Fax: 708-202-7998
www.hines.med.va.gov

John Cline, Acting Chief

Hospital administration, medicine, nursing, allied health sciences.

8532 University of Chicago Social Services Administration Library
1100 E 57th Street
Chicago, IL 60637-2677
773-702-8740
Fax: 773-702-0874
www.lib.uchicago.edu

Eileen Libby, Librarian

Social services, American and foreign social work, public welfare, mental health, social and urban policy, social problems, child welfare, health care, aged, psychotherapy.

8533 Voices of Vision Talking Book Center
Dupage Library System Building
127 S 1st Street
Geneva, IL 60134-2771
630-232-8457
Fax: 630-232-0699
kodean@dupagels.lib.il.us
www.dupagels.lib.il.us

Karen Odean, Manager

Large Print, audio cassette, or computer diskette.

Indiana

8534 Allen County Public Library
900 Library Plaza
Fort Wayne, IN 46802
260-421-1200
Fax: 260-421-1386
ask@acpl.info
www.acpl.lib.in.us

Joyce Misner, Librarian
Mark Allen, Vice President

Summer reading programs, braille writer, magnifiers, closed-circuit TV, large-print photocopier, cassette books and magazines, children's books on cassette, home visits and other reference materials on blindness and other handicaps.

8535 Allen County Public Library of New Haven
648 Green Street
New Haven, IN 46774-1681
260-421-1345
Fax: 260-493-0130
ask@acpl.info
www.acpl.lib.in.us/newhaven

Linda Jeffrey, Manager

Magazines, large print books, educational videos, books on tape, and books on CD.

8536 Allen County Public Library of Woodburn
4701 State Road 101 North
Woodburn, IN 46797
260-421-1370
Fax: 260-632-0101
ask@acpl.info
www.acpl.lib.in.us/woodburn

Genie Bishop, Manager

Books on tape, educational videos, software; CDRoms.

8537 Allen County Public Library, Aboite Branch
5630 Coventry Lane
Fort Wayne, IN 46804-7140
260-421-1310
Fax: 260-432-2394
ask@acpl.info
www.acpl.lib.in.us/aboite

Susan Hunt, Manager

Collection of books and other materials such as magazines, large print books and books on cassette and CD.

8538 Allen County Public Library, Pontiac Branch
2215 S Hanna Street
Fort Wayne, IN 46803-2431
260-421-1350
Fax: 260-744-5372
ask@acpl.info
www.acpl.lib.in.us/pontiac

Ann Hoehn, Manager

Large print books, books on tape and CD, educational videos, movies on DVD, music CDs, and CD-ROMs.

8539 American Legion
National Headquarters Library
700 N Pennsylvania Street
Indianapolis, IN 46204-1172
317-630-1200
Fax: 317-630-1223
library@legion.org
www.legion.org

Howard Trace, Librarian
Daniel S Wheeler, CEO

Veterans' affairs, children and youth, national defense, patriotism, American Legion.

8540 American United Life Insurance Company Library
1 American Square
Po Box 368
Indianapolis, IN 46282
317-285-1877
Fax: 317-263-1979
www.aul.com

Dayton H Molendorp, CEO

Insurance on life and health; pensions.

8541 Bartholomew County Public Library
536 5th St
Columbus, IN 47201
812-379-1255
www.barth.lib.in.us

Sharon Thompson, Librarian
Beth Poor, Executive Director

Summer reading programs, braille writer, magnifiers, closed-circuit TV, large-print photocopier, cassette books and magazines, children's books on cassette, home visits and other reference materials on blindness and other handicaps.

8542 Evansville-Vanderburgh County Public Library
Allen County Public Library
PO Box 2270
Fort Wayne, IN 46801-2270
219-424-7241

Joyce Misner, Contact

Offers books on disc and cassette.

8543 Indiana School for the Deaf: Alumni Hall Library
1200 E 42nd Street
Indianapolis, IN 46205-2004
317-550-4800
Fax: 317-923-2853
www.deafhoosiers.com

Laura Kesterke, Librarian
David Geeslin III, Superintendent/CEO

American sign language, deaf studies, Bi-Bi education.

8544 Michigan City Public Library: Indiana Rooom/Genealogy
100 East 4th Street
Michigan City, IN 46360-3302
219-873-3044
Fax: 219-873-3068
reference@mclib.org
www.mclib.org

Don Glossinger, Director

Provides a center for information, education, culture, and recreation for all patrons throughout thier life span.

8545 Northwest Indiana Subregional Library for Blind and Physically Handicapped
1919 W Lincoln Highway
Merrillville, IN 46410-5332
219-769-3541
Fax: 219-756-9358
www.lakeco.lib.in.us/talkingbooks.htm

Renee Lewis, Contact
Larry Acheff, Manager

Summer reading programs, braille writer, magnifiers, closed-circuit TV, large-print photocopier, cassette books and magazines, children's books on cassette, home visits and other reference materials on blindness and other handicaps.

8546 Purdue University: Humanities, Social Science, Education Library
Purdue University
504 West State St
West Lafayette, IN 47907
765-494-4600
Fax: 765-494-0156; *Toll Free:* 800-825-4264
hsselib@purdue.edu
www.lib.purdue.edu/hsse/

J Mark Tucker, Librarian

English and American literature, US history, North American Indians, education.

8547 Special Services Division: Indiana State Library
140 N Senate Avenue
Indianapolis, IN 46204-2207
317-232-3684
Fax: 317-232-3728; *Toll Free:* 800-622-

Lissa Shanahan, Librarian

Circulates a collection of fourty thousand titles in braille, large print and on cassette and the special equipment needed to play the recorded materials to anyone in Indiana who cannot read regular print due to a visual or physical disability. This is a free library service. The Division maintains a small reference collection and provides reference and referral services on disabilities and services available to people with disabilities

8548 US Department of Veterans Affairs, Medical Center Library Service
2121 Lake Avenue
Fort Wayne, IN 46805-5100
219-460-1490
Fax: 219-460-1364
www.martinsburg.va.gov

Laveta J Diem, Librarian

Medicine, nursing, patient education.

8549 US Department of Veterans Affairs: Indiana Health Care System
1700 E 38th Street
Marion, IN 46953-4568
765-677-3120
Fax: 765-677-3111

Scott Pierce, Manager Education
Patrick H Lau, DO

Medicine, with special emphasis on psychiatry and psychology.

8550 US Deprtment of Veterans Affairs: Center Library
1481 W 10th Street
Indianapolis, IN 46202-2803
317-554-0000
www.martinsburg.va.gov

Linda J Bennett, Chief Library Service

General medicine, surgery, nursing, psychiatry, allied health sciences.

Iowa

8551 Ames Public Library Ames and Iowa History Collection
515 Douglas Avenue
Ames, IA 50010-6291
515-239-5630
Fax: 515-232-4571
www.ames.lib.ia.us

Gina Millsap, Executive Director

8552 Calhoun County Historical Museum Library
301 S. Ann
Port Lavaca,, TX 77979

712-297-8139
www.calhouncountymuseum.org

8553 Iowa Library For The Blind And Physically Handicapped
524 4th Street
Des Moines, IA 50309-2364
515-281-1333
Fax: 515-281-1263
library@blind.state.ia.us

Karen Keninger, Librarian
Allen C Harris, Executive Director

Summer reading programs, braille writer, magnifiers, closed-circuit TV, cassette books and magazines, children's books on cassette, home visits and other reference materials on blindness and other handicaps.

8554 US Department of Veterans Affairs: Central Iowa Health Care System
1515 W Pleasant Street
Knoxville, IA 50138-3399
641-828-5127
www.centraliowa.va.gov/contact/

Judy Gottshall, Manager

Psychiatry, psychology, medicine, nursing.

Kansas

8555 Bukovina Society of the Americas Library
PO Box 81
Ellis, KS 67637
785-625-9492
info@bukovinasociety.org
www.bukovinasoiety.org

Martha McLelland, President

8556 Cherokee County Genealogical Historical Society
PO Box 33
100 S Tennessee
Columbus, KS 66725
620-429-2992
skyways.lib.ks.us

Marilyn Schmidt, Manager

8557 Kansas State Historical Society: Library & Archives Division
6425 SW 6th Avenue
Topeka, KS 66615-1099
785-272-8681 Toll free: 785-272-8682
www.kshs.org

Patricia A Michaelis, Division Director
Margaret Knecht, Librarian Section Head
Susan Forbes, Western Hist. Cat.
1975

8558 Kansas State Library Talking Book Service ESU Memorial Union
1200 Commercial Street
PO Box 4055
Emporia, KS 66801-5057
620-343-7124
Fax: 620-343-7124

KSLIB_talking_books@library.ks.gov
www.kslib.info/talking

Toni Harrell, Librarian

Summer reading programs, braille, cassette books and magazines, children's books on cassette, home visits and other reference materials on blindness and other handicaps.

8559 Leavenworth County Genealogical Society Library
PO Box 362
Leavenworth, KS 66048
913-682-8181

Nettie Graden, Book Community Chairman
1984

8560 Manhattan Public Library
629 Poyntz Avenue
Manhattan, KS 66502-6131
785-776-4741
Fax: 785-776-1545; *Toll Free:* 800-432-2796
www.manhattan.lib.ks.us

Marion Rice, Librarian
Fred Atchison, Manager

Cassette books and magazines, children books on cassette, summer reading program braille writer, magnifiers, closed-circuit TV, large-print photocopier, Community Assistive Technology Center, home visits and other reference materials aon blindness and other disabilities.

8561 Northwest Kansas Library System Talking Books
2 Washington Square
PO Box 446
Norton, KS 67654
785-877-5148
Fax: 785-877-5697; *Toll Free:* 800-432-2858
nwkls.mykansaslibrary.org

Clarice Howard, Librarian
Leslie Bell, Executive Director

Offers books on cassette and DVS videos to qualified individuals.

8562 Old Fort Genealogical Society Of Southeastern Kansas Inc
At 3rd And National
Po Box 786
Fort Scott, KS 66701
620-223-3300
Fax: 913-367-2717
ofgs@pbxmail.com
skyways.lib.ks.us

Roxanna Tosterud, President
P J Capps, Manager
Cova Chambers, VP

A non profit volunteer organization to explore and research family ancestry.

8563 South Central Kansas Library System
321 A North Main St
South Hutchinson, KS 67505
620-663-5441
Fax: 620-663-9797; *Toll Free:* 800-234-0529
www.sckls.info

Karen Socha, Talking Books
Cheryl Canfield, Reference Librarian
Leroy Gattin, Director

Summer reading programs, braille writer, magnifiers, closed-circuit TV, large-print books, photocopier, cassette books and magazines, children's books on cassette, home visits and other reference materials on blindness and other handicaps.

8564 Talking Books Service

1515 SW 10th Avenue
Topeka, KS 66604-1304
785-231-0574
Fax: 785-231-0579

Suzanne Bundy, Librarian

Summer reading programs, braille writer, magnifiers, closed-circuit TV, large-print photocopier, cassette books and magazines, children's books on cassette, home visits and other reference materials on blindness and other handicaps.

8565 US Department of Veterans Affairs: Dwight D. Eisenhower Center Medical Library

4101 S 4th Street
Leavenworth, KS 66048-5014
913-682-2000
www.va.gov

Jan Gosselin, Medical Librarian
Edgar Tucker, Manager

Medicine, allied health sciences, psychology.

8566 US Department of Veterans Affairs: Medical & Regional Office Center Library Service

5500 E Kellogg Drive
Wichita, KS 67218-1607
www.va.gov

Alice H Schad, Chief Library Service

Medicine, nursing, allied health sciences, patient health education, veterans affairs.

8567 Wichita Public Library

223 S Main Street
Wichita, KS 67202-3795
316-261-8500
Fax: 316-262-4540
admin@wichita.lib.ks.us
www.wichita.lib.ks.us

Roger Woods, President

Offers a variety of programs and services to older adults and their caregivers. Nine convenient locations throughout the Wichita community.

8568 Young Historical Library

PO Box 55
Little River, KS 67457
620-897-6236
info@visityoung.com.au
www.getitalldoneinyoung.com.au

Doris Cory, Librarian
Lillie Whiteman, Manager
1990

8569 Kentucky Historical Society-Thomas D Clark Research Library

100 W Broadway Street
Frankfort, KY 40601-1931
502-564-1792
Fax: 502-696-3846
history.ky.gov

Kent Whitworth, Executive Director
Shirley Ackerman, Technical Services Librarian

The Thomas D Clark Research Library of the Kentucky Historical Society houses over 90,000 published works, dealing primarily with history and genealogy, as well as over 12,000 reels of microfilm, and over 20,000 vertical files of collected and contributed research.

8570 Kentucky Talking Book Library

PO Box 537
Frankfort, KY 40602-0537
502-564-8300
Fax: 502-564-5773
kdla.ky.gov/collectionsktbl.htm

Barbara Penegor, Head Librarian

Children's and adult cassette books and magazines, Braille books, and descriptive videos and DVDs for the blind and physically handicapped.

8571 Louisville Talking Book Library
Louisville Free Public Library

301 York Street
Louisville, KY 40203-2257
502-574-1611
www.lfpl.org/tbl.tbl.asp

Linda Atzinger, Head Librarian

Braille transcription, computer workstation with magnifier, children's and adult cassette books and magazines, Braille books, and descriptive videos and DVDs for the blind and physically handicapped.

8572 Northern Kentucky Talking Book Library

502 Scott Street
Covington, KY 41011-1530
859-962-4095
Fax: 859-655-7960
www.kentonlibrary.org

Clif Mayhew, Head Librarian

Children's and adult cassette books and magazines and Braille books for the blind and physically handicapped.

8573 US Department of Veterans Affairs: Hospital Library

800 Zorn Avenue
Louisville, KY 40206-1433
502-894-6240
Fax: 502-894-6134
www.louisville.va.gov

James F Kastner, Chief Librarian

Clinical medicine, surgery, nursing, psychiatry, social work.

8574 US Department of Veterans Affairs: Medical Center Libraries

810 Vermont Avenue
Washington, DC 20420
859-281-4916
Fax: 859-281-4808
www.va.gov

Robert Bradley, Contact

Psychology, psychiatry, nursing, medicine, surgery, social sciences, patient health education.

Louisiana

8575 Mary Bird Perkins Cancer Center Community Library

4950 Essen Lane
Baton Rouge, LA 70809-3432
225-767-0847
Fax: 225-215-1215
www.marybird.org

Todd Stevens, CEO/President
Tom J Meek, Secretary
Randolph Waes, Treasurer

Cancer; coping.

8576 New Orleans Public Library: Louisiana Division

219 Loyola Avenue
New Orleans, LA 70112-2007
504-596-2570
Fax: 504-596-2609
www.nutrias.org/~nopl/welcome.htm

Stephen Kuehling, Louisiana Division Librarian
Greg Osborn, Louisiana Division Librarian
Irene Wainwright, Louisiana Division Archivist

The Louisiana Division is a reference division which collects all types of printed, manuscript, graphic, and oral resources relating to the study of Louisiana and its citizens and to the city of New Orleans and New Orleanians. Other areas of concentration are the Mississippi River, the Gulf of Mexico, and the South. Included within the Division's collections are books by or about Louisianians; city, regional, and state documents; manuscripts, maps, newspapers, periodicals, microfilms, photographs, slides, motion pictures, sound recordings, video tapes, postcards, and ephemera of every sort.

1946

8577 Tulane University: Howard-Tilton Memorial Library-Louisiana Collection

Tulane Libraries, Jones Hall
Tulane University
New Orleans, LA 70118
504-865-5685
Fax: 504-865-5761
meneray@tulane.edu
specialcollections.tulane.edu/

Wilbur E Meneray, Special Collections Librarian
Jessica Jones, Special Collections Librarian
Kenneth Owen, Special Collections Librarian

The Library houses nearly 2 million print volumes, more than 7,750 current serials, nearly a million government documents, more than three linear miles of manuscripts, hundreds of thousands of microforms, as well as collections of photographs and recordings. In addition, the Library is serving a new role as a gateway to digital resources. Located within the Howard-Tilton building are many important departments and collections with librarians andstaff who work to maintain the library's resources and to provide an array of useful library services. The general collections of the Library, its Latin American Library, the Maxwell Music Library, and a federal Government Documents depository reside in the main building. Special Collections includes the Hogan Jazz Archive, Louisiana collections, Manuscripts, Rare Books, University Archives, and the Southeastern Architectural Archive. The Special Collections were moved to the adjacent Jones Hall building in 1999.

8578 US Deparment of Veterans Affairs: Center Library

810 Vermont Avenue
Washington, DC 20420
504-589-5272
Fax: 504-589-5916
www.va.gov

Mark Petersen, Manager

Medicine, nursing, dentistry, surgery, allied health sciences.

8579 US Department of Veterans Affairs: Medical Center Medical Library

810 Vermont Avenue
Washington, DC 20420
318-473-0010
Fax: 318-473-9491
www.va.gov

Charles T Cooker, Library Manager

Medicine, employee development, patient education and recreation.

8580 US Department of Veterans Affairs: Overton Brooks Medical Center Library

510 E Stoner Avenue
Shreveport, LA 71101-4243
318-221-8411
Fax: 318-424-6156; *Toll Free:* 800-863-7441
www.shreveport.va.gov

Dixie Jones, Manager

General medicine.

8581 University of Southwestern Louisiana: Jefferson Caffery Louisana Room-Southwestern Archives and Manuscripts Collection

302 East Saint Mary Boulevard
Lafayette, LA 70503-2038
337-482-5702
Fax: 337-482-5702
www.usl.edu/Departments/Library

Dr. I Bruce Turner, Special Collections Director
Jean S Kiesel, Louisiana Room Librarian
Jane Vidrine, Archives Specialist

The Special Collections department is composed of the Louisiana Room, the Rare Book Collection, the University Archives and Acadiana Manuscripts Collection, the Cajun and Creole Music Collection, the University Records Management Program, and the Microforms Room. The Louisiana Room provides access to materials pertaining to Louisiana, including books, periodicals, state government documents, genealogical materials, rare books, newspapers, and other special collections. Most Louisiana newspapers are housed in the Louisiana Room. The University Archives and Acadiana Manuscripts Collection houses the archival records of the University starting in 1900. There are also over 300 collections of personal or family papers, business or organizational records, photograph collections, and much more related to the Acadiana region.

1962

Maine

8582 Bangor Public Library

145 Harlow Street
Bangor, ME 04401-4900
207-947-8336
Fax: 207-945-6694
www.bpl.lib.me.us

Judith Leighton, Librarian
Barbara McDade, Manager

Summer reading programs, braille writer, magnifiers, closed-circuit TV, large-print photocopier, cassette books and magazines, children's books on cassette, home visits and other reference materials on blindness and other handicaps.

8583 Governor Baxter School for the Deaf Library

PO Box 799
One Mackworth Island
Falmouth, ME 04105
207-781-6237
Fax: 207-781-6240
www.gbsd.org/pages/MEDHH_library/index

Leone Anderson, Manager

Deafness, sign language, deaf education, professional education.

8584 Jackson Laboratory: Joan Staats Library

600 Main Street
Bar Harbor, ME 04609-1523
207-288-6000
Fax: 207-288-6079
library@jax.org
www.jax.org/library

Douglas T Macbeth, Librarian
Rick Woychik, Executive Director

Inbred strains of mice, genetics, cancer, growth, animal health and husbandry, immunology, aging, cell biology, molecular genetics.

8585 Lewiston Public Library

200 Lisbon St
Lewiston, ME 04240-7203
207-513-3004
Fax: 207-784-0135
lplonline.org
Richard Speer, Director

Summer reading programs, braille writer, magnifiers, closed-circuit TV, large-print photocopier, cassette books and magazines, children's books on cassette, home visits and other reference materials on blindness and other handicaps.

8586 Maine State Library

64 State House Station
230 State St
Augusta, ME 04333-0064
207-287-5600
Fax: 207-287-5624
benitad@ursus3.ursus.maine.edu
maine.gov/msl/index.shtml

J Gary Nichols, Librarian

Summer reading programs, braille writer, magnifiers, closed-circuit TV, large-print photocopier, cassette books and magazines, children's books on cassette, home visits and other reference materials on blindness and other handicaps.

8587 Portland Public Library

5 Monument Square
Portland, ME 04101-4072
207-871-1700
Fax: 207-871-1703
www.portlandlibrary.com

Janice Littlefield, Librarian
Claire Hannan, Manager

Summer reading programs, braille writer, magnifiers, closed-circuit TV, large-print photocopier, cassette books and magazines, children's books on cassette, home visits and other reference materials on blindness and other handicaps.

8588 US Department of Veterans Affairs: Medical & Regional Office Center

810 Vermont Avenue
Washington, DC 20420
207-623-5773
Fax: 207-623-5766
www.va.gov

Judy Littlefield, Team Leader

Social sciences/psychiatry, medicine, alcoholism, nursing, dentistry, hospital administration.

8589 Waterville Public Library

73 Elm Street
Waterville, ME 04901-6078
207-872-5433
Fax: 207-873-4779
www.waterville.lib.me.us

Meta Vigue, Librarian
Sarah Sugden, Executive Director

Summer reading programs, braille writer, magnifiers, closed-circuit TV, large-print photocopier, cassette books and magazines, children's books on cassette, home visits and other reference materials on blindness and other handicaps.

Maryland

8590 American College of Cardiology

2400 N Street NW
Washington, DC 20037
202-375-6000
Fax: 202-375-7000
www.acc.org

James T Dove MD, FACC, President

Cardiovascular disease and surgery.

8591 Friends of Libraries for Deaf Action
2930 Craiglawn Road
Silver Spring, MD 20904-1816
301-572-5168
folda86@aol.com
www.folda.net/

Alice Hagemeyer, Founder/President

Library services for people that are deaf impaired.

8592 Maryland State Library for the Blind and Physically Handicapped
415 Park Avenue
Baltimore, MD 21201-3638
410-230-2424
Fax: 410-333-2095; *Toll Free:* 800-964-9209
www.lbph.lib.md.us
TDD 410-333-8679

Sharron McFarland, Librarian
Nancy Grasmick, Manager

Summer reading programs, braille writer, magnifiers, large-print photocopier, cassette books and magazines, children's books on cassette, and other reference materials on blindness and other handicaps.

8593 Special Needs Library Montgomery County Department of Public Libraries
6400 Cemocracy Boulevard
Bethesda, MD 20817
301-897-2212
TDD 301-897-2217

Charlette Stinnett, Contact

8594 Spring Dell Center
6040 Radio Station Road
La Plata, MD 20646-3368
301-934-4561
Fax: 301-870-2439
www.springdellcenter.org

Reed Walker, Transportation Director
Donna Retzlaff, Executive Director

Since 1967, Spring Dell center has been, 'bridging the gap' to enhance the lives of developmentally disabled people. Spring Dell's goal is to empower people in every aspect of their lives through the implementation of two programs, employment/vocational services and residential services including transportation. Spring Dell offers transportation door-to-door for persons with developmental disabilities, including day care programs, supportive envvironment, residential and other transportation.

8595 US Army: Medical Command Center for Health Promotion & Preventive Medicine
Aberdeen Proving Ground
Building E1570
Aberdeen, MD 21001
410-671-4236
Fax: 410-671-3665

Krishan S Goel, Librarian

Occupational medicine, safety and health; chemistry and toxicology; audiology; medical entomology; laser, microwave, and radiological safety and health; air and water pollution; sanitary engineering.

8596 US Department of Veterans Affairs Hospitl: Fort Howard Hospital Library
9600 N Point Road
Fort Howard, MD 21052-3050
410-477-1800
Fax: 410-477-7207
www.maryland.va.gov

Joanne M Bennett, Chief Librarian
Dennis H Smith, Executive Director

Medicine.

8597 US Department of Veterans Affairs: Baltimore Medical Center Library Service
10 N Greene Street
Baltimore, MD 21201-1524
410-605-7092
Fax: 410-605-7905
stout.deborah@baltimore.va.gov
www.maryland.va.gov

Deborah A Stout, Chief Library Service
Joanna Lin, Manager

Medicine, surgery, nursing.

8598 US National Institutes of Health: National Cancer Institute-Scientific Library
Bldg. 427, Rm. 1
PO Box B
Frederick, MD 21702-1124
301-846-1093
Fax: 301-846-6332
ncifrederick.cancer.gov/

Susan W Wilson, Director

Cancer biology, biological and chemical carcinogenesis, acquired immunodeficiency syndrome, biomedical research.

8599 US Social Security Administration Library & Records Management Branch
Altmeyer Building
Room 570
Baltimore, MD 21235
410-962-3311
Fax: 410-966-2027

Bill Vitek, Director/Librarian

Social insurance, medical and hospital economics, operations research, management, personnel administration, supervision and training, electronic data processing, law, health insurance, business and management.

Massachusetts

8600 Boston College: Social Work Library
McGuinn Hall
Room B38
Chestnut Hill, MA 02467
617-552-3233
Fax: 617-552-3199

Donna L Ferullo, Head Librarian

Clinical social work; child welfare and families, individuals, and groups; ethnic studies and special populations; gerontology; human behavior; mental health; social policy; administration and research; social planning.

8601 Caption Center
125 Western Avenue
Boston, MA 02134-1008
617-300-3600
Fax: 617-300-3600
www.icdri.org/dhhi/ccowgbh.htm

Lori Kay, Co-Director
Tom Apone, Co-Director

Provides closed captioning for videos, including training, safety, instructional and educational films. Maintains a consumer information service for overcoming communications barriers in the workplace.

8602 Caritas Southwood Hospital Medical Library
111 Dedham Street
Norfolk, MA 02056-1666
508-668-0385
Fax: 781-769-9622
schnuha@ma.ultranet.com
mblc.state.ma.us/

8603 Dana-Farber Cancer Institute Library
44 Binney Street
Boston, MA 02115-6084
617-632-3000
Fax: 617-632-2488
www.dana-farber.org

Christine W Fleuriel, Librarian
Edward Benz, President

Cancer research, AIDS research.

8604 Deaconess Hospital Horrax Library
185 Pilgrim Road
Boston, MA 02215-5324
617-632-9202

Paul Vaiginas, Librarian
Carl A Rasumssen, Manager

General medicine, diabetes, cancer, renal disease, cardiology, surgery.

8605 Framingham Public Library: Framingham Room
49 Lexington Street
Framingham, MA 01702-8218
508-532-5570
Fax: 508-820-7210
www.framinghamlibrary.org

Tom Gilchrist, Contact

1955

8606 Laboure College Library
303 Adams Street
Milton, MA 02186
617-202-3491
www.laboure.edu

Maryann O'Toole, Director
Andrew Callo, Manager

Offers information on physical disabilities, independent living, peer counseling and advocacy.

8607 Perkins School for the Blind: Samuel P Hayes Research Library
175 N Beacon Street
Watertown, MA 02472-2751
617-972-7250
hayeslibrary@perkins.org
www.perkins.org/researchlibrary

Jennifer Arnott, Research Librarian

Nonmedical aspects of blindness and deaf-blindness, including education, rehabilitation, welfare.

8608 US Department of Veterans Affairs Bedford: Edith Nourse Rogers Memorial Veterans Hospital Medical Library
200 Springs Road
Bedford, MA 01730-1114
781-687-2000
Fax: 781-687-2102
www.bedford.va.gov

Arlene Devlin, Chief Library Service

Psychiatry, geriatrics.

8609 US Department of Veterans Affairs Medical Center Library
N Main Street
Northampton, MA 01060
413-584-4040
Fax: 413-582-3039

Dorothy E Young, Chief Library Service
Joanne Carney, Manager

Neurology, psychiatry, psychology, nursing, medicine, gerontology.

8610 US Department of Veterans Affairs Outpatient Clinic Learning Resources Service
251 Causeway Street
Boston, MA 02114-2148
617-248-1170
Fax: 617-248-1406
www.boston.va.gov/bwropc_caus.asp

Irmeli Kilburn, Acting Chief Library Service

Health sciences, patient health education.

8611 US Department of Veterans Affairs: Boston Hospital Medical Library
150 S Huntington Avenue
Boston, MA 02130-4817
617-232-9500
Fax: 617-278-4508
www.va.gov

Irmeli Kilburn, Contact
Michael Lawson, President

General medicine, surgery, allied health sciences, patient education.

8612 US Department of Veterans Affairs: Medical Center Library
940 Belmont Street
Brockton, MA 02301-5596
508-583-4500
Fax: 508-895-0074
www.va.gov/valnet/

Suzanne N Noyes, Chief Library Service
Christine Croteau, Manager

Psychiatry, psychology, hospital administration, nursing, alcoholism, drug abuse.

8613 Worcester Public Library
3 Salem Square
Worcester, MA 01608-2074
508-799-1655
Fax: 508-799-1652
www.worcpublib.org
Penelope B Johnson, Head Librarian

Summer reading programs, braille writer, magnifiers, closed-circuit TV, large-print photocopier, cassette books and magazines, children's books on cassette, home visits and other reference materials on blindness and other handicaps.

Michigan

8614 Area Agency on Aging Library
29100 Northwestern Highway
Southfield, MI 48034-1046
248-213-6704
Fax: 248-948-9691; *Toll Free:* 800-852-7795
www.aaa1b.org

Jenny Jarvis, Director of Communications
Sandra Reminga, Executive Director

Older adult issues.

8615 Downtown Detroit Subregional Library for the Blind
121 Gratiot Avenue
Detroit, MI 48226-2203
313-965-3830
Fax: 313-965-1977
www.detroit.lib.mi.us
TDD 313-224-0584

Deborah Evans, Librarian
George Saad, Owner

Summer reading programs, braille writer, magnifiers, closed-circuit TV, large-print photocopier, cassette books and magazines, children's books on cassette, home visits and other reference materials on blindness and other handicaps.

8616 Grand Traverse Area Library for the Blind and Physically Handicapped
610 Woodmere Avenue
Traverse City, MI 49686-2339
231-995-8558
Fax: 231-932-8578; *Toll Free:* 877-931-8558
lbph@tadl.tcnet.org
www.tadl.org/lbph/about
TDD 231-932-8507

Evelyn Welty, Contact
Daniel Truckey, Manager

8617 Herman Miller Research Corporation
3971 Research Park Drive
Ann Arbor, MI 48108-2219
734-994-0200

Dallas Moore, Librarian
Robert Logeman, Partner

Library on aging and disability.

8618 Karmanos Cancer Institute Research Library
4100 John R
Detroit, MI 48201-1312

313-833-0710
Fax: 313-831-8714

CJ Glodek, Head Librarian
April Allen, Manager

Cancer research, allied health sciences.

8619 Kent County Library for the Blind
775 Ball Avenue NE
Grand Rapids, MI 49503-1397
616-336-3265
Fax: 616-336-3256
www.kentcountylibrary.org/index.php

Claudya Muller, Librarian

Summer reading programs, braille writer, magnifiers, closed-circuit TV, large-print photocopier, cassette books and magazines, children's books on cassette, home visits and other reference materials on blindness and other handicaps.

8620 Library of Michigan Service for the Blind
PO Box 30007
Lansing, MI 48909-7507
517-373-5614
Fax: 517-373-5865

Nancy Robertson, Manager

Summer reading programs, braille writer, magnifiers, closed-circuit TV, large-print photocopier, cassette books and magazines, children's books on cassette, home visits and other reference materials on blindness and other handicaps.

8621 Macomb Library for the Blind and Physically Handicapped
16480 Hall Road
Clinton Township, MI 48038-1132
586-286-1580
Fax: 810-286-0634
www.libcoop.net/macspe/

Linda Champion, Librarian
Beverlee Babcock, Executive Director

Summer reading programs, braille writer, magnifiers, closed-circuit TV, large-print photocopier, cassette books and magazines, children's books on cassette, home visits and other reference materials on blindness and other handicaps.

8622 Mideastern Michigan Library Co-op
G-4195 W Pasadena Avenue
Flint, MI 48504
810-732-1120
Fax: 810-732-1715
www.thegdl.org

Kelly Richards, Librarian

Summer reading programs, braille writer, magnifiers, closed-circuit TV, large-print photocopier, cassette books and magazines, children's books on cassette, home visits and other reference materials on blindness and other handicaps.

8623 Northland Library Cooperative
316 E Chisholm Street
Alpena, MI 49707-2892
989-356-1622
Fax: 989-354-3939
www.nlc.lib.m.us

Catherine Glomski, Librarian
Christine Johnston, Executive Director

Summer reading programs, braille writer, magnifiers, closed-circuit TV, large-print photocopier, cassette books and magazines, children's books on cassette, home visits and other reference materials on blindness and other handicaps.

8624 Oakland County Library for the Blind and Physically Handicapped
1200 N Telegraph Road
Dept 482
Pontiac, MI 48341
248-858-5050
Fax: 248-452-9145
www.oakland.lib.mi.us/oakllbph.htm

Betty Ramey, Contact
David Conklin, Manager

8625 Senior Alliance Area Agency on Aging
3850 2nd Street
Suite 201
Wayne, MI 48184-1755
734-722-2830
Fax: 734-722-2836
info@tsalink.org
www.thesenioralliance.org

Bob Brown, Executive Director
Lori Vail, Program Manager

To coordinate a comprehensive network of services in Western and Southern Wayne County to enable older persons to function as independently as possible in the community environment which best suits their needs. To provide the advocacy, programming, planning, contracting, funding, and personnel necessary to accomplish the foregoing purpose.

8626 St Clark County Library for the Blind and Physically Handicapped
210 McMorran Boulevard
Port Huron, MI 48060-4098
810-982-3600
Fax: 800-272-8570
lbph@sccl.lib.mi.us
www.sccl.lib.mi.us

Jackie Skinner, Librarian
James Warwick, Executive Director

Offers library services to the blind and visually impaired.

8627 US Department of Veterans Affairs: Ann Arbor Hospital Library
2215 Fuller Road
Ann Arbor, MI 48105-2335
734-769-7100
Fax: 734-845-3260; *Toll Free:* 800-361-8387
www.va.gov

Vickie Smith, Chief Librarian
Aishe Haimour, Manager

Medicine, patient education.

8628 US Department of Veterans Affairs: Battle Creek Medical Center Library Service
5500 Armstrong Road
Battle Creek, MI 49016

269-966-5600
Fax: 269-966-5483
www.va.gov

Linda S Polardin, Contact

Psychiatry, neurology, psychology, post traumatic stress disorder, substance abuse, geropsychiatry.

8629 US Department of Veterans Affairs: Detroit Medical Center Library Service
4646 John R Street
Detroit, MI 48201-1916
313-576-1000
Fax: 313-576-1025
tubolino.karen_m@forun.va.gov
www.va.gov

Karen M Tubolino, Librarian Head

Surgery, oncology, internal medicine, psychiatry, psychology, health management.

8630 US Department of Veterans Affairs: Iron Mountain Medical Center Library
325 E H Street
Iron Mountain, MI 49801
906-774-3300
Fax: 906-779-3188
Durocher.Jeanne@Iron-Mtn.VA.gov
www.va.gov

Jeanne M Durocher, Chief Library Service

Medicine, surgery, nursing, patient education, allied health.

8631 US Department of Veterans Affairs: Saginaw Aleda E Lutz Medical Center Library
1500 Weiss Street
Saginaw, MI 48602-5251
989-497-2500
Fax: 989-321-4903; *Toll Free:* 800-406-5143
www.saginaw.va.gov

Debbie Zapolski, Program Specialist

Medicine, surgery, nursing, health education.

8632 Washtenaw County Library
PO Box 8645
4135 Washtenaw Avenue
Ann Arbor, MI 48107-8645
734-973-4359
Fax: 734-973-4963
lbpd@ewashtenaw.org
www.ewashtenaw.org

Margoret Wolfe, Librarian
Julie McClellan, Manager

Summer reading programs, braille writer, magnifiers, closed-circuit TV, large-print photocopier, cassette books and magazines, children's books on cassette, home visits and other reference materials on blindness and other handicaps.

8633 Wayne County Regional Library for the Blind
33030 Van Born Road
Wayne, MI 48184-2453
734-727-7088
Fax: 734-326-3008
www.waynecountylbph.wordpress.com
TDD 313-326-3008

Pat Klemans, Librarian
Betty McCoy, Manager

Summer reading programs, braille writer, magnifiers, closed-circuit TV, large-print photocopier, cassette books and magazines, children's books on cassette, home visits and other reference materials on blindness and other handicaps.

Minnesota

8634 Duluth Public Library
520 W Superior Street
Duluth, MN 55802-1578
218-730-4200
www.duluth.lib.mn.us

Dean Casperson, President

Adapted access to Apple computer, adapted toys and adapted library equipment.

8635 Minnesota Library for the Blind
388 6th Avenue SE
Faribault, MN 55021-6300
507-333-4828
Fax: 507-333-4832; *Toll Free:* 800-722-0550
www.msab.state.mn.us
Catherine Durivage, Library Program Director

Summer reading programs, braille writer, magnifiers, closed-circuit TV, large-print photocopier, cassette books and magazines, children's books on cassette, home visits and other reference materials on blindness and other handicaps.

8636 US Department of Veterans Affairs: Minneapolis Medical Center Library Service
1 Veterans Drive
Minneapolis, MN 55417-2309
612-725-2000
Fax: 612-725-2049; *Toll Free:* 866-414-5058
www.va.gov

A Sinha, Chief
Howard Ansel, MD

General medicine, psychology, geriatrics, biomedical research, biomedical ethics, nursing, brain science, neuroscience.

Mississippi

8637 Mississippi (State) Department of Mental Health Library and Division of Professional Development
1101 Robert East Lee Bldg
239 North Lamar Street
Jackson, MS 39201-1325
601-359-1288
Fax: 601-359-6295
www.dmh.state.ms.us/

Margueritte Ransom, Librarian

The Mental Health Library lending service was established primarily for use by the personnel of the Department of Mental Health, and other mental health/mental retardation service agencies, but its holdings are also available to the public through the Interlibrary Loan service of any public

library. Information about this service can be obtained from the Mississippi Department of Mental Health Library.

1975

8638 Mississippi Library Commission
3881 Eastwood Drive
Jackson, MS 39211-6439
601-354-7208
Fax: 601-432-4484
www.mlc.lib.ms.us
TDD 601-354-6411

Blair Booker, Reference Librarian

Summer reading programs, braille writer, magnifiers, closed-circuit TV, large-print photocopier, cassette books and magazines, children's books on cassette, home visits and other reference materials on blindness and other handicaps.

Missouri

8639 Bonne Terre Memorial Library
5 Southwest Main Street
Bonne Terre, MO 63628-1741
573-358-2260
Fax: 573-358-5941
btml@bonneterre.net
library.bonneterre.net/

Doris Smither, Librarian

The mission of the Bonne Terre Memorial Library is to provide access to informational, educational, cultural and recreational library materials and services in a variety of formats and technologies; to be responsive to the public library needs of the community; and to uphold the public's freedom of access to information. Community needs drive our services and we take a personal interest in ensuring that they are delivered in a welcoming, convenient and responsive manner.

8640 US Department of Veterans Affairs, John Cochran Division Library
915 N Grand Boulevard
Saint Louis, MO 63106-1621
314-652-4100
Fax: 314-289-6557; *Toll Free:* 800-228-5459
www.stlouis.va.gov

Donna S Locke, Contact
Ann Repetto, Manager

Medicine and allied health sciences.

8641 US Department of Veterans Affairs: Kansas Medical Center Library
4801 E Linwood Boulevard
Kansas City, MO 64128-2226
816-861-4700
Fax: 816-922-3303; *Toll Free:* 800-525-1483
g.library@kansas_city.va.gov
www.va.gov

Shirley C Ting, Chief Library Service
John McDonald, Manager

Medicine, surgery, neurology, nursing, psychology, psychiatry.

8642 US Department of Veterans Affairs: Poplar Bluff Library Service
Medical Center
1500 N Westwood Blvd
Poplar Bluff, MO 63901
573-686-4151
Fax: 573-778-4559
www.visn15.med.va.gov

Genise E Denton, Chief Lirary Service
Nancy Arnold, Manager

Medicine.

8643 Wolfner Memorial Library for the Blind
600 West Main Street
Jefferson City, MO 65102
573-751-4936
Fax: 573-526-2985; Toll Free: 800-392-2614
Info@sos.mo.gov
www.sos.mo.gov
TDD 800-347-1379

Elizabeth Eckles, Librarian
Richard J Smith, Executive Director

Summer reading programs, braille writer, magnifiers, closed-circuit TV, large-print photocopier, cassette books and magazines, children's books on cassette, home visits and other reference materials on blindness and other handicaps.

Montana

8644 Montana State Library
1515 E 6th Avenue
Po Box 201800
Helena, MT 59620-1800
406-444-3115
Fax: 406-444-5612
www.montanastatelibrary.org
TDD 406-444-5431

Darlene Staffeldt, State Librarian

Summer reading programs, braille writer, magnifiers, closed-circuit TV, large-print photocopier, cassette books and magazines, children's books on cassette, home visits and other reference materials on blindness and other handicaps.

8645 St. Patrick Hospital and Health Sciences Center: Library Center
500 W Broadway
Missoula, MT 59802
406-543-7271
Fax: 406-329-5688
library@saintpatrick.org
www.saintpatrick.org

Marianne Farr, Medical Librarian

Access to medical and consumer health related information.

8646 US Department of Veterans Affairs: Fort Harrison Medical Center Library
Library Services 142d
Fort Harrison, MT 59636
406-442-6410
Fax: 406-447-7948
www.va.gov

Charles Grasmick, Chief Library Service
Medicine, internal medicine, surgery.

8647 US Department of Veterans Affairs: Miles City Medical Center Library
3687 Veterans Drive
P.O. Box 1500
Fort Harrison, MT 59301-4742
877-468-8387
Fax: 406-442-6410
www.montana.va.gov

Gail Shaw Wilkerson, Chief Library Service
Medicine; nursing; geriatrics.

8648 William K. Kohrs Memorial Library
501 Missouri Avenue
Deer Lodge, MT 59722
406-846-2622Toll free: 888-872-2622
kohrslibrary.org/

Nancy Silliman, Library Director
Materials and resources on adult education and classes that the library sponsors.

Nebraska

8649 Nebraska School for the Visually Handicapped Library
824 10th Avenue
Nebraska City, NE 68410-1370
402-873-5513
Fax: 402-873-3463

Sally Giittinger, Administrator
Education, the blind and visually impaired.

8650 North Platte Public Library
120 W 4th Street
North Platte, NE 69101-3901
308-535-8036
Fax: 308-535-8296
library@ci.north-platte.ne.us
www.ci.north-platte.ne.us/library

Brenda Behsman, Librarian
Cecelia Lawrence, Executive Director

Summer reading programs, braille writer, magnifiers, closed-circuit TV, large-print photocopier, cassette books and magazines, children's books on cassette, home visits and other reference materials on blindness and other handicaps.

8651 US Department of Veterans Affairs: Grand Island Greater Nebraska Health Care System Library
2201 N Broadwell Avenue
Grand Island, NE 68803-2153
308-382-3660
Fax: 308-389-5148; Toll Free: 866-580-1810
www.nebraska.va.gov

Patricia Petersen, Technician
Medicine, nursing.

8652 US Department of Veterans Affairs: Omaha Hospital Library
4101 Woolworth Avenue
Omaha, NE 68105-1850
402-346-8800
Fax: 402-449-0692; *Toll Free:* 800-451-5796
www.nebraska.va.gov

Medicine and allied health sciences.

Nevada

8653 Las Vegas-Clark County Library District
833 Las Vegas Blvd N
Las Vegas, NV 89101
702-734-7323
Fax: 702-733-1567
www.lvccld.org

Mary Anne Morton, Librarian
Laura Golod, Manager

Summer reading programs, braille writer, magnifiers, closed-circuit TV, large-print photocopier, cassette books and magazines, children's books on cassette, home visits and other reference materials on blindness and other handicaps.

8654 Nevada State Library and Archives
Capitol Complex
100 North Stewart Street
Carson City, NV 89710
775-684-3360
Fax: 775-684-3330
nslref@clan.lib.nv.us
dmla.clan.lib..nv.us/docs/nsla
TDD 702-687-8338

Kevin E Putnam, Librarian

Summer reading programs, braille writer, magnifiers, closed-circuit TV, large-print photocopier, cassette books and magazines, children's books on cassette, home visits and other reference materials on blindness and other handicaps.

8655 Nevada State Library: Talking Book Services
100 N Stewart Street
Carson City, NV 89701-4285
775-684-3310
Fax: 775-684-3330
nslref@clan.lib.nv.us
dmla.clan.lib.nv.us
TDD 775-687-8338

Keri E Putnam, Regional Librarian

Services to blind, visually or physically handicapped individuals. Books and magazines are available on cassette, disc or in Braille. Recorded books and magazines and special playback equipment are loaned to eligible readers free of charge.

8656 US Department of Veterans Affairs: Reno Medical Center Library Services
975 Kirman Avenue
Reno, NV 89502
775-786-7200
Fax: 775-328-1464
simpson@equinox.unr.edu
www.reno.va.gov/

Christine J Simpson, Chief Library Service

Clinical medicine, gerontology.

New Hampshire

8657 Dartmouth College Biomedical Libraries: Dana Biomedical Library
6168 Dana Biomedical Library
Hanover, NH 03755-3880
603-646-1110
Fax: 603-650-1354
contact@dartmouth.edu
www.dartmouth.edu

William F Garrity, Director Biomedical Librarie

Medicine, life sciences, nursing.

8658 New Hampshire State Library
117 Pleasant Street
Concord, NH 03301-3852
603-271-3429
www.nh.gov/nhsl

Betty Clark, Library Technician

Summer reading programs, braille writer, magnifiers, closed-circuit TV, large-print photocopier, cassette books and magazines, children's books on cassette, home visits and other reference materials on blindness and other handicaps.

8659 US Department of Veterans Affairs: Manchester Medical Center Library
718 Smyth Road
Manchester, NH 03104-7004
603-624-4366
Fax: 603-626-6579; *Toll Free:* 800-892-8384
www.manchester.va.gov

Martha Roberts, Chief Library Service

Medicine, surgery, nursing.

New Jersey

8660 Cytogen Corporation R&D Library
307 College Road E
Princeton, NJ 08540-6608
609-750-8200
Fax: 609-987-8640

Michael D Becker, CEO

Cancer research, biotechnology.

8661 New Jersey Department of Environmental Protection
PO Box 402
Trenton, NJ 08625-0402
609-984-2249
Fax: 609-292-3298
mbarattn@dep.state.nj.us
www.nj.gov

Maria Baratta, Library Manager
Mary Kearns-Kaplan, Manager

Toxic substances; hazardous waste; pollution - water, air, soil; carcinogens; drinking water; water resources.

8662 New Jersey Library for the Blind and Physically Handicapped
2300 Stuyvesant Avenue
Trenton, NJ 08618-3226
609-530-4000
Fax: 609-530-6384; *Toll Free:* 800-792-8322
njlbh@njstatelib.org
www.njlbh.org
TDD 609-633-7250

Vianne Connor, Librarian

Summer reading programs, braille writer, magnifiers, closed-circuit TV, large-print photocopier, cassette books and magazines, children's books on cassette, home visits and other reference materials on blindness and other handicaps.

8663 Princeton University Industrial Relations Library
Firestone Library
1 Washington Rd
Princeton, NJ 08544
609-258-4040
Fax: 609-258-2907
kpbarry@princeton.edu
www.princeton.edu

Kevin P Barry, Librarian
Andrew Golden, President

8664 Sandoz Pharmaceuticals Corporate Library
Rr 10
East Hanover, NJ 07936
973-503-7500
Fax: 973-503-6357

Medicine, chemistry, oncology, pharmacology, toxicology, biochemistry, business, management.

8665 UMDNJ and Coriell Research Library
401 Haddon Avenue
Camden, NJ 08103-1505
856-757-7740
Fax: 856-757-7713
swartz@umdnj.edu
www.umdnj.edu

Betty Jean Swartz, Librarian

Cancer, immunology, genetics, microbiology, cell biology, cytogenetics, molecular biology.

8666 US Department of Veterans Affairs: East Orange Medical Center Library
385 Tremont Avenue
East Orange, NJ 07018-1023
973-676-1000
Fax: 973-395-7062
www.eastorange.va.gov

Sophie Winston, Chief Library Service
Samuel Greene, President

General medicine.

New Mexico

8667 Capitan Public Library
101 E 2nd Street
PO Box 1169
Capitan, NM 88316

505-354-3035
Fax: 505-354-3223
www.capitanlibrary.org

Pat Sullivan, President
George Hinch, VP

For the older adults there is a speaker once a month that talks about issues pertaining to seniors, free computer classes are offered and there is a literacy program.

8668 New Mexico State Library: Blind and Physically Handicapped
1209 Camino Carlos Rey
Santa Fe, NM 87503
505-476-9700
Fax: 505-476-9701
lbph@state.nm.us
www.nmstatelibrary.org/lbph

Glee Wenzel, Librarian

Books, magazines, and other material in alternate format (cassette, Braille, and electronic text), playback equipment, and some production of print materials in alternative media.

8669 Roswell Public Library
301 N Pennsylvania
Roswell, NM 88201
505-622-7101
rplref@roswellpubliclibrary.org
www.roswellpubliclibrary.org

Variety of books and other materials to inform and entertain adults. Audio books are available on cassette and CD. Video cassettes and DVD's cover a wide range of topics, including how-to, history, drama and travel.

8670 US Department of Veterans Affairs: Albuquerque Medical Center Library
2100 Ridgecrest Drive SE
Albuquerque, NM 87108-5128
505-256-2786
Fax: 505-256-2870
www.albuquerque.va.gov/about/hist

Phyllis L Kregstein, Contact

Medicine, surgery, nursing, psychiatry.

New York

8671 Albany Talking Book Center
300 Pine Avenue
Albany, NY 10103
229-431-2900
Fax: 229-430-4020

Kathryn Sinquefield, Librarian

Offers discs, cassettes, reference materials on blindness and other handicaps, large-print photocopiers, summer reading programs, cassette books and more.

8672 Braille Book Bank
3 Townline Circle
Rochester, NY 14623-2537
585-427-8260
Fax: 585-427-0263
nbaoffice@nationalbraille.org
www.nationalbraille.org

David Shaffer, *Executive Director*
Diane Spence, *President*

Contains over 1,800 titles and braille music scores which are constantly updated and enlarged by transcriptions from BTAS and RTR.

8673 Calvary Hospital Medical Library
1740 Eastchester Road
Bronx, NY 10461-2392
718-518-2229
Fax: 718-518-2686

Dorothy M Maucione, Medical Librarian
Irina Pulatova, Manager

Medicine, cancer, nutrition, nursing.

8674 Center for Thanatology Research Library
391 Atlantic Avenue
Brooklyn, NY 11217-1701
718-858-3026
Fax: 718-852-1846
thanatology@pipeline.com
www.thanatology.org

Roberta Halporn, Executive Director

Aging, dying, death, bereavement, gravestone studies.

8675 Center for the Study of Aging Library
706 Madison Avenue
Albany, NY 12208-3695
518-462-1331
Fax: 518-462-1339
hs.boisestate.edu/csa

Sara Harris, Executive Director

Gerontology and geriatrics, physical activity and aging, mental health and illness, environment, social work, housing, medicine, social sciences, caregiving, nutrition, housing, prevention, long term care.

8676 Cold Spring Harbor Laboratory
1 Bungtown Road
Cold Spring Harbor, NY 11724-2209
516-367-8800
Fax: 516-367-6843
www.cshl.org/library
Bruce Stillman, *President*

Biological sciences, genetics, cancer research, cell biology, molecular biology, neurobiology, virology.

8677 Columbia University Oral History Research Office
801 Butler Library Box 20
535 W 114th St MC1129
New York, NY 10027
212-854-7083
Fax: 212-854-5378
www.columbia.edu/cu/lweb/indiv/oral/

Ronald J Grele, Director

National affairs, New York history, international relations, culture and the arts, social welfare, business and labor, philanthropy, African-American community, law, medicine, education, journalism, religion.

8678 Columbia University: Augustus C Long Health Sciences Library
701 West 168th Street
New York, NY 10032-2704

212-305-3605
Fax: 212-234-0595
hs-library@columbia.edu
library.cpmc.columbia.edu/hsl/

Mel Rodriguez, Departmental Administrator
Michael Koehn, Acting Library Director

The Augustus C. Long Health Sciences Library is the medical library responsible for serving students, faculty and staff at Columbia University's College of Physicians and Surgeons, College of Dental Medicane, Mailman School of Public Health, School of Nursing and the New york Presbyterian Hospital. The library provides a robust permanent reserve collection for student support. It also maintains a deep collection of current and historic monographs and serials, supporting both immediate medical needs and long-term research needs. Nearly all current serials are taken in electronic format only.

8679 Columbia University: Whitney M Young, Jr Memorial Library of Social Work
535 West 114th Street
New York, NY 10027
212-854-2271
Fax: 212-854-9099
www.columbia.edu

Social work; community organization; social policy development and administration; health, mental health, mental retardation; social services - family and children, day care, legal; aging; corrections and court services - probation, parole, diversionary treatment; alcoholism and drug addiction; psychoanalysis; industrial social welfare; intergroup relations; social and physical rehabilitation.

8680 Cornell University School of Industrial and Labor Relations
309 Ives Hall
Ithaca, NY 14853
607-254-7250
Fax: 607-255-2741
www.ilr.cornell.edu

Gordon Law, Director

Labor-management relations, labor law and legislation, labor organization, industrial and labor conditions, labor economics, human resources, social security, personnel administration, supervision, occupational safety and health, international labor conditions and problems, organizational behavior.

8681 Hasting Center Library
Rr 9d
21 Malcolm Gordon Road
Garrison, NY 10524
845-424-4040
Fax: 845-424-4545
www.thehastingscenter.org

Thomas H Murray, President/CEO

Hasting Center pursues interdisciplinary research and education that includes both theory and practice. The center, as a private not-for-profit institute addresses fundamental ethical issues in the area of health, medicine and the environment as they affect individuals, communities and societies. Publishes The Hastings Center Report.

8682 Highland Hospital: John R Williams, Sr Health Sciences Library
1000 South Avenue
Rochester, NY 14620-2733
585-341-6761
Fax: 716-758-1796
adixon@highland.rochester.edu
www.urmc.rochester.edu

Angela Dixon, Head Science Librarian
Yvonne Thorne, Executive Director

Medicine, surgery, family medicine, nursing, hematology/oncology, radiation therapy, obstetrics, gynecology.

8683 Hunter College of the City University of New York: Health Professional Library
425 E 25th Street
New York, NY 10010-2547
Fax: 212-481-5116
library.wexler.hunter.cuny.edu

Laura Cobus, Head
Yat Ping Wong, Deputy Head

Nursing, medicine, speech and hearing pathology, physical therapy, dance therapy, medical laboratory sciences, environmental health sciences, allied health services administration, community health education, nutrition, occupational health.

8684 International Ladies' Garment Workers Union Research Department Library
227 Ives Hall
Ithaca,, NY 14853
212-265-7000
Fax: 212-489-7238
rmc.library.cornell.edu

Walter Mankoff, Associate Director Research
Bruce Raynor, President

Earnings and hours, employment and payrolls, fringe benefits, labor and labor statistics, old-age insurance, social insurance, trade unions, unemployment insurance, union agreements, wearing apparel industry, women's clothing industry.

8685 Lighthouse: Ruth M Shellens Library
111 E 59th Street
New York, NY 10022-1202
212-821-9200
Fax: 212-821-9707; Toll Free: 800-829-0500
www.lighthouse.org

Tara A Cortes, President/CEO

Blindness and visual impairment, handicaps.

8686 MC Migel Memorial Library and Helen Keller Archives
11 Penn Plaza
Suite 300
New York, NY 10001-2006
212-502-7600
Fax: 212-502-7777
afbinfo@afb.net
www.afb.org

Carl R Augusto, President/CEO

The history, education, sociology and rehabilitation of individuals who are blind or visually impaired; Helen Keller's papers, personal library, memorabilia and photography collection.

8687 Monroe Community Hospital: TF Williams Health Sciences Library
435 E Henrietta Road
Rochester, NY 14620-4684
585-760-6500
Fax: 585-760-6066
www.monroehosp.org

Marilyn Rosen, Library Director
Frank Tripodi, CEO

Geriatrics, gerontology, long-term care, medicine, nursing, administration.

8688 Montefiore Medical Center Health Sciences Library: Tishman Learning Center
111 E 210th Street
Bronx, NY 10467-2401
718-920-4321
Fax: 212-920-4658
www.montefiore.org

Steven M Safyer, President/CEO

Medicine, health sciences administration, geriatrics, psychology, psychiatry, nursing.

8689 Nassau Library System
900 Jerusalem Avenue
Uniondale, NY 11553
516-292-8920
Fax: 516-481-4777
outreach@nassaulibrary.org
www.nassaulibrary.org

Jackie Tresher, Director

Information about public library services in Nassau County, including services for people with disabilities and the Senior Connections volunteer project (information and referral for seniors and their families). Co-sponsor of the Long Island Talking Book Library.

8690 National Association for Visually Handicapped Library
22 W 21st Street
New York, NY 10010-6904
212-889-3141
Fax: 212-727-2931
www.navh.org

Lorianie Marchi, CEO

General collection for the visually impaired.

8691 New York Office of Mental Health Binghamton Psychiatric Center Library Services Department
425 Robinson Street
Binghamton, NY 13904-1775
607-724-1391
Fax: 607-773-4387
www.omh.state.ny.us

Psychiatry, adolescent psychiatry, community mental health, psychology, child psychology, group psychotherapy, mental illness, general medicine, psychoanalysis, social services, family therapy, gerontology, geriatric nursing, geriatric psychiatry, quality improvement, managed mental health care.

8692 New York Public Library
40 W 20th Street
New York, NY 10011-4211

212-206-5400
Fax: 212-206-5418
www.nypl.org
TDD 212-206-5458

Bonnie Birdman, Librarian
Kevin Winkler, Manager

Offers assistive devices for the visually impaired and books on cassette.

8693 New York Public Library General Reference & Advisory Services: Accessibility Services
455 5th Avenue
New York, NY 10016
212-340-0849
Fax: 212-576-0048
www.nypl.org
TDD 212-340-0931

Wol Sue Lee, Department Head
Fu Mei Yang, Supervising Librarian

The disabled - vision impaired, hearing impaired, learning and mobility impaired.

8694 New York State Talking Book & Braille Library
Empire State Plaza CEC
Albany, NY 12230
518-474-5935
Fax: 518-474-5786
TBBL@mail.nysed.gov
www.nypl.org
TDD 518-474-7121

Jane Somers, Director

Books on audio cassette, cassette players, braille books, summer reading programs, braille writer, magnifiers, closed-circuit TV, large-print photocopier, cassette books and magazines, children's books on cassette, reference materials on blindness and other handicaps.

8695 Program Planners: Library/Information Center
230 W 41st Street
Floor 19
New York, NY 10036-7207
212-840-2609
Fax: 212-764-4094
ppi@bway.net

Burt Lazarin, Resources Director

Collective bargaining, public employee pensions/retirement systems, local government, urban affairs, health care, insurance, sanitation.

8696 Rochester Institute of Technology Library
90 Lomb Memorial Drive
Rochester, NY 14623-5604
585-475-2562
Fax: 585-475-7007
wally.rit.edu

Chandra V McKenzie, Director
Albert J Simone, President

Academic library for art, business, criminal justice, printing, micro-optics, computer science, imaging science, photography, social work, engineering, science, liberal arts, food, hotel tourism.

8697 Roosevelt Hospital Medical Library
428 W 59th Street
New York, NY 10019-1105
212-523-8500
Fax: 212-523-6108
www.roosevelthospitalnyc.org

Paul E Barth, Librarian

Medicine, surgery, gerontology, geriatrics, hospital administration, pediatrics, anesthesia.

8698 Sea View Hospital Rehabilitation Center Health Sciences Library
460 Brielle Avenue
Staten Island, NY 10314-6427
718-317-3000
Fax: 718-980-7182

Danial Mulligan, Director Education
Thomas Matteo, Executive Director

Medicine, nursing, geriatrics, hospital administration, social service, rehabilitation, dentistry.

8699 Sisters of Life: Dr Joseph R Stanton Human Life Issues Library and Resource Center
1955 Needham Avenue
Bronx, NY 10466-5824
718-881-7286
Fax: 718-881-7287
www.sistersoflife.org

Josamarie Perpetua, SV Director

A library and resource center providing books, videos, audiotapes, pamphlets and other information about the threat posed by assisted suicide and euthanasia to the chronically ill, the frial, and the vulnerable. Also covers abortion and beginnng of life issues. Also contains the archives of the pro life movement in America, and many resources from around the world.

1970

8700 St Mary's School for the Deaf Library Information Center
2253 Main Street
Buffalo, NY 14214-2392
716-834-7200
Fax: 716-834-2720
www.smsdk12.org

Bill Johnson, Superintendent Of The School
Pat Brant, Administrative Assistant

Deafness, audiology, speech, special education, ASL, sign language, deaf culture, deaf history.

8701 Suffolk Cooperative Library System
627 Sunrise Service Road N
Bellport, NY 11713-1554
631-286-1600
Fax: 631-286-1647
www.suffolk.lib.ny.us

Kevin Verbesey, Director

Talking Books Plus provides specialized resources, services, and information to help member libraries serve people with disabilities, their family members, and service providers. Some of these resources, like talking books, are provided directly to patrons by mail or in person. Other materials, such as print books, videotapes, programming kits, and TTYs, are loaned through member libraries

8702 Syracuse University Center for Policy Research
426 Eggers Hall
Syracuse, NY 13244-1020
315-443-3114
Fax: 315-443-1081
ctrpol@syr.edu
www.pr.maxwell.syr.edu/index.htm

Timothy M Smeeding, Director

Aging and long-term care, development studies, domestic urban and regional studies, public finance, social welfare, poverty, income security and microsimulation.

8703 Teachers College Milbank Memorial Library
Columbia University
525 W 120th St
New York, NY 10027
212-678-3494
Fax: 212-678-3092
library.tc.columbia.edu

Jane P Franck, Director
Gary Natriello, Executive Director

Education, psychology, health sciences, nutrition, nursing, communications, computing, technology, speech and language pathology, audiology.

8704 Towers Perrin Corporate Information Center
100 Summit Lake Drive
Valhalla, NY 10595-1339
914-745-4000
Fax: 914-745-4555
www.towerspervin.com

Jack Borbely, Director Information Service
Ann Farquhar, Manager

Compensation, retirement/pensions, employee benefits, US companies and industries, international business, insurance.

8705 US Department of Veterans Affairs: Bath Medical Center Library Service
76 Veterans Avenue
Bath, NY 14810
607-664-4000
Fax: 877-845-3247
www.va.gov

Sally Ann Hillegas, Chief Librarian

Geriatrics, chronic diseases, general internal medicine, long term care.

8706 US Department of Veterans Affairs: Bronx Medical Center Library
130 W Kingsbridge Road
Bronx, NY 10468-3904
718-584-9000
Fax: 718-741-4269; *Toll Free:* 800-877-6976
www.bronx.va.gov

Sumitte De Soyza, Chief Librarian

Medicine and allied health sciences.

8707 US Department of Veterans Affairs: Brooklyn Medical Center Library
800 Poly Place
Brooklyn, NY 11209-7104
718-836-6600
Fax: 718-630-3573
www.brooklyn.va.gov

Francine Tidona, Library Service

Medicine, surgery, psychiatry, psychology, nursing, social work.

8708 US Department of Veterans Affairs: Buffalo Medical Center Library Service
3495 Bailey Avenue
Buffalo, NY 14215-1129
716-834-9200
Fax: 716-862-8759
www.va.gov

Betty A Withrow, Chief Librarian

Medicine, surgery, nursing, management.

8709 US Department of Veterans Affairs: Castle Point Department of Medicine and Surgery Library Service
Rt 9D
Castle Point, NY 12511
845-831-2000
Fax: 845-838-5193
www.hudsonvalley.va.gov

Jeffrey Nicholas, Chief Library Service

Spinal cord injuries, surgery, nursing education, geriatric medicine, dentistry.

8710 US Department of Veterans Affairs: Montrose Medical Library
Veterans Medical Center
2094 Albany Post Rd. Rt 9A Po Box 100
Montrose, NY 10548
914-737-4400
Fax: 914-788-4244
www.hudsonvalley.va.gov

Bruce S Delman, PhD Chief Library Service

Psychiatry, psychology, medicine, social work, nursing, geriatrics.

8711 US Department of Veterans Affairs: New York Harbour Healthcare System, New York Campus Library
423 E 23rd Street
New York, NY 10010-5011
212-686-7500
Fax: 212-951-3487
www.manhattan.va.gov

Karin Wiseman, Chief Librarian
Tom Waugh, Librarian
Judy Steerle, Librarian

Medicine, surgery, neurology, psychiatry, nursing.

8712 US Department of Veterans Affairs: Northport Medical Center-Medical Library
79 Middleville Road
Northport, NY 11768-2200
631-261-4400
Fax: 631-754-7992; *Toll Free:* 800-551-3996
www.northport.va.gov

Caryl Kazen, Chief Library Service

Medicine, allied health sciences, psychiatry, and dentistry.

8713 W Alton Jones Cell Science Center: George and Margaret Gey Library
10 Old Barn Road
Lake Placid, NY 12946-1009
518-523-1267
Fax: 518-523-4385

Teresa B Wilmes, MLIS

Cell culture, organ culture, cytology, cancer research, virology, biochemistry, immunology.

8714 Wallace Memorial Library
90 Lomb Memorial Drive
Rochester, NY 14623-5604
585-424-4606
Fax: 585-475-7007
wally.rit.edu

Melanie Norton, Reference Librarian
Dwight Wallace, Manager

Information on physical disabilities and deafness.

8715 Xavier Society for the Blind
154 E 23rd Street
New York, NY 10010-4595
212-473-7800
Fax: 212-473-7801; *Toll Free:* 800-637-9193
info@xaviersocietyfortheblind.org
www.xaviersocietyfortheblind.org

Kathleen Lynch, Executive Director
Margie Montenegro, Client Services Manager
Bathleen

Provides spiritual and inspirational reading material to visually impaired persons in suitable format: braille, large print and audio cd, throughout the USA and Canada. Services provided by way of regular periodicals which are non-returnable, and through our lending library where books are returned. All services are provided free of charge, and interested persons can write, phone or email.

North Carolina

8716 Duke University Center for Demographic Studies Library
2117 Campus Drive
Durham, NC 27708
919-477-9292
Fax: 919-684-3861
www.duke.edu

Sue P Hicks, Librarian
Michael Duke, Owner

Demography; human ecology; census, vital statistics, other data sources; methods of research and analysis; population dynamics; urban and regional studies; economics of population size and distribution; migration studies; gerontology.

8717 Family Health International
PO Box 13950
Research Triangle Park, NC 27709-3950
919-544-7040
Fax: 919-544-7261
broinson@fhi.org
www.fhi.org

Dr. Willard Cates Jr, President
Albert J Siemens, Chairman/CEO

Reproductive medicine, family planning, contraception, population, developing countries.

8718 North Carolina Library for the Blind
109 East Jones Street
Raleigh, NC 27635
919-807-7450
Fax: 919-733-6910; *Toll Free:* 888-388-2460
nclbph@ncmail.net
www.statelibrary.ncdcr.gov
TDD 919-733-1462

Francine Martin, Librarian

Free laon of books on tape, in braille, and in large print to north Carolinians who caanot read standard print due to a visual or physical disability. Materials mailed to and from library via Free Matter for the Blind mailing privileges. Certified application required.

8719 US Department of Veterans Affairs: Asheville Medical Center Library
1100 Tunnel Road
Asheville, NC 28805-2043
828-298-7911
Fax: 828-299-2502; *Toll Free:* 800-932-6408
www.visn6.va.gov

Peggy Patterson, Acting Chief
Dan Potter, Manager

General and cardiopulmonary medicine, thoracic surgery, nursing.

8720 US Department of Veterans Affairs: Durham Medical Center Library
508 Fulton Street
Durham, NC 27705-3875
919-286-0411
Fax: 919-286-6859; *Toll Free:* 888-878-6890
kager.durham@ncdur.va.gov
www.durham.va.gov

Jeffrey F Kager, Chief Library Service

Clinical medicine, pre-clinical sciences, allied health sciences, management, research, patient health education.

8721 US Department of Veterans Affairs: Fayettville Medical Center Library Service
810 Vermont Avenue,
Washington, DC 20420
910-488-2120
Fax: 910-822-7093; *Toll Free:* 800-771-6106
www.visn6.va.gov

Pamela A Jackson, Chief Library Service
Karen March, Manager

Medicine, nursing, dentistry, patient education, allied health sciences.

8722 US Department of Veterans Affairs: Salisbury Medical Center Library
1601 Brenner Avenue
Salisbury, NC 28144-2515
704-638-9000
Fax: 704-638-3395; *Toll Free:* 800-469-8262
medical@interpath.com
www.visn6.va.gov

Nancy J Stine, Learning Research Service

Psychology, psychiatry, nursing, internal medicine, alcoholism, surgery, gerontology, dentistry.

North Dakota

8723 North Dakota State Library: Disability Services
604 E Boulevard Avenue
Bismarck, ND 58505
701-328-2492
Fax: 701-328-2040; *Toll Free:* 800-472-2104
tbooks@state.nd.us
ndsl.lib.state.nd.us/

Stella Cone, Head Local Library Disability
Sue Bicknell, Department Manager

Provides talking book service to the print impaired citizens
of North Dakota.

8724 US Department of Veterans Affairs: Fargo Medical Center Library
2101 Elm Street N
Fargo, ND 58102-2417
701-451-4600
Fax: 701-451-4690
www.va.gov

Diane Nordeng, Manager

Medicine, dentistry, nursing, social work, hospital administration.

Ohio

8725 Benjamin Rose Institute Library
11890 Fairhill Road
300
Cleveland, OH 44120-1053
216-791-8000
Fax: 216-231-7323
info@benrose.org
www.benrose.org

Karen Bensing, Librarian

Aged - research, home care, long-term care, nursing homes,
social work, nursing.

8726 Cleveland Public Library
325 Superior Ave
Cleveland, OH 44114
216-623-2800
Fax: 330-623-7036
www.cpl.org/index.php?q=node/17

Barbara Mates, Librarian

Summer reading programs, braille writer, magnifiers,
closed-circuit TV, large-print photocopier, cassette books
and magazines, children's books on cassette, home visits
and other reference materials on blindness and other
handicaps.

8727 Frank Reed Memorial Library
PO Box 760
Steubenville, OH 43952-5760
740-282-3810
Fax: 740-282-0769

Rita Marker, Executive Director

8728 Harris Library, MSASS, Case Western Reserve University
Mandel School of Applied of Applied Social Sciences
11235 Belliflower Road
Cleveland, OH 44106-7164

216-368-2302
Fax: 216-368-2106
harrisref@case.edu
www.msass.case.ed/harrislibrary

Samantha C Skutnik, Library Director

Social work, social welfare, poverty, alcoholism, aging,
child welfare, minorities, community organization, mental
health.

8729 Lourdes College Duns Scotus Library
6832 Convent Boulevard
Sylvania, OH 43560-4805
419-885-3211
Fax: 419-882-3786
truffing@lourdes.edu
www.lourdes.edu/library

Mary Tho Ruffing, Library Director
Robert Helmer, President

Religious studies, health sciences, psychology, occupational therapy, gerontology, art.

8730 Miami University Humanities and Social Sciences Department
King Library
Oxford, OH 45056
513-529-1809
Fax: 513-529-1682
quayrch@lib.muohio.edu
www.lib.muohio.edu

Richard H Quay, Head Hum/Social Science Dept

Business, history, education, American literature, political
science, geography, sociology, anthropology, gerontology,
military and naval science, foreign language, theater, economics, philosophy, psychology, religion, area studies,
black world studies, women's studies, American studies.

8731 Ohio Regional Library for the Blind and Physically Handicapped
800 Vine Street Library Square
Cincinnati, OH 45202
513-369-6900
Fax: 513-369-3111
www.cincinnatilibrary.org
TDD 513-665-3384

Deliaan A Gettler, President

Summer reading programs, braille writer, magnifiers,
closed-circuit TV, large-print photocopier, cassette books
and magazines, children's books on cassette, home visits
and other reference materials on blindness and other
handicaps.

8732 Ohio School for the Deaf Library
500 Morse Road
Columbus, OH 43214-1899
614-995-1566
Fax: 614-995-1567
www.ohioschoolforthedeaf.org

Ada Kent, Manager

General collection, deafness, professional education.

8733 Public Library of Cincinnati and Hamilton Outreach Services Department
800 Vine Street
Cincinnati, OH 45202-2071

513-369-6900
Fax: 513-369-4586
www.cincinnatilibrary.org

Elizabeth Zuelke, Head Outreach Services
Kimber L Fender, Executive Director

Programs and materials for children with special needs, books by mail for the homebound, delivery service to nursing homes and other facilities, extensive collection of large print books.

8734 State Library of Ohio: Talking Book Program
274 E 1st Avenue
Suite 100
Columbus, OH 43201-3692
614-644-7061
Fax: 614-995-2186; *Toll Free:* 800-686-1531
winslo.state.oh.us

Roger Verny, Deputy State Librarian
Jo Budler, Librarian

A machine-lending agency for the visually and physically impaired.

8735 US Department of Veterans Affairs: Brecksville Medical Center Library
10000 Brecksville Road
Brecksville, OH 44141-3204
440-526-3030
Fax: 440-838-6045
www.va.gov

Janet Monk Gillette, Chief Regional Library Service

Psychology, nursing, psychiatry, social work, clinical medicine.

8736 US Department of Veterans Affairs: Chillicothe Medical Library
17273 State Route 104
Chillicothe, OH 45601-8608
740-773-1141
Fax: 740-773-1141; *Toll Free:* 800-358-8262
www.chillicothe.va.gov

Jennifer Gray, Chief Library Service
Douglas Moorman, Executive Director

Psychiatry, nursing, medicine, allied health.

8737 US Department of Veterans Affairs: Cincinati Learning Resources Service
3200 Vine Street
Cincinnati, OH 45220-2213
513-861-3100
Fax: 513-475-6500; *Toll Free:* 888-267-7873
www.cincinnati.va.gov

Sandra Mason, Chief

Medicine, mental health, nursing, surgery.

8738 US Department of Veterans Affairs: Dayton Medical Center Library Service
4100 W 3rd Street
Dayton, OH 45428-9000
937-268-6511
Fax: 937-262-2179; *Toll Free:* 800-368-8262
www.dayton.va.gov

Niki B Conca, Chief Library Service
Kathleen Mannix, Manager

Medicine, nursing, hospital administration, patient education, local VA history.

8739 University of Cincinnati Medical Center Libraries
3110 Vine Street
Po Box 210033
Cincinnati, OH 45221-0033
513-556-1424
Fax: 513-558-9102
libraries.uc.edu

Doris A Haag, Director

Nursing, clinical medicine, gerontology, education, sociology.

Oklahoma

8740 Integris Baptist Medical Center: Wann Langston Memorial Library
3300 NW Expressway
Oklahoma City, OK 73112-4999
405-949-3011
Fax: 405-945-3883
www.integris-health.com

Cheryl Suttles, Director Medical Library
Stanley F Hupfeld, CEO

Geriatrics, medicine, nursing, hospital management.

8741 Oklahoma Library for the Blind & Physically Handicapped
300 NE 18th Street
Oklahoma City, OK 73105-3212
405-521-3514
Fax: 405-521-4582
library@drs.state.ok.us
www.library.state.ok.us

Geraldine Adams, Librarian

Summer reading programs, braille writer, magnifiers, closed-circuit TV, large-print photocopier, cassette books and magazines, children's books on cassette, home visits and other reference materials on blindness and other handicaps.

8742 Tulsa City-County Library System
400 Civic Center
Tulsa, OK 74103-3830
918-596-7977
www.tulsalibrary.org

Ellen Ontko, Librarian
Linda Saferite, Executive Director

Summer reading programs, braille writer, magnifiers, closed-circuit TV, large-print photocopier, cassette books and magazines, children's books on cassette, home visits and other reference materials on blindness and other handicaps.

8743 US Department of Veterans Affairs: Oklahoma City Medical Center Library
921 NE 13th Street
Oklahoma City, OK 73104-5007
405-270-0501
Fax: 405-270-1560; *Toll Free:* 866-835-5273
www.oklahoma.va.gov

Charles T Coker, Chief
Tom Duchene, Plant Manager
Medicine, patient health education.

Oregon

8744 Oregon School for the Blind Media Center
700 Church Street SE
Salem, OR 97301-3714
503-378-3820
Fax: 503-373-7537
www.ode.state.or.us

Margie C Jordan, Media Specialists
Visual and hearing impairment; multihandicapped.

8745 Oregon State Library
250 Winter Street NW
Salem, OR 97310
503-378-4243
Fax: 503-585-8059
www.oregon.gov
TDD 503-378-4276

Mary Mohr, Librarian
Jim Scheppke, Manager

Summer reading programs, braille writer, magnifiers,
closed-circuit TV, large-print photocopier, cassette books
and magazines, children's books on cassette, home visits
and other reference materials on blindness and other
handicaps.

**8746 US Department of Veterans Affairs: Portland
Medical Library**
3710 SW US Veterans Hospital Rd
Portland, OR 97239
503-220-8262
Fax: 503-273-5319; *Toll Free:* 800-949-1004
www.portland.va.gov

Mara R Wilhelm, Chief Library Service
Kim Winn, Manager

Medicine, nursing, allied health sciences, psychology, basic
sciences.

**8747 US Department of Veterans Affairs: White City
Library**
8495 Crater Lake Highway
White City, OR 97503-3011
541-826-2111
Fax: 541-830-3500
sandy.darland@va.gov
www.va.gov

Max E McIntosh PhD MBA, Director
Rehabilitation Center & Clinics

Pennsylvania

8748 Carnegie Library of Pittsburgh
4400 Forbes Ave
Pittsburgh, PA 15213-1389
412-622-3114
Fax: 412-687-2442
clbph@clpgh.org
www.carnegielibrary.org

Barbara Mistick, President/Director

Provides on loan recorded books and magazines, large print
books, and described videos to Western Pennsylvannia residents unable to use standard printed materials due to visual,
physical, or physically-based reading disabilities. Also
loans special cassette and disc machines; does not loan
equipment to play described videos. Information about disabilities and related agencies is also available.

8749 Center for Information Resources
4025 Chestnut Street
Floor 3
Philadelphia, PA 19104-3046
215-898-8108

Kristen MacLeod, Publications Coordinator

Information on physical disabilities and computer-related
vocational rehabilitation.

**8750 Fair Acres Center
Medical Library**
340 N Middletown Road
Lima, PA 19037-0496
610-891-5700
Fax: 610-891-2705
Joseph Doughterty, Administrator

Medicine, nursing, geriatrics, allied health sciences.

8751 Free Library of Philadelphia
1901 Vine Street
Philadelphia, PA 19103
215-686-5322
Fax: 215-928-0856
flpblind@library.phila.gov
www.freelibrary.org

Vickie Lange Collins, Librarian

Summer reading programs, braille writer, magnifiers,
closed-circuit TV, large-print photocopier, cassette books
and magazines, children's books on cassette, home visits
and other reference materials on blindness and other
handicaps.

8752 Overbrook School for the Blind Library
6333 Malvern Avenue
Philadelphia, PA 19151-2597
215-877-0313
Fax: 215-877-2709
www.obs.org

Julia A Flinchbaugh, Librarian
Bernadette Kappen, Executive Director

Standard, large print, and braille books for kindergarten
through high school; general library of braille, tape, and
print titles for primary, elementary, and high school; library
of print for faculty members.

**8753 Pennsylvania Department of Public Welfare
Norristown State Hospital**
Building 11
Norristown, PA 19401
610-313-5369
Fax: 610-313-5370
www.dpw.state.pa.us

Frieda Liem, Librarian

Psychiatry and neurology; clinical psychology; psychiatric
nursing; psychiatric and clinical social work; activities
therapy - recreational, music, occupational, vocational; aging; geriatrics; gerontology.

8754 Pennsylvania State University: Human Development Collection
201 Henderson Building
University Park, PA 16802-6506
814-865-1428
Fax: 814-865-3282
healthhd@psu.edu
www.hhdev.psu.edu

Gerontology, adolescent and child psychology, marriage and family.

8755 Philadelphia Corporation for Aging Library
642 N Broad Street
Philadelphia, PA 19130-3049
215-765-9000
Fax: 215-765-9066
sspencer@pcaphl.org
www.pcacares.org

Scott Spencer, Librarian
Rodney Williams, President
Octavia Greene, Library Assistant

Provides information resources to employees and others in the Philadelphia area. Provides services tot the elderly and adult disabled.

8756 Polisher Research Institute Library: Philadelphia Geriatric Center
5301 Old York Road
Philadelphia, PA 19141-2912
215-456-2981
Fax: 215-456-2017
www.pgc.org

Sheryl Panka-Bryman, Librarian
Mary McCaffrey, Library Assistant

Gerontology, geriatrics, long-term care industry, psychology, sociology, housing, long-term care administration, anthropology, research methods, death and dying.

8757 Talbot Cancer Research Library
333 Cottman Avenue
Philadelphia, PA 19111
215-728-2710
Fax: 215-728-3655; *Toll Free:* 888-369-2427
www.fccc.edu/facilities/library/talbot

Karen M Albert, Librarian

Biochemistry, cancer, cell biology, chemistry, clinical research, experimental pathology, genetics.

8758 US Deparment of Veterans Affairs: Philadelphia Medical Center Library
University & Woodland Avenues
Philadelphia, PA 19104
215-823-5860
Fax: 215-823-5108
www.va.gov

Mark Marchino, Chief Library Service
Bob Lye, Manager

Medicine and allied health sciences.

8759 US Department of Veterans Affairs: Altoona James E Van Zandt Medical Center Library Service
2907 Pleasant Valley Boulevard
Altoona, PA 16602-4305

814-943-8164
Fax: 814-940-7895

Gerald Williams, Executive Director

Medicine, patient education, management.

8760 US Department of Veterans Affairs: Butler Medical Center Library
325 New Castle Road
Butler, PA 16001-2480
724-287-4781
Fax: 724-282-4408; *Toll Free:* 800-362-8262
www.butler.va.gov

Mary Ann Wagner, Library Technician
David Wood, Executive Director

Nursing, general medicine.

8761 US Department of Veterans Affairs: Coatesville Medical Center Library
1400 Blackhorse Hill Road
Coatesville, PA 19320-2096
610-394-7711
Fax: 610-860-2135; *Toll Free:* 800-290-6172
vamc@hslc.org
www.coatesville.va.gov

Andrew Henry, Librarian

Psychiatry, neurology, medicine, nursing, psychology, geriatrics.

8762 US Department of Veterans Affairs: Erie Medical Center Library
135 E 38th Street
Erie, PA 16504-1559
814-868-8661
Fax: 814-860-2135; *Toll Free:* 800-274-8387
www1.va.gov/erie

Mary Nourse, Director

Medicine, nursing, geriatrics, quality assurance.

8763 US Department of Veterans Affairs: Lebanon Medical Center Library
1700 S Lincoln Avenue
Lebanon, PA 17042-7529
717-272-6621
Fax: 717-228-6045; *Toll Free:* 800-409-8771
www.va.gov/lebanonvamc/

Medicine, aging and geriatrics, psychiatry.

8764 US Department of Veterans Affairs: Pittsburgh Education, Media and Reference Service
University Drive
Pittsburgh, PA 15240
Fax: 412-688-6121; *Toll Free:* 866-482-7488
www.va.gov/pittsburgh/

Terrie R Wheeler, Chief MLS

Medicine, surgery, gerontology, and allied health sciences.

8765 US Department of Veterans Affairs: Wilkes-Barre Medical Center Library
1111 E End Boulevard
Wilkes Barre, PA 18711
570-824-3521
www.va.gov

Jay Suffren, Librarian
Roland Moore, CEO

Medicine, allied health sciences.

8766 Wistar Institute of Anatomy & Biology Library
3601 Spruce Streets
Philadelphia, PA 19104
215-898-3700
www.wistar.upenn.edu

Russel E Kaufman, President/CEO

Cancer, virus diseases, molecular immunology, molecular genetics, biochemistry.

Rhode Island

8767 Drug & Alcohol Treatment Association of Rhode Island: In-Rhodes Resource Center Library
90 Dean Street
Providence, RI 02903-1504
401-273-3731
Fax: 401-273-6349
www.dataofri.org

8768 US Department of Veterans Affairs: Providence Health Sciences Library
830 Chalkstone Avenue
Providence, RI 02908-4799
401-273-7100
Fax: 401-457-3097; *Toll Free:* 866-590-2976
www.providence .gov

Nicola F Pallotti, Contact
Kipp Hartmann, Executive Director

Medicine, nursing, and allied health sciences.

South Carolina

8769 Captioned Media Program: National Association of the Deaf
1447 E Main Street
Spartanburg, SC 29307-2240
864-585-1778
Fax: 864-585-2611
info@dcmp.org
www.dcmp.org
TTY: 864-585-2617

Max Duckler, President/Founder Of Caption Max

Free loans of educational and entertainment captioned films and videos for deaf and hard of hearing people.

8770 South Carolina State Library
PO Box 11469
Columbia, SC 29202
803-734-8666
Fax: 803-734-8676
reference@statelibrary.sc.gov
www.statelibrary.sc.gov
TDD 803-734-7298

David S Goble, Director/State Librarian

Summer reading programs, braille writer, magnifiers, closed-circuit TV, large-print photocopier, cassette books and magazines, children's books on cassette, home visits and other reference materials on blindness and other handicaps.

8771 US Deparment of Veterans Affairs: Columbia William Jennings Bryan-Dorn Veterans Hospital Library
Va Medical Center
6439 Garners Ferry Road
Columbia, SC 29209-1639
803-776-4000
Fax: 803-695-6739
www.va.gov/columbia/sc

Florence D Mays, Staff Librarian

Medicine, surgery, nursing, dentistry, psychiatry.

South Dakota

8772 South Dakota Human Services Center Medical Library
PO Box 76
Yankton, SD 57078
605-668-3165
Fax: 605-668-3222

Mary Lou Kostel, Librarian

Psychiatry, psychology, psychiatric nursing, gerontology, social work, medicine.

8773 South Dakota State Library: Braille and Talking Book Program
800 Governors Drive
Pierre, SD 57501-2235
605-773-3131
Fax: 605-773-6962; *Toll Free:* 800-423-6665
library@state.sd.us
library.sd.gov
TDD 605-773-4950

Dan Siebersma, State Librarian
Quynn Verhelst, Sr. Secretary
Barb Templeton, Support Staff

Summer reading programs, braille writer, magnifiers, closed-circuit TV, large-print books, scripture videos, cassette books and magazines, children's books on cassette, home visits and other reference materials on blindness and other handicaps. Publishes quarterly newsletter for adults and children.

8774 US Department of Veterans Affairs: For Meade VA Black Hills Health Care System Medical Library
113 Comanche Road
Fort Meade, SD 57741-1002
605-347-2511
Fax: 605-720-7171; *Toll Free:* 800-743-1070
www.blackhills.va.gov

Gene Stevens, Chief Librarian

Medicine and allied health sciences.

Tennessee

8775 LRC for Students with Disabilities: MSU Library Reference Department
Memphis State University
Memphis, TN 38152
901-678-2208

Ross Johnson, Reference Librarian

Information on physical disabilities, blindness and visual impairments.

8776 Tennessee Library for the Blind and Physically Handicapped
403 7th Avenue N
Nashville, TN 37243-1409
615-741-2764
Fax: 615-532-9293; *Toll Free:* 800-342-3308
reference.tsla@tn.gov
www.tennessee.gov/tsla/

Ruth Hemphill, Director
Donna Cirenza, Assistant Director

Offers free public library services to those unable to hold, read or turn the pages of ordinary books and magazines due to physical or visual impairment. Special library materials are provided by the Library of Congress, and free mailing privileges for these materials is provided through the US Post Office. Playback equipment is also provided.

8777 US Department of Veterans Affairs: Johnson City Medical Center Library
Corner Of Lamont And Sydney Streets
Mountain Home, TN 37684
423-926-1171
Fax: 423-979-3519
www.mountainhome.va.gov

Medicine and allied health sciences.

8778 US Department of Veterans Affairs: Memphis Medical Center Library
1030 Jefferson Avenue
Memphis, TN 38104-2127
901-523-8990
Fax: 901-577-7251; *Toll Free:* 800-636-8262
www.memphis.va.gov

Patricia Pittman, Director/CEO

Medicine, dentistry, nursing.

8779 US Department of Veterans Affairs: Murfreesboro Medical Center Library Service
3400 Lebanon Pike
Murfreesboro, TN 37129
615-741-2764
Fax: 615-532-9293; *Toll Free:* 800-342-3308
reference.tsla@tn.gov
www.tennessee.gov/tsla/

Pamela Howell, Chief Librarian Services

Psychiatry, medicine, nursing, geriatrics.

8780 US Department of Veterans Affairs: Nashville Medical Center Library Service
1310 24th Avenue South
Nashville, TN 37212-2637
615-741-2764
Fax: 615-532-9293; *Toll Free:* 800-342-3308
reference.tsla@tn.gov
www.tennessee.gov/tsla/

Medicine, nursing, dentistry, surgery.

8781 University of Memphis Libraries: Audiology, Speech Language, Pathology Branch
807 Jefferson Avenue
Memphis, TN 38105-5042

901-678-5846
Fax: 901-525-1282
exlibris.memphis.edu

John Swearengen, Library Assistant

Audiology, speech pathology.

Texas

8782 American Heart Association National Center Library
National Center Library
7272 Greenville Avenue
Dallas, TX 75231-4596
214-373-6300
Fax: 214-706-1211
vanessap@heart.org
www.americanheart.org

Vanessa S Perez, Reference Consultant
M Cass Wheeler, CEO

Cardiovascular and cerebrovascular diseases.

8783 Christian Education for the Blind
4200 S Freeway Drive
Suite 702
Fort Worth, TX 76115
817-920-0444
Fax: 817-920-0777
www.bcebonline.org

Rodger Dyer, Executive Director

Offers braille and large print books and cassettes for the visually impaired.

8784 Houston Public Library: Access Center
500 McKinney Street
Houston, TX 77002-5000
713-236-1313Toll free: 832-393-1313
www.houstonlibrary.org

Mary Crocker, Supervisor

Offers Kurzweil Reading Machine 400, closed-circuit TV, braille writer, reference materials on visual impairments and other handicaps.

8785 Houston Public Library: Acres Homes Branch
8501 W Montgomery Road
Houston, TX 77088-7118
832-393-1700
Fax: 832-393-1701
www.houstonlibrary.org

Johnson Dweban, Manager

8786 Houston Public Library: Bracewell Branch
9002 Kingspoint Dr
Houston, TX 77075-3409
832-393-2580
Fax: 832-393-2581
www.houstonlibrary.org

8787 Houston Public Library: Carnegie Branch
1050 Quitman Street
Houston, TX 77009-7858
832-393-1720
Fax: 832-393-1721
www.houstonlibrary.org

8788 Houston Public Library: Collier Regional Branch
6200 Pinemont Drive
Houston, TX 77092-3204
832-393-1740
Fax: 832-393-1741
www.houstonlibrary.org

T R Lynch, Manager

8789 Houston Public Library: Dixon Branch
8002 Hirsch Road
Houston, TX 77016-5602
832-393-1760
Fax: 832-393-1768
www.houstonlibrary.org

Chris Hu, Manager

8790 Houston Public Library: Flores Branch
110 N Milby Street
Houston, TX 77003-1931
832-393-1780
Fax: 832-393-3178
www.houstonlibrary.org

Elvia Pillado, Manager

8791 Houston Public Library: Hillendahl Branch
2436 Gessner Drive
Houston, TX 77080-5012
832-393-1940
Fax: 832-393-1941
www.houstonlibrary.org

8792 Houston Public Library: Moody Branch
9525 Irvington Boulevard
Houston, TX 77076-5247
832-393-1950
Fax: 832-393-1951
www.houstonlibrary.org

Sergio Tineda, Manager

8793 Houston Public Library: Park Place Regional Branch
8145 Park Place Boulevard
Houston, TX 77017-3032
832-393-1970
Fax: 832-393-1971
www.houstonlibrary.org

Regina Stemmer, Manager

8794 Houston Public Library: Pleasantville Branch
1520 Gellhorn
Houston, TX 77029
832-393-2330
Fax: 832-393-2331
www.houstonlibrary.org

8795 Houston Public Library: Robinson-Westchase Branch
3223 Wilcrest Drive
Houston, TX 77042-3349
832-393-2011
Fax: 832-393-2021
www.houstonlibrary.org

8796 Houston Public Library: Scenic Woods Regional Branch
10677 Homestead Road
Houston, TX 77016-2703
832-393-2030
Fax: 832-393-2031
www.houstonlibrary.org

Ande Tensae, Manager

8797 Houston Public Library: Smith Branch
3624 Scott Street
Houston, TX 77004-4744
832-393-2050
Fax: 713-747-1924
www.houstonlibrary.org

Lori Smith, Manager

8798 Houston Public Library: Tuttle Branch
702 Kress Street
Houston, TX 77020-4912
832-393-2100
Fax: 713-674-0093
www.houstonlibrary.org

Beatriz Deangulo, Manager

8799 Houston Public Library: Young Branch
5260 Griggs Road Palm Center
Houston, TX 77021
832-393-2140
Fax: 832-393-2141
www.houstonlibrary.org

8800 Kerrville State Hospital Professional Library
721 Thompson Drive
Kerrville, TX 78028-5199
512-458-7111
www.dshs.state.tx.us
Geriatrics, psychology, medicine, nursing, social studies.

8801 Mind Science Foundation Library
117 W El Prado Drive
San Antonio, TX 78212-2024
210-821-6094
Fax: 210-821-6199
info@mindscience.org
www.mindscience.org

Joseph Dial, Executive Director

Parapsychology, psychology, mind-made health, creativity, traditional healing, self-esteem, brain mapping.

8802 REACH/Resource Center on Independent Living
1205 Lake Street
Fort Worth, TX 76102-4501
817-870-9082
Fax: 817-877-1622
reachftw@reachcils.org
www.reachcils.org

Charlotte Stewart, Director
Anne Ancy, Case Manager

Information and referral services, peer counseling, independent living skills training, loaner equipment, advocacy assistance, ADA technical assistance and social/recreational activities.

8803 Texas Department of Health Library
1100 W 49th Street
Austin, TX 78756-3101
512-458-7355
Fax: 512-458-7474; *Toll Free:* 888-963-7111
www.dshs.state.tx.us
TDD 512-458-7708

Cindy Milam Faries, Program Administrator
Lesa Walker, MD

Public health, infectious diseases, laboratory methods, environmental health, dental health, pediatrics, nursing, hospitals, heart, cancer, health promotion, health funding.

8804 Texas State Library
PO Box 12927
Austin, TX 78711-2927
512-463-5458
Fax: 512-936-0685; *Toll Free:* 800-252-9605
tbp.services@tsl.state.tx.us
www.texastalkingbooks.org

Ava Smith, Director

8805 Texas State Library Talking BookProgram
PO Box 12927
Austin, TX 78711
512-463-5458
Fax: 512-936-0685; *Toll Free:* 800-252-9605
tbp.services@tsl.texas.gov
www.texastalkingbooks.org

Ava Smith, Director

Reading materials (recorded cartridge, large print, braille) and download equipment for persons who cannot read standard print, Talking Book Program is part of the national library service. Patrons must meet eligibility requirements.

Year Founded: 1931

8806 Texas State Library Talking Book Program
PO Box 12927
Austin, TX 78711-2927
512-463-5458
Fax: 512-936-0685; *Toll Free:* 800-252-9605
tbp.services@tsl.state.tx.us
www.texastalkingbooks.org

Ava M Smith, Director

Free library services to Texas residents for persons with vision, physical and learning impairments.

8807 Texas State Technical College: Waco Library
3801 Campus Drive
Waco, TX 76705-1696
254-799-3611Toll free: 800-792-8784
walib.tstc.edu

Linda S Koepf, Library Director
Elton Stuckly, President

Laser electro-optics, electronics, air pilot training, aviation maintenance, automotive mechanics, biomedical equipment operation.

8808 US Department of Veterans Affairs Medical Center Library Service
7400 Merton Minter Street
San Antonio, TX 78229-4404
210-617-5300
Fax: 210-617-5246; *Toll Free:* 888-686-6350
www.vasthcs.med.va.gov

Janean Garrett, Medical Librarian
Charles Sepich, CEO

Medicine, allied health sciences.

8809 US Department of Veterans Affairs: Temple Medical Center Medical Library
Olin E Teague Veterans Admini
1901 Veterans Memorial Drive
Temple, TX 76504
254-778-4811
Fax: 254-743-2338
www.va.gov

Joann Greenwood, Chief Library Service

Medicine, surgery, nursing, dentistry.

8810 US Department of Veterans Affairs: Amarillo Hospital Library
6010 Amarillo Blvd, West
Amarillo, TX 79106
806-355-9703
Fax: 806-354-7860; *Toll Free:* 800-687-8262
www.amarillo.va.gov

General medicine, surgery, nursing, dentistry.

8811 US Department of Veterans Affairs: Big Spring Hospital Library
300 Veterans Blvd
Big Spring, TX 79720
915-263-7361
Fax: 915-264-4834; *Toll Free:* 800-472-1365
www.bigsprings.va.gov

Samie Pequeno, Contact

General medicine, surgery.

8812 US Department of Veterans Affairs: Kerrville South Texas Veterans Health Care System
3600 Memorial Boulevard
Kerrville, TX 78028-5768
830-896-2020
www.vasthcs.med.va.gov

Lois A Johnson, Division Manager Library Service

Medicine and allied health sciences.

8813 US Department of Veterans Affairs: Waco Medical Center Library
4800 Memorial Drive
Waco, TX 76711-1329
254-752-6581
Fax: 254-297-3161; *Toll Free:* 800-423-2111
www.centraltexas.va.gov

JoAnn Greenwood, Site Manager
Paul Batterton, CEO

Psychiatry, neurology, psychology, nursing, gerontology, posttraumatic stress.

Utah

8814 US Department of Veterans Affairs: Salt Lake City Hospital Medical Library
500 Foothill Drive
Salt Lake City, UT 84148

801-582-1565
Fax: 801-584-1289; *Toll Free:* 800-613-4012
www.saltlakecity.va.gov

Carl Worstell, Chief Librarian
Kirk Davis, Manager

Medicine, surgery, psychiatry, emergency medicine, research, allied health sciences.

8815 Utah State Library: Blind and Disabled Services
250 N 1950 West
Suite A
Salt Lake City, UT 84116-7901
801-715-6789Toll free: 800-662-5540
blind@utah.gov
www.blindlibrary.utah.gov
TDD 801-715-6721

Bessie Oakes, Program Manager
Julie Anderson, Executive Secretary

Braille, large print, and audio books; specialized playback equipment, and a radio will be loaned by the library to eligible registered readers without charge.

Vermont

8816 Austine School: Library Media Center
209 Austine Drive
Brattleboro, VT 05301-6818
802-258-9500
Fax: 802-254-3921
vcdhh.org

Anne Potter, Director

Education of the deaf.

8817 US Department of Veterans Affairs: White River Junction Medical & Regional Office CenterLibrary Service
215 North Main Street
White River Junction, VT 05009
Fax: 802-296-5150; *Toll Free:* 800-827-1000
www.va.gov

Richard Haver, Chief Library Service

Medicine, surgery, psychiatry, nursing.

8818 Vermont Department of Libraries
PO Box 1870
109 State Street
Montpelier, VT 05602
802-828-3261
Fax: 802-828-2199
dol.state.vt.us

Summer reading programs, braille writer, magnifiers, closed-circuit TV, large-print photocopier, cassette books and magazines, children's books on cassette, home visits and other reference materials on blindness and other handicaps.

Virginia

8819 Alexandria Library Talking Book Service
5005 Duke Street
Alexandria, VA 22304-2903

703-746-1702
www.alexandria.lib.va.vs
TDD 703-746-1763

Rose T. Dawson, Library Director
Kimberly Nathaniel, Communication Officer
Joseph Yuen, IT Manager

Summer reading programs, braille writer, magnifiers, closed-circuit TV, large-print photocopier, cassette books and magazines, children's books on cassette, home visits and other reference materials on blindness and other handicaps.

8820 Alexandria Library: Special Collections
717 Queen Street
Alexandria, VA 22314-2420
703-746-1703
Fax: 703-746-1708
www.alexandria.lib.va.us

Rose T. Dawson, Library Director
Kimberly Nathaniel, Communication Officer
Joseph Yuen, IT Manager
1994

8821 Amelia Historical Society: Amelia Historical Library
PO Box 113
Amelia Court House, VA 23002
804-561-3180
www.ameliava.com

Dorothy Eppes, President
Jerry Morris, VP
1957

8822 American College of Health Care Administrators: Information Center
12100 Sunset Hills Road
Suite 130
Reston, VA 20190
703-739-7900
Fax: 703-435-4390
info@achca.org
www.achca.org

Marianna Kern Grachek, President/CEO

Long-term care, gerontology.

8823 American Life League Library
PO Box 1350
Stafford, VA 22555-1350
540-659-4171
Fax: 540-659-2586
sysop@all.org
www.all.org

Judie Brown, President

8824 Arlington County Department of Libraries
1015 N Quincy Street
Arlington, VA 22201-4603
703-358-5990
Fax: 703-358-5962
library.arlingtonva.us/
TDD 703-358-6320

Roxanne Barnes, Librarian

Summer reading programs, braille writer, magnifiers, closed-circuit TV, large-print photocopier, cassette books and magazines, children's books on cassette, home visits and other reference materials on blindness and other handicaps.

8825 Central Rappahannock Regional Library

1201 Caroline Street
Fredericksburg, VA 22401-3701
540-372-1144
Fax: 540-373-9411
TDD 540-371-9165

Nancy Schiff, Librarian
Donna Cote, Executive Director

Offers reference materials on blindness and other disabilities.

8826 Division for the Visually Handicapped

1901 N. Du Pont Highway
Biggs Bldg.
New Castle, DE 19720
302-255-9800
Fax: 302-255-4441
dhss.delaware.gov

Daniel Madrid, Director

Members are teachers, college faculty members, administrators, supervisors and others concerned with the education and welfare of visually handicapped and blind children and youth. This is a division of the Council For Exceptional Children.

8827 Fairfax County Public Library

12000 Government Center Parkway
Suite 324
Fairfax, VA 22035
703-324-3185
Fax: 703-765-5893
www.fairfaxcounty.gov/library
TDD 703-660-8524

Jeanette Studley, Librarian
Lindsey Culin, Manager

Summer reading programs, braille writer, magnifiers, closed-circuit TV, large-print photocopier, cassette books and magazines, children's books on cassette, home visits and other reference materials on blindness and other handicaps.

8828 Roanoke City Public Library System

706 South Jefferson St
Roanoke, VA 24017-5333
540-853-2473
Fax: 540-853-1030

Rebecca Cooper, Librarian
Wendy Allen, Manager

Summer reading programs, braille writer, magnifiers, closed-circuit TV, large-print photocopier, cassette books and magazines, children's books on cassette, home visits and other reference materials on blindness and other handicaps.

8829 Staunton Public Library Talking Book Center

1 Churchville Avenue
Staunton, VA 24401-3229
540-885-6215
Fax: 540-332-3906; *Toll Free:* 800-995-6215
talkingbooks@ci.staunton.va.us
www.staunton.va.us

Oakley Pearson, Librarian

Sub-regional library for those who are unable to use standard print materials due to visual, physical, or reading disability.

8830 Thomas Balch Library

208 W Market Street
Leesburg, VA 20176-2709
703-737-7195
Fax: 703-737-7150
balchlib@leesburgva.gov
www.leesburgva.gov/thomasbalchlibrary

Alexandra S Gressitt, Library Director

A history and genealogy owned and operated by the Town of Leesburg. Collections focus on Loudoun County, regional and Virginia history, genealogy, ethnic history, and military history with special emphasis on the American Civil War. Collection materials include books, periodicals, maps, visual items, newspapers, and manuscripts.

8831 US Department of Veterans Affairs: Hampton Medical Center Library and Educational Resources

300 W. Morgan St
Suite 700
Durham, NC 27701
757-722-9961
Fax: 757-723-6620
www.visn6.va.gov

Jacqueline Bird, Director
Joseph Williams Jr, Executive Director

Surgery, medicine, nursing, psychology, patient education.

8832 US Department of Veterans Affairs: Richmond Hospital Library

1201 Broad Rock Boulevard
Richmond, VA 23249
804-675-5000
Fax: 804-675-5142
www.richmond.va.gov

Eleanor Rollins, Chief Library Service
Paul Phillips, Manager

Medicine, psychology, sociology.

8833 US Department of Veterans Affairs: Salem Medical Center Library

1970 Roanoke Boulevard
Salem, VA 24153-6404
540-982-2463
Fax: 540-983-1079; *Toll Free:* 888-982-2463
www.salem.va.gov

Jean A Kennedy, Chief Librarian

Medicine, psychiatry, nursing, allied health sciences.

Washington

8834 Fred Hutchinson Cancer Research Center: Arnold Digital Library

1100 Fairview Ave North
Seattle, WA 98109
206-288-7222
Fax: 206-667-5826
aclark@fhcrc.org
www.fhcrc.org/library

Leukemia, immunology, molecular biology, cancer research, genetics, cancer prevention, soft tissue tumors, biostatistics, epidemiology.

8835 Lutheran Bible Institute of Seattle Library
2802 Wetmore Avenue
Everett, WA 98201
425-249-4800
Fax: 425-249-4801; *Toll Free:* 800-843-5659
www.tlc.edu

Irene A Hausken, Head Librarian
John Stamm, President

Bible; theology - doctrinal, moral, pastoral, devotional; religion and philosophy; Christian church; missions; psychology; social sciences; Christian education; youth work; gerontology; Pacific Northwest Indians.

8836 Northwest Geriatric Education Center
PO Box 358123
1910 Fairview Ave E, Suite 203
Seattle, WA 98195-8123
206-685-7478
Fax: 206-685-3436
sgural@u.washington.edu
depts.washington.edu

Susan Guralnick, Associate Director

Geriatrics.

8837 US Department of Veterans Affairs: Seattle Puget Sound Health Care System
1660 S Columbian Way
Seattle, WA 98108-1532
206-762-1010
Fax: 206-764-2224; *Toll Free:* 800-329-8387
www.puget-sound.med.va.gov

Elizabeth L Serha, Chief Library Service

Medicine.

8838 US Department of Veterans Affairs: Spokane Medical Center Library
4815 N Assembly Street
Spokane, WA 99205-6185
509-434-7000
Fax: 509-434-7119; *Toll Free:* 800-325-7940
www.visn20.med.va.gov

Mary Curtis-Kellett, Chief Library Service

Medicine and allied health sciences.

8839 US Department of Veterans Affairs: Tacoma/Puget Sound Health Care System
96000 Veterans Drive
Tacoma, WA 98493
253-582-8440
Fax: 253-589-4029; *Toll Free:* 800-329-8387
www.va.gov

Elizabeth L Serha, Chief Library Service

Psychiatry, psychology, general medicine, nursing, patient health.

8840 US Department of Veterans Affairs: Walla Walla Jonathan M Wainwright Memorial VA Medical Library
77 Wainwright Drive
Walla Walla, WA 99362-3975

509-525-5200
Fax: 509-527-3452; *Toll Free:* 888-687-8863
www.va.gov

Darlene Fleming, Chief Librarian

Medicine, nursing, allied health sciences.

8841 Washington Library for the Blind and Physically Handicapped
821 Lenora Street
Seattle, WA 98129
206-464-6930
Fax: 206-464-0247
wtbbl@spl.lib.wa.us
www.spl.lib.wa.us

Jan Ames, Librarian

Summer reading programs, braille writer, magnifiers, closed-circuit TV, large-print photocopier, cassette books and magazines, children's books on cassette, home visits and other reference materials on blindness and other handicaps.

West Virginia

8842 Kanawha County Public Library
123 Capitol Street
Charleston, WV 25301-2686
304-343-4646
Fax: 304-348-6530
kanawha.lib.wv.us

Dixie Smith, Librarian
Linda Wright, Manager

Summer reading programs, braille writer, magnifiers, closed-circuit TV, large-print photocopier, cassette books and magazines, children's books on cassette, home visits and other reference materials on blindness and other handicaps.

8843 Parkersburg and Wood County Public Library
3100 Emerson Avenue
Parkersburg, WV 26104-2414
304-420-4587
Fax: 304-420-4589
www.parkersburg.lib.wv.us

Michael Hickman, Contact
Brian E Raitz, Manager

Services for the bind and physically handicapped.

8844 US Department of Veterans Affairs: Beckley Library Service
200 Veterans Avenue
Beckley, WV 25801-6444
304-255-2121
Fax: 304-255-2431
www.beckley.va.gov

Lois M Watson, Chief Library Service
Debbie Coloski, Manager

Medicine, nursing, surgery.

8845 US Department of Veterans Affairs: Clarkburg Loouis A Johnson VA Medical Center Library
1 Med Center Drive
Clarksburg, WV 26301-4155

304-623-3461
Fax: 304-626-7026
www.va.gov

Wanda F Kincaid, Chief Library Service
Mary McCloud, Manager

Medicine.

8846 US Department of Veterans Affairs: Huntinington Learning Resource Center
1540 Spring Valley Drive
Huntington, WV 25704-9300
304-429-6741
Fax: 304-429-6713; *Toll Free:* 800-827-8244
www.hungington.va.gov

Ronald Maynard, Chief LRC
Philip S Elkins, Executive Director

Clinical medicine.

8847 US Department of Veterans Affairs: Martinsburg Learning Resources Service
510 Butler Ave
Martinsburg, WV 25401
304-263-0811
Fax: 304-262-7433; *Toll Free:* 800-817-3807
www.martinsburg.va.gov

Eric Vance, Cheif Learning Resources Service

Medicine, surgery, allied health sciences.

8848 West Virginia Library Commission
1900 Kanawha Boulevard E
Charleston, WV 25305
304-558-2041
Fax: 304-558-2044
librarycommission.lib.wv.us

J.D. Waggoner, State Librarian

Summer reading programs, braille writer, magnifiers, closed-circuit TV, large-print photocopier, cassette books and magazines, children's books on cassette, home visits and other reference materials on blindness and other handicaps.

8849 West Virginia School for the Blind
301 E Main Street
Romney, WV 26757-1828
304-822-4800
Fax: 304-822-3370
wvsdb2.state.k12.wv.us

Cynthia Johnson, Librarian
Jane McBride, Administrator

Summer reading programs, braille writer, magnifiers, closed-circuit TV, large-print photocopier, cassette books and magazines, children's books on cassette, home visits and other reference materials on blindness and other handicaps.

Wisconsin

8850 Gateway Technical College Learning Resource Center
3520 30th Avenue
Kenosha, WI 53144-1690
262-564-2200
Fax: 262-656-8768
www.gtc.edu

Gerald F Perona, Distribution Librarian
Samuel Borden, President

Office education, law enforcement, nursing and allied health sciences, horticulture, aeronautics, electronics, physical therapy, data processing.

8851 Marquette University Libraries Special Collections and University Archives
1355 W Wisconsin Avenue
Milwaukee, WI 53233-2287
414-288-7256
Fax: 414-288-6709
www.marquette.edu

Matt Blessing, Head Special Collections/Archive
Janice Walburn, Dean of Librarians

Catholic social thought and action, Catholic Indian ministry, Marquette University history, recent US political history, Catholic religious formation and vocation ministries.

8852 Rock County Health Care Center Staff Library
PO Box 351
Janesville, WI 53547
608-757-5150
Fax: 608-757-5010

Ruth Beyer, Inservice Director

Psychiatry, psychiatric social work, geriatrics and nursing.

8853 Sentry Insurance Company Library
1800 N Point Drive
Stevens Point, WI 54481-1283
715-346-6000
Fax: 715-946-7560; *Toll Free:* 800-301-3366
ww.sentry.com

John Carlson, Library Services Coordinator
Dale Schuh, CEO

Insurance - property/casualty and life; pensions; law; business management.

8854 US Department of Veterans Affairs: Tomah Health Sciences Library
500 E Veterans Street
Tomah, WI 54660-3105
608-372-3971
Fax: 608-372-1670; *Toll Free:* 800-872-8662
www.va.gov

Phyllis Goetz, Manager

Psychiatry, neurology, general medicine, psychology, nursing, geriatrics, gerontology.

8855 Wisconsin Regional Library for the Blind: Talking Book Program
813 W Wells Street
Milwaukee, WI 53233-1436
414-286-3045
Fax: 414-286-3102; *Toll Free:* 800-242-8822
lbph@milwaukee.gov
www.talkingbooks.dpi.wi.gov
TDD 414-286-3548

Marsha Valance, Regional Librarian
Judith Glover, Assistant Librarian

Circulates recorded materials, playback equipment and braille materials to print-handicapped Wisconsin residents.

8856 Wisconsin Veterans Museum & Research Center
30 W Mifflin Street
Madison, WI 53703-2589
608-267-1790
Fax: 608-264-7615
veterans.museum@dva.state.wi.us
museum.dva.state.wi.us/

Dr Richard Zeitlin, Director
Came Bohman, Reference Archivist
Gayle Martinson, Manager

Military and veterans history.

Wyoming

8857 US Department of Veterans Affairs: Cheyenne Medical and Regional Office Center
Learning Resources
2360 E Pershing Boulevard
Cheyenne, WY 82001-5356
Toll Free: 800-827-1000
www.va.gov

Kerry Skidmore, Chief LRS

Medicine, nursing.

8858 US Department of Veterans Affairs: Sheridan Medical Center Library
1898 Fort Road
Sheridan, WY 82801
307-672-3473
Fax: 307-672-1900; *Toll Free:* 866-822-6714
www.sheridan.va.gov

Pat Carlson, Chief Library Service

Psychiatry, psychology, medicine, nursing, administration, post-traumatic stress disorder.

8859 Wyoming Services for the Visually Disabled
State Department of Education
2300 Capitol Avenue
Cheyenne, WY 82002-2060
307-777-7690
Fax: 307-777-6234
www.k12.wy.us

Kent Jensen, Contact

Eligible readers of Wyoming receive library service from the regional library in Salt Lake City, Utah.

Print Resources for Older Americans

Publishers

8860 Activity Factory
2227 Rock Island Court
Roswell, GA 30278
770-979-5727
Fax: 770-979-7010
www.activityfactory.biz

Dennis Goodwin, Owner

Publishes books on recreation ideas for nursing home activity programs.

8861 Alliance Press
3911 5th Avenue
Suite 202
San Diego, CA 92103-3146
858-454-3610
Fax: 858-454-2432
www.alliance-press.com

Joe Casciani PhD, President

Self-publishes a book on aging and mental health. Offers audio cassettes. Reaches market through direct mail. Presently inactive.

8862 American Association of Homes and Services for the Aging
901 E Street NW
Suite 500
Washington, DC 20004-2037
202-661-5700
Fax: 202-783-2255
www.leadingage.org

Patricia A McGinn, Contact
Daniel Smith, Vice President

Publishes paperback books about homes for the aging. Offers video cassettes. Does not accept unsolicited manuscripts.

8863 American Foundation for the Blind
11 Penn Plaza
Suite 300
New York, NY 10001-2018
212-502-7600
Fax: 212-620-2105

Carl Augusto, President

Publishes pamphlets, books, and other informational materials pertaining to the blind and visually impaired.

8864 Association for Gerontology in Higher Education
1001 Connecticut Avenue NW
Suite 410
Washington, DC 20036-5529
202-289-9806
Fax: 202-429-6097

Derek Stepp, Manager

Nonprofit association of 320 institutions of higher education committed to gerontology education, training, and research. Publishes a national directory, a series of brief bibliographies, research reports, and annual meeting abstracts. Offers a quarterly newsletter, AGH Exchange, and a national database on gerontology. Reaches market through direct mail.

8865 Briggs Corporation
PO Box 1698
Des Moines, IA 50306-1698
515-327-6400
Fax: 800-222-1996; *Toll Free:* 800-247-2343
www.briggscorp.com

Kristin Keeline, Prof. Resources Product Manager
Merwyn Dan, CEO

Publishes on health care related subjects. Reaches market through direct mail and telephone sales.

8866 Calyx Books & Calyx Journal
PO Box B
Corvallis, OR 97339
541-753-9384
Fax: 541-753-0515
www.calyxpress.org

Margarita Donnelly, Director

Publishes books by women query for guidelines. Distributed by Consortium Book Sales and Distributes small press, Distributors, and others.

8867 Caresource Healthcare Communications
230 N. Main St.
Dayton, OH 45402
937-224-3300
Fax: 206-682-2901; *Toll Free:* 800-448-5213
service@caresource.com
www.caresource.com

Diane Kenny, Contact

Specializes in print and electronic publications for senior care and healthcare. We serve consumers and senior care and healthcare professionals and provider organizations. Products and services include: healthy aging books, booklets, and brochures; videotapes; websites; web based education; and custom publishing.

8868 Center for Bio-Gerontology
PO Box 11097
Pensacola, FL 32524-1097
904-484-0595
Fax: 850-474-5255

Kum-Ja Chae, Marketing Director

Publishes books related to biological aging, aging retardation, and life extension. Accepts unsolicited manuscripts. Reaches market through direct mail and wholesalers.

8869 Center for Public Representation
22 Green Street
PO Box 260049
Northampton, MA 1060
608-251-4008
Fax: 413-586-5711; *Toll Free:* 800-369-0388
info@cpr-ma.org
www.centerforpublicrep.org
TDD 413-586-6024

Melissa Hoberg, Publications Assistant

Publishes materials relevant to the elderly and health care providers, and consumer publications on guardianship and health care.

8870 Center for Thanatology Research & Education
391 Atlantic Avenue
Brooklyn, NY 11217-1701
718-858-3026
Fax: 718-858-3026
hdporn@mindspring.com

Roberto Halton, Contact

Objective is to distribute and promote all publications on aging, dying, and death and gravestones studies, and release relevant titles in these subjects. Offers audio cassettes, video cassettes, a newsletter and a journal. Reaches market through direct mail and trade sales. Does not accept unsolicited manuscripts.

8871 Center for the Study of Human Rights
1108 Iab
New York, NY 10027
212-854-2479
Fax: 212-316-4578
cshr@columbia.edu

J Paul Martin, Executive Director

Promotes teaching and research in international human rights. Publishes occasional papers, reports, proceedings, and course syllabi. Reports and documents copyrighted.

8872 Educare Press
PO Box 17222
Seattle, WA 98127
206- 70- 410
Fax: 206-784-7556
educarepress@educarepress.com
www.educarepress.com

Kieran O'Mahony, Publisher

Publishes educational, geography and aging titles. Reaches market through direct mail and trade sales. Does not accept unsolicited manuscripts.

8873 Edward Feil Productions
4614 Prospect Avenue
Cleveland, OH 44103-4394
216-881-0040
Fax: 216-751-6434
naomifeil@aol.com
www.vfvalidation.org

Edward R Feil, President

Publishes a book helping the aging using the Validation Method. Also offers films and video cassettes. Reaches market through direct mail and telephone sales. Produces Videos (VHS) helping caregivers communicate with older people who are diagnosed with a dementia.

8874 Elder Book Store
Elder Books
2115 Elliston Place
Nashville, TN 37203-5289
615-327-1867
Fax: 415-488-4720
info@eldersbookstore.com
www.eldersbookstore.com

Randy Elder, Manager

8875 Elder Books
PO Box 490
Forest Knolls, CA 94933
415-488-9002
Fax: 415-488-4720; *Toll Free:* 800-909-COPE

Susan Sullivan, Director

Publishes how-to books for families and caregivers looking after Alzheimer's patients and books of Celtic interest. Accepts unsolicited manuscripts. Reaches market through direct mail, trade sales, and wholesalers.

8876 Employee Benefit Research Institute
2121 K Street NW
Suite 600
Washington, DC 20037-1800
202-659-0670
Fax: 202-775-6312
publications@ebri.org
www.ebri.org

Cheri Meyer, Contact
Dallas Salisbury, President

Publishes to contribute to the development of effective and responsible public policy in the employee benefit field. Also publishes newsletters, abstracts, journals, and speeches. Reaches market through direct mail.

8877 Gateway Books
2023 Clemens Road
Oakland, CA 94602-1915
510-530-0299
Fax: 510-530-0497
www.sfgateway.com

Judith Merwin, Publisher

Publishes a series of books aimed at those interested in retirement living in the US and abroad. Accepts proposals for manuscripts. Reaches market through direct mail and Publishers Group West.

8878 Gerontological Society of America
1220 L Street NW,
Suite 901
Washington, DC 20005-4083
202-842-1275
Fax: 202-842-1150
geron@geron.org
www.geron.org

Jennifer Campi, Production Editor
Carol Schutz, Executive Director

Publishes five print journals on aging. Offers a database, a calendar online only, and both a print and an online newsletter. Accepts unsolicited manuscripts. Reaches market through trade sales.

8879 Gibbs Associates
PO Box 706
Boulder, CO 80306
303-444-6032
Fax: 303-444-6032; *Toll Free:* 800-378-5089

Betty Gibbs, President

Publishes a book on Alzheimer's disease, and a book of poetry. Reaches market through direct mail and internet.

8880 Grey House Publishing
4919 Route 22
PO Box 56
Amenia, NY 12501
518-789-8700
Fax: 845-373-6390; *Toll Free:* 800-562-2139

books@greyhouse.com
www.greyhouse.com

Richard Gottlieb, President & Co-Founder
Leslie Mackenzie, Publisher & Co-Founder
Laura Mars, Editorial Director

Publisher of numerous consumer health directories, including Complete Directory for People with Chronic Illness, Complete Directory for People with Disabilities, Medical Device Market Place, and the biennial Complete Mental Health Directory; in addition to numerous other directories and reference works.

Year Founded: 1981

8881 Human Growth & Development Associates

6780 S Adams Way
Centennial, CO 80122-1802
303-771-8424
Fax: 303-773-1264

Mary K Kouri, Co-Owner

Self-publisher of workbook for life planning for older adults. Presently inactive.

8882 Hunter House Publishing

PO Box 2914
1515« Park Street
Alameda, CA 94501
510-865-5282
Fax: 510-865-4295; Toll Free: 800-266-5592
ordering@hunterhouse.com
www.hunterhouse.com

Christina Sverdrup, Customer Service Manager
David Spero RN, Author

8883 Idyll Arbor

PO Box 720
Ravensdale, WA 98051
360-825-7797
Fax: 425-432-3726
sales@idyllarbor.com
www.IdyllArbor.com

Tom Blaschko, Contact

Publishes books for activity professionals, recreational therapists and allied therapists. Reaches market through direct mail, catalogs, reviews and listings, professional conferences and general book stores. Accepts unsolicited manuscripts from experienced professionals in health care. Catalog of approximately 200 books, assessments and games are available.

8884 Impact Publishers

PO Box 910
San Luis Obispo, CA 93406
805-543-5911
Fax: 805-543-4093

Connie Magee, Marketing Manager

Publishes books on human development. Accepts unsolicited manuscripts from human service professionals. Reaches market through direct mail and trade sales.

8885 Legal Counsel for the Elderly

601 E Street NW
Washington, DC 20049
202-434-2170
Fax: 202-434-6464

Sally Balch Hurme, Publications Coordinator
Jan May, Manager

Disseminates legal information on the problems of the elderly to attorneys, paralegals, other advocates, and consumers. Offers two newsletters, the bimonthly Elder Law Forum and a quarterly, Trainingworks. Reaches market through direct mail. Does not accept unsolicited manuscripts.

8886 Leisure Living

83 Cimitiere Street
Launceston, MO 7250
036-334-3145
Fax: 036-334-3146
simon@leisureliving.com.au
www.leisureliving.com.au

Robert S Tillman, President

Publishes video cassettes of retirement locations throughout the US Reaches market through direct mail, Quality Books, New Age Video, Unique Books, and Edu-Tech Corp. Accepts unsolicited manuscripts.

8887 National Citizens' Coalition for Nursing Home Reform

1828 L Street NW
Suite 801
Washington, DC 20036-5104
202-332-2275
Fax: 202-332-2949

Laurie Demsey, Contact
Alice Hedt, Executive Director

Publishes on nursing home reform.

8888 Otterbein Homes Program Department

1 South Grove Street
Westerville, OH 43081
614-890-3000
Fax: 513-932-5159
www.otterbein.edu

Charles W Peckham, Author/Educator

Publishes books on and for the elderly. Reaches market through direct mail. Does not accept unsolicited manuscripts.

8889 Potentials Development

P.O. Box 55339
Seattle, WA 98155-0339
716-691-6601
Fax: 716-691-6620; Toll Free: 800-691-6602
www.potentialsdevelopment.com

Patricia Maurer, Administrative Associate

Established by two occupational therapists who had seen the need for educational materials in the field of aging. Their philosophy is that age is not an event, it is an ongoing process. Provides resources to the elderly, their families and caregivers. Materials on Alzheimer's, resources for social workers, family support groups, etc.

8890 Resources for Rehabilitation

33 Bedford Street
Suite 19a
Lexington, MA 02420-4330
781-862-6455
Fax: 781-861-7517
orders@rfr.org

Susan L Greenblatt, Treasurer

Publishes books and large print brochures designed to help seniors and people with disabilities function independently. Offers desk references for professionals. Reaches market through direct mail. Does not accept unsolicited manuscripts.

8891 Richard W. Waring

845 Heathermoor Lane
Perrysburg, OH 43551-2980
419-244-6711
Fax: 419-244-4791

Provides financial and estate planning resource materials for individuals, professional, financial, and estate planners, and pre-retirement programs. Conducts seminars for non-profit organizations. Offers The Collection Basket, a fund raising newsletter, and Presenting and Extending Our Catholic Heritage, a pamphlet. Reaches market through direct mail and trade sales.

8892 SCENE

Braille Institute
741 N Vermont Avenue
Los Angeles, CA 90029-3514
310-234-0339 Toll free: 800-BRA-ILLE

Serial Beccai, Owner

Offers information on the organization, question and answer column, articles on the newest technology and more for visually impaired persons.

8893 Scripps Ranch Publications

10301 Scripps Lake Drive
San Diego, CA 92131-1258
858-538-8158
Fax: 858-538-8154

Nancy Assaf, Manager

Publishes for working adults who are concerned about their future retirement. Presently inactive.

8894 Senior Fitness Productions

1780 Penfield Road
Penfield, NY 14526-2104
585-586-7548
Fax: 585-385-9581; *Toll Free:* 800-306-3137
bpc@senior-fitness.com
www.senior-fitness.com

Betty Perkins-Carpenter, President

Publishes books and guides for senior citizens. Does not accept unsolicited manuscripts. Reaches market through direct mail trade sales and workshops/keynotes.

8895 Sequoia Retirement Services

1911 San Ysidro Drive
Beverly Hills, CA 90210-1520
310-859-1961
Fax: 310-859-7077

T Lan, Owner

Publishes materials on retirement and retirement planning. Offers a personal computer-based program that is used in conjunction with the materials. Accepts unsolicited manuscripts. Reaches market through seminar sales.

8896 Southern California Senior Life

6500 Wilshire Boulevard
Suite 1200
Los Angeles, CA 90048-4932
213-427-3200
Fax: 323-933-9261
www.seniorlifeusa.com

Micheal Carpernter, Advertising Director
Laurence Vittes, Editor
Dirk Stoehr, Manager

Publishes a directory of special services, help lines, medical care, legal and financial information, etc., for seniors. Offers a monthly newspaper, Southern California Senior Life. Reaches market through direct mail. Does not accept unsolicited manuscripts.

8897 Springer Publishing Company

536 Broadway
New York, NY 10012-3915
212-431-4370
Fax: 212-941-7842
www.springerpub.com

Ursula Springer, President

Publishers of scholarly books and journals in fields of psychology, social work, medicine/public health, gerontology and geriatrics, nursing, and rehabilitation. Reaches market through direct mail, Baker & Taylor, Login Brothers, and J. A. Majors. Does not accept unsolicited manuscripts.

8898 Third Age Press

1075 NW Murray Road
Suite 277
Portland, OR 97229-5501
503-690-3251
Fax: 503-669-5325
www.thirdagepress.co.uk

Al Tauber, VP

Publishes on aging and discrimination against the aged. Does not accept unsolicited manuscripts. Reaches market through trade sales and wholesalers, including Bookpeople, Quality Books, Unique Books, Pacific Pipeline, Baker & Taylor Books, and Upper Access.

8899 Thornapple Publishing Company

450 Springfield Avenue Summit
Ada, MI 49301
616-676-1583
Fax: 616-676-1583

Robert Redd, President

Publishes on retirement and non royalty short plays. Does not accept unsolicited manuscripts. Distributes for Gateway Books, Bristol, Contemporary Books, and Goldfish. Reaches market through direct mail.

8900 Transaction Publishers

390 Campus Drive
Somerset, NJ 08873-1102
732-445-1245
Fax: 732-748-9801; *Toll Free:* 888-999-6778
www.transactionpub.com

Periodic updates on new large print titles.

Travel & Recreation

Transportation

8901 America West Airlines/US Airways
4000 E Sky Harbor Blvd.y
Phoenix, AZ 85034
480-693-0800 Toll free: 800-235-9292
www.usairways.com

J Scott Kirby, Executive VP Sales/Marketing
Tom Cartwright, Manager

Senior saver pack: book of 4 or 8 one way coupons. Tickets require 14 day advance purchase; other restrictions apply. 10% off regular priced air fares for people 62 years and older.

8902 American Airlines
PO Box 619616
dFW Airport
Fort Worth, TX 75261-9616
817-963-1234
Fax: 817-967-4162
www.aa.com
TDD 800-543-1586

Greg Clark, Managing Director
Gerard J Arpey, CEO

Senior Traveler Coupon Books contain either four or eight one-way tickets for anywhere in the 48 continental states or the Carribean. Tickets are good for 1 year, are nontransferable, and must be reserved 14 days in advance; and there is a $25 fee to change reservations. There is also a 10% discount on regular priced fares. For people 62 years and older.

8903 Amtrak Railways
PO Box 2709
Washington, DC 20013-2709
Toll Free: 800-872-7245
www.amtrak.com

David L Gunn, President/CEO

15% off travel Monday through Thursday for people 62 years and older.

8904 British Airways
7520 Astoria Boulevard
Flushing, NY 11370-1190
718-335-0464
Fax: 718-397-4204; *Toll Free:* 800-403-0882
www.britishairways.com

John Lampl, VP Communications

Privileged Traveler Program: 10% off regular priced air fares, cars, hotels, etc., also includes other benefits. For people 60 years and older. Companion must be 50 years or older.

8905 CEH
4457 63rd Circle
Charleston, SC 29410
727-522-0364
Fax: 727-522-9024; *Toll Free:* 877-926-4162
info@liftsandramps.com
www.liftsandramps.com

Andrew E Manatos, President
Phillip Faas, Owner

New vans, used vans, rental vans; specializing in quad conversions, all types of handicap equipment. Celebrating 25 years in business.

8906 Continental Airlines
1600 Smith Street
Houston, TX 77002-7362
713-324-5000 Toll free: 800-525-0280
www.continental.com

Lawrence W Kellner, President/CEO

Check website for occasional Senior discounts.

8907 Continental Airlines - Senior Programs
1600 Smith Street
Houston, TX 77002-7362
713-324-5000 Toll free: 800-525-0280
www.continental.com

General information about special discounts for senior citizens flying with Continental Airlines are available on this site.

8908 Delta Shuttle
Po Box 20706
Atlanta, GA 30320
404-715-2600 Toll free: 800-933-5935
www.delta-air.com

Gerald Grinstein, CEO

Senior Pass: half-price tickets to and from New York, Washington D.C., and Boston. Flight times and days vary: Monday through Friday 10:00 a.m. to 2:30 p.m.; 7:30 p.m. to 11:59 p.m.; all day Saturday and Sunday. For people 65 years and older.

8909 Dollar Rent-a-Car
5330 E 31st Street
Tulsa, OK 74153-1167
918-669-3000
Fax: 918-669-8563; *Toll Free:* 800-800-4000
www.dollar.com

Gary Paxton, President/CEO
Steven Hildebrand, Senior Executive VP

Discounts vary among locations.

8910 El Al Israel Airlines
15 E 26th Street
New York, NY 10010
212-768-9200
Fax: 212-852-0793; *Toll Free:* 800-223-6700
www.elal.com

David Hermesh, President
Michael Mayer, Manager

Golden Age fare: 15% off regular apex fare to Israel. Must purchase tickets 14 days in advance. For people 60 years and older.

8911 Greyhound Bus
PO Box 660691
MS 470
Dallas, TX 75266-0691
214-849-8000 Toll free: 800-231-2222
www.greyhound.com
TDD 800-345-3109
TTY: 800-345-3109

Dave Leach, President & CEO
Bill Blankenship, Chief Operating Officer

Five percent discount to Seniors on all fares.

Year Founded: 1914

8912 Greyhound Bus Info Senior Discounts

PO Box 660691
MS 470
Dallas, TX 75266-0691
214-849-8100
Fax: 214-849-8000; Toll Free: 800-231-2222
www.greyhound.com
TDD 800-345-3109
TTY: 800-345-3109

Greyhound Bus Senior Discounts.

8913 Hawaiian Airlines

3375 Koapaka Street
Honolulu, HI 96819-1800
808-835-3700
Fax: 808-835-3690; Toll Free: 800-367-5320
www.hawaiianair.com

Mark B Dunkerley, President/CEO
Keoni Wagner, VP Public Affairs

10% off excursion fares from the islands to the mainland.
No discounts for flights between islands. For people 60
years and older.

8914 Horizon Air

19521 Pacific Highway S
Seattle, WA 98188-5499
206-241-6757
Fax: 203-248-6200; Toll Free: 800-547-9308
www.horizonair.com

Jeff Pinneo, President/CEO
Cheryl Temple, Public Affairs
Dan Russo, Director Mktging/Communications

Book of four or eight one way coupons. 14 day advance
purchase required; other restrictions apply. For people 62
years and older.

8915 Housing and Transportation of the Handicapped

William Hein & Company
1285 Main Street
Buffalo, NY 14209-1911
716-882-2600
Fax: 716-883-8100; Toll Free: 800-828-7571
mail@wshein.com
www.wshein.com

Kevin Marmion, President

National laws, recognizing the problems encountered by
the handicapped in the areas of Housing and Transportation
and providing assistance in an effort to surmount those
problems. Microfilm.

8916 Iberia Airlines of Spain

6100 Blue Lagoon Drive
Miami, FL 33126-2079
902-400-500
Fax: 305-262-8763; Toll Free: 800-772-4642
iberiaus@iberia.com
www.iberia.com

Fernando Conte, President
Luis Tirad, Plant Manager

10% off regular priced fares. Must belong to the United Silver Wings Plus travel club.

8917 KLM Royal Dutch/Northwest Airlines

565 Taxter Road
Elmsford, NY 10523-2312
914-784-2000
Fax: 612-726-0776; Toll Free: 800-374-7747
www.klm.com

L M Van Wijk, President/CEO

Discount varies. Call for details. For people 60 years and
older and spouses. Must be a member of the United Silver
Wings Plus travel club.

8918 Mesa Airlines

410 N. 44th Street,
Ste. 700
Phoenix, NM 85008
602-685-4000
Fax: 602-685-4350; Toll Free: 800-326-3338
www.mesa-air.com

John Ornstein, Chairman/CEO
Michael J Lotz, President/COO
Brian S Gillman, Executive Vice President

Discount varies depending on time of year and destination.
For people 62 years and older.

8919 Midwest Express Airlines

6744 S Howell Avenue
Oak Creek, WI 53154-1402
414-570-4000
Fax: 414-570-9922; Toll Free: 800-452-2022
www.midwestexpress.com

Timothy E Hocksema, Chairman/President/CEO
Scott R Dickson, Senior VP/CMO

10% off regular fares. For people 62 years and older.

8920 National Car Rental

6929 North Lakewood Avenue
Suite 100
Tulsa, OK 74117-1808
918-401-6000
Fax: 843-767-5526; Toll Free: 800-468-3334
www.nationalcar.com

Bill Lobeck, Executive Director
Howard Schwartz, General Counsel

Discounts vary among locations, usually 5 to 10 percent for
Seniors.

8921 Northwest Limousine Service

9950 Lawrence Avenue
Schiller Park, IL 60176-1310
847-671-5482
Fax: 847-671-5482
www.northwestlimo.com

Kathleen Maloney, Manager
Ann Walsh, Office Reservations

Offers wheelchair accessible mini vans, sedans, stretch and
super stretch limousines for hourly or daily rental.

8922 PALAESTRA

Challenge Publications
PO Box 508
Macomb, IL 61455
309-833-1902
Fax: 309-833-1902
www.palaestra.com

David P Beaver, Editor in Cheif

Journal focusing on sports, physical education, and recreation for persons with disabilities.

60 pages Frequency: Quarterly

8923 Rollx Vans
6591 Highway 13 W
Savage, MN 55378-1177
440-322-5804
Fax: 952-890-1903; *Toll Free:* 800-335-5804
questions@rollxvans.com
www.rollxvans.com

Mike Harris, President
Scott Andrews, Marketing

Luxury wheelchair conversion vans equipped with fully automatic liffts with tie-downs. Trade ins accepted for vehicles of all types, conversions and long term leasing available.

8924 Spa
Waterfront Press Company
5305 Shilshole Avenue NW
Suite 200
Seattle, WA 98107-4021
206-826-4000
Fax: 206-789-9193
wfpress@wolfenet.com

Janet Thomas, Editor
Laurie Munnis, Advertising Director

Magazine containing articles on travel, well-being, and renewal.

Frequency: Quarterly

8925 Swiss International Airlines
445 Broadhollow Road
Suite 419
Melville, NY 11747
Fax: 631-956-9200; *Toll Free:* 888-715-5551
www.swiss.com

Pieter Bouw, CEO
Daniel Wede, Marketing/Services

Some Senior discounts available, please inquire for specifics.

8926 Thrifty Rent-a-Car
5330 E 31st Street
Tulsa, OK 74135-5028
918-660-7700
Fax: 918-669-2060; *Toll Free:* 800-367-2277
www.thrifty.com

Gary L Paxton, CEO

Discounts vary by location, usually 5% for those over 55 years of age.

8927 USAir
2345 Crystal Drive
Arlington, VA 22227
703-418-7000
Fax: 336-661-8031; *Toll Free:* 800-428-4322
www.usairways.com

Bruce Lakefield, President/CEO

Senior Discount Books contain four or eight one-way coupons. Tickets are transferable to grandchildren between the ages of 2-17. There is a $25 penalty to change reservations. Other restrictions apply. For people 62 years and older.

8928 USAirways Shuttle
PO Box 1501
Winston Salem, NC 27102-1501
336-661-0061
Fax: 336-661-8031; *Toll Free:* 800-428-4322
www.usairways.com

Bruce Lakefield, CEO USAirways Group

Senior discounts vary by market, also works with AARP for discounts. Call for your best rate.

8929 United Airlines
PO Box 66100
Chicago, IL 60666
773-601-5180Toll free: 877-228-1327
www.united.com

Glenn Tilton, CEO
Diane Soucy Bergan, Director Customer Relations

Silver Wings Plus: pay $75 and receive a three-year membership that includes three $25 coupons, or pay $150 for a lifetime membership and receive three $50 coupons. Membership also includes discounts for hotels, car rentals, and more. Receive 10% off regular priced fares. Silver Travel Pac Program: book of four or eight one-way coupons. Some restrictions apply. For people 62 years and older.

8930 Wheelchair Getaways Accessible Van Rentals
PO Box 5591
Lynnwood, WA 98046
859-873-4973
Fax: 859-873-8039; *Toll Free:* 800-536-5518
corporate@wheelchairgetaways.com
www.wheelchair-getaways.com

Richard Gatewood, President/CEO

Rents wheelchair/scooter accessible vans by the day, week, month or longer and offers delivery to major airports and other convenient locations in more than 200 cities in 42 states. Also offers full size and mini vans with automatic lifts and ramps. Some vans are equipped with hand controls, six-way power seats and remote controls for powered door operation and lifts. Discount may apply depending on location.

1921

8931 Wheeler's Accessible Van Rentals
6614 W Sweetwater Avenue
Glendale, AZ 85304-1040
623-878-3540Toll free: 456-137-

Judy Jordan, Reservations Manager
Gery King, Operations Developer

Offers customized van rentals to the disabled persons allowing them freedom and independence in their travel.

8932 Wheelers Accessible Van Rentals
6614 West Sweetwater
Glendale, AZ 85304
Fax: 623-412-9920; *Toll Free:* 800-456-1371
info@wheelersvanrentals.com
www.wheelersvanrentals.com

Offers delivery to airports at 60 locations throughout the country. Wheelers offers a variety of van configurations with capacity for up to three wheelchairs, automatic ramps or lifts and nylon tie-downs, hand controls or other modifications.

1987

State Programs

8933 Alabama Bureau of Tourism and Travel
401 Adams Avenue Suite 126
Po Box 4927
Montgomery, AL 36103-4927
334-242-4169
Fax: 334-242-4554; *Toll Free:* 800-252-2262
info@touralabama.org
www.touralabama.org

Lee Sentell, Director
Frances Smiley, Welcome Center Manager

8934 Alaska Division of Tourism
2600 Cordova Street
Suite 201
Anchorage, AK 99503
907-465-2017
Fax: 907-465-3767
www.travelalaska.com

Tom Gerrett, Manager

8935 Arizona Office of Tourism
1110 W Washington St.
Suite 155
Phoenix, AZ 85007
Fax: 602-240-5432; *Toll Free:* 800-842-8257
www.arizonaguide.com

8936 Arkansas Department of Parks & Tourism
1 Capitol Mall
Little Rock, AR 72201-1087
501-682-7777
Fax: 501-682-1364; *Toll Free:* 800-NAT-URAL
www.1800natural.com

Richard Davies, Executive Director

8937 California Division of Tourism
PO Box 1499
Sacramento, CA 95812-1499
916-444-4429
Fax: 916-322-3402; *Toll Free:* 800-862-2543
www.gocalif.ca.gov

8938 Colorado Travel & Tourism Authority
1127 Pennsylvania Street
Denver, CO 80203-2502
Fax: 303-832-6174; *Toll Free:* 800-COL-ORAD
www.colorado.com

8939 Connecticut Office of Tourism
One Financial Plaza
755 Main Street
Hartford, CT 06106-7107
860-256-2800
Fax: 860-270-8077; *Toll Free:* 888-288-4748
ct.travelinfo@ct.gov
www.tourism.state.ct.us

Ed Dombroskas, Executive Director

8940 Delaware Tourism Office
99 Kings Highway
Dover, DE 19901-7305
302-739-4271
Fax: 302-739-5749; *Toll Free:* 866-284-7483
www.visitdelaware.com

8941 District of Columbia
DC Committee to Promote Washington
901 7th Street NW
4th Floor
Washington, DC 20001-3719
202-789-7000
Fax: 202-789-7037
mp.washington.org

The Golden Washingtonian Club provides discounts to residents from about 1,800 merchants listed in the Gold Mine. The directory includes restaurants, hotels, and retail stores. Call for a free copy. For people 60 years and older.

8942 Georgia Department of Industry Trade & Tourism
75 Fifth Street NW
Suite 1200
Atlanta, GA 30308
404-962-4000
Fax: 404-651-9063; *Toll Free:* 800-847-4842
www.georgia.org/itt/tourism

8943 Golden Buckeye Program
Ohio Department of Aging
50 W Broad Street
9th Floor
Columbus, OH 43215-3363
614-466-6191
Fax: 614-466-5741; *Toll Free:* 800-266-4346
ODAMail@age.state.oh.us
www.goldenbuckeye.com

Cindy Clark, Golden Buckeye Program Manager

The Golden Buckeye Card provides holders discounts on goods and services from over 20,000 participating businesses throughout the state. The program also provides cardholders with significant discounts on prescription drugs. For Ohio residents 60 years and older. For people 18-59 with total and permanent disabilities.

8944 Hawaii Tourism Office
2270 Kalakaua Avenue
Suite 801
Honolulu, HI 96815-1513
808-973-2255
Fax: 808-973-2253; *Toll Free:* 800-464-2924
info@hvcb.org
www.gohawaii.com

Rex Johnson, Manager

8945 Idaho Division of Tourism Development
700 West State Street
Po Box 83720
Boise, ID 83720-0093
208-334-2470
Fax: 208-334-2631; *Toll Free:* 800-406-6418
www.visitid.org

Carl Wilgus, Administrator

Dedicated to the growth of the tourism industry in Idaho and provides information for consumers and assistance to our tourism partner businesses across the state. We market the state's travel opportunitites throughout the West and the world with a variety of programs and partnerships.

8946 Illinois Bureau of Tourism
100 W Randolph Street
Chicago, IL 60601-3218
312-814-4732
Fax: 312-814-6581; *Toll Free:* 800-406-6418
ceo.enjoyillinois@illinois.gov
www.enjoyillinois.com

Jan Kostner, Manager

8947 Indiana Tourism Division
1 N Capitol Avenue
Suite 600
Indianapolis, IN 46204-2040
317-232-8860
Fax: 317-233-6887; *Toll Free:* 888-ENJ-OYIN
www.ai.org/tourism

Anicia Richardson, Marketing & Tourism Sales Mgr.
Juana Johnson, Administrations Manager
Carrie Lambert, Marketing Director

8948 Iowa Tourism Office/Iowa Travel Guide
200 E Grand Avenue
Des Moines, IA 50309
515-242-4700
Fax: 515-242-4809; *Toll Free:* 888-472-6035
www.traveliowa.com

Mike Tramontina, Director

The Travel Guide lists Iowa destinations, attractions, lodging and campling.

184 pages Frequency: Annually

8949 Kansas Travel & Tourism
534 S Kansas Avenue
Suite 1210
Topeka, KS 66603
785-296-2009
Fax: 785-296-5563; *Toll Free:* 800-452-6727
www.state.ks.us
TDD 785-296-3487

Scott D Allegrucci, Executive Director

8950 Kentucky Department of Travel
500 Mero Street
22nd Floor
Frankfort, KY 40601-1957
502-564-4930
Fax: 502-564-5695; *Toll Free:* 800-225-8747
www.kentuckytourism.com

8951 Louisiana Office of Tourism
1051 N 3rd Street
Baton Rouge, LA 70802-5239
225-342-8100
Fax: 225-342-8390; *Toll Free:* 800-334-9626
www.lousianatravel.com

Darienne Wilson, Manager

8952 Maine Office of Tourism
59 State House Station
Augusta, ME 04333-0059
207-287-5710
Fax: 207-287-8070; *Toll Free:* 888-624-6345
www.visitmaine.com
TDD 877-624-6331

8953 Maryland Office of Tourism Development
217 E Redwood Street
9th Floor
Baltimore, MD 21202-3316
410-767-3400
Fax: 410-333-6643; *Toll Free:* 866-639-3526
info@mdisfun.org
www.mdisfun.org

Dennis Castleman, Manager

8954 Massachusetts Office of Travel & Tourism
10 Park Plaza
Suite 4510
Boston, MA 02116-3981
617-973-8500
Fax: 617-973-8525; *Toll Free:* 800-277-6277
vacationinfo@state.ma.us
www.mass-vacation.com

Mary Jane McKenna, Executive Director

8955 Michigan Travel Bureau
PO Box 30226
Lansing, MI 48909-7726
517-373-0670
Fax: 517-373-0059; *Toll Free:* 800-543-2937
www.michigan.org

8956 Minnesota Office of Tourism
121 7th Place E
Metro Square Suite 100
Saint Paul, MN 55101
651-296-5029
Fax: 651-296-2800; *Toll Free:* 800-868-7476
explore@state.mn.us
www.exploreminnesota.com

John Edman, Executive Director

8957 Mississippi Division of Tourism Development
PO Box 849
Jackson, MI 39205
601-359-3297
Fax: 601-359-5757; *Toll Free:* 800-927-6378
tourdiv@mississippi.org
www.decd.state.ms.us

8958 Missouri Division of Tourism
PO Box 1055
Jefferson City, MO 65102-1055
573-751-4133
Fax: 573-751-5160; *Toll Free:* 800-877-1234
tourism@ded.mo.gov
www.visitmo.com

Becky Hereen, Marketing Executive

8959 Nebraska Division of Travel & Tourism
301 Centennial Mall South, 4th Floor
Lincoln, NE 68509-8907
402-471-3796
Fax: 402-471-3026; *Toll Free:* 877-632-7275
tourism@visitnebraska.org
www.visitnebraska.org

Sarah Baker, PR Coordinator

Free vacation guide The Nebraska Traveler. The Traveler includes a listing of all accomidations for hotels, motels, bed and breakfasts, guest ranches, and campgrounds. Outfitters and attractions.....more than 140 pages.

8960 Nevada Commission on Tourism
401 N Carson Street
Carson City, NV 89701-4221
775-687-4322
Fax: 702-687-6779; Toll Free: 800-638-2328
ncot@travelnevada.com
www.travelnevada.com

Bruce Bommarito, Executive Director

8961 New Hampshire Office of Travel & Tourism Development
PO Box 1856
172 Pembroke Road
Concord, NH 03302-1856
603-271-2343
Fax: 603-271-6870; Toll Free: 800-FUN-INNH
travel@dred.state.nh.us
www.visitnh.gov

8962 New Jersey Tourism Division
20 W State Street
Trenton, NJ 08608-1206
609- 59- 654
Fax: 609-633-7418; Toll Free: 800-JER-SEY7
www.state.nj.us/travel

Nancy Bryne, Executive Director

8963 New Mexico Department of Tourism
491 Old Santa Fe Trl
Santa Fe, NM 87503
505-827-7400
Fax: 505-827-7402; Toll Free: 800-545-2040
www.newmexico.org

Michael Cerletti, Manager

8964 New York Division of Tourism
1 Commerce Plaza
Albany, NY 12245
518-474-4116
Fax: 518-486-6416; Toll Free: 800-225-5697
www.iloveny.com

8965 North Carolina Division of Tourism
301 N Wilmington Street
Raleigh, NC 27601-1058
919-733-4171
Fax: 919-715-3097; Toll Free: 800-847-4863
www.visitnc.com

Gordon Clapp, Executive Director

8966 Ohio Division of Travel and Tourism
PO Box 1001
Columbus, OH 43216-1001
614-466-8844
Fax: 614-466-6744; Toll Free: 800-282-5393
www.ohiotourism.com

8967 Oklahoma Tourism & Recreation Department
120 N Robinson Avenue
6th Floor
Oklahoma City, OK 73102-5405
405-230-8400
Fax: 405-522-5257; Toll Free: 800-652-6552
www.otrd.state.ok.us

Hardy Watkins, Executive Director

8968 Oregon Tourism Commission
775 Summer Street NE
Salem, OR 97310
503-986-0000
Fax: 503-986-0001; Toll Free: 800-547-7842
info@traveloregon.com
www.traveloregon.com

8969 Pennsylvania Center for Travel, Tourism & Film
400 North Street
4th Floor
Harrisburg, PA 17120-0225
717-787-5453
Fax: 717-787-0687; Toll Free: 800-847-4872
www.visitpa.com

Tom Corbett, Governvor

8970 South Carolina Department of Parks, Transportation & Tourism
1205 Pendleton Street
Columbia, SC 29201-3756
803-734-1700
Fax: 803-734-0133; Toll Free: 866-224-9339
www.scpit.com

8971 South Dakota Department of Tourism
711 E Wells Avenue
Pierre, SD 57501-3385
605-773-3301
Fax: 605-773-3256; Toll Free: 800-732-5682
travelsd@state.sd.us
www.travelsd.com

Billie Jo Waara, Manager

8972 State of Florida
Greater Ft Lauderdale Convention &
1850 Eller Drive
Fort Lauderdale, FL 33316-4202
954-765-4466
Fax: 954-765-4467; Toll Free: 800-22S-UNNY
www.sunny.org

Nicki Grossman, President

Write for the complete Greater Fort Lauderdale Super Senior Savers. Information includes lodging discounts, attraction discounts, calander of events, and visitors guide.

8973 State of Illinois
Department of Commerce & Community Affairs
620 E Adams Street
Springfield, IL 62701-1615
217-782-7500
Fax: 217-785-6336; Toll Free: 800-226-6632
www.commerce.state.il.us
TDD 800-785-6055

The Golden Age Hunting and Fishing License provides free hunting and fishing. For people 65 years and older.

8974 State of Missouri
Missouri Department of Social Services
221 West High Street
Po Box 1527
Jefferson City, MO 65102-1337
573-634-5165
Fax: 573-751-4386; Toll Free: 800-235-5503
www.dss.mo.gov

Josh Campbell, Manager

Silver Citizen Discount Card entitles holders to discounts at restaurants, stores, services, and other businesses throughout the state. For people 60 years and older.

8975 State of Rhode Island
Department of Elderly Affairs
160 Pine Street
Providence, RI 02903-3708
401-462-4000
Fax: 401-222-1490
www.dea.ri.gov

Noreen Shawcross, Executive Director

Free admission to state parks. For people 65 years and older.

8976 State of Texas Office of the Governor Economic Development and Tourism
PO Box 12428
Austin, TX 78711-2428
512-936-0100
Fax: 512-936-0450
www.governor.state.tx.us

David Teel, Executive Director

8977 State of Utah
Park City Convention & Visitors Bureau
1910 Prospector Avenue
Park City, UT 84060-7211
435-649-6100
Fax: 801-649-4132; *Toll Free:* 800-453-1360
www.2chambers.com/utah_state

William Malone, Executive Director

The Silver Card entitles holders to special discounts May through September. Restrictions do apply. Call for details. For people 50 years and older.

8978 State of Vermont
Vermont Deptartment of Aging
103 S Main Street
Weeks Building
Waterbury, VT 05671-1601
802-241-2388
Fax: 802-241-1363
www.vermont.gov/dial

Patrick Flood, Manager

The Green Mountain Passport entitles Vermont residents free day use admission to any state park and its programs. Other benefits are included. For people 62 years and older.

8979 State of West Virginia
West Virginia Commission on Aging
1900 Kanawha Blvd East
Charleston, WV 25305
304-558-3317
Fax: 304-558-5609
www.wvseniorservices.gov

The Golden Mountaineer Discount Card provides discounts to over 3,500 participating merchants and professionals in the state. For people 60 years and older.

8980 Tennessee Department of Tourist Development
312 Rosa L. Parks Avenue
13th Floor
Nashville, TN 37243

615-741-2159
Fax: 615-741-7225; *Toll Free:* 888-836-6200
tourdev@state.tn.us
state.tn.us/tourdev

Susan Whitaker, Commissioner
Laura Heatherly, Exec. Assistant To Commissioner
Cindy Dupree, Public Information Officer

8981 Utah Travel Council
300 N State Street
Council Hall/Capitol Hill
Salt Lake City, UT 84114
801-538-1030
Fax: 801-538-1399; *Toll Free:* 800-200-1160
travel@utah.com
www.utah.com

Leigh Von Der Esch, Managing Director
David Williams, Deputy Dir./Marketing Research
Tracie Cayford, Dep. Dir./ Comm. & Operations

The Utah Office of Tourism promotes tourism into the state through advertising and media contacts. We are an office within the Governor's office of Economic Development. Our mission is to improve the quality of life of Utah citizens through revenue and tax relief, by increasing the quality and quantity of tourism visits and spending.

8982 Virginia Department of Economic Development Division of Tourism
901 E Byrd Street
Richmond, VA 23219-4052
804-771-9500
Fax: 804-786-1919; *Toll Free:* 800-847-4882
vainfo@helloinc.com
www.virginia.org

Gina M Burgin

8983 Washington State Tourism
PO Box 42500
Olympia, WA 98504-2500
360-753-5601
Fax: 360-753-4470; *Toll Free:* 800-544-1800
tourism@cted.wa.gov
www.tourism.wa.gov

Kristin Jacobson, Public Relations

8984 West Virginia Division of Tourism
90 MacCorkle Ave. SW
Charleston, WV 25305-2216
304-558-2200
Fax: 304-558-0108; *Toll Free:* 800-225-5982
www.state.wv.us/tourism

Mission is to cultivate a world-class travel and tourism industry in West Virginia through creation of jobs, stimulation of investment, expansion of current tourism attractions and promotion of a postive state image, thereby improving the way of life for West Virginians.

8985 Wisconsin Department of Tourism
201 W Washington Avenue
Po Box 8690
Madison, WI 53708-8690
608-266-2161
Fax: 608-266-3403; *Toll Free:* 800-432-8747
tourinfo@travelwisconsin.com
www.tourism.state.wi.us

Mary Burke, Manager

8986 Wyoming Division of Tourism
I-25 & College Drive
Cheyenne, WY 82002
307-777-7777
Fax: 307-777-2877; *Toll Free:* 800-225-5996
www.wyomingtourism.org

Alan Dibberley, Manager

Tours & Services

8987 Accessible Journeys
35 West Sellers Avenue
Ridley Park, PA 19078-2113
610-521-0339
Fax: 610-521-6959; *Toll Free:* 800-846-4537
www.disabilitytravel.com

Howard Mccoy III, Director
Deborah Hoover, Associate Director

Tour operator for slow walker and wheelchair travelers offering tours to culturally intriguing destinations like Africa, China, Brazil, Alaska and Hawaii. Also offers a quarterly newsletter.

8988 Addie's You & I Travel Service
7545 NE Sandy Boulevard
Portland, OR 97213-6461
503-282-7545
Fax: 503-828-2479; *Toll Free:* 800-342-5500
www.addiesyouanditravel.com

Addie Lindstrom, Contact

Arrange travel for all special needs.

8989 America West/US Airways Airline
4000 E Sky Harbor Boulevard
Phoenix, AZ 85034-3802
480-693-0800
www.usairways.com

Diana Lawson, Contact
W Douglas Parker, CEO

This airline trains employees to make sure that passengers with disabilities enjoy convenient, safe and comfortable travel.

8990 American Hotel and Motel Association
1201 New York Avenue NW
Washington, DC 20005-3931
202-289-3100
Fax: 202-289-3199
eiinfo@ahla.com
www.ahla.com

Joseph McInerney, President/CEO
Pam Inman, Executive VP/COO
Joori Jeon, Executive VP/CFO

Will disseminate information, develop and conduct a series of seminars for the hotel and motel industry at state-level association conferences, and develop and distribute an ADA Compliance handbook for use by the lodging industry.

8991 Anglo California Travel Service
4250 Williams Road
San Jose, CA 95129-3344

408-257-2257
Fax: 408-257-2664
www.anglocalifornia.com

Helen Jones, Contact
Audrey Cooper, President

Plans for one and two week accessible tours.

8992 B&A Travel
701 S University Avenue
Carbondale, IL 62901-2894
618-549-7347
Fax: 618-457-0241
www.batravel.com

Dave Coracy, Contact

Arranges wheelchair travel.

8993 Bill Dvorak Kayak & Rafting
17921 Us Highway 285
Nathrop, CO 81236-9701
719-539-6851
Fax: 719-539-3378; *Toll Free:* 800-824-3795
info@dvorakexpeditions.com
www.dvorakexpeditions.com

Bill Dvorak, Contact
Jaci Dvorak, Contact

Rafting and kayak trips for mobility limitations.

8994 Charlie Brown's Goodtime Travel
1465 North Union Blvd.
Colorado Springs, CO 80909
719-635-8992
Fax: 719-635-0045
www.cbgt.com

Sandy Stern, Contact
Charlie Brown, Owner

Arranges travel for all limitations.

8995 Classic Hawaii
5893 Rue Ferrari
San Jose, CA 95138
408-287-4550
Fax: 408-287-9272; *Toll Free:* 800-635-1333
www.classicvacations.com

Paula Schneider, Contact
Greg Brockway, President

Offer accessible tours to Hawaii.

8996 Diabetic Cruise Desk
Hartford Holiday Travel
129 Hillside Avenue
Williston Park, NY 11596
516-746-6670
Fax: 516-746-6690; *Toll Free:* 800-828-4813
www.hartfordholidays.com

Offers a seven-day cruise to Alaska for people with diabetes. Includes seminars on diabetes, self management, planning, special guidance for exercise classes and individual dietary advice.

8997 Easter Seals Project ACTION
1425 K Street NW
Suite 200
Washington, DC 20005-3956
202-347-3066
Fax: 202-737-7914; *Toll Free:* 800-659-6428

project_action@easterseals.com
www.projectaction.org
TDD 202-347-7385
TTY: 202-347-7385

Alan Abeson, Director
Liz Moore, Communication/Mktging Mgr
Joseph Romer, Vice President

A national technical assistance program designed to improve access to transportation services for people with disabilities and assist transit providers in implementing the Americans with Disabilities Act.

8998 Elderhostel
11 Avenue de Lafayette
Boston, MA 02111
877-426-8056
Fax: 877-426-2166; Toll Free: 800-454-5768
www.elderhostel.org

Non-profit organization dedicated to providing exceptional learning opportunities to adults at a remarkable value. As the nation's first, and the world's largest, edcuational travel organiztion primarily for adults, we believe that learning is an integral part of a healthy and fulfilling life.

8999 Elderhostel Institute Network
PO Box 1959
Wakefield, MA 01880-5959
617-426-7788
Fax: 617-426-0549
www.elderhostel.org

Elderhostel Institute Network is a voluntary association of over 200 Institutes for Learning in Retirement (I.L.R.). An I.L.R. is a community based organization of retirement age learners dedicated to meeting the educational interests of its members.

9000 Empress Directions Unlimited (Acccessible Tours)
123 Green La
Bedford Hills, NY 10507-1534
914-241-1700
Fax: 914-241-0243; Toll Free: 800-533-5343
lawebmaster@la.gov

Lois Bonanni, Director

Arranges vacations throughout the world for all disabilities including accessible cruises, African safari, rafting and scuba diving.

9001 Environmental Traveling Companions
Fort Mason Center Building
San Francisco, CA 94123
415-474-7662
Fax: 415-474-3919
info@etctrips.org
www.etctrips.org

Diane Poslosky, Executive Director
Deb Glazer, Development Director
Davido Crow, River Program Manager

Aids travelers regardless of physical or financial limitations to experience the beauty and challenge of the wilderness.

9002 Flying Wheels Travel
143 W Bridge Street
Owatonna, MN 55060-2917

507-451-5005 Toll free: 800-535-6790
bjacobson@ll.net
www.flyingwheelstravel.com

Barbara Jacobson, Contact

Arranges travel for persons with mobility limitations.

9003 Galludet University/Alumni House
800 Florida Avenue NE
Washington, DC 20002-3600
202-250-2590
Fax: 202-651-5062
www.gallaudet.edu

Erving King Jordan, President

Offers tours with ASL interpreters for the deaf and hearing-impaired.

9004 General Motors Mobility Program for Travelers with Disabilities
GM Mobility Program
PO Box 09011
Detroit, MI 48209
Toll Free: 800-323-9935

9005 Green Tortoise Adventure Travel
494 Broadway
San Francisco, CA 94133-4515
415-834-1000
Fax: 415-956-4900; Toll Free: 800-867-8647

Gardner Kent, Owner

Bus travel with experience for travelers who have mobility impairments.

9006 Handi-Cabs of the Pacific
PO Box 22428
Honolulu, HI 96823-2428
808-946-6666
Fax: 808-946-6676
www.handicabs.com

Craig Kimura, General Manager
Nick Comsa, Owner

Wheelchair taxi and tour company. All vehicles have ramps.

9007 Hinsdale Travel Service
201 E Ogden Avenue
Hinsdale, IL 60521-3633
630-325-1335
Fax: 630-325-1342; Toll Free: 888-325-1357
inquiries@hinsdaletravel.com
www.hindsdaletravel.com

Laurie Karhun, Owner
Cindy Kovacik, Agent

Offers specialized assistance for independent travel or tours for persons with disabilities including cruises and travel in the USA and abroad.

9008 House of Travel
1107 L Street
Sacramento, CA 95814-3995
916-442-0743
Fax: 916-442-5656; Toll Free: 800-444-9996
www.houseoftravel.co.nz

Ann Hilderbrand, Contact
Anita Van Der Zanden, Owner

Arranges travel for all limitations.

9009 Journeys East
2443 Fillmore Street
289k
San Francisco, CA 94115-1814
415-647-9565
Fax: 510-601-1977; Toll Free: 800-527-2612

Davis Everett, Co-Director

Specializes in backcountry trips to Japan with hands on experience staying in Japanese inns and temples. All trips open to persons with disabilities but type of disability may preclude joining certain trips.

9010 Kayak and Rafting Expeditions
17921 U.S. Highway 285
Nathrop, CO 81236
719-539-6851
Fax: 719-539-3378; Toll Free: 800-824-3795
info@dvorakexpeditions.com
www.dvorakexpeditions.com

Bill Dvorak, President
Jaci Dvorak, VP

This organization does river trips for people who are deaf, visually impaired, physically or mentally disabled. Rafting trips with groups and families and whitewater instruction.

9011 Kon Tiki Travel Agency
7906 5th Avenue
Brooklyn, NY 11209-4510
718-748-7400
Fax: 718-238-3604; Toll Free: 800-822-5838
gerd@kontiki-travel.com
www.norhouse.com/kontiki.asp

Mary Mosleh, Contact
Gerd Bjorgan, Owner

Tours for hearing-impaired. Interpreters available.

9012 MedEscort International
ABE International Airport
PO Box 8766
Allentown, PA 18105-8766
610-791-3111
Fax: 610-791-9189; Toll Free: 800-255-7182
medescort@fast.net
www.medescort.com

Diane Horvath, Director
Craig Poliner, President

Offers specially trained escorts for individuals who cannot travel alone due to age or disability.

9013 Melwood Access Adventures
5606 Dower House Road
Upper Marlboro, MD 207772
301-599-8000
Fax: 301-599-0180
services@melwood.org
www.melwood.org

Andrew V Colevas, Chairman Of The Board
Frank O Coombs, Business Executive
Stanley J Botts, Director

A year round recreation facility that serves mentally and physically disabled individuals, offers a variety of vacations, outdoor recreation, travel and respite care.

9014 Monte Travel
4127 Hylan Boulevard
Staten Island, NY 10308-3308
718-987-6900
Fax: 718-980-2158

Ann Marie Colombo, Owner

Arranges travel for all special needs.

9015 Nantahala Outdoor Center
13077 Highway 19 W
Bryson City, NC 28713-9165
828-488-2176
Fax: 828-488-2498; Toll Free: 800-232-7238
rafting@noc.com
www.noc.com

Jennifer Petosz, Advertising Coordinator
Payson Kennedy, CEO

Nantahala Outdoor Center, the leader in outdoor recreation and education for over 27 years, strongly encourages and supports participants with disabilities. We offer whitewater rafting adventures on six rivers in the Southeast for all skill and thrill levels, also kayak and canoe adaptive instruction. NOC will tailor a whitewater program to your skill and ability level, modify the gear, and pace instruction for you.

9016 National Association of Traveling Nurses
PO Box 35189
Chicago, IL 60707-189
708-453-0080
Fax: 708-453-0083

Richard Johnson, President

Members of the medical profession. Provides travel information. Offers substantial discounts for members at major hotels, resorts, and car rental agencies. Provides members with complete list of approved travel industry suppliers, including travel agents, vendors, airlines, cruise ship companies, and hotels.

9017 National Tour Association: Travel Division
546 East Main Street
Lexington, KY 40508-2342
859-226-4444
Fax: 859-226-4414; Toll Free: 800-682-8886
joinnta@ntastaff.com
www.ntaonline.com

Provides callers with a list of tour companies who can accomodate the disabled on their escorted tours. Hours: 8:00 a.m. to 5:00 p.m. Monday-Friday.

9018 Northridge Travel
9700 Reseda Boulevard
Northridge, CA 91324-2099
818-886-2000
Fax: 818-885-8229; Toll Free: 800-842-8880
www.northridgetravel.com

Helen Reiter, Contact
Teresa Tsent, Owner

One of the leading Travel Management Companies in the San Fernando Valley. It was established in 1962 and has grown from 2 to more than 48 employees.

9019 Odyssey Club
2950 SE Stark Street
Portland, OR 97214-3082
503-233-9961 Toll free: 800-452-4100

Provides tours all over the world for people over age 55. Member of the Society for the Advancement of Travel for the Handicapped.

9020 Professional Respite Care
Act for Health
1385 S Colorado Boulevard
Denver, CO 80222-3304
303-757-4808
Fax: 303-757-3821

Kevin Volmer, Owner

Offers travel accompaniment services for disabled persons or senior citizens.

9021 Reid & Hurley Travel
710 West Street
Braintree, MA 02184-3833
617-380-8778
Fax: 617-380-7809

Susan Packenham, Contact

Annual tour for those with severe breathing disorders.

9022 River Odysseys West (Row)
314 E Garden Avenue
Po Box 579
Coeur D Alene, ID 83814
208-765-0841
Fax: 208-667-6506; Toll Free: 800-451-6034
info@rowadventures.com
www.rowadventures.com

Peter Grubb, Owner

Offers one to six day rafting trips to physically disadvantaged people. Designs custom itineraries, or trips with a special focus for small groups. For those with special dietary needs, they prepare special meals. Free brochure upon request.

9023 Rodeway Inns
10750 Columbia Pike
Silver Spring, MD 20901-4427
301-592-5000Toll free: 800-228-2000

Marni Altschuler, Contact
Charles A Ledsinger Jr, CEO

This organization has a limited number of rooms for the handicapped with extra wide doors and special bathroom assist bars.

9024 Sheridan Travel Service
7200 W Alameda Avenue
W4
Lakewood, CO 80226-3210
303-238-7111Toll free: 800-444-4334
sheridantravel@vacation.com
www.sheridantravel.com
TDD 303-936-8599

Tuttles Manley, Contact
Thea Foley, Owner

Travel and tours for hearing-impaired.

9025 Shilo Inns & Resorts
11707 NE Airport Way
Portland, OR 97220-1075
503-252-7500
Fax: 503-254-0794; Toll Free: 800-222-2244
www.shiloinns.com

Offers handicapped-assist rooms including larger bathrooms equipped with assistance railings and wheelchair access. Please call for property specifics.

9026 Sports 'n Spokes
Paralyzed Veterans of America
2111 E Highland Avenue
Suite 180
Phoenix, AZ 85016-4756
602-224-0500
Fax: 602-224-0507; Toll Free: 888-888-2201

Cliff Crase, Editor
Sherri Shea, Advertising Manager

Magazine covering wheelchair sports and recreation news.
Frequency: Bimonthly

9027 Sue Smith Travel Service
3806 Jfk Boulevard
North Little Rock, AR 72116-8248
501-771-0987
Fax: 501-984-6191
www.suesmithvacations.com

Donna Brown, Owner
Mike Wilkinson, Owner

Established library service for disabled travelers in the area.

9028 Sundial Special Vacations
Sundial Tours
2609 Highway 101 N
Suite 103
Seaside, OR 97138-6845
503-738-3324
Fax: 503-738-3369; Toll Free: 800-547-9198
www.sundialtour.com

Jill Conner Ross, Tour Operations Director/Owner
Patsy Conner, Owner
Nancy Wyse, Tour Leader

Provides special vacations for developmentally disabled persons. Provides quality vacations for persons with developmental disabilities. Ratio is 1 for 7 or 1 for 5 depending on tour. Only two people to a room. Exciting destinations. 3 to 4 star properties.

9029 Travel Companion Exchange
PO Box 633
Amityville, NY 11701-633
631-454-0880
www.whytravelalone.com

Eul Lee, Contact

Networks divorced, widowed and single individuals in the US and Canada for leisure activities and travel.

9030 Travel Trends
9500 Topega Boulevard
Chatsworth, CA 91311
818-576-0500
Fax: 818-576-0520
www.traveltrends.biz
TDD 818-993-5250

Kevin Mills, Contact

Tours for hearing-impaired.

9031 Travelers Aid Society
1612 K Street NW
Suite 506
Washington, DC 20006-2849
202-546-0599
Fax: 202-546-1625
www.travelersaid.org

Raymond M Flint, President
Michael S Oring Esq., VP Local Programs
Martha A Morris, Dir. Development & Comm.

Provides crisis intervention and casework services, limited financial assistance, protective travel assistance and information and referrals for travelers, transients and newcomers.

9032 Travelfair
320 Main Street
Islip, NY 11751-3414
631-581-4040
Fax: 631-581-4044

Kenneth Reinert, Contact

Arranges travel for all disabilities.

9033 Travelin' Talk Newsletter
PO Box 3534
Clarksville, TN 37043-3534
931-552-6670
Fax: 931-552-1182

Rick Crowder, Founder

Updates members on the progress of the Travelin' Talk network. A network which introduces numerous sources to travelers, shares tips and stories of ways people are helping travelers with disabilities, and helps members get to know each other better and establish new-found friendships.

8 pages Frequency: Quarterly

9034 US SERVAS
1125 16th Street
Suite 201
Arcata, CA 95521-5585
707-825-1714
Fax: 707-825-1762
info@usservas.org
www.usservas.org

Nancy Mitchell, Board Chair
Judy Sears, Office Staff

International network that links travelers with hosts in 130+ countries with the hope of building world peace through understanding and friendship.

9035 Wheelchair Getaways
7276 Narcoossee Rd
Orlando, FL 32822
407-281-8369Toll free: 800-536-5518
www.wheelchairgetaways.com

Mike Nilan, Contact
Joe Bobalik, Owner

Van rentals.

9036 Wilderness Inquiry
808 14th Ave SE
Minneapolis, MN 55414-1516
612-676-9400
Fax: 612-676-9401; *Toll Free:* 800-728-0719
info@wildernessinquiry.org
www.wildernessinquiry.org

Greg Lais, Executive Director
Greta Arnquist, Registration Manager

Allows people of all ages and abilities to share the adventure of wilderness travel. This nonprofit organization was formed in 1978 and conducts tours to some of the most beautiful and remote parts of the world.

9031 **Travelers Aid Society**
1612 K Street NW
Suite 506
Washington, DC 20006-2808
202-546-0500
Fax 202-546-1625
www.travelersaid.org

Ramona M. Finn, President
Manuel S. Ortiz, Esq., VP Board Programs
Martha A. Morris, Dir. Development & Const.

Provides crisis intervention and casework services, limited financial assistance, protective travel assistance and information and referrals for travelers, runaways and newcomers.

9032 **Travelout**
320 Main Street
Islip, NY 11251-3414
631-581-3414
631-581-4040
Fax 631-581-4049

Kenneth Rivera, Contact

Arranges travel for all disabilities.

9033 **Travelin' Talk Newsletter**
PO Box 8534
Clarksville, TN 37040-3534
931-552-6670
Fax 931-552-1182

Rick Crowder, Founder

Updates members on the progress of the Travelin' Talk network. A network which introduces numerous sources to travelers, shares tips and stories of ways people are helping travelers with disabilities, and helps members get to know each other better and establish a new found friendship.

9034 **US SERVAS**
1125 16th Street
Suite 201
Arcata, CA 95521-5585
707-825-1714
Fax 707-825-1704
info@usservas.org
www.usservas.org

Nancy Ziegler, Board Chair
... Sowle, Office Mgr.

International network that links travelers with hosts in 130+ countries with the hope of building world peace through understanding and friendship.

9035 **Wheelchair Getaways**
7970 Narcoossee Rd
Orlando, FL 32822
407-281-8850 Toll free, 800-536-5518
www.wheelchairgetaways.com

Mike, Tran, Contact
Joe Bobula, Owner

Rentals.

9036 **Wilderness Inquiry**
808 14th Ave SE
Minneapolis, MN 55414-1516
612-676-9400
Fax 612-676-9401, Toll free 800-728-0719
info@wildernessinquiry.org
www.wildernessinquiry.org

Greg Lais, Executive Director
Gavin Vaughn, Reservation Manager

Allows people of all ages and abilities to share the adventure of wilderness travel. This nonprofit organization was formed in 1978 and conducts tours to some of the most beautiful and remote parts of the world.

Glossary of Health & Medical Terms

DISEASES

Abnormal PAP Smear: The Papanicolaou (Pap) smear is the most effective screening test for cervical cancer. The Pap smear is usually performed by a physician during a gynecologic examination. A wooden instrument is used to collect brushings from the cervix, which are then analyzed for abnormal cells that could be early signs of cervical cancer. An abnormal pap smear is one that has cells on it that are suspicious for infection, inflammation, or cancer.

Acute Stress Reaction: An Acute Stress Reaction or Nervous Breakdown is an emotional event that causes a significant, and at times prolonged, physiologic response felt by the body. Constant Stress can contribute to and create medical illness and physical consequences.

Asthma: Asthma or Reactive Airway Disease is a medical disease that is caused by airway inflammation and hyperactivity in the lungs. Reactive Airway Disease is a more general category that includes allergic and occupational triggers for this airway inflammation and reactivity.

Breast Cancer: A common disease of women where a portion of the breast tissue transforms into cancer, and then the cancer can spread to other parts of the body. Breast cancer can be detected early with routine physical examination and surveillance mammograms.

Cervical Cancer: Cervical cancer is a condition where a cancerous growth (also called a malignancy) arises on of the lower portion of the uterus. Cervical cancer only occurs in women. Cervical cancer can be prevented through screening Pap Smears.

Colon Cancer: Colon cancer is a condition where a cancerous growth (also called a malignancy) arises out of the large intestine. Colon cancer is a common cancer in both men and women. Screening tests for Colon cancer include colonoscopies, flexible sigmoidoscopies, and fecal occult blood cards. Colon cancer is many cases can be prevented by identifying precancerous colon polyps and removing them.

Colon Polyps: Colon polyps are growths that form in the large intestine that can be precancerous. There are many types of polyps and not all of them are the type that lead to colon cancer. Colon polyps are quite often

hereditary and can cause microscopic bleeding into the bowels.

Coronary Artery Disease: A disease where cholesterol-like plaque builds up in the heart blood vessels leading to restricted blood flow and oxygen delivery and thus resulting in heart attacks. The predominate risk factors for CAD are high blood pressure, smoking, diabetes, family history of CAD, and elevated cholesterol levels.

Depression: Depression or Mood-related disorder is a medical disease of mood problems stemming from changes in brain chemistry resulting in significant relationship, occupational, and lifestyle consequences. Other mood disorders are bipolar disorder and mania.

Diabetes: A disease where the body loses the ability to control blood sugar levels. Diabetics are at high risk for heart attacks, blindness, kidney failure, and nerve damage. Diabetics can control their disease with diet, exercise, and medications.

Diabetes of Pregnancy: A condition of abnormal blood sugar regulation that occurs only during pregnancy. Individuals with this diagnosis during pregnancy are at higher risk to develop adult onset diabetes in the future.

Diabetic Protein loss in urine: Diabetes is a condition where the blood sugar is not regulated appropriately by the body resulting in increased blood glucose levels. Overtime, diabetes can cause eye disease, kidney disease, and nerve disease. An early sign of diabetic kidney disease is protein loss in the urine. This can be tested on a routine urinalysis.

Gastric Cancer: Gastric cancer is a condition where a cancerous growth (also called a malignancy) arises in the stomach. Gastric cancer risk factors include both dietary and infectious causes.

Glaucoma: Glaucoma is a condition of increased pressure in the eye. More specifically, the Intraocular pressure is elevated, which can lead to nerve damage and blindness. Glaucoma does run in families. Glaucoma can be treated to reduce the eye pressures and prevent vision loss.

Hearing Deficiency: Hearing deficiency is a common, under diagnosed condition. Routine audiogram tests can measure baseline hearing ability. Hearing loss can result from infection, age, trauma, and noise exposure.

Heavy Menstrual Flow: Heavy menstrual flow is a difficult condition to measure. Every woman's monthly cycle is different in frequency and amount of blood flow. Heavy menstrual flow is defined as bleeding for more than 6 days straight and more than 4-6 pads per day, but a physician's judgment of the flow pattern defines it more subjectively as light, moderate, or heavy.

High Blood Pressure: High blood pressure (also called Hypertension) is a condition of elevated pressures in the blood vessels. The blood pressure measurement is composed of a systolic (top number) and a diastolic (bottom number). High blood pressure is defined as a pressure above 140/90. High blood pressure is a significant risk factor for heart disease.

High Cholesterol: High cholesterol (also called Hyperlipidemia) is a condition of elevated cholesterol in the blood. The blood total cholesterol panel is composed of the LDL-cholesterol (bad cholesterol), the HDL-cholesterol (good cholesterol), the cholesterol ratio (Total cholesterol/HDL), and the triglycerides. The goal cholesterol value depends on the medical history, family history, and health status, but is generally accepted as an LDL -cholesterol of less than 130.

High Risk Pregnancy: A pregnancy, where because of a specific health history of the mother or child, the risk of birth defects or complications is increased. Prenatal interventions can lessen this risk in some cases.

Hypogonadal: Hypogonadism is a condition where the body does not produce adequate amounts of sex hormone. For example, men that have a testosterone deficiency are hypogonadal. Women can also suffer from hypogonadism.

Iron Deficiency Anemia: Anemia is a condition where the body's red blood cell count is low. The most common cause of anemia is Iron Deficiency. This condition is much more common in women than men. Women with heavy menstrual flows are at risk for developing Iron Deficiency Anemia.

Medically Overweight: Medically overweight is defined as being more than 10% above your ideal body weight. A formula called the Body Mass Index (BMI) offers a numeric BMI score based on height and weight variables. BMI scores over 26 are suggestive of being medically overweight.

Melanoma: Melanoma is a dangerous cancer arising from cells in the skin, usually from a nevus (also called a mole). Pigmented skin lesions that change in size, color, borders, or shape should be evaluated by a physician.

Osteoporosis: Osteoporosis is a condition where an excessive loss of calcium from the bones results in an increased risk of fractures. Osteoporosis usually affects the hips and spine of both men and women. Exercise, calcium supplements, and some medications can help prevent osteoporosis.

Prostate Cancer: A common disease of men where the prostate gland transforms into cancerous tissue, and then the cancer can spread to other parts of the body. Prostate cancer can be detected early by screening strategies with digital rectal exams (DRE) and prostate specific antigen (PSA) testing.

Skin Cancer: Skin cancer is a condition where a cancerous growth arises out of the skin. The most common type is called a basal cell carcinoma which commonly occurs on the face or back. Most Skin cancers are related directly to sun exposure. Melanoma and squamous cell carcinoma are other common skin cancers.

Stroke: A stroke (also called a cerebral vascular accident (CVA)) is a condition where an area of the brain does not get the blood flow it needs resulting in permanent brain damage in that area. Strokes can be life threatening. Smoking, diabetes, and high blood pressure increase the risk of stroke.

Testicular Cancer: Testicular cancer is a condition where a cancerous growth (also called a malignancy) arises out of the male testes. This cancer occurs usually in young men and is picked up by self examination. Testicular cancer can be cured with surgery and radiation if it is caught early.

Thyroid Disease: Thyroid disease results from too much or too little thyroid hormone. The thyroid gland manufactures all of the body's thyroid hormone. Any condition that affects the thyroid gland can also affect the secretion of thyroid hormone. Thyroid diseases can run in families.

SCREENINGS

5-Day Blood Pressure Check: A five-day blood pressure check is a series of blood pressure readings performed on 5 different days in both arms to get an average as to a person's blood pressure readings. Usually individuals, who take a high blood pressure medication, get a five-day blood pressure check done once a year to make sure that their medication(s)work to control their blood pressure.

Blood Pressure: A qualified healthcare provider can use a blood pressure cuff and a stethoscope to measure a person's blood pressure.

Blood Thyroid Level: The TSH (Thyroid Stimulating Hormone) blood test is a measure of thyroid gland function. The TSH level helps physicians evaluate the body's overall thyroid status.

Bone Density Scan: Bone Density scanning can be performed by many different machines. These machines screen a person's bones for their calcium content and overall strength. The DXA Scan (also called Dual X-ray Absorptionmetry) is the most accurate and reliable measure for osteoporosis.

Cholesterol: A fasting blood test that measures the cholesterol levels in the blood. This measurement includes the total cholesterol value as well as the break down of good (HDL) and bad (LDL) cholesterols and triglyceride level.

Clinical Breast Exam: A complete manual examination of both breasts looking for suspicious nodules or masses performed by an experienced healthcare provider. This exam includes examination of all the breast tissue and the surrounding lymph nodes.

Clinical Testicular Exam: A clinical testicular exam is a full examination of the testicles for any suspicious masses by a qualified healthcare provider.

Colonoscopy: A Colonoscopy is a procedure performed by a gastroenterologist where a fiber optic tube with a camera on the end is inserted into the large intestine. The colonoscopy helps to prevent colon cancer by identifying any polyps or lesions that could become cancerous.

Complete Blood Count: A complete blood count (CBC) is a measure of the quantity and the concentration of the white blood cells, red blood cells, hemoglobin, and platelets found in the bloodstream.

Dental Exam: A dental examination is performed by a licensed dentist who exams the mouth for cavities, injured teeth and gum disease. Often a dental x-ray Is part of this routine examination.

Diabetic Foot Exam: A frequently neglected portion of the physical examination where the soles and forefoot of diabetes are examined for signs of infection, nerve disease, or other diabetic problems.

Digital Rectal Exam: A part of the physical examination where a healthcare provider inserts a gloved finger into the anus. This exam can detect prostate nodules, prostate cancer, and also rectal polyps and hemorrhoids.

EKG: An electrocardiogram, or EKG (also called an ECG by some), is a tracing of a 12 lead electronic signature of the heart. The heart emits an electronic impulse with each contraction and this registers on the EKG tracing as a waveform. These EKG "waves" can show evidence of heart enlargement, asynchrony, and even heart attacks.

Exercise Treadmill Test: A treadmill cardiac stress test is a procedure used to diagnose coronary artery disease (CAD...also called heart disease) or measure a person's functional status. The treadmill test involves walking on a exercise treadmill while being hooked up to an EKG and vital sign monitoring.

Fasting Blood Glucose: The Fasting Blood Glucose Test (FBGT) is a measurement of the amount of sugar in the blood stream at baseline. Glucose is the primary source of energy for our body. The liver can manufacture glucose, but most sugar molecules are taken in through the diet. The muscles, brain, and other vital organs require a constant glucose source to function. Individuals with high fasting glucose levels are likely to be diabetic.

Fecal Occult Blood Test: An excellent screening test for colon cancer where a small sample of stool is examined for hidden blood content. Hidden blood loss in to the bowels could be an early sign of colon cancer or polyps.

Flexible Sigmoidoscopy: A flexible sigmoidoscopy is a procedure where a fiber optic tube with a camera on the end is inserted into the large intestine. This ""Flex Sig"" scope helps to prevent colon cancer by identifying any polyps or lesions that could become cancerous.

Hearing Test: A hearing test is a specialized audiogram performed in a hearing booth to measure bilateral hearing acuity.

Helicobacter Pylori Antibody Blood Test: The Helicobacter Pylori antibody blood test measures a person's blood for the presence of an antibody to the Helicobacter Pylori bacteria. Having this antibody suggests ongoing infection with this bacteria. Helicobacter Pylori infection has been associated with peptic ulcer disease and some forms of stomach cancer.

Hemoglobin A1C: A blood test for diabetics that reveals the average blood sugar values over the past 3 months. This test is used to monitor patients with diabetes and assess their level of disease control. The goal Hemoglobin A1C should be less than 7.

Intraocular Pressure (IOP) Test: Intraocular pressure (IOP) can be measured by the primary care physician or the eye doctor. There are several different methods of measuring the eye pressure depending on equipment. An elevated eye pressure can be a sign of glaucoma.

Mammogram: A compression X-Ray of the breast tissue looking for suspicious calcifications, lesions, masses or other early signs of breast cancer. Baseline mammograms are usually initiated on women age 35-40 years old.

Pap Smear: A gynecologic examination by a healthcare provider where the female reproductive tract is examined manually for abnormalities. At the same time, a small sample of tissue is removed from the cervix using a small wooden spatula (called the PAP Smear). This cervical tissue specimen is then examined for suspicious cell types that could be the early stages of cervical cancer.

Prostate Specific Antigen: A blood test, called a PSA (Prostate Specific Antigen), can be used to detect the presence of prostate cancer in early stages. In the right situation, this test can help to diagnose prostate cancer before it becomes life threatening.

Retinal Eye Exam: A mandatory annual examination for all diabetics where the back of the eye (Retina) is examined for diabetic changes that could lead to blindness. Diabetic eye disease is the number one cause of blindness in our country.

Self Breast Exam: A complete manual examination of both breasts looking for suspicious masses. This self-exam is to be performed each month by the individual.

Self Testicular Exam: A self testicular exam is a full examination of the testicles for any suspicious masses by the individual. Self Testicular examination should be done monthly.

Total Body Skin Exam: A full skin exam is a complete examination of all of a person's skin for suspicious skin lesions that could be skin cancer or precancerous growths. This full exam is usually performed by either a primary care physician or a dermatologist.

Urinalysis: A simple test run on a urine sample looking for the presence of glucose, protein, blood, or any signs of infection in the urine.

MEDICATIONS

ACE Inhibitor: ACE (Angiotensin Converting Enzyme) Inhibitors are a family of medications used to control high blood pressure. ACE Inhibitors have been found to be very beneficial in diabetes for preventing kidney disease and in heart disease for remodeling heart muscle after heart attacks.

Anti-Anxiety Medication: Medications in this category include Valium, Xanax, Ativan to name a few. Anti-anxiety medications assist in re-establishing ideal brain chemistry to control anxiety and counterproductive emotions of panic and fear.

Anti-Depressant Medication: Medications in this category include antidepressants, which assist in re-establishing ideal brain chemistry to aid in recovering from mood disorders, anti-anxiety medications, and other mood stabilizers (some examples include Prozac, Zoloft, Celexa, Xanax, Lithium, and Depakote).

Aspirin: Aspirin is an anti-inflammatory medication used to treat sore muscles, arthritis, and headaches. Aspirin also plays a critical role in heart disease prevention by thinning the blood for people at risk for heart attack.

Asthma Inhaler: Common Asthma medications include Albuterol, Proventil, Advair, and Asmacort meter dose inhalers (MDI's). These preparations are inhaled into the lungs periodically to dilate the airways. Some preparations include an anti-inflammatory component as well. Individuals with aggressive disease may additionally need nebulizer treatments or by mouth medications like steroids or Singular.

Calcium (1500 mg each day): Calcium is a mineral that is found in our body predominantly in our bones. Calcium is found in most dairy products and in fortified cereals and fruit juices. Men and women should take in at least 1000mg to 1500mg of calcium every day.

Contrast Dye: Iodine was a large component of contrast dye used in the past for intravenous contrast during CAT Scans and X-rays. Today, contrast dye has much less iodine and generally is very well tolerated by most people.

Folate (1mg each day): A vitamin, also known as Folic Acid, in the B vitamin family that is associated with reduced risk of birth defects, cardiac events, and improved cognitive function.

High Blood Pressure Medication: Medications used to treat hypertension. There are numerous families of high blood pressure medicines (i.e. diuretics, beta blockers, calcium blockers, ACE Inhibitors, etc.) Each family works quite well with rather few significant side effects.

High Cholesterol Medication: Medications used to control blood cholesterol levels. The family of medicines most commonly used is the STATINs of which there are several different varieties (i.e. atorvastatin, simvastatin, lovastatin, pravastatin, etc.) The goal is to have your LDL level, the bad cholesterol, under good control.

Iodine: Iodine was a large component of imaging dye used in the past for intravenous contrast during CAT Scans and X-rays. Today, these imaging dyes have much less iodine in them and generally are very well tolerated by most people. Some people, who are allergic to iodine will react to lobster, shrimp, and some shellfish.

Morphine: Morphine is a strong narcotic pain medication. This medication is usually given into the veins during a hospital stay to treat pain. Morphine can be given by injection for severe pain.

Penicillin: Penicillin is an antibiotic medication used to treat certain infections like strep throat and syphilis.

Prednisone: A steroid medication that functions as an anti-inflammatory for some specific medical conditions. It is frequently used in the short term for asthma, poison ivy, and some forms of arthritis. Long term therapy with prednisone increases the risk of diabetes, cataracts, and osteoporosis.

Sulfa Drugs: Sulfa drugs are a group of medications made up of mostly antibiotics, although a few diuretics are also in this family. Some people are allergic to sulfa, and thereby need to stay away from these sulfa based products.

Tamoxifen: A medication that is a hormonal treatment used to reduce the potential development of breast cancer in women with high-risk family histories of the disease. This medication is also used at times to treat breast cancer.

Testosterone: Testosterone is the male sex hormone. Too much or too little testosterone can cause medical problems. Women have trace amounts of testosterone manufactured in their bodies.

Tetracycline: Tetracycline is an antibiotic usually used for rosacea. Tetracycline is in the same family as doxycycline.

Vitamin D (400mg each day): Vitamin D is manufactured in our skin from a sunlight reaction. Vitamin D is found in the recommended daily allowance in most multivitamins and in conjunction with calcium supplements.

Vitamin E (400iu each day): Vitamin E is a well known anti-oxidant that is found in the recommended daily allowance in most multivitamins.

Glossary of Legal Terms

Activities of daily living (ADL)

Activities usually performed for oneself in the course of a normal day. Although definitions differ, ADLs are usually considered to be mobility (e.g., transfer from bed to chair), dressing, bathing, self-feeding and toileting.

People may need assistance with ADLs regardless of their living arrangements. Assistance to a person limited in his/her ADLs is customarily performed by a family member, a home health aide or attendant, or a nurse's aide in a nursing facility. The assistance is of a nonmedical nature, commonly characterized as personal care, custodial care or physical care. Assistance provided in a home setting may extend beyond ADLs and include such nonmedical activities as housekeeping (e.g., cleaning, cooking), laundry and shopping.

Medicare cannot be looked to, except to a limited extent, for coverage of assistance with ADLs. Medicare pays for acute care services and does not provide coverage for chronic personal or custodial care.

Medicaid, unlike Medicare, will cover Medicaid-eligible persons for many home care services including personal care, and in certain cases ancillary services such as housekeeping.

Adult guardian

The person appointed by a court, usually a probate court under a modern protective services statute, to perform the court-ordered tasks of caring for an incapacitated adult's financial affairs and/or personal needs.

Three different types of guardians have varying degrees of authority:

- *Plenary guardian* with total authority over personal and property matters;

- *Guardian of the person* with authority only over personal matters such as medical decisions and residential questions; and

- *Guardian of the estate* with authority over property only

Assisted living facility

Provides a combination of housing and personalized health care in a professionally managed group-living environment designed to respond to the individual needs of persons who require assistance with activities of daily living.

This type of facility is specifically designed to promote maximum independence and dignity in the most residential and homelike setting possible. It may be all or part of a building that houses a few or several hundred persons, or a distinct part of a residential campus. It traditionally serves the more frail resident who cannot or chooses not to live alone, but who does not require the 24-hour skilled or custodial care of a nursing home.

Generally, residents of this type of housing pay privately in the form of rent, rent plus service charge, and sometimes a deposit or entry fee. In some states, Medicaid will pay for certain ADL services under home and community-based service waivers. Medicaid will not pay for room and board charges. Private long-term care insurance may also be used for some of the provided services.

Licensure of this housing type varies by state, depending upon each state's own regulatory requirements. These facilities sometimes are called residential care homes, domiciliary care homes, personal care homes, adult congregate living facilities, homes for the aged, catered living facilities, or board and care homes.

Balance billing/Medicare

This term refers to health care providers charging patients for amounts above the Medicare-approved charge. By Federal law antedating the Balanced Budget Act of 1997, the maximum allowable charge (charge limit) may not exceed 115% of the Medicare-approved charge. A number of states — Connecticut, Massachusetts, Minnesota, New York, Ohio, Pennsylvania, Rhode Island and Vermont — have by state statute banned the practice of balance billing. Although the statutes have been challenged in Federal courts on preemption grounds, each has withstood the challenge.

Under the Balanced Budget Act of 1997 which created Medicare+Choice plans, health care providers may or may not be permitted to engage in the practice of balance billing — depending upon the type of plan, and whether or not the provider has a contract with the plan.

Providers under contract - Under all Medicare+Choice plans, except private fee-for-service (PFFS) plans, physicians and other health care providers who contract with a plan may not balance bill. However, a contracting physician or other health care provider under a PFFS contract that establishes a payment rate for services may balance bill (i.e., charge) for their services an amount not to exceed, including deductibles, coinsurance, copayments or other balance billing, 115% of such payment rate.

Providers not under contract - Under all Medicare+ Choice plans, except Medicare+ Choice medical savings accounts (MSA) and PFFS plans, noncontracting physicians or other health care providers may not balance bill, but must accept as payment in full from a Medicare+Choice plan enrollee, the amount that would have been paid under traditional Medicare fee-for-service arrangement. However, a noncontracting physician or other health provider under an MSA or PFFS plan may balance bill without limitation.

Bed hold/Medicaid, Medicare

Preservation of a nursing home bed when a nursing home resident is temporarily hospitalized or out of the facility on therapeutic leave. State Medicaid programs may pay for bed holds, but are not required to. Nursing facility residents on Medicaid have a right to return to the first available bed in the facility which they temporarily left, even if the state has not paid to hold their original bed.

Medicare does not itself pay to hold a bed; moreover, it prohibits facilities from taking payment from beneficiaries to hold a bed if the date of return is certain. If it is not certain, beneficiaries may pay.

Community spouse's resource allowance (CSRA)/Medicaid

The CSRA is an amount of resources that states must protect for the spouse of an institutionalized person seeking Medicaid coverage. It is determined by application of a formula, or, as explained below, through a fair hearing, or by court order. The CSRA may not be counted in determining the eligibility of an individual seeking Medicaid.

The CSRA is determined as follows:

(1) All nonexempt resources belonging to either member of the married couple will be pooled together regardless of who owns them, and regardless of marital property laws (e.g., equitable distribution laws, community property laws).

(2) The community spouse is entitled to an amount (community resource allowance), subject to paragraph 3 below, equal to the greater of:

- $19,824 (2000), as adjusted annually for inflation, or more, if a greater minimum amount is set by the state, or

- One-half the total resources of the couple to a maximum of $16,824 (2000), as adjusted annually for inflation.

(3) A state may establish a dollar amount which is both the minimum and maximum resource amount. Under the foregoing formula, $84,120 represents a maximum and $16,392 represents a minimum on the CSRA. A state, by opting to use the maximum resource amount, can establish $84,120 as both a maximum and minimum. A state may opt to select a spousal share amount which, in the alternative, is that sum (e.g., New York, $74,820) or a greater figure equal to one-half of the couple's resources, but not to exceed the maximum figure of $84,120.

(4) The CSRA amount is determined according to resources owned by the couple on the first day of a continuous period of institutionalization regardless of whether the institutionalized spouse applied for Medicaid at the time. Either spouse may ask the Medicaid agency to complete an assessment of their resources as of that time.

The CSRA can be increased above the formula amount in two ways:

- Either spouse can request a fair hearing in which to demonstrate that a larger amount of resources must be protected (i.e., transferred to the community spouse from the institutionalized spouse) to generate income needed to bring the community spouse's income up to the minimum monthly maintenance needs allowance.

- A court order granting a larger amount of resources for the community spouse; the order must be honored by the Medicaid agency.

Continuing care retirement community (CCRC)

This type of housing alternative, sometimes called a life care community, generally requires that an individual be able to live independently upon becoming a resident in the community. As a resident begins to need more assistance, specific additional services are made available. Most CCRCs offer three basic levels of housing on an as-needed basis: fully independent living, assisted living (personal care services) and skilled nursing care.

The basic idea of a CCRC is that once an individual becomes a resident, he/she never has to move again because any housing type and personal care services he/she will probably ever need are provided within the single campus setting. A CCRC guarantees housing and care across the continuum in that one community.

Generally, a CCRC will charge an entrance fee as well as a monthly payment for its residential, leisure and nursing services. In some cases, health care and personal care services can be paid for on an as-needed basis. The entrance fee, formerly nonrefundable, now is generally refundable on departure under a variety of specified conditions.

Basically, there are three types of CCRC contracts:

- *Extensive contract* - Covers shelter and residential services, amenities (e.g., swimming pool, possibly tennis courts and other types of recreation facilities) and unlimited long-term nursing care. The entrance fees and the monthly costs are usually higher than those under modified or fee-for-service contracts.

- *Modified or fee-for-service contract* - Provides shelter, residential services and amenities, plus a specified amount of nursing care, which the resident can obtain on an unlimited basis provided he/she pays for it at a daily or monthly nursing care rate.

- *Fee-for-service continuing care contract* - Covers shelter, meals, residential services and amenities, and in addition emergency and short-term nursing care. Access to long-term nursing care is provided only upon a daily nursing care rate.

Discharge planning

This service is usually performed by a social worker on staff in connection with a discharge of a patient from a hospital, nursing home or like institution. Discharge planning involves the social worker assessing the patient's level of functioning and needs following his/her discharge, including a smooth transition in moving from one level of care to another, for example from a hospital to a nursing home or from a hospital to home care. The discharge planner also contacts home health agencies to assist the patient in connection with his/her home care.

Estate recovery/Medicaid

Federal law mandates that each state place into effect an estate recovery program which provides for recovery of medical assistance to a Medicaid recipient. Mandated recovery centers mostly around the receipt by chronically ill individuals of long-term care services, although states may opt to recover Medicaid payments for other services rendered. The individuals and the assets subject to mandated recovery are set forth below.

1. Individuals subject to recovery - Recovery must be sought by the state from the following three categories of persons:

A. Permanently institutionalized individuals - These are individuals in nursing facilities, intermediate care facilities for the mentally retarded or other medical institutions where the state has determined that the individual cannot reasonably be discharged from the facility and return home.

B. Individuals age 55 and over - These individuals received from the state, through Medicaid, nursing home facility care, home and community-based services and related hospital and prescription drug services.

C. Individuals with certain state authorized insurance programs - These individuals received Medicaid assistance under provisions of a state law (not recognized by Medicaid law) that permits a disregard by Medicaid of assets because of purchase of long-term care insurance, known as a Robert Wood Johnson Foundation insurance plan. Exempted are those individuals in five states with such state laws, recognized by Medicaid law, that were in effect on May 14, 1993. These states are California, Connecticut, Indiana, Iowa and New York.

2. Assets subject to recovery - The assets of these three categories of individuals which are subject to state recovery are set forth below.

Recovery must be sought from the estates of these individuals, as the term is defined by state probate law. States may adopt a broader definition of estate than is defined in state probate laws to include jointly held property and other property in which the recipient had a legal interest at the time of death. All states, except the five states mentioned in section 1C above, are mandated to apply this broader definition to any individual who received Medicaid nursing facility and other long-term care services under a Robert Wood Johnson insurance plan.

Recovery cannot occur against an individual's assets until after the death of the surviving spouse, and until there are no blind or disabled children or children under age 21.

If a lien has been properly imposed upon a Medicaid recipient's homestead, the state must seek recovery upon the sale of the liened property, or from the estate of the recipient after he/she dies. In either case, the state may not seek recovery if the Medicaid recipient's spouse is alive, if blind or disabled children or children under age 21 are alive, nor if certain siblings or caretaker children reside in the house.

Recovery from a spouse who survived the Medicaid recipient is neither required nor authorized by Medicaid law. However, some state laws do authorize recovery from a surviving spouse's estate, though these laws have been challenged as being beyond the scope of and inconsistent with the Federal law.

In situations where recovery would work undue hardship, Federal law requires states to waive it.

Hospice care/Medicare

Hospice care is designed for terminally ill persons and is covered by Medicare Part A. Hospice programs will care for patients in a hospice facility or whenever possible in their homes and emphasize relieving pain and managing symptoms rather than undertaking curative procedures. An individual may elect to receive hospice care rather than regular Medicare benefits for the management of his/her illness. For routine home care, Medicare coverage is available for the level of care that is reasonable and necessary. For periods of crisis, Medicare will cover continuous home care, including nursing for up to 24 hours per day. The beneficiary need not be homebound. During a person's lifetime, Medicare pays for up to two 90-day periods of hospice care followed by an unlimited number of 60-day periods that the individual elects to receive hospice, provided the following four conditions are met:

- The attending physician — either in the employ of the hospice, or under contract with the hospice as an independent physician or part of an independent physicians group — and the medical director of the hospice must establish and periodically review a written plan for hospice care and at the beginning of each of the successive periods mentioned above, certify that a patient is terminally ill, i.e., that the patient's life expectancy is six months or less.

- The patient must elect to receive care from a hospice instead of standard Medicare medical benefits for the terminal illness. A patient may elect to revert to standard Medicare benefits, but will then be required to pay any applicable deductibles and copayments.

- Care must be provided by a Medicare-certified hospice program.

- The individual must be eligible for Part A benefits.

If these conditions are met, Medicare will pay for the following services:

- nursing services;

- doctors' services;

- drugs, including outpatient drugs for pain relief and symptom management;

- physical, occupational and speech-language therapy;

- home health aides and homemaker services;

- medical social services;

- medical supplies (including drugs and biologicals) and appliances;

- short-term inpatient care including respite care, procedures necessary for pain control, and acute and chronic symptom management;

- training and counseling for the patient and family members; and

- any other item or service which is specified in the plan mentioned above and for which payment may otherwise by paid by Medicare.

There is no deductible for these hospice care benefits. Copayments, however, are required for two benefits:

- prescription drugs for pain relief and symptom management, for which patients can be charged 5% of the reasonable cost, but no more than $5 per prescription; and

- respite care, for which a patient can be charged about $5 per day, depending on the area of the country.

Medicare+Choice organizations are not required to provide hospice services but may do so on a voluntary basis

Income cap states/Medicaid

Several states, referred to as income cap states, do not have a medically needy program serving nursing facility residents. In these states individuals are not allowed to spend down to the SSI income level (i.e., cap) to become eligible for Medicaid-covered nursing home care.

These states avail themselves of an optional Medicaid program termed the optional categorically needy program under which individuals are provided limited nursing facility coverage. Under this program individuals qualify for Medicaid nursing home coverage if their countable income does not exceed a cap of a prescribed percentage, usually 300%, of the SSI benefit for one person. The cap is categorically fixed and severe: one dollar of excess income above the cap will disqualify the individual. An individual is not permitted to spend down for medical expenses, nor can he/she forego collection of a pension, Social Security benefits or interest income in order to fall within the income cap.

A possible method for reducing the income of an individual seeking to qualify under the optional categorically needy program, also commonly referred to as the 300% program, is to obtain from a state court a Qualified Domestic Relations Order which allocates pension payments to the community spouse. The community spouse as the payee under such order arguably is the beneficiary of the pension, and payments to him/her would constitute his/her income under the name-on-the-check rule, not income of the institutionalized spouse who was the original pensioner.

Another method of qualifying for the optional categorically needy program is available under the provisions of OBRA '93. With this law Congress allowed individuals in income cap states to become eligible for Medicaid nursing home assistance by putting their income (e.g., pension, Social Security benefits) into a so-called Miller trust. During the Medicaid recipient's lifetime, all but a small portion of the money in the trust must go toward paying the nursing home bill. If any money remains in the trust after the recipient's death, it must be paid to the state, up to the amount of Medicaid assistance that was rendered.

The income cap states are Alabama, Alaska, Colorado, Delaware, Idaho, Mississippi, Nevada, New Mexico, Ohio, South Dakota and Wyoming.

Nursing home reform law

Sometimes referred to as OBRA '87, this Federal law regulating aspects of nursing homes is contained in the Omnibus Budget Reconciliation Act of 1987. It is the most comprehensive Federal nursing home law since the passage of Medicare and Medicaid in 1965. It sets Federal standards of care, including one stipulating that nursing homes may use physical and chemical restraints only in very specific circumstances and only after other interventions have been tried. The bill also establishes certain rights for patients and requires states and the Federal government to inspect nursing homes and to enforce standards through the use of a range of sanctions designed to promote compliance without forcing the relocation of residents due to the closing of facilities.

The resident's bill of rights, mandated in the nursing home reform law, includes a resident's rights to:

- admit and discharge oneself;

- control one's own medical care and be informed of all aspects of one's health;

- choose his/her own physician of own choice and refuse treatment;

- self-administer drugs;

- be free of restraints (physical or chemical);

- see all his/her medical records;

- receive notice of any decision to transfer or discharge or change a roommate;

- manage own financial affairs;

- receive visitors of one's choice as well as refuse visitors; and

- have access to a private telephone.

Transfers or discharges are permitted only under three situations:

- if necessary for the resident's welfare and if her/his needs cannot be met in the facility;

- if a resident's health has improved and he/she no longer needs care; or

- if a resident's presence or nonpayment of charges endangers the health and safety of other residents in the facility.

All residents, whether private pay or receiving Medicaid assistance or Medicare benefits, are entitled to due process, namely, a fair hearing. In this connection, the procedures for Medicaid fair hearings apply to nursing home transfers and discharges. The right to a pretransfer hearing is mandated except for emergency transfers subject to a resident's right to a bedhold pending a post-transfer hearing.

The law requires every resident to undergo a process known as preadmission, screening, and annual resident review. Prior to admission there is to be a functional evaluation, and at the time of admission a comprehensive care plan must be developed. This plan must be prepared annually with a physician and nursing team.

The law contains a number of other significant requirements. Nursing homes may not require as a condition for admission or for continuing stay a guarantee of payment from a third party. They must provide coverage by a registered nurse, not less than eight hours a day, seven days a week. Aides must go through a training program and pass a nursing aide registry certification. States are required to create a nursing aide registry to train, certify and maintain a listing of all approved workers.

Pourover will

The testator provides in his/her will that designated assets will be paid over and distributed to a previously established trust.

Program for all-inclusive care for the elderly (PACE)

Based on a model created by On Lok Senior Services in San Francisco, this program began as a Medicare and Medicaid demonstration project initially tested at ten sites. The Balanced Budget Act expanded PACE to become an option open to all states. PACE targets frail elderly persons living at home who are eligible for nursing home care. The program integrates health and long-term care services in an adult day care setting and uses a multidisciplinary case management team of providers, including physicians, nurses, social workers, nu-

tritionists, occupational and speech therapists, and health and transportation personnel. PACE participants are required to attend an adult day care center regularly.

Unlike the Social Health Maintenance Organization project, PACE providers in the demonstration project receive most of their funding from Medi-caid. The funding is allocated according to a fixed monthly capitated fee for each participant based on the frailty of enrollees. The project represents a test to link acute care under Medicare and long-term care under Medicaid.

The Balanced Budget Act of 1997 established PACE as a state option to furnish comprehensive health care to persons who are enrolled with an organization that has contracted to operate the PACE program, who are eligible for Medicaid, and who receive Medicaid solely through the PACE program. The salient characteristics of PACE offered as a state option are set forth below.

PACE providers may be public or private not-for-profit entities, except for those entities (up to 10) participating in the demonstration to test the operation of PACE by private, for-profit entities. During the three-year period beginning August 5, 1997, the Secretary of HHS is required to give priority to entities operating a PACE demonstration waiver program, and then to entities that have applied to operate a program as of May 1, 1997. The number of PACE program agreements that may be effective on August 5 of each year is limited. HCFA authorized up to 80 in 1999 and has limited increases by 20 for each following year.

Persons eligible for PACE must be 55 years of age or older; require nursing facility level of care that would be covered under a state's Medicaid program; reside in the service area of the PACE program; and meet such other eligibility conditions as may be imposed under the PACE program agreement. Eligible individuals include both Medicare and Medicaid beneficiaries. Medicare participants not enrolled in the PACE program through Medicaid must pay premiums equal to Medicaid capitation. PACE enrollees will be reevaluated annually to determine if they continue to need nursing facility level of care.

Under a PACE agreement, a provider at a minimum must provide eligible persons all care and services covered under Medicare and Medicaid. The services must be provided without any limitation or condition as to amount, duration and scope and without application of deductibles, copayments, coinsurance or other cost sharing that would otherwise apply under Medicare or Medicaid. The services must be provided 24 hours per day, every day of the year through a comprehensive multi-disciplinary health and social services delivery system which integrates acute and long-term services.

Primary medical care for a PACE enrollee must be furnished by a primary care physician who serves as a gatekeeper for access to treatment by specialists. HCFA may grant waivers of this requirement. A primary care physician, registered nurse, medical director, program director, other health professionals and a governing body to guide the operation must be part of the multi-disciplinary team.

States will make a prospective monthly capitation payment for each enrollee in an amount specified in the PACE agreement. PACE agreements are for one year, but may be extended for additional contract years at the discretion of the Secretary of HHS.

Qualified long-term care insurance contract

The Health Insurance Portability and Accountability Act of 1996 extends certain tax advantages to a qualified long-term care insurance contract, sometimes informally called a tax-qualified policy. The law defines such a contract as a guaranteed renewable life insurance contract or as a rider to a life insurance contract, under which the only insurance protection provided is coverage of qualified long-term care services. A qualified LTCI contract does not pay or reimburse expenses reimbursable by Medicare, except for coinsurance or deductible amounts. Nor may a qualified LTCI contract provide for a cash surrender value or other money that can be paid, pledged or borrowed. Further, certain consumer protection provisions set forth in the Long-term Care Services Model Regulations and Model Act of the National Association of Insurance Commissioners must be part of the contract.

To be qualified, LTCI contracts sold after January 1, 1997 must meet Federal standards explained above. Policies issued prior to this date that have met existing state standards are considered qualified policies though they may not meet the Federal requirements.

Qualified long-term care services

The Health Insurance Portability and Accountability Act of 1996 defines qualified long-term services as necessary diagnostic, preventive, therapeutic, curing, treating, mitigating and rehabilitative services and maintenance or personal care services which are required by a chronically ill individual and provided pursuant to a plan of care prescribed by a licensed health care provider. The phrase "maintenance or personal care services" means any care the primary purpose of which is the provision of needed assistance with any of the disabilities as a result of which the individual is chronically ill, including severe cognitive impairment. The cost of qualified long-term services can be counted as a medical expense deduction for income tax purposes.

Remainderman

This is a person or other entity designated in a trust as the beneficiary entitled to the principal or corpus of the trust after the income-paying stage comes to an end, that is after the income beneficiary of the trust has been paid in full in accordance with the terms of the trust.

Representative payee

Under Federal laws a representative payee may act as a surrogate on behalf of an individual who is not capable of making cognitive decisions, for the purpose of receiving and handling cash benefit checks of a Social Security or Supplemental Security Income recipient. The legal authority of the surrogate is usually limited to merely managing the benefits received for the well-being of the original beneficiary. A representative payee can be a public agency, nonprofit organization, bank or an individual.

The designation of a representative payee generally is a protective arrangement for incapacitated persons. It is less restrictive, simpler and less expensive than alternative protective arrangements such as guardianship or conservatorship and does not require a judicial finding of incompetency or incapacity. The arrangement can be terminated if the recipient regains cognitive ability to handle the government benefits to which he/she is entitled.

Reverse mortgage

A reverse equity mortgage allows senior citizens who are house rich and cash poor to obtain a loan based on the equity in their home. They retain title to their home as long as they continue to live there and receive nontaxable income which they can flexibly use for their own needs. According to the terms of most mortgages currently available, the loan, interest and other costs such as origination fees do not have to be paid back until the owner vacates the property through a move or death. Almost all reverse mortgages now provide a guarantee of lifetime tenancy. Most reverse mortgages are nonrecourse loans which means the lender can look only to the value of the home for repayment.

Payments to a home owner from a reverse mortgage can be in the form of a single lump sum of cash, regular monthly advances or a line of credit. New mortgage plans allow a combination of payment methods. The amount of the loan is seldom for the full value of the property; most lenders place minimum and maximum limits on the size of mortgages they are willing to establish. Loan periods can vary.

Some mortgages combine a reverse mortgage with an annuity, thereby guaranteeing individuals monthly income for their lifetime regardless of whether they continue to live in their homes or not. The monthly payments are considered annuity advances and thus partially taxable. For purposes of Medicaid edibility these payments may be counted as income.

Reverse mortgages are currently available in all states, except Texas, and the District of Columbia. Several different plans are available, some more widely than others. Plan features offered by the same lender can vary from state to state. The Home Equity Conversion Mortgage is federally insured through the U.S. Department of Housing and Urban Development and is the most widely available plan. In 1995 the Federal National Mortgage Association began a program called Home Keeper. The three main private for-profit plans are offered by Transamerica HomeFirst, Freedom House Equity Partners, and Household Senior Services.

Roth IRA

The Roth IRA, named after Senator Roth who created it under the Taxpayer Relief Act of 1997, is a nondeductible individual retirement account. Several significant differences exist between a traditional or deductible IRA and a Roth IRA:

- eligibility to contribute to a Roth IRA is subject to special adjusted gross income limits;

- contributions to a Roth IRA are not deductible;

- Roth IRA contributions may be made after the owner has attained the age of 70½; and,

- qualified distributions from a Roth IRA are not included in gross income or subject to the minimum distribution rules if certain conditions are met.

As with a traditional IRA, the income earned on the assets of a Roth IRA is tax free prior to distribution.

Contributions to a Roth IRA are subject to two limitations:

- *Dollar limitation* - Under this a contribution cannot exceed the maximum amount allowed after the deduction for a regular IRA (the lesser of $2,000 or 100% of an individual's compensation), reduced by any contributions that an individual may have made for a taxable year to any other individual retirement plan(s) maintained for the individual's benefit.

- *Adjusted gross income limitation* - This is based upon an individual's modified adjusted gross income. The Roth IRA contribution for a taxable year is phased out after adjusted gross income reaches certain levels. The amount an individual can contribute to a Roth IRA declines when his/her income reaches $95,000 and phases out entirely when the adjusted gross income reaches $110,000. For married individuals filing jointly, the phase out occurs when their adjusted gross income is between $150,000 and $160,000, and for married individuals filing separately, the phase out occurs when the adjusted gross income is between $0 and $10,000.

An individual may make a regular contribution to both a traditional IRA and a Roth IRA for a taxable year. In this case a maximum contribution limit for a Roth IRA is the lesser of the amount determined under the dollar limitation reduced by the amount contributed to a traditional IRA for the taxable year; or, the amount determined under the adjusted gross income limitation. Eligible taxpayers may contribute to both a Roth IRA and a deductible IRA by dividing their contribution between the two. But in no event may an individual's combined total annual contributions exceed $2,000.

Withdrawals from a Roth IRA are tax exempt only if: the account has been in existence for at least five years and the taxpayer is at least age 59½ or disabled; or a distribution of no more than $10,000 is made to finance the first-time home buying expenses of a taxpayer, his/her spouse or children, grandchildren, or ancestors of a taxpayer or spouse.

Skilled nursing care

The term refers to a level of care which must be furnished by or under direct supervision of licensed nursing personnel and under the general direction of a physician in order to assure the safety of the patient and achieve the medically desired result. The service involves observation and assessment of the total needs of the patient, planning and management of a treatment plan, and rendering direct services to the patient. As long as a patient needs skilled nursing care, it makes no difference whether his/her condition is acute, chronic or terminal.

Examples of skilled nursing care are:

- intravenous injections,
- tube feeding,
- kidney dialysis,
- colostomy care,
- the use of medical gases,
- observation and monitoring of a patient's unstable condition, and
- changing sterile dressings.

Expressly excluded from the term is any service that could be safely and effectively performed (or self-administered) by the average nonmedical personnel without the direct supervision of a licensed nurse.

In determining whether the level of care required by a patient is custodial care, which is not Medicare-covered, or skilled nursing care, which is covered by Medicare, the courts have applied several accepted legal principles:

- The primary responsibility determining a patient's need for skilled nursing care rests with the physician.
- While the opinion of a physician about the need for skilled nursing care is not binding on Medicare, when there is no conflicting evidence, his decision is required to be given great weight.
- The courts will avoid using a technical approach but rather use a common sense meaning and a consideration of the needs and underlying conditions affecting the patient as a whole.

Skilled nursing facility/Medicare

A skilled nursing facility is specially staffed and equipped to provide intensive nursing and rehabilitative care to patients. Care is provided by registered and other licensed nurses or licensed therapists under the supervision of a doctor. Medicare's requirement for admission to a skilled nursing facility, the benefits covered and the period of coverage are set forth below.

Supplemental needs trust

This type of trust, also known as a special needs trust, is an irrevocable trust, sometimes funded by assets of a third party, created for a disabled beneficiary, and intended to supplement government benefits. The trust prohibits the trustee from spending trust assets in diminution of government benefits. The beneficiary has no power to control distributions.

For SSI and generally for Medicaid, disbursements from the trust are governed by SSI income principles. If payments are made for food, clothing or shelter, or if payments are made directly to the beneficiary, the amounts are counted as income to the beneficiary for purposes of eligibility. The more common arrangement with such trusts is for the trustee to make direct payments to vendors of services or goods that are not food, clothing or shelter; such payments are not considered income to the beneficiary.

In addition to these general rules, Medicaid has special rules governing the treatment of trusts established by and for a Medicaid recipient or his/her spouse during their lifetime. These rules are discussed under the entry Trust, Medicaid eligibility rules.

Terminally ill

See also *Hospice care/Medicare*

An illness, disease or injury where recovery can no longer be reasonably expected. For purposes of Medicare-covered hospice care, a person with a terminal illness has a life expectancy of six months or less, as certified by a physician, if the illness runs a normal course. In the context of tax regulations governing accelerated benefits, a terminally ill person has a reasonable life expectancy of 24 months or less.

Testator

The person who creates a will.

The glossary is reprinted with permission and made up of selections from the Dictionary of Eldercare Terminology *by Walter Feldesman (2nd edition, National Information Services Corporation).*

N

Alabama

Alabama Bureau of Tourism and Travel, 11653

Alabama Client Assistance Program, 326

Alabama Department of Education: Disability Determination Service, 327

Alabama Department of Public Health, 328

Alabama Department of Rehabilitation Services, 329

Alabama Department of Retirement Systems, 330

Alabama Department of Revenue, 331

Alabama Department of Senior Services, 332, 10687

Alabama Department of Veteran Affairs, 333

Alabama Developmental Disability Council, 334

Alabama Disabilities Advocacy Program, 335

Alabama Disabilities Advocacy Program (ADAP), 10688

Alabama Division of Mental Illness and Substance Abuse Community Programs, 6875

Alabama Industries for the Blind, 7238

Alabama Institute for Deaf and Blind, 11026

Alabama Protection & Advocacy for Persons with Mental Illness, 336

Alabama Radio Reading Service Network, 337

Alabama Regional Library for the Blind and Physically Handicapped, 11027

Alabama State Bar: Elder Law, 10689

Alabama State Department of Human Resources, 338

Alabama Tombigbee Regional Commission, 339

Alabama Workers Compensation Division, 340

American Diabetes Association: Upstate Alabama Area Office, 5948

Auburn University: Special Collections& Archives, 11028

Birmingham Independent Living Center, 10340

Cardiovascular Research and Training Center: University of Alabama, 6602

Diabetes Research and Training Center: University of Alabama at Birmingham, 6059

East Alabama Commission: Agency on Aging, 341

Fair Haven Retirement Community, 7786

Gardens of Clanton, 7787

Gordon Oaks Convalescent Center, 7788

Governor's Committee on Employment of Persons with Disabilities, 342

Home Care Association of Alabama, 343

Homestead Village of Fairhope, 7789

Houston-Love Memorial Library, 11029

Huntsville Subregional Library for the Blind, 11030

Independent Living Center-Jasper, 10342

Jefferson County Office of Senior Citizens, 344

Jefferson County Office of Senior Citizens Services (OSCS), 10690

Kirkwood by the River, 7790

Knowlwood Assisted Living, 7791

Lee Russell Council of Governments: Area Agency on Aging, 345

Legal Services for the Elderly: Area Agency on Aging, 10691

Library for the Blind & Handicapped: Public Library-Anniston/Calhoun Counties, 11031

Liveoak Village, 7792

Mitchell Hollingsworth Annex, 7793

Mobile Association for the Blind, 7387

Montgomery Area Council on Aging, 346

Montgomery Independent Living Center, 10343

Morningside of Decatur, 7794

Mount Royal Towers, 7795

Murray House, 7796

North Central Alabama Regional Council of Governments: Area Agency on Aging, 347

North Mobile Retirement Center, 7797

Northwest Alabama Council of Governments: Area Agency on Aging, 348

Plantation Manor Assisted Living I, 7798

Protection & Advocacy for Persons with Developmental Disabilities, 349

RSVP Athens Limestone County, 350

RSVP Baldwin County, 351

RSVP Birmingham Area, 352

RSVP Calhoun County, 353

RSVP Dallas County, 354

RSVP Escambia County, 355

RSVP Etowah County, 356

RSVP Houston Henry Geneva Counties, 358

RSVP Lee & Russell Counties, 359

RSVP Marshall County, 360

RSVP Mobile, 361

RSVP Monroe/Cone-Cuh County, 362

RSVP Pike County, 363

RSVP Southwest Alabama, 364

RSVP Tallapossa & Coosa Counties, 365

Railroad Retirement Board: Alabama District Office, 366

Saint Martins in the Pines, 7799

Samford University Library Special Collections, 11032

Somerby at Jones Farm, 7800

Somerset Assited Living Facility, 7801

South Central Alabama Development Commission: Area Agency on Aging, 367

Specialized Center of Research in Ischemic Heart Disease, 6628

Stroke Research and Treatment Center, 6804

TARCOG: Area Agency on Aging, 368

US Deptartment of Veterans Affairs: Central Alabama Veterans Health Care System, 11033

US Deptartment of Veterans Affairs: Medical Center Library, 11034

US Deptartment of Veterans Affairs:Alabama Veterns Health Care System, 11035

University of Alabama at Birmingham: Congenital Heart Disease Center, 6629

University of Alabama at Birmingham: Parkinson's Disease Center, 6793

University of Alabama: Speech and Hearing Center, 6557

Village at Cook Springs, 7802

Volunteer Center of Morgan County, 369

Volunteers of America Southeast, 370

West Alabama Planning and Development Council: Area Agency on Aging, 371

West Alabama Regional Commission's Senior Programs: Legal Counsel for the Elderly (WARC), 10692

Alaska

AK Division of Vocational Rehabilitation State Vocational Rehabilitation Committee, 372

Access Alaska-Anchorage, 10344

Access Alaska-Fairbanks, 10345

Alaska Client Assistance Program (CAP), 373

Alaska Commission on Aging, 374

Alaska Commission on Aging: Alaska Department of Health & Social Services, 10693

Alaska Department of Military and Veterans Affairs, 375

Alaska Department of Revenue, 376

Alaska Disability Law Center, 377

Alaska Division of Mental Health and Developmental Disabilities, 378

Alaska Division of Retirement & Benefits, 379

Alaska Division of Tourism, 11654

Alaska Division of Vocational Rehabilitation, 380

Alaska Legal Services Corporation: Senior Legal Services Project, 10694

Alaska State Library Talking Book Center, 11036

Alaska Statewide Independent Living Council, 381

Alaska Welcomes You, 382

Alaska Workers Compensation Board, 383

Alaskans Commission on Aging, 384

Amazing Grace Family Living, 7804

American Diabetes Association: Alaska Area Office, 5898

Anchorage Pioneers' Home, 7805

Arctic Hearth Assisted Living Homes, 7806

Arkansas Office of Alcoholism and Substance Abuse, 6886

Assistive Technology of Alaska, 385

Bear Mountain Manor, 7807

Chugiak-Eagle River Senior Center, 7808

Dignified Home Life Care, 7809

Disability Law Center Of Alaska, 10695

Downtown Care, 7810

Easy Living Adult Care, 7811

Elderlaw Project, 10696

Fairbanks Senior Center, 387

Farthest North Club of the Deaf, 388, 6131

Graceful Living Assisted Living Home, 7812

Health Care Bridges, 7813

Hidden Heights Assisted Living Home, 7814

Holy Family Adult Foster Home, 7815

Holy Family Assisted Living Home, 7816

Immaculate Conception Home, 7817

Juneau Pioneers Home, 7818

Kat's Eldercare, 7819

Kenai Peninsula Independent Living Center-Homer, 10346

Kenai Peninsula Independent Living-Central Peninsula, 10347

Kenai Senior Connection, 389

Marlow Manor/Manor Management, 7820
Palmer Pioneers' Home, 7821
Respect Your Elders Tender Loving Adult Care, 7822
Saint Augustine Assisted Living Home, 7823
Saint Augustine Assisted Living Home II, 7824
Scott Manor, 7825
Seward Independent Living Center, 10348
Shirley's Assisted Living Home, 7826
Social Security: Juneau Disability Determination Services, 390
Southeast Alaska Independent Living (SAIL), 10349
Southeast Alaska Independent Living Center (SAIL), 10350
Southeast Alaska Living Center (SAIL), 10351
State of Alaska, Department of Health & Social Services, 391
Summer Shades Residential Care, 7827
Thania's Assisted Living Home, 7828
Tranquility Manor, 7829
Turnagain Adult Foster Home, 7830
University of Alabama: Center for Alcohol and Addiction Studies, 7219

Arizona

ALC Copper Hills House, 7834
Advocates for the Disabled, 10697
America West Airlines/US Airways, 11616
America West/US Airways Airline, 11710
American Council on Alcoholism, 6882
American Diabetes Association: Arizona Area Office, 5899
American Diabetes Association: Border Area Office, 5903
American Holistic Nurses Association, 43
Arizona Aging and Adult Administration, 392
Arizona Alcoholism and Drug Abuse, 6883
Arizona Area Agency on Aging: Region One, 393
Arizona Bridge to Independent Living, 10352
Arizona Center for Disability Law, 10698
Arizona Center for the Blind and Visually Impaired, 7260
Arizona Center on Aging, 394
Arizona Commission for the Deaf & Hard of Hearing, 6103
Arizona Department of Aging, 395
Arizona Department of Economic Security, 396
Arizona Department of Economic Security: Division of Aging and Community Services, 10699
Arizona Department of Family Health Services, 397
Arizona Department of Revenue, 398
Arizona Department of Veterans Services, 399
Arizona Disability Determination Services, 400
Arizona Elder Abuse and Fraud Taskforce Committee, 10700
Arizona Heart Institute, 6575
Arizona Industries for the Blind, 7261
Arizona Inter Tribal Council, 401

Arizona Office of Substance Abuse & General Mental Health, 6885
Arizona Office of Tourism, 11655
Arizona Protection and Advocacy Agency: Arizona Center for Disability Law, 10701
Arizona Public Safety Personnel Retirement System, 402
Arizona Rehabilitation State Services for the Blind and Visually Impaired, 7262
Arizona Retirement System, 403
Arizona State Braille and Talking Book Library, 11037
Arizona Workers Compensation Board, 404
Bee Hive Homes of Yuma, 7835
Bethesda Gardens, 7836
Big Print Address Book, 3315
Book Holder, 3317
Broadway Proper, 7837
C & C Adult Care Home, 7838
Capable Hands Adult Care Home, 7839
Capscrew, 3189
Care Concepts, 2825
Care with Love, 7840
Cypress Court at Tucson, 7841
DIRECT Independent Living Center, 10353
DNA People's Legal Services, 10702
Desert Point-La Reserve, 7842
Do It Now Foundation, 6897
Emerald Springs Retirement & Assisted Living Community, 7843
Emeritus at Catalina Foothills, 7844
Flagstaff City-Coconino County Library for the Visually & Physically Impaired, 11038
Folding Dressing Stick, 3096
Forum at Tucson, 7845
Fountain Hills Lioness Braille Service, 11039
Geronimo, 3384
Hand/Nail Brush, 3115
Handy Reacher, 3163
Helping Handle, 2904
La Casa Asperanza Assisted Living, 7846
La Posada, 7847
La Siena, 7848
Large Print Typewriter, 2994
Legal Advocate Program: Pinal-Gila Council for Senior Citizens, 10703
McDowell Village, 7849
Mesa Arizona Regional Family History Center, 11040
Mr. Escort Manual Wheelchair Carrier, 2852
National Association of Professional Geriatric Care Managers (PGCM), 180
Navajo Area Agency on Aging: Division of Health, 406
New Horizons Independent Living Center - Prescott Valley, 10354
Northern Arizona Council of Governments Area Agency on Aging, 407
Parkinson Association of Arizona, 6709
Phoenix Public Library: Special Needs Center, 11041
Pill Splitter, 3124
Pima Council on Aging, 408, 11042
Pinal/Gila Council for Senior Citizens, 409
Power for Off-Pavement, 3394
Prescott Talking Book Library, 11043
RSVP East Valley Retired & Senior Volunteer Program, 410
RSVP Gila Pinal, 411
RSVP Maricopa County, 412

RSVP Northern Arizona, 413
RSVP Southeastern Arizona, 414
RSVP Tucson, 415
RSVP Western Arizona, 416
Redman Apache, 3395
Redman Crow Line, 3396
Retired Activities Office: Phoenix Affairs Office, 417
Ruth E Golding Clinical Pharmacokinetics Laboratory, 7215
SEAGO Area: Agency on Aging, 418
Senior Citizens of Patagonia, 419
Services Maximizing Independent Living and Empowerment (SMILE), 10355
Southern Arizona Legal Aid (SALA), 10705
Spatial Tilt Custom Chair, 2915
Sports 'n Spokes, 11750
Statewide Independent Living Council (SILC), 10356
SunQuest Village of Yuma, 7850
Travis L Williams Family Services Center, 11044
Tucson Family History Center, 11045
U.S. Railroad Retirement Board, 420
US Department of Veterans Affairs: Northern Arizona VA Health Care System, 11046
US Department of Veterans Affairs: Phoenix Medical Center Library, 11047
US Department of Veterans Affairs: Tucson Medical Center Library, 11048
US Travel Systems, 11760
Verde Valley Senior Citizens Association, 421
Villa Hermosa, 7851
Western Arizona Council of Governments: Area Agency on Aging, 422
Westown Adult Care Home, 7852
Wheeler's Accessible Van Rentals, 2863, 11651
Wheelers Accessible Van Rentals, 11652
White Bench, 2898
William E Morris Institute for Justice, 10706

Arkansas

American Diabetes Association: Arkansas, 5900
Arizona Bureau of Alcohol and Drug Abuse, 6884
Arkansas Advocates for Nursing Home Residents, 423
Arkansas Aging Foundation, 424
Arkansas Aging Foundation Information Center, 11049
Arkansas Assistive Technology Projects, 425
Arkansas Department of Aging, 426
Arkansas Department of Finance and Administration, 427
Arkansas Department of Health & Human Services: Division of Aging and Adult Services, 10707
Arkansas Department of Human Services: Division of Aging and Adult Services, 428
Arkansas Department of Parks & Tourism, 11656
Arkansas Department of Public Employees Retired Systems, 429

California

California Protection and Advocacy Agency (PAI), 10716

California Public Employees' Retirement System, 488

California Seniors Council, 489

California State Bar Committee on Legal Problems of Aging, 10717

California State Board of Equalization, 490

California State Independent Living Council (SILC), 10365

California State Library: Braille & Talking Book Library, 11057

California State Teachers Retirement System, 491

California Women's Commission on Alcohol and Drug Dependencies, 6890

California Workers Compensation Board, 492

Californian Retirement Residence, 7885

Campbell Adult Center, 7886

Canine Companions for Independence, 7296

Caregiver Alliance, 86

Center for Independence of the Disabled (CID), 10366

Center for Independence of the Disabled-North Branch, 10367

Center for Independent Living (CIL), 10368

Center for Independent Living - Central Coast/Hollister (CCCIL), 10369

Center for Independent Living-Merced Outreach, 10370

Center for Independent Living-Oakland, 10371

Central California Legal Services, 10718

Central Coast Commission for Senior Citizens, 493

Chancellor Health Care, 7887

Chancellor Place of Chino Hills, 7888

Chancellor Place of Lodi, 7889

Chancellor Place of Murrieta, 7890

Chancellor Place of Pasadena, 7891

Chancellor Place of Windsor, 7892

Chaplains Religious Enrichment Program Southwest, 494

Charles R Drew Hypertension Research Center, 6660

CiminoCare, 7893

City of Hope, 96

City of Los Angeles Department of Aging, 495

Classic, 2826

Classic Hawaii, 11716

Clearinghouse for Specialized Media and Technology, 7307

Coalition for Economic Survival, 101

Cocaine Anonymous, 6892

Community Access Center, 10372

Community Resources for Independence (CRI) Napa, 10373

Community Resources for Independence - CRI/Santa Rosa, 10374

Community Resources for Independent Living, 10375

Compax 12, 3373

Contra Costa County Office on Aging, 496

Convaid Products, 3374

Convention of American Instructors of the Deaf, 6120

Cordia Senior Living, 7894

Costa Mesa Senior Center, 497

Council on Aging of Silicon Valley, 498

Council on Aging of Sonoma County, 10719

Country Villa Terrace Assisted Living, 7895

Country Villa West Assisted Living Center, 7896

Country Village Senior Services, 7897

Courtyards at Pine Creek, 7898

Crown Cove, 7899

Cruiser Bus Buggy 4MB, 3285

Cypress Court Escondido, 7900

Damaco D90, 3377

Dayle McIntosh Center for the Disabled, 10376

Dayle McIntosh Center-Clubhouse, 10377

Dayle McIntosh-South County, 10378

Deaf Adults Education Access Program, 6122

Deaf Counseling, Advocacy & Referral Agency, 6124

Deaf and Hard of Hearing Services Center, 6128

Departments of Neurology & Neurosurgery: University of California, 6864

Diabetes Hands Foundation, 5958

Diablo Valley Foundation for the Aging, 499

Disability Determination Services: Los Angeles West Branch, 500

Disability Determination Services: Central Support Services Branch, 501

Disability Determination Services: La Jolla Branch, 502

Disability Determination Services: Los Angeles South Branch, 503

Disability Determination Services: Oakland Branch, 504

Disability Determination Services: Roseville Branch, 505

Disability Determination Services: Sacramento Branch, 506

Disability Determination Services: San Diego Branch, 507

Disability Evaluations Division: Sierra Branch, 508

Disability Rights Education and Defense Fund, 10720

Driving Systems, 2878

Drug Abuse Resistance Education of America, 6898

Drugs Anonymous, 6900

East Los Angeles Service Center, 509

El Dorado County Area: Agency on Aging, 510

Elder Care Alliance, 511

Elderly People or Persons with Disabilities Housing, 113

Emeritus at Alhambra, 7901

Emeritus at Garden Manor, 7902

Emeritus at Orange, 7903

Emeritus at Valley View, 7904

Emeritus at Victorian Court, 7905

Emeritus at Villa De Anza, 7906

Environmental Traveling Companions, 11723

Ernest Gallo Clinic and Research Center, 7197

Eskaton Cameron Park Lodge, 7907

Eskaton Gold River Lodge, 7908

Eureka Ward Family History Center, 11058

Extensions for Independence, 7324

Fairwinds-Ivey Ranch, 7909

Fairwinds-West Hills, 7910

Fairwinds-Woodward Park, 7911

Fifty-Plus Lifelong Fitness, 124

Fighting Back, 6902

Font-Tools BIGFONT, 2981

Foundation Aiding the Elderly, 128

Fountaingrove Lodge, 7912

Fountains at Sea Bluffs, 7913

Fresno County Free Library: Talking Book Library for the Blind, 11059

Fresno Madera Area: Agency on Aging, 512

Friday Night Live, 6904

Garden of Palms, 7914

Gardens at Hillsborough Village, 7915

Gardens at Park Balboa, 7916

Gardens of Santa Monica, 7917

Gardens of Tarzana, 7918

General Clinical Research Center: University of California at Los Angeles, 6608

Glaucoma Research Foundation, 7766

Glaucoma Support Network, 7334

Glen Bollinger Humanitarian Award, 2508

Governor's Policy Council on Drug & Alcohol Abuse, 6906

Gray Panthers of Central Contra Costa, 513

Gray Panthers of East Bay/Berkeley, 514

Gray Panthers of Long Beach, 515

Gray Panthers of Marin County, 516

Gray Panthers of Orange County, 517

Gray Panthers of Sacramento, 518

Gray Panthers of San Fernando Valley, 519

Gray Panthers of San Francisco, 520

Gray Panthers of Santa Barbara, 521

Gray Panthers of South Bay, 522

Gray Panthers of Southern Alameda County, 523

Greater Valley Physicians Medical Group, 524

Green Tortoise Adventure Travel, 11727

Grossmont Gardens, 7919

Guide Dogs for the Blind, 7339

HEAR Center, 6135

Hacienda, 7920

Hawkins Center of Law and Services for the Disabled, 10721

Hearing Education and Awareness for Rockers, 6139

Heart Research Foundation of Sacramento, 6612

Helping Hands for the Blind, 7345

Heritage Estates, 7921

Heritage Estates Senior Apartments, 7922

Heritage Pointe, 7923

Hollenbeck Palms, 7924

HomeAid Orange County, 525

House Ear Institute, 6144

House Ear Institute: Athalie Irvine Clarke Library, 11060

House Ear Institute: Care Center Parent Resource Library, 11061

House of Travel, 11730

IL Resources of Contra Costa County-Fairfield, 10379

Imperial County: Area Agency on Aging, 526

Independent Living Center of Kern County, 10380

Independent Living Center of Southern California (ILCSC), 10381

Independent Living Center-Lancaster, 10382

Independent Living Center-Santa Clarita, 10383

Independent Living Resource Center (ILRCSF), 10384

Stanislaus County Department of Aging and Veteran Services, 587
Steven Motor Chair, 3403
Summerville at Main Place, 7948
Sunny View Manor, 7949
Sunrise at Yorba Linda, 7950
Sunset Hall, 588
Sunshine Care Mountain Vistas, 7951
Synthetic Sheep-Skin Pads, 3086
Systems 2000, 3306
Torso Support, 3425
Travel Trends, 11755
Trinity House, 7952
U-Control II, 3040
US Department of Veteran Affairs: Palo Alto Health Care and Medical Information Service, 11069
US Department of Veterans Affairs: H Earl Gordon Medical Library, 11070
US Department of Veterans Affairs: Loma Linda Medical Center Library Service, 11071
US Department of Veterans Affairs: Long Beach Medical Center Library Service, 11072
US Department of Veterans Affairs: San Diego Medical Center Library Service, 11073
US Department of Veterans Affairs: San Francisco Medical Center Library Service, 11074
US SERVAS, 11759
University of California, Irvine: UCI Diabetes Research Program, 6070
University of California: Cardiovascular Research Laboratory, 6631
University of California: Los Angeles Department of Medicine, 6869
University of California: Los Angeles Jules Stein Eye Institute, 7779
University of California: Mount Zion Medical Center, 11075
University of California: San Diego General Clinical Research Center, 6632
University of California: San Francisco Cardiovascular Research Institute, 6633
University of California: San Francisco Center on Deafness Library, 11076
University of California: San Francisco General Clinical Research Center, 6630
University of Southern California: Coronary Care Research, 6638
University of Southern California: Division of Nephrology, 6670
VA Central California Health Care System, 11077
Vacaville Public Library: Town Square, 11078
Ventura County Area: Agency on Aging, 589
Vertical Home Lift Sales, 3276
Villa Capri at Varenna, 7953
Villa Santa Barbara, 7954
Visually Impaired Veterans of America, 7503
Volunteer Center, 590
Volunteer Center Orange County, 591
Volunteer Center of Kern County, 592
Volunteer Exchange, 593
Volunteer Lawyers Project for the Elderly, 10733
Volunteers of America Bay Area, 594

Weitbrecht Communications, 3048
West Hollywood Senior Center: Jewish Family Service, 595
Western Law Center for Disability Rights, 10734
Westside Center for Independent Living, 10399
Whisper 2000, 3049
Whittier Institute for Diabetes & Endocrinology, 6088
Words+ IST (Infrared, Sound, Touch), 3051
World Institute on Disability, 313
Yuba-Sutter Legal Center for Seniors, 10735

Canada

Abbotsford Seniors' Association, 314
Advocacy Centre for the Elderly, 315
Age & Opportunity, 316
Association of Mature Canadians, 317
Canada Association for Retired Persons, 318
Carefirst Seniors & Community Services Association, 319
Help the Aged, 320
Institute for Life Course and Aging, 321
National Institute for the Care of the Elderly, 322
National Pensioners & Senior Citizens Federation, 323
Older Women's Network, 324
Seniors' Society, 325
Tapestry at Village Gate West, 10320

Colorado

AMC Cancer Research Center Medical Library, 11079
Administration on Aging: Region VIII, 596
Agency on Aging: Region 10, 597
Air Liftunlimited, 3409
Alpine: Area Agency on Aging, 598
American Academy of Oral & Maxillofacial Radiology, 11
American Diabetes Association: Mountain States & Pacific/Northwest Regional Office, 5930
American Diabetes Association: Wyoming District Office, 5953
American Society of General Surgeons, 59
Anam Chara Homes, 7955
Argyle Square, 7956
Atlantis Community, 10400
Atria Inn at Lakewood, 7957
Beatrice Hover Assisted Living, 7958
Beyond Sight, 3314
Bill Dvorak Kayak & Rafting, 11714
Boulder County Aging Services Division, 599
Boulder County Aging Services Division: Elder Rights Program, 10736
Broadmoor Court, 7959
Bye-Bye Decubiti (BBD), 3056
Bye-Bye Decubiti Air Mattress Overlay, 2900
Center For People With Disabilities, 10401
Center for Applied Prevention Research, 7195
Center for Independence, 10402
Charlie Brown's Goodtime Travel, 11715
Collinwood, 7960
Colorado Aging and Adult Services, 600

Colorado Association of Homes & Services for the Aging, 601
Colorado Client Assistance Program, 602
Colorado Department of Aging, 603
Colorado Department of Human Services: Division of Aging and Adult Services, 10737
Colorado Department of Revenue, 604
Colorado Department of Social Service, 11080
Colorado Department of Social Services: Division of Older American Programs, 605, 606
Colorado Developmental Disability Council, 607
Colorado Disability Determination Services, 608
Colorado Division of Mental Health, 609
Colorado Mountain College Senior Nutrition Program, 610
Colorado Protection & Advocacy for Persons with Disabilities, 611
Colorado Protection and Advocacy Agency: The Legal Center at Grand Junction, 10738
Colorado Public Employees Retirement Association, 612
Colorado School for the Deaf and Blind, 11081
Colorado Springs Independence Center, 10403
Colorado Talking Book Library, 11082
Colorado Travel & Tourism Authority, 11658
Colorado Workers Compensation Board, 613
Denver Regional Council of Governments: Area Agency on Aging, 614
Devonshire Acres Nursing and Rehabilitation Center, 109
East Central Colorado: Area Agency on Aging, 615
Eastern Colorado Services for the Disabled, 616
Easy Pivot Transfer Machine, 3235
Elderhaus, 617
Emeritus at Highline, 7961
Golden Pond, 7962
Grand Villa, 7963
Granville Assisted Living Center, 7964
Harvard Square, 7965
Hemlock Society USA, 136
Huerfano Las Animas: Area Agency on Aging, 618
International Hearing Dog, 6147
Jay Cushion, 3068
Kayak and Rafting Expeditions, 11732
Kit Carson and Lincoln Counties RSVP, 619
Larimer County Office on Aging (LCOA), 10739
Legal Center for People with Disabilities and Older People, 10740
Longmont Meals on Wheels, 620
Lumbo-Posture Back Support, 3071
Lyons Golden Gang, 621
MacKenzie Place: Colorado Springs, 7966
MacKenzie Place: Fort Collins, 7967
Museum of Western Colorado: Research Center & Special Library, 11083
National Association of Blind Lawyers, 7392

National Jewish Medical and Research Center, 215
National Stroke Association, 6802
Nightingale Suites at Springwood, 7968
Oval Window Audio, 3142
Over the Hill Gang International, 255
Penrose Hospital: Webb Memorial Library, 11084
Pikes Peak Area Council of Government: Agency on Aging, 622
Professional Respite Care, 11744
RSVP Adams-Arapahoe, 623
RSVP Boulder County, 624
RSVP Colorado West, 625
RSVP High County, 626
RSVP Otero Bent-Crowley Counties, 628
RSVP Pueblo, 629
RSVP Rural Resort Region, 630
RSVP San Luis Valley, 631
RSVP VOA Colorado Branch, 632
RSVP VOA Denver, 633
RSVP Weld County, 634
Railroad Retirement Board: Colorado District Office, 635
Rand-Scot, 3352
Reclining Power Wheelchairs, 3423
Retired Enlisted Association, 276
Retirees Club International Associationof Ironworkers, 636
Rocky Mountain Heart Research Institute, 6626
San Juan Basin Area: Agency on Aging, 637
Sheridan Travel Service, 11748
South Central Colorado Seniors, 638
Sterling House of Arvada, 7969
Sunrise of Boulder, 7970
Superarm Lift, 2858
Telephone Pioneers of America, 7482
Teller Senior Coalition, 639
US Department of Veterans Affairs: Denver Medical Center Library, 11085
US Department of Veterans Affairs: Grand Junction Medical Center Library Service, 11086
US Department of Veterans Affairs: Southern Colorado Healthcare System, 11087
United States Association for Blind Athletes, 7490
University of Colorado: Boulder Communication Disorders Clinic, 6559
University of Colorado: Science Libaray, 11088
Upper Arkansas Area: Agency on Aging, 640
View Pointe, 7971
Weld Library District: Lincoln Park Branch Library, 11089
Winslow Court, 7972

Connecticut

AMI Aquamassage, 3102
Academy Point at Mystic, 7973
American Diabetes Association: Connecticut, 5910
Arbors at Hop Brook, 7974
Atria Crossroads Place, 7976
Atria at Stratford, 7977
BESB Industries, 7273
Bellmarie, 7978

Bridges at Lake Whitney, 7979
Bridges at the Green, 7980
Bureau of Rehabilitation Services: Disability Determination Services, 641
Center for Disability Rights, 10404
Center for Independent Living of Northwestern Connecticut, 10405
Center for Medicare Advocacy, 10741
Chester Village West, 7981
Connecticut Association of Not-for-Profit Providers for the Aging, 642
Connecticut Bar Association: Section on Legal Problems of the Elderly, 10742
Connecticut Board of Education and Services for the Blind, 643
Connecticut Braille Association, 7312
Connecticut Client Assistance Program, 644
Connecticut Commission on Deaf and Hearing Impaired, 6119
Connecticut Commisson on Aging, 645
Connecticut Council On Developmental Disabilities, 646
Connecticut Department of Aging, 647
Connecticut Department of Mental Health and Addiction Services, 6893
Connecticut Department of Revenue, 648
Connecticut Department of Social Services: Elderly Services Division, 10743
Connecticut Disability Determination Serices, 649
Connecticut Lawyers' Legal Aid to the Elderly Program (CLLAEP), 10744
Connecticut Military Retired Activities Office, 650
Connecticut Office of Tourism, 11659
Connecticut Protection & Advocacy for Persons with Disabilities, 651
Connecticut Protection and Advocacy Agency: Office of Protection and Advocacy for Persons with Disabilities, 10745
Connecticut Society to Prevent Blindness, 11090
Connecticut State Library for the Blindand Physically Handicapped, 11091
Connecticut State of Veterans Affairs Department of Rocky Hill: Hospital Services Program, 652
Connecticut Teachers Retirement Board, 653
Crescent Point at Niantic, 7982
Curtis Home, 7983
Disability Resource Center of Fairfield County (DRCFC), 10406
East Coast Assistance Dogs, 654
East Hill Woods, 7984
Eastern Connecticut Area: Agency on Aging, 655
Edgehill Health Center, 7985
Elim Park Baptist Home, 7986
Emeritus at Litchfield Hills, 7987
Emeritus at Rocky Hill, 7988
Essex Meadows, 7989
Evergreen Woods, 7990
Fidelco Guide Dog Foundation, 7327
Gables at Farmington, 7991
Gables at Guilford, 7992
Gardenside Terrace, 7993
Greens at the Greenwich, 7994
Hamilton Heights Place of West Hartford, 7995
Hartford Area Social Security Office, 656

Hartford Hospital Health Science Libraries, 11092
Hartford Hospital: Gerontology Resource Center, 11093
Heights at Avery Heights, 7996
Independence Unlimited Inc., 10407
Laurel Gardens at Milford, 7997
Laurel Gardens of Avon, 7998
Laurel Gardens of Orange, 7999
Laurel Gardens of Woodbridge, 8000
Legal Assistance for Elders in Connecticut, 10746
Legal Services Programs for Elders: Bridgeport, 10747
Legal Services Programs for Elders: Hartford, 10748
Legal Services Programs for Elders: Waterbury, 10749
Legal Services Programs for Elders: Willimantic, 10750
Lockwood Lodge at Ashlar of Newtown, 8001
Maple Woods at Hamden Benchmark Assisted Living, 8002
Marriott's Brighton Gardens of Stamford, 8003
McAuley, 8004
Middlewoods of Farmington, 8005
Middlewoods of Newington, 8006
Miller Memorial Community, 8007
Mulberry Gardens of Southington, 8008
National Theatre of the Deaf, 6179
New Haven Legal Assistance Association (LAA), 10751
North Central Area Agency on Aging, 657
Orchards at Southington, 8009
PRIDE Foundation, 256
Pomperaug Woods, 8010
Prevent Blindness America New York City Division, 1741
Prevent Blindness Connecticut, 7451
Prevent Blindness New Jersey, 1615
Prevent Blindness Tri-State, 7459
RSVP Central Connecticut, 658
RSVP Central Naugatuck Valley, 659
RSVP Eastern Fairfield County, 660
RSVP Greater Bristol, 661
RSVP Greater Hartford, 662
RSVP Mid State, 663
RSVP Northern Fairfield County, 664
RSVP Southern New London, 665
RSVP Southwestern Connecticut, 666
RSVP Windham-Tolland Counties, 667
Rosedale of Glastonbury, 8011
Rosedale of Trumbull Assisted Living Community, 8012
Shady Oaks Assisted Living, 8013
South Central Connecticut: Agency on Aging, 668
Spring Meadows at Trumbull, 8014
State of Vermont Division of Disabilityand Aging Services, 10998
Stony Brook Court, 8015
Suffield by the River, 8016
Summerville at South Windsor, 8017
Sunrise Assisted Living of Stamford, 8018
Sunrise Assisted Living of Wilton, 8019
Tower One/Tower East, 8020
US Department of Veterans Affairs, Health & Science Library, 11094
US Department of Veterans Affairs: Healthcare System in West Haven, 11095

Florida

Georgia

Hawaii

Kansas

Aeroquip Wheelchair Securement System, 2821

Alterra Sterling House of Abilene, 8475

Alterra Sterling House of Abilene II, 8476

Alterra Sterling House of Arkansas, 8477

Alterra Sterling House of Augusta, 8478

Alterra Sterling House of Derby, 8479

Alterra Sterling House of Dodge City, 8480

Alterra Sterling House of Emporia, 8481

Alterra Sterling House of Fairdale, 8482

Alterra Sterling House of Great Bend, 8483

Alterra Sterling House of Hays, 8484

Alterra Sterling House of Junction, 8485

Alterra Sterling House of Lawrence, 8486

Alterra Sterling House of Leawood, 8487

Alterra Sterling House of Lenexa II, 8488

Alterra Sterling House of McPherson, 8489

Alterra Sterling House of Olathe, 8490

Alterra Sterling House of Olathe II, 8491

Alterra Sterling House of Salina, 8492

Alterra Sterling House of Topeka, 8493

Alterra Sterling House of Wichita, 8494

Alterra Sterling House of Woodland, 8495

American Academy of Addiction Psychiatry, 7192

American Diabetes Association: Kansas Area Office, 5920

Andover Court Assisted Living, 8496

Assisted Lifestyles Of KS Inc., 8497

Assisted Living at Windsor Place, 8498

Atria Assisted & Retirement Living, 8499

Beach Center on Families and Disability, 1024

Brookside Assisted Living, 8500

Bukovina Society of the Americas Library, 11214

Butler County Department on Aging, 1025

Carriage House of Greensburg, 8501

Cedar Lake Village, 8502

Cedarview Assisted Living, 8503

Center for Independent Living for Southwest Kansas, 10477

Center for Independent Living of Southwest Kansas, 10478

Central Plains: Area Agency on Aging, 1026

Chaucer Estates-Retirement, 8504

Cherokee County Genealogical Historical Society, 11215

Cherry Creek Village Retirement Center, 8505

Cornerstone Assisted Living, 8378, 8506

Cornerstone Ridge Plaza, 8507

Disability Rights Center of Kansas, 1027

East Central Kansas: Area Agency on Aging, 1028

Elm Grove Estates, 8508

Evergreen Gardens of Garden City, 8509

Fort Scott Presbyterian Village, 8510

Georgetown Village, 8511

Gran Villas, 8512

Gran Villas-Atchison, 8513

Gran Villas-Eureka, 8514

Gran Villas-Fredonia, 8515

Gran Villas-Hiawatha, 8516

Gran Villas-Neodesha, 8517

Gran Villas-Osage City, 8518

Gran Villas-Wamego, 8519

Grand Court of Overland Park II, 8520

Gravity Down Platform Lift, 3243

Great Bend Homestead, 8521

Great Plains Region Helen Keller National Center, 7335

Halstead Place, 8522

Harvey County Department on Aging, 1029

Homestead of Auburn Assisted Living, 8523

Homestead of Garden City, 8524

Hutchinson Homestead, 8525

Hutchinson Independent Living Center, 10479

Independence, Inc., 10480

Independent Connection, 10481

Independent Living of Northeast Kansas, 10483

Kansas Alcohol and Drug Abuse Services, 6919

Kansas Association for the Blind and Visually Impaired, 7361

Kansas Client Assistance Program, 1030

Kansas Commission for the Deaf and Hard of Hearing, 6153

Kansas Commission on Disability Concerns, 1031

Kansas Commission on Veterans Affairs, 1032

Kansas Department for Aging and Disability Services, 1033

Kansas Department of Aging: Legal Assistance Services for Older Adults (KDOA), 10837

Kansas Department of Human Resources: Commission on Disabilities Concern, 1034

Kansas Department of Social and Rehabilitation Services, 1035

Kansas Department on Aging, 1036

Kansas Developmental Disability Council, 1037

Kansas Division of Services for the Blind, 7363

Kansas Employment Services and Job Training Program Liaison, 1038

Kansas Hearing Aid Association, 6154

Kansas Hearing Society, 6155

Kansas Masonic Home, 8526

Kansas Mental Health & Retardation Service, 1039

Kansas Protection and Advocacy Agency & Disability Rights Center of Kansas, 10838

Kansas Public Employees Retirement System, 1040

Kansas Specialty Dog Service, 1041

Kansas State Historical Society: Library & Archives Division, 11216

Kansas State Library Talking Book Service, 11217

Kansas Travel & Tourism, 11669

Leavenworth County Genealogical Society Library, 11218

Leavenworth Homestead, 8527

Linwood Place I & II, 8528

Living Independently in Northwest Kansas (LINK), 10484

Manhattan Homestead Assisted, 8529

Manhattan Public Library, 11219

Marquis Place, 8530

National Federation of the Blind of Kansas, 1042, 7409

National Organization of HIV over Fifty, 224

National Silver-Haired Congress: Kansas Department on Aging, 1043

North Central Flint Hills: Area Agency on Aging, 1044

Northeast Kansas: Area Agency on Aging, 1045

Northwest Kansas Library System Talking Books, 11220

Northwest Kansas: Area Agency on Aging, 1046

Old Fort Genealogical Society Of Southeastern Kansas Inc, 11221

Overland Park Place, 8532

Pace Saver Plus II, 3291

Park View Assisted Living, 8533

Parkinson Association of Greater Kansas City, 6710

Parkwood Village, 8534

Peterson Assisted Living, 8535

RSVP Barton County, 1047

RSVP Butler County, 1048

RSVP Finney County, 1049

RSVP Ford County, 1050

RSVP Harvey County, 1051

RSVP Johnson County: Coming of Age, 1052

RSVP Northwest Kansas, 1053

RSVP Pratt County, 1054

RSVP Reno County, 1055

RSVP Riley County, 1056

RSVP Saline County, 1057

RSVP Southeast Kansas, 1058

RSVP Wyandotte County, 1059

Railroad Retirement Board: Kansas, 1060

Redbud Plaza, 8536

Rolling Hills Assisted Living Apartments, 8537

Sealye House, 8538

Shawnee Heartland Assisted Living, 8539

South Central Kansas Library System, 11222

South Central Kansas: Area Agency on Aging, 1061

Southeast Kansas Independent Living (SKIL), 10486

Southeast Kansas: Area Agency on Aging, 1062

St John's New Horizons, 8540

Statewide Independent Living Council of Kansas, 10487

Super Scout Three Wheeler, 3305

Talking Books Service, 11223

Three Rivers, 10488

Three Rivers-Manhattan, 10489

Topeka Independent Living Resource Center, 10490

Twin Oaks Assisted Living, 8541

US Department of Veterans Affairs: Dr Karl Menninger Medical Library, 11224

US Department of Veterans Affairs: Dwight D. Eisenhower Center Medical Library, 11225

University of Kansas: Regional Diabetes Center, 6074

Village East, 8542

Village of Ninnescah, 8543

Vintage Park at Lenexa, 8544

Vintage Park of Atchison, 8545

Vintage Park of Baldwin City, 8546

Vintage Park of Gardner, 8547

Vintage Park of Louisburg, 8548

Vintage Park of Paola, 8549

Vintage Place of Derby, 8550

Vintage Place of Russell, 8551

Maine

Maryland

National Kidney Disease Program (NKDEP), 5966

National Kidney and Urologic Diseases Information Clearinghouse, 6681

National Prevention Resource Center, 6938

National Rehabilitation Information Center, 230, 6177, 6801, 6801

National Support Awards, 2532

National Volunteer Training Center for Substance Abuse Prevention, 6939

Nelson Cruikshank Award, 2534

Neurology Institute, 6803

Newel Perry Award, 2536

Oakcrest Village, 8644

Office of Applied Studies, 7210

Office of Disability: Social Security Administration, 250

Office of Retirement and Survivors, 1213

Office of Supplemental Security Income, 251

Office of Supplemental Security Income: Social Security Administration, 1214

Office of Women's Services, 6949

Outstanding Newsletter Recognitions, 2539

Outstanding Service Medallion, 2540

Potomac Technology, 3017

President's Award for Exceptional and Innovative Leadership in Adult and Continuing Education, 2544

Prince George's County Bureau of Aging, 1215

Professional Advisory Support Award, 2545

Providence Assisted Living, 8645

Pulmonary Hypertension Association, 6650

Queen Anne's County Department of Aging, 1216

RADAR Network, 6958

RP Foundation Fighting Blindness (RPFFB), 7461

RSVP Allegany County, 1217

RSVP Baltimore City, 1218

RSVP Hagerstown, 1219

RSVP Lower Eastern Shore, 1220

RSVP Prince George's County, 1222

RSVP St. Mary's County, 1223

Railroad Retirement Board: Maryland District Office, 1224

Renaissance Gardens at Charlestown, 8646

Renaissance Gardens at Oak Crest, 8647

Renaissance Gardens at Riderwood, 8648

Resources for Independence, 10503

Retirement Industry Trust Association, 279

Rodeway Inns, 11747

Ronald Park Place, 8649

Rubens-Alcais Challenge, 2552

Self-Help for Hard of Hearing People, Cleveland West Chapter, 6195

Senior Service America, 283

Setting Priorities for Retirement YearsFoundation, 284

Sexual Function Health Council, 6687

Social Security Administration, 286

Social Security: Baltimore Disability Determination, 1225

Social Security: Retirement Insurance, 287

Social Security: Special Benefits for Persons Aged 72 & Older, 288

Southern Maryland Center for LIFE, 10504

Special Friend of Hearing Impaired People Award, 2553

Special Needs Library Montgomery County Department of Public Libraries, 11255

Spirit of SHHH Award, 2554

Spring Dell Center, 11256

St. Mary's County Office on Aging, 1226

Substance Abuse & Mental Health ServicesAdministration, 6962

Substance Abuse and Mental Health Services Administration, 7218

Ticket Counter, 11753

US Army: Medical Command Center for Health Promotion & Preventive Medicine, 11257

US Department of Veterans Affairs Hospitl: Fort Howard Hospital Library, 11258

US Department of Veterans Affairs: Baltimore Medical Center Library Service, 11259

US National Institutes of Health: National Cancer Institute-Scientific Library, 11260

US Social Security Administration Library & Records Management Branch, 11261

Urban Cardiology Research Center, 6642

Vascular Disease Foundation, 6643

Volunteers for the Visually Handicapped, 7504

Walter T. Ridder Award, 2558

Warren Grant Magnuson Clinical Center, 6086, 6644, 7783, 7783

Washington County Commission on Aging, 1227

Washington Ear, 7506

Wheelchair and Mattress Pads, 3089

Workplace Program, 6973

Massachusetts

AD LIB Incorporated, 10505

Adams Council on Aging, 1228

Administration on Aging: Region I, 1229

Alden Place, 8650

Allerton House at Central Park, 8651

Allerton House at Hancock Park, 8652

Allerton House at Harbor Park, 8653

Allerton House at the Village at Duxbury, 8654

American Inn at Sawmill, 8655

American Macular Degeneration Foundation, 7255

Arbors at Amherst, 8656

Artia in Falmouth, 8657

Assistive Technology, 2944

Atrium at Cardinal Drive, 8658

Atrium at Drum Hill Alzheimer's Dementia Assisted Living, 8659

Atrium at Faxon Woods, 8660

Atrium at Veronica Drive, 8661

Avery Crossing, 8662

Bay State Council of the Blind, 7274

Baypath Senior Citizens Services, 1230

Berman-Gund Laboratory for the Study of Retinal Degenerations, 7761

Bernardston Council on Aging, 1231

Bertram House of Swampscott, 8663

Beverly Council on Aging, 1232

Billerica Crossings, 8664

Bookholder: Roberts, 3318

Boston Center for Independent Living, 10506

Boston College Legal Assistance Bureau, 10863

Boston College: Social Work Library, 11262

Boston Commission on Affairs of the Elderly, 1233

Boston University Laboratory of Neuropsychology, 7193

Boston University: General Clinical Research Center, 6600

Boston University: Whitaker Cardiovascular Institute, 6601

Briarwood Continuing Care Retirement Community, 8665

Brighton Gardens of Dedham, 8666

Brighton Gardens of North Shore by Marriott, 8667

Bristol Elder Services, 1234, 10864

Cadbury Commons at Cambridge, 8668

Cambridge Homes, 8669

Cameron House, 8670

Cape & Islands Senior Corps, 1235

Cape Organization for Rights of the Disabled (CORD), 10507

Caption Center, 11263, 6108

Caritas Southwood Hospital Medical Library, 11264

Carmel Terrace, 8671

Carroll Center for the Blind, 7298

Center for Living and Working, 10508

Central Massachusetts Agency on Aging, 1236

Chelmsford Crossings, 8672

Chelsea-Revere-Winthrop: Area Agency onAging, 1237

Christopher Heights Assisted Living, 8673

Christopher Heights of Webster, 8674

Coastline Elderly Services, 1238

Cohen Florence Levine Estates, 8675

Commonwealth of Massachusetts Executive Office of Elder Affairs, 10865

Community Action Commission of Cape Cod & Islands, 1239

Concord Park Assisted Living, 8676

Country Club Heights, 8677

DEAF Inc., 10509

Dalton Council on Aging, 1240

Dana-Farber Cancer Institute Library, 11265

Davis Manor, 8678

Deaconess Hospital Horrax Library, 11266

Decatur House, 8679

Deluxe Sock and Stocking Aid, 3092

Digi-Flex, 3107

Disability Law Center (DLC), 10866

Draper Place at Hopedale, 8680

Duxbury Braille Translator, 2973

Duxbury Systems, 2974

Eaton-Peabody Laboratory of Auditory Physiology, 6130

Elastic Shoelaces, 3094

Elder Service Plan of the North Shore, 1241

Elder Services of Berkshire County, 1242

Elder Services of Cape Cod and the Islands, 1243

Eldercare Initiative in Consumer Law, 111

Elderhostel, 11720

Elderhostel Institute Network, 11721

Electric Leg Bag Emptier and Tub Slide Shower Chair, 2879

Emmanuel House Residence, 8681

Eye Relief Word Processing Software, 2978

Falls at Cordingly Dam, 8682

Featherweight Reachers, 3095

Ferguson Industries for the Blind, 7326

Finger Print Pen, 3326

Forge Hill Senior Living Community, 8683

Mulligan Foundation, 6783
Nek-Lo, Nek-Lo Hot and Cold,
    Pillow-Perfect, Body Buddy, 3077
Northeast Michigan: Agency on Aging,
    1329
Northland Library Cooperative, 11286
Northpointe Woods Assisted Living, 8786
Oakland County Library for the Blind and
    Physically Handicapped, 11287
Park Village Pines, 8787
Parkinson Association of Michigan, 6712
Personal Amplifier, 3170
Personal FM Systems, 3012
Personal Infrared Listening System, 3013
Pilgram Manor, 8788
Plymouth Inn, 8789
Porter Hills Presbyterian Village, 8790
Presbyterian Village Redford, 8791
RSVP Genesee-Shiawassee Counties, 1330
RSVP Ingham, 1331
RSVP Kent County, 1333
RSVP Macomb, 1334
RSVP Marquette County, 1335
RSVP Mecosta/Lake/Osceola, 1336
RSVP Oakland County, 1337
RSVP Ostego County, 1338
RSVP Wayne County, 977, 1339
Railroad Retirement Board: Michigan
    District Office, 1340
Region Seven: Area Agency on Aging, 1341
Region Two: Area Agency on Aging, 1342
Renaissance Gardens at Henry Ford Village,
    8792
Rest Haven Home, 8793
Right to Life of Michigan, 1343
Riverview Manor, 8794
Room Valet Visual-Tactile Alerting System,
    3022
Rose Garden Home, 8795
Saginaw Geriatrics Home, 8796
Senior Alliance Area Agency on Aging,
    11288
Senior Companion Program of Macomb,
    1344
Senior Services, 1345
Sixty Plus Elderlaw Clinic, 10879
Speech Discrimination Unit, 3024
St Ann's Home, 8797
St Anne's Mead Retirement Home, 8798
St Clark County Library for the Blind and
    Physically Handicapped, 11289
St Joesph's Home for the Aged, 8799
State Bar of Michigan: Senior Justice
    Committee, 10880
State of Michigan Travel Resources, 11694
Strobe Light Signalers, 3029
Sunrise Assisted Living at Farmington Hills,
    8800
Sunrise Assisted Living at Northville, 8801
Sunrise Assisted Living of Ann Arbor, 8802
Sunrise Assisted Living of Rochester, 8803
Sunrise Assisted Living of Troy, 8804
Sunrise Assisted Living of West Bloomfield,
    8805
TTY's-Telephone Device for the Deaf, 3033
Tactile Smoke Detector, 3174
Talking Clocks, 3035
Telephone Signaler, 3175
The Chatter Vox - Speech Amplifier, 3038
The Senior Alliance: Area Agency on Aging
    1-C, 1346
Thurston Woods Village: The Villa, 8806

Tinnitus Masker, 3176
Tri-County Office on Aging, 1347
US Department of Veterans Affairs: Ann
    Arbor Hospital Library, 11290
US Department of Veterans Affairs: Battle
    Creek Medical Center Library Service,
    11291
US Department of Veterans Affairs: Detroit
    Medical Center Library Service, 11292
US Department of Veterans Affairs: Iron
    Mountain Medical Center Library, 11293
US Department of Veterans Affairs:
    Saginaw Aleda E Lutz Medical Center
    Library, 11294
University of Michigan Alcohol Research
    Center, 7221
University of Michigan: Communicative
    Disorders Clinic, 6560
University of Michigan: Division of
    Hypertension, 6668
University of Michigan: Kresge Hearing
    Research Institute, 6561
University of Michigan: Tecumster Mental
    Health Study, 5888
Valley: Area Agency on Aging, 1348
Vibrating Personal Pager, 3178
Vibrating Watch, 3179
Vibrotactile Personal Alerting System, 3046
Visual Smoke Detector, 3180
Visually Impaired Center, 7501
WINVISION, 3047
Waltonwood of Royal Oak, 8807
Washtenaw County Library, 11295
Waterford Senior Center, 1349
Wayne County Regional Library for the
    Blind, 11296
Weather Alert Systems, 3181
William T Gossett Parkinson's Disease
    Center, 6796
Woodhaven Retirement Community, 8808
Woodside at Friendship Village, 8809

Minnesota

Ability Research, 2925
AbleNet, 2929
Agape Senior Homes, 8810
Aging Service of Minnesota, 1350
Alliance Assisted Living Services, 8811
Almond House, 8812
Alterra Clare Bridge Cottage of West St
    Paul, 8813
Alterra Clare Bridge Cottage-Coon Rapids,
    8814
Alterra Clare Bridge Cottage-Owatonna,
    8815
Alterra Clare Bridge of Eagan, 8816
Alterra Clare Bridge of North Oaks, 8817
Alterra Clare Bridge of Plymouth, 8818
Alterra Sterling House of Apple Valley,
    8819
Alterra Sterling House of Blaine, 8820
Alterra Sterling House of Coon Rapids,
    8821
Alterra Sterling House of Faribault, 8822
Alterra Sterling House of Inver Grove
    Heights, 8823
Alterra Sterling House of West St Paul, 8824
Alterra Sterling House-Brooklyn Center,
    8825
Alterra Sterling House-Mankato, 8826

Alterra Sterling House-Sauk Rapids, 8827
Alterra Sterling House-Willmar, 8828
Alterra Sterling House-Winona, 8829
Alterra Sterling-Owatonna, 8830
Alterra Wynwood of Rochester, 8831
American Academy of Neurology, 6797
American Diabetes Association: Minnesota
    Area Office, 5926
Arlington Place, 8832
Arrowhead Senior Living Community, 8833
Arrowhead: Area Agency on Aging, 1351
Assisted Living in Heritage Hall, 8834
Assumption Court, 8835
Assured Care, 8836
Auburn Courts, 8837
BIGmack Communication Aid, 2947
Barrett Assisted Living Community, 8838
Barross House, 8839
Battery Device Adapter, 3131
Big Red Switch, 2949
Brickford Cottage, 8366, 8840
Brookridge, 8841
Brooks of St Paul, 8842
Bryant House, 8843
Bureau of Naval Personnel: Minnesota
    Retired Activities Office, 1352
Burnsdale Extended Care, 8844
Callista Court, 8845
Care Pointe, 8846
Care-Age Country Home, 8847
Carefree Living America-Brainerd, 8848
Carefree Living America-Burnsville, 8849
Carefree Living of America-St Cloud, 8850
Carric Manor, 8851
Cartens Harbour, 8852
Cass County Council on Aging, 1353
Catholic Eldercare at Home, 8853
Cedar Crest Estate, 8854
Cedars of Austin, 8855
Centennial Villa Assisted Living, 8856
Central Minnesota Council on Aging, 1354
Central Todd County Care Center, 8857
Chandler Place, 8858
Chappys Golden Shore, 8859
Claddagh House, 8860
Clearwater Suites Assisted Living, 8861
Commons on Marice, 8862
Communicating for Seniors, 1355
Community Assisted Living, 8863
Computer Switch Interface, 2965
Copperfield Hill Phase II, 8864
Cordless Big Red Switch, 2966
Cordless Receiver, 3154, 3191
Country Care Homes, 8215, 8865
Country Neighbors, 8866
Country Neighbors-Lake Crystal, 8867
Country Neighbors-Le Center, 8868
Country Oaks Elder Care, 8869
Country Villa, 8870
Dentists Concerned for Dentists, 6896
Department of Employment and Economic
    Development, 1356
Dignified Living, 8871
Dignified Living-Prior Lake, 8872
Dual Switch Latch and Timer, 3157
Duluth Lighthouse for the Blind, 7318
Duluth Public Library, 11297
East Central Regional Development
    Commission Area on Aging, 1358
Easy Stand, 3236
Edgewood Vista-Virginia, 8874
Elder Haven Homes, 8875

Mississippi

Missouri

Excel Stair Lift, 3240
Fairwinds-River's Edge, 9051
Foam Decubitus Bed Pads, 2902
Gateway Older Adult Legal Services, 10890
Greater St. Louis Association of the Deaf, 1437
Independent Living Center, 10341, 10537
Independent Living Resource Center, 10482, 10538
International Lutheran Deaf Association, 6151
Kansas City Association for the Blind, 7362
Legal Aid of Western Missouri: Kansas City, 10891
Living Independently for Everyone (LIFE), 10539
Long Term Care Ombudsman Program, 1438
Lutheran Library for the Blind, 11306
McKnight Place Assisted Living, 9053
Mid-America Regional Council of Aging Services, 1439
Mid-East: Area Agency on Aging, 1440
Midland Empire Resources for Independent Living (MERIL), 10540
Minivator Residential Elevator, 3252
Missouri Assisted Living Association, 1441
Missouri Council of the Blind, 1442
Missouri Department of Mental Health, 1443
Missouri Department of Revenue, 1444
Missouri Division of Senior & Disability Services, 10892
Missouri Division of Tourism, 11678
Missouri Division on Aging, 1445
Missouri Employees Retirement System, 1446
Missouri Planning Council For Developmental Disabilities, 1447
Missouri Protection & Advocacy Services, 1448
Missouri Protection and Advocacy, 10893
Missouri Rehabilitation Services for the Blind, 7386
National Rural Health Association, 234
NorthEast Independent Living Services (NEILS), 10541
On My Own, 10542
Ozark Independent Living, 10543
Paraquad, 10544
Pony Express Association of the Blind, 7449
Porch-Lift Vertical Platform Lift, 3254
RSVP Heartland, 1449
RSVP Andrew County, 1450
RSVP Boone County, 1451
RSVP Douglass Community Services, 1452
RSVP Dunklin County, 1453
RSVP Grundy/Sullivan Counties, 1454
RSVP Harrison-Daviess Counties, 1455
RSVP Jackson-Platte Counties, 1456
RSVP Jasper County, 1457
RSVP Livingston County, 1458
RSVP Mississippi County, 1459
RSVP Northwest Missouri/Northeast Kansas, 1460
RSVP Pemiscot County, 1461
RSVP Pettis-Saline Counties, 1462
RSVP Poplar Bluff-Altrusa Club, 1463
RSVP Quad Lakes, 1464
RSVP Scott-Cape Counties, 1465
RSVP Springfield, 1466

RSVP St. Charles-Lincoln-Warren Counties, 1467
RSVP St. Louis, 1468
Railroad Retirement Board: Kansas City Missouri District Office, 1469
Railroad Retirement Board: St. Louis, 1470
Region Ten: Area Agency on Aging, 1471
Rural Advocates for Independent Living (RAIL), 10545
SEMO Alliance for Disability Independence (SADI), 10546
Saint Louis Altenheim, 9054
Side-to-Side Folding Chair, 3399
Silver Glide Stairway Lift, 3260
Southwest Center for Independent Living (SCIL), 10548
Southwest Missouri Office on Aging, 1472
St. Louis Society for the Blind, 7478
St. Louis Society for the Blind and Visually Impaired, 1473
St. Louis University: Department of Psychiatry, 5887
St. Louis: Area Agency on Aging, 1474
Stair & Glide Stairway Lift, 3264
State of Missouri, 11695
Stretch-View Wide-View Rectangular Illuminated Magnifier, 3027
Sunrise Senior Living, 9055
Tower Club of the Blind, 7487
Tri-County Center for Independent Living, 10549
UMKC Institute for Human Development, 1475
US Department of Veterans Affairs, John Cochran Division Library, 11307
US Department of Veterans Affairs: Kansas Medical Center Library, 11308
US Department of Veterans Affairs: Poplar Bluff Library Service, 11309
US Department of Veterans Affairs:, Columbus Hospital Library, 11310
University of Missouri: Columbia Cosmopolitan Diabetes Center, 6077
University of Missouri: Columbia Division of Cardiothoracic Surgery, 6636
University of Missouri: Kansas City Drug Information Service, 7223
VPL Series Vertical Wheelchair Lift, 3274
VantAge Point: Area Agency on Aging-Region Ten, 1476
Washington University School of Medicine, 6873
Washington University: Diabetes Research and Training Center, 6087
Wecolator Stairway Lift, 3278
West Central Independent Living Solutions (WCILS), 10550
Wolfner Memorial Library for the Blind, 11311
Workers Compensation Board Missouri, 1477
Ziggy Medi-Chair, 3280

Montana

Action for Eastern Montana, 1478
American Diabetes Association: Montana, 5929
Area 1 Agency on Aging, 461, 1479
Area 2 Agency on Aging, 1480
Area 4 Agency on Aging, 463, 1481

Area 5 Agency on Aging, 1482
Area 7 Agency on Aging, 1483
Area 8 Agency on Aging, 1484
Area 9 Agency on Aging, 1485
Ashley Manor Medley I, 9056
Aspen Meadows Retirement Community, 9057
Bee Hive Homes of Flathead County, 9058
Bee Hive Homes of Helena, 9059
Buffalo Hill Terrace, 9060
Edgewood Vista, 8873, 9061
Grand Park Assisted Living Community, 9062
Hamilton House, 9063
Harmony House, 9064
Hawthorne House, 9065
Heritage Acres Assisted Living, 9066
Heritage Retirement Home, 9067
Highwood Senior Citizens, 1487
Hillside Place, 9068
Hunters Glen at Grizzly Peak, 9069
Kathy's Place, 9070
Living Independently for Today & Tomorrow (LIFTT), 10551
Lodge at Lone Tree Creek, 9071
Lodge at Mission River Manor, 9072
Loveland Acres, 9073
Missoula Aging Services, 1488
Montana Advocacy Program, 1489, 10894
Montana Department of Administration: Teacher's Retirement System, 1490
Montana Department of Military Affairs: Division of Veteran's Affairs, 1491
Montana Department of Public Health & Human Services, 1492
Montana Department of Retirement Administration, 1493
Montana Department of Revenue, 1494
Montana Department of Social and Rehabilitation Services, 1495
Montana Developmental Disability Council, 1496
Montana Division of Addictive & Mental Disorders, 6929
Montana Independent Living Project, 10552
Montana Legal Services Association: Helena, 10895
Montana Legal Services Developer Program & Office on Aging, 10896
Montana Masonic Home, 9075
Montana Protection & Advocacy Agency, 1497
Montana State Library, 11312
Next Best Place, 9076
North Central Independent Living Services, 10553
North Central Montana: Area Agency on Aging, 1498
Northern Rocky Mountain Retiree Association, 1499
Prestige Assisted Living at Kalispell, 9077
Prevention Resource Center, 6956
RSVP Butte School District No 1, 1500
RSVP Cascade County, 1501
RSVP Dawson-Wibaux, 1502
RSVP Fallon County, 1503
RSVP Helena, 1504
RSVP Hill County, 1505
RSVP Miles City, 1506
RSVP Roosevelt County, 1507
RSVP South Central Montana, 1508
RSVP Southwest Montana, 1509

RSVP Yellowstone County, 1510
Railroad Retirement Board: Montana District Office, 1511
Ravalli County Council on Aging, 1512
River Ridge, 9078
Springmeadows, 9079
St. Patrick Hospital and Health Sciences Center: Library Center, 11313
Summit Independent Living Center-Kalispell, 10554
Summit Independent Living Center-Missoula, 10555
Summit Independent Living Center-Ronan, 10556
US Department of Veterans Affairs: Fort Harrison Medical Center Library, 11314
US Department of Veterans Affairs: Miles City Medical Center Library, 11315
Waterford on Elizabeth Warren, 9080
Waterford on Saddle Drive, 9081
William K. Kohrs Memorial Library, 11316
Workers Compensation Court Montana, 1513

Nebraska

Aging Office of Western Nebraska, 1514
Aging Partners, 1515
Ambassabor Nebraska City Assisted Living, 9310
American Diabetes Association: Nebraska/South Dakota Area Office, 5931
An Angels Touch, 9311
Bell View Rehabilitation Center, 9312
Belle Aims Assisted Living Facility, 9313
Berverly Square Franklin, 9314
Bethany Home, 9315
Betty's House, 9316
Betty's House-Maple Street, 9317
Beverly Health Oak Grove, 9318
Beverly Healthcare Norfolk Chateau, 9319
Beverly Square Cozad, 9320
Beverly Square Fullerton, 9321
Beverly Square Nebraska City, 9322
Beverly Square Scottsbluff, 9323
Blue Rivers: Area Agency on Aging, 1516
Blue Valley Riverside Apartments, 9324
Brighton Gardens of Omaha, 9325
Cambridge Court, 9326
Carter House, 9327
Centennial Park Retirement Village, 9328
Center for Independent Living of Central Nebraska, 10562
Chancellor Place at Aspen Park, 9329
Chapion Home of Hastings, 9330
Chrisoma West Assisted Living, 9331
Christian Homes Assisted Living Center, 9332
Christian Record Services, 7305
Circus House, 9333
Clara-Ellen House, 9334
Clark Jeary Home, 9335
Comfortcare Homes of Nebraska, 9336
Community Action Partnership of Mid-Nebraska Volunteer Services, 1517
Community Memorial Health Center, 9337
Community Pride Care Center, 9338
Cornor Cottage, 9339
Cottonwood House, 9340
Cottonwood Villa, 9341

Countryside Home, 9342
Creighton University Cardiac Center, 6605
Creighton University: Midwest Hypertension Research Center, 6661
Crossroads Assisted Living, 9343
Crowell Home Health Services, 9344
Crown Villa, 9345
Custer Care Center, 9346
Diability Rights Nebraska, 1518
Division of Aging & Disability Services, 1520
Division of Aging and Disability Services: Legal Services for Older Adults, 10897
East Park Villa, 9347
Eastern Nebraska Office on Aging, 1521
Eastmont Towers, 9348
Edgewood Vista Columbus, 9349
Edgewood Vista Grand Island, 9350
Edgewood Vista Norfolk, 9351
Edgewood Vista of Fremont, 9352
Edgewood Vista of Hastings, 9353
Edgewood Vista of Omaha, 9354
El Dorado Manor Nursing Home, 9355
Emerald Court, 9356
Florence Home Assisted Living, 9357
Garden Square of Crete, 9358
Gateway Manor, 9359
Gold Crest Retirement Center, 9360
Golden Manor Assisted Living, 9361
Good Samaritan Society-Prairie View Gardens, 9362
Good Samaritan Towers, 9363
Good Shepherd Lutheran Home, 9364
Gordon Countryside Care, 9365
Grabd Island Sterling House, 9366
Gramercy Hill, 9367
Grand Court Seward Retirement Community Assisted Living, 9368
Grand Court Seward Retirment Community Assisted Living, 9369
Grand Island Veterand Home, 9370
Greeley Assisted Living, 9371
Greene House, 9372
Hastings Homestead, 9373
Haven Manor Assisted Living, 9374
Haven Manor College View, 9375
Heather and Shamrock Apartments, 9376
Hester Memorial Home, 9377
Hickory Villa, 9378
Hidden Pines Assisted Living Community, 9379
Highland House, 9380
Homestead, 9381
Hospice House, 9382
Immanuel Lakeside Terrace, 9383
Immanuel Trinity Village, 9384
Imperial Manor Nursing Home, 9385
Improved Living, 9386
Improved Living House II, 9387
Improved Living II, 9388
Kimball County Manor Nusing Home, 9389
Kirkwood House, 9390
League of Human Dignity Independent Living Center, 10563
Lebensraum Retirement Residence, 9391
Legacy, 9392
Legacy Terrace, 9393
Lester Dual-Mode Battery Charger, 3418
Lestronic II, 3419
Longs Creek Village, 9394
Madison House, 9395
Madonna Assisted Living, 9396

Mahoney House, 9397
Meadows, 8424, 8531, 8946, 8946, 9398
Merrick Manor Assisted Living, 9399
Methodist Memorial Homes, 9400
Midland: Area Agency on Aging, 899, 1522
Midwest Geriatrics, 1523
Morton House, 9401
National Federation of the Blind: Writers Division, 7420
National Organization of the Senior Blind, 7423
Nebraska Advocacy Services, 10898
Nebraska Assistive Technology Partnership, 1524
Nebraska Association Area Agencies on Aging, 1525
Nebraska Bar Association: Elderlaw Committee, 10899
Nebraska Client Assistance Program, 1526
Nebraska Commission for the Blind & Visually Impaired, 7426
Nebraska Commission for the Blind and Visually Impaired, 1527
Nebraska Commission for the Deaf & Hard of Hearing, 6180
Nebraska Department of Aging, 1528
Nebraska Department of Revenue, 1529
Nebraska Department of Veterans Affairs, 1530
Nebraska Division of Alcoholism and Drug Abuse, 6940
Nebraska Division of Travel & Tourism, 11679
Nebraska Library Commission: Talking Book & Braille Service, 11317
Nebraska School for the Visually Handicapped Library, 11318
New Cassel Retirement Center, 9402
Norfolk Homestead, 9403
North Platte Public Library, 11319
Northeast Nebraska: Area Agency on Aging, 1531
Northridge Retirement Community, 9404
Nye Square Retirement Community, 9405
Oakland Heights, 8432, 9406
Oaks Retirement Center, 9407
Omaha Department of Veteran Affairs Medical Center Research Service, 6069
Orchard Park, 9408
Our Homes, 9409
Paddock Kensington, 9410
Papillion Senior Citizen Center, 1532
Park Avenue Estates, 9411
Parkview Lodge Asssited Living, 9413
Parsons House on Eagle Run, 9414
Pathfinder House, 9415
Pawnee Hills, 9416
Pender Care Center, 9417
Pine Lane of Hartington, 9418
Plum Creek Care Center, 9419
Ponderosa Villa, 9420
Prairie Pines Lodge, 9421
Prairie Village Retirement, 9422
Prairie Winds, 9423
Precious Time, 9424
Premier Estates, 8440, 9425
Premier Estates Senior Living Community, 9426
Prescott Place, 9427
Prevent Blindness Nebraska, 7453
Princess Anne Residential Care, 9428
Quality Living, 9429

Nevada

New Hampshire

New Jersey

Soft-Touch Gel Flotation Cushion, 3082
Somerset County Office on Aging, 1636
Somerset Manor North, 9519
Somerset Manor South, 9520
Spring Hills at Morristown, 9521
Spring Meadows at Summit, 9522
St Marys Assisted Residence at Morris Hill, 9523
Stop-Leak Gel Flotation Cushion, 3084
Summerville at Hillsborough, 9524
Summerville at Stafford, 9525
Summerville at Voorhees, 9526
Sunnyside Manor, 9527
Sunrise Assisted Living East Brunswick, 9528
Sunrise Assisted Living of Edgewater, 9529
Sunrise Assisted Living of Morris Plains, 9530
Sunrise Assisted Living of Mt Laurel, 9531
Sunrise Assisted Living of Paramus, 9532
Sunrise Assisted Living of Wall, 9533
Sunrise Assisted Living of West Essex, 9534
Sunrise Assisted Living of Westfield, 9535
Sunrise of Old Tappan, 9536
Sunrise of Wayne, 9537
Sunrise of Woodbury Lake, 9538
Surnise of Woodcliff Lake, 9539
Sussex County Office on Aging, 1637
Total Living Center (TLC), 10573
Transportation Equipment for People with Disabilities, 2860
Transportation Made Easier, 2861
Twin Cedars, 9540
Twin-Rest Seat Cushion & Glamour Pillow, 3087
UMDNJ and Coriell Research Library, 11335
US Department of Veterans Affairs: East Orange Medical Center Library, 11336
US Department of Veterans Affairs: Lyon New Jersey Health Care System - Lyons Campus Hospital Library, 11337
Ultra-Lite XL Hand Control, 2862
Ultratec-Auto Answer TTY, 3041
Union County Division on Aging, 1638
Van Dyke Valley Assisted Living, 9541
Victoria Mews Assisted Living, 9542
Volunteer Center of Camden County, 1639
Volunteer Center of Monmouth County, 1640
Warren County Division of Senior Services, 1641
Waterproof Sheet-Topper Mattress and Chair Pad, 2906
Whispering Knoll Assisted Living, 9543
Willows at Holmdel Assisted Living Community, 9544
Wings & Wheels Greeting Cards, 3337
Wound, Ostomy and Continence Nurses Society, 6697

New Mexico

Ability Center for Independent Living, 10574
Acantilado Vista, 9545
American Diabetes Association: New Mexico Area Office, 5933
Beverly Foundation, 84
CHOICES Center for Independent Living, 10575

Capitan Public Library, 11338
City of Albuquerque-Bernalillo County: Department of Senior Affairs, 1642
Eastern New Mexico: Area Agency on Aging, 1644
Indian Health Services (IHS), 5960
Mesa Airlines, 11636
National Indian Council on Aging, 207
Native American Disability Law Center, 10915
New Mexico Aging & Long-Term Services Department: Elderly and Disability Services Division, 10916
New Mexico Behavioral Health Services, 6943
New Mexico Client Assistance Program, 1645
New Mexico Commission for the Blind, 7433
New Mexico Committee on Concerns of the Handicapped, 1646
New Mexico Department of Aging, 1647
New Mexico Department of Taxation and Revenue, 1648
New Mexico Department of Tourism, 11683
New Mexico Educational Retirement Board, 1649
New Mexico Governor's Committee on Concern of the Handicapped, 1650
New Mexico Protection & Advocacy for Persons with Disabilities, 1651
New Mexico Protection and Advocacy Agency, 10917
New Mexico Public Employees Retirement Association, 1652
New Mexico State Library: Blind and Physically Handicapped, 11339
New Mexico Technology Assistance Program, 1653
New Mexico Veterans Service Commission, 1654
New Mexico Workers Compensation Board, 1655
New Vistas Independent Living Center, 10576
North Central New Mexico: Area Agency on Aging, 1656
Office of Indian Affairs: Area Agency on Aging, 1657
Quality Senior Services, 1658
RSVP Alamogordo City, 1659
RSVP Artesia, 1660
RSVP Carlsbad City, 1661
RSVP Chaves County, 1662
RSVP Grant County, 1664
RSVP Los Alamos, 1665
RSVP Luna County, 1666
RSVP McKinley County, 1667
RSVP Metropolitan, 1668
RSVP Mid Rio Grand, 1669
RSVP San Juan County, 1670
RSVP Sandoval, 1671
RSVP Santa Fe City, 1672
RSVP Sierra County, 1673
RSVP Village of Ruidoso, 1674
RSVP-Rio Grande Valley, 1675
Railroad Retirement Board: New Mexico, 1676
Rampvan, 2854
Roswell Public Library, 11340
Senior Citizens Law Office, 10918

Southwestern New Mexico: Area Agency onAging, 1677
State Bar of New Mexico: Elder Law Section, 10919
State Bar of New Mexico: Lawyer Referral for the Elderly Program, 10920
US Department of Veterans Affairs: Albuquerque Medical Center Library, 11341
University of New Mexico: General Clinical Research Center, 6078

New York

3M Brailler, 2918
3M Large Printed Labeler, 2919
Academy of Rehabilitative Audiology, 6093
Access USA, 2930
Access to Independence and Mobility (AIM, 10577
Access to Independence and Mobility-Bath (AIM), 10578
Access to Independence of Cortland County, 10579
Access to Travel Magazine, 11615
Action Toward Independence, 10580
Adjustable Raised Toilet Seat, 2866
Adjustable Toilet Safety Rails, 2867
Administration on Aging (AoA): Regions II & III, 2378
Albany County Department for Aging and the Handicapped, 1678
Albany Talking Book Center, 11342
Alcoholics Anonymous, 6879
Allegany County Office for the Aging, 1679
Altria Plainview, 9546
Aluminum Adjustable Support Canes for the Blind, 3339
Aluminum Crutches, 3340
Aluminum Walking Canes, 3341
American Assembly for Men in Nursing, 14
American Board of Perianesthesia Nursing Certification, 31
American College of Clinical Pharmacology, 33
American Council for Drug Education, 6880
American Diabetes Association: Eastern Regional Office, 5914
American Diabetes Association: New York City Area Office, 5935
American Foundation for the Blind, 7247
American Parkinson's Disease Association, 6701
American Psychoanalytic Association, 54
American Society of Hypertension, 6645
American Thoracic Society, 65
Anna Erika Home for Adults, 9547
Arthwriter, 2941
Associated Blind, 7264
Association for Macular Diseases, 7267
Association for the Blind & Visually Impaired of Greater Rochester, 7269
Association of Belltel Retirees, 1680
Association of Personal Historians, 80
Association of the Bar of the City of New York: Committee for Senior Volunteer Lawyers, 10921
Atria Forest Hills, 9548
Auburn Options for Independence, 10581
Audio Recordings, 3313
Aurora of Central New York, 7272

North Carolina

North Dakota

Ohio

Oklahoma

Oregon

Lakeside Assisted Living Community, 9834
Lakewood Pointe Assisted Living, 9835
Lancaster Assisted Living, 9836
Lancaster Village, 9837
Lancaster Woods, 9838
Lane Council of Governments: Senior and Disabled Services Division, 1959
Lane County Law and Advocacy Center: Senior Law Service, 10951
Laurelhurst House Assisted Living Community, 9839
Legal Aid Services of Oregon: Senior Law Project, 10952
Lincolnshire Retirement & Assisted Living, 9840
Linkville House, 9841
Lone Oak Assisted Living, 9842
MacDonald Residence, 9843
Macklyn House, 9844
Magnolia Gardens Assisted Living Facilities, 9845
Markham House, 9846
Marquis Vintage Suites at Forest Grove, 9847
Mary's Woods at Marylhurst, 9848
McAuley Terrace, 9849
McKillop Residence Assisted Living Facility, 9850
McLoughlin Place, 9851
Meadow Creek Village Assisted Living Residence, 9852
Meadowbrook Place, 9853
Mid-Columbia Senior and Disabled Services, 1960
Mt Saint Joseph, 9854
Multnomah County Aging Services Division, 1961
Neawanna by the Sea, 9855
New Breakthroughs, 3009
Northridge Center, 9856
Oaks at Lebanon, 9857
Ocean Crest Retirement & Assisted Living Facility, 9858
Odyssey Club, 11741
Oregon Advocacy Center, 1962
Oregon Advocacy Center (OAC), 10953
Oregon Alliance of Senior & Health Services, 1963
Oregon Cascades West Senior Services, 1964
Oregon Commission on Disabilities, 1965
Oregon Council on Developmental Disabilities, 1966
Oregon Department of Addictions and Mental Health Services, 5841
Oregon Department of Aging, 1967
Oregon Department of Revenue, 1968
Oregon Department of Veterans Affairs, 1969
Oregon Health Sciences University, 6786
Oregon Health Sciences University: Oregon Hearing Research Center, 6548
Oregon Hearing Society, 1970
Oregon Office of Alcohol and Drug Abuse Programs, 6953
Oregon Protection & Advocacy for Persons with Disabilities, 1971
Oregon Public Employees Retirement System, 1972
Oregon School for the Blind Media Center, 11429
Oregon Senior Services, 1973

Oregon State Bar: Rights of Persons with Disabilities Section, 10954
Oregon State Commission for the Blind, 7444
Oregon State Library, 11430
Oregon Tourism Commission, 11688
Outback Ranch Outfitters, 11742
Park Place Assisted Living Residence, 9859
Parkhurst House, 9860
Parkland Village Assisted Living Facility, 9861
Pheasant Pointe Assisted Living, 9862
Pilot Rock Senior Center, 1974
Powell Valley ASL & ALZ Care Community, 9863
Prairie House Retirement & Assisted Community, 9864
Princeton Village, 9865
Providence Benedictine Orchard House, 9866
Providence Brookside Manor, 9867
Quail Run Assisted Living at Mennonite Village, 9868
RSVP Clackamus, 1975
RSVP Columbia County, 1751, 1976
RSVP Coos County, 1578, 1977
RSVP Curry County, 1663, 1978
RSVP Deschutes County, 1979
RSVP Jackson County, 1332, 1980
RSVP Josephine County, 1981
RSVP Lincoln County, 1982
RSVP Linn Benton County, 1983
RSVP Marion County, 752, 1984
RSVP Multonamah County, 1985
RSVP Roseburgburg, 1986
RSVP Washington County, 1906, 1987
Rackleff House, 9869
Railroad Retirement Board: Oregon District Office, 1988
Redwood Heights, 9870
Redwood Terrace, 9871
Regent at Regency Park Assisted Living, 9872
Regional Resource Center on Deafness, 6191
Ridgeview Assisted Living, 9873
River Road Assisted Living Residence, 9874
Riverwood Assisted Living, 9875
Rogue Valley Council of Governments: Senior and Disability Services Division, 1989
Rose Arbor Assisted Living, 9876
Rose Valley Assisted Living Facility, 9877
Rosewood Park, 9878
Russellville Park, 9879
SPOKES Unlimited, 10626
Sawyer House, 9880
Settler's Park Assisted Living & Memory Care, 9881
Shilo Inns & Resorts, 11749
Shore Pines Assisted Living, 9882
Silver Creek Assisted Living, 9883
Skylark Assisted Living, 9884
Southern Hills Assisted Living Community, 9885
Spencer House, 9886
Spring Meadows, 9887
Spring Valley Assisted Living Residence, 9888
Spring Village, 9889
Spruce Point, 9890
St Anthony Village, 9891

Summit Assisted Living, 9892
Summit Springs Assisted Living Facility, 9893
Sun Terrace Hermiston, 9894
Sundial Special Vacations, 11752
Suzanne Elise Assisted Living, 9895
Tanner Spring, 9896
Terwilliger Plaza, 9897
Timberhill Place, 9898
US Department of Veterans Affairs: Portland Medical Library, 11431
US Department of Veterans Affairs: Roseburg Medical Center Library Service, 11432
US Department of Veterans Affairs: White City Library, 11433
Valley View Assisted Living, 8290, 9899
Vestibular Disorders Association, 305
Vintage Suites, 9900
Vintage Suites at Hope Village, 9901
Vocational Rehabilitation Division, 1990
Washington County: Area Agency on Aging, 1991
Well Springs Assisted Living Facility, 9902
Wiley Creek Community, 9903
Willamette Manor, 9904
Willamette View, 9905
Willamette View Health Center, 9906
Wilsonville, 9907
Woodland Heights, 9908
Woodside Assisted Living Community, 9909

Pennsylvania

Accessibility Lift, 3221
Accessible Journeys, 11708
Active Aging, 1992
Adams County Office for Aging, 1993
Address Book, 3311
Adjustable Bed, 2899
Aging Services, 1994
Allegheny County Area Agency on Aging, 10955
Allegheny County Department of Aging, 1995
Alterra Wynnwood of Northampton Manor, 9910
Alzheimer Treatment Research Center Library, 11434
American Baptist Homes and Hospitals Association, 27
American Board of Internal Medicine, 30
American Board of Ophthalmology, 7244
American College of Physicians, Internal Medicine, 35
American Diabetes Association: Central Pennsylvania Area, 5908
American Diabetes Association: Western Pennsylvania Area Office, 5952
Anthracite Region Center for Independent Living, 10627
Armstrong: Area Agency on Aging, 1996
Artman Lutheran Home, 9911
Associated Services for the Blind and Visually Impaired, 7265
Beaver County Association for the Blind, 7275
Beaver County Office on Aging, 1997
Behan Health Science Library, 11435

Rhode Island

Tennessee

Inn at Los Patios, 10194
Inn at Orchard Park, 10195
Internet Stroke Center, 6799
Jefferson Place Assisted Living, 10196
Kensington Cottages at Quail Creek, 10197
Kensington Cottages by Centex, 10198
Kerrville State Hospital Professional
 Library, 11491
Kilroy House, 10199
Kings Manor Methodist Retirement System,
 2213
Kings Manor Personal Care Home, 10200
Kingsley Place at Oakwell, 10201
Kingsley Place at Stonebridge Ranch, 10202
Lakeridge Place, 10203
Lakewood 24 Hour Personal Care, 10204
Lakewood Village: Cummings Assisted
 Living Apartments, 10205
Leading Age Texas, 2214
Lexington Place, 10206
Lighthouse for the Blind of Houston, 7370
Lodge at Leon Springs, 10207
Lower Rio Grande Valley: Area Agency
 onAging, 2215
Magnolia Place, 9074, 10208
Marbridge Ranch, 10209
Meadow View Family Service, 10210
Memorial Oaks by Marriott, 10211
Merrill Gardens at Denton, an Assisted
 Living Community, 10212
Merrill Gardens at North Richland Hills,
 10213
Merrill Gardens at Round, 10214
Merrill Gardens at San Antonio, 10215
Merrill Gardens at San Marcos, 10216
Middle Rio Grande: Area Agency on Aging,
 2216
Mind Science Foundation Library, 11492
Morningside Manor, 10217
National Academy for Teaching and
 Learning About Aging, 165
National Federation of the Blind of Texas:
 Austin Chapter, 7412
New Life Outreach Boarding Home, 10218
Nissi Care Homes, 10219
North Central Texas: Area Agency on
 Aging, 2217
Northwest Oaks, 10220
Oak Park Retirement Center, 10221
Oak Shadows Allendale, 10222
Oak Wood Acres, 10223
Oak Wood Place, 10224
Oaktree Assisted Living, 10225
PROPATH, 6707
Pafford Place, 10226
Panhandle: Area Agency on Aging, 2218
Park Place Retirement, 10227
Park Place Retirement Residence of
 Friendswood, 10228
Park Place Retirement Residence of
 Stafford, 10229
Park at Beckett Meadows, 10230
Parkwood Place, 10231
Performance Gel Cushions, 3078
Permian Basin: Area Agency on Aging,
 2219
Pine Tree Cottage, 10232
Pointe at Cedar Park, 10233
Presbyterian Hospital of Dallas, 6789
Prevent Blindness Texas, 7458
Prevent Blindness Texas Central Regional,
 6189

Quality Personal Care Home, 10234
Quality of Living Residential Home, 10235
RDL Supply, 3257
REACH of Plano Resource Center on
 Independent Living, 10649
REACH/Resource Center on Independent
 Living, 11493
RSVP Bexar County, 2220
RSVP Big Country, 2221
RSVP Big Spring, 2222
RSVP Brazos Valley, 2223
RSVP Chisholm Trail County, 2224
RSVP Concho Valley, 2225
RSVP Concho Valley Texas, 2226
RSVP Corpus Christi, 2227
RSVP Dallas, 2228
RSVP Deep East Texas, 2229
RSVP El Paso City, 2230
RSVP Galveston County, 2231
RSVP Golden Triangle, 2232
RSVP Heart of Texas, 2233
RSVP Hockley County, 2234
RSVP Houston County, 2235
RSVP Lubbock, 2236
RSVP Metro Tarrant, 2237
RSVP Midland, 2238
RSVP North Texas, 2239
RSVP Red River Valley, 1383, 2240
RSVP Rio Grande Valley, 2241
RSVP Runningwater Draw, 2242
RSVP Swisher County, 2243
RSVP Texas Panhandle, 2244
RSVP Texoma, 2245
RSVP Travis County, 2246
Railroad Retirement Board: Fort Worth,
 Texas District Office, 2247
Railroad Retirement Board: Houston, Texas
 District Office, 2248
Reach Resource Center on Independent
 Living, 10650
Reach of Denton Resource Center on
 Independent Living, 10651
Regal Estates Senior Living, 10236
Regency of El Paso, 10237
Regent at Hamilton House Assisted Living,
 10238
Regent at Parmer Woods Assisted Living,
 10239
Remington Park, 10240
Rio Grande: Area Agency on Aging, 2249
Round Rock Volunteer Center, 2250
Royal Estates of El Paso, 10241
Royal Estates of San Angelo, 10242
SAILS, 10652
Sabine House, 10243
Saddleridge Lodge, 10244
Senior Citizens of Earth: Springlake Area,
 2251
Serenity Gardens Personal Care, 10245
Shallowater Senior Citizens, 2252
Signature Pointe on the Lake, 10246
Silicone Padding, 3081
Silverado Senior Living-Cypresswood,
 10247
Silverado Senior Living-Sugarland, 10248
Smooth Mover, 3263
South Plains Association of Governments
 Area: Agency on Aging, 2253
South Texas Lighthouse for the Blind, 7472
South Texas: Area Agency on Aging, 2254
Southeast Texas: Area Agency on Aging,
 2255

Southern Knights Assisted Living Center,
 10249
Spenco Medical Group, 3083
St Joesph Haven, 10250
State Bar of Texas: Texas Young Lawyers
 Association, 10987
State of Texas Office of the Governor
 Economic Development and Tourism,
 11697
Sugar Land Oaks Guest Home, 10251
Summer Glen Senior Living, 10252
Summer Ridge Assisted Living &
 Retirement Community, 10253
Summit at Lakeway, 10254
Summit at Northwest Hills, 10255
Taping for the Blind, 7480
Tarrant County Association for the Blind,
 7481
Texas Association of Area Agencies on
 Aging, 2256
Texas Association of Coordinators and
 Hearing Officers, 6197
Texas Association of Directors of Volunteer
 Services, 2257
Texas Association of Retinitis Pigmentosa,
 7484
Texas Commission for the Blind, 7485
Texas Commission on Alcohol and Drug
 Abuse, 6964
Texas Comptroller of Public Accountants,
 2258
Texas Council for Developmental Disabilities,
 2259
Texas Department of Aging and Disability
 Services (DAD), 2260, 10988
Texas Department of Health Library, 11494
Texas Department of Mental Health &
 Mental Retardation, 5845
Texas Geriatrics Society, 2261
Texas Governor's Committee for People
 With Disabilities, 2262
Texas Heart Institute, 6581
Texas Legal Services Center: Legal Hotline
 for Older Texans, 10989
Texas Protection & Advocacy Services for
 Disabled Persons, 2263
Texas Protection and Advocacy Agency
 North Texas Regional Office: Dallas,
 10990
Texas Society to Prevent Blindness, 7486
Texas State Library, 11495
Texas State Library Talking Book Program,
 11496
Texas State Technical College: Waco
 Library, 11497
Texas Tech University:
 Speech-Language-Hearing Clinic, 6555
Texas Tech University: Tarbox Parkinson's
 Disease Institute, 6792
Texas Veterans Commission, 2264
Texas Workers Compensation Commission,
 2265
Texoma: Area Agency on Aging, 2266
The Chandler Senior Center, 2267
Touch of Home, 10256
Travis Association for the Blind, 7488
Travis County Services for the Deaf and
 Hard of Hearing, 6198
Trinity Towers, 10257
Twelve Oaks Irving Assisted Living Center,
 10258

Utah

Vermont

Virginia

Washington

Abuse, Elder

Clearinghouse on Abuse and Neglect of the Elderly, 84
International Network for the Preventionof Elder Abuse, 2621
National Center on Elder Abuse, 2630
National Clearinghouse on Abuse in Later Life, 2632
National Committee for the Prevention of Elder Abuse, 155
T.A.S.A. Taskforce Against Senior Abuse, 8149

Abuse, Substance: See Substance Abuse

The Council on Alcohol and Drugs, 5385
Fresh Start Alcohol and Drug Recovery Group, 5340
SMART Recovery, 5378

Acquired Immunodeficiency Syndrome: See AIDS

American Civil Liberties Union: HIV, 3249
HIV Wisdom for Older Women, 3252
Life Force: Women Fighting AIDS, 3256

Active Elderly

ACE Fitness Matters, 2801
Assisted Living Federation of America, 65
Buena Vida, 2813
Center for Positive Aging, 2616
Center for Social Gerontology, 2617
Central Vermont Council on Aging (CVCOA), 1716
Diabetic's Guide to Health and Fitness, 4625
Digi-Flex, 2280
Elder Fit: A Health and Fitness Guide, 2674
Exercise and Your Heart, 5104
Experience Works, 102, 2619
Fairwinds-Woodward Park, 6229
Fitness Diet and Exercise Guide, 2832
Functional Fitness Assessment for Adults, 2680
General Fitness, 3039
Gentle Path Through the Twelve Steps, 5412
Jefferson's Garden, 7485
Mini-Max Cushion, 2262
National Senior Games Association, 190
Over the Hill Gang International, 198
Stay Fit Video, 3010
Suggested Exercise Program for People with Parkinson's Disease, 5222
Therapy Putty, 2298

Adult Children

Advanced Sign Language Vocabulary, 4785
Aging Children & Aging Parents, 2654
Al-Anon Family Groups - Classic Edition, 5401
Alabama Developmental Disability Council, 260
Allergy and Asthma Network Mothers of Asthmatics, 3457
Choices in Deafness, 4794

Colorado School for the Deaf and Blind, 8450
Disability Rights Education and Defense Fund, 8161
Endeavor, 4935
Family Guide - Growth & Development of the Partially Seeing Child, 6048
Food Allergy and Atopic Dermatitis, 3451
If Your Parents Drink Too Much, 5514
Immune Deficiency Foundation, 3255
Legal Center for People with Disabilities and Older People, 8177
Lessons in Laughter: The Autobiography of a Deaf Actor, 4838
Lisa and Her Soundless World, 4840
My Mother, My Father, 3001
NAD Broadcaster, 4889

Adult Day Care

Elderhaus, 405
National Adult Day Services Association, 139

Aging

AARP, 2525, 3015
AARP Bulletin, 2799
AARP The Magazine, 2800
AgainCare.org, 2600
Age in place, 3017
Agency on Aging: Region 10, 391
Aging in America, 3091
Aging Research Institute, 3089
Alameda County Area: Agency on Aging, 337
Alaskans Commission on Aging, 288
Albemarle Commission, 1342
Alliance for Aging, 454
Alliance for Aging Research, 2601, 3092
Alliance for Retired Americans, 2602
Alpine: Area Agency on Aging, 392
American Aging Association, 3093
American Federation for Aging Research, 3094
American Society on Aging, 2606
Area 1 Agency on Aging, 339
Area 12 Agency on Aging, 340
Area 4 Agency on Aging, 341
Arizona Center on Aging, 296, 2609
Arkansas Department of Human Services: Division of Aging and Adult Services, 317
Art of Getting Well, 2660
Association for Adult Development and Aging, 2610
Boston Commission on Affairs of the Elderly, 841
Brookdale Center for Healthy Aging and Longevity, 2612, 3102
Butler County Department on Aging, 667
California Agency of Health and Welfare: Department of Aging, 344
California Association of Area Agencies on Aging, 345
California Commission on Aging, 346
California Department of Aging, 347
California Department of Aging and Adult Services, 348
Capital: Area Agency on Aging, 1625
Center for Benefits Access, 2613

Center for Healthy Aging, 2614
Central Savannah River Regional: Area Agency on Aging, 502
Coastal Bend: Area Agency on Aging, 1627
Colorado Aging and Adult Services, 394
Commission on Law and Aging, 87
Concho Valle: Area Agency on Aging, 1628
Connecticut Commission On Again, 423
Denver Regional Council of Governments:Area Agency on Aging, 402
East Alabama Commission: Agency on Aging, 266
East Arkansas Area: Agency on Aging, 327
East Central Illinois: Area Agency on Aging, 563
Eastern Connecticut Area: Agency on Aging, 428
Egyptian: Area Agency on Aging, 564
ElderCareMatters.com, 3030
Elderhostel, 8998
Experimental Aging Research, 2831
Florida Department of Aging, 462
Genesis Institute, 110
Georgia Department of Aging, 506
Georgia Office of Aging, 511
Golden Crescent: Area Agency on Aging, 1633
Harvey A. Friedman Center for Aging, 2620, 3133
Henry County Council on Aging, 517
Houston-Galveston: Area Agency on Aging, 1638
Huerfano Las Animas: Area Agency on Aging, 407
Hunter House Publishing, 8882
Imperial County: Area Agency on Aging, 368
Jefferson Council on Aging, 751
Jewish Council for the Aging of GreaterWashington, 2622
Journal of American Aging Association, 2851
Journey to Pain Relief, 2685
Kern County Aging and Adult Services, 369
Kings Tulare Area: Agency on Aging, 370
Lafourche Council on Aging, Inc., 752
Leadership Council of Aging Organizations, 2623
Leading Age Texas, 1640
LeadingAge, 450, 2624
Los Angeles County: Area Agency on Aging, 372
Lower Rio Grande Valley: Area Agency onAging, 1641
Merced County: Area Agency for Aging, 374
Mid-Carolina: Area Agency on Aging, 1354
Middle Rio Grande: Area Agency on Aging, 1642
Midland: Area Agency on Aging, 583
Minnesota Board on Aging, 968
National Association of Area Agencies on Aging, 144
National Association of States United for Aging and Disabilities, 149
National Center for Creative Aging, 2629
National Council on Aging, 2634
National Indian Council on Aging (NICOA), 171
National Institute of Senior Centers, 2636
National Older Worker Career Center, 2638

AIDS

Allergies

Alzheimer's Disease, See also Dementia

American Cancer Society: Beaumont, 3897
American Cancer Society: Bethlehem, 3898
American Cancer Society: Billings, 3899
American Cancer Society: Birmingham, 3900
American Cancer Society: Blue Bell, 3901
American Cancer Society: Boise, 3902
American Cancer Society: Bowling Green, 3903
American Cancer Society: Brockton, 3904
American Cancer Society: Bronx, 3905
American Cancer Society: Brooklyn, 3906
American Cancer Society: Burbank, 3907
American Cancer Society: Campbell, 3908
American Cancer Society: Canfield, 3909
American Cancer Society: Cedar Knolls, 3910
American Cancer Society: Cedar Rapids, 3911
American Cancer Society: Charleston, 3912
American Cancer Society: Charlotte, 3913
American Cancer Society: Charlottesville, 3914
American Cancer Society: Chattanooga, 3915
American Cancer Society: Cherry Hill, 3916
American Cancer Society: Chicago, 3917
American Cancer Society: Chico, 3918
American Cancer Society: Cincinnati, 3919
American Cancer Society: Clearfield, 3920
American Cancer Society: Cleveland, 3921
American Cancer Society: Colorado Springs, 3922
American Cancer Society: Columbia, 3923
American Cancer Society: Columbus, 3924
American Cancer Society: Corpus Christi, 3925
American Cancer Society: Culver City, 3926
American Cancer Society: Cumberland, 3927
American Cancer Society: Dallas, 3928
American Cancer Society: Daytona Beach, 3929
American Cancer Society: Denver, 3930
American Cancer Society: Des Moines, 3931
American Cancer Society: Dublin, 3932
American Cancer Society: Duluth, 3933
American Cancer Society: Eagan, 3934
American Cancer Society: East Lansing, 3935
American Cancer Society: East Syracuse, 3936
American Cancer Society: El Centro, 3937
American Cancer Society: El Paso, 3938
American Cancer Society: Eldersburg, 3939
American Cancer Society: Erie, 3940
American Cancer Society: Eugene, 3941
American Cancer Society: Eureka, 3942
American Cancer Society: Evansville, 3943
American Cancer Society: Everett, 3944
American Cancer Society: Fairlawn, 3945
American Cancer Society: Fargo, 3946
American Cancer Society: Flint, 3947
American Cancer Society: Flushing, 3948
American Cancer Society: Fort Lauderdale, 3949
American Cancer Society: Fort Myers, 3950
American Cancer Society: Fort Walton Beach, 3951
American Cancer Society: Fort Wayne, 3952
American Cancer Society: Fort Worth, 3953

American Cancer Society: Frackville, 3954
American Cancer Society: Framingham, 3955
American Cancer Society: Fresno, 3956
American Cancer Society: Gainesville, 3957
American Cancer Society: Gainesville, FL, 3958
American Cancer Society: Glen Allen, 3959
American Cancer Society: Grand Junction, 3960
American Cancer Society: Greater Tampa, 3961
American Cancer Society: Greater Ventura, 3962
American Cancer Society: Greeley, 3963
American Cancer Society: Green Bay, 3964
American Cancer Society: Greenbelt, 3965
American Cancer Society: Greensboro, 3966
American Cancer Society: Greensburg, 3967
American Cancer Society: Greenville, 3968
American Cancer Society: Greenville, NC, 3969
American Cancer Society: Greenwood, 3970
American Cancer Society: Harrisonburg, 3971
American Cancer Society: Hershey, 3972
American Cancer Society: Hilo, 3973
American Cancer Society: Hollidaysburg, 3974
American Cancer Society: Holyoke, 3975
American Cancer Society: Honolulu, 3976
American Cancer Society: Houston, 3977
American Cancer Society: Huntsville, 3978
American Cancer Society: Indianapolis, 3979
American Cancer Society: Jackson, 3980
American Cancer Society: Jackson, TN, 3981
American Cancer Society: Jacksonville, 3982
American Cancer Society: Jefferson City, 3983
American Cancer Society: Johnson City, 3984
American Cancer Society: Kansas City, 3985
American Cancer Society: Kearney, 3986
American Cancer Society: Kennesaw, 3987
American Cancer Society: Knoxville, 3988
American Cancer Society: Lafayette, 3989
American Cancer Society: Lake County, 3990
American Cancer Society: Lakeland, 3991
American Cancer Society: Lakes Region, 3992
American Cancer Society: Lancaster, 3993
American Cancer Society: Las Vegas, 3994
American Cancer Society: Latham, 3995
American Cancer Society: Lawton, 3996
American Cancer Society: Lexington, 3997
American Cancer Society: Lihue, 3998
American Cancer Society: Lincoln, 3999
American Cancer Society: Little Rock, 4000
American Cancer Society: Long Beach, 4001
American Cancer Society: Louisville, 4002
American Cancer Society: Lubbock, 4003
American Cancer Society: Lufkin, 4004
American Cancer Society: Lynchburg, 4005
American Cancer Society: Macon, 4006
American Cancer Society: Madison, 4007
American Cancer Society: Manasquan, 4008

American Cancer Society: Manhattan, 4009
American Cancer Society: Marco Island, 4010
American Cancer Society: Marion, 4011
American Cancer Society: Martinsville, 4012
American Cancer Society: Maryville, 4013
American Cancer Society: McAllen, 4014
American Cancer Society: Medford, 4015
American Cancer Society: Melbourne, 4016
American Cancer Society: Memphis, 4017
American Cancer Society: Miami, 4018
American Cancer Society: Midland, 4019
American Cancer Society: Mishawaka, 4020
American Cancer Society: Missoula, 4021
American Cancer Society: Mobile, 4022
American Cancer Society: Modesto, 4023
American Cancer Society: Montgomery, 4024
American Cancer Society: Morgantown, 4025
American Cancer Society: Myrtle Beach, 4026
American Cancer Society: Naples, 4027
American Cancer Society: Nashville, 4028
American Cancer Society: New Castle, 4029
American Cancer Society: New Hampshire, 4030
American Cancer Society: New Orleans, 4031
American Cancer Society: New Windsor, 4032
American Cancer Society: Newport News, 4033
American Cancer Society: North Charleston, 4034
American Cancer Society: Norwalk, 4035
American Cancer Society: Oak Brook Terrace, 4036
American Cancer Society: Oklahoma City, 4037
American Cancer Society: Omaha, 4038
American Cancer Society: Onalaska, 4039
American Cancer Society: Orange County Region, 4040
American Cancer Society: Osage Beach, 4041
American Cancer Society: Paducah, 4042
American Cancer Society: Palm Beach, 4043
American Cancer Society: Palm Desert, 4044
American Cancer Society: Panama City, 4045
American Cancer Society: Pasadena, 4046
American Cancer Society: Pensacola, 4047
American Cancer Society: Peoria, 4048
American Cancer Society: Perrysburg, 4049
American Cancer Society: Philadelphia, 4050
American Cancer Society: Phoenix, 4051
American Cancer Society: Pittsburgh, 4052
American Cancer Society: Portland, 4053
American Cancer Society: Raleigh, 4054
American Cancer Society: Reno, 4055
American Cancer Society: Rhode Island, 4056
American Cancer Society: Riverside, 4057
American Cancer Society: Roanoke, 4058
American Cancer Society: Rochester, 4059
American Cancer Society: Rocky Hill, 4060
American Cancer Society: Rogers, 4061

American Cancer Society: Sacramento, 4062

American Cancer Society: Saint Cloud, 4063

American Cancer Society: Saint Louis, 4064

American Cancer Society: Salinas, 4065

American Cancer Society: Salisbury, 4066

American Cancer Society: Salt Lake City, 4067

American Cancer Society: San Antonio, 4068

American Cancer Society: San Diego, 4069

American Cancer Society: Santa Barbara, 4070

American Cancer Society: Santa Rosa, 4071

American Cancer Society: Sarasota, 4072

American Cancer Society: Savannah, 4073

American Cancer Society: Seattle, 4074

American Cancer Society: Sioux Falls, 4075

American Cancer Society: Southfield, 4076

American Cancer Society: Spokane, 4077

American Cancer Society: Springfield, 4078

American Cancer Society: State College, 4079

American Cancer Society: Staten Island, 4080

American Cancer Society: Statesboro, 4081

American Cancer Society: Stockton, 4082

American Cancer Society: Stroudsburg, 4083

American Cancer Society: Suffolk Region, 4084

American Cancer Society: Suisun City, 4085

American Cancer Society: Tacoma, 4086

American Cancer Society: Tallahassee, 4087

American Cancer Society: Taylor, 4088

American Cancer Society: Tinley Park, 4089

American Cancer Society: Topeka, 4090

American Cancer Society: Topsham, 4091

American Cancer Society: Tucson, 4092

American Cancer Society: Tulsa, 4093

American Cancer Society: Tuscon, 4094

American Cancer Society: Tyler, 4095

American Cancer Society: Utica, 4096

American Cancer Society: Valencia, 4097

American Cancer Society: Vermont, 4098

American Cancer Society: Vero Beach, 4099

American Cancer Society: Vienna, 4100

American Cancer Society: Villages, 4101

American Cancer Society: Virginia Beach, 4102

American Cancer Society: Waco, 4103

American Cancer Society: Wailuku, 4104

American Cancer Society: Walnut Creek, 4105

American Cancer Society: Waukesha, 4106

American Cancer Society: West Palm Beach, 4107

American Cancer Society: White Pines, 4108

American Cancer Society: Wichita, 4109

American Cancer Society: Williamsport, 4110

American Cancer Society: Wilmington, 4111

American Cancer Society: Winter Park, 4112

American Cancer Society: Wyoming, 4113

American Institute for Cancer Research, 4346

American Lung Association, 3023, 3376, 3459, 4114

American Lung Association: Alabama, 3377, 4115

American Lung Association: Alaska, 3378, 4116

American Lung Association: Arizona, 3379, 4117

American Lung Association: Arkansas, 3380, 4118

American Lung Association: California, 3381, 4119

American Lung Association: Colorado, 3382, 4120

American Lung Association: Connecticut, 3383, 4121

American Lung Association: Delaware, 3384, 4122

American Lung Association: District of Columbia, 3385, 4123

American Lung Association: Florida, 3386, 4124

American Lung Association: Georgia, 3387, 4125

American Lung Association: Hawaii, 3388, 4126

American Lung Association: Idaho, 3389, 4127

American Lung Association: Illinois, 3390, 4128

American Lung Association: Indiana, 3391, 4129

American Lung Association: Iowa, 3392, 4130

American Lung Association: Kansas, 3393, 4131

American Lung Association: Kentucky, 3394, 4132

American Lung Association: Louisiana, 3395, 4133

American Lung Association: Maine, 3396, 4134

American Lung Association: Maryland, 3397, 4135

American Lung Association: Massachusetts, 3398, 4136

American Lung Association: Michigan, 3399, 4137

American Lung Association: Minnesota, 3400, 4138

American Lung Association: Mississippi, 3401, 4139

American Lung Association: Missouri, 3402, 4140

American Lung Association: Montana, 3403, 4141

American Lung Association: Nebraska, 3404, 4142

American Lung Association: Nevada, 3405, 4143

American Lung Association: New Hampshire, 3406, 4144

American Lung Association: New Jersey, 3407, 4145

American Lung Association: New Mexico, 3408, 4146

American Lung Association: New York, 3409, 4147

American Lung Association: North Carolina, 3410, 4148

American Lung Association: North Dakota, 3411, 4149

American Lung Association: Ohio, 3412, 4150

American Lung Association: Oklahoma, 3413, 4151

American Lung Association: Oregon, 3414, 4152

American Lung Association: Pennsylvania, 3415, 4153

American Lung Association: Rhode Island, 3416, 4154

American Lung Association: South Carolina, 3417, 4155

American Lung Association: South Dakota, 3418, 4156

American Lung Association: Tennessee, 3419, 4157

American Lung Association: Texas, 3420, 4158

American Lung Association: Utah, 3421, 4159

American Lung Association: Vermont, 3422, 4160

American Lung Association: Virginia, 3423, 4161

American Lung Association: Washington, 3424, 4162

American Lung Association: West Virginia, 3425, 4163

American Lung Association: Wisconsin, 3426, 4164

American Lung Association: Wyoming, 3427, 4165

American Prostate Society, 3024

American Thoracic Society, 59, 4166

Aptium Oncology, 4167

Arizona State University: Cancer Research Institute, 4347

Ask the Doctor: Breast Cancer, 4262

Association for the Cure of Cancer of the Prostate, 4168

Association of Community Cancer Centers, 4169

Boston University Cancer Research Center, 4350

Breast Cancer: Understanding Treatment Options, 4282

Brigham Young University: Cancer Research Center, 4351

Brown University: Division of Biology and Medicine, 4352

California Institute for Medical Research, 5224

Calvary Hospital Medical Library, 8673

Cancer and Leukemia Group B, 4177

Cancer Care, 4171

Cancer Caring Center, 4172

Cancer Center of Wake Forest University: Bowman Gray School of Medicine, 4353

Cancer Control Society and Cancer Book House, 4173

Cancer Dictionary, 4263

Cancer Facts and Figures, 4264

Cancer Federation, 4174

Cancer of the Bladder: Research Report, 4283

Cancer of the Colon and Rectum: Research Report, 4284

Cancer of the Ovary: Research Report, 4285

Cancer of the Pancreas: Research Report, 4286

Cancer of the Uterus: Research Report, 4287

Cancer Prevention Institute of California, 4175

Cancer Rates and Risks, 4265

Cancer Research Center, 4354

Caregivers

Civil Rights, See also Legal Aid

Community Services

Computer Hardware, Software

Assistive Software Products, 2159
Dorma Architectural Hardware, 2318
Duxbury Braille Translator, 2182
Gibbs Associates, 8879
GW Micro, 2190
Vantage Plus, 2243

Consumer Rights, Protection

Coalition for Independent Living Options, 457
Council of Better Business Bureaus, 91
Eldercare Initiative in Consumer Law, 95
Vision World Wide, 6119

Continuing Education, See also Education

Adult Education, 1929
Association for Gerontology in Higher Education, 66, 8468, 8864
ASU Continuing Education, 1919
The Continuing Education Institute of Illinois, 1977
Grandparents Rights Organization, 111
Idaho State Continuing Education & Workforce Training, 1973
Institute for Integrative Healthcare, 2015
Milestone Continuing Education, 1980
Purchase College: School of Liberal Studies & Continuing Education, 2024
UA College of Continuing Studies, 1916
UAA Continuing Education Program, 1917
UD Professional & Continuing Studies, 1959
University of Alaska Southeast Campus: Adult Education Program, 1918
University of Arizona Continuing and Professional Education, 1926
University of Colorado Continuing Education, 1953
University of Phoenix Continuing Education, 1927

Day Care Centers

Division of Aging and Adult Services - Elder Choices, 7874
Florida Dog Guides F.T.D., 469
Rachel's Place Adult Day Care, 592
Senior Services of Northern Kentucky, 735

Deafness: See Hearing Impaired

ALDA News, 6021
American Cochlear Implant Alliance, 4703
Association of Late-Deafened Adults, 4708
National Federation of the Blind: Deaf-Blind Division, 5833

Death & Dying, See also Bereavement and Grief

Compassion and Choices, 4444
On Death and Dying, 4458

Talking About Death, 4461
United States Naval Academy Alumni Association: Register of Alumni, 2792

Dementia, See also Alzheimer's Disease

ABC's of Dementia, 3574
Activities for the Elderly: Volume 2-Working with Residents with Significant Physical and Cognitive,
Activity Programming for Persons with Dementia: A Sourcebook, 3575
Aegis at Shadowridge, 6175
Aegis of Carmichael, 6177
Aegis of Concord, 6179
Aegis of Pleasant Hill, 6187
Broadview Residential Care Center, 6204
Copper Ridge, 6682
Edward Feil Productions, 8873
Feil Method, VALIDATION, 2677
Garden of Palms, 6232
Gardens at Park Balboa, 6234
Guidelines for Dignity, 3590, 3628
Harvard Brain Tissue Resource Center, 3131
Key Elements of Dementia Care, 3595
Lewy Body Dementia Association, 4490
Marlow Manor/Manor Management, 6156
University of Wisconsin-Madison Neuropsychology Laboratory, 3237

Depression

Anxiety & Depression in Adults & Children, 4528
Anxiety and Depression Association of America, 4474
Depression & Antidepressents: A Guide, 4529
Depression and Bipolar Support Alliance, 4481
Depression and Recovery From Chemical Dependency, 4545, 5489
Depression in Older Adults, 2991
Depression in the Elderly: Multimedia Sourcebook, 4538
The Mindful Way through Depression: Freeing Yourself from Chronic Unhappiness, 4537
Mood Apart, 4533
Overcoming Depression, 4535
Plain Talk About Depression, 2957
Questions & Answers About Depression & Its Treatment, 4536
Understanding Depression and Addiction, 5569

Diabetes

American Diabetes Association, 4559
American Diabetes Association: Alabama, 4560
American Diabetes Association: Alaska, 4561
American Diabetes Association: Arizona, 4562
American Diabetes Association: Arkansas, 4563
American Diabetes Association: Central Florida, 4564

American Diabetes Association: Central Ohio, 4565
American Diabetes Association: Central Texas, 4566
American Diabetes Association: Colorado, 4567
American Diabetes Association: Connecticut & Western Massachusetts, 4568
American Diabetes Association: Districtof Columbia, 4569
American Diabetes Association: Eastern Pennsylvania & Delaware, 4570
American Diabetes Association: Georgia, 4571
American Diabetes Association: Hawaii, 4572
American Diabetes Association: Iowa, 4573
American Diabetes Association: Kansas, 4574
American Diabetes Association: Kentucky, 4575
American Diabetes Association: Louisiana & Mississippi, 4576
American Diabetes Association: Maryland, 4577
American Diabetes Association: Massachusetts, Maine, Rhode Island, New Hampshire, Vermont & Connecti, 4578
American Diabetes Association: Michigan, 4579
American Diabetes Association: Minnesota & North Dakota, 4580
American Diabetes Association: Missouri, 4581
American Diabetes Association: Montana, 4582
American Diabetes Association: Nebraska& South Dakota, 4583
American Diabetes Association: New Jersey, 4584
American Diabetes Association: New York, 4585
American Diabetes Association: No. California, 4586
American Diabetes Association: North Carolina, 4587
American Diabetes Association: North Texas, 4588
American Diabetes Association: Northeast Ohio, 4589
American Diabetes Association: Oklahoma, 4590
American Diabetes Association: Oregon, 4591
American Diabetes Association: So. California, 4592
American Diabetes Association: Tennessee, 4593
American Diabetes Association: Utah & Nevada, 4594
American Diabetes Association: Virginia, 4595
American Diabetes Association: Washington, 4596
American Diabetes Association: West Texas & New Mexico, 4597
American Diabetes Association: West Virginia, 4598
American Diabetes Association: Western Pennsylvania, 4599

Digestive Disorders

Disabled, See also Handicapped

Discrimination

Electronic Resources

Emergency Help

Employment, See also Occupations

Estate Planning: See Legal Aid

Euthanasia: See Assisted Suicide

Excercise, See also Physical Therapy

Family Relations

Pulmonary Hypertension Association, 5124
Wake Forest School of Medicine
 Hypertension and Vascular Research
 Center, 5125

Impotence

American Association of Sexuality
 Educators, Counselors & Therapists, 5138
American Urological Association, 5139
Family Meds, 3034
Impotence Causes and Treatments, 2933
Impotence Resource Center, 5144
Urology Care Foundation, 5141
UrologyHealth extra, 5143

Incontinence

American Association of Clinical Urologists,
 5148
American Association of Kidney Patients,
 5149
American Board of Urology, 5150
American Urological Association (AUA),
 5151
Female Urinary Incontinence, 5155
Informer, 2842, 2934
International Foundation for
 FunctionalGastrointestinal Disorders,
 5152
Managing Incontinence: A Guide to Living
 with Loss of Bladder Control, 5156
Pennsylvania State University Gerontology
 Center, 3165
Priva Inc., 2129
Quality Care, 2962
Simon Foundation for Continence, 2970,
 5158
Solution Starts with You, 3009
Wound, Ostomy & Continence Nurses
 Society, 5154

Independence

Abbotswood at Irving Park Assisted Living,
 7003
Access to Independence, 8117
Aegis of Napa, 6186
Aging in Stride: A Practical Guide for Older
 Adults & Their Families, 2656
Aiken Area Council on Aging, 1573
Alaska Commission on Aging, 280
Alaska Statewide Independent Living
 Council, 285
American Printing House for the Blind,
 5656, 5971, 6109
Appalachian Independence Center, 8109
Area 1 Northwest Indiana Community
 Action Corp., 609
Auburn Options for Independence, 8049
Bethlehem Woods Retirement Community,
 6460
Brooklyn Center for Independence of the
 Disabled, 8051
California Seniors Council, 356
Catskill Center for Independence, 8053
Center for Disability Rights, 7907
Center for Independence, 7906
Center for Independence of Disabled in New
 York (CIDNY), 8054
Citizens for Independence and Access, 8086

Clarity, 2173
Colorado Developmental Disability Council,
 398
Community Resources for Independence,
 8087
Costa Mesa Senior Center, 363
Country House in Westchester, 7340
Cumberland County Office of Aging, 1506
DBC-1 DU-IT Bed Control, 2126
Elder Services of Berkshire County, 850
Elderwise, 2064
Electric Leg Bag Emptier and Tub Slide
 Shower Chair, 2111
Finger Lakes Independence Center, 8055
Fountains at Crystal Lake-The Inn, 6464
Fountains at the Albemarle Inn, 7079
Gardens at Hillsborough Village, 6233
Grand Residence at Upper St. Clair, 7621
Greatest of Ease Company Catalog, 2751
Harvey County Department on Aging, 671
Heightened Independence & Progress (HIP),
 8041
Heightened Independence &
 Progress-Hudson (HIP Hudson), 8042
Illinois Department on Aging, 577
IMPACT, 7932
Independence, 8034
Independence Court of Hyattsville, 6692
Independence First, 8120
Independence Hill Assisted Living, 7765
Independence Manor at Hunterdon, 7301
Independence Now, 7979
Independence Place, 7971
Independence Unlimited Inc., 7910
Life and Independence for Today, 8091
Life Stream Services, 630
Linda Valley Villa, 6246
Living Independence for Everyone (LIFE)
 Center for Independent Living, 7927
Lumex's Cushions and Mattresses, 2261
Maine Department of Labor: Bureau of
 Rehabilitation Services, 793
Maryfield, 7104
Michigan Department of Human Services,
 923
North Carolina Council on Developmental
 Disabilities, 1360
North Country Center for Independence,
 8063
North Florida: Area Agency on Aging, 477
Northampton County: Area Agency on
 Aging, 1522
Oak Park Place-Albert Lea, 6927
Oklahoma Developmental Disability
 Council, 1448
OPTIONS for Independence-Northern Utah
 Center For Independent Living, 8105
Outdoor Independence, 2423
Palmer Independence, 2425
Plantation South at Duluth, 6386
Progressive Independence, 8079
Provena Fox Knoll Retirement, 6473
Push-Button Quad Cane, 2475
Regency at Glen Cove, 7350
Residence at Glen Riddle, 7624
Seniors First, 493
Southeast Texas: Area Agency on Aging,
 1676
Southeastern Illinois: Area Agency on
 Aging, 600
Southern Maine: Area Agency on Aging,
 802

Southern Nevada Center for Independent
 Living, 8038
Southwestern Illinois: Area Agency on
 Aging, 601
Sure Hands International, 2406
Texas Governor's Committee for People
 With Disabilities, 1683
Utah Statewide Independent Living Council,
 8108
Waterford Senior Center, 952
Woodside at Friendship Village, 6838

Information Centers,
See also Libraries

AARP Alabama, 2526
AARP Arizona, 2527
AARP Arkansas, 2528
AARP California: Pasadena, 2529
AARP California: Sacramento, 2530
AARP California: San Francisco, 2531
AARP Colorado, 2532
AARP Connecticut, 2533
AARP Delaware, 2534
AARP Florida: Doral, 2535
AARP Florida: St. Petersburg, 2536
AARP Florida: Tallahassee, 2537
AARP Georgia, 2538
AARP Hawaii, 2539
AARP Idaho, 2540
AARP Illinois, 2541
AARP Indiana, 2542
AARP Iowa, 2543
AARP Kansas, 2544
AARP Kentucky, 2545
AARP Louisiana, 2546
AARP Maine, 2547
AARP Maryland, 2548
AARP Massachusetts, 2549
AARP Michigan, 2550
AARP Minnesota, 2551
AARP Mississippi, 2552
AARP Missouri, 2553
AARP Montana, 2554
AARP Nebraska, 2555
AARP Nevada, 2556
AARP New Hampshire, 2557
AARP New Jersey, 2558
AARP New Mexico, 2559
AARP New York: Albany, 2560
AARP New York: New York, 2561
AARP New York: Rochester, 2562
AARP North Carolina, 2563
AARP North Dakota, 2564
AARP Ohio, 2565
AARP Oklahoma, 2566
AARP Oregon, 2567
AARP Pennsylvania: Harrisburg, 2568
AARP Pennsylvania: Philadelphia, 2569
AARP Rhode Island, 2570
AARP South Carolina, 2571
AARP South Dakota, 2572
AARP Tennessee, 2573
AARP Texas: Austin, 2574
AARP Texas: Dallas, 2575
AARP Texas: Houston, 2576
AARP Utah, 2577
AARP Vermont, 2578
AARP Virgin Islands, 2579
AARP Virginia, 2580
AARP Washington, 2581

Insurance

Large Print

Legal Aid

Libraries, See also Information Centers

Long Term Care

Lung Disease

Marketing

Medicaid

Medicare

Medicine

Minority Elderly

Mobility Aids

Money Management, See also Investments

Myths, Aging

Nursing Homes

Nutrition, See also Food

Older Americans Act

Orthopedics

Osteoporosis

Parkinson's Disease

Pensions

Physical Therapy, See also Exercise

Central Massachusetts Agency on Aging, 844

Directory of Community Care Facilities, 2732

Gray Panthers Metro Detroit, 914

HIV Disease in People with Hemophilia: Your Questions Answered, 3304

International Society for Sexual Medicine, 5146

Living and Loving: Information About Sexuality and Intimacy, 3836

National Civil Rights Clearinghouse Library, 8479

Patient Perspectives on Parkinson's, 5218

Protection & Advocacy for People with Disabilities, 1579

Selling to Seniors, 2968

Sexual Intimacy and the Alcoholic Relationship, 5556

Sexuality & Aging, 3007

A Thousand Tomorrows, 3653

Tonight's the Night, 3011

Unisex Low Vision Watch, 2240

University of North Carolina: General Clinical Research Center, 3365

Safety

Adjustable Bed, 2124

Alabama State Department of Human Resources, 263

Aluminum Walking Canes, 2471

Arizona Public Safety Personnel Retirement System, 303

Caption Center, 8601

Cornell Communications, 2177

Easy Pour Locking Lid Pot, 2343

Evacu-Trac, 2492

Great Big Safety Tub Mat, 2112

Home Safety for the Alzheimer's Patient, 3629

Illinois Society for the Prevention of Blindness, 5740

Just One Little Bite Can Hurt! Important Facts About Anaphylaxis, 3452

Luminaud Inc., 2203

Mat Factory, 2521

Mr. Escort Manual Wheelchair Carrier, 2091

Plums Award Winning Protects Hip, 2294

PowerLink 2 Control Unit, 2328, 2355

Prevent Blindness Connecticut, 5868

Prevent Blindness News, 6081

Prevent Blindness Northern California, 5872

Prevent Blindness Texas, 5875

ProtectaCap+PLUS, ProtectaHip, 2296

Savannah Court, 6389

Schoharie County Office for the Aging, 1326

Sierra 3000/4000, 2433

Transfer Bench with Back, 2138

US Army: Medical Command Center for Health Promotion & Preventive Medicine, 8595

Wyoming Workers Safety & Compensation Division, 1848

Ziggy Medi-Chair, 2415

Senility, See also Alzheimer's Disease

Center for Senility Studies: Alzheimer's Disease Treatment Research, 3682

UCSF Memory and Aging Center, 3187

Social Issues

Addiction and Responsibility, 5397

Addictive Personality, 5399

Aging Research: National Institute on Aging, Public Health Service, 3090

Asian Americans Advancing Justice, 64

Boston College: Social Work Library, 8600

Brain Research Institute University of California, Los Angeles, 3099

CARF Directory of Organizations with Accredited Programs, 2719

Center for the Study of Aging of Albany, 1239

Central Michigan University: Center for Adult Longitudinal Studies, 3112

Choice & Challenge: Caring for Aggressive Older Adults Across Levels of Care, 2990

Clinical Program for Evaluating and Managing Stroke-at-Risk Patients, 5251

Complete Directory for People with Disabilities, 2722

Complete Mental Health Directory, 2725

Cornell University School of Industrial and Labor Relations, 8680

Dartmouth College Center for Evaluative Clinical Sciences, 3117

Duke University Center for the Study of Aging and Human Development, 3118

Educational Gerontology, 2829

Ethel Percy Andrus Gerontology Center, 3122

Families Anonymous, 5338

Georgia Consortium on the Psychology of Aging, 3127

Hazelden, 3044

Hazelden Betty Ford Foundation, 5343

ILRU Insights, 2932

Institute for Retired Professionals at Syracuse, 2016

Journal of Aging and Health, 2849

Kent State University Exercise Physiology Lab, 3143

Massachusetts Alzheimer's Disease Research Center, 3693

Massachusetts Institute of Technology General Clinical Research Center, 3147

Maximizing the Role of Nutrition in Diabetes Management, 4629

National Institute on Aging, 3068, 3151

National Institute on Aging Gerontology Research Center, 3152

New York State Institute for Basic Research in Developmental Disabilities, 3155

Oregon Research Institute, 3162

Pennsylvania State University Center for Developmental and Health Genetics, 3164

Portland State University Institute on Aging, 3169

Quality Care Conference, 1976, 3005

Research Institute of the Hebrew Home of Greater Washington, 3172

Richard Kalish Innovative Publication Award, 1902

Rockefeller University Laboratory of Neuroendocrinology, 3174

RSVP Scott-Cape Counties, 1068

Rutgers University Institute for Health, Health Care Policy: and Aging Research, 3177

Southern California Research Institute, 5624

St. Louis University: Department of Psychiatry, 4551

Steps to Understanding Challenging Behaviors, 3644

University of California, San Francisco Center for Social and Behavioral Sciences, 3191

University of Kentucky: Sanders-Brown Center on Aging, 3209

University of Miami: Center on Adult Development and Aging, 3216

University of Michigan Center for Human Growth and Development, 3217

University of Michigan: Institute of Gerontology, 3219

University of Tennessee: Knoxville Society for the Study of Social Problems, 3231

University of Texas-Houston Health Science Center Mental Sciences Institute, 3232

University of Wisconsin: Milwaukee Institute on Aging and Environment, 3239

US Department of Veteran Affairs: Palo Alto Health Care and Medical Information Service, 8439

Wayne State University Center for Health Research, 3242

Workers at Risk: Drugs and Alcohol on the Job, 5584

Social Security

Austin Disability Determination Services, 1622

Bureau of Disability Adjudication, 1143

Bureau of Disability Determination, 1394

Bureau of Rehabilitation Services: Disability Determination Services, 421

Charleston Disability Determination Services, 1801

Chicago Social Security Management Association, 910

Department for Disability Determination Services, 706

Disability Determination Branch, 531

Disability Determination Division, 1439

Disability Determination Unit, 1155

Disability Determinations, 1122

Disability Workbook for Social Security Applicants, 5280

Division of Disability Determination Services, 1181

Georgia Department of Labor: Disability Adjudication Section, 507

Massachusetts Disability Determination Services, 864

Massachusetts Social Security Region 1 Administration, 869

Mental Health Law Reporter, 4546

National Academy of Social Insurance, 8477

National Committee to Preserve Social Security & Medicare, 156, 2633

National Council of Social Security Management Associations, 158

National Organization of Social Security Claimants' Representatives, 8328

Nolo's Guide to Social Security Disability: Getting and Keeping Your Benefits, 2693

Social Security Administration, 218

Social Security Bulletin, 2972

Social Security for Public Employees, 1557

Social Security, Medicare and Pensions, 2701

Social Security: Atlanta Disability Determination, 526

Social Security: Baltimore Disability Determination, 836

Social Security: Disability Determination Services, 293

Social Security: Louisville Disability Determination, 736

Social Security: Tallahassee Disability Determination, 494

Social Security: West Columbia Disability Determination, 1584

Spiringfield Social Security DisabilityDetermination, 602

State of Alaska, Department of Health & Social Services, 294

University of Pennsylvania Institute on Aging, 3226

US Social Security Administration Library & Records Management Branch, 8599

US Social Security Administration: Washington Library, 8485

Speech Impairments

Parkinson Handbook: A Guide for Patients and Their Families, 5212

Phoenix Public Library: Special Needs Center, 8419

Providence Speech and Hearing Center, 4773

Washington Hearing and Speech, 4783

Sports, See also Hobbies, Recreation

Activity Factory, 8860

Community Recreation and People with Disabilities for Inclusion, 2670

Community Service Program of Van Nuys, 1937

Eagle Sportschairs, 2491

Eskaton Cameron Park Lodge, 6225

Eskaton Gold River Lodge, 6226

Exercise for Older Adults, 2675

Falls Church Senior Center, 1744

Idyll Arbor, 8883

Jewish Association for Services for the Aged, 1257

Lazy Days RV Center, 2084

Marin Senior Coordinating Council (Whistlestop), 373

Massillon Senior Citizens' Center, 1406

Mattoon Area Senior Center: Coles Council on Aging, 582

Mature Health, 2863

Michigan City Public Library: Indiana Rooom/Genealogy, 8544

Modern Maturity, 2867

Modern Maturity Center, 444

Nantahala Outdoor Center, 9015

New Bedford Council on Aging, 872

Northern Rocky Mountain Retiree Association, 1102

PALAESTRA, 8922

Pennsylvania Department of Public Welfare Norristown State Hospital, 8753

Ranger, 2428

Scooter, Power Chair and Wheelchair Lifts, 2396

Senior Action in a Gay Environment, 1329

Senior Adult Activities Center of Montgomery County, 1556

Senior Citizens of Patagonia, 312

Senior Times Magazine, 2879

Sports 'n Spokes, 9026

Strength Training for Seniors, 2703

SureHands Lift & Care Systems, 2407

Travis County Services for the Deaf and Hard of Hearing, 4779

University of Connecticut in Storrs: Homer Babbidge Library, 8463

USA Deaf Sports Federation, 4781, 4887, 5073

William Beardall Senior Center, 499

WinSCAN-The Single Switch Interface for PCs with Windows, 2248

Stroke

Adaptive Resources Guide, 5248

African-Americans and Stroke, 5268

Alzheimer's, Stroke and 29 Other Neurological Disorders Sourcebook, 3583

American Academy of Neurology, 3565, 5301

American Brain Foundation, 5241

American Stroke Association, 5242

The American Stroke Foundation, 5247

Atrial Fibrillation and Stroke, 5270

Be Stroke Smart, 5271

Be Stroke Smart - Communication, 5272

Be Stroke Smart - Emotional Aspects, 5273

Be Stroke Smart - Home and Work Adaptation, 5274

Be Stroke Smart - Prevention and Warning Signs, 5275

Be Stroke Smart - Rehabilitation Guidelines and Resources, 5276

Be Stroke Smart Series, 5277

Brain at Risk: Understanding and Preventing Stroke, 5299

Cerebral Blood Flow Laboratories, 5302

Clinical Trials Participation, 5279

Columbia University Irving Center for Clinical Research, 3113

Comprehensive Stroke Center of Oregon, 5303

Dana Foundation and the Dana Alliance for Brain Initiatives, 5305

Discovery Circles, 5252

Guide to Understanding Stroke, 5281

Heart and Stroke Facts, 5282

Heart and Stroke Risk Factors, 5283

High Blood Pressure and Stroke, 5284

Home Exercises for Stroke Survivors, 5285

Internet Stroke Center, 5243

Introduction to Stroke, 5254

Invaluable Guide to Life After Stroke: An Owner's Manual, 5255

Journal of Stroke and Cerebrovascular Diseases, 5267

Living at Home After a Stroke, 5286

Living with Stroke: A Guide for Families, 5257

National Institute of Neurological Disorders & Stroke, 5244

National Institute of Neurological Disorders and Stroke, 3067

National Rehabilitation Information Center, 184, 4766, 5245

National Stroke Association, 5246

November Days, 5258

NSA Audio Tape Series, 5300

NSA's Guide to Stroke, 5287

Pathways: Moving Beyond Stroke and Aphasia, 5259

Recovery After a Stroke, 5288

Recurrent Stroke, 5289

Road Ahead: A Stroke Recovery Guide, 5260

Rush University Neuroscience Institute, 3175

Stroke Book, 5261

Stroke Connection, 5291

Stroke Council, 5309

Stroke is a Brain Attack!, 5293

Stroke Treatment and Recovery, 5292

Stroke: Clinical Updates, 5294

Stroke: Putting the Pieces Back Together, 5263

Stroke: Questions & Answers, 5295

Stroke: Reducing Your Risk (Spanish), 5296

Stroke: Your Complete Exercise Guide, 5264

Symbi-Key Computer Switch Interface, 2231

University of Chicago Brain Research Institute, 3195

University of Florida Brain Institute, 3198

University of Miami Center for Neurological Diseases, 3214

US Stroke Club Listing, 5266

Winning Over Stroke, 5265

Substance Abuse

Adler School of Professional Psychology, 8518

AHA Guide to the Health Care Field, 2712

Alcohol Alert #17: Treatment Outcome Research, 5465

American Council on Addiction and Alcohol Problems, 5321

American Psychological Association, 5322

Arizona Substance Abuse Task Force, 5323

Art of Living with Change: Turning Your Good Intentions Into Progress..., 5588

Betty Ford Center, 5325

Brandeis University Institute for Health Policy, 3100

Breaking the Chain of Substance Abuse and Hearing Loss, 4905, 5480

Caring for Ourselves: Hope for Healthy Relationships, 5591

Center for Alcohol & Addiction Studies, 5608

Center for Substance Abuse Prevention, 5327, 5597

Center for Substance Abuse Research, 5328

Center of Alcohol Studies, 5329

DrugAbuse.com, 5599

Dual Disorders Recovery Book, 5409

Getting Started in AA, 5413

Suicide, See also Assisted Suicide

Travel Agencies, Clubs, Tours

Travel Trends, 9030
Travelers Aid Society, 9031
Travelfair, 9032
Travelin' Talk Directory, 2789
Travelin' Talk Newsletter, 9033
Tub Slide Shower Chair, 2123
United Airlines, 8929
United States Department of the Interior:
National Park Service, 2978
University of Connecticut Health Center:
Center on Aging, 8462
US SERVAS, 9034
Utah Travel Council, 8981
Washington State Tourism, 8983
West Virginia Division of Tourism, 8984
Wheeler's Accessible Van Rentals, 2101,
8931
Wilderness Inquiry, 9036
Wisconsin Department of Tourism, 8985
A World of Options: A Guide to
International, Educational, Exchange,
Community Service...for Persons,
Wyoming Division of Tourism, 8986

Veterans

Alabama Department of Veteran Affairs,
259
Alaska Department of Military and Veterans
Affairs, 281
American Legion, 8539
American Legion Magazine, 2809
Arkansas Department of Veterans Affairs,
319
Association of the United States Army, 74
Blind Rehabilitation Services, 5679
Blinded Veterans Association, 5681, 6110
California Department of Veterans Affairs,
350
Delaware Commission of Veterans Affairs,
435
Diplomatic and Consular Officers, Retired,
94
Directory of Department of Veterans Affairs
Facilities, 2733
Disabled American Veterans, 708
Disabled American Veterans Magazines,
2824
Federal Benefits for Veterans and
Dependents, 2743
Financial Aid for Veterans, Military
Personnel and Their Dependents, 2744
Florida Department of Veterans Affairs, 466
Georgia Department of Veterans Service,
509
Illinois Department of Veterans Affairs, 576
Indiana Department of Health Veteran's
Home, 622
Indiana Department of Veterans Affairs, 624
Iowa Commission of Veterans Affairs, 643
Irving Diener Award, 1867
Jewish Veteran, 2894
Kansas Commission on Veterans Affairs,
676
Kentucky Department of Veterans Affairs,
715
Life Insurance for Veterans: Veterans
Benefits Administration, 1515
Living with Low Vision: A Resource Guide
for People with Sight Loss, 5940, 5966

Louisiana Department of Veterans Affairs,
756
Maine Department of Defense, Veterans and
Emergency Management, 792
Major General Melvin J. Maas Achievement
Award, 1875
Maryland Veterans Commission, 825
Military Officers Association of America,
133
Military Order of the World Wars, 134
Minnesota Department of Veterans Affairs,
972
Mississippi State Veterans Affairs Board,
1013
National Active and Retired Federal
Employees Association, 138
National Association of Blind Veterans,
5773
National Association of State Veterans
Homes, 148
National Association of Veterans' Program
Administrators, 150
Navy Seabee Veterans of America Inc., 194
Nebraska Department of Veterans Affairs,
1133
New Hampshire Veterans Council, 1168
New Mexico Veterans Service Commission,
1228
New York Division of Veterans Affairs,
1270
North Dakota Department of Veterans
Affairs, 1378
Ohio Disabled American Veterans, 1416
Oklahoma Department of Veterans Affairs,
1447
Omaha Department of Veteran Affairs
Medical Center Research Service, 4682
Oregon Department of Veterans Affairs,
1474
Paralyzed Veterans of America (PVA), 8201
South Carolina Department of Veterans
Affairs, 1588
Tennessee Department of Veterans Affairs,
1614
Texas Veterans Commission, 1684
U.S. Department of Veterans Affairs, 231
US Deparment of Veterans Affairs: Center
Library, 8578
US Deparment of Veterans Affairs:
Columbia William Jennings Bryan-Dorn
Veterans Hospital Library, 8771
US Deparment of Veterans Affairs:
Philadelphia Medical Center Library,
8758
US Department of Veterans Affairs and
Center Learning Resources Service
Library, 8500
US Department of Veterans Affairs Bedford:
Edith Nourse Rogers Memorial Veterans
Hospital Medical Li, 8608
US Department of Veterans Affairs Hospital
Libraries, 8428
US Department of Veterans Affairs Hospitl:
Fort Howard Hospital Library, 8596
US Department of Veterans Affairs Medical
Center Library Service, 8429, 8514, 8609,
8808
US Department of Veterans Affairs Medical
Library, 8499
US Department of Veterans Affairs
Outpatient Clinic Learning Resources
Service, 8610

US Department of Veterans Affairs,
Hospital Library, 8501
US Department of Veterans Affairs, John
Cochran Division Library, 8640
US Department of Veterans Affairs, Medical
Center Library Service, 8483, 8548
US Department of Veterans Affairs:
Albuquerque Medical Center Library,
8670
US Department of Veterans Affairs: Altoona
James E Van Zandt Medical Center
Library Service, 8759
US Department of Veterans Affairs:
Amarillo Hospital Library, 8810
US Department of Veterans Affairs: Ann
Arbor Hospital Library, 8627
US Department of Veterans Affairs:
Asheville Medical Center Library, 8719
US Department of Veterans Affairs:
Baltimore Medical Center Library
Service, 8597
US Department of Veterans Affairs: Bath
Medical Center Library Service, 8705
US Department of Veterans Affairs: Battle
Creek Medical Center Library Service,
8628
US Department of Veterans Affairs: Beckley
Library Service, 8844
US Department of Veterans Affairs: Big
Spring Hospital Library, 8811
US Department of Veterans Affairs: Boston
Hospital Medical Library, 8611
US Department of Veterans Affairs:
Brecksville Medical Center Library, 8735
US Department of Veterans Affairs: Bronx
Medical Center Library, 8706
US Department of Veterans Affairs:
Brooklyn Medical Center Library, 8707
US Department of Veterans Affairs: Buffalo
Medical Center Library Service, 8708
US Department of Veterans Affairs: Butler
Medical Center Library, 8760
US Department of Veterans Affairs: Carl
Vinson Medical Center Library, 8515
US Department of Veterans Affairs: Castle
Point Department of Medicine and
Surgery Library Service, 8709
US Department of Veterans Affairs: Central
Iowa Health Care System, 8554
US Department of Veterans Affairs:
Cheyenne Medical and Regional Office
Center, 8857
US Department of Veterans Affairs: Chicago
Health Care System-West Side Division,
8529
US Department of Veterans Affairs:
Chillicothe Medical Library, 8736
US Department of Veterans Affairs:
Cincinati Learning Resources Service,
8737
US Department of Veterans Affairs:
Clarkburg Loouis A Johnson VA Medical
Center Library, 8845
US Department of Veterans Affairs:
Coatesville Medical Center Library, 8761
US Department of Veterans Affairs: Dayton
Medical Center Library Service, 8738
US Department of Veterans Affairs: Denver
Medical Center Library, 8452
US Department of Veterans Affairs: Detroit
Medical Center Library Service, 8629

US Department of Veterans Affairs: Durham Medical Center Library, 8720

US Department of Veterans Affairs: Dwight D. Eisenhower Center Medical Library, 8565

US Department of Veterans Affairs: East Orange Medical Center Library, 8666

US Department of Veterans Affairs: Erie Medical Center Library, 8762

US Department of Veterans Affairs: Fargo Medical Center Library, 8724

US Department of Veterans Affairs: Fayettville Medical Center Library Service, 8721

US Department of Veterans Affairs: For Meade VA Black Hills Health Care System Medical Library, 8774

US Department of Veterans Affairs: Fort Harrison Medical Center Library, 8646

US Department of Veterans Affairs: Grand Island Greater Nebraska Health Care System Library, 8651

US Department of Veterans Affairs: Grand Junction Medical Center Library Service, 8453

US Department of Veterans Affairs: H Earl Gordon Medical Library, 8440

US Department of Veterans Affairs: Hampton Medical Center Library and Educational Resources, 8831

US Department of Veterans Affairs: Health Administration Medical Center, 8465

US Department of Veterans Affairs: Hospital Library, 8530, 8573

US Department of Veterans Affairs: Huntinington Learning Resource Center, 8846

US Department of Veterans Affairs: Indiana Health Care System, 8549

US Department of Veterans Affairs: Iron Mountain Medical Center Library, 8630

US Department of Veterans Affairs: Johnson City Medical Center Library, 8777

US Department of Veterans Affairs: Kansas Medical Center Library, 8641

US Department of Veterans Affairs: Kerrville South Texas Veterans Health Care System, 8812

US Department of Veterans Affairs: Lebanon Medical Center Library, 8763

US Department of Veterans Affairs: Library Services, 8531

US Department of Veterans Affairs: Loma Linda Medical Center Library Service, 8441

US Department of Veterans Affairs: Long Beach Medical Center Library Service, 8442

US Department of Veterans Affairs: Manchester Medical Center Library, 8659

US Department of Veterans Affairs: Martinsburg Learning Resources Service, 8847

US Department of Veterans Affairs: Medical & Regional Office Center, 8566, 8588

US Department of Veterans Affairs: Medical Center Library, 8516, 8517, 8574, 8579, 8612

US Department of Veterans Affairs: Medical Library, 8502, 8503

US Department of Veterans Affairs: Memphis Medical Center Library, 8778

US Department of Veterans Affairs: Miles City Medical Center Library, 8647

US Department of Veterans Affairs: Minneapolis Medical Center Library Service, 8636

US Department of Veterans Affairs: Montrose Medical Library, 8710

US Department of Veterans Affairs: Murfreesboro Medical Center Library Service, 8779

US Department of Veterans Affairs: Nashville Medical Center Library Service, 8780

US Department of Veterans Affairs: New York Harbour Healthcare System, New York Campus Library, 8711

US Department of Veterans Affairs: Northern Arizona VA Health Care System, 8423

US Department of Veterans Affairs: Northport Medical Center-Medical Library, 8712

US Department of Veterans Affairs: Oklahoma City Medical Center Library, 8743

US Department of Veterans Affairs: Omaha Hospital Library, 8652

US Department of Veterans Affairs: Overton Brooks Medical Center Library, 8580

US Department of Veterans Affairs: Phoenix Medical Center Library, 8424

US Department of Veterans Affairs: Pittsburgh Education, Media and Reference Service, 8764

US Department of Veterans Affairs: Poplar Bluff Library Service, 8642

US Department of Veterans Affairs: Portland Medical Library, 8746

US Department of Veterans Affairs: Providence Health Sciences Library, 8768

US Department of Veterans Affairs: Reno Medical Center Library Services, 8656

US Department of Veterans Affairs: Richmond Hospital Library, 8832

US Department of Veterans Affairs: Saginaw Aleda E Lutz Medical Center Library, 8631

US Department of Veterans Affairs: Salem Medical Center Library, 8833

US Department of Veterans Affairs: Salisbury Medical Center Library, 8722

US Department of Veterans Affairs: Salt Lake City Hospital Medical Library, 8814

US Department of Veterans Affairs: San Diego Medical Center Library Service, 8443

US Department of Veterans Affairs: San Francisco Medical Center Library Service, 8444

US Department of Veterans Affairs: Seattle Puget Sound Health Care System, 8837

US Department of Veterans Affairs: Sheridan Medical Center Library, 8858

US Department of Veterans Affairs: Southern Colorado Healthcare System, 8454

US Department of Veterans Affairs: Spokane Medical Center Library, 8838

US Department of Veterans Affairs: Tacoma/Puget Sound Health Care System, 8839

US Department of Veterans Affairs: Temple Medical Center Medical Library, 8809

US Department of Veterans Affairs: Tomah Health Sciences Library, 8854

US Department of Veterans Affairs: Tucson Medical Center Library, 8425

US Department of Veterans Affairs: Waco Medical Center Library, 8813

US Department of Veterans Affairs: Walla Walla Jonathan M Wainwright Memorial VA Medical Library, 8840

US Department of Veterans Affairs: White City Library, 8747

US Department of Veterans Affairs: White River Junction Medical & Regional Office CenterLibrary Serv, 8817

US Department of Veterans Affairs: Wilkes-Barre Medical Center Library, 8765

US Deprtment of Veterans Affairs: Center Library, 8550

US Deptartment of Veterans Affairs: Central Alabama Veterans Health Care System, 8412

US Deptartment of Veterans Affairs: Medical Center Library, 8413

US Deptartment of Veterans Affairs:Alabama Veterns Health Care System, 8414

VA Central California Health Care System, 8446

Vermont Veterans Affairs, 1734

Veterans & Military Organizations Directory, 2794

Veterans Administration Medical Center: Research Service, 5635

Veterans Affairs Medical Center: Geriatric Research, Education and Clinical Center, 3240

Washington Department of Veterans Affairs, 1796

Wisconsin Department of Veterans Affairs, 1840

Wisconsin Veterans Museum & Research Center, 8856

Visually Impaired

ACB Government Employees, 5056, 5637, 6104

ACB Radio Amateurs, 5057, 5638, 6105

ACB Social Service Providers, 5058, 6106

Achromatopsia Network, 5639

AER Report, 2802

AFB Directory of Services for Blind and Visually Impaired Persons in the US, 5913, 5956

After a Stroke: 300 Tips to Making Life Easier, 5249

Aging Eye and Low Vision, 5917

Alliance on Aging and Vision Loss, 5640

Aluminum Adjustable Support Canes for the Blind, 2469

American Academy of Ophthalmology, 5641

American Action Fund for Blind Children and Adults, 5642

American Association of the Deaf-Blind, 5645

American Association of Visually Impaired Attorneys, 5644

Volunteerism

Widowhood, See also Bereavement, Death & Dying

Wills, See also Probate, Legal Aid

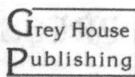
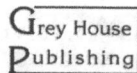
General Reference
America's College Museums
American Environmental Leaders: From Colonial Times to the Present
Encyclopedia of African-American Writing
Encyclopedia of Constitutional Amendments
Encyclopedia of Human Rights and the United States
Encyclopedia of Invasions & Conquests
Encyclopedia of Prisoners of War & Internment
Encyclopedia of Religion & Law in America
Encyclopedia of Rural America
Encyclopedia of the Continental Congress
Encyclopedia of the United States Cabinet, 1789-2010
Encyclopedia of War Journalism
Encyclopedia of Warrior Peoples & Fighting Groups
The Environmental Debate: A Documentary History
The Evolution Wars: A Guide to the Debates
From Suffrage to the Senate: America's Political Women
Gun Debate: An Encyclopedia of Gun Rights & Gun Control in the U.S.
Opinions throughout History: National Security vs. Civil and Privacy Rights
Opinions throughout History: Immigration
Opinions throughout History: Drug Abuse & Drug Epidemics
Political Corruption in America
Privacy Rights in the Digital Era
The Religious Right: A Reference Handbook
Speakers of the House of Representatives, 1789-2009
This is Who We Were: 1880-1900
This is Who We Were: A Companion to the 1940 Census
This is Who We Were: In the 1900s
This is Who We Were: In the 1910s
This is Who We Were: In the 1920s
This is Who We Were: In the 1940s
This is Who We Were: In the 1950s
This is Who We Were: In the 1960s
This is Who We Were: In the 1970s
This is Who We Were: In the 1980s
This is Who We Were: In the 1990s
This is Who We Were: In the 2000s
U.S. Land & Natural Resource Policy
The Value of a Dollar 1600-1865: Colonial Era to the Civil War
The Value of a Dollar: 1860-2014
Working Americans 1770-1869 Vol. IX: Revolutionary War to the Civil War
Working Americans 1880-1999 Vol. I: The Working Class
Working Americans 1880-1999 Vol. II: The Middle Class
Working Americans 1880-1999 Vol. III: The Upper Class
Working Americans 1880-1999 Vol. IV: Their Children
Working Americans 1880-2015 Vol. V: Americans At War
Working Americans 1880-2005 Vol. VI: Women at Work
Working Americans 1880-2006 Vol. VII: Social Movements
Working Americans 1880-2007 Vol. VIII: Immigrants
Working Americans 1880-2009 Vol. X: Sports & Recreation
Working Americans 1880-2010 Vol. XI: Inventors & Entrepreneurs
Working Americans 1880-2011 Vol. XII: Our History through Music
Working Americans 1880-2012 Vol. XIII: Education & Educators
Working Americans 1880-2016 Vol. XIV: Industry Through the Ages
Working Americans 1880-2017 Vol. XV: Politics & Politicians
World Cultural Leaders of the 20th & 21st Centuries

Education Information
Charter School Movement
Comparative Guide to American Elementary & Secondary Schools
Complete Learning Disabilities Directory
Educators Resource Handbook
Special Education: Policy and Curriculum Development

Health Information
Comparative Guide to American Hospitals
Complete Directory for Pediatric Disorders
Complete Directory for People with Chronic Illness
Complete Directory for People with Disabilities
Complete Mental Health Directory
Diabetes in America: Analysis of an Epidemic
Guide to Health Care Group Purchasing Organizations
Guide to U.S. HMO's & PPO's
Medical Device Market Place
Older Americans Information Directory

Business Information
Complete Television, Radio & Cable Industry Directory
Directory of Business Information Resources
Directory of Mail Order Catalogs
Directory of Venture Capital & Private Equity Firms
Environmental Resource Handbook
Financial Literacy Starter Kit
Food & Beverage Market Place
Grey House Homeland Security Directory
Grey House Performing Arts Directory
Grey House Safety & Security Directory
Hudson's Washington News Media Contacts Directory
New York State Directory
Sports Market Place Directory

Statistics & Demographics
American Tally
America's Top-Rated Cities
America's Top-Rated Smaller Cities
Ancestry & Ethnicity in America
The Asian Databook
Comparative Guide to American Suburbs
The Hispanic Databook
Profiles of America
"Profiles of" Series – State Handbooks
Weather America

Financial Ratings Series
Financial Literacy Basics
TheStreet Ratings' Guide to Bond & Money Market Mutual Funds
TheStreet Ratings' Guide to Common Stocks
TheStreet Ratings' Guide to Exchange-Traded Funds
TheStreet Ratings' Guide to Stock Mutual Funds
TheStreet Ratings' Ultimate Guided Tour of Stock Investing
Weiss Ratings' Consumer Guides
Weiss Ratings' Financial Literary Basic Guides
Weiss Ratings' Guide to Banks
Weiss Ratings' Guide to Credit Unions
Weiss Ratings' Guide to Health Insurers
Weiss Ratings' Guide to Life & Annuity Insurers
Weiss Ratings' Guide to Property & Casualty Insurers

Bowker's Books In Print® Titles
American Book Publishing Record® Annual
American Book Publishing Record® Monthly
Books In Print®
Books In Print® Supplement
Books Out Loud™
Bowker's Complete Video Directory™
Children's Books In Print®
El-Hi Textbooks & Serials In Print®
Forthcoming Books®
Law Books & Serials In Print™
Medical & Health Care Books In Print™
Publishers, Distributors & Wholesalers of the US™
Subject Guide to Books In Print®
Subject Guide to Children's Books In Print®

Canadian General Reference
Associations Canada
Canadian Almanac & Directory
Canadian Environmental Resource Guide
Canadian Parliamentary Guide
Canadian Venture Capital & Private Equity Firms
Canadian Who's Who
Financial Post Directory of Directors
Financial Services Canada
Governments Canada
Health Guide Canada
The History of Canada
Libraries Canada
Major Canadian Cities

2018 Title List

Visit www.SalemPress.com for Product Information, Table of Contents, and Sample Pages

Science, Careers & Mathematics

Ancient Creatures
Applied Science
Applied Science: Engineering & Mathematics
Applied Science: Science & Medicine
Applied Science: Technology
Biomes and Ecosystems
Careers in the Arts: Fine, Performing & Visual
Careers in Building Construction
Careers in Business
Careers in Chemistry
Careers in Communications & Media
Careers in Environment & Conservation
Careers in Financial Services
Careers in Green Energy
Careers in Healthcare
Careers in Hospitality & Tourism
Careers in Human Services
Careers in Law, Criminal Justice & Emergency Services
Careers in Manufacturing
Careers in Outdoor Jobs
Careers in Overseas Jobs
Careers in Physics
Careers in Sales, Insurance & Real Estate
Careers in Science & Engineering
Careers in Sports & Fitness
Careers in Social Media
Careers in Sports Medicine & Training
Careers in Technology Services & Repair
Computer Technology Innovators
Contemporary Biographies in Business
Contemporary Biographies in Chemistry
Contemporary Biographies in Communications & Media
Contemporary Biographies in Environment & Conservation
Contemporary Biographies in Healthcare
Contemporary Biographies in Hospitality & Tourism
Contemporary Biographies in Law & Criminal Justice
Contemporary Biographies in Physics
Earth Science
Earth Science: Earth Materials & Resources
Earth Science: Earth's Surface and History
Earth Science: Physics & Chemistry of the Earth
Earth Science: Weather, Water & Atmosphere
Encyclopedia of Energy
Encyclopedia of Environmental Issues
Encyclopedia of Environmental Issues: Atmosphere and Air Pollution
Encyclopedia of Environmental Issues: Ecology and Ecosystems
Encyclopedia of Environmental Issues: Energy and Energy Use
Encyclopedia of Environmental Issues: Policy and Activism
Encyclopedia of Environmental Issues: Preservation/Wilderness Issues
Encyclopedia of Environmental Issues: Water and Water Pollution
Encyclopedia of Global Resources
Encyclopedia of Global Warming
Encyclopedia of Mathematics & Society
Encyclopedia of Mathematics & Society: Engineering, Tech, Medicine
Encyclopedia of Mathematics & Society: Great Mathematicians
Encyclopedia of Mathematics & Society: Math & Social Sciences
Encyclopedia of Mathematics & Society: Math Development/Concepts
Encyclopedia of Mathematics & Society: Math in Culture & Society
Encyclopedia of Mathematics & Society: Space, Science, Environment
Encyclopedia of the Ancient World
Forensic Science
Geography Basics
Internet Innovators
Inventions and Inventors
Magill's Encyclopedia of Science: Animal Life
Magill's Encyclopedia of Science: Plant life
Notable Natural Disasters
Principles of Artificial Intelligence & Robotics
Principles of Astronomy
Principles of Biology
Principles of Biotechnology
Principles of Chemistry
Principles of Climatology
Principles of Physical Science
Principles of Physics
Principles of Programming & Coding
Principles of Research Methods
Principles of Sustainability
Science and Scientists
Solar System
Solar System: Great Astronomers

Solar System: Study of the Universe
Solar System: The Inner Planets
Solar System: The Moon and Other Small Bodies
Solar System: The Outer Planets
Solar System: The Sun and Other Stars
World Geography

Literature

American Ethnic Writers
Classics of Science Fiction & Fantasy Literature
Critical Approaches: Feminist
Critical Approaches: Multicultural
Critical Approaches: Moral
Critical Approaches: Psychological
Critical Insights: Authors
Critical Insights: Film
Critical Insights: Literary Collection Bundles
Critical Insights: Themes
Critical Insights: Works
Critical Survey of American Literature
Critical Survey of Drama
Critical Survey of Graphic Novels: Heroes & Super Heroes
Critical Survey of Graphic Novels: History, Theme & Technique
Critical Survey of Graphic Novels: Independents/Underground Classics
Critical Survey of Graphic Novels: Manga
Critical Survey of Long Fiction
Critical Survey of Mystery & Detective Fiction
Critical Survey of Mythology and Folklore: Heroes and Heroines
Critical Survey of Mythology and Folklore: Love, Sexuality & Desire
Critical Survey of Mythology and Folklore: World Mythology
Critical Survey of Novels into Film
Critical Survey of Poetry
Critical Survey of Poetry: American Poets
Critical Survey of Poetry: British, Irish & Commonwealth Poets
Critical Survey of Poetry: Cumulative Index
Critical Survey of Poetry: European Poets
Critical Survey of Poetry: Topical Essays
Critical Survey of Poetry: World Poets
Critical Survey of Science Fiction & Fantasy
Critical Survey of Shakespeare's Plays
Critical Survey of Shakespeare's Sonnets
Critical Survey of Short Fiction
Critical Survey of Short Fiction: American Writers
Critical Survey of Short Fiction: British, Irish, Commonwealth Writers
Critical Survey of Short Fiction: Cumulative Index
Critical Survey of Short Fiction: European Writers
Critical Survey of Short Fiction: Topical Essays
Critical Survey of Short Fiction: World Writers
Critical Survey of World Literature
Critical Survey of Young Adult Literature
Cyclopedia of Literary Characters
Cyclopedia of Literary Places
Holocaust Literature
Introduction to Literary Context: American Poetry of the 20th Century
Introduction to Literary Context: American Post-Modernist Novels
Introduction to Literary Context: American Short Fiction
Introduction to Literary Context: English Literature
Introduction to Literary Context: Plays
Introduction to Literary Context: World Literature
Magill's Literary Annual 2018
Masterplots
Masterplots II: African American Literature
Masterplots II: American Fiction Series
Masterplots II: British & Commonwealth Fiction Series
Masterplots II: Christian Literature
Masterplots II: Drama Series
Masterplots II: Juvenile & Young Adult Literature, Supplement
Masterplots II: Nonfiction Series
Masterplots II: Poetry Series
Masterplots II: Short Story Series
Masterplots II: Women's Literature Series
Notable African American Writers
Notable American Novelists
Notable Playwrights
Notable Poets
Recommended Reading: 600 Classics Reviewed
Short Story Writers

History and Social Science

The 2000s in America
50 States
African American History
Agriculture in History
American First Ladies
American Heroes
American Indian Culture
American Indian History
American Indian Tribes
American Presidents
American Villains
America's Historic Sites
Ancient Greece
The Bill of Rights
The Civil Rights Movement
The Cold War
Countries, Peoples & Cultures
Countries, Peoples & Cultures: Central & South America
Countries, Peoples & Cultures: Central, South & Southeast Asia
Countries, Peoples & Cultures: East & South Africa
Countries, Peoples & Cultures: East Asia & the Pacific
Countries, Peoples & Cultures: Eastern Europe
Countries, Peoples & Cultures: Middle East & North Africa
Countries, Peoples & Cultures: North America & the Caribbean
Countries, Peoples & Cultures: West & Central Africa
Countries, Peoples & Cultures: Western Europe
Defining Documents: American Revolution
Defining Documents: American West
Defining Documents: Ancient World
Defining Documents: Asia
Defining Documents: Civil Rights
Defining Documents: Civil War
Defining Documents: Court Cases
Defining Documents: Dissent & Protest
Defining Documents: Emergence of Modern America
Defining Documents: Exploration & Colonial America
Defining Documents: Immigration & Immigrant Communities
Defining Documents: LGBTQ
Defining Documents: Manifest Destiny
Defining Documents: Middle Ages
Defining Documents: Middle East
Defining Documents: Nationalism & Populism
Defining Documents: Native Americans
Defining Documents: Political Campaigns, Candidates & Discourse
Defining Documents: Postwar 1940s
Defining Documents: Reconstruction
Defining Documents: Renaissance & Early Modern Era
Defining Documents: Secrets, Leaks & Scandals
Defining Documents: 1920s
Defining Documents: 1930s
Defining Documents: 1950s
Defining Documents: 1960s
Defining Documents: 1970s
Defining Documents: The 17th Century
Defining Documents: The 18th Century
Defining Documents: The 19th Century
Defining Documents: The 20th Century: 1900-1950
Defining Documents: Vietnam War
Defining Documents: Women
Defining Documents: World War I
Defining Documents: World War II
Education Today
The Eighties in America
Encyclopedia of American Immigration
Encyclopedia of Flight
Encyclopedia of the Ancient World
Fashion Innovators
The Fifties in America
The Forties in America
Great Athletes
Great Athletes: Baseball
Great Athletes: Basketball
Great Athletes: Boxing & Soccer
Great Athletes: Cumulative Index
Great Athletes: Football
Great Athletes: Golf & Tennis
Great Athletes: Olympics

Great Athletes: Racing & Individual Sports
Great Contemporary Athletes
Great Events from History: 17th Century
Great Events from History: 18th Century
Great Events from History: 19th Century
Great Events from History: 20th Century (1901-1940)
Great Events from History: 20th Century (1941-1970)
Great Events from History: 20th Century (1971-2000)
Great Events from History: 21st Century (2000-2016)
Great Events from History: African American History
Great Events from History: Cumulative Indexes
Great Events from History: LGBTG
Great Events from History: Middle Ages
Great Events from History: Secrets, Leaks & Scandals
Great Events from History: Renaissance & Early Modern Era
Great Lives from History: 17th Century
Great Lives from History: 18th Century
Great Lives from History: 19th Century
Great Lives from History: 20th Century
Great Lives from History: 21st Century (2000-2017)
Great Lives from History: American Women
Great Lives from History: Ancient World
Great Lives from History: Asian & Pacific Islander Americans
Great Lives from History: Cumulative Indexes
Great Lives from History: Incredibly Wealthy
Great Lives from History: Inventors & Inventions
Great Lives from History: Jewish Americans
Great Lives from History: Latinos
Great Lives from History: Notorious Lives
Great Lives from History: Renaissance & Early Modern Era
Great Lives from History: Scientists & Science
Historical Encyclopedia of American Business
Issues in U.S. Immigration
Magill's Guide to Military History
Milestone Documents in African American History
Milestone Documents in American History
Milestone Documents in World History
Milestone Documents of American Leaders
Milestone Documents of World Religions
Music Innovators
Musicians & Composers 20th Century
The Nineties in America
The Seventies in America
The Sixties in America
Sociology Today
Survey of American Industry and Careers
The Thirties in America
The Twenties in America
United States at War
U.S. Court Cases
U.S. Government Leaders
U.S. Laws, Acts, and Treaties
U.S. Legal System
U.S. Supreme Court
Weapons and Warfare
World Conflicts: Asia and the Middle East

Health

Addictions & Substance Abuse
Adolescent Health & Wellness
Cancer
Complementary & Alternative Medicine
Community & Family Health
Genetics & Inherited Conditions
Health Issues
Infectious Diseases & Conditions
Magill's Medical Guide
Nutrition
Nursing
Psychology & Behavioral Health
Psychology Basics

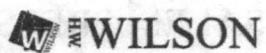
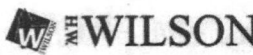
Current Biography
Current Biography Cumulative Index 1946-2013
Current Biography Monthly Magazine
Current Biography Yearbook: 2003
Current Biography Yearbook: 2004
Current Biography Yearbook: 2005
Current Biography Yearbook: 2006
Current Biography Yearbook: 2007
Current Biography Yearbook: 2008
Current Biography Yearbook: 2009
Current Biography Yearbook: 2010
Current Biography Yearbook: 2011
Current Biography Yearbook: 2012
Current Biography Yearbook: 2013
Current Biography Yearbook: 2014
Current Biography Yearbook: 2015
Current Biography Yearbook: 2016
Current Biography Yearbook: 2017

Core Collections
Children's Core Collection
Fiction Core Collection
Graphic Novels Core Collection
Middle & Junior High School Core
Public Library Core Collection: Nonfiction
Senior High Core Collection
Young Adult Fiction Core Collection

The Reference Shelf
Aging in America
Alternative Facts: Post Truth & the Information War
The American Dream
American Military Presence Overseas
The Arab Spring
Artificial Intelligence
The Brain
The Business of Food
Campaign Trends & Election Law
Conspiracy Theories
The Digital Age
Dinosaurs
Embracing New Paradigms in Education
Faith & Science
Families: Traditional and New Structures
The Future of U.S. Economic Relations: Mexico, Cuba, and Venezuela
Global Climate Change
Graphic Novels and Comic Books
Guns in America
Immigration
Immigration in the U.S.
Internet Abuses & Privacy Rights
Internet Safety
LGBTQ in the 21st Century
Marijuana Reform
The News and its Future
The Paranormal
Politics of the Ocean
Prescription Drug Abuse
Racial Tension in a "Postracial" Age
Reality Television
Representative American Speeches: 2008-2009
Representative American Speeches: 2009-2010
Representative American Speeches: 2010-2011
Representative American Speeches: 2011-2012
Representative American Speeches: 2012-2013
Representative American Speeches: 2013-2014
Representative American Speeches: 2014-2015
Representative American Speeches: 2015-2016
Representative American Speeches: 2016-2017
Representative American Speeches: 2017-2018
Rethinking Work
Revisiting Gender
Robotics
Russia
Social Networking
Social Services for the Poor
South China Seas Conflict
Space Exploration & Development
Sports in America

The Supreme Court
The Transformation of American Cities
U.S. Infrastructure
U.S. National Debate Topic: Educational Reform
U.S. National Debate Topic: Surveillance
U.S. National Debate Topic: The Ocean
U.S. National Debate Topic: Transportation Infrastructure
Whistleblowers

Readers' Guide
Abridged Readers' Guide to Periodical Literature
Readers' Guide to Periodical Literature

Indexes
Index to Legal Periodicals & Books
Short Story Index
Book Review Digest

Sears List
Sears List of Subject Headings
Sears: Lista de Encabezamientos de Materia

Facts About Series
Facts About American Immigration
Facts About China
Facts About the 20th Century
Facts About the Presidents
Facts About the World's Languages

Nobel Prize Winners
Nobel Prize Winners: 1901-1986
Nobel Prize Winners: 1987-1991
Nobel Prize Winners: 1992-1996
Nobel Prize Winners: 1997-2001

World Authors
World Authors: 1995-2000
World Authors: 2000-2005

Famous First Facts
Famous First Facts
Famous First Facts About American Politics
Famous First Facts About Sports
Famous First Facts About the Environment
Famous First Facts: International Edition

American Book of Days
The American Book of Days
The International Book of Days

Monographs
American Reformers
The Barnhart Dictionary of Etymology
Celebrate the World
Guide to the Ancient World
Indexing from A to Z
Nobel Prize Winners
The Poetry Break
Radical Change: Books for Youth in a Digital Age
Speeches of American Presidents

Wilson Chronology
Wilson Chronology of Asia and the Pacific
Wilson Chronology of Human Rights
Wilson Chronology of Ideas
Wilson Chronology of the Arts
Wilson Chronology of the World's Religions
Wilson Chronology of Women's Achievements